Topley & Wilson's

MICROBIOLOGY AND MICROBIAL INFECTIONS

First published in Great Britain 1929
Second edition 1936
Third edition 1946
Fourth edition 1955
Fifth edition 1964
Sixth edition 1975
Seventh edition 1983 and 1984
Eighth edition 1990
Ninth edition published in Great Britain 1998
by Arnold, a member of the Hodder Headline Group,
338 Euston Road, London NW1 3BH

Co-published in the United States of America by
Oxford University Press, Inc.,
198 Madison Avenue, New York, NY 10016
Oxford is a registered trademark of Oxford University Press

Whilst the advice and information in this book is believed to be true and
accurate at the date of going to press, neither the authors nor the publisher
can accept any legal responsibility or liability for any errors or omissions
that may be made. In particular (but without limiting the generality of the
preceding disclaimer) every effort has been made to check drug dosages;
however it is still possible that errors have been missed. Furthermore,
dosage schedules are constantly being revised and new side-effects
recognized. For these reasons the reader is strongly urged to consult the
drug companies' printed instructions before administering any of the drugs
recommended in this book.

British Library Cataloguing in Publication Data
A catalogue record for this book is available from the British Library

Library of Congress Cataloging-in-Publication Data
A catalog record for this book is available from the Library of Congress

ISBN 0 340 663162 (Volume 1)
ISBN 0 340 614706 (Set)

Publisher:	Georgina Bentliff
Project Editor:	Sophie Oliver
Project Coordinator:	Melissa Morton
Production Controller:	Helen Whitehorn
Copy Editor:	Gillian Clarke
Proofreader:	Elizabeth Weaver
Indexer:	Jan Ross

Typeset in 9.5/11pt New Baskerville by Photo·graphics
Printed and bound in Great Britain at The Bath Press, Avon

Topley & Wilson's

MICROBIOLOGY AND MICROBIAL INFECTIONS

NINTH EDITION

Leslie Collier
Albert Balows • Max Sussman

VOLUME 1

VIROLOGY

VOLUME EDITORS
Brian WJ Mahy • Leslie Collier

A member of the Hodder Headline Group
LONDON • SYDNEY • AUCKLAND
Co-published in the USA by Oxford University Press, Inc., New York

Editor-in-Chief

Leslie Collier MD, DSc, FRCP, FRCPath

Professor Emeritus of Virology, The London Hospital Medical College, London; formerly Director, Vaccines and Sera Laboratories, The Lister Institute of Preventive Medicine, Elstree, Hertfordshire, UK

General Editors

Albert Balows AB, MS, PhD, ABMM

Professor Emeritus, Emory University School of Medicine and Georgia State University; Former Director at The Center for Infectious Diseases, Centers for Disease Control and Prevention, Atlanta, Georgia, USA

Max Sussman BSc, PhD, CBiol, FIBiol, FRCPath

Professor Emeritus of Bacteriology, Department of Microbiology, The Medical School, Newcastle upon Tyne, UK

Volume Editors

Brian WJ Mahy PhD, ScD

Director, Division of Viral and Rickettsial Diseases, Centers for Disease Control and Prevention, Atlanta, Georgia, USA; formerly Director, The Animal Virus Research Institute, Pirbright, Surrey, UK

Leslie Collier MD, DSc, FRCP, FRCPath

Professor Emeritus of Virology, The London Hospital Medical College, London; formerly Director, Vaccines and Sera Laboratories, The Lister Institute of Preventive Medicine, Elstree, Hertfordshire, UK

Contents of Volume 1
Virology

PART IV: SYNDROMES CAUSED BY A RANGE OF VIRUSES

PART V: PRINCIPLES OF DIAGNOSIS AND CONTROL

CONTENTS OF VOLUMES 2, 3, 4 AND 5

VOLUME 4: MEDICAL MYCOLOGY

PART I: BACKGROUND AND BASIC INFORMATION

CONTRIBUTORS

Masamichi Aikawa MD, PhD
Professor, The Research Institute of Medical Sciences, Tokai University, Boseidai, Isehara, Kanagawa, Japan

Libero Ajello PhD
Adjunct Professor, Department of Ophthalmology, Emory University Eye Center, Atlanta, Georgia, USA

RP Allaker BSc, PhD
Lecturer in Oral Microbiology, Department of Oral Microbiology, St Bartholomew's and the Royal London School of Medicine and Dentistry, London, UK

Stephen D Allen MA, MD
Director, Division of Clinical Microbiology, Director of Laboratories, Department of Pathology and Laboratory Medicine, Indiana University School of Medicine, and Director, Disease Control Laboratories, Indiana State Department of Health, Indianapolis, Indiana, USA

Martin Altwegg PhD
Professor of Medical Microbiology, Head of Molecular Diagnostics Unit, Department of Medical Microbiology, University of Zurich, Zurich, Switzerland

Daniel Amsterdam PhD
Professor of Microbiology and Pathology, Associate Professor of Medicine, Director of Clinical Microbiology and Immunology, Director, Department of Laboratory Medicine, Erie County Medical Center, University of Buffalo Medical School, Buffalo, New York, USA

Larry J Anderson MD
Chief, Respiratory and Enteric Viruses Branch, Centers for Disease Control and Prevention, Atlanta, Georgia, USA

Roy M Anderson BSc, PhD, FRS
Director, Wellcome Trust Centre for the Epidemiology of Infectious Disease; Linacre Professor and Head, Department of Zoology, University of Oxford, Oxford, UK

Jørn Andreassen PhD
Assistant Professor, Department of Population Biology, Zoological Institute, University of Copenhagen, Copenhagen, Denmark

Masanori Aoki MS
Professor of Physics, School of Health Sciences, Faculty of Medicine, Kanazawa University, Kanazawa, Ishikawa, Japan

Sarath N Arseculeratne MB BS, DipBact, DPhil
Professor of Microbiology, Faculty of Medicine, University of Peradeniya, Sri Lanka

RW Ashford PhD, DSc
Professor of Medical Zoology, The Liverpool School of Tropical Medicine, Liverpool, UK

Hazel M Aucken MA, PhD
Clinical Microbiologist, Laboratory of Hospital Infection, Central Public Health Laboratory, Colindale, London, UK

L Andrew Ball D Phil
Professor of Microbiology, Department of Microbiology, University of Alabama at Birmingham, Birmingham, Alabama, USA

Albert Balows AB, MS, PhD, ABMM
Emeritus Professor and Emeritus Director, National Center for Infectious Diseases, Centers for Disease Control and Prevention, Atlanta, Georgia, USA

Jangu E Banatvala MA, MD, FRCP, FRCPath, DCH, DPH
Professor of Clinical Virology, Department of Virology, United Medical and Dental Schools of Guy's and St Thomas's, St Thomas's Hospital, London, UK

PA Bates BA, PhD
Lecturer in Medical Parasitology, The Liverpool School of Tropical Medicine, Liverpool, UK

Derrick Baxby BSc, PhD, FRCPath, FRSA
Senior Lecturer in Medical Microbiology, Department
of Medical Microbiology and Genitourinary Medicine,
Liverpool University, Liverpool, UK

Norman T Begg MBCLB, DTM&H, FFPHH
Consultant Epidemiologist, Public Health Laboratory
Service Communicable Diseases Surveillance Centre,
London, UK

William J Bellini PhD
Chief, Measles Virus Section, Respiratory and
Enterovirus Branch, Centers for Disease Control and
Prevention, Atlanta, Georgia, USA

PM Bennett BSc, PhD
Reader in Bacteriology, Department of Pathology and
Microbiology, School of Medical Sciences, University of
Bristol, Bristol, UK

Ruth L Berkelman MD
Deputy Director, National Center for Infectious
Diseases, Centers for Disease Control and Prevention,
Atlanta, Georgia, USA

Jennifer M Best PhD, FRCPath
Reader in Virology, Department of Virology, United
Medical and Dental Schools of Guy's and St Thomas's,
St Thomas's Hospital, London, UK

Jochen Bockemühl MD, PhD
Head, Division of Bacteriology, Institute of Hygiene,
Hamburg, Germany

SP Borriello BSc, PhD, FRCPath
Director, Central Public Health Laboratory, Colindale,
London, UK

Edward J Bottone PhD
Director, Consultative Microbiology, Division of
Infectious Diseases, Department of Medicine, Mount
Sinai Hospital, Mount Sinai School of Medicine, New
York, New York, USA

George HW Bowden PhD
Professor, Department of Oral Biology, Faculty of
Dentistry, University of Manitoba, Winnipeg, Manitoba,
Canada

Janet M Bradbury BSc, MSc, PhD
Reader, Department of Veterinary Pathology, University
of Liverpool, Leahurst, Neston, South Wirral, UK

William J Britt MD
Professor, Department of Pediatrics, University of
Alabama at Birmingham, Birmingham, Alabama, USA

B Kay Buchanan PhD
Microbiology and Immunology Director, Microbiology
Laboratory, Sarasota Memorial Hospital, Sarasota,
Florida, USA

Donald E Burgess PhD
Associate Professor, Veterinary Molecular Biology
Laboratory, College of Agriculture, Agricultural
Experiment Station, Montana State University,
Bozeman, Montana, USA

James P Burnie MD, PhD, MSc, MA, MRCP,
FRCPath
Head of Department, Department of Medical
Microbiology, Manchester Royal Infirmary, Manchester,
UK

Colin K Campbell BSc, MSc, PhD
Clinical Scientist, Mycology Reference Laboratory,
Bristol, UK

Richard Campbell BSc, MSc, PhD
Senior Lecturer, School of Biological Sciences, Bristol,
UK

Michael Cappello MD
Assistant Professor, Pediatric Infectious Diseases,
Laboratory of Epidemiology and Public Health, Yale
University School of Medicine, New Haven,
Connecticut, USA

Keith AV Cartwright MA, BM, FRCPath
Group Director, Public Health Laboratory Service,
South West, Gloucester Royal Hospital, Gloucester, UK

Pascal Cassinotti PhD
Deputy Head, Molecular Biology Division, Institute for
Clinical Microbiology and Immunology, St Gallen,
Switzerland

E Owen Caul FIBMS, PhD, FRCPath
Deputy Director, Head of Virology, Regional Virus
Laboratory, Public Health Laboratory, Bristol, UK

Glenn H Chambliss BSc, MSc, PhD
Professor and Chair, Department of Bacteriology,
Madison, Wisconsin, USA

Francis W Chandler DVM, PhD
Professor of Pathology, Department of Pathology,
Medical College of Georgia, Augusta, Georgia, USA

Ken Charlton DVM, PhD
Formerly Research Scientist, Animal Diseases Research
Institute, Nepean, Ontario, Canada

T Cheasty BSc
Head, *E. coli* and *Shigella* Reference Unit, Laboratory of
Enteric Pathogens, Central Public Health Laboratory,
Colindale, London, UK

Ian L Chrystie TD, PhD
Lecturer, Department of Virology, United Medical and
Dental Hospitals of Guy's and St Thomas's, St
Thomas's Hospital, London, UK

Ian N Clarke BSc, PhD
Senior Lecturer in Microbiology, Molecular
Microbiology, University Medical School, Southampton
General Hospital, Southampton, UK

Jill E Clarridge PhD, ABMM
Chief, Microbiology Section, Veterans Administration
Medical Center; Associate Professor, Baylor College of
Medicine, Houston, Texas, USA

Timothy J Cleary PhD
Director of Clinical Microbiology, Department of Pathology, University of Miami, Jackson Memorial Hospital, Miami, Florida, USA

J Barklie Clements BSc, PhD, FRSE
Professor of Virology, Department of Virology, Institute of Virology, University of Glasgow, Glasgow, UK

Leslie Collier MD, DSc, FRCP, FRCPath
Professor Emeritus of Virology, The London Hospital Medical College, London; formerly Director, Vaccines and Sera Laboratories, The Lister Institute of Preventive Medicine, Elstree, Hertfordshire, UK

Michael J Corbel PhD, DSc, MRCPath, CBiol, FIBiol
Head, Division of Bacteriology, National Institute for Biological Standards and Control, Potters Bar, Hertfordshire, UK

CS Cox BSc, PhD
Research Leader, DERA, Chemical and Biological Defence, Porton Down, Salisbury, Wiltshire, UK

Francis EG Cox PhD, DSc
Professor of Parasite Immunology, School of Life, Basic Medical and Health Sciences, King's College London, London, UK

Gary M Cox MD
Assistant Professor of Medicine, Duke University Medical Center, Durham, North Carolina, USA

Nancy J Cox PhD
Chief, Influenza Branch, Division of Viral and Rickettsial Disease, Centers for Disease Control and Prevention, Atlanta, Georgia, USA

Marie B Coyle PhD
Professor of Laboratory Medicine and Microbiology, Department of Laboratory Medicine, Harbor View Medical Center, University of Washington, Seattle, Washington, USA

Dorothy H Crawford PhD, MD, MRCPath, DSc
Professor of Microbiology, Department of Medical Microbiology, University of Edinburgh, Medical School, Edinburgh, UK

DWT Crompton MA, PhD, ScD, FRSE
John Graham Kerr Professor of Zoology, Division of Environmental and Evolutionary Biology, Institute of Biomedical and Life Sciences, University of Glasgow, Glasgow, UK

William L Current BS, MS, PhD
Senior Research Scientist, Infectious Diseases Research, Lilly Research Laboratories, Eli Lilly and Company, Indianapolis, Indiana, USA

A Curry BSc, PhD
Top Grade Clinical Scientist, Public Health Laboratory, Withington Hospital, Manchester, UK

Melanie T Cushion PhD
Associate Professor of Medicine, Division of Infectious Diseases, Department of Internal Medicine, University of Cincinnati College of Medicine, Cincinnati, Ohio, USA

William Cushley BSc, PhD
Senior Lecturer, Division of Biochemistry and Molecular Biology, Institute of Biomedical and Life Sciences, University of Glasgow, Glasgow, UK

David AB Dance MB ChB, MSc, FRCPath, DTM&H
Director/Consultant Microbiologist, Public Health Laboratory Service, Derriford Hospital, Plymouth, UK

Gregory A Dasch BA, PhD
Senior Microbiologist, Viral and Rickettsial Diseases Program, Infectious Diseases Department, Naval Medical Research Institute, Bethesda, Maryland, USA

AJ Davison MA, PhD
Senior Scientist, MRC Virology Unit, Institute of Virology, Glasgow, UK

Martin Day BSc, PhD
Reader in Microbial Genetics, School of Pure and Applied Biology, University College Wales, Cardiff, UK

DD Despommier BS, MS, PhD
Professor of Public Health and Microbiology, Division of Environmental Health Sciences, Faculty of Medicine, School of Public Health, Columbia University, New York, New York, USA

Ulrich Desselberger MD, FRCPath, FRCP
Director, Clinical Microbiology and Public Health Laboratory, Addenbrooke's Hospital, Cambridge, UK

Arthur F DiSalvo MD
Director, Nevada State Health Laboratory, Reno, Nevada, USA

Edouard Drouhet MD
Professor of Mycology, Pasteur Institute, Mycology Unit, Pasteur Institute, Paris, France

JP Dubey MVSC, PhD
Senior Scientist/Microbiologist, Parasite Biology and Epidemiology Laboratory, US Department of Agriculture, Beltsville, Maryland, USA

Brian I Duerden BSc, MD, FRCPath
Professor and Head, Department of Medical Microbiology, University of Wales College of Medicine, Cardiff; Deputy Director, Public Health Laboratory Service, London, UK

Lee M Dunster PhD
Co-ordinator, Viral Haemorrhagic Fever/Arbovirus Surveillance, Kenya Medical Research Institute, Virus Research Centre, Nairobi, Kenya

Daniel Elad DVM, PhD
Head, General Bacteriologic and Mycologic Diagnostics Division, Kimron Veterinary Institute, Beit Dagan, Israel

David B Elkins MSPH, PhD
Senior Research Fellow, Australian Centre for
International and Tropical Medicine and Nutrition,
Queensland Institute of Medical Research, Brisbane,
Queensland, Australia

David H Ellis BSc, MSc, PhD
Associate Professor, Department of Microbiology and
Immunology, University of Adelaide and Head,
Mycology Unit, Women's and Children's Hospital,
North Adelaide, Australia

Gisela Enders MD
Professor Dr, Institut für Virologie und Epidemiologie,
Stuttgart, Germany

Sir MA Epstein CBE, MA, MD, PhD, DSc, FRCPath,
FRS
Professor, Nuffield Department of Clinical Medicine,
University of Oxford, John Radcliffe Hospital, Oxford,
UK

Martha Espinosa Cantellano MD, DSc
Associate Professor, Department of Experimental
Pathology, Center for Research and Advanced Studies,
Mexico City, Mexico

SJ Eykyn FRCP, FRCS, FRCPath
Reader (Hon Consultant) in Clinical Microbiology,
Division of Infection, United Medical and Dental
School of Guy's and St Thomas's, St Thomas's Hospital,
London, UK

Richard R Facklam PhD
Chief, Streptococcus Laboratory, Centers for Disease
Control and Prevention, Atlanta, Georgia, USA

S Faine MD, DPhil, FRCPA, FASM
Emeritus Professor, Department of Microbiology,
Monash University, Melbourne, Australia Armadale,
Victoria, Australia

Heinz Feldmann MD
Assistant Professor, Institut für Virologie, Philipps
University Marburg, Marburg, Germany

Hugh J Field ScD, FRCPath
Lecturer in Virology, Centre for Veterinary Science,
University of Cambridge, Cambridge, UK

Roger G Finch FRCP, FRCPath, FFPM
Professor of Infectious Diseases, Department of
Microbiology and Infectious Diseases, Nottingham City
Hospital, University of Nottingham, Nottingham, UK

Sydney M Finegold MD
Professor of Medicine; Professor of Microbiology and
Immunology, UCLA School of Medicine; Staff
Physician, Infectious Diseases Section, Veteran Affairs
Medical Center, Los Angeles, California, USA

Michelle Nett Fiordalisi PhD
Fellow, William W McLendon Clinical Immunology
Laboratory, University of North Carolina Hospitals,
Chapel Hill, North Carolina, USA

Ana Flisser BS, PhD
Director, National Institute for Epidemiological
Diagnosis and Reference, Ministry of Health, Carpio,
Mexico City, Mexico

James D Folds PhD
Professor, Pathology and Laboratory Medicine;
Director, McLendon Clinical Laboratories, University of
North Carolina Hospitals, Chapel Hill, North Carolina,
USA

Thomas M Folks BA, MS, PhD
Chief, HIV/Retrovirus Diseases Branch, DASTLR,
Centers for Disease Control and Prevention, Atlanta,
Georgia, USA

Edward AC Follett BSc, PhD, FRCPath
Adviser in Microbiology, Scottish National Blood
Transfusion Service, Regional Virus Laboratory, Ruchill
Hospital, Glasgow, UK

Jocelyn RL Forsyth MB ChB, Dip Bact, MD,
FRCPA
Senior Associate, Department of Microbiology, The
University of Melbourne, Parkville, Victoria, Australia

Hisashi Fujioka PhD
Assistant Professor of Pathology, Institute of Pathology,
Case Western Reserve University, Cleveland, Ohio, USA

Guido Funke MD, FAMH
Consultant in Medical Microbiology, Department of
Medical Microbiology, University of Zurich, Zurich,
Switzerland

Kenneth L Gage PhD
Plague Section Chief, Bacterial Zoonoses Branch,
Division of Vector-Borne Infectious Diseases, Centers
for Disease Control and Prevention, Fort Collins,
Colorado, USA

N Spence Galbraith CBE, MB, FRCP, FFPHM,
DPH
Formerly Director, Public Health Laboratory Service,
Communicable Disease Surveillance Centre, Colindale,
London, UK

Lynne S Garcia MS, F(AAM)
Manager, UCLA Brentwood Facility Laboratory,
Pathology and Laboratory Medicine, University of
California at Los Angeles Medical Center, Los Angeles,
California, USA

Nigel J Gay MA, MSc
Mathematical Modeller, Immunisation Division, Public
Health Laboratory Service, Communicable Disease
Surveillance Centre, London, UK

Edwin E Geldreich AB, MS
Microbiology Consultant in Drinking Water, Cincinnati,
Ohio, USA

Caroline Attardo Genco PhD
Associate Professor, Department of Microbiology and
Immunology, Morehouse School of Medicine, Atlanta,
Georgia, USA

Wolfram H Gerlich PhD
Professor, Institute of Medical Virology, Giessen, Germany

Saheer E Gharbia BSc, PhD
Research Fellow (Hon), National Collection of Type Cultures, Public Health Laboratory Service, Colindale, London, UK

David I Gibson PhD, DSc
Head, Parasitic Worms Division, Department of Zoology, The Natural History Museum, London, UK

RJ Gilbert MPharm, PhD, DipBact, FRCPath
Director, Food Hygiene Laboratory, Central Public Health Laboratory, London, UK

Herbert M Gilles MSc, MD, DSc, DMedSc, FRCP, FFPHM
Emeritus Professor, Liverpool School of Tropical Medicine, Liverpool, UK

Youri Glupczynski MD, PhD
Head, Department of Clinical Microbiology, Centre Hospitalier Universitaire André Vésale, Montigny-le-Tilleul, Belgium

Robert C Good BA, MS, PhD
Guest Researcher, TB/Mycobacteriology Branch, Division of AIDS, STD and TB Laboratory Research, Centers for Disease Control and Prevention, Atlanta, Georgia, USA

Michael Goodfellow PhD, DSc, CBiol, FIBiol
Professor of Microbial Systematics, Department of Microbiology, The Medical School, Newcastle upon Tyne, UK

Norman L Goodman PhD
Professor and Director of Clinical Microbiology Laboratory, Department of Pathology, College of Medicine, University of Kentucky, Lexington, Kentucky, USA

Michael C Goodnough PhD
Assistant Scientist, Department of Food Microbiology and Toxicology, University of Wisconsin, Madison, Wisconsin, USA

Alexander WC von Graevenitz MD
Professor of Medical Microbiology; Director, Department of Medical Microbiology, Department of Medical Microbiology, Zurich University, Zurich, Switzerland

JM Grange MD, MSc
Reader in Clinical Microbiology, Imperial College School of Medicine, National Heart and Lung Institute, London, UK

John R Graybill MD
Chief, Infectious Diseases Division, Audie Murphy Veterans, Administration Hospital; and University of Texas Health Science Center, San Antonio, Texas, USA

David Greenwood PhD, DSc, FRCPath
Professor of Antimicrobial Science, Division of Microbiology and Infectious Diseases, Department of Clinical Laboratory Sciences, University Hospital, Queen's Medical Centre, Nottingham, UK

Duane J Gubler ScD, MS
Director, Division of Vector-Borne Infectious Diseases, Centers for Disease Control and Prevention, Fort Collins, Colorado, USA

Eveline Guého PhD
Researcher at INSERM, Unité de Mycologie, Institut Pasteur, Paris, France

Jacques Guillot DVM, PhD
Assistant Professor of Parasitology-Mycology, Unité de Parasitologie-Mycologie, URA-INRA Immunopathologie Cellulaire et Moleculaire, Ecole National Vétérinaire d'Alfort, Maisons-Alfort, France

Stephen C Hadler MD
Director, Epidemiology and Surveillance Division, National Immunization Program, Centers for Disease Control and Prevention, Atlanta, Georgia, USA

Thomas L Hale PhD
Department Chief, Department of Enteric Infections, Walter Reed Army Institute of Research, Washington DC, USA

Pekka E Halonen MD
Emeritus Professor of Virology, Medicity and Department of Virology, University of Turku, Turku, Finland

JM Hardie BDS, PhD, DipBact, FRCPath
Professor of Oral Microbiology, Department of Oral Microbiology, St Bartholomew's and the Royal London School of Medicine and Dentistry, London, UK

Melissa R Haswell-Elkins BA, MSc, PhD
Senior Research Fellow, Indigenous Health Programme, Australian Centre for International and Tropical Health and Nutrition, University of Queensland, Royal Brisbane Hospital, Brisbane, Queensland, Australia

Charles L Hatheway PhD
Chief, Botulism Laboratory, Centers for Disease Control and Prevention, Atlanta, Georgia, USA

Harald zur Hausen MD, DSc
Managing Director, Deutsches Krebsforschungszentrum, Heidelberg, Germany

Sir David L Hawksworth CBE, DSc, FDhc, CBiol, FIBiol, FLS
President, International Union of Biological Sciences; Visiting Professor, Universities of Kent, London and Reading; Director, International Mycological Institute, Egham, Surrey, UK

Roderick J Hay DM, FRCP, FRCPath
Mary Dunhill Professor of Cutaneous Medicine, St John's Institute of Dermatology, United Medical and Dental Schools of Guy's and St Thomas's, Guy's Hospital, London, UK

John C Hierholzer PhD
Former Supervisory Research Microbiologist, Centers
for Disease Control and Prevention, Atlanta, Georgia,
USA

Tor Hofstad MD, PhD
Professor of Medical Microbiology, Department of
Microbiology and Immunology, The Gade Institute,
University of Bergen, Bergen, Norway

John J Holland PhD
Professor Emeritus, Biology Department, University of
California at San Diego, La Jolla, California, USA

Barry Holmes PhD, DSc, FIBiol
Clinical Scientist, National Collection of Type Cultures,
Central Public Health Laboratory, Colindale, London,
UK

Stanley C Holt PhD
Professor of Microbiology, Department of Microbiology,
University of Texas Health Science Center at San
Antonio, San Antonio, Texas, USA

Marcel Hommel MD, PhD
Alfred Jones and Warrington Yorke Professor of
Tropical Medicine, Liverpool School of Tropical
Medicine, Liverpool, UK

GS de Hoog PhD
Professor of Mycology, Centraalbureau voor
Schimmelcultures, Baarn, The Netherlands

Douglas B Hornick MD
Associate Professor of Pulmonary and Critical Care
Medicine, Department of Medicine, University of Iowa
School of Medicine, Iowa City, Iowa, USA

Peter J Hotez MD, PhD
Associate Professor, Department of Pediatrics and
Epidemiology, Yale University School of Medicine, New
Haven, Connecticut, USA

TGB Howe MD, PhD
Senior Lecturer in Bacteriology, Department of
Pathology and Microbiology, School of Medical
Sciences, University of Bristol, Bristol, UK

TJ Humphrey BSc, PhD, MRCPath
Professor; Head of Public Health Laboratory Service
Food Microbiology Research Unit, Heavitree, Exeter,
Devon, UK

Hilary Humphreys MD, FRCPI, FRCPath
Consultant Microbiologist, Federated Dublin Voluntary
Hospitals, Dublin, Ireland

Charles J Hunter MD
Fellow, Department of Pathology, Division of Infectious
Diseases, University of Virginia Health Science Center,
Charlottesville, Virginia, USA

Thomas J Inzana PhD
Professor of Microbiology, Department of Biomedical
Sciences and Pathobiology, Virginia-Maryland Regional
College of Veterinary Medicine, Blacksburg, Virginia,
USA

Michael J Janda BSc, MS, PhD
Chief, Enterics and Special Pathogens Section,
Microbial Diseases Laboratory, California Department
of Health Services, Berkeley, California, USA

AE Jephcott MA, MD, FRCPath, DipBact
Director, Public Health Laboratory, Bristol, UK

Robert C Jerris PhD
Assistant Professor, Department of Pathology and
Laboratory Medicine, Emory University School of
Medicine, Atlanta, Georgia, USA

David T John MSPH, PhD
Professor of Microbiology/Parasitology; Associate Dean
for Basic Sciences, Department of Biochemistry and
Microbiology, Oklahoma State University, College of
Osteopathic Medicine, Tulsa, Oklahoma, USA

Elizabeth M Johnson BSc, PhD
Clinical Scientist, Mycology Reference Laboratory,
Bristol, UK

Eric A Johnson ScD
Professor of Food Microbiology and Toxicology, Food
Research Institute, College of Agricultrual and Life
Sciences, University of Wisconsin, Madison, Wisconsin,
USA

Russell C Johnson PhD
Professor of Microbiology, Department of Microbiology,
University of Minnesota, Minneapolis, Minnesota, USA

Dorothy Jones BSc, MSc, PhD, DipBact
Honorary Fellow, Department of Microbiology and
Immunology, University of Leicester, Leicester, UK

J Zoe Jordens BSc, PhD
Clinical Scientist/Honorary Senior Lecturer,
Haemophilus Reference Laboratory, Oxford Public
Health Laboratory and Nuffield Department of
Pathology & Bacteriology, John Radcliffe Hospital,
Headington, Oxford, UK

Stephen L Josephson PhD
Director, Microbiology/Virology, APC 1136, Rhode
Island Hospital, Providence, Rhode Island, USA

Kimberly L Kane BSc, PhD
Postdoctoral Fellow, Clinical Microbiology–Immunology
Laboratories, University of North Carolina Hospitals,
Chapel Hill, North Carolina, USA

Michael Kann MD
Research Fellow, Institute of Medical Virology, Justus-
Liebig-Universität Giessen, Giessen, Germany

SHE Kaufmann PhD
Professor and Head of Immunology, Department of
Immunology, University of Ulm, Ulm, Germany

Yoshihiro Kawaoka PhD
Professor, Department of Pathobiological Science,
School of Veterinary Medicine, University of Wisconsin-
Madison, Madison, Wisconsin, USA

Masako Kawasaki PhD
Instructor, Department of Dermatology, Kanazawa
Medical University, Uchinada, Ishikawa, Japan

Rima F Khabbaz MD
Associate Director for Medical Science, Division of Viral
and Rickettsial Diseases, National Center for Infectious
Diseases, Centers for Disease Control and Prevention,
Atlanta, Georgia, USA

Michael P Kiley BS, MS, PhD
Senior Scientific Adviser, Federal Laboratories for
Health Canada and Agriculture and Agri-Food Canada,
Winnipeg, Manitoba, Canada

Mogens Kilian DMD, DSc
Professor of Microbiology, Head, Department of
Medical Microbiology and Immunology, University of
Aarhus, Aarhus, Denmark

Hans-Dieter Klenk MD
Professor of Virology, Head, Department of Hygiene
and Medical Microbiology, Institute for Virology,
Philipps-University Marburg, Marburg, Germany

Wesley E Kloos PhD
Professor of Genetics and Microbiology, Department of
Genetics, North Carolina State University, Raleigh,
North Carolina, USA

Somei Kojima MD, PhD
Professor of Parasitology, Department of Parasitology,
University of Tokyo, Minato-ku, Tokyo, Japan

Paul E Kolenbrander PhD
Research Microbiologist, National Institute of Dental
Research, National Institutes of Health, Bethesda,
Maryland, USA

Myriam S Künzi PhD
Postdoctoral Fellow, John Hopkins Oncology Center,
Baltimore, Maryland, USA

Ralph Lainson OBE, FRS, AFTWAS, DSc
Professor (Honoris Causa), Federal University of Pará,
ex Director, The Wellcome Belém Leishmaniasis Unit,
Departamento de Parasitologia, Instituto Evandro
Chagas, Belém, Pará, Brazil

Paul R Lambden BSc, PhD
Senior Research Fellow, Molecular Microbiology,
University Medical School, Southampton General
Hospital, Southampton, UK

Sandra A Larsen MS, PhD
Guest Researcher, Bacterial STD Branch, Division of
AIDS, Sexually Transmitted Diseases and Tuberculosis
Laboratory Research, National Center for Infectious
Diseases, Centers for Disease Control and Prevention,
Atlanta, Georgia, USA

Edward R Leadbetter PhD
Professor of Microbiology, Department of Molecular
and Cell Biology, University of Connecticut, Storrs,
Connecticut, USA

James W LeDuc PhD
Associate Director, Global Health, National Center for
Infectious Diseases, Centers for Disease Control and
Prevention, Atlanta, Georgia, USA

Paul F Lehmann PhD
Professor of Microbiology and Immunology,
Microbiology Department, Medical College of Ohio,
Toledo, Ohio, USA

Stanley M Lemon MD
Professor of Microbiology and Immunology and
Internal Medicine, Chairman, Department of
Microbiology and Immunology, University of Texas
Medical Branch at Galveston, Galveston, Texas, USA

Lony Chong-Leong Lim PhD
Fellow, William W McLendon Clinical Immunology
Laboratory, University of North Carolina Hospitals,
Chapel Hill, North Carolina, USA

Graham Lloyd BSc, MSc, PhD
Head of Diagnosis, Centre for Applied Microbiology
and Research, Porton Down, Salisbury, Wiltshire, UK

Alberto T Londero MD
Emeritus Professor, Department of Microbiology,
Session Medical Mycology, School of Medicine, Federal
University of Santa Maria, Santa Maria, RS, Brazil

Francisco J López-Antuñano MD, MPH
Consultant, Instituto Nacional de Salud, Morelos,
Mexico

Mario Lozano Chiu PhD
Postdoctoral Fellow, University of Texas Medical
School, Houston, Texas, USA

David M MacLaren MA, MD, FRCP, FRCPath
Emeritus Professor of Medical Bacteriology, Moidart
House, Bodicote, Banbury, Oxford, UK

Alastair P MacMillan BVSc, MSc, MRCVS
Head, FAO/WHO Collaborating Centre for Reference
and Research on Brucellosis, Central Veterinary
Laboratory, Addlestone, Surrey, UK

CR Madeley MD, FRCPath
Consultant Virologist, Public Health Laboratory Service,
Institute of Pathology, Newcastle General Hospital,
Newcastle upon Tyne, UK

John T Magee PhD, MSc, FIMLS
Top Grade Scientific Officer, Department of Medical
Microbiology and Public Health Laboratory, University
of Wales College of Medicine, Cardiff, UK

Brian WJ Mahy PhD, ScD
Director, Division of Viral and Rickettsial Diseases,
National Center for Infectious Diseases, Centers for
Disease Control and Prevention, Atlanta, Georgia, USA

Scott A Martin BS, MS, PhD
Professor, Department of Animal and Dairy Science,
College of Agriculture, Livestock and Poultry,
University of Georgia, Athens, Georgia, USA

William J Martin PhD
Director, Scientific Resources Program, National Center
for Infectious Diseases, Centers for Disease Control and
Prevention, Atlanta, Georgia, USA

Adolfo Martínez-Palomo MD, DSc
Director General, Centro de Investigación y de Estudios
Avanzados, Mexico City, Mexico

Tadahiko Matsumoto MD, DMSc
Director, Department of Dermatology, Toshiba
Hospital, Higashi-oi, Shinagawa-ku, Tokyo, Japan

Ruth Matthews MD, PhD, MSc, FRCPath
Reader in Medical Microbiology, Department of
Medical Microbiology, Manchester Royal Infirmary,
Manchester, UK

Joseph E McDade PhD
Associate Director for Laboratory Science, National
Center for Infectious Diseases, Centers for Disease
Control and Prevention, Atlanta, Georgia, USA

Michael R McGinnis PhD
Director, Medical Mycology Research Center, Associate
Director, University of Texas at Galveston-WHO
Collaborating Center for Tropical Diseases, and
Professor, Department of Pathology, University of Texas
Medical Branch at Galveston, Galveston, Texas, USA

Jim McLauchlin PhD
Clinical Scientist, Central Public Health Laboratory,
Colindale, London, UK

Heinz Mehlhorn PhD
Professor of Parasitologie, Institut für Zoomorphologie,
Zellbiologie und Parasitologie, Heinrich-Heine-
Universität, Düsseldorf, Germany

A Leonel Mendoza MS, PhD
Assistant Professor, Department of Microbiology,
Medical Technology Program, Michigan State
University, East Lansing, Michigan, USA

Volker ter Meulen MD
Chairman, Institute for Virology and Immunobiology,
University of Würzberg, Würzberg, Germany

Gillian Midgley BSc, PhD
Lecturer in Medical Mycology, Department of Medical
Mycology, St John's Institute of Dermatology, United
Medical and Dental School of Guy's and St Thomas's,
St Thomas's Hospital, London, UK

Michael A Miles MSc, PhD, DSc
Professor of Medical Parasitology and Head, Applied
Molecular Biology Unit, Department of Medical
Parasitology, London School of Hygiene and Tropical
Medicine, London, UK

J Michael Miller PhD, ABMM
Chief, Diagnostic Microbiology Section, Hospital
Infections Program, National Center for Infectious
Diseases, Centers for Disease Control and Prevention,
Atlanta, Georgia, USA

P Minor BA, PhD
Head, Division of Virology, National Institute for
Biological Standard and Control, Potters Bar,
Hertfordshire, UK

AC Minson BSc, PhD
Professor of Virology, Virology Division, Department of
Pathology, University of Cambridge, Cambridge, UK

DH Molyneux MA, PhD, DSc
Director, Professor of Tropical Health Sciences,
Liverpool School of Tropical Medicine, Liverpool, UK

Arnold S Monto MD
Professor of Epidemiology, School of Public Health,
University of Michigan, Ann Arbor, Michigan, USA

Stephen A Morse MSPH, PhD
Associate Director for Science, Division of AIDS, STD
and Tuberculosis Laboratory Research, Centers for
Disease Control and Prevention, Atlanta, Georgia, USA

RP Mortlock BS, PhD
Professor of Microbiology, Section of Microbiology,
Cornell University, Ithaca, New York, USA

Ralph Muller DSc, PhD, BSc, FIBiol
Formerly Director, International Institute of
Parasitology, St Albans, Hertfordshire, UK

David A Murdoch MA, MBBS, MSc, MD, MRCPath
Honorary Clinical Research Fellow, Department of
Microbiology, Southmead Health Services NHS Trust,
Westbury-on-Trym, Bristol, UK

Frederick A Murphy DVM, PhD
Professor, School of Veterinary Medicine, University of
California, Davis, California, USA

RP Murray PhD
Professor, Division of Laboratory Medicine,
Departments of Pathology and Medicine, Washington
University School of Medicine, St Louis, Missouri, USA

David Mutimer MBBS
Senior Lecturer, Birmingham University Department of
Medicine; Honorary Consultant Physician, Liver and
Hepatobiliary Unit, Queen Elizabeth Hospital,
Edgbaston, Birmingham, UK

Irving I Nachamkin PhD
Professor of Pathology and Laboratory Medicine,
Department of Pathology and Laboratory Medicine,
University of Pennsylvania School of Medicine,
Philadelphia, Pennsylvania, USA

Francis E Nano PhD
Associate Professor, Department of Biochemistry and
Microbiology, University of Victoria, Victoria, British
Columbia, Canada

AA Nash BSc, MSc, PhD
Professor, Department of Veterinary Pathology,
University of Edinburgh, Edinburgh, UK

Neal Nathanson MD
Professor and Chair Emeritus, Department of
Microbiology, University of Pennsylvania Medical
Center, Philadelphia, Pennsylvania, USA

James C Neil BSc, PhD
Professor of Virology and Molecular Oncology,
Department of Veterinary Pathology, University of
Glasgow, Glasgow, UK

WC Noble DSc, FRCPath
Professor of Microbiology, Department of Microbial
Diseases, St John's Institute of Dermatology, United
Medical and Dental Schools of Guy's and St Thomas's,
St Thomas's Hospital, London, UK

Steven J Norris PhD
Professor of Pathology and Laboratory Medicine,
Microbiology and Molecular Genetics, Department of
Pathology, University of Texas Health Science Center,
Houston, Texas, USA

David C Old PhD, DSc, FIBiol, FRCPath
Reader in Medical Microbiology, Department of
Medical Microbiology, Ninewells Hospital and Medical
School, Dundee, UK

Arvind A Padhye PhD
Chief, Fungus Reference Laboratory, Emerging
Bacterial and Mycotic Diseases Branch, Division of
Bacterial and Mycotic Diseases, Centers for Disease
Control and Prevention, Atlanta, Georgia, USA

Norberto J Palleroni PhD
Professor of Microbiology, Center for Agricultural
Molecular Biology, Cooke College, Rutgers University,
New Brunswick, New Jersey, USA

Stephen R Palmer MA, MB, BChir, FFPHM
Professor & Director, Welsh Combined Centres for
Public Health, University of Wales College of Medicine;
Head, Communicable Disease Surveillance Centre
Welsh Unit, Cardiff, UK

Demosthenes Pappagianis PhD, MD
Professor of Medical Biology and Immunology,
Department of Medical Microbiology and Immunology,
University of California, Davis, California, USA

M Thomas Parker MD, FRCPath, DipBact
Formerly Director, Cross-Infection Reference
Laboratory, Central Public Health Laboratory,
Colindale, London, UK

D Parratt MD, FRCPath
Senior Lecturer, Department of Medical Microbiology,
Ninewells Hospital, Dundee, UK

Roger Parton BSc, PhD
Senior Lecturer, Division of Infection and Immunity,
Institute of Biomedical and Life Sciences, University of
Glasgow, Glasgow, UK

Thomas F Patterson MD
Associate Professor of Medicine, Division of Infectious
Diseases, Department of Medicine, University of Texas
Health Science Center, San Antonio, Texas, USA

Charles W Penn BSc, PhD
Reader in Microbiology, School of Biological Sciences,
University of Birmingham, Edgbaston, Birmingham, UK

T Hugh Pennington MB, BS, PhD, FRCPath, FRSE
Professor of Bacteriology, Department of Medical
Microbiology, University of Aberdeen, Aberdeen, UK

John R Perfect MD
Professor of Medicine, Duke University Medical Center,
Durham, North Carolina, USA

William A Petri Jnr MD, PhD
Professor, Department of Infectious Diseases, University
of Virginia Health Sciences Center, Charlottesville,
Virginia, USA

Paula M Pitha BS, MS, PhD
Professor of Oncology, Oncology Center and
Department of Molecular Biology and Genetics,
Baltimore, Maryland, USA

Tyrone L Pitt MPhil, PhD
Deputy Director, Laboratory of Hospital Infection,
Central Public Health Laboratory, Colindale, London,
UK

Tanja Popovic MD, PhD
Principal Investigator, Diphtheria Research Project,
Childhood and Respiratory Diseases Branch, Division of
Bacterial and Mycotic Diseases, National Center for
Infectious Diseases, Centers for Disease Control and
Prevention, Atlanta, Georgia, USA

R Scott Pore PhD
Professor of Microbiology and Immunology,
Department of Microbiology and Immunology, West
Virginia University School of Medicine, Morgantown,
West Virginia, USA

Roger Pradinaud MD
Directeur, Service de Dermato-Vénéreo-Leprologie,
Centre Hospitalier de Cayenne, Guyane Française

Craig R Pringle BSc, PhD
Professor of Biological Sciences, Biological Sciences
Department, University of Warwick, Coventry,
Warwickshire, UK

Stanley B Prusiner AB, MD
Professor of Neurology, Biochemistry and Biophysics,
Department of Neurology, University of California, San
Francisco, California, USA

Thomas J Quan PhD, MPH
Microbiologist, Imu-Tek Animal Health Inc, Fort
Collins, Colorado, USA

CP Quinn BSc, PhD
Head, Biotherapy Unit, Centre for Applied
Microbiology and Research, Porton Down, Salisbury,
Wiltshire, UK

Sharath K Rai PhD
Postdoctoral Fellow, Department of Molecular
Immunology, Bristol Myers Squibb PRI, Seattle,
Washington, USA

Anita Rampling MA, PhD, MB ChB, FRCPath
Director, Public Health Laboratory, Department of
Pathology, West Dorset Hospital, Dorchester, UK

Robert C Read MD, MRCP
Senior Clinical Lecturer in Infectious Diseases,
Department of Medical Microbiology, University of
Sheffield Medical School, Sheffield, UK

Stephen C Redd MD
Chief, Measles Elimination Activity, Epidemiology and
Surveillance Division, Centers for Disease Control and
Prevention, Atlanta, Georgia, USA

Sanjay G Revankar MD
Infectious Diseases Fellow, Department of Medicine,
Division of Infectious Diseases, University of Texas
Health Science Center, San Antonio, Texas, USA

John H Rex MD
Associate Professor, University of Texas Medical School,
Houston, Texas, USA

Malcolm D Richardson BSc, PhD, CBiol, MIBiol,
FRCPath
Director, Regional Mycology Reference Laboratory,
Department of Dermatology, Glasgow, UK

Geoffrey L Ridgway MD, BSc, MRCP, FRCPath
Consultant Microbiologist, Department of Clinical
Microbiology, University College London Hospitals;
Honorary Senior Lecturer, University College Hospital,
London, UK

Glenn D Roberts PhD
Director, Clinical Mycology and Mycobacteriology
Laboratories; Professor of Microbiology and Laboratory
Medicine, Mayo Medical School, Division of Clinical
Microbiology, Mayo Clinic, Rochester, Minnesota, USA

Betty H Robertson PhD
Chief, Virology Section, Hepatitis Branch, Division of
Viral and Rickettsial Diseases, Centers for Disease
Control and Prevention, Hepatitis Branch, Atlanta,
Georgia, USA

Frank G Rodgers PhD
Professor of Microbiology; Editor, Journal of Clinical
Microbiology, Department of Microbiology, Rudman
Hall, University of New Hampshire, Durham, New
Hampshire, USA

John T Roehrig PhD
Chief, Arbovirus Diseases Branch, Division of Vector-
Borne Infectious Diseases, National Center for
Infectious Diseases, Centers for Disease Control and
Prevention, Fort Collins, Colorado, USA

MJ Rosovitz BSc
Research Assistant, Department of Bacteriology,
University of Wisconsin-Madison, Madison, Wisconsin,
USA

Paul A Rota PhD
Research Microbiologist, Measles Virus Section, Centers
for Disease Control and Prevention, Atlanta, Georgia,
USA

Andrew H Rudolph MD
Clinical Professor of Dermatology, Dermatology
Department, Baylor College of Medicine, Houston
Texas, USA

Kathryn L Ruoff PhD
Assistant Professor of Pathology, Harvard Medical
School; Assistant Director, Microbiology Laboratories,
Massachusetts General Hospital, Boston, Massachusetts,
USA

A Denver Russell BPharm, PhD, DSc, FRCPath,
FRPharmS
Professor, Welsh School of Pharmacy, University of
Wales at Cardiff, Cardiff, UK

WC Russell BSc, PhD, FRSE
Emeritus Research Professor, School of Biological and
Medical Sciences, University of St Andrews, St Andrews,
Fife, UK

Maria S Salvato PhD
Assistant Professor, Department of Pathology and
Laboratory Medicine, Services Memorial Institute,
University of Wisconsin Medical School, Madison,
Wisconsin, USA

Anthony Sanchez PhD
Special Pathogens Branch, Division of Viral and
Rickettsial Diseases, National Center for Infectious
Diseases, Centers for Disease Control and Prevention,
Atlanta, Georgia, USA

Klaus P Schaal MD
Director, Professor of Medical Microbiology, Institute
for Medical Microbiology and Immunology, University
of Bonn, Bonn, Germany

Julius Schachter PhD
Professor of Laboratory Medicine, World Health
Organization Collaborating Centre for References and
Research on Chlamydia, Chlamydia Research
Laboratory, Department of Laboratory Medicine, San
Francisco General Hospital, San Francisco, California,
USA

Wiley A Schell MSc
Research Associate, Department of Medicine, Duke
University Medical Center, Durham, North Carolina,
USA

Walter F Schlech III MD
Professor of Medicine, Faculty of Medicine, Dalhousie
University, QE II HSC, Halifax, Nova Scotia, Canada

L Schlesinger MD
Associate Professor of Medicine, Department of
Medicine, Division of Infectious Diseases, University of
Iowa, Iowa City, Iowa, USA

Connie S Schmaljohn PhD
Chief, Department of Molecular Virology, US Army
Medical Research Institute of Infectious Diseases, Fort
Detrick, Maryland, USA

Gabriel A Schmunis MD, PhD
Coordinator, Communicable Diseases Program, Pan
American Health Organization, Washington, DC, USA

Sibylle Schneider-Schaulies PhD
Lecturer, Institut für Virologie und Immunbiologie,
Universität Würzberg, Würzberg, Germany

John Richard Seed PhD
Professor, Department of Epidemiology, School of
Public Health, University of North Carolina, Chapel
Hill, North Carolina, USA

Esther Segal PhD
Professor of Microbiology/Mycology, Department of
Human Microbiology, Sackler School of Medicine, Tel
Aviv University, Ramat Aviv, Tel Aviv, Israel

Bernard W Senior BSc, PhD, FRCPath
Lecturer in Medical Microbiology, Department of
Medical Microbiology, Dundee University Medical
School, Ninewells Hospital and Medical School,
Dundee, UK

Haroun N Shah BSc, PhD, FRCPath
Head, Identification Services Unit, National Collection
of Type Cultures, Central Public Health Laboratory,
Colindale, London, UK

Jeffrey J Shaw PhD, DSc
Professor, Departamento de Parasitologia, Instituto de
Ciências Biomédicas, Universidade de São Paulo, São
Paulo, Brazil

Thomas M Shinnick PhD
Chief, Tuberculosis/Mycobacteriology Branch, Centers
for Disease Control and Prevention, Atlanta, Georgia,
USA

Stuart G Siddell BSc, PhD
Professor of Virology, Institute of Virology, University
of Würzburg, Würzburg, Germany

Gunter O Siegl PhD
Professor and Head, Institute for Clinical Microbiology
and Immunology, St Gallen, Switzerland

Lynne Sigler MSc
Curator and Associate Professor, University of Alberta
Microfungus Collection and Herbarium, Devonian
Botanic Garden, Edmonton, Alberta, Canada

RB Sim BSc, DPhil
MRC Scientific Staff, MRC Immunochemistry Unit,
Department of Biochemistry, University of Oxford,
Oxford, UK

Peter Simmonds BM, PhD, MRCPath
Senior Lecturer, Department of Medical Microbiology,
University of Edinburgh Medical School, Edinburgh,
UK

Anthony Simmons MA, MB, BChir, PhD, FRCPath
Senior Medical Specialist, Infectious Diseases
Laboratories, Institute of Medical and Veterinary
Science, Adelaide, Australia

Martin B Skirrow MB, ChB, PhD, FRCPath, DTM&H
Consultant Medical Microbiologist, Public Health
Laboratory, Gloucestershire Royal Hospital, Gloucester,
UK

Mary PE Slack MA, MB, FRCPath
Lecturer (Honorary Consultant) in Bacteriology,
Haemophilus Reference Laboratory, Oxford Public
Health Laboratory and Nuffield Department of
Pathology and Bacteriology, John Radcliffe Hospital,
Oxford, UK

Henry R Smith MA, PhD
Deputy Director, Laboratory of Enteric Pathogens,
Central Public Health Laboratory, Colindale, London,
UK

Eric J Snijder PhD
Assistant Professor, Department of Virology, Institute of
Medical Microbiology, Leiden University, Leiden, The
Netherlands

Phyllis H Sparling DVM, MS
Liaison, Centers for Disease Control and Prevention,
Atlanta, Georgia, USA

David CE Speller MA, BM, BCh, FRCP, FRCPath
Emeritus Professor of Clinical Microbiology, University
of Bristol, Bristol, UK

Carol A Spiegel PhD
Associate Professor, Department of Pathology and
Laboratory Medicine, University of Wisconsin, Madison,
Wisconsin, USA

Andrew Spielman ScD
Professor of Tropical Public Health, Department of
Tropical Public Health, Harvard School of Public
Health, Boston, Massachusetts, USA

Bret M Steiner PhD
Chief, Treponemal Pathogenesis, Division of Sexually
Transmitted Diseases, Centers for Disease Control and
Prevention, Atlanta, Georgia, USA

Scott J Stewart BS
Formerly of National Institute of Allergies and
Infectious Diseases; 344 Roaring Lion Road, Hamilton,
Montana, USA

Max Sussman BSc, PhD, CBiol, FIBiol, FRCPath
Emeritus Professor of Bacteriology, Department of
Microbiology, The Medical School, Newcastle upon
Tyne, UK

Roland W Sutter MD, MPH, TM
Deputy Chief for Technical Affairs, Polio Eradication
Activity, National Immunization Program, Centers for
Disease Control and Prevention, Atlanta, Georgia, USA

Bala Swaminathan PhD
Chief, Foodborne and Diarrhoeal Diseases Laboratory
333 Section, Foodborne and Diarrhoeal Diseases
Branch, Centers for Disease Control and Prevention,
Atlanta, Georgia, USA

Robert V Tauxe MD, MPH
Chief, Foodborne and Diarrhoeal Diseases Branch,
Division of Bacterial and Mycotic Diseases, Centers for
Disease Control and Prevention, Atlanta, Georgia, USA

David J Taylor MA, VetMB, PhD, MRCVS
Reader in Veterinary Microbiology, Department of
Veterinary Pathology, University of Glasgow, School of
Veterinary Medicine, Bearsden, Glasgow, UK

John M Taylor PhD
Senior Member, Fox Chase Cancer Center,
Philadelphia, Pennsylvania, USA

David Taylor-Robinson MD, MRCP, FRCPath
Emeritus Professor of Microbiology and Genitourinary
Medicine, Department of Genitourinary Medicine, St
Mary's Hospital, London, UK

Lucia Martins Teixeira PhD
Associate Professor, Universidade Federal do Rio de
Janeiro, Instituto de Microbiologia, Rio de Janeiro,
Brazil

Sam Rountree Telford III DSc
Lecturer in Tropical Health, Department of Tropical
Public Health, Harvard University, Boston,
Massachusetts, USA

Ram P Tewari PhD
Professor of Microbiology, Department of Medical
Microbiology and Immunology, Southern Illinois
University, Springfield, Illinois School of Medicine,
Springfield, Illinois, USA

E John Threlfall BSc, PhD
Grade C Clinical Scientist, Laboratory of Enteric
Pathogens, Central Public Health Laboratory,
Colindale, London, UK

Richard C Tilton BS, MS, PhD
Senior Vice President, Chief Scientific Director, BBI
Clinical Laboratories, New Britain, Connecticut, USA

Noel Tordo PhD
Head, Laboratoire de Lyssavirus, Institut Pasteur, Paris,
France

Anna Maria Tortorano PhD
Associate Professor of Hygiene, Laboratory of Medical
Microbiology, Institute of Hygiene and Preventive
Medicine, School of Medicine, Università degli Studi di
Milano, Milano, Italy

Kevin J Towner BSc, PhD
Consultant Clinical Scientist, Public Health Laboratory,
University Hospital, Queen's Medical Centre,
Nottingham, UK

JG Tully BS, MS, PhD
Chief, Mycoplasma Section, Laboratory of Molecular
Microbiology, National Institute of Allergy and
Infectious Diseases, National Institutes of Health,
Frederick, Maryland, USA

Peter C B Turnbull BSc, MS, PhD
Head, Anthrax Section, Centre for Applied
Microbiology and Research, Porton Down, Salisbury,
Wiltshire, UK

Kenneth L Tyler MD
Professor of Neurology, Medicine, Microbiology and
Immunology, Department of Neurology, University of
Colorado Health Sciences Center, and Chief,
Neurology Service Denver Veteran Affairs Medical
Center, Denver, Colorado, USA

Edward J Usherwood MA, PhD
Research Fellow, Department of Veterinary Pathology,
Edinburgh, UK

Maria Anna Viviani MD
Associate Professor of Hygiene, Laboratory of Medical
Microbiology, Institute of Hygiene and Preventive
Medicine, School of Medicine, Università degli Studi di
Milano, Milano, Italy

Martin I Voskuil BA
Research Scientist, Department of Bacteriology,
University of Wisconsin-Madison, Madison, Wisconsin,
USA

William G Wade BSc, PhD
Richard Dickinson Professor of Oral Microbiology,
Head of Oral Biology Unit, Department of Oral
Medicine and Pathology, United Medical and Dental
Schools of Guy's and St Thomas's, Guy's Hospital,
London, UK

Derek Wakelin BSc, PhD, DSc, FRCPath
Professor of Zoology, Department of Life Science,
University of Nottingham, Nottingham, UK

Alexander Wandeler MSc, PhD
Head of Rabies Unit, Animal Diseases Research
Institute, Nepean, Ontario, Canada

Audrey R Wanger PhD
Assistant Professor, Department of Pathology and
Laboratory Medicine, University of Texas Medical
School at Houston, Houston, Texas, USA

Bodo Wanke PhD, MD
Head of Laboratório de Micologia Médica, Laboratório
de Micologia, Hospital Evandro Chagas, Rio de Janeiro,
Brazil

ME Ward BSc, PhD
Professor of Medical Microbiology, Molecular
Microbiology, Southampton University School of
Medicine, Southampton General Hospital,
Southampton, UK

MFR Waters OBE, MB, FRCP, FRCPath
Formerly Consultant Leprologist and Physician,
Hospital for Tropical Diseases, London, UK

Emilio Weiss BS, MS, PhD
Emeritus Chair of Science, Naval Medical Research
Institute, Bethesda, Maryland, USA

Irene Weitzman PhD
Assistant Director, Clinical Microbiology Service, and
Associate Professor of Clinical Pathology in Medicine,
Columbia Presbyterian Medical Center, New York, New
York, USA

Lawrence J Wheat MD
Professor of Medicine, Infectious Disease Division,
Wishard Memorial Hospital, Indianapolis, Indiana, USA

Richard J Whitley MD
Professor of Pediatrics, Microbiology and Medicine,
Department of Pediatrics, University of Alabama at
Birmingham, Birmingham, Alabama, USA

James Whitworth MD, FRCP, DTM&H
Team Leader, MRC Programme on AIDS, Entebbe,
Uganda

Louis A Wilson BS, MSc, MD, FACS
Professor of Ophthalmology, Emory University School
of Medicine and Adjunct Professor of Microbiology,
Georgia State University, Atlanta, Georgia, USA

John A Wyke MA, VetMB, PhD, MRCVS, FRSE
Director of Research, Beatson Institute, Honorary
Professor at University of Glasgow, Beatson Institute for
Cancer Research, Glasgow, UK

Kentaro Yoshimura BVM, DVM, PhD
Professor of Parasitology, Chairman, Department of
Parasitology, Akita University School of Medicine, Akita,
Japan

Viqar Zaman MBBS, DSc, DTM&H, FRCPath
Professor, Department of Microbiology, The Aga Khan
University, Karachi, Pakistan

Stephen H Zinder BA, MS, PhD
Professor of Microbiology, Section of Microbiology,
Cornell University, Ithaca, New York, USA

EDITOR-IN-CHIEF'S PREFACE

The period since publication of the first edition in 1929 has seen various modifications in the form and content of *Topley and Wilson*, perhaps the most important of which was the change with the 7th edition to a multi-author work in four volumes. This, the 9th edition, marks three spectacular departures from past policy.

First, and most obviously, the work now covers every class of pathogen: viruses, bacteria, fungi and parasites, including the helminths. The arrangement is in order of complexity, ranging from *Virology* in Volume 1 through *Systematic Bacteriology* and *Bacterial Infections* in Volumes 2 and 3, *Medical Mycology* in Volume 4 and *Parasitology* in Volume 5. Each has its own index, and a general index to the entire work is provided in Volume 6.

This major expansion called for a change in authorship, which previously was almost entirely British. Clearly, the range of expertise now needed to cover every aspect of medical microbiology, including mycology and parasitology, can no longer be provided from any one country and we have been fortunate in recruiting leading experts from many parts of the world for this expanded edition. In all, there are 234 chapters, of which the USA has provided 45% and the UK 35%; the remainder come from 20 other countries.

The third important new feature is the appearance of an electronic version alongside the printed work, which will facilitate information retrieval, cross-referencing and, most important, a continual programme of revision and updating.

During the planning phase, surveys of known and potential readers indicated a majority demand for more detailed referencing than hitherto, and the provision of factual material rather than the more speculative and discursive treatment characteristic of the early editions. This trend has become increasingly apparent with successive editions, and there is now no justification for retaining the word 'Principles' in the title. Despite this change in emphasis, the readership

for whom the work is intended remains the same; it comprises primarily microbiologists working in research, diagnostic and public health laboratories and those teaching both undergraduates and postgraduates. Although it is first and foremost a treatise on microbiology, the comprehensive coverage of the clinical and pathological features of infection makes it also an invaluable source of reference for physicians dealing with infective disease.

The 8th edition comprised four volumes of text, of which the first covered *General Bacteriology and Immunity*, and was intended to service those dealing with the more specialized topics. This arrangement did not, however, prove satisfactory; the 9th edition is therefore designed to make the volumes more self-contained, and descriptions of the immune response as it relates respectively to viruses, bacteria and the eukaryotic parasites are provided in the appropriate volumes.

The arrangement of the *Virology* volume is similar to that in the 8th edition, except that it is divided into five rather than two parts. Accounts of the general characteristics of bacteria and of bacteria in the environment will now be found in Volume 2 (*Systematic Bacteriology*). Both this and Volume 3 (*Bacterial Infections*) can be read individually, but, as in past editions, they obviously complement each other. The quantity of information now available has meant a further increase in size of Volumes 1, 2 and 3, which now contain about 30% more material than did the whole of the 8th edition. The two new volumes, dealing respectively with *Medical Mycology* and *Parasitology*, greatly enhance the value of the work as a whole. Whether to include the helminths under the title *Microbiology and Microbial Infections* was a debatable point, which succeeded on the grounds that to omit them would impair coverage of the entire gamut of infection, and that a separate mention in the title would have made it unwieldy.

Some points of editorial policy deserve mention. As in previous editions, the emphasis throughout is on infections of humans; animal diseases are given much less prominence, usually receiving mention only when they cause zoonoses, serve as models of pathogenesis or are of economic importance. Sections likely to be of interest only to the more specialized reader are indicated by the use of a small typeface, and the location and cross-referencing of specific sections are now made easier by numbering them.

The standard of the illustrations, many of which are now in colour, is considerably higher than in previous editions; in particular, there is a wealth of excellent drawings and photographs in Volumes 4 and 5. The quality of the references has been greatly improved by providing the titles of papers and both first and last pages; and the international provenance of the contributors has resulted in broader surveys of the world literature than is usual in predominantly British or American texts.

In conclusion, I take this opportunity of saying how much I appreciate the efforts of all those concerned with bringing this large and complex work to fruition. Almost by definition, the more distinguished the author, the more he or she will have other pressing commitments, a consideration that applies to most of our contributors. Sincere thanks are due to them for their participation and for providing the huge fund of learning and expertise that is apparent throughout the edition. I gladly take this opportunity of expressing my gratitude to all my colleagues on the editorial team for the intensive and sustained effort they have devoted to bringing this large and complex publication to fruition. It would be invidious to single out individuals among the copy-editors and the staff at Arnold who have laboured so devotedly behind the scenes, but to each of them my gratitude is also due for their competent help and unfailing support during the preparation of this edition.

LC

VOLUME EDITORS' PREFACE

The profound influence of molecular techniques on all branches of biomedical science is nowhere more apparent than in virology. The rate of accretion of knowledge within the lifetime of the last two editions has been exponential, and has had profound effects not only on our understanding of the basic properties of viruses, but of the pathogenesis, immunology and epidemiology of viral infections. These considerations are reflected in the size, scope and arrangement of this volume. The 34 chapters in the 8th edition have been increased to 47 and are now arranged in five parts: 1. General Characteristics of Viruses; 2. General Characteristics of Viral Infections, 3. Specific Viruses and Viral Infections; 4. Syndromes caused by a Range of Viruses; and 5. Principles of Diagnosis and Control.

Readers familiar with the 8th edition of *Topley and Wilson* will recognize a number of previous contributors to the Virology volume and will appreciate how thoroughly it has been updated, both by them and by the many new authors recruited for this edition.

As might be expected, a number of topics are new, or have been considerably expanded since the last edition. In Parts 1 and 2, there are now chapters on the origin and evolution of viruses, virus–host cell interactions and the role of cytokines in viral infections. Whereas the herpesviruses were previously considered in one chapter, there are now four, dealing respectively with their general properties and with the three subfamilies individually. Likewise, the single monograph on the hepatitis viruses has also been expanded to four, the previous umbrella group 'non-A non-B' viruses now being differentiated into hepatitis C, E and G viruses. Part 3 also contains new articles on the corona- and reoviruses. The increase in our understanding of prions and their aetiological role in the spongiform encephalopathies of animals and humans is well reflected in another important contribution; and for the first time there is a chapter on safety in the virology laboratory. The final article, on the emergence and re-emergence of virus infections, opens a vista of future trends in the study of viruses and their infections, ranging widely from the molecular basis for the emergence of new variants to the influence of increased day care facilities on the spread of viruses.

The editorial policies are similar to those for the 8th edition. Inevitably, there are some overlaps in subject matter within this volume and occasionally between this and the bacteriological volumes. The latitude permitted was a matter of editorial judgement; we hope that, within individual chapters, we have struck a reasonable balance between the tedium of repetition and the benefit of self-sufficiency.

In general, little prominence is given to infections of non-human species, except where they bear upon human infections in terms of, for example, zoonoses, models of pathogenesis or economic importance.

As in the 8th edition, we have preferred anglicized to latinized names of viruses, and for nomenclature have relied heavily on the Sixth Report of the International Committee on Taxonomy of Viruses (Murphy et al. 1995).

With the increasingly rapid move from morphological to genetic descriptions of viruses, we shall continue to define new virus species, genera and families. Many newly identified viruses now known to cause significant disease are being diagnosed using molecular techniques, even though they have not been characterized by the traditional methods of cell culture and infection of animal hosts. As a consequence, the inestimable value of research on viruses in the treatment and prevention of many human diseases will continue to be recognized; we hope that, not least among its functions, this volume will provide a valuable guide to those who become involved in these developments.

BM
LC

Reference

Murphy FA, Fauquet CM et al., 1995, Virus Taxonomy: Sixth Report of the International Committee on Taxonomy of Viruses, *Arch Virol*, **Suppl. 10**, Springer-Verlag, New York.

ABBREVIATIONS

aa	amino acid	BRSV	bovine respiratory syncytial virus
AAAV	avian adenoassociated virus	BRV	Breda virus
AaDNV	*Aedes albopictus* densovirus	BSE	bovine spongiform encephalopathy
AAV	adenoassociated virus	BSL	biosafety level
AChR	acetylcholine receptor	BTV	bluetongue virus
ACV	aciclovir, acyclovir	BVaraU	bromovinyl arabinosyl-uracil
ACV-DP	ACV diphosphate	BVDU	bromovinyl deoxyuridine
ACV-MP	ACV monophosphate	BVDV	bovine viral diarrhoea virus
ACV-TP	ACV triphosphate	C	core [protein]
ADC	AIDS dementia complex	C/H	cysteine–histidine rich motif
ADCC	antibody-dependent cell cytotoxicity	ca	cold-adapted
ADE	antibody-dependent enhancement	CAAV	canine adenoassociated virus
AFP	α-fetoprotein	CAM	cell adhesion molecule; chorioallantoic membrane
AGMK	African green monkey kidney		
AHC	acute haemorrhagic conjunctivitis	CAR	congenitally acquired rubella
AHDV	African horse sickness virus	CAV	canine adenovirus; Coxsackie A virus
AIDS	acquired immmunodeficiency syndrome	ccc	covalently closed circular [DNA]
ALV	avian leucosis virus	CCHF	Crimean–Congo haemorrhagic fever
AM	alveolar macrophage; aseptic meningitis	CCV	canine coronavirus; channel catfish virus
AMDV	Aleutian mink disease parvovirus	CEA	carcinoembryonic antigen
AMP-RT	amplified reverse transcriptase	CEE	Central European encephalitis
APD	average pore diameter	CF	complement fixation
AraA	adenine arabinoside	CFT	complement fixation test
ARDS	adult respiratory distress syndrome	CHO	Chinese hamster ovary
ARIMA	autoregressive integrated moving average	ChPV	chicken parvovirus
ARV	Adelaide river virus	CI	complementation index
ATL	adult T cell leukaemia/lymphoma	CID	cytomegalic inclusion disease
AZT	azidothymidine	CIN	cervical intraepithelial neoplasia
B19V	B19 virus	CJD	Creutzfeldt–Jakob disease
BAAV	bovine adenoassociated virus	CLP	core-like particle
BBB	blood–brain barrier	CMI	cell-mediated immunity
BCG	bacillus Calmette–Guérin	CMV	cytomegalovirus
BCV	bovine coronavirus	CNS	central nervous system
BDV	Borna disease virus	COSHH	Control of Substances Hazardous to Health
BEFV	bovine ephemeral fever virus		
BEV	Berne virus	CPE	cytopathic effect
BHA	bromelain-cleaved soluble haemagglutinin	CPMV	cowpea mosaic virus
BKV	BK virus	CPV	canine parvovirus
BL	biosafety level	CR	cellular receptor
BLV	bovine leukaemia virus	cRNA	complementary sense RNA
BmDNV	*Bombyx mori* densovirus	CSF	cerebrospinal fluid; colony-stimulating factor
bp	base pair		
BPIV	bovine parainfluenza virus	CTC	cytotoxic T cell
BPL	β-propiolactone	CTD	carboxy-terminal domain
BPV	bovine parvovirus	CTFV	Colorado tick fever virus

CTL	cytotoxic T lymphocyte		**GM**	growth medium
CV	coronavirus		**GM-CSF**	granulocyte macrophage colony stimulating factor CSF
CVB	Coxsackievirus B			
CVS	Challenge Virus Standard; congenital varicella syndrome		**GmDNV**	*Galleria mellonella* densovirus
			GP	glycoprotein; growth protein
D4T	2′,3′-didehydro-2′-deoxythymidine		**GPI**	glycophosphatidylinositol
DAF	decay accelerating factor		**GPV**	goose parvovirus
DBP	DNA-binding protein		**GSHV**	ground squirrel hepatitis virus
DDC	2′,3′-dideoxycytidine		**GSS**	Gerstmann–Sträussler–Scheinker [disease]
DDI	2′,3′-dideoxyinosine		**H-1PV**	H-1 virus
DHBV	Pekin duck hepatitis virus		**H-Ast2**	human astrovirus serotype 2
DHF	dengue haemorrhagic fever		**HA**	haemagglutination; haemagglutinin; heterophile antibody
DHF/DSS	dengue haemorrhagic fever/dengue shock syndrome			
			HAI	haemagglutination inhibition
DI	defective interfering		**HAM/TSP**	HTLV-I-associated myelopathy/tropical spastic paraparesis
DIC	disseminated intravascular coagulation			
DMSO	dimethyl sulphoxide		**HAV**	hepatitis A virus
DNApol	DNA polymerase		**HBIG**	hepatitis B immunoglobulin
dNTP	deoxyribonucleoside triphosphate		**HBsAg**	hepatitis B surface antigen
dPyK	deoxypyrimidine kinase		**HBV**	hepatitis B virus
DR	direct repeat		**HCC**	hepatocellular carcinoma
ds	double-stranded		**HCV**	hepatitis C virus; human coronavirus
dsRF	double-stranded replicative form		**HD**	Hodgkin's disease
DTH	delayed-type hypersensitivity		**HDCS**	human diploid cell strain
dUTPase	deoxyuridine triphosphatase		**HDV**	hepatitis D virus/hepatitis delta virus
E	envelope [protein]		**HE**	haemagglutinin–esterase
EA	early antigen		**HEF**	haemagglutinin–esterase fusion [protein]
EAAV	equine adenoassociated virus		**HEK**	human embryo kidney
EAE	experimental allergic encephalitis/encephalomyelitis		**HEL**	NTP binding/helicase domain
			HEPT	hydroxyethoxymethylphenylthiothymine
EAV	equine arteritis virus		**HEV**	haemagglutinating encephalomyelitis virus; hepatitis E virus
EBER	Epstein–Barr virus-encoded early RNA			
EBNA	Epstein–Barr viral nuclear antigen		**HF**	host factor
EBOV	Ebola virus		**HFMD**	hand-foot-and-mouth disease
EBV	Epstein–Barr virus; European bat virus		**HFRS**	haemorrhagic fever with renal syndrome
EDTA	ethylenediaminetetraacetic acid		**HFV**	human foamy virus
EEE	eastern equine encephalitis		**HGH**	human growth hormone
EEV	extracellular enveloped virus		**HGV**	hepatitis G virus
EGF	epidermal growth factor		**HHBV**	grey heron hepatitis B virus
EHDV	epizootic haemorrhagic disease virus		**HHV**	human herpesvirus
EHV	equine herpesvirus		**HI**	haemagglutination inhibition
EI	erythema infectiosum		**Hib**	*Haemophilus influenzae* type b
EIA	enzyme immunoassay		**HIV**	human immunodeficiency virus
EIAV	equine infectious anaemia virus		**HMEC**	human microvascular endothelial cell
EIPV	enhanced potency inactivated polio vaccine		**HNIG**	human normal immunoglobulin
			HPIV	human parainfluenza virus
ELISA	enzyme-linked immunosorbent assay		**HPMPC**	hydroxyphosphonylmethoxycytosine
EM	electron microscope/microscopy		**HPS**	hantavirus pulmonary syndrome
EMCV	encephalomyocarditis virus		**HPV**	human papillomavirus
EMV	equine morbillivirus		**HRIG**	rabies immunoglobulin of human origin
ER	endoplasmic reticulum		**HRV**	human rhinovirus
EV	epidermodysplasia verruciformis		**HSK**	HSV-induced keratitis
FcR	Fc receptor		**HSV**	herpes simplex virus
FCV	famciclovir; feline calicivirus		**HTLV**	human T cell leukaemia virus
FECV	feline enteric coronavirus		**HuCV**	human calicivirus
FeLV	feline leukaemia virus		**HUVEC**	human umbilical cord vein endothelial cell
FFI	fatal familial insomnia			
ffu	focus-forming unit		**HVS**	*Herpesvirus saimiri*
FIPV	feline infectious peritonitis virus		**IAHA**	immune adherence assay
FMDV	foot-and-mouth disease virus		**IBV**	infectious bronchitis virus
FPV	feline panleucopenia virus; feline parvovirus		**ICA**	islet cell antibody
			ICAM	intercellular adhesion molecule
FTIR	Fourier transform infrared [spectroscopy]		**ICE**	interleukin-1β-converting enzyme
GACRIA	IgG-capture radioimmunoassay		**IDDM**	insulin-dependent diabetes mellitus
GAPDH	glyceraldehyde-3-phosphate dehydrogenase		**IDU**	idoxuridine; injecting drug user
			IE	immediate early
GCV	ganciclovir		**IEM**	immunoelectron microscopy
GF	growth factor		**IF**	immunofluorescence

IFA	immunofluorescence assay	**MMR**	measles/mumps/rubella
IFN	interferon	**MMTV**	mouse mammary tumour virus
Ig	immunoglobulin	**MMV**	mice minute virus
IHA	indirect haemagglutination	**moi**	multiplicity of infection
IL	interleukin	**MPGN**	membranoproliferative glomerulonephritis
IM	infectious mononucleosis	**mRNA**	messenger RNA
iNOS	inducible nitric oxide synthetase	**MuLV**	murine leukaemia virus
INV	intracellular naked virus	**MuV**	mumps virus
IP	immunoperoxidase	**MV**	measles virus
IPA	immunoperoxidase assay	**MVC**	minute virus of canine
IPV	inactivated polio vaccine	**MVE**	Murray Valley encephalitis
IR	inverted repeat	**NA**	neuraminidase
IRES	internal ribosome entry site	**NAAT**	nucleic acid amplification technique
ISCOM	immuno-stimulating complex	**NANB**	non-A, non-B [hepatitis]
ISG	immune serum globulin; interferon-stimulated gene	**NASBA**	nucleic acid sequence-based amplification
ISRE	interferon-specific response element	**NDV**	Newcastle disease virus
ISVP	intermediate subviral particle	**NFT**	neurofibrillary tangles
ITR	inverted terminal repeat/repetition	**NGF**	nerve growth factor
IVDU	intravenous drug user	**NK**	natural killer
IVIG	intravenous immunoglobulin	**NLS**	nuclear localization site
JAK	Janus kinase	**NNSV**	non-segmented negative-strand [RNA] virus
JcDNV	*Junonia coenia* densovirus	**NP**	nucleoprotein
JCV	JC virus	**NPC**	nasopharyngeal carcinoma
JE	Japanese encephalitis	**NPS**	nasopharyngeal secretion
JHMV	murine coronavirus JHM	**NSI**	non-syncytia inducer
JLP	juvenile laryngeal papillomatosis	**NSP**	non-structural protein
kDa	kilodalton	**nt**	nucleotide
KRV	Kilham rat virus	**NTR**	non-translated region; non-translated RNA
KSHV	Kaposi's sarcoma herpesvirus	**OAAV**	ovine adenoassociated virus
LA	latex agglutination	**2′,5′-OAS**	2′,5′-oligoadenylate synthetase
LAT	latency-associated transcript	**OPV**	oral poliovirus
LAV	lymphadenopathy-associated virus	**ORF**	open reading frame
LCL	lymphoid cell line	**ORS**	oral rehydration salt
LCMV	lymphocytic choriomeningitis virus	**P & I**	pneumonia and influenza
LCR	ligase chain reaction	**PAGE**	polyacrylamide gel electrophoresis
LDL	low density lipoprotein	**PBMC**	peripheral blood mononuclear cell
LDV	lactate dehydrogenase-elevating virus	**PBS**	phosphate-buffered saline; primer binding site
LIP	lymphoid interstitial pneumonitis	**PCP**	papain-like cysteine proteinase; *Pneumocystis carinii* pneumonia
LMP	last menstrual period; latent membrane protein	**PCR**	polymerase chain reaction
LNYV	lettuce necrotic yellows virus	**PCV**	penciclovir
LOD	logarithm of odds	**PEDV**	porcine epidemic diarrhoea virus
LPD	lymphoproliferative disease	**PFA**	phosphonoformate
LPV	lapine parvovirus	**pfu**	plaque-forming unit
LSD	lumpy skin disease	**PHA**	phytohaemagglutinin
LTR	long terminal repeat	**PHC**	primary hepatocellular carcinoma
LUIIV	LUIII virus	**pHSA**	polymerized human serum albumin
M	matrix/membrane [protein]	**PK**	[cytoplasmic] protein kinase
M-MuLV	Moloney murine leukaemia virus	**PKC**	cellular protein kinase
MAb	monoclonal antibody	**PKR**	protein kinase dsRNA
MACRIA	M-antibody capture radioimmunoassay	**PMKC**	primary [cynomolgus/rhesus] monkey kidney cell
MADT	morphological alteration and disintegration test	**PML**	progressive multifocal leucoencephalopathy
MAI	*Mycobacterium avium* intracellular [infection]	**PPD**	purified protein derivative
MAR	monoclonal antibody-resistant	**PPV**	porcine parvovirus
MBP	mannose-binding protein; myelin basic protein	**PRCV**	porcine respiratory coronavirus
MDCK	Madin–Darby canine kidney [cell]	**PRRSV**	porcine reproductive and respiratory syndrome virus
ME	myalgic encephalomyelitis	**PTA**	phosphotungstic acid
MEV	mink enteritis virus	**PTB**	polypyrimidine tract binding [protein]
MGF	myxoma growth factor	**pTP**	precursor of terminal protein
MHC	major histocompatibility complex	**PVR**	poliovirus receptor
MHV	murine hepatitis virus; murine herpesvirus	**RbCV**	rabbit coronavirus
MIBE	measles inclusion body encephalitis	**RCV**	rat coronavirus
MK	monkey kidney	**RdRp**	RNA-dependent RNA polymerase
MM	maintenance medium		

REA	restriction enzyme analysis
RER	rough endoplasmic reticulum
RF	replicative form
RHDV	rabbit haemorrhagic disease virus
RI	replicative intermediate
RIA	radioimmunoassay
RIPA	radioimmunoprecipitation assay
RK	receptor kinase
RNP	ribonucleoprotein
RPV	raccoon parvovirus
RR	ribonucleotide reductase; Ross River
RRE	rev-responsive element
RREID	rapid rabies enzyme immunodiagnosis
RRV	rhesus rotavirus
RSSV	Russian spring–summer encephalitis
RSV	respiratory syncytial virus; Rous sarcoma virus
RT	reverse transcriptase
RT-PCR	reverse transcriptase polymerase chain reaction
RTPV	RT parvovirus
RV	rabies virus; rubella virus
SAR	secondary attack rate; structure–activity relationship
SCID	severe combined immunodeficiency
SCR	short consensus repeat
SDAV	sialodacryoadenitis virus
SDS-PAGE	sodium dodecyl sulphate–polyacrylamide gel electrophoresis
sec	secretion factor
serpin	serine protease inhibitor
SF	Semliki Forest
SFGF	Shope fibroma growth factor
SFV	Semliki Forest virus
SHFV	simian haemorrhagic fever virus
SI	syncytia inducer
SIRSV	swine infertility and respiratory syndrome virus
SIV	simian immunodeficiency virus
SKIF	specific PKR inhibitory factor
SLE	St Louis encephalitis
SN	serum neutralization
SNV	Sin Nombre virus
SP-A	surfactant protein A
SP-D	surfactant protein D
SPIEM	solid phase immunoelectron microscopy
SRH	single radial haemolysis
SRP	signal recognition particle
SRSV	small round structured virus
SRV	small round virus
ss	single-stranded
SSPE	subacute sclerosing panencephalitis
Stat	signal transducers and activators of transcription
STD	sexually transmitted disease
STLV	simian T cell leukaemia virus
SV	subvirion
SV40	simian virus 40
SVD	swine vesicular disease
SVDV	swine vesicular disease virus
SVP	subviral particle
SYNV	sonchus yellow net virus
T1L	type 1 Lang [virus]
T3D	type 3 Dearing [virus]

TAC	transient aplastic crisis
TAP	transporter associated with antigen processing
TBEV	tick-borne encephalitis virus
Tc	cytotoxic T cell
3TC	2′-deoxy-3′-thiacytidine
TCID50	median tissue culture infectious dose
TCR	T cell receptor
TCV	turkey coronavirus
TF	transcription factor
TFT	trifluorothymidine
Tg	transgenic
TGEV	transmissible gastroenteritis virus
TGF	transforming growth factor
Th	T helper [cell]
TIBO	tetrahydro-imidazo[4,5,1-jk][1,4]-benzodiazepin-2H(1H)-thione
α-TIF	α-*trans*-inducing factor
TK	thymidine kinase
TMEV	Theiler's murine encephalomyelitis virus
TMV	tobacco mosaic virus
TNF	tumour necrosis factor
TP	terminal protein
TR-FIA	time-resolved fluoroimmunoassay
TRIS	tris(hydroxymethyl)amino-methane
TRTV	turkey rhinotracheitis virus
ts	temperature sensitive
TS	thymidylate synthase
TSP/HAM	tropical spastic paraparesis/HTLV-I-associated myelopathy
TTP	thymidine triphosphate
TUT	terminal uridylate transferase
TVX	tumour virus X
UTR	untranslated region
V-RG	vaccinia-rabies glycoprotein
VA	virus associated
VACV	valaciclovir
VAP	virus attachment protein
VCA	viral capsid antigen
VCAM	vascular cell adhesion molecule
VEE	Venezuelan equine encephalitis
VETF	viral early transcription factor
VEV	vesicular exanthem virus
vIL	viral interleukin
VLA	very late antigen
VLP	virus-like particle
VN	virus neutralization
VNA	virus-neutralizing antibody
vRNA	virion RNA
VSV	vesicular stomatitis virus
VV	vaccinia virus
VZIG	varicella-zoster immune globulin
VZV	varicella-zoster virus
WB	Western blot
WEE	western equine encephalitis
WG	week of gestation
WHV	woodchuck hepatitis virus
WKA	Wistar–King–Aptekman
WV	whole virus
XLA	X-linked agammaglobulinaemia
XLPS	X-linked lymphoproliferative syndrome (Duncan syndrome)
YFV	yellow fever virus
ZIG	zoster immunoglobulin

Part I

General characteristics of viruses

Chapter 1

A SHORT HISTORY OF RESEARCH ON VIRUSES

L Collier

1 INTRODUCTION

Virus (Latin, from Greek φιος): a poisonous or slimy fluid

I have not called this chapter 'The history of virology' because it pertains almost entirely to viruses themselves, and not to the whole subject, which includes epidemiology, diagnosis, immune responses, pathogenicity and many other topics. Such extended coverage would have demanded a chapter of inappropriate length. The survey deals with the period from the end of the nineteenth century to about 1975, and includes references to papers that are now seen to have provided points of departure for major advances.

2 THE FOUNDATIONS

THE DISCOVERY OF VIRUSES

Bacteria were seen and cultivated before their association with disease was determined. By contrast, the nature of viruses was not elucidated until well after it was realized that certain diseases of plants and animals could be transmitted by an invisible infective principle that differed considerably from the known parasites. This discovery was made amid the ferment of ideas and experimentation on microbes that took place in the closing decades of the nineteenth century; the technical advance on which it was based was the invention by Charles Chamberland (1884), a colleague of Louis Pasteur, of a porcelain filter originally designed to sterilize drinking water. In 1892, Iwanowski in Russia showed that such a filter allowed passage of the agent causing mosaic disease of tobacco. Somewhat

diffidently, he suggested that the infective principle might be a toxin elaborated by bacteria, but did not pursue the matter. In 1898 Beijerinck independently made similar observations on this infection, but extended them much further (Beijerinck 1899). To exclude the possibility that his porcelain filter was letting through a very small bacterium he used the then novel device of diffusing sap through agar gel, after which it still retained infectivity. He also observed that the agent multiplied only in dividing cells, and that it withstood desiccation but was inactivated by boiling. Having failed with the means at his disposal to demonstrate its particulate nature, he termed it a *contagium vivum fluidum*. In the same year, Loeffler and Frosch (1898), both associates of Robert Koch, reported passage of the agent of foot-and-mouth disease through a bacteria-retaining filter. They ruled out the idea of an inert toxin on the basis of the dilution factors involved, and concluded, first, that the agent must be able to replicate, and, second, that it must be smaller than the smallest bacterium then known, and thus beyond the resolving power of the best available microscopes. Although the great majority of viruses were beyond the bounds of resolution of the light microscope, Buist (1887) visualized one of the largest, vaccinia, after staining it with aniline methyl violet. He also assigned it the remarkably accurate measurement of 100–500 nm.

PROPAGATION IN TISSUE CULTURE

By the end of the nineteenth century, viruses had been defined solely in terms of their infectivity, filterability and, as a result of Beijerinck's percipience, their requirement for living cells as a substrate for growth. Hitherto, viruses had been propagated only in intact animals or plants. Further progress demanded a much more simple and controllable system, the foundation of which was laid by Harrison (1906–7) who devised the first tissue culture, not for propagating viruses but for studying the growth of frog nervous tissue in clotted lymph. Steinhardt, Israeli and Lambert (1913) exploited Harrison's technique to grow vaccinia in fragments of guinea-pig cornea embedded in clotted plasma. They could not demonstrate the virus directly in these preparations, but concluded from the results of serial subcultures that replication had taken place.

In 1928, Maitland and Maitland propagated vaccinia in suspensions of minced hens' kidneys. Their method was not widely used and its potential was not fully realized until a quarter of a century later, when flask cultures of trypsinized fragments of monkey kidney were used to grow poliovirus on a large scale for vaccine production.

QUANTIFICATION

Guérin (1905) found that the number of vesicles produced by a suspension of vaccinia inoculated into scarified rabbit skin was roughly proportional to its dilution. This method was used by Steinhardt, Israeli and Lambert (1913) in their tissue culture experiments, and was the precursor of many later and more accurate methods of assaying viral infectivity.

HOST RANGE AND PATHOGENICITY: EFFECTS ON CELLS

The discovery of animal and plant viruses was soon followed by the finding of others that affected insects and bacteria. Oncogenic viruses were discovered by Ellerman and Bang (1908) and by Rous (1911), who respectively showed that a leukaemia and a sarcoma of fowls could be transmitted by filterable agents. Another category, bacterial viruses (Twort 1915, d'Herelle 1917), was also to prove of the first importance, particularly for the study of viral replication and bacterial genetics.

In the early years of this century various workers described intracellular inclusion bodies in the tissues of animals and humans infected with viruses (e.g. rabies, cytomegalovirus and vaccinia). As the only obvious manifestation of viral activity within cells, inclusions were for long the objects of intense study and speculation; they were categorized in terms of staining properties (eosinophilic or basophilic), location (intranuclear or cytoplasmic) and morphology (Cowdry 1934). They are now largely of academic interest.

IMMUNE RESPONSES

It was long ago appreciated that certain infectious illnesses were followed by resistance to a second attack. This observation prompted the inoculation of material from cases of smallpox (variolation), which was for centuries practised in eastern countries. The practice was associated with significant mortality (c. 2%) and was eventually superseded by the use of cowpox as the result of astute observations in the eighteenth and early nineteenth centuries by Edward Jenner (1801) and by lesser known figures such as Benjamin Jesty, a farmer in Dorset. The last two decades of the nineteenth century saw the pioneering work of Louis Pasteur and his associates on immunization against both bacterial and viral infections, the most dramatic example being rabies. Meanwhile, the mechanisms of immunity underlying these somewhat empirical observations were being unravelled in the laboratory. Elias Metchnikoff (1891) demonstrated the importance of phagocytes in combating certain bacterial infections, and thus founded the concept of cell-mediated immunity. This line of investigation was for long overshadowed by work on humoral factors. Around the turn of the century, the quantitative and qualitative aspects of antigen–antibody reactions and their specificity were under intensive study by von Behring, Kitasato, Ehrlich, Landsteiner and others; and Nuttall and Bordet discovered a heat-labile factor in blood, later to be designated **complement**, that was bactericidal in the presence of specific antibody. For a more detailed account of early research on immunology, see Volume 3, Chapter 13.

THE END OF THE BEGINNING

By the end of the first world war, therefore, the foundations of virology had been laid. It had been established that viruses are much smaller than bacteria, and appeared to be capable of growing only in living cells, sometimes leaving evidence of their presence in the form of inclusion bodies. The main categories of viruses affecting respectively vertebrates, invertebrates, bacteria and plants had been identified, the existence of oncogenic viruses was established, and the outlines of the immune response to viruses and other microbes were beginning to take shape.

3   PROPAGATION OF VIRUSES IN THE LABORATORY

Before discussing work on the properties of viruses, mention must be made of their propagation outside the intact animal, because such techniques are essential for studying them and most other micro-organisms.

CHICK EMBRYOS

Before the advent of antibiotics, tissue culture methods depended mostly on the growth of explants in clotted plasma, and freedom from contamination was difficult to maintain. The removal of these constraints, which impeded both quantitative work and large scale cultivation, was signalled in 1931 with the finding by Woodruff and Goodpasture that fowlpox virus inoculated on to the chorioallantoic membrane of 10–15 day embryos produced discrete lesions (pocks). Within the next few years other viruses, including herpes simplex, Newcastle disease of fowls and louping ill, had been propagated in this way and infectivity titrations by the pock-counting method were being carried out (Burnet 1936). Later, the allantoic and amniotic routes of inoculation were used to grow a range of viruses (Beveridge and Burnet 1946), and some, notably yellow fever and influenza, were grown in large quantities for vaccine production.

CELL CULTURES

The tedious method of growing tissue fragments in plasma clot was quite unsuited to the propagation of viruses in any quantity. In the early 1950s it was largely replaced by true cell cultures as a result of several technical advances, given impetus by the celebrated discovery of Enders, Weller and Robbins (1949) that poliomyelitis virus would grow in non-neural tissues. The technical advances were (1) the introduction of antibiotics to control bacterial and fungal contamination, (2) the use of trypsin to obtain suspensions of single cells that could then be grown as monolayers on glass or plastic surfaces, and (3) the production of lines of cells that could be propagated by serial passage, which fell into two main groups. Some were derived either from malignant tumours, for example the HeLa line (Scherer, Syverton and Gey 1953), or from cells that had acquired malignant characteristics, including aneuploidy, during serial transfer or after infection with certain viruses; these 'continuous' cell lines would grow indefinitely. Others were derived from normal tissues, and retained their diploid karyotype for a limited number of transfers. Monolayer cultures had the great advantage, *inter alia*, that the effects of viruses in terms of cell destruction (cytopathic effect) could be readily observed by low power microscopy.

QUANTITATIVE METHODS

The use of cell cultures greatly improved the accuracy of infectivity titrations, for which two principal methods were developed. The first was analogous to the counting of bacterial colonies obtained from a known dilution of suspension, and, as we have seen, was applied to infectivity titrations of viruses that produced discrete lesions on the chick embryo chorioallantoic membrane. Suitably diluted suspensions of bacteriophage produced cleared areas ('plaques') in confluent lawns of bacteria on solid media, and, likewise, some animal viruses produced foci of destruction in cell monolayers overlaid with gel (Dulbecco and Vogt 1954). Because each plaque resulted, in theory at least, from the replication of one virus particle, the infectivity of the suspension could be accurately assayed as the mean of a number of replicate counts.

The second method was useful when plaque counting was impracticable. It depended on ascertaining the highest dilution of suspension producing a certain endpoint, for example the death of an animal or a cytopathic effect in a cell culture. The precision of the method was much enhanced by estimating the dilution producing the endpoint in 50% of the animals or cultures inoculated. The earliest and perhaps best known method for doing so was that of Reed and Muench (1938).

4 THE PROPERTIES OF VIRUSES

4.1 Physical characteristics

SIZE

Probably because of the difficulty of propagating them in the laboratory, research on the sizing of viruses by filtration and centrifugation was, *faut de mieux*, an important focus of attention until well into the 1940s.

In 1929, Elford described a method of making series of collodion membrane filters of known average pore diameter (APD); with the proviso that the conditions of filtration had to be carefully controlled, their availability greatly assisted the measurement of viruses. Thus by 1940 the sizes of about 25 animal viruses, ranging from the enteroviruses (c. 20 nm) to poxviruses (c. 250 nm) had been measured with fair accuracy (see van Rooyen and Rhodes 1940a). Such studies were further advanced by the use of high speed centrifuges, notably of the Sharples and Svedberg varieties (reviewed by van Rooyen and Rhodes 1940b), to estimate size as a function of the sedimentation characteristics.

Centrifugation was also useful for purifying viruses and became more so with the introduction by Brakke (1953) of sucrose density gradients, in which particles within a mixture can be separated according to their sedimentation rates. Later, caesium chloride and other salts were used with great success in high speed centrifuges to separate viruses from contaminating material on the basis of their differing buoyant densities.

MORPHOLOGY

Until 1939, next to nothing was known about the structure of viruses because of the constraints imposed by the limited resolving power of light, even of short wavelengths in the ultraviolet range. In that year Kausche, Pfannkuch and Ruska visualized a virus with the newly invented electron microscope (EM), in which beams of electrons travelling in a vacuum are focused on the object with electromagnetic fields. Given the then current interest in crystalline tobacco mosaic virus (TMV) (see Section 4.2, p. 6), it is not surprising that this was the first virus to be examined. Kausche and his colleagues employed the technique of shadow-casting, whereby the objects on the specimen grid were coated with gold particles generated by heating the metal in a vacuum; they defined the size of the crystals as about 25×300 nm.

After the interruption of the second world war, new techniques were introduced to exploit the potential of the EM; they are well reviewed by Almeida (1984). In brief, shadow-casting revealed important morphological features of viruses, including the fact that some have an icosahedral structure. Negative staining, in which the background, but not the virus, is stained with an electron-dense salt of tungsten, uranium or osmium, found wide application, not least in the diagnostic laboratory, and demonstrated that the outer surfaces of virus particles are composed of subunits.

Methods were developed for cutting ultrathin sections in the 2 nm range, which, alone or treated with labelled antibodies, yielded much information about virus–host cell relationships.

These techniques, together with x-ray diffraction studies, showed that most viruses fall into one of two groups: the icosahedral viruses with so-called cubic symmetry; and those with helical symmetry, in which the outer subunits are arranged like the treads in a spiral staircase.

4.2 Chemical composition: the role of the nucleic acids

The demonstration by Stanley (1935) that TMV could be obtained in an apparently crystalline form further stimulated the active, but ultimately sterile, debate on whether viruses are living entities. More important, it prompted study of the chemical composition of such preparations; and in 1937, Bawden and Pirie showed that they were not, as Stanley at first thought, pure proteins but also contained a nucleic acid, probably RNA. From this observation stemmed the realization that viruses consist of a nucleic acid contained within a protein coat; by the end of the decade, it was also clear that some viruses contain DNA rather than RNA. Following the demonstration by Avery, MacLeod and McCarty (1944) that the genetic information determining the type specificity of pneumococci resides in their DNA, Hershey and Chase (1952) confirmed the crucial role of the nucleic acid in viral replication by showing that, after attachment of bacteriophage T2, the DNA, but not the protein coat, enters the bacterial cell. A further major step was the demonstration by Gierer and Schramm (1956) and Fraenkel-Conrat (1956) that RNA in infective form could be extracted from TMV.

The concept of the virion

Not long after Watson and Crick (1953) solved the structure of DNA, they suggested that viral nucleic acid is protected by a shell of identical protein subunits (Crick and Watson 1956). This notion, based on the limited coding capacity of viral nucleic acid, proved essentially correct. All viruses were found to have this basic architecture (Klug and Caspar 1960, Caspar and Klug 1962), the nucleic acid being, with few exceptions, double-stranded DNA or single-stranded RNA. Caspar et al. (1962) proposed the following terminology: the complex of protein shell (**capsid**) and nucleic acid is the **nucleocapsid**; the mature nucleocapsid, surrounded in some viruses by an outer envelope, is referred to as the **virion**.

4.3 Replication

For well over half a century after their discovery, nothing was known of the way in which viruses reproduce themselves. From about 1940 onwards, however, research by Delbrück, Luria, Hershey, Lwoff and many others elucidated the basic mechanisms. Much of the work was done with bacteriophages, which had the advantages over animal viruses of easy propagation in vitro, accurate quantification and growth cycles measured in minutes rather than hours; considerable use was made of radiolabelling to trace the synthesis of nucleic acids and proteins. The mechanisms of viral attachment, penetration and uncoating were defined, as was that of the coding of enzymic and structural proteins by messenger RNA.

By 1957 André Lwoff was able to crystallize the essential features that distinguish viruses from all other organisms: they are strictly intracellular and potentially pathogenic entities with an infectious phase and (1) possess only one type of nucleic acid, (2) multiply in the form of their genetic material, (3) are unable to grow and undergo binary fission, and (4) are devoid of a Lipmann system of enzymes for energy production.

4.4 'Unconventional' viruses

Two groups of viruses or virus-like agents stand apart from the generality of animal viruses: they are the **retroviruses** and the **prions**.

Retroviruses

The finding by Ellerman and Bang (1908) and Rous (1911) that certain malignancies of fowl are caused by a transmissible agent was followed by the observation that many others in birds and animals, both of the solid tissues and of blood, can be transmitted vertically, from parents to offspring, as well as horizontally. The oncogenic effects of the viruses concerned are characterized by unusually long incubation periods. Temin argued for many years that the persistence of these RNA-containing viruses was due to a DNA 'provirus' that had become integrated into infected cells. This was finally confirmed when it was discovered that their RNA is transcribed to a DNA copy by means of an enzyme, reverse transcriptase (Temin and Mituzani 1970, Baltimore 1970), thus called because it reverses the usual flow of genetic information from DNA to RNA.

Fatal infections, also with long incubation periods but otherwise dissimilar, appeared among sheep in Iceland following the importation of Karakul sheep from Germany in 1933; known as **maedi** and **visna**, they respectively affected the lungs and central nervous system (Sigurdsson 1954a). Other viruses, the so-called 'foamy agents', were first detected in monkey kidney cells used for polio vaccine production during the 1950s and later in the kidneys of other species, including humans; these agents appear not to cause disease.

The viruses concerned have now been grouped into the *Retroviridae* family. The insertion and integration of viral DNA (provirus) into the host cell genome accounts both for the chronicity of these infections and for the oncogenic potential of many of the viruses in the family. Later, retroviruses were discovered that cause infections of humans, notably leukaemias and acquired immunodeficiency syndrome, and viruses of other families, notably hepatitis B, were found to utilize reverse transcription during replication; but these developments are outside the scope of this chapter.

PRION DISEASES

For the past 200 years a widespread disease of sheep and goats has been recognized that affects the central nervous system, has an incubation period of several years and is always fatal; it is known as **scrapie** because the severe itching impels affected animals to rub against posts and fences. The disease could be transferred between sheep by injection of brain tissue (Cuillé and Chelle 1936); its transfer to mice (Chandler 1961) and hamsters, with an incubation period of less than a year, greatly facilitated experimental work. A similar disease, **rida**, was reported in sheep in Iceland (Sigurdsson 1954b) and such infections were later identified in other animals, notably cattle in the UK. All were characterized by, *inter alia*, severe neuronal degeneration and vacuolation (spongiform encephalopathy) and by the presence in the brain of tangles of fibrils (scrapie-associated fibrils, or SAF). Analogous infections were found in humans, in the form of Creutzfeldt–Jakob disease (Creutzfeldt 1920, Jakob 1921), Gerstman–Sträussler–Scheinker syndrome and kuru (Gajdusek and Zigas 1957), a now extinct disease of the Fore tribe in Papua New Guinea spread by endocannibalism.

The causal agents of these infections differ in many respects from 'conventional' viruses and cannot be classified on similar criteria. They are very small and highly resistant to heat and ionizing radiation. Even so, they can reproduce themselves and some at least can undergo genetic variation. Prusiner (1982) marshalled the evidence suggesting that these agents are protein and devoid of nucleic acid; he termed them **prions** (proteinaceous infectious particles). His view that they are an aberrant form (PrP^Sc) of a protein (PrP) normally found in the brain is now gaining wide acceptance. The mode of reproduction has not been finally established but may be explained by repetitive conformational changes induced by PrP^Sc in the normal protein.

5 CLASSIFICATION OF VIRUSES

Now that the story of research on the properties of viruses has been described, it is appropriate to consider how they have been applied to viral classification. The early history of this topic was reviewed by Brown (1984); here, there is space to refer only to the main events.

The earliest attempts at grouping viruses were necessarily based on what they do rather than on what they are: the criteria included clinical effects, pathological changes and tissue tropisms. The inadequacies of such systems were apparent, and in 1950 a Subcommittee on Virus Nomenclature under the chairmanship of C H Andrewes was set up at the International Congress of Microbiology held at Rio de Janeiro; it recommended use of a system based on the physical,

chemical and antigenic properties of the viruses themselves, and allotted names to some of the better known (e.g. Poxvirus, Herpesvirus, Myxovirus). In 1961, Cooper proposed, *inter alia*, the fundamentally important grouping by type of nucleic acid. Soon afterwards, Lwoff, Horne and Tournier (1962) put forward a universal system that has contributed much to the modern classification. The criteria were: (1) the type of nucleic acid (DNA or RNA); (2) symmetry of the virus; (3) presence or absence of an envelope; and (4) diameter of the nucleocapsid for helical viruses or the number of capsomeres for cubic viruses. On the basis of these and other criteria, viruses are assigned to families (and sometimes subfamilies), genera and species. Baltimore (1971) provided a basis for further refining classification that takes into account genome conformation and strategies for mRNA synthesis, characteristics that are being used on an increasing scale (Murphy et al. 1995).

6 IMMUNIZATION AND ANTIVIRAL THERAPY

At the beginning of this chapter I stated that it would not be possible to cover applied virology. Nevertheless, at a time when major successes are being scored both by virus vaccines and antiviral drugs, it is only right to include mentions of these topics, brief though they must be.

VIRAL VACCINES

Smallpox vaccine was the first to come into general use and the first to eradicate an infectious disease world-wide (Fenner et al. 1988), the last natural case having occurred in Somalia in 1977. The conquest of smallpox is set fair to be repeated with other vaccines, notably poliomyelitis and measles. The development of viral vaccines reflects the advances in virological techniques over the past two centuries, ranging successively from animal inoculation to the use of chick embryos, cell cultures and finally recombinant DNA technology (Table 1.1).

ANTIVIRAL THERAPY

Because of the intimate association between viruses and their host cells, the development of antiviral agents lagged behind that of compounds active against other microbes. Since the replication of viruses was not well understood, its basis was at first purely empirical and depended largely on random screening of many potentially useful compounds; the devising of compounds directed against specific target activities such as attachment to the host cell, nucleic acid synthesis and release of mature virus is of more recent origin.

An early development in antiviral therapy was the discovery by Isaacs and Lindenmann (1957) of interferon (IFN), a low molecular weight protein produced by cells in response to infection with viruses, some bacteria, double-stranded nucleic acids and other biological compounds. (See also Isaacs, Lindenmann and

Table 1.1 Vaccines for human use developed in the past two centuries

Decade in which introduced	Vaccine	Live (L) or inactivated (I)	Derivation
1800–09	Smallpox	L	Animals
1880–89	Rabies	I	
1940–49	Yellow fever	L	Chick embryos
	Influenza	I	
1950–59	Polio (Salk type)	I	Cell cultures
1960–69	Rabies	I	Cell cultures
	Polio (Sabin type)	L	
	Measles	L	
	Mumps	L	
	Rubella	L	
1980–89	Hepatitis B	I	Human plasma
	Hepatitis B	I	Yeast[a]
	Japanese B encephalitis	I	Mice or cell cultures
	Varicella	L	Cell cultures
1990–99	Hepatitis A	I	Cell cultures

[a]Genetically engineered antigen.

Valentine 1957.) Three classes of IFN (α, β and γ) with differing properties are now recognized. The early finding that IFN inhibited a wide range of viruses raised hopes that it would be in the nature of a universal panacea for viral infections. This expectation was not fulfilled but, more recently, IFNs have proved useful in treating some cases of chronic hepatitis B. The large doses required can be produced by recombinant DNA techniques.

The precursor of all synthetic antiviral compounds was *p*-amino-benzaldehyde,3-thiosemicarbazone (Brownlee and Hamre 1951) which inhibited vaccinia virus. A related compound, methisazone, appeared to have a prophylactic effect in smallpox contacts, but was rendered superfluous by the success of the vaccine eradication campaign. However, a more profitable approach was becoming apparent. By 1955, Matthews and Smith were able to write:

> There is a growing body of evidence suggesting that the genetic properties of viruses may reside largely in their nucleic acids, and a number of recent observations show that virus multiplication can be delayed by compounds which interfere with nucleic acid metabolism. As a class, analogues of the puridine and pyrimidine bases may inhibit growth by a variety of mechanisms.

This prediction was fulfilled; the greatest achievements have in fact been the therapy and prophylaxis of herpesvirus infections with nucleoside analogues, at first idoxuridine (5-iodo-2'-deoxyuridine) and latterly acyclovir (9-(2-hydroxyethoxymethyl)guanine (Table 1.2). Another such compound, zidovudine, has had a limited measure of success against infection with human immunodeficiency virus. It is, however, clear that our successors will regard this era as still part of the early history of antiviral therapy.

The benefits of molecules designed to block specific receptors, drugs accurately aimed at defined targets within the replication cycle, synthetic antigens, DNA vaccines and novel delivery systems lie still in the future.

7 CONCLUSION

The virologist will readily appreciate how much has had to be omitted from this brief account; but I hope that it will convey to the non-specialist something of the many and complex strands that have combined to make the study of viruses such a leading influence in microbiology. From its beginnings, virology has provided a high degree of intellectual challenge that has attracted many leading minds, not least through its contributions to our knowledge of biological processes at the molecular level. The reader who wishes to study the fascinating story in more detail will find good

Table 1.2 Representative antiviral compounds developed since 1960

Year[a]	Compound	Virus(es) inhibited
1960	Methisazone	Poxviruses
1962	Idoxuridine	Herpesviruses
1963	Amantadine	Influenza A
1972	Ribavirin	Respiratory syncytial virus Lassa fever
1978	Acyclovir	Herpesviruses
1978	Foscarnet	Herpes simplex HIV-1
1985	Zidovudine	HIV-1

[a]Approximate only. Indicates an early description rather than when licensed for clinical use.

accounts in the books by Lechevalier and Solotorovsky (1965) and Waterson and Wilkinson (1978).

REFERENCES

Almeida JD, 1984, Morphology: virus structure, *Topley and Wilson's Principles of Bacteriology, Virology and Immunity*, 7th edn, eds Wilson GS, Miles AA, Parker MT, Edward Arnold, London, 14–48.

Avery OT, MacLeod CM, McCarty M, 1944, Studies on the chemical nature of the substance inducing transformation of pneumococcal types. Induction of transformation by a desoxyribonucleic acid fraction isolated from Pneumococcus Type III, *J Exp Med*, **79**: 137–57.

Baltimore D, 1970, RNA-dependent DNA polymerase in virions of RNA tumour viruses, *Nature (London)*, **226**: 1209–11.

Baltimore D, 1971, Expression of animal virus genomes, *Bacteriol Rev*, **35**, 235–41.

Bawden FC, Pirie NW, 1937, The isolation and some properties of liquid crystalline substances from solanaceous plants infected with three strains of tobacco mosaic virus, *Proc Roy Soc London, B*, **123**: 274–320.

Beijerinck MW, 1899, Ueber ein Contagium vivum fluidum als Ursache der Fleckenkrankheit der Tabaksblätter, *Zentralbl Bakteriol Parasitenkd Infektionskr Hyg Abt 2*, **5**: 27–33 (First published in Dutch in 1898. Cited by Waterson and Wilkinson, 1978, p 27).

Beveridge WIB, Burnet FM, 1946, *The cultivation of viruses and rickettsiae in the chick embryo: Special Report Series No 256*, Medical Research Council/HMSO, London.

Brakke ML, 1953, Zonal separations by density-gradient filtration, *Arch Biochem Biophys*, **45**: 275–90.

Brown F, 1984, Classification of viruses, *Topley and Wilson's Principles of Bacteriology, Virology and Immunity*, 7th edn, eds Wilson GS, Miles AA, Parker MT, Edward Arnold, London, 5–13.

Brownlee KA, Hamre D, 1951, Studies on chemotherapy of vaccinia virus, *J Bacteriol*, **61**: 127–34.

Buist JB, 1887, *Vaccinia and Variola: a study of their life history*, Churchill, London.

Burnet FM, 1936, *The use of the developing egg in virus research: Special Report Series No 220*, Medical Research Council/HMSO, London.

Caspar DLD, Klug A, 1962, Physical principles in the construction of regular viruses, *Cold Spring Harbor Symp Quant Biol*, **27**: 1–24.

Caspar DLD, Dulbecco R et al., 1962, Proposals, *Cold Spring Harbor Symp Quant Biol*, **27**: 49.

Chamberland, C, 1884, Sur un filtre donnant de l'eau physiologiquement pure, *C R Acad Sci*, **99**: 247–8.

Chandler RL, 1961, Encephalopathy in mice produced by inoculation with scrapie brain material, *Lancet*, **1**: 1378–9.

Cooper PD, 1961, A chemical basis for the classification of animal viruses, *Nature (London)*, **190**: 302–5.

Cowdry EV, 1934, The problem of intra-nuclear inclusions in virus diseases, *Arch Pathol*, **18**: 527–42.

Creutzfeldt HG, 1920, Über die eigenartige herdförmige Erkrankung des Zentralnervensystems, *Z ges Neurol Psychiat*, **57**: 1–18.

Crick FHC, Watson JD, 1956, Structure of small viruses, *Nature (London)*, **177**: 473–5.

Cuillé J, Chelle, P-L, 1936, La maladie dite tremblante du mouton est-elle inoculable?, *C R Acad Sci*, **203**: 1552–4.

Dulbecco R, Vogt M, 1954, Plaque formation and isolation of pure lines with poliomyelitis viruses, *J Exp Med*, **99**: 167–82.

Elford WJ, 1929, Ultra-filtration methods and their application in bacteriological and pathological studies, *Br J Exp Pathol*, **10**: 126–44.

Ellerman V, Bang O, 1908, Experimentelle leukämie bei Hühnerin, *Zentralbl Bakteriol Parasitenkd Infetktionskr Hyg Abt 1 Orig*, **46**: 595–609.

Enders JF, Weller TH, Robbins FC, 1949, Cultivation of the Lansing strain of poliomyelitis virus in cultures of various human embryonic tissues, *Science*, **109**: 85–7.

Fenner F, Henderson DA et al., 1988, *Smallpox and its Eradication*, World Health Organization, Geneva.

Fraenkel-Conrat H, 1956, The role of the nucleic acid in the reconstitution of active tobacco mosaic virus [Correspondence], *J Am Chem Soc*, **78**: 882–3.

Gajdusek DC, Zigas V, 1957, Degenerative disease of the central nervous system in New Guinea: the endemic occurrence of 'kuru' in the native population, *N Engl J Med*, **257**: 974–8.

Gierer A, Schramm G, 1956, Infectivity of ribonucleic acid from tobacco mosaic virus, *Nature (London)*, **177**: 702–3.

Guérin MC, 1905, Contrôle de la valeur des vaccins Jenneriens par la numération des éléments virulents, *Ann Inst Pasteur (Paris)*, **15**: 317–20.

Harrison RG, 1906–7, Observations on the living developing nerve fibre, *Proc Soc Exp Biol Med*, **4**: 140–3.

d'Herelle F, 1917, Sur un microbe invisible antagoniste des bacilles dysentériques, *C R Acad Sci*, **165**: 373–5.

Hershey AD, Chase M, 1952, Independent functions of viral protein and nucleic acid in growth of bacteriophage, *J Gen Physiol*, **36**: 39–56.

Isaacs A, Lindenmann J, 1957, Virus interference. I. The interferon, *Proc Roy Soc London B*, **147**: 258–67.

Isaacs A, Lindenmann J, Valentine RC, 1957, Virus interference. II. Some properties of interferon, *Proc Roy Soc London, B*, **147**: 268–73.

Ivanowski DI, 1892, Ueber die Mosaikkrankheit der Tabakspflanze, *St Petersburg Acad Imp Sci Bull*, **35**: 67–70.

Jakob A, 1921, Über eigenartigen Erkrankungen des Zentralnervensystems mit bermerkenswertem anatomische Befunde, *Z ges Neurol Psychiat*, **64**: 147–228.

Jenner E, 1801, *An inquiry into the causes and effects of the* Variolae Vaccinae, *a disease discovered in some of the Western counties of England, particularly Gloucestershire, and known by the name of the Cow-pox*, Edward Jenner, London.

Kausche GA, Pfannkuch E, Ruska H, 1939, Die Sichtbarmachung von pflanzlichem Virus im Übermikroskop, *Naturwissenschaften*, **27**: 292–9.

Klug A, Caspar DLD, 1960, The structure of small viruses, *Adv Virus Res*, **7**: 225–325.

Lechevalier HA, Solotorovsky M, 1965, *Three Centuries of Microbiology*, McGraw-Hill, New York.

Loeffler [F], Frosch [P], 1898, Berichte der Kommission zur Erforschung der Maul und Klauenseuche bei dem Institut für Infektionskrankheiten in Berlin, *Zentralbl Bakteriol Parasitenkd Infektionskr Hyg Abt 1 Orig*, **23**: 371–91.

Lwoff A, 1957, The concept of virus, *J Gen Microbiol*, **17**: 239–53.

Lwoff A, Horne R, Tournier P, 1962, A system of viruses, *Cold Spring Harbor Symp Quant Biol*, **27**: 51–5.

Maitland HB, Maitland MC, 1928, Cultivation of vaccinia virus without tissue culture, *Lancet*, **2**: 596–7.

Matthews REF, Smith JD, 1955, The chemotherapy of viruses, *Adv Virus Res*, **3**: 49–148.

Metchnikoff E, 1891, Lecture on phagocytosis and immunity, *Br Med J*, **1**: 213–17.

Murphy FA et al. (eds) 1995, Virus taxonomy: sixth report of the International Committee on Taxonomy of Viruses, Springer-Verlag, New York.

Prusiner SB, 1982, Novel proteinaceous particles cause scrapie, *Science*, **216**: 136–44.

Reed LJ, Muench H, 1938, A simple method of estimating fifty-percent end points, *Am J Hyg*, **27**: 493–7.

van Rooyen CE, Rhodes AJ, 1940a, The particulate nature of

viruses – a summary of results, *Virus Diseases of Man*, Oxford University Press, London, 52–7.

van Rooyen CE, Rhodes AJ, 1940b, The centrifugalisation of elementary bodies, *Virus Diseases of Man*, Oxford University Press, London, 44–51.

Rous P, 1911, Transmission of a malignant new growth by means of a cell-free filtrate, *JAMA*, **56**: 198.

Scherer WF, Syverton JT, Gey GO, 1953, Studies on the propagation in vitro of poliomyelitis viruses. IV. Viral multiplication in a stable strain of human malignant cells (strain HeLa) derived from an epidermoid carcinoma of the cervix, *J Exp Med*, **97**: 695–709.

Sigurdsson B, 1954a, Maedi, a slow progressive pneumonia of sheep: an epizoological and a pathological study, *Br Vet J*, **110**: 255–70.

Sigurdsson B, 1954b, Rida, a chronic encephalitis of sheep; with general remarks on infections which develop slowly and some of their special characteristics, *Br Vet J*, **110**: 341–54.

Stanley WM, 1935, Isolation of a crystalline protein possessing the properties of tobacco-mosaic virus, *Science*, **81**: 644–5.

Steinhardt E, Israeli C, Lambert RA, 1913, Studies on the cultivation of the virus of vaccinia, *J Infect Dis*, **13**: 294–300.

Temin HM, Mituzani S, 1970, RNA-dependent DNA polymerase in virions of Rous sarcoma virus, *Nature (London)*, **226**: 1211–13.

Twort FW, 1915, An investigation on the nature of ultra-microscopic viruses, *Lancet*, **2**: 1241–3.

Waterson AP, Wilkinson L, 1978, *An Introduction to the History of Virology*, Cambridge University Press, Cambridge.

Watson JD, Crick FHC, 1953, Molecular structure of nucleic acids: a structure for deoxyribonucleic acid, *Nature (London)*, **171**: 737–8.

Woodruff AM, Goodpasture EW, 1931, The susceptibility of the chorio-allantoic membrane of chick embryos to infection with the fowl-pox virus, *Am J Pathol*, **7**: 209–2.

Chapter 2

THE ORIGIN AND EVOLUTION OF VIRUSES

J J Holland

| 1 Origin(s) of viruses | 2 Virus evolution and mechanisms involved |

1 ORIGIN(S) OF VIRUSES

As with the origin of life, the origin of viruses is necessarily a matter for speculation. Even if the polymerase chain reaction (PCR) and other molecular techniques eventually enable recovery of virus sequences from well-preserved animal and plant fossils, it is likely that such sequences will often be incomplete, cryptic and difficult to relate to modern viruses because of their rapid evolution. There has been speculation that viruses evolved as (and with) primordial life forms during the earliest life on earth (Gilbert 1986, Robertson 1992, Gesteland and Atkins 1993, Illangasekare et al. 1995); that they have evolved from cellular DNA or RNA (Jakob and Wollman 1961, Hayes 1968, Alberts et al. 1983, Cech 1986); or that they evolved by degeneration of cellular parasitic forms (Lwoff 1959). The most fanciful theories even envisage that viruses were seeded on earth from extraterrestrial sources in deep space (Hope-Simpson 1978, Hoyle and Wickramasinghe 1979). Rigorous proof or disproof of any theory for the early origins of present-day viruses is probably not attainable. It is likely that simple, self-replicating virus-like or viroid-like RNA molecules were involved in primordial life on earth, and that some present-day viruses evolved from these. It is equally plausible that viruses have derived many of their genes – and in some cases *all* their genes – from cellular genes. It is commonplace for viral DNA genes to integrate to become part of cellular chromosomes, and viruses (particularly defective viruses) can acquire cellular genes as part of their genomes (Hayes 1968, Monroe and Schlesinger 1983, Harrison, Thompson and Davison 1991). Regardless of the details of early evolution of life on earth, and of the earliest origins of viruses, it is clear that cellular nucleic acid interacts with, exchanges with and co-evolves with the DNA and RNA of viruses, plasmids, transposons, retrotransposons and other mobile genetic elements. Cell interactions with viruses and other mobile genetic elements play a major role in the evol-

ution of both the host cells and the mobile infectious elements (Hayes 1968, Monroe and Schlesinger 1983, Shapiro 1983, Watson et al. 1987, Boeke 1988, Berg and Howe 1989, Doolittle et al. 1989, Harrison, Thompson and Davison 1991, Coffin 1992, Doolittle and Feng 1992, Syvanen 1994, Lodish et al. 1995). Novel viruses are among the 'new' life forms that evolve from such interactions, and the 'origination' of viruses is therefore a never-ending process (Brown 1989). Their ubiquity, mobility and capacity to recombine put viruses (and other mobile elements) in the mainstream of all evolution on earth.

1.1 DNA viruses

DNA viruses are probably the most likely to have derived from new combinations of cellular genes. However, some DNA viruses, and many genes of DNA viruses, may have arisen by reverse transcription of RNA molecules. It is not yet clear, for example, whether a hepadnavirus (such as hepatitis B virus) was formerly a DNA virus that has acquired a reverse transcriptase to allow replication via RNA transcripts or if it was a retrovirus that has evolved to encapsidate DNA replication intermediates instead of the RNA 'genome' (Doolittle et al. 1989, Doolittle and Feng 1992). Regardless of ultimate origins, any DNA virus has the potential to capture useful genes from cell chromosomes via DNA recombination.

1.2 DNA viruses as mobile DNA replicons

The distinction between DNA viruses and other autonomously replicating DNA replicons is sometimes tenuous. Plasmids, insertion sequences, transposons and retrotransposons are mobile autonomous DNA replicons (Shapiro 1983, Watson et al. 1987, Boeke 1988, Berg and Howe 1989, Doolittle et al. 1989, Coffin 1992, Doolittle and Feng 1992, Syvanen 1994) that resemble viruses in many respects, but they lack the capsid protein coats (and lipid/glycoprotein envelopes) that package viral genomes, protect them and deliver them to appropriate receptors on susceptible host cells. It is this extracellular infectious stage that distinguishes viruses from other mobile DNA elements. Bacteriophage Mu is an example of a virus that is also a transposon (Watson et al. 1987, Berg and Howe 1989). It is a temperate phage, which, unlike phage 1 λ, can insert its DNA into numerous sites in the host bacterial chromosome. Copies of Mu DNA then transpose to many thousands of other chromosomal sites, thereby causing an enormous increase in mutation frequency. Mu therefore differs from the more common transposons because it encodes phage coat proteins which enable efficient transfer as a virus. As suggested by Botstein (1981), it is likely that virus genomes undergo 'modular evolution' in which 'new' viruses can be created by a combination of genes or gene clusters derived from multiple sources, including chromosomes, defective viruses, plasmids, transposable elements, etc.

1.3 Viroids and circular satellite RNAs

Of all the infectious virus-like mobile genetic elements, the viroids and related circular satellite RNAs (Maramorosch 1991, Robertson 1992) are the most primitive, and the most likely to have descended directly from primordial RNAs during the early evolution of life on earth. The viroids are small, naked RNA molecules several hundred nucleotides in length. They are covalently closed circular strands of RNA with extensive secondary structure, which replicate autonomously when introduced into susceptible plants, frequently causing characteristic signs of disease. They have intrinsic ribozyme self-splicing activity related to group 1 introns, and apparently replicate via a rolling circle mechanism by interaction with plant cell transcription components. They do not require a protein coat for transmission and do not encode capsid proteins, so genome transmission and disease progression can be very slow, but effective. However, there are related satellite viruses (sometimes termed 'virusoids') that depend on co-infection of plants with an infectious helper virus to provide them with capsid proteins for efficient transmission. As yet, there are no known viroids (or viroid diseases) of animals or humans. Robertson (1992) has, however, pointed out the close similarity between human hepatitis D virus (delta (δ) agent) and viroids. Delta agent contains a self-cleavage viroid domain joined to a protein-coding domain that encodes the δ antigen. Furthermore, the δ agent RNA is a defective circular 'satellite' RNA that depends on co-infection with hepatitis B virus as a helper virus to provide capsid protein. This striking similarity to viroids or circular satellite RNAs led Robertson (1992) to postulate mechanisms of evolution of early self-replicating RNA genomes to form various 'conjoined' RNA replicons that ultimately evolved into mosaic DNA systems. These plausible speculations envisage early RNA replicons as progenitors of both present day viroids and the intricate DNA-based life forms which now predominate. It should be noted that naked viroid RNAs and circular satellite RNAs thereby bear a relationship to RNA viruses similar to that of naked DNA replicons, including plasmids and transposons, to DNA viruses. In both cases, viruses are distinguished as autonomously replicating nucleic acid mobile elements with the capacity to encode capsid proteins.

1.4 RNA viruses

RNA viruses are the most ubiquitous and diverse viruses, and they include 2 major groups, the riboviruses and the retroviruses. Both have very high mutation rates, and even clones form diverse 'quasi-species' populations or 'mutant swarms'. The extreme mutability of RNA viruses and the biological consequences are discussed in detail in section 2.3 of this chapter (p. 15).

RIBOVIRUSES

The ordinary non-retrovirus RNA viruses that replicate their RNA genomes entirely via RNA templates are called riboviruses. Their ultimate origins are uncertain, and are probably quite varied. Some may be directly descended from early primordial RNA replicons, whereas others may have originated more recently by recombination, reassortment or mutation of cellular RNAs. Regardless of ultimate origins, it is likely that most riboviruses have exchanged RNA sequences with cellular RNAs (and other virus RNAs) and so their genomes are mosaics of sequences from multiple sources. RNA genetic exchange is discussed below. Finally, 'new' riboviruses may frequently arise by recombination of genome segments from 2 or more different riboviruses. One example is western equine encephalitis virus, which is a recombinant virus derived from parental genomes of eastern equine encephalitis virus and from New World relatives of Sindbis virus (Hahn et al. 1988, Weaver et al. 1993). Genetic recombination in riboviruses may be common on evolutionary time scales (Strauss and Strauss 1988, 1994, Zimmern 1988). A striking laboratory example of the creation of a new virus by recombination of unrelated riboviruses has recently been reported. Rolls et al. (1994), using recombinant DNA intermediates, created a remarkable infectious virus in which the surface glycoprotein of vesicular stomatitis virus (VSV) is expressed from a replicon of Semliki Forest virus (SFV). The SFV replicon encodes only the SFV replicase, and no structural proteins. When the VSV glycoprotein gene was inserted by molecular genetic techniques, infectious virus particles were formed by budding of plasma membrane vesicles containing the VSV glycoproteins enclosing RNA replicons. Because VSV is a negative-strand ribovirus and SFV is a positive-strand ribovirus, a highly unexpected 'hybrid virus' was created. This demonstrates not only that novel viral genome matings can be productive but also that enveloped infectious viruses can be much simpler than virologists had expected.

RETROVIRUSES

Retroviruses, hepadnaviruses and calimoviruses have a unique capacity for their genomes to participate regularly as part of both the RNA and the DNA worlds. Although their ultimate origins are uncertain, it is probable that they have evolved from retroid transposable elements, as originally proposed in Temin's (1970) 'protovirus' hypothesis. There is a wide variety of 'viral' and 'non-viral' retrotransposons and related elements, including Gypsy, Copia, LINES and LINE-like elements, mitochondrial introns, mitochondrial retroplasmids and bacterial reverse transcriptase DNA (Boeke 1988, Doolittle et al. 1989, Temin 1989, Coffin 1992, Doolittle and Feng 1992). The so-called 'viral' retrotransposons more closely resemble retrovirus genomes. All these elements have in common the presence of reverse transcriptase, but most lack envelope genes which allow cell-to-cell and organism-to-organism transmission as mature virus particles (virions). Other retroviral genes and domains such as LTR, capsid protein, ribonuclease, integrase and protease are variably present in various 'viral' and 'non-viral' retroid elements (Boeke 1988, Doolittle et al. 1989, Temin 1989, Coffin 1992, Doolittle and Feng 1992). Most of these retroid elements may represent little more than 'selfish' jumping genes which sometimes cause useful rearrangements of host cell DNA sequences and sometimes damage or kill their hosts via DNA alterations. At least some of them may, however, perform essential functions. For example, a LINE-like retrotransposon, TART in *Drosophila*, apparently preferentially retrotransposes to the termini of chromosomes in an essential process by which *Drosophila* telomeres are maintained (Sheen and Levis 1994). The telomerases involve reverse transcription to elongate chromosome termini (telomeres), a process required for indefinite periods of cell division in mammals (Kim et al. 1994).

Over all, there is very strong evidence that retroid elements have been around for aeons, that they can acquire additional genes, and that these 'protoviruses' of Temin (1970) can become retroviruses only if they can acquire envelope genes to confer infectivity. Even now, 'new' retroviruses are continuously born (or reborn) by recombinational acquisition of cellular genes (e.g. proto-oncogenes in the case of some transforming retroviruses). Another source is acquisition of genes from other retroviruses (e.g. LTR sequences, or altered *env* genes from proviruses in the case of mouse lymphoma viruses) (Coffin 1992). High mutation rates can also play a major role in the creation of 'new' retroviruses.

2 VIRUS EVOLUTION AND MECHANISMS INVOLVED

Because they can replicate rapidly with high yields of progeny, and readily mutate, recombine and reassort their genomes, most viruses can exhibit great genetic plasticity and adaptability. This provides the possibility for extremely rapid evolution, but does not dictate constant rapid genome evolution. Viruses, like other living things, can have periods of relative evolutionary stasis, punctuated by periods of evolutionary disequilibrium and rapid genetic change (Holland 1992).

2.1 Recombination

Recombination affords rapid, major rearrangements of viral genomes, and this mechanism for evolution is widespread among DNA viruses, RNA viruses and retroviruses. Both homologous and heterologous recombination are very common, and the latter has the potential to produce quite extensive genome alterations and bizarre phenotypes.

DNA VIRUS RECOMBINATION

Mechanisms of DNA recombination and transposition have been widely studied, are well characterized (Kucherlapati and Smith 1988) and will not be reviewed here. Recombination or transposition allows DNA viruses to acquire new genes from other viruses; to integrate into, and excise from, host cell chromosomes; to generate defective virus genomes and to rescue genes from them; and to capture host cell genes or to transfer them to new host cells. In short, DNA virus genomes have available to them all the recombinatorial mechanisms extant in the DNA-based world, and this gives them the potential for profound genome rearrangements and for extensive genetic interactions with DNA-based hosts. Many DNA virus genomes contain genes that have been captured (or rescued) from earlier hosts. For example, the thymidine kinase (TK) genes of herpesviruses exhibit broad substrate specificity, and have apparently evolved from cellular deoxycytidine kinase enzymes (Harrison, Thompson and Davison 1991), whereas poxvirus TK genes were apparently derived from cellular TK genes (Boyle et al. 1987). Defective viruses produced by recombination are ubiquitous among DNA viruses and may often help shape their evolution by maintaining functional (and rescuable) gene modules. Botstein (1981) suggested that the product of virus evolution 'is not a given virus but a family of interchangeable genetic elements (modules) each of which carries out a particular biological function. Each virus encountered in nature is a favorable combination of modules . . .' This plausible theory allows recombination to generate useful new combinations of modules at frequent intervals to produce 'new' viruses. It also allows the evolution of viral genes to occur within differing viral genomes, host chromosomes, defective viruses, plasmids, transposons, etc. Viral genes can not only associate with plasmids and episomes and other replicons, but they can also become episomes or plasmids (autonomous, non-infectious replicons). Examples are bacteriophage F1 selected for 'benevolent' interactions with host *Escherichia coli* (Bull and Molineux 1992) and Epstein–Barr (EB) virus 'episomal' circular genomes within transformed (immortalized) B lymphocytes (Lindahl et al. 1976, Lawrence, Villnave and Singer 1988, Middleton et al. 1991, Kirchmaier and Sugden 1995). The 'benevolent'

F1 plasmids eventually lost viral genes, and infectivity, but replicated efficiently within host bacteria, and the EB episome genomes in EB-immortalized B cell lines are generally non-infectious or poorly infectious unless 'induced' (Weigel and Miller 1983).

RETROVIRUS RECOMBINATION

Retroviruses, of course, have the potential to recombine at the proviral DNA level (as for any other DNA). However, they have the additional capacity to undergo recombination as a result of the tendency for reverse transcriptases to switch from one template to another (copy choice) during DNA chain elongation. This occurs at an extremely high frequency, is responsible for most retrovirus recombination events and can play a major role in retrovirus evolution (Coffin 1992).

RIBOVIRUS RECOMBINATION

Riboviruses can also exhibit very high rates of genome recombination due to frequent copy choice switching from one template RNA strand to another by RNA replicase. The RNA replicase carries the growing RNA chain to another RNA template and can align it precisely by base pairing. Therefore, most recombination is homologous ('legitimate') for positive-strand RNA viruses, which replicate their genomes as naked RNA (King 1988, Lai 1992, Wimmer, Hellen and Cao 1993). This is analogous to the high frequency homologous recombination of retrovirus reverse transcriptase (Coffin 1992). Such homologous recombination is clearly important for RNA virus evolution. For example, recombinants between different serotypes of poliovirus vaccine strains occur frequently in vaccinated humans and can be rather strongly selected in their intestinal tract (Kew et al. 1981, Minor et al. 1986, Minor 1992, Georgescue et al. 1994). Frequent homologous recombination helps to shape the evolution of numerous other riboviruses such as coronaviruses (Lai 1992) and brome mosaic virus of plants (Rao and Hall 1990, Nagy and Bujarski 1995). Even though copy choice recombination is much more common than non-homologous ('illegitimate') recombination among positive-stranded riboviruses (and retroviruses), non-homologous recombination can occasionally produce major genome changes of great evolutionary importance. For example, mouse hepatitis virus, a coronavirus, appears to have acquired its haemagglutinin-esterase gene by recombination with influenza C virus, a negative-strand virus (Luytjes et al. 1988). Likewise, western equine encephalitis virus was produced by recombination between an eastern equine encephalitis virus and a Sindbis-like parent virus. Several cross-overs and some non-homologous recombination events were involved (Hahn et al. 1988, Weaver et al. 1993, Strauss and Strauss 1994). Finally, mucosal disease variants of bovine viral diarrhoea virus (BVDV), a positive-strand pestivirus, are cytopathogenic defective viruses generated by recombination of parental, non-defective, non-cytopathogenic BVDV genomes with cellular mRNAs (Meyers et al. 1991, Tautz et al. 1994).

Negative-strand riboviruses, which replicate their genomes as ribonucleoprotein strands rather than naked RNAs, only very rarely undergo homologous recombination. Replicase template switching occurs frequently, but this nearly always produces non-homologous recombination because the growing RNA strands, being ribonucleoprotein, are not able to anneal and align the growing RNA chain precisely on homologous segments of the new template (Barrett and Dimmock 1986, Roux, Simon and Holland 1991). Nevertheless, recombination of negative-strand riboviruses regularly produces biologically important variant genomes, particularly defective interfering (DI) particles. These can exert significant modulatory effects on parental virus infections (Barrett and Dimmock 1986, Huang 1988, Kaper and Collmer 1988, Roux, Simon and Holland 1991). Occasionally, quite bizarre recombinants between cellular RNAs and viral RNA genomes arise. For example, when a 54 nucleotide segment of 28S ribosomal RNA was inserted into the haemagglutinin gene segment of influenza A virus (by recombination during growth in chick embryo cells) the resulting recombinant virus was much more virulent, causing systemic lethal infections in chickens (Katchikian, Orlich and Rott 1989). Similarly, a number of isolates of potato leafroll virus have acquired a 119 nucleotide segment from plant chloroplast DNA (Mayo and Jolly 1991), and cell culture replication of well characterized strains of poliovirus (Charini et al. 1994) and Sindbis virus (Monroe and Schlessinger 1983) led to acquisition of a short ribosomal RNA segment and a tRNA respectively. Thus, although major heterologous recombination events are probably infrequent in ribovirus evolution, they occur sufficiently often to have significant evolutionary effects. They might even influence the results of biotechnological manipulations in which resistance to virus is conferred on transgenic plants expressing viral mRNA segments. For example, recombination between a defective plant virus genome and a viral mRNA transcript expressed in transgenic plants restored infectivity to the defective viral genome (Green and Allison 1994).

2.2   Reassortment of ribovirus genome segments

A number of ribovirus families have segmented genomes: their genomes consist of a number of specific segments, each of which encodes one or more gene products. Each specific segment must be included in a virion together with all other segments in order for that virion to be infectious and to replicate infectious progeny. As expected, the various genomic segments from genetically different (but related) viruses can recombine to produce recombinant viruses. This 'sexual' exchange process is called reassortment, and it is equivalent to the reassortment of maternal and paternal chromosomes that occurs during meiotic gametogenesis in diploid eukaryotic organisms. Ribovirus gene reassortment occurs when two distinct viruses simultaneously infect the same cell(s). Gene reassortment can cause major genome alterations during evolution of segmented riboviruses. The most striking examples are the influenza A viruses. Both the 1957 Asian and the 1968 Hong Kong influenza pandemics began in south China. These 'new' human viruses arose by reassortment of gene segments apparently derived from circulating avian viruses and from circulating human virus sources. Domestic pigs were suggested as the probable hosts in which the reassortment events took place ('mixing vessels') (Gorman, Bean and Webster 1992, Webster et al. 1992); in fact, it has recently been shown that European children have become infected with avian–human reassortment H3N2 influenza A viruses currently circulating in European swine (Claas et al. 1994). It is probable that the next major influenza A pandemic will emerge some time during the next few decades, and that it will be due to reassortment events occurring in swine or humans or another 'mixing vessel'. Influenza C viruses, which usually circulate as multiple, independently evolving lineages in humans, have recently undergone gene reassortment in man (Peng et al. 1994). Major gene reassortment events between avian and human influenza A viruses are rare. This is undoubtedly because the currently circulating gene segments are co-evolving (and selected) for optimal interactions with each other. Therefore, only rare events could create a new virus with optimally interacting gene segments derived from widely divergent sources. Reassortment is common; it is the low probability for efficient interactions among diversely derived gene segments that greatly restricts the emergence of new influenza A pandemics. Reoviruses and many other segmented riboviruses also readily undergo genetic reassortment of segments from related lineages, and similar principles apply (Ramig, Ahmed and Fields 1983). There is, for example, evidence for segment reassortment in nature among viruses related to hantavirus pulmonary syndrome (Li et al. 1995), and for interspecific segment reassortment in the evolution of cucumoviruses of plants (White, Morales and Roosinck 1995).

2.3 Mutation of virus genomes

Mutation is the primary driving force for all evolution, and it occurs inevitably and inexorably in all life forms, including viruses. In the RNA viruses (both riboviruses and retroviruses), a combination of small genomes, high mutation rates, high virus yields and very rapid replication can produce spectacular rates of evolution. DNA viruses apparently mutate and evolve at lower rates, but they can nevertheless be quite mutable and biologically adaptable.

MUTATION AND EVOLUTION OF DNA AND RNA VIRUSES

The mutation rates of DNA bacteriophages have been characterized much more thoroughly than have those of the DNA viruses of humans and animals. Although mutation rates vary widely at individual genome sites, Drake (1991) has shown that there is a rather constant rate of spontaneous mutations per genome per replication in DNA-based microbes (including bacteria, yeasts, moulds and 3 DNA bacteriophages). Their genomic mutation rates per replication varied only about 2.5-fold around an average value of 0.0033 mutations per genome per replication round. Because the genome sizes of these diverse DNA-based microbes vary by thousands-fold, their average mutation rates per base pair also vary by thousands-fold. Drake (1993) later calculated the genomic rates of spontaneous mutation among RNA viruses (the only known life forms with RNA genomes) and found them to be consistently higher. Animal lytic viruses (riboviruses) and RNA bacteriophages have an average genomic mutation rate per replication in the neighbourhood of 1, and retroviruses average slightly (about 10-fold) lower genomic mutation rates (Drake 1993). Over all, Drake's calculations tell us that **genomic** mutation rates do not vary markedly. They are remarkably fixed for DNA-based organisms, and are also fairly constant, but higher for RNA-based life forms (riboviruses and retroviruses). Obviously, as Drake (1993) has pointed out, evolutionary forces must be shaping genomic mutation rates.

Despite the quite constant nature of genomic mutation rates there is enormous variation in the mutation rates per nucleotide, per genome replication. This difference arises from the huge variation in genome sizes among living things (Drake 1991, 1993). RNA viruses, which are among the smallest genomes, have maximal mutation rates per nucleotide (which exceed by millions-fold the base misincorporation rates of their eukaryotic hosts). This allows (but does not necessitate) rates of RNA virus evolution to proceed millions of times faster than that of their animal and human hosts. This topic has been comprehensively reviewed (Holland et al. 1982, Smith and Inglis 1987, Domingo, Holland and Ahlquist 1988, Eigen and Biebricher 1988, Domingo et al. 1992, Domingo and Holland 1994, Duarte et al. 1994a). A clear example of this was given by Gojobari and Yokoyama (1985), who showed that the Moloney sarcoma virus, a retrovirus of mice, evolves at a rate a millionfold higher than the rate of its integrated cellular homologue, c-*mos*.

Extremely high mutation rates generate 'mutant swarms' or 'quasispecies' populations of RNA viruses, and can provide great adaptability. This factor must be balanced against the inevitable high levels of lethality when the rates are too high. Eigen and Biebricher (1988) have shown by computer simulation that when mutation rates increase they suddenly exceed an 'error threshold' at which there is a 'melting' of genome information or 'error catastrophe'. They have proposed that RNA virus quasispecies generally adapt to the error threshold at which the misincorporation rate per nucleotide per replication will be in the neighbourhood of $1/v$ where v is the length (in bases) of the genome. This figure can vary somewhat, depending on a selectivity factor for the most fit 'master' sequences within a quasispecies population (Eigen and Biebricher 1988). This threshold limit dictates that genomic mutation rates generally cannot exceed values of about 1. Drake's (1993) calculations indicate that most RNA virus mutation rates are in fact close to 1. Strong chemical mutagenesis of RNA viruses (inducing high lethality in progeny) increases only slightly mutation rates in viable progeny (Holland et al. 1990). This indicates that RNA viruses are at or near to their error threshold. As Eigen and Biebricher (1988) have pointed out, occasional, short duration violations of the error threshold can provide brief evolutionary advantages, but persistent violations are lethal for viral genomes. One mechanism for radical mutational changes in RNA viruses is biased hypermutation (Cattaneo et al. 1988, Wain-Hobson 1992, Cattaneo 1994, Martinez, Vartanian and Wain-Hobson 1994). Biased hypermutation can produce long segments of viral genome in which certain bases are substituted in a regular, recurring pattern. There are two major mechanisms, one of which involves deamination of adenosines to inosines by a cellular RNA editing enzyme (Cattaneo et al. 1988, Cattaneo 1994). The other mechanism involves reverse transcriptase errors in retrovirus replication due to biased deoxyribonucleotide triphosphate pool concentrations (Wain-Hobson 1992, Martinez, Vartanian and Wain-Hobson 1994). Either can produce sudden, massive genome changes.

In general, most RNA viruses are life forms that replicate and evolve near the extreme limits of mutability and adaptability. Genomic mutation rates in the range around 0.1–1 dictate that even clones of riboviruses and retroviruses are quasispecies, or mutant swarms, rather than collections of identical virus genomes. This quasispecies nature of RNA virus populations has numerous biological consequences, some of which are outlined below.

Biological significance of virus quasispecies

First and foremost, quasispecies populations endow RNA viruses with enormous environmental adaptability and capacity for extremely rapid evolution. This subject has been reviewed extensively (Holland et al. 1982, Smith and Inglis 1987, Domingo, Holland and Ahlquist 1988, Eigen and Biebricher 1988, Domingo et al. 1992, Eigen and Winkler-Oswatitsch 1992, Domingo and Holland 1994, Duarte et al. 1994a).

Certain regions of an RNA virus genome (and certain single base sites) may be much less variable (more highly conserved) than others and therefore evolve at much slower rates, but even highly conserved regions evolve much more rapidly in RNA viruses. For example, sequence comparisons among all influenza viruses or all rhabdoviruses show that, eventually, nearly all sites can undergo viable mutations. However, in any currently circulating human strain of influenza A virus, evolution is gradual, and virus surface antigens evolve much more rapidly than do internal proteins (Webster et al. 1992). Likewise, influenza A virus strains apparently evolve much more slowly in birds than in humans, even though these human strains have been derived from avian sources (Webster et al. 1992). Clearly, even RNA virus populations can reach adaptive equilibrium with host spec-

ies, and relative evolutionary stasis results, whereas the same virus genes in a new host can be driven to disequilibrium and rapid evolution when introduced into different selective environments (Holland et al. 1982, Domingo, Holland and Ahlquist 1988, Domingo and Holland 1994). Apparently, influenza viruses replicating in the intestinal tract of wildfowl are well adapted and subject to far fewer selective pressures than are their human counterparts facing a new selective environment.

Similarly, many arthropod-borne RNA viruses such as alphaviruses evolve about an order of magnitude more slowly in nature than do most other RNA viruses (Weaver, Rico-Hesse and Scott 1992, Strauss and Strauss 1994, Weaver et al. 1994). Presumably, adaptive constraints necessary for efficient replication in two quite different environments (animal and insect tissues) can limit the rate of arbovirus evolution. But it is the evolutionary adaptability of RNA viruses that allows insect vector–host transmission cycles to evolve in the first instance. With very few exceptions, viruses that infect both insects and animals (or insects and plants) are RNA viruses. Generally, only RNA virus quasispecies have the diversity and adaptability to move readily back and forth between quite diverse selective environments. Very often only one, or several mutational changes can allow a virus to gain virulence, change its tissue tropism, or become resistant to an antiviral drug, or a monoclonal antibody, etc. (Holland et al. 1982, Smith and Inglis 1987, Domingo, Holland and Ahlquist 1988, Eigen and Biebricher 1988, Domingo et al. 1992, Eigen and Winkler-Oswatitsch 1992, Domingo and Holland 1994, Duarte et al. 1994a). Compared with the average (consensus) genome sequence, a large RNA virus quasispecies population will usually already contain almost every possible single base change and many double and triple base change combinations required for significant biological changes, so population selection rather than further mutation will often be sufficient. This is clearly illustrated by a study of HIV-infected individuals in whom AZT-resistant mutants were already present in the complete absence of current or prior drug treatment (Nájera et al. 1995). Following antiviral drug treatment of influenza-infected (Hayden and Hay 1992) or HIV-infected (Richman 1992) individuals, a substantial proportion of drug-resistant variants can emerge within days or a week. Quantitative studies of RNA virus fitness gains in either new or constant environments reveal a remarkable exponential process of environmental adaptation, even when starting from a single infectious virus particle (Chao 1990, 1994, Duarte et al. 1992, 1994b, Clarke et al. 1993).

Selective forces do not act only on single virions; it is the quasispecies mutant swarm that is the main target of selection, as proposed by Eigen and Biebricher (1988) and Eigen and Winkler-Oswatitsch (1992). Individual virions quickly generate swarms of variants as they replicate, so it is inescapable that groups of many related, but different, subsets of the quasispecies are subjected to simultaneous selection. As any particular quasispecies 'swarm' or 'cloud' of mutants evolves, its genomes generally move through those areas of 'sequence space' (Eigen and Biebricher 1988, Eigen and Winkler-Oswatitsch 1992) that offer the most biologically fit genotypes and phenotypes. The vastness of sequence space staggers human imagination. For a typical RNA virus genome of approximately 10 000 bases, there are $4^{10\,000}$ coding alternatives (even if addition and deletion mutations and recombination are ignored). Most areas of sequence space are, of course, 'dead space'; i.e. they do not encode viable life forms. There is no possibility that a random exploration of sequence space could produce highly fit, rapidly evolving life forms in the absence of guiding principles or 'laws'. As Eigen and Biebricher (1988) elegantly elaborated, these guiding principles are to be found in natural selection, coupled with the high connectivity of sequence space. For a 10 kb RNA genome, no sequence among the $4^{10\,000}$ possibilities is farther away than the sequence length v (in this case 10^4). This distance, the Hamming distance, between any two sequences will often be much shorter (it is equal to the number of positions at which the two sequences differ).

Natural selection of most-fit genomes can 'guide' a quasispecies cloud of mutants along many productive evolutionary paths through the hostile vastness of sequence space. The quasispecies clouds produced near the edge of error catastrophe evolve most rapidly because higher error rates produce extinction, whilst very low mutation rates or error-free replication would strongly dampen or prevent evolution. It is not possible to generalize about the relative contributions of positive or negative selection (or neutral drift) to RNA virus quasispecies evolution, but all occur. The usual preponderance of 'silent' base substitution rates over non-synonymous (amino acid-replacing) substitutions suggests that a large proportion of mutations are selectively neutral, but non-coding and synonymous base substitutions can frequently be strongly selected. Such selection has often been observed with poliovirus, for example (Skinner et al. 1989, Andino, Riechof and Baltimore 1990, de la Torre et al. 1992, Borzakian et al. 1993). Conclusive proof for or against neutral theory is lacking (Gillespie 1993). Neutral drift is inevitable at some level (Kimura 1989), but darwinian selection for improved fitness occurs in constant and changing environments (Holland et al. 1982, Smith and Inglis 1987, Domingo, Holland and Ahlquist 1988, Eigen and Biebricher 1988, Coffin 1992, Domingo et al. 1992, Eigen and Winkler-Oswatitsch 1992, Clark et al. 1993, Domingo and Holland 1994, Duarte et al. 1994b, Novella et al. 1995). Conversely, the rather regular fitness losses that occur during genetic bottleneck transfers of RNA viruses demonstrate that many members of a viral quasispecies are unfit and are subject to elimination during competition (Chao 1990, 1994, Duarte et al. 1992, 1994b, Clark et al. 1993). It seems obvious that positive and negative darwinian selection and neutral drift all occur during virus evolution.

Thus, chance (random sampling) events that occur during host-to-host transmissions (and some trans-missions within an infected host) act together with stochastic mutational variation and selection to shape the evolution of RNA virus populations. This means that RNA virus evolution is variable and unpredictable. No two quasispecies populations in different hosts could possibly be identical, even if both were infected from the same clonal source. This confers a certain randomness to the disease processes that accompany RNA virus infections. Variations in viral quasispecies composition can often influence the nature and severity of viral disease. This is not widely recognized among physicians and scientists who often tend to view measles, AIDS, hepatitis C or poliomyelitis as single disease entities to which different patients respond differently. Such a view ignores the fundamental nature of RNA viruses. Similar arguments apply to variations in epidemiological patterns of RNA virus outbreaks, to differences in responses to vaccine programmes or antiviral drug regimens, to γ-globulin prophylaxis, to the sensitivity and specificity of diagnostic reagents, and so on (Domingo, Holland and Ahlquist 1988, Duarte et al. 1994a). The extremely heterogeneous, transient, indeterminate, random and unpredictable nature of RNA virus quasispecies populations creates a counter-intuitive RNA genetics with which many scientists are both unfamiliar and uncomfortable. But it is the basis for the ubiquity of RNA viruses, and it is at the heart of the problems they pose for the control of RNA virus diseases. Where RNA virus vaccines have been successful (e.g. polio, measles, mumps), it was because certain antigenic epitopes within virus proteins have low probability for significant change without severely compromising virus viability or fitness. Identifying and exploiting such poorly variable (but immunizing) epitopes in other RNA viruses such as foot-and-mouth disease virus, HIV-1 and hepatitis C virus will sometimes pose severe challenges owing to the fleeting nature of quasispecies swarms.

The rapidity of RNA virus evolution mandates that 'new' viruses will appear, and 'old' viruses will suffer extinction at rates exceeding by millions-fold the emergence and extinction of new species among their DNA-based eukaryotic hosts. Most RNA viruses undergo evolutionary divergence at rates ranging from c. 10^{-4} to c. 10^{-2} base substitutions per nucleotide site per year, but these changes do not generally represent a regular 'molecular clock' dominated by continuous neutral drift as envisaged by neutralists (Kimura 1989, Gojobori, Moriyama and Kimura 1990). Rather, the evidence over all favours periods of relative evolutionary stasis punctuated by disequilibrium and saltatory change (Holland et al. 1982, Smith and Inglis 1987, Domingo, Holland and Ahlquist 1988, Eigen and Biebricher 1988, Strauss and Strauss 1988, 1994, Domingo et al. 1992, Eigen and Winkler-Oswatitsch 1992, Weaver, Rico-Hesse and Scott 1992, Webster et al. 1992, Gillespie 1993, Nichol, Rowe and Fitch 1993, Weaver et al. 1993, Domingo and Holland 1994, Duarte et al. 1994a). Punctuated equilibrium is expected from adaptive landscape theories of evolution (Lande 1985, Newman, Cohen and Kipnis 1985,

Eigen and Biebricher 1988). In fact, Nichol, Rowe and Fitch (1993) have shown evidence for a 'geographical clock' rather than a 'temporal clock' in the evolution of vesicular stomatitis virus in nature. Virus genome sequences diverged increasingly with distance (but not time of isolation) from endemic foci in Central America, perhaps owing to associations with distinct insect vector hosts (sandflies and blackflies in different geographic zones). Similarly, each of the 8 characterized hantaviruses is associated with different primary rodent reservoirs (Morzunov et al. 1995, Schmaljohn et al. 1995). Rapid evolutionary change is expected whenever viruses are adapting to new hosts or during any other major change in the selective environment. In fact, it is very likely that most of today's human RNA viruses 'emerged' in their present form quite recently (during the last few thousand to tens of thousands of years), and some are probably much more recent arrivals. Virus extinctions are as inevitable as emergences, even though preservation of some stable viruses by freezing or drying could 'resurrect' extinct viruses.

The re-emergence, after 2 decades, of H1N1 influenza A viruses in the human population is an example (Nakajima, Desselberger and Palese 1978). This re-emerged H1N1 strain could have come from a live vaccine programme freezer, but its source is not known. Regardless of its source, its subsequent success in the human population was due, in part at least, to the birth of many millions of susceptible humans during its absence (Gorman, Bean and Webster 1992, Webster et al. 1992), and its earlier extinction presumably resulted from strong immune selection in a largely immune population. Both HIV-1 and HIV-2 have emerged into the human population independently and recently, although how recently is uncertain (Doolittle 1989, Myers, MacInnes and Myers 1993). Many additional human RNA virus emergences in the future are a certainty (Holland et al. 1982, Smith and Inglis 1987, Domingo, Holland and Ahlquist 1988, Eigen and Biebricher 1988, Domingo et al. 1992, Eigen and Winkler-Oswatitsch 1992, Morse 1993, Domingo and Holland 1994, Duarte et al. 1994a). Some will be due to contact with 'old' viruses of animals and others will arise from recombinations or reassortments or mutation–hypermutation, but successful emergence in every case will involve rapid RNA quasispecies evolution and adaptation to the human host. This adaptation will sometimes lead to epidemic/pandemic transmission in humans, as occurs with influenza A and HIV-1, but it will often involve humans as sporadic 'dead end' hosts, as usually occurs with hantaviruses (Morzunov et al. 1995, Schmaljohn et al. 1995), filoviruses (Peters et al. 1993), haemorrhagic fevers (Johnson 1993) and others. At rare intervals, viral quasispecies evolution enables viruses to adapt well to 'dead end' hosts and they then effectively become transmitting hosts able to initiate outbreaks.

Slow co-evolution of some DNA viruses with their hosts

Most DNA viruses have mutation rates lower than those of RNA viruses (Drake 1991, 1993) but surprisingly little is known about the mutability of DNA viruses of animals. Smith and Inglis (1987) have reviewed the rather high mutability and adaptability of some eukaryotic DNA viruses. Herpesviruses, for example, can become resistant to antiviral drugs rather efficiently and this creates clinical problems. Bacteriophage T7, a classic DNA virus, exhibits clear evolution in a growing plaque (Yin 1993). On the other hand, many small DNA viruses clearly do not form quasispecies, and their evolution is tied to that of their hosts. For example, the polyomaviruses and papillomaviruses, which generally cause benign persistent infections, co-evolve with their hosts, and their capsid coding sequences yield phylogenetic trees similar to those of their host species (Shadan and Villarreal 1993). Shadan and Villarreal (1993) have proposed that this exceedingly slow co-evolution is linked to conserved domains of viral regulatory proteins that must interact with a restricted, crucial set of host regulatory proteins. Thus, virus and host evolution are tightly linked.

A remarkable study of the co-evolution of human papillomavirus types 16 and 18 has revealed an ancient phylogenetic root in Africa, and viral genetic drift correlates with ethnic groups and the migrations of ancient human populations (Ho et al. 1993, Ong et al. 1993). Diversity within these human papillomavirus types has evolved slowly over a period of more than 200 000 years whereas diversity between the papillomavirus types evolved over several million years. Rather unexpectedly, subtypes of a human retrovirus, human T-lymphotropic virus type I (HTLV-I), are related to anthropological backgrounds and to human migrations during the prehistoric (and recent) past (Miura et al. 1994, Vidal et al. 1994). At first glance, it would seem to be impossible for retroviruses (which can form quasispecies) to be so slowly evolving. However, HTLV-I is transmitted extremely inefficiently (by cell-associated infections), and mainly by mother to child. The adult T cell leukaemias that are triggered by HTLV-I are due not to extensive virus replication but to clonal expansion of tumour cells and of non-malignant T cells in carriers containing integrated HTLV-I provirus (Yoshida et al. 1984, Wattel et al. 1995). Thus, this retrovirus exhibits exceptional genetic stability because it seldom, if ever, produces quasispecies populations in humans. It replicates its genome mainly by division of cell clones carrying integrated provirus DNA.

Another type of intimate, slow co-evolution of DNA viruses and their hosts occurs in endoparasitic wasps whose eggs develop within injected host insect larvae (Stolz 1993, Beckage et al. 1994, Harwood and Beckage 1994, Harwood et al. 1994). Polydnaviruses are transmitted vertically as chromosomal proviruses in these wasps; they replicate in wasp ovarian calyx cells and their virions are injected into host larvae during parasitization. In the parasitized host larvae the multi-segment viral DNA circles do not replicate, but they express mRNAs and viral proteins that suppress host immune responses and affect pupal development. This exquisite virus–host relationship is observed in many lines of wasps, indicating that such virus–wasp co-evolution is important in wasp ecology.

Over all, virus evolution can range from RNA virus quasispecies swarms, evolving millions-fold more rapidly than their hosts, to small persistently infecting DNA viruses (and integrated proviruses) co-evolving slowly with their hosts. The former are primitive but effective, often involving massive replication with severe consequences for many hosts. The latter are usually subtle, elegantly regulated, and benign. Both are intimately involved with the genetics and the evolution of their host species.

REFERENCES

Alberts B, Bray D et al., 1983, *Molecular Biology of the Cell*, Garland, New York, 239–40.

Andino R, Riechof GE, Baltimore D, 1990, A functional ribonucleoprotein complex forms around the 5′ end of poliovirus RNA, *Cell*, **63:** 369–80.

Barrett AD, Dimmock NJ, 1986, Defective interfering viruses and infections of animals, *Curr Top Microbiol Immunol*, **128:** 55–84.

Beckage NE, Tan FF et al., 1994, Characterization and biological effects of *Cotesia congregata* polydnavirus on host larvae of the tobacco hornworm *Manduca sexta*, *Arch Insect Biochem Physiol*, **26:** 165–95.

Berg DE, Howe MH, 1989, *Mobile DNA*, American Society for Microbiology, Washington DC.

Boeke JD, 1988, Retrotransposons, *RNA Genetics*, vol 2, eds Domingo E, Holland JJ, Ahlquist P, CRC Press, Boca Raton FL, 59–103.

Borzakian S, Pelletier I et al., 1993, Precise missense and silent mutations are fixed in the genomes of poliovirus mutants from persistently infected cells, *J Virol*, **67:** 2914–17.

Botstein D, 1981, A modular theory of virus evolution, *Animal Virus Genetics*, eds Fields BN, Jaenisch R, Fox CF, Academic Press, New York, 363–84.

Boyle DB, Coupar BEH et al., 1987, Fowlpox virus thymidine kinase: nucleotide sequence and relationships to other thymidine kinases, *Virology*, **156:** 355–65.

Brown F, 1989, Classification and nomenclature of viruses: summary of results of meetings of the international committee on taxonomy of viruses in Edmonton, Canada, 1987, *Intervirology*, **30:** 181–6.

Bull JJ, Molineux IJ, 1992, Molecular genetics of adaptation in an experimental model of cooperation, *Evolution*, **46:** 882–3.

Cattaneo R, 1994, RNA editing. RNA duplexes guide base conversions, *Curr Biol*, **4:** 134–6.

Cattaneo R, Schmid A et al., 1988, Biased hypermutation and other genetic changes in defective measles viruses in human brain infections, *Cell*, **55:** 255–65.

Cech TR, 1986, RNA as an enzyme, *Sci Am*, **255:** 64–75.

Chao L, 1990, Fitness of RNA virus decreased by Muller's ratchet, *Nature (London)*, **348:** 454–5.

Chao L, 1994, Evolution of genetic exchange in RNA viruses, *The Evolutionary Biology of Viruses*, ed Morse SS, Raven Press, New York, 233–50.

Charini WA, Todd S et al., 1994, Transduction of a human RNA sequence by poliovirus, *J Virol*, **68:** 6547–52.

Claas EC, Kawaoka Y et al., 1994, Infection of children with avian–human reassortant influenza virus from pigs in Europe, *Virology*, **204:** 453–7.

Clarke D, Duarte E et al., 1993, Genetic bottleneck and population passages cause profound fitness differences in RNA viruses, *J Virol*, **67:** 222–8.

Coffin JH, 1992, Genetic diversity and evolution of retrovirus, *Curr Top Microbiol Immunol*, **176:** 143–64.

Domingo E, Holland JJ, 1994, Mutation rates and rapid evolution of RNA viruses, *Emerging Viruses*, ed Morse S, Oxford University Press, Oxford, 203–18.

Domingo E, Holland JJ, Ahlquist P, 1988, *RNA Genetics*, vols 1, 2, 3, CRC Press, Boca Raton FL.

Domingo E, Escarmis C et al., 1992, Foot-and-mouth disease virus populations are quasispecies, *Curr Top Microbiol Immunol*, **176:** 33–48.

Doolittle RF, 1989, Immunodeficiency viruses: the simian–human connection, *Nature (London)*, **339:** 338–9.

Doolittle RF, Feng DF, 1992, Tracing the origin of retroviruses, *Curr Top Microbiol Immunol*, **176:** 195–211.

Doolittle RF, Feng DF et al., 1989, Origins and evolutionary relationships of retroviruses, *Q Rev Biol*, **64:** 1–30.

Drake JW, 1991, A constant rate of spontaneous mutation in DNA-based microbes, *Proc Natl Acad Sci USA*, **88:** 7160–4.

Drake JW, 1993, Rates of spontaneous mutation among RNA viruses, *Proc Natl Acad Sci USA*, **90:** 4171–5.

Duarte E, Clarke D et al., 1992, Rapid fitness losses in mammalian RNA virus clones due to Muller's ratchet, *Proc Natl Acad Sci USA*, **89:** 6015–19.

Duarte E, Novella IS et al., 1994a, RNA virus quasispecies: significance for viral disease and epidemiology, *Infect Agents Dis*, **3:** 201–14.

Duarte E, Novella IS et al., 1994b, Subclonal components of consensus fitness in an RNA virus clone, *J Virol*, **68:** 4295–301.

Eigen M, Biebricher CK, 1988, Sequence space and quasispecies distribution, *RNA Genetics*, vol 3, eds Domingo E, Holland JJ, Ahlquist P, CRC Press, Boca Raton FL, 211–45.

Eigen M, Winkler-Oswatitsch R, 1992, *Steps Toward Life. A Perspective on Evolution*, Oxford University Press, Oxford.

Georgescu M-M, Delpeyroux F et al., 1994, High diversity of poliovirus strains isolated from the central nervous system from patients with vaccine-associated paralytic poliomyelitis, *J Virol*, **68:** 8089–101.

Gesteland RF, Atkins JF, 1993, *The RNA World*, Cold Spring Harbor Laboratory Press, Cold Spring Harbor NY.

Gilbert W, 1986, The RNA world, *Nature (London)*, **319:** 618.

Gillespie JH, 1993, Episodic evolution of RNA viruses, *Proc Natl Acad Sci USA*, **90:** 10411–12.

Gojobori T, Yokoyama S, 1985, Rates of evolution of the retroviral oncogene of Moloney murine sarcoma virus and of its cellular homologues, *Proc Natl Acad Sci USA*, **82:** 4198–201.

Gojobori T, Moriyama EN, Kimura M, 1990, Molecular clock of viral evolution and the neutral theory, *Proc Natl Acad Sci USA*, **87:** 10015–18.

Gorman OT, Bean WJ, Webster RG, 1992, Evolutionary processes in influenza viruses: divergence, rapid evolution and stasis, *Curr Top Microbiol Immunol*, **176:** 75–97.

Green AE, Allison RF, 1994, Recombination between viral RNA and transgenic plant transcripts, *Science*, **263:** 1423–5.

Hahn CS, Lustig S et al., 1988, Western equine encephalitis virus is a recombinant virus, *Proc Natl Acad Sci USA*, **85:** 5997–6001.

Harrison PT, Thompson R, Davison AJ, 1991, Evolution of herpesvirus thymidine kinases from cellular deoxycytidine kinase, *J Gen Virol*, **72:** 2583–6.

Harwood SH, Beckage NE, 1994, Purification and characterization of an early-expressed polydnavirus-induced protein from the hemolymph of *Manduca sexta* larvae parasitized by *Cotesia congregata*, *Insect Biochem Mol Biol*, **24:** 685–98.

Harwood SH, Grosovsky AJ et al., 1994, An abundantly expressed hemolymph glycoprotein isolated from newly parasitized *Manduca sexta* larvae is a polydnavirus gene product, *Virology*, **205:** 381–92.

Hayden FG, Hay AJ, 1992, Emergence and transmission of influenza A viruses resistant to amantadine and rimantadine, *Curr Top Microbiol Immunol*, **176:** 119–30.

Hayes W, 1968, *The Genetics of Bacteria and their Viruses*, 2nd edn, Wiley, New York.

Ho L, Chan SY et al., 1993, The genetic drift of human papillomavirus type 16 is a means of reconstructing prehistoric viral spread and the movement of ancient human populations, *J Virol*, **67**: 6413–23.

Holland JJ, ed, 1992, Genetic diversity of RNA viruses, *Curr Top Microbiol Immunol*, **176**: 1–226.

Holland JJ, Spindler K et al., 1982, Rapid evolution of RNA genomes, *Science*, **215**: 1577–85.

Holland JJ, Domingo E et al., 1990, Mutation frequencies at defined single codon sites in vesicular stomatitis virus can be increased only slightly by chemical mutagenesis, *J Virol*, **64**: 3960–2.

Hope-Simpson RE, 1978, Sunspots and influenza – a correlation, *Nature (London)*, **275**: 86.

Hoyle F, Wickramasinghe C, 1979, *Diseases from Space*, Dent, London.

Huang AS, 1988, Modulation of viral disease processes by defective interfering particles, *RNA Genetics*, vol 3, eds Domingo E, Holland JJ, Ahlquist P, CRC Press, Boca Raton FL, 195–208.

Illangasekare M, Sanchez G et al., 1995, Aminoacyl-RNA synthesis catalyzed by an RNA, *Science*, **267**: 643–7.

Jakob F, Wollman EL, 1961, *Sexuality and the Genetics of Bacteria*, Academic Press, New York, 327–32.

Johnson KM, 1993, Emerging viruses in context: an overview of viral hemorrhagic fevers, *Emerging Viruses*, ed Morse SS, Oxford University Press, New York, 46–57.

Kaper JM, Collmer CW, 1988, Modulation of viral plant diseases by secondary RNA agents, *RNA Genetics*, vol 3, eds Domingo E, Holland JJ, Ahlquist P, CRC Press, Boca Raton FL, 171–94.

Katchikian D, Orlich M, Rott R, 1989, Increased viral pathogenicity after insertion of a 28S ribosomal RNA sequence into the haemagglutinin gene of an influenza virus, *Nature (London)*, **340**: 156–7.

Kew O, Nottay MBK et al., 1981, Multiple genetic changes can occur in the oral poliovaccines upon replication in humans, *J Gen Virol*, **56**: 337–47.

Kim NW, Piatyszek MA et al., 1994, Specific association of human telomerase activity with immortal cells and cancer, *Science*, **266**: 2011–15.

Kimura M, 1989, The neutral theory of molecular evolution and the world view of the neutralists, *Genome*, **31**: 24–31.

King AMQ, 1988, Recombination in positive strand RNA viruses, *RNA Genetics*, vol 2, eds Domingo E, Holland JJ, Ahlquist P, CRC Press, Boca Raton, FL, 149–65.

Kirchmaier AL, Sugden B, 1995, Plasmid maintenance of derivatives of *ori* P of Epstein–Barr virus, *J Virol*, **69**: 1280–3.

Kucherlapati RS, Smith GR, 1988, *Genetic Recombination*, American Society for Microbiology, Washington DC.

Lai MMC, 1992, Genetic recombination in RNA viruses, *Curr Top Microbiol Immunol*, **176**: 21–32.

Lande R, 1985, Expected time for random genetic drift of a population between stable phenotypic states, *Proc Natl Acad Sci USA*, **82**: 7641–5.

Lawrence JB, Villnave CA, Singer RH, 1988, Sensitive, high-resolution chromatin and chromosome mapping in situ: presence and orientation of two closely integrated copies of EBV in a lymphoma line, *Cell*, **52**: 51–61.

Li D, Schmaljohn AL et al., 1995, Complete nucleotide sequence of the M and S segments of two hantavirus isolates from California: evidence for reassortment in nature among viruses related to hantavirus pulmonary syndrome, *Virology*, **206**: 973–83.

Lindahl T, Adams A et al., 1976, Covalently closed circular duplex DNA of Epstein–Barr virus in a human lymphoid cell line, *J Mol Biol*, **102**: 511–30.

Lodish H, Baltimore D et al., 1995, *Molecular Cell Biology*, 3rd edn, Freeman, New York, 320–344.

Luytjes W, Bredenbeek PJ et al., 1988, Sequence of mouse hepatitis virus A59 mRNA 2: indications for RNA recombination between coronaviruses and influenza C virus, *Virology*, **166**: 415–22.

Lwoff A, 1959, Factors influencing the evolution of virus diseases at the cellular level and in the organism, *Bacteriol Rev*, **23**: 109–24.

Maramorosch K, 1991, *Viroids and Satellites: molecular parasites at the frontier of life*, CRC Press, Boca Raton FL.

Martinez MA, Vartanian J-P, Wain-Hobson S, 1994, Hypermutagenesis of RNA using human immunodeficiency virus type 1 reverse transcriptase and biased dNTP concentrations, *Proc Natl Acad Sci USA*, **91**: 11787–91.

Mayo M, Jolly CA, 1991, The 5′ terminal sequence of potato leafroll virus RNA: evidence of recombination between virus and host RNA, *J Gen Virol*, **72**: 2591–5.

Meyers G, Tautz N et al., 1991, Viral cytopathicity correlated with integration of ubiquitin-coding sequences, *Virology*, **180**: 602–6.

Middleton T, Gahn TA et al., 1991, Immortalizing genes of Epstein–Barr virus, *Adv Virus Res*, **40**: 19–55.

Miura T, Fukunaga T et al., 1994, Phylogenetic subtypes of human T-lymphotropic virus type I and their relations to the anthropological background, *Proc Natl Acad Sci USA*, **91**: 1124–7.

Minor PD, 1992, The molecular biology of poliovaccines, *J Gen Virol*, **73**: 3065–77.

Minor PD, John A et al., 1986, Antigenic and molecular evolution of the vaccine strain of type 3 poliovirus during the period of excretion by a primary vaccine, *J Gen Virol*, **67**: 693–706.

Monroe SS, Schlesinger S, 1983, RNAs from two independently isolated defective interfering particles of Sindbis virus contain cellular tRNA sequence at their 5′ ends, *Proc Natl Acad Sci USA*, **80**: 3279–83.

Morse SS, ed, 1993, *Emerging Viruses*, Oxford University Press, New York.

Morzunov SP, Feldmann H et al., 1995, A newly recognized virus associated with a fatal case of hantavirus pulmonary syndrome in Louisiana, *J Virol*, **69**: 1980–3.

Myers G, MacInnes K, Myers L, 1993, Phylogenetic moments in the AIDS epidemic, *Emerging Viruses*, ed Morse SS, Oxford University Press, New York, 120–37.

Nagy PD, Bujarski JJ, 1995, Efficient system of homologous recombination in brome mosaic virus: sequence and structure requirements and accuracy of crossovers, *J Virol*, **69**: 131–40.

Nájera I, Holguín A et al., 1995, *Pol* gene quasispecies of human immunodeficiency virus: mutations associated with drug resistance in virus from patients undergoing no drug therapy, *J Virol*, **69**: 23–31.

Nakajima K, Desselberger U, Palese P, 1978, Recent human influenza A (H1N1) viruses are closely related genetically to strains isolated in 1950, *Nature (London)*, **274**: 334–9.

Newman CM, Cohen JE, Kipnis C, 1985, Neo-darwinian evolution implies punctuated equilibria, *Nature (London)*, **315**: 400–1.

Nichol ST, Rowe JE, Fitch WM, 1993, Punctuated equilibrium and positive Darwinian evolution in vesicular stomatitis virus, *Proc Natl Acad Sci USA*, **90**: 10424–8.

Novella IS, Duarte EA et al., 1995, Exponential increases of RNA virus fitness during large population transmissions, *Proc Natl Acad Sci USA*, **92**: 5841–4.

Ong CK, Chan SY et al., 1993, Evolution of human papillomavirus type 18: an ancient phylogenetic root in Africa and intratype diversity reflect coevolution with human ethnic groups, *J Virol*, **67**: 6424–31.

Peng G, Hongo S et al., 1994, Genetic reassortment of influenza C viruses in man, *J Gen Virol*, **75**: 3619–22.

Peters CJ, Johnson ED et al., 1993, Filoviruses, *Emerging Viruses*, ed Morse SS, Oxford University Press, New York, 159–75.

Ramig RF, Ahmed R, Fields BN, 1983, A genetic map of reovirus:

assignment of the newly defined mutant groups H, I and J to genome segments, *Virology*, **125:** 299–313.

Rao ALN, Hall TC, 1990, Requirement for a viral transacting factor encoded by brome mosaic virus RNA-2 provides strong selection *in vivo* for functional recombinants, *J Virol*, **64:** 2437–41.

Richman DD, 1992, Selection of zidovudine-resistant variants of human immunodeficiency virus by therapy, *Curr Top Microbiol Immunol*, **176:** 131–42.

Robertson HD, 1992, Replication and evolution of viroid-like pathogens, *Curr Top Microbiol Immunol*, **176:** 213–19.

Rolls MM, Webster P et al., 1994, Novel infectious particles generated by expression of the vesicular stomatitis virus glycoprotein from a self-replicating RNA, *Cell*, **79:** 497–506.

Roux L, Simon AE, Holland JJ, 1991, Effects of defective interfering viruses on virus replication and pathogenesis *in vitro* and *in vivo*, *Adv Virus Res*, **40:** 181–211.

Schmaljohn AL, Li D et al., 1995, Isolation and initial characterization of a newfound hantavirus from California, *Virology*, **206:** 963–72.

Shadan FF, Villarreal LP, 1993, Coevolution of persistently infecting small DNA viruses and their hosts linked to host-interactive regulatory domains, *Proc Natl Acad Sci USA*, **90:** 4117–21.

Shapiro JA, 1983, *Mobile Genetic Elements*, Academic Press, New York.

Sheen F-M, Levis RW, 1994, Transposition of the LINE-like retrotransposon TART to *Drosophila* chromosome termini, *Proc Natl Acad Sci USA*, **91:** 12510–14.

Skinner MA, Racaniello VR et al., 1989, New model for the secondary structure of the 5′ non-coding RNA of poliovirus is supported by biochemical and genetic data that also show that RNA secondary structure is important in neurovirulence, *J Mol Biol*, **207:** 379–92.

Smith DB, Inglis SC, 1987, The mutation rate and variability of eukaryotic viruses: an analytical review, *J Gen Virol*, **68:** 2729–40.

Stolz DB, 1993, The polydnavirus life cycle, *Parasites and Pathogens of Insects*, vol 1, eds Beckage NE, Thompson SN, Frederici BA, Academic Press, New York, 167–225.

Strauss JH, Strauss EG, 1988, Evolution of RNA viruses, *Annu Rev Microbiol*, **42:** 657–83.

Strauss JH, Strauss EG, 1994, The alphaviruses: gene expression, replication and evolution, *Microbiol Rev*, **58:** 491–562.

Syvanen M, 1994, Horizontal gene transfer: evidence and possible consequences, *Annu Rev Genet*, **28:** 237–61.

Tautz N, Thie HJ et al., 1994, Pathogenesis of mucosal disease: a cytopathogenic pestivirus generated by an internal deletion, *J Virol*, **68:** 3289–97.

Temin HM, 1970, Malignant transformation of cells by viruses, *Perspect Biol Med*, **14:** 11–26.

Temin HM, 1989, Retrons in bacteria, *Nature (London)*, **339:** 254–5.

de la Torre JC, Giachetti C et al., 1992, High frequency of single base transitions, and extreme frequency of precise, multiple-base reversion frequencies in poliovirus, *Proc Natl Acad Sci USA*, **89:** 2531–5.

Vidal AU, Gessain A et al., 1994, Phylogenetic classification of human T cell leukaemia/lymphoma virus type I genotypes in five major molecular and geographical subtypes, *J Gen Virol*, **75:** 3655–66.

Wain-Hobson S, 1992, Human immunodeficiency virus type 1 quasispecies *in vivo* and *ex vivo*, *Curr Top Microbiol Immunol*, **176:** 181–94.

Watson J, Hopkins NH et al., 1987, *Molecular Biology of the Gene*, 4th edn, Benjamin Cummings, Menlo Park, CA.

Wattel E, Vartanian J-P et al., 1995, Clonal expansion of HTLV-I infected cells in asymptomatic and symptomatic carriers without malignancy, *J Virol*, **69:** 2863–70.

Weaver SC, Rico-Hesse R, Scott TW, 1992, Genetic diversity and slow rates of evolution in new world alphaviruses, *Curr Top Microbiol Immunol*, **176:** 99–117.

Weaver SC, Hagenbaugh A et al., 1993, A comparison of the nucleotide sequences of eastern and western equine encephalomyelitis viruses with those of other alphaviruses and related RNA viruses, *Virology*, **197:** 375–90.

Weaver SC, Hagenbaugh A et al., 1994, Evolution of alphaviruses in the eastern equine encephalomyelitis complex, *J Virol*, **68:** 158–69.

Webster RG, Bean WJ et al., 1992, Evolution and ecology of influenza A viruses, *Microbiol Rev*, **56:** 152–79.

Weigel R, Miller G, 1983, Major EB virus-specific cytoplasmic transcripts in a cellular clone of the HR-1 Burkitt lymphoma line during latency and after induction of viral replicative cycle by phorbol esters, *Virology*, **125:** 287–98.

White PS, Morales F, Roosinck MJ, 1995, Interspecific reassortment of genomic segments in the evolution of cucumoviruses, *Virology*, **207:** 334–7.

Wimmer E, Hellen CUT, Cao X, 1993, Genetics of poliovirus, *Annu Rev Genet*, **27:** 353–435.

Yin J, 1993, Evolution of bacteriophage T7 in a growing plaque, *J Bacteriol*, **175:** 1272–7.

Yoshida M, Seiki M et al., 1984, Monoclonal integration of human T-cell leukemia provirus in all primary tumors of adult T-cell leukemia suggests causative role of human T-cell leukemia virus in the disease, *Proc Natl Acad Sci USA*, **81:** 2534–7.

Zimmern D, 1988, Evolution of RNA viruses, *RNA Genetics*, vol 3, eds Domingo E, Holland JJ, Ahlquist P, CRC Press, Boca Raton FL, 211–40.

Chapter 3

THE NATURE AND CLASSIFICATION OF VIRUSES

T H Pennington

1 VIRUS CLASSIFICATION

1.1 History

The urge to classify things is a powerful human trait. Lack of knowledge or understanding of the objects of classification has never been an impediment to the exercise and many viruses, through their diseases, were categorized and arranged in taxonomic schemes long before information about their physical nature became available. The vernacular names of virus diseases given at this time live on in the modern taxonomic scheme, of course. Viruses are unique in this respect, all other living things having binomial systems of nomenclature with Latin names. The use of English for viruses marks its emergence as the current *lingua franca* of science, an event that took place after the Second World War just before the development of techniques that allowed virus taxonomy to become established as a mature subject in its own right. Another feature of viruses that distinguishes them from other organisms is the smallness of their genomes. For classification the important corollary of this is the limit that it puts on the number of taxonomically useful phenotypic properties. It explains why the development of a new technique for virus characterization has usually been closely followed by its vigorous exploitation by taxonomists.

The research methods available up to the mid-1970s are described in Chapter 1. The succeeding 2 decades saw a considerable increase in the techniques of molecular biology, among which the following are particularly worthy of note.

GEL ELECTROPHORESIS

The introduction of polyacrylamide gel as a supporting and sieving medium during electrophoresis (Ornstein 1964) provided a method, at once rapid, cheap and capable of high resolution, for the quantitative separation and characterization of proteins and nucleic acids. This is a key method in modern molecular biology and an essential element in all polypeptide characterization and nucleic acid sequencing techniques. Nucleic acid sequence analysis makes use of a combination of specific enzymes – particularly DNA polymerases – and fluorescent or radioactive-labelled deoxyribonucleotides together with a chain-terminating dideoxyribonucleotide to yield fragments of increasing length. The subsequent analysis of radioactive-labelled fragments by gel electrophoresis allows the rapid and accurate sequencing of large DNA molecules.

RECOMBINANT DNA TECHNIQUES AND THE POLYMERASE CHAIN REACTION

Fragments of DNA that result from digestion by restriction enzymes, or DNA transcripts of mRNA, can be isolated and amplified by inserting them into a vector (i.e. a plasmid or a phage), which can be grown in a bacterial or other host. The fragments can then be sequenced (see above) or further manipulated, rearranged and expressed. The polymerase chain reaction has become an important taxonomic tool because it facilitates the rapid detection, amplification and sequencing of specific nucleic acid sequences.

2   WHAT IS A VIRUS?

Science distinguishes itself from other human enterprises in that it aims to express itself in a language of fixed and unambiguous meanings. Thus 'scientific terms are intended to mean neither more nor less than what they say, and to say neither more nor less than what they mean' (Keller and Lloyd 1992). In practice, things are not so straightforward. As an example the term 'gene' illustrates the difficulties faced by those who aspire to define biological entities concisely and unambiguously, because justice cannot be done to it whether as a unit of selection or as a segment of nucleic acid or as a functional unit controlling and affecting phenotype, or as all these things together (which it is) without an essay-length description. 'Virus' presents similar difficulties to the lexicographer. The definition and descriptions of 'virus' by the French virologist and Nobel laureate, André Lwoff, illustrate them. All serve as useful introductions to the subject. His statements that 'a virus is a virus' and 'whether or not viruses should be regarded as organisms is a matter of taste' (Lwoff et al. 1962) emphasize their uniqueness and the difficulty of a simple, clear definition. He also acknowledged the probability that viruses are polyphyletic (i.e. that different groups of viruses have evolved independently). In practical terms he defined viruses as strictly intracellular and potentially pathogenic entities with an infectious phase and (1) possessing only one type of nucleic acid, (2) multiplying in the form of their genetic material, (3) unable to grow and to undergo binary fission, and (4) devoid of a Lipmann system (a series of enzymes for energy production) (Lwoff 1957). This definition emphasizes one of the features unique to a virus, which is that, at a point during its growth in a host cell, its specific material is reduced to a genetic element, i.e. a nucleic acid. It also stresses the non-cellular nature of viruses and their dependence on host cell metabolism. An equally useful way of describing viruses is the definition of Luria and Darnell (Luria et al. 1978): 'viruses are entities whose genomes are elements of nucleic acid that replicate inside living cells, using the cellular synthetic machinery and causing the synthesis of specialized elements that can transfer the viral genome to other cells'. This description emphasizes one of the central roles of the virus particle – the virion – which is to enable the transfer of the viral genome from one cell to another.

A very clear and singularly influential demonstration of this genome–virion relationship was provided by the 'Waring blender' experiment of Hershey and Chase (1952). Bacteria, recently infected with phage T2, of which the protein was labelled with ^{35}S and DNA with ^{32}P, were spun in a blender to strip virus coats from the surface of the bacteria and then centrifuged. Most of the phage protein was found in the supernatant fluid. In Hershey's own words, the 'empty phage coats . . . may therefore be thought of as passive vehicles for the transport of DNA from cell to cell, . . . which, having performed that task, play no further role in phage growth'. Such a clear demonstration is possible only in bacterial systems, in which the rigid cell wall serves as a tough and effec-

tive barrier which can be breached only by macromolecules in specialized ways. In the case of phage T2, for example, specialized virion structures in the tail inject the virus DNA through the cell wall into the bacterium. Animal cells are very different from bacteria in that they lack rigid cell walls. Consequently, the membrane that forms their external boundary can be crossed quite easily by large structures such as virus particles or virus nucleocapsids. In a number of virus families the initial stages of virus macromolecular synthesis in the infected cell are catalysed by enzymes in the virion or in the virus nucleocapsid, which must therefore pass into the cell for infection to be initiated.

One of the reasons why it has proved difficult to formulate a concise commonsense definition of viruses is that different groups show considerable heterogeneity in the structure and composition of both virion and genome. Nevertheless, the functions of the virion can be summarized concisely under three headings.

1   Transmissibility by the provision of structures that absorb to specific host cell receptors and interact with cell membranes to facilitate the subsequent entry of the genome into the host cell.
2   Protection of the genome from hostile environmental factors such as nucleases and ultraviolet (UV) radiation.
3   In some, but not all, virus groups the provision of nucleoprotein structures, enzymes and other proteins essential for the early stages of virus macromolecular synthesis in the infected cell.

The structures that carry out these functions are relatively easy to detect morphologically and biochemically, and are illustrated by the example of vesicular stomatitis virus, a rhabdovirus, shown in Fig. 3.1. Also indicated in this Figure are features of the virion constructed using host genome information – a mode of exploitation additional to the dependence of the virus on the protein-synthesizing and energy-producing systems of the host cell.

2.1   Structure and composition of the virion

A virion is a complex multicomponent macromolecule. Built round the virus genome, which consists of one or more nucleic acid molecules, is either a spherical shell or a helical structure made of **protein subunits**. In some viruses these structures are in turn surrounded by a membrane or **envelope** made from host lipids and virus proteins. The latter are modified by glycosylation. As predicted by Crick and Watson (1956), viruses, because of their limited amount of genetic material, are parsimonious in their use of information, and their particles tend to be constructed from a rather small number of different subunits, of which many copies are present in a single virion.

The details of virus structure are considered further in Chapter 4.

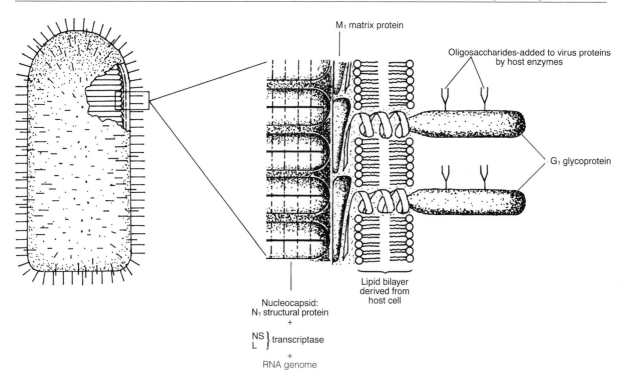

Fig. 3.1 Diagrammatic representation of the structure of vesicular stomatitis virus. Infection is initiated by the binding of the G glycoprotein spikes to receptors on the surface of the host cell. After entry into the cytoplasm the transcriptase in the virion is activated and synthesizes virus mRNA using building blocks already available in the cell.

2.2 The viral genome

Viruses are unique in that many families use RNA as the permanent repository of their genetic information and in order to bridge the informational gap between one replication cycle and the next. The genomes of many RNA viruses, and of the DNA-containing circoviruses or parvoviruses, can also be sharply distinguished from those of prokaryotes and eukaryotes in that they are single-stranded. In addition, in some RNA viruses the genomes consist of several different molecules (**segmentation**).

Larger viral nucleic acid molecules are usually DNA whereas smaller viral genomes may be either DNA or RNA. Viral RNA molecules range in molecular weight from 2000 to 15 000 kDa whereas the limits for DNA viruses are much wider – from 1000 to 200 000 kDa. Finally, the nucleic acid of most, although not all, viruses consists of a single molecule, and so, in genetic terms, the majority of viruses, like bacteria, are haploid with a single chromosome. Retroviruses, which have a diploid genome, are a notable exception.

Within this framework there is considerable variety and there are important exceptions to the general pattern.

Consideration and comparison of the virions of a very large virus (vaccinia virus, a poxvirus) and a very small virus (poliovirus, a picornavirus) (Fig. 3.2) illustrate well the very different ways in which viruses achieve their common objective, i.e. replication of progeny particles. Both viruses are typical members of families that contain many genera, and although a few

viruses have smaller virions and genomes than poliovirus, and a few have longer genomes than vaccinia, these 2 can be taken as fair examples of the extremes of complexity in virions, those of most other families falling in an intermediate position.

3 THE CLASSIFICATION OF VIRUSES

In the absence of detailed knowledge of the aetiological agents, early classifications of viruses were based on the symptomatology and pathology of the diseases they caused. Such schemes have been supplanted by a system of classification based largely on the morphology and biochemistry of virions and their behaviour in cells. This system has a high predictive value, serves well the dual purposes of a classification – the practical and the general – and is associated with a stable and generally agreed nomenclature. Its origins are well described by Brown (1984) in the 7th edition of this book. Its most up to date version appeared in 1995 (Murphy et al. 1995) and should be referred to for a comprehensive overview of the principles and details of virus taxonomy and the internationally agreed official scheme for virus nomenclature.

3.1 Philosophy of classification: the species concept

Biologists agree that the entities that are assembled

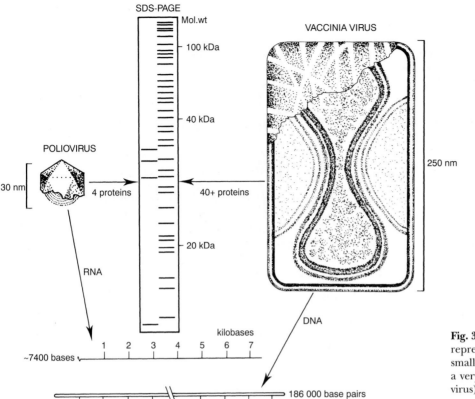

Fig. 3.2 Diagrammatic representation of a very small virus (poliovirus) and a very large virus (vaccinia virus). Virion protein composition, genome size and virion morphology are shown.

into genera and higher taxa in a classification form the species. They represent the lowest level of real discontinuity above the level of the individual. However, biologists have never agreed on a common definition of this entity, and there is probably no other concept in biology that has remained so consistently controversial as the concept of the species (Mayr 1982). Indeed, the longest, most animated and most abstract controversies of mediaeval philosophy stemmed from consideration of this problem. The starting point of these controversies was the apparently unobjectionable statement: 'as regards families and species I will refrain from saying whether they have independent reality or exist as mere motions . . .' in the introduction by the Greek commentator Porphyry to the *Categories* of Aristotle. Different positions were taken by the rival mediaeval schoolmen, the realists and the nominalists. Realists such as the followers of Thomas Aquinas and Duns Scotus believed that species consisted of individuals sharing in the same essence. On the other hand, William of Ockham and his fellow nominalists held that species were man-made constructs grouped on the basis of similarities. Echoes of their controversies have come from modern virologists. Those who have wished to designate groups of viruses as species without being altogether sure how to define the term (Mathews 1982) have been, perhaps, closer to the realists, whereas the proponents of cryptograms and numerical taxonomy (Gibbs et al. 1966) can be regarded as nominalists. In fact, some virologists have found it difficult to agree that viruses form

species at all, and most have been very slow to arrive at a common definition of a virus species. Consensus on these topics was recently arrived at, however (Murphy et al. 1995), when, in 1991, the International Committee on Taxonomy of Viruses accepted a definition that runs: 'A virus species is defined as a polythetic class of viruses that constitutes a replicating lineage and occupies a particular ecological niche'. van Regenmortel (1990) has provided theoretical justifications and explanations for this definition, which is his. He has stressed its breadth and catholicity and emphasized that it is not an operational definition. Thus although incorporating the notion of a polythetic class – one defined by a combination of multiple characteristics – it does not specify what these characteristics are, neither does it say what proportion of such characteristics have to differ between viruses to cause them to be considered different species. He also admits that his definition 'does not address the problem of how to define the terms virus lineage or niche which is a different issue altogether' (van Regenmortel 1990). That the breadth of this definition should render it impractical as an identification guide, or that it relies heavily on terms that some regard as tautological (thus one classical definition of 'niche' is itself set in terms of the space occupied by a particular species in relationship to a set of other species (Hutchinson 1978)) is not surprising. After all, Darwin's *The Origin of Species* convinced the world of the concept of evolution without offering a clear definition of the term used in its title! Darwin took a pragmatic view in *The Origin*: 'In determining whether a form should be ranked as a species or a variety, the opinion of naturalists having sound judgement and wide experience seems the only guide to follow.'

Most virologists adopt a similarly pragmatic view of the status of their objects of study.

3.2 Classification of viruses: the universal system

The basis for the modern scheme of virus classification was laid down by Lwoff, Horne and Tournier in 1962. Their pragmatic scheme gave weight to characteristics considered to be important. These were the nature of the **virion nucleic acid** – whether RNA or DNA – and the structure of the virion, including its **symmetry**, the presence or absence of a lipid **envelope** and its **size**. The pathways of virus messenger RNA synthesis also form a central feature of the modern scheme of virus classification. They are summarized in Baltimore's (1971) scheme, which is described in more detail in Chapter 6.

Although we are primarily concerned here with animal viruses, any account of virus classification would be incomplete without a brief discussion of the taxonomic position of viruses that infect bacteria, plants and insects. Many of the viruses that infect these hosts are distinguished by special features that not only are taxonomically important but also clearly refer to aspects of their natural history that are linked to properties of their hosts or their modes of spread. Allusion has already been made (section 2, p. 24) to the specialized structures that the T2 bacteriophage virion uses for adsorption and the injection of its DNA through the tough cell wall of *Escherichia coli*. Such structures are found only in bacteriophages. Plant viruses have adopted a different strategy for penetrating the rigid cell walls of plant cells. They rely, passively, on insect or nematode vectors to perform the mechanical process of penetration and transport for them. A unique feature of these viruses is the occurrence of species in which virus genome components are distributed among more than one virion, so that the successful initiation of infection requires the entry into the cell of more than one virus particle, an event optimized by the transmission of particles by vectors.

A consideration of some plant pathogens pushes the concept of infectious nucleic acid to its limit. Viroids (e.g. cadang-cadang disease of coconut palms and the 'planta macho' disease of tomatoes) consist of circular RNAs made up of 250–575 bases. They have no structural components, do not code for any proteins and use the machinery of the cell for replication (Diener 1993).

A distinctive feature of many insect viruses is the inclusion of their virions at the end of infection in large paracrystalline structures. Although made of protein, these bodies are extremely resistant to environmental factors. Alkaline conditions trigger their breakdown and the release of the virions occluded in them; such conditions are found in the insect gut.

Fewer than half the families so far described by virus taxonomists contain viruses of humans and animals, and many of the remaining families have members that infect only bacteria or plants or insects. Important exceptions occur, however. Thus members of the *Togaviridae* and *Flaviviridae*, which are transmitted from animals to humans by insect vectors, multiply in both animal and insect hosts. Less versatile in terms of the width of host range shown by individual members, but still versatile as a group, is the family *Rhabdoviridae*, which contains some species that grow in vertebrate hosts, some in arthropods and some in plants. Another good example of a family with a wide host range is the *Reoviridae*, which contains some members (orbiviruses) that grow in both vertebrate and insect hosts, some (reoviruses, rotaviruses) that grow only in vertebrates and others that grow only in plants (phytoreoviruses, fijiviruses and cypoviruses).

Key branch points in the classification of viruses at family level include the characteristics used in the Lwoff–Horne–Tournier scheme. Virion morphology provides a series of taxonomically important features. Thus DNA viruses with icosahedral symmetry – a mode of construction adopted by all animal viruses with spherical shells made of repeating protein subunits – can be assigned unequivocally to families solely on the basis of subunit number per virion (Fig. 3.3). This assignment is reinforced when features unique to each family are considered; thus the possession of a single-stranded DNA genome is diagnostic of the *Parvoviridae*, the occurrence of projecting fibres at the vertices (corners) of the protein shell is restricted to members of the *Adenoviridae*, and a membrane containing virus proteins surrounding the icosahedral particle is a universal feature of members of the *Herpesviridae*. Simple quantitative measures are not found as easily among the viruses that have virions composed of membranes and internal nucleoprotein structures. However, special morphological features define the taxonomic position of these viruses in a very satisfactory manner. Thus the bullet-shaped virion of the *Rhabdoviridae*, the shape and dimensions of the external spikes and the nucleocapsid morphology of the *Orthomyxoviridae* and the morphology of the external spikes of the virions of *Coronaviridae* (illustrated in Fig. 3.3) are all features characteristic of and exclusive to members of these families.

The commonsense approach adopted by Wildy and others in their contributions to the work of the International Committees on Nomenclature and Taxonomy of Viruses has meant that virology has been spared the bitter arguments and controversies that have been distinctive byproducts of the taxonomic endeavours of other biologists. Particularly contentious has been the issue raised by the desires of some taxonomists – and most users of taxonomic schemes – to erect schemes of classification based on those characteristics considered, in their judgement, to be 'important'. The weighting of these features contrasts with the proposition, strongly held by other taxonomists, that stable classificatory schemes are best based on an analysis of a large number of characteristics

	MORPHOLOGY	GENOME
Poxviridae	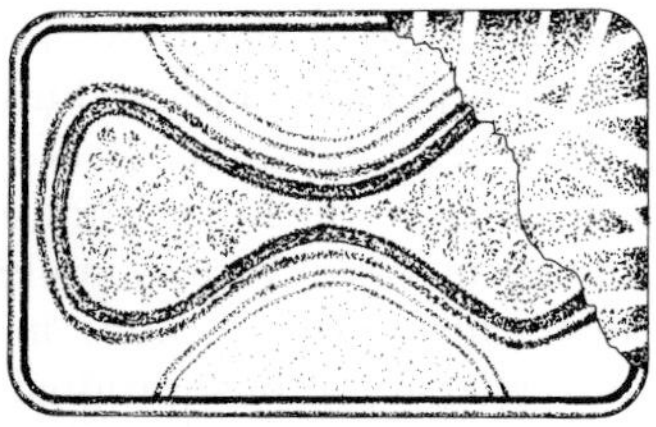 Brick-shaped or ovoid, (300 – 450) × (170 – 260) nm External coat with lipid enclosing a core which contains the genome >40 particle polypeptides	dsDNA 1 molecule Mol. wt 80 – 240 × 10⁶ Associated with virion transcriptase
Herpesviridae	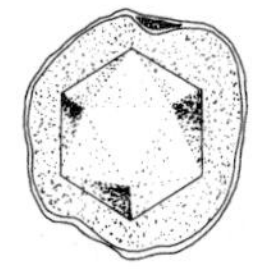 Envelope, 120 – 150 nm diam. Icosahedral capsid >20 particle polypeptides	dsDNA 1 molecule, linear Mol. wt 80 – 150 × 10⁶ No virion transcriptase
Adenoviridae	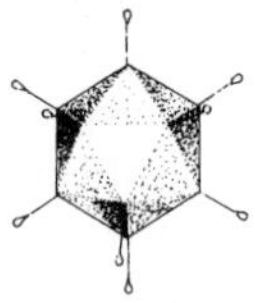 No envelope, icosahedral, 70 – 90 nm diam. Fibres at vertices >10 particle polypeptides	dsDNA 1 molecule, linear Mol. wt 20 – 30 × 10⁶ No virion transcriptase
Papovaviridae	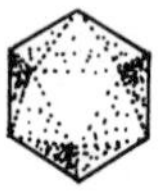 No envelope, icosahedral, 45 – 55 nm diam. About 5 particle polypeptides	dsDNA 1 molecule, circular Mol. wt 3 – 5 × 10⁶ No virion transcriptase
Hepadnaviridae	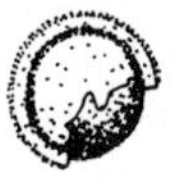 Envelope, 42 nm diam. Spherical nucleocapsid Several particle polypeptides	DNA, mostly ds 1 molecule, circular Mol. wt 1.6 × 10⁶ Associated with DNA polymerase in virion
Parvoviridae	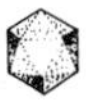 No envelope, icosahedral, 18 – 26 nm diam. 3 particle polypeptides	ssRNA 1 molecule Mol. wt 1.5 – 2.2 × 10⁶ No virion transcriptase
Paramyxoviridae	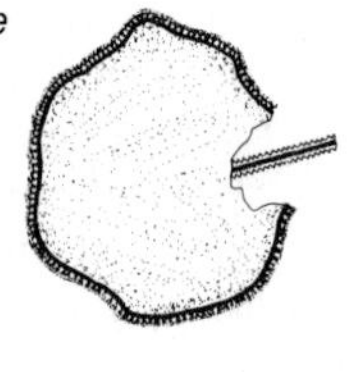 Envelope, 150 nm diam. Helical nucleocapsid 5 – 7 particle polypeptides	ssRNA 1 molecule, −ve stranded Mol. wt 5 – 7 × 10⁶ Associated with virion transcriptase
Filoviridae	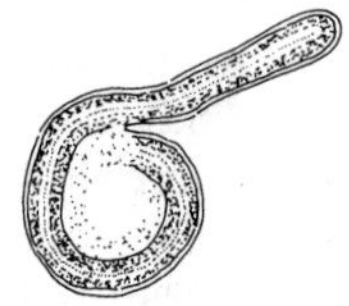 Envelope, tubular, 80 nm diam., up to 14 000 nm long Helical nucleocapsid At least 5 particle polypeptides	ssRNA 1 molecule, −ve stranded Mol. wt 5 – 7 × 10⁶
Rhabdoviridae	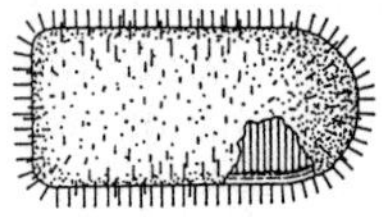 Envelope, bullet-shaped, 50 – 95 nm diam., 130 – 380 nm long 5 – 6 particle polypeptides	ssRNA 1 molecule, −ve stranded Mol. wt 3.5 – 4.5 × 10⁶ Associated with virion transcriptase

Fig. 3.3   The main characteristics that define the families of viruses infecting humans. Schematic drawings of virions, to scale with the exception of *Filoviridae*, are accompanied by information on virion size; the presence or absence of a membranous envelope; the structural arrangement of the nucleocapsid (constructed from protein subunits which complex with the nucleic acid genome to form a structure with icosahedral, helical or complex symmetry); the complexity of the virion as judged by the number of different polypeptides in its structure; and special features. The genomes of the different families

		MORPHOLOGY	GENOME
Bunyaviridae		Envelope, 90 – 100 nm diam. Helical nucleocapsids At least 4 particle polypeptides	ssRNA 3 molecules, −ve stranded Mol. wts 3, 2, 0.6 $\times 10^6$ Associated with virion transcriptase
Reoviridae		No envelope, icosahedral inner and outer shells, 60 – 80 nm diam. Up to 10 particle polypeptides	dsRNA linear, 10 – 12 pieces Total mol. wt 12 – 20 $\times 10^6$ Associated with virion transcriptase
Flaviviridae		Envelope, 40 – 70 nm diam. Icosahedral nucleocapsid 3 – 4 particle polypeptides	ssRNA 1 molecule, linear, +ve stranded Mol. wt 4 $\times 10^6$ No poly (A) at 3′ end No virion transcriptase
Togaviridae		Envelope, 40 –70 nm diam. Icosahedral nucleocapsid 3 – 4 particle polypeptides	ssRNA 1 molecule, linear, +ve stranded Mol. wt 4 $\times 10^6$ Poly (A) at 3′ end No virion transcriptase
Coronaviridae		Envelope, 75 – 160 nm diam. Helical nucleocapsid 4 – 6 particle polypeptides	ssRNA 1 molecule, linear, +ve stranded Mol. wt 5.5 – 6.1 $\times 10^6$ No virion transcriptase
Orthomyxoviridae		Envelope, 80 – 120 nm diam. Helical nucleocapsid 7 – 9 particle polypeptides	ssRNA −ve stranded, 8 pieces, Total mol. wt 5 $\times 10^6$ Associated with virion transcriptase
Arenaviridae		Envelope, 50 – 300 nm diam. At least 4 particle polypeptides Particles usually contain some host ribosomes	ssRNA −ve stranded 2 molecules, linear or circular Total mol. wt 3.2 – 4.8 $\times 10^6$ Associated with virion transcriptase
Retroviridae		Envelope, 80 – 100 nm diam. Icosahedral capsid, nucleocapsid may be helical 7 particle polypeptides	ssRNA +ve stranded, linear, inverted dimer Mol. wt 6 $\times 10^6$ Associated with virion reverse transcriptase
Picornaviridae		No envelope, icosahedral, diam. 22 – 30 nm 4 particle polypeptides	ssRNA +ve stranded 1 molecule Mol. wt 2.5 $\times 10^6$
Caliciviridae		No envelope, icosahedral, diam. 35 – 39 nm 1 major particle polypeptide with trace of another	ssRNA +ve stranded 1 molecule Mol. wt 1.8 – 2.8 $\times 10^6$

are characterized in terms of strandedness (either double (ds) or single (ss) stranded); nucleic acid type (DNA or RNA); size and number of nucleic acid molecules (mol) in each virion (a measure of information content); and the presence or absence in the virion of enzymes that are essential for virus growth and which use the genome as a template to make messenger RNA (transcriptases), DNA copies of RNA (reverse transcriptases) or DNA copies of DNA (polymerases).

given more or less equal weight. Virologists have been forced into a pragmatic position by the relative paucity of taxonomically suitable characters and have adopted a position in the middle ground. So, although much weight is given to the Lwoff–Horne–Tournier and Baltimore characteristics, all features find some place in the present scheme of virus taxonomy.

Under the guidance of the International Committee on Nomenclature of Viruses and its successor, the International Committee on Taxonomy of Viruses, this scheme has been steadily extended and associated with a stable binomial system of nomenclature (Matthews 1982) (see also Brown (1984) and Murphy et al. (1995) for a detailed account of these developments). Three main hierarchical levels – **family**, **genus** and **species** – and a subsidiary grouping at **subfamily** level are recognized. Despite the very loose and imprecise definitions given to these groups ('the genus is a group of species of viruses that share common characteristics and are distinct from the member viruses of other genera'; 'a family is a group of genera of viruses that share common characteristics and are distinct from the member viruses of other families'), their application in practice has presented little difficulty.

3.3   Taxonomy and the evolution of viruses

The insecure nature of the genetic basis of most characteristics used to classify animals and plants has provided a powerful catalyst for controversy and debate, often bitter, about the relationship between traditional systematic schemes and the phylogeny (the evolutionary history) of these organisms. Virus taxonomists have avoided such difficulties. This is because they have, until recently, exercised a self-denying ordinance on debate about the phylogenetic significance of their schemes of classification. This has partly been due to the absence of a fossil record, partly because of the paucity of characteristics available for analysis and partly because of the early realization of the high probability that key features common to different virus groups might be the product of convergent evolution. A good example of the last-mentioned is the accurate prediction by Crick and Watson (1956) that spherical viruses would essentially be built of identical protein subunits arranged with cubic symmetry, an argument stemming not from evolutionary considerations but from the application of Occam's razor – that the coding of the coat protein in the form of identical molecules would be the most efficient way of using the limited information contained in the virus nucleic acid.

The ease with which nucleic acids can be sequenced, and the development of statistical methods for the identification and measurement of sequence similarity, have in recent years revolutionized approaches to virus phylogeny. It is now possible to ask meaningful questions about virus evolutionary trees, including the order of branching (the splitting of lineages), branch lengths (the changes of

lineages through time), and the possibility of genetic transfer between branches and the incorporation of genetic information from the host (see Chapter 2). The creation of the order *Mononegavirales*, on the basis of nucleocapsid gene sequence similarity and similarities in gene arrangement and gene products, comprising the families *Paramyxoviridae*, *Rhabdoviridae* and *Filoviridae* (Pringle 1991), marks the first formal taxonomic outcome of these new phylogenetic approaches at the suprageneric level. At the other extreme, the study of virus evolution in real time at the subspecific level has grown to become a major field of study and is making major contributions to our understanding of the natural history of viruses such as influenza (Chapter 22) and HIV (Chapter 38).

4   THE IDENTIFICATION OF VIRUSES

The identification of a virus to family and, very often, genus level can nearly always be made unequivocally on the grounds of virion morphology, usually determined by negative staining and transmission electron microscopy. Considerations of host and tissue specificity and antigenic structure usually then suffice for identification to species level. The full panoply of characteristics used in the formal classification of viruses – characterization of genome type, size, arrangement and sequences, the characterization of virus polypeptides, and so on – are usually brought into play only when a novel or previously undescribed virus is under consideration. Chapter 5 describes the methods of identifying viruses, and Chapter 44 their application for diagnostic purposes.

5   VIRUS NOMENCLATURE

For more than 30 years the International Committee on Taxonomy of Viruses (ICTV) and its precursor, the International Committee on Nomenclature of Viruses, has provided the framework of rules that govern the officially recognized names of viruses. The founders of this scheme deliberately set out to create a scheme that would not generate the unseemly and unproductive disputes about priority that have dogged the traditional binomial Latin nomenclational systems adopted by zoologists and others, disputes that often stemmed from the rigorous application of rules invented to maintain stability but which in practice have seemed to have the opposite effect. In this the ICTV has been successful. A stable scheme using English virus family, subfamily, genus and species names has evolved: family names have the suffix *viridae*, subfamily *virinae* and genera *virus*. Over the years, it has become evident that the criteria used to define these categories have been well chosen, because the taxonomic scheme has not only been stable but also easy to use in practice. The ICTV's role in taxonomic affairs as well as in matters concerning nomenclature has been important. It is another feature that distinguishes the virological from other nomenclatorial controlling bodies, the latter restricting themselves almost exclusively to oversight of the process of naming and the regulation of semantics.

REFERENCES

Baltimore D, 1971, Expression of animal virus genomes, *Bacteriol Rev*, **35**: 235–41.

Brown F, 1984, Classification of viruses, *Topley and Wilson's Principles of Bacteriology, Virology and Immunity*, 7th edn, eds Brown F, Wilson G, Edward Arnold, London, 5–13.

Brown F, Wilson G (eds), 1984, *Topley and Wilson's Principles of Bacteriology, Virology and Immunity*, 7th edn, Edward Arnold, London.

Crick FHC, Watson JD, 1956, The structure of small viruses, *Nature (London)*, **177**: 473–5.

Diener TO, 1993, The viroid: big punch in a small package, *Trends Microbiol*, **1**: 289–94.

Fenner F, Ratcliffe FN, 1965, *Myxomatosis*, Cambridge University Press, Cambridge.

Gibbs AJ, Harrison BD et al., 1966, What's in a virus name?, *Nature (London)*, **209**: 450–4.

Hershey AD, Chase M, 1952, Independent functions of viral protein and nucleic acid in growth of bacteriophage, *J Gen Physiol*, **36**: 39–56.

Hutchinson, 1978, *An Introduction to Population Ecology*, Yale University Press, New Haven.

Luria SE, Darnell JE Jr et al., 1978, *General Virology*, 3rd edn, John Wiley, New York.

Lwoff A, 1957, The concept of virus, *J Gen Microbiol*, **17**: 239–53.

Lwoff A, Horne J, Tournier P, 1962, A system of viruses, *Cold Spring Harbor Symp Quant Biol*, **27**: 51–5.

Mathews REF, 1982, Classification and nomenclature of viruses, *Intervirology*, **17**: 1–199.

Mayr E, 1982, *The Growth of Biological Thought*, Belknap Press, Cambridge MA.

Murphy FA, Fauquet CM et al., 1995, *Virus Taxonomy*, Springer-Verlag, Vienna.

Ornstein L, 1964, Disk electrophoresis. 1. Background and theory, *Ann NY Acad Sci*, **121**: 321–49.

van Regenmortel MHV, 1990, Virus species, a much overlooked but essential concept in virus classification, *Intervirology*, **31**: 241–54.

Chapter 4

THE MORPHOLOGY AND STRUCTURE OF VIRUSES

I L Chrystie

1 **Techniques used in the study of viral morphology**
2 **Virus structure**

3 **Morphological types of viruses**
4 **Conclusions**

Since its invention in the late 1950s (Brenner and Horne 1959), the negative staining technique has enabled the characterization of viruses to be based on morphology. Although the future of virus taxonomy is increasingly dependent on genome sequence data, some newly discovered viruses being identified without having been visualized under the electron microscope (EM) (e.g. hepatitis C virus: Choo et al. 1989; and hepatitis G virus: Linnen et al. 1996), the continuing importance of EM examination for both research and diagnostic purposes cannot be overstated.

This chapter first describes the techniques employed in studies of viral morphology; then discusses viral structure; and finally presents a classification based on morphological features.

The use of EM techniques in the diagnosis of viral infections is covered in Chapter 44.

1 TECHNIQUES USED IN THE STUDY OF VIRAL MORPHOLOGY

1.1 Negative contrast EM

In the transmission EM, a beam of electrons is focused onto the specimen and an image is formed on a phosphorescent viewing screen by a series of electromagnetic lenses. Electrons pass through biological material without significant deviation, and the contrast necessary to make structures visible is provided by electron-dense salts of heavy metals. In negative contrast EM, virus particles are mixed with a suitable heavy metal solution and dried onto a support film. The stain then provides an electron-opaque background against which the virus can be visualized. The penetration of the stain into the particle can reveal

further details of its morphology. Negative stains must contain an electron-dense element (a heavy metal such as uranium, tungsten, molybdenum); be water soluble; and, on drying, must produce an amorphous, non-crystalline, sheet. Ideally such stains should not react with virus particles.

Because of their smaller effective size, uranium salts are devoid of visible structure, even at high magnifications, and can also enter the interstices of the virus surface more readily: such salts are therefore useful in high resolution work. However, the pH of most uranyl salts can be altered only over a very narrow range (at or about pH 4.4) and they provide relatively poor contrast compared to tungsten salts. The commonest stain used by animal virologists is potassium or sodium phosphotungstate (pH 5.0–8.0). Although this stain can have a detrimental effect on some viruses, its high contrast and its ability to tolerate high concentrations of salts in the virus suspension make it a good, all-purpose stain.

The preparation of viruses for negative contrast examination is simple. An aqueous suspension of the virus is mixed with the stain and the mixture placed on the microscope grid. All but a small amount is then drawn off with filter paper and the residual virus–stain mixture allowed to dry. The dried grid is then inserted in the microscope and the virus particles are examined at high magnification. When specimens contain high concentrations of salts, or when prolonged adsorption times might be necessary to improve sensitivity, the virus suspension alone can be applied to the grid (for up to several hours if necessary). The grid is then washed gently with distilled water and then negative stain before removal of most of the stain with filter paper, drying and examination. It should be noted that only a small quantity of the virus-containing material remains on the grid and that, to visualize the virus, a minimum concentration of 10^6 virions/ml is required. Although most viruses have a characteristic morphology, others, such as rubella virus, have few details helping identification and are therefore difficult to recognize. (For more detailed descriptions of methodology, see Doane and Anderson 1987, Nermut, Hockley and Gelderblom 1987, Chrystie 1996.)

1.2   Thin section electron microscopy

Although negative staining techniques provide the resolution necessary to study viral morphology, the many interactions between viruses and cells (adsorption, uptake, morphogenesis, release) are best studied by thin section methods. In addition, viruses that do not demonstrate a well defined structure by negative staining are often more readily studied in thin section (e.g. rubella virus or members of the *Retroviridae*).

In essence, virus-containing material (cells, tissues, etc.) is fixed to preserve fine structure (e.g. with glutaraldehyde/osmium tetroxide). After washing and dehydration, the material is embedded in a resin (e.g. Araldite) and polymerized. Thin sections are cut on an ultramicrotome and then positively stained with an electron-dense stain to provide contrast. Lead, uranium or osmium salts are the most commonly used stains, their affinity with protein being exploited to make virus and cellular structures visible (Fig. 4.1). (For more detailed descriptions of methodology, see Glauert 1975, Reid 1975, Nermut, Hockley and Gelderblom 1987, Chrystie 1996.)

1.3   Immunoelectron microscopy

Immunoelectron microscopy (IEM) is the visualization of the reaction between an antigen (usually a virus) and an antibody, and may be used to detect either component of this reaction. Combined with negative staining, the technique has been used to

detect serological responses to such viruses as Norwalk virus (Kapikian et al. 1972); has assisted in the identification of rubella virus (Best et al. 1967); and has been used diagnostically to identify hepatitis B virus infection (Kelen, Hathaway and McLeod 1971) and viruses associated with diarrhoea. The technique is also used routinely by some workers to serotype such viruses as rotaviruses, enteroviruses and adenoviruses. At its simplest the technique involves mixing virus and antibody, incubating for 60 min at 37°C and detecting virus–antibody complexes by standard negative staining; clumping of virus particles indicates a positive result (Fig. 4.2).

Identification of the immune reaction can be enhanced by labelling antibody molecules with electron-dense markers. Such markers include ferritin or colloidal gold (which is available in a variety of well defined sizes). Although the primary antibody may be labelled, it is more usual, and more efficient, for a secondary anti-immunoglobulin to be labelled (see Doane and Anderson 1987).

With thin section EM, the visualization of the immune reaction is widely used for the detection of virus particles and antigens, and is of particular value in determining stages of viral morphogenesis. Both gold- and ferritin-labelled antibody may be employed. In addition, enzyme-labelled antibody may be detected by visualizing the reaction product. There are 2 basic techniques, labelling either before or after embedding procedures (Chrystie 1996).

1.4   Electron cryomicroscopy

Both negative staining and thin section EM techniques inevitably introduce artefacts into the specimen by the use of fixatives, dehydration and staining. The technique of electron cryomicroscopy (cryo-EM) (Dubochet et al. 1988) eliminates such artefacts and has revealed far greater detail than had been possible with resolutions of 0.9 nm being reported.

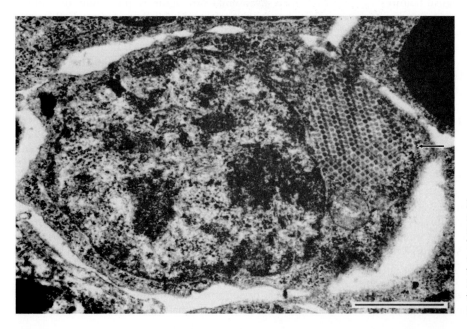

Fig. 4.1 Thin sectioning allows virus to be visualised in relation to the host cell. The cell shown here has a crystalline arrangement of virus particles (arrow). Infectious bursal disease virus in chicken bursal tissue.

(a)

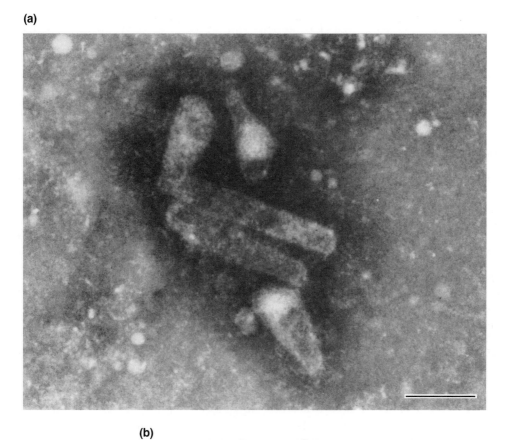

(b)

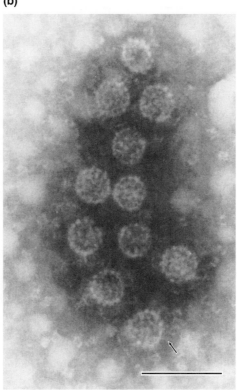

Fig. 4.2 (a) Clump of isolated HIV-2 cores following incubation with serum from an HIV-2-infected man. Negative staining with PTA, pH 6.5. (b) Clump of BK virus following reaction with the IgM fraction of anti-BK positive human serum. IgM molecules are clearly visible (arrow). Negative staining with PTA, pH 6.5. Bar = 100 nm.

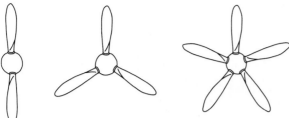

Fig. 4.3 Two-, 3- and 5-bladed propellers illustrating rotational symmetry. Each can rotate about its axis (the shaft) and will have 2, 3 or 5 identical positions respectively in one rotation.

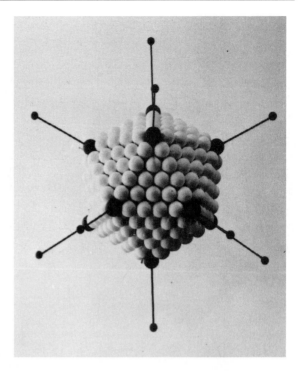

Fig. 4.5 Model of the most typically icosahedral animal virus – the adenovirus. The capsid is composed of 252 morphological units of similar size: 240 hexons (with 6 neighbouring units, white in the model); and 12 apical pentons (with 5 neighbouring units, black in the model). Each penton bears a fibre with a terminal knob. (Model by the late Dr RC Valentine.)

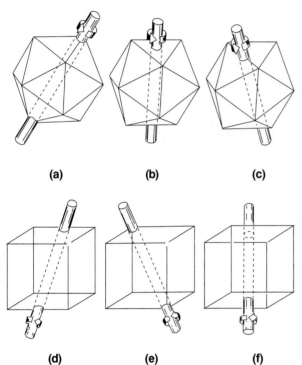

Fig. 4.4 Drawings of (a–c) icosahedra and (d–f) cubes, showing their axes of rotational symmetry. (Reproduced, with permission of Churchill Livingstone, from Madeley and Field 1988.)

Essentially, high-titre virus suspensions ($>10^{10}$ particles/ml) are placed on holey carbon grids and rapidly frozen in liquid ethane. This embeds virions in a thin layer of amorphous ice within the holes in the carbon. Grids are then examined in a cryo-EM stage. To prevent radiation damage, specimens are examined and images recorded using low electron dose techniques. Micrographs are digitized and 3-dimensional reconstruction performed (Crowther et al. 1994).

1.5   X-ray diffraction

Higher resolutions may be obtained from x-ray diffraction methodologies. However, such techniques require the preparation of single crystals of the relevant virus or viral component. In outline the tech-

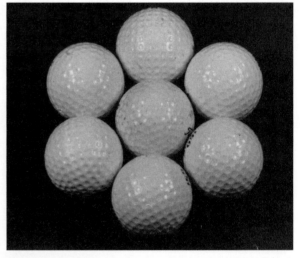

Fig. 4.6 Six golf balls arranged about a seventh to illustrate the relationship between a hexon and its neighbours. All can lie on a flat surface or, depending on the flexibility of binding sites, on a cylindrical one.

nique involves: the production of a sufficient quantity of pure virus/viral component; crystal growth and assessment; x-ray diffraction and data collection; and, finally, data processing. Viruses that have been studied in this way include poliovirus, rhinovirus, foot-and-mouth disease virus and canine parvovirus (Tsao et al.

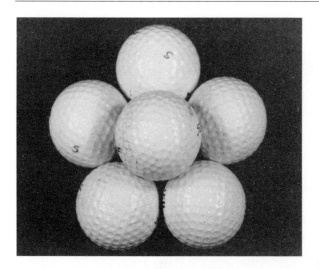

Fig. 4.7 Five golf balls surrounding a sixth to illustrate the relationship between a penton and its neighbours. If the 5 have to remain in contact with the central one, it must be lifted slightly. The structure cannot, therefore, lie on a flat or curved surface but must lie at an apex.

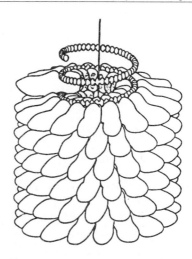

Fig. 4.9 Model of tobacco mosaic virus. Clog-like protein subunits are inserted between the turns of the helical single strand of RNA. (Drawing by Dr DLD Caspar and reproduced by permission of J B Lippincott Co.)

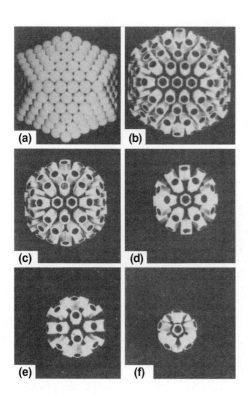

Fig. 4.8 Model of regular icosahedra constructed from varying numbers of subunits: (a) 252 (adenovirus); (b) 162 (herpesvirus capsid); (c) 92; (d) 42; (e) 32; and (f) 12 (picornavirus). Note that only the larger models (a) and (b) look icosahedral. (Models and picture from Horne and Wildy 1961.)

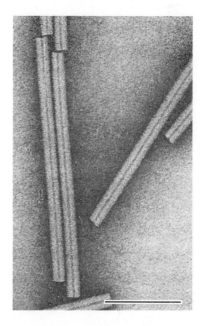

Fig. 4.10 Tobacco mosaic virus as visualized by negative staining. The central axis and the 2.3 nm pitch are clearly resolved. Bar = 100 nm. (Micrograph courtesy of Dr J T Finch.)

1.6 Additional techniques

Also of interest in the study of viral morphology, but not discussed here, are such techniques as: shadowing virus particles, especially with platinum or tungsten using electron beam evaporators; freeze drying and freeze-fracturing; the use of ultrathin frozen sections, especially when combined with immunoelectron microscopy; and scanning electron microscopy.

Finally, advances in data processing have permitted the development of advanced image analysis and image processing techniques that may be applied to most of the techniques listed above.

1991). The technique has also been employed to study such viral components as the adenovirus hexon (Roberts et al. 1986), and influenzavirus neuraminidase and haemagglutinin.

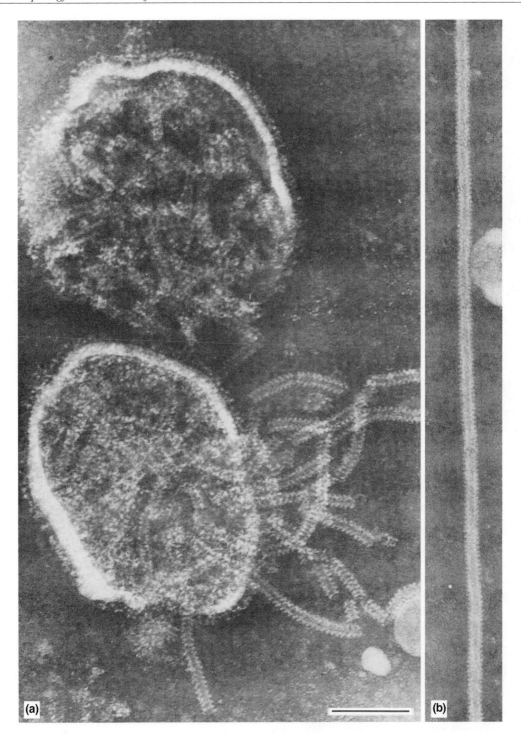

Fig. 4.11 Paramyxovirus. (a) Two partially disrupted paramyxovirus particles. The cell-derived lipoprotein envelope has a fringe of virus-specific glycoprotein surface projections. Note also the distinctive herring-bone pattern of the ribonucleoprotein. Bar = 100 nm. (b) Very long lengths of ribonucleoprotein can occasionally be seen; this one measured over 2 μm. Bar = 100 nm. (Micrographs by Dr J D Almeida.)

2 VIRUS STRUCTURE

2.1 Definitions

The complete, fully assembled, infective virus is the virion. It may or may not have an envelope, a lipid bilayer with associated glycoprotein projections or peplomers forming a fringe, surrounding the capsid, the protein shell enclosing the genome. The capsid is composed of morphological units or capsomer(e)s, which, in icosahedral capsids, will be either pentamers or hexamers. Capsomers consist of assembly units that often comprise a set of structure units or protomers. The nucleic acid–protein complex that comprises the

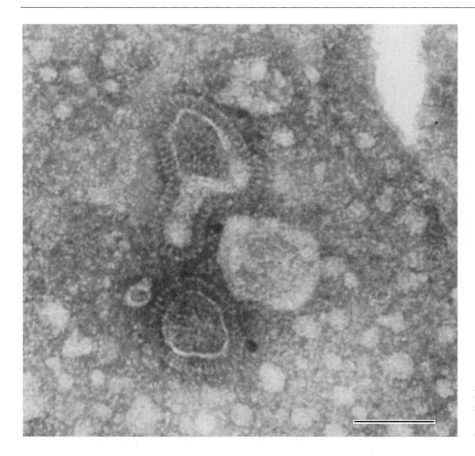

Fig. 4.12 Respiratory syncytial virus (RSV). Note the pronounced fringe. Bar = 100 nm.

genome is often termed the nucleocapsid. The nucleocapsid is often enclosed in a core within the capsid.

2.2 Limitations of current technology

Although the EM provides the most useful means of determining virus morphology, it has many limitations. Even the thinnest of sections limits the resolution of thin section EM to about 5–10 nm (often higher), and basic negative staining techniques, although having a theoretical resolution of 1.5–2.0 nm, suffer from such problems as radiation damage, grain size of the stain, and optical aberrations. In addition, the recorded image is a composite of the information provided by both top and bottom surfaces and, in some cases, also by the interior of the particle. The depth of field of a transmission EM is substantially greater than the thickness of the particle, so the information from all 3 levels is equally in focus and this can make interpretation of the image far from straightforward. The application of image analysis techniques to negative-stained and cryo-EM images can improve resolution somewhat, and resolution at the molecular level is possible with x-ray diffraction.

Thus, the understanding of how any particular virus is constructed is based on a careful analysis of all available data from a variety of techniques. Considerable knowledge of virus structure has been obtained but only a small part of it will be visible on a single micrograph.

Detailed interpretations based on data from such different sources are not beyond dispute, especially in the case of viruses that cannot be obtained in sufficiently purified preparations. Nevertheless, the following general principles of virus construction have emerged.

1. Viruses carry sufficient genetic information for their specification. Space for the genome is limited and efficient use of the information it contains is essential. Such genetic economy requires that structures be composed of identical copies of one or a few different subunits. Such construction leads to a symmetrical arrangement which, among viruses, is nearly always either helical or icosahedral (see section 2.3, below).

2. Nucleic acid, whether DNA or RNA, is helical. It may be protected by a 3-dimensional container or by insertion of protein units between the turns of the helix. Both forms of protection are found with different viruses and are characteristic for each virus family.

2.3 Symmetry

The 2 halves of the human body, split vertically from head to toe, would, although not mirror images of each other, look superficially very similar. They may therefore be considered to be symmetrical on either side of an imaginary central plane traversed by the vertical split. In a similar way, objects may be symmetrical about axes of symmetry as well as planes. In the case of an axis, the object may be rotated about it and

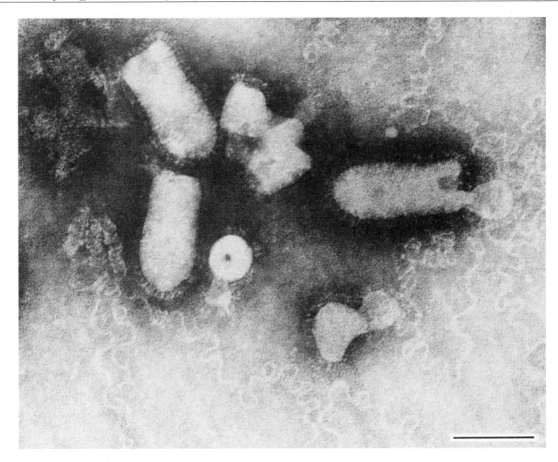

Fig. 4.13   Rhabdovirus: vesicular stomatitis virus. Note the 10 nm fringe and the ribonuclear protein helix. Bar = 100 nm. (Micrograph by Dr J D Almeida.)

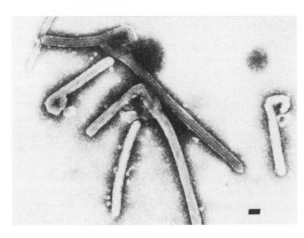

Fig. 4.14   Ebola virus. Bar = 100 nm. (Courtesy of Dr C D Humphrey.)

there will be 2 or more positions at which it will seem identical. If there are 2 such positions, it is said to be an axis of 2-fold symmetry; if three, 3-fold; etc. This is illustrated in Fig. 4.3, which shows 2-, 3- and 5-bladed propellers viewed along their axes, in this case the propeller shafts. Solid figures may have several such axes of symmetry (Fig. 4.4). Because of the general similarity in concept, icosahedral viruses are often referred to as having cubic symmetry. The helical symmetry of,

for example, a spiral staircase is described by the number of units per turn and the axial rise per unit (which together define the pitch).

2.4   **Icosahedral symmetry**

Most animal viruses are spherical or icosahedral. The regular icosahedron, which is optimal for constructing a closed shell from identical subunits, comprises 20 equilateral triangular faces, 30 edges and 12 vertices, and exhibits 2-, 3- and 5-fold symmetry. The minimum number of capsomers required to form an icosahedron is 12, each composed of 5 identical subunits. But many virus particles are composed of more than 12 capsomers. These are organized according to the principle of triangulation in which each face of the icosahedron is subdivided into identical equilateral triangles with the capsomers located at the apices of such triangles. T, the triangulation number (1, 4, 9, 16, 25, etc.), specifies the number of such triangular subdivisions. Capsomers at the apices of the icosahedron are surrounded by 5 capsomers and are termed pentons or pentamers; additional capsomers, where T>1, are each surrounded by 6 capsomers and are termed hexamers or hexons.

Figure 4.5 is a model of an adenovirus capsid and shows the latter features. In this model the every white capsomer

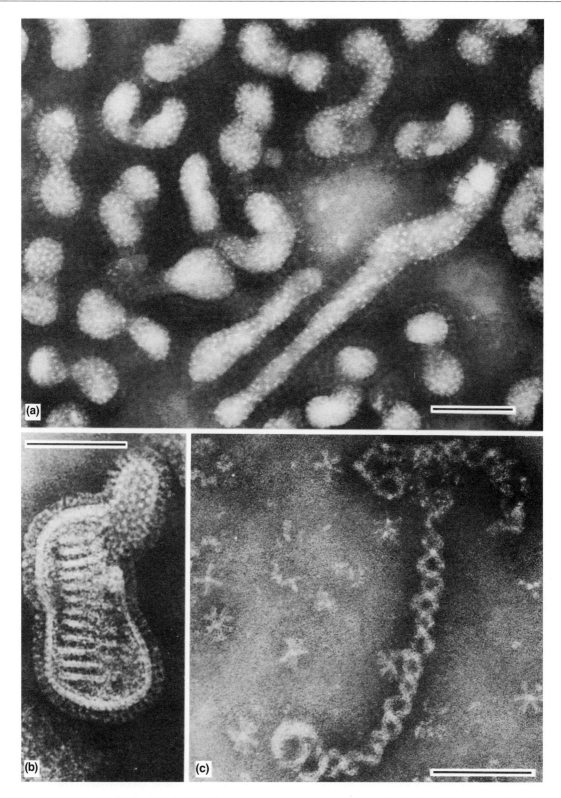

Fig. 4.15 (a) A field of influenza A particles showing the heterogeneous nature of this virus. The characteristic feature of influenza is the prominent 10 nm projections on the surface. These projections represent the haemagglutinin and neuraminidase of the virus. In this micrograph no internal component is visible. (b) One influenza virus particle which has been penetrated by stain to reveal the internal helix. This helix is formed from a strand 6 nm wide and the diameter of the helix is approximaely 50 nm. (c) Detergent treatment degrades the influenza virus and allows the internal helix to be visualized on its own. As can be seen, it is a double helix formed from the 6 nm diameter ribonucleoprotein strand. During the detergent treatment the surface haemagglutinin re-forms to give the stars and rosettes seen in the background of this micrograph. Bar = 100 nm. (Micrograph by Dr J D Almeida.)

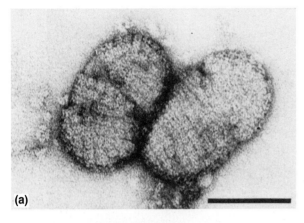

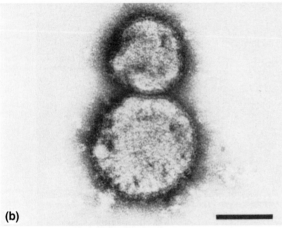

Fig. 4.16   Hantavirus. Bar = 100 nm. (Courtesy of (a) Dr M L Martin and (b) Dr C D Humphrey.)

is surrounded by 6 other subunits so that each, presumably, has 6 sites with which it may interact or link with another similar subunit: the black subunits, on the other hand, are each surrounded by 5 white subunits and have only 5 reactive sites. The white subunits (hexons) can lie on a flat surface closely surrounded by the 6 others (Fig. 4.6); in contrast, the black subunits with their 5 hexon neighbours cannot each touch their neighbours on a flat surface. Experimentation soon shows that the centre ball must be lifted slightly before all the balls can touch a neighbour (Fig. 4.7) and thus the pentons, the black subunits in Fig. 4.4, must always lie at the apex of the icosahedron. This also shows that an icosahedron can be constructed from only 2 kinds of subunit. Experimentation with various numbers and sizes of spherical units soon reveals that a variety of composite particles can be made within the bounds of icosahedral construction. Figure 4.8 illustrates some of these varieties, constructed from spheres or hollow prisms, and confirms that only those with a large number of subunits actually look icosahedral. As the number of subunits decreases, the particles seem more spherical.

However, for many virions the simple explanation above is insufficient. As has been stated, each face of the icosahedron can be subdivided into a number of identical equilateral triangles – this being the triangulation number (T) – and thus accommodate subunits in multiples of 60. But this subdivision can be made in different ways or classes, designated P, and can be parallel to the edge (P = 1), bisect the angle between adjacent edges (P = 3), or be unrelated to the edge, termed skew.

In general, $P = h^2 + hk + k^2$ where h and k are non-negative integers with no common factor. Thus for h = 1, k = 0 – P = 1; for h = 1, k = 1 – P = 3; etc. (all other values are of the skew class and can occur as either left- or right-handed enantiomorphs). The triangulation number can be defined as $T = f^2P$, where f^2 denotes the number of triangular subdivisions of each face of the icosahedron.

There are also other complications. For example, the capsid of the polyomavirus SV40 is composed of 72 capsomers. For many years it was assumed that there were 12 pentamers and 60 hexamers; however, it is now evident that all 72 are pentamers but with 60 surrounded by 6 rather than 5 other pentamers (Rayment et al. 1982). A similar all-pentamer construction has also been observed in human and bovine papillomaviruses (Baker et al. 1991).

Icosahedral symmetry is easier to visualize in naked rather than enveloped viruses. However, many enveloped viruses contain icosahedral cores or capsids. In addition, surface patterns suggestive of icosahedral symmetry are evident on the envelopes of many other viruses (e.g. HIV (Özel, Pauli and Gelderblom 1988)). It is likely that distortions of virions when subject to conventional techniques such as negative staining preclude the identification of underlying symmetry in more flexible structures; the more recently developed techniques (e.g. cryo-EM) may provide more definitive information.

2.5   Helical symmetry

The helical nucleocapsid is relatively simple to understand. There is an obvious axis down the centre of the helix but, unless individual subunits can be seen, the number of positions during rotation in which it will seem to be the same may be infinite. The pitch of the helix (P) is described in terms of the number of subunits per turn (u) and the axial rise per subunit (p) such that $P = u \times p$. Figure 4.9 shows a model of a typical nucleocapsid of this kind, that of tobacco mosaic virus. The central axis is clear, with protein subunits placed between the turns of the nucleic acid. An electron micrograph of the virus appears in Fig. 4.10.

2.6   Viral envelopes

Most enveloped viruses bud from a cellular membrane (e.g. plasma or nuclear membrane). The viral envelope comprises cellular lipid/protein bilayer into which has been inserted virus-encoded glycoproteins. The envelope can be relatively amorphous, as for herpesvirions, or have a definite and distinctive organization, as in, for example, the alphaviruses and myxoviruses. As discussed in Chapter 22, the full 3-dimensional structures of influenza virus haemagglutinin and neuraminidase have now been determined, and the proteins responsible for all membrane-

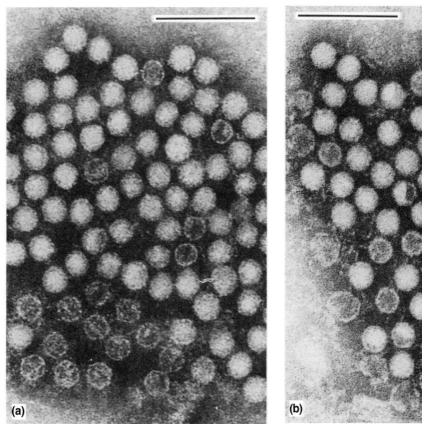
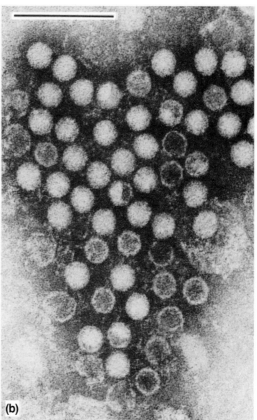

Fig. 4.17 (a) Picornavirus. Immune complex of poliovirus virions. Bar = 100 nm. (b) Rhinovirus. Immune complex of rhinovirus virions. Bar = 100 nm. (Micrographs by Dr J D Almeida.)

associated functions of that virus have also been described.

2.7 Conclusions

As demonstrated in the following pages, viruses are diverse in their detailed structure. If those infecting other phyla are included, the diversity is widened. Viruses have in common the possession of a single species of nucleic acid and at least one covering protein coat but little else. To some extent their structure probably reflects adaptation to their ecology and to selection pressures, but possibly owes more to the economies necessitated by limited genetic information. Their structures and their variations are elegant and efficient. During the last decade our understanding of virus structure has increased enormously – due mainly to the development of new examination techniques combined with powerful image analysis programmes. Such advances are likely to continue but, perhaps more important, advances in our understanding of viral morphology may generate novel strategies for the synthesis of antiviral agents.

3 MORPHOLOGICAL TYPES OF VIRUSES

On the following pages viruses are listed according to

morphology and illustrated with relevant electron micrographs.

3.1 Helical viruses

MONONEGAVIRALES

Although the universal scheme of viral classification has resisted attempts to use hierarchical levels higher than the family, the creation of this order (Pringle 1991) has recently been approved (Murphy et al. 1995). This recognizes the common gene sequences and gene arrangements of the *Paramyxoviridae*, *Rhabdoviridae* and *Filoviridae*. The *Orthomyxoviridae* form a separate family outside this order.

Paramyxoviridae

The family *Paramyxoviridae* contains 2 subfamilies: the *Paramyxovirinae*, with 3 genera (*Paramyxovirus*, *Morbillivirus* and *Rubulavirus*); and the *Pneumovirinae*, with a single genus (*Pneumovirus*). The pleomorphic virions are 100 nm or more in diameter and comprise a fringed, lipid envelope (derived from the host cell) and a nucleocapsid (a single molecule of linear, negative-sense ssRNA plus associated proteins).

Paramyxovirus Although the intact paramyxovirus particle has a diameter of c. 100 nm and is roughly spherical, most particles examined by negative staining show some degree of breakdown and frequently

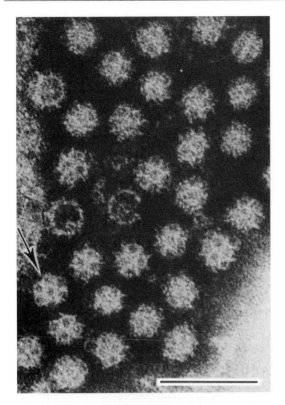

Fig. 4.18 Feline calicivirus particles showing the characteristic cup-shaped depressions. Bar = 100 nm. (Micrograph by Dr J D Almeida.)

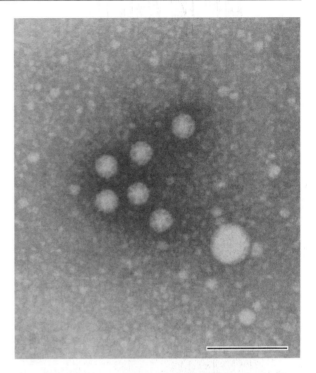

Fig. 4.20 Human astrovirus showing distinctive stellate appearance. Bar = 100 nm. (Micrograph by Dr C D Humphrey.)

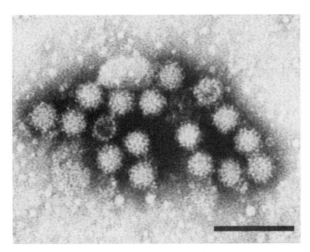

Fig. 4.19 Norwalk virus. Bar = 100 nm. (Micrograph by Dr C D Humphrey.)

look flattened on the grid with diameters of up to 500 nm (Fig. 4.11a). The nucleocapsid helix is c. 18 nm in diameter with a length of up to 1 μm (Fig. 4.11b); however, most micrographs show the helix broken into numerous short lengths. The helix can be seen at various stages of degradation, varying from a tightly arranged rigid structure similar to a tobacco mosaic virus (TMV) particle to a completely opened-up arrangement revealing the underlying single ribonucleoprotein strand of which the helix is formed. It is also possible to see single turns of the helix that has

broken off and the radiating subunits of the central canal of the helix. Most micrographs show the helix slightly extended, revealing its herring-bone pattern. The lipoprotein envelope carries short glycoprotein projections, c. 8 nm long, on the surface of the particle.

Members of the genus possess a neuraminidase. There is intermediate sequence relatedness with the morbilliviruses but little with the rubulaviruses.

Viruses include human parainfluenza viruses 1 and 3, Sendai virus and bovine parainfluenza virus type 3.

Morbilliviruses (measles virus, canine distemper virus, rinderpest virus) and rubulaviruses (mumps virus, human parainfluenza viruses 2, 4a, 4b) are morphologically indistinguishable from paramyxoviruses.

Pneumonovirus Although morphologically similar to the paramyxoviruses, members of the genus differ from the *Paramyxovirinae* in several ways, including smaller average gene size, smaller nucleocapsid diameter of 13–14 nm and glycoprotein projections 10–12 nm long (Fig. 4.12). Members lack a neuraminidase.

Viruses include human respiratory syncytial virus and bovine respiratory syncytial virus.

Rhabdoviridae

Rhabdoviruses are bullet-shaped, enveloped particles, 100–430 nm long and 45–100 nm in diameter, rounded at one end and flat at the other (Fig. 4.13). The flat end frequently has a 'tail' of cell-derived, but virally altered, membrane. The outer surface of the particle bears fine projections 5–10 nm long, which are viral glycoprotein and are set in the cell-derived

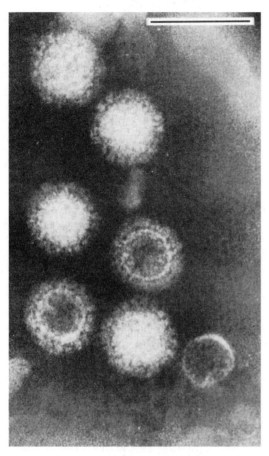

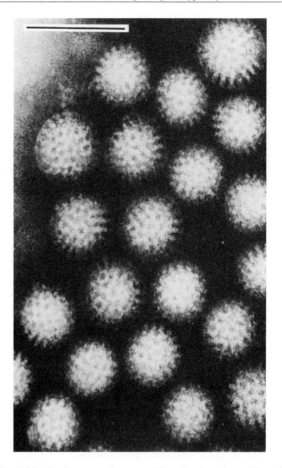

Fig. 4.21 Reovirus virions showing the 45 nm core and the apparently loose attachment of the outer subunits. Bar = 100 nm. (Micrograph by Dr J D Almeida.)

Fig. 4.22 Bovine rotavirus particles showing 'rough' and 'smooth' particles. Bar = 100 nm. (Micrograph by Dr J D Almeida.)

lipoprotein membrane. Within this membrane the nucleocapsid forms a regular helical structure with a periodicity of 4.5 nm and a diameter of c. 50 nm. When particles are either spontaneously or deliberately degraded, the nucleocapsid uncoils revealing a morphology not dissimilar to that of the paramyxoviruses. Nucleic acid is a single molecule of linear, negative-sense ssRNA.

All viruses have a similar morphology although rabies virions have less prominent surface projections which, when suitably orientated, have a honeycomb arrangement.

Viruses include *Vesiculovirus* (vesicular stomatitis virus, Chandipura virus, Piry virus) and *Lyssavirus* (rabies virus).

Filoviridae

Filovirus These are large, enveloped, pleomorphic viruses consisting of fringed 80 nm diameter filaments that vary in length up to 14 000 nm. Surface projections are 7 nm long at 10 nm intervals. Virions may be filamentous, branching, U-shaped or circular (Fig. 4.14). The 50 nm diameter helical nucleocapsid has a central 20 nm axis and a 5 nm periodicity. The nucleic acid is a single molecule of linear, negative-strand ssRNA.

Viruses include Marburg and Ebola viruses.

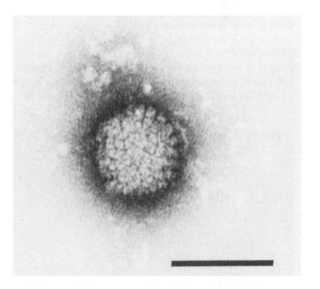

Fig. 4.23 Coltivirus. Colorado tick fever virus. Bar = 100 nm. (Courtesy of Professor F A Murphy.)

Orthomyxoviridae

These have highly pleomorphic lipoprotein-bound particles, with very distinct surface projections 10–14 nm long. The form encountered most frequently is

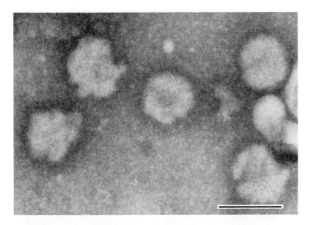

Fig. 4.24 Rubellavirus. Rubella virus particles. Bar = 100 nm.

a roughly spherical particle of 80–120 nm diameter, although curved forms are also common (Fig. 4.15). However, considerable variation both in shape and in size occurs and filamentous forms of the virus are common, especially following passage in culture. Rod-shaped haemagglutinin spikes and mushroom-shaped neuraminidase spikes are present in influenza viruses A and B but are rarely visualized in intact particles; influenza C virions have only a single type of spike. Unlike the *Paramyxoviridae*, influenza particles are physically stable and the internal component is not visible in most particles. The genome is segmented, linear ssRNA and has helical symmetry. The number of RNA segments varies (influenza A and B: 8 segments; influenza C: 7 segments; Thogoto virus group: 6 or 7 segments).

Viruses include influenzavirus A and B, influenzavirus C and Thogoto-like viruses.

Bunyaviridae

Virions are spherical or pleomorphic (Fig. 4.16), 80–120 nm in diameter, with 5–10 nm projections emanating from the surface of the bilayered envelope. Brief

negative staining, especially at acidic pH, often reveals on the surface of particles structural detail suggestive of an icosahedral arrangement of the glycoprotein projections. Similar information is provided by freeze etching studies. Viral nucleocapsids are 2–2.5 nm in diameter (10–12 nm when coiled) and display helical symmetry. The genome comprises 3 molecules of negative or ambisense ssRNA

Viruses include *Bunyavirus*, *Hantavirus*, *Nairovirus* and *Phlebovirus*.

3.2 Cubic viruses

Unlike animal helical viruses, cubic viruses may contain either RNA or DNA as their nucleic acid. Also unlike helical viruses, animal cubic viruses may or may not have an additional lipoprotein membrane enclosing the symmetry-bearing component. It is therefore convenient to divide cubic viruses, first by nucleic acid and then according to their possessing a lipoprotein outer membrane. Those without an outer membrane are described as simple, or naked; those with a membrane are either compound or enveloped.

Simple cubic RNA viruses

Picornaviridae

Picornaviruses are small, unenveloped, icosahedral particles. Viruses can be sensitive to pH, and negative staining solutions should be adjusted to values of pH 7–8 before satisfactory preparations can be obtained. By negative staining EM, viruses display no detectable subunit structure. All appear as smooth, round structures of c. 25–30 nm diameter. The few particles that are penetrated by stain show that the outer shell is some 2.5 nm thick (Fig. 4.17a). Occasionally, some particles show a hexagonal outline, providing

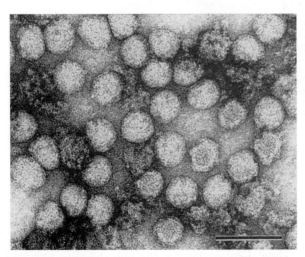

Fig. 4.25 Flavivirus. Yellow fever virus. Bar = 100 nm. (Courtesy of Dr M L Martin.)

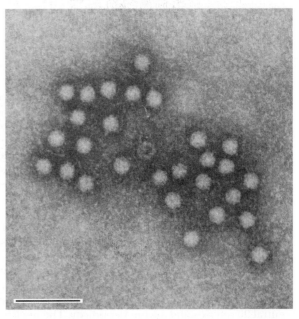

Fig. 4.26 Clump of human parvovirus from the serum of an HIV-positive man with negative staining. PTA, pH 6.5. Bar = 100 nm.

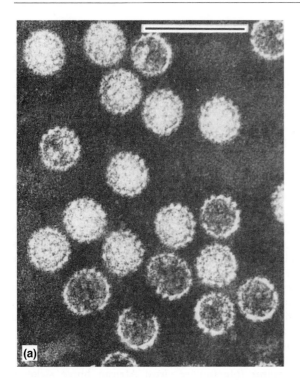 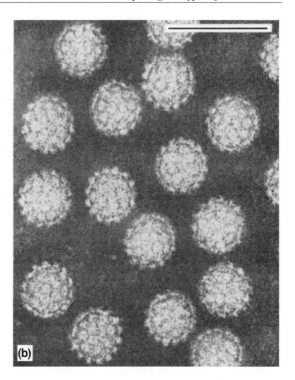

Fig. 4.27 (a) Polyomavirus particles. Bar = 100 nm. (b) Papillomavirus. Human wart virus particles. Bar = 100 nm. (Micrographs by Dr J D Almeida.)

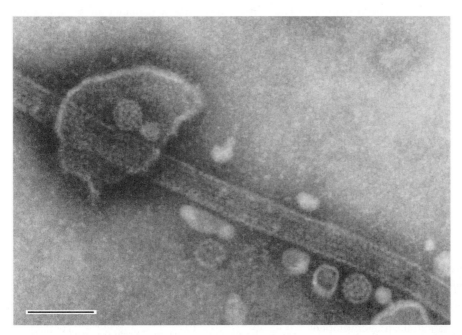

Fig. 4.28 Papillomavirus. On occasions papillomavirus capsomers aggregate into long tubules. Bar = 100 nm.

additional evidence of the underlying but unresolved cubic symmetry. For practical purposes it is often an advantage to use IEM to visualize these viruses. The enteroviruses are pH-stable and are negatively stained by the routine phosphotungstic acid solution adjusted to pH 6. Rhinoviruses (Fig. 4.17b), on the other hand, are labile below pH 6 and must be visualized with a negative stain adjusted to above this value; pH 8 is normally used. Genome is linear ssRNA.

X-ray crystallographic analysis has confirmed that the protein shell is composed of 60 subunits arranged as 12 pentamers, each subunit comprising 4 proteins.

Viruses include *Enterovirus, Cardiovirus, Rhinovirus, Hepatovirus* and *Aphthovirus*.

Caliciviridae

Calicivirus Caliciviruses are distinctive particles of 35–39 nm diameter with 32 cup-shaped depressions in icosahedral symmetry. The 'diagnostic' patterns seen are one subunit surrounded by 6 (resembling a star

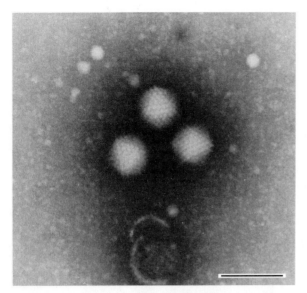

Fig. 4.29 Human adenovirus showing characteristic icosahedral symmetry. Bar = 100 nm.

of David), a pattern of 4 hollows or a circular particle with 10 surface projections (Fig. 4.18). The characteristic cup-shaped depressions are not seen in many species (e.g. Norwalk virus; Fig. 4.19), but the icosahedral architecture of such viruses has been demonstrated by image processing and cryo-EM techniques (Prasad, Matson and Smith 1994). The nucleic acid is linear, positive-sense ssRNA.

Viruses include vesicular exanthema of swine, feline calicivirus, human calicivirus (including Norwalk virus) and hepatitis E virus.

Astroviridae

***Astrovirus* (human astrovirus)**   Astrovirus particles are non-enveloped and 28–30 nm in diameter with a smooth margin. A variable number of virions display a characteristic surface morphology of 5- or 6-pointed stars (Fig. 4.20). The genome is a single molecule of linear ssRNA.

Birnaviridae

These icosahedral, non-enveloped, single-shelled viruses are c. 60 nm in diameter. The genome comprises 2 segments of dsRNA.

Reoviridae

This family comprises icosahedral, non-enveloped virions, 60–80 nm in diameter, which consist of an internal icosahedral core surrounded by several protein layers. Within the *Reoviridae* there are subtle, but distinct, morphological differences between the genera. The reoviruses (Fig. 4.21) are larger than rotaviruses (Fig. 4.22) and have separate, radiating, external subunits. Orbiviruses display a less distinct structure than the other members. The genome is segmented, linear dsRNA.

***Orthoreovirus* (mammalian reovirus 1, 2 and 3)**   Reoviruses contain a genome of dsRNA in 10

segments. The capsid consists of a double-shelled construction of protein subunits on a smooth-walled internal core (see Fig. 4.21). The diameter of the core is 49 nm, the internal capsid 60 nm and the complete particle 81 nm. Cryo-EM has shown that both the internal capsid and the complete virion exhibit 5-, 3- and 2-fold axes of symmetry and have subunits that project separately round the edge of the particle (Metcalf, Cyrklaff and Adrian 1991).

Rotavirus The rotavirus particle consists of a triple-layered icosahedral capsid containing 11 segments of dsRNA. There is an inner core 45 nm in diameter, an internal capsid 50 nm in diameter, described as 'rough' because of the projecting subunits, and an external capsid 65 nm in diameter. The external capsid is described as smooth because there seems to be a continuous line round the periphery of the particle. Cryo-EM has shown that both the inner and the outer capsid have icosahedral symmetry with short (6 nm) surface spikes (Prasad et al. 1988). The internal capsid bears the group-specific antigens, the type-specific antigens being on the external capsid.

***Orbivirus* (bluetongue virus; African horse sickness virus)**   Orbiviruses demonstrate a basic construction similar to other members of the *Reoviridae*, an internal 60 nm capsid showing distinct subunit construction. The outer capsid has a diameter of 80 nm and a slightly 'fuzzy' appearance that distinguishes this group from the other 2. Icosahedral symmetry and surface projections are visualized when specimens are examined by cryo-EM (Hewat, Booth and Roy 1992). The genome consists of 10 segments of dsRNA.

Coltivirus   Coltiviruses, previously classified as orbiviruses, are double layered, icosahedral, 80 nm particles possessing a relatively smooth surface (Fig. 4.23). The genome consists of 12 dsRNA segments.

Viruses include Colorado tick fever virus.

CUBIC RNA VIRUSES WITH LIPOPROTEIN ENVELOPES

Togaviridae

Togaviruses are more or less spherical particles of 70 nm diameter consisting of a lipid envelope containing a 40 nm icosahedral nucleocapsid. The surface of the lipoprotein envelope bears fine projections seen as a halo around the particle. Cryo-EM has shown that these glycoprotein projections are arranged in an icosahedral lattice (Paredes et al. 1993).

Rubivirus virions are pleomorphic and show little, if any, structure by negative staining (Fig. 4.24). In thin section the virus exhibits an electron-dense core c. 30 nm in diameter and an electron-lucent area between this core and the lipoprotein envelope. The genome is linear, positive-sense ssRNA.

Viruses include *Alphavirus* (Sindbis virus, eastern equine encephalomyelitis, western equine encephalomyelitis, Venezuelan equine encephalomyelitis; Semliki Forest virus) and *Rubivirus* (rubella).

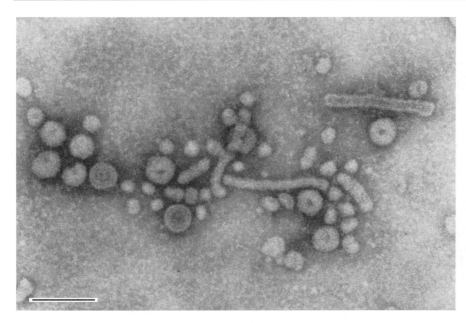

Fig. 4.30 Hepatitis B virus showing the 42 nm double-shelled virion (the Dane particle) and the 22 nm spherical and tubular HBsAg. Bar = 100 nm.

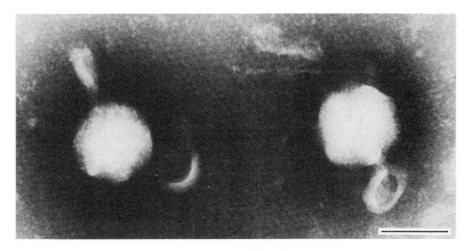

Fig. 4.31 Intact herpes virus particles in which the outer envelope has not been penetrated by the negative stain. Bar = 100 nm. (Micrograph by Dr J D Almeida.)

Flaviviridae

Flavivirus virions comprise a 40–60 nm enveloped spherical particle with an indistinct, 6 nm fringe and a 30 nm viral core (Fig. 4.25). The pestivirus envelope has 10–12 nm ring-like subunits on its surface. Further structural details are not currently known. The genome comprises a single molecule of positive-sense ssRNA. Unless very pure preparations are available, it is advisable to use IEM for their identification because only when they are present in the form of complexes is it possible to be certain of their nature.

Viruses include *Flavivirus* (yellow fever virus, tick-borne encephalitis virus group, Japanese encephalitis group, dengue virus group), *Pestivirus* (bovine viral diarrhoea virus) and hepatitis C-like viruses.

Simple cubic DNA viruses

Parvoviridae: *Parvovirinae*

The parvoviruses are small, unenveloped, icosahedral virions 18–26 nm in diameter containing linear ssDNA. Particles often have a hexagonal outline; stain-penetrated empty particles are common (Fig. 4.26).

Viruses include *Parvovirus* (bovine and canine parvoviruses), *Erythrovirus* (B19 virus) and *Dependovirus* (adeno-associated viruses).

Papovaviridae

Papovavirus particles are non-enveloped and icosahedral with 72 pentameric capsomers in a skewed arrangement (Rayment et al. 1982, Baker et al. 1991). (The lack of hexameric capsomers in an icosahedral capsid requires flexible intercapsomeric attachment at the apices of the particle.) Polyomaviruses (Fig. 4.27a) are 45 nm in diameter compared to the larger (55 nm) papillomaviruses (Fig. 4.27b). Aberrant tubular forms are common (Fig. 4.28). The genome is circular dsDNA.

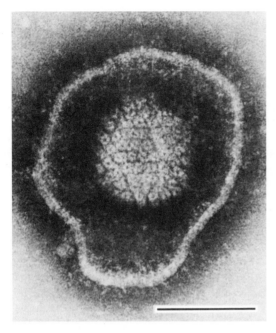

Fig. 4.32   Herpes simplex virus. Note that the stain has penetrated the envelope and that the icosahedral capsid is visible. Bar = 100 nm. (Micrograph by Dr J D Almeida.)

Polyomavirus   The polyomaviruses have distinctive rough-surfaced particles of 45 nm diameter (see Fig. 4.27a). Capsomers are readily resolved but, because of the comparatively small size of the virus and the fact that it maintains a 3-dimensional structure rather than flattening on the grid, it is not easy to determine the arrangement of these subunits.

Viruses include murine polyomavirus, SV40, BK virus and JC virus.

Papillomavirus   Although the difference in size between papillomaviruses and polyomaviruses does not seem great, the wart viruses appear as considerably larger, more robust particles in the electron microscope (see Fig. 4.27b). Papillomaviruses may be skewed to the left or the right. Human wart virus is right-handed whereas rabbit papilloma is left-handed.

Viruses include cottontail rabbit papillomavirus (Shope) and human papillomaviruses.

Adenoviridae

Of all viruses examined by negative staining, the adenoviruses provide the best example of icosahedral structure (Fig. 4.29). The non-enveloped capsid has 252 morphological subunits comprising 240 non-vertex capsomers, 8–10 nm in diameter, and 12 vertex capsomers (pentons). Each penton has a 9–30 nm fibre attached to it and this fibre terminates in a spherical knob. The apical fibres are seen only very rarely in routine preparations. The genome is linear dsDNA.

Cryo-EM techniques have produced 3-dimensional images at below 3.5 nm resolution (Stewart, Fuller and Burnett 1993).

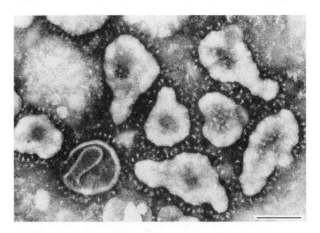

Fig. 4.33   Avian infectious bronchitis virus – a coronavirus – showing the characteristic club-shaped peplomers. Bar = 100 nm. (Micrograph by Dr J D Almeida.)

CUBIC DNA VIRUSES WITH LIPOPROTEIN ENVELOPES

Hepadnaviridae

Hepadnavirions are spherical, double-shelled particles, 40–48 nm in diameter, with no surface projections. The outer, 7 nm thick, lipoprotein envelope encloses a 27–35 nm, icosahedral nucleocapsid core; 22 nm diameter filamentous structures and spherical particles, comprising envelope material alone, are often visualized. The genome is a single molecule of partially double-stranded and partially single-stranded circular DNA. Orthohepadnavirus (hepatitis B virus – HBV) virions are 42 nm in diameter and contain a 27 nm core. Considerable quantities of core-less 22 nm spheres and filaments are formed (HBsAg) (Fig. 4.30). Duck hepatitis B virus virions are 46–48 nm spheres containing a 35 nm core.

Also present in HBV-positive patients may be hepatitis delta virus (HDV) particles. These are of similar size to HBV virions but have a smaller, 19 nm, core. HDV is considered to be a satellite virus of HBV and comprises a floating genus '*Deltavirus*'.

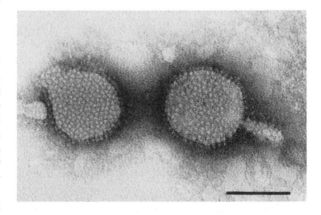

Fig. 4.34   Arenavirus. Tacaribe virus. Bar = 100 nm. (Courtesy of Dr E L Palmer.)

Herpesviridae

All the herpesviruses are composed of a geometric capsid (containing a core) with a surrounding amorphous material (the tegument) and an outer lipoprotein membrane. The 100–110 nm icosahedral capsid comprises 162 capsomers (150 hexamers, 12 pentamers), each of which displays a distinct central hole. Cryo-EM techniques have demonstrated 320 triplexes, which provide intercapsomeric connections (Zhou et al. 1994). In intact particles the surrounding envelope is closely applied and itself reproduces the hexagonal or pentagonal outline of the underlying icosahedral structure (Fig. 4.31). However, more often the envelope is disrupted and the particle resembles a fried egg with the capsid as yolk and the envelope as the white (Fig. 4.32). The outer envelope carries poorly resolved fine projections 12 nm long. The core of the mature virus is occasionally visualized as a torus. The genome is linear dsDNA.

Viruses include herpes simplex viruses 1 and 2, human cytomegalovirus Epstein–Barr virus, human herpesvirus 6, 7 and 8, and varicella-zoster virus.

3.3 Viruses not yet accorded symmetry properties or of complex symmetry

Although all the viruses described so far have either definite or presumptive symmetry, there remain some with less definite or no evidence of symmetry.

RNA VIRUSES

Coronaviridae

The fringed, enveloped virions are 120–160 nm in diameter. The family comprises two genera: the coronaviruses and the toroviruses.

Coronavirus Coronavirus virions are enveloped and predominantly spherical with a particle diameter range of 75–160 nm. The outstanding physical feature is the distinctive club- or leaf-shaped projections (peplomers) on the surface (Fig. 4.33), 12–24 nm long, which, in many instances, readily detach themselves from the virus surface. Some species have both short and long projections. Coronaviruses without surface projections are almost impossible to identify, as their lipoprotein envelopes look like cell fragments. The viral nucleocapsid is helical (14–16 nm diam.). The genome is linear, positive-sense, ssRNA.

Morphologically, this is one of the most difficult viruses to identify. Many fringed particles, particularly in faecal specimens, have been put forward as coronaviruses although they do not possess the true characteristics of this virus group. Their classification as coronaviruses (and even their identity as viruses) remains controversial.

Viruses include avian infectious bronchitis virus, human coronavirus, murine hepatitis virus and porcine transmissible gastroenteritis.

Torovirus Torovirus virions are fringed, enveloped, 120–140 nm in diameter, and disc-, kidney- or rod-shaped. The nucleocapsid is tubular.

Viruses include Berne virus and Breda virus.

Arenaviridae

Arenavirus Arenaviruses are pleomorphic, often spherical, enveloped particles 50–300 nm in diameter covered with 8–10 nm long club-shaped projections. Electron-dense, 20–25 nm ribosomes are visualized within the particles by thin section EM (Fig. 4.34). Isolated nucleocapsids are organized as closed circles of varying length (450–1300 nm) displaying an array of nucleosomal subunits. The genome consists of 2 ssRNA molecules.

Viruses include lymphocytic choriomeningitis virus, Lassa virus, Junin virus and Pichinde virus.

Retroviridae

Early morphological studies employing thin section EM classified the retroviruses into 4 groups (A–D) on the basis of structure and morphogenesis. Although now obsolete, elements of this classification are still used, as follows. Group A particles are small intracellular, double-layered ring-like structures, some of which are now known to be fully formed cores of B- and D-type retroviruses and spumaviruses. Group B particles are extracellular, fringed, enveloped particles with an eccentric, condensed core; budding of the virus occurs around preformed group A particles at the cell membrane. Group C particles are also formed at the cell surface, with budding and core assembly occurring virtually simultaneously, and with mature particles resembling B particles but with a less well defined fringe and a centrally placed core. Group D particles have a morphology similar to that of group B particles but often have a conical core and a C-type fringe.

In general, members of the *Retroviridae* are enveloped and spherical (80–100 nm diam.) with more or less prominent surface projections. Internal cores are spherical or icosahedral. The nucleocapsid is eccentric (type B), concentric (type C, 'BLV-HTLV' and spumaviruses) or rod/cone shaped (lentiviruses). The genome is a dimer of linear, positive-sense ssRNA.

Mammalian type B oncovirus group These pleomorphic lipoprotein-bound particles are roughly spherical in shape and c. 90–112 nm in diameter. Particles penetrated by stain show an eccentric, condensed core 40–60 nm in diameter (Fig. 4.35). The external surface of the particle bears distinct 10 nm long projections that closely resemble those on the influenza virus particle and which sometimes display as a hexagonal array. Capsid assembly occurs within the cytoplasm prior to budding from the plasma membrane.

Viruses include Bittner mouse mammary tumour virus.

Mammalian type C oncovirus group Virus particles are 100–120 nm in diameter and comprise a fringed envelope, an inner coat and a centrally located, con-

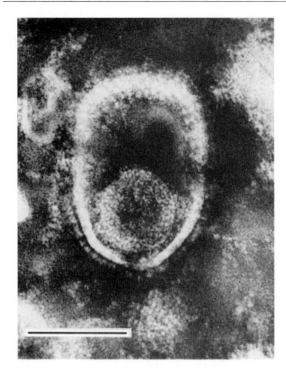

Fig. 4.35 The Bittner mouse mammary tumour virus showing fringed envelope and eccentric core. Bar = 100 nm. (Micrograph by Dr J D Almeida.)

densed core. The knob-like surface spikes are c. 10 nm in diameter and are often lost during preparative techniques. Virus assembly occurs at the inner membrane surface during budding. Multi-cored virions and aberrant tubular cores are sometimes observed.

Viruses include murine leukaemia virus and feline leukaemia virus.

Type D retroviruses Virions are 100–130 nm in diameter and consist of a fringed envelope enclosing a 75 nm long tubular or conical core containing a 40 nm electron-dense ribonucleoprotein complex. The virus lacks prominent surface spikes but 5 nm long projections can be revealed by negative staining. The virus buds around preformed 75 nm cores, which exhibit a fringe.

Viruses include Mason–Pfizer monkey virus and simian type D virus 1.

'BLV-HTLV' retroviruses Virions of this genus have a morphology similar to that of C-type retroviruses.

Viruses include bovine leukaemia virus and human lymphotropic viruses 1 and 2.

Lentivirus Virions are roughly spherical particles, 90–120 nm in diameter, comprising a fringed envelope, an inner coat and a conical nucleocapsid 100 nm long attached to the virus envelope at its narrow end (Fig. 4.36). Multi-cored particles and aberrant cores are sometimes visualized (Chrystie and Almeida 1989). The icosahedral arrangement of the glycoprotein knobs forming the fringe (Özel et al. 1988) and computer simulations from thin section electron micrographs (Marx, Munn and Joy 1988, Nermut, Pauli and Gelderblom 1993) together with image

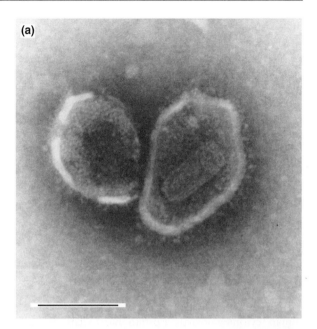

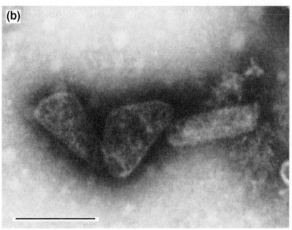

Fig. 4.36 Human immunodeficiency virus showing (a) fringed envelope and conical core, and (b) 3 isolated viral cores. Bar = 100 nm.

analysis of cryo-EM images are all suggestive of an icosahedral architecture for the virus. Virus budding and core formation occur simultaneously at the cell membrane.

Viruses include human and simian immunodeficiency viruses and visna-maedi viruses of sheep.

Spumavirus Spumavirus virions are 100–130 nm in diameter, have prominent surface spikes 15 nm long and a central, condensed, 50 nm core (Fig. 4.37). Capsid assembly occurs in the cytoplasm prior to budding. Multi-cored particles are frequently seen.

Viruses include human spumavirus, simian foamy virus and bovine syncytial virus.

DNA VIRUSES WITH COMPLEX SYMMETRY
Poxviridae

Poxvirus particles are ovoid or brick-shaped. The genome consists of a single, linear molecule of dsDNA.

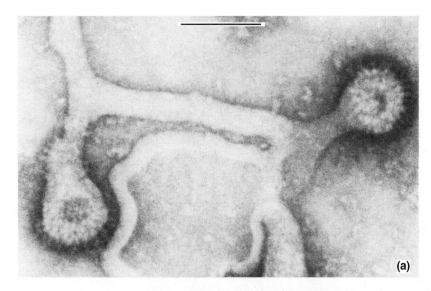

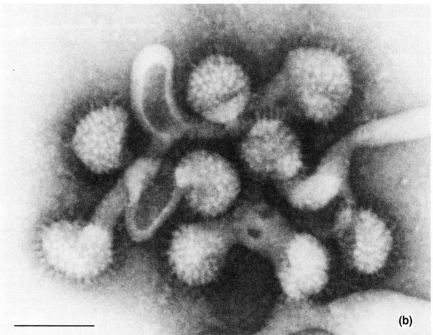

Fig. 4.37 A foamy virus (spumavirus) isolated from an orang-utan. The distinctive fringe and core are apparent. Bar = 100 nm.

Orthopoxvirus Virions are brick-shaped; 200 × 200 × 250 nm. The lipoprotein outer membrane has a rough appearance with tubules randomly wrapped around the particle (Fig. 4.38). Negative staining reveals that the outer membrane encloses a biconcave core with a lateral body in each concavity.

Viruses include vaccinia virus, cowpox virus, monkeypox virus and variola virus.

Many other poxviruses – for example *Avipoxvirus* (fowlpox virus, canarypox virus) *Capripoxvirus* (sheeppox virus, goatpox virus), *Leporipoxvirus* (myxoma virus), *Suipoxvirus* (swinepox virus) and *Molluscipoxvirus* (molluscum contagiosum virus) – have morphology very similar to that of the orthopoxviruses but with slight differences in size.

Parapoxvirus Virions are ovoid, 220–300 × 140–170 nm, with a single surface filament appearing, because both sides of the particle are visible, as a cross-hatched coil spiralling around the particle (Fig. 4.39).

Viruses include orf virus and pseudocowpox virus

4 CONCLUSIONS

The advent of the negative contrast technique for visualizing viruses in the electron microscope in 1959 revealed viruses in all their beauty and diversity. Seeing them gives them a reality not found with other techniques and often allows diagnosis of infection to be made with certainty directly on clinical specimens, particularly those from the skin, stools and urine. But the electron microscope also helps to confirm other tests and to recognize dual, triple or quadruple infections, which would be tedious to unravel by other techniques.

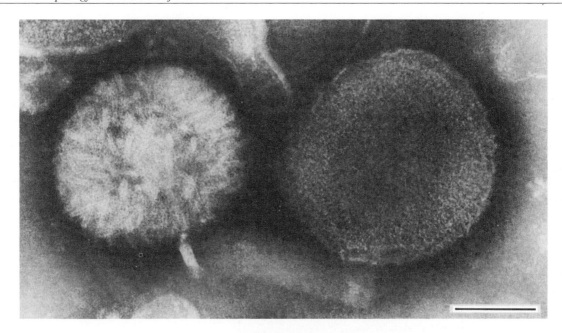

Fig. 4.38 Orthopoxvirus. Vaccinia virions showing filamentous appearance of the surface. Bar = 100 nm. (Micrograph by Dr J D Almeida.)

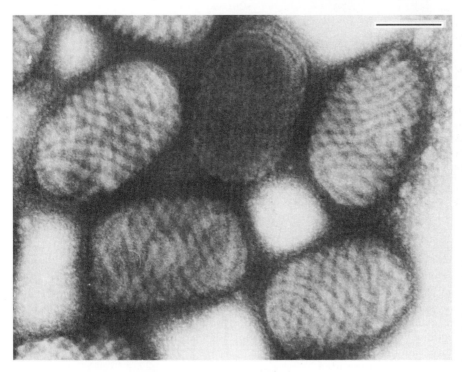

Fig. 4.39 Orf virus, a parapoxvirus. The distinctive helical pattern on the surface results from visualizing both sides of the virus. Bar = 100 nm. (Micrograph by Dr J D Almeida.)

Electron microscopy is a 'catch-all' technique that holds an endless fascination for those who are interested in visual appearances. It is also practical in providing information on how viruses are constructed and how they come apart. It is the yardstick against which deductions about virus structure and theories of assembly must be measured. That it also reveals such elegance of form among viruses is an added bonus and a constant delight.

REFERENCES

Baker TS, Newcombe WW et al., 1991, Structures of bovine and human papillomaviruses. Analysis by cryoelectron microscopy and three-dimensional image reconstruction, *Biophys J*, **60**: 1445–6.

Best JM, Banatvala JE et al., 1967, Morphological characteristics of rubella virus, *Lancet*, **2**: 237–9.

Brenner S, Horne RW, 1959, A negative staining method for high resolution electron microscopy of viruses, *Biochim Biophys Acta*, **34**: 103–10.

Choo Q-L, Kuo G et al., 1989, Isolation of a c-DNA clone derived from a blood-borne non-A, non-B viral hepatitis genome, *Science*, **244**: 359–62.

Chrystie IL, 1996, Electron microscopy, *Virology Methods Manual*, eds Mahy BWJ, Kangro HO, Academic Press, London, 91–106.

Chrystie IL, Almeida JD, 1989, Recovery of antigenically reactive HIV-2 cores, *J Med Virol*, **27**: 188–95.

Crowther RA, Kiselev NA et al., 1994, Three-dimensional structure of hepatitis B virus core particles determined by electron cryomicroscopy, *Cell*, **77**: 943–50.

Doane FW, Anderson N, 1987, *Electron Microscopy in Diagnostic Virology: a practical guide and atlas*, Cambridge University Press, Cambridge.

Dubochet J, Adrian M et al., 1988, Cryo-electron microscopy of vitrified specimens, *Q Rev Biophysics*, **21**: 129–228.

Glauert AM (ed), 1975, *Practical Methods in Electron Microscopy*, vol 3, part 1, *Fixation, Dehydration and Embedding of Biological Specimens*, Elsevier, Amsterdam.

Hewat EA, Booth TF, Roy P, 1992, Structure of bluetongue virus-like particles by cryo-electron microscopy, *J Struct Biol*, **109**: 61–9.

Horne RW, Wildy P, 1961, Symmetry in virus architecture, *Virology*, **15**: 348–73.

Kapikian AZ, Wyatt RG et al., 1972, Visualization by immune electron microscopy of a 27 nm particle associated with acute infectious non-bacterial gastroenteritis, *J Virol*, **10**: 1075–81.

Kelen AE, Hathaway AE, McLeod DA, 1971, Rapid detection of Australia/SH antigen and antibody by a simple and sensitive technique of immunoelectron microscopy, *Can J Microbiol*, **17**: 993–1000.

Linnen J, Wages J et al., 1996, Molecular cloning and disease association of hepatitis G virus: a transfusion-transmissible agent, *Science*, **271**: 505–8.

Madeley CF, Field AM, 1988, *Virus Morphology*, 2nd edn, Churchill Livingstone, Edinburgh, 295.

Marx PA, Munn RJ, Joy KI, 1988, Computer emulation of thin section electron microscopy predicts an envelope-associated icosadeltahedral capsid for human immunodeficiency virus, *Lab Invest*, **58**: 112–18.

Metcalf P, Cyrklaff M, Adrian M, 1991, The three-dimensional structure of reovirus obtained by cryoelectron microscopy, *EMBO J*, **10**: 3129–36.

Murphy FM, Fauquet CM et al., 1995, Virus Taxonomy. Sixth Report of the International Committee on Taxonomy of Viruses. *Arch Virol*, **suppl 10**.

Nermut MV, Hockley DJ, Gelderblom H, 1987, Electron microsopy: methods for 'structural analysis' of the virion, *Animal Virus Structure*, eds Nermut MV, Steven AC, Elsevier, Amsterdam, 21–56.

Nermut MV, Grief C et al., 1993, Further evidence of icosahedral symmetry in human and simian immunodeficiency virus, *AIDS Res Hum Retroviruses*, **9**: 929–38.

Ozel M, Pauli G, Gelderblom HR, 1988, The organisation of the envelope projections on the surface of HIV, *Arch Virol*, **100**: 255–66.

Paredes AM, Brown DT et al., 1993, Three-dimensional structure of a membrane-containing virus, *Proc Natl Acad Sci USA*, **90**: 9095–9.

Prasad BVV, Matson DO, Smith AJ, 1994, Three-dimensional structure of caliciviruses, *J Mol Biol*, **240**: 256–64.

Prasad BVV, Wang GJ et al., 1988, Three-dimensional structure of rotavirus, *J Mol Biol*, **199**: 269–75.

Pringle CR, 1991, The order *Mononegavirales*, *Arch Virol*, **117**: 137–40.

Rayment I, Baker TS et al., 1982, Polyoma virus capsid structure at 22.5 Å resolution, *Nature (London)*, **295**: 110–15.

Reid N, 1975, *Practical Methods in Electron Microscopy*, ed Glauert AM, vol 3, part 2, *Ultramicrotomy*, ed Glauert AM, Elsevier, Amsterdam.

Roberts MM, White JL et al., 1986, Three-dimensional structure of the adenovirus major coat protein hexon, *Science*, **232**: 1148–51.

Stewart PL, Fuller SD, Burnett RM, 1993, Difference imaging of adenovirus: bridging the resolution gap between X-ray crystallography and electron microscopy, *EMBO J*, **12**: 2589–99.

Tsao J, Chapman MS et al., 1991, The three-dimensional structure of canine parvovirus and its functional implications, *Science*, **251**: 1456–64.

Zhou ZH, Prasad BVV et al., 1994, Protein subunit structures in the herpes simplex virus A-capsid determined from 400 kV spot-scan electron cryomicroscopy, *J Mol Biol*, **242**: 456–69.

Chapter 5

PROPAGATION AND IDENTIFICATION OF VIRUSES

J C Hierholzer

1 Systems for propagating viruses	3 Isolation and identification of viruses from
2 Preparation of reagents for virus	clinical specimens
identification	

This chapter gives an overview of the main techniques used for propagating and identifying viruses. Detailed descriptions will be found in the appropriate journal citations and in Chapter 44. In some instances, more general references are made to textbooks of laboratory methods, without necessarily citing specific sections.

1 SYSTEMS FOR PROPAGATING VIRUSES

Viruses can replicate only in living cells. An essential first step in propagating them in the laboratory is thus the provision of cells in one form or another. Nowadays, the most widely used method is **cell culture**, but older techniques such as **tissue** or **organ culture** may still be used for specialized purposes, as may **chick embryo** and **animal inoculation**.

1.1 Cell cultures

GENERAL

Cell cultures are prepared either as single layers (monolayers), on a glass or plastic surface, or as suspensions, the choice depending on their proposed use. Another choice to be made is the type of cell needed for a particular study, as over 3000 cell lines are now available. Several international repositories can serve as the starting point for reference cell lines and for microbiological reagents; they include the European Collection of Animal Cell Cultures (Salisbury, Wiltshire, England), the American Type Culture Collection (Rockville, Maryland, USA) (ATCC 1985), Statens Seruminstitut (Copenhagen), Institut Pasteur (Paris) and the World Health Organization

(Geneva). Detailed information on culture media and specialized techniques is also available from these centres, and in other reference works (Lennette et al. 1988, 1995, NJ Schmidt 1989, Freshney 1993, Murray et al. 1995).

SAFETY

All procedures involving cell lines should be performed in a class II biological safety cabinet under strict aseptic conditions, both to minimize the risk of contaminating cells with bacteria, yeasts and mycoplasmas and to protect the worker. Cell lines should be considered potentially hazardous; although continuous (transformed) cell lines are assumed to be free of infective agents, they may in fact harbour latent viruses that could infect the worker (Barkley 1979). Safety precautions should include the general measures reviewed by Fleming et al. (1995), Lennette et al. (1995), Sewell (1995) and in Chapter 43.

CELL CULTURE MEDIA

Most of the basic media in use today are chemically defined, but must be supplemented with 5–20% serum; this is usually obtained from calf fetuses and must be carefully checked for contamination by viruses, mycoplasma, bacteria and specific viral antibodies. Cells generally grow well at pH 7.0–7.4. Phenol red is often used as an indicator in the medium, changing progressively from purple at pH 7.8 through red at pH 7.4 to yellow at pH 6.5 (Freshney 1993).

Culture media require careful buffering to stabilize the pH under all conditions. In plastic dishes with unsealed lids, in which exposure to oxygen causes the pH to rise, exogenous CO_2 is required by cell lines, particularly at low cell concentrations, to prevent total loss of dissolved CO_2 and bicarbonate from the medium. In tubes or flasks with tight caps, pH can be adjusted by loosening the caps, changing the medium or placing the vessels in a CO_2 incubator with a gas-permeable cap, as dictated by the indicator. The CO_2 level is critical and can be monitored by a gas analyser; a 1% increase can result in cell death.

Medium components should be prepared with endotoxin-free water. Water systems are available to produce type I reagent grade water, which minimizes metal and organic ions leaching from storage containers and prevents bacterial and yeast contamination by being used immediately.

Media, media components and reagents are sterilized by autoclaving if they are heat-stable (e.g. water, salt solutions, amino acid hydrolysates) or by membrane filtration if they are not (e.g. protein or sugar solutions). The type of membrane is important; cellulose acetate membranes are best for applications involving low protein binding, and cellulose nitrate membranes for general purpose filtration. Cotton pads, membranes of larger pore size or commercial prefilters should be used for prefiltering, and membranes of 0.22 μm average pore diameter (APD) for sterilization.

TYPES OF CELL CULTURE

Cell cultures may be either **primary** or **continuous**. Primary cultures contain mixtures of cells freshly derived from the tissue of origin, which may be obtained either from laboratory animals or from human material procured in the course of surgery. Some specimens (e.g. foreskin) are not pathological. Tissues from young or embryonic animals give better results than those from adults. They are minced into 3 mm pieces. The cells are disaggregated by one or more treatments with a solution of 0.22% trypsin and 0.02% versene, filtered through sterile gauze and washed by centrifugation in cold growth medium (GM). They are finally suspended in GM and the concentration of viable cells is determined by counting a sample diluted in trypan blue, which selectively stains dead or damaged cells. Tubes or flasks are seeded at c. 3×10^5 viable cells/ml.

Cell lines are also derived from primary cells, but can be repeatedly subcultured. They fall into two categories. **Euploid** cells, such as normal human fibroblasts, retain their normal karyotype throughout their culture life-span, rarely give rise to continuous lines and, after c. 50 generations, stop dividing (Hayflick 1973). They are sometimes called semicontinuous lines. By contrast, **aneuploid** cells, such as those from many human and animal tumours, may give rise to true continuous cell lines that can be subcultured indefinitely. Aneuploid cell lines have a chromosome complement between that of diploid and tetraploid cells.

Insect cell lines are continuous cultures derived from, for example, the SF9 ovary (fall armyworm, *Spodoptera frugiperda*) and from mosquitoes (e.g. *Aedes aegypti* and *Ae. albopictus*). The SF9 line, which is grown in special media, is highly susceptible to infection with baculoviruses and can be used for baculovirus expression vectors and other needs. Mosquito lines are used as suspension cultures for the replication of many mosquito-borne viruses; they have special media and subculturing requirements (Lennette et al. 1995).

Suspension cultures can be prepared from many mouse and human leukaemias and ascites tumours. They are incubated on shakers or in roller drums or allowed to settle to the bottom of a large culture flask such as a roller bottle. Alternatively, a spinner apparatus is available which forces normally adherent cells to grow in suspension in a special medium.

Shell vial cultures contain a cell monolayer grown on one side of a coverslip in a tube of the Leighton type. The tube is then inoculated and centrifuged at low speed, which apparently distorts the cell surface and renders it more susceptible to viral attachment. After 1–3 days of incubation, irrespective of any cytopathic effects (CPE), the coverslip is washed briefly, and tested by immunofluorescence assay (IFA), nucleic acid hybridization or other test for whichever viruses are suspected. The method can be used as a rapid test for adenovirus (Espy, Hierholzer and Smith 1987), cytomegalovirus (CMV) (Gleaves et al. 1989, Buller et al. 1992), varicella-zoster virus (VZV) (Schirm et al. 1989), respiratory syncytial virus (RSV) (Smith, Creutz and Huang 1991) and other respiratory viruses (Matthey et al. 1992, Schirm et al. 1992, Olsen et al. 1993).

Microcultures are cost-efficient systems which have recently become popular, having overcome earlier problems with cross-contamination between wells, over-oxygenation and toxic plastics. Microcultures in the 4- to 8-well format in plates with sealable lids (or snug lids for CO_2 incubators) are now commonplace for plaque assays. In 96-well microtitre plates with flat well bottoms, microcultures are ideal for neutralization tests, tissue culture enzyme-linked immunosorbent assay (ELISA), monoclonal antibody testing and many screening assays (Hierholzer and Bingham 1978, Anderson et al. 1985, Lennette et al. 1995, Murray et al. 1995). Macrocultures in standard tubes, however, are still preferred for primary virus isolation because of the ease of setting up stationary or roller cultures in ordinary incubators, of reading the monolayers for CPE and of obtaining sufficient volume of virus culture to use for subpassaging, identification tests, viral genetic analyses and storage.

Specialized culture systems have been devised to satisfy particular needs. For example, suspension cultures of human peripheral blood lymphocytes are sensitive to the Epstein–Barr herpesvirus, where it is detected by a transformation assay, and, under co-cultivation procedures, to the human T cell leukaemia virus (HTLV) and human immunodeficiency viruses (HIV) (Lennette et al. 1988, 1995, Fields et al. 1990, Isenberg 1992). Immortalized human microvascular endothelial cell cultures derived from foreskin are sensitive to a wide variety of viruses under special culture conditions, and have potential use as a model to study the biology of these important cells (Ades et al. 1992). Extracellular matrix systems support the 3-dimensional growth of cells as opposed to monolayer cultures; the Matrigel Invasion Chamber (Collaborative Biomedical Products, Bedford MA), for instance, can support fastidious cell types and is currently being explored for its use in viral culture and alterations in cell physiology following viral infection (Bissell et al. 1990, Thompson et al. 1991). Finally, large-volume culture systems, such as suspension culture vats, cells on the surfaces of Sephadex beads or other microcarriers, and cells on spirals of Sterilin or other plastic film are used extensively in industry to prepare vaccines, interferons and monoclonal antibodies (White and Ades 1990).

QUALITY CONTROL

Contamination by bacteria, yeasts and fungi is a readily apparent problem in cell culture work. Most are detected visually by turbidity and pH changes in the culture medium, and more definitively by examining the cultures microscopically. Detailed protocols for the detection of most bacteria and fungi that would be expected to survive in cell cultures in the presence of the customary antibiotics may be found elsewhere (ATCC 1985). The same methods should be incorporated into the quality control programme of the media production laboratory to preclude the contamination of cells by detecting organisms in the GM intended for cell cultures.

Contamination by mycoplasmas and viruses is more difficult to detect, because these organisms usually do not cause turbidity or pH changes, and may not cause a CPE in the cells. Thus, they may be passaged with the cells indefinitely without detection unless specific testing is performed. Primary rhesus monkey kidney (MK), primary African green monkey kidney (AGMK) and primary bovine embryonic kidney cell cultures are particularly notorious for adventitious virus contamination (Hull 1968, Crandell et al. 1978, Schmidt 1989, Eberle and Hilliard 1995). Commercial testing services are available for mycoplasmas and viruses. Two common methods for mycoplasma detection in the cell culture laboratory are culture and fluorescent staining, and both should be incorporated into the quality control programme. The DNA-specific fluorescent stain (Chen 1977) may be used as the presumptive test and the culture method (Hayflick 1973) as the confirmatory test. Commercially produced kits such as the MycoTect test (GIBCO) are available for detecting mycoplasmas.

Contamination by other cell lines may also occur, the intrusion of HeLa cells into many other lines giving the most problems. Precautions to prevent this include working with only one cell line at a time; keeping bottles of medium, trypsin/versene etc. separate for each cell line; allowing a 'resting' period of c. 30 min between manipulation of different cell lines in a biological safety cabinet; and decontaminating cabinet surfaces before introducing another cell line to the work area. The species of origin of a cell line can be determined by various immunological, isoenzyme and cytogenetic tests (ATCC 1985). Such testing requires expertise not commonly available, however, and so commercial testing services may need to be used. Thus, quality control programmes for cell culture laboratories must incorporate periodic searches for contaminants of microbiological and cellular origin, because the contaminants may cause irreversible changes in the cell cultures and can completely confound the interpretation of diagnostic tests.

PROPAGATION OF CELLS

Propagating cells by **scraping** is a physical method of removing adherent cells from the surface of a culture vessel, and is used when enzymatic removal may be toxic to the cells or may destroy receptors or other important cell surface molecules. The GM is discarded, the cells are physically scraped from the vessel surface with a disposable cell scraper into fresh GM, and the cells are then dispersed by vigorously pipetting the mixture to obtain a suspension of single cells. The cells are counted and appropriately diluted for passage to new flasks or other vessels.

Cell counts are used to quantify viable cells for passaging and seeding. They are best performed in the presence of a vital stain, which is excluded by living cell membranes and is incorporated only into dead cells. In the trypan blue vital stain procedure, a sample of the cell suspension is mixed with 0.4% dye in physiological saline, placed in the counting chamber of a haemocytometer and the cells counted at $\times 100$ magnification. The stained (dead) cells and the unstained (living) cells can be counted separately to determine percentage viability if this is desired. Trypan blue and erythrosin B are the dyes most commonly used for dye exclusion tests; others (e.g. methylene blue, acridine orange, eosin, nigrosin and safranin) have also been used (Evans, Perry and Vincent 1975). Dyes such as crystal violet stain both living and dead cells and are best used to clarify morphology.

Cells can also be propagated by **enzyme treatment**, a chemical method of detaching adherent cells from the culture vessel with enzymes such as trypsin, pronase or collagenase, together with chelating agents such as versene (tetrasodium ethylenediaminetetraacetic acid, EDTA). After washing the monolayer with phosphate-buffered saline (PBS), it is covered with a solution of 0.05% trypsin and 0.53 mM versene and placed at room temperature with cell surface down until the cells detach. After vigorously pipetting to break up clumps the cells are resuspended at the desired concentration in fresh GM.

Cells in suspension cultures are propagated by adding a sample to sufficient GM to give the desired concentration.

For lymphocyte cultures, fresh mononuclear cells can be isolated from whole blood by Ficoll–Hypaque gradient centrifugation and cultured in suspension. Their uses for diagnosis, evaluation of immunity and detection of disease are numerous, as are the procedures for isolating particular subpopulations of cells from peripheral blood or lymphoid tissues (Markham and Salahuddin 1987, Castro et al. 1988, Coligan et al. 1991).

MAINTENANCE OF CULTURES

Once cells have been passaged, routine medium changes are necessary to encourage their viability by feeding them with fresh amino acids, vitamins, glucose and other metabolic constituents. The initial cell concentration and the metabolic rate of the cells will determine the feeding schedule. Feeding is done with a maintenance medium (MM), which is the regular medium with only 1–2% serum rather than the 10–20% used in GM. MM may hold untransformed cell lines at a single cell layer for an extended period, even 2–3 weeks, because it tends not to stimulate mitosis. Diploid cells, with a finite life-span, can thus be maintained without using up the limited number of cell generations available to them.

Cells can also be maintained by subculturing, particularly important for transformed cells, which continue to divide under MM and thus cannot be successfully fed. Transformed (heteroploid) epithelial cells such as HeLa and HEp-2 metabolize rapidly and should be subcultured twice a week; alternatively, the seeding concentration of such rapidly proliferating cells may be lowered to reduce subculturing to once a week. Diploid fibroblast cells such as MRC5 and WI-38 metabolize slowly and require subculturing only once a week, with a feeding at least once during that week. Suspension cultures must be subcultured, or the volume of medium increased as the cell population reaches c. 2×10^6 cells/ml, because the viability of suspended cells drops rapidly at higher concentrations.

STORAGE OF CELLS

Cells may be stored by cryopreservation, which provides a ready stock if any is lost through contamination, malfunction of an incubator, natural senescence or a genetic drift that may affect their ability to exhibit the expected response in routine assays. They are packed by low-speed centrifugation and resuspended in a freeze medium containing serum and dimethylsulphoxide (DMSO) (NJ Schmidt 1989, Freshney 1993, Mahy and Kangro 1996). One ml volumes are dispensed into cryovials frozen slowly at c. 1°C per min, preferably in a controlled-rate freezer and stored in liquid nitrogen (–165°C).

Cells are recovered from storage by rapidly thawing in a 37°C water bath, diluting the cells with the appropriate medium and placing them in a cell culture flask. The medium is replaced after 24 h to remove all traces of DMSO. The medium exchange for a suspension culture requires centrifugation and resuspension in fresh medium.

1.2 Tissue and organ cultures

Laboratory cultures of pieces of human embryonic lung, kidney, intestine and other organs have proven essential to the discovery of many viruses, such as the respiratory coronaviruses and rhinoviruses. Organ cultures are explants of whole tissue (c. 1 mm³), so many cell types are present in their natural form, and feeding medium must be perfused through the explants to maintain viability. The human enteric coronaviruses – whose existence is still in dispute – may replicate in primary human fetal intestinal organ cultures containing trypsin. Once inoculated with a clinical specimen, virus may be detected by cessation of ciliary movement (in lung) or by specific tests for the viral products accumulated in the medium (McIntosh et al. 1967, Tyrrell and Blamire 1967, Caul and Egglestone 1977).

1.3 Chick embryos

The chick embryo is a versatile host system in diagnostic virology, although its use has been diminished in recent years by the development of highly sensitive direct detection methods. It is still vital to the isolation of influenza viruses, and the size and appearance of pocks on the chorioallantoic membrane (CAM) afford a quick diagnostic criterion for poxviruses. The advantages of eggs include ease of handling, production of large amounts of infectious amniotic or allantoic fluids, and lack of antibody production by the host which might hinder virus identification. Disadvantages include the need to obtain sterile eggs of known age (certified germ-free eggs can be virtually unobtainable in some countries) and the need to eliminate all viable bacteria, yeasts and mycoplasmas from the patient's specimen before inoculation.

Fertile eggs must be incubated at 37°C in 40–70% humidity and rotated about every 4 h to keep the embryo floating in the centre of the egg. For influenza virus isolation in amniotic or allantoic cavities, 9- to 11-day old eggs are needed; for poxvirus isolation in the CAM, 12-day-old eggs are best. For details of chick embryo techniques, see 'Chick embryos' (p. 64).

1.4 Laboratory animals

Many animal systems have been developed to serve as models of human infection and to produce high-titre antisera for diagnostic tests. Others have been developed for propagating viruses that do not grow in cell cultures. Suckling mice (see Gould and Clegg 1985) are required for the recovery of some Coxsackie A enteroviruses, and suckling mice, suckling hamsters, rabbits, mosquitoes or ticks are needed for some arboviruses. Primates are the most sensitive systems for the hepatitis viruses, with ducks, woodchucks and mice as alternatives for hepatitis B and mice and piglets for hepatitis E. In addition, newborn mice or hamsters, young adult guinea-pigs and primates are required for some of the biosafety level (BSL)-4 agents (e.g. filoviruses, arenaviruses); these highly specialized and dangerous systems are beyond the reach of most laboratories, and the reader should consult other works for details (Lennette et al. 1988, 1995, Isenberg 1992, Murray et al. 1995).

Animals should be purchased from companies specializing in the breeding of laboratory animals, so that the strain of the species is documented, immunizations for known adventitious organisms are given and the quality of care (housing, temperature, air filtraton, food and water) are within the appropriate national guidelines for animal care. The strains of mice and guinea-pigs may be important; often, only a single strain is suitable for a particular virus. Housing of animals in the receiving laboratory is also critical, not only to conform with national regulations on the humane use of animals but also to minimize the introduction of exogenous micro-organisms and cross-contamination.

2 PREPARATION OF REAGENTS FOR VIRUS IDENTIFICATION

2.1 Preparation of antigens

Viral antigens may be structural or non-structural proteins or glycoproteins produced during viral replication, and may be located internally in the virion or be part of the external capsid components. Many are produced in excess during replication and are released into the supernatant fluid as 'soluble' antigens. For some tests, the antigen may simply be the supernatant fluid from the cell culture in which the virus was propagated. For others, intact virus is required at the highest titres achievable, so several freeze–thaw or sonication cycles are applied to the virus culture to disrupt any remaining cells. Again, a particular viral product may need to be enriched in proportion to other products, but not purified in the biochemical sense. For still others, only a specific viral protein can be used in the test, so it must be purified, concentrated and preserved after removing interfering viral products and medium components; alternatively, it may be specifically produced by a eukaryotic or prokaryotic gene expression system.

The two most basic concepts are microbiological purity of the starting viral culture and laboratory safety. For **purity**, starting cultures and final virus products should be proven free of viable bacterial, fungal and mycoplasmal contamination by appropriate culturing in thioglycolate broth, trypticase soy broth, neopeptone infusion agar streak/pour plates with 5% defibrinated sheep blood, Sabouraud glucose agar slants for yeasts and Hayflick's biphasic medium for mycoplasma. Depending on the test and the day-to-day usage, many antigens can be preserved by adding thiomersal (thimerosal) or sodium azide to the final product to final concentrations of 0.01% and 0.1% respectively. For **safety**, the routine laboratory precautions already discussed (p. 57) and in Chapter 43 must be followed throughout.

For every virus antigen, a parallel 'dummy antigen' should be prepared as a negative control. Dummy antigens are prepared by sham-inoculating cell cultures, eggs or animals with normal medium and thereafter treating them exactly as for the active preparation.

RELEASING VIRUS FROM CULTURE CELLS

Starting with the highest titres of infectious virus achievable is essential for antigen preparations. Freeze–thaw cycles, sonication and chemical treatments are the most widely used techniques for liberating virus from the host cells and for disrupting virions to expose particular antigens (Mahy and Kangro 1996).

For **freeze–thawing**, cultures with maximal CPE are frozen at −70°C or below, then thawed to a slush and agitated to dislodge the cells. The procedure is repeated twice and the final material is clarified by centrifugation.

For **sonication**, either the cultures may be freeze–thawed but not centrifuged or the cells may be scraped off the vessel surface with a rubber 'policeman'. The energy level and time are determined in pilot tests; 30–70 watts output for 1–3 min with multiple pulses per minute will generally disrupt the cells without denaturing the antigen. The sonicated material is clarified by low-speed centrifugation.

Chemical treatments may also be used. Alkaline glycine extraction exposes intracellular antigens useful for complement fixation (CF), indirect haemagglutination (IHA) and radioimmunoassay (RIA) tests for many viruses, particularly those that are membrane-associated (Mahy and Kangro 1996). Treating with trypsin or trypsin–versene, followed by sonicating and centrifuging, produces high-titre antigens useful for ELISA and haemagglutination (HA) tests for many viruses. Antigens for use in immunofluorescence tests may be prepared from infected cells disaggregated with trypsin and washed.

VIRUS INACTIVATION PROCEDURES

Most viral antigens are effective after inactivation and then have the advantage of safety. The 3 principal methods of virus inactivation are sonication, β-propiolactone (BPL) treatment and radiation (Mahy and Kangro 1996).

Sonication can disrupt virus particles and cleave macromolecules if sufficient energy is applied. The optimum power, number of cycles and length of time must be determined for each virus and test.

BPL treatment is widely used to inactivate viruses because it generally does not interfere with antigen test systems. Cultures are clarified by centrifugation and mixed with BPL in the presence of tris-(hydroxymethyl)amino-methane (TRIS) buffer, the final BPL concentration and incubation time having been previously determined in pilot tests. They are then clarified again, adjusted to pH 7.3–7.4 as needed and preserved with thiomersal or sodium azide.

Radiation can be carried out only by people trained and certified for such procedures. The clarified virus/antigen is exposed in an unbreakable container in an ice bath to a ^{60}Co γ source. The dosage required for complete inactivation of the virus (Table 5.1) is estimated from dose–response curves. The product is tested for residual infectivity and for potency (Gamble, Chappel and George 1980).

Other virus inactivation methods are useful for specific purposes. For immunoperoxidase assays (IPA) and IFA, infected cells may be fixed with acetone for 10 min at 4°C, which inactivates the virus, stabilizes

Table 5.1 Dosage of ^{60}Co γ-irradiation required for complete inactivation of viruses

Mrad*	Viruses inactivated
0.5	Cytomegalovirus
1.5	Influenza
1.6	Herpes simplex virus-1, 2
1.7	Respiratory syncytial virus
2.0	Newcastle disease, rabies
2.2	Rotavirus
3.4	Lymphocytic choriomeningitis

*Megarad, or 10^6 rad (rad, radiation absorbed dose).

proteins by partial denaturation and preserves morphological structure and immunological reactivity. Alternatively, they can be inactivated with 10% formalin at pH 7.0; methanol or ethanol (4 min at 4°C); acetone/methanol 50 : 50 (Lennette et al. 1995); 80% acetone (Anderson et al. 1985); or photochemically with psoralen and related compounds (Hanson, Riggs and Lennette 1978). Copper-catalysed sodium ascorbate preserves CF and IHA antigens of herpes simplex virus (White et al. 1986); certain detergents (e.g. 1% Nonidet P-40, 0.1–0.5% sodium lauryl sulphate, Tween-20 or Tween-80) can break up virus envelopes without destroying antigenic activity.

ANTIGEN EXTRACTION PROCEDURES

Extraction procedures can free antigens of non-specific inhibitors, anticomplementary reactions, competing proteins and lipoproteins, and undesired reactions related to the viral host system. For example, HA antigens must be free of serum antibodies, host cell components and microbial contaminants which may agglutinate the erythrocytes used in the assay. Some antigens are enhanced in reactivity by treatment with freeze–thaw cycles, sonication, Tween-80, fluorocarbon, ether or other organic solvents (Norrby 1962, Chappell, White and Gamble 1984). The Tween-80–ether extraction method is found in Mahy and Kangro (1996). The sucrose–acetone–BPL and fluorocarbon methods are briefly described here, by way of example. Alternatively, non-ionic detergents such as Nonidet P-40, high concentrations of salts in the presence of EDTA and β-mercaptoethanol, and other extracting agents can be used to prepare viral antigens (Isenberg 1992, Mahy and Kangro 1996).

The **sucrose–acetone–BPL extraction** method is useful for the CF and HA antigens of some viruses, including togaviruses (Venezuelan equine encephalomyelitis) and flaviviruses (dengue, Japanese B encephalitis, Rocio, St Louis encephalitis, yellow fever and other formerly group B arboviruses) (Schmidt and Lennette 1971, Chappell, White and Gamble 1984). A 40% suspension of infected tissue (e.g. mouse brain) is homogenized in borate-saline, pH 9.0 in ice; 1 M TRIS/borate-saline equal to 1/10 the volume of suspension is added, followed by cold BPL drop-wise to a final concentration of 0.1–0.3%. After mixing for 1 day in the cold, an equal volume of 17% sucrose in distilled water is added, together with 20 volumes of cold acetone chilled to –20°C per volume of homogenate, still in ice and with mixing. After vigorous shaking the tissue is allowed to settle out at –20°C for 30 min, and the supernatant acetone is aspirated. The preparation is again extracted with acetone, keeping the 20 : 1 ratio. The antigen may be preserved best as a freeze-dried powder, but should be reconstituted in borate-saline and centrifuged at 10 000 *g* for 1 h before use.

For **fluorocarbon extraction**, the centrifuged starting material is placed in a stainless steel vessel in an ice bath for high-speed homogenization. Sufficient fluorocarbon (e.g. Genetron; CF_3CCl_3) is added to obtain a 2 : 1 ratio of antigen to fluorocarbon and the mixture is homogenized at full speed for 4–6 min. The aerosol is allowed to settle in the closed container for 1 h in ice. The suspension is then decanted into bottles or tubes for layer separation at 1000 *g* for 20 min at 4°C; the supernatant is the treated antigen (Gessler, Bender and Parkinson 1956).

Viral antigens can be partially purified by adsorption/elution from erythrocytes or from calcium phosphate gels (Mahy and Kangro 1996). More effective purification is achieved by various types of solid-phase immunological adsorption/elution techniques and by affinity chromatography. Antigens may be immunoaffinity-purified by passing viral cultures (usually after SLS or enzyme treatment to disrupt virions and liberate proteins) through columns containing gel beds coated with specific antibody, or beds of monoclonal antibody-bound protein A–sepharose beads, etc. Other types of affinity chromatography use enzyme- or substrate-bound matrices. The reader is referred to other sources for detailed methods of affinity chromatography (Eisenberg et al. 1982, Wilchek, Miron and Kohn 1984, Chong and Gillum 1985, Harlow and Lane 1988).

EXPRESSION OF ANTIGENS

Expressed antigens are usually small amino acid sequences, and thus may not possess the secondary and tertiary structure needed for an active antigen. This problem can sometimes be overcome by further modifications in the gene expression system or by manipulation after the product has been expressed. Prokaryotic expression systems are convenient and inexpensive, but possess different processing pathways which prevent the amino terminal modifications, disulphide bond formation and glycosylation required for many viral antigens to be active. Eukaryotic expression systems are more complex and expensive, but are closer to the natural mode of replication of the virus; thus, post-translational modifications necessary for antigenicity are more likely to take place. Many viruses can serve as expression vectors in eukaryotic systems, but the baculovirus is particularly useful because it can be 'engineered' to incorporate various tag genes which make it possible to purify and identify the virus or its expressed products. Once the gene for the desired antigen has been inserted into the recombinant baculovirus, the virus is grown at 27°C in SF9 or SF21 fall armyworm ovary cells and the desired antigen identified by IFA, radioimmunoprecipitation, electrophoresis or western blot. The reader is referred to other sources for the details and methods of gene expression systems (Smith and Johnson 1988, Bennink and Yewdell 1990, Vialard et al. 1990, Ausubel et al. 1991, Jarvis 1991, Taylor et al. 1992, Cox, Tartaglia and Paoletti 1993, Alberts et al. 1994).

2.2 Preparation of high-titre antisera

High-titre antisera to viruses and viral antigens are readily produced in animals for use in diagnostic tests. Such antisera were the backbone of early virology, being widely used to distinguish between strains and serotypes and to study the antigenic make-up of viruses. They were prepared by repeatedly injecting a virus or viral antigen into, for example, rabbits, mice and guinea-pigs, or larger animals such as goats and horses. By such methods, polyclonal antisera of high titre ('hyperimmune sera') were produced. The general procedure is to clarify the preparation by centrifugation, mix it with an equal volume of Freund's incomplete adjuvant or a synthetic muramyl dipeptide adjuvant, inject the mixture into suitable sites 2–4 times biweekly, and obtain a blood sample 10–14 days after the last injection. The pre- and post-immunization sera are then tested for the desired antibody. Use of other adjuvants, injection in multiple sites with or without adjuvant, techniques to minimize the development of host cell antibodies, and the binding of antigens to solid matrices such as *Staphylococcus aureus* are described in other sources (Hierholzer, Stone and Broderson 1991, Lennette et al. 1995, Murray et al. 1995, Mahy and Kangro 1996).

2.3 Preparation of monoclonal antibodies

Monoclonal antibodies have become a vital immunological reagent since their inception in 1975 (Scharff, Roberts and Thammana 1981, Peter and Baumgarten 1992, Lennette et al. 1995, Murray et al. 1995). Many variations in their production have been described, including immunization in vitro and EBV-transformation techniques (Seigneurin et al. 1983, Boss 1986, Foung, Engelman and Grumet 1986, Treanor, Madore and Dolin 1988). Suitable methods are described by Anderson et al. (1985) and Hierholzer et al. (1993a).

3 ISOLATION AND IDENTIFICATION OF VIRUSES FROM CLINICAL SPECIMENS

3.1 Appropriate specimens for virus isolation

To avoid misleading results, it is of the utmost importance that adequate specimens are taken from sites appropriate to the clinical findings and then correctly stored and processed. In case of doubt, it is always best to consult the virology laboratory sooner rather than later.

COLLECTION

The type of specimen and the manner of collection depend on the laboratory methods to be used and on the sites clinically affected (Johnson 1990, Hierholzer 1991, 1993, Lennette et al. 1995). Specimens should be collected within 2 days of the onset of symptoms, because most viruses are shed only in the initial stages of illness. Nasal and throat swabs are placed in 2 ml of transport medium (e.g. tryptose phosphate broth with 0.5% gelatin, veal heart infusion broth or trypticase soy broth), preferably without antibiotics to allow the culture of bacteria and mycoplasmas. Nasopharyngeal aspirates are also excellent specimens for respiratory viruses and are collected with a neonatal mucus extractor and mucus trap to which transport medium is added (Waris et al. 1990). According to the circumstances, other specimens may include urine, stool, whole blood, serum, cerebrospinal fluid, biopsy and autopsy specimens, and swabs or scrapings of ves-

icular lesions. Specimens are placed on wet ice and transported to the laboratory for immediate culturing. If testing is not possible within 5 days of collection, they are frozen on dry ice and stored at –70°C until they can be processed, although this may reduce the amount of viable virus.

TREATMENT

Before inoculation into the appropriate host system, specimens are treated with antibiotics, mixed vigorously, and clarified by centrifuging at 1000 *g* for 3 min at 4°C to remove cell debris and bacteria. Most viruses require one or more subpassages for recovery.

3.2 Procedures for isolating viruses

IN CELL CULTURES

Cell cultures should include a continuous human epithelial line (e.g. HEp-2 (Johnston and Siegel 1990) KB, A549 (Woods and Young 1988), HeLa), a human embryonic lung diploid cell strain (e.g. HLF, HELF, MRC5, WI38), human lung mucoepidermoid cells (NCI-H292) to replace MK cells for most applications (Castells, George and Hierholzer 1990, Hierholzer et al. 1993b) and human rhabdomyosarcoma cells (RD) for the broadest coverage of viruses within practical limitations (Matthey et al. 1992). Treated specimens are adsorbed onto cell monolayers whose GM has been decanted; MM is added and cultures are incubated at 35–36°C up to several weeks, with subpassaging as required. Toxic specimens (urine, stool, tissue homogenates) should be decanted before medium is added.

Some cell types and certain viruses require roller cultures, whereas others do best as stationary cultures during their incubation period. In general, all tube cultures of MK, AGMK and their derivative cell lines (Vero, BSC-1, LLC-MK2, etc.), all diploid fibroblast cell cultures and NCI-H292 cells should be rolled in roller drums or agitated on rocker platforms to remove toxic byproducts from the cell surface and to replenish critical nutrients to the cells more quickly. Cultures of HEK, HEp-2, KB, A549 and HeLa do not need to be rolled, except for the isolation of RSV and measles virus.

Small variations in media composition and incubation temperature are also important for the isolation of certain viruses. For instance, viruses may require prior treatment with trypsin (Almeida et al. 1978, Sanchez-Fauquier et al. 1994), or the cells may require trypsin in the MM to render them sensitive to certain viruses (Itoh et al. 1970, Frank et al. 1979, Agbalika, Hartemann and Foliguet 1984, Castells, George and Hierholzer 1990). Cooler temperatures (33–35°C) are best for less invasive viruses such as coronaviruses, rhinoviruses and the enteroviruses that cause haemorrhagic conjunctivitis. Finally, whenever MK or AGMK cells are used (e.g. for influenza, measles or rubella, one should presume that simian adventitious agents are present and may confound the isolation and identification of human viruses (Hull 1968, Eberle and Hilliard 1995).

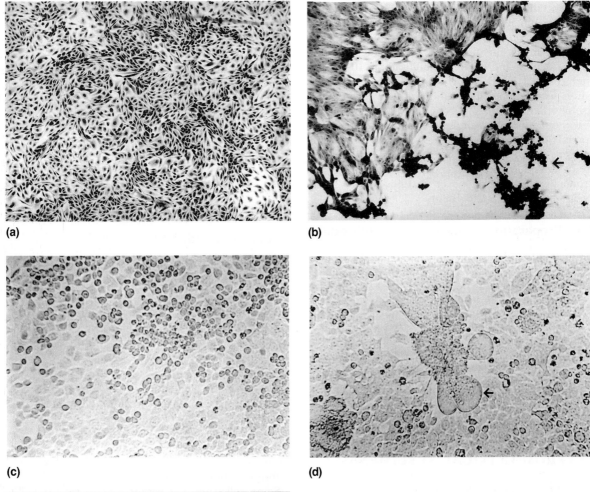

(a)

(b)

(c)

(d)

(e)

Fig. 5.1 Low power views of various cytopathic effects. (a) Uninfected monkey kidney cells. (b) Adenovirus in monkey kidney cells; note the grape-like clusters of dead cells. (c) Picornavirus in HEp-2 cells producing rounded, degenerative cells (top of field). (d) Respiratory syncytial virus in HEp-2 cells producing large syncytia (arrow). (e) A line of human lymphoid cells infected with human immunodeficiency virus (HIV-1). Note syncytia (arrowed). (Part (e) from Collier and Oxford, *Human Virology*, 1993, by permission of Oxford University Press.)

CHICK EMBRYOS

Except for influenza and poxviruses, chick embryos have been largely superseded by cell cultures for virus isolation and identification.

Amniotic and allantoic routes

The **amniotic** route of inoculation is used mainly for primary isolation of influenza viruses, and the **allantoic** route for serial passages and for obtaining large quantities of virus. Embryos c. 10 days old are inoculated by well established methods and the fluids are harvested 2–4 days later.

The **chorioallantoic membrane** (CAM) method is used mainly for poxviruses. The membranes of 12 day old embryos are inoculated through an opening in the shell about halfway along the long axis of the egg, the CAM having first been pulled away from the shell by

Viral growth is usually detected as CPE in the infected cell monolayer by scanning at ×40–100 magnification and observing in greater detail at ×200–400 magnification (Fig. 5.1). The type of CPE and the time required for it to appear in a particular cell type are suggestive of the type of virus present. Thus, careful observation of the monolayers is important for applying the proper identification tests.

applying negative pressure to a second hole drilled over the natural air sac. The CAM is inspected for the appearance of pocks after further incubation for 2–4 days.

For a detailed account of chick embryo methods, see Barrett and Inglis (1985) and Lennette et al. (1995).

LABORATORY ANIMALS

Like chick embryos, animals have largely been superseded by other systems; they are occasionally used for special purposes, such as the isolation and partial characterization of coxsackieviruses in suckling mice, which can be inoculated both intracerebrally and intraperitoneally (Gould and Clegg 1985).

For use of other animal systems, the reader is referred to chapters dealing with the relevant virus groups in this volume and elsewhere (Lennette et al. 1988, 1995, Murray et al. 1995).

3.3 Recovery and identification of viruses

Table 5.2 summarizes the relative value of a range of methods for isolating and propagating human viruses. Further details may be found in Isenberg (1992), Lennette et al. (1995) and Murray et al. (1995).

PARVOVIRUSES

The human parvovirus B19 (see Chapter 14) causes 'fifth disease' (erythema infectiosum) and is easily spread by aerosolized droplets and fomites in schools, and vertically to the fetus during the first trimester of pregnancy (see Chapter 41). The virus may grow in specialized erythropoietic stem cell cultures, but not in standard culture systems. Thus, B19 infection is established by EIA testing of a sample of the patient's acute-phase serum, in which both virus and antibodies are sought; electron microscopy (EM), Western blots, DNA hybridization probes and polymerase chain reaction (PCR) have also been used extensively (Anderson 1987, Durigon et al. 1993).

PAPOVAVIRUSES

The papovaviruses (see Chapter 16) consist of 2 genera, but members of only one can be isolated in cell culture. Polyoma BK virus can be recovered in HEK, NCI-H292 and diploid fibroblast cells, and the polyoma JC virus replicates in primary human fetal glial cells, but both viruses may be missed because their CPE develops slowly and may be ill-defined. It is a granular, degenerative, slowly lytic CPE, similar to that caused by reoviruses. BK virus is identified by haemagglutination inhibition (HI) tests at 4°C with human 'O' erythrocytes and specific antiserum; BK and JC viruses are identified by EIA, serum neutralization (SN), PCR and hybridization probes. The other genus, papillomaviruses, cannot be propagated in cell culture so are identified in biopsied tissues by anti-peptide EIAs and by DNA hybridization and PCR techniques (Eklund and Dillner 1995, Ylitalo, Bergstrom and Gyllenstein 1995).

ADENOVIRUSES

Adenoviruses (see Chapter 15) are associated with diverse clinical syndromes. They are spread by droplets, fomites and the faecal–oral route; some serotypes are also spread venereally. Most serotypes replicate readily in HEK, HEp-2, KB, A549 and NCI-H292 cells, with or without rolling, producing grape-like clusters of round, refractile, enlarged cells. Thus, adenoviruses grow in most of the same cells as herpes simplex, but more slowly (3–14 days), depending on serotype, and make more discrete, irregularly shaped cell clusters. Adenoviruses can be adapted to replicate in fibroblast cells, but the CPE develops slowly and infectivity titres are low. Types 40 and 41, associated with infant gastroenteritis, grow best in an Ad5-transformed HEK line (Graham-293 cells) or in HEp-2 under a fortified Opti-MEM medium containing 0.4% fetal calf serum and 0.1% 2-mercaptoethanol. The adenoviruses are among the easier viruses to identify because they are unique in producing in cell culture very large quantities of soluble antigens with many type- and group-specific properties that lend themselves to a wide variety of diagnostic tests. Adenoviruses are distinguished from other viruses by EM, CF, latex agglutination (LA), IFA, IPA, EIA, time-resolved fluoroimmunoassay (TR-FIA) (Hierholzer et al. 1987, Brown et al. 1990), DNA probes, restriction enzyme analysis (REA) (Adrian et al. 1986), PCR (Hierholzer et al. 1993c), and cytological and inclusion-body staining methods; they are then serotyped by HI and SN tests (Hierholzer 1992).

HERPESVIRUSES

The herpesviruses (see Chapters 17, 18, 19 and 20) are spread by aerosolized droplets, fomites and direct contact, and cause a wide range of ocular, oropharyngeal, genital and generalized disease in humans. They have 3 types of CPE in cell culture. HSV-1 and 2 grow well in many cell types, producing grape-like clusters of round, refractile, enlarged cells often identical to adenovirus CPE in HEK, HEp-2, KB, HeLa, A549, HLF, NCI-H292, primary rabbit kidney, and other cells. At complete CPE, all cells become lysed and detached from the vessel surface. HSV-1 grows fast (1–2 days), makes fewer clusters, and may produce ballooned, multinucleate giant cells with granulated cytoplasm. HSV-2, usually a genital isolate, grows more slowly than type 1. HSV does not require roller cultures, but HEp-2, NCI-H292 and fibroblast cells will probably be on roller or rocker apparatus for the benefit of other viruses to which these cells are susceptible.

CMV is notably labile; the only herpesvirus that is shed in great amounts in the urine, it replicates slowly (12–30 days) in roller cultures of diploid fibroblast cells. CMV produces giant-cell CPE resembling elongated foci of refractile, swollen cells, somewhat akin to measles CPE.

VZV, the cause of chickenpox and herpes zoster (shingles), also grows slowly in fibroblasts on roller culture. It produces a CPE characterized by enlarged, round, glassy cells in small foci in 2–10 days, which is

Table 5.2   Isolation and propagation systems for human viruses

Virus family/group	Cell cultures					Organ culture	Embry. eggs		Laboratory animals		
	Primary	Epithelial	Fibroblast	Vero	Other		amn./all.	CAM	Rodents	Primates	Other
Parvoviridae											
Parvovirus B19	−	−	−	−	±	−	−	−	−	−	−
Papovaviridae											
Papillomaviruses	−	−	−	−	−	−	−	−	−	−	−
Polyomavirus BK, JC	+	−	±	±	−	−	−	−	−	−	−
Adenoviridae											
Adenovirus 1–49	+	+	±	+	+	+	−	−	−	−	−
Hepadnaviridae											
Hepatitis B	±	−	−	−	±	−	−	−	±	+	+
Herpesviridae											
Herpes simplex 1, 2	+	+	+	+	+	+	−	+	+	−	−
Varicella-zoster (VZ)	+	+	+	±	±	−	−	+	−	+	−
Cytomegalovirus (CMV)	−	−	+	−	−	−	−	−	−	+	+
Epstein–Barr (EBV)	−	−	−	−	+	−	−	−	−	−	−
HHV-6, HHV-7	−	−	−	−	+	−	−	−	−	−	−
Poxviridae											
Vaccinia	+	+	+	+	+	+	+	+	+	−	+
Smallpox	+	+	+	+	+	+	+	+	−	+	−
Parapoxviruses	+	−	±	−	+	−	−	+	+	+	+
Molluscum contagiosum	−	−	−	−	±	−	−	−	−	−	−
Picornaviridae											
Poliovirus 1, 2, 3	+	+	+	+	+	+	−	−	+	+	−
Coxsackie A (23 types)	±	−	±	−	+	±	−	−	+	±	−
Coxsackie B (6 types)	+	+	+	+	+	+	−	−	+	−	−
Echovirus (31 types)	+	±	±	±	+	+	−	−	−	−	−
Enterovirus 68–71	+	±	±	±	+	+	−	−	−	±	−
Hepatitis A	±	−	±	±	±	−	−	−	−	+	−
Rhinoviruses (~125)	+	±	+	−	+	+	−	−	−	+	−
Caliciviridae											
Caliciviruses	+	−	−	−	+	−	−	−	−	−	−
Norwalk	−	−	−	−	−	−	−	−	−	±	−
Hepatitis E(?)	±	−	−	−	±	−	−	−	+	+	+

Family / Virus								
Reoviridae								
Reovirus 1, 2, 3	+	+	+	−	−	+	+	±
Colorado tick fever	−	−	+	−	−	±	±	−
Rotaviruses	±	±	−	−	−	+	−	−
Togaviridae								
Sindbis, EEE, WEE, Simliki Forest & other arboviruses	+	±	+	+	−	+	±	+
Rubella	+	±	±	−	−	+	+	±
Flaviviridae								
Dengue 1–4, JE, SLE, West Nile, yellow fever, other arboviruses	+	±	+	−	−	+	±	+
Hepatitis C	−	+	−	−	−	+	−	−
Orthomyxoviridae								
Influenza A, B, C	+	−	±	−	+	+	+	−
Paramyxoviridae								
Parainfluenza 1–4B	+	±	±	±	±	+	±	±
Mumps	+	±	+	+	+	+	+	±
Measles	+	+	+	+	+	+	+	+
Resp. syncytial (RSV)	+	+	+	−	−	+	+	+
Arenaviridae								
LCM, Lassa, others	−	+	+	−	−	±	+	−
Rhabdoviridae								
Rabies	+	+	±	−	−	±	+	+
VSV, other arboviruses	±	+	+	+	+	±	±	+
Filoviridae								
Marburg, Ebola	−	+	+	+	+	+	+	+
Coronaviridae								
Coronaviruses	±	−	±	−	−	+	−	−
Bunyaviridae								
CE, La Crosse	±	±	+	+	+	+	±	±
Hantaviruses	−	−	±	−	−	−	−	±
Other arboviruses	±	±	+	+	+	+	+	±
Retroviridae								
HIV, HTLV	−	−	−	−	−	+	±	−

+ = suitable for growth of virus; ± = partly suitable, i.e. some strains do not grow, or titres are low; − = unsuitable.
Embry, embryonate; CE, California encephalitis; EEE, eastern equine encephalitis; all., allantoic cavity; amn., amniotic cavity; CAM, chorioallantoic membrane; HIV, human immunodeficiency virus; HTLV, human T cell leukaemia/lymphoma virus; JE, Japanese encephalitis; LCM, lymphocytic choriomeningitis; SLE, St Louis encephalitis; VSV, vesiculovirus; WEE, western equine encephalitis.

thus distinct from that caused by CMV. VZV can produce large foci of multinucleate giant cells when the individual foci coalesce.

Epstein–Barr virus (EBV) is associated with infectious mononucleosis, Burkitt's lymphoma and nasopharyngeal carcinoma; human herpesvirus type 6 (HHV-6), the cause of roseola infantum (exanthema subitum or 'fourth disease') in children; and HHV-7, the probable cause of some roseola cases. EBV requires special conditions and cells for successful cultivation in the laboratory. In culture, it infects both B lymphocytes and epithelial cells with the CD21 receptor; HHV-6 grows best in primary CD4+ T lymphocytes rendered more susceptible by the presence of antibody to CD3 (Pellett, Black and Yamamoto 1992, Yasukawa et al. 1993, Hall et al. 1994) and HHV-7 also replicates in CD4+ T-lymphocytes (Black and Pellett 1993, Lusso et al. 1994, Tanaka et al. 1994).

Herpesviruses are readily visualized by EM, the icosahedral nucleocapsid and the baggy envelope being prominent. The viruses are commonly speciated by IFA, IPA, EIA, LA and SN tests and by DNA probes and PCR (Buller et al. 1992, Drew 1992, Perez et al. 1995).

POXVIRUSES

Vaccinia and certain other poxviruses (see Chapter 21) can be isolated in MK, Vero, NCI-H292 and diploid fibroblast cells. Their CPE is characterized as cell fusion with plaques. Plaques ranging from 1 to 6 mm in diameter (depending on the virus) are formed in 2–4 days, during which the infected cells fuse, form cytoplasmic bridging and then disintegrate. Some poxviruses produce plaques on the CAM of 12-day chick embryos. Identification is accomplished from the type and size of plaques formed and by EM, CF, HI, EIA, IFA, RIA and RE and other DNA tests.

PICORNAVIRUSES

This large family (see Chapter 25) includes the enteroviruses (poliovirus 1–3; 23 Coxsackie A viruses; 6 Coxsackie B viruses; 31 echoviruses; and 5 more recent enteroviruses), and the rhinoviruses (c. 125 serotypes). The enteroviruses are spread by aerosolized droplets, fomites and the faecal–oral route, whereas the rhinoviruses are spread by aerosols and fomites only (Agbalika, Hartemann and Foliguit 1984, Dick et al. 1987, Mandell, Douglas and Bennett 1990). These viruses produce a 'shrunken cell degeneration' CPE in NCI-H292, MK, RD, trypsin-treated MA-104 and diploid fibroblast cells, preferably in roller cultures although some Coxsackie A viruses grow only in the brain of suckling mice. The CPE is often observed as tadpole-shaped, shrunken cells with pyknotic nuclei, beginning in patches at the edges of the monolayer and progressing inward. CPE for polioviruses and some Coxsackie B viruses is quite rapid, becoming complete in 1–3 days with all cells detached from the glass. CPE for the remaining enteroviruses and the rhinoviruses generally requires 4–7 days or longer, is often characterized by individual small, rounded and sometimes refractile cells or by a degenerative appear-

ance across the monolayer, and may never become complete. Subpassaging is helpful. The variable CPE found in enterovirus- or rhinovirus-infected cells is not diagnostically confusing, however, because these viruses do not haemadsorb, rarely haemagglutinate with any species of erythrocytes, and do not interfere with test systems for other viruses. Enteroviruses are distinguished from rhinoviruses by acid- and chloroform-lability tests in which both genera are chloroform-stable but only enteroviruses are acid-stable, or by group-specific PCR and hybridization tests (Abebe et al. 1992, Hyypia and Stanway 1993, Egger et al. 1995, Halonen et al. 1995). The viruses can be serotyped only by type-specific SN tests.

REOVIRUSES

Reoviruses 1–3 can be isolated from throat and rectal specimens in NCI-H292, MK and HeLa cells under stationary or roller conditions after 5–14 days of culture, but, unlike other members of the *Reoviridae* family (see Chapter 27), have never been clearly associated with human disease. In cell culture they cause a slow lytic degeneration with granulation of the cytoplasm, similar to polyomavirus CPE. MK cultures should be rolled. Reoviruses are easily seen by EM and serotyped by SN and HI tests with human 'O' erythrocytes.

RUBELLA

Rubellavirus, a togavirus (see Chapter 28), was originally detected because of its ability to prevent another virus from infecting the cells in which it was replicating. Current diagnostic testing for rubella may employ specialized cultures in which CPE may become evident; rubella can, under certain conditions, cause an ill-defined and variable CPE in rabbit cornea, rabbit kidney and Vero cells. Usually, however, rubella is detected by the interference test, in which replication of another virus (e.g. echovirus-11 or coxsackievirus-A9) is inhibited by prior inoculation of the test material. A positive result may be confirmed by HI, EIA, LA, TR-FIA and PCR tests (Shankaran et al. 1990).

ORTHOMYXOVIRUSES

Influenza A, B and C viruses (see Chapter 22) are spread by aerosol droplets and fomites, and are best recovered in roller cultures of MK and MDCK cells and in intact chick embryos. Chick embryo cells, MDCK and other cells require rolling and a fortified medium containing trypsin 2 µg/ml for optimal sensitivity; the CPE may be seen as a combination of syncytia, rounding and degeneration. The syncytia caused by influenza B may be accompanied by vacuolation. Influenza CPE may develop in 4–7 days, but cultures should be blind-passaged and held an additional week. Because the cells rarely become detached and may not have an obvious CPE, virus detection in MK cultures is verified by haemadsorption with chicken or guinea-pig erythrocytes, and in MDCK cells by HA. Some strains of influenza A and B can be isolated only in 9- to 11-day chick embryos. The viruses are then typed by HI, IFA, IPA, EIA, TR-FIA or PCR tests (Frank et al. 1979, Grandien et al. 1985, Walls et al. 1986, Bucher et al. 1991, Ziegler et al. 1995).

Haemadsorption is a fast and convenient method for detecting orthomyxoviruses (influenza A, B, C) and non-RSV paramyxoviruses (parainfluenza 1, 2, 3, 4A, 4B; mumps; measles) in cell cultures. It is even used in the presence of CPE to obtain a quick distinction from other virus groups that may cause similar CPE in the same types of cultures. The supernatant fluid from the cell culture is decanted into a sterile tube at the end of the incubation period (7–10 days), to conserve virus and viral antigens for passaging and testing. The monolayer is washed twice with 2–3 ml of plain Hank's balanced salt solution (HBSS) at room temperature; 1 ml of fresh HBSS is added, followed by 0.2 ml of 0.4% mammalian erythrocyte suspension from the appropriate species. The tube is incubated stationary with the fluid covering the monolayer. The test is read 3 times at 20 min intervals by agitating the tube in a sideways motion and then observing at ×40–100 magnification for erythrocytes firmly attached to the cultured cells (positive) or floating free in the fluid (negative).

PARAMYXOVIRUSES

The human paramyxoviruses (Chapter 23) are parainfluenza types 1, 2, 3, 4A, 4B, mumps, measles (rubeola) and RSV. The parainfluenza and mumps viruses replicate well in roller cultures of NCI-H292 cells under a fortified medium containing trypsin 1.5 µg/ml for optimal sensitivity, and in MK cells without trypsin (Meguro et al. 1979, Castells, George and Hierholzer 1990). The CPE induced by these viruses may develop in 4–7 days, and is a combination of syncytia and rounding. The syncytia may be accompanied by a granular degeneration with parainfluenzavirus types 1–4; mumps virus often gives rise to large syncytia. The cultures must generally be blind-passaged and held an additional week to ensure viral growth. The cells rarely become detached, and may not show obvious CPE at all, so NCI-H292 or MK cultures for these viruses must be haemadsorbed with guinea-pig, human or monkey erythrocytes at the end of the culture period and the viruses then typed by HI, IFA, EIA or TR-FIA tests (Grandien et al. 1985, Van Tiel et al. 1988, Hierholzer et al. 1989, 1993a, Takimoto et al. 1991, Moscona and Peluso 1992).

Measles virus produces classic multinucleate giant cell CPE in AGMK, Vero and HEK cells after 7–14 days of roller culture. This CPE is characterized by fusion of the cells, with the formation of multinucleate giant cells. But, because the CPE usually develops slowly and may not be recognized, the monolayers should be haemadsorbed with vervet monkey erythrocytes to ensure detection of the virus. Measles is further identified by HI tests with vervet erythrocytes, IFA, EIA, SN, RNA probes or PCR tests (Erdman et al. 1991, Naniche et al. 1993, Nakayama et al. 1995).

RSV produces a distinct syncytial CPE in HEp-2, HeLa and NCI-H292 cells in 5–12 days in roller cultures. The balled-up syncytia usually become detached from the glass surface and float freely in the medium. Some strains of RSV, particularly of group B, produce more cellular degeneration than syncytia in HEp-2

and NCI-H292 cells. Group A and B strains of RSV are readily identified by IFA, EIA and TR-FIA tests (Freymuth et al. 1991, Waris 1991, Cane, Matthews and Pringle 1992, Hierholzer et al. 1994b). Details on paramyxovirus typing are found elsewhere (Popow-Kraupp et al. 1986, Ahluwalia et al. 1987, Akerlind et al. 1988, Anderson et al. 1991).

CORONAVIRUSES

The human coronaviruses (see Chapter 24) cause a significant proportion of 'common colds' and are spread by droplets, but are best identified directly in nasal and throat specimens by FA, EIA and TR-FIA because the viruses are extremely labile and difficult to recover in the laboratory. The viruses growing in diploid fibroblast cells (229E virus) or in RD cells (OC43 virus) do not cause discernible CPEs during their replication phases. Only when viral replication is complete and the virus titre has peaked (at c. 10^7 tissue culture infective doses (TCID50)/0.1 ml), after 26–30 hours of roller incubation, do changes begin to be evident in the monolayer. For the next several days, CPE develops as an even degeneration across the monolayer. The CPE becomes complete concomitant with autolysis of the newly formed virions; by this time, little infectious virus is left in the culture (Hierholzer 1976, Schmidt, Cooney and Kenny 1979). The peplomers constitute the primary antigen detected in all tests, including the HI test for strain OC43 (Schmidt, Cooney and Kenny 1979, Hierholzer et al. 1994a). Alternatively, the RNA can be identified by hybridization tests (Myint, Siddell and Tyrrell 1989, Myint et al. 1990).

RETROVIRUSES

The HIV and HTLV viruses (see Chapter 38) also require specialized systems for isolation and identification, and will not be recovered by standard culture methods. They are identified by Western blots, EIA and PCR (Isenberg 1992, Persing et al. 1993, Signoret et al. 1993).

HEPATITIS VIRUSES

Hepatitis A virus, a picornavirus (see Chapter 34), replicates in MK cultures in 1–4 weeks but is non-cytolytic; it is detected by EIA or hybridization tests. The hepatitis B (see Chapter 36), C (Chapter 35), D (Chapter 37) and E (Chapter 34) viruses do not grow in routine cell cultures and must be detected by specific protein EIA or RIA tests or nucleic acid-based tests (Siitari et al. 1983, Balayan 1993, Wilber 1993, Kurstak et al. 1995).

GASTROENTERITIS VIRUSES

These viruses (see Chapters 26 and 27) also belong to diverse families and have unique requirements for culture. Rotaviruses, after treatment with trypsin, will replicate in BSC-1, MA104 and AGMK cells under roller conditions. Caliciviruses and astroviruses may replicate in HEK or LLC-MK2 cells under a fortified medium with trypsin (Sanchez-Fauquier et al. 1994). The human enteric coronaviruses, whose existence is doubtful, the toroviruses and the Norwalk-like viruses cannot be isolated in the laboratory (Koopmans and Horzinek 1994, Lennette et al. 1995). The adenoviruses were discussed above (see p. 65). The gastroenteritis viruses can be distinguished by EM, LA, EIA, RIA, TR-FIA and PCR tests (Hughes et al. 1984, Pereira et al. 1985, Erdman, Gary and Anderson 1989, Sanekata et al. 1990, Siitari 1990).

'ARBOVIRUSES'

The **togaviruses**, **flaviviruses** (see Chapter 29), **arenaviruses** (Chapter 31), **rhabdoviruses**, **filoviruses** (Chapter 32) and **bunyaviruses** (Chapter 30) contain most of the agents covered by the term 'arboviruses' and many rare and unusual viruses that cause disease in geographically distinct parts of the world; they often have special isolation requirements. Certain arboviruses can be isolated in primary hamster kidney cells, primary chick or duck embryo cells, or derivative cell lines such as AP61 mosquito cells, BHK-21 hamster kidney cells, Vero (African green monkey kidney cells) and LLC-MK2 rhesus monkey kidney cells, after 2–10 days of culture. The CPE may not be apparent at first, but becomes generalized in subpassages or forms plaques under agarose. Other arboviruses grow best in mosquito suspension cell cultures at 20–30°C, in which replication is detected by subpassaging to monolayer cultures, in which CPE may be evident, or by HA/HI, EIA, CF, IFA, RIA, neutralization or nucleic acid tests for the specific viruses suspected. Still other arboviruses can be recovered only in whole animal systems such as chick embryos, suckling mice or hamsters, or mosquitoes. Fortunately, most diagnostic laboratories will not encounter these viruses, either because of their rarity in most parts of the world or because of their requirement for BSL-3 or 4 containment facilities. The reader is therefore referred to other works that detail the isolation requirements and systems, the specific identification tests and the laboratory precautions for these viruses (Fields et al. 1990, Lennette et al. 1988, 1995, Murray et al. 1995).

Of particular interest is the isolation in deer mice of the causative agent of the newly described hantavirus pulmonary syndrome. The virus, named Sin Nombre hantavirus, is a bunyavirus and can be propagated in the Vero–E6 cell line after growth in deer mouse lungs (Feldmann et al. 1993, Elliott et al. 1994).

The interpretation of any culture isolation result or of any test used to identify the isolate depends on the methods employed, but viral growth alone should never be considered pathognomonic. The association of an isolate with disease depends on the clinical data obtained with the specimen and on the known epidemiology of the virus. Thus, careful virus isolation and identification test results coupled with sound epidemiological data are the key to accurate diagnosis of viral infections.

REFERENCES

Abebe A, Johansson B et al., 1992, Detection of enteroviruses in faeces by polymerase chain reaction, *Scand J Infect Dis*, **24:** 265–73.

Ades EW, Hierholzer JC et al., 1992, Viral susceptibility of an immortalized human microvascular endothelial cell line, *J Virol Methods*, **39:** 83–90.

Adrian T, Wadell G et al., 1986, DNA restriction analysis of adenovirus prototypes 1 to 41, *Arch Virol*, **91:** 277–90.

Agbalika F, Hartemann P, Foliguet JM, 1984, Trypsin-treated MA-104: a sensitive cell line for isolating enteric viruses from environmental samples, *Appl Environ Microbiol*, **47:** 378–80.

Ahluwalia G, Embree J et al., 1987, Comparison of nasopharyngeal aspirate and nasopharyngeal swab specimens for respiratory syncytial virus diagnosis by cell culture, indirect immunofluorescence assay, and enzyme-linked immunosorbent assay, *J Clin Microbiol*, **25:** 763–7.

Akerlind B, Norrby E et al., 1988, Respiratory syncytial virus: heterogeneity of subgroup B strains, *J Gen Virol*, **69:** 2145–54.

Alberts B, Bray D et al., 1994, *Molecular Biology of the Cell*, 3rd edn, Garland, New York.

Almeida JD, Hall T et al., 1978, The effect of trypsin on the growth of rotavirus, *J Gen Virol*, **40:** 213–18.

Anderson LJ, 1987, Role of parvovirus B19 in human disease, *Pediatr Infect Dis J*, **6:** 711–18.

Anderson LJ, Hierholzer JC et al., 1985, Microneutralization test for respiratory syncytial virus based on an enzyme immunoassay, *J Clin Microbiol*, **22:** 1050–2.

Anderson LJ, Hendry RM et al., 1991, Multicenter study of strains of respiratory syncytial virus, *J Infect Dis*, **163:** 687–92.

ATCC, 1985, *ATCC Quality Control Methods for Cell Lines*, American Type Culture Collection, Rockville MD.

Ausubel FM, Brent R et al., eds, 1991, *Current Protocols in Molecular Biology*, Green Publ and Wiley-Interscience, New York.

Balayan MS, 1993, Hepatitis E virus infection in Europe: regional situation regarding laboratory diagnosis and epidemiology, *Clin Diagn Virol*, **1:** 1–9.

Barkley WE, 1979, Safety considerations in the cell culture laboratory, *Methods Enzymol*, **58:** 36–43.

Barrett T, Inglis SC, 1985, Growth, purification and titration of influenza viruses, *Virology: a practical approach*, ed Mahy BWJ, IRL Press, Oxford, 119–50.

Bennink JR, Yewdell JW, 1990, Recombinant vaccinia viruses as vectors for studying T lymphocyte specificity and function, *Curr Top Microbiol Immunol*, **163:** 153–84.

Bissell DM, Caron JM et al., 1990, Transcriptional regulation of the albumin gene in cultured rat hepatocytes: role of basement-membrane matrix, *Mol Biol Med*, **7:** 187–97.

Black JB, Pellett PE, 1993, Human herpesvirus 7, *Rev Med Virol*, **3:** 217–23.

Boss BD, 1986, An improved in vitro immunization procedure for the production of monoclonal antibodies, *Methods Enzymol*, **121:** 27–33.

Brown M, Shami Y et al., 1990, Time-resolved fluoroimmunoassay for enteric adenoviruses using the europium chelator 4,7-bis(chlorosulfophenyl)-1,10-phenanthroline-2,9-dicarboxylic acid, *J Clin Microbiol*, **28:** 1398–402.

Bucher DJ, Mikhail A et al., 1991, Rapid detection of type A influenza viruses with monoclonal antibodies to the M protein (M1) by enzyme-linked immunosorbent assay and time-resolved fluoroimmunoassay, *J Clin Microbiol*, **29:** 2484–8.

Buller RS, Bailey TC et al., 1992, Use of a modified shell vial technique to quantitate cytomegalovirus viremia in a population of solid-organ transplant recipients, *J Clin Microbiol*, **30:** 2620–4.

Cane PA, Matthews DA, Pringle CR, 1992, Analysis of relatedness of subgroup A respiratory syncytial viruses isolated worldwide, *Virus Res*, **25:** 15–22.

Castells E, George VG, Hierholzer JC, 1990, NCI-H292 as an alternative cell line for the isolation and propagation of the human paramyxoviruses, *Arch Virol*, 115: 277–88.

Castro BA, Weiss CD et al., 1988, Optimal conditions for recovery of the human immunodeficiency virus from peripheral blood mononuclear cells, *J Clin Microbiol*, 26: 2371–6.

Caul EO, Egglestone SI, 1977, Further studies on human enteric coronaviruses, *Arch Virol*, 54: 107–17.

Chappell WA, White LA, Gamble WC, 1984, *Production Manual for Viral, Rickettsial, Chlamydial, Mycoplasmal Reagents*, 6th edn, Centers for Disease Control, Atlanta GA.

Chen TR, 1977, In situ detection of mycoplasma contamination in cell cultures by fluorescent Hoechst 33258 stain, *Exp Cell Res*, 104: 255–62.

Chong P, Gillam S, 1985, Purification of biologically active rubella virus antigens by immunoaffinity chromatography, *J Virol Methods*, 10: 261–8.

Coligan JE, Kruisbeek AM et al., eds, 1991, *Current Protocols in Immunology*, vol 1, Green Publ and Wiley-Interscience, New York.

Collier LH, Oxford JO, 1993, *Human Virology*, Oxford University Press, Oxford.

Cox WI, Tartaglia J, Paoletti E, 1993, Induction of cytotoxic T lymphocytes by recombinant canarypox (ALVAC) and attenuated vaccinia (NYVAC) viruses expressing the HIV-1 envelope glycoprotein, *Virology*, 195: 845–50.

Crandell RA, Hierholzer JC et al., 1978, Contamination of primary embryonic bovine kidney cell cultures with parainfluenza type 2 simian virus 5 and infectious bovine rhinotracheitis virus, *J Clin Microbiol*, 7: 214–18.

Dick EC, Jennings LC et al., 1987, Aerosol transmission of rhinovirus colds, *J Infect Dis*, 156: 442–8.

Drew WL, 1992, Nonpulmonary manifestations of cytomegalovirus infection in immunocompromised patients, *Clin Microbiol Rev*, 5: 204–10.

Durigon EL, Erdman DD et al., 1993, Multiple primer pairs for polymerase chain reaction (PCR) amplification of human parvovirus B19 DNA, *J Virol Methods*, 44: 155–65.

Eberle R, Hilliard J, 1995, The simian herpesviruses, *Infect Agents Dis*, 4: 55–70.

Egger D, Pasamontes L et al., 1995, Reverse transcription multiplex PCR for differentiation between polio- and enteroviruses from clinical and environmental samples, *J Clin Microbiol*, 33: 1442–7.

Eisenberg RJ, Ponce de Leon M et al., 1982, Purification of glycoprotein gD of herpes simplex virus types 1 and 2 by use of monoclonal antibody, *J Virol*, 41: 1099–104.

Eklund C, Dillner J, 1995, A two-site enzyme immunoassay for quantitation of human papillomavirus type 16 particles, *J Virol Methods*, 53: 11–23.

Elliott LH, Ksiazek TG et al., 1994, Isolation of the causative agent of hantavirus pulmonary syndrome, *Am J Trop Med Hyg*, 51: 102–8.

Erdman DD, Gary GW, Anderson LJ, 1989, Development and evaluation of an IgM capture enzyme immunoassay for diagnosis of recent Norwalk virus infection, *J Virol Methods*, 24: 57–66.

Erdman DD, Anderson LJ et al., 1991, Evaluation of monoclonal antibody-based capture enzyme immunoassays for detection of specific antibodies to measles virus, *J Clin Microbiol*, 29: 1466–71.

Espy MJ, Hierholzer JC, Smith TF, 1987, The effect of centrifugation on the rapid detection of adenovirus in shell vials, *Am J Clin Pathol*, 88: 358–60.

Evans VJ, Perry VP, Vincent MM, eds, 1975, *TCA Manual*, vol 1, Tissue Culture Association, Rockville MD.

Feldmann H, Sanchez A et al., 1993, Utilization of autopsy RNA for the synthesis of the nucleocapsid antigen of a newly recognized virus associated with hantavirus pulmonary syndrome, *Virus Res*, 30: 351–67.

Fields BN, Knipe DM et al., eds, 1990, *Virology*, 2nd edn, vols 1 and 2, Raven Press, New York.

Fleming DO, Richardson JH et al., eds, 1995, *Laboratory Safety: principles and practices*, 2nd edn, American Society for Microbiology Press, Washington DC.

Foung SK, Engleman EG, Grumet FC, 1986, Generation of human monoclonal antibodies by fusion of EBV-activated B cells to a human–mouse hybridoma, *Methods Enzymol*, 121: 168–74.

Frank AL, Couch RB et al., 1979, Comparison of different tissue cultures for isolation and quantitation of influenza and parainfluenza viruses, *J Clin Microbiol*, 10: 32–6.

Freshney RI, 1993, *Culture of Animal Cells: a manual of basic technique*, 3rd edn, Wiley–Liss, New York.

Freymuth F, Petitjean J et al., 1991, Prevalence of respiratory syncytial virus subgroups A and B in France from 1982 to 1990, *J Clin Microbiol*, 29: 653–5.

Gamble WC, Chappell WA, George EH, 1980, Inactivation of rabies diagnostic reagents by gamma radiation, *J Clin Microbiol*, 12: 676–8.

Gessler AE, Bender CE, Parkinson MC, 1956, A new and rapid method for isolating viruses by selective fluorocarbon deproteinization, *Trans N Y Acad Sci*, 2: 701–3.

Gleaves CA, Hursh DA et al., 1989, Detection of cytomegalovirus from clinical specimens in centrifugation culture by in situ DNA hybridization and monoclonal antibody staining, *J Clin Microbiol*, 27: 21–3.

Gould EA, Clegg JCS, 1985, Growth, titration and purification of alphaviruses and flaviviruses, *Virology: a practical approach*, ed Mahy BWJ, IRL Press, Oxford, 44–78.

Grandien M, Pettersson CA et al., 1985, Rapid viral diagnosis of acute respiratory infections: comparison of enzyme-linked immunosorbent assay and the immunofluorescence technique for detection of viral antigens in nasopharyngeal secretions, *J Clin Microbiol*, 22: 757–60.

Hall CB, Long CE et al., 1994, Human herpesvirus-6 infection in children: a prospective study of complications and reactivation, *N Engl J Med*, 331: 432–8.

Halonen P, Rocha E et al., 1995, Detection of enteroviruses and rhinoviruses in clinical specimens by PCR and liquid-phase hybridization, *J Clin Microbiol*, 33: 648–53.

Hanson CV, Riggs JL, Lennette EH, 1978, Photochemical inactivation of DNA and RNA viruses by psoralen derivatives, *J Gen Virol*, 40: 345–8.

Harlow E, Lane D, 1988, *Antibodies – A Laboratory Manual*, Cold Spring Harbor Laboratory, Cold Spring Harbor NY.

Hayflick L, 1973, Fetal human diploid cells, *Tissue Culture Methods and Applications*, eds Kruse PF, Patterson MK, Academic Press, New York, 43–5.

Hierholzer JC, 1976, Purification and biophysical properties of human coronavirus 229E, *Virology*, 75: 155–65.

Hierholzer JC, 1991, Rapid diagnosis of viral infection, *Rapid Methods and Automation in Microbiology and Immunology*, eds Vaheri A, Tilton RC, Balows A, Springer-Verlag, Berlin, 556–73.

Hierholzer JC, 1992, Adenoviruses in the immunocompromised host, *Clin Microbiol Rev*, 5: 262–74.

Hierholzer JC, 1993, Viral causes of respiratory infections, *Immunol Allergy Clin N Am*, 13: 27–42.

Hierholzer JC, Bingham PG, 1978, Vero microcultures for adenovirus neutralization tests, *J Clin Microbiol*, 7: 499–506.

Hierholzer JC, Stone YO, Broderson JR, 1991, Antigenic relationships among the 47 human adenoviruses determined in reference horse antisera, *Arch Virol*, 121: 179–97.

Hierholzer JC, Johansson KH et al., 1987, Comparison of monoclonal time-resolved fluoroimmunoassay with monoclonal capture-biotinylated detector enzyme immunoassay for adenovirus antigen detection, *J Clin Microbiol*, 25: 1662–7.

Hierholzer JC, Bingham PG et al., 1989, Comparison of monoclonal antibody time-resolved fluoroimmunoassay with monoclonal antibody capture-biotinylated detector enzyme immunoassay for respiratory syncytial virus and parainfluenza virus antigen detection, *J Clin Microbiol*, **27**: 1243–9.

Hierholzer JC, Bingham PG et al., 1993a, Time-resolved fluoro-immunoassays with monoclonal antibodies for rapid identification of parainfluenza type 4 and mumps viruses, *Arch Virol*, **130**: 335–52.

Hierholzer JC, Castells E et al., 1993b, Sensitivity of NCI-H292 human lung mucoepidermoid cells for respiratory and other human viruses, *J Clin Microbiol*, **31**: 1504–10.

Hierholzer JC, Halonen PE et al., 1993c, Detection of adenovirus in clinical specimens by polymerase chain reaction and liquid-phase hybridization quantitated by time-resolved fluorometry, *J Clin Microbiol*, **31**: 1886–91.

Hierholzer JC, Halonen PE et al., 1994a, Antigen detection in human respiratory coronavirus infections by monoclonal time-resolved fluoroimmunoassay, *Clin Diagn Virol*, **2**: 165–79.

Hierholzer JC, Tannock GA et al., 1994b, Subgrouping of respiratory syncytial virus strains from Australia and Papua New Guinea by biological and antigenic characteristics, *Arch Virol*, **136**: 133–47.

Hughes JH, Tuomari AV et al., 1984, Latex immunoassay for rapid detection of rotavirus, *J Clin Microbiol*, **20**: 441–7.

Hull RN, 1968, The simian viruses, *Virol Monogr*, **2**: 1–66.

Hyypia T, Stanway G, 1993, Biology of coxsackie A viruses, *Adv Virus Res*, **42**: 343–73.

Isenberg HD, ed, 1992, *Clinical Microbiology Procedures Handbook*, vol 2, American Society for Microbiology, Washington DC.

Itoh H, Morimoto Y et al., 1970, Effect of trypsin on viral susceptibility of Vero cell cultures – *Cercopithecus* kidney line, *Jpn J Med Sci Biol*, **23**: 227–35.

Jarvis DL, 1991, Baculovirus expression vectors, *Ann N Y Acad Sci*, **646**: 240–7.

Johnson FB, 1990, Transport of viral specimens, *Clin Microbiol Rev*, **3**: 120–31.

Johnston SL, Siegel CS, 1990, Presumptive identification of enteroviruses with RD, HEp-2, and RMK cell lines, *J Clin Microbiol*, **28**: 1049–50.

Koopmans M, Horzinek MC, 1994, Toroviruses of animals and humans: a review, *Adv Virus Res*, **43**: 233–73.

Kurstak E, Kurstak C et al., 1995, Current status of the molecular genetics of hepatitis C virus and its utilization in the diagnosis of infection, *Clin Diagn Virol*, **3**: 1–15.

Lennette EH, Halonen P, Murphy FA, eds, 1988, *Laboratory Diagnosis of Infectious Diseases: principles and practice*, vol II, *Viral, Rickettsial, and Chlamydial Diseases*, Springer-Verlag, New York.

Lennette EH, Lennette DA, Lennette ET, eds, 1995, *Diagnostic Procedures for Viral, Rickettsial and Chlamydial Infections*, 7th edn, American Public Health Assn, Washington DC.

Lusso P, Secchiero P et al., 1994, CD4 is a critical component of the receptor for human herpesvirus 7: interference with human immunodeficiency virus, *Proc Natl Acad Sci USA*, **91**: 3872–6.

McIntosh K, Halonen P, Ruuskanen O, 1993, Report of a workshop on respiratory viral infections: epidemiology, diagnosis, treatment, and prevention, *Clin Infect Dis*, **16**: 151–64.

McIntosh K, Dees JH et al., 1967, Recovery in tracheal organ cultures of novel viruses from patients with respiratory disease, *Proc Natl Acad Sci USA*, **57**: 933–40.

Mahy BWJ, Kangro H, eds, 1996, *Virology Methods Manual*, Academic Press, London.

Mandell GL, Douglas RG, Bennett JE, eds, 1990, *Principles and Practice of Infectious Diseases*, Churchill Livingstone, New York.

Markham PD, Salahuddin SZ, 1987, In vitro cultivation of human leukocytes: methods for the expression and isolation of human viruses, *BioTechniques*, **5**: 432–43.

Matthey S, Nicholson D et al., 1992, Rapid detection of respiratory viruses by shell vial culture and direct staining by using pooled and individual monoclonal antibodies, *J Clin Microbiol*, **30**: 540–4.

Meguro H, Bryant JD et al., 1979, Canine kidney cell line for isolation of respiratory viruses, *J Clin Microbiol*, **9**: 175–9.

Moscona A, Peluso RW, 1992, Fusion properties of cells infected with human parainfluenza type 3: receptor requirements for viral spread and virus-mediated membrane fusion, *J Virol*, **66**: 6280–7.

Murray PR, Baron EJ et al., eds, 1995, *Manual of Clinical Microbiology*, 6th edn, American Society for Microbiology Press, Washington DC.

Myint S, Siddell S, Tyrrell D, 1989, Detection of human coronavirus 229E in nasal washings using RNA:RNA hybridisation, *J Med Virol*, **29**: 70–3.

Myint S, Harmsen D et al., 1990, Characterization of a nucleic acid probe for the diagnosis of human coronavirus 229E infections, *J Med Virol*, **31**: 165–72.

Nakayama T, Mori T et al., 1995, Detection of measles virus genome directly from clinical samples by reverse transcriptase-polymerase chain reaction and genetic variability, *Virus Res*, **35**: 1–16.

Naniche N, Varior-Krishnan G et al., 1993, Human membrane cofactor protein (CD46) acts as a cellular receptor for measles virus, *J Virol*, **67**: 6025–32.

Norrby E, 1962, Hemagglutination by measles virus: a simple procedure for production of high potency antigen for hemagglutination-inhibition (HI) tests, *Proc Soc Exp Biol Med*, **111**: 814–18.

Olsen MA, Shuck KM et al., 1993, Isolation of seven respiratory viruses in shell vials: a practical and highly sensitive method, *J Clin Microbiol*, **27**: 2107–9.

Palmer EL, Martin ML, 1988, *Electron Microscopy in Viral Diagnosis*, CRC Press, Boca Raton FL.

Pellett PE, Black JB, Yamamoto M, 1992, Human herpesvirus 6: the virus and the search for its role as a human pathogen, *Adv Virus Res*, **41**: 1–52.

Pereira HG, Azeredo RS et al., 1985, A combined enzyme immunoassay for rotavirus and adenovirus (EIARA), *J Virol Methods*, **10**: 21–8.

Perez JL, Niubo J et al., 1995, Comparison of three commercially available monoclonal antibodies directed against pp65 antigen for cytomegalovirus antigenemia assay, *Diagn Microbiol Infect Dis*, **21**: 21–5.

Persing DH, Smith TF et al., eds, 1993, *Diagnostic Molecular Microbiology: principles and applications*, American Society for Microbiology, Washington DC.

Peter JH, Baumgarten H, 1992, *Monoclonal Antibodies*, Springer-Verlag, Berlin.

Popow-Kraupp T, Kern G et al., 1986, Detection of respiratory syncytial virus in nasopharyngeal secretions by enzyme-linked immunosorbent assay, indirect immunofluorescence, and virus isolation: a comparative study, *J Med Virol*, **19**: 123–34.

Sanchez-Fauquier A, Carrascosa AL et al., 1994, Characterization of a human astrovirus serotype 2 structural protein (VP26) that contains an epitope involved in virus neutralization, *Virology*, **201**: 312–20.

Sanekata T, Taniguchi K et al., 1990, Detection of adenovirus type 41 in stool samples by a latex agglutination method, *J Immunol Methods*, **127**: 235–9.

Scharff MD, Roberts S, Thammana P, 1981, Monoclonal antibodies, *J Infect Dis*, **143**: 346–51.

Schirm J, Meulenberg J et al., 1989, Rapid detection of varicella-zoster virus in clinical specimens using monoclonal antibodies on shell vials and smears, *J Med Virol*, **28**: 1–6.

Schirm J, Luijt DS et al., 1992, Rapid detection of respiratory viruses using mixtures of monoclonal antibodies on shell vial cultures, *J Med Virol*, **38**: 147–51.

Schmidt NJ, 1989, Cell culture procedures for diagnostic virology, *Diagnostic Procedures for Viral, Rickettsial and Chlamydial Infections*, 6th edn, eds Schmidt NJ, Emmons RW, American Public Health Assn, Washington DC, 51–100.

Schmidt OW, Cooney MK, Kenny GE, 1979, Plaque assay and improved yield of human coronaviruses in a human rhabdomyosarcoma cell line, *J Clin Microbiol*, **9**: 722–8.

Schmidt NJ, Lennette EH, 1971, Comparison of various methods for preparation of viral serological antigens from infected cell cultures, *Appl Microbiol*, **21:** 217–26.

Seigneurin JM, Desgranges C et al., 1983, Herpes simplex virus glycoprotein D: human monoclonal antibody produced by bone marrow cell line, *Science*, **221:** 173–5.

Sewell DL, 1995, Laboratory-associated infections and biosafety, *Clin Microbiol Rev*, **8:** 389–405.

Shankaran P, Reichstein E et al., 1990, Detection of immunoglobulins G and M to rubella virus by time-resolved immunofluorometry, *J Clin Microbiol*, **28:** 573–9.

Signoret N, Poignard P et al., 1993, Human and simian immunodeficiency viruses: virus–receptor interactions, *Trends Microbiol*, **1:** 328–32.

Siitari H, 1990, Dual-label time-resolved fluoroimmunoassay for the simultaneous detection of adenovirus and rotavirus in faeces, *J Virol Methods*, **28:** 179–88.

Siitari H, Hemmila I et al., 1983, Detection of hepatitis-B surface antigen using time-resolved fluoroimmunoassay, *Nature (London)*, **301:** 258–60.

Smith DB, Johnson KS, 1988, Single-step purification of polypeptides expressed in *Escherichia coli* as fusions with glutathione S-transferase, *Gene*, **67:** 31–40.

Smith MC, Creutz C, Huang YT, 1991, Detection of respiratory syncytial virus in nasopharyngeal secretions by shell vial technique, *J Clin Microbiol*, **29:** 463–5.

Takimoto S, Grandien M et al., 1991, Comparison of enzyme-linked immunosorbent assay, indirect immunofluorescence assay, and virus isolation for detection of respiratory viruses in nasopharyngeal secretions, *J Clin Microbiol*, **29:** 470–4.

Tanaka K, Kondo T et al., 1994, Human herpesvirus 7: another causal agent for roseola (exanthem subitum), *J Pediatr*, **125:** 1–5.

Taylor J, Weinberg R et al., 1992, Nonreplicating viral vectors as potential vaccines: recombinant canarypox virus expressing measles virus fusion (F) and hemagglutinin (HA) glycoproteins, *Virology*, **187:** 321–8.

Thompson EW, Nakamura S et al., 1991, Supernatants of acquired immunodeficiency syndrome-related Kaposi's sarcoma cells induce endothelial cell chemotaxis and invasiveness, *Cancer Res*, **51:** 2670–6.

Treanor JJ, Madore HP, Dolin R, 1988, Development of a monoclonal antibody to the Snow Mountain agent of gastroenteritis, *Proc Natl Acad Sci USA*, **85:** 3616–17.

Tyrrell DA, Blamire CJ, 1967, Improvements in a method of growing respiratory viruses in organ cultures, *Br J Exp Pathol*, **48:** 217–27.

Van Tiel FH, Kraaijeveld CA et al., 1988, Enzyme immunoassay of mumps virus in cell culture with peroxidase-labelled virus-specific monoclonal antibodies and its application for determination of antibodies, *J Virol Methods*, **22:** 99–108.

Vialard J, Lalumiere M et al., 1990, Synthesis of the membrane fusion and hemagglutinin proteins of measles virus, using a novel baculovirus vector containing the B-galactosidase gene, *J Virol*, **64:** 37–50.

Walls HH, Johansson KH et al., 1986, Time-resolved fluoroimmunoassay with monoclonal antibodies for rapid diagnosis of influenza infections, *J Clin Microbiol*, **24:** 907–12.

Waris M, 1991, Pattern of respiratory syncytial virus epidemics in Finland: two-year cycles with alternating prevalence of groups A and B, *J Infect Dis*, **163:** 464–9.

Waris M, Ziegler T et al., 1990, Rapid detection of respiratory syncytial virus and influenza A virus in cell cultures by immunoperoxidase staining with monoclonal antibodies, *J Clin Microbiol*, **28:** 1159–62.

White LA, Ades EW, 1990, Growth of Vero E6 cells on microcarriers in a cell bioreactor, *J Clin Microbiol*, **28:** 283–6.

White LA, Freeman CY et al., 1986, In vitro effect of ascorbic acid on infectivity of herpesviruses and paramyxoviruses, *J Clin Microbiol*, **24:** 527–31.

Wilber JC, 1993, Development and use of laboratory tests for hepatitis C infection: a review, *J Clin Immunoassay*, **16:** 204–7.

Wilchek M, Miron T, Kohn J, 1984, Affinity chromatography, *Methods Enzymol*, **104:** 3–55.

Woods GL, Young A, 1988, Use of A-549 cells in a clinical virology laboratory, *J Clin Microbiol*, **26:** 1026–8.

Yasukawa M, Yakushijin Y et al., 1993, Specificity analysis of human CD4+ T-cell clones directed against human herpesvirus 6 (HHV-6), HHV-7, and human cytomegalovirus, *J Virol*, **67:** 6259–64.

Ylitalo N, Bergstrom T, Gyllenstein U, 1995, Detection of genital human papillomavirus by single-tube nested PCR and type-specific oligonucleotide hybridization, *J Clin Microbiol*, **33:** 1822–8.

Ziegler T, Hall H et al., 1995, Type- and subtype-specific detection of influenza viruses in clinical specimens by rapid culture assay, *J Clin Microbiol*, **33:** 318–21.

THE REPLICATION OF VIRUSES

T H Pennington

1 Initiation of infection	**3 Genome replication**
2 Virus macromolecular synthesis: viral genome strategies	**4 Virion assembly**

Viruses are obligate intracellular parasites. At all stages of replication their virions, genomes and genome-coded macromolecules interact with cellular structures, and their pathways of macromolecular synthesis make extensive use of host organelles, structures, enzymes and host cell pools of building blocks for macromolecular synthesis.

These events can be divided into a number of stages. Thus after the binding of surface components of the virus to receptors on the surface of the host cell the virus crosses or fuses with the cell membrane to enter the cytoplasm. Expression of the virus genome then follows either in cytoplasm or in nucleus; this may require transcription, i.e. the synthesis of virus messenger RNA (mRNA) with postsynthetic processing of the mRNA molecules by either host- or virus-directed mechanisms. Although universal, the type and extent of processing differs from virus to virus. Translation of mRNA to form virus proteins then follows. Protein synthesis resembles mRNA synthesis in that further processing of the macromolecular product is very common, virus proteins often being modified by proteolytic cleavage or the addition of sugar groups, for example. Host mechanisms are often used to carry out the various processing steps. Whereas the signals for postsynthetic processing of RNA and proteins often reside in their nucleotide or amino acid sequences, the processing events themselves are often carried out by host machinery. The last category of virus-induced macromolecular synthesis – genome synthesis – is clearly very distinct from that of the uninfected host in its scale, timing and, in many cases, cellular site, a considerable number of viruses undergoing their entire growth cycle in the cytoplasm, although some virus genomes do enter into very close relationships with host chromosomes. Virion assembly and release ends the virus growth cycle. Even in the simplest case of automatic self-assembly, the concentration of virion precursor mol-

ecules in particular parts of the cell and the provision of a controlled intracellular environment play key roles in optimizing the process. All enveloped viruses incorporate cell membrane into their virions, and all viruses gain release from the cell through disruptive or more subtle interactions with the cell membrane.

1 INITIATION OF INFECTION

1.1 Viral ligands

The first event in the infection of a cell by a virus is the attachment of the virus particle to the cell surface. Attachment is specific, and is mediated by the binding of virion surface structures, ligands, to receptors on the cell surface. Virions are much simpler than cell surfaces, and in consequence more is known about the virion ligands than the cell receptors. For enveloped viruses the classic and best understood model is the influenza virus (Wiley and Skehel 1987). A virion surface glycoprotein, the haemagglutinin, binds specifically to sialic acid residues of cell membrane glycoproteins. The arrangement of the haemagglutinin in the virus particle and its sequence have been established, and its 3-dimensional structure has been studied in detail down to the atomic level. The receptor-binding site is a pocket composed of the side chains of amino acids. It is located near the tip of the rod-shaped molecule. The amino acid sequence of this region of the haemagglutinin is largely conserved in different virus strains, unlike the residues in other parts of the molecule. Other enveloped viruses resemble influenza in that their surface glycoproteins also serve as ligands.

The concentration of research activity on human immunodeficiency virus (HIV) has made this one of the best-characterized viruses. It is enveloped, and conforms to the general rule in that its exposed surface glycoprotein, gp120, acts as the ligand when attachment to the host cell surface takes place. It binds to the CD4 60 kDa glycoprotein on the surface of mature T lymphocytes, the interaction with CD4 being with a region or regions in the carboxy terminal half of gp120.

The ligands of non-enveloped viruses have in general proved to be difficult to study, and in the case of some of the larger DNA viruses have not yet been fully characterized at the molecular level. As a general rule, the receptor-binding structures of icosahedral viruses are situated at the vertices of the icosahedron, either as easily identifiable discrete structures, such as the fibres of adenoviruses, or as less morphologically obvious structural entities, such as the α1 polypeptide of reoviruses. This polypeptide has been identified as a ligand by genetic and biochemical techniques. The x-ray crystallographic determination of the 3-dimensional virion structure of human rhinovirus and poliovirus at the atomic resolution level has shown that the peak at each of the 12 vertices of the icosahedral virion is surrounded by a pronounced groove, 2.4 nm deep and 1.2–1.3 nm wide, and termed a 'canyon' by its describers. It has been proposed that the receptor-binding sites for these viruses are located on the walls and floor of the canyon.

1.2   Cell surface receptors

A very wide range of cell surface structures serve as virus receptors (Table 6.1) (Wimmer 1994). Some generalizations can be made: many viruses have been shown to use structures that have physiological roles in the normal host, including cell recognition and adhesion and hormone receptors. Members of the same virus family do not always use similar receptors, and some species use more than one type of cell receptor for attachment. Most receptors so far described are glycoproteins. The presence of the appropriate receptors on the cell surface is a prerequisite for virus attachment and subsequent infection, and receptor availability and distribution often play a key role in pathogenesis. A classic demonstration of their importance has been provided by the observation that the inability of poliovirus to infect non-primate cells – which is determined by a lack of receptors on these cells – can be overcome if the cells are infected with intact virion RNA. Infectious in its own right, poliovirus RNA crosses cell membranes without showing any particular specificity (Nomoto, Koikes and Aoki 1994).

The initial attachment of virus to cell is largely temperature- and energy-independent. Attachment rates vary over a wide range according to the virus–cell system under study but can be very rapid. The effect of ionic composition on attachment indicates that electrostatic attraction is important in enhancing the optimum binding of virus to cell. In the case of influenza virus, hydrogen bonding and van der Waals contacts are involved. Dissection of subsequent events at the cell surface has shown that the initial interaction is followed by secondary changes in which binding

Table 6.1   Cell receptors for viruses

Family and virus	Receptor
Adenoviridae	
Adenovirus type 2	Integrins $\alpha_v\beta_3$, α_v, β_s
Coronaviridae	
Human coronavirus	Aminopeptidase N
Mouse hepatitis virus	N-acetyl-9-O-acetylneuraminic acid Carcinoembryonic antigens
Herpesviridae	
Herpes simplex virus	Heparan sulphate moeity of proteoglycans
Cytomegalovirus	
Pseudorabies virus	
Epstein–Barr virus	Type 2 complement receptor
Orthomyxoviridae	
Influenza A, B	Sialic acid on glycoproteins and gangliosides
Influenza C	N-acetyl-9-O-acetylneuraminic acid
Paramyxoviridae	
Paramyxoviruses	Sialic acid on glycoproteins and gangliosides
Measles	Membrane co-factor protein (CD46 antigen), moesin
Parvoviridae	
Parvovirus B19	Erythrocyte P antigen
Picornaviridae	
Echovirus type 1	Integrin VLA-2 (α_2 β_1)
Rhinoviruses	ICAM-1
Poxviridae	
Vaccinia virus	EGF receptor
Retroviridae	
HIV	CD4 glycoprotein, galactosyl ceramide
Gibbon ape leukaemia virus	Phosphate permease
Rhabdoviridae	
Rabies virus	Acetycholine receptor (α-1)
Togaviridae	
Sindbis	High affinity laminin receptor

becomes irreversible. These are usually temperature-sensitive in that they occur optimally at physiological temperatures. They are often characterized by conformational changes in viral ligands. Thus in HIV alterations occur in the antibody-binding sites and protease sensitivity of gp120. Similar postadsorption changes in the polio virion are termed eclipse, when it changes its antigenic structure and protease sensitivity, loses a minor polypeptide component, VP4, and extrudes the amino terminus of VPI, another virion polypeptide.

1.3 Entry into the host cell

Attachment is followed by penetration and uncoating. Viruses use one of 4 mechanisms to enter cells. Some non-enveloped viruses enter by translocation of the whole virus particle across the cell membrane. They are then uncoated in the cytoplasm. More commonly, viruses enter cells by endocytosis (engulfment by the invagination of a section of plasma membrane) with the accumulation of virus particles in cytoplasmic vesicles and their subsequent uncoating. Enveloped viruses can also enter by endocytosis of the virion, but differ from non-enveloped viruses in that their envelopes then fuse with the membranes of the endosomes. Direct fusion of the virion envelope with the surface membrane of the cells also takes place with some viruses.

It is not understood how intact virus particles move directly through cell membranes. It is possible that endocytosis leading to the accumulation of virions in vesicles in the cytoplasm may be mediated by the same mechanisms that are responsible for receptor-mediated endocytosis. This occurs with a wide range of non-viral ligands, including hormones and lipoproteins. Ligand binding to a specific receptor is followed by migration of the ligand–receptor complex to particular regions of the cell membrane (coated pits) and the internalization of the complexes in specialized vesicles coated with a protein called clathrin. Clathrin is a large multicomponent molecule made up of one heavy and several light chains. These molecules form a cage-like lattice around the vesicle, which, however, breaks down shortly after endocytosis. The multi-step nature of binding and internalization is illustrated by adenovirus (Fig. 6.1). Its initial high-affinity bonding to a 50 kDa cell surface protein is mediated by the fibre protein. The penton base then interacts with cell α_v integrins through its RGD sequences (Arg–Gly–Asp). Internalization follows. Integrins are divalent cation-dependent heterodimeric cell surface receptors that mediate cell–cell and cell–extracellular matrix interactions and communications between the extracellular environment and the cytoskeleton.

1.4 Fusion with cell membranes

After attachment, the genome of an enveloped virus is separated from the cytoplasm of the cell by 2 membranes, that of the virus and that of the cell. Virion envelope glycoproteins with fusion activity mediate the penetration of these barriers by causing melding of the 2 phospholipid bilayers and mixing of the aqueous compartments previously separated by them. In some viruses a specialized glycoprotein is responsible for fusion. The Sendai virus F protein is the best understood model of this type. It is synthesized as an inactive precursor, F_0, which becomes active after proteolytic cleavage to 2 chains, F_1 and F_2. A conformational change then takes place that increases the hydrophobicity of the molecule. The cleavage is catalysed by host proteases, and their availability in cells is important in determining the pathogenicity of paramyxoviruses. The fusion activity of these viruses is distinctive in that it is active externally and does not require prior endocytosis. Retroviruses and herpesviruses also fuse directly with the plasma membrane. For orthomyxoviruses, rhabdoviruses, alphaviruses and flaviviruses, endocytosis and engulfment in vesicles comprise a necessary precursor to fusion, its onset being triggered by a reduction of pH in the vesicle, or endosome. This type of fusion activity is not mediated by a protein with a single specialized activity but is carried out by the virion glycoprotein, which also acts as the ligand during attachment to the cell. Thus, for example, the influenza virus haemagglutinin also mediates fusion. As in the case of the Sendai virus F polypeptide, cleavage of this molecule into 2 chains, HA_1 and HA_2, is a prerequisite for fusion activity. Exposure of HA_2 to the low pH of the endosomal interior, produced by a vesicular proton ATPase which pumps protons into the endosome, causes a conformational change that leaves the hydrophobic portion more exposed and more interactive with membranes. The sequence of this region is analogous to the N terminal sequence of the Sendai virus F_1 fusion peptide. It is not known how fusion proteins work. Any general explanation will have to account for the fact that their interaction with membrane bilayers overcomes the hydration force which in normal circumstances causes membranes to repel each other vigorously when they approach at distances less than 2 nm.

1.5 Uncoating

The uncoating of non-enveloped viruses in the cell cytoplasm or in vesicles is also a poorly understood process (Greber, Singh and Helenius 1994). This is because the events are difficult to study experimentally. It is assumed that interaction of the virion with host components and enzymes leads to a breakdown of the virion and exposure of the genome in a form suitable for primary transcription. Proteolytic enzymes within lysosomes probably play a key role. Their effects can be mimicked in vitro in experimental systems, and the uncoating of reovirus illustrates this particularly well. In the lysosome, 2 virion proteins are removed and one is partially degraded, transcription then being activated. The same sequence of events follows the treatment of virions with chymotrypsin in vitro.

The uncoating of enveloped viruses can readily be mimicked in vitro by treating the virions with non-ionic detergents. These reagents rupture and solubilize the virion envelope by interacting with the hydrophobic parts of the proteins and lipids, causing them to become inserted into detergent micelles. The virion nucleocapsid is thus released. If it possesses a transcriptase, the enzyme becomes active and will start to synthesize virus mRNA as soon as nucleoside triphosphates are added.

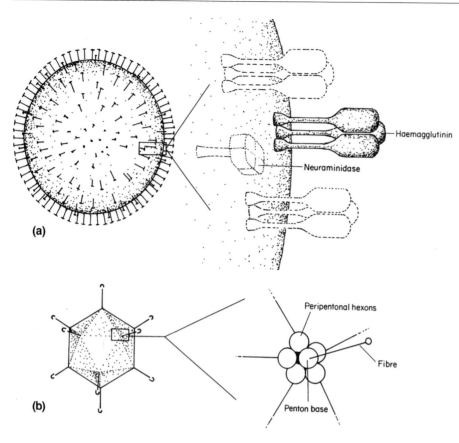

(a)

(b)

— Haemagglutinin

— Neuraminidase

Peripentonal hexons

Fibre

Penton base

Fig. 6.1 Diagrammatic representation of structures that act as ligands during virus attachment. (a) The influenza virus haemagglutinin binds to sialic acid molecules on host cell surface glycoproteins and is a typical example of the spike-like proteins that are found on the surface of all enveloped viruses. (b) The adenovirus fibre is a particularly striking example of a ligand situated at the vertex of an icosahedral virus particle; other examples of similarly situated ligands are the 'canyons' that surround the vertices of picornavirus particles and the σ1 polypeptides of reoviruses.

2   VIRUS MACROMOLECULAR SYNTHESIS: VIRAL GENOME STRATEGIES

Viruses have adopted a number of different strategies for the expression of their genes and the replication of their genomes. Certain cellular mechanisms and pathways are used by some but not by other viruses: thus most DNA viruses use cell transcriptases located in the nucleus to generate mRNAs, and similarly situated DNA polymerases for genome replication, whereas other DNA viruses, notably the poxviruses, use a different strategy which includes mRNA synthesis by virion-bound transcriptases and polymerases, allowing them to synthesize both mRNAs and genomes in the cytoplasm. Most RNA viruses, with the exception of retroviruses whose genomes can be copied into DNA, synthesize virus-specific mRNAs in the cytoplasm using virus-encoded enzymes.

The relationship between viral mRNA and the virus genome is a central one in virus replication and forms one of the key points in the classification of viruses. Baltimore's (1971) scheme for the grouping of viruses divides them into classes based on the pathways of mRNA synthesis and the nature of the virus genome. A modified version is presented in Fig. 6.2. For RNA viruses a central feature of this scheme is the assignment of viruses with single-stranded genomes to positive- or negative-strand classes. In the former the genome sequence can be translated directly into virus proteins, the virion genomes being mRNA in sense. Negative-strand genomes are anti-mRNA in sense and

must be transcribed into complementary form for information transfer into protein to occur. Because cells cannot synthesize RNA molecules from RNA templates, negative-strand viruses undertake this task themselves and their virions contain transcriptases that are taken into the cell to initiate virus macromolecular synthesis.

2.1   DNA viruses

Viruses with complete double-stranded DNA fall into 2 groups. The majority of viruses belong to families (*Papovaviridae, Adenoviridae, Herpesviridae*) whose members use the host nucleus for mRNA synthesis and genome replication, relying on host enzymes for transcription. After entry of the virus and uncoating, virus DNA moves into the nucleus from the cytoplasm without modification. One family of viruses with complete double-stranded DNA, the poxviruses, is distinct in that replication takes place in the cytoplasm. The virus codes for its own RNA and DNA polymerases and produces functional mRNAs without requiring any cell nuclear functions. RNA polymerase molecules are incorporated into virions as they are assembled and are used for early macromolecular synthesis during the next cycle of infection. The presence of RNA polymerase in the virion is an obligatory requirement for the initiation of infection, and naked poxvirus DNA – unlike that of papovaviruses, adenoviruses and herpesviruses – is not infectious when extracted from virions.

The DNA of the hepadnaviruses is incorporated into virions in a partially double-stranded form.

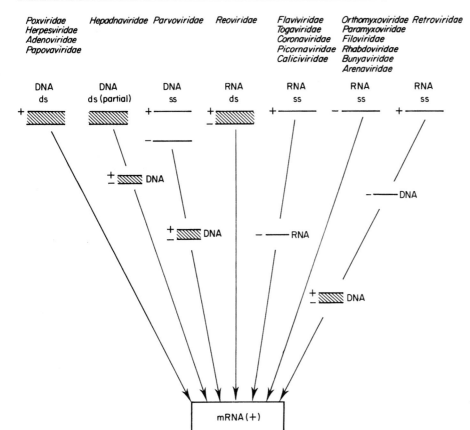

Fig. 6.2 Grouping of viruses by genome composition and pathway of mRNA synthesis.

Completion of the duplex molecule by a virion-associated DNA polymerase enzyme occurs in the cytoplasm before the mature DNA enters the nucleus to be transcribed by host transcriptase. Circovirus and parvovirus virions contain a single-stranded DNA molecule that moves directly into the nucleus after uncoating. It is then converted into duplex molecules and transcribed by host enzymes.

2.2 RNA viruses

Reoviruses contain a genome consisting of double-stranded segmented RNA. Messenger RNA is produced by conservative transcription catalysed by a set of virion enzymes. Virus replication takes place in the cytoplasm and has no host enzyme requirements.

Picornaviruses, togaviruses and flaviviruses contain a single strand of positive-strand RNA that has mRNA activity. This RNA is infectious by itself and is translated into protein immediately after uncoating in the cytoplasm. Picornaviruses use complete virus RNA as mRNA throughout the virus growth cycle, the individual protein being first synthesized as a single long polypeptide strand which is then cleaved to give the different functional proteins. Togaviruses synthesize at least 2 forms of mRNA, one being the same length as the virion RNA and the other being equivalent to the third of the virion RNA at the 3' end.

Most RNA viruses with single-stranded negative-sense genomes replicate in the cytoplasm. The RNA of these viruses is incapable of initiating infection by itself and the virions contain a transcriptase that starts to synthesize functional mRNA soon after the virion envelope has fused with cell membranes, allowing the virus nucleocapsid to enter the cytoplasm. The genomes of these viruses may consist of a single molecule (paramyxoviruses, filoviruses and rhabdoviruses) or may be segmented (arenaviruses, bunyaviruses and influenza viruses). All viruses with segmented negative-strand genomes require a functional cell nucleus for replication, and initiate transcription by using capped oligonucleotide primers derived from the 5' ends of cell mRNA or mRNA precursors, which are spliced onto the 5' end of the virus mRNA. This phenomenon, known as 'cap-snatching', occurs also during the replication of certain plant viruses (e.g. the tenuiviruses, which have a segmented negative-strand RNA genome).

Retroviruses resemble DNA viruses in that transcription takes place from double-stranded virus DNA molecules situated in the nucleus and requires cellular DNA-dependent RNA polymerases. Virions possess a reverse transcriptase that copies the diploid RNA genome into a single DNA strand, which it then converts into a duplex molecule. These double-stranded DNA molecules then enter the nucleus and integrate into host chromosomes. Transcription by host enzymes then occurs.

2.3 Messenger RNA synthesis and processing

Cellular mRNA is synthesized in the nucleus. Primary transcripts undergo a good deal of modification there before they move into the cytoplasm for translation. Viruses differ in the use that they make of host enzymes for transcription and transcript modification. Viruses that use the nucleus for replicative processes have access to the enzymes there, whereas viruses that replicate exclusively in the cytoplasm must adopt alternative strategies because RNA-directed RNA synthesis and cytoplasmic transcription and transcript processing do not occur in the eukaryotic cell. Despite these constraints the structure of viral mRNAs closely resembles that of normal eukaryotic cells. Viruses have played a key role as model systems in elucidation of the mechanisms responsible for mRNA synthesis and processing, their relative simplicity and ease of biochemical access contrasting sharply with the complexity of the cell nucleus. Noteworthy examples of viruses that have served as particularly useful paradigms are SV40 and adenovirus (for the study of nuclear events) and vaccinia virus, which, as a large DNA virus with a largely cytoplasmic replication cycle and a great degree of enzymatic independence from host macromolecular synthesis pathways, has been aptly described a 'wandering nucleus'.

In summary, the main features of the production of biologically active fully processed cell and virus mRNA are:

1   The initiation of transcription by a DNA-dependent or RNA-dependent RNA polymerase, the first nucleotide of the primary transcript becoming the first nucleotide of the mRNA.
2   The addition of a methylated cap structure or a virus-specific protein (VPg) at the 5′ end of the primary transcript.
3   The addition of a poly(A) sequence at the 3′ hydroxyl end of the transcript.
4   For some mRNAs produced in the cell nucleus, the removal of one or more parts of the transcript known as introns – and the splicing together of the remaining parts known as exons – to form the biologically active mRNA molecule.

2.4 Capping and polyadenylation of mRNAs

For the synthesis of an mRNA molecule in the uninfected cell the RNA polymerase in the nucleus is guided by the promoter (see section 2.5) to start transcription at the nucleotide to which the methylated cap is added. The cap consists of a terminal nucleotide, 7-methylguanylate (m^7G) in a 5′–5′ linkage with the initial nucleotide of the mRNA chain. It probably plays an important role in the translation of mRNA to protein; the precise details of this have not yet been fully worked out. The biosynthesis of the cap is catalysed by a series of enzymes, which include methyltransferases. Viruses that replicate in the cytoplasm

use their own enzymes to cap their mRNA; indeed one virus, vaccinia virus, has for technical reasons played a key role as a particularly suitable model for the study of cap biosynthesis (Moss 1995). Vaccinia virus is a large DNA virus which itself codes for the individual enzymes needed for processing of the termini of mRNA molecules. Its mRNA capping enzyme also illustrates the general principle that virus gene products are often multifunctional because it also acts as a transcription termination factor in early mRNA synthesis and an initiation factor during the transcription of intermediate genes. Other viruses with much smaller genomes have adopted different strategies for mRNA processing. Vesicular stomatitis virus (VSV), for example, has a single-stranded 11 kb RNA genome that is transcribed by a ribonucleoprotein complex. This contains only one protein with enzyme activity, the L protein, which, it is thought, catalyses transcription as well as possessing methyltransferase activity and poly(A) polymerase activity.

The location of the poly(A) addition site in mRNA molecules is probably determined by sequences both upstream and downstream of the site itself. Particularly important are the strongly conserved consensus sequence AAUAAA situated 15–30 nucleotides (nt) upstream and sequences starting c. 12 nt downstream. Termination of transcription by RNA polymerase in uninfected cells occurs downstream of all these sequences and is probably determined by other conserved sequences.

2.5 The control of mRNA synthesis

The array of mRNA molecules in a cell determines the kind and amount of different proteins synthesized in that cell. Control of the synthesis of these macromolecules is exerted in a number of different ways, transcriptional control playing a central role. Promoters in DNA molecules are sequences situated within 100 base pairs (bp) upstream of the mRNA start site. The integrity of these sequences is important in determining the precise site of transcription initiation and its frequency. Often 2 or 3 short sequences, sequence elements, act as promoters. The most important of these is the highly conserved TATA sequence – the TATA box (Fig. 6.3). This usually starts about 30 bases upstream of the initiation site. If the TATA box is moved, the initiation site also moves so that the 30 bp separation is maintained, showing that a link exists between the position of these sites on the DNA molecule in terms of transcriptional control. Removal or alteration of the sequence of parts of the TATA box stops, or drastically decreases, transcription. Other sequences upstream of the TATA box, including CCAAT and GC boxes, also act as promoters.

Enhancers resemble promoters at the molecular level in that they are made up of arrays of conserved sequence elements, or motifs. They differ from them in that their influence on transcription is essentially independent of position or orientation relative to the initiation site of transcription. In a sense, although *cis-*

-30   -20   -10 mRNA start site

TATA box

GGGCTATAAAGGGGGTGGGGGGGCGTTCGTCCTCA

Fig. 6.3 The adenovirus major late promoter.

acting (influencing transcription from the molecule in which they are situated), they exert remote control. Enhancers are typically about 200 bp long, even in viruses, where genome size is clearly restricted by structural constraints. Indeed, cytomegalovirus enhancers 400–700 bp in length are the strongest in terms of influence and the longest found so far. Length seems to be an important feature of enhancers, and they are often constructed in modular fashion, the complete structure being made up of a combination of different sequence elements or multiple copies of the same element. Much of our knowledge of enhancers has been obtained by work on viruses, one in the SV40 genome being the first to be discovered. It is made up of two 72 bp repeat sequences situated next to the SV40 early promoter. Manipulation of these sequences has shown that one of the two 72 bp elements can be removed without loss of activity and that enhancement is produced whether the elements are inserted in a 5'–3' or a 3'–5' orientation. How enhancers exert their remote control is not known. Experimental work with the adenoviruses has shown, however, that the enhancer function can be replaced by a protein. The adenovirus early gene *E1A* is the first gene to be expressed during infection, and its products are required for the expression of the other mRNAs that are synthesized early in infection. If genes normally requiring an enhancer for their expression are introduced without the enhancer sequence into cells expressing gene *E1A,* gene expression occurs as efficiently as if the enhancer were present. Indeed, during the normal process of infection, gene *E1A* not only plays its role in the control of adenovirus gene expression but also causes the activation of normal host genes, including, for example, the 70 kDa heat shock gene.

Interactions between promoter and enhancer sequences and proteins such as RNA polymerases and those with enhancer-like functions play central roles in transcriptional control. Although a good deal is known about the nucleic acid sequences and the proteins, particularly in certain model systems, the basic rules that underlie their interactions are still proving to be elusive and difficult to understand.

2.6 Virus mRNA synthesis: RNA polymerases

Two categories of enzyme catalyse the synthesis of virus mRNA. Host RNA polymerase II is used by viruses whose duplex DNA genomes are transcribed in the nucleus. Cytoplasmic transcription from RNA genomes, the DNA genome of poxviruses, and the transcription of orthomyxovirus genomes are carried out by viral RNA polymerases.

Sequence analysis of RNA polymerases from eukaryotic cells and from DNA and RNA viruses shows homologies between these diverse enzymes, including the canonical GDD (Gly–Asp–Asp) sequence. Sequence homologies are not uniform, conserved domains being interspersed with non-homologous regions. The GDD tripeptide sequence is also found in plant and bacterial virus RNA polymerases and reverse transcriptases, and it has been suggested that it plays a role in the recognition of template nucleic acids. Comparison of the amino acid sequence of the largest subunit of the vaccinia virus RNA polymerase shows homologies in 5 domains with yeast RNA polymerases II and III and *Escherichia coli* RNA polymerase, and another homology just with yeast. The most highly conserved sequence is NADFDGD (Asn–Ala–Asp–Phe–Asp–Gly–Asp), which has also been found in the largest subunit of *Drosophila* RNA polymerase II.

Smaller viruses use a significant proportion of their genomes to code for RNA polymerases. Thus 19.5% of the poliovirus genome, 49.3% of the influenza virus genome, 54.5% of the Sendai virus genome and 62.7% of the VSV genome is used for this purpose (Ishihama and Nagata 1988). The RNA-dependent RNA polymerase of VSV was the first enzyme of this type to be discovered as a virion component and has been studied in detail (Banerjee 1987). Treatment of the virus with a non-ionic detergent strips off its envelope and leaves a ribonucleoprotein that actively engages in transcription if provided with the 4 ribonucleoside 5'-triphosphates. The ribonucleoprotein is composed of 1200 molecules of polypeptide N, which has a structural role, 500 molecules of polypeptide NS, which is a phosphoprotein known to serve a stoichiometric but otherwise undefined role in RNA synthesis, and 50 molecules of polypeptide L, the RNA polymerase itself. L also possesses methyltransferase and poly(A) polymerase activities and thereby can synthesize mature biologically active mRNA molecules without any host cell enzyme requirement. The host cytoskeleton seems to play an enhancing role in RNA synthesis, however, in that tubulin and microtubule-associated protein promote transcription in vitro. L has 2109 amino acid residues and a mol. wt of 241 kDa, and so is about 5 times larger than the average-sized polypeptide. Other negative-strand viruses have RNA polymerases of similar sizes.

An even greater degree of complexity is shown by the vaccinia virus RNA polymerase, which has 7 subunits and a mol. wt in excess of 500 kDa.

2.7 Patterns of information transfer from viral genome via mRNA to protein

Not long after the firm establishment of nucleic acids as the repositories of genetic information, Crick and Watson predicted that viruses would use information in a parsimonious fashion when constructing their virions, and would do so by the use of repeating identical protein subunits. Unsuspected at that time was the extent to which some viruses exploit the triplet genetic code for information storage and retrieval by using overlapping genes, gene splicing at mRNA level and different translational reading frames. A virus that employs all 3 devices is the small DNA virus, SV40. Early in infection 2 SV40 proteins are synthesized, large T antigen (81 kDa) and small T antigen (20 kDa). The mRNAs coding for these proteins share sequences for the first 246 bases. Large T mRNA undergoes splicing at this point, the next 345 bases forming an intron that is removed to allow the mature molecule to be formed by joining the 5′ exon with a 3′ 1879-base exon synthesized in a different reading frame. The synthesis of small T mRNA continues uninterrupted past the splice point until it terminates 276 bases downstream.

Overlapping genes and gene splicing are characteristic of many DNA viruses (Sharp 1994). The mRNA splicing machinery is located in the nucleus and, as no virus seems to have evolved the ability to carry out this process independently, it is restricted to viruses with a nuclear phase in replication. Gene splicing is universal among adenovirus mRNAs, and most papovavirus mRNAs are processed similarly. Only a minority of herpesvirus mRNAs seem to undergo splicing. Among RNA viruses, some retrovirus and influenza virus mRNAs are also spliced. Influenza virus also has overlapping genes and uses more than one reading frame to synthesize proteins from 2 of its 8 RNA segments. In each case one protein is encoded in a continuous reading frame extending for much of the length of the RNA segment, whereas the other protein shares only a short sequence run at the 5′ end of the gene, this portion of the mRNA being spliced to another molecule copied from the 3′ end in a different reading frame.

Some viruses further exploit and expand the limited coding potential of their genomes by using a single mRNA to code for more than one protein. Thus the mRNA specifying the polymerase-associated Sendai virus P protein contains the information for a small non-structural component, protein C, embedded within its sequence in a different reading frame. Other RNA and DNA viruses also synthesize bifunctional mRNAs. The ability of one mRNA to direct the synthesis of 2 proteins has been explained by proposing that the initiation of translation can occur at 2 sites. It has been suggested (Kozak 1986) that the 40S ribosomal subunit binds at the 5′ end of the mRNA and migrates to the first AUG triplet. Initiation of synthesis takes place on some but not all mRNAs because this first initiation site is set in a less than optimal sequence context. The remaining ribosomes continue their migration down the molecule to initiate synthesis of the second protein at the next AUG triplet.

A frameshift change during translation is another mechanism that some viruses use to code for more than one protein from a single mRNA. In avian retroviruses, for example, the pol (reverse transcriptase) protein is produced by the cleavage of a precursor *gag–pol* polyprotein coded for by a single mRNA. The *gag* and *pol* sequences do not directly follow each other in the mRNA, however, but overlap and are in different reading frames. Most ribosomes translate the *gag* region only, but about 5% seem to shift reading frames near the end of the *gag* sequences and then continue translation, producing small amounts of the *gag–pol* protein. A similar process occurs during infection with the human immunodeficiency virus (HIV-1). Again, the viral *pol* gene and the upstream *gag* gene lie in different reading frames, with *pol* in the −1 frame with reference to *gag* and with the 3′ end of *gag* overlapping the 5′ end of *pol* by 205 nt. Efficient ribosomal frameshifting occurs at a UUA leucine codon near the 5′ end of the overlap, leading to the production of *gag* and *gag–pol* fusion proteins in the ratio of about 8:1, indicating a frameshifting efficiency of 11%. It occurs as a random event in normal eukaryotic mRNA at a frequency less than 5×10^{-5} per codon. High frequency specific frameshifting is primarily a viral phenomenon although it also happens in prokaryotes. Two mRNA structural features are essential for it to occur: a homopolymeric 'slippery sequence' of the general form XXXYYYZ; and a region a few nucleotides downstream which arranges itself as a stem–loop or a pseudoknot – a quasi-continuous double helix joined by single-strand connecting loops. A simple example is the overlap region between the 1a–1b open reading frames of human astrovirus serotype 1 (Fig. 6.4).

Most viral mRNAs are monocistronic. Several different mechanisms are used to achieve the punctuation of these mRNAs and the proteins whose synthesis they direct. Transcription in viruses with segmented genomes (reoviruses, orthomyxoviruses, bunyaviruses) is usually from end to end of the individual segments, or nearly so. Punctuation at transcriptional level with internal start and stop signals is common (poxviruses, herpesviruses, rhabdoviruses, paramyxoviruses), the size of an mRNA generally corresponding to the size of its protein.

Subgenomic truncated mRNAs are also common. In retroviruses, papovaviruses, parvoviruses and adenoviruses they are produced by splicing. Coronaviruses synthesize a family of 6 progressively shorter subgenomic mRNAs, with common 3′ sequences, and initiation at an internal promoter in togaviruses and parvoviruses produces subgenomic RNAs. Arenaviruses contain 2 genome RNA segments, each of which encodes a gene in the positive sense and an additional gene in the negative sense. For example,

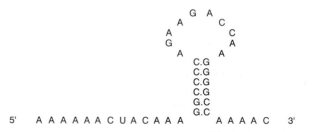

Fig. 6.4 Overlap region between the 1a–1b open reading frames of human astrovirus serotype 1.

from their S RNA genome segment, the virus glyco-protein is coded from the 5′ half of the segment with its mRNA in the positive sense, and the virus N protein is coded from the 3′ half with its mRNA in the negative sense.

Post-translational punctuation by proteolysis is used by picornaviruses. The genome of these viruses is translated entirely without punctuation into a polyprotein which, in a series of steps, is cut into functional proteins.

2.8 Patterns of viral mRNA and protein synthesis: quantitative and temporal controls

DNA VIRUSES

Wide variations in the amounts of different virus proteins are found when the infected cell is examined. Much, but not all, of this variation stems from comparable differences in the amount of functional mRNAs produced during infection. DNA viruses have much more complex patterns of mRNA synthesis and processing than RNA viruses, and the well studied model of adenovirus type 2 illustrates most of the important control mechanisms used by these viruses.

Adenovirus transcription is divided into 2 phases, early and late, by the time of onset of virus DNA replication. In the early phase, mRNAs are produced from 5 distinct regions of virus DNA: in 3 of these regions one strand of virus DNA is used as template; in the other 2 regions the opposite strand is transcribed. Transcription of each region leads to the production of several species of mRNA that have common capped 5′ termini differing in length and sequence as a result of splicing and polyadenylation of the primary transcript at different positions.

Most mRNAs produced late in infection also fall into 5 groups. In these cases, however, the groupings are based on the sharing of common sites of polyadenylation. All the RNAs seem to share a common 5′ terminal sequence formed by the splicing of 3 short regions of the primary transcript. This situation is shown diagrammatically in Fig. 6.5. The primary transcripts are initiated at position 16 and extend beyond the polyadenylation sites on occasions to the end of the genome at position 100. They are then nucleolytically processed, polyadenylated at one of the 5 specified sites, each of which is near an AAUAAA sequence, and finally spliced to generate the multiple messenger RNAs, all of which contain the same capped 5′ terminal sequence.

Virtually all the steps in the production line of mRNA synthesis are used by adenovirus as control points (Flint 1986). Thus the frequency of transcriptional initiation during the early phases of infection is controlled by the E1A protein. This is the first virus gene product to be synthesized in the infected cell, and has been termed a pre-early gene. Its presence greatly facilitates the transcription of the early transcription units.

Structural features of the DNA template from infecting virions prevent the transcription of late genes until DNA replication – and the production of new templates – has occurred. Individual mRNAs are selectively processed after synthesis by polyadenylation and splicing. Some early mRNAs have different degrees of stability. Finally, there is some evidence that the transport of mRNAs from nucleus to cytoplasm is selectively controlled in the infected cell; newly synthesized and processed host mRNA fails to leave the nucleus late in infection, in contrast to the viral mRNAs made at that time. The molecular basis of these control mechanisms is not understood, and, although obvious parallels for most of them exist with other DNA viruses, it is not possible to make generalizations except at the descriptive level. Thus the herpes simplex virus 4 gene plays a role similar to the adenovirus E1A protein as a transcriptional regulator. Its gene product, IE175, is expressed early in infection and is required for the expression of subsequent genes. It also has a negative effect on the expression of other early genes. It binds to promoter-regulatory domains and to the 5′ transcribed non-coding sequences of most viral genes. The details of how it works are not fully understood but it is known that a target sequence for its interaction with the genome is an AT-rich motif with the consensus sequence TAAT-GARATTC (R = purine).

As with adenovirus, an early–late switch activated by DNA replication is also a marked feature of gene expression in cells infected with papovaviruses and poxviruses, and some herpesvirus genes also stringently require viral DNA synthesis for their expression. In general, virus-coded gene products needed for virus DNA replication are synthesized early, and virion structural proteins are synthesized late.

Selective gene splicing is not a marked feature of herpesvirus mRNA synthesis, and is not available to poxviruses, which replicate only in the cytoplasm.

Herpesviruses and poxviruses resemble each other in possessing large genomes, in coding for many enzymes and in showing particularly complex patterns of gene expression superimposed on the early–late switch. With herpes simplex virus, for example, the sequential appearance of the α, β and γ classes of gene products during infection has been described as a cascade, α genes being switched on by a virion component, the α-*trans*-inducing factor, α gene products then inducing β genes, β gene products shutting off the expression of α genes and inducing the expression of γ genes, and γ gene products shutting off the expression of β genes. Of all gene products, only a subset of the γ genes fails to be expressed if viral DNA synthesis is blocked. β gene products are mostly involved in nucleic acid metabolism. A few of them, designated β_1, are expressed earlier than the majority, which fall into the β_2 class; γ proteins are heterogeneous with respect to the timing of their appearance. Most of them are virion structural components.

In the case of vaccinia virus, uncoating releases a virus core into the cytoplasm, activating the virion RNA polymerase which immediately starts to synthe-

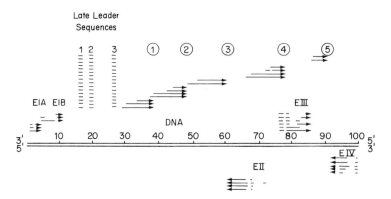

Fig. 6.5 Adenovirus messenger RNA (mRNA) synthesis. Different mRNAs are produced during the 'early' and 'late' stages of virus replication, before and after the onset of virus DNA synthesis respectively. The 'early' mRNAs are in 5 transcription units, designated E1A, E1B, EII, EIII and EIV, from each of which several different mRNAs are produced by splicing at different sites in the primary transcripts. 'Late' mRNAs form 5 groups (①–⑤) with the members of each group sharing a common poly(A) addition site. In addition, the mRNAs in all 5 groups have a common 5' capped sequence. The adenovirus genome can be divided into 100 units as shown and the common 5' capped sequence is derived from sequences at positions 16, 19 and 27, which together, by splicing, form the tripartite 5' leader sequences.

size functional capped and polyadenylated early mRNAs. About half the genome is transcribed before DNA replication starts. Some early genes are described as delayed because their expression requires prior virus protein synthesis. Early transcripts are initiated 10–15 bp upstream of the AUG start codon, and terminated at discrete sites downstream of the coding sequence, the sequence T_5NT (where N is any nucleotide) being an essential *cis*-acting element in this process. Termination occurs 50–70 bp downstream of this element. After DNA replication a dramatic change occurs in that nearly the whole genome is transcribed. Concatemeric intermediates are synthesized, resolved into unit length genomes and used as templates for the successive expression of intermediate and late genes. Late mRNAs seem to run through early genes, these late transcripts not having defined 3' ends, and mRNAs coding for a single protein vary enormously in length. Two temporal classes of late proteins have been identified, one being synthesized almost immediately after DNA synthesis and the other being delayed. Each temporal class of genes has its own distinctive promoter sequence that is recognized by specific viral proteins. Regulatory factors that act late include mRNA stability, which decreases during the course of infection, and a suppressor protein that acts at the translational level. Vaccinia virus genes are closely packed in the genome, transcription regulatory sequences for one gene being embedded in the coding sequences of adjacent genes. Early genes are often intermixed with late genes, and each DNA strand is able to serve as a template strand.

Vaccinia ranks as one of the largest viruses in terms of coding potential and of structural complexity of its virion, and enjoys more autonomy from host functions than do other viruses. Parvoviruses occupy a position at the opposite extreme. Some will grow only in cells already infected with another virus and are known as dependoviruses. Others are autonomous. DNA replication and gene expression by these viruses are entirely dependent on one or more cellular functions

transiently expressed during the S phase of the cell cycle. Their genomes are single-stranded, contain about 5000 bases and have only 2 major coding regions. These overlap and produce mRNAs that undergo splicing.

RNA VIRUSES

The pattern of gene expression of RNA viruses with positive-strand, negative-strand, segmented and entire genomes varies considerably both between and within these groups, and generalizations are difficult to make.

Positive-strand viruses

The 49S capped and polyadenylated genome of the positive-strand togaviruses (Fig. 6.6b) functions as an mRNA as it dissociates from the nucleocapsid in the cell cytoplasm at the beginning of infection. Translation proceeds for about two-thirds of the length of the RNA. The polyprotein that is produced is cleaved by proteases to form proteins that catalyse the replication of the genome RNA and the transcription from this molecule of further capped and polyadenylated 49S plus-strand molecules and a similarly processed subgenomic 26S mRNA which functions as the message for virus structural proteins. Temporal and quantitative regulation occur. The non-structural proteins coded by 49S RNA are mostly made early in infection. The bulk of virus-specific proteins made during infection are structural, however, and a 3-fold excess of 26S–49S RNA exists through most of the infectious cycle. As much of the 49S RNA becomes sequestered into nucleocapsids, the ratio of translationally active 26S to 49S molecules approaches 10:1.

Coronaviruses are also positive stranded but use subgenomic RNA molecules on a grander scale than do togaviruses (Fig. 6.6c). As in the coronaviruses, the capped and polyadenylated genome codes for RNA polymerase as the first synthetic event during infection. The negative-strand RNA synthesized by this enzyme then serves as a template for the synthesis of

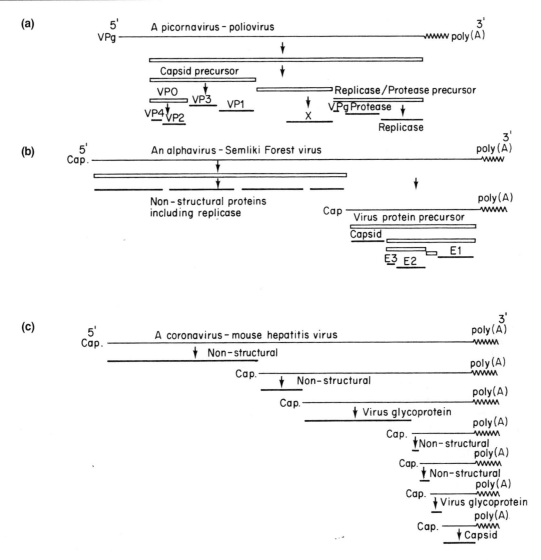

Fig. 6.6 Translation of plus-strand RNA virus mRNAs. (a) The genome RNAs of picornaviruses are translated into polypeptide precursors which are proteolytically processed to generate the enzymes and capsid proteins required for virus replication. The proteases involved seem to be virus-coded. (b) Alphavirus protein synthesis requires 2 mRNAs: virus RNA and a 3' terminal short RNA which contains the information for virion protein synthesis. The enzymes involved in virus RNA synthesis are produced by direct translation of virus RNA. (c) In coronavirus replication distinct mRNAs are produced for each virus-specific protein.

a nested set of 6 overlapping subgenomic RNAs with common 3' ends. These molecules are capped and polyadenylated but only their 5' ends are translated. Unequal amounts of these mRNAs are synthesized, but their relative proportions do not change during the infectious cycle.

The picornavirus positive strand is polyadenylated but carries a covalently linked small virus-encoded protein at its 5' end (Fig. 6.6a). It contains a single long reading frame encoding a long polypeptide chain. This polyprotein is cleaved during translation so that the full length protein is not generally formed. A cascade of cleavages catalysed by at least 2 different virus-coded proteases follows, generating about 12 proteins. Subsequent RNA synthesis increases the number of plus strands in the cell. They are either used as mRNA or are packaged into virions. Subgenomic RNAs are not synthesized by picornaviruses.

Negative-strand viruses

Vesicular stomatitis virus, a rhabdovirus, possesses a virion transcriptase that works particularly well in vitro, so this virus has been widely studied as a model negative-strand virus with cytoplasmic replication (Banerjee 1987). Entry of the ribonucleoprotein of the virus into the cytoplasm leads to the onset of transcription. The synthesis of a 47 nt leader RNA is followed by the sequential synthesis of capped and polyadenylated mRNAs coding for proteins N, NS, M, G and L, an order corresponding to the order of genes on the genome. The transcription of each gene requires the transcription of all 3' proximal genes, and the amount synthesized decreases with increasing distance from the 3' end of the genome. This pattern of synthesis is followed throughout infection and no translational controls have been described.

Influenza virus transcription involves both host and virus RNA polymerases. Transcription of the 8 RNAs occurs in the nucleus; the mRNAs produced are capped and polyadenylated. However, although virus particles contain RNA transcriptase activity, they do not have enzymes responsible for capping. Instead, they contain an endonuclease that seems to generate capped primers c. 12 nt in length from nuclear DNA transcripts synthesized by RNA polymerase II. These primers are used to initiate the virus transcripts and, as a consequence, each virus mRNA contains a capped 5′ terminal extension, heterogeneous in sequence and derived from nuclear DNA transcripts. As in VSV transcription, polyadenylation at the 3′ terminus of mRNAs is signalled by U-rich sequences that are present 16 nt before the 5′ terminus of the template RNAs. In addition to 8 mRNAs, which are co-linear with their 8 RNA templates, 3 more capped and polyadenylated virus-specific mRNAs are produced from transcripts of the 2 smallest virus RNAs by splicing. Primary transcription from the infecting influenza virus gene is unregulated. Secondary transcription from newly synthesized template RNAs shows a degree of temporal regulation in that mRNAs coding for internal proteins are preferentially synthesized early in replication and surface protein mRNAs are more prominent in the late stages. Polypeptide abundances are similar. It is not known how these changes are regulated.

Double-stranded RNA viruses

Reoviruses are the best studied. Their segmented genomes are transcribed by a virion polymerase, the mRNAs being complete transcripts of each segment. These mRNAs are capped by a virion enzyme. mRNAs active in eukaryotic cells are extremely unusual in not being polyadenylated. Transcription frequency is in general inversely related to the size of the genome segments. The amounts of protein synthesized in the infected cell are controlled by the amount of mRNA and also by differences in the frequency with which each mRNA is translated. The mRNAs synthesized early by the virion polymerase of infecting viral particles are capped whereas those synthesized at later times by progeny virions are uncapped. There seems to be a host cell shift from cap-dependent to cap-independent mRNA translation, thus favouring virus protein synthesis.

2.9   Protein synthesis, transport and processing

Effect of viruses on host protein synthesis

Viruses make full use of the host cell machinery for protein synthesis and exploit the pathways provided by the cell for protein transport and post-translational modification. In using the cellular machinery for these events viruses compete with their host, and many viruses have developed mechanisms that allow them to dominate and usurp the cellular apparatus. Subver-

sion of the cell by the virus in this way is of particular interest to the medical virologist because the lethal consequences for the cell account in many instances for the ability of the virus to cause disease, as in the classic example of poliovirus which causes paralysis by killing anterior horn cells in the spinal cord and other parts of the CNS. On the other hand, cells have evolved defence mechanisms against viruses that are designed to inhibit the translation of virus proteins, and these are also of considerable interest both as naturally occurring defence mechanisms and as examples of pathways that the designer of antiviral strategies might follow. Viruses use many different mechanisms to turn off host cell protein synthesis selectively (Schneider and Shenk 1987). These can be divided into 2 main types: mechanisms that attack host-specific factors, and others that selectively favour the virus.

Large DNA viruses such as poxviruses and herpesviruses directly affect host mRNA by coding for factors that rapidly degrade these macromolecules. Herpes simplex virus virions, for example, contain one or more factors that shut off host protein synthesis, causing the disruption of host polyribosomes and accelerating the turnover of cellular mRNA. It is not known how such factors discriminate between virus and host mRNA. The translation of normal host mRNA requires initiation factors, and some viruses cause these to be completely or partially inactivated. As the virus mRNA in these cases either does not need the factor in question or is inherently translated very efficiently, the virus gains with respect to the cell.

Viruses with mRNAs that are similar to those of the host and are not handled in any special way by host ribosomes can effectively compete by being abundant; well studied examples of this simple way of achieving dominance have been described. Some virus mRNAs have structural features that favour them over host molecules. The messengers of some picornaviruses, for example, initiate translation more efficiently than do host molecules, and the influenza virus messenger competes effectively for the translation initiation factor eIF-2.

Protein transport

All ribosomes in the eukaryotic cell are functionally equivalent. Those that are bound to the endoplasmic reticulum and the others that are not membrane-bound have the same structure and composition, their location being determined by the amino acid sequence of the protein that they are synthesizing. Thus membrane-bound ribosomes are engaged in synthesizing membrane proteins and glycoproteins, and membrane-free ribosomes synthesize enzymes and other soluble proteins. The determinant of this differential location of ribosomes is an amino acid sequence at the N terminal end of the polypeptide, the signal sequence. The signal sequences of more than 200 different polypeptides are known, and all have as a common feature a stretch of at least 7 hydrophobic amino acid residues.

Other polypeptide sequences and substituents added after synthesis serve to direct proteins to various locations in the cell to be processed further, to enter the nucleus, to insert into membranes, and so on. These determinants are known as sorting signals. They are specific and consist of quite short amino acid sequences. Proteins are not only directed to particular types of cell organelle but can also be sorted and transported to different regions of the cell. Thus the surface glycoprotein of VSV is mainly inserted into the basolateral plasma membrane of epithelial cells, whereas the equivalent proteins of influenza virus behave as apical membrane proteins. It is thought that the sorting process occurs in the Golgi apparatus, where recognition of a sorting signal is followed by segregation of the proteins into separate vesicles. Transport and final fusion of the carrier vesicle with the appropriate cell surface domain then follows (Simons and Fuller 1985).

PROCESSING OF PROTEINS

Proteolytic cleavage during protein maturation

Many virus proteins are cleaved by proteolytic enzymes either during or after their synthesis. Such cleavages can be mediated by host enzymes and occur in ways similar to the processing steps undergone by normal host proteins. Thus host and viral membrane proteins both lose their N terminal signal sequence while the nascent chain is still growing as part of the normal process of membrane protein synthesis. Many proteolytic cleavages have no host counterpart, however. Although not always mediated by virus-specified enzymes, such steps often play key roles in the production of functional virus-induced proteins both before and after virion assembly and release. It has already been noted that picornavirus proteins undergo a complex series of cleavages mediated by virus-coded enzymes. These cleavages start before the synthesis of the single large virus-induced protein is complete, and continue thereafter, leading to the cutting of this molecule into a considerable number of protein molecules. Some of these are enzymes and others serve as structural components of the virion.

In some viruses polypeptide cleavages occur at the time of virion assembly, and may play roles similar to those identified during the assembly of the head of bacteriophage T4. The assembly of this virus takes place in a series of steps. Component proteins of the head assemble to form a rather unstable prohead. When this assembly process is complete, most of the component proteins are cleaved, the prohead being converted into the chemically resistant virus capsid.

In many viruses the biological activity of virion proteins, and in particular those surface proteins of enveloped viruses that are responsible for fusion of the membranes of virus and host cell, requires proteolytic cleavage for activation. This cleavage is carried out by host cell proteases and constitutes an important determinant of pathogenicity in that the ability of the virus to grow in particular cells, tissues and hosts is determined by the availability of the appropriate proteolytic enzyme.

Protein glycosylation

Many eukaryotic proteins contain one or more carbohydrate groups, and are termed glycoproteins. Cell surface proteins and secretory proteins are often modified in this way. The cellular machinery that adds sugars to polypeptides – a post-translational event – is used, unmodified, by many viruses. Most proteins exposed on the surface of enveloped viruses are glycosylated, for example. Although it is not yet possible to give a full explanation of the function of the carbohydrate on glycoproteins, it is clear that its role is connected with the location of the proteins, and may be important in protecting proteins from attack by extracellular environmental factors. Internal cytoplasmic proteins differ from externally exposed membrane proteins in that they are never glycosylated. Likewise, internal virion proteins are never glycosylated.

The sugar residues of both host cell and viral glycoproteins fall into 2 classes: N-linked, joined to asparagine; and O-linked, joined to serine or threonine. N-linked sugar residues are often quite complex, and contain the sequence $Man^{1,4}$–$GlcNac^{1,4}$–GlcNac linked to asparagine. O-linked sugar residues are often simpler, frequently being only 1–3 sugar residues long.

The glycosylation of glycoproteins with N-linked sugar residues is a complex process. It starts at the time of synthesis of the polypeptide on the endoplasmic reticulum with the addition *en bloc* of a precursor oligosaccharide made up of a number of glucose, mannose and N-acetylglucosamine molecules linked to an unsaturated long chain lipid carrier molecule known as dolichol. A complex sequence of steps then follows in which various sugars are removed and others are added. These processes are catalysed by sugar transferase and sugar-cleaving enzymes situated in the endoplasmic reticulum and the Golgi apparatus; during the processing period the protein moves from the former to the latter organelle. The outcome of the glycosylation process is determined by the input of cellular enzymes, the amino acid sequence and the conformation of the protein being glycosylated, this determining the type of modifications undergone during processing of the oligosaccharide.

O-linked sugar residues are nearly always added to proteins in the Golgi apparatus. The various sugars in the oligosaccharide moiety are added one at a time, each reaction being catalysed by a different glycosyltransferase.

Other post-translational modifications of virus proteins

A variety of other modifications of viral proteins have been identified by biochemical methods. The functional significance of most of these modifications is not yet absolutely clear, although clues can often be found in the class of protein modified and the kind of molecule that becomes covalently linked to the protein. Thus phosphorylation is a common modification, and the virus proteins modified usually interact with nucleic acids, playing a role in transcription (e.g.

the VSV NS protein) or binding to nucleic acids and playing other roles in virus replication (e.g. the large T antigen of SV40). Another common modification is acylation, whereby fatty acids become covalently linked to virus proteins. As with the glycoproteins of enveloped viruses, which are often acylated, the proteins in question usually interact with cell membranes in the hydrophobic portion of the molecule and where it seems possible that the covalently linked fatty acid may play a role in the insertion or anchoring of the proteins into membranes. A capsid protein of picornaviruses and papovaviruses is also acylated; it has been suggested that this modification might be important in virus–membrane interaction at the beginning (during entry) or at the end (during assembly or release) of the virus growth cycle. Other modifications that have been detected biochemically include poly(ADP) ribosylation, sulphation and myristylation.

3   GENOME REPLICATION

Virus RNAs are either single stranded or double stranded, linear or circular, and the replication processes are somewhat different for each type. The small linear single-stranded DNAs of parvoviruses are replicated by cellular polymerases most effectively in rapidly dividing cells. They are initially converted into double-stranded molecules (replicative forms) in a reaction primed by the 3′ terminus of the infecting DNA, which is presented in a loop structure formed by base pairing with the neighbouring sequence (Fig. 6.7). It is suggested that the hairpin-like double-stranded intermediate is then nicked at a position opposite the initiation site to generate a 3′-hydroxyl from which the chain is elongated to complete the replicative form. Single-stranded DNA replication subsequently necessitates copying of the template strand of the replicative form, with concomitant displacement of virus DNA.

Replication of the linear double-stranded adenovirus DNA also requires specialized terminal structures. Replication can be initiated at either end of the double strand and is primed by an early adenovirus protein, part of which remains covalently attached to the 5′ terminus of the new DNA strand. Synthesis from 5′ to 3′ then proceeds continuously with displacement of the parental strand of the same polarity. In turn the displaced strands serve as templates in the formation of double-stranded molecules by synthesis of complementary DNA strands.

The adenovirus DNA polymerase carries out chain elongation; another virus-specified protein with affinity for single-stranded DNA is also required for this process.

For viruses containing circular double-stranded DNAs, the papovavirus SV40 may be taken as an example. In this case replication begins at a unique site at which an early virus protein, the T antigen, seems to promote unwinding of the DNA helix. DNA synthesis by host polymerases proceeds in both

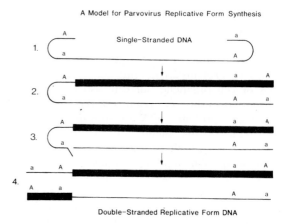

A Model for Parvovirus Replicative Form Synthesis

Fig. 6.7   The first stage in the replication of single-stranded DNA virus genomes consists of the synthesis of double-stranded replicative form (RF) DNA molecules. (1) Synthesis of the DNA strand complementary to virus DNA is initiated by self-priming at the 3′ terminus. (2) 'A' and 'a' represent regions of complementary sequence in virus DNA at both 5′ and 3′ termini which allow terminal loop structures to form. DNA synthesis proceeds to the 5′ terminus of virus DNA to produce the hairpin structure. (3) The virus DNA strand of this duplex is nucleolytically cleaved opposite the site of initiation, and (4) DNA synthesis reinitiates at the 3′-OH group so produced to complete the synthesis of the replicative form DNA.

directions from this origin and both strands are copied simultaneously. Because all nucleic acid biosynthesis proceeds in a 5′ to 3′ terminal direction, the simultaneous synthesis of both strands requires that one must grow in the direction opposite to the movement of the other (Fig. 6.8). This is accomplished by repeated initiation and synthesis of short DNA segments complementary to one strand of the template, followed by ligation of the segments to produce a complete strand. Replication is therefore semi-discontinuous; in each direction one strand is produced as a continuous polymer, the other in a discontinuous fashion in segments up to 300 deoxynucleotides long. As in cellular DNA replication, discontinuous synthesis is primed by short RNA molecules c. 10 nt in length, and ligation of the DNA products is preceded by primer removal and DNA segment extension to fill the resulting discontinuity.

Retrovirus replication also needs the synthesis of double-stranded DNA, in this case by reverse transcription of virus RNA, but unlike other virus DNAs this replicative intermediate has to be integrated into cellular chromosomes to function in replication (Levy 1992). Initiation of DNA synthesis by reverse transcriptase is primed by host transfer RNA molecules packaged in virus particles that contain sequences complementary to and associated with a short region of virus RNA near the 5′ terminus (Fig. 6.9). Reverse transcription proceeds from this site of initiation to the 5′ end of virion RNA. The diagram of virus RNA structure in Fig. 6.9 shows that at the 5′ terminus there is a sequence about 80 nt long that is repeated exactly at the 3′ terminus; the next stage in reverse transcrip-

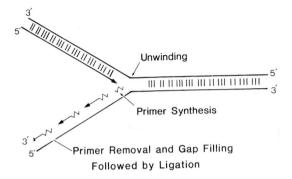

Fig. 6.8 A summary of the processes involved in discontinuous DNA replication. In this scheme one strand of the double-stranded DNA template is supposed to be copied continuously, the other discontinuously. Discontinuous synthesis is primed by small RNA molecules 9–10 nt long, which are removed when the length of the nascent DNA fragments is between 100 and 200 nt. The gaps produced are then filled in before ligation to complete the new DNA strand.

tion seems to involve displacement of the DNA–enzyme complex from this 5′ terminal repeat and its transfer to form a similar association with the 3′ terminal repeat. Synthesis of the complementary DNA strand then proceeds by reverse transcription toward the 5′ terminus of the template virion RNA. Synthesis of the second DNA strand is initiated once reverse transcription has proceeded beyond a specific site near the 3′ terminus of the RNA template. In this case the template for double-stranded DNA synthesis is the nascent reverse transcript, and extension of the second strand beyond the site of initiation of this template occurs after completion of reverse transcription. Synthesis of the first strand does not, however, terminate at this point but is continued by copying the second DNA strand to the position equivalent to the terminus of virus RNA. In this way the completed double-stranded DNA product contains copies of the 5′ terminal RNA sequence, the terminal repeat and the 5′ terminal RNA sequence at both ends (Fig. 6.9). Minor modifications occasioning the removal of 2 bp from each end complete the structure of the provirus, which is found integrated in many different regions of the cell genome, and transcription of provirus DNA leads to the production of virus RNA.

By comparison, the replication of other virus RNAs seems much less tortuous. Reoviruses replicate their double-stranded RNA by encapsulating mRNAs and copying each of them once to form double-stranded molecules within the subviral particle. All other RNA viruses replicate their genomes by forming complete transcripts of virion RNA which are then used as templates or RNA replication. In many cases details of the enzymes responsible are not known but, for example in poliovirus RNA synthesis, it seems that initiation of replication involves the covalent linkage of the 5′ terminal nucleotide to a virus polypeptide. The polypeptide is subsequently proteolytically cleaved, possibly to release the replicase required for RNA elongation, leaving a short peptide attached to the 5′ terminus of the newly synthesized RNA chain.

Consequently, in this process each replicase would produce a single virus RNA. For negative-strand RNA viruses the mechanism of distinction between complete transcript production and the synthesis of the subgenomic or incomplete transcripts that function as mRNA is not known. It has been suggested that certain virus proteins interact with specific sequences in virus RNAs to influence the course of transcription, and that the choice between complete or incomplete transcript formation may depend on the abundance of such proteins in infected cells at different times after infection. With regard to selection of the correct transcript as a template for replication, it is certainly a common observation that terminal RNA sequences are conserved within groups of viruses, which suggests that they have a functional importance. They might serve as recognition signals for the replicase molecules.

Parvoviruses and papovaviruses use the cellular DNA polymerase for DNA synthesis. The larger DNA viruses code for their own DNA polymerases. These are large polypeptides, the adenovirus polymerase having a molecular weight of 120 kDa, herpesvirus 136 kDa and vaccinia 109 kDa. These enzymes exhibit intrinsic 3′ to 5′ exonuclease activity, which is likely to be concerned with proofreading functions. They show a pronounced degree of sequence homology, and each has a highly conserved 14 amino acid sequence with YGDTDS (Tyr–Gly–Asp–Thr–Asp–Ser) in its centre. This sequence occurs at residue 864 in the adenovirus enzyme, residue 880 in the herpesvirus enzyme and residue 938 in the poxvirus enzyme. It may be a DNA-binding domain.

4 VIRION ASSEMBLY

The assembly of animal viruses has proved to be a difficult subject for experimental investigation. This can be partly explained by the complexity of most of the viruses and of the cellular environment in which assembly takes place. Elucidation of the rules and principles governing virus assembly has largely come, so far, from studies of bacterial and plant viruses, aided by the relative ease with which assembly-defective mutants can be generated and studied in the former, and, in the latter, by the success that has attended the biochemical studies in vitro of assembly of their simple virions.

In general, virus particles are assembled in stepwise fashion from distinct subassemblies. These subassemblies are themselves constructed from protein subunits, which may form spontaneously by the aggregation of individual polypeptides. Genome coding constraints determine that virion substructures are made from many identical copies of a few kinds of protein. These are arranged symmetrically with specific intersubunit bonding.

The incorporation of genome nucleic acid molecules into virion substructures and virions is specific. However, with the exception of short defined nucleic acid 'packaging sequences' in helical viruses

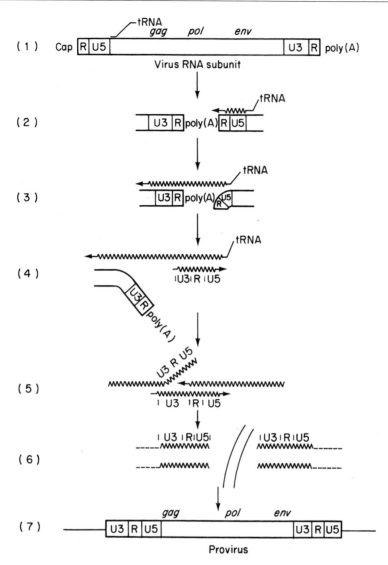

Fig. 6.9 Reverse transcription of retrovirus RNA to produce double-stranded DNA. (1) One of the 2 identical subunits of a retrovirus genome to show the 5′ terminal cap and the 3′ terminal poly(A); R, a short sequence about 80 nt long present at both ends of the subunit; U5 and U3, sequences unique to the 5′ and 3′ ends of virus RNA respectively, which vary in length from c. 80 to 1000 nt in different viruses; transfer RNA bound to the site near U5 at which DNA synthesis begins; and the location of the genes for the virus specific proteins, *gag*, *pol* and *env*, which encode the virus core proteins, the reverse transcriptase and the virus membrane proteins respectively. (2) Complementary DNA (cDNA) synthesis is initiated from the host tRNA primer bound at a site adjacent to U5, and reverse transcription proceeds to the 5′ terminus of the virus RNA subunit. (3) The nascent cDNA strand, indicated by associates with the repeat sequence R at the 3′ terminus of either the same virus RNA subunit or possibly the other subunit of the diploid genome. This requires displacement of the 5′ terminal R sequence, and is followed by extension of the reverse transcript using the newly associated region of RNA as template. (4) Synthesis of the second DNA strand begins when reverse transcription has passed the U3 region. The primer for initiation of this strand is not known. Using the newly synthesized cDNA as template, the second strand is extended to the tRNA primed initiation site of cDNA. (5) cDNA synthesis is completed but is extended using the second DNA strand as template so that it contains R3–R–U5 sequences at both ends. Second strand synthesis continues using the completed cDNA as template. The primer tRNA is removed. (6) Double-stranded DNA synthesis is complete with the linear molecule having identical sequences at both ends. (7) Double-stranded DNA is integrated into cell chromosomes at many sites as provirus DNA, which lacks only 2 base pairs from each end of linear double-stranded DNA.

such as tobacco mosaic virus (TMV), which play a key role at the start of the assembly process, nucleic acids and proteins interact in a sequence-independent way. A similar non-specific interaction takes place in icosahedral viruses, in which the condensation of nucleic acid is sequence-independent.

Sometimes subviral protein structures may be assembled before nucleic acid association. Such a situation seems to occur in poliovirus replication, in which a procapsid is formed that subsequently binds and encapsidates virus RNA. Proteolytic cleavage of specific procapsid polypeptides, which is required for the formation of infectious virus particles, follows RNA encapsidation. Similarly, DNA-free protein shells serve as precursors to virions in the nuclei of adenovirus-infected cells, and a number of proteins are processed by proteolysis during virus maturation.

The membranes of enveloped viruses are derived from the host cell. Membranes in general grow by expansion of existing membranes, and this constraint may explain why these viruses use host membranes for their virions rather than inducing independent synthesis of their own envelopes *de novo*.

Cell membranes are modified by the insertion of virus-specific transmembrane glycoproteins. In the budding of viruses from cell membranes it is surmised that subviral particles containing nucleic acid interact with the cytoplasmic domains of the glycoproteins and, in so doing, induce the modified membrane to envelope them. The specificity of these reactions seems to vary between groups of viruses. The icosahedral nucleocapsids of alphaviruses, for example, interact specifically with their membrane-associated glycoproteins to yield virus particles containing equal numbers of virus capsid proteins and membrane glycoproteins. The interaction between the helical nucleocapsids of myxo-, paramyxo- and rhabdoviruses, on the other hand, is mediated by additional virus proteins, the M proteins, and, although M protein–nucleocapsid associations are virus-specific, in mixed infections viruses can be obtained containing the glycoprotein components of unrelated viruses. This implies that M protein–glycoprotein interactions are less specific. Nevertheless, it is striking that cellular membrane glycoproteins are excluded from the virus assembly process. In the final maturation of a number of membrane-containing viruses proteolytic cleavage of specific virus glycoproteins is also required to generate infectious virus particles. Examples of glycoproteins processed in this way are the fusion glycoprotein of parainfluenza viruses and the haemagglutinin of influenza viruses.

REFERENCES

Baltimore D, 1971, Expression of animal virus genomes, *Bacteriol Rev*, **35**: 235–41.

Banerjee AK, 1987, The transcription complex of vesicular stomatitis virus, *Cell*, **48**: 363–4.

Flint SJ, 1986, Regulation of adenovirus in RNA formation, *Adv Virus Res*, **31**: 169–228.

Greber UF, Singh I, Helenius A, 1994, Tissue tropism and species specificity of poliovirus infection, *Trends Microbiol*, **2**: 52–6.

Ishihama A, Nagata K, 1988, Viral RNA polymerases, *CRC Crit Rev Biochem*, **23**: 27–76.

Kozak M, 1986, Regulation of protein synthesis in virus-infected animal cells, *Adv Virus Res*, **31**: 229–92.

Levy JA, 1992, *The Retroviridae*, Plenum Press, New York.

Moss B, 1995, Vaccinia virus transcription, *Transcription: Mechanisms and Regulation* eds Conaway RC and Conaway JW, Raven Press, New York, 185–205.

Nomoto A, Koikes S, Aoki J, 1994, Tissue tropism and species specificity of poliovirus infection, *Trends Microbiol*, **2**: 47–51.

Schneider RJ, Shenk T, 1987, Impact of virus infection on host cell protein synthesis, *Annu Rev Biochem*, **56**: 317–32.

Sharp PA, 1994, Split genes and RNA splicing, *Cell*, **77**: 805–15.

Simons K, Fuller SD, 1985, Cell surface polarity in epithelia, *Annu Rev Cell Biol*, **1**: 243–88.

Wiley DC, Skehel JJ, 1987, The structure and function of the hemagglutinin membrane glycoprotein of influenza virus, *Annu Rev Biochem*, **56**: 365–94.

Wimmer E, 1994, *Cellular Receptors for Animal Viruses*, Cold Spring Harbor Laboratory, Cold Spring Harbor NY.

FURTHER READING

Bouloy M, 1991, *Bunyaviridae*: genome organization and replication strategies, *Adv Virus Res*, **40**: 235–66.

Chambers TJ, Hahn CS et al., 1990, Flavivirus genome organization, expression, and replication, *Annu Rev Microbiol*, **44**: 649–88.

Cullen BR, 1993, *Human Retroviruses*, IRL Press, Oxford.

Elliott RM, Schmaljohn CS, Collett MS, 1991, *Bunyaviridae*: genome structure and gene expression, *Curr Top Microbiol Immunol*, **169**: 91–141.

Fields BN, Knipe DM et al. (eds), 1995, *Fields' Virology*, 3rd edn, Raven Press, New York.

Frey TK, 1994, Molecular biology of rubella virus, *Adv Virus Res*, **44**: 69–160.

Kingsbury DW, 1991, *The Paramyxoviruses*, Plenum Press, New York.

Koopmans M, Horzinek MC, 1994, Toroviruses of animals and humans. A review, *Adv Virus Res*, **43**: 233–73.

Lai MM, 1990, Coronavirus: organization, replication and expression of genome, *Annu Rev Microbiol*, **44**: 303–33.

Luciw PA, Leung NJ, 1992, Mechanisms of retrovirus replication, *The* Retroviridae, ed Levy JA, Plenum Press, New York.

Morrow WJW, Haigwood NL, 1993, *HIV Molecular Organization, Pathogenicity and Treatment*, Elsevier, Amsterdam.

Nakhasi HL, Singh NK et al., 1993, Identification and characterization of host factor interactions with *cis*-acting elements of rubella virus RNA, *Proceedings of the 3rd International Positive Strand RNA*, eds Brinton MA, Rueckert R, American Society for Microbiology, Washington DC.

Salvato MS (ed), 1993, *The* Arenaviridae, Plenum Press, New York.

Weiss R, Teich N et al., 1982, *RNA Tumor Viruses*, Cold Spring Harbor Laboratory, Cold Spring Harbor NY.

C h a p t e r   7

GENETICS

C R Pringle

1 Genetic systems and the origin of viruses	4 Applications of genetic analysis in virology
2 The strategy of the virus genome	5 Immune evasion
3 Methods of genetic analysis	

1 GENETIC SYSTEMS AND THE ORIGIN OF VIRUSES

The major concerns of virus genetics are the elucidation of the detailed structure of the genomes of the various types of viruses found in nature and the extent to which the individual components of the virus genome determine the biological and disease-producing potential of viruses. Virus genetics is also concerned with understanding the pattern and origin of the variability of viruses, in terms both of virus evolution (see Strauss, Strauss and Levine 1990) and of the temporal changes in antigenicity and pathogenicity of viruses that determine the prevalence and course of the virus-mediated infectious diseases of humans and animals. Although virus genetics impinges on all aspects of virology, this account of virus genetics will be limited to consideration of genome strategy and the methodology of genetic analysis.

Viruses display a diversity of genetic systems unparalleled in any other group of organisms. The viruses considered in this chapter are those that infect humans and higher animals. The genetic systems described do not include all the known categories and only occasional reference is made to the viruses infecting invertebrates, plants, fungi, protozoa, algae, mycoplasmas and bacteria. With the determination of the complete sequences of the genomes of many plant and animal viruses, previously unsuspected phylogenetic relationships are being revealed. Cowpea mosaic virus (CPMV), a plant comovirus with a bipartite positive-sense RNA genome, shows organizational similarity and local sequence homology with the monopartite vertebrate picornaviruses. Tobacco mosaic virus, a monopartite positive-sense RNA virus, and alfalfa mosaic virus and brome mosaic virus, both tripartite genome viruses, show sequence relationships with the animal alphaviruses. It is clear now on the basis of genome organization and comparison of RNA-dependent RNA polymerase sequences that most plant positive-sense RNA viruses can be classified into 2 supergroups comprising the picornavirus-like plant viruses (como-, nepo- and potyviruses), and the alphavirus-like plant viruses (tobamo-, bromo-, carla-, clostero-, cucumo-, furo-, gordei-, ilar-, potex-, tymo- and tobraviruses) (Koonin and Dolja 1993). The picornavirus-like plant viruses and the animal picornaviruses resemble each other in encoding a number of non-structural proteins that exhibit similar functions and show some degree of amino acid homology. The alphavirus-like plant viruses are more diverse, but again they encode genes in the same relative order that specify proteins exhibiting significant sequence homology to the 3 non-structural proteins of the vertebrate Sindbis virus. There is also an apparent genetic link between the potyviruses of plants and the flaviviruses of animals in that the putative helicase protein of potyviruses exhibits closer resemblance to the NS3 protein of flaviviruses, which contains a nucleotide-binding motif, than to the helicases of picornaviruses (Goldbach and de Haan 1993).

Although most viruses are restricted in their host range, several groups of viruses are characteristically unrestricted by taxonomic barriers and may multiply in hosts of quite different origin. For example, some of the arthropod-borne bunyaviruses and rhabdoviruses that infect vertebrates or plants are also able to multiply in their arthropod vector. Despite the apparent phylogenetic relationships described above, however, no contemporary virus exists that is able to multiply in both vertebrates and plants.

The existence of plant and animal RNA viruses with similarly ordered genomes encoding proteins with similar amino acid sequences suggests common ancestry. However, the common ancestors from which these viruses diverged probably appeared subsequent to the separation of the plant and animal kingdoms some

10^9 years ago, and divergent evolution alone cannot account for certain features of these relationships. The coupling of common genes to unique genes in various of these genomes suggests a recombinational polyphyletic origin. Many viral genomes can best be regarded as different assemblages of modules of conserved genes that have arisen by a process of modular evolution (Goldbach 1987).

The application of molecular phylogeny analysis to the large DNA-containing herpesviruses has confirmed the ancient origin of these viruses and provided a timescale for their evolution. The branching pattern of the 3 subfamilies of the mammalian herpesviruses is congruent with that of their corresponding host lineages (McGeoch et al. 1995). Assuming a constant molecular clock, these authors have estimated that the *Alphaherpesvirinae*, *Betaherpesvirinae* and *Gammaherpesvirinae* subfamilies diverged $1.8–2.2 \times 10^8$ years ago, about the time of emergence of mammals from mammal-like reptiles, and that the major sublineages within these subfamilies probably arose before the radiation of placental mammals some $6–8 \times 10^7$ years ago. Palaeontological dating of host lineages has suggested that the contemporary virus lineages within the *Alphaherpesvirinae* have evolved by a process of cospeciation of viruses with their mammalian hosts (McGeoch and Cook 1994). The extreme sequence divergence of fish herpesviruses from mammalian and avian herpesviruses (Davison 1992, Bernard and Mercier 1993), on the other hand, is indicative of an earlier phase in the evolution of the herpesviruses which places the origin of the herpesviruses earlier than 220 million years before the present.

2 THE STRATEGY OF THE VIRUS GENOME

The 'strategy of the virus genome' is a phrase that has been used to describe collectively the organization and function of the genetic information content of viruses (see also Chapter 6). The mammalian viruses fall into 3 major categories: the DNA-containing viruses, the RNA and DNA reverse transcribing viruses and the RNA-containing viruses. The encoding of genetic information in RNA is unique to viruses (animal, plant and bacterial), and RNA is the predominant molecular form of the genome in animal and plant viruses. The genomes of >90% of plant viruses consist of single- or double-stranded RNA. The reverse transcribing viruses alternate between RNA and DNA forms of the genome; in the retroviruses (and retroid elements, p. 100), the genome exists as proviral DNA integrated into the host cell genome and as RNA in the extracellular virion. By contrast, in the DNA-containing hepadnaviruses and the plant caulimoviruses the DNA form is present as partially or completely double-stranded DNA in the virion, the RNA form acting as a replicative intermediate in the infected cell. The DNA viruses range from viruses with small genomes, such as the parvoviruses and the papovaviruses, which depend on host cell functions for their repli-cation, to large genome viruses such as the herpesviruses and poxviruses, which have acquired a battery of additional genes that function (among other things) to subvert the immune response of the host.

2.1 The coding potential of viruses

The molecular sizes of the genomes of the DNA viruses extend over a 200-fold range, from the 1000 kDa of hepatitis B virus to the 195 000 kDa of fowlpox virus. In contrast, the RNA viruses are more uniform, varying within a 30-fold range from the 500 kDa of deltavirus to the 15 000 kDa of reovirus. This circumstance has been interpreted as a reflection of the low fidelity of viral RNA polymerases, which lacks proofreading capability. The consequent high mutability of RNA viruses may impose an upper limit on the size of informational RNA molecules (Reanney 1984). The viruses with the smallest genomes are hepatitis B virus and porcine circovirus, which possess circular genomes of some 1700 kilobases (kb) of partially double-stranded DNA and single-stranded RNA, respectively.

Table 7.1 lists the currently recognized mammalian viruses according to the taxonomy defined in the VIth Report of the International Committee on Taxonomy of Viruses (Murphy et al. 1995). The first column shows that mammalian virus genomes, according to virus family, may be linear or circular, single- or double-stranded, covalently linked to small terminal proteins, or may exist as a unique complement of subunits. The minimum information content of a viral genome can be estimated from the number of non-overlapping coding triplets if the sequence is known, or, if not, from the ratio of the molecular mass of the genome and the gene products. As a rule of thumb the ratio of the molecular mass of genome and gene products is approximately 10:1 for single-stranded genomes and 20:1 for double-stranded genome viruses. Thus, for example, the 4000 kDa of the genome of the rhabdovirus vesicular stomatitis virus (VSV) is sufficient to code for polypeptides with a total mass of 400 kDa, which approximates closely to the 396 kDa of the 5 gene products of VSV. This is a special case, however, because the non-coding regions are limited to the di- or trinucleotide intergenic junctions and short leader and trailer regions. The relationship between linear length and coding capacity is maintained in the larger DNA viruses, but the coding capacity of small virus genomes is greatly expanded by a number of devices, some of which are listed in the final column of Table 7.1: for example, overlapping reading frames (many viruses), transcription from both strands (adenoviruses), mRNA splicing and alternate splicing (many viruses), accessing of multiple open reading frames by RNA editing (paramyxoviruses), ribosomal frameshifting (retroviruses and coronaviruses), use of alternate start sites (paramyxoviruses) and alternate initiation codons (adenoviruses and paramyxoviruses), post-translational cleavage (picornaviruses and togaviruses), usurpation of host factors (several viruses), and transactivation of host genes (lentiviruses).

Ribosomal frameshifting is virtually confined to RNA viruses and usually involves the expression of replicases. Slippage of ribosomes into the −1 reading frame (in a 5′ direction) occurs at a specific site comprising 2 essential elements; a homopolymeric slippage sequence separated by 5–8 bases from an RNA a pseudoknot structure (see Chapter 6 and Brierley 1995). Ribosomal frameshifting may be a strategy to achieve stoichiometry of gene products or to ensure inclusion of replicative enzymes in virions (e.g. by production of gag–pol fusions in retroviruses). Figure 7.1 summarizes diagrammatically some of the modes of multiple expression of genetic information from viral genomes.

2.2 Diversity of organization of the viral genome

The diverse nature of the viral genome can be rationalized by regarding the genome as an intermediate stage in the cycle of replication of virus nucleic acid that has been sequestered in an extracellular particle (Fig. 7.2). It is conventional to designate a single-stranded RNA molecule as positive-sense if it functions as mRNA in protein synthesis, and its complement as the negative-sense strand or antimessage. The retroviruses and some RNA viruses encapsidate the positive-sense RNA strand in the virion, whereas other RNA viruses encapsidate the negative-sense strand or the double-stranded form in the virion. The DNA viruses may be single- or double-stranded, the positive and negative strands being encapsidated in separate particles in the defective parvoviruses. The only stage in the replication cycle of viral nucleic acids (excluding the replicative intermediates) not represented in known viruses is the RNA : DNA intermediate in the reverse transcription pathway. A small proportion of hepatitis B virus particles, however, do contain DNA/RNA hybrid molecules.

2.3 Segmentation of the viral genome

Figure 7.2 excludes consideration of the segmentation of the genome seen in the arena-, bunya-, orthomyxo- and reoviruses. A consequence of segmentation of the genome is the possibility of increasing genetic heterogeneity by reassortment of subunits during replication and morphogenesis; the evolution of segmentation in RNA viruses has been equated somewhat fancifully with the evolution of sex, allowing the participation of 2, 3 or more parents in the production of offspring (Chao 1994). Segmentation and the consequent facility for reassortment may allow the rapid elimination of deleterious mutations and defective genomes. It has been suggested also that segmentation may be a device to circumvent the inferred restriction on the absolute size of informational RNA molecules imposed by their high mutability (Reanney 1984). This argument is difficult to sustain, however, because the total genome sizes of the segmented genome viruses are in the same range as those of non-segmented genome viruses, and the genome of the largest segmented genome viruses (the 19 kb of the nairovirus Congo–Crimean haemorrhagic fever virus) is less than that of the largest non-segmented genome virus (the 30 kb of the coronavirus mouse hepatitis virus). Segmentation of the genome may more often be a device to obtain greater control of transcription.

Among mammalian viruses segmentation of the genome is confined to the negative-stranded and double-stranded RNA viruses where the complete complement of genome subunits is contained within a single particle and the infectious unit is a single virion. Segmentation of the genome is common, however, among the positive-sense single-stranded RNA viruses of plants. These are all multicomponent viruses, however, in which the individual genome subunits are contained in different particles and the infectious unit is a full complement of particles. Genetic reassortment can accompany the maturation of multicomponent viruses and is termed pseudorecombination by plant virologists (Pringle 1996).

2.4 Ambisense encoding of information

Also omitted from Fig. 7.2 is the phenomenon of ambisense encoding of genetic information, which is exhibited by viruses of the family *Arenaviridae* and some members of the family *Bunyaviridae*. Ambisense encoding is illustrated diagrammatically in Fig. 7.3. In Punta Toro virus (family *Bunyaviridae*, genus *Phlebovirus*) the N polypeptide is encoded in a viral complementary subgenomic RNA corresponding to the 3′ half of the S RNA, whereas the presumptive NS protein is encoded in a subgenomic viral sense RNA corresponding to the 5′ half of the genome; i.e. the S RNA of Punta Toro virus is both positive and negative sense. Ambisense encoding of information is common to members of the genus *Phlebovirus*, but is not observed in the other genera of the *Bunyaviridae*. In the *Arenaviridae* both segments of the bipartite genome exhibit ambisense encoding of information. The large subunit encodes the L gene in the 3′ half and the Z gene in opposite sense in the 5′ half, and the small subunit the N gene in the 3′ half and the G gene in opposite sense in the 5′ half. Ambisense encoding seems to be a device to obtain temporal control of transcription rather than a means of expanding coding capacity.

2.5 Site of multiplication

RNA viruses replicate in the cytoplasm, with the exception of the segmented genome orthomyxoviruses and the monopartite negative-stranded bornaviruses which have nuclear phases (Schneemann et al. 1995). Some others fail to replicate in enucleated cells and depend on the presence of a functional nucleus (Pringle 1977). The genome of the positive-sense single-stranded RNA viruses is infectious because it can function directly on entry as mRNA for the entire complement of viral proteins, which include the RNA replicase required for replication of the viral genome. The genome of the negative-sense single-stranded

Table 7.1 Properties of the genomes of mammalian viruses

Nucleic acid type	Family (subfamily)	Genus (species)	Genome size in nucleotides	Special features
The DNA viruses				
ssDNA, linear	Parvoviridae	Erythrovirus (B 19 virus)	5 kb	Nuclear −ve and +ve sense molecules encapsidated separately Cell division dependent Inverted terminal repeats (383 b) with a palindromic region (365 b)
		Dependovirus (adenoassociated 1 virus)	4.7 kb	Nuclear −ve and +ve sense molecules encapsidated separately Helper virus dependent Inverted terminal repeats (145 b) with a palindromic region (125 b)
ssDNA, circular	Circoviridae	Circovirus (porcine circovirus)	1.7–2.3 kb	3 ORFs, 1 virion protein S growth phase dependent
dsDNA, circular	Papovaviridae	Polyomavirus (SV40 virus)	5 kbp	Nuclear Early and late mRNA transcribed from opposite strands ORFs overlap Induce host DNA synthesis
		Papillomavirus (papillomavirus 16)	8 kbp	Nuclear Early and late mRNA transcribed from the same strand ORFs may overlap Episomal replication Restricted to differentiating epithelial tissue
dsDNA, linear	Adenoviridae	Mastadenovirus (adenovirus type 2)	36 kbp	Nuclear Inverted terminal repeats (103 bp) Covalently linked protein at 5′ and 3′ termini Temporal control of transcription; early genes modulate host's transcription apparatus Intricate mRNA splicing generating c. 40 proteins 70–200 ORFs
	Herpesviridae (Alphaherpesvirinae)	Simplexvirus (human herpesvirus 1)	152 kbp	Nuclear No terminally associated protein Long and short unique regions separated by repeats of both termini, producing 4 isomers on internal replication Splicing of mRNA rare Becomes latent in sensory ganglia
	(Betaherpesvirinae)	Cytomegalovirus (human herpesvirus 5)	235 kbp	Nuclear Splicing of mRNA frequent

	(*Gammaherpes-virinae*)	*Lymphocryptovirus* (human herpesvirus 4)	170 kbp	Site of latency may be lymphoreticular cells Nuclear Unique sequences interrupted by direct repeat sequences Splicing of mRNA frequent Latent in B lymphocytes of oropharynx
	Poxviridae (*Chordopoxvirinae*)	*Orthopoxvirus* (Vaccinia virus)	170–250 kbp	Cytoplasmic Linear dsDNA with covalently linked ends Two isomeric terminal inverted complementary sequences (hairpin) structures
		Parapoxvirus	130–150 kbp	
		Capripoxvirus	145 kbp	
		Leporipoxvirus	160 kbp	Cytoplasmic inclusions (factories) Encodes 150–300 proteins, c. 100 present in virion, including RNA polymerase and other enzyme activities
		Suipoxvirus	175 kbp	
		Molluscipoxvirus	188 kbp	
		Yatapoxvirus	146 kbp	Temporal control of gene expression Genetic recombination within genera

The DNA and RNA reverse transcribing viruses

Non-covalently linked circular dsDNA	*Hepadnaviridae*	*Orthohepadnavirus* (hepatitis B virus)	6.6 kbp	Nuclear –ve sense strand complete, +ve strand variable Circularized by base-pairing of cohesive ends Covalently attached protein at 5' end of –ve strand 4 partially overlapping genes; the P gene overlaps the other 3 and encodes a reverse transcriptase, DNA polymerase and RNase H
Positive sense dimeric ssRNA	*Retroviridae*	Mammalian retrovirus B	10 kb (M)	Nuclear Monomers held together by hydrogen bonding RNA not infectious, DNA provirus infectious
		Mammalian retrovirus C	8.3 kb (M)	Primary translation products are polyproteins
		retrovirus D	8.0 kb (M)	tRNA base paired to 5' primer region
		BLV/HTLV retrovirus	8.3 kb (M)	5' *gag–pro–pol–env* 3' basic genome order with additional regulatory genes in some genera
		Lentivirus	9.2 kb (M)	In some host sequences inserted into complete genomes or in defective genomes as substitutions for deleted gene sequences
		Spumavirus	11 kb (M)	Access of some ORFs by ribosomal frameshifting

The RNA viruses: positive-sense ssRNA viruses

ssRNA, linear	*Picornaviridae*	*Enterovirus* (poliovirus 1)	7–8.5 kb	All cytoplasmic Genomic RNA and cDNA infectious

Table 7.1 Continued

Nucleic acid type	Family (subfamily)	Genus (species)	Genome size in nucleotides	Special features
		Rhinovirus *Hepatovirus* *Cardiovirus* *Aphthovirus*		Post-translationally cleaved polyprotein One or 2 non-structural proteins have proteolytic activity Virus-encoded 5' terminal covalently linked protein (VPg) Long 5' non-coding region with internal ribosome entry site; poly(C) tract in some; poly(A) tail Low frequency recombination
	Caliciviridae	*Calicivirus* (VEV)	7.4–7.7 kb	5' covalently linked VPg in some Non-structural proteins translated as polyprotein Capsid protein translated from second ORF in some and from subgenomic RNA in others
	Astroviridae	*Astrovirus* (human astrovirus 1)	6.8–7.9 kb	Subgenomic 2.8 kb polyadenylated RNA
	Coronaviridae[a]	*Coronavirus* (mouse hepatitis virus)	30 kb	Genomic RNA acts as mRNA for RNA polymerase Pol encoded as two 5' proximal overlapping ORFs, the second accessed by ribosomal frameshifting Genome length –ve strand acts as template for synthesis of 'nested set' of 3' co-terminal subgenomic mRNAs High frequency genetic recombination Replication of mRNAs
		Torovirus	20 kb	
	Arteriviridae[a]	*Arterivirus*	13 kb	Genome strategy similar to coronaviruses
	Flaviviridae	*Flavivirus* (yellow fever virus)	10.7 kb	Single ORF encoding a polyprotein proteolytically cleaved co- and post-translationally
		Pestivirus	12.5 kb	
		Hepacivirus	9.5 kb	5' end of genome encodes structural proteins, protease, helicase and polymerase at 3' end
	Togaviridae	*Alphavirus* (Sindbis virus)	11–12 kb	Capped genomic RNA serves as mRNA for precursor of non-structural proteins encoded in 5' two-thirds of the genome Structural proteins translated from a –ve strand copy of the genome; cleavage of polyprotein by virus and host proteases
		Rubivirus	9.8 kb	Structural proteins translated from a subgenomic mRNA

The RNA viruses: negative-sense ssRNA viruses

Nucleic acid type	Family (subfamily)	Genus (species)	Genome size in nucleotides	Special features
ssRNA, circular	Unassigned	*Deltavirus*	1.7 kb	Forms rod-shaped structure by intramolecular base-pairing Site-specific autocatalytic cleavage and ligation Single mRNA encoding delta antigen (HDAg) Defective, dependent on HBV helper Cytoplasmic 5(6) ORFs, single 3' proximal promoter
ssRNA, linear	*Rhabdoviridae*[b]	*Vesiculovirus* (VSV) *Lyssavirus* *Ephemerovirus*	11.2 kb 11.9 kb 14.6 kb	Virion RNA polymerase Recombination not recorded

			Genome size	Features
	Paramyxoviridae[b] (Paramyxovirinae)	Paramyxovirus (NDV)	15.2 kb	Cytoplasmic, single 3' proximal promoter; Virion RNA polymerase
		Rubulavirus	15.4 kb	6–7 ORFs
		Morbillivirus	15.9kb	Recombination not recorded
	(Pneumovirinae)	Pneumovirus	15.2 kb	8–10 ORFs; Recombination not recorded
	Filoviridae[b]	Filovirus (Ebola virus)	19.0 kb	Cytoplasmic; 7 ORFs, some overlaps; Virion RNA polymerase
	Bornaviridae[b]	Bornavirus (Borna disease virus)	8.9 kb	Nuclear; 5 ORFs with low homology to other NNSVs; Gene overlap; mRNA splicing
ssRNA, segmented	Arenaviridae	Arenavirus (LCM)	7.6 kb	Cytoplasmic; 2 subunits, ambisense encoding in both; High frequency reassortment; Ribosomal and other RNAs variably present in virion; Virion RNA polymerase
	Bunyaviridae	Bunyavirus (Bunyamwera virus)	12.3 kb	Cytoplasmic; 3 subunits, ambisense encoding in S RNA of phleboviruses, circular nucleocapsids
		Hantavirus	11.8 kb	4 structural proteins
		Nairovirus	18.9 kb	High frequency reassortment
		Phlebovirus	12.2 kb	Virion RNA polymerase
	Orthomyxoviridae	Influenzavirus A, B	13.6 kb	Nuclear phase; 7–8 subunits, some mRNAs bicistronic with overlapping ORFs or with alternate gene products derived by splicing
		Influenzavirus C	10 kb	High frequency reassortment; Virion RNA polymerase
dsRNA viruses	Reoviridae	Orthoreovirus (reovirus 3)	23.7 kb	Cytoplasmic; 10 subunits, mostly monocistronic; High frequency reassortment; Virion RNA polymerase
		Orbivirus	19.2 kb	10 subunits
		Rotavirus	18.6 kb	11 subunits
		Coltivirus	No data	12 subunits

[a]Constituent families of the order *Nidovirales*.

[b]Constituent families of the order *Mononegavirales*.

BLV, bovine leukaemia virus; HTLV, human T cell lymphotropic virus; LCM, lymphocytic choriomeningitis virus; M, monomer; NDV, Newcastle disease virus; NNSVs, non-segmented negative-strand RNA viruses; ORF, open reading frame; VEV, vesicular exanthema virus; VSV, vesicular stomatitis virus.

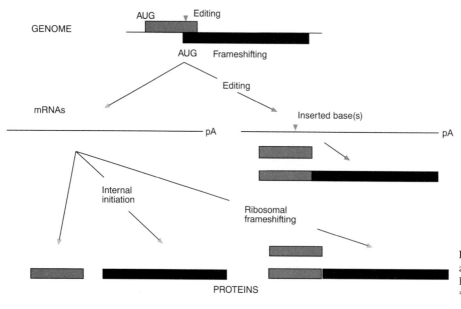

Fig. 7.1 Three mechanisms allowing expression of hidden reading frames. *Cattaneo, 1989.

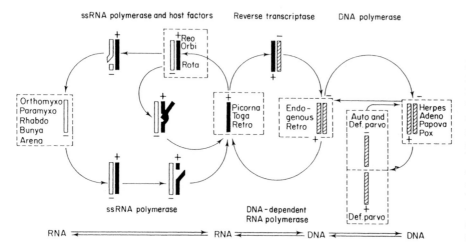

Fig. 7.2 The stages of the replication cycle of viral nucleic acid sequestered in virions. RNA replication follows a 5 intermediate model; positive-sense strands are indicated in black and negative-sense strands in white; DNA strands are cross-hatched. The stages sequestered in virions are indicated by the dashed boxes. Auto, autonomous; Def., defective.

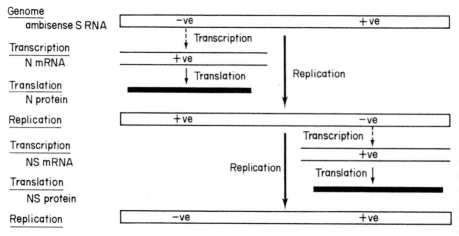

Fig. 7.3 The ambisense encoding of genetic information in the S RNA of the Punta Toro phlebovirus (family *Bunyaviridae*). (After Ihara, Akashi and Bishop 1984.)

RNA viruses, on the other hand, is not infectious because it cannot function as mRNA or be replicated. Mammalian cells do not contain enzymes that can transcribe or replicate RNA templates, so transcription can be initiated only if the requisite RNA polymerase is introduced into the host cell together with the infecting genome in the form of a nucleocapsid structure. The genome of retroviruses is not infectious, probably because it depends on preformed virion-associated reverse transcriptase for its replication, whereas the proviral DNA form is infectious because it can be transcribed by the host cell DNA-dependent RNA polymerase. The genomic DNA of the nuclear DNA viruses is generally infectious, but that of the cytoplasmic poxviruses is not. The poxviruses exhibit the greatest level of independence of host cell activities and the virion contains several enzyme activities, which include a viral DNA-dependent RNA polymerase whose presence seems to be essential for infectivity (see also Chapter 6). The discovery of this enzyme by Kates and McAuslan (1967) was crucial to understanding the nature of viral genomes and led ultimately to the independent discovery and characterization of the reverse transcriptase of retroviruses by Temin and Mitzutani (1970) and Baltimore (1970), which is perhaps the greatest single contribution of virology to general biology and which greatly accelerated the exploitation of recombinant DNA technology.

2.6 The retroviruses and retroid elements

The retrovirus genome is present in the virion in a diploid form. Two identical subunits of c. 3000 kDa are linked by hydrogen bonding between short repeats at their 5′ ends. As a result of reverse transcription a single copy of the viral genome with direct terminal repeats becomes stably integrated into the host cell genome as proviral DNA. At the cell–virus junction there is a 5 bp direct repeat of cellular DNA next to a 3 bp inverted repeat of viral DNA, a structure similar to that present at the termini of several bacterial transposons. A major distinction between the retroviruses and other nuclear DNA viruses is that the former maintain productive infections but do not usually kill the host cell, whereas the latter invariably destroy their host cell and can only become stably integrated in a non-productive form. (Further study of the phenomenon of latency in herpesviruses, however, may blur this distinction.) Endogenous retroviruses are defective or non-defective retroviruses transmitted from one generation to the next via the germline, and which probably evolve in synchrony with their hosts to establish multigenic families (Coffin 1982). About 0.01–0.1% of the genomic DNA of laboratory mice may comprise retroviral sequence, and it is probable that the genomes of primates contains a similar amount of retroviral genetic information. Many of these endogenous retroviruses seem to have originated from cross-infections at an earlier stage in the evolution of their host. For example, the endogenous feline virus RD114 is thought to have originated as a result of horizontal transfer of an endogenous primate retrovirus, possibly as far back as the Pliocene Age. High frequency recombination is an inherent property of retroviruses. The diploid nature of the genome means that heterozygous genomes can exist and may be intermediates in the generation of stable recombinants. In crosses of exogenous retroviruses, recombination has been detected both between and within genes and between exogenous and endogenous viruses. In the replication of retroviruses, the location of the tRNA primer for DNA synthesis near the 5′ ends

of the tandemly associated monomers means that the reverse transcriptase must transfer from the 5′ end of one monomer to the 3′ end of the same or the other monomer soon after the initiation of synthesis (see Chapter 6). Thus every round of synthesis becomes a replication event. Comparison of the inferred amino acid sequences of retroviral proteins suggests that recombination has played an important role in the diversification of the envelope proteins of retroviruses, whereas the polymerase gene seems to have been protected from recombinational events (McClure et al. 1988). The extreme variability of the surface proteins of HIV-1 seems to be mediated by progressive mutational change rather than by recombinational events (Williams and Loeb 1992). It should be emphasized, however, that enhanced mutability is not confined to HIV-1. Two distinct types of hypermutation have been described: the phenomenon of biased A → I hypermutation in measles virus, possibly due to post-transcriptional enzymatic misreading of A residues (Billeter and Cattaneo 1991); and the G → A hypermutation observed in HIV-1 and other retroviruses, possibly due to reverse transcriptase-mediated substitution of dCTP by dTTP due to local intracellular depletion of dCTP (Martinez, Vartanian and Wain-Hobson 1994). High frequency mutation mediated by error-prone polymerases has been described also for VSV (Pringle et al. 1981) and respiratory syncytial virus (Cane, Matthews and Pringle 1993).

Reverse transcription is not uniquely associated with viruses belonging to the families *Retroviridae* and *Hepadnaviridae*. Comparative analysis of the organization of the RNA associated with vertebrate genetic elements, such as the intracisternal A particles, VL30 genes and LIMd, and a variety of transposable elements from yeast (Ty), *Drosophila* (*copia*), *Dictyostelium* (DIRS-1) and maize (B1) revealed structural similarities with the integrated form of the retrovirus genome. Furthermore, the RNA form of the nucleic acid component of *D. copia* and Ty is present within virus-like particles that have associated reverse transcriptase activity. Comparative maps of the genomes and transcripts of 2 hepadnaviruses (ground squirrel hepatitis virus and cauliflower mosaic virus), 5 retroviruses (Rous sarcoma virus, Moloney murine leukaemia virus, human T cell lymphotropic virus type II, human immunodeficiency virus type I, human spumavirus) and 3 transposon or transposon-like elements (the yeast Ty element, the *D. copia* and 17.6 *copia*-like elements) are presented in Fig. 7.4. The common features are the terminal redundancies, which can range from the 17–21 nucleotides of Rous sarcoma virus to the 1123 nucleotides of the human spumavirus, the partial or complete *gag–pol–env* order, and the domain structure of the polymerase. In the *gag–pol* region the retrotransposons conform to the retrovirus pattern, apart from the inversion of the integrase and reverse transcriptase domains in *D. copia* and Ty. It has been proposed that, during the evolution of these agents, cassettes of genes were added to the basic *gag–pol* core to facilitate adaptation to specific host environments (Hull and Covey 1986, McClure 1991). For example, the *env* gene of vertebrate retroviruses is required for protection of the core complex and for cell-to-cell spread, whereas the caulimoviruses have acquired additional genes to facilitate plant-to-plant transmissibility and movement within the plant.

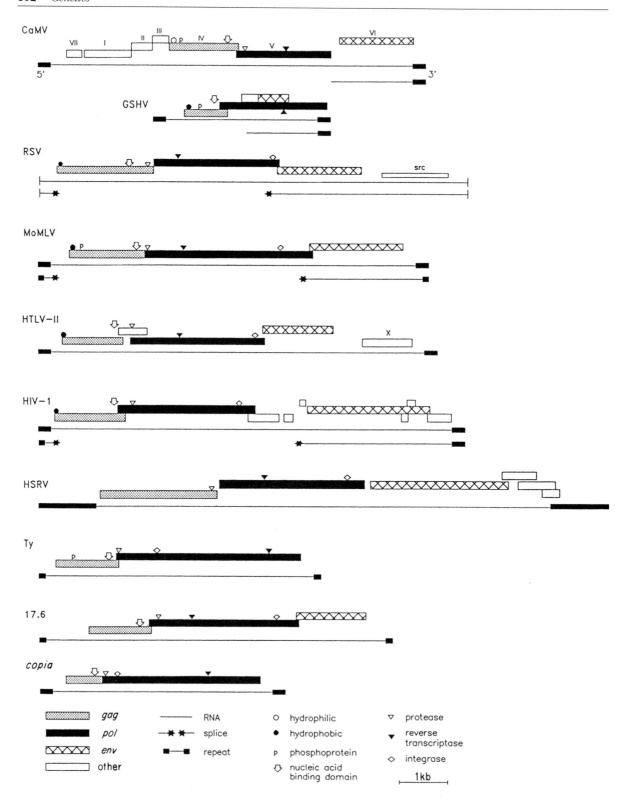

Fig. 7.4 Genome organization of retroviruses and retroid agents; cauliflower mosaic virus (CaMV), ground squirrel hepatitis virus (GSHV), Rous sarcoma virus (RSV), Moloney murine leukaemia virus (MoMLV), human T cell lymphotropic virus type II (HTLV-II), human immunodeficiency virus type 1 (HIV-1), human spumavirus (HSRV), yeast Ty element, *Drosophila copia*-like element 17.6, and *Drosophila copia* element. Each is shown as the genome-length RNA (—), the terminal repeats being indicated by black boxes, and the subgenomic RNA for the *env* gene or its equivalent is shown below the genomic RNA. (Reproduced by courtesy of R Hull and S Covey.)

3 METHODS OF GENETIC ANALYSIS

Classic genetic analysis of viruses depended on the isolation of spontaneously occurring mutants or the induction of mutations by random mutagenesis followed by non-selective isolation of mutants exhibiting a single conditional lethal phenotype. Further selective screening procedures or laborious characterization of individual mutants were required to identify useful mutations in specific viral genes. Nevertheless, despite the imperfections, many well defined mutations were identified which played significant roles in the molecular characterization of mammalian viruses, and provisional genetic and physical maps of many viral genomes have been obtained (see Pringle 1990, Ramig 1990).

3.1 Conditional lethal mutants

Conditional lethal phenotypes (temperature sensitivity and host range) were the favoured phenotypes for the isolation of mutations in essential genes. Other phenotypes such as plaque morphology, drug resistance, enzyme deficiencies and spontaneous deletions (sometimes presenting as defective interfering particles) had application in specific circumstances. The conditional lethal mutants employed in animal virology have been temperature-sensitive mutants, cold-sensitive mutants or temperature-dependent host range mutants (Pringle 1987, 1990, Ramig 1990). Host range conditional lethal mutants analogous to the suppressible chain-terminating mutants of bacteriophage (amber or non-sense mutations) have played virtually no role in animal virus genetics, although such mutants allow direct identification of the mutated gene product, because a truncated gene product may be present in the non-permissive host cell and an intact protein in the permissive cell. Host restriction in animal cells is probably due to the absence of a specific receptor, and permissive mammalian cells naturally able to suppress amber mutations by insertion of an amino acid at an amber stop codon have not been identified. Mammalian cells expressing amber-suppressible tRNAs have been engineered, however, and these have been used successfully to isolate mutations of VSV following random mutagenesis (White and McGeoch 1987) and by mutagenesis of poliovirus cDNA in vitro (Sedivy et al. 1987).

3.2 Spontaneous mutants and random mutagenesis

Spontaneous mutants occur at low frequency, and a variety of mutagens have been employed to increase the frequency of recovery of mutants. Mutagens that have proved effective with human and animal viruses include base analogues (e.g. 5-fluorouracil and 5-azacytidine for RNA viruses and 5-bromodeoxyuridine for DNA viruses), alkylating agents (e.g. ethylmethane sulphonate, diethyl sulphate), intercalating agents (e.g. proflavine and *N*-nitro-*N*-nitrosoguanidine), deaminating agents (e.g. nitrous acid), hydroxylamine and ultraviolet light irradiation. The base analogues are incorporated into the viral genome and mutations are produced by miscoding during replication. The other mutagens induce mutations by direct chemical action. The majority of induced mutations seem to be missense mutations whereby substitution of an amino acid modifies the functional activity of a gene product. Frameshift and non-sense mutations of animal viruses are rare. Practical protocols for random mutagenesis and isolation of mutants are described by Leppard and Pringle (1995).

It is generally accepted that mutation frequencies in most RNA viruses are very high, ranging from 10^{-3} to 10^{-6} and usually in the range 10^{-4} to 10^{-5} (Holland, de la Torre and Steinhauer 1992). Consequently, a 10 kb RNA genome will on average carry one or more mutations, and any population of RNA viruses will comprise a heterogeneous swarm of diverse mutants. The term quasispecies has been introduced to take account of this phenomenon and the consequent difficulty of defining a viral species (Eigen and Biebricher 1988). A single 'master' sequence may predominate at any one time during replication in a defined environment, but its existence will be transient and dependent on maintenance of strong external selective forces. The high mutation frequencies of RNA viruses are attributed to the inherent error proneness of RNA-dependent RNA polymerase and reverse transcriptase and to the lack of a proofreading function. Paradoxically some RNA viruses exhibit great sequence stability during replication in vivo or during propagation in cultured cells. Even the highly variable HIV-1 is more stable during replication in cell culture than the error proneness of the purified polymerase would predict, indicating the existence of cellular stabilizing factors (Mansky and Temin 1995).

3.3 Site-specific and directed mutagenesis

These empirical methods have been largely superseded by the development of in vitro methods of site-specific mutagenesis. The methodology for constructing such mutants is similar for all DNA and positive-stranded RNA viruses, although there is an operational distinction between viruses whose genome is small enough to be cloned (as a cDNA in the case of RNA viruses) in its entirety (parvoviruses, polyomaviruses, picornaviruses, retroviruses) and those in which mutagenesis must be carried out with a fragment that, after genetic manipulation, is incorporated into a complete genome, generally by recombination in vivo (adenoviruses, herpesviruses, poxviruses) (Coen 1990, Leppard and Pringle 1996).

GENERAL METHODOLOGY

A prerequisite for directed mutagenesis is a source of molecularly cloned viral nucleic acid. RNA genomes must be first converted to cDNA by reverse transcription and the larger genomes cleaved with an appropriate restriction endonuclease to generate a library of fragments. Once cloned, directed mutagenesis may make use of existing fortuitous restriction sites or employ synthetic oligonucleotides with specific mismatches flanked by regions of complementarity. Oligonucleotide-directed mutagenesis can be used to obtain precisely located deletions. This is achieved by cloning wild type genomic DNA into a single-stranded bacteriophage vector (e.g. M13mp19). Single-stranded phage DNA is isolated and annealed to the mutagenizing oligonucleotide that comprises 2 non-contiguous complementary sequences flanking the region to be looped out to produce the required deletion, or a mismatched base for the production of point mutations. The annealed oligonucleotide acts as a primer for DNA synthesis in vitro and the resulting double-stranded DNA is circularized with DNA ligase. A mutated genome is recovered by repair synthesis on a single-stranded DNA template or, increasingly, by polymerase chain reaction (PCR). A generalized protocol for directed mutagenesis has been described by Leppard and Pringle (1995).

PCR-based directed mutagenesis has gained the ascendency in practice because of its greater flexibility. Synthetic primers are designed to locate on opposite strands on either side of the target site. The region targeted for mutagenesis can be defined further by 2 opposing internal primers, one of which generates the desired mutation while the other eliminates one of 2 restriction sites flanking the target site. Two-stage amplification yields DNA that can be cleaved at the sites flanking the target site; only mutated DNA should retain the dispensable restriction site. The recovered fragment can then be ligated into an appropriately cleaved plasmid or M13 vector, a process that is facilitated if the restriction sites in the amplified fragment are also unique to the recipient genomic clone. In the case of parvoviruses, polyomaviruses, picornaviruses and retroviruses, infectious progeny can be generated by direct rescue, i.e. by direct transfection of the reconstructed DNA into susceptible host cells.

Transfection of nucleic acid is mediated variously by calcium phosphate precipitation, lipofection, electroporation, etc. Although picornaviruses can be rescued by transfection of cloned DNA (Racaniello and Baltimore 1981), the process is more efficient if RNA transcribed in vitro is transfected by electroporation (van der Werf et al. 1986). For viruses with larger genomes (adeno-, herpes- and poxviruses), rescue of the mutated fragment into infectious virus is achieved by co-transfection of the mutated sequence and intact viral genomic DNA into permissive cells. Recombination will occur provided the flanking sequences on either side of the mutated site are sufficient to permit homologous recombination. With the intermediate-sized adenoviruses, viral genomic DNA can be inactivated by cleavage with a single-cutting restriction enzyme such that the genome fragments overlap with the mutant-carrying fragment. In this situation infectious virus can be generated only by a process of homologous recombination and most of the progeny virus will contain the mutation. In the herpesviruses

and poxviruses, rescue of directed mutations is mostly confined to genes with phenotypes that are amenable to selection (e.g. enzyme deficiencies, drug resistance, cytopathology), on account of the high background of unmutated virus in the absence of selection.

DELETION MUTANTS

Operationally, deletion mutants are the simplest to obtain. However, deletion of sequences from a specific protein-coding gene does not always produce a 'null' phenotype. For example, the carboxy terminal region of the attachment (G) protein of respiratory syncytial virus can be deleted without affecting the attachment function or viability. Similarly, the herpesvirus thymidine kinase retains substantial activity despite loss of the first 45 amino acids. Deletion mutant analysis is particularly useful in defining promoter regions. Specific deletions can be engineered by digesting cloned single-stranded DNA from a single-stranded DNA bacteriophage vector with one or 2 restriction enzymes and recircularizing to generate 2 circular molecules, the extent and type of deletion obtained depending on the availability of restriction enzyme sites. Sets of deletion mutations can be obtained by restriction enzyme cleavage of a circular DNA molecule followed by progressive extension of a deletion using an exonuclease and recircularization.

LINKER SCANNING MUTAGENESIS

Linker scanning mutagenesis introduces clustered sets of point mutations at desired locations and allows more refined analysis of *cis*-acting control sequences and characterization of protein-binding sites. This procedure allows rapid screening for mutations and their immediate localization as a result of the appearance of a new restriction site (McKnight and Kinsbury 1982). A limitation of deletion mutant analysis is that if the deletion is large it may cause non-specific effects; for example, steric interactions in proteins, or spacing constraints on promoter function.

LINKER INSERTION MUTAGENESIS

Linker insertion mutagenesis does not involve deletion; a linker is inserted at restriction sites within an open reading frame and many sites can be mutagenized by limiting digestion by a frequent cutting restriction enzyme. A linker of 3 bp (or multiples of 3) will maintain the reading frame beyond the insertion, whereas chain termination can be produced in all 3 reading frames by insertion of other linkers.

REVERSE GENETICS OF NEGATIVE-STRAND RNA VIRUSES

A recent development that foreshadows the application of reverse genetics to the negative-strand RNA viruses is the rescue of synthetic RNA molecules into infectious influenza A virus (Garcia-Sastri and Palese 1993) and rabies virus (Schnell, Mebatsion and Conzelmann 1994). The genomic RNA of negative-strand RNA viruses is not infectious because the negative-strand is not translated. However, Luytjes et al. (1989) achieved amplification, transcription and rescue of synthetic RNA molecules by reconstitution of a biologically active nucleoprotein complex using synthetic RNA and purified core proteins in the presence of helper influenza virus. The problem of packaging of the much larger genomic RNAs of the non-segmented genome viruses (the *Mononegavirales*) has been solved by the construction of complete cDNA clones of rabies virus (Schnell, Mebatsion and Conzelmann 1994) and VSV (Lawson et al. 1995) genomes, which can be transcribed by bacteriophage T7 polymerase in permissive cells into a complete positive-sense copy of the RNA genome. Expression of such RNA in cells also expressing the L, N and P nucleocapsid proteins results in the rescue of infectious virus. It is presumed that expression of the antigenomic RNA, rather than genomic RNA, avoids sequestration and functional loss of the L, M and P mRNAs by annealing to genomic-sense RNA. Lawson et al. (1995) produced a recombinant virus by this route in which the glycoprotein gene was derived from another serotype of VSV. This is the first example of recombination in negative-strand viruses and it opens the way to the use of these viruses as vectors for use in vaccine development and gene therapy. Early results indicate that negative strand viruses can tolerate insertion of foreign sequences and gross rearrangements of gene order (Ball A, Wertz G et al., personal communication).

3.4 Genetic and non-genetic interactions

Interactions between viruses can be classified broadly as either genetic or non-genetic. Genetic interactions include recombination, subunit reassortment and multiplicity reactivation. Their characterization provides information about the evolutionary potential of viruses as well as means of their experimental manipulation. Non-genetic interactions include complementation, phenotypic mixing and interference.

COMPLEMENTATION

Complementation is the ability of the defective gene product of one virus to be substituted by the normal gene product of another, when both viruses are present in the same host cell. Complementation provides a test for non-identity, whereby mutants of similar phenotype (e.g. temperature-sensitivity) can be assigned to different genes without prior knowledge of the existence or function of the genes. Operationally, a complementation index (CI) can be used to assess the efficiency of complementation; i.e. in the case of temperature-sensitive mutants,

$$CI = yield\ (A + B)^{RT}/yield\ A^{RT} + yield\ B^{RT}$$

where A and B are any 2 mutants and RT is the restrictive temperature of incubation. Progeny virus produced as a consequence of complementation between viruses retains the mutant genotype, because the interaction between viruses occurs at the level of gene products only. Consequently, assay of the progeny from a complementation experiment is carried out at the permissive temperature and a positive CI indicates non-identity of function. Complementation is normally intergenic in nature, but in the case of multifunctional gene products intragenic complementation may be observed.

Complementation analysis has had a prominent role in defining gene function in the papovaviruses, adenoviruses, herpesviruses, poxviruses, retroviruses, alphaviruses, flaviviruses, paramyxoviruses, rhabdoviruses, arenaviruses, bunyaviruses, orthomyxoviruses and reoviruses (see Pringle 1990).

PHENOTYPIC MIXING AND PSEUDOTYPE FORMATION

Phenotypic mixing is a form of non-genetic interaction between viruses whereby the structural components (capsid or envelope) may be interchanged partially or completely when 2 different viruses multiply in the same cell. Phenotypic mixing normally occurs between related viruses, but heterologous phenotypic mixing can occur between unrelated viruses (Zavada 1982). Viruses that are enveloped on exit from the host cell are prone to phenotypic mixing. The mixing of genomes and structural proteins results in the production of progeny virus particles in which the phenotype does not reflect the genotypic properties of the virus. Phenotypic mixing is thus a transient phenomenon.

Pseudotype formation, the complete investment of the core of one virus by the envelope of another, has provided a convenient means of rapid assay of non-cytopathic or fastidious viruses. For example, some of the progeny virus released from cells co-infected with the non-fastidious and rapidly cytopathic rhabdoviruses, VSV or Chandipura virus, and a host-restricted and non-cytopathic or slowly cytopathic retrovirus will possess the genome of the lytic virus contained within the envelope of the retrovirus. The pseudotype yield, detected as rapidly plaque-forming virus resistant to neutralization by antiserum to the parental lytic virus, provides a means of detection and rapid assay of its non-lytic partner. This technique has been used successfully for studying the host range and assay of HIV-1, HTLV-I and II, mouse mammary tumour virus, bovine leukaemia virus and several avian retroviruses (Weiss and Bennett 1980, Clapham, Nagy and Weiss 1984).

INTERFERENCE AND DEFECTIVE INTERFERING PARTICLES

Many of the oncogenic avian and mammalian retroviruses exist as replication-defective viruses and are dependent on helper leukaemia-associated retroviruses. These oncogenic retroviruses often exist as pseudotypes because their envelope glycoproteins are supplied by the helper virus. Other examples of asymmetrical complementation or phenotypic mixing are the association of hepatitis D and B viruses and the adenovirus helper-dependent parvoviruses. The ubiquity of non-genetic interactions such as complementation and phenotypic mixing is responsible for the prevalence of defective viruses. Defective viruses accumulate in most laboratory-propagated stocks of viruses, and are dependent on the presence of their non-defective progenitor for their survival. It is a characteristic of most defective viruses that they specifically interfere with the replication of their helper or closely related viruses. Interference occurs at the level of transcription and replication, and is not interferon-mediated. The mechanism of interference varies between viruses belonging to different families and between different defective viruses of the same virus (see Holland 1990). For example, the majority of the defective interfering (DI) particles of VSV, known as panhandle or hairpin DIs, which contain genomes with complementary 5′ ends and incomplete L gene sequences, interfere with the replication of viruses of homologous serotype only, whereas the DI particles that contain internal deletions of the L gene interfere with VSV of both homologous and heterologous serotypes. In formal terms, a single mutant or nucleotide substitution can constitute a DI genome, and deletion of sequence is not an essential characteristic (Youngner and Quagliana 1976). The hypothesis has been advanced that the generation of DI virus is a natural phenomenon that moderates the course of viral disease and contributes to the self-limiting nature of most viral disease (Huang and Baltimore 1970). It has been difficult, however, to obtain evidence of the presence of DI virus in natural infections, although in a few instances the administration of DI particles can alter the outcome of an infection. Mice can be protected from an influenza virus-induced immune-mediated pneumonia by administration of DI particles. However, the DI particles do not reduce the replication of virus in the lung, but seem to act by preventing the virus-induced T cell response that is responsible for consolidation (Morgan and Dimmock 1992).

Persistent infection

DI particles have been implicated in the initiation, although not necessarily the maintenance, of persistent infection in vivo and in vitro. For example, a DI particle associated with the tsG31 mutant of VSV, possessing a 90% deletion of the genome, was a good inducer of persistent infection (Holland 1987). It has been hypothesized from in vitro experimentation that persistent infection may be a driving force in evolution, and may play an important role in maintaining the variability of negative-strand RNA viruses that cannot acquire variation by genetic recombination. The generation of DI virus is a spontaneous mutational event, which in due course forces a mutational response in the parental virus to counteract the DI-mediated interference, and a cyclical phenomenon of alternating generation of new DI and specific DI interference-resistant viruses ensues. Progressive and extensive mutational change over the whole genome was observed to accompany the propagation of the normally lytic VSV as a persistent non-lytic infection in cultured cells, whereas the virus is genetically stable during cycles of lytic infection. The extensive mutation of the measles virus genome observed in the defective virus recovered from the brain of people with subacute sclerosing panencephalitis (SSPE) may be a natural example of this phenomenon.

Recombination in DNA and positive-strand RNA viruses

Recombination occurs as a consequence of the physical interaction of viral genomes in the infected cell. It is a phenomenon common to all DNA-containing viruses, the RNA-containing retroviruses and some positive-strand RNA viruses. It is presumed that the DNA-containing reverse-transcribing viruses can interact in this way, but as yet there is no direct evidence. Recombination between DNA genomes is probably a conventional intramolecular mechanism involving a breakage and reformation of covalent bonds, whereas recombination between RNA genomes is a process unique to viral RNA and mediated by a template switching ('copy-choice') mechanism during minus-strand synthesis (Kirkegaard and Baltimore 1986). The probability of occurrence of a recombinational event between 2 genes is proportional to the physical distance separating them on the genome, and genetic maps can be constructed on the basis of recombination frequencies. Temperature-sensitive (ts) mutants have formed the framework for most genetic maps. The recombination frequency (RF) between any 2 temperature-sensitive mutants, A and B, is measured as a frequency (percentage), such that

$$RF = 2 \times 100 \times \text{yield } (A + B)^{RT} - (\text{yield } A^{RT} + \text{yield } B^{RT})/\text{yield } (A + B)^{PT}$$

where RT is the restrictive temperature and PT the permissive temperature. The single and mixed infections are carried out at the permissive temperature and yields assayed at the temperatures indicated by the superscript. The factor 2 is included because only the wild type recombinant is measured by this assay and it is assumed that the reciprocal recombinant (the double ts mutant) occurs with equal frequency. Using a quantitative PCR assay, Jarvis and Kirkegaard (1992) have confirmed that frequencies of the reciprocal recombinants in poliovirus recombination are equivalent, but only when the parental input multiplicities are identical. Linear genetic maps of several DNA viruses (adeno-, herpes-, pox- and picornaviruses) have been constructed on the basis of 2 factor crosses to establish relative proximity and 3 factor crosses to confirm orientation (for a detailed account, see Ramig 1990).

Mutants classified in the same complementation group cluster in the map, and the greatest distance separating mutants in the cluster defines the minimum size of the gene. In the adenoviruses and herpesviruses intertypic crosses with the parental ts mutants derived from viruses of different serotype have been employed to confirm the linear order of the genetic map and to show that the genetic and physical maps of the genome, constructed on the basis of restriction endonuclease fragment analysis or direct sequencing, are co-linear. Natural recombinants between herpesvirus types 1 and 2 have been isolated from patients, but their infrequency suggests that there are selective constraints preventing such interactions. Paradoxically, although the frequency of recombination is generally lower, natural recombinants occur more frequently in RNA viruses. For example, intertypic recombinants are prominent in the virus recovered from children after vaccination with the trivalent Sabin vaccine, although none of these recombinants has as yet escaped the immune response of the host to become established in nature. Rare heterologous recombinants also occur: for example, the alphavirus known as Western equine encephalitis virus seems to be a recombinant of another alphavirus, Eastern equine encephalitis virus, and a New World relative of Sindbis virus (Hahn et al. 1988).

Recombination in RNA viruses is not universal (reviewed by Lai 1992, Wimmer, Hellen and Cao 1993). Low frequency genetic recombination (up to 0.9%) occurs in viruses with positive-strand genomes and linear genetic maps have been derived for both poliovirus and foot-and-mouth disease virus which have been shown to be co-linear with physical maps. Homologous recombination does not seem to be site-specific, although intertypic recombination in poliovirus and foot-and-mouth disease virus may be influenced by local structural features. The 3 poliovirus types differ by c. 15% in their nucleotide sequences, and the frequency of recombination observed between viruses of different subtypes, as expected by a template switching (copy-choice) mode of recombination, is about 100-fold less than between isogenic viruses.

Large genome sections can be transposed as a result of natural recombination in vivo, and the characterization of the phenotypic properties of recombinants has played a prominent role in the mapping of attenuating mutations in the Sabin poliovirus vaccine strains. Transposition of segments of any size can now be achieved in a more controlled manner by exchange of segments between existing or engineered restriction sites in infectious cDNA clones. This approach also provides a means of direct verification of the association of particular mutations with a specific phenotype. For example, a poliovirus mutant carrying a 4 base insertion at position 70 within the 5' untranslated leader region has a small plaque ts phenotype and is deficient in RNA synthesis. Revertants of this mutant retained the 4 base insert, and mix-and-match experiments with cDNA located these second site suppressor mutations to a site within the 3C protease gene (Andino et al. 1990). The isolation and characterization of revertants is an essential feature of the characterization of any mutant. The same approach can be used to produce chimaeric viruses in order to study the homology and functional compatibility of genetic elements. For example, it has been shown that the 5' untranslated leader regions of poliovirus and a Coxsackie B virus can be interchanged.

The 5' untranslated region of the genome of picornaviruses contains an internal ribosomal entry site (IRES), and poliovirus can be transformed into a vector by insertion of a foreign gene between tandemly arranged IRES sequences, in which one is derived from a non-homologous IRES (e.g. from encephalomyocarditis virus, EMCV) to prevent loss by homologous recombination. A dicistronic virus mimicking the genetic organization of the plant picornavirus CPMV can be created by insertion of an IRES from EMCV between the capsid precursor coding region and the non-structural protein coding region of the poliovirus genome. Unlike CPMV, however, the 2 transcriptional units are linked and contained within the same particle.

Exceptionally, high frequency genetic recombination is observed in mixed infections of coronaviruses, but a linear map of the coronavirus genome has not been produced. This may be a consequence of the complexity of the organization of the coronavirus genome with its unique 'nested set' configuration of genetic information, whereby subgenomic RNAs with a common 3' terminus and differential extensions in a 5' direction are intermediates in mRNA transcription. In addition, the polymerase protein of coronaviruses is encoded in 2 large open reading frames from which the gene product is derived by translational frameshifting (ribosomal slippage). The largest coronavirus genome (c. 31 kb) is much larger than the picornavirus genome (c. 7.5 kb), but the rate of recombination per nucleotide is similar and c. 0.1% per 100 nucleotides (Lai 1992).

MULTIPLICITY REACTIVATION AND CROSS-REACTIVATION

Multiplicity reactivation occurs when cells are infected with parental viruses, which are themselves non-infectious (usually as a result of UV irradiation). At higher multiplicities of infection progeny virus may be released from susceptible cells that contains markers contributed by both parents. Infectivity has been restored by replacement of defective genes by recombination (or reassortment). Multiplicity reactivation is observed only if the inactivating lesions in the 2 parental viruses are located in different genes. Multiplicity reactivation has been observed between strains of the same virus and also between viruses of different serotype. Reactivation between an inactivated parent and an infectious parent is termed cross-reactivation, or marker rescue, and is likewise mediated by recombination (or reassortment). Cross-reactivation can be exploited to increase the yield of recombinants (or reassortants) by infecting susceptible cells with a non-plaque-forming virus and a UV-inactivated plaque-forming virus.

These forms of reactivation have to be distinguished from the non-genetic reactivation observed with some poxviruses, in which infectivity is restored as a result of complementation of the defective DNA-dependent RNA polymerase of one parent by the functional DNA-dependent RNA polymerase of another.

ABSENCE OF INTRAMOLECULAR RECOMBINATION IN NEGATIVE-STRAND AND DOUBLE-STRANDED RNA VIRUSES

True intramolecular recombination has not been demonstrated unequivocally for any RNA virus with a negative-strand or double-stranded genome, with the exception of the tripartite genome double-stranded RNA phage phi6 (Mindich 1995). It is likely that recombination can occur as a rare event; otherwise it is difficult to account for the origin of some of the DI viruses of VSV, influenza A virus and rotavirus which have truncated and juxtaposed genes, or the rare phenomena such as the inversion of genes in the mammalian pneumoviruses, which departs from the otherwise invariant paramyxovirus pattern.

RECOMBINATION WITH HOST TRANSCRIPTS

Functions essential to replication and maturation can be attributed to no more than half the genes of the herpes simplex virus genome (McGeoch 1989). It is likely that some of the excess coding capacity of the large DNA viruses represents accretion and modification of host genetic material by recombination. It is clear also that the oncogenic retroviruses have acquired their oncogenic potential by incorporation of cellular oncogenes with concomitant loss of viral genetic information by a recombinational mechanism. It is perhaps surprising, in view of the obligatory proviral phase in the multiplication cycle of these viruses, that these events have been so rare and restricted to experimental propagation of viruses in an inappropriate host. Although conventional RNA viruses might not be expected to interact with the host cell genome, there are isolated reports of such interactions: a variant of influenza A virus exists whose N gene subunit has an additional sequence homologous with host ribosomal RNA sequences; and several independently isolated strains of the pestivirus bovine viral diarrhoea virus (BVDV) seem to have acquired a cytopathic and virulent phenotype as a consequence of insertion of one or more cellular ubiquitin gene monomer sequences into a large duplicated region of the viral genome. A mechanism based on template switching of the viral polymerase during negative-strand synthesis has been proposed to explain this phenomenon (Meyers et al. 1991). Interactions between cellular RNAs and replicating viral RNA have also been demonstrated in plant viruses, where a replication-competent deletion mutant of CPMV was rescued by recombination in transgenic plants expressing the deleted sequences (Greene and Allison 1994).

SUBUNIT REASSORTMENT

All the segmented genome RNA viruses of animals, which are ambisense, negative-strand or double-stranded, are able to exchange genetic information by a process of subunit reassortment. Reassortment occurs at high frequency between related viruses; for example, all influenza A viruses are able to exchange genome subunits, but influenza A, B and C viruses do not interact. In the bunyaviruses and the reoviruses restriction on reassortment of genome subunits closely parallels the serological and sequence divergence of the viruses, and does not correlate with the geographic origin of the isolates (see Pringle 1996). In the orthomyxoviruses it is asserted that there is random (i.e. unlinked) association of genome subunits and that the low electron microscope particle/plaque-forming unit ratio is a reflection of the imprecision of the maturation process whereby only some particles receive the essential complement of 8 unique subunits.

In the bunyaviruses with their tripartite genomes it is possible to undertake complete progeny analysis, because there are only 6 ($2^3 - 2$) non-parental reassortant genotypes in contrast to the 254 ($2^8 - 2$) of influenza A virus to be assayed. Independent studies have concluded that reassortment is not random and that there are preferred associations of subunits even in the case of closely related viruses (Iroegbu and Pringle 1981, Urquidi and Bishop 1992). The mechanism of restriction seems to operate at the level of gene products, because the terminal sequences of the subunits are identical and do not exhibit the specificity required for non-random reassortment. However, in crosses of Bunyamwera and Maguari viruses, which belong to the Bunyamwera serogroup, once a parental subunit configuration had been broken by reassortment, the restriction on reassortment was relaxed.

In the reoviruses, where maturation is efficient and precise, and particle/infectivity ratios are close to unity, reassortment seems to be random. In sharp contrast, if cells were infected (by lipofection) with reovirus infectious cores rather than virions, the progeny comprised almost exclusively monoreassortant virus (i.e. virus with 9 subunits from one parent and 1 from the other). Lipofection of cells with naked RNA permitted only assortment (i.e. recovery of parental virus), not reassortment (Joklik and Roner 1995). These observations emphasize the complexity of the reassortment process and suggest again that protein–protein interactions rather than RNA sequence recognition determine the specificity of reassortment. A complicating factor in the analysis of reassortment, described in rotavirus progeny analysis but probably true for all segmented genome viruses, is that the phenotype of the reassortants recovered may be modified by the genetic background of the recipient (Chen et al. 1989).

In general, reassortment is restricted to taxonomically related viruses: in the *Orthomyxoviridae* the boundaries are defined by species, and by serogroups within species in other virus families. Conversely, genetic compatibility as measured by the ability to reassort genome subunits, may be a useful approach to equating taxons in different virus families. All segmented genome viruses have the potential for rapid adaptation to new hosts, for abrupt generation of viruses with new antigenic characteristics and for sudden extensions of host range and virulence. Transmission by vectors and multiplication in alternate hosts are also common features of these viruses.

GENETIC REASSORTMENT AND THE EPIDEMIOLOGY OF INFLUENZA

Genetic reassortment plays a major role in the epidemiology of human influenza. Mutation accounts for the progressive genetic and antigenic variation (antigenic drift) of influenza A virus during interpandemic periods, but the appearance of new pandemic strains requires the introduction of new genes by reassortment (antigenic shift). Avian viruses seem to provide the reservoir of antigenic variation from which new pandemic strains can be generated. Much evidence suggests that the pig provides the 'mixing vessel' in which avian and human viruses can interact, generating progeny with new antigenic properties and the constellations of genes required to allow transmission to and spread within human hosts (Castrucci et al. 1993). In South China the domestic duck may be the intermediate host carrying viruses from feral ducks to the pig, whereas in North America domesticated turkeys may be a more important intermediate host. Reassortant influenza A viruses seem to have been responsible for the major pandemics afflicting the human population since the beginning of the twentieth century. However, a recent outbreak of a lethal antigenically novel avian-like virus in horses in the Far East indicates that avian viruses can spread directly to animals without the need for reassortment.

SUPERINFECTION EXCLUSION AND GENE CAPTURE

The 3 serotypes of reovirus exchange genome segments freely during mixed infection both in vitro and in vivo, but little is known about the role of reassortment in the evolution of these viruses. In some segmented genome viruses (e.g. some bunyaviruses and bluetongue virus) but not in others (e.g. the rotaviruses), a phenomenon of superinfection exclusion is observed whereby a superinfecting virus is able to participate in subunit reassortment for only a short period after primary infection. Superinfection exclusion is also host-dependent. For example, reassortment of the genome subunits of the orbivirus bluetongue virus is inhibited if the introduction of the second virus is delayed by more than 4 hours, whereas there is no interference for a period of at least 5 days in asynchronously infected midges.

Natural reassortants of rotaviruses are probably of frequent occurrence, and there is ample evidence for gene capture by the interaction of segmented genome viruses present in alternate hosts. For example, the Au-1 strain of human rotavirus has a VP-4-coding subunit encoding a feline rotavirus-like VP-4, suggesting that genetic interaction between feline and human rotaviruses is not infrequent. Other rotaviruses recovered from humans seem to be reassortants of human, bovine and a third unidentified parental rotavirus. Likewise, it has been inferred that the 5 serotypes of bluetongue virus present in North America are derived from 3 distinct gene pools, and that serotype 17 has evolved by a combination of reassortment and genetic drift.

4 APPLICATIONS OF GENETIC ANALYSIS IN VIROLOGY

A genetic approach has many actual and potential applications in virology: for example, the analysis of antigenic properties (epitope mapping) and receptor interactions, identification of determinants of virulence and drug resistance, interpretation of molecular epidemiology, and the engineering of live virus vaccines.

4.1 Epitope analysis

Neutralization escape mutants can be isolated following exposure to, or growth in the presence of, a specific antiserum or an appropriate monoclonal antibody. Specific epitopes can be identified by analysis of the reactivity of neutralization escape mutants with panels of monoclonal antibodies. These epitopes can then be located by nucleotide sequencing of the escape mutants and physical mapping of the mutational changes. Optimally, these changes can then be located on the 3-dimensional structure of viral attachment proteins (e.g. the HA protein of influenza A virus – see Chapter 22) or the whole virion (e.g. poliovirus – see Chapter 25).

Non-neutralizing monoclonal antibody escape mutants can be obtained by a modification of the selection technique. Infected cell monolayers are reacted with an appropriate murine monoclonal antibody and then treated with an enzyme-linked second antibody (e.g. a horseradish peroxidase rabbit anti-mouse polyclonal serum). Plaques that are unstained represent monoclonal antibody-resistant (MAR) mutants, which can be employed in analysing the antigenic properties of non-structural and internal components of viruses.

4.2 Drug resistance

The isolation of drug resistance mutants can identify the site of action of an antiviral agent and assist in analysing both the mechanism of action of the drug and the function of the target protein. For example, identification of the function of the M2 protein of influenza virus and confirmation of its presence in the virion were direct results of the isolation of amantidine-resistant mutants of influenza A virus (Haydon and Hay 1992).

The isolation of drug resistance mutants can also provide information of relevance in the treatment of viral disease. For example, molecular analysis of mutants of HIV-1 virus resistant to 3′-azido-3′-deoxythymidine (AZT), nucleoside analogues and other non-nucleoside RT inhibitors revealed unpredicted interaction between drugs in patients. In particular, suppression of phenotypic AZT resistance was observed in some viruses with mutations in the RT gene, which conferred resistance to other antiretroviral drugs. Other combinations of mutations conferred co-resistance. A conclusion from such analyses is that certain combinations of antivirals are more likely than others to induce multidrug resistance in the patient, and that it may be possible to design treatment schedules to reduce this possibility, and even perhaps to reverse loss of efficacy of AZT (Larder 1994).

4.3 Identification of virulence determinants

Analysis of the determinants of the virulence of the 3 Sabin poliovirus vaccine strains, which were produced by a process of adaptation to growth in non-neural tissue in vitro, provides one of the best examples of the potential of genetic analysis (see Almond 1987, Wimmer, Hellen and Cao 1993). Determination of the complete sequence of the type 1 Sabin vaccine strain and its Mahoney virulent progenitor revealed that 56 single-site mutations, resulting in 21 amino acid substitutions, differentiated the 2 strains. Production of intratypic and intertypic recombinants generated by in vivo recombination experiments, construction of in vitro clones from cDNA clones and site-directed mutagenesis led to the conclusion that several mutations, mapped to VP1, VP3 ,VP4, 3D^{pol} and the 3′ non-coding region, contributed to the attenuation and temperature-sensitive phenotypes. Although there was a strong correlation between the rct (temperature sensitivity) phenotype and loss of neurovirulence, assay of these recombinants and mutants in transgenic mice expressing the human poliovirus receptor revealed that the determinants of temperature sensitivity and attenuation were separable genetically (Bouchard, Lam and Racaniello 1995). A similar analysis was not possible with the type 2 virus, because the progenitor was already avirulent in monkeys. Recognition of virulence determinants in this case relied on comparison of the vaccine virus with a neurovirulent revertant isolated from a vaccine recipient. It was concluded that 2 major attenuating mutations resided in the 5′NTR (non-coding region) and in VP1. A similar conclusion was derived from analysis of the type 3 vaccine strain in which the wild type (Leon) progenitor and a neurovirulent revertant from a patient were available for comparison. Remarkably, only 10 single-site mutations, resulting in 43 amino acid substitutions, differentiated the vaccine strain from its virulent progenitor. Two mutations, one located at site 472 in the 5′NTR and the other a ts mutation in the VP3 region, contributed to the attenuation phenotype. Later a third mutation located in the VP1 region was identified as an additional attenuating factor. The C → U mutation at 472 associated with the attenuated phenotype was observed to revert at high frequency following vaccination. Virus recovered from the gut of a human infant as early as 47 hours after vaccination had reverted, and exhibited increased neurovirulence in monkeys. The role of mutation in the 5′NTR region in attenuation was confirmed by mix-and-match type in vitro recombination experiments. Subsequently, mutations at positions 480 and 481 of poliovirus types 1 and 2, respectively, were similarly shown to be involved in the attenuation phenotype (Fig. 7.5). The 5′NTR mutations locate to different bases in the same inferred secondary structure and may act by destabilizing this stem–loop structure, possibly affecting the translation efficiency of the viruses (Macadam et al. 1994). The other mutations affecting attenuation show no common features and it is considered that 5′NTR mutations may be responsible for the greater stability of the 3 Sabin vaccines over their earlier rivals. A mutation in the 5′ non-coding region of Coxsackie B3 virus has been identified as a determinant of cardiovirulence in mice (Tu et al. 1995)

4.4 Natural chimaeras, transgenes and genetically engineered vectors

In addition to the homologous intra- and inter-recombinants of influenza viruses, rotaviruses and picornaviruses frequently encountered in nature, an ever-increasing list of genetically engineered heterologous recombinant viruses is being described: for example, Sindbis/VSV, influenza A/B, VSV Indiana/VSV New Jersey. There are rare examples, however, of natural heterologous recombination. Thogoto virus, a tick-borne orthomyxovirus with a baculovirus-like glycoprotein, may be an extreme example of this phenomenon (Morse, Marriott and Nutall 1992). The best documented chimaeras are the adeno/SV40 hybrid viruses, which were isolated inadvertently during the 'adaptation' of adenovirus type 7 to growth in non-permissive SV40-contaminated African green monkey kidney cells (Grodzicher 1981). Hybrid viruses were obtained in which adenovirus and SV40 virus genetic material was covalently linked. A few adeno-SV40 hybrids were isolated in which an intact adenovirus or SV40 genome was present, whereas others were incomplete and dependent for their propagation on an adenovirus helper. Subsequently, helper-dependent and helper-independent adeno2-SV40 hybrids were produced in the same way. The ad2ND1 hybrid contained a non-defective, though incomplete, adenovirus genome covalently linked to SV40 sequence. The SV40 sequence, which conferred the ability to multiply in monkey cells, varied from 7% to 43%, and the dispensable amount of adenovirus genome deleted varied from 4.5% to 7.6%. In all the adeno2-SV40 hybrids the insertion point was the same, namely at a site 14% from one end of the adenovirus genome.

Continuous passage of papovaviruses at high multiplicity of infection generates particles that have lower buoyant density than competent virions and contain less DNA. The DNA in these particles is circular and may have 10–50% of the papovavirus genome deleted. The segment deleted may be substituted by reiterated or non-reiterated host cell DNA sequences, which may be larger than the segment deleted. These phenomena show that the genome of papovaviruses, and presumably other DNA viruses, can be modified by the incorporation of host DNA sequences, and on rare occasions can contribute DNA sequences, either by homologous or by illegitimate recombination, to other DNA-containing viruses.

An additional dimension has been added to genetic analysis by the ability to introduce foreign DNA into fertilized murine ova and to raise to maturity transgenic animals that have the foreign DNA integrated

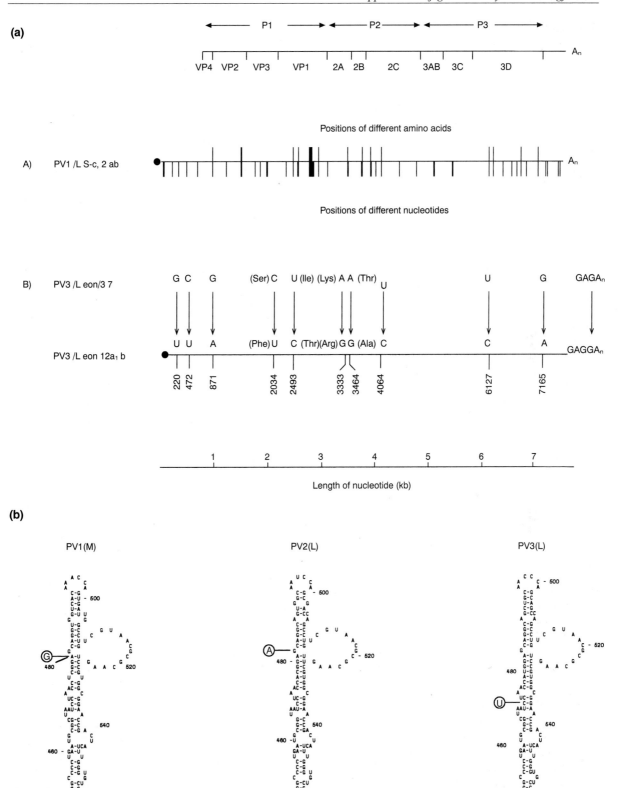

Fig. 7.5   (a) Location of attenuating mutations in the Sabin strains of poliovirus types 1 and 3: (A) the 21 amino acid and 56 nucleotide differences between the virulent parental (P1/Mahomey/41) and vaccine (P1/LSs, Zab) type 1 strains: (B) the 4 amino acid and 10 nucleotide differences between virulent parental (P3/Leon 37) and vaccine (P3/Leon 12a1b) type 3 strains. (b) Domain V of the 5′ non-coding region of poliovirus types 1, 2 and 3. The attenuating mutations are circled. (Reproduced with permission from *Annual Review of Genetics*, vol 27, © 1993 by Annual Reviews Inc.)

chromosomally. Among other things, this technique enables the determinants of tissue specificity to be investigated directly. For example, comparison of the pattern of tumour development in mice transgenic for genes from SV40, JC and BK viruses indicated that tissue specificity is determined by early genes.

The construction of recombinant viruses for use as vaccines and gene vectors probably is the most obvious practical outlet for genetic technology. Vaccines of proven worth and safety (e.g. vaccinia virus, poliovirus, adenovirus) can be employed as vectors for heterologous antigens. This approach to vaccine development has the advantages of inherent safety, speed, ease of delivery and the likelihood of obtaining a balanced immune response. The potential limitation of pre-existing or induced immunity to the vector has not been a major problem in experimental trials. Control of rabies in wildlife by oral vaccination of red fox populations in Europe using a bait laced with a vaccinia virus/rabies G protein gene recombinant virus is the first successful application of this approach (Aubert et al. 1994).

5   IMMUNE EVASION

Characterization of the vaccinia virus genome in the interests of ameliorating residual virulence and promoting its use as a vector has resulted in the identification of a number of genes that interfere with the immune response of the host. The genome of vaccinia virus comprises c. 200 genes, about one-third of which are dispensable for propagation of the virus in cultured cells. These genes map in the extensive dispensable terminal regions of the vaccinia virus genome together with host range and virulence markers. Some of these dispensable genes seem to contribute to the survival of the virus in vivo by interfering with specific arms of the immune system, such as complement, interferon, inflammation, cytokines and cytotoxic T lymphocyte recognition (Smith 1993, 1994). The vaccinia virus genome encodes several proteins that have amino acid similarity to components of the complement system, and may prevent complement activation by competitively binding either complement control factors or complement receptors. Analogous genes are present in some herpesviruses.

At least 4 poxvirus genes interfere with interferon action. The type I interferon response is inhibited by the vaccinia virus E3L and K3L genes, which encode proteins competitively binding double-stranded RNA and double-stranded RNA-activated protein kinase, respectively. The K3L protein is a homologue of the eukaryotic initiation factor eIF-α. Other viruses achieve the same end by different routes; for example, the virus-associated RNAs transcribed from the adenovirus genome block the double-stranded RNA-activated protein kinase activity. A third vaccinia virus gene blocks interferon action by synthesis of a soluble type I interferon receptor (Symons, Alcami and Smith 1995), and some poxviruses also synthesize a type II interferon receptor. Synthesis of cytokine and growth factor homologues or their receptors is a strategy also employed by other large DNA viruses (Smith 1994). Other genes moderate inflammation by producing proteins that interfere intracellularly with cytokine synthesis and function.

Down-regulation of MHC class I antigens to counteract cytotoxic T cell responses is another device for confounding the immune response common to several viruses (Maudsley 1995). Several genes in the adenovirus genome subvert host defences (Wold, Hermiston and Tollefson 1994): virus-associated RNA inhibits interferon-mediated shut-off of protein synthesis, and at least 5 proteins interfere with interferon action, cytotoxic T cell activity, tumour necrosis factor activity and apoptosis. Herpes simplex virus encodes a gene that blocks presentation of peptides by inhibition of peptide translocation (Fruh et al. 1995, Hill et al. 1995). The Epstein–Barr virus-encoded nuclear antigen-1 (EBNA-1) directly inhibits antigen processing and enables EBNA-1-expressing cells to escape immunosurveillance, thereby ensuring the persistence of Epstein–Barr virus in the host without resort to indiscriminate immunosuppression (Levitskaya et al. 1995). Specific suppression of the cell-mediated immune response may be a determining factor in the persistence and latency associated with many of the large DNA viruses in particular, and a determining factor in pathogenesis.

REFERENCES

Almond JW, 1987, The attenuation of poliovirus neurovirulence, *Annu Rev Microbiol*, **41:** 153–80.

Andino R, Reickhof GE et al., 1990, Substitutions in the protease (3C^{pro}) gene of poliovirus can suppress a mutation in the 5′ noncoding region, *J Virol*, **64:** 607–12.

Aubert MFA, Masson E et al., 1994, Oral wildlife rabies vaccination field trials in Europe with recent emphasis on France, *Curr Top Microbiol Immunol*, **187:** 219–44.

Baltimore D, 1970, RNA-dependent DNA polymerase in the virions of RNA tumour viruses, *Nature (London)*, **226:** 1209–11.

Bernard J, Mercier D, 1993, Sequence of two *Eco*R1 fragments from Salmonid herpesvirus 2 and comparison with Ictalurid herpesvirus 1, *Arch Virol*, **132:** 437–42.

Billeter MA, Cattaneo R, 1991, Molecular biology of defective measles viruses persisting in the human central nervous system, *The Paramyxoviruses*, ed Kingsbury DW, Plenum Press, New York and London, 323–46.

Bouchard MJ, Lam D-H, Racaniello VR, 1995, Determinants of attenuation and temperature-sensitivity in the type 1 poliovirus Sabin vaccine, *J Virol*, **69:** 4972–8.

Brierley I, 1995, Ribosomal frameshifting on viral RNAs, *J Gen Virol*, **76:** 1885–92.

Cane PA, Matthews DA, Pringle CR, 1993, Frequent polymerase errors observed in a restricted area of clones derived from the attachment (G) gene of respiratory syncytial virus, *J Virol*, **67:** 1090–3.

Castrucci MR, Donatelli I et al., 1993, Genetic reassortment between avian and human influenza A viruses in Italian pigs, *Virology*, **193:** 503–6.

Chao L, 1994, Evolution of genetic exchange in RNA viruses, *The Evolutionary Biology of Viruses*, ed Morse SS, Raven Press, New York, 233–50.

Chen D, Burns JW et al., 1989, Phenotypes of rotavirus reassortants depend upon the recipient genetic background, *Proc Natl Acad Sci USA*, **86:** 3743–7.

Clapham P, Nagy K, Weiss RA, 1984, Pseudotypes of human T-cell leukaemia virus types 1 and 2: neutralization by patients' sera, *Proc Natl Acad Sci USA*, **81**: 2886–9.

Coen DM, 1990, Molecular genetics of animal viruses, *Fields' Virology*, 2nd edn, ed Fields BN, Knipe DM et al., Raven Press, New York, 123–49.

Coffin JC, 1982, Endogenous viruses, *RNA Tumor Viruses*, 2nd edn, ed Weiss R, Teich N et al., Cold Spring Harbor Laboratory, Cold Spring Harbor NY, 1109–204.

Davison AJ, 1992, Channel catfish virus: a new type of herpesvirus, *Virology*, **186**: 9–14.

Eigen M, Biebricher CK, 1988, Sequence space and quasispecies distribution, *RNA Genetics*, vol 3, eds Domingo E, Holland JJ, Ahlquist P, CRC Press, Boca Raton FL, 211–45.

Fruh K, Ahn K et al., 1995, A viral inhibitor of peptide transporter for antigen presentation, *Nature (London)*, **375**: 415–18.

Garcia-Sastri A, Palese P, 1993, Genetic manipulation of negative-strand RNA virus genomes, *Annu Rev Microbiol*, **47**: 765–90.

Goldbach R, 1987, Genome similarities between plant and animal RNA viruses, *Microbiol Sci*, **4**: 197–202.

Goldbach R, de Haan PT, 1993, RNA viral supergroups and the evolution of RNA viruses, *The Evolutionary Biology of Viruses*, ed Morse SS, Raven Press, New York, 105–19.

Greene AE, Allison RF, 1994, Recombination between viral RNA and transgenic plant transcripts, *Science*, **263**: 1423–5.

Grodzicher T, 1981, Adenovirus-SV40 hybrids, *DNA Tumor Viruses*, 2nd edn, ed Tooze J, Cold Spring Harbor Laboratory, Cold Spring Harbor NY, 577–614.

Hahn CS, Lustig S et al., 1988, Western equine encephalitis virus is a recombinant virus, *Proc Natl Acad Sci USA*, **85**: 5997–6001.

Hayden FG, Hay AJ, 1992, Emergence and transmission of influenza A viruses resistant to amantadine and remantadine, *Curr Top Microbiol Immunol*, **176**: 119–30.

Hill A, Jugovic P et al., 1995, Herpes simplex virus turns off the TAP to evade host immunity, *Nature (London)*, **375**: 411–15.

Holland JJ, 1987, Defective interfering rhabdoviruses, *The Rhabdoviruses*, ed Wagner RR, Plenum Press, New York and London, 297–360.

Holland JJ, 1990, Defective viral genomes, *Fields' Virology*, 2nd edn, ed Fields BN, Knipe DM et al., Raven Press, New York, 151–65.

Holland JJ, de la Torre JC, Steinhauer DA, 1992, RNA virus populations as quasispecies, *Curr Top Microbiol Immunol*, **176**: 1–19.

Huang AS, Baltimore D, 1970, Defective virus particles and viral disease processes, *Nature (London)*, **226**: 325–7.

Hull R, Covey SN, 1986, Genome organisation and expression of reverse transcribing elements: variations and a theme, *J Gen Virol*, **67**: 1751–8.

Ihara T, Akashi H, Bishop DHL, 1984, Novel coding strategy (ambisense genomic RNA) revealed by sequence analysis of Punta Toro phlebovirus S-RNA, *Virology*, **136**: 293–306.

Iroegbu CU, Pringle CR, 1981, Genetic interactions among viruses of the Bunyamwera complex, *J Virol*, **37**: 383–94.

Jarvis TC, Kirkegaard K, 1992, Poliovirus recombination: mechanistic studies in the absence of selection, *EMBO J*, **11**: 3135–45.

Joklik WR, Roner MR, 1995, What reassorts when reovirus genome segments reassort?, *J Biol Chem*, **270**: 4181–4.

Kates JR, McAuslan BR, 1967, Poxvirus DNA-dependent RNA polymerase, *Proc Natl Acad Sci USA*, **58**: 134–41.

Kirkegaard K, Baltimore D, 1986, The mechanism of RNA recombination in poliovirus, *Cell*, **47**: 433–43.

Koonin EV, Dolja W, 1993, Evolution and taxonomy of positive-strand RNA viruses: implications of comparative analysis of amino acid sequences, *Crit Rev Biochem Mol Biol*, **28**: 375–430.

Lai MMC, 1992, RNA recombination in animal and plant viruses, *Microbiol Rev*, **56**: 61–79.

Larder BA, 1994, Interactions between drug resistance mutations in human immunodeficiency virus type 1 reverse transcriptase, *J Gen Virol*, **75**: 951–7.

Lawson ND, Stillman EA et al., 1995, Recombinant vesicular stomatitis virus from DNA, *Proc Natl Acad Sci USA*, **92**: 4477–81.

Leppard KN, Pringle CR, 1996, Virus mutants, *Virology Methods Manual*, eds Mahy BWJ, Kangro H, Academic Press, London, 231–49.

Levitskaya J, Coram M et al., 1995, Inhibition of antigen processing by the internal repeat region of the Epstein–Barr virus nuclear antigen-1, *Nature (London)*, **375**: 685–8.

Luytjes W, Krystal M et al., 1989, Amplification, expression and packaging of a foreign gene by influenza virus, *Cell*, **59**: 1107–13.

Macadam AT, Stone DM et al., 1994, The 5′ noncoding region and virulence of poliovirus vaccine strains, *Trends Microbiol*, **2**: 449–54.

McClure MA, 1991, Evolution of retrotransposons by acquisition or deletion of retrovirus-like genes, *Mol Biol Evol*, **8**: 835–56.

McClure MA, Johnson MS et al., 1988, Sequence comparisons of retroviral proteins: relative rates of change and general phylogeny, *Proc Natl Acad Sci USA*, **85**: 2469–73.

McGeoch DJ, 1989, The genomes of human herpesviruses: contents, relationships and evolution, *Annu Rev Microbiol*, **43**: 235–65.

McGeoch DJ, Cook S, 1994, Molecular phylogeny of the *Alphaherpesvirinae* subfamily and a proposed evolutionary timescale, *J Mol Biol*, **238**: 9–22.

McGeoch DJ, Cook S et al., 1995, Molecular phylogeny and evolutionary timescale for the family of mammalian herpesviruses, *J Mol Biol*, **247**: 443–58.

McKnight SL, Kingsbury R, 1982, Transcriptional control signals of a eukaryotic protein-coding gene, *Science*, **217**: 316–24.

Mansky LM, Temin HM, 1995, Lower in vivo mutation rate of human immunodeficiency virus type 1 than that predicted from the fidelity of purified reverse transcriptase, *J Virol*, **69**: 5087–94.

Martinez MA, Vartanian J-P, Wain-Hobson S, 1994, Hypermutagenesis of RNA using human immunodeficiency virus type 1 reverse transcriptase and biased dNTP concentrations, *Proc Natl Acad Sci USA*, **91**: 11787–91.

Maudsley DJ, 1995, Modulation of MHC antigen expression by viruses, *Modulation of MHC Antigen Expression and Disease*, eds Blair GE, Pringle CR, Maudsley DJ, Cambridge University Press, Cambridge, 133–49.

Meyers G, Tautz N et al., 1991, Viral cytopathogenicity correlated with integration of ubiquitin-coding sequences, *Virology*, **180**: 602–16.

Mindich L, 1995, Heterologous recombination in the segmented dsRNA genome of bacteriophage 6, *Semin Virol*, **6**: 75–83.

Morgan DI, Dimmock NJ, 1992, Defective interfering virus inhibits immunopathological effects of infectious virus in the mouse, *J Virol*, **66**: 1188–92.

Morse MA, Marriott AC, Nuttall PA, 1992, The glycoprotein of Thogoto virus (a tick borne orthomyxo-like virus) is related to the baculovirus glycoprotein gp64, *Virology*, **186**: 640–6.

Murphy FA, Fauquet C et al., 1995, *Virus Taxonomy: Classification and nomenclature of viruses*, Springer-Verlag, Vienna.

Pringle CR, 1977, Enucleation as a technique in the study of virus–host interactions, *Curr Top Microbiol Immunol*, **76**: 49–82.

Pringle CR, 1987, Rhabdovirus genetics, *The Rhabdoviruses*, eds Fraenkel H, Wagner RR, Plenum Press, New York and London, 167–243.

Pringle CR, 1990, The genetics of viruses, *Topley and Wilson's Principles of Bacteriology, Virology and Immunity*, 8th edn, vol 4, eds Collier LH, Timbury MC, Edward Arnold, London, 69–103.

Pringle CR, 1996, Bunyavirus genetics, *The Bunyaviruses*, ed Elliott RME, Plenum Press, New York and London, 189–226.

Pringle CR, Devine V et al., 1981, Enhanced mutability associated with a temperature-sensitive mutant of vesicular stomatitis virus, *J Virol*, **39**: 377–89.

Racaniello VR, Baltimore D, 1981, Molecular cloning of poliovirus DNA and determination of the complete nucleotide sequence of the viral genome, *Proc Natl Acad Sci USA*, **78**: 4887–91.

Ramig RF, 1990, Principles of animal virus genetics, *Fields' Virology*, 2nd edn, eds Fields BH, Knipe DM et al., Raven Press, New York, 95–122.

Reanney D, 1984, The molecular evolution of viruses, *The Microbe 1984*, Society for General Microbiology symposium 36, vol I, Viruses, eds Mahy BWJ, Pattison JR, Cambridge University Press, Cambridge, 175–96.

Schneemann A, Schneider PA et al., 1995, The remarkable coding strategy of Borna disease virus: a new member of the nonsegmented negative strand RNA viruses, *Virology*, **210**: 1–8.

Schnell MJ, Mebatsion T, Conzelmann KK, 1994, Infectious rabies virus from cloned cDNA, *EMBO J*, **13**: 4195–203.

Sedivy JM, Capone JP et al., 1987, An inducible mammalian amber suppressor: propagation of a poliovirus mutant, *Cell*, **50**: 379–89.

Smith GL, 1993, Vaccinia virus glycoproteins and immune evasion, *J Gen Virol*, **74**: 1725–40.

Smith GL, 1994, Virus strategies for evasion of the host response to infection, *Trends Microbiol*, **2**: 81–8.

Strauss EG, Strauss JH, Levine AJ, 1990, Virus evolution, *Fields' Virology*, 2nd edn, eds Fields BN, Knipe, DN et al., Raven Press, New York, 167–90.

Symons JA, Alcami A, Smith GL, 1995, Vaccinia virus encodes a soluble type 1 interferon receptor of novel structure and broad species specificity, *Cell*, **81**: 551–60.

Tu Z, Chapman NM et al., 1995, The cardiovirulent phenotype of Coxsackie B3 is determined at a single site in the genomic 5' nontranslated region, *J Virol*, **69**: 4607–18.

Urquidi V, Bishop DHL, 1992, Non-random reassortment between the tripartite RNA genomes of La Crosse and snowshoe hare viruses, *J Gen Virol*, **73**: 2255–65.

Weiss RA, Bennett PLP, 1980, Assembly of membrane glycoproteins studied by phenotypic mixing between mutants of vesicular stomatitis virus and retroviruses, *Virology*, **100**: 252–74.

van der Werf S, Bradley J et al., 1986, Synthesis of infectious poliovirus RNA by purified T7 RNA polymerase, *Proc Natl Acad Sci USA*, **83**: 2330–4.

White BT, McGeoch DJ, 1987, Isolation and characterisation of conditional lethal nonsense mutants of vesicular stomatitis virus, *J Gen Virol*, **68**: 3033–44.

Williams KJ, Loeb LA, 1992, Retroviral reverse transcriptases: error frequencies and mutagenesis, *Curr Top Microbiol Immunol*, **176**: 165–80.

Wimmer E, Hellen CU, Cao X, 1993, Genetics of poliovirus, *Annu Rev Genet*, **27**: 353–436.

Wold WSM, Hermiston TW, Tollefson AE, 1994, Adenovirus proteins that subvert host defenses, *Trends Microbiol*, **2**: 437–43.

Youngner JS, Quagliana DO, 1976, Temperature-sensitive mutants of vesicular stomatitis virus are conditionally defective particles that interfere with and are rescued by wild type virus, *J Virol*, **19**: 102–7.

Zavada J, 1982, The pseudotype paradox, *J Gen Virol*, **63**: 15–24.

*Cattaneo R, 1989, How hidden reading frames are expressed, *Trans Biochem Sci*, **14**: 165–7.

Chapter 8

VIRUS–HOST CELL INTERACTIONS

L Andrew Ball

1 INTRODUCTION

As obligate intracellular parasites, viruses depend on their host cells at all stages of their infectious cycles. Different viruses impinge on almost every aspect of host cell metabolism, so virus–host cell interactions are diverse and complex. The details of these interactions have been shaped during the co-evolution of individual viruses and their hosts, and they can be fully understood only within that context. In fact, examination of the defences mounted by cells and organisms against viral infection, and of the various mechanisms that different viruses have evolved to help them evade these defences, provides a revealing glimpse into the heart of the host–parasite relationship (Smith 1994).

Experimental studies of virus–cell interactions are usually performed in cell culture, by using purified viruses to infect cultured cells that may be a different type or even a different species from those in which the viruses evolved. Because the consequences of infection can vary greatly from one cell type to another, the link between laboratory studies of virus–cell interactions and the behaviour of viruses in their natural state is sometimes tenuous. Nevertheless, experimental studies of virus–host cell interactions have not only enriched our understanding of viral infection but also illuminated many areas of molecular and cellular biology. Among these areas are the mechanisms of receptor function (Nomoto 1992, Haywood 1994, Wimmer 1994) and membrane fusion (White 1992, Bentz 1993); the pathways and control of macromolecular synthesis, processing and transport (Nevins 1989, Ehrenfeld 1993); the regulation of cell cycling (Levine 1993, Weinberg 1995); and oncogenic transformation (Teich 1991, Jansen-Durr 1996). This chapter presents a survey of this complex and far-reaching subject, and refers the reader to more detailed coverage of specific topics in other chapters. It also contains an extensive bibliography that includes many review articles to guide those interested in reading further.

1.1 Cytopathic effects of viral infection

Infection of susceptible cells with an animal virus usually causes cytological changes that are visible by light microscopy and collectively referred to as the cytopathic effect (CPE) of the virus. The nature of the CPE differs between viruses and from one type of virus–cell interaction to another (described in section 3, p. 117). In the case of a cytocidal virus infecting a cell monolayer, for example, the CPE frequently includes cell rounding and loss of adherence to the tissue-culture plate, visible consequences of the perturbations of cellular metabolism that presage the death of the cell (Fig. 8.1a). In contrast, cells infected with a tumour virus, where the outcome is not cell death but neoplastic transformation, undergo more subtle changes in morphology, although the overall consequences of infection both in cell culture and in animals can be at least as profound (Fig. 8.1c).

Viral CPEs are not due simply to the increased load on cellular protein synthesis (which is usually insignificant) nor even to its inhibition, because translation in uninfected cells can be blocked by drugs without inducing a CPE. On the contrary, some aspects of viral CPEs are directly due to the action of specific viral proteins: for example, detachment of adenovirus-infected cells from cell-culture plates results from the penton-base protein of the virion binding to cellular integrins during entry and thereby disrupting their interaction with vitronectin that was responsible for cellular adherence (Wickham et al. 1993). Similarly, some retroviral proteases cause cell rounding by disrupting the cytoskeleton (Luftig and Lupo 1994). However, it also seems that cells can respond to viral infection by launching a specific

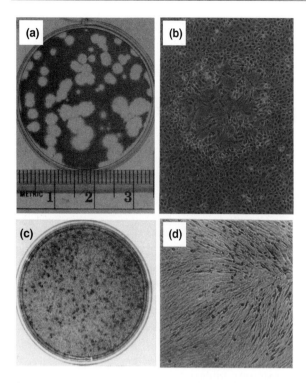

Fig. 8.1 (a) Plaque assay of a lytic virus (vesicular stomatitis virus). (b) Microphotograph of the typical cytopathic effect (CPE) of a lytic virus (vaccinia virus). (c) Focus-forming assay of a transforming retrovirus. (d) Microphotograph of part of a focus of transformed cells. Thanks to Drs Donald Blair and Karen Joyce Dunn (NIH, NCI) for the photographs shown in (c) and (d).

genetic programme that leads to cell death (apoptosis: see section 7.3, p. 140), which indicates that some of the consequences of infection are self-inflicted (Razvi and Welsh 1995, Steller 1995). The benefit to the organism of thus limiting the spread of infection outweighs the cost in sacrificed cells (Williams 1994).

2 QUANTITATIVE ASPECTS OF VIRUS–CELL INTERACTIONS

2.1 Multiplicity of infection

Infection is an encounter between 2 populations: the virus particles and the host cells. The average number of infectious virus particles per cell is called the multiplicity of infection (moi). When the moi is very low (10^{-4}, say), only a correspondingly small fraction of the cell population will be infected initially, although the infection can then spread through the cell culture as the virus multiplies. If the spread is contained, by an agarose overlay for example, areas of infected cells (plaques) will develop around each initial infection site, allowing the number of infectious particles (or plaque-forming units, pfu) in the virus inoculum to be calculated. This is the basis of the plaque assay, an example of which is shown in Fig. 8.1a and b. In contrast, when the moi is high, essentially all the cells will be infected at the outset and the virus will be limited

to a single round of synchronous replication. Tumour viruses, which transform cells rather than killing them, produce local foci of transformed cells in culture (Fig. 8.1c and d) and can therefore be quantified by an analogous assay that measures the number of infectious particles (or focus-forming units, ffu) in a tumour virus preparation.

2.2 Poisson distribution

The distribution of virus particles among a population of cultured cells is random and can be described mathematically by the Poisson distribution. This formula relates the average moi (m) to the fraction of cells (P) that actually receive any given number (k) of infectious particles. It shows that an moi of 1.0 pfu per cell will result in the infection of only 63.2% of the population, and that a moi of ≥5 is required to infect at least 99% of the cells (Table 8.1).

2.3 Ratios of physical particles to plaque-forming units

Not all virus particles in a preparation are capable of forming a plaque; indeed, the particle : pfu ratios for most animal viruses are seldom lower than 10 and sometimes much higher. There are several explanations for this surprising and often overlooked result. First, infection is a multi-step process in which the probability of successful completion of each step may be less than 100% even for an intrinsically infectious particle. Secondly, the apparent homogeneity of a virus preparation can conceal a substantial level of microheterogeneity: differences in the age of individual particles, their protein composition and even their genome sequences can influence infectivity. Among the RNA viruses, the high polymerase error rate that results from the absence of proofreading during RNA replication creates a population of genomes whose sequences compose a molecular swarm or quasispecies distribution around a consensus sequence (Smith and Inglis 1987, Holland, de la Torre

Table 8.1 Poisson distribution: percentage of cells receiving 0, 1 and >1 particles at different mois

Multiplicity of infection (pfu/cell)	Uninfected cells (%)	Singly infected cells (%)	Multiply infected cells (%)
0.0	100.0	0.0	0.0
0.5	60.7	30.3	9.0
1.0	36.8	36.8	26.4
2.0	13.5	27.0	59.5
3.0	5.0	15.0	80.0
5.0	0.67	3.35	96.0
10.0	0.0045	0.045	99.95

$P(k) = (e^{-m} \cdot m^k) \cdot 1/k!$
$P(0) = e^{-m}$
$P(1) = m \cdot e^{-m}$
$P(>1) = 1 - e^{-m}(m+1)$

and Steinhauer 1992, Drake 1993, Eigen 1993, Duarte et al. 1994). This concept has profound implications for our understanding of RNA virus evolution (Chapter 2).

Non-infectious virions can nevertheless participate in infection under both natural and experimental conditions. Typically, the number of particles that can undergo receptor binding and other early stages of infection will far exceed the infectious titre, a fact that complicates the study of early events in virus–cell interaction because it is difficult to identify the minority of particles that are on the pathway to productive infection (Wilson 1992). In many cases the genomes of non-infectious particles can engage in complementation and recombination with one another and thus contribute to the outcome of infection. Moreover, some of the most important physiological effects of infection, such as killing of the host cell and the induction of interferon (see section 7.1, p. 138, and Chapter 11), do not depend on the production of viral progeny and can therefore be accomplished by more virus particles than are needed to demonstrate full infectivity (Marcus and Sekellick 1974). The situation is further complicated by the fact that most animal viruses generate defective particles, particularly on repeated passage at high moi. As their name implies, defective particles are incapable of replication except when supported by co-infection with their parent virus with which they often interfere, thus earning the name defective interfering (DI) particles. Under experimental conditions DI particles can play critical roles in maintaining persistent infections, modulating viral pathogenesis (Chapter 9) and guiding virus evolution (Chapter 2), and it seems likely that they exert similar effects in nature (Dimmock 1985, Barrett and Dimmock 1986, Whitaker-Dowling and Youngner 1987, Roux, Simon and Holland 1991, Bangham and Kirkwood 1993).

2.4 Single-hit relationships

The fact that preparations of animal viruses have high particle : pfu ratios does not mean that more than one particle per cell is required to initiate a productive infection. The quantitative relationship between virus inoculum and infectivity is generally linear rather than exponential, which shows that infection is a single-hit phenomenon. Combining this observation with a demonstration that the inoculum contains only monomeric virus particles proves that under normal conditions a single virion suffices to infect a cell, although infections that depend on complementation or recombination between viral mutants provide exceptions to this rule. For viruses that have naturally segmented genomes, the quantitative dependence of infectivity on inoculum can supply information on the distribution of genome segments among the individual virus particles.

3 TYPES OF VIRUS–HOST CELL INTERACTIONS

Viral infections fall into 2 categories, productive and non-productive, depending on whether or not viral progeny are produced from the infected cells (Table 8.2). In reality, cellular permissiveness covers a wide spectrum from total non-productivity, through cases where very low numbers of virions are released, to fully productive situations in which each cell makes hundreds or thousands of infectious particles. Moreover, in the case of latent infections in animals (e.g. by members of the herpesvirus family), infectious virus can re-emerge several years after a non-productive interaction in one cell type as a fully productive infection in another (Chapters 17 and 18). As far as the host cell is concerned, its survival is determined not simply by whether the infection is productive but by the interplay between its genetic programme and that of the virus, as described in section 7 (p. 138) (and see Table 8.2).

3.1 Productive infections

The steps in a typical productive viral infection are as follows: (1) adsorption of the virus to specific cellular receptors; (2) its penetration across the plasma membrane and into the cell; (3) virus disassembly resulting in partial or complete uncoating of its genome; (4) transcription, translation and replication of the viral nucleic acid (the order and subcellular location of these steps reflecting the genome strategy of the family to which the virus belongs); (5) assembly of progeny virus particles; and (6) their release from the cell.

CYTOCIDAL INFECTIONS

Whether these events kill the host cell depends on the type of virus. For a typical, non-enveloped, cytocidal virus such as poliovirus (Chapter 25) which is released when the cell membrane disintegrates, cell death coincides with virus release, although some lytic viruses may be released by an unknown mechanism before the cells burst (Tucker and Compans 1993). In contrast, the release of cytocidal enveloped viruses such as vesicular stomatitis virus (VSV) (see Chapter 33), which mature by budding, occurs in a more prolonged manner and precedes the death of the host cell.

PRODUCTIVE TRANSFORMATION

This ability of enveloped viruses to bud from cells without necessarily killing them is exploited by the RNA tumour viruses (Chapter 38), which establish productive infections in which the host cells undergo neoplastic transformation rather than death (Chapter 12). By integrating their entire genome into that of the host cell and expressing oncogenes, RNA tumour viruses transform cells to a state of uncontrolled cell division and continuous release of infectious viral progeny.

Table 8.2   Classification of virus–cell interactions

| Consequences for the: | | Classification | Specific example | Chapter |
Virus	Cell			
Productive	lethal	Cytolysis	Poliovirus in human cells	058
	Non-lethal	Transformation	Rous sarcoma virus in chicken cells	096
		Persistence	Lymphocytic choriomeningitis virus in mouse cells	018
Non-productive	Lethal	Apoptosis	Vaccinia virus in Chinese hamster ovary cells	008
	Non-lethal	Transformation	Simian virus 40 in mouse cells	052
		Latency	Herpes simplex virus in neural cells	090

PERSISTENCE

Persistent infections in cell culture provide situations that are intermediate between these 2 extremes, and several mechanisms of persistence have been identified (Mahy 1985). These include carrier cultures, in which for some reason only a specific subpopulation of cells is susceptible to infection; cases in which virus spread is restricted because it can occur only by cell-to-cell contact; and steady states in which infected cells coexist with the virus because they have similar rates of multiplication. In cell culture, temperature-sensitive mutants, DI particles and interferon have all been implicated in maintaining persistence; the situation in animals is even more complex because it also involves interactions with different cell types, cytokines and the immune system (Oldstone 1991, Levine, Hardwick and Griffin 1994, ter Meulen 1994). These aspects are described in detail elsewhere (Chapters 10 and 11).

3.2   Non-productive infections

Counterintuitively, non-productive infections are often more challenging than productive ones, both intellectually and medically. In cells that carry receptors for a virus, the initial stages of a non-productive infection are the same as those listed above for productive situations: receptor binding, penetration and uncoating. In contrast, cells that lack appropriate receptors are usually not susceptible to infection, although some exceptions to this rule are described in section 4.3 (p. 122). After these initial stages, however, non-productive infections can have several different causes, courses and consequences (see Table 8.2).

APOPTOSIS

In some cases, the early steps of infection trigger the onset of the cell's apoptotic response, resulting in prompt cell death without either virus replication or the production of progeny (Razvi and Welsh 1995). Infection of Chinese hamster ovary cells by vaccinia virus provides a good example of this. Several viral genes have been identified whose actions delay the onset of apoptosis (E White 1993, Clem and Miller 1994, Ink, Gilbert and Evan 1995), which suggests that anti-apoptotic mechanisms may be widespread among animal viruses (see section 7.3, p. 140).

NON-PRODUCTIVE TRANSFORMATION

Replication of the smaller DNA viruses such as those in the papovavirus family (Chapter 16) depends on viral oncogenes that coax the infected cell into the S phase of the cell cycle and thus establish conditions that are conducive for DNA synthesis. This is particularly critical for papillomaviruses, which replicate only in terminally differentiated, non-cycling cells of the epidermis. In this situation, any block in virus replication that allows the cell to survive the infection can lead to integration of the viral oncogenes and consequent neoplastic transformation of the cell (see Table 8.2).

LATENCY

Of all the types of virus–host interactions, those that result in latency are the most perplexing (Garcia-Blanco and Cullen 1991). Members of the alpha-herpesvirus family (Chapter 18) typically progress from primary productive interactions, often with epithelial cells, to secondary latent infections, usually in neural cells, from which they can re-emerge periodically throughout the life of the infected individual (Wagner 1994). The viral genome remains intact during latency and is maintained as an episome in the nucleus, with at most a small subset of the viral genes being expressed. This situation is best understood for latent infections established by Epstein–Barr virus in B lymphocytes (Masucci and Ernberg 1994, Farrell 1995), which can be examined in cell culture. The general mechanisms by which herpesviruses establish, maintain and re-emerge from latency are subjects of intense investigation, but the scarcity of cell culture systems in which these processes can be duplicated renders them difficult to study.

4   ADSORPTION OF VIRUSES TO HOST CELLS

The first step in virus–cell interaction is a specific non-covalent binding between attachment sites on the surface of the virion and receptors on the plasma membrane of the host cell. Unlike some bacteriophages, all animal viruses carry multiple copies of their attachment proteins or sites, usually arranged in symmetrical or regular arrays on the surface of the virion (Chapter 4). Even the small picornaviruses have 60 receptor-binding sites per virion, and influenza virus has several hundred. What fraction of these sites must be occupied for successful virus binding and uptake is unknown although it is probably much less than 100% and may vary widely among different viruses. Indeed, a current model for the early stages of virus uptake proposes that the initial interaction with one or a few receptor molecules is followed by the recruitment of more receptors that can diffuse laterally in the plasma membrane. This would strengthen the binding, cause invagination of the membrane around the virus particle, and initiate what used to be called viropexis but is now generally referred to as receptor-mediated endocytosis (Fig. 8.2). See Wimmer (1994) for several reviews on all aspects of this subject.

The receptor–virus interaction can fulfil 2 distinct functions: positioning the virus particle for uptake by the cell and, at least in some cases, promoting virion disassembly. Virus structures have evolved to serve as metastable intermediates between successive cycles of replication, and some receptors not only bind the incoming virus particle but also act as keys to unlock its structure (section 4.4, p. 122). Of course, the presence of cell surface components that can perform these functions is not due to natural selection of cells for their ability to be infected, but rather to opportunism by viruses whose potential for faster evolution allows them to take advantage of existing host cell molecules with other functions. A remarkable variety of cell surface molecules have been co-opted by different viruses to enable them to bind and enter cells (Table 8.3), and these receptors are described further in section 4.2 (p. 121).

The presence of an appropriate receptor is usually necessary but not always sufficient to allow a particular virus to infect a cell or organism. For example, poliovirus naturally infects only humans and closely related primates because certain cells of these species have a receptor (the poliovirus receptor, PVR) to which the virus can attach, but the host range of the virus can be extended to mice if they are engineered to express the human gene for PVR (Ren et al. 1990, Nomoto, Koike and Aoki 1994). In contrast, mouse cells

expressing CD4, the receptor for human immunodeficiency virus (HIV), can bind the virus but are not infected by it, showing that in some cases there is more to uptake and penetration than simple binding (see section 4.5, p. 124). Similarly, although receptor distribution is a major determinant of viral tissue tropism, the susceptibility of different tissues in an organism does not simply reflect the tissue distribution of the receptor, because productive infection often requires accessory factors for virus entry (section 4.5, p. 124) as well as a hospitable intracellular environment for replication. The overall relationship between viral entry mechanisms examined in cell culture and virus spread during a natural infection is a difficult and contentious area of virology.

4.1 Viral attachment proteins and sites

In the simplest cases, the task of binding to the host cell has been assigned by evolution to a single species of viral surface protein, such as the haemagglutinin (HA) of influenza virus (Weis et al. 1988) or gp120 of HIV (Weiss 1992), although such attachment proteins usually function as oligomers. In more complex situations such as the picornaviruses, receptor-binding sites on the virion surface are created at the interfaces between 2 or more viral polypeptides (Colonno 1992, Olson et al. 1993). Larger viruses may show a still higher level of complexity, in which 2 or more viral surface proteins are involved in a series of progressively tighter interactions with different cell surface components. For example, glycoprotein C of herpes simplex virus (HSV) binds the abundant heparan sulphate moieties of cell surface proteoglycans whereas glycoprotein D binds to mannose-6-phosphate receptors (Spear 1993, Brunetti et al. 1994). Strictly speaking, such downstream components of a multi-step entry pathway are best considered 'entry accessory factors' (section 4.5, p. 124) rather than viral receptors. Nevertheless, the idea of a rapid, relatively low-affinity interaction being followed by a slower, tighter binding, either to a secondary component or to newly recruited primary receptors, is reminiscent of the mechanism by which circulating leucocytes adhere to vascular endothelial cells, by rolling across weak recep-

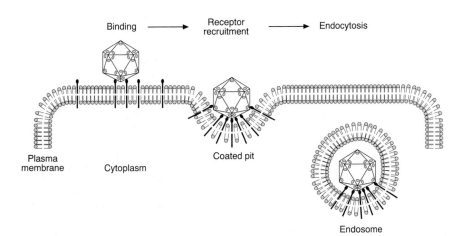

Fig. 8.2 Receptor-mediated endocytic uptake of a virus particle.

Table 8.3   Some examples of virus receptors

Virus family	Viruses	Receptors
Coronaviridae	Mouse hepatitis virus	Carcinoembryonic antigen family member
	Human coronavirus 229E	Aminopeptidase *N*
	Human coronavirus OC43	*N*-acetyl-9-*O*-acetylneuraminic acid
Herpesviridae	Epstein–Barr virus	B lymphocyte C3d complement receptor (CD21)
	Herpes simplex virus	Heparan sulphate moieties of proteoglycans
Orthomyxoviridae	Influenza A and B viruses	*N*-acetylneuraminic acid (sialic acid) on glycoproteins and glycolipids
	Influenza C virus	*N*-acetyl-9-*O*-acetylneuraminic acid
Paramyxoviridae	Sendai virus	Sialoglycoprotein GP2
	Measles virus	Complement regulator CD46
Picornaviridae	Poliovirus	Poliovirus receptor (immunoglobulin superfamily member)
	Rhinoviruses (major group)	Intercellular adhesion molecule 1 (ICAM-1)
	Rhinoviruses (minor group)	LDL receptor
	Foot-and-mouth disease virus	Integrin (RGD-binding protein)
Reoviridae	Reovirus type 3	β-Adrenergic receptor
Retroviridae	Human immunodeficiency viruses	T cell surface glycoprotein CD4, and galactosyl ceramide
	Ectropic murine leukaemia virus	Cationic amino acid transporter
	Gibbon ape leukaemia virus	Sodium-dependent phosphate symporter
	Feline leukaemia virus	Sodium-dependent phosphate symporter
Rhabdoviridae	Vesicular stomatitis virus	Phosphatidylserine and phosphatidylinositol
Togaviridae	Sindbis virus	High-affinity laminin receptor

For references to the original work that described these receptors, see Lentz (1990), Haywood (1994) and Wimmer (1994).

tors (selectins) before binding irreversibly to integrins (Lawrence and Springer 1991). The speed of the initial binding in 3 dimensions that is required to capture a passing particle is combined with a slower, 2-dimensional search for the interactions that give the overall process its necessary high affinity.

GLYCOPROTEIN SPIKES

Many enveloped viruses display their attachment proteins as surface spikes that project perpendicularly from the viral envelope. These spikes are visible in electron micrographs and consist of oligomers of virus-specified integral membrane glycoproteins. In some, perhaps many, cases, the arrangement of the surface spikes reflects the symmetry of the nucleocapsid underlying the viral envelope (Paredes et al. 1993, Cheng et al. 1995). The 3-dimensional structure of one viral attachment glycoprotein, the influenza virus HA, was determined at near-atomic resolution in 1981 and has been influential in shaping ideas of the structure and function of such proteins (Fig. 8.3; see also Plate 8.3) (Wiley and Skehel 1987). It consists of a bundle of 3 identical monomers extending 135 Å

from the surface of the viral envelope, arranged around a symmetry axis that is parallel to its length. Each monomer contains 2 disulphide-linked polypeptides, HA1 and HA2, produced by cleavage of the 550 amino acid primary translation product. The globular top of the trimeric bundle has 3 concave binding sites for sialic acid, the cellular receptor for influenza virus, as well as several antigenic sites that elicit and react with antibodies that neutralize the infectivity of the virus. At its bottom, HA2 anchors the protein by passing through the viral membrane, although the protein whose structure was determined was first made soluble by removal of the transmembrane domain.

A very different picture is presented by glycoprotein E of the flavivirus tick-borne encephalitis virus (TBEV) (Chapter 28), the only other attachment glycoprotein whose structure has been determined (Rey et al. 1995). Like influenza virus HA, this is a type I integral membrane protein that is anchored in the viral envelope by its C terminus. However, rather than forming a protruding spike, the TBEV glycoprotein forms an elongated homodimer that lies flat on the surface of the viral envelope with a symmetry axis that is perpen-

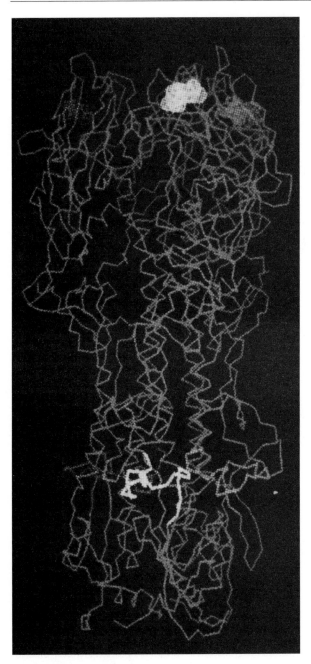

Fig. 8.3 The influenza virus haemagglutinin (HA). The α-carbon backbone of the HA trimer is displayed in blue with the 3 fusion peptides, located in the stem of the molecule, highlighted in red, yellow and green. The molecular surfaces of 3 sialic acid residues are shown (red, yellow, green) in the receptor-binding sites of the globular head domains. The 3 monomers would be anchored in the viral membrane at the bottom. See also Plate 8.3. (From White 1992.)

Capsid attachment sites

In non-enveloped viruses, the receptor-binding sites are built into the architecture of the particles and are thus displayed in a symmetry determined by that of the capsid. A technical consequence of this is that individual virus particles with receptors bound at each site can be visualized using cryoelectron microscopy and image reconstruction methods to achieve a resolution of about 25 Å. Figure 8.5a shows a rhinovirus particle decorated with its receptor, intercellular adhesion molecule 1 (ICAM-1) (Olson et al. 1993, Rossmann et al. 1994). Sixty receptor molecules are bound to each virion, arranged in groups of 5 around each of the 12 axes of 5-fold symmetry in the icosahedral particle. The receptors thus occupy chemically identical binding sites which, in this and some other picornaviruses, lie in a trench-like depression called the canyon that encircles each 5-fold axis. A higher resolution image that shows how a single receptor molecule fits into the canyon has been generated by combining the crystal structure of the rhinovirus particle with the predicted structure of ICAM-1 (Fig. 8.5b; see also Plate 8.5b). It shows that the binding site is created and protected by the juxtaposition of the capsid proteins VP1, VP2 and VP3, parts of which form the walls of the canyon. Ultimately, it may prove possible to co-crystallize a virus–receptor protein complex and directly examine the molecular contacts at atomic resolution.

The specific contacts by which a viral attachment protein binds to its receptor, and hence the amino acid residues involved, are largely fixed by the requirement that they must create a binding surface with steric, electronic and hydropathic complementarity for the receptor. It is important, therefore, that these residues avoid immune surveillance, because an antibody directed specifically and exclusively against the receptor-binding site would create a barrier to infection that the virus could not circumvent by mutation. This problem has been solved in different ways by different viruses (Chapman and Rossmann 1993). For example, location of the receptor-binding sites in the canyon of rhino- and polioviruses protects them from reach by antibodies which are much bulkier than the receptors (Rossmann 1989). In contrast, the receptor-binding site in foot-and-mouth disease virus is in a surface loop that may avoid antigenic scrutiny by being structurally mobile. Finally, there may be cases where the receptor-binding site mimics the structure of the natural ligand so precisely that the immune system does not recognize it as foreign.

4.2 Cellular receptors for viruses

A wide variety of cell surface molecules can be used as receptors by different viruses (Table 8.3). In some cases, a ubiquitous carbohydrate modification is recognized, such as sialic acid or heparan sulphate on a glycoprotein or glycolipid, whereas in other cases it is a specific protein that may be present on the surface of only certain cell types (such as CD4 on T lymphocytes), which thus directs and restricts the tro-

dicular to its length (Fig. 8.4; see also Plate 8.4). The receptor that the protein recognizes is not known, but its receptor-binding domain has an immunoglobulin-like folded structure that presents the binding site on the surface of the virion.

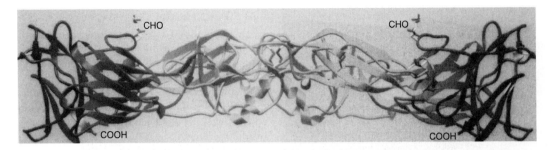

Fig. 8.4   Three-dimensional structure of glycoprotein E of tick-borne encephalitis virus. The dimer is viewed from the side, as it would lie on the surface of the viral membrane. For colour, see Plate 8.4. (From Rey et al. 1995.)

pism of the virus (Lentz 1990, Wimmer 1994). The receptors for poliovirus (PVR), rhinovirus (ICAM-1) and HIV (CD4), among others, belong to the immunoglobulin superfamily of proteins, and contain 3–5 repeats of the 'immunoglobulin fold', a structural domain that is characteristic of the immunoglobulins (White and Littman 1989). The 3-dimensional structure of 2 such domains in a fragment of CD4 that includes the HIV binding site is illustrated in Fig. 8.6 (see also Plate 8.6) (Harrison et al. 1992, Signoret et al. 1993). Since members of this protein superfamily have been naturally selected for cell surface expression and the ability to bind protein ligands with high specificity, it is easy to understand why they should have been commandeered as viral receptors. Indeed, 2 very different viruses, HIV and human herpes virus type 7, both use CD4 as their receptor, and the malaria parasite also uses ICAM-1 for cell attachment. The versatility of the immunoglobulin fold as a protein-binding domain is further illustrated by the fact that it sometimes occurs in the other partner in the interaction, the viral attachment protein (Rey et al. 1995).

Just as dissimilar viruses can share the same receptor, so can closely related viruses use different receptors. Human rhinoviruses, of which there are over 100 serotypes, divide into a major group that use ICAM-1 and a minor group that use the low density lipoprotein (LDL) receptor. In this case, the use of different receptors does not seem to influence the outcome of infection, but there are examples where the use of alternative receptors by a single virus can have profound consequences. The ability of HIV to use galactosyl ceramide instead of CD4 to enter cells may be responsible for its infection of the brain and the resulting AIDS-related dementia (Weiss 1992).

Infection of animals is usually initiated in epithelial cells, which are naturally polarized and express different sets of proteins on their apical and basolateral surfaces (Tucker and Compans 1993, Eaton and Simons 1995). Interaction of viruses with polarized cells whose receptors are distributed asymmetrically can occur only at the cell surface that expresses the receptor, because the intercellular tight junctions prevent access of the virus to the other face of the polarized cell layer. For example, SV40 infection can occur only from the apical surface. Since virus release also often occurs in a polarized manner from epithelial cells, asymmetric

receptor distribution can greatly influence the course of infection and the pathway of virus spread in an infected animal (Tucker, Wimmer and Compans 1994).

4.3   Antibody-mediated enhancement

Although the presence of a cognate receptor is usually a prerequisite for infection, some virus–cell interactions can occur through intermediate molecules for which both the virus and the cell have affinity. Paradoxically, virus-specific antibodies can play this role and actually promote virus uptake because some cells express a receptor for the Fc portion of the antibody molecule (Porterfield 1986, Halstead 1994). In this way, the immune system can collaborate in the spread of infection by circumventing the requirement for a virus-specific receptor (Mason, Rieder and Baxt 1994). The pathogenesis of infections by both dengue virus and HIV can be exacerbated by antibody-mediated enhancement of infectivity, but the phenomenon is probably irrelevant for viruses such as polio in which interaction with the cognate receptor mediates an essential structural change in the virion (section 4.4, p. 122).

4.4   Consequences of receptor binding

As mentioned at the start of section 4 (p. 118), receptor binding initiates virus entry into the cell and, at least in some cases, destabilizes the structure of the virion so that it begins to disassemble. Before binding to the receptor, poliovirus is stable at pH 2 and can therefore enter the body through the strongly acidic environment of the stomach. However, reaction with PVR causes a major conformational change in the capsid that involves swelling, loss of a small internal protein (VP4) and extrusion of the hydrophobic N terminus of VP1 in preparation for its interaction with membranes (Flore et al. 1990, Racaniello 1992, Gomez Yafal et al. 1993). But only a few of the poliovirus particles that interact with the receptor are internalized. Substantial numbers of these antigenically altered particles, which can no longer bind the receptor and have therefore lost their infectivity, dissociate from cells during poliovirus infection and may play a role in decoying the immune response. In the case of some rhinoviruses, reaction with the recep-

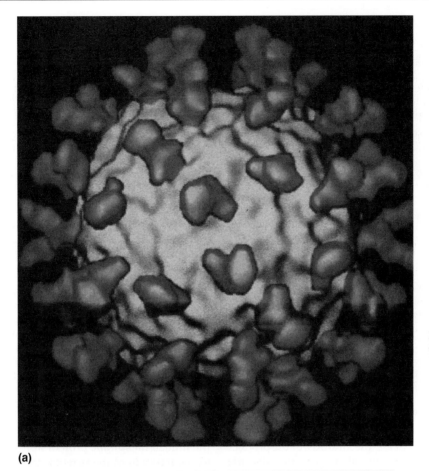

(a)

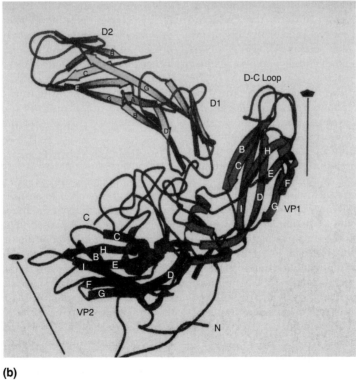

(b)

Fig. 8.5 Interaction of rhinovirus with its receptor ICAM-1. (a) Cryo-EM reconstruction of a virus particle complexed with 60 receptor molecules (orange). (b) High-resolution image of a single receptor-binding site interaction. For colour, see Plate 8.5. (From Olson et al. 1993.)

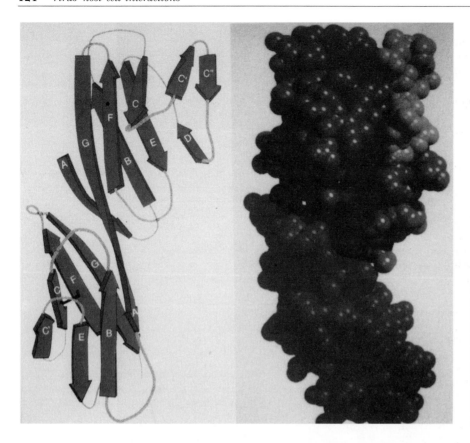

Fig. 8.6 Backbone and solid representations of the 3-dimensional structure of CD4 (D1D2 domains). The D1 domain is in red, the D2 domain is in blue and the region of D1 implicated in the binding HIV gp120 is yellow. For colour, see Plate 8.6. (From Wang et al. 1990.)

tor is sufficient to release the viral RNA and produce empty capsids, whereas in other cases this requires exposure to mildly acidic conditions such as those encountered during passage through the endocytic pathway into the cytoplasm (Giranda et al. 1992, Greve and Rossmann 1994) (see section 5). These observations suggest that receptor binding and acid pH may co-operate to initiate picornavirus disassembly. In the case of HIV, binding to the receptor CD4 causes the release of the viral attachment protein gp120 from the particle, exposing a hydrophobic fusion peptide whose interaction with membranes mediates the next step in viral entry (section 5).

When the natural function of the receptor is transmembrane signalling, virus binding can trigger a physiological response even without internalization. It is thought that Epstein–Barr virus can activate B lymphocytes by binding to the C3d complement receptor (Hutt-Fletcher 1987). Moreover, this type of effect can be widely disseminated because infected cells often secrete soluble forms of the viral attachment protein. Some of the complex effects of HIV on T lymphocyte function may be mediated directly by the phosphorylation of CD4 and the consequent transmembrane signalling that is caused by the binding of gp120.

4.5 Entry accessory factors

There are many instances in which the ability of a virus to bind to the surface of a cell is sufficient for uptake but there are others where something else is needed. For example, rodent cells that express human CD4 fail to become infected with HIV unless they also express the human membrane protein fusin, which is required for penetration of the virus-receptor complex into the cell (Feng et al. 1996). In the case of adenovirus, initial receptor binding by the fibre protein must be followed by an interaction between the penton base protein of the virus and cellular integrins in order for internalization to occur (Wickham et al. 1993). The distinction between secondary receptors and entry accessory factors, and the roles that each plays in virus uptake are unclear and will probably remain so until more details of this multi-step process are known.

4.6 Release from receptors

For viral progeny to spread most effectively, some mechanism is needed to ensure release from receptors expressed by the primary infected cells. In general, a combination of virus-mediated receptor down-regulation and the inhibition of protein synthesis contribute to this requirement, but viruses that bind to sialic acid also carry specific 'receptor-destroying enzymes' that remove terminal sialic acid residues from oligosaccharides. Along with the HA protein described in section 4.1 (p. 119), particles of influenza A and B virus have a second surface glycoprotein (NA) that has neuraminidase (sialidase) activity. Although the presence of this enzyme may allow infecting virions to 'browse' the cell surface during entry, its only essential roles in infection are to prevent infected cells from trapping progeny virus particles and to eliminate the self-aggregation that would otherwise result from HA binding to its own oligosaccharides (Liu et al. 1995). Particles of influenza C virus and some coronaviruses, whose attachment proteins bind to *N*-acetyl-9-*O*-acetylneuraminic acid, carry an esterase that likewise mediates destruction of receptors. In the latter case, and in some paramyxoviruses, the receptor-binding and receptor-destroying activities are both present in the same molecule (HE and HN, respectively), raising interesting questions about their interrelationship and regulation.

5 PENETRATION AND UNCOATING

Virus particles assemble in cells as very stable structures that are able to withstand harsh extracellular environments, but when re-exposed to intracellular conditions they spontaneously disassemble. In some cases, binding to the receptor contributes to this dramatic change in virion stability (section 4.4), but an important role is played by the paths that viruses follow as they enter cells. Depending on the type of virus, its genome must cross one, 2 or 3 lipid bilayers between binding to the receptor at the plasma membrane and reaching its intracellular destination. During infection, all viral genomes must penetrate the plasma membrane; those of enveloped viruses must also cross the viral membrane, and those that replicate in the nucleus also need to traverse the nuclear membrane. Virion proteins play active roles in these transmembrane passages, and have been sculpted by natural selection to transfer the viral genome to the appropriate cellular compartment. Some stages of virion disassembly and genome uncoating invariably accompany membrane penetration (Hoekstra and Kok 1989, Marsh and Helenius 1989, Carrasco 1994, Greber, Singh and Helenius 1994, Lanzrein, Schlegel and Kempf 1994).

5.1 Two pathways of virus entry

Although some viral receptors naturally transport small molecules (see Table 8.3) (Dautry-Varsat and Lodish 1984), it seems that not even the smallest virus is directly carried across the plasma membrane by its receptor. Instead, enveloped viruses transfer their nucleocapsids across membranes by fusing with them, a reaction that achieves simultaneous envelope removal and cell entry. Fusion is mediated by specific virion surface proteins that can fuse lipid bilayers (section 5.2), and some non-enveloped viruses probably achieve the same result by inserting capsid proteins into a cellular membrane (section 5.4, p. 127). For many viruses, both with and without envelopes, activation of the ability to fuse with membranes requires exposure to a mildly acidic environment (pH 5–6); such viruses enter cells by receptor-mediated endocytosis (see Fig. 8.2) into endosomes whose contents then become acidified by an ATP-driven proton pump. The result is fusion of the virus with the membrane of the endosome and release of the viral genome into the cytoplasm. Other viruses can fuse without being exposed to low pH, and can therefore enter the cytoplasm directly by fusion with the plasma membrane (Fig. 8.7).

Infection by viruses that enter through endosomes can be inhibited by lysosomotropic agents such as ammonium chloride or chloroquine which raise the endosomal pH, whereas viruses that enter at the plasma membrane are insensitive to these reagents. The pathway of entry that leads to a productive infection is thus determined largely by the properties of the viral protein responsible for membrane fusion: whether exposure to low pH is required to activate it. In general, viruses in the herpes-, papova-, paramyxo-, retro- and rotavirus families can enter cells by fusion with the plasma membrane in a pH-independent manner, whereas those in the adeno-, alpha-, bunya-, flavi-, orthomyxo-, picorna-, reo- and rhabdovirus families need to pass through an acidic endosome. However, there are several individual exceptions to these family rules.

The ability of many viruses to fuse with cellular membranes is responsible for a common cytopathic effect of viral infection: the formation of multi-nucleated syncytia by cell-to-cell fusion. This is due to the abundant expression of the viral proteins that cause membrane fusion (section 5.2) on the surface of infected cells, where they can interact with both infected and uninfected neighbours ('fusion from within'). Cell fusion creates a pathway for the local spread of an infection by which a virus can partly elude the immune system. For respiratory syncytial virus, a member of the paramyxovirus family, the extensive syncytium formation that accompanies infection both in the respiratory tract and in cell culture was used in naming the virus and in diagnosing infections. Another paramyxovirus, Sendai virus, has been widely used by cell biologists as a laboratory reagent to induce the formation of heterokaryons by 'fusion from without'.

5.2 Viral fusion proteins

Some viruses (e.g. the paramyxoviruses) have separate envelope glycoproteins for receptor binding and membrane fusion; others (e.g. influenza and the retroviruses) combine the 2 functions into a single viral protein. Despite their variety of structures, however, the fusion proteins of enveloped viruses have features in common. They all contain 2 hydrophobic regions: a transmembrane domain by which they are anchored in the viral envelope, and a fusion peptide of 16–26 non-polar amino acids in the ectodomain of the protein that interacts with the target membrane (Schlesinger and Schlesinger 1987, White 1990, 1992, Doms et al. 1993). Formation of a bridge between the viral and cellular membranes by means of divalent anchoring is thought to mediate membrane apposition (Fig. 8.8), an essential step in fusion (Bentz 1993).

The hydrophobic nature of the fusion peptide must remain masked, both during translation, to allow it to pass through the membrane of the endoplasmic reticulum (ER), and during virus assembly and release, to prevent premature activation of its fusogenic potential. For these reasons, fusion peptide sequences are

Fusion at
the plasma
membrane
Cytoplasm
Plasma membrane
Endosome
Fusion after
endocytosis
Endocytosis
H+

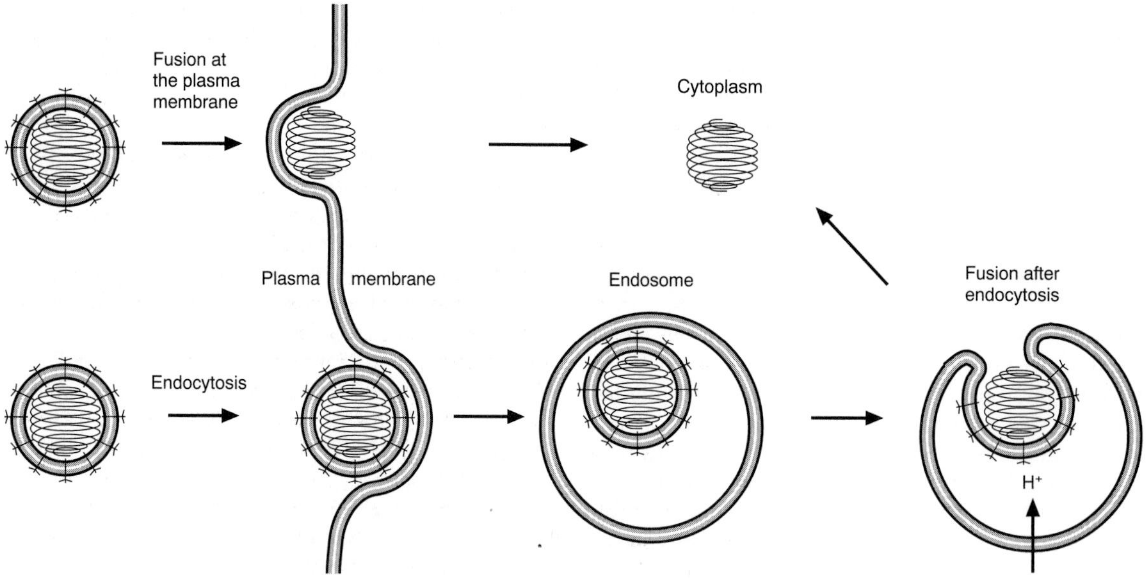

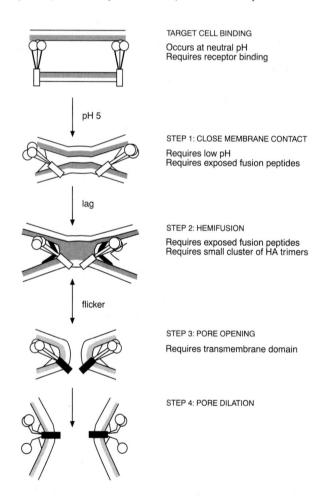

Fig. 8.7 Two pathways of enveloped virus entry: fusion at the plasma membrane or fusion after endocytosis.

TARGET CELL BINDING
Occurs at neutral pH
Requires receptor binding
pH 5
STEP 1: CLOSE MEMBRANE CONTACT
Requires low pH
Requires exposed fusion peptides
lag
STEP 2: HEMIFUSION
Requires exposed fusion peptides
Requires small cluster of HA trimers
flicker
STEP 3: PORE OPENING
Requires transmembrane domain
STEP 4: PORE DILATION

Fig. 8.8 Steps in HA-mediated membrane fusion. (From White 1994.)

initially buried, both in the primary sequences and in the oligomeric structure of fusion proteins. A maturational cleavage event, which sometimes occurs after virus release, places the fusion peptide sequence at a newly created N terminus, as in the influenza HA structure where it forms the N terminus of HA2 (see Fig. 8.3 and Plate 8.3) or in the HIV gp120/gp41 structure in which it is the N terminus of gp41. However, the 2 cleavage products remain associated with one another, sometimes by disulphide bonds, in an oligomeric structure that continues to mask the fusion peptide. In the case of influenza HA, rearrangement of the subunits of the trimer is necessary to expose their fusion peptides to the target membrane, and it is likely that a major conformational change of this sort is a common feature of the activation of fusion proteins (section 5.3).

Different viruses prevent premature activation of their fusion proteins in different ways. For Sendai virus, the required cleavage of the fusion protein precursor is mediated by a protease at the membrane of the target cell. For HIV, receptor binding dissociates gp120 and thereby exposes the hydrophobic N terminus of gp41. For Semliki Forest virus, the fusion protein monomer is maintained as an inactive heterodimer with the viral attachment protein until receptor binding and exposure to low pH release it to form the homotrimer that is fusogenic (Kielian 1995). For some paramyxoviruses, fusion requires both the attachment protein HN and the fusion protein F, because binding of HN to its receptor somehow activates the fusion protein, its partner in the viral envelope (Lamb 1993). For influenza A virus, where exposure to low pH triggers the conformational change that activates HA, the protein is chaperoned during its synthesis and maturation by the viral M2 protein, which acts a transmembrane proton channel to regulate the pH in the cellular compartments through which the maturing HA must pass (Pinto, Holsinger and Lamb 1992). Another role for the influenza virus M2 protein as an ion channel is described in section 5.5 (p. 128).

5.3 Mechanisms of membrane fusion

The 3-dimensional structure of the neutral form of HA (see Fig. 8.3 and Plate 8.3) raised some perplexing questions about how it mediated membrane fusion. Because the receptor-binding site is 135 Å from the transmembrane domain and about 100 Å from the fusion peptide, it was not clear how, after receptor binding, the protein could closely juxtapose the viral envelope in which it was anchored with the target membrane for insertion of the fusion peptide. Some of these problems were solved when it was discovered that a region of HA2 underwent a massive conformational change at the pH of membrane fusion, resulting in a 100 Å relocation of the fusion peptide to one apex of the molecule (Fig. 8.9; see also Plate 8.9) (Carr and Kim 1993, Bullough et al. 1994).

In this new location, membrane insertion of the N terminus of HA2 is easy to envisage, although it is not clear whether this and other fusion peptides are inserted into their target membranes vertically, obliquely or horizontally, as random coils or perhaps as amphipathic α-helices. Unfortunately, the new HA2 structure does not reveal the relative positions of the fusion peptide and the anchor domain, so the way that these regions and the receptor-binding site collaborate to mediate membrane fusion is still unclear (Carr and Kim 1994, Stegman 1994, Hughson 1995). When last seen in the low pH structure, the C terminus of HA2 was heading in the direction of the fusion pep-

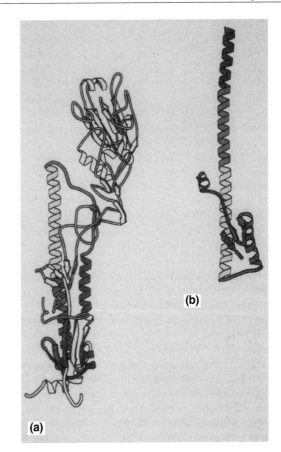

Fig. 8.9 The conformational change induced by low pH in influenza virus HA. The neutral pH form of the HA1,2 monomer is shown on the left in the same orientation as in the HA trimer shown in Fig. 8.3. The low pH form of the HA2 monomer is shown on the right. Corresponding regions are coloured identically. For colour, see Plate 8.9. (From Bullough et al. 1994.)

tide (Fig. 8.9), raising the possibility that the acid-induced conformational change brings the anchor and fusion peptides (and hence perhaps the viral and cellular membranes) into close proximity with one another. However, there is much yet to be discovered about the mechanism of membrane fusion and several models have been proposed that involve hemi-fused intermediates (Fig. 8.8), inverted micelles, proteinaceous pores or intermembrane stalks (Stegman 1994). It is interesting that an engineered mutant of HA that is anchored only in the outer membrane leaflet rather than traversing the lipid bilayer mediates only hemifusion, showing that the anchor domain plays different roles in mixing the lipids of the 2 leaflets (Kemble, Danieli and White 1994).

5.4 Uncoating of non-enveloped viruses

Non-enveloped viruses are also destabilized during cell entry, by interactions with their receptors (section 4.4, p. 122) and in some cases by exposure to endosomal pH, reducing conditions or low intracellular calcium ion concentrations. Although entry of non-enveloped viruses into the cytosol cannot be achieved by membrane fusion, it is possible that the hydrophobic N terminus of VP1 of some picornaviruses may play the role of a fusion peptide. It is buried in the capsid structure but becomes exposed when the virus binds to its receptor, and may perhaps be inserted into the cell membrane as a pentamer derived from one of the 12 5-fold axes of the icosahedral virion. The internal protein VP4, which exits the virus particle after receptor binding, is myristylated at its N terminus, and could thereby also interact with membranes. Such a complex might form a hydrophilic transmembrane channel through which the viral RNA could pass into the cytosol (Fig. 8.10) (Mosser, Sgro and Rueckert 1994, Johnson 1996). Despite the external protein symmetry of icosahedral virions and nucleocapsids, it is possible that the asymmetry of the nucleic acid inside confers different properties on some of the capsomers and that these differences are exploited during virion disassembly. Whether the RNA enters the cytosol in a polar manner as depicted in Fig. 8.10 remains to be determined. However, the capsid proteins of infecting alphavirus particles are transferred to 28S ribosomal RNA (Singh and Helenius 1992), thus releasing the viral RNA genome for translation. The disassembly of tobacco mosaic virus and cowpea chlorotic mottle virus in plants also occurs co-translationally, by ribosomes displacing capsid proteins from the viral RNA during the initial round of protein synthesis (Verduin 1992), and a similar possibility exists for extraction of the RNA from positive-strand RNA animal viruses.

For adeno- and reoviruses, whose genomes do not interact directly with ribosomes, partially disassembled subviral particles exit the endosome by lysis or permeabilization of the vesicle membrane. As in the examples described above, it is the acidic environment, sometimes in conjunction with proteolytic cleavage of viral structural proteins, that activates the virus particles to disrupt the endosomal membrane (Dryden et al. 1993).

5.5   Transit to the nucleus

Viral genomes that replicate in the nucleus need to travel there from where they entered the cytosol. For a herpesvirus particle infecting a neuron, this may be a journey of several centimetres during which the viral nucleocapsid is transported by axonal flow (Chapter 18). In less extreme cases, transport mechanisms that are thought to involve interactions with the cytoskeleton deliver the viral genome or nucleocapsid to the cytoplasmic face of pores in the nuclear membrane. For adeno- and herpesviruses, whose nucleocapsids are too large to enter the nucleus intact, a final stage of uncoating occurs at the nuclear pores to release the viral DNA into the nucleus. In contrast, most retroviruses require the natural breakdown of the nuclear membrane that occurs during mitosis, and they are therefore restricted to infection of dividing cells.

Influenza virus replicates in the nucleus but assembles its progeny in the cytoplasm and therefore faces unusual problems of compartmentation. The binding of viral nucleocapsids to the matrix protein (M1), which is responsible for their transport out of the nucleus in preparation for virus assembly, must be disrupted at the start of infection in order to permit the incoming viral genome to migrate into the nucleus. This is another function of the viral M2 protein; it creates acid-activated ion channels in the viral envelope which open at the low pH of the endosome to admit ions into the interior of the virion, thereby releasing the viral nucleocapsids from their association with the matrix protein (Hay 1992, Helenius 1992, Marsh 1992). The anti-influenza drug amantadine inhibits this process by blocking the ion channel activity of the M2 protein.

5.6   Poxvirus uncoating requires viral gene expression

In the uncoating mechanisms described above,

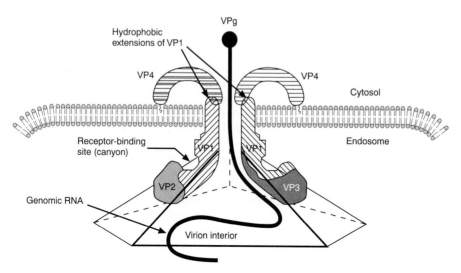

Fig. 8.10 Possible model for the exit of picornavirus RNA into the cytoplasm. (Adapted from Mosser, Sgro and Rueckert 1994.)

components of the infecting virions played active and essential roles, but the expression of new viral genes was not necessary. Members of the poxvirus family, however, uncoat by a 2-stage process in which the second stage depends on viral gene expression (Chapter 21). Vaccinia virus, for example, is taken up by receptor-mediated endocytosis, although the identity of its receptor is uncertain (Hugin and Hauser 1994, Chang et al. 1995). On release of the nucleocapsid core into the cytosol, a viral DNA-dependent RNA polymerase that is part of the core begins to transcribe several viral genes, among them one for a protease that triggers the second stage of uncoating that releases the viral DNA into the cytosol in preparation for genome replication.

6 EFFECTS ON HOST CELL METABOLISM

An incoming virus particle faces a formidable challenge in subverting the metabolism of the host cell to its own ends. Depending on the virus, a single copy of its genetic programme dominates one that is 10^4–10^6 times larger and already being expressed. To meet this challenge, viruses have evolved a wide variety of ways to manipulate the intracellular environment so that it can better support their replication. These include changes in intermediary metabolism, particularly of deoxyribonucleotides, as well as effects on the synthesis, processing, transport and turnover of cellular macromolecules. Viruses achieve dominance by combining mechanisms that enhance the expression of viral genes with those that interfere with the host. Many of the latter perturbations have detrimental effects on the infected cell that result in viral pathogenesis and disease (Chapter 9), but it seems that few if any of them evolved with the primary purpose of causing cellular damage. On the contrary, viruses, like all successful parasites, survive not because they kill the host but because they avoid inducing its premature demise.

The nature of the initial biosynthetic reaction – DNA, RNA or protein synthesis – and where it occurs in the infected cell depend on the genome strategy of the virus (Table 8.4). Most DNA genomes replicate in the nucleus, whereas most RNA genomes replicate in the cytoplasm, although the pox- and orthomyxoviruses are notable exceptions to this generalization. The retro- and hepadnaviruses are difficult to classify in this regard because their genomes alternate between RNA and DNA during each replication cycle. Whatever the initial biosynthetic reaction, a mechanism that most viruses use to help them attain dominance over the cell is to differentiate their infectious cycles into an early phase, when the viral genomes are present in low copy-number and direct the synthesis of catalytic amounts of viral replication proteins, and a late, post-replicative phase, when the abundant progeny genomes direct the synthesis of stoichiometric amounts of structural proteins.

6.1 DNA metabolism

Host cell DNA replication occurs only during the S phase of the cell cycle, in a tightly regulated manner that is co-ordinated with the cell cycle as a whole. It requires pools of deoxyribonucleotides, replication enzymes, continuous protein synthesis and access to appropriate anchor points on the nuclear matrix (Challberg and Kelley 1989, Echols 1990, Challberg 1991, Stillman et al. 1992). Viruses perturb this process to different degrees, depending on how much they rely on it for their own replication. Retroviruses, for example, which integrate DNA copies of their genomes into host chromosomes, ensure their replication by the expression of oncogenes that drive the cell relentlessly through the cell cycle, but do not otherwise affect cellular DNA replication (Chapter 38). At the other end of the spectrum, the elaborate genomes of herpes- and poxviruses replicate with almost complete autonomy, to the extent that infection by HSV blocks cells from progressing to S phase, and infection by vaccinia virus even causes cellular DNA degradation (Kelly, Wold and Li 1988).

DEOXYRIBONUCLEOTIDE BIOSYNTHESIS

Most cells in the body continue to make RNA and protein throughout their lives, but many terminally differentiated cells stop dividing and therefore suppress DNA synthesis. For a virus with a DNA genome to be able to replicate in such cells, it must not only circumvent this suppression or provide the necessary enzymes for DNA replication (or both) but also restore the cellular pools of deoxyribonucleoside triphosphates (dNTPs). Even in dividing cells, the metabolic load imposed by viral DNA synthesis can exceed the capacity of the cell and require continuous replenishment of the dNTP pools. This problem is particularly acute for the poxviruses, which replicate their DNA in the cytoplasm (Chapter 21).

Two distinct mechanisms have evolved to relieve this constraint: DNA viruses with relatively small genomes, such as the papova- and adenoviruses, induce cells to enter S phase, when the cellular genes for the necessary enzymes are naturally expressed. This is the basis for the oncogenic potential of viruses in these families (Jansen-Durr 1996), which is described in Chapter 12. In contrast, larger DNA viruses in the herpes- and poxvirus families have genomes with sufficient capacity to encode viral versions of some of the critical enzymes of nucleotide metabolism. Figure 8.11 shows the major pathways of dNTP biosynthesis in animal cells, with the enzymes encoded by either herpes- or poxviruses (or both) underlined. It is presumed that the genes for these enzymes were acquired from the host during viral evolution and serve to liberate these viruses from dependence on S phase. However, the genes are usually dispensable for virus replication in cultured cells, which are metabolically active and cycling.

Although these virus-specified enzymes catalyse the same reactions as their cellular counterparts, their substrate specificities and regulatory properties are

Table 8.4   Initial biosynthetic events in animal virus infections

Initial biosynthetic event	Virus families	Subcellular location	Origin of enzymes
DNA-dependent DNA synthesis	*Parvo*	Nucleus	Cell
	Hepadna	Nucleus	Virion
RNA-dependent DNA synthesis	*Retro*	Cytoplasm	Virion
DNA-dependent RNA synthesis	*Papova*	Nucleus	Cell
	Adeno	Nucleus	Cell
	Herpes	Nucleus	Cell
	Baculo	Nucleus	Cell
	Irido	Nucleus	Cell
	Pox	Cytoplasm	Virion
RNA-dependent RNA synthesis	*Orthomyxo*	Nucleus	Virion
	Delta agent	Nucleus	Cell (RNA pol II)
	Paramyxo	Cytoplasm	Virion
	Rhabdo	Cytoplasm	Virion
	Filo	Cytoplasm	Virion
	Bunya	Cytoplasm	Virion
	Reo	Cytoplasm	Virion
	Arena	Cytoplasm	Virion
Protein synthesis	*Picorna*	Cytoplasm	Cell (ribosomes)
	Toga	Cytoplasm	Cell (ribosomes)
	Flavi	Cytoplasm	Cell (ribosomes)
	Corona	Cytoplasm	Cell (ribosomes)
	Calici	Cytoplasm	Cell (ribosomes)
	Noda	Cytoplasm	Cell (ribosomes)

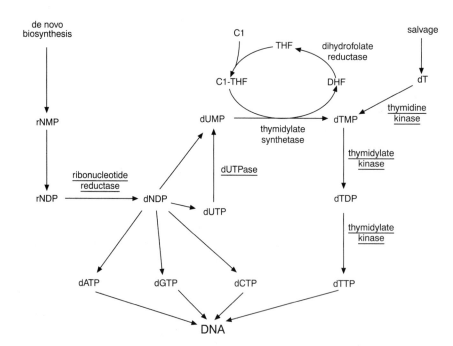

Fig. 8.11   Pathways of deoxyribonucleotide biosynthesis. Underlined enzymes are encoded by some herpes- or poxviruses.

often somewhat different, which makes them feasible targets for the development of antiviral agents (Chapter 46). For example, the antiherpetic drugs acyclovir and ganciclovir are analogues of guanosine that can be phosphorylated by the thymidine kinase enzyme of HSV but not by that of the host. Because the 5'-triphosphates of these drugs act as chain terminators during DNA synthesis, they block DNA repli-

cation specifically in HSV-infected cells. However, the propensity of viral genomes for mutation and the facile selection of drug-resistant mutants create problems for the long-term use of antiviral agents that are similar to those encountered with antibiotics. For example, suppression of vaccinia virus replication by hydroxyurea, which inhibits ribonucleotide reductase by a radical scavenging mechanism, readily selects for resistant mutants that contain multiple copies of the gene for one of the subunits of the viral enzyme (Slabaugh, Roseman and Mathews 1989). Nevertheless, the virus-specific enzymes of nucleotide metabolism that are encoded by the larger DNA viruses provide versatile genetic tools as well as possible targets for the development and testing of antiviral agents. The possibility is also being explored of incorporating the HSV thymidine kinase gene into suicide vectors targeted to tumour cells to render them sensitive to acyclovir (Morgan and Anderson 1993).

DNA REPLICATION

As described above, DNA viruses with small genomes stimulate the host cell to provide them with many of the enzymes they need for DNA replication. Papovaviruses such as SV40 induce S phase in infected cells by the action of a single viral gene product, large T antigen, which is expressed early in the infectious cycle (Fanning and Knippers 1992). This viral protein binds to the cellular tumour-suppressor protein pRb (Wiman 1993), displacing transcription factors of the E2F family to which it is normally bound (Nevins 1992). These transcription factors switch on several cellular genes involved in cell cycle control and DNA replication, including the genes for DNA polymerase α, the enzyme that replicates the viral genome. T antigen also binds to another tumour-suppressor protein, p53, and relieves the cell cycle block that is normally imposed by this protein (Ludlow 1993, Ludlow and Skuse 1995). Thus by expressing a single viral protein, SV40 prepares the cell for DNA replication and gains access to the enzymes necessary to catalyse it. During a productive infection, viral DNA replication will ensue, but the properties of large T antigen are those of an oncogene, and expressed on its own it will transform cells and cause tumours (whence it derives the name of **T**umour antigen). In the related papilloma viruses, the inactivation of pRb and p53 is delegated to 2 viral proteins, E7 and E6 respectively (Vousden 1993, Farthing and Vousden 1994).

With DNA genomes 3–6 times larger than those of the papovaviruses, adenoviruses (Chapter 15) have sufficient genetic capacity to encode 3 of the proteins necessary for DNA replication: DNA polymerase, a genome-linked terminal protein involved in the initiation of viral DNA synthesis, and a single-stranded DNA binding protein. But they still need to push the cell into S phase to establish supportive conditions. This push is mediated by 2 early viral gene products, E1A and E1B, which together perform the functions described above for SV40 T antigen: binding to the tumour-suppressor proteins pRb and p53, respectively (Moran 1993).

In addition to the enzymes of nucleotide metabolism (Fig. 8.11), HSV encodes 7 proteins that are directly involved in DNA replication (Chapter 18). By providing so much of the replication apparatus itself, HSV gains independence from the cell cycle and attains a degree of autonomy that lets it replicate in highly differentiated cells such as neurons. Similarly,

encoding most or all of their replication machinery enables poxviruses to replicate their DNA in the cytoplasm (Chapter 21).

Two families of animal viruses synthesize DNA by a pathway that has no cellular counterpart, that of reverse transcription of RNA. Retro- and hepadnaviruses both encode an RNA-dependent DNA polymerase (reverse transcriptase) that catalyses this unique reaction which is central to their mechanisms of genome replication (Chapters 38 and 36, respectively). The enzyme is a structural component of virus particles from both families and it catalyses the initial biosynthetic reactions of their infectious cycles, the synthesis of viral DNA. Retroviruses also encode an integrase enzyme that recombines the proviral DNA into the genome of the host.

Because cellular DNA replication depends on continuous protein synthesis, it is inhibited by many DNA and RNA viruses as a consequence of their effects on translation (section 6.3, p. 134). The viruses probably benefit from the increased availability of nucleotides. Inhibition also results from the ability of viral DNA molecules to displace cellular DNA from anchor points on the nuclear matrix that are thought to provide the necessary structural framework for DNA replication. It has been suggested that competition for these sites may modulate the interaction between viral and host cell DNA replication (Cook 1991), and, in accordance with this idea, components of the cell's replication machinery are also redistributed within the nucleus following HSV infection (de Bruyn Kops and Knipe 1988).

DNA MAINTENANCE AND TRANSFER

Viral DNAs can be stably maintained in the host cell either by integration into a cellular chromosome, as with the retroviruses, or in the form of extrachromosomal circular episomes, as with papilloma and hepadnavirus DNAs and during latent infections with herpesviruses. In the integrated state, retroviral DNAs use both the origins and the enzymes of the cell for replication, but episomal DNAs contain their own *cis*-acting replication origins and usually express *trans*-acting viral proteins to assist in their replication and maintenance. In general, the long-term coexistence of viral and host DNAs in the same cellular compartment creates possibilities for the transfer of genetic information in both directions. Transfers from virus to cell are exemplified by the many instances of cellular transformation mediated by the incorporation of oncogenes from DNA tumour viruses (Teich 1991). Transfers from cell to virus are considered to have been responsible for the acquisition of proto-oncogenes during evolution of the RNA tumour viruses and for the integration of a cellular retrotransposon into baculovirus DNA (Friesen and Nissen 1990).

DNA MODIFICATION AND DEGRADATION

Unlike bacteria, eukaryotic cells do not generally contain DNA restriction/modification enzyme systems to protect themselves against invading DNA, although a few examples have been found of such enzymes being induced or encoded by viruses of eukaryotes. A family of DNA viruses that infect the green alga *Chlorella* encode DNA methyltransferases and sequence-specific endonucleases that resemble restriction enzymes of prokaryotes (van Etten et al. 1988, van Etten, Lane and Meints 1991). Cells infected by frog virus 3, an iridovirus, express a cytosine methyltransferase that protects the viral DNA against degradation by a virus-encoded DNase (Murti, Goorha and Granoff 1985). Poxviruses, on the other hand, rely on subcellular compartmentation to achieve specific degradation of host DNA. Vaccinia virus particles contain a DNase that enters the host cell nucleus early in infection and degrades the cellular DNA. The liberated nucleotides are recycled into viral DNA to such an extent that the incorporation of exogenous thymidine via the thymidine kinase pathway is almost completely suppressed during the later stages of viral DNA synthesis. Degradation of cellular DNA also occurs as a result of the induction of apoptosis in response to infection by some viruses (section 7.3, p. 140). During this process, internucleosomal cleavage of chromatin produces a characteristic ladder of DNA fragments that can be resolved by agarose gel electrophoresis. Finally, the genomes of vaccinia virus and HSV encode uracil DNA glycosylases that are thought to be involved in viral DNA base excision repair (Dodson, Michaels and Lloyd 1994, Millns, Carpenter and DeLange 1994).

6.2 RNA metabolism

Whatever the initial biosynthetic event in infection, sooner or later every virus has to deliver mRNA to the cytoplasm to direct viral protein synthesis. Because the nature of the problem varies with the genetic strategy of the virus, virus families have evolved different mechanisms to ensure efficient transcription of viral genes and to disrupt the expression of host cell genes (Nevins 1989, Tevethia and Spector 1989).

PREFERENTIAL SYNTHESIS OF VIRAL RNAS

Three general mechanisms have been identified that promote transcription of viral genes at the start of infection: (1) seduction of the cellular RNA polymerase (pol II) by means of a strong promoter/enhancer sequence in the viral DNA (e.g. papova- and adenoviruses); (2) import of a new transcription factor that redirects pol II to the viral DNA (e.g. HSV); and (3) import of a new RNA polymerase with specificity for the viral genome (e.g. poxviruses and all negative-strand and double-stranded RNA viruses). These 3 distinct mechanisms are described below.

Enhancers

Studies of the early SV40 promoter, which directs pol II to transcribe the viral T antigen gene, were the first to discover the *cis*-acting DNA element now known as an enhancer which increases the level of transcription from a minimal promoter on a DNA molecule (Tjian and Maniatis 1994). Enhancers work by recruiting cellular transcription factors which are often differentially expressed in different cell types, so the properties of the viral enhancer can determine which types of cell are able to support replication of the virus (Drapkin, Merino and Reinberg 1993). For example, human papilloma virus (Chapter 16) is restricted to replication in keratinocytes partly because the enhancer for its E6 and E7 oncogenes must be recognized by a keratinocyte-specific transcription factor.

Transcription factors

In HSV infection, the viral DNA enters the nucleus together with a virion structural protein called α-*trans*-inducing factor (α-TIF or VP16) which is necessary for efficient transcription of the α class of viral genes that are expressed immediately after infection. α-TIF works in conjunction with the cellular transcription factor Oct-1 to recruit pol II to the Oct-1-binding sites (ATGCAAAT) that are present in the promoters for the α-genes (Kristie and Sharp 1993). Among the products of α-gene expression are at least 2 other transcription factors that change the specificity of the cellular polymerase to prepare it for the next stage of viral gene expression, transcription of the β-genes (Chapters 17 and 18). In general, DNA viruses switch transcription from one temporal class of genes to the next by the synthesis of viral factors that act directly or indirectly on the corresponding RNA polymerases. Some of the properties of the SV40 T antigen and the E1A/E1B proteins of adenovirus that provide examples of this were described in section 6.1 (p. 129). Transcription factors for immediate early genes (e.g. HSV α-TIF) are synthesized late in the preceding infectious cycle because they themselves are encoded in late viral genes. It is not yet known what prevents them from becoming active until the start of the next infection.

RNA polymerases

Many virus families have genomes that cannot be transcribed by any cellular polymerase and must therefore be presented to the cell in conjunction with a functional virus-specific transcriptase. For example, although poxvirus genomes are composed of double-stranded DNA, infection delivers them to the cytoplasm, which lacks RNA polymerase activity, and anyway their promoter sequences are unrecognizable by the nuclear RNA polymerases (Chapter 21). To ensure transcription of their genes under these conditions, infecting poxvirus particles contain a multi-subunit transcription complex that is activated once the viral core reaches the cytoplasm. It is guided specifically to the early viral genes by a viral early transcription factor (VETF) that is bound to early promoters, in conjunction with a polymerase-associated protein (rap94) that is responsible for recruiting the subunits of the transcription complex during virus assembly in the previous infection (Zhang, Ahn and Moss 1994).

RNA viruses whose genomes consist of either double-stranded RNA or single-stranded negative- or ambisense RNA face the same problem and solve it in the same manner: infection delivers the genome complexed with a virus-encoded RNA-dependent RNA polymerase that transcribes the viral genes (Ishihama and Barbier 1994). In many cases, virion-associated enzymes then cap, methylate and polyadenylate the primary transcripts to produce functional mRNAs. The following virus families use this strategy: reo-, orthomyxo-, paramyxo-, rhabdo-, filo-, bunya- and arenaviruses (see Table 8.4).

PERTURBATIONS OF CELLULAR RNA METABOLISM

Every step of cellular RNA metabolism is disrupted by one virus family or another: transcription, processing, transport from the nucleus to the cytoplasm, translation and RNA degradation. These effects usually give the viral genes a competitive advantage, although in some cases the advantage may be too slight to be demonstrable during a single infectious cycle. Effects on translation are described in section 6.3 (p. 134), the others below.

RNA synthesis

The expression of oncogenes by tumour viruses results in a stimulation of cellular RNA synthesis as a consequence of cell cycling. In contrast, most non-oncogenic viruses inhibit cellular transcription, although the mechanisms, which are largely unknown, may be consequences of the inhibition of protein synthesis or the rearrangement of cellular chromatin, or both. The benefit to the virus is presumed to be decreased competition for ribonucleoside triphosphates, and in some cases the increased availability of pol II. Curiously, VSV, a rhabdovirus that replicates entirely in the cytoplasm (Chapter 33), also inhibits cellular transcription. The 46 nucleotide (nt) VSV leader RNA migrates into the nucleus early in infection, associates with the cellular La protein and can inhibit pol II. However, the idea that leader RNA is responsible for the inhibition of transcription in infected cells has been challenged, and the physiological significance of these effects is unclear.

Influenza virus disrupts cellular RNA synthesis in an unusual manner that is directly related to its own mechanism of transcription (Chapter 22). By endonucleolytic cleavage, the viral RNA polymerase removes 10–13 nt fragments that include the cap from the 5′ ends of newly made cellular transcripts, and uses these fragments to prime the synthesis of viral mRNAs in the nucleus of infected cells (Lamb and Krug 1996). The effect is to transfer the caps from cellular mRNA precursors to viral messages, thereby labilizing the former and ensuring the translatability of the latter. Bunyaviruses (Chapter 30) use a similar cap-snatching mechanism to derive the 5′ ends of their mRNAs, except in this case the cap donors are mature cellular messages that are already in the cytoplasm (Kolakofsky and Hacker 1991).

RNA processing and transport

For viruses that replicate in the nucleus, RNA splicing is usually an important control point in gene expression. In the interests of genetic economy, DNA viruses with small genomes frequently splice their primary transcripts in several different ways, both to derive multiple mRNAs from a single promoter and to access 2 overlapping reading frames in the same region of the viral genome. Retroviruses use alternative splicing patterns too, but they also need a mechanism to allow the export to the cytoplasm of unspliced RNA to encode some of the viral structural proteins and to be encapsidated into progeny virions. Complex retroviruses such as HIV achieve this by the interaction between a viral protein rev, itself the translation product of a spliced message, and a specific RNA sequence in the viral genome (the rev-response element, RRE). This interaction allows the export of viral RNAs that still contain complete introns and would otherwise be retained in the nucleus (Gait and Karn 1993, Cullen 1994). In simpler retroviruses such as Mason–Pfizer monkey virus, the function of the rev/RRE complex is performed instead by a small *cis*-acting RNA element that somehow promotes the export of unspliced viral RNAs to the cytoplasm (Bray et al. 1994).

The NS1 protein of influenza virus inhibits splicing of both viral and cellular mRNA precursors by binding to their poly(A) tails and blocking spliceosome function, but in this case the unspliced host cell transcripts are retained in the nucleus, where they provide a source of the capped oligonucleotides that are needed as primers for viral transcription. Phosphorylation of NS1 regulates this inhibition to permit the release of viral mRNAs to the cytoplasm (Lamb and Krug 1996). Yet another variation is provided by adenovirus, the system by which splicing was originally discovered (Berget, Moore and Sharp 1977, Chow et al. 1977). Splicing is not inhibited in infected cells, and indeed primary adenovirus transcripts are extensively and differentially spliced to access many different open reading frames from a few promoter sites (Chapter 15). However, 2 of the early proteins (E1B and E4) specifically inhibit the export of processed cellular mRNAs from the nucleus and promote that of late viral mRNAs, resulting in the preferential synthesis of viral proteins. It is likely that further studies of the ways that different viruses impinge on the processing and transport of cellular transcripts will deepen our understanding both of virus–cell interactions and of the regulation of mRNA synthesis in uninfected cells (Krug 1993).

RNA degradation

The pathways and control of mRNA degradation in eukaryotic cells are poorly understood (Katze and Agy 1990) but, as with RNA processing and transport, viral genetics provide powerful experimental tools to assist research in this area. Both HSV and vaccinia virus infections increase the rate of host mRNA degradation and thereby inhibit cellular protein synthesis (Rice and Roberts 1983, Strom and Frenkel 1987). The effects are not specific for cellular messages, because viral mRNAs are turned over equally fast, but the greater vigour of viral transcription is better able to compensate for the short mRNA half-lives, which also facilitate the rapid transitions from expression of one temporal class of viral genes to the next. For HSV-1, the ability to induce mRNA labilization has been mapped to the *vhs* gene (for **v**iral **h**ost **s**hut-off), which encodes a virus structural protein. The vhs protein in the virion is sufficient to trigger mRNA degradation in some cells, although it is not known whether it works directly as a nuclease or by activating a host cell degradative mechanism. In vaccinia virus, the gene responsible for enhanced mRNA turnover has not been mapped, but mutations that subtly affect the function of the viral RNA polymerase can cause massive non-specific RNA degradation by producing abundant double-stranded RNA which activates the cellular 2-5A system for RNA breakdown (Bayliss and Condit 1993) (see section 7.1, p. 138, and Chapter 11). It will be interesting to see whether the nuclease activity that generates the 3′ end of a late cowpox mRNA is also involved in the enhanced turnover of cellular mRNA (Antczak et al. 1992).

6.3 Protein metabolism

The synthesis, processing and transport of viral proteins lie at the heart of the overlap between viral and cellular metabolism, because, whereas most viruses encode specific enzymes or factors that participate in viral transcription and genome replication, they all depend on the host cell for the entire machinery of protein synthesis and transport. One consequence of this is that translation, which is such an effective target for antibacterial agents, is not available as a target for the development of antiviral drugs.

PROTEIN SYNTHESIS

The rate of protein synthesis from a particular mRNA is influenced by many factors (Lodish 1976). In eukaryotic cells, most translational control is exerted at initiation (Merrick 1990), and a schematic picture of this multi-step reaction is shown in Fig. 8.12. Because of its complexity, the regulation of this process is not yet fully understood, but the following factors all play a part: the abundance of the mRNA, its 5′ cap structure, the local nucleotide sequence context and secondary structure surrounding its initiation codon, whether it is translated on free or membrane-bound polysomes, and the availability and activity of cellular initiation factors (Hershey 1990, 1993, Kozak 1991a, Wek 1994). Two prominent control points among the latter are eIF-4F, the cap-binding complex, and eIF-2, which binds the initiator met-tRNA to the 40S ribosomal subunit. Both of these initiation factors are altered in some virus-infected cells, as described below (Kozak 1986, Schneider and Shenk 1987).

Initiation in uninfected eukaryotic cells usually involves recognition by eIF-4F of the 7-methylguanylate cap at the 5′ end of cellular mRNA, followed by association of the mRNA with a complex that contains the 40S ribosomal subunit, met-tRNA$_i$ and eIF-2 (Fig. 8.12). eIF-4F is a cap-dependent RNA helicase that is required for the translation of almost all capped messages. On a very small number of cellular mRNAs

and on picornaviral RNAs (see p. 135), initiation occurs at an internal ribosome entry site (IRES), in a manner that is independent of the 5′ cap and eIF-4F. In both cases, the 40S subunit then scans in a 3′ direction until it encounters the first AUG codon. If the local sequence context of this AUG is favourable for initiation, the 60S ribosomal subunit joins the complex, eIF-2 dissociates and the synthesis of the polypeptide chain begins. Initiation efficiency is influenced most by the identity of the nucleotides in the −3 and +4 positions relative to the AUG, the sequence . . . **CRCCAUGG** . . . being optimal for initiation, but other features of the mRNA 5′ end including its secondary structure can also exert effects (Kozak 1989, 1991a, 1991b, 1992a, 1992b, 1994). Although eukaryotic protein synthesis usually starts at the first AUG codon, if its context is unfavourable for initiation the 40S subunit can continue scanning until it finds the next and start there instead. In rare instances, alternative initiation codons, including non-AUG codons, are used to derive more than one translation product from a single mRNA, as in the case of the P mRNA of some paramyxoviruses (Curran, Richardson and Kolakofsky 1986) (see Chapter 23). When eIF-2 dissociates from the initiation complex it is bound to GDP, but before it can form another met-tRNA$_i$–40S subunit complex for another round of initiation, it must exchange this GDP for GTP, a reaction that requires initiation factor eIF-2B (Fig. 8.12). In several metabolic situations including viral infection, this exchange reaction is a major site at which protein synthesis is regulated, as described below (p. 136) (Hershey 1993).

Host shut-off and the preferential translation of viral mRNAs

The inhibition of host cell protein synthesis is one of the most obvious metabolic consequences of viral infection, and it has been the focus of much research using several different virus systems (see Ehrenfeld 1993 for some recent reviews). Unfortunately, although it is easy to demonstrate the phenomenon, it has proved difficult to elucidate its mechanisms, because, somewhat surprisingly, viruses shut off host protein synthesis in different ways and even closely related viruses can use completely different mechanisms (Table 8.5). Cytocidal viruses such as polio and vaccinia inhibit host translation profoundly, but retroviruses, which depend on the cell's continued growth and survival, scarcely perturb host protein synthesis at all. Many other viruses lie between these 2 extremes. Some of the conflicts in the literature on this subject may be because some viruses use more than one mechanism or use different mechanisms when infecting different cell types.

Because viral and host mRNAs compete directly for translation, viruses have evolved mechanisms that favour the synthesis of their own proteins, often at the expense of the cell's. However, the total amount of translation occurring in infected cells is almost always less than that in uninfected cells, because infection generally reduces the overall capacity of the cell for protein synthesis. Rather than simply displacing host mRNAs, viral messages are preferentially translated against the background of a progressive inhibition of total protein synthesis to which they are relatively resistant. For this reason, how viruses inhibit host protein synthesis and the mechanisms they use to achieve

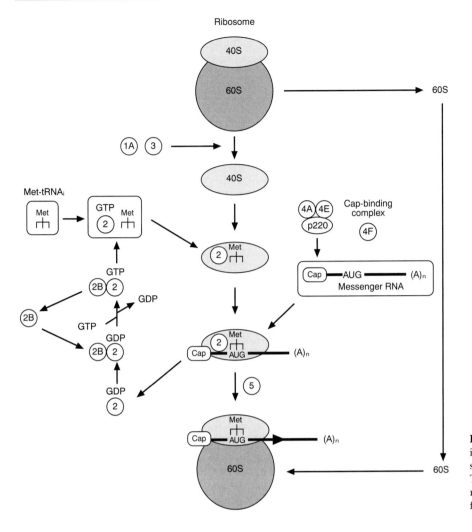

Fig. 8.12 Mechanism of initiation of protein synthesis in animal cells. The numbered circles represent the initiation factors.

Table 8.5 Mechanisms of inhibition of host cell protein synthesis

Virus	Mechanism	Reference
Herpes simplex	Degradation of host (and viral) mRNAs	Strom and Frenkel 1987
Vaccinia	Degradation of host (and viral) mRNAs	Rice and Roberts 1983
Polio	Inactivation of eIF-4F-γ by cleavage	Etchison et al. 1982
Rhino	Inactivation of eIF-4F-γ by cleavage	Etchison and Fout 1985
Adeno	Inactivation of eIF-4F-α by under-phosphorylation	Huang and Schneider 1991
	Inactivation of eIF-2B-β by phosphorylation	O'Malley et al. 1989
Vesicular stomatitis	mRNA abundance	Lodish and Porter 1981
	Not mRNA abundance	Schnitzlein et al. 1983
	Affinity for ribosomes	Nuss, Oppermann and Koch 1975
	Interference with eIF-2 function	Centrella and Lucas-Lenard 1982
	Interference with eIF-3/4B function	Thomas and Wagner 1983

preferential translation of their own mRNAs are interdependent.

Several such mechanisms have been identified (Table 8.5). To begin with, the abundance of individual viral mRNAs is usually greater than that of most cellular mRNAs, because of vigorous viral transcription and the high gene copy-number that results from viral genome replication. In the herpes- and poxviruses, this effect is magnified by an increased rate of mRNA breakdown (section 6.2, p. 132). In addition, many viral mRNAs have a competitive advantage whose structural basis is not fully understood (Garfinkel and Katze 1993, Kozak 1994). Part of the answer lies in the nucleotide sequence context of their initiation codons, but strong contexts, although common, are not ubiquitous in viral mRNAs (Kozak 1986). Their 5′ untranslated regions are usually shorter than those of host mRNAs, and the resulting proximity of the cap to the initiation codon and other undefined structural features of their 5′ ends may also favour translation.

For polio- and rhinoviruses, the mechanism is clear and elegant (Sonenberg 1987, Jackson, Howell and Kaminski 1991, Wycoff 1993): infection results in the expression of a viral protease (2A) which, directly or indirectly, mediates cleavage of a component (p220 or the γ subunit) of the cellular cap-binding complex, eIF-4F (Etchison et al. 1982, Etchison and Fout 1985). The result is inactivation of the initiation factor and consequent inhibition of translation of capped mRNAs. Viral RNA is immune to this inhibition because it is translated from an IRES and naturally lacks a 5′ cap (Meerovitch and Sonenberg 1993). In virions, polio- and rhinovirus RNAs carry a covalently attached viral protein (VPg) at their 5′ ends, while the translated form of the viral RNA starts with a 5′-monophosphate, pUp . . . (Chapter 25). The efficacy of eIF-4F-γ cleavage as a shut-off mechanism for capped mRNAs is illustrated by the fact that expression of functional poliovirus 2A protein from a recombinant vaccinia virus is lethal for the vector.

It is surprising that cleavage of the cap-binding protein is unique to polio- and rhinoviruses, and does not occur in cells infected with other picornaviruses, despite the fact that all their RNAs contain IRES elements, are translated in a cap-independent manner, and mostly shut off host protein synthesis (Duncan 1990). Because it is incontrovertible that picornaviruses are all descended from a common ancestor, their use of different shut-off mechanisms suggests either that an ancestral mechanism was replaced in some but not other descendants or that the ancestor did not inhibit host translation and that the present-day mechanisms evolved separately after divergence. Taken with the fact that polio- and herpesvirus mutants that cannot shut off host translation are only partly debilitated for growth (Bernstein, Sonenberg and Baltimore 1985, Strom and Frenkel 1987), this evidence suggests that inhibition of host protein synthesis, though beneficial, is not essential for virus replication. Indeed, a general selection method has been developed for the isolation of non-conditional viral mutants that are deficient in host protein shut-off (Francoeur, Poliquin and Stanners 1987).

The activity of the cap-binding complex is also reduced in adenovirus-infected cells, but in this case it is by reduced phosphorylation of the α subunit (eIF-4A, which is the cap-binding protein itself) rather than by cleavage of p220 (Huang and Schneider 1991, Zhang and Schneider 1993). Because adenovirus mRNAs are capped, the rationale for eIF-4F inactivation is less obvious than with the picornaviruses. However, it seems that the tripartite leader, a 200 nt RNA segment that is common to the 5′ end of all late adenovirus mRNAs (Chapter 15), renders them less dependent for translation on the helicase activity of eIF-4F than are cellular messages.

Changes in the level of phosphorylation of another initiation factor, eIF-2, are responsible for the regulation of protein synthesis under many different conditions of cellular stress, but in this case it is increased phosphorylation that interferes with initiation. As shown in Fig. 8.12, eIF-2 needs to exchange its bound GDP for GTP between each round of initiation, and this exchange requires the formation of a complex with eIF-2B. Phosphorylation of the α subunit of eIF-2 prevents the dissociation of this complex, and, because

eIF-2B is scarce relative to eIF-2, a modest increase in the level of phosphorylation inhibits initiation profoundly. As described in section 7.1 (p. 138), this mechanism is part of the cell's response to viral infection that is enhanced by treatment of cells with interferon. Increases in the phosphorylation of eIF-2-α occur in cells infected with adeno- and reoviruses, but it is unclear whether these are part of the virus-mediated inhibition of host mRNA translation or the cell-mediated inhibition of the virus. Nevertheless, this regulatory mechanism is a key point in the balance between viral and cellular protein synthesis, as shown by the fact that vaccinia virus encodes a homologue of eIF-2-α, and several other viruses perturb the phosphorylation of eIF-2-α in other ways (section 7.4, p. 141)

Access to alternative open reading frames

In addition to alternative RNA splicing (section 6.2, p. 132) and transcriptional editing (Cattaneo 1991, Jacques and Kolakofsky 1991), some viruses use translational frameshifting to express open reading frames that would otherwise be inaccessible in an mRNA. Retroviruses in particular use this mechanism to make proteins that they require only in small amounts, like the gag–pol precursor to the reverse transcriptase in Rous sarcoma virus (Jacks and Varmus 1985). Frameshifting is promoted by specific 'slippery' sequences in the mRNA, which, often in conjunction with adjacent 'hungry' codons and strong RNA secondary structure, persuade ribosomes occasionally to switch reading frames during translation (Brierley 1993). Whether viral infection modulates the intrinsic propensity of the ribosomes for frameshifting is not yet clear. In other retroviruses, synthesis of the gag–pol precursor is achieved by suppression of the termination codon at the end of the *gag* gene (Chapter 38).

Protein processing

During and after their synthesis, viral proteins are processed along many of the same reaction pathways as cellular proteins, and, because they offer such attractive experimental subjects, they have been widely used as model systems for the study of these pathways. There are also several cases in which protein processing reactions are mediated by viral enzymes or modified by viral proteins, and this is a frequent cause of CPEs.

Folding and oligomerization

Viral proteins must adopt the correct tertiary and quaternary structures before they become functional and, in many cases, before they can be transported to their ultimate destinations in the cell. These reactions have been examined in particular detail for viral envelope glycoproteins such as influenza HA, which must undergo glycosylation, folding and trimerization before it can move from the ER, via the compartments of the Golgi apparatus, to the cell surface in preparation for virus assembly (Gething, McCammon and Sambrook 1986, Doms et al. 1993). Folding is facilitated by interaction with a cellular protein BiP which resides in the lumen of the ER and binds transiently to newly made glycoproteins. BiP belongs to the hsp70 family of cellular proteins that are induced by heat shock and other types of stress, and it functions both to catalyse protein unfolding/refolding and to target misfolded and mutant proteins for degradation (Pelham 1988, Hartl 1996).

Proteolytic cleavage

Many viral proteins are cleaved during maturation, by either cellular or viral proteases. For example, the activation of viral fusion proteins by cleavage (section 5.2, p. 125) is often catalysed by members of the furin family of cellular proteases (Klenk and Garten 1994a). However, viral proteolysis is used most extensively by the non-segmented, positive-strand RNA viruses of the picorna-, toga- and flavivirus families (Chapters 25, 28 and 29). These viruses synthesize large polyprotein precursors that undergo multiple co- and post-translational cleavages catalysed by several viral proteases to yield the mature viral proteins (Krausslich and Wimmer 1988, Strauss 1990, Dougherty and Semler 1993). They are forced into this strategy of gene expression by a combination of their need to make several different viral proteins from a single mRNA and the reluctance of eukaryotic ribosomes to initiate at more than one site on a message. In contrast, viruses whose transcriptional mechanisms allow them to synthesize individual mRNAs and those with segmented genomes rely less heavily on proteolytic processing.

The assembly of icosahedral and more complex viral structures is also often accompanied by cleavage of structural protein precursors, which imposes a rigid order on the assembly process and can result in large-scale conformational changes in the maturing virion, often coincident with the acquisition of stability and infectivity (Guo 1994). Both in picorna- and in nodaviruses, the final maturational cleavage event occurs inside the assembled virion, and is catalysed by the interior of the capsid itself. It is interesting that the assembly of helical nucleocapsids generally seems not to involve protein cleavage.

Glycosylation

All enveloped viruses carry surface glycoproteins whose glycosylation is mediated by the normal cellular pathways of carbohydrate attachment and processing. Both *N*- and *O*-linked oligosaccharides are found but viral proteins with the former modification are more common.

Whether glycosylation is required for glycoprotein transport and function varies from one case to another, and probably reflects the different roles that oligosaccharides can play in determining the native structures of individual proteins. In certain cases, however, the influence of glycosylation can be dramatic: the presence or absence of a particular *N*-linked oligosaccharide in influenza HA that partially obstructs the HA1–HA2 cleavage site can have a profound effect on viral virulence because it determines which proteases can cleave the HA precursor, and hence how the virus can spread in the infected animal (Deshpande et al. 1987).

Phosphorylation

Viruses and cells interact with one another by phosphorylation in both directions: the phosphorylation of cellular proteins by viral kinases and the phosphorylation of viral proteins by cellular kinases. Prominent among the former are reactions catalysed by the tyrosine kinases that are encoded by the oncogenes of Rous sarcoma virus (*v-src*) and its relatives. In these cases, the major targets of kinase action are cellular proteins involved in cell cycle regulation whose activities are perturbed by phosphorylation. Conversely, cellular kinases can phosphorylate viral proteins and thereby modify their activities. For example, phosphorylation of the P protein of VSV by cellular casein kinase II enables it to form oligomers, which is an essential step in viral transcription (Gao and Lenard 1995).

Other covalent modifications

A wide variety of other covalent modifications of viral proteins have been described in different virus–cell systems, including N terminal acetylation, acylation (with both palmitate and N terminal myristate), ADP ribosylation, isoprenylation, methylation and sulphation. In most cases the cellular enzymes that catalyse these reactions are widely distributed and therefore do not restrict virus replication, but the effects of many of the modifications on the properties of viral proteins have yet to be fully explored.

PROTEIN TRANSPORT

Viral proteins are transported to the appropriate intracellular sites for replication and assembly by interaction with cellular protein trafficking pathways: to the plasma membrane via the ER and Golgi apparatus, to the nucleus, and to other organelles. Despite the disruption of the cytoskeleton and the extensive changes in cell morphology that often accompany infection, these trafficking pathways are generally not disrupted. Many viral proteins contain signals that define their destination in the cell, such as the hydrophobic signal sequences of integral membrane glycoproteins which, by binding to the signal recognition particle, commit the proteins to ER membrane insertion and transport along the exocytic pathway. Nuclear localization signals, which were first identified in the SV40 T antigen (Kalderon et al. 1984), target the corresponding viral proteins to the nucleus for replication and assembly. Proteins that contain *cis*-acting signals such as these are transported to the appropriate cellular compartment even when they are expressed from a vector in the absence of other viral proteins. In contrast, proteins that lack signals of their own can co-localize by binding with targeted proteins. A striking example of the influence of such signals on virus assembly is provided by the observation that a point mutation in a retroviral matrix protein determines whether the viral nucleocapsids assemble in the cytoplasm or at the plasma membrane (Rhee and Hunter 1990).

PROTEIN DEGRADATION

As described above, viruses in many families encode proteases with new specificities that can cleave cellular as well as viral polypeptides. It is likely that the resulting exposure of new N termini (Varshavsky 1992) to the protein degradation pathways (Hershko and Ciechanover 1992, Rubin and Finley 1995) will enhance the rate of turnover of specific proteins in cells infected with these viruses, although, apart from the cleavage of eIF-4F described above (p. 136), few specific examples have yet been described.

7 CELLULAR RESPONSES TO VIRAL INFECTION

Because viruses are a threat to the survival of cells and organisms, it is inevitable that cells and organisms should have evolved defence mechanisms to counteract them. It is similarly inevitable that those viruses with sufficient genetic capacity should have evolved counter-measures to circumvent these defences. In higher vertebrates, the major defence of organisms against infection is provided by the mucosal, humoral and cell-mediated arms of the immune system, which are described in Chapter 10. The major defences at the cellular level are the interferon (IFN) system (see below and Chapter 11) and the mechanisms of stress response and apoptosis. The interplay between the processes of virus replication, these cellular responses and the corresponding viral evasion mechanisms determines the outcome of infection at the cellular level.

7.1   Induction and actions of interferons

The IFNs are a family of cytokines that elicit profound physiological changes in the cells with which they interact, including the development of resistance to viral infection. In higher vertebrates, the IFN system acts within a few hours of infection, long before the onset of the immune response, to limit the spread of the infection and thus to diminish its severity. Indeed, many of the familiar early symptoms of a viral infection in humans are attributable to IFN action. IFNs are synthesized and secreted by most cell types in response to infection and some other stimuli, and they exert their effects by inducing the expression of several IFN-responsive genes. Understanding the system as a whole therefore requires knowledge of the IFN genes, how they are induced, the IFN proteins themselves and how they interact with their target cells, how these interactions trigger expression of the IFN-inducible genes and, finally, how the products of these latter genes render the cell resistant to viral infection and mediate their other effects. Although much remains to be learned about this complex and multifunctional regulatory system, intense research in recent years has clarified many important aspects. Here is presented only an overview of the IFN system; for more details the reader should consult Chapter 11 or a review article (Revel and Chebath 1986, Pestka et al. 1987, Samuel 1988, Staeheli 1990, Samuel 1991, Sen and Lengyel 1992, Sen and Ransohoff 1993, Johnson et al. 1994).

INTERFERONS

Four distinct types of IFNs have been identified and characterized: α, β, γ and ω. Although their properties overlap to the extent that they are all recognized as IFNs, they are secreted by different cell types in response to different inducers and they exert somewhat different physiological effects on different target cells. In the context of virus–host cell interactions, α, β and γ IFNs are the most relevant because α and β induce a virus-resistant state in most cell types whereas IFN-γ primarily modulates aspects of the cell-mediated immune response via its effects on macrophages. α IFNs, which are encoded in a multi-gene family, are homologous to IFN-β and interact as monomers with the same receptor on the surface of target cells. In contrast, IFN-γ has little homology with the other types and binds as a dimer to 2 copies of a different cell surface receptor (Walter et al. 1995).

INTERFERON INDUCTION

α and β IFNs are induced and secreted from many different cell types in response to infection by most viruses as well as some other assaults, and these cytokines act as an early warning system that alerts other cells in the body that infection is imminent. In contrast, IFN-γ is produced only by T lymphocytes and natural killer cells, in response to induction by cognate antigens and other T cell activators. Induction of IFNs occurs by transcriptional activation of the IFN genes, and, although many of the mechanistic details remain obscure, a satisfying picture is emerging for the induction of IFN-β. It has long been known that IFN-β can be induced by treating cells with double-stranded RNA, and indeed the production of double-stranded RNA may be a general mechanism by which viruses induce IFNs. Among the cellular targets for double-stranded RNA is a cytoplasmic protein kinase called PKR, which is also involved in the mechanism of IFN action (see below). On activation by binding to double-stranded RNA, PKR phosphorylates I-κB, the inhibitory subunit of the transcription factor NF-κB (Karin and Hunter 1995). Phosphorylation of I-κB allows NF-κB to enter the nucleus where it recognizes specific DNA binding sites and thereby activates the transcription of several genes, including that for IFN-β (Proud 1995).

INTERFERON ACTION

The binding of IFNs to their corresponding receptors initiates signals that are transmitted to the nucleus of the IFN-treated cell via the JAK/STAT pathway. Signal transduction occurs by the activation of a family of tyrosine kinases (Janus kinases or JAKs) that are associated with the cytoplasmic domains of the transmembrane IFN receptors and activated when the receptors are occupied by binding to IFNs. The activated JAKs phosphorylate a family of transcription factors (signal transducing activators of transcription, or STATs), which then migrate from the cytoplasm to the nucleus. Here they form active complexes that bind to interferon-specific response elements (ISREs) present in the promoter sites upstream of IFN-inducible genes, thereby activating their transcription (Williams 1991, Pellegrini and Schindler 1993). It is remarkable that many other polypeptide ligands that exert a wide variety of physiological effects on cells also transmit their signals to the nucleus via the JAK/STAT pathway. The specificity of the ligand/response relationship seems to be maintained by subtle quantitative, qualitative and temporal differences in the spectra of JAK activation and STAT phosphorylation that are elicited by the different ligands, although much more work is needed to define fully how the integrity of different signals is maintained (Schindler and Darnell 1995).

Although the IFN system was first discovered by the observation that IFN-treated cells are resistant to viral infection, it has since become clear that this is only one aspect of their altered physiology. IFNs can also have profound antiproliferative and immunomodulatory effects, so the physiology of the IFN response in whole animals is complex. The multiple effects of IFNs are mediated by the IFN-inducible proteins of which more than 30 have been identified, but the roles that many of them play in the altered physiology of the IFN-treated cell are still unknown. Best understood are 2 inducible enzymes that are responsible, at least in part, for the resistance of cells to infection by several different viruses. These are the protein kinase (PKR) that is also implicated in the induction of IFN-β (see above), and a family of enzymes called 2′,5′-oligoadenylate (2-5A) synthetases (Fig. 8.13).

PKR, a double-stranded RNA-dependent protein kinase

The protein kinase now known as PKR is a 68 kDa polypeptide that is induced by IFN treatment of most types of cultured vertebrate cells. The enzyme is active only when bound to double-stranded RNA, whereupon it phosphorylates and activates itself, and also phosphorylates the translational initiation factor eIF-2-α. This interferes with the initiation of protein synthesis (as described in section 6.3 (p. 134) and Fig. 8.12), which limits viral replication (Hershey 1990, 1993). Untreated cells contain only basal levels of PKR and the enzyme is largely inactive because of the absence of double-stranded RNA. IFN-treated cells contain substantial levels of PKR, but it remains inactive until viral infection produces double-stranded RNA, either as an intermediate of RNA replication or as a byproduct of overlapping transcription. In this way, the effects of IFN are fully manifested only after viral infection, a mechanism that restricts the major physiological consequences to the cells where they will have the greatest effect. Viruses have evolved numerous ways to counteract the effects of IFN in general and PKR in particular (see section 7.4, p. 141), implying not only that the IFN response significantly restricts virus replication in nature but also that PKR is a central component in the mechanism of resistance to many viruses.

2-5A synthetases

The 2-5A synthetases that are also induced by IFN treatment catalyse the template-independent oligomerization of ATP to form a series of 2′-5′-linked oligomers that are referred to collectively as 2-5A (Ball 1982). Like PKR, the 2-5A synthetases depend on double-stranded RNA for enzyme activity, so full development of this aspect of the IFN response also requires viral infection of IFN-treated cells. The 2-5A oligomers have the general structure $ppp(A^{2'}p^{5'})_nA_{OH}$, and in cells the trimer and tetramer predominate. In general, 2′,5′-phosphodiester bonds are a biochemical rarity, although single such bonds are formed during RNA splicing (Sharp 1994) and also during the priming of cDNA synthesis by bacterial reverse transcriptase (Shimamoto, Inouye and Inouye 1995). The only known function of 2-5A oligomers is to activate an endoribonuclease, RNase L, which is present as a constitutive but latent enzyme in most cell types. On activation by 2-5A, RNase L degrades mRNAs and ribosomal RNAs, and thereby inhibits protein synthesis. The degradation of 2-5A itself by a 2′-phos-

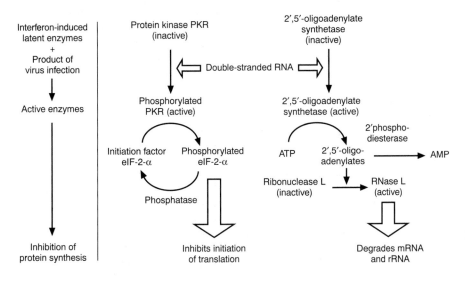

Fig. 8.13 Mechanisms of the antiviral action of interferons.

phodiesterase restores RNase L to its latent state. Thus in IFN-treated virus-infected cells, PKR and 2-5A synthetase collaborate to restrict virus replication by inhibiting both the initiation and the elongation of polypeptides.

Specificity of IFN action

Although IFN treatment generally induces resistance to a wide range of viruses, the induced gene products play quantitatively different roles in combating infection by different viruses. For example, the 2-5A system seems to be particularly important in the resistance to picornavirus infection, but much less so in the resistance to several other virus families. The murine *Mx* gene is a more extreme example of an IFN-induced resistance mechanism that is effective only against a specific virus family because the Mx protein product makes mice and murine cells resistant to infection by influenza virus but not by other viruses (Staeheli 1990, Samuel 1991). However, a broader and more complex question is whether IFN action can discriminate generally between viral and cellular events and, if so, how this is achieved. IFN treatment clearly enables organisms and cell cultures to survive viral challenges that would otherwise be lethal, and yet the properties of PKR and 2-5A synthetase provide only a partial explanation for this apparent selectivity. The recognition by these enzymes of double-stranded RNA as a signature of viral infection establishes a mechanism for discriminating between infected and uninfected cells rather than between viral and cellular mRNAs, and in some cases the infected cells are sacrificed to prevent viral replication. In other cases, enzyme activation imposes an indiscriminate but transient suppression of protein synthesis, a situation from which the cell can recover but the virus cannot. Finally, in some situations, the IFN-induced enzymes seem to be preferentially activated in cytoplasmic microenvironments surrounding the viral double-stranded RNA molecules that are responsible for their activation, thus achieving selectivity on the basis of compartmentalization.

It seems likely that combinations of these effects enable PKR and 2-5A synthetase/RNase L, which have no demonstrable specificity for viral mRNAs, nevertheless to discriminate between cellular and viral processes.

VIRAL FACILITATION BY INHIBITION OF THE IFN SYSTEM

Viruses differ in their sensitivity to IFNs, in part because some of them have evolved effective countermeasures against one or more components of the IFN system (see section 7.4, p. 141). Accordingly, a virus such as vaccinia, which is relatively insensitive, can in some circumstances facilitate the replication of a co-infecting IFN-sensitive virus such as VSV by inhibiting the action of IFN. This contrasts with the more common situation in which co-infecting viruses interfere with one another by a variety of mechanisms that are unrelated to the IFN system (Whitaker-Dowling and Youngner 1987).

7.2 Induction and actions of cellular stress proteins

Although viral infection suppresses the synthesis of most cellular proteins by the mechanisms described in section 6.3 (p. 134), some host cell genes are induced by infection and their proteins are relatively resistant to shut-off. These include the genes that encode the IFNs (see section 7.1, p. 138) and also those for a set of proteins that are generally induced by conditions of metabolic stress, including heat-shock (Jindal and Malkovsky 1994). Some of the cellular stress proteins normally function as molecular chaperones, and certain viruses exploit these properties to assist their own replication and assembly. This is true of some bacteriophages and has also been suggested for several eukaryotic viruses. For example, the cytoplasmic hsp70 protein binds transiently to the poliovirus capsid precursor, perhaps facilitating its folding and assembly. Similarly, BiP protein, which resides in the lumen of the rough endoplasmic reticulum, binds briefly to newly synthesized integral membrane proteins such as viral glycoproteins and assists their maturation (Hartl 1996). In addition to these roles, however, the display of virus-induced stress proteins or their peptide fragments on the surface of infected cells may stimulate immune recognition and participate in the activation of the immune response.

7.3 Apoptosis

Metazoan organisms have evolved a highly conserved and tightly regulated cellular pathway called apoptosis which, once triggered, leads irreversibly to cell death (Martin, Green and Cotter 1994, Martin and Green 1995, Steller 1995). Apoptosis is the mechanism by which unwanted cells are eliminated during development, but it is also triggered in response to infection by a wide variety of cytocidal viruses (Vaux, Haecker and Strasser 1994, Razvi and Welsh 1995). It is characterized by cell rounding, condensation of chromatin and fragmentation of cellular DNA, blebbing of the plasma membrane, and finally breakup of the cell contents into membrane-bound apoptotic bodies that are suitable for ingestion by phagocytes. In the context of viral infection, apoptosis serves as an effective defence mechanism for the organism whereby a relatively small number of cells die altruistically to limit virus spread (Williams 1994). This is reminiscent of the self-sacrifice of some IFN-treated infected cells that was described in section 7.1 (p. 138). The mechanisms by which viruses induce apoptosis have yet to be clearly defined, but changes in membrane permeabilities leading to Ca^{2+} influx, the expression of viral proteases with new specificities and perturbation of the functions of the cellular tumour-suppressor proteins p53 and pRb may all be involved in different situations.

The most persuasive evidence that the effects of apoptosis in virus–host cell interactions are, on balance, detrimental to the virus comes from the observation that several viruses have evolved countermeasures that delay or prevent the onset of apoptosis

(Ink, Gilbert and Evan 1995, Razvi and Welsh 1995, Gillet and Brun 1996). For example, cowpox virus expresses an inhibitor of an enzyme that is thought to be involved in the apoptotic pathway, the interleukin-1β-converting enzyme (ICE) (Kumar 1995), and it thereby blocks both apoptosis and inflammation (Ray et al. 1992). In the absence of an effective apoptotic response, a normally cytocidal virus such as Sindbis can instead establish a persistent infection (Griffin et al. 1994). Conversely, suppression of apoptosis by the adenovirus E1B oncogene is necessary to allow the induction of cell proliferation that is mediated by the E1A oncogene to result in the transformation of adenovirus-infected cells (E White 1993).

7.4 Viral mechanisms to evade cellular defences

During co-evolution with their hosts, different viruses have adopted several different methods of counteracting the various defence mechanisms, an observation that provides compelling evidence for the efficacy of the corresponding host defences themselves (Smith 1993, 1994). As might be expected, inactivation or deletion of the viral genes involved in these evasion mechanisms generally reduces the virulence of the virus. This aspect of the study of virus–host interactions is particularly informative because it provides a window on the relationships as they exist in nature. Moreover, some of the evasion mechanisms have involved the viral acquisition and adaptation of host genes that benefit the virus in much the same way as the acquisition of an oncogene benefits a retrovirus by ensuring cell cycling and concomitant viral replication. These host-derived genes and their products can provide insight into the heart of the virus–host relationship as well as potential reagents for the experimental and therapeutic manipulation of the host's defence mechanisms (McFadden 1995).

EVASION OF IMMUNE RESPONSES

Many RNA viruses continually evade the immune responses of the host by mutation. The inability of RNA polymerases to correct their mistakes leads to heterogeneous virus populations or quasispecies from which antibody-escape mutants are readily selected (Smith and Inglis 1987, Duarte et al. 1994). For viruses that have segmented genomes (e.g. influenza), this effect is reinforced by the potential for reassortment of RNA segments between viruses with different pedigrees (see Chapter 22). With HIV, the continuous generation of antigenic variants within each infected individual eventually overwhelms the ability of the immune system to respond and contributes to the onset of AIDS (see Chapter 38). In contrast, viruses with double-stranded DNA genomes are usually replicated with much greater fidelity and have therefore resorted to other methods of immune evasion. For example, herpesviruses are hidden from immune surveillance during latent infections (Masucci and Ernberg 1994, Wagner 1994, Lewin 1995), and during lytic growth they specifically inhibit the intracellular

transport mechanism by which viral peptide fragments are presented to the cell-mediated immune system (York et al. 1994, Fruh et al. 1995). Adeno-, cytomegalo- and poxviruses also interfere with peptide presentation, by down-regulating the expression of the major histocompatibility complex class I protein (Smith 1993, 1994). In addition, poxviruses encode a variety of soluble cytokine 'receptors' that are secreted from infected cells to intercept immunostimulatory cytokines (Pickup 1994, Spriggs 1994) (see also Chapter 11).

EVASION OF COMPLEMENT

The complement system is a major host defence mechanism which, on activation, attacks and permeabilizes the surface membranes of enveloped viruses and infected cells. Complement is activated by 2 tightly regulated pathways: the classical pathway, which requires an antibody response to the infecting virus, and the alternative pathway, which is antibody-independent. Several members of the pox- and herpesvirus families express cell surface or secreted proteins that interfere either with the complement activation pathways or with the formation of the membrane attack complex itself, which attests to the potential efficacy of complement against these viruses (Isaacs, Kotwal and Moss 1992, Smith 1994).

EVASION OF INTERFERON

In contrast to the ease with which antibody-resistant mutants can be isolated, IFN-resistant mutants seldom arise even when they are deliberately selected for (Novella et al. 1996), probably because IFNs induce several distinct and overlapping antiviral mechanisms. Nevertheless, viruses vary considerably in their intrinsic sensitivities to IFNs, not only because they differentially activate the IFN-induced enzymes but also because some of them deploy specific IFN evasion mechanisms (McNair and Kerr 1992). For example, among the soluble cytokine receptors secreted from poxvirus-infected cells are proteins that decoy both α and γ IFNs (Smith 1993, Pickup 1994, Spriggs 1994, Alcami and Smith 1996). Intracellularly, reovirus and vaccinia virus express double-stranded RNA-binding proteins that interfere with the activation of PKR, whereas adenovirus and Epstein–Barr virus (EBV) synthesize abundant small RNAs (called virus-associated (VA) RNAs and EBV-encoded early RNAs (EBERs), respectively) that compete with double-stranded RNA for PKR binding but which fail to activate the kinase (Mathews and Shenk 1991, Mathews 1993). Yet other mechanisms are used by poliovirus, which degrades the activated PKR, and by influenza virus, which activates a latent cellular inhibitor of PKR (Katze 1993, 1995). Its role in uninfected cells has yet to be determined. Finally, vaccinia virus expresses a homologue of eIF-2-α, which decoys the kinase and protects the authentic initiation factor against phosphorylation. The variety of mechanisms that have evolved to circumvent the PKR system argues strongly that it can potentially restrict the replication of a wide range of viruses. Viral mechanisms to evade the 2-5A system also exist but they remain to be fully characterized.

8 SUMMARY

Their large population sizes and high mutation rates allow viruses to evolve much faster than the host organisms on which they depend for replication. For this reason, they will continue to threaten the health of the rest of the biosphere and to shape the evolution of their hosts. But, as described in this chapter, exam-

ination of the intricacies of virus–host interactions provides unique insights into these competitive relationships and illuminates almost every aspect of the biology of the host organisms. The future promises an even richer harvest of experimental and conceptual advances in this area, both enhancing our ability to control and prevent viral diseases and increasing our understanding of the mechanistic and evolutionary relationships between viruses and their hosts.

REFERENCES

Alcami A, Smith GL, 1996, Receptors for gamma-interferon encoded by poxviruses: implications for the unknown origin of vaccinia virus, *Trends Microbiol*, **4**: 321–6.

Antczak JB, Patel DD et al., 1992, Site-specific RNA cleavage generates the 3′ end of a poxvirus late mRNA, *Proc Natl Acad Sci USA*, **89**: 12033–7.

Ball LA, 1982, 2′,5′-oligoadenylate synthetase, *The Enzymes*, vol XV, Nucleic Acids, part B, 3rd edn, ed Boyer PD, Academic Press, New York, 281–313.

Bangham CR, Kirkwood TB, 1993, Defective interfering particles and virus evolution, *Trends Microbiol*, **1**: 260–4.

Barrett AD, Dimmock NJ, 1986, Defective interfering viruses and infections of animals, *Curr Top Microbiol Immunol*, **128**: 55–84.

Bayliss CD, Condit RC, 1993, Temperature-sensitive mutants in the vaccinia virus A18R gene increase double-stranded RNA synthesis as a result of aberrant viral transcription, *Virology*, **194**: 254–62.

Bentz J (ed), 1993, *Viral Fusion Mechanisms*, CRC Press, Boca Raton FL.

Berget SM, Moore C, Sharp PA, 1977, Spliced segments at the 5′ terminus of adenovirus 2 late mRNA, *Proc Natl Acad Sci USA*, **74**: 3171–5.

Bernstein HD, Sonenberg N, Baltimore D, 1985, Poliovirus mutant that does not selectively inhibit host protein synthesis, *Mol Cell Biol*, **5**: 2913–23.

Bray M, Prasad S et al., 1994, A small element from the Mason–Pfizer monkey virus genome makes human immunodeficiency virus type 1 expression and replication Rev-independent, *Proc Natl Acad Sci USA*, **91**: 1256–60.

Brierley I, 1993, Probing the mechanism of ribosomal frameshifting on viral RNAs, *Biochem Soc Trans*, **21**: 822–6.

Brunetti CR, Burke RL et al., 1994, Herpes simplex virus glycoprotein D acquires mannose-6-phosphate residues and binds to mannose-6-phosphate receptors, *J Biol Chem*, **269**: 17067–74.

de Bruyn Kops A, Knipe DM, 1988, Formation of DNA replication structures in herpes virus-infected cells requires a viral DNA-binding protein, *Cell*, **55**: 857–68.

Bullough PA, Hughson FM et al., 1994, Structure of influenza haemagglutinin at the pH of membrane fusion, *Nature (London)*, **371**: 37–43.

Carr CM, Kim PS, 1993, A spring-loaded mechanism for the conformational change of influenza hemagglutinin, *Cell*, **73**: 823–32.

Carr CM, Kim PS, 1994, Flu virus invasion: halfway there, *Science*, **266**: 234–6.

Carrasco L, 1994, Entry of animal viruses and macromolecules into cells, *FEBS Lett*, **350**: 151–4.

Cattaneo R, 1991, Different types of messenger RNA editing, *Annu Rev Genet*, **25**: 71–88.

Centrella M, Lucas-Lenard J, 1982, Regulation of protein synthesis in vesicular stomatitis virus-infected mouse L-929 cells by decreased protein synthesis initiation factor 2 activity, *J Virol*, **41**: 781–91.

Challberg M (ed), 1991, Animal virus DNA replication, *Semin Virol*, **2**: 247–304.

Challberg MD, Kelly TJ, 1989, Animal virus DNA replication, *Annu Rev Biochem*, **58**: 671–717.

Chang W, Hsiao J-C et al., 1995, Isolation of a monoclonal antibody which blocks vaccinia virus infection, *J Virol*, **69**: 517–22.

Chapman MS, Rossmann MG, 1993, Comparison of surface properties of picornaviruses: strategies for hiding the receptor site from immune surveillance, *Virology*, **195**: 745–56.

Cheng RH, Kuhn RJ et al., 1995, Nucleocapsid and glycoprotein organization in an enveloped virus, *Cell*, **80**: 621–30.

Chow LT, Gelinas RE et al., 1977, An amazing sequence arrangement at the 5′ ends of adenovirus 2 messenger RNA, *Cell*, **12**: 1–8.

Clem RJ, Miller LK, 1994, Control of programmed cell death by the baculovirus genes p35 and iap, *Mol Cell Biol*, **14**: 5212–22.

Colonno RJ, 1992, Molecular interactions between human rhinoviruses and their cellular receptors, *Semin Virol*, **3**: 101–8.

Cook P, 1991, The nucleoskeleton and the topology of replication, *Cell*, **66**: 627–35.

Cullen BR, 1994, RNA-sequence-mediated gene regulation in HIV-1, *Infect Agents Dis*, **3**: 68–76.

Curran JA, Richardson C, Kolakofsky D, 1986, Ribosomal initiation at alternate AUGs on the Sendai virus P/C mRNA, *J Virol*, **57**: 684–7.

Dautry-Varsat A, Lodish HF, 1984, How receptors bring proteins and particles into cells, *Sci Am*, **250**: 52–8.

Deshpande KL, Fried VA et al., 1987, Glycosylation affects cleavage of an H5N2 influenza virus hemagglutinin and regulates virulence, *Proc Natl Acad Sci USA*, **84**: 36–40.

Dimmock NJ, 1985, Defective interfering viruses: modulators of infection, *Microbiol Sci*, **2**: 1–7.

Dodson ML, Michaels ML, Lloyd RS, 1994, Unified catalytic mechanism for DNA glycosylases, *J Biol Chem*, **269**: 32709–12.

Doms RW, Lamb RA et al., 1993, Folding and assembly of viral membrane proteins, *Virology*, **193**: 545–62.

Dougherty WG, Semler BL, 1993, Expression of virus-encoded proteinases: functional and structural similarities with cellular enzymes, *Microbiol Rev*, **57**: 781–822.

Drake JW, 1993, Rates of spontaneous mutation among RNA viruses, *Proc Natl Acad Sci USA*, **90**: 4171–5.

Drapkin R, Merino A, Reinberg D, 1993, Regulation of RNA polymerase II transcription, *Curr Opin Cell Biol*, **5**: 469–76.

Dryden KA, Wang G et al., 1993, Early steps in reovirus infection are associated with dramatic changes in supramolecular structure and protein conformation: analysis of virions and subviral particles by cryo-electron microscopy and image reconstruction, *J Cell Biol*, **122**: 1023–41.

Duarte EA, Novella IS et al., 1994, RNA virus quasispecies: significance for viral disease and epidemiology, *Infect Agents Dis*, **3**: 201–14.

Duncan RF, 1990, Protein synthesis initiation factor modifications during viral infections: implications for translational control, *Electrophoresis*, **11**: 219–27.

Eaton S, Simons K, 1995, Apical, basal, and lateral cues for epithelial polarization, *Cell*, **82**: 5–8.

Echols H, 1990, Nucleoprotein structures initiating DNA replication, transcription, and site-specific recombination, *J Biol Chem*, **265**: 14697–700.

Ehrenfeld E (ed), 1993, Translational regulation in virus-infected cells, *Semin Virol*, **4**: 199–268.

Eigen M, 1993, Viral quasispecies, *Sci Am*, **269**: 42–9.

Etchison D, Fout S, 1985, Human rhinovirus 14 infection of HeLa cells results in the proteolytic cleavage of the p220 cap-binding complex subunit and inactivates globin translation in vitro, *J Virol*, **54**: 634–8.

Etchison D, Milburn SC et al., 1982, Inhibition of HeLa cell protein synthesis following poliovirus infection correlates with the proteolysis of a 220,000 dalton polypeptide associated with eukaryotic initiation factor 3 and a cap binding protein complex, *J Biol Chem*, **257**: 14806–10.

Fanning E, Knippers R, 1992, Structure and function of simian virus 40 large tumor antigen, *Annu Rev Biochem*, **61**: 55–85.

Farrell PJ, 1995, Epstein–Barr virus immortalizing genes, *Trends Microbiol*, **3**: 105–9.

Farthing AJ, Vousden KH, 1994, Functions of human papilloma virus E6 and E7 oncoproteins, *Trends Microbiol*, **2**: 170–4.

Feng Y, Broder CC et al., 1996, HIV-1 entry cofactor: functional cDNA cloning of a seven-transmembrane, G protein-coupled receptor, *Science*, **272**: 872–7.

Flore O, Fricks CE et al., 1990, Conformational changes in poliovirus assembly and cell entry, *Semin Virol*, **1**: 429–38.

Francoeur AM, Poliquin L, Stanners CP, 1987, The isolation of interferon-inducing mutants of vesicular stomatitis virus with altered viral P function for the inhibition of total protein synthesis, *Virology*, **160**: 236–45.

Friesen PD, Nissen MS, 1990, Gene organization and transcription of TED, a lepidopteran retrotransposon integrated within the baculovirus genome, *Mol Cell Biol*, **10**: 3067–77.

Fruh K, Ahn K et al., 1995, A viral inhibitor of peptide transporters for antigen presentation, *Nature (London)*, **375**: 415–18.

Gait MJ, Karn J, 1993, RNA recognition by the human immunodeficiency virus Tat and Rev proteins, *Trends Biochem Sci*, **18**: 255–9.

Gao Y, Lenard J, 1995, Multimerization and transcriptional activation of the phosphoprotein (P) of vesicular stomatitis virus by casein kinase-II, *EMBO J*, **14**: 1240–7.

Garcia-Blanco MA, Cullen BR, 1991, Molecular basis of latency in pathogenic human viruses, *Science*, **254**: 815–20.

Garfinkel MS, Katze MG, 1993, How does influenza virus regulate gene expression at the level of mRNA translation? Let us count the ways, *Gene Expr*, **3**: 109–18.

Gething MJ, McCammon K, Sambrook J, 1986, Expression of wild-type and mutant forms of influenza hemagglutinin: the role of folding in intracellular transport, *Cell*, **46**: 939–50.

Gillet G, Brun G, 1996, Viral inhibition of apoptosis, *Trends Microbiol*, **4**: 312–17.

Giranda VL, Heinz BA et al., 1992, Acid-induced structural changes in human rhinovirus 14: possible role in uncoating, *Proc Natl Acad Sci USA*, **89**: 10213–17.

Gomez Yafal A, Kaplan G et al., 1993, Characterization of poliovirus conformational alteration mediated by soluble cell receptors, *Virology*, **197**: 501–5.

Greber UF, Singh I, Helenius A, 1994, Mechanisms of virus uncoating, *Trends Microbiol*, **2**: 52–6.

Greve JM, Rossmann MG, 1994, Interaction of rhinovirus with its receptor ICAM-1, *Cellular Receptors for Animal Viruses*, ed Wimmer E, Cold Spring Harbor Laboratory, Cold Spring Harbor NY, 195–213.

Griffin DE, Levine B et al., 1994, The effects of alphavirus infection on neurons, *Ann Neurol Suppl*, **35**: S23–7.

Guo P (ed), 1994, Viral assembly, *Semin Virol*, **5**: 1–83.

Halstead SB, 1994, Antibody-dependent enhancement of infection: a mechanism for indirect virus entry into cells, *Cellular Receptors for Animal Viruses*, ed Wimmer E, Cold Spring Harbor Laboratory, Cold Spring Harbor NY, 493–516.

Harrison SC, Wang J et al., 1992, Structure and interactions of CD4, *Cold Spring Harbor Symp Quant Biol*, **57**: 541–8.

Hartl FU, 1996, Molecular chaperones in cellular protein folding, *Nature (London)*, **381**: 571–80.

Hay AJ, 1992, The action of adamantanamines against influenza A viruses: inhibition of the M2 ion channel protein, *Semin Virol*, **3**: 21–30.

Haywood AM, 1994, Virus receptors: binding, adhesion strengthening, and changes in viral structure, *J Virol*, **68**: 1–5.

Helenius A, 1992, Unpacking the incoming influenza virus, *Cell*, **69**: 577–8.

Hershey JWB, 1990, Overview: phosphorylation and translation control, *Enzyme*, **44**: 17–27.

Hershey JWB, 1993, Introduction to translational initiation factors and their regulation by phosphorylation, *Semin Virol*, **4**: 201–8.

Hershko A, Ciechanover A, 1992, The ubiquitin system for protein degradation, *Annu Rev Biochem*, **61**: 761–807.

Hoekstra D, Kok JW, 1989, Entry mechanisms of enveloped viruses. Implications for fusion of intracellular membranes, *Biosci Rep*, **9**: 273–305.

Holland JJ, de la Torre JC, Steinhauer DA, 1992, RNA virus populations as quasispecies, *Curr Top Microbiol Immunol*, **176**: 1–20.

Huang J, Schneider RJ, 1991, Adenovirus inhibition of cellular protein synthesis involves inactivation of cap binding protein, *Cell*, **65**: 271–80.

Hughson FM, 1995, Structural characterization of viral fusion proteins, *Curr Biol*, **5**: 265–74.

Hugin AW, Hauser C, 1994, The epidermal growth factor receptor is not a receptor for vaccinia virus, *J Virol*, **68**: 8409–12.

Hutt-Fletcher LM, 1987, Synergistic activation of cells by Epstein–Barr virus and B-cell growth factor, *J Virol*, **61**: 774–81.

Ink BS, Gilbert CS, Evan GI, 1995, Delay of vaccinia virus-Lamb induced apoptosis in non-permissive chinese hamster ovary cells by the cowpox *CHOhr* and adenovirus *E1B 19K* genes, *J Virol*, **69**: 661–8.

Isaacs SN, Kotwal GJ, Moss B, 1992, Vaccinia virus complement-control protein prevents antibody-dependent complement-enhanced neutralization of infectivity and contributes to virulence, *Proc Natl Acad Sci USA*, **89**: 628–32.

Ishihama A, Barbier P, 1994, Molecular anatomy of viral RNA-directed RNA polymerases, *Arch Virol*, **134**: 235–58.

Jacks T, Varmus HE, 1985, Expression of the Rous sarcoma virus *pol* gene by ribosomal frameshifting, *Science*, **230**: 1237–42.

Jackson RJ, Howell MT, Kaminski A, 1991, The novel mechanism of initiation of poliovirus RNA translation, *Trends Biochem Sci*, **15**: 477–83.

Jacques JP, Kolakofsky D, 1991, Pseudo-templated transcription in prokaryotic and eukaryotic organisms, *Genes Dev*, **5**: 707–13.

Jansen-Durr P, 1996, How viral oncogenes make the cell cycle, *Trends Genet*, **12**: 270–5.

Jindal S, Malkovsky M, 1994, Stress responses to viral infection, *Trends Microbiol*, **2**: 89–91.

Johnson JE, 1996, Functional implications of protein–protein interactions in icosahedral viruses, *Proc Natl Acad Sci USA*, **93**: 27–33.

Johnson HM, Bazer FW et al., 1994, How interferons fight disease, *Sci Am*, **270**: 68–75.

Kalderon D, Roberts BL et al., 1984, A short amino acid sequence able to specify nuclear location, *Cell*, **39**: 499–509.

Karin M, Hunter T, 1995, Transcriptional control by protein phosphorylation: signal transmission from the cell surface to the nucleus, *Curr Biol*, **5**: 747–57.

Katze MG, 1993, Games viruses play: a strategic initiative against the interferon-induced dsRNA-activated 68,000 Mr protein kinase, *Semin Virol*, **4**: 258–68.

Katze MG, 1995, Regulation of the interferon-induced PKR: can viruses cope?, *Trends Microbiol*, **3**: 75–8.

Katze MG, Agy MB, 1990, Regulation of viral and cellular RNA turnover in cells infected by eukaryotic viruses including HIV, *Enzyme*, **44**: 332–46.

Kelly TJ, Wold MS, Li J, 1988, Initiation of viral DNA replication, *Adv Virus Res*, **34**: 1–42.

Kemble GW, Danieli T, White JM, 1994, Lipid-anchored influenza hemagglutinin promotes hemifusion, not complete fusion, *Cell*, **76**: 383–91.

Kielian M, 1995, Membrane fusion and the alphavirus life cycle, *Adv Virus Res*, **45**: 113–51.

Klenk HD, Garten W, 1994a, Host cell proteases controlling virus pathogenicity, *Trends Microbiol*, **2**: 39–43.

Klenk HD, Garten W, 1994b, Activation cleavage of viral spike proteins by host proteases, *Cellular Receptors for Animal Viruses*, ed Wimmer E, Cold Spring Harbor Laboratory, Cold Spring Harbor NY, 241–80.

Kolakofsky D, Hacker D, 1991, Bunyavirus RNA synthesis: genome transcription and replication, *Curr Top Microbiol Immunol*, **169**: 143–59.

Kozak M, 1986, Regulation of protein synthesis in virus-infected animal cells, *Adv Virus Res*, **31**: 229–92.

Kozak M, 1989, The scanning model for translation: an update, *J Cell Biol*, **108**: 229–41.

Kozak M, 1991a, An analysis of vertebrate mRNA sequences: intimations of translational control, *J Cell Biol*, **115**: 887–903.

Kozak M, 1991b, Structural features in eukaryotic mRNAs that modulate the initiation of translation, *J Biol Chem*, **266**: 19867–70.

Kozak M, 1992a, Regulation of translation in eukaryotic systems, *Annu Rev Cell Biol*, **8**: 197–225.

Kozak M, 1992b, A consideration of alternative models for the initiation of translation in eukaryotes, *Crit Rev Biochem Mol Biol*, **27**: 385–402.

Kozak M, 1994, Determinants of translational fidelity and efficiency in vertebrate mRNAs, *Biochimie*, **74**: 815–21.

Krausslich H-G, Wimmer E, 1988, Viral proteinases, *Annu Rev Biochem*, **57**: 701–54.

Kristie TM, Sharp PA, 1993, Purification of the cellular C1 factor required for the stable recognition of the oct-1 homeodomain by the herpes simplex virus α trans-inducing factor (VP16), *J Biol Chem*, **268**: 6526–34.

Krug RM, 1993, The regulation of export of mRNA from nucleus to cytoplasm, *Curr Opin Cell Biol*, **5**: 944–9.

Kumar S, 1995, ICE-like proteases in apoptosis, *Trends Biochem Sci*, **20**: 198–202.

Lamb RA, 1993, Paramyxovirus fusion: a hypothesis for changes, *Virology*, **197**: 1–11.

Lamb RA, Krug RM, 1996, *Orthomyxoviridae*: the viruses and their replication, *Fields' Virology*, 3rd edn, eds Fields BN, Knipe DM et al., Raven Press, New York, 1353–95.

Lanzrein M, Schlegel A, Kempf C, 1994, Entry and uncoating of enveloped viruses, *Biochem J*, **302**: 313–20.

Lawrence MB, Springer TA, 1991, Leukocytes roll on a selectin at physiologic flow rates: distinction from and prerequisite for adhesion through integrins, *Cell*, **65**: 859–73.

Lentz TL, 1990, The recognition event between virus and host cell receptor: a target for antiviral agents, *J Gen Virol*, **71**: 751–66.

Levine AJ, 1993, The tumor suppressor genes, *Annu Rev Biochem*, **62**: 623–51.

Levine B, Hardwick JM, Griffin DE, 1994, Persistence of alphaviruses in vertebrate hosts, *Trends Microbiol*, **2**: 25–8.

Lewin DI, 1995, Herpes, EBV survive by antigenic stealth, *J NIH Res*, **7**: 49–53.

Liu C, Eichelberger MC et al., 1995, Influenza type A virus neuraminidase does not play a role in viral entry, replication, assembly, or budding, *J Virol*, **69**: 1099–106.

Lodish HF, 1976, Translational control of protein synthesis, *Annu Rev Biochem*, **45**: 39–72.

Lodish HF, Porter M, 1981, Vesicular stomatitis virus mRNA and inhibition of translation of cellular mRNA. Is there a P function in vesicular stomatitis virus?, *J Virol*, **38**: 504–17.

Ludlow JW, 1993, Interactions between SV40 large-tumor antigen and the growth suppressor proteins pRB and p53, *FASEB J*, **7**: 866–71.

Ludlow JW, Skuse GR, 1995, Viral oncoprotein binding to pRB, p107, p130, and p300, *Virus Res*, **35**: 113–21.

Luftig RB, Lupo LD, 1994, Viral interactions with the host-cell cytoskeleton: the role of retroviral proteases, *Trends Microbiol*, **2**: 178–82.

McFadden G (ed), 1995, *Viroceptors, Virokines and Related Immune Modulators Encoded by DNA Viruses*, Demos Publications, New York.

McNair AN, Kerr IM, 1992, Viral inhibition of the interferon system, *Pharmacol Ther*, **56**: 79–95.

Mahy BWJ, 1985, Strategies of virus persistence, *Br Med Bull*, **41**: 50–5.

Marcus PI, Sekellick MJ, 1974, Cell killing by viruses. I. Comparison of cell-killing, plaque-forming, and defective-interfering particles of vesicular stomatitis virus, *Virology*, **57**: 321–38.

Marsh M, 1992, Keeping the viral coat on, *Curr Biol*, **2**: 379–81.

Marsh M, Helenius A, 1989, Virus entry into animal cells, *Adv Virus Res*, **36**: 107–51.

Martin SJ, Green DR, 1995, Protease activation during apoptosis: death by a thousand cuts?, *Cell*, **82**: 349–52.

Martin SJ, Green DR, Cotter TG, 1994, Dicing with death: dissecting the components of the apoptosis machinery, *Trends Biochem Sci*, **19**: 26–30.

Mason PW, Rieder E, Baxt B, 1994, RGD sequence of foot-and-mouth disease virus is essential for infecting cells via the natural receptor but can be bypassed by an antibody-dependent enhancement pathway, *Proc Natl Acad Sci USA*, **91**: 1932–6.

Masucci MG, Ernberg I, 1994, Epstein–Barr virus: adaptation to a life within the immune system, *Trends Microbiol*, **2**: 125–30.

Mathews MB, 1993, Viral evasion of the cellular defense mechanisms: regulation of the protein kinase DAI by RNA effectors, *Semin Virol*, **4**: 247–57.

Mathews MB, Shenk T, 1991, Adenovirus virus-associated RNA and translational control, *J Virol*, **65**: 5657–62.

Meerovitch K, Sonenberg N, 1993, Internal initiation of picornavirus RNA translation, *Semin Virol*, **4**: 217–28.

Merrick WC, 1990, Mechanism of translation initiation in eukaryotes, *Enzyme*, **44**: 7–16.

ter Meulen V (ed), 1994, Pathogenesis of persistent virus infections, *Semin Virol*, **5**: 259–324.

Millns AK, Carpenter MS, DeLange AM, 1994, The vaccinia virus-encoded uracil DNA glycosylase has an essential role in viral DNA replication, *Virology*, **198**: 504–13.

Moran E, 1993, Interaction of adenoviral proteins with pRB and p53, *FASEB J*, **7**: 880–5.

Morgan RA, Anderson WF, 1993, Human gene therapy, *Annu Rev Biochem*, **62**: 191–217.

Mosser AG, Sgro J-Y, Rueckert RR, 1994, Distribution of drug resistance mutations in type 3 poliovirus identifies three regions involved in uncoating functions, *J Virol*, **68**: 8193–201.

Murti KG, Goorha R, Granoff A, 1985, An unusual replication strategy of an animal iridovirus, *Adv Virus Res*, **30**: 1–19.

Nevins JR, 1989, Mechanisms of viral-mediated trans-activation of transcription, *Adv Virus Res*, **37**: 35–83.

Nevins JR, 1992, E2F: a link between the Rb tumor suppressor protein and viral oncoproteins, *Science*, **258**: 424–9.

Nomoto A (ed), 1992, Cellular receptors for virus infection, *Semin Virol*, **3**: 77–133.

Nomoto A, Koike S, Aoki J, 1994, Tissue tropism and species specificity of poliovirus infection, *Trends Microbiol*, **2**: 47–51.

Novella IS, Cilnis M et al., 1996, Large population transmissions of vesicular stomatitis virus in interferon-treated cells select variants of only limited resistance, *J Virol*, **70**: 6414–17.

Nuss DL, Oppermann H, Koch G, 1975, Selective blockage of

initiation of host protein synthesis in RNA virus-infected cells, *Proc Natl Acad Sci USA*, **72**: 1258–62.

Oldstone MB, 1991, Molecular anatomy of viral persistence, *J Virol*, **65**: 6381–6.

Olson NH, Kolatkar PR et al., 1993, Structure of a human rhinovirus complexed with its receptor molecule, *Proc Natl Acad Sci USA*, **90**: 507–11.

O'Malley RP, Duncan RF et al., 1989, Modification of protein synthesis initiation factors and the shut-off of host protein synthesis in adenovirus-infected cells, *Virology*, **168**: 112–18.

Paredes AM, Brown DT et al., 1993, Three-dimensional structure of a membrane-containing virus, *Proc Natl Acad Sci USA*, **90**: 9095–9.

Pelham H, 1988, Heat shock proteins: coming in from the cold, *Nature (London)*, **332**: 776–7.

Pellegrini S, Schindler C, 1993, Early events in signalling by interferons, *Trends Biochem Sci*, **18**: 338–42.

Pestka S, Langer JA et al., 1987, Interferons and their actions, *Annu Rev Biochem*, **56**: 727–77.

Pickup DJ, 1994, Poxviral modifiers of cytokine response to infection, *Infect Agents Dis*, **3**: 116–27.

Pinto LH, Holsinger LJ, Lamb RA, 1992, Influenza virus M2 protein has ion channel activity, *Cell*, **69**: 511–28.

Porterfield JS, 1986, Antibody-dependent enhancement of viral infectivity, *Adv Virus Res*, **31**: 335–55.

Proud CG, 1995, PKR: a new name and new roles, *Trends Biochem Sci*, **20**: 241–6.

Racaniello VR, 1992, Interaction of poliovirus with its cell receptor, *Semin Virol*, **3**: 473–82.

Ray CA, Black RA et al., 1992, Viral inhibition of inflammation: cowpox virus encodes an inhibitor of the interleukin-1β converting enzyme, *Cell*, **69**: 597–604.

Razvi ES, Welsh RM, 1995, Apoptosis in viral infections, *Adv Virus Res*, **45**: 1–60.

Ren R, Costantini F et al., 1990, Transgenic mice expressing a human poliovirus receptor: a new model for poliomyelitis, *Cell*, **63**: 353–62.

Revel M, Chebath J, 1986, Interferon-activated genes, *Trends Biochem Sci*, **11**: 166–70.

Rey FA, Heinz FX et al., 1995, The envelope glycoprotein from tick-borne encephalitis virus at 2Å resolution, *Nature (London)*, **375**: 291–8.

Rhee SS, Hunter E, 1990, A single amino acid substitution within the matrix protein of a type D retrovirus converts its morphogenesis to that of a type C retrovirus, *Cell*, **63**: 77–86.

Rice AP, Roberts BE, 1983, Vaccinia virus induces cellular mRNA degradation, *J Virol*, **47**: 529–39.

Rossmann MG, 1989, The canyon hypothesis. Hiding the host cell receptor attachment site on a viral surface from immune surveillance, *J Biol Chem*, **264**: 14587–90.

Rossmann MG, Olson NH et al., 1994, Crystallographic and cryo EM analysis of virion–receptor interactions, *Arch Virol Suppl*, **9**: 531–41.

Roux L, Simon AE, Holland JJ, 1991, Effects of defective interfering viruses on virus replication and pathogenesis in vitro and in vivo, *Adv Virus Res*, **40**: 181–211.

Rubin DM, Finley D, 1995, The proteasome: a protein-degrading organelle?, *Curr Biol*, **5**: 854–8.

Samuel CE, 1988, Mechanisms of the antiviral action of interferons, *Prog Nucleic Acid Res Mol Biol*, **35**: 27–72.

Samuel CE, 1991, Antiviral actions of interferon: interferon-regulated cellular proteins and their surprisingly selective antiviral activities, *Virology*, **183**: 1–11.

Schindler C, Darnell JE Jr, 1995, Transcriptional responses to polypeptide ligands: the JAK-STAT pathway, *Annu Rev Biochem*, **64**: 621–51.

Schlesinger MJ, Schlesinger S, 1987, Domains of virus glycoproteins, *Adv Virus Res*, **33**: 1–44.

Schneider RJ, Shenk T, 1987, Impact of virus infection on host cell protein synthesis, *Annu Rev Biochem*, **56**: 317–32.

Schnitzlein WM, O'Banion MK et al., 1983, Effect of intracellular

vesicular stomatitis virus mRNA concentration on the inhibition of host cell protein synthesis, *J Virol*, **45**: 206–14.

Sen GC, Lengyel P, 1992, The interferon system. A bird's eye view of its biochemistry, *J Biol Chem*, **267**: 5017–20.

Sen GC, Ransohoff RM, 1993, Interferon-induced antiviral actions and their regulation, *Adv Virus Res*, **42**: 57–102.

Sharp PA, 1994, Split genes and RNA splicing, *Cell*, **77**: 805–15.

Shimamoto T, Inouye M, Inouye S, 1995, The formation of the 2′,5′-phosphodiester linkage in the cDNA priming reaction by bacterial reverse transcriptase in a cell-free system, *J Biol Chem*, **270**: 581–8.

Signoret N, Poignard P et al., 1993, Human and simian immunodeficiency viruses: virus–receptor interactions, *Trends Microbiol*, **1**: 328–33.

Singh I, Helenius A, 1992, Nucleocapsid uncoating during entry of enveloped animal RNA viruses into cells, *Semin Virol*, **3**: 511–18.

Slabaugh MB, Roseman NA, Mathews CK, 1989, Amplification of the ribonucleotide reductase small subunit gene: analysis of novel joints and the mechanism of gene duplication in vaccinia virus, *Nucleic Acids Res*, **12**: 7073–88.

Smith DB, Inglis SC, 1987, The mutation rate and variability of eukaryotic viruses: an analytical review, *J Gen Virol*, **68**: 2729–40.

Smith GL, 1993, Vaccinia virus glycoproteins and immune evasion, *J Gen Virol*, **74**: 1725–40.

Smith GL, 1994, Virus strategies for evasion of the host response to infection, *Trends Microbiol*, **2**: 81–8.

Sonenberg N, 1987, Regulation of translation by poliovirus, *Adv Virus Res*, **33**: 175–204.

Spear PG, 1993, Entry of alphaherpesviruses into cells, *Semin Virol*, **3**: 167–80.

Spriggs M, 1994, Poxvirus-encoded soluble cytokine receptors, *Virus Res*, **33**: 1–10.

Staeheli P, 1990, Interferon-induced proteins and the antiviral state, *Adv Virus Res*, **38**: 147–200.

Stegman T, 1994, Anchors aweigh, *Curr Biol*, **4**: 551–4.

Steller H, 1995, Mechanisms and genes of cellular suicide, *Science*, **267**: 1445–9.

Stillman B, Bell SP et al., 1992, DNA replication and the cell cycle, *CIBA Found Symp*, **170**: 147–56.

Strauss JH (ed), 1990, Viral proteinases, *Semin Virol*, **1**: 307–84.

Strom T, Frenkel N, 1987, Effects of herpes simplex virus on mRNA stability, *J Virol*, **61**: 2198–207.

Teich N (ed), 1991, Viral oncogenes, Parts I and II, *Semin Virol*, **2**: 305–409.

Tevethia MJ, Spector DJ, 1989, Heterologous transactivation among viruses, *Prog Med Virol*, **36**: 120–90.

Thomas JR, Wagner RR, 1983, Inhibition of translation in lysates of mouse L-cells infected with vesicular stomatitis virus: presence of a defective ribosome-associated factor, *Biochemistry*, **22**: 1540–6.

Tjian R, Maniatis T, 1994, Transcriptional activation: a complex puzzle with few easy pieces, *Cell*, **77**: 5–8.

Tucker SP, Compans RW, 1993, Virus infection of polarized epithelial cells, *Adv Virus Res*, **42**: 187–247.

Tucker SP, Wimmer E, Compans RW, 1994, Expression of viral receptors and the vectorial release of viruses in polarized epithelial cells, *Cellular Receptors for Animal Viruses*, ed Wimmer E, Cold Spring Harbor Laboratory, Cold Spring Harbor NY, 323–40.

van Etten JL, Lane LC, Meints RH, 1991, Viruses and viruslike particles of eukaryotic algae, *Microbiol Rev*, **55**: 586–620.

van Etten JL, Xia YN et al., 1988, Chlorella viruses code for restriction and modification enzymes, *Gene*, **74**: 113–15.

Varshavsky A, 1992, The N-end rule, *Cell*, **69**: 725–35.

Vaux DL, Haecker G, Strasser A, 1994, An evolutionary perspective on apoptosis, *Cell*, **76**: 777–9.

Verduin BJM, 1992, Early interactions between viruses and plants, *Semin Virol*, **3**: 423–32.

Vousden K, 1993, Interactions of human papillomavirus transforming proteins with the products of tumor suppressor genes, *FASEB J*, **7:** 872–9.

Wagner EK (ed), 1994, Herpesvirus latency, *Semin Virol*, **5:** 189–258.

Walter MR, Windsor WT et al., 1995, Crystal structure of a complex between interferon-γ and its soluble high-affinity receptor, *Nature (London)*, **376:** 230–5.

Wang J, Yan Y et al., 1990, Atomic structure of a fragment of human CD4 containing two immunoglobulin domains, *Nature (London)*, **348:** 411–18.

Weinberg RA, 1995, The retinoblastoma protein and cell cycle control, *Cell*, **81:** 323–30.

Weis W, Brown JH et al., 1988, Structure of the influenza virus haemagglutinin complexed with its receptor, sialic acid, *Nature (London)*, **333:** 426–31.

Weiss RA, 1992, Human immunodeficiency virus receptors, *Semin Virol*, **3:** 79–84.

Wek RC, 1994, eIF-2 kinases: regulators of general and gene-specific translation initiation, *Trends Biochem Sci*, **19:** 491–6.

Whitaker-Dowling P, Youngner JS, 1987, Viral interference-dominance of mutant viruses over wild-type virus in mixed infections, *Microbiol Rev*, **51:** 179–91.

White E, 1993, Regulation of apoptosis by the transforming genes of the DNA tumor virus adenovirus, *Proc Soc Exp Biol Med*, **204:** 30–9.

White JM, 1990, Viral and cellular membrane fusion proteins, *Annu Rev Physiol*, **52:** 675–97.

White JM, 1992, Membrane fusion, *Science*, **258:** 917–24.

White JM, 1994, Fusion of influenza virus in endosomes: role of the hemagglutinin, *Cellular Receptors for Animal Viruses*, ed Wimmer E, Cold Spring Harbor Laboratory, Cold Spring Harbor NY, 281–301.

White JM, Littman DR, 1989, Viral receptors of the immunoglobulin superfamily, *Cell*, **56:** 725–8.

Wickham TJ, Mathias P et al., 1993, Integrins $\alpha_v\beta_3$ and $\alpha_v\beta_5$ promote adenovirus internalization but not virus attachment, *Cell*, **73:** 309–19.

Wiley DC, Skehel JJ, 1987, The structure and function of the hemagglutinin membrane glycoprotein of influenza virus, *Annu Rev Biochem*, **56:** 365–94.

Williams BR, 1991, Transcriptional regulation of interferon-stimulated genes, *Eur J Biochem*, **200:** 1–11.

Willams GT, 1994, Programmed cell death: a fundamental protective response to pathogens, *Trends Microbiol*, **2:** 464–4.

Wilson TMA (ed), 1992, Early events in RNA virus infection, *Semin Virol*, **3:** 419–527.

Wiman KG, 1993, The retinoblastoma gene: role in cell cycle control and cell differentiation, *FASEB J*, **7:** 841–5.

Wimmer E (ed), 1994, *Cellular Receptors for Animal Viruses*, Cold Spring Harbor Laboratory, Cold Spring Harbor NY.

Wycoff EE, 1993, Inhibition of host cell protein synthesis in poliovirus-infected cells, *Semin Virol*, **4:** 209–16.

York IA, Roop C et al., 1994, A cytosolic herpes simplex virus protein inhibits antigen presentation to CD8[+] T lymphocytes, *Cell*, **77:** 525–35.

Zhang Y, Ahn BY, Moss B, 1994, Targeting of a multicomponent transcription apparatus into assembling vaccinia virus particles requires rap94, an RNA polymerase-associated protein, *J Virol*, **68:** 1360–70.

Zhang Y, Schneider RJ, 1993, Adenovirus inhibition of cellular protein synthesis and the specific translation of late viral mRNAs, *Semin Virol*, **4:** 229–36.

Part II

General characteristics of viral infections

THE PATHOGENESIS OF VIRAL INFECTIONS

Neal Nathanson and Kenneth L Tyler

1 INTRODUCTION

Viral pathogenesis deals with the interaction between a virus and its host. Included within the scope of pathogenesis are the stepwise progression of infection from virus entry through dissemination to shedding, the defensive responses of the host and the mechanisms of virus clearance or persistence. Pathogenesis also encompasses the disease processes that result from infection, variations in viral pathogenicity and the genetic basis of host resistance to infection or disease. A subject this broad cannot be treated in a single chapter, so this presentation reviews the dissemination of viruses and their pathogenicity; other aspects of pathogenesis are dealt with in Chapters 8, 10, 11 and 12. Several detailed reviews of viral pathogenesis have recently been published (Nathanson 1996, Tyler and Fields 1996).

2 DISSEMINATION IN THE ANIMAL HOST

One of the cardinal differences between viral infection of a simple cell culture and infection of an animal host is the structural complexity of the multicellular organism. The virus must overcome a number of barriers to accomplish the stepwise infection of the host, beginning with entry, followed by dissemination, localization in a few target tissues, shedding and transmission to other hosts (Fig. 9.1).

2.1 Entry

SKIN AND MUCOUS MEMBRANES

Some viruses (such as papillomaviruses, poxviruses and herpes simplex viruses) will replicate in cells of the skin or mucous membranes. It is likely that infections with these viruses are initiated at breaks in the epithelium, just as the skin must be scratched to facilitate a 'take' by vaccinia virus. Mucous membranes represent a minimal physical barrier to infection but are bathed in mucus that contains immunoglobulin and provides protection by virtue of its viscous nature. Following infection of skin, viruses may spread further by passage of intact virions or virus-infected macrophages and dendritic cells to the regional lymph nodes.

The epidermis consists of several layers of cells, including, from the deepest to most superficial, the basal germinal layer of dividing cells (malpighian stratum), the granular layer of dying cells (stratum granulosum), and the superficial layer of keratin (stratum corneum). Most viruses that replicate in the skin grow in the germinal cells, and some viruses, such as papillomaviruses, have a selective tropism for these cells (Shah and Howley 1990). Poxviruses and herpes simplex viruses also replicate in fibroblasts and macrophages in the dermis (Blank et al. 1951, Roberts 1962a). Some adenoviruses, coxsackievirus A24, and enterovirus type 70 are regularly associated with conjunctivitis, and the conjunctiva may represent a primary portal of entry in such instances.

UROGENITAL TRACT

A considerable number of viruses cause sexually transmitted disease, which is usually acquired by exposure to virus-containing secretions. Infection is initiated either by penetration through breaks in the skin or by direct invasion of the superficial epithelium of the mucous membranes. For papillomaviruses and herpes simplex viruses the initial sites of replication are the germinal layer of the epidermis and the fibroblasts and phagocytes in the dermis.

Some sexually transmitted viruses, such as hepatitis B and human immunodeficiency virus (HIV), give rise to persistent viraemia, and may invade by mechanisms different from those used by viruses that replicate in skin and membranes. Thus, contaminated blood,

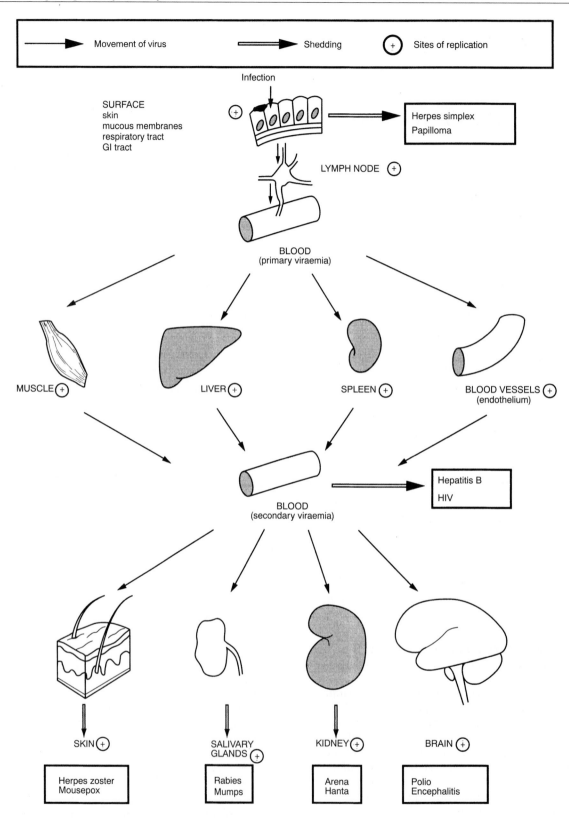

Fig. 9.1   A generalized scheme of the virus life cycle in the infected host to show entry, dissemination and shedding of blood-borne viruses, with a few representative examples. This scheme represents many but not all viruses, and does not illustrate neural spread. (Revised after Mims 1987.)

semen or secretions may introduce virus or virus-infected cells directly into the circulation via breaks in skin and membranes. Alternatively, HIV may establish initial infection in dendritic macrophages (Langerhans cells) in the epidermis, or in epithelial cells of the cervix, although the latter cells lack the CD4 receptor (Pomerantz et al. 1988, Langhoff et al. 1991, Tan, Pearce-Pratt and Phillips 1993).

TRANSCUTANEOUS AND INTRAVENOUS INJECTION

Although the skin is a formidable barrier, mechanical injection that breaches the barrier is a 'natural' route of entry for many viruses.

Arboviruses

Many animal viruses are maintained in nature by a cycle that involves a vector and a vertebrate host (Monath 1988), including over 500 individual viruses mainly in the families *Bunyaviridae*, *Flaviviridae*, *Togaviridae* (see Chapters 29 and 30), *Reoviridae* and *Rhabdoviridae*. When the infected vector takes a blood meal, virus contained in the salivary gland is injected. Although most viruses that are transmitted by an insect vector replicate in the vector, there are a few instances in which the vector acts only as a 'flying pin' and apparently carries the virus mechanically from one vertebrate host to another; examples are myxoma virus of rabbits and rabbit papillomatosis virus (Dalmat 1958, Fenner 1983).

Intramuscular injection: rabies

Rabies is the only virus that is maintained in many of its natural cycles by the bite of a sick animal (Baer 1991). Following transcutaneous and intramuscular injection, the virus may either enter the processes of peripheral nerves directly or replicate in striated muscle. It can then cross the neuromuscular junction and spread along peripheral nerves to the central nervous system.

Injection or transfusion

Virus may be transmitted accidentally by repeated use of contaminated needles, injection of a virus-contaminated therapeutic substance, or transfusion with virus-contaminated blood or blood products. The agents most frequently involved are those that produce persistent viraemias, such as hepatitis B, C or D, cytomegalovirus and human immunodeficiency virus. Contaminated needles play a major role in transmission, either by parenteral injection of drugs by abusers in developed countries or by re-use of needles in developing countries. Following parenteral injection, virus appears to be widely disseminated, reaching those cells for which it has a tropism.

OROPHARYNX AND GASTROINTESTINAL TRACT

The oropharynx and gastrointestinal tract is an important portal of entry for many viruses, and enteric viruses may invade the host in a variety of sites from the oral cavity to the colon. Some viruses produce localized infections that remain confined to the gastrointestinal tract whereas others disseminate to produce systemic infection. Most enteric viruses, such as rotaviruses, infect the epithelium of the small or large intestine (Little and Shadduck 1982, Saif 1990), but some enteroviruses, such as poliovirus, also can replicate in the lymphoid tissue of the gut and nasopharynx.

There are numerous barriers to infection via the enteric route. First, much of the ingested inoculum will remain trapped in the luminal contents and never reach the wall of the gut. Secondly, the lumen constitutes a hostile environment because of the acidity of the stomach, the alkalinity of the small intestine, the digestive enzymes found in saliva and pancreatic secretions, and the lipolytic action of bile. Thirdly, the mucus that lines the intestinal epithelium presents a physical barrier protecting the intestinal surface. Fourthly, phagocytic scavenger cells and secreted antibodies in the lumen can reduce the titre of infectious virus.

Acid-labile viruses, such as rhinoviruses, cannot infect by the intestinal route. Viruses that are successful in using the enteric portal tend to be resistant to acid pH, proteolytic attack and bile, and some may actually exploit the hostile environment to enhance their infectivity (Clark, Roth and Clark 1981, Estes, Graham and Mason 1981). Hepatitis A and B viruses illustrate this point – both viruses are excreted in the bile into the intestinal tract but hepatitis A virus survives and is excreted in an infectious form in the faeces whereas hepatitis B virus is inactivated. As a consequence, only hepatitis A is transmitted as an enterovirus.

Lower gastrointestinal tract

The importance of anal intercourse as a risk factor for hepatitis B and HIV infection has led to the recognition that some viruses can gain entry through the lower gastrointestinal tract. HIV has been detected in bowel epithelium (Levy 1994), but the exact mechanism of HIV infection through the anocolonic portal remains to be determined.

RESPIRATORY TRACT

Respiratory infection may be initiated either by virus contained in aerosols that are inhaled by the recipient host or by virus that is contained in nasopharyngeal fluids and is transmitted by hand-to-hand contact. Important groups of viruses transmitted by the respiratory route include rhinoviruses, myxoviruses, adenoviruses, herpesviruses and poxviruses.

Aerosolized droplets are deposited at different levels in the respiratory tract depending upon their size: those over 10 μm diameter are deposited in the nose, those 5–10 μm in the airways and those <5 μm in the alveoli (Lippmann et al. 1980). Once deposited, the virus must bypass several effective barriers to initiate infection. These barriers include phagocytic cells in the respiratory lumen, a covering layer of mucus and ciliated epithelial cells that clear the respiratory tree of foreign particles. The temperature of the respiratory tract varies from 33°C in the nasal passages to 37°C (core body temperature) in the alveoli. Viruses (such as rhinoviruses) that can replicate well at 33°C but not at 37°C are limited to the upper respiratory tract and, conversely, viruses that replicate well at 37°C but not at 33°C (such as influenza virus) mainly infect the lower respiratory tract. Most respiratory viruses initiate infection by replicating in epithelial cells lining the alveoli or the respiratory tree, but some viruses also replicate in phagocytic cells located either in the respiratory lumen or in subepithelial spaces (Roberts 1962b, Douglas et al. 1966).

2.2 Spread

Once infection is established at the site of entry, most viruses spread locally by cell-to-cell transmission of infection. Some viruses remain localized near their site of entry whereas others spread widely. One determinant of dissemination is the pattern of viral release from polarized epithelial cells. Viruses that are released only at the apical surface of infected cells tend to remain localized, whereas those that are released at the basal surface tend to disseminate (Tucker and Compans 1992). Usually, the first step in dissemination of the infection is the transport of virus via the efferent lymphatic drainage from the initial site of infection to the regional lymph nodes, either as free virions or in virus-infected phagocytic cells.

Viraemia

The single most important route of dissemination is the circulation, which can potentially carry viruses to any site in the body. There are several sources of viraemia. Virus may enter with the efferent lymphatic flow, or may be shed from infected endothelial cells or circulating mononuclear leucocytes. Viruses can circulate either free in the plasma phase of the blood ('plasma' viraemia) or associated with formed elements ('cell-associated' viraemia), and these 2 types of viraemia have quite different characteristics and implications.

'Passive' viraemia is used to describe the entry of a virus inoculum directly into the circulation following injection, without any preceding replication (Fig. 9.2). Passive viraemia typically occurs 3–6 hours after injection and disappears within 12–24 hours. It has been estimated that about 0.1% of the virus in a subcutaneous inoculum enters the blood stream (Griot et al 1993, Pekosz et al. 1995).

'Active' viraemia is used to designate viraemia caused by the active replication of virus in the host. In some instances, active viraemia may occur in 2 phases, a 'primary' viraemia in which virus spreads from a focal site of entry and a 'secondary' viraemia generated after infection has occurred and virus has initially replicated in peripheral tissues such as endothelium, tissue macrophages, liver, muscle or other sites (see Fig. 9.1). An example of an active viraemia is shown in Fig. 9.3, in which the virus appears in the plasma a few days after infection and lasts for about one week. The initial lag period is the interval

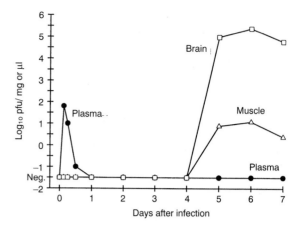

Fig. 9.2 Passive viraemia, after injection of La Crosse virus in weanling mice. Viraemia appears as a sharp peak limited to the first 12 hours and stands out in profile because there is no active viraemia in mice of this age. Even this transient viraemia was sufficient to deliver enough virus to the target organ to initiate a lethal encephalitis. (Data from Pekosz et al. 1995.)

required for tissue replication and shedding into the circulation. Termination of viraemia is often quite abrupt and coincides with the appearance of neutralizing antibody in the serum. When an infected animal is treated with an immunosuppressive regimen, the viraemia may not be cleared quickly but persist for longer periods (Nathanson and Cole 1971).

Plasma viraemia reflects a dynamic process in which virus continually enters the circulation and is removed. The rate of turnover of virus within the plasma compartment is best expressed as transit time, the average duration of a virion in the blood compartment. Typically, transit times range from 1 to 60 minutes and tend to decrease as the size of the virions increases (Mims 1964). Circulating viruses are removed by the phagocytic cells of the reticuloendothelial system, principally in the liver (Kupffer cells) and to a lesser extent in the lung, spleen and lymph nodes. The fate of viruses that are ingested by Kupffer

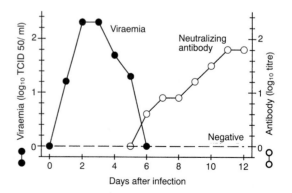

Fig. 9.3 Active plasma viraemia after intramuscular injection of poliovirus in monkeys. Viraemia lasts for about one week, and the clearance of viraemia coincides with the appearance of neutralizing antibody in the serum. (Data from Nathanson and Bodian 1961.)

cells is quite variable and may be an important determinant of pathogenesis. Ingested virions may be degraded, may transit within macrophages to underlying parenchyma without replicating, or may replicate in macrophages with or without spread of infection to underlying parenchymal cells. Once the host has developed circulating antibody, plasma virus is very rapidly neutralized in the circulation (Fig. 9.3), and virus–antibody complexes bind to Fc receptors, facilitating removal by sessile macrophages lining the circulation. In these circumstances, it may be assumed that transit time is greatly reduced below the ranges described above.

Although plasma viraemias are usually short-lived, there are notable exceptions. Some viruses are bound by antibody but the immune complex retains infectivity. In these instances, such as Aleutian disease virus (a parvovirus) and lactic dehydrogenase virus (a togavirus), plasma infectivity may resist neutralization with exogenous antibody but may be reduced by the addition of anti-Ig antibodies (Notkins et al. 1966, Porter and Larsen 1976). Other exceptions are instances in which the infected host is 'tolerant' of the viral antigens and fails to develop enough antibody to clear viraemia. Examples are hepatitis B virus and lymphocytic choriomeningitis virus (Fig. 9.4).

A number of viruses replicate in cells that are found in the circulation, particularly monocytes, B or T lymphocytes or (rarely) erythrocytes (Table 9.1). In these circumstances, the viraemia is 'cell-associated' although some virus may also be found free in the plasma compartment. Cell-associated viraemias may be of short duration, as in the case of ectromelia and other poxviruses. However, in many instances of cell-associated viraemia, virus titres are low, virus may be difficult to isolate from the blood and viraemia persists

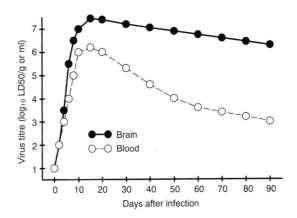

Fig. 9.4 Persistent plasma viraemia associated with immunological hyporesponsiveness to the viral antigens. Adult mice were infected with lymphocytic choriomeningitis virus (LCMV) intracerebrally and were immunosuppressed with aminopterin on days 4 and 6 after infection. Mice infected in the same way but not treated with aminopterin died of acute choriomeningitis about 8 days after infection. (Data from Hotchin 1962.)

for the life of the host rather than terminating when neutralizing antibody appears (Fig. 9.5).

Human immunodeficiency virus (HIV) provides an important instance of cell-associated viraemia (Hsia and Spector 1991, Bagasra et al. 1993, Levy 1994). HIV infects both CD4+ T lymphocytes and monocytes in the blood, mostly the former. The proportion of infected peripheral blood CD4+ T lymphocytes varies from 0.2–10% in asymptomatic people to 2–60% in symptomatic patients, and 50–90% of infected T lymphocytes contain the genome in a latent state. In typical asymptomatic individuals there are about 5000 infected cells per millilitre of blood. In addition to

Table 9.1 Viruses that replicate in circulating blood cells: a representative list

Cell type	Virus family	Example	Duration of viraemia	References
Monocytes	*Flaviviridae*	Dengue	Acute	Halstead and O'Rourke 1977
	Togaviridae	Rubella	Acute	Chantler and Tingle 1982
	Paramyxoviridae	Measles	Acute	Esolen et al. 1993
	Arenaviridae	LCMV	Persistent	Matloubian et al. 1993
	Retroviridae	HIV	Persistent	Collman et al. 1989
		Ovine visna maedi	Persistent	Gendelman et al. 1985
	Herpesviridae	Cytomegalovirus	Persistent	Taylor-Weideman et al. 1991
	Poxviridae	Mousepox	Acute	Fenner 1949
		Rabbit myxoma	Acute	Fenner 1983
B lymphocytes	*Retroviridae*	Murine leukaemia	Persistent	Kozak and Ruscetti 1992
	Herpesviridae	Epstein–Barr virus	Persistent	Ho 1981
T lymphocytes	*Retroviridae*	HIV	Persistent	Bagasra et al. 1993
		HTLV-I	Persistent	Depper et al. 1984
	Herpesviridae	Human herpes 6, 7	Acute	Takahashi, Sonoda and Higashi 1989
Erythroblasts	*Reoviridae*	Colorado tick fever	Acute	Oshiro et al. 1978

HIV, human immunodeficiency virus; HTLV, human T cell leukaemia virus; LCMV, lymphocytic choriomeningitis virus.

infected cells, free infectious HIV is also present in the plasma, the amount varying with the stage of disease. In typical asymptomatic individuals, it has been estimated that there are about 100 tissue culture infectious doses (TCIDs) per millilitre of plasma, considerably fewer than the number of infected cells.

Antibody-dependent enhancement of infection is a special aspect of cell-associated viraemia, which has been described mainly for dengue and other flaviviruses (Halstead and O'Rourke 1977, Gollins and Porterfield 1984). Dengue virus replicates primarily in monocytes, but it does not enter these cells readily. However, in the presence of low concentrations of antibody, infection is markedly enhanced, presumably because the virus–antibody complex is bound to the Fc receptors on monocytes, enhancing viral entry.

Tissue invasion from the blood

There are several ways in which a virus might cross the vascular wall (Johnson and Mims 1968), but the precise mechanism for penetrating the blood–tissue barrier is unknown in most instances.

1   In many tissues, the capillary endothelial cells are not joined by tight junctions, and viruses can pass between them. One example is the fenestrated capillaries of the choroid plexus of the central nervous system. Penetration at this site provides access to the epithelial cells of the choroid plexus and can be followed by entry into the cerebrospinal fluid and spread to the ependymal cells lining the ventricles (Herndon, Johnson and Davis 1974).

2   Virus may be transported through endothelial cells by a process of endocytosis, translocation of virus-containing vesicles and subsequent release by exocytosis at the basal surface of the endothelial cell (Johnson and Mims 1968, Pathek and Webb 1974).

3   Some viruses are capable of replicating within endothelial cells and are released from these cells into the surrounding tissues. Examples include certain picornaviruses, retroviruses, alphaviruses and parvoviruses (Johnson 1965, Baringer and Nathanson 1972, Friedman, Macarek and MacGregor 1981, Pitts, Powers and Billelo 1987).

4   Viruses that cause a cell-associated viraemia may invade by an alternative mechanism, namely, as 'passengers' in infected lymphocytes or monocytes, a mechanism that has been suggested for tissue invasion of HIV and other lentiviruses (Haase 1986). Infected mononuclear cells can cross the blood–tissue barrier as part of their normal trafficking pattern, or may be actively recruited into sites of inflammation.

NEURAL SPREAD

Some viruses can disseminate by spreading along peripheral nerves (Table 9.2). Although less important than viraemia, neural spread plays an essential role for certain viruses (such as rabies viruses and several herpesviruses) whereas other viruses (such as poliovirus and reovirus) can utilize both mechanisms of spread. Different strains of the same virus may differ markedly in their ability to use the neural route (Nathanson and Bodian 1961, Tyler, McPhee and Fields 1986, Ren et al. 1990), as shown in Table 9.3.

It seems that viruses enter neurons by mechanisms similar to those involving entry into other cell types. The uncoated nucleocapsid is then carried passively along axons or dendrites, probably by fast axoplasmic flow. After the transport process the virus may replicate in the perikaryon, but this is a much slower process and is not required for neural spread. There are several lines of evidence for this reconstruction of neural spread.

1   Neural transection will block neural spread (Table 9.3) and the rate of movement (>5 cm per day) is similar to the rate of axoplasmic transport (>10 cm per day) (Kristensson, Lycke and Sjostrand 1971, Tyler, McPhee and Fields 1986, Tsiang 1993).

2   Drugs, such as colchicine, that block fast axoplasmic transport also block the transport of viral genomes (Tsiang 1979).

3   Temperature-sensitive strains of herpesvirus (which cannot replicate at body temperature) are able to move from a peripheral site of inoculation to a sensory ganglion, such as the trigeminal ganglion, and may be recovered by culturing the explanted ganglion at temperatures that are permissive for temperature-sensitive clones (Sederati, Margolis and Stevens 1993).

4   Several days after initiation of neural spread, viruses such as rabiesvirus, herpes simplex virus and pseudorabies (an alphaherpes virus) virus may be seen replicating within axons as shown in Fig.

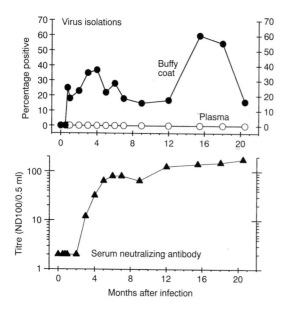

Fig. 9.5   Cell-associated viraemia in sheep infected with visna-maedi virus, a lentivirus. Virus was isolated by co-cultivation of buffy coat cells with indicator cells and was never isolated from the plasma. The frequency of virus isolations was unrelated to the appearance or titre of neutralizing antibody. (Data from Petursson et al. 1976.)

Table 9.2 Viruses that spread by the neural route: a representative list

Virus family	Example	Notes	References
Picornaviridae	Poliovirus	Neuroadapted clones only; natural isolates are viraemogenic	Nathanson and Bodian 1961 Bodian 1955
Flaviviridae	Yellow fever	Neuroadapted clones only; natural isolates are viraemogenic	Strode 1951
Alphaviridae	VEE	Haematogenous invasion of peripheral nerves	Charles et al. 1995
Coronaviridae	Mouse hepatitis	Neural spread after intranasal infection	Perlman, Jacobsen and Afifi 1989 Barnett and Perlman 1993
Rhabdoviridae	Rabies	Exclusively neural	Baer 1991
Reoviridae	Reovirus	Type 3 uses neural route Type 1 spreads by the haematogenous route	Tyler, McPhee and Fields 1986 Morrison, Sidman and Fields 1991
Herpesviridae	Herpes simplex 1, 2 Pseudorabies	Exclusively neural in adults; pantropic in newborns Used for neural pathways	Cook and Stevens 1973 Enquist 1994

VEE, Venezuelan equine encephalitis.

9.6 (Rabin, Jenson and Melnick 1968). Also, see Chapter 40.

2.3 Localization or tropism

One of the salient features that distinguishes viruses is their localization within the animal host (see Fig. 9.1). The names of individual viral diseases often reflect the organs or tissues that are involved; thus, poliomyelitis and hepatitis each have their characteristic features. Localization of infection, or viral tropism, is regulated both by viral dissemination and by cellular susceptibility. Disease localization may not correspond to the distribution of infection because it reflects both the spread of the virus and the host response to infection.

VIRAL DISSEMINATION

The localization of a virus is determined at several phases of infection, including penetration at the portal of entry, systemic spread by viraemia or the neural route, and the invasion of local organs or tissues.

Portal of entry

The physical characteristics of a virus that influence its ability to survive in the external environment play a role in circumscribing the portal of entry. Thus, many picornaviruses are enteroviruses that are capable of surviving in the hostile environment of the enteric tract, but some picornaviruses, such as the rhinoviruses, are acid-labile, cannot survive gastric acidity and are confined to the respiratory tract. The biological characteristics of the virus also play a role in its initial localization. Again, the rhinoviruses replicate well at 33°C, the temperature of the nasopharynx, whereas influenza virus has a replication optimum of 37°C that permits it to infect the lower respiratory tract. These limiting factors are particularly important for the localization of viruses that fail to spread systemically.

Table 9.3 Different mode of dissemination of a neurotropic and a pantropic strain of the same virus*

	Neuroadapted MV strain		Pantropic Mahoney strain	
	Control	**Block**	**Control**	**Block**
Paralysis	25/26	0/11	19/19	18/20

Site of initial paralysis:
   injected leg
   other
	
	24
	1
		
		–
		–
			
			3
			16
				
				5
				13

Incubation to paralysis	5 days	–	7 days	7.5 days

*Comparison of a neuroadapted and a natural pantropic isolate of poliovirus following intramuscular injection in cynomolgus macaques. The neuroadapted virus spreads only by the neural route, causes initial paralysis in the injected limb and fails to paralyse after a nerve block, whilst the pantropic strain spreads by viraemia, does not cause localized initial paralysis, and is not impeded by nerve block. (Data from Nathanson and Bodian 1961.)

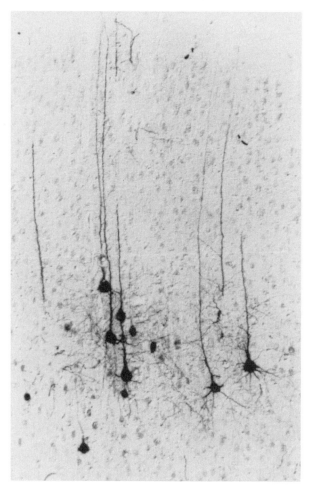

Fig. 9.6 The intraneuronal spread of a virus. Pseudorabies virus is seen in neurons in the perirhinal cortex of a rat following virus injection into the prefrontal cortex. Peroxidase staining has been used to visualize viral antigen (Card and Enquist 1994). (Photomicrograph kindly provided by Patrick Card and Lynn Enquist.)

Viraemia and neural spread

Viraemia plays a key role in the systemic spread of most viruses (see Fig. 9.1), and the viraemogenicity of the specific viral strain determines its likelihood of reaching target organs. Conversely, the inability to initiate viraemia explains the local nature of the infections caused by many respiratory and enteric viruses. The importance of viraemia in determining localization is illustrated in Table 9.4, which indicates that in adult mice La Crosse virus (a bunyavirus) can initiate a lethal encephalitis after intracerebral injection of a minimal dose (c. 1 pfu) but fails to cause illness after subcutaneous injection of $>10^7$ pfu because no viraemia is produced. Likewise, poliovirus, in spite of its high potential for causing paralysis, is estimated to cause only one paralytic case per 150 human infections, presumably because it rarely generates sufficient viraemia to reach the spinal cord (Fig. 9.7).

For viruses that spread primarily by the neural route the ability to disseminate is also an important determinant of localization. For instance, herpes simplex virus

is capable of initiating a very severe encephalitis in humans if the virus reaches the central nervous system. However, most infections are either silent or limited to mucocutaneous lesions, and encephalitis occurs at a rate of less than one case per 1000 primary infections, indicating that the virus rarely reaches its potential target in sufficient dose to localize in the brain.

CELLULAR RECEPTORS

Most viruses are quite selective in the cell types that are infected in vivo and this selectivity plays a significant role in localization. A major determinant of cellular susceptibility is the presence of viral receptors, i.e. molecules on the cellular surface that act as receptors for the specific virus, usually by binding a protein on the virion surface (the viral attachment protein). From studies of many viral receptors, several generalizations can be made (Wimmer 1994).

1 Although receptors have been identified for only a small proportion of viruses, it is generally thought that specific receptors are necessary for efficient infection by most viruses. Presumably, viruses have evolved to utilize, as receptors, cellular surface molecules that subserve other functions required for normal cellular activity.
2 Although viral receptors are often proteins, other cellular surface molecules, such as sialic acid residues that bind the haemagglutinin of influenza virus, can also act as receptors.
3 Many viruses are capable of utilizing more than a single cellular molecule as a receptor.
4 Entry of a virus into a potential host cell is a multi-step process in which binding to the receptor is only one of the first steps, and successful binding does not always lead to productive infection (Haywood 1994).

A representative list of viral receptors is given in Table 9.5.

These generalizations are illustrated by human immunodeficiency virus, HIV (Levy 1994, Weiss 1994). The CD4 molecule is a type I protein, which is expressed by certain subsets of T lymphocytes and monocytes/macrophages, and subserves signalling between lymphoid and monocytic cells. CD4 has 4 immunoglobulin-like domains in its extracellular amino terminus, and the outermost of these domains contains a region that binds a specific domain on gp120, the surface glycoprotein of HIV. The primary cellular targets of HIV are CD4+ T lymphocytes and monocytes/macrophages, and the distribution of CD4 explains this cellular localization. However, the expression of CD4 on the surface of a cell is not sufficient to ensure viral entry (Maddon et al. 1986). When CD4– cells are stably transfected with CD4, they may become permissive for HIV if they are primate cells but not if they are rodent cells, suggesting that there are other accessory molecules that must act in concert with CD4 for successful viral entry. Finally, some CD4– human cells can be infected with HIV, and at least one alternative receptor (galactosyl ceramide) has been identified on a subset of these CD4– permissive cell lines (Harouse et al. 1991). Galactosyl ceramide, a glycosphingolipid that is expressed on CD4– oligodendroglia and certain neuroglial cell lines

Table 9.4 The relative virulence of viruses depends on the context within which they are assessed*

Virus clone	pfu : LD50			
	Intracerebral infection: suckling mice*	Subcutaneous infection: suckling mice	Intracerebral infection: adult mice	Subcutaneous infection: adult mice
Wild type La Crosse original	~1	~1	~1	>10^7
Attenuated B.5 clone	~1	>10^5	>10^6	>10^7

*Illustrated by two variants of La Crosse virus, a bunyavirus, when injected by different routes in suckling and adult mice. One clone, La Crosse/original, is a wild type isolate and the other clone, B.5, is a laboratory-derived attenuated strain. Note that the two viruses have striking differences in virulence upon intracerebral injection of adult mice or subcutaneous injection of suckling mice, but that they appear similar both in their high virulence for suckling mice inoculated intracerebrally and in their low virulence for adult mice inoculated subcutaneously. Virulence is expressed as the ratio of pfu : LD50; the lower the number the more virulent the virus. (Data from Endres et al. 1990.)

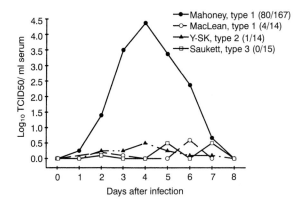

Fig. 9.7 Viraemia as a determinant of viral virulence. Type 1 Mahoney virus produced the highest level of viraemia and the highest frequency of paralysis (48%) while the other 3 (low viraemia) strains produced an aggregate paralytic rate of 12% (the frequency of paralysis is shown in parentheses). (Data from Bodian 1954.)

(Nathanson et al. 1994), has been shown to bind HIV via the V3 loop on the surface protein, a region different from the domain on the surface protein that binds to CD4.

Poliovirus offers another example of localization determined by receptors (Freistadt et al. 1994, Wimmer 1994). It had long been known that poliovirus would replicate only in primate tissues, and it had been deduced that this was because a putative poliovirus receptor (PVR) was expressed only by primate cells, since non-primate mammalian cells would support poliovirus replication if transfected with viral RNA, thereby bypassing the requirement for a viral receptor. Using this concept the PVR was cloned and sequenced, and when transfected into rodent cells it rendered them permissive for the virus (Mendelsohn, Wimmer and Racaniello 1989). Furthermore, when transgenic mice were created that expressed the PVR, the animals developed typical clinical and pathological poliomyelitis after intracerebral injection of human poliovirus (Ren and Racaniello 1992).

However, the relationship of the PVR to viral localization appears to be more complex, because the PVR alone may not confer cellular susceptibility. Thus, the PVR is expressed in most or all human tissues, but

most of these tissues are not infected by the virus. Also, PVR transgenic mice cannot be readily infected via the oral route (the natural route of infection in primates), and pantropic strains of poliovirus that are viraemogenic in primates fail to cause viraemia in mice (Ren and Racaniello 1992). Furthermore, there is evidence that CD44H, a cellular transmembrane protein, is involved in the entry of poliovirus (Shepley 1994). CD44H seems to act as an accessory molecule since cells that are CD44+ but PVR– are neither susceptible to poliovirus infection nor able to bind the virus to their surface, and yet a monoclonal antibody against CD44H will protect PVR+ cells from infection with the virus. Furthermore, CD44H has a distribution in the nervous system that corresponds with the location of cells susceptible to the virus whereas the PVR has a wider distribution.

OTHER MECHANISMS OF CELLULAR LOCALIZATION

Cellular susceptibility may be determined at post-entry steps in the replication cycle. Some viruses are quite fastidious and can replicate only in selected cell types, thus accounting for their localization. For example, some of the murine leukaemia viruses seem to require enhancers or promoters that are supplied only in certain cell types (Evans and Morrey 1987). In these instances, genetic studies have mapped the viral determinants of replication to the unique 3' (U3) non-coding region of the viral genome (Hopkins, Golemis and Speck 1989).

LOCALIZATION OF VIRAL PATHOLOGY

Pathological lesions initiated by viral infections do not always co-localize at the sites of viral replication. Some viruses kill all cells in which they replicate, and in such instances viral disease tends to mirror the localization of viral replication. However, certain viruses destroy some but not all of the cells in which they replicate. For instance, viruses that are cytocidal because they trigger a cascade of events leading to cellular apoptosis may replicate in a non-cytocidal fashion in cells in which apoptosis is blocked by the protective effect of the *bcl 2* proto-oncogene (Griffin et al. 1994).

A number of viruses initiate immune-mediated cellular pathology in which CD8+ T lymphocytes

Table 9.5 Cellular receptors for animal viruses: a selected list

Type of molecule	Receptor (binding domain)	Virus family	Virus	References
Immunoglobulin-like molecules	VCAM-1	*Picornaviridae*	EMC-D	Huber 1994
	ICAM-1 (first domain)	*Picornaviridae*	HRV (major group)	Tomassini, Maxson and Colonno 1989
	PVR (first domain)	*Picornaviridae*	Poliovirus	Mendelsohn, Wimmer and Racaniello 1989
	CD4 (first domain)	*Retroviridae*	HIV, SIV	Maddon et al. 1986
	CEA (first domain)	*Coronaviridae*	Mouse hepatitis virus	Williams, Jiang and Holmes 1991
Integrins	VLA-2 (α chain)	*Picornaviridae*	Echovirus 1, 8	Bergelson et al. 1993
	Vibronectin	*Picornaviridae*	CAV 9, echovirus 22	Roivainen et al. 1994
Signalling receptors	LDL receptor family	*Picornaviridae*	HRV (minor group)	Hofer et al. 1994
	LDL receptor family	*Retroviridae*	ALV subgroup A	Bates, Young and Varmus 1993
Other proteins	Aminopeptidase N	*Coronaviridae*	HCV 229E, TGEV	Yeager et al. 1992
	Complement receptor CR2	*Herpesviridae*	EBV	McClure 1992
	CD46	*Morbilliviridae*	Measles virus	Dorig et al. 1993
Carbohydrates	Sialic acid	*Orthomyxoviridae*	Influenza virus	Weis et al. 1988
	Galactosyl ceramide	*Retroviridae*	HIV, SIV	Harouse et al. 1991

ALV, avian leukosis virus; CAV, Coxsackie A virus; CEA, carcinoembryonic antigen; EMC, encephalomyocarditis virus; HCV, human coronavirus; HIV, human immunodeficiency virus; HRV, human rhinovirus; ICAM, intercellular adhesion molecule; LDL, low density lipoprotein; PVR, poliovirus receptor; SIV, simian immunodeficiency virus; TGEV, transmissible gastroenteritis virus; VCAM, vascular cell adhesion molecule; VLA, very late antigen. (Adapted from Wimmer 1994.)

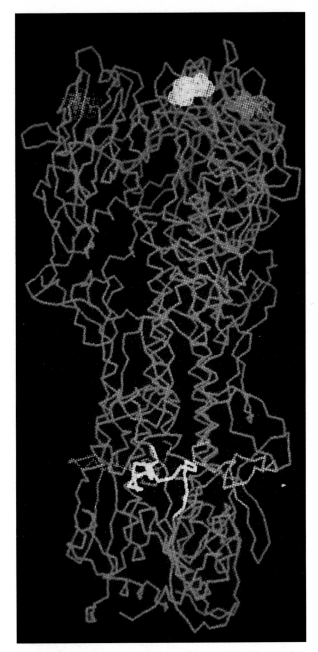

Plate 8.3 The influenza virus haemagglutinin (HA). The α-carbon backbone of the HA trimer is displayed in blue with the 3 fusion peptides, located in the stem of the molecule, highlighted in red, yellow and green. The molecular surfaces of 3 sialic acid residues are shown (red, yellow, green) in the receptor-binding sites of the globular head domains. The 3 monomers would be anchored in the viral membrane at the bottom. (From White 1992.)

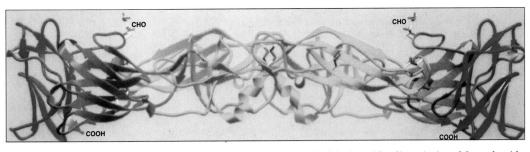

Plate 8.4 Three-dimensional structure of glycoprotein E of tick-borne encephalitis virus. The dimer is viewed from the side, as it would lie on the surface of the viral membrane. (From Rey et al. 1995.)

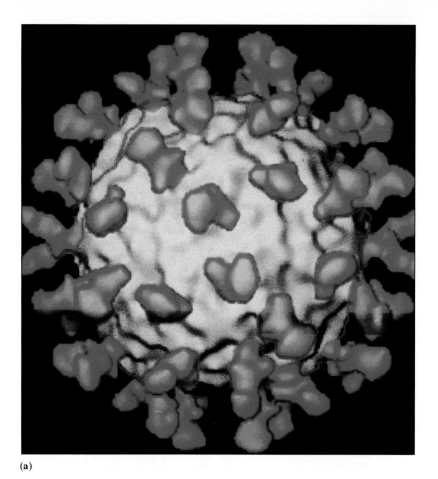

(a)

(b)

Plate 8.5 Interaction of rhinovirus with its receptor ICAM-1. (a) Cryo-EM reconstruction of a virus particle complexed with 60 receptor molecules (orange). (b) High-resolution image of a single receptor-binding site interaction. (From Olson et al. 1993.)

attack cells that present viral peptides associated with MHC class I proteins. If the virus infects both cells that do and cells that do not express MHC class I molecules, the MHC-negative cells are not attacked. This phenomenon is thought to explain the sparing of neurons after infection by certain viruses, because neurons do not express class I molecules (Rall, Mucke and Oldstone 1995). Immune-mediated lesions may be even more indirect, such as those that are caused by antigen–antibody complexes. In this instance, the lesions are seen in locations such as the glomerulus of the kidney, which cannot handle the large accumulations of macromolecular complexes, while the virus has replicated at sites distant from the kidney (Oldstone 1975).

2.4 Shedding

Acute viral infections are characterized by brief periods of intensive virus shedding into respiratory aerosols, faeces, urine or other bodily secretions or fluids (see Fig. 9.1). Persistent viruses are often shed at relatively low titres, but this may be adequate for transmission over the prolonged duration of infection.

GASTROINTESTINAL AND RESPIRATORY TRACTS

The course of shedding of enteric viruses can be readily followed. For instance, poliovirus is shed in the pharynx for 2–4 weeks and in the faeces for 1–2 months after infection, although viraemia lasts only about one week (see Fig. 9.3). Respiratory viruses may be transmitted by aerosols generated by coughing or sneezing or by virus-containing nasopharyngeal fluids that are transmitted by hand-to-hand contact. Most acute respiratory viruses are excreted over a relatively short period and infected people are potential transmitters for only about one week (Fig. 9.8); transmission may begin a few days before onset of symptoms (Douglas et al. 1966).

SKIN, MUCOUS MEMBRANES, ORAL AND GENITAL FLUIDS, SEMEN AND MILK

Although many viruses replicate in the skin, relatively few are spread from skin lesions. Exceptions are herpes simplex (labial transmission), varicella zoster (rarely, spread from zoster to cause chickenpox), papillomaviruses, molluscum contagiosum and Ebola, a filovirus that causes haemorrhagic fever (Peters 1996). Those viruses, such as herpes simplex type 2 and papillomaviruses, which cause sexually transmitted disease, are often shed from lesions of the genital mucous membranes. In addition, some viruses, such as rabies, mumps and Epstein–Barr viruses, replicate in the salivary glands and are discharged into the saliva to enter the oral cavity.

Several viruses are shed in the semen, including hepatitis B and human immunodeficiency virus (Alter, Purcell and Gerin 1977, Levy 1994). A number of viruses are excreted in colostrum and milk, including cytomegalovirus, mumps, rubella and ovine visna-maedi virus (de Boer and Houwers 1979).

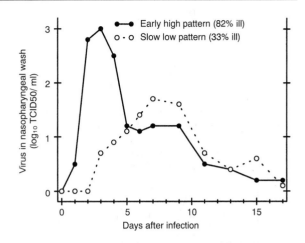

Fig. 9.8   The excretion of a typical respiratory virus, rhinovirus type 15, following inoculation of human volunteers by the transnasal route. The subjects had either an early-onset high-concentration pattern associated with a high frequency of respiratory symptoms or a late-onset low-concentration pattern associated with a low frequency of symptoms. (Data from Douglas et al. 1966.)

BLOOD AND URINE

Blood is also an important source of transmitted virus, particularly for those viruses that produce persistent plasma or cell-associated viraemias. Hepatitis B, C and D viruses, HIV, HTLV-I, HTLV-II and cytomegalovirus are among the important human pathogens 'shed' in this manner. Arboviruses usually cause short-term acute viraemias, and are transmissible only if an appropriate vector ingests a blood meal during this brief interval. In view of the limited amount of blood taken, the viraemia must reach considerable levels if it is to be transmitted.

A number of viruses have been isolated from the urine but viruria is probably not important for the transmission of most viruses. Special exceptions are certain zoonotic viruses, such as the arenaviruses and the hantaviruses, which cause lifelong virurias in their natural rodent hosts, leading to human infection through exposure to aerosolized dried urine (Gonzalez-Scarano and Nathanson 1990), and cytomegalovirus, which spreads readily among young children in environments contaminated by urine (e.g. crèches and play centres).

SURVIVAL IN THE ENVIRONMENT

The probability that a virus will be transmitted depends both on the intensity and duration of shedding and on its ability to survive in the environment. Viruses differ in their ability to survive in aerosols and, somewhat surprisingly, under conditions of low humidity, enveloped viruses seem to be better able to retain viability than are non-enveloped viruses (deJong and Winkler 1968). To be excreted in an infectious form, enteric viruses must survive the harsh environment of the lower gastrointestinal tract.

2.5   Transmission

Once shed, there are several means by which a virus is transmitted from host to host in a propagated chain of infection. Probably the most important mechanism is contamination of the hands of the infected transmitter from faeces, oral fluids or respiratory secretions expelled during coughing or sneezing. The virus is then passed by hand-to-hand contact, leading to oral, gastrointestinal or respiratory infection. A second common route is inhalation of aerosolized virus. A third significant mechanism involves direct person-to-person contact (oral–oral, genital–genital, oral–genital or skin–skin). Finally, indirect person-to-person transmission can occur via blood or contaminated needles. Common source transmissions are less frequent but can produce dramatic outbreaks, via contaminated water, food products or biologicals such as blood products and vaccines.

The success of a virus, as a life form, can be defined as its ability to be perpetuated over the millennia. In turn, perpetuation of a virus depends in part on its efficient transmission, particularly for viruses that cause only acute infections. The relative transmissibility of a virus in different populations is reflected in the age-specific profile of immune individuals, as illustrated in Fig. 9.9 for hepatitis A virus. For viruses that can persist in individual hosts, perpetuation is determined by transmission over the lifetime of the host and, in some instances, by the ability to be passed vertically to offspring of the host, either by transplacental or perinatal routes or as germline genes. If transmissibility is reduced sufficiently, a given virus will disappear from a defined population. This can happen in nature when a virus spreads so widely in a specific population that it eliminates most susceptibles and 'burns out'. Transmissibility can also be reduced by immunization which, under certain circumstances, can be used to eradicate a virus from its host population. Smallpox is the seminal example of planned eradication (Fenner et al. 1988), and the elimination of wild poliovirus from the western hemisphere is another important illustration.

3   VIRULENCE OF VIRUSES

Virulence refers to the ability of a virus to cause illness or death in an infected host, relative to other isolates or variants of the same agent. From the beginnings of experimental virology it has been recognized that different strains of a given virus may vary in their ability to cause disease. The study of virulence variants can provide important insights into pathogenesis, and variation in viral phenotype must be given consideration in design and interpretation of in vivo studies of the dissemination, localization and pathological consequences of viral infection. Study of virulence also has practical implications because it carries the potential for development of attenuated live virus variants that can be used as vaccines, a principle that was initially recognized by Jenner in 1798 when he intro-

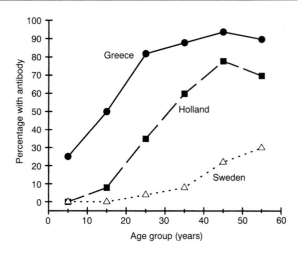

Fig. 9.9   Differences in transmissibility of hepatitis A virus in three European countries, as reflected in the different age-specific profiles of antibody prevalence. (Data from Frosner et al. 1979.)

duced vaccinia virus for the prevention of smallpox (Fenner et al. 1988).

There are 2 distinct approaches to the study of virulence. If virulence is regarded as a property of the virus, it is possible to map the genetic determinants that underlie the virulence phenotype. The other approach is through a study of pathogenesis, which describes the differences in infections with viral variants of different virulence. Pathogenic measures of virulence may be quantitative, involving the rate of viral replication or number of cells infected. Alternatively, differences in virulence may be qualitative, because variants of a single virus may differ markedly in their cellular tropism, their mode of dissemination in the infected host or the disease phenotype that they produce.

3.1   Measures of viral virulence

RELATIVE NATURE OF VIRAL VIRULENCE

Virulence is not an absolute property of a virus strain but depends on the dose of virus, the route of infection and the age, gender and genetic susceptibility of the host. Two viruses that differ in virulence in one experimental paradigm may have similar degrees of virulence in another paradigm. This point is illustrated in Table 9.4, which compares a virulent wild type clone with a laboratory-derived attenuated clone of California serogroup bunyaviruses. When the 2 viruses are injected intracerebrally in adult mice, the differences in their virulence are striking; one plaque forming unit (pfu) of the wild type virus initiates a fatal encephalitis whereas 10^6 pfu of attenuated clone B.5 fails to cause any illness. On the other hand, both viruses are highly virulent when injected intracerebrally in suckling mice (~1 pfu of either virus is lethal) and cannot be distinguished.

CLINICAL, PATHOLOGICAL AND FUNCTIONAL INDICATORS OF DISEASE

The conventional measure of viral virulence is the production of disease in the host, using as an endpoint either death or some specific constellation of signs and symptoms caused by the infection. This is illustrated in Table 9.6, which compares the paralysis rate following primary infection with wild type virus with the rate following oral poliovirus vaccine. An alternative measure of virulence is an assessment of virus-induced pathological lesions. Laboratory tests that reflect virus-induced pathophysiological changes can also be used as surrogate markers of virulence. For instance, the severity of hepatitis can be assessed by the serum titre of alanine aminotransferase that signals release of hepatocellular proteins, and the severity of HIV infection by the reduction in the blood concentration of CD4+ T lymphocytes.

For a precise estimate of virulence it is important to adjust for virus dose, which can conveniently be done by titrating different virus strains in a permissive cell culture system as well as in animals. The number of plaque-forming units per 50% lethal dose (pfu per LD50) can then be compared for different virus variants (Fig. 9.10).

3.2 Experimental manipulation of virulence

A prerequisite to the study of virulence is the availability of viral variants differing in their virulence phenotype. In some instances natural isolates may differ in virulence, for example serotype 1 and serotype 3 reoviruses, which vary remarkably in their biological properties even though reassortants between them are readily constructed. In many instances, laboratory manipulation must be used to obtain virulence variants.

PASSAGE IN ANIMAL HOSTS

In general, passage by a defined route in a particular species enhances the virulence of the virus when assessed under the conditions of passage, but often reduces the virulence in other animals or by other routes of infection. Human polioviruses have, on occasion, been adapted to mice; repeated mouse passage of monkey neurovirulent isolates produces variants that often have high intracerebral and intraspinal virulence for mice but may have relatively low intracerebral virulence for monkeys (Racaniello 1988).

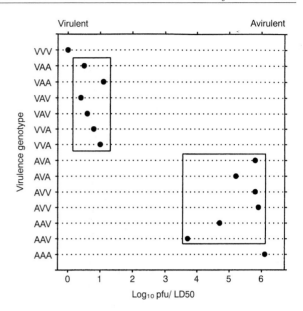

Fig. 9.10 Quantitative comparison of virulence using a panel of California serogroup viruses. Virulence is expressed as the number of plaque-forming units per 50% lethal dose (pfu per LD50) plotted on a log scale. Reassortants were made between a virulent (genotype VVV for the large, intermediate and small gene segments, respectively) and an avirulent clone (genotype AAA). Reassortants bearing a large gene segment derived from the virulent parent had a virulent phenotype and those bearing a large segment derived from the avirulent parent had an avirulent phenotype. (Data from Griot et al. 1994.)

PASSAGE IN CELL CULTURE

Passage in cell culture frequently leads to the selection of attenuated virus strains. A prominent example was Theiler's successful search for an attenuated variant of yellow fever virus, culminating in the selection of the 17D strain (Theiler and Smith 1937). Experience with cell passage has led to several common observations: (1) apparently identical passage protocols can yield stocks with different degrees of attenuation so that there is an element of unpredictability in this approach to attenuation; (2) viral stocks often represent a 'swarm' of genetically diverse variants that differ in their degree of attenuation (see Chapter 2, section 2.3, p. 15); and (3) attenuated variants may be temperature sensitive even when they were not selected for this phenotype.

Table 9.6 Virulence expressed as the comparative ability of different strains of a virus to produce clinical illness

Virus	Paralytic case rate per 1 000 000 primary infections (range)	Relative rates	Study period
Wild type (mainly type 1)	7000 (2000–20 000)	~10 000	1931–1954
OPV (mainly type 3)	0.62	1	1961–1978

The paralytic rate following infection with wild type polioviruses is compared with the rate following infection with attenuated oral polioviruses (OPV). (Data from Schonberger, McGown and Gregg 1976, Nathanson and Martin 1979, Nathanson 1984, Nkowane et al. 1987.)

Mutagenesis and temperature-sensitive mutants

A standard strategy for the production of attenuated variants is the treatment of a virus with a mutagen. One convenient way to select mutants is to look for viral variants that are temperature sensitive (*ts*), and that will replicate well at the permissive temperature of 33–37°C but not at an elevated non-permissive temperature, such as 40°C, when the non-mutagenized parent virus will still replicate well. Many *ts* mutants have reduced virulence in animals. Reduced virulence is not necessarily a direct consequence of temperature sensitivity, as the body temperature of the host is frequently within the range of permissive temperatures. It is more likely that such *ts* mutants are also host range restricted in certain cell types even at the permissive temperature, thus explaining their in vivo attenuation. Although random mutagenesis is a convenient way to produce attenuated viruses, it has the drawback that there may be mutations in several viral genes that are 'silent' in cell culture but influence behaviour in vivo, complicating conclusions about the mechanism of attenuation.

Many viruses can be 'cold adapted' by passage at a reduced temperature (traditionally 25°C) and such variants are often attenuated in animals (Maassab and DeBorde 1985). Cold-adapted variants of influenza virus replicate as well at 37°C and much better at 25°C than wild type virus, but are usually temperature sensitive at 40°C, and have markedly reduced pneumopathogenicity when tested intranasally in ferrets. Cold-adapted influenza viruses have mutations in many or all of their 8 gene segments but reassortant viruses bearing only a few segments from cold-adapted variants have the cold-adapted attenuated phenotype.

Designed mutations

With the development of methods for introducing mutations into DNA, it has become possible to design mutants of many DNA and RNA viruses. Several kinds of mutation can be introduced, including point mutations that result in substitution of a single or several individual amino acids, construction of genetic chimaeras between 2 viral variants by exchange of genetic sequences, or inactivation of an open reading frame by introduction of a stop codon, by insertion of a selectable marker cassette, or by deletion of part of the open reading frame. In some instances, non-coding domains of the viral genome carry major determinants of virulence, which can be mapped by similar methods (Almond 1991, Minor 1993, Racaniello, Ren and Bouchard 1993).

An example of the use of these methods is provided by human and simian immunodeficiency viruses (HIV and SIV), in which genetic modifications have been utilized to address various aspects of virulence (Levy 1994). For example, chimaeric viruses have been used to map macrophage tropism to the *env* gene and point mutations have been used to map tropism within the fine structure of the V3 loop of the surface (gp120) glycoprotein. Introduced stop codons and deletions have been used to explore the role of the *nef* gene of SIV, with the finding that *nef* deletions do not affect the ability of the virus to replicate in cell culture but markedly reduce the ability of a virulent clone, 239, to induce AIDS in rhesus monkeys.

Selection of attenuated variants

In selecting variants of reduced virulence, several points should be kept in mind. First, as noted above, most virus pools consist of a mixture of variants, which may differ markedly in their biological phenotype. Thus it is necessary to plaque-purify and characterize a number of stocks before selecting virus variants for study. Secondly, the mutations of greatest interest are those that specifically impair virulence in vivo without affecting the ability of a virus to replicate in a defined reference cell culture system. Such mutants can be considered to be 'host range' variants, in contrast to 'global' mutants with impaired replication in all cell hosts.

With the development of panels of monoclonal antibodies for most viruses, it has become possible to select variants that escape neutralization. Such variants often represent point mutations and occur naturally at a frequency of about 10^{-5} depending on the virus (Steinhauer and Holland 1987). When a panel of such monoclonal antibody-resistant (MAR) variants are tested in vivo it is often observed that a few of the escape mutants are attenuated. Variants selected in this manner generally have mutations in the viral attachment protein because this is the typical target of neutralizing monoclonal antibodies.

3.3 Pathogenic mechanisms of virulence

There are many steps in a viral infection, and a difference in the comparative replication of 2 virus variants at any one of these steps could explain their relative degrees of virulence. In practice, attenuated variants usually replicate or spread less briskly in one or several tissues associated with the pathogenic process. Also, variant viruses may differ qualitatively in their cell and tissue tropism or in their mode of dissemination.

Viraemia

A reduction in viraemia can be an important mechanism for the reduction in virulence. An example is shown in Fig. 9.7, which compares poliovirus strains of different virulence. The Mahoney strain of type 1 poliovirus caused a much higher viraemia and paralysis rate than did several other strains that were less viraemogenic.

Neural spread

Rabies viruses are obligatory neurotropes and disseminate only by neural spread. The attenuation of rabies virus has been investigated using MAR mutants. Some of the MAR variants in one epitope group were markedly attenuated, and one attenuating mutation was mapped to a single amino acid residue (at position 333) in the rabies glycoprotein (Tuffereau et al. 1989). After intramuscular injection, an attenuated mutant spread to the brain at a rate similar to virulent parent CVS virus, but within the central nervous system the attenuated clone spread to relatively few neurons whereas the virulent virus spread rapidly to many contiguous neurons (Jackson 1991). The difference between virulent and attenuated MAR viruses lay in their relative efficiency of entry into neuronal cells, probably associated with differences in the binding of their glycoproteins to cellular receptors (Dietzschold et al. 1983).

Tropism and host range

Different variants of a single virus can exhibit differences in their tropism for organs, tissues and cell types, which gives virulence a multidimensional character. Thus, a variant virus may be reduced in its ability to cause one type of pathology but enhanced in its ability to cause another. Human immunodeficiency virus (HIV) presents an example of tropism differences (Table 9.7). Most strains of HIV can be classified into 2 categories, according to their ability to replicate in T cell lines (T-tropic) or in primary macrophages (M-tropic). Tropism has been mapped to the envelope (gp120 or surface) protein, and studies of the initial steps in infection suggest a difference in the efficiency of virus entry (Levy 1994). The role of the 2 tropism biotypes of HIV in disease pathogenesis is only partly understood, but it is known that M-tropic strains dominate during the prolonged period of clinical latency, whereas the T-tropic strains are isolated more frequently from the blood of patients with clinical AIDS.

Virulence for target organs

Different variants of a specific virus may have different degrees of virulence for a key target organ. The 3 attenuated strains of poliovirus used in the oral poliovirus vaccine provide an example (Table 9.8). The type 3 strain has the greatest virulence because it causes more cases of paralytic poliomyelitis in vaccine recipients than does either the type 1 or the type 2 strain. The type 2 strain is clearly the most viraemogenic in children. However, after intracerebral injection of monkeys, the type 3 strain produces very severe spinal cord lesions at a higher frequency than do type 1 or type 2 strains. In this instance, virulence for the target organ (the spinal cord), rather than viraem-

ogenicity, seems to be the most important determinant of virulence after virus feeding.

Tumorigenesis

When applied to tumour viruses, virulence can be expressed in several different ways. The most common differences among the oncogenic viruses involve either the latent period from infection to development of a neoplasm or the cell type that is transformed. In general, the transforming retroviruses can be divided into 2 major classes, according to whether they cause tumours with a long latency or are acutely transforming. The long latency viruses are often replication-competent and do not carry a transduced oncogene. They act as insertional mutagens when their proviruses are integrated into the host DNA. On rare occasions, insertion occurs at a site where the promoter, enhancer or terminator sequences in the viral genome can influence the transcriptional rate of a proto-oncogene. Up-regulation of such a proto-oncogene then leads to transformation of the infected cell, which can result in neoplasia, usually after a long latency.

Murine leukaemia viruses (MuLVs) are replication-competent long-latency oncogenic retroviruses. Different MuLV isolates induce different kinds of neoplasms, involving T lymphocytes, B lymphocytes or erythroid or myeloid precursor cells. Genetic studies, including the production of viral chimaeras, have mapped the genetic determinants to the viral U3 region, a non-coding part of the viral genome that is just upstream from the transcriptional start site and has a domain that contains a number of transcriptional enhancer sites (Hopkins, Golemis and Speck 1989). Tropism is thought to correlate with relative ability to replicate in different potential target cells, and this has been borne out, at least in part, by studies in vivo of the relative replication rates of different MuLVs in different tissues (Evans and Morrey 1987).

3.4 Genetic determinants of virulence

Viral virulence is encoded in the viral genome and expressed through structural proteins, non-structural proteins or non-coding sequences. A large body of information about virus variants has established several important points.

Table 9.7 Isolates of a single virus may vary in their host range

Viral biotype	HIV-1 isolate	Growth in each cell type		
		Peripheral blood leucocytes	Monocyte-derived macrophages	T cell line Sup-T1
T tropic	IIIB	++++	+	++++
	DV	++++	++	++++
M-tropic	SF162	++++	+++	−
	89.6	++++	+++	−

HIV (human immunodeficiency virus) strains can be classified into two major biotypes: M-tropic (replicating in macrophages) and T-tropic (replicating in T lymphocytes), as shown for several different virus strains. (Data from Collman et al. 1989, Collman and Nathanson 1992.)

Table 9.8   Virulence for the target organ appears to be the major determinant of the relative virulence in vivo of the three oral poliovirus vaccine strains

	Type 1	Type 2	Type 3
Virulence in vivo (poliomyelitis in OPV recipients)	22	13	62
Viraemogenicity (frequency of viraemia)	0/16	17/19	0/16
Neurovirulence (percentage severe lesions)	0.05%	...	1.15%

Top line The type 3 vaccine strain causes paralytic poliomyelitis at a rate that is about 3-fold higher than the type 1 and 5-fold higher than the type 2 strain. Cases of paralytic poliomyelitis in recipients of oral poliovirus vaccine (OPV), USA, 1961–1984. (Data from Schonberger et al. 1976, Nkowane et al. 1987.)
Middle line The type 2 strain is much more viraemogenic than either of the other strains, indicating that it has a much higher potential for invading the spinal cord. Frequency of viraemia in infants fed oral poliovirus vaccine. (Data from Horstmann et al. 1964.)
Bottom line On direct intraspinal injection of monkeys, the type 3 strain causes severe spinal cord lesions at a rate that is much higher than the rate associated with type 1 strain. (Data from Nathanson and Horn 1992.)

1   The use of mutants has made it possible to identify the role of individual genes and proteins as determinants of the biological behaviour of many viral variants.

2   There is no 'master' gene or protein that determines virulence, and attenuation may be associated with changes in any of the structural or non-structural proteins, or in the non-coding regions of the genome.

3   The virulence phenotype can be altered by very small changes in the genome, if they occur at 'critical sites'. At such sites, a single point mutation leading to the substitution of a specific amino acid or base is often sufficient to alter virulence. For most viruses with small genomes (<20 kb) only a few discrete 'critical sites' have been discovered, usually fewer than 10 per genome.

4   It is possible to create variants with attenuating mutations at several critical sites and these may be more attenuated than single point mutants. Also, reversion to virulence is less frequent in variants with several discrete attenuating mutations.

5   Attenuating mutations are often host range mutations that affect replication in some cells but not in others. This is partly a reflection of the fact that most well characterized mutants have been deliberately selected because they replicate well in a standard cell culture system.

6   Although many attenuating mutations have been sequenced, relatively few have been characterized as to their mechanism of action at a biochemical or structural level. These generalizations may be illustrated with examples from a few selected virus groups.

POLIOVIRUSES

Polioviruses are single-stranded RNA viruses of positive polarity, with a genome that contains a relatively long 5' and a shorter 3' nontranslated region (NTR) flanking a single open reading frame of about 7 kb encoding a single polyprotein that is cleaved into 4 structural proteins (VP1–VP4) and several non-structural proteins.

Virulence studies have focused on the 3 attenuated strains of types 1, 2 and 3 poliovirus that constitute the OPV originally developed by Sabin (1985). The 3 vaccine strains are about 10 000-fold less virulent than wild type poliovirus (see Table 9.6), and they can be compared with the wild type viruses from which they were derived. However, the genomes of wild type parental viruses and their vaccine progeny differ at a considerable number of sites (reflecting their complex passage history) and many of these differences are not relevant to the attenuated phenotype. Virulent revertants of the vaccine strains occur on passage in humans or in cell culture, and are better suited to genetic analysis, because there are relatively few sequence differences between them and the vaccine strains. Using 'reverse genetics' (Racaniello and Baltimore 1981), infectious DNA clones of poliovirus genomes can be used to construct chimaeric viruses, and these clones can then be transfected into permissive cells to reconstitute mutated infectious virus.

The 5' non-translated region

The attenuation of the vaccine strains of poliovirus is due to critical sites, both in the 5' non-translated region (NTR) upstream from the long open reading frame and in selected structural and non-structural proteins (Racaniello 1988, Almond 1991, Minor 1992, 1993, Racaniello et al. 1993). Each of the 3 strains of OPV carry point mutations in the 5' NTR, at positions 480, 481 or 472, in types 1, 2 and 3, respectively. Attenuating mutations at these sites are associated with reduced neurovirulence in monkeys and reduced ability to replicate in the central nervous system of transgenic mice bearing the poliovirus receptor. Attenuated variants are temperature-sensitive host range mutants that replicate well in primate fibroblast cell lines such as HeLa cells, but have reduced ability to replicate in neuroblastoma cells (La Monica and Racaniello 1989). The bases at attenuating sites in the 5' NTR are thought to be involved in an RNA stem–loop based on computer models of their predicted secondary structure. It is believed that the stem structure at positions 470–540 is involved in the binding of ribosomal complexes at the initiation of translation. Presumably, initiation factors must differ, either quantitatively or qualitatively, in different cell types to explain the cellular host range restriction of the vaccine strains.

Structural or non-structural proteins

Each of the OPV strains carries at least one mutation that is associated with an alteration in a viral structural or non-structural protein and confers temperature sensitivity and reduced neurovirulence, and these mutations involve different proteins for the 3 OPV strains. For type 1 OPV, mutations associated with increased virulence are found in the virus capsid proteins, and in the non-structural 3D polymerase (Bouchard, Lam and Racaniello 1995, Georgescu et al. 1995). For type 2 OPV it seems that neurovirulence in the mouse is associated with virus capsid protein VP1 (Ren, Moss and Racaniello 1991, Macadam et al. 1993). For type 3 OPV, sites in virus capsid proteins VP3 and VP1 confer temperature sensitivity and neuroattenuation (Tatem et al. 1992). It is not clear how mutations in the structural proteins produce attenuation, but it has been suggested that these are involved in structural transitions that occur during either virion assembly or virion uncoating.

BUNYAVIRUSES

Bunyaviruses are negative-stranded (or ambisense) RNA viruses with a tri-segmented genome. The large (L) RNA segment encodes the viral polymerase; the middle (M) RNA segment encodes 2 glycoproteins (G1 and G2) and a non-structural protein, NS_m; the small (S) segment encodes the nucleoprotein (N) and a non-structural protein, NS_s. Most studies of virulence have used members of the California serogroup that will reassort readily with each other. Beginning with 2 parent viruses, panels of reassortants containing all possible combinations of gene segments can be constructed. In addition, MAR mutants have been used to identify variants in the major G1 glycoprotein that are associated with differences in virulence. Attenuation can involve either the ability of the virus to replicate in the central nervous system (neurovirulence) or its ability to cause viraemia and reach the central nervous system (neuroinvasiveness).

The middle RNA segment and glycoprotein G1

A detailed comparison has been made of 2 California serogroup viruses, wild type La Crosse virus and a laboratory passaged strain of Tahyna virus which had reduced neuroinvasiveness but high neurovirulence (Griot, Gonzalez-Scarano and Nathanson 1993). The reduction in neuroinvasiveness of the attenuated virus is associated with low viraemogenicity which, in turn, is associated with a reduced ability to replicate in striated muscle, the major extraneural site of replication of this group of viruses. Attenuation maps to the M RNA segment encoding the viral glycoproteins, indicating that there is an alteration in the entry phase of infection of myocytes (but not of neurons). These viruses formed plaques equally well on BHK-21 cells; however, on a murine myocyte cell line (C2C12), viral variants bearing the M RNA segment of the attenuated parent failed to produce plaques, whereas variants bearing the M RNA segment of the virulent parent did so readily (Griot et al. 1994).

MAR mutants of La Crosse virus are readily obtained, using antibodies directed against the major (G1) glycoprotein, and a mutant at one epitope site (but not at other sites) had reduced neuroinvasiveness with wild type neurovirulence (Gonzalez-Scarano et al. 1985). Furthermore, the attenuated clone had strikingly reduced fusion efficiency at acid pH compared with parental wild type La Crosse virus. These observations suggested that attenuation might be associated with an alteration in glycoprotein G1 that reduced efficiency in the infection of myocytes.

The large RNA segment and the viral polymerase

An attenuated California serogroup virus clone, B.5, obtained by passage in BHK-21 cells, showed a striking reduction in its ability to replicate in the central nervous system of adult mice. Using reassortant analysis (see Fig. 9.10) clone B.5 was shown to bear an attenuated L RNA segment (Endres et al. 1990). This clone is a temperature-sensitive host range mutant that replicates poorly in C1300 NA neuroblastoma and other murine cell lines, although it grows well in BHK-21 cells. Presumably, clone B.5 has a mutant polymerase that restricts viral replication in neurons and certain other cell types.

REOVIRUSES

Reoviruses are double-stranded 10-segmented RNA viruses. The gene segments and the proteins that they encode have been characterized in detail. The large number of segments has made reoviruses an attractive model system for study of the genetic determinants of viral phenotypes (Virgin, Tyler and Dermody 1996). These studies have been facilitated by major differences in the biological phenotypes of naturally occurring reovirus serotypes, particularly serotypes 1 and 3. Table 9.9 illustrates the use of reassortants to map virulence phenotypes to reovirus gene segments.

Biological functions have been ascribed to many of the reovirus genes and proteins. Most of the virulence determinants represent qualitative differences between type 1 Lang and type 3 Dearing (T1L and T3D) in tissue and organ tropism rather than quantitative differences in disease severity.

1   The S1 segment encodes the σ1 protein, which is the viral attachment protein that binds to receptors on permissive cells, and is a major target for neutralizing and haemagglutination-inhibiting (HI) antibodies. T1L and T3D viruses differ markedly in the disease that they cause in suckling mice. T1L disseminates through the blood and causes an ependymitis in the brain whereas T3D disseminates through the neural route and causes a neuronotropic encephalitis in the brain. The S1 segment is the major determinant of dissemination and brain cell tropism (Table 9.9). In addition, the S1 segment is a determinant of replication in cardiac myocytes and myocarditis, and of replication levels in the intestine.
2   The M1 segment encoding the μ2 protein influences replication in cardiac myocytes and myocarditis.
3   The M2 segment encoding the μ1 protein affects the protease sensitivity of the virion, and quantitative neurovirulence.
4   The L1 segment encoding the λ3 protein influences replication in cardiac myocytes and myocarditis.

Table 9.9 Mapping virulence to a specific viral gene segment

Pattern of spread	Outer capsid gene segments			Core gene segments					Non-structural gene segments		Clone
	M2	S1	S4	L2	L1	L3	M1	S2	M3	S3	
Viraemia	L	L	L	L	L	L	L	L	L	L	T1L
	D	L	L	L	L	L	L	L	D	D	R
	L	L	L	D	D	D	D	D	L	D	R
	L	L	D	L	L	L	L	L	L	L	R
	D	L	D	D	D	D	D	D	D	D	R
	D	L	L	D	D	D	L	D	D	D	R
	L	L	D	D	D	D	D	D	L	D	R
Neural	D	D	D	D	D	D	D	D	D	D	T3D
	D	D	D	D	D	D	D	D	D	L	R
	L	D	L	L	D	L	L	L	L	L	R
	L	D	L	L	L	L	L	L	L	L	R
	L	D	L	D	L	L	L	L	L	L	R

The S1 gene segment of reovirus determines whether the virus spreads by viraemia or by the neural route, because it was the only gene segment that co-segregated with the mode of spread. Two viruses, type 1 Lang (T1L) and type 3 Dearing (T3D), were used to derive reassortment clones (R) that were genotyped (L or D indicates the origin of each segment) and were tested for their mode of spread. (Adapted from Tyler, McPhee and Fields 1986.)

5 The L2 segment encoding the λ2 protein acts as a guanylyl transferase in cell culture and influences replication levels in the intestine, titres of shed virus, and horizontal transmission between mice.

3.5 Viral virulence genes of cellular origin

Since 1985 a new class of virus-encoded proteins has been recognized that contributes to the virulence of viruses by mimicking normal cellular proteins (McFadden 1995). This group of 'cell-derived' genes has been identified primarily within the genomes of large DNA viruses, which probably have a greater capacity to maintain accessory genes than do viruses with small genomes. Because these genes are homologues of cellular genes, it is hypothesized that they were acquired by recombination and modification. Thus, from an evolutionary viewpoint, they resemble viral oncogenes.

Cell-derived viral genes encode proteins that enhance virulence by many different mechanisms. 'Virokines' are secreted from virus-infected cells and mimic cytokines, thereby perturbing normal host responses. 'Viroceptors' resemble cellular receptors for cytokines (including antibodies or complement components) that are thereby diverted from their normal cellular targets. Some virus-encoded proteins interfere with antigen presentation and immune induction, whereas others prevent apoptosis or interrupt intracellular signalling initiated by cytokines or interferons. A brief review of selected cell-derived genes that have been described for pox- and herpesviruses will serve as examples of this group of viral genes and illustrate how they contribute to viral virulence.

Poxviruses

Tumour induction

Several poxviruses cause either benign or malignant tumours. However, it seems that the mechanism of oncogenesis is different from that associated with classic DNA or RNA tumour viruses, because there is no evidence that viral sequences are incorporated into the genome of transformed cells. Virus strains may gain or lose tumorigenicity quite independent of their ability to replicate, and continued productive replication of the virus seems to be required for tumour growth. It was postulated in the 1960s that these viruses might produce a growth factor that accounted for their induction of tumours (Kato, Miyamoto and Takahashi 1963). A large body of research has now shown that several poxviruses encode a protein that can be classified as a member of the EGF-like (epidermal growth factor) family of growth factors (McFadden, Graham and Opgenorth 1995). Both Shope fibroma virus and malignant rabbit fibroma virus encode a very similar protein (Shope fibroma growth factor, SFGF) and myxoma virus encodes a related myxoma growth factor (MGF). These proteins contain the functional domains (6 characteristically spaced cysteines) shared by members of the EGF family. Furthermore, when these genes are deleted from the virus genomes, the MGF– or SFGF– viruses replicate normally in cell culture but have a much reduced ability to induce tumours in rabbits (Opgenorth, Strayer and Upton 1992).

Receptors for tumour necrosis factor

Tumour necrosis factor (TNF) is a potent proinflammatory cytokine that is produced by activated macrophages and T cells. TNF acts by binding to a class of cellular receptors that are type 1 integral membrane proteins characterized by multiple cysteine-rich exodomains. Through their receptors on myeloid and lymphoid cells, the TNFs exert complex pleiotropic effects on immune networks and host responses to infection. A number of poxviruses encode a protein, designated T2, that is a soluble form of the cellular p75 TNF receptor (Smith and Goodwin 1995). It is presumed that this protein binds free TNF, thereby modulating TNF-mediated cellular responses to infection. It is postulated that T2 could enhance replication of poxviruses in vivo by down-modulating the antiviral defences of the infected host, although T2 might simultaneously favour the host by reducing the severity of virus-induced inflammatory lesions.

Vaccinia virus complement control protein

The complement system is a complex group of proteins that act in a cascade that forms one of the initial host defences against microbial pathogens. The system is a potent one that, uncontrolled, has the potential to cause severe damage, and is therefore tightly regulated by several different mechanisms, including C4-BP, a plasma protein that binds C4b2a, one of the complexes formed in the course of complement activation. Vaccinia virus encodes a protein, vaccinia virus complement control protein, or VCP, that is homologous to C4-BP (Isaacs and Moss 1995). VCP binds human C4b, and a VCP– mutant of vaccinia virus fails to inhibit complement-mediated lysis of sensitized sheep erythrocytes whereas wild type vaccinia virus has an inhibitory effect (Kotwal et al. 1990). When wild type and VCP– vaccinia viruses were compared in vivo, the VCP– mutant was less virulent when injected intracerebrally into mice and, as shown in Fig. 9.11, produced smaller skin lesions after intradermal inoculation in rabbits (Isaacs, Kotval and Moss 1992).

HERPES SIMPLEX VIRUSES

Herpes simplex virus complement receptors

The importance of the complement cascade and its regulation have already been mentioned. C3b, one of the intermediates in the cascade, plays a key role in initiating the formation of the membrane attack complex (the last part of the complement cascade), so its regulation is important. A number of cell types,

including monocytes/macrophages, neutrophils and some T cells, express receptors for C3b, that down-modulate the complement cascade by reducing the levels of C3b and enhancing its inactivation by cleavage to iC3b. Glycoprotein C (gC) of HSV-1 binds C3b and iC3b, thereby providing protection against complement-mediated neutralization of HSV, and against complement-mediated lysis of HSV-infected cells (Harris, Frank and Lee 1990, York and Johnson 1995). Although it has not yet been demonstrated that gC– mutants are less virulent in vivo, the conservation of gC in natural isolates of HSV suggests that this protein (and its complement-binding activity) plays a role in HSV survival in nature.

HSV Fc receptors

HSV-infected cells express receptors (FcR) for the Fc domain of the immunoglobulin (IgG) molecule (Baucke and Spear 1979). A considerable body of work (York and Johnson 1995) has identified glycoproteins gE and gI of HSV as the molecules that bind IgG. It has been suggested that the presence of Fc receptors on the HS virion or on the surface of virus-infected cells would lead to bipolar bridging of the IgG molecule that might reduce secondary effects of antibody binding, such as the ability to initiate the complement cascade. Comparison of an FcR-deficient mutant, expressing an altered gE protein, with wild type HSV, has shown that FcR-deficient virus is more susceptible to complement-mediated neutralization and lysis of virus-infected cells, as shown in Fig. 9.12 (Frank and Friedman 1989, Dubin, Socolof and Frank 1991). Furthermore, gE– HSV has reduced virulence in mice (Rajcani, Herget and Kaerner 1990).

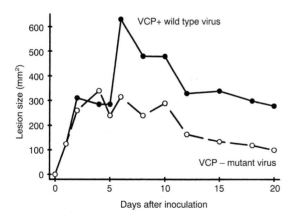

Fig. 9.11 Cell-derived viral genes can act as virulence factors. The skin lesions produced by a wild type vaccinia virus expressing the vaccinia complement control gene (VCP+) are more extensive than the lesions caused by the same virus from which the gene had been deleted (VCP–). (Data [median of three rabbits] from Isaacs, Kotwal and Moss 1992.)

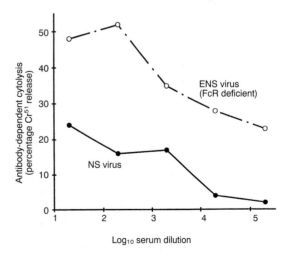

Fig. 9.12 Cell-derived viral genes can act as virulence factors. Glycoprotein gE of herpes simplex virus, which functions as an Fc receptor (FcR), influences the susceptibility of HSV-infected cells to antibody-dependent cell-mediated cytotoxity (ADCC). Target cells infected with the NS (FcR+) strain of HSV show lower percentage lysis than cells infected with an FcR-deficient mutant of NS virus (strain ENS), indicating that the viral-encoded FcR can reduce the susceptibility of HSV-infected cells to ADCC. (Data from Dubin et al. 1991.)

4 HOST DETERMINANTS OF SUSCEPTIBILITY AND RESISTANCE

The outcome of the virus–host interaction is determined in part by host variables that can be conveniently considered under 2 categories: physiological factors and genetic determinants.

4.1 Physiological factors

The host response to a viral infection may be influenced by a variety of physiological variables such as age, sex, stress and pregnancy, all of which have been shown to affect the outcome of infection with some viruses (Brinton 1996). Age is perhaps the most consistently important variable in this category.

In general, very young animals are more susceptible than adult hosts to acute viral infections and are more likely to undergo severe or fatal illness. However, it is important to recognize that, in most mammalian species, young animals born of immune mothers receive maternal antibody either in utero by the transplacental route or postnatally in colostrum and milk, or both. Furthermore, newborns have a special transport system that permits them to absorb intact immunoglobulin from the gut lumen into the circulation. The innate high susceptibility of infants born of non-immune mothers is revealed only in those rare instances when a virus has disappeared from an isolated community, so all age groups lack immune protection. A classic example is measles, which can be a devastating disease with a mortality of up to 25% in non-immune infants (Panum 1940) but which is relatively benign in most societies where almost all women of childbearing age have acquired active immunity from natural infection or from measles vaccine. The mechanisms of enhanced susceptibility of newborn animals have been obscure, but recently it has been shown that an alphavirus induces apoptosis in neurons of newborn mice but does not kill neurons from older mice in which enhanced expression of the cellular oncogene, *bcl 2*, blocks apoptosis (Levine et al. 1993).

Less commonly, advanced age can also be associated with increased susceptibility to viral infection. St Louis encephalitis is an example of this phenomenon (Table 9.10); in one epidemic the ratio of encephalitis cases to infections was about 0.2 per 1000 for children aged 0–9 years and about 3.0 per 1000 for adults aged 60 or over. Another example is varicella-zoster virus, which usually produces primary infections in childhood, followed by latent infections of the spinal ganglia. Reactivations of latent infections, in the form of herpes zoster, rarely occur before the age of 50 (except in individuals with other debilitating illnesses) but are much more common over 60 years of age.

Table 9.10 Age is one of the physiological variables that can determine host susceptibility

Age group	Encephalitis per 100 000	Case-fatality rate per 100	Percentage with SLE antibody
0–9	8	0	41
10–19	13	0	29
20–29	15	0	38
30–39	14	0	36
40–49	17	0	26
50–59	28	13	38
60+	78	27	25

The age distribution of St Louis encephalitis shows that attack rates increased strikingly in the older age groups although the frequency of infection was similar for all ages. (Data from Luby et al. 1967, Henderson et al. 1970.)

Table 9.11 Genetic determinants of host susceptibility can be delineated in inbred strains of mice

Mouse strain	Genotype (R: resistant; r: susceptible)	Mortality: dead/total	Log$_{10}$ virus titre in blood
Not treated			
A/J	r/r	4/4	6.0
A2G	R/R	0/4	3.7
F1 (A/J × A2G)	R/r	0/4	3.5
Treated with anti-interferon antiserum			
A/J	r/r	4/4	6.0
A2G	R/R	4/4	6.3
F1 (A/J × A2G)	R/r	4/4	6.5

A/J mice are susceptible and A2G mice are resistant to a hepatotropic strain of influenza virus and the F1 hybrid is also resistant, indicating that a single dominant autosomal gene determines resistance. In addition, treatment with anti-interferon antiserum abrogates resistance, suggesting that the effect is mediated through the action of interferon. (Data from Haller et al. 1980.)

4.2 Host genes

Studies with inbred animals have shown that the outcome of infections often varies in different strains of mice (Brinton 1996), and genetic analyses have been conducted to determine the form of inheritance of susceptibility and to map the chromosomal location of the responsible genetic loci. Several generalizations may be made, based on numerous studies of a wide variety of viruses.

1   Most genetic loci control susceptibility to a specific family of viruses and not to all viruses.
2   Susceptibility can often be mapped to a single autosomal locus, but multiple loci have been identified in some instances.
3   When a single genetic locus has been identified, susceptibility may be either dominant or recessive.
4   Where loci have been mapped, they are usually distant from the major histocompatibility locus and in most instances the mechanism of susceptibility is not immunological.
5   The exact mechanism of susceptibility has not been well defined in most instances.

An example of genetically determined host suscepti-bility is shown in Table 9.11, in which there is a single autosomal genetic locus and resistance is dominant (Haller et al. 1980). In this instance, the genetic determinant, called the *Mx* locus, has been shown to influence the response to influenza viruses and is related to differential ability to mount an interferon response (Pavlovic, Haller and Staeheli 1992, Staeheli, Pitossi and Pavlovic 1993). Thus, treatment with anti-interferon antibody abolishes resistance and renders all strains of mice equally susceptible.

It is difficult to investigate whether genetic determinants of host susceptibility occur in outbred populations. Classic studies of myxoma virus in outbred rabbit populations (Fenner 1983) have clearly demonstrated that there are genetic determinants of host susceptibility that can become manifest under the selective pressure of a virulent virus. If it is assumed that there are human homologues for most mouse genes, then it may be inferred that the outcome of viral infections in humans is also influenced by genetic determinants. Consistent with this presumption are observations that human responses to standardized virus inocula may be somewhat variable (see Table 9.6 and Fig. 9.8).

REFERENCES

Almond JW, 1991, Poliovirus neurovirulence, *Semin Neurosci*, **3**: 101–8.

Alter HJ, Purcell RH, Gerin JL, 1977, Transmission of hepatitis B surface antigen positive saliva and semen, *Infect Immun*, **16**: 928–33.

Baer GM, ed, 1991, *The Natural History of Rabies*, CRC Press, Boca Raton FL.

Bagasra O, Seshamma T et al., 1993, High percentages of CD4-positive lymphocytes harbor the HIV-1 provirus in the blood of certain infected individuals, *AIDS*, **7**: 1419–25.

Baringer JR, Nathanson N, 1972, Parvovirus hemorrhagic encephalopathy of rats: electron microscopic observations of the vascular lesions, *Lab Invest*, **27**: 514–22.

Barnett EM, Perlman S, 1993, The olfactory nerve and not the trigeminal nerve is the major site of CNS entry for mouse hepatitis virus, strain JHM, *Virology*, **194**: 185–91.

Bates P, Young JA, Varmus HE, 1993, A receptor for subgroup A Rous sarcoma virus is related to the low density lipoprotein receptor, *Cell*, **74**: 1043–52.

Baucke RB, Spear PG, 1979, Membrane proteins specified by herpes simplex virus. V. Identification of an Fc-binding glycoprotein, *J Virol*, **32**: 779–89.

Bergelson JM, St John N et al., 1993, Infection by echoviruses 1 and 8 depends on the alpha2 subunit of human VLA-2, *J Virol*, **67**: 6847–54.

Blank H, Burgoon CF et al., 1951, Cytologic smears in diagnosis of herpes simplex, herpes zoster, and varicella, *JAMA*, **146**: 1410–12.

Bodian D, 1954, Viremia in experimental poliomyelitis. I. General aspects of infection after intravascular inoculation with strains of high and low invasiveness, *Am J Hyg*, **60**: 339–57.

Bodian D, 1955, Emerging concepts of poliomyelitis infection, *Science*, **122**: 105–8.

de Boer GF, Houwers DJ, 1979, Aspects of slow and persistent virus infections, *Epizootology of Maedi/Visna in Sheep*, ed Tyrrell DAJ, Martinus Nijhoff, The Hague, 198–220.

Bouchard MJ, Lam D-H, Racaniello VR, 1995, Determinants of attenuation and temperature sensitivity in the type 1 poliovirus Sabin vaccine, *J Virol*, **69**: 4972–8.

Brinton MA, 1996, Host factors controlling susceptibility to viral diseases, *Viral Pathogenesis*, ed Nathanson N, Lippincott–Raven, Philadelphia, 303–328.

Card JP, Enquist LW, 1994, Use of pseudorabies virus for definition of synaptically linked populations of neurons, *Methods Mol Genet*, **4**: 363–82.

Chantler JK, Tingle AJ, 1982, Isolation of rubella virus from human lymphocytes after acute natural infection, *J Infect Dis*, **145**: 673–7.

Charles PC, Walters E et al., 1995, Mechanism of neuroinvasion of Venezuelan equine encephalitis virus in the mouse, *Virology*, **208**: 662–71.

Clark SM, Roth JR, Clark ML, 1981, Tryptic enhancement of rotavirus infectivity: mechanism of enhancement, *J Virol*, **39**: 816–22.

Collman R, Nathanson N, 1992, Human immunodeficiency virus type-1 infection of macrophages, *Semin Virol*, **3**: 185–202.

Collman R, Hassan NF et al., 1989, Infection of monocyte-derived macrophages with human immunodeficiency virus type 1 (HIV-1). Monocyte- and lymphocyte-tropic strains of HIV-1 show distinctive patterns of replication in a panel of cell types, *J Exp Med*, **170**: 1149–63.

Cook ML, Stevens JG, 1973, Pathogenesis of herpetic neuritis and ganglionitis in mice: evidence of intra-axonal transport of infection, *Infect Immun*, **7**: 272–88.

Dalmat H, 1958, Arthropod transmission of rabbit papillomatosis, *J Exp Med*, **108**: 9–20.

DeJong JG, Winkler KC, 1968, The inactivation of poliovirus in aerosols, *J Hyg*, **66**: 557–65.

Depper JM, Leonard WJ et al., 1984, Augmented T cell growth factor receptor expression in HTLV-1-infected human leukemic T cells, *J Immunol*, **133**: 1691–5.

Dietzschold B, Wunner WH et al., 1983, Characterization of an antigenic determinant of the glycoprotein that correlates with pathogenicity of rabies virus, *Proc Natl Acad Sci USA*, **80**: 70–4.

Dorig RE, Marcil A et al., 1993, The human CD46 molecule is a receptor for measles virus (Edmonton strain), *Cell*, **75**: 295–304.

Douglas RG Jr., Cate TR et al., 1966, Quantitative rhinovirus shedding patterns in volunteers, *Am Rev Respir Dis*, **94**: 159–67.

Dubin G, Socolof E, Frank I, 1991, Herpes simplex virus type 1 Fc receptor protects infected cells from antibody-dependent cellular cytotoxicity, *J Virol*, **65**: 7046–50.

Endres MJ, Valsamakis A et al., 1990, Neuroattenuated bunyavirus variant: derivation, characterization, and revertant clones, *J Virol*, **64**: 1927–33.

Enquist LW, 1994, Infection of the mammalian nervous system by pseudorabies virus (PRV), *Semin Virol*, **5**: 221–31.

Esolen LM, Ward BJ et al., 1993, Infection of monocytes during measles, *J Infect Dis*, **168**: 47–52.

Estes MK, Graham DY, Mason BB, 1981, Proteolytic enhancement of rotavirus infectivity: molecular mechanisms, *J Virol*, **39**: 879–88.

Evans L, Morrey J, 1987, Tissue-specific replication of Friend and Moloney mouse leukemia viruses in infected mice, *J Virol*, **61**: 1350–7.

Fenner F, 1949, Mousepox (infectious ectromelia of mice): a review, *J Immunol*, **63**: 341–73.

Fenner F, 1983, Biological control as exemplified by smallpox eradication and myxomatosis, *Proc Roy Soc London, B*, **218**: 259–85.

Fenner F, Henderson DA et al., 1988, *Smallpox and its Eradication*, World Health Organization, Geneva.

Frank I, Friedman H, 1989, A novel function of the herpes simplex virus type 1 Fc receptor: participation of bipolar bridging of antiviral immunoglobulin, *J Virol*, **63**: 4479–88.

Freistadt M, 1994, Distribution of the poliovirus receptor in human tissue, *Cellular Receptors for Animal Viruses*, ed Wimmer E, Cold Spring Harbor Laboratory Press, Cold Spring Harbor NY, 445–62.

Friedman H, Macarek E, MacGregor RA, 1981, Virus infection of endothelial cells, *J Infect Dis*, **143**: 266–73.

Frosner GG, Papaevangelou G et al., 1979, Antibody against hepatitis A in seven European countries. I. Comparison of prevalence data in different age groups, *Am J Epidemiol*, **110**: 63–9.

Gendelman HE, Narayan O et al., 1985, Slow, persistent replication of lentiviruses: role of tissue macrophages and macrophage precursors in bone marrow, *Proc Natl Acad Sci USA*, **82**: 7082–90.

Georgescu M-M, Tardy-Panit M et al., 1995, Mapping of mutations contributing to the temperature sensitivity of the Sabin 1 vaccine strain of poliovirus, *J Virol*, **69**: 5278–86.

Gollins SW, Porterfield JS, 1984, Flavivirus infection enhancement in macrophages: radioactive and biological studies on the effect of antibody on viral fate, *J Gen Virol*, **65**: 1261–72.

Gonzalez-Scarano F, Nathanson N, 1990, Bunyaviruses, *Fields' Virology*, 2nd edn, eds Fields BN, Knipe DM, Raven Press, New York, 1195–228.

Gonzalez-Scarano F, Janssen R et al., 1985, An avirulent G1 glycoprotein variant of La Crosse bunyavirus with defective fusion function, *J Virol*, **54**: 757–63.

Griffin DE, Levine B et al., 1994, Age-dependent fatal encephalitis: alphavirus infection of neurons, *Arch Virol*, **9S**: 31–9.

Griot C, Gonzalez-Scarano F, Nathanson N, 1993, Molecular determinants of the virulence and infectivity of California serogroup bunyaviruses, *Annu Rev Microbiol*, **47**: 117–38.

Griot C, Pekosz A et al., 1993, Polygenic control of neuroinvasiveness in California serogroup viruses, *J Virol*, **67**: 3861–7.

Griot C, Pekosz A et al., 1994, Replication in cultured C2C12 muscle cells correlates with the neuroinvasiveness of California serogroup bunyaviruses, *Virology*, **201**: 399–403.

Haase AT, 1986, Pathogenesis of lentivirus infections, *Nature (London)*, **322**: 130–6.

Haller O, Arnheiter H et al., 1980, Host gene influences sensitivity to interferon action selectively for influenza virus, *Nature (London)*, **283**: 660–2.

Halstead SB, O'Rourke EJ, 1977, Dengue viruses and mono-nuclear phagocytes. I. Infection enhancement by non-neutralizing antibody, *J Exp Med*, **146**: 201–17.

Harouse JM, Bhat S et al., 1991, Inhibition of entry of HIV-1 in neural cell lines by antibodies against galactosyl ceramide, *Science*, **253**: 320–3.

Harris SL, Frank I, Yee A, 1990, Glycoprotein C of herpes simplex virus type 1 prevents complement-mediated cell lysis and virus neutralization, *J Infect Dis*, **162**: 331–7.

Haywood AM, 1994, Virus receptors: binding, adhesion strengthening, and changes in viral structure, *J Virol*, **68**: 1–5.

Henderson BE, Pigford CA et al., 1970, Serologic survey for St Louis encephalitis and other group B arbovirus antibodies in residents of Houston, Texas, *Am J Epidemiol*, **91**: 87–98.

Herndon RM, Johnson RT, Davis LE, 1974, Ependymitis in mumps virus meningitis: electron microscopic studies of the cerebrospinal fluid, *Arch Neurol*, **30**: 475–9.

Ho M, 1981, The lymphocyte in infections with Epstein–Barr virus and cytomegalovirus, *J Infect Dis*, **143**: 857–62.

Hofer F, Grunberger M et al., 1994, Members of the low density lipoprotein receptor family mediate cell entry of a minor group common cold virus, *Proc Natl Acad Sci USA*, **91**: 1839–45.

Hopkins N, Golemis E, Speck N, 1989, Role of enhancer regions in leukemia induction by nondefective murine C type retroviruses, *Concepts in Viral Pathogenesis*, eds Notkins AL, Oldstone MBA, Springer-Verlag, New York, 41–9.

Horstmann DM, Opton EM et al., 1964, Viremia in infants vaccinated with oral poliovirus vaccine (Sabin), *Am J Hyg*, **79**: 47–63.

Hotchin J, 1962, The biology of lymphocytic choriomeningitis infection: virus-induced immune disease, *Cold Spring Harbor Symp Quant Biol*, **27**: 479–500.

Hsia K, Spector SA, 1991, Human immunodeficiency virus DNA is present in a high percentage of CD4+ lymphocytes of seropositive individuals, *J Infect Dis*, **164**: 470–5.

Huber SA, 1994, VCAM-1 is a receptor for encephalomyocarditis virus on murine endothelial cells, *J Virol*, **68**: 3453–9.

Isaacs SN, Moss B, 1995, Inhibition of complement activation by vaccinia virus, *Viroceptors, Virokines, and Related Immune Modulators Encoded by DNA Viruses*, ed McFadden G, RG Landes, Austin TX, 55–66.

Isaacs SN, Kotwal GJ, Moss B, 1992, Vaccinia virus complement-control protein prevents antibody-dependent complement-enhanced neutralization of infectivity and contributes to virulence, *Proc Natl Acad Sci USA*, **89**: 628–32.

Jackson A, 1991, Biological basis of rabies virus neurovirulence in mice: comparative pathogenesis study using the immunoperoxidase technique, *J Virol*, **65**: 537–40.

Johnson RT, 1965, Virus invasion of the central nervous system. A study of Sindbis virus infection in the mouse using fluorescent antibody, *Am J Pathol*, **46**: 929–43.

Johnson RT, Mims CA, 1968, Pathogenesis of virus infections of the nervous system, *N Engl J Med*, **278**: 23–92.

Kato S, Miyamoto H, Takahashi M, 1963, Shope fibroma and rabbit myxoma viruses. II. Pathogenesis of fibromas in domestic rabbits, *Biken J*, **6**: 135–43.

Kotwal GJ, Isaacs SN et al., 1990, Inhibition of the complement cascade by the major secretory protein of vaccinia virus, *Science*, **250**: 827–30.

Kozak CA, Ruscetti S, 1992, Retroviruses in rodents, *The Retroviridae*, ed Levy JA, Plenum Press, New York, 405–81.

Kristensson K, Lycke E, Sjostrand J, 1971, Spread of herpes simplex virus in peripheral nerves, *Acta Neuropathol*, **17**: 44–53.

La Monica N, Racaniello VR, 1989, Differences in replication of attenuated and neurovirulent polioviruses in human neuroblastoma cell line SH-SY5Y, *J Virol*, **63**: 2357–60.

Langhoff E, Terwilliger EF, Bos J et al., 1991, Replication of human immunodeficiency virus type 1 in primary dendritic cell cultures, *Proc Natl Acad Sci USA*, **88**: 7998–8002.

Levine B, Huang Q et al., 1993, Conversion of lytic to persistent alphavirus infection by the *bcl 2* cellular oncogene, *Nature (London)*, **361:** 739–42.

Levy JA, 1994, *HIV and the Pathogenesis of AIDS*, ASM Press, Washington.

Lippmann M, Yeates DB, Albert RE, 1980, Deposition, retention, and clearance of inhaled particles, *Br J Indust Med*, **37:** 337–62.

Little LM, Shadduck JA, 1982, Pathogenesis of rotavirus infection in mice, *Infect Immun*, **38:** 755–63.

Luby JP, Miller G et al., 1967, The epidemiology of St. Louis encephalitis in Houston, Texas, *Am J Epidemiol*, **86:** 584–97.

McClure JE, 1992, Cellular receptor for Epstein–Barr virus, *Prog Med Virol*, **39:** 116–38.

McFadden G, ed, 1995, *Viroceptors, Virokines, and Related Immune Modulators Encoded by DNA Viruses*, RG Landes, Austin TX.

McFadden G, Graham K, Opgenorth A, 1995, Poxvirus growth factors, *Viroceptors, Virokines, and Related Immune Modulators Encoded by DNA Viruses*, ed McFadden G, RG Landes, Austin TX, 1–16.

Macadam AJ, Pollard SR et al., 1993, Genetic basis of the attenuation of the Sabin type 2 vaccine strain of poliovirus in primates, *Virology*, **192:** 18–26.

Maddon PJ, Dalgleish AG et al., 1986, The T4 gene encodes the AIDS virus receptor and is expressed in the immune system and brain, *Cell*, **47:** 333–48.

Matloubian N, Kolhekar SR et al., 1993, Molecular determinants of macrophage-tropism and viral persistence: importance of single amino acid changes in the polymerase and glycoprotein of lymphocytic choriomeningitis virus, *J Virol*, **67:** 7340–9.

Mendelsohn CL, Wimmer E, Racaniello VR, 1989, Cellular receptor for poliovirus: molecular cloning, nucleotide sequence, and expression of a new member of the immunoglobulin superfamily, *Cell*, **56:** 855–69.

Mims CA, 1964, Aspects of the pathogenesis of virus diseases, *Bacteriol Rev*, **28:** 30–71.

Mims CA, 1987, *The Pathogenesis of Infectious Disease*, Academic Press, London.

Minor PD, 1992, The molecular biology of poliovaccines, *J Gen Virol*, **73:** 3065–77.

Minor PD, 1993, Attenuation and reversion of the Sabin strains of poliovirus, *Dev Biol Stand*, **78:** 17–26.

Monath TR, ed, 1988, *The Arboviruses: epidemiology and ecology*, CRC Press, Boca Raton FL.

Morrison LA, Sidman RL, Fields BN, 1991, Direct spread of reovirus from intestinal lumen to the central nervous system through the autonomic vagal nerve fibers, *Proc Natl Acad Sci USA*, **88:** 2852–6.

Nathanson N, 1984, Eradication of poliomyelitis in the United States, *Rev Infect Dis*, **4:** 940–5.

Nathanson N, ed, 1996, *Viral pathogenesis*, Lippincott–Raven, Philadelphia.

Nathanson N, Bodian D, 1961, Experimental poliomyelitis following intramuscular virus injection. I. The effect of neural block on a neurotropic and a pantropic strain, *Bull Johns Hopkins Hosp*, **108:** 308–19.

Nathanson N, Cole GA, 1971, Immunosuppression: a means to assess the role of the immune response in acute virus infection, *Fed Proc*, **30:** 1822–30.

Nathanson N, Horn SD, 1992, Neurovirulence tests of type 3 oral poliovirus vaccine manufactured by Lederle Laboratories 1964–1988, *Vaccine*, **10:** 469–75.

Nathanson N, Martin JR, 1979, The epidemiology of poliomyelitis: enigmas surrounding its appearance, epidemicity, and disappearance, *Am J Epidemiol*, **110:** 672–92.

Nathanson N, Cook DG et al., 1994, Pathogenesis of HIV encephalopathy, *Ann N Y Acad Sci*, **724:** 87–106.

Nkowane BM, Wassilak SGF et al., 1987, Vaccine-associated paralytic poliomyelitis, United States: 1973 through 1984, *JAMA*, **257:** 1335–40.

Notkins AL, Mahar S et al., 1966, Infectious virus–antibody complexes in the blood of chronically infected mice, *J Exp Med*, **124:** 81–97.

Oldstone MBA, 1975, Virus neutralization and virus-induced immune complex disease, *Prog Med Virol*, **19:** 84–119.

Opgenorth A, Strayer D, Upton C, 1992, Deletion of the growth factor gene related to EGF and TGFa reduces virulence of malignant rabbit fibroma virus, *Virology*, **186:** 175–91.

Oshiro LS, Dondero DV et al., 1978, The development of Colorado tick fever virus within cells of the haemopoietic system, *J Gen Virol*, **39:** 73–9.

Panum PL, 1940, *Observations made during the Epidemic of Measles on the Faroe Islands in the Year 1846*, American Public Health Association, New York.

Pathak S, Webb HE, 1974, Possible mechanisms for the transport of Semliki Forest virus into and within mouse brain: an electron microscopic study, *J Neurol Sci*, **23:** 175–84.

Pavlovic J, Haller O, Staeheli P, 1992, Human and mouse Mx proteins inhibit different steps of the influenza virus multiplication cycle, *J Virol*, **66:** 2564–9.

Pekosz A, Griot C et al., 1995, Protection from La Crosse virus encephalitis with recombinant glycoproteins: role of neutralizing anti-G1 antibodies, *J Virol*, **69:** 3475–81.

Perlman S, Jacobsen G, Afifi A, 1989, Spread of a neurotropic murine coronavirus into the CNS via the trigeminal and olfactory nerves, *Virology*, **170:** 556–60.

Peters CJ, 1996, Viral hemorrhagic fevers, *Viral Pathogenesis*, ed Nathanson N, Lippincott–Raven, Philadelphia, 779–800.

Petursson G, Nathanson N et al., 1976, Pathogenesis of visna. I. Sequential virologic, serologic, and pathologic studies, *Lab Invest*, **35:** 402–12.

Pitts O, Powers M, Billelo J, 1987, Ultrastructural changes associated with retroviral replication in central nervous system capillary endothelial cells, *Lab Invest*, **56:** 401–9.

Pomerantz RJ, de la Monte SM, et al., 1988, Human immunodeficiency virus (HIV) infection of the uterine cervix, *Ann Intern Med*, **108:** 321–7.

Porter DD, Larsen AE, 1967, Aleutian disease of mink: infectious virus–antibody complexes in the serum, *Proc Soc Exp Biol Med*, **126:** 680–2.

Rabin E, Jenson A, Melnick J, 1968, Herpes simplex virus in mice: electron microscopy of neural spread, *Science*, **162:** 126–9.

Racaniello VR, 1988, Poliovirus neurovirulence, *Adv Virus Res*, **34:** 217–46.

Racaniello VR, Baltimore D, 1981, Cloned poliovirus complementary DNA is infectious in mammalian cells, *Science*, **214:** 914–19.

Racaniello VR, Ren R, Bouchard MJ, 1993, Poliovirus attenuation and pathogenesis in a transgenic mouse model for poliomyelitis, *Dev Biol Stand*, **78:** 109–16.

Rajcani J, Herget U, Kaerner HC, 1990, Spread of herpes simplex virus (HSV) strains SC16, ANG, ANGpath and its glyC minus and GlyE minus mutants in DBA-2 mice, *Acta Virol*, **34:** 305–20.

Rall GF, Mucke L, Oldstone MBA, 1995, Consequences of cytotoxic T lymphocytes interaction with major histocompatibility complex Class I-expressing neurons in vivo, *J Exp Med*, **182:** 1201–12.

Ren R, Racaniello VR, 1992, Poliovirus spreads from muscle to the central nervous system by neural pathways, *J Infect Dis*, **166:** 747–52.

Ren R, Moss EG, Racaniello VR, 1991, Identification of two determinants that attenuate vaccine-related type 2 poliovirus, *J Virol*, **65:** 1377–82.

Ren R, Constantini FJ et al., 1990, Transgenic mice expressing a human poliovirus receptor: a new model for poliomyelitis, *Cell*, **63:** 353–62.

Roberts JA, 1962a, The histopathogenesis of mousepox. II. Cutaneous infection, *Br J Exp Pathol*, **43:** 462–70.

Roberts JA, 1962b, Histopathogenesis of mousepox. I. Respiratory infection, *Br J Exp Pathol*, **43:** 451–61.

Roivainen M, Piirainen L et al., 1994, Entry of Coxsackie A9 into host cells: specific interactions with alphanubeta3 integrin, *Virology*, **203**: 357–70.

Sabin AB, 1985, Oral poliovirus vaccine: history of its development and use and current challenge to eliminate poliomyelitis from the world, *J Infect Dis*, **151**: 420–36.

Saif LJ, 1990, Comparative aspects of enteric virus infection, *Viral Diarrheas of Man and Animals*, eds Saif LJ, Theil KW, CRC Press, Boca Raton FL, 9–31.

Schonberger LB, McGowan JE Jr, Gregg MB, 1976, Vaccine-associated poliomyelitis in the United States, 1961–1972, *Am J Epidemiol*, **104**: 202–11.

Sederati F, Margolis TP, Stevens JG, 1993, Latent infection can be established with drastically restricted transcription and replication of the HSV-1 genome, *Virology*, **192**: 687–91.

Shah KV, Howley PM, 1990, Papillomaviruses, *Fields' Virology*, 2nd edn, eds Fields BN, Knipe DM, Raven Press, New York, 1651–78.

Shepley MP, 1994, Lymphocyte homing receptor CD44 and poliovirus attachment, *Cellular Receptors for Animal Viruses*, ed Wimmer E, Cold Spring Harbor Laboratory Press, Cold Spring Harbor NY, 481–92.

Smith CA, Goodwin RG, 1995, Tumor necrosis factor receptors in the poxvirus family: biological and genetic implications, ed McFadden G, *Viroceptors, Virokines and Related Immune Modulators Encoded by DNA Viruses*, RG Landes, Austin TX, 29–40.

Staeheli P, Pitossi F, Pavlovic J, 1993, Mx proteins: GTPases with antiviral activity, *Trends Cell Biol*, **3**: 268–72.

Steinhauer DA, Holland JJ, 1987, Rapid evolution of RNA viruses, *Annu Rev Microbiol*, **41**: 409–33.

Strode GK, ed, 1951, *Yellow Fever*, McGraw-Hill, New York.

Takahashi K, Sonoda S, Higashi K, 1989, Predominant CD4 T-lymphocyte tropism of human herpes 6-related virus, *J Virol*, **63**: 3161–3.

Tan X, Pearce-Pratt R, Phillips DM, 1993, Productive infection of a cervical epithelial cell line with human immunodeficiency virus: implications for sexual transmission, *J Virol*, **67**: 6447–52.

Tatem JM, Weeks-Levy C et al., 1992, A mutation present in the amino terminus of Sabin 3 poliovirus VP1 protein is attenuating, *J Virol*, **66**: 3194–7.

Taylor-Wiedeman J, Sissons JGP et al., 1991, Monocytes are a major site of persistence of human cytomegalovirus in peripheral blood mononuclear cells, *J Gen Virol*, **72**: 2059–64.

Theiler M, Smith HH, 1937, Effect of prolonged cultivation in vitro upon pathogenicity of yellow fever virus, *J Exp Med*, **65**: 767–86.

Tomassini JE, Maxson TR, Colonno RJ, 1989, Biochemical characterization of a glycoprotein required for rhinovirus attachment, *J Biol Chem*, **264**: 1656–62.

Tsiang H, 1979, Evidence for an intraaxonal transport of fixed and street rabies virus, *J Neuropathol Exp Neurol*, **38**: 286–95.

Tsiang H, 1993, Pathophysiology of rabies virus infection of the nervous system, *Adv Virus Res*, **42**: 375–412.

Tucker SP, Compans RW, 1992, Virus infection of polarized epithelial cells, *Adv Virus Res*, **42**: 187–247.

Tuffereau C, Leblois H et al., 1989, Arginine or lysine in position 333 of ERA and CVS glycoprotein is necessary for rabies virulence in adult mice, *Virology*, **172**: 206–12.

Tyler KL, Fields BN, 1996, Viral pathogenesis, *Fields' Virology*, 3rd edn, eds Fields BN, Knipe DM et al., Lippincott–Raven, Philadelphia, 173–218.

Tyler K, McPhee D, Fields BN, 1986, Distinct pathways of viral spread in the host determined by reovirus S1 gene segment, *Science*, **233**: 770–4.

Virgin HW IV, Tyler KL, Dermody TS, 1996, Reovirus, *Viral Pathogenesis*, ed Nathanson N, Lippincott–Raven, Philadelphia, 669–702.

Weis W, Brown JH et al., 1988, Structure of the influenza virus haemagglutinin complexed with its receptor sialic acid, *Nature (London)*, **333**: 426–32.

Weiss RA, 1994, Human receptors for retroviruses, *Cellular Receptors for Animal Viruses*, ed Wimmer E, Cold Spring Harbor Laboratory Press, Cold Spring Harbor NY, 15–32.

Williams RK, Jiang G-S, Holmes KV, 1991, Receptor for mouse hepatitis virus is a member of the carcinoembryonic antigen family of glycoproteins, *Proc Natl Acad Sci USA*, **88**: 5533–8.

Wimmer E, 1994, Introduction, *Cellular Receptors for Animal Viruses*, ed Wimmer E, Cold Spring Harbor Laboratory Press, Cold Spring Harbor NY, 1–15.

Wimmer E, ed, 1994, *Cellular Receptors for Animal Viruses*, Cold Spring Harbor Laboratory Press, Cold Spring Harbor NY.

Wimmer E, Harber JJ et al., 1994, Poliovirus receptors, *Cellular Receptors for Animal Viruses*, ed Wimmer E, Cold Spring Harbor Laboratory Press, Cold Spring Harbor NY, 101–28.

Yeager CL, Ashmun RA et al., 1992, Human aminopeptidase N is a receptor for human coronavirus 229E, *Nature (London)*, **357**: 420–3.

York IA, Johnson DC, 1995, Inhibition of humoral and cellular immune recognition by herpes simplex viruses, *Viroceptors, Virokines, and Related Immune Modulators Encoded by DNA Viruses*, ed McFadden G, RG Landes, Austin TX, 89–110.

Chapter 10

THE IMMUNE RESPONSE TO VIRAL INFECTIONS

A A Nash and E J Usherwood

1 **Innate immune defences**	5 **Examples of immune responses to specific viruses**
2 **T lymphocytes and immunity to viruses**	
3 **The role of antibodies in immunity to viruses**	6 **Viral strategies for evading the immune response**
4 **Immunopathology in virus infection**	7 **Concluding remarks**

Viruses and the immune system are continually involved in a sophisticated game of hide and seek. Whereas many virus infections are readily controlled by the immune response, some have evolved strategies to evade detection and persist in their host. This balance in the host–pathogen relationship is maintained by the immune system; a breakdown in immune surveillance can lead to recurrent infections and clinical disease.

The immune system employs a variety of strategies to combat virus infection. These can be divided into innate or 'non-specific' defences, which include interferon, natural killer (NK) cells and macrophages, and adaptive or specific immunity that involves T cells and antibodies. The evolution of T cell and antibody receptor diversity has probably been critical for the survival of higher vertebrates; it has enabled the host to match evolutionary mutations in structure used by viruses to evade host defences (Janeway 1989, 1992, Zinkernagel 1995).

Immunological defences are marshalled at strategic areas in the body where entry of virus is favoured. For example, IgA at mucosal surfaces functions by blocking virus adsorption and penetration, macrophages are located throughout the body in various tissues and interferon is produced by most cells in response to viral infection. Once the outer defences are breached, viruses and viral antigens become channelled into the lymphoid system where they encounter T and B cells. A critical event in this process is the uptake and presentation of antigens by specialized antigen-presenting cells, which include dendritic cells, macrophages and B lymphocytes. From such encounters antiviral T cells are generated that target and rapidly destroy infected cells, and antiviral antibodies are produced that protect the host from viraemia. How the immune response recognizes and kills virus-infected cells, how virus is neutralized by antibodies and complement and how these responses can have pathological outcomes will be discussed. These events will be contrasted with the evasion strategies employed by viruses.

1 INNATE IMMUNE DEFENCES

The innate defences restrict early infection and limit spread to other tissues. Because this first line defence is mobilized within minutes or a few hours, it may hold the balance in the host response to virus infection. Restricting the early infection is the province of interferons α and β, natural killer cells and macrophages. The inflammatory response that follows this early encounter with viruses signals its location to the specific immune system, which becomes effective after a few days to a week. Only then will T cells home to the site of infection and antibody be active in limiting virus spread. A time scale for the evolution of the immune response is shown in Fig. 10.1.

1.1 Antiviral properties of interferon

In many ways interferon is the first line of defence against viruses. There are 2 major families of interferon (IFN): type I, which includes IFN-α (leucocyte-type) encoded by c. 20 genes on human chromosome 9, IFN-β (fibroblast-type) encoded by a single gene on chromosome 9, IFN-ω and IFN-τ (trophoblast); and type II, which includes IFN-γ (immune), encoded by

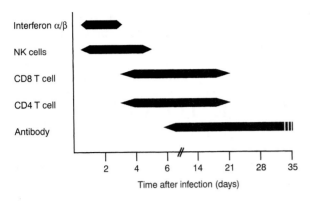

Fig. 10.1 Time-scale of the innate and adaptive immune response.

a single gene on human chromosome 12. Interferon is induced within hours of infection and exerts its antiviral action via an IFN-α/β receptor on neighbouring cells, which become activated to synthesize new protein (Vilcek and Sen 1996) (see also Chapter 11).

The mechanism by which IFN induces the antiviral state depends upon the virus, the cell type and the type of interferon induced. Generally, inhibition of virus replication involves disruption of mRNA translation. This can be achieved by the induction of a 67 kDa protein kinase (Hovanessian 1989) which phosphorylates eIF-2, causing inhibition of protein synthesis (this mechanism is active against adenovirus, vaccinia and influenza viruses) and/or the production of 2'5'-oligoadenylate synthetase and a 'latent' endonuclease (Sen and Ransohoff 1992), which results in the degradation of viral RNA (active against picornaviruses). Other mechanisms involve the selective inactivation of influenza virus transcription by the induction of the Mx protein (Staeheli 1990). The *Mx* gene is activated only by IFN-α/β and not by IFN-γ. Other properties of IFN include interference with penetration and uncoating of some retroviruses and the inhibition of maturation and release of herpes simplex virus (HSV) and vesicular stomatitis virus (VSV). In both cases the mechanisms involved are unknown. Interferon can also lead to the activation of NK cells and to the up-regulation of MHC molecules, proteosomes and transporter associated with antigen processing (TAP) proteins involved in antigen presentation. Although IFN-γ can exert direct antiviral activity, it is more readily identified with cell activation in the immune system where it occupies a pivotal role in the activation of macrophages and in the induction of other cytokines and defence molecules. It is also associated with the terminal differentiation of B and T cells.

The importance of type I IFN in antiviral immunity stems from 3 experimental approaches: (1) the local administration of IFN to sites such as the nasal passage which protects against rhinovirus infection (Merigan et al. 1973); (2) the administration of anti-IFN antibodies to neutralize IFN-α/β in mice which leads to an increased susceptibility to infection with VSV and HSV (Gresser et al. 1976); and (3) the use of IFN

receptor gene knock out mice. The last demonstrates quite dramatically the importance of IFN in arresting viral replication in vivo. A variety of RNA viruses (lymphocytic choriomeningitis virus (LCMV), VSV, Theiler's murine encephalomyelitis virus) and DNA viruses (vaccinia, herpesviruses) show increased replication and pathogenic effects in IFN-α/β receptor knock-out mice (van den Broek et al. 1995).

1.2 NK cells in antiviral immunity

NK cells are large granular lymphocytes distinct from T and B cell lineages. Human NK cells are characterized by the presence of CD16 and CD56 markers. Mouse NK cells have NK1 or NK2 and asialo-GM1 markers that are used to study their function in vivo. They also express the α chain of the interleukin 2 (IL-2) receptor, which means they can be activated directly by IL-2. NK cells produce a number of cytokines involved in antiviral immunity (see Chapter 11), including IFN-γ, tumour necrosis factor α (TNF-α), tumour growth factor β1 (TGF-β1), GM-CSF and IL-1β (Trinchieri 1989, Perussia 1991). Recently, a population of NK1.1, CD8-positive cells has been described, which have important regulatory functions in the immune response (Vicari and Zlotnik 1996).

Functionally, NK cells are characterized by their ability to kill certain tumour cell lines in vitro (e.g. K562). What NK cells recognize on the surface of tumour cells or virus-infected cells is not known. However, there is an inverse correlation between the expression of major histocompatibility complex (MHC) class I antigens and NK cell killing (Liao et al. 1991). Because some viruses (e.g. herpesviruses and adenovirus) down-regulate MHC class I expression, such virus-infected cells are likely targets for NK cells. As we shall see later (section 5.4, p. 185), this appears to be the case. There is also the implication that normal or increased MHC class I expression may protect cells from NK cell killing. The presence of Ly49 (mouse) and p58 (human) on NK cells protects 'self' cells from NK cell destruction by interacting with particular MHC class I molecules; for example, p58 targets HLA-C (Colonna 1996). This is an important safeguard for the host and means that only abnormal cell phenotypes are likely to attract the attention of NK cells.

NK cells can also recognize IgG antibody-coated cell surfaces via FcγRIII (CD16) and kill target cells. This process, known as antibody-dependent cell cytotoxicity (ADCC), is a highly efficient mechanism for activating NK cells and precipitating rapid destruction of virus-infected cells. Cell killing seems to be mediated by a perforin-dependent mechanism (Kagi et al. 1994).

NK cells seem to be rapidly mobilized following virus infection. They are detected at sites of infection within 2 days of virus entry, and their appearance is related to a rise in type I interferon levels in the blood. Viruses with pronounced susceptibility to NK cells in vivo include the herpesviruses, in particular murine cytomegalovirus (CMV). Experiments demonstrating this include the depletion of NK cells by antiasialo-

GM1 or NK1.1 antibodies in vivo (Shanley 1990) and the use of beige mutant mice, which have an impaired NK cell response (Shellam et al. 1981); both approaches increase the susceptibility of mice to the virus.

Mice vary in susceptibility to murine CMV. Resistance to infection is controlled by both *H-2* and non-*H-2* genes. The latter was identified as a single autosomal dominant gene called *Cmv-1* (Scalzo et al. 1992). This gene is located on chromosome 6 and is linked to the NK cell complex, which includes *NK1.1* and *Ly49* genes. Depletion of NK cells in mice bearing the *Cmv-1* gene increases viral replication, proving the link between this gene and NK cell activity (Scalzo et al. 1990).

An interesting series of experiments involves the role of NK cells in immunity to vaccinia. Athymic nude mice are highly susceptible to vaccinia but are resistant to vaccinia virus expressing the *IL-2* gene. The mechanism of resistance in this instance involves activation of NK cells by IL-2 to produce IFN-γ, which mediates protection, probably via macrophage activation (Karupiah, Blanden and Ransgaw 1990).

In humans, NK cells are considered to play an important role in immunity to herpesvirus infections. A single NK cell-deficient patient has been reported with severe herpesvirus infections, including CMV and varicella-zoster virus (VZV) (Biron, Byron and Sullivan 1989).

1.3 The key role of macrophages in immunity to viruses

Macrophages are strategically placed throughout the body as a first line of defence against infectious agents. Their importance in virus infections is often underestimated; nevertheless, they have potent antiviral activity and serve to limit virus spread. Macrophage antiviral activity can be broadly divided into intracellular and extracellular defence mechanisms. Macrophages are the major producers of IFN-α found in the blood stream following infection. Other antiviral molecules produced by macrophages include:

1 TNF-α, which functions either by inducing genes coding for 2'5'-A synthetase and Mx, or by selectively lysing virus-infected cells, probably via apoptosis (Wong and Goeddel 1986).
2 Arginase, which depletes local arginine concentrations and effectively aborts HSV infection (Bonina et al. 1984).
3 Nitric oxide synthase, which is induced following IFN-γ activation of macrophages and leads to the generation of nitric oxide which inhibits the replication of vaccinia virus and HSV (Karupiah et al. 1993).

For many viruses the hostile environment of a phagolysosome leads to a loss of infectivity. Here both oxygen-dependent and oxygen-independent mechanisms are likely to contribute to the inactivation of certain viruses. Viruses can be targeted for intracellular destruction by phagocytosis of infected cells or by opsonization of virus–antibody complexes via the Fc receptor; the latter is an efficient way of removing virus from the blood stream. Macrophages can also kill virus-infected cells either by direct contact or, more efficiently, by ADCC through recognition of IgG antibody. In herpesvirus infections neutrophils have also been implicated in the destruction of infected cells via ADCC.

Despite the hostile nature of macrophages some viruses selectively exploit these cells for growth and survival; they include lactate dehydrogenase virus, maedi-visna virus, human immunodeficiency virus (HIV) and CMV.

1.4 Collectins and the complement system

Collectins are soluble proteins found in serum, lung and nasal secretions that can act as a first line of defence against infectious agents (Epstein et al. 1996). They include mannose-binding protein (MBP), conglutinin and lung surfactant proteins A and D (SP-A, SP-D). The basic structural unit is composed of a collagen stalk and a globular head with a lectin-binding domain. Each unit exists as a trimer or multimeric complex. These structural features are similar to the first complement protein C1q. The collectins constitute a primitive antibody-like defence able to target diverse carbohydrate structures on pathogens and yet distinguish self from non-self structures. MBP interacts with HIV, influenza virus and HSV, and is capable of activating the classical complement pathway to neutralize the virus (Malhotra and Sim 1995).

Complement proteins can also directly target viruses or virus-infected cells. Human serum is particularly efficient in the neutralization of certain retroviruses (e.g. murine leukaemia virus, MLV). Human C1q binds the p15E protein of MLV, resulting in activation of the complement system and neutralization of the virus by a process termed virolysis, i.e. damage to the virion envelope (Bartholomew, Esser and Muller-Eberhard 1978). Sindbis virus is also able to activate the classical complement pathway, but can also directly activate the alternative pathway, i.e. via C3. Other important roles for complement involve interaction with antibody: these events are discussed in section 3 (p. 179). A summary of the complement activation pathways and their functions is shown in Fig. 10.2.

The significance of the complement system in antiviral immunity has been difficult to evaluate. In humans and animals natural deficiencies of complement components do not predispose the host to severe virus infection (Lachmann and Rosen 1979). Experimental approaches have involved the administration of cobra venom factor to exhaust endogenous C3 and hence incapacitate the complement system. Although most virus infections studied were not affected by depletion of C3, with Sindbis virus an increased viraemia was observed in the depleted mice (Hirsch, Winkelstein and Griffin 1980).

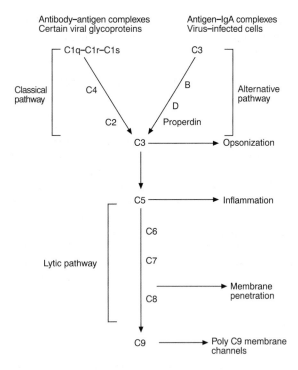

Fig. 10.2   Activation of the complement cascade by virus infection.

1.5   Summary of innate immunity

Innate immunity performs an essential role in the early stages of virus infection. Components of the system act rapidly and initiate the cascade of events that focus the specific immune response on the infected area. Factors released in the processes described above lead to an up-regulation of adhesion and MHC molecules on local blood vessels, which enable lymphocytes to extravasate and enter the parenchyma. Chemoattractants produced by mast cells, macrophages, NK cells and complement components recruit lymphocytes, which can then interact with antigen-presenting cells both at the site of infection and in the local lymph nodes.

2   T LYMPHOCYTES AND IMMUNITY TO VIRUSES

T lymphocytes are central for inducing immunological responses and, in many instances, for the recognition and destruction of virus-infected cells. A deficiency or complete absence of T cells in a host often predisposes to severe or fatal disease. This is particularly so in patients who are severely immunocompromised during organ transplantation. These individuals are at particular risk from reactivating herpesviruses, such as CMV and Epstein–Barr virus (EBV). The complex interrelationship between HIV and humans is another example of an apparent selective immunodeficiency of CD4 T cells leading inexorably to opportunistic infection in which CMV becomes a life-threatening infection.

Our understanding of the importance of T cells in viral infections stems from studies in animal models.

In mice, selective immunodeficiency states can be 'manufactured' using gene knock-out technology (Doherty 1993a). These enable specific questions to be addressed on the function of different T cell populations and their products (e.g. cytokines and receptors). A similar approach involves the use of monoclonal antibodies to interfere selectively with the function of lymphocytes and other cells and cytokines. The advantage of these techniques is that cell activity can be interrupted before or during an infection, thus permitting examination of the induction and effector capacity of the immune response. The inbred nature of laboratory mice also enables specific T cell populations and clones to be adoptively transferred to syngeneic recipients and their function monitored. This approach has implications for immunotherapy in humans, in whom protection of high risk transplant patients from CMV disease can be achieved by the transfer of selective anti-CMV T cell clones derived from the patient prior to immunosuppression (Riddell and Greenberg 1994).

These powerful techniques emphasize the importance of α/β T cell receptor populations, in particular the role of CD8 T cells in immunity and immunopathology of virus infections. The significance of γ/δ T cells in antiviral immunity is still unclear although they are found at sites of virus infection, suggesting a role in defence (Born et al. 1991). They have a more restricted receptor repertoire than α/β T cells and are thought to recognize different restriction elements, including CD1 molecules (Sciammas et al. 1994). In this section we focus on the activities of α/β T cells.

2.1   Central role for CD4 T cells in the induction of the immune response to viruses

As with any antigenic challenge the initial events in the induction of immunity involve the uptake of virus or viral proteins by dendritic cells and processing to peptides for presentation by MHC class II molecules (Germain 1994). Briefly, antigen is internalized in endosomes and subjected to proteolytic degradation. These endosomal compartments then fuse with vesicles carrying MHC class II molecules to the cell membrane. MHC class II arises in the endoplasmic reticulum (ER) complexed with the invariant chain. The invariant chain serves 2 important functions: (1) to target MHC class II to the trans Golgi and (2) to block the MHC class II cleft from binding peptides prematurely in the ER. On fusing with endosomes a combination of the acidic pH and MHC class II M molecules (a non-classic MHC class II molecule) dissociates the invariant chain and allows peptides of c. 15 amino acids in length to associate with MHC molecules (Busch and Mellins 1996). Recognition of this structure on the antigen-presenting cell is by the T cell receptor (TCR) and CD4 molecule on T cells. Additional secondary interactions between cell surface receptors, e.g. B7 and CD28, LFA-1 and ICAM 1/2, LFA-3 and CD2, lead to signal transduction and the production of IL-2 and IL-2 receptors, resulting in clonal expansion of the interacting CD4 T cell (Dustin and Springer 1991). These events initiate the T helper cell response, which catalyses the induction of CD8 cytotoxic T cells, activates NK cells and macrophages, and is critical for induction of the T-dependent antibody response. Many of these amplifying events involve cytokines and the interaction with key cell surface molecules CD40 and CD40L (T cell ligand) and B7.1 and CD28. B lymphocytes are the other major antigen-presenting cells in the immune system. There is current debate as to whether they are active in the induction of T cell responses; they are, however, highly effective at presenting to memory T cells. Figure 10.3 outlines the various helper interactions mediated by CD4 T cells.

2.2 Recognition of virus-infected cells by CD8 T lymphocytes

CD8+ T cells recognize a complex of MHC class I with a foreign (virus) peptide on infected cells. The process by which viral antigens are processed and presented is referred to as the endogenous antigen-presenting pathway (Lehner and Cresswell 1996). Briefly, newly synthesized viral proteins are degraded in part by a complex of proteolytic enzymes called the proteosome. Small peptides generated by this process are actively transported via peptide transporters (TAP1 and 2) to the ER where they associate with the MHC class I heavy chain. Peptides may be trimmed by enzymes in order to fit snugly into the MHC cleft which accommodates peptides of c. 9 amino acids. The light chain (β2-microglobulin) associates with the heavy chain and the trimolecular complex is transported to the cell surface. The evolutionary advantage of this process is that peptides derived from intracellular pathogens can be processed at an early stage in the

infection, well before replication or assembly of new virions has occurred. If they can be recognized by the immune system the infectious agent can be rapidly eliminated. The fact that viral immediate early and early antigens can be recognized by T cells supports this view.

Selection for the relevant peptides can occur at 3 stages in this processing pathway: (1) the proteosome, i.e. where peptide cleavage occurs according to the enzymatic specificity within the proteosome; (2) the peptide transporters that show a preference for selecting certain C terminus amino acids; and (3) the MHC molecule for which many allelic forms exist, all differing at the peptide-binding groove/cleft.

Because MHC class I molecules occur on virtually all nucleated cells, viruses will have difficulty avoiding the attentions of cytotoxic CD8 T cells. They have, however, evolved some intriguing strategies to disrupt antigen presentation, discussed below.

FAILURE OF VIRAL PROTEINS TO BE DEGRADED

It now appears that EBNA-1, the major genome maintenance protein in latent EBV-infected B cells, cannot be processed by proteosomes because of the presence of Gly–Ala repeats. Removal of these from EBNA-1 enables processing to proceed (Levitskaya et al. 1995).

INHIBITION OF PEPTIDE TRANSPORT TO THE ER

Another way to blockade MHC class I expression is by interfering with the uptake of peptides from the cytosol. An immediate early protein of HSV-1, ICP47, interacts with the TAP proteins inhibiting peptide transport (York et al. 1994, Hill et al. 1995).

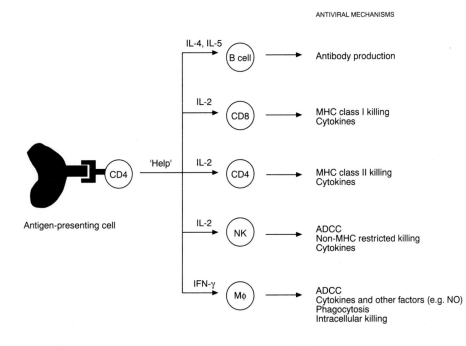

ANTIVIRAL MECHANISMS

Fig. 10.3 CD4 T cell 'help' for other arms of the immune response. ADCC, antibody-dependent cell cytotoxicity; IL, interleukin; MHC, major histocompatibility complex; Mϕ, macrophage.

ATTACKING MHC CLASS I MOLECULES IN THE ER

An excellent way to block transport of MHC molecules to the cell surface is to anchor them in the ER. The E3 19 kDa protein of certain strains of adenovirus has an ER retention motif and a high affinity for MHC class I molecules. This protein–protein interaction firmly anchors MHC class I in the ER (Burgert and Kvist 1985). A similar mechanism may exist during murine CMV infection in which a failure to transport the trimolecular complex to the middle compartment of Golgi was observed (del Val et al. 1992, Thale et al. 1995). A novel method used by human CMV entails proteolysis of MHC class I products. The mechanism involves a virus-encoded ER resident type 1 transmembrane glycoprotein which dislocates newly synthesized MHC class I molecules to the cytosol where they become rapidly targeted for degradation (Wiertz et al. 1996).

ANTIGENIC VARIATION AND T CELL RECEPTOR ANTAGONISM

Mutation in antigenic peptides is a feature of some viral infections, notably HIV. Changes can arise that affect (1) peptide binding to MHC class I molecules, (2) peptide recognition by the TCR, and (3) peptide processing by proteosomes. In (3), alterations to amino acids flanking either side of an antigenic peptide could alter peptide processing. Altered peptides affecting TCR recognition can antagonize the T cell response to the unmutated antigenic peptides (Klenerman, Phillips and McMichael 1996).

2.3 T cells in antiviral immunity

The importance of particular T cell subsets in immunity to viruses depends on several, often interrelated, factors, including the nature of the infecting virus, dose of infecting agent, route of infection and age of the host. Since 1976 a vast amount of information has been generated on the role of T cells in a number of virus infections, including the well studied examples of influenza virus, LCMV, vaccinia virus, HSV and hepatitis B virus. A more detailed analysis of the immune response to selected virus families is provided in section 5 (p. 182). These studies indicate a direct role for CD4 and CD8 T cells in recovery from infection, which is emphasized in studies on mice deficient in MHC class I and II genes.

Targeted disruption of β2-microglobulin resulted in low levels of MHC class I expression. (These mice have normal CD4 T cells but are severely lacking in CD8 T cells.) Such deficient mice infected with LCMV had an impaired ability to clear the infection, stressing the importance of CD8 T cells in this process. In contrast, when these mice were infected with influenza, Sendai or vaccinia viruses they cleared the infection normally. This was surprising, because previous experiments on the adoptive transfer of CD4 or CD8 T cells from infected mice had indicated that CD8 T cells were central to recovery and that CD4 T cells contributed to

pathology of the lung infection (Leung and Ada 1982).

Mice deficient in MHC class II molecules had a deficient CD4 response but normal numbers of CD8 T cells. Infection of these animals with influenza virus resulted in the generation of a virus-specific CD8 T cell response and recovery from infection (Bodmer et al. 1993). This and previous observations on HSV infection in CD4 T cell-deficient mice (Nash et al. 1987) indicate that virus-specific CD8 T cells can be induced in a 'helperless' environment. It is interesting that, in mice with a CD4 disrupted gene, there is a failure to maintain a LCMV-specific CD8 T cell response, leading to persistence of the virus (Battegay et al. 1994). These data argue in favour of a role for CD4 T cells in the maintenance of a continuing CD8 T cell response and of T cell memory.

How do CD4 and CD8 T cells mediate antiviral immunity in vivo? Following recognition of the relevant restriction element (MHC class I or II molecules) and T cell activation, the effector activity of T cells involves cytolysis of the infected cell or control of infection by cytokines, or both. Cytolysis can occur via perforin and the fragmentins, e.g. granzymes, Fas–Fas ligand interaction and tumour necrosis factor (TNF) (Doherty 1993b). The key cells in cytolysis are the CD8 T cells; 'killer' CD4 T cells have been described in measles and HSV infections but are clearly limited to target cells expressing MHC class II molecules (Yasukawa and Zarling 1984). The major cytokines in antiviral immunity include IL-2, IFN-γ and TNF.

The importance of cytolytic mechanisms in vivo has been demonstrated by targeted gene disruption. Mice deficient in perforin expression are susceptible to LCMV infection. Susceptibility is correlated with a considerably reduced ability of CD8 T cells to lyse infected target cells in vivo. However, some lytic activity is still detected which is attributed to Fas-mediated cell death (Kagi et al. 1994). In murine gammaherpesvirus infection perforin does not seem to be essential for antiviral immunity mediated by CD8 T cells (Nash and Usherwood 1996, unpublished observations).

In many virus infections the destruction of certain tissue cells by cytolytic mechanisms may be an unacceptable price for the host to pay. Consequently, nondestructive mechanisms that eliminate the virus but spare the cell are biologically advantageous. Cytokines clearly fulfil this role and are now viewed in a much more positive light as effector molecules in viral infections (Ramshaw et al. 1992, Ramsey, Ruby and Ramshaw 1993) (see also Chapter 11). Perhaps the best characterized is IFN-γ. In mice with disruption of the IFN-γ receptor gene, susceptibility to vaccinia is increased and replication of LCMV is enhanced. A more striking illustration of cytokine-mediated antiviral immunity is seen in hepatitis B virus transgenic mice (Guidotti et al. 1996) (see also section 5.3, p. 184).

3 THE ROLE OF ANTIBODIES IN IMMUNITY TO VIRUSES

In general, antibodies appear 5–7 days after virus infection. The first antibody class to appear is IgM, which is usually of low affinity. Such antibodies are effective in controlling the spread of virus in the blood stream. As the antibody response evolves and affinity maturation proceeds (a process involving B cell proliferation leading to somatic mutation of immunoglobulin V regions and immunoglobulin class switching) IgG becomes the dominant class in serum and is characterized by increased affinity for viral antigens (Wabl and Steinberg 1996). Such antibodies are the major defence against reinfection by virus, which become neutralized by a variety of mechanisms (see section 3.1, below). The main antibody defence at mucosal surfaces involves IgA, which occurs as a dimeric immunoglobulin with a secretory piece which protects them against the hostile environment of the gut and other mucosal sites. As discussed in section 3.3 (p. 180), antibodies form an important link with the innate immune response where they focus and activate the complement system and interact with a variety of phagocytic cells and lymphocytes via receptors for the Fc region of IgG (FcγR) and complement (CR). This combined response leads to neutralization of virus or lysis of virus-infected cells or phagocytosis.

3.1 Mechanisms of antibody-mediated neutralization of virus

The process whereby antibody neutralizes a virus is extremely varied and depends on the nature of the viral epitope, the class of antibody and the nature of the infected cell (for review, see Dimmock 1995). This process falls into 2 parts: neutralization at the cell surface and neutralization within the cell. A summary of the various antiviral mechanisms involving antibody is shown in Fig. 10.4.

An obvious mechanism involves the blockade of virus ligand–cell receptor interaction. However, this event is quite rare, because a build-up of antibody on the virion surface is necessary in order to occupy all the available attachment sites, thus making the process inefficient from the viewpoint of the host defences. Steric hindrance of receptor–anti-receptor interaction occurs with antibody neutralization of rhinoviruses. Here the antibodies attach to the rim of a 'canyon' or pit on the virion which is the site for binding to ICAM-1 on the cell membrane (Rossman 1989). In the early stages of the immune response when antibodies have a low affinity for viral antigens, activation of the complement system can augment neutralization. This is illustrated with monoclonal antibodies that neutralize only in the presence of complement. The rapid build-up of complement on the virion membrane can lead to steric hindrance of virus–cell interaction or lysis of the virion envelope.

Another form of antibody-mediated neutralization involves inhibition of penetration of the virion. This might involve interfering with the fusion of the virion envelope with the cell membrane, as seen with HIV (Dimmock 1995). This process is probably the main mechanism of neutralization of paramyxoviruses and herpesviruses.

Even when a virus has entered the cell it is still subject to neutralization by antibody. For example, fusion with the endosome is a key mechanism used by influenza virus to enter the cytoplasm. To achieve this the haemagglutinin undergoes a major conformational rearrangement to engage and fuse with the endosomal membrane. Antibodies have been implicated in inhibiting this process (Wharton et al. 1995). Certain non-enveloped viruses enter the cell by adsorptive endocytosis, and changes in local pH lead to acidification and eventual uncoating. Poliovirus undergoes a series of changes resulting in a reduced sedimentation coefficient from 160S to 140S to 80S. Several neutralizing antibodies have been defined that inhibit this pro-

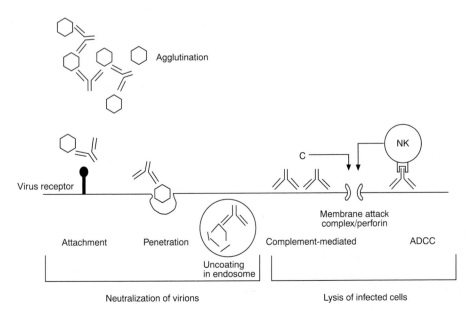

Fig. 10.4 Antiviral effector mechanisms mediated by antibodies. ADCC, antibody-dependent cell cytotoxicity; C, complement; NK, natural killer.

gression, blocking uncoating (Vrijsen, Mosser and Boeye 1993). A similar process occurs with adenovirus, in which the anti-hexon antibody inhibits the pH-dependent changes required for fusion with the endosome and infectivity (Wohlfart 1988). In rare instances antibody can neutralize infectivity after uncoating has taken place. With influenza virus, transcription is blocked by a failure of the ribonucleoprotein to function (Armstrong and Dimmock 1992).

3.2 Other direct effects of antibody

In neurons infected with Sindbis virus replication is inhibited following antibody binding to viral glycoproteins on the cell membrane. This occurs with neutralizing and non-neutralizing monoclonal antibodies and is independent of complement and ADCC. The mechanism is unclear but may involve up-regulation of some cytoplasmic defence system (Levine et al. 1991, Levine and Griffin 1992).

Neutralization by IgA is a highly effective method of inhibiting virus invasion at mucosal surfaces. This can take place at 2 levels: extracellular and intracellular neutralization of virus. The latter is thought to occur in polarized cells in which IgA passes through them via the poly-Ig receptor from the luminal to the apical surface. It is speculated that, during this process, vesicles containing IgA interact with those containing virus, leading to neutralization (Mazanec et al. 1992, 1993).

Antibodies can inhibit the release of some viruses from the infected cell. Examples include the herpesviruses in which antibodies to glycoprotein H of HSV-1 can block virus egress. Antibodies are also effective in blocking virus-induced cell fusion, thereby inhibiting syncytial (giant cell) formation.

3.3 Destruction of infected cells

Antibody can contribute to the destruction of virus-infected cells in 2 ways: complement-dependent lysis and ADCC.

Usually a high density of membrane-bound antibody (calculated to be of the order of 5×10^6 IgG molecules/cell) is required for complement-mediated lysis of measles virus-infected cells. Clearly, such mechanisms are likely to be effective late in the infectious cycle. It is interesting that in most cases of antibody-targeted complement-mediated lysis it is the alternative complement pathway that becomes activated and not the classical pathway as one might have predicted (Sissons 1984).

ADCC is a highly efficient process, requiring only small quantities of bound IgG (10^3 molecules/cell). With HSV-1-infected cells ADCC is effective early on, before new progeny virus is assembled and released (Kohl 1991). The types of cell involved in this process have been discussed in sections 1.2 and 1.3 (pp. 174 and 175).

3.4 Significance of antiviral antibody mechanisms in vivo

It is likely that all the antibody mechanisms discussed above contribute to immunity in the host. Studies with monoclonal antibodies have allowed dissection of the role of specific mechanisms. Antibodies that neutralize viruses in vitro are also effective at inhibiting their replication in vivo. This is illustrated by the inactivation of respiratory syncytial virus (RSV) by Fab fragments directed against the F protein of the virus (Crowe et al. 1994). Currently, 'humanized' anti-F protein antibodies are undergoing clinical trials to treat RSV infections.

Non-neutralizing monoclonals against some viruses (e.g. HSV-1) can also protect against infection when passively administered to mice. The antibodies function in the absence of an active complement system (i.e. in C5-deficient mice), indicating a likely role for ADCC (Kohl 1991).

Passive delivery of antibody is an important natural process in the protection of the newborn. Transplacental transport of IgG antibodies offers an important initial defence against microbial invasion, allowing the infant's immune system time to develop. Likewise, antibodies delivered via colostrum are a major defence against rotavirus infections.

Despite the obvious advantages of antiviral antibodies in preventing infection, individuals with natural deficiencies in antibody are generally not prone to severe virus infections. Exceptions include echovirus infections, in which individuals with X-linked agammaglobulinaemia (XLA) are prone to chronic infections of the central nervous system (CNS) and muscles that can prove fatal (McKinney, Katz and Wilfert 1987).

3.5 Summary of T and B cell immunity

T and B lymphocytes form an integrated system that tailors the immune response specifically to the relevant virus infection. In addition to specificity, the system retains a memory of the viruses to which it has been exposed, so that the host can be protected better on subsequent encounter. Central to the specific response is the CD4 T cell, which produced growth factors that induce the proliferation and differentiation of both T and B lymphocytes to magnify an immune response. In addition, 'help' from CD4 T cells enables B cells to produce higher affinity antibodies as the response progresses, which are more potent in binding to virus proteins. Such antiviral antibodies can neutralize free virions, and are therefore effective in infections in which there is a cell-free viraemia. Cytotoxic T cells then complement antibody by destroying cells that have already been infected. In influenza virus infection, cytotoxic T cells are necessary to resolve an initial infection; however, antiviral antibody prevents virus spreading in the body and provides subsequent protection from reinfection with the same virus strain.

4 IMMUNOPATHOLOGY IN VIRUS INFECTION

In any virus infection there is a likelihood of pathological damage to tissues by the immune system. The mechanisms associated with damage are varied and depend on the nature of the virus, its tissue tropism and the antigenic load associated with the infection. Examples of virus-induced immunopathology are listed in Table 10.1.

4.1 Antibody-mediated pathology

Antibody-mediated damage can be divided into immune complex diseases and enhancement of virus infectivity. In flavivirus infection subneutralizing antibody concentrations may enhance infectivity in macrophages through FcR-mediated uptake of virus–antibody complexes (Porterfield 1986). This phenomenon, termed antibody-dependent enhancement of virus infectivity (ADE), is illustrated by dengue virus infection. Children aged <1 year are particularly susceptible, probably because of waning maternal antibody and consequent exacerbation of infection. This enhancement of infectivity can lead to dengue haemorrhagic fever or dengue shock syndrome (Halstead 1988), the latter resulting in excessive procoagulant release by monocytes. ADE can also be seen in individuals subsequently infected with another dengue virus subtype to which there are cross-reactive antibodies.

In immune complex disease there is usually a large excess of virus antigen which circulates as complexes with antibody and becomes deposited in tissues such as the kidney or blood vessels, leading to complement activation and inflammation. In persistent LCMV infection only a weak neutralizing antibody response is generated and immune complexes become lodged in the kidney, resulting in glomerulonephritis (Oldstone et al. 1975). Chronic hepatitis B virus carriers are also prone to glomerulonephritis and polyarteritis nodosa, an inflammatory disease of blood vessels initiated by deposition of virus–antibody complex (Lai et al. 1991).

4.2 T cell-mediated immune pathology

Damage mediated by T cells can occur via cytolysis of infected cells or by cytokine liberation. The widely used example of T cell-mediated pathology in virus infection involves LCMV. In adult mice, infection of the CNS results in severe pathological changes mediated by CD8 T cells. Treatment of mice with anti-CD8 antibodies protects against disease. The damage is not related to massive cell destruction, but is attributed to cerebral oedema arising from damage to the blood–brain barrier (Buchmeier et al. 1980). CD8 cytotoxic T cells are thought to underlie the damage to hepatocytes seen in chronic hepatitis B virus carriers.

Delayed type hypersensitivity mediated by CD4 T cells (Th1 cells) has been associated with several types of virus-triggered immunopathology; for example, lung damage in experimental influenza virus infection (Leung and Ada 1982) and deep stromal disease of the eye in HSV-1 infection (Doymaz and Rouse 1992). CD4 T cells have also been implicated in RSV vacci-

Table 10.1 Examples of antibody and T cell-mediated immune pathology in virus infections

Virus	Host	Comments
T cell-mediated effects		
LCMV	Mouse	CD8 T cell damage during virus infection of CNS
Hepatitis B	Humans	CD8 T cell destruction of chronically virus-infected hepatocytes
HSV	Mouse	CD4 T cell-mediated stromal keratitis
EBV	Humans	Infectious mononucleosis
Alcelaphine herpes	Cattle	Malignant catarrhal fever
Murine encephalomyelitis	Mouse	CD4 T cell-mediated demyelination
Measles	Humans	Rash dependent on T cell immunity
Immune complex disease		
Aleutian mink disease	Mink	High risk of immune complex disease in kidney and blood vessels
LCMV	Mouse	Non-neutralizing antibody in a persisting virus infection leads to glomerulonephritis
Hepatitis B	Humans	Rash, glomerulonephritis, polyarteritis nodosa
Feline peritonitis	Cat	Disseminated intravascular coagulation triggered by immune complexes
Other antibody effects		
Dengue	Humans	Antibody-dependent enhancement of infection leads to dengue haemorrhagic fever
Rabies	Humans/animals	Antibody enhancement linked to early death syndrome

EBV, Epstein–Barr virus; HSV, herpes simplex virus; LCMV, lymphocytic choriomeningitis virus.

nation pathology. Vaccination of mice with the G protein of RSV induces a CD4 Th2 cell response, which, on challenge with RSV, initiates eosinophilic infiltration in the lung (Alwan, Kozlowska and Openshaw 1994). This type of pathology was identified in patients who received an ineffective formalin-inactivated RSV vaccine and subsequently became infected with RSV.

In EBV-induced infectious mononucleosis there is amplification of lymphocytes and an outpouring of cytokines (see section 5.4, p. 185). An exaggerated form of infectious mononucleosis is malignant catarrhal fever seen in cattle infected with alcelaphine herpesvirus-1. This fatal disease is associated with intense proliferation of T cells resulting from a dysregulation of the cytokine response (Reid et al. 1984).

Immune-mediated pathology is a feature of infection of the CNS by a number of different viruses. Theiler's murine encephalomyelitis virus, a picornavirus, establishes a chronic infection in glial cells and induces a chronic delayed-type hypersensitivity response. Activated macrophages recruited to the CNS are believed to secrete factors such as TNF-α that kill local glial cells and result in areas of demyelination around infected cells (Chamorro, Aubert and Brahic 1986, Clatch, Lipton and Miller 1986). Similarly, Semliki Forest virus (an alphavirus) causes demyelinating immunopathology, but in this case the culprit is believed to be virus-specific CD8 T cells that kill infected oligodendrocytes (Subak-Sharpe, Dyson and Fazakerley 1993). Sheep infected with the maedi-visna retrovirus often develop a chronic inflammatory condition that can result in accumulation of mononuclear cells and accompanying pathological changes in various organs, including the CNS, respiratory tract, bones and joints (Sigurdsson, Palsson and van Bogaert 1962, Oliver et al. 1981).

4.3 Summary of immunopathology

The immune system is often likened to a double-edged sword, capable of efficient protection from infectious agents but sometimes causing damage to healthy tissue in the process. When the intricate series of checks and balances that regulate immune control of the host–virus relationship is upset (e.g. by excessive secretion of a viral protein in a persistent infection), an inappropriate response can often be deleterious. In some virus infections (e.g. hepatitis B, see below, see Section 5.3, p. 184) the disease has a large immunopathological component, and therapy for such diseases is the focus of much research.

5 EXAMPLES OF IMMUNE RESPONSES TO SPECIFIC VIRUSES

General mechanisms of immunity to viruses have been outlined above; however, it is useful to consider certain 'case histories' to illustrate how different components of the immune response are integrated. Picornaviruses are chosen as examples of acute virus infections in which antibody plays an important role. The other 3 virus families cause persistent and chronic infections in which the immune system has failed to clear the virus and the infection continues in the face of a continuing immune response. With herpesviruses and retroviruses the expression of viral genes is restricted, presenting fewer targets for the immune system, and in addition the viruses have numerous subtle strategies for evading the immune response. Hepatitis B virus is an example of a chronic viral infection in which the equilibrium with the infected individual is biased toward an immune response that is deleterious to the host. Immunopathological damage ensues, manifest as chronic liver disease. These 4 examples broadly cover the spectrum of viral diseases ranging from acute self-limiting infections to life-long, chronic conditions.

5.1 Immune response to retroviruses

Retroviruses (Chapter 38) have several unique characteristics that make recognition by the host particularly difficult. Their life cycle involves reverse transcription of viral RNA into DNA, which is then integrated into the host genome. Once integrated, the virus may remain transcriptionally inactive and become methylated along with the surrounding cellular DNA. This ability to exist in the host genome without expressing viral protein makes the retrovirus invisible to the immune system. Indeed, it is estimated that 5–10% of the mammalian genome consists of elements introduced by reverse transcription, 10% of which are retrovirus-like. Most of these endogenous retroviruses cause no harm to their host, but coexist and are propagated along with host DNA and inherited by any offspring.

Vertical transmission via the germ cells is a mode of spread unique to retroviruses, and enables the virus to influence the host's immune system in early development. For example, certain mouse mammary tumour viruses (MMTV) encode superantigens capable of stimulating T lymphocytes expressing particular V_β chains of the T cell receptor. These MMTV proteins are recognized as 'self' by the developing immune system, and the responding T cells are purged from the immune repertoire. The adult animal does not therefore possess lymphocytes capable of recognizing and eliminating infected cells expressing this antigen. In a different murine retrovirus system Ronchese and colleagues (1984) showed that mice carrying endogenous Moloney murine leukaemia virus (M-MuLV) did not develop antibody or cytotoxic T lymphocyte (CTL) responses to the antigenically cross-reactive murine sarcoma virus. Mice infected with M-MuLV had a lower than normal complement of CTL precursor cells, suggesting that clonal deletion of virus-specific cells had taken place.

Much effort has been expended in recent years on the investigation of immune responses to human retroviruses, research that has been driven partly by the HIV epidemic. HIV, a retrovirus of the *Lentivirus* genus, is therefore the most intensively studied retrovirus, although care must be taken when extrapolating from HIV to other retrovirus infections. This section deals with the importance of antibodies and T cells in protection from retrovirus infection and disease, taking examples from a variety of animal and human retroviruses.

As may be expected for a family of viruses in which the survival strategy is to integrate into the cellular genome, infectivity is largely cell-associated. The recognition of infected cells rather than free virus is therefore vitally important if an infection of this kind is to be controlled in the host. CTLs perform this function, and there is a growing body of evidence underlining their importance. In Gambian female prostitutes who were repeatedly exposed to HIV yet remained seronegative there were good CTL responses in half the group, suggesting that this may constitute protective immunity to HIV (Rowland-Jones et al. 1995). Cytotoxic cells seem unable to clear HIV infection once it has become established, since persistently infected individuals often have demonstrably strong HIV-specific CTLs in their blood but the infection continues unabated. Similarly, in sheep infected with maedi-visna virus, an ovine lentivirus, CTLs are readily detectable (Blacklaws et al. 1994) but the virus is not cleared. A recent study of HIV virus dynamics (Wei et al. 1995) showed that the turnover rate of plasma virus and virus-producing cells is very fast (half-life 2 days); this, coupled with the brisk antiviral CTL response, leads to the conclusion that there is a complex equilibrium between the production of virus and the destruction of infected cells by the immune system, which drives the evolution of novel virus populations within the host. Mutations in CTL epitopes have been reported (reviewed by Klenerman, Phillips and McMichael 1996), which allow the virus to escape immune recognition, at least until the next wave of effector T cells recognizes the different epitope.

Many retroviruses are capable of transforming the cells they infect, and the cell-mediated immune system is important in the destruction of potentially malignant cells. Balb/B mice are usually able to reject cells transformed with Gross murine leukaemia virus, but when the cytotoxic T cell response is suppressed the cells survive long enough to grow into tumours (Plata 1985). In another system the transfer of a murine sarcoma virus-specific CTL line was able to protect T cell-deficient mice from virus-induced tumours (Cerundolo et al. 1987).

Antibodies also have a role in some retrovirus infections. A classic example of this is equine infectious anaemia virus (EAIV). Episodes of disease coincide with viraemia, which is brought under control by the antibody response. Disease then remits until a new virus variant emerges that cannot be neutralized by the previous antibodies; there follows another disease episode. With time the episodes of disease become less severe, until the horse enters an asymptomatic carrier state. In this phase the disease is under effective immune control, as demonstrated by the fact that immunosuppression induces relapse.

Evasion of the antibody response is an interesting feature of HIV infection. The receptor-binding protein of HIV, gp120, is a prime target for a neutralizing antibody response; however, it is very heavily glycosylated, which restricts the access of antibodies to the important functional domains of the protein. One of the exposed loops, thought to contain an important neutralizing determinant, is exceptionally variable, enabling rapid escape from any effective neutralizing antibody response. Soluble gp120 is secreted in large amounts during infection, and it has been suggested that this may act as a 'decoy' to raise an antibody response, but the conformation of gp120 on the virion is different, so the antibodies are not neutralizing. This may explain why there is a large amount of virus-specific antibody in infected individuals but the vast majority is not neutralizing.

In many retrovirus infections there is a detectable neutralizing antibody response, but it is generally ineffective in controlling the infection. Virus-specific antibodies can contribute to limiting the disease process. For example, in Rous sarcoma virus (RSV) infection of chickens there seems to be a correlation between the levels of antiviral antibody and the regression of tumours.

In conclusion, the cytotoxic T cell response seems to be more important than the antibody response in protection against most retrovirus infections. The antibody response may affect the course of disease or influence the evolution of the virus population within the host animal.

5.2   Immune response to picornaviruses

Picornaviruses are small non-enveloped RNA viruses with a relatively simple structure consisting of an icosahedral capsid comprising 4 proteins and a single strand of positive-sense RNA. Members of this family are very diverse and can cause a wide range of diseases, which are usually acute infections in which the virus replicates in the host over a short time and does not persist. There are some exceptions: for example, Theiler's murine encephalomyelitis virus can remain in the CNS for the lifetime of the host (Lipton et al. 1984). Others do not generally persist but can do so on rare occasions; for example, some cattle infected with foot-and-mouth disease virus go on to become chronic virus secretors.

Most picornavirus infections occur at mucosal surfaces, so the first line of defence for the host lies in the acidic mucus, which contains a number of proteases. Sensitized B cells may secrete antibody of the IgA isotype, which is transported through mucosal cells and secreted from the luminal surface. Attempted reinfection with virus of a strain previously encountered by the immune system will result in neutralization of the virus by secreted antibody before it is able to gain access to the epithelial surface. Stimulation of IgA is the rationale behind the oral polio vaccine; it is more effective than the inactivated virus given systemically because it stimulates gut immunity directly, leading to an effective mucosal antibody response.

The replication of rhinoviruses is confined to the

epithelial surface of the upper respiratory tract, and occurs so quickly that by the time the immune system has raised a response the infection has already resolved. The object of the immune system here is to prevent reinfection. Rhinoviruses exist in hundreds of different serotypes, so there is little chance of preventing reinfection with viruses other than the initial strain. This explains the high incidence of, and poor protection against, the common cold.

In the course of systemic picornavirus infections the virus penetrates the mucosal surface and can invade the blood stream. The viraemia is not cell-associated, making the virions particularly susceptible to neutralization by serum antibody. Poliovirus infection illustrates this very well. After initial replication in the small intestine and mucosal-associated lymphoid tissue (tonsils, Peyer's patches and lymph nodes of the neck), poliovirus can be detected in the blood. The relatively rare neurological disease (poliomyelitis) occurs following virus invasion of the CNS via the blood or through retrograde transport inside neurons. The experimental administration of neutralizing antibody can prevent the paralytic disease in both monkeys and humans.

Both B and T cells are involved in the generation of an effective antibody response, because in the absence of T cell help only low affinity antibodies can be made, and there is no immunological memory. In recent years the contribution made by T lymphocytes in immunity to picornavirus infections has been studied extensively. CD4 T cells involved in providing immunological 'help' for the antibody response are often cross-reactive between virus serotypes, and sometimes between different members of the picornavirus family.

The importance of T cell help can be illustrated by experiments performed in the mouse poliovirus model. Poliovirus does not normally infect mice, but when the human poliovirus receptor is introduced into transgenic mice they become susceptible to infection of the CNS. T cell clones have been raised against poliovirus proteins, and the transfer of these cell lines with immune B cells was able to protect the mice from lethal infection (Mahon et al. 1995). Transfer of immune B cells alone had no effect, however, emphasizing the importance of T cells in protection. The T cell lines secreted interferon-γ, and this seemed to stimulate the preferential secretion of the IgG2a antibody isotype.

There have been several reports of CTLs in picornavirus infections (reviewed by Usherwood and Nash 1995). These are usually of the CD8 phenotype, although specific CD4 cytotoxic T cells are also known to exist. Their role in the protection against picornaviruses is unclear at present, although CD8 cells are known to influence the susceptibility of mice to chronic Theiler's virus infection (Pullen et al. 1993). Whether this effect is due to cytotoxic CD8 T cells or CD8 cells acting in a suppressive capacity is under investigation. In coxsackievirus infection CTLs can contribute to the disease process as they recognize and destroy heart muscle cells.

Because of their small genome size (7–8.5 kb) it has been possible to map mutations that affect antibody-binding sites and T cell recognition elements for a number of picornaviruses (Usherwood and Nash 1995). In several members of the family antibody-binding sites are present on all 3 external capsid proteins (e.g. poliovirus, human rhinovirus), whereas in others only 2 proteins are thought to be involved (e.g. hepatitis A virus). There does not seem to be a close association between the position of T and B cell epitopes on a given virus protein.

5.3 Immune response to hepatitis B virus

Hepatitis B virus (HBV) infects c. 5% of the world's population. Most adults subsequently clear the infection but it persists in 5–10% of cases. Neonatal infection also occurs, resulting in a degree of immunological tolerance to the virus; over 90% of such children become chronically infected. The risk of developing liver cirrhosis and hepatocellular carcinoma is greatly increased in individuals chronically infected with HBV. Reports indicate that the lifetime risk to males infected with HBV at birth developing hepatocellular carcinoma approaches 40% (Beasley et al. 1981). The immunological response to HBV illustrates the varied effects of alterations in the equilibrium between virus replication and the antiviral immune response.

During acute, self-limiting viral hepatitis antibodies can be detected that are specific for the viral envelope, nucleocapsid antigens and the viral polymerase (Chisari and Ferrari 1995). Anti-envelope antibodies are thought to play an important role in virus clearance by binding to cell-free virus and preventing spread to other susceptible cells. Antibodies recognizing nucleocapsid antigens cannot function in the same way, as these proteins are not exposed on the intact virion. Passively administered anti-nucleoprotein antibodies can protect chimpanzees against HBV infection but the mechanism remains obscure (Stephan, Prince and Brotman 1984). CD4+ and CD8+ T cell responses against all the viral proteins are strong in acute hepatitis, the only exception being a weak CD4+ T cell response to the viral envelope. Cytotoxic T cells are believed to be crucial in the control of the infection, as a vigorous polyclonal response is detectable against envelope, nucleocapsid and polymerase antigens during the acute disease (Penna et al. 1991, Nayersina et al. 1993). Thus it seems that the infection is self-limiting when a rapid, strong T cell and antibody response is induced; in some cases, however, the immune response is inadequate, allowing the virus to persist.

Both the antibody and the T cell responses are weak during chronic HBV infection. Antiviral T cells can be detected in the liver, but in small numbers. Consistent with their inability to clear the virus infection, CTL responses are also weak, although, as in the acute infection, they are specific for all the virus antigens. Recent studies aimed at developing an immunotherapy for chronic HBV infection have focused on stimulating the CTLs in an attempt to mimic the response seen in the acute infection, which can clear the virus from the liver (Vitiello et al. 1994). A potential problem with this approach is that, in addition to their antiviral activities, CTLs can also cause immunopathological changes as a result of the destruction of liver tissue. This prompts chronic liver repair, which is thought to increase the chances of oncogenic mutations that may lead to hepatocellular carcinoma.

HBV does not infect mice or rats, which has hampered experimentation in vivo designed to elucidate the roles of different factors in HBV-induced disease and immunity. The advent of transgenic mouse technology has, however, provided several transgenic lines with the entire HBV sequence integrated into the host's genome that constitutively produce HBV and mimic chronic liver infection. Transfer of virus-specific CTL lines into these mice has shown that the immunopathology caused by CTLs can be divided into 3 stages (Chisari and Ferrari 1995). Initially, CTLs induce apoptosis of infected liver cells, which, however, causes little damage to the liver as whole. Activated CTLs then release a variety of chemoattractants, resulting in the recruitment of large numbers of leucocytes to the liver, which increases focal necrosis in the vicinity of the infiltrated CTLs. Liver disease does not proceed beyond this point in most transgenic animals, but lines that overexpress and retain HBsAg intracellularly progress to more severe disease. Liver cells in these animals are very sensitive to IFN-γ (Gilles et al. 1992), so the IFN-γ produced by infiltrating cells leads to widespread necrosis, resembling fulminant hepatitis in humans. IFN-γ also seems to be important in suppressing virus replication, as CTLs that secrete it can suppress virus gene expression and replication when transferred into HBV-transgenic mice, an action that is independent of cellular destruction by CTLs (Guidotti et al. 1996).

Current evidence suggests that both the T cell and the antibody responses to HBV are necessary to clear the virus, and that CTLs may act not only by lysing infected cells but also by releasing cytokines such as IFN-γ that reduce the intracellular virus load without killing the infected cell. The immune system also seems to contribute to the chronic liver pathology by causing chronic destruction of hepatocytes, resulting in a high rate of mitosis and therefore an increased risk of damaging mutations.

5.4 Immune response to herpesviruses

There are 3 subfamilies in the *Herpesviridae*, each with different biological and genetic characteristics (see Chapters 18, 19 and 20). A central feature of the biology of these viruses is their epitheliotropic nature and their ability to establish latent infections in either the nervous or the immune system.

HSV is the prototype of the alphaherpesviruses. The natural history of HSV involves infection at mucosal surfaces followed by transmission to the peripheral nervous system where the virus remains latent in neurons. Periodic reactivation occurs with reinfection of epithelial cells, which may present as recrudescent dis-

ease. The primary infection is readily controlled by T lymphocytes. Antibody has been shown experimentally to interfere with virus entry to and movement from the nervous system (Simmons and Nash 1985). A clear role for CD4 T cells is identified by their clearing of virus from the mouse epidermis. The mechanism of protection involves IFN-γ and macrophages, and resembles a delayed hypersensitivity response (Nash and Cambouropoulos 1993). It is interesting that in the nervous system CD8 T cells assume a more important role, and regulate virus replication in neurons without destroying these cells (Simmons and Tscharke 1992). During recurrences in humans CD4 T cells localize to sites of infection where IFN-γ production is evident (Cunningham and Merigan 1983). The importance of CD4 T cells as effectors in this infection is probably influenced by the down-regulation of MHC class I molecules via the effects of ICP47 and thus the activity of CD8 T cells. In terms of protective immunity the glycoproteins gD and gB are dominant antigens and have been used successfully to vaccinate experimental animals against the establishment of latent infections. Both stimulate neutralizing antibodies and CD4 T cells (Th1), and gB induces a CD8 T cell response (Blacklaws and Nash 1990).

The betaherpesviruses are typified by human and murine cytomegaloviruses, but also include human herpesviruses 6 and 7. The initial infection by CMV is via epithelial surfaces and involves a persistent or latent phase, probably in monocytes (Taylor-Wiedeman et al. 1991). Recovery from the primary infection is dominated by CD8 T cells. In murine CMV the CD8 T cell response is against an immediate early (IE) antigen, pp89. A single antigenic peptide is recognized in the context of H-2L^d (MHC class I restriction molecule) of Balb/c mice. Immunization with this peptide is sufficient to confer protection against CMV infection. Likewise, adoptive transfer of T cell clones specific for the antigenic peptide also eliminate productive infection in most tissues (Koszinowski, del Val and Reddechasse 1990). As discussed in section 6 (p. 186), CMV carries genes that code for proteins able to disrupt MHC class I expression, giving the virus an advantage in evading host T cell defences. However, NK cells are highly effective in targeting cells with reduced MHC class I expression and are particularly active against CMV infections.

The principal feature of the gammaherpesviruses is a tropism for either B or T lymphocytes. The best studied member is EBV, which targets B cells in which a latent infection is established. This virus also, has the ability to transform B cells in vitro and is associated with lymphoproliferative disease. The main immunological surveillance is by CD8 T cells, which target predominantly B cells expressing the latent viral antigens EBNA-3 and LMP (Rickinson and Kieff 1996). Immunosuppression as seen in transplantation affects this balance by reducing the number of EBV-specific CD8 T cells, which results in the appearance of B cell lymphomas.

Recently, an important viral model has been identified with biological properties similar to those of EBV. Murine gammaherpesvirus (MHV-68) also establishes a latent infection in B cells and is associated with lymphoproliferative disease in infected mice. During the primary infection the virus replicates in alveolar epithelial cells. CD8 T cells clear the productive infection in the lung and also regulate the number of latently infected B cells detected in the spleen (Nash, Usherwood and Stewart 1996). A critical event in the primary infection is the induction of splenomegaly. This also occurs in infectious mononucleosis and is mediated by latently infected B cells and CD4 T cells (Usherwood et al. 1996). The biological significance of splenomegaly is unclear, but a transient increase in the number of latently infected B cells is observed.

6 VIRAL STRATEGIES FOR EVADING THE IMMUNE RESPONSE

In order to survive in the host for a prolonged period a virus must either hide from or evade the antiviral immune response. As mentioned in section 5.1 (p. 182), viruses such as MMTV that contain a superantigen can induce a state of tolerance against themselves. A similar situation has been reported with lymphocytic choriomeningitis virus infection, in which an overwhelming infection is thought to 'exhaust' the immune response; the virus then infects the thymus so that newly emerging T lymphocytes are tolerant to virus antigens (Moskophidis, Laine and Zinkernagel 1993). Some sites in the body are regarded as immunologically privileged, meaning that the ability of the immune system to respond to foreign proteins present in them is impaired. Some viruses have exploited such shelters, and preferentially infect sites such as the CNS (Fazakerley and Buchmeier 1993).

As with any rapidly replicating organism, viruses can evolve quickly in response to a changing environment. In the case of eukaryotic viruses the immune system is a potent selective pressure, so, in order to survive, many viruses have acquired ways either of evading recognition or of obstructing the effector arms of the immune response. Most RNA viruses have high mutation rates due to errors produced by virus polymerases that lack proofreading functions. A mutation rate of 10^{-4}–10^{-5} per base per replication cycle is typical (Holland, de la Torre and Steinhauer 1992). Any mutant virus that is recognized less efficiently by the immune system will dominate the virus population in the face of a stringent immune response. For example, the retrovirus HIV has a highly variable surface protein, gp120, which is the target for antiviral antibodies. Many serotypes of influenza virus exist, which have been selected by their ability to evade neutralizing antibody responses. Periodically an antigenic shift occurs, when reassortment between 2 distinct influenza virus isolates results in antigenically distinct progeny that may give rise to pandemics as the virus replicates in a non-immune population (Webster et al. 1992).

DNA viruses have less plastic genomes, often of sufficient size to accommodate genes acquired from host cells that may allow them to subvert immune attack strategies. There are also examples of convergent evolution whereby viral genes have apparently evolved to mimic cellular genes involved in immune regulation. As should be clear from the preceding sections of this chapter, many facets of the immune system are involved in the antiviral response, and the following section and Table 10.2 detail how each part of the immune network may be subverted by viruses.

6.1 Non-specific defences

Inflammation is the first response to virus-induced tissue damage, which releases many cytokines necessary to attract immune cells. Vaccinia virus encodes a steroid-synthesizing enzyme, 3β-hydroxysteroid dehydrogenase, which is transcribed early in infection. It is not known which steroids are synthesized by this enzyme; several glucocorticoids are, however, antiinflammatory and it is known that this gene contributes to viral virulence. Several poxviruses possess serine protease inhibitors (serpins), which are thought to interfere with the pathways leading to the production of lipoxygenase metabolites and IL-1β production, both of which are important pro-inflammatory factors.

Type I interferon released from infected cells can both induce enzymes that destroy intracellular viral nucleic acid and prevent translation of viral mRNA. Proteins made by reovirus and vaccinia virus can complex with double-stranded RNA (dsRNA) and inhibit dsRNA-dependent protein kinase (PKR) activation. Small RNAs made by adenovirus, HIV-1 and EBV are able to bind to PKR and inhibit its activation. Another protein produced by vaccinia virus acts as an alternative substrate for PKR, preventing it from phosphorylating eIF-2a. The normal cellular control mechanisms for PKR regulation are subverted by influenza virus, resulting in the repression of PKR by another cellular factor, p58. By contrast, poliovirus induces the phosphorylation and degradation of PKR.

6.2 Complement

As mentioned in section 1.4 (p. 175), the complement cascade is activated by a C3-convertase that can be induced by either cross-linked antibody or the surface of particular pathogens, the end result being the deposition of a membrane attack complex that causes lysis of cells or virus. Proteins encoded by some poxviruses and herpesviruses contain short consensus repeats (SCRs), which are present in many complement control proteins. One such protein from vaccinia virus is secreted and binds to C3b and C4b, inhibiting the C4b2a C3 convertase. Purified EBV virions have also been reported to accelerate the decay of C3 convertase. An additional vaccinia protein is present on the cell surface; its ability to bind complement components is unknown but the virus is atten-

Table 10.2 Examples of viral encoded genes involved in immune evasion

Virus	Virus factor	Mechanism of inhibition	Reference
Non-immune defences			
Vaccinia	Steroid synthesizing enzyme	?Synthesis of anti-inflammatory steroids	Moore and Smith 1992
Myxoma	Serpins	Reduce inflammation	Upton et al. 1990
Interferon			
Reovirus	Binds dsRNA	Inhibits IFN-dependent PKR activation	Imani and Jacobs 1988
Vaccinia	Binds dsRNA	Inhibits IFN-dependent PKR activation	Akkaraju et al. 1989
Adenovirus	Small RNAs	Inhibits dsRNA-dependent PKR	Mathews and Shenk 1991
EBV	Small RNAs	Inhibits dsRNA-dependent PKR	Swaminathan, Tomkinson and Kieff 1991
HIV-1	Small RNAs	Inhibits dsRNA-dependent PKR	Roy et al. 1990
Influenza	Unknown	Prevents PKR autophosphorylation	Katze et al. 1988
Poliovirus	Unknown	Accelerates PKR degradation	Black et al. 1989
Vaccinia	Alternative PKR substrate	Prevents PKR phosphorylation of eIF-2α	Beattie, Tartaglia and Paoletti 1991
Complement			
HVS	CD59 homologue	Inhibits membrane attack complex	Albrecht et al. 1992
HVS	SCRs	?Mimics complement regulatory proteins	Albrecht and Fleckenstein 1992
Vaccinia	SCRs, binds C3b and C4b	Blocks activation of complement cascade	Kotwal and Moss 1988
Vaccinia	SCRs	Unknown	Engelstad, Howard and Smith 1992
EBV	Virions	Accelerates decay of C3 convertase	Mold et al. 1988
HSV-1	gC	Binds C3b, inhibits complement cascade	Friedman et al. 1984
Antibody			
HCMV	Fc receptor	Prevents complement fixation or opsonization by phagocytes	Frey and Einsfelder 1984
HSV-1	Fc receptor gE–gI	Prevents complement fixation or opsonization by phagocytes	Bell et al 1990
MHC I interference			
Adenovirus	Binds MHC I	Prevents MHC I expression on cell surface	Anderson, McMichael and Peterson 1987
Adenovirus	Inhibits MHC I enhancer	Down-regulates MHC I transcription	Schrier et al. 1983
MCMV	Unknown	Prevents MHC I expression on cell surface	del Val et al. 1992
HCMV	MHC-I-like molecule	Complexes with β_2 microglobulin	Browne et al. 1990

uated if the gene is deleted. Similarly, *Herpesvirus saimiri* (HVS) possesses a protein with 4 SCRs that is both secreted by and present on infected cells and virions. HVS also has a homologue of CD59, a cellular factor that accelerates the decay of the membrane attack complex. A protein present on the infected cell and on the virion of HSV-1, glycoprotein C, can bind C3b and C3bi, inhibiting initiation of the complement cascade.

6.3 Antibody

Two herpesviruses, human CMV and HSV-1, are known to code for Fc receptor homologues. It is thought that these bind antibody molecules in such a way that their Fc portion cannot activate the classical complement pathway or be available for engagement by Fc receptors on phagocytes. The presence of bound immunoglobulin on the cell surface may also hinder

Table 10.2   Continued

Virus	Virus factor	Mechanism of inhibition	Reference
Cytokines			
Vaccinia	IL-1β receptor	Blocks IL-1 function	Spriggs et al. 1992
Myxoma	TNF receptor	Blocks TNF function	Upton et al. 1991
Myxoma	IFN-γ receptor	Blocks IFN-γ function	Upton et al. 1992
Cowpox	Serpin	Inhibits intracellular IL-1 processing	Ray et al. 1992
HCMV	C–C chemokine receptor	Blocks C–C chemokine function	Neote et al. 1993
HVS	IL-17	Unknown	Yao et al. 1995
HVS	IL-8 receptor	Unknown	Albrecht et al. 1992
EBV	IL-10	Reduces IFN-γ production	Moore et al. 1990
EHV-2	IL-10	Unknown	Rode et al. 1993
HBV	Pre-S2 protein	?Sequestration of IL-6	Neurath, Strick and Sproud 1992
Adenovirus	E1B	Protects cells from TNF-induced lysis (human)	Gooding et al. 1991a
Adenovirus	E3	Protects cells from TNF-induced lysis (mouse)	Gooding et al. 1988
Adenovirus	E3	Protects cells from TNF-induced lysis (mouse)	Gooding et al. 1991b

EBV, Epstein–Barr virus; HBV, hepatitis B virus; HCMV, human cytomegalovirus; HIV, human immunodeficiency virus; HSV, herpes simplex virus; LCMV, lymphocytic choriomeningitis virus; MCMV, murine cytomegalovirus.

the attachment of antibodies specific for virus antigens.

6.4   MHC class I-directed cytolysis

As described in section 2.2 (p. 177), cytotoxic lymphocytes recognizing MHC class I in association with a viral peptide represent an important defence mechanism against several viruses. It has recently been postulated that some viruses can overwhelm the immune system by replicating to very high titres within a short period, resulting in a rapid expansion in the number of specific CTLs, which then enter apoptosis and die. This may be true in some situations; some viruses, however, have more subtle ways of manipulating the CTL response, by interfering with normal antigen presentation mechanisms through MHC class I. Adenovirus encodes a protein that binds to MHC class I complexed with β$_2$-microglobulin (β$_2$M), resulting in its retention in the endoplasmic reticulum. A lack of surface MHC–peptide complexes leads to a failure in CTL recognition of infected cells. Adenovirus type 12 also down-regulates the transcription of MHC class I genes by inhibiting a transcriptional enhancer element. Another virus that blocks MHC transport to the cell surface is murine CMV. Unlike adenovirus, murine CMV arrests MHC transport in the medial Golgi compartment, and the block occurs only during the early (but not immediate early) phase of the infection. An HSV-1 protein has been identified with homology to MHC class I , which complexes with β$_2$M, and without which cellular MHC class I cannot reach the cell surface. The significance of this protein in CTL evasion is still unclear.

6.5   Cytokines and cytokine receptors

The cytokine system represents the communication network co-ordinating the character and magnitude of the immune response. Some viruses synthesize proteins capable of binding to cytokines, preventing them from acting on their intended target cells. A soluble protein from vaccinia virus binds IL-1β, and a serpin encoded by cowpox virus inhibits the IL-1β precursor-converting enzyme, suggesting that IL-1β plays an important role in poxvirus infections. Other poxviruses encode proteins that are secreted and bind TNF or IFN-γ. C–C chemokines are potent chemoattractants for leucocytes, and a receptor encoded by human CMV may sequester chemokines and limit the range of their action. *Herpesvirus saimiri* possesses a molecule with sequence similarity to the low-affinity human IL-8 receptor. A protein on the virion of hepatitis B virus (pre-S2 protein) can bind to IL-6, and it has been proposed that the large numbers of free virions present in a chronically infected individual may act as a sink for IL-6.

Some viruses express homologues of cytokine genes, which may have a role in deviating the immune response to the advantage of the virus. EBV produces a homologue of human IL-10, a cytokine that both inhibits the action of IFN-γ and promotes the EBV-mediated transformation of B lymphocytes. Equine herpesvirus 2 also possesses an IL-10-like protein, and HVS encodes a novel cytokine, tentatively labelled IL-17, although the function of these cytokine homologues is not yet known. Rather than encoding cytokine or receptor homologues, adenovirus encodes 3 proteins capable of protecting infected cells from lysis by TNF. These proteins may act by inhibiting the activation of cytoplasmic phospholipase A$_2$. (See also Chapter 11.)

7 CONCLUDING REMARKS

Viruses of humans and animals and their immune systems have evolved together over millions of years, each shaping the other. As protective mechanisms become more efficient and sophisticated, so do the strategies used by viruses to favour their survival. Because of their short replication time and their ability to mutate and evolve rapidly, viruses have been able to exploit niches inaccessible to immune cells. Some viruses have appropriated cellular genes coding for proteins that have a role in immune regulation, whereas others synthesize their own mimics to fool the hapless lymphocyte.

In most cases, however, the immune system can limit the damage caused during virus infections. From the perspective of the virus it is a distinct advantage if the host remains healthy, as this will assist its dissemination. Thus acute infections (e.g. rhinoviruses) may replicate quickly, causing a mild, self-limiting disease that can spread to a new host before the immune system eliminates it. The strategy adopted by viruses causing chronic infections is different: the virus can be disseminated over a much longer period of time but it must evade the immune response. Some herpesviruses (e.g. HHV-6) seem to have mastered the art of persisting in a large proportion of the population for long periods without causing disease except in special circumstances. Infections such as these can be considered to have reached an amicable compromise with the host's immune system, causing little disease yet enabling the virus to spread. Viruses causing more severe disease may be those that have recently spread to their host species and have not yet evolved a mutually acceptable relationship.

REFERENCES

Akkaraju GR, Whitaker-Dowling P et al., 1989, Vaccinia specific kinase inhibitory factor prevents translational inhibition by double stranded RNA in rabbit reticulocyte lysate, *J Biol Chem*, **264:** 10321–5.

Albrecht JC, Fleckenstein B, 1992, New member of the multigene family of complement control proteins in *Herpesvirus saimiri*, *J Virol*, **66:** 3937–40.

Albrecht JC, Nicholas J et al., 1992, Primary structure of the *Herpesvirus saimiri* genome, *J Virol*, **66:** 5047–58.

Alwan WH, Kozlowska WJ, Openshaw PJ, 1994, Distinct types of lung disease caused by functional subsets of antiviral T cells, *J Exp Med*, **179:** 81–9.

Andersson M, McMichael A, Peterson PA, 1987, Reduced allorecognition of adenovirus-2 infected cells, *J Immunol*, **138:** 390–6.

Armstrong SJ, Dimmock NJ, 1992, Neutralization of influenza virus by low concentrations of HA-specific polymeric IgA inhibits viral fusion activity but activation of the ribonucleoprotein is also inhibited, *J Virol*, **66:** 3823–32.

Bartholomew RM, Esser AF, Muller-Eberhard HJ, 1978, Lysis of oncornaviruses by human serum isolation of the viral complement (CI) and identification as p15E, *J Exp Med*, **147:** 844–53.

Battegay M, Moskophidis D et al., 1994, Enhanced establishment of a virus carrier state in adult CD4+ T cell-deficient mice, *J Virol*, **68:** 4700–4.

Beasley RP, Lin C-C et al., 1981, Hepatocellular carcinoma and hepatitis B virus: a prospective study of 22,707 men in Taiwan, *Lancet*, **2:** 1129–33.

Beattie E, Tartaglia J, Paoletti E, 1991, Vaccinia virus-encoded eIF-2α homolog abrogates the antiviral effect of interferon, *Virology*, **183:** 419–22.

Bell S, Cranage M et al., 1990, Induction of immunoglobulin G Fc receptors by recombinant vaccinia viruses expressing glycoproteins E and I of herpes simplex virus type 1, *J Virol*, **64:** 2181–6.

Biron CA, Byron KS, Sullivan JA, 1989, Severe herpesvirus infections in an adolescent without natural killer cells, *N Engl J Med*, **320:** 1731–5.

Black TL, Safer B et al., 1989, The cellular 68,000 Mr protein kinase is highly autophosphorylated and activated yet significantly degraded during poliovirus infection: implications for translational regulation, *J Virol*, **63:** 2244–51.

Blacklaws BA, Nash AA, 1990, Immunological memory to herpes simplex virus type 1 glycoproteins B and D in mice, *J Gen Virol*, **71:** 863–71.

Blacklaws B, Bird P et al., 1994, Circulating cytotoxic T lymphocyte precursors in maedi-visna virus-infected sheep, *J Gen Virol*, **75:** 1589–96.

Bodmer H, Obert G et al., 1993, Environmental modulation of the autonomy of cytotoxic T lymphocytes, *Eur J Immunol*, **23:** 1649–54.

Bonina L, Nash AA et al., 1984, T-cell macrophage interaction in arginase mediated resistance to herpes simplex virus, *Virus Res*, **1:** 501–5.

Born WK, Harshen K et al., 1991, The role of g/d T lymphocytes in infection, *Curr Opin Immunol*, **3:** 455–9.

van den Broek MF, Muller U et al., 1995, Immune defence in mice lacking type I and/or type II interferon receptors, *Immunol Rev*, **148:** 8–18.

Browne H, Smith G et al., 1990, A complex between the MHC class I homologue encoded by human cytomegalovirus and β2 microglobulin, *Nature (London)*, **347:** 770–2.

Buchmeier MJ, Welsh RM et al., 1980, The virology and immunology of lymphocytic choriomeningitis virus infection, *Adv Immunol*, **30:** 275–331.

Burgert H-G, Kvist S, 1985, An adenovirus type 2 glycoprotein blocks cell surface expression of human histocompatibility class I antigens, *Cell*, **41:** 987–97.

Busch R, Mellins ED, 1996, Developing and shedding inhibitions: how MHC class II molecules block maturity, *Curr Opin Immunol*, **8:** 51–8.

Cerundolo V, Lahay T et al., 1987, Functional activity in vivo of effector T cell populations. III. Protection against Moloney murine sarcoma virus (M-MSV)-induced tumours in T cell deficient mice by the adoptive transfer of a M-MSV-specific cytolytic T lymphocyte clone, *Eur J Immunol*, **17:** 173–8.

Chamorro M, Aubert C, Brahic M, 1986, Demyelinating lesions due to Theiler's virus are associated with ongoing central nervous system infection, *J Virol*, **57:** 992–7.

Chisari FV, Ferrari C, 1995, Hepatitis B virus immunopathogenesis, *Annu Rev Immunol*, **13:** 29–60.

Clatch RJ, Lipton HL, Miller SD, 1986, Characterisation of Theiler's murine encephalomyelitis virus (TMEV)-specific delayed-type hypersensitivity responses in TMEV-induced demyelinating disease: correlation with clinical signs, *J Immunol*, **136:** 920–7.

Colonna M, 1996, Natural killer cell receptors specific for MHC class I molecules, *Curr Opin Immunol*, **8:** 101–7.

Crowe JE, Murphy BR et al., 1994, Recombinant human respiratory syncytial virus (RSV) monoclonal antibody Fab is effective therapeutically when introduced directly into the lungs of RSV-infected mice, *Proc Natl Acad Sci USA*, **91:** 1386–90.

Cunningham AL, Merigan TC, 1983, Gamma-interferon production appears to predict time of recurrence of herpes labialis, *J Immunol*, **130:** 2397–400.

Dimmock NJ, 1995, Update on the neutralisation of animal viruses, *Rev Med Virol*, **5:** 165–79.

Doherty PC, 1993a, Virus infections in mice with targeted gene disruption, *Curr Opin Immunol*, **5:** 479–83.

Doherty PC, 1993b, Cell-mediated cytotoxicity, *Cell*, **75:** 607–12.

Doymaz MZ, Rouse BT, 1992, Immunopathology of herpes simplex virus infections, *Curr Top Microbiol Immunol*, **179:** 121–36.

Dustin ML, Springer TA, 1991, Role of adhesion receptors in transient interactions and cell locomotion, *Annu Rev Immunol*, **9:** 27–66.

Engelstad M, Howard ST, Smith GL, 1992, A constitutively expressed vaccinia gene encodes a 42 kDa glycoprotein related to complement control factors that forms part of the extracellular virus envelope, *Virology*, **188:** 801–10.

Epstein J, Eichbaum Q et al., 1996, The collectins in innate immunity, *Curr Opin Immunol*, **8:** 29–35.

Fazakerley JK, Buchmeier MJ, 1993, Pathogenesis of virus-induced demyelination, *Adv Virus Res*, **42:** 249–324.

Frey J, Einsfelder B, 1984, Induction of surface IgG receptors in cytomegalovirus-infected human fibroblasts, *Eur J Biochem*, **138:** 213–16.

Friedman HM, Cohen GH et al., 1984, Glycoprotein C of herpes simplex virus 1 acts as a receptor for the C3b complement component on infected cells, *Nature (London)*, **309:** 633–5.

Germain RN, 1994, MHC-dependent antigen processing and peptide presentation: providing ligands for T lymphocyte activation, *Cell*, **76:** 287–99.

Gilles PN, Guerrette DL et al., 1992, Hepatitis B surface antigen retention sensitizes the hepatocyte to injury by physiologic concentrations of gamma interferon, *Hepatology*, **16:** 655–63.

Gooding LR, Elmore LW et al., 1988, A 14,700 MW protein from the E3 region of adenovirus inhibits cytolysis by tumor necrosis factor, *Cell*, **53:** 341–6.

Gooding LR, Aquino L et al., 1991a, The E1B 19,000-molecular weight protein of group C adenoviruses prevents tumor necrosis factor cytolysis of human cells but not of mouse cells, *J Virol*, **65:** 3083–94.

Gooding LR, Ranheim TS et al., 1991b, The 10,400 and 14,500-Dalton proteins encoded by region E3 of adenovirus function together to protect many but not all mouse cell lines against lysis by tumor necrosis factor, *J Virol*, **65:** 4144–23.

Gresser I, Tovey MG et al., 1976, Role of interferon in the pathogenesis of virus diseases as demonstrated by the use of anti-interferon serum. II. Studies with herpes simplex, Moloney sarcoma, vesicular stomatitis, Newcastle disease and influenza viruses, *J Exp Med*, **144:** 1316–24.

Guidotti LG, Ishikawa T et al., 1996, Intracellular inactivation of the hepatitis B virus by cytotoxic T lymphocytes, *Immunity*, **4:** 25–36.

Halstead SB, 1988, Pathogenesis of dengue: challenges to molecular biology, *Science*, **239:** 476–81.

Hill A, Jugovic P et al., 1995, Herpes simplex virus turns off the TAP to evade host immunity, *Nature (London)*, **375:** 411–15.

Hirsch GL, Winkelstein JA, Griffin DE, 1980, The role of complement in viral infections, *J Immunol*, **124:** 2507–10.

Holland JJ, de la Torre JC, Steinhauer DA, 1992, RNA virus populations as quasispecies, *Curr Top Microbiol Immunol*, **176:** 1–20.

Hovanessian A, 1989, The double stranded RNA activated protein kinase induced by interferon, *J Interferon Res*, **9:** 641–7.

Imani F, Jacobs BL, 1988, Inhibitory activity for the interferon-induced protein kinase is associated with the reovirus serotype 1 σ3 protein, *Proc Natl Acad Sci USA*, **85:** 7887–91.

Janeway CA, 1989, A primitive immune system, *Nature (London)*, **351:** 108.

Janeway CA, 1992, The immune system evolved to discriminate self from non-infectious self, *Immunol Today*, **13:** 11–16.

Kagi D, Lederman B, 1994, Cytoxicity mediated by T cells and natural killer cells is greatly impaired in perforin-deficient mice, *Nature (London)*, **369:** 31–7.

Karupiah G, Blanden RV, Ramshaw IA, 1990, Interferon-γ is involved in the recovery of athymic nude mice from recombinant vaccinia virus/IL-2 infection, *J Exp Med*, **172:** 1495–502.

Karupiah G, Xie Q-W et al., 1993, Inhibition of viral replication by interferon γ-induced nitric oxide synthase, *Science*, **261:** 1445–8.

Katze MG, Tomita J et al., 1988, Influenza virus regulates protein synthesis during infection by repressing autophosphorylation and activity of the cellular 68,000 Mr protein kinase, *J Virol*, **62:** 3710–17.

Klenerman P, Phillips R, McMichael A, 1996, Cytotoxic T cell antagonism in HIV-1, *Semin Virol*, **7:** 31–40.

Kohl S, 1991, Role of antibody-dependent cellular cytotoxicity in defense against herpes simplex virus infections, *Rev Infect Dis*, **13:** 108–14.

Koszinowski UH, del Val M, Reddehasse MJ, 1990, Cellular and molecular basis of the protective immune response to cytomegalovirus infection, *Curr Top Microbiol Immunol*, **154:** 189–220.

Kotwal GJ, Moss B, 1988, Vaccinia virus encodes a secretory polypeptide structurally related to complement control proteins, *Nature (London)*, **335:** 176–8.

Lachmann PJ, Rosen FS, 1979, Genetic defects of complement in viral infection, *Semin Immunopathol*, **1:** 339–53.

Lai KN, Li PKY et al., 1991, Membranous nephropathy related to hepatitis B in adults, *N Engl J Med*, **324:** 1457–63.

Lehner PJ, Cresswell P, 1996, Processing and delivery of peptides presented by MHC class I molecules, *Curr Opin Immunol*, **8:** 59–67.

Leung KN, Ada GL, 1982, Different functions of subsets of effector T cells in murine influenza virus infection, *Cell Immunol*, **67:** 312–24.

Levine B, Griffin DE, 1992, Persistence in mouse brains after recovery from acute alphavirus encephalitis, *J Virol*, **66:** 6429–35.

Levine B, Hardwick JM et al., 1991, Antibody-mediated clearance of alpha virus infection from neurons, *Science*, **254:** 856–60.

Levitskaya J, Coram M et al., 1995, Inhibition of antigen processing by the internal repeat region of the Epstein–Barr virus nuclear antigen-1, *Nature (London)*, **375:** 685–8.

Liao NS, Bix M et al., 1991, MHC class I deficiency: susceptibility to natural killer (NK) cells and impaired NK activity, *Science*, **253:** 199–202.

Lipton H, Kratchovil J et al., 1984, Theiler's virus antigen detected in mouse spinal cord $2\frac{1}{2}$ years after infection, *Neurology*, **34:** 1117–19.

McKinney RE Jr, Katz SL, Wilfert CM, 1987, Chronic enteroviral meningoencephalitis in agammaglobulinaemic patients, *Rev Infect Dis*, **9:** 334–56.

Mahon BP, Katrak K et al., 1995, Poliovirus-specific CD4 Th1 clones with both cytotoxic and helper activity mediate protective humoral immunity against a lethal poliovirus infection in transgenic mice expressing the human poliovirus receptor, *J Exp Med*, **181:** 1285–92.

Malhotra R, Sim RB, 1995, Collectins and viral infection, *Trends Microbiol*, **3:** 240–4.

Mathews MB, Shenk T, 1991, Adenovirus virus-associated RNA and translational control, *J Virol*, **65:** 5657–62.

Mazanec M, Kaetzel CS et al., 1992, Intracellular neutralization of virus by immunoglobulin A antibodies, *Proc Natl Acad Sci USA*, **89:** 6901–5.

Mazanec MB, Nedrud JG et al., 1993, A three-tiered view of the role of IgA in mucosal defence, *Immunol Today*, **14:** 430–5.

Merigan TC, Reed SE et al., 1973, Inhibition of respiratory virus infection by locally applied interferon, *Lancet*, **1:** 563.

Mold C, Bradt BM et al., 1988, Epstein–Barr virus regulates acti-

(a)   **(b)**   **(c)**

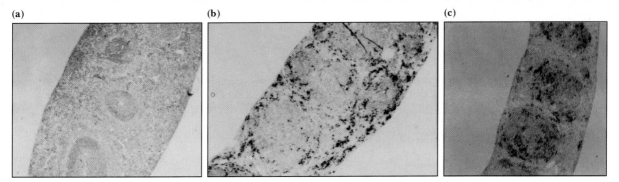

Plate 31.10 Localization of LCMV nucleic acids in murine spleen by in situ hybridization with ^{35}S riboprobe specific for NP mRNA. (a) Spleen section from an uninfected control mouse (BALB/c ByJ). (b) Spleen section from a mouse infected i.v. with LCMV Armstrong for 3 days. (c) Spleen section from a mouse infected i.v. with the clone 13 variant of LCMV Armstrong for 3 days. (Reproduced from Borrow et al. 1995.)

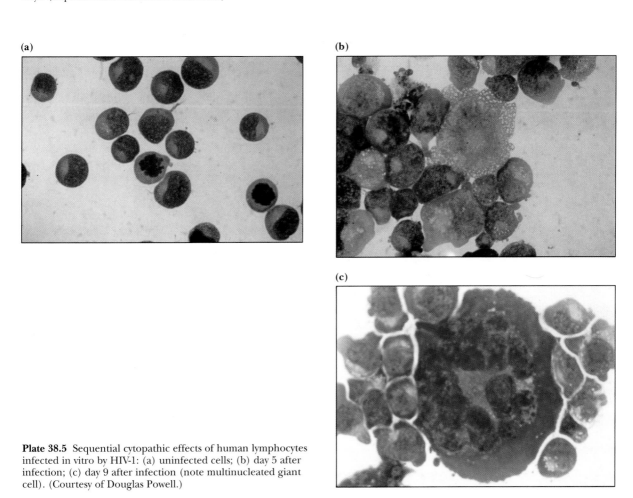

Plate 38.5 Sequential cytopathic effects of human lymphocytes infected in vitro by HIV-1: (a) uninfected cells; (b) day 5 after infection; (c) day 9 after infection (note multinucleated giant cell). (Courtesy of Douglas Powell.)

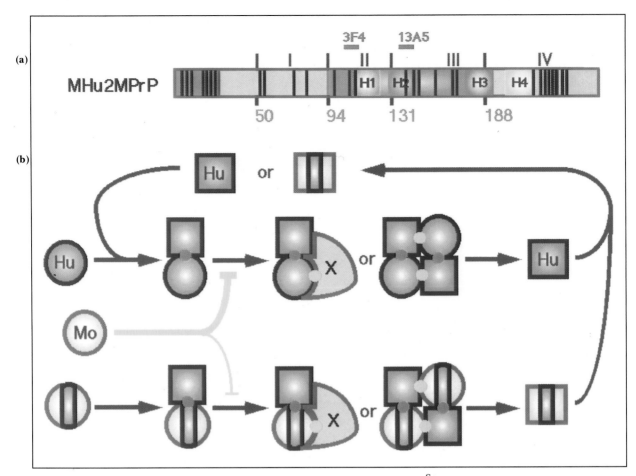

Plate 39.5 The chimaeric Hu/Mo PrP transgene and a model for the formation of PrP^{Sc}. (a) Schematic representation of the open reading frame (ORF) of the PrP gene, showing the 28 differences between the Hu and Mo PrP (vertical blue lines). The ORF of HuPrP encoded a protein of 253 amino acids, and that of MoPrP 254 residues. The 4 putative α-helical regions of PrP^C are designated H1 (red), H2 (green), H3 (light blue) and H4 (yellow). In segments II and III, a DNA fragment from the HuPrP gene (cyan rectangle) was substituted for MoPrP (mauve rectangle). The signal peptide at the N terminus is denoted by the purple rectangle. The signalling sequence at the C terminus, which is removed on addition of the GPI anchor, is denoted by the yellow rectangle. (b) A possible model for the formation of PrP^{Sc}. PrP^C is represented by circles and PrP^{Sc} by squares. HuPrP is cyan and MoPrP is mauve. The site for binding of PrP^{Sc} to PrP^C is denoted by the orange disk and the site for binding of PrP^C to protein X by the yellow disk. When present, MoPrP^C inhibits the formation of HuPrP^{Sc} more than it inhibits the production of MHu2MPrP^{Sc} as denoted by the yellow effector lines. An alternative model for the formation of PrP^{Sc} is shown where protein X is PrP^{Sc}. If this is the case, the yellow disk designates the binding of the C terminal domain of PrP^C to PrP^{Sc}. Although a tetrameric intermediate is shown, a dimeric intermediate is also possible where the same molecule of PrP^{Sc} binds a molecule of PrP^C at 2 sites.

vation and processing of the third component of complement, *J Exp Med*, **168:** 949–69.

Moore JB, Smith GL, 1992, Steroid hormone synthesis by a vaccinia enzyme: a new type of virus virulence factor, *EMBO J*, **11:** 1973–80.

Moore KW, Vieira P et al., 1990, Homology of cytokine synthesis inhibitory factor (IL-10) to the Epstein–Barr virus gene *BCRF-1*, *Science*, **248:** 1230–4.

Moskophidis D, Laine E, Zinkernagel RM, 1993, Peripheral clonal deletion of antiviral memory CD8+ T cells, *Eur J Immunol*, **23:** 3306–11.

Nash AA, Cambouropoulos P, 1993, The immune response to herpes simplex virus, *Semin Virol*, **4:** 181–6.

Nash AA, Usherwood EJ, Stewart JP, 1996, Immunological features of murine gammaherpesvirus infection, *Semin Virol*, **7:** 125–30.

Nash AA, Jayasuriya A et al., 1987, Different roles for L3T4+ and Lyt2+ T cell subsets in the control of an acute herpes simplex virus infection of the skin and nervous system, *J Gen Virol*, **68:** 825–33.

Nayerina R, Fowler P et al., 1993, HLA-A2-restricted cytotoxic T lymphocyte responses to multiple hepatitis B surface antigen epitopes during hepatitis B virus infection, *J Immunol*, **150:** 4659–71.

Neote K, DiGregorio D et al., 1993, Molecular cloning, functional expression and signalling characteristics of a C–C chemokine receptor, *Cell*, **72:** 415–25.

Neurath AR, Strick N, Sproud P, 1992, Search for hepatitis B virus cell receptors reveals binding sites for interleukin 6 on the virus envelope protein, *J Exp Med*, **175:** 461–9.

Oldstone MB, Welsh RM, Joseph BS, 1975, Pathogenic mechanisms of tissue injury in persistent viral infections, *Ann NY Acad Sci*, **256:** 65–72.

Oliver RE, Gorham JR et al., 1981, Ovine progressive pneumonia: pathologic and virologic studies on the naturally occurring disease, *Am J Vet Res*, **42:** 1554–9.

Penna A, Chisari FV et al., 1991, Cytotoxic T lymphocytes recognise and HLA-A2-restricted epitope within the hepatitis B virus nucleocapsid antigen, *J Exp Med*, **174:** 1565–70.

Perussia B, 1991, Lymphokine activated killer cells, natural killer cells and cytokines, *Curr Opin Immunol*, **3:** 49–55.

Plata F, 1985, Enhancement of tumour growth correlates with suppression of the tumour-specific cytolytic T lymphocyte response in mice chronically infected by *Trypanosoma cruzi*, *J Immunol*, **134:** 1312.

Porterfield JS, 1986, Antibody dependent enhancement of viral infectivity, *Adv Virus Res*, **31:** 335–55.

Pullen LC, Miller SD et al., 1993, Class-I deficient resistant mice intracerebrally inoculated with Theiler's virus show an increased T cell response to virus antigens and susceptibilty to demyelination, *Eur J Immunol*, **23:** 2287–93.

Ramsey AJ, Ruby J, Ramshaw IA, 1993, A case for cytokines as effector molecules in the resolution of virus infection, *Immunol Today*, **14:** 155–7.

Ramshaw IA, Ruby J et al., 1992, Expression of cytokines by recombinant vaccinia viruses: a model for cytokines in virus infections in vivo, *Immunol Rev*, **127:** 157–82.

Ray CA, Black RA et al., 1992, Viral inhibition of inflammation: cowpox virus encodes an inhibitor of the interleukin 1β-converting enzyme, *Cell*, **69:** 597–604.

Reid HW, Buxton D et al., 1984, Malignant catarrhal fever, *Vet Rec*, **114:** 581–4.

Rickinson AB, Kieff E, 1996, Epstein–Barr virus, *Fields' Virology*, 3rd edn, eds Fields BN, Knipe DM et al., Lippincott-Raven, New York, 2397–446.

Riddell SR, Greenberg PD, 1994, Therapeutic reconstitution of human viral immunity by adoptive transfer of cytotoxic T lymphocyte clones, *Curr Top Microbiol Immunol*, **189:** 9–34.

Rode HJ, Janssen W et al., 1993, The genome of equine herpesvirus type 2 harbours an interleukin 10 (IL-10)-like gene, *Virus Genes*, **7:** 111–16.

Ronchese F, D'Andrea E et al., 1984, Tolerance to viral antigens in Mov-13 mice carrying endogenized Moloney-murine leukaemia virus, *Cellular Immunol*, **83:** 379.

Rossman MG, 1989, The canyon hypothesis. Hiding the host cell receptor attachment site on a viral surface from immune surveillance, *J Biol Chem*, **264:** 14587–90.

Rowland-Jones S, Sutton J et al., 1995, HIV-specific cytotoxic T-cells in HIV-exposed but unifected Gambian women, *Nature Med*, **1:** 59–64.

Roy S, Katze MG et al., 1990, Control of the interferon-induced 68-kilodalton protein kinase by the HIV-1 tat gene product, *Science*, **247:** 1216–19.

Scalzo AA, Fitzgerald NA et al., 1990, *Cmv-1*, a genetic locus that controls murine cytomegalovirus replication in the spleen, *J Exp Med*, **171:** 1469–83.

Scalzo A, Fitzgerald NA et al., 1992, The effect of the *Cmv-1* resistance gene, which is linked to the natural killer cell gene complex, is mediated by natural killer cells, *J Immunol*, **149:** 581–9.

Schrier PI, Bernards R et al., 1983, Expression of class I major histocompatibility antigens switched off by highly oncogenic adenovirus 12 in transformed cells, *Nature (London)*, **305:** 771–5.

Sciammas R, Johnson RM et al., 1994, Unique antigen recognition by a herpesvirus-specific TCR-gamma delta cell, *J Immunol*, **152:** 5392–7.

Sen GC, Ramsohoff RM, 1992, Interferon induced anti-viral actions and their regulation, *Adv Virus Res*, **42:** 57–102.

Shanley JD, 1990, In vivo administration of monoclonal antibody to NK11 antigen of natural killer cells: effect on acute murine cytomegalovirus infection, *J Med Virol*, **30:** 58–60.

Shellam GR, Allan JE et al., 1981, Increased susceptibility to cytomegalovirus infection in beige mice, *Proc Natl Acad Sci USA*, **78:** 5104–9.

Sigurdsson B, Palsson PA, van Bogaert L, 1962, Pathology of visna transmissible demyelinating disease in sheep in Iceland, *Acta Neuropathol*, **1:** 343–62.

Simmons A, Nash AA, 1985, Role of antibody in primary and recurrent herpes simplex infection, *J Virol*, **53:** 944–8.

Simmons A, Tscharke DC, 1992, Anti-CD8 impairs clearance of HSV from the nervous system: implications for the rate of virally infected neurons, *J Exp Med*, **175:** 1337–44.

Sissons JGP, 1984, Antibody and complement lysis of virus infected cells, *Concepts in Viral Pathogenesis*, vol 39, eds Oldstone MBA, Notkins AL, Springer-Verlag, New York.

Spriggs MK, Hruby DE et al., 1992, Vaccinia and cowpox viruses encode a novel secreted interleukin-1-binding protein, *Cell*, **71:** 145–52.

Staeheli P, 1990, Interferon-induced proteins and the antiviral state, *Adv Virus Res*, **38:** 147–200.

Stephan W, Prince AM, Brotman B, 1984, Modulation of hepatitis B infection by intravenous application of an immunoglobulin preparation that contains antibodies to hepatitis B e and core antigens but not to hepatitis B surface antigen, *J Virol*, **51:** 420–4.

Subak-Sharpe I, Dyson H, Fazakerley JK, 1993, In vivo depletion of CD8 T cells prevents lesions of demyelination in Semliki Forest virus infection, *J Virol*, **67:** 7629–33.

Swaminathan S, Tomkinson B, Kieff E, 1991, Recombinant Epstein–Barr virus with small RNA (EBER) genes deleted transforms lymphocytes and replicates in vitro, *Proc Natl Acad Sci USA*, **85:** 7887–91.

Taylor-Wiedman J, Sissons JG et al., 1991, Monocytes are a major site of persistence of human cytomegalovirus in peripheral blood mononuclear cells, *J Gen Virol*, **72:** 2059–64.

Thale R, Szepan U et al., 1995, Identification of the mouse cytomegalovirus genomic region affecting major histocompatibility complex class I molecule transport, *J Virol*, **69:** 6098–105.

Trinchieri G, 1989, Biology of natural killer cells, *Adv Immunol*, **47:** 187–376.

Upton C, Mossman K, McFadden G, 1992, Encoding of a homolog of the IFN-γ receptor by myxoma virus, *Science,* **258:** 1369–72.

Upton C, Macen JL et al., 1990, Myxoma virus and malignant rabbit fibroma virus encode a serpin-like protein important for virus virulence, *Virology,* **179:** 618–31.

Upton C, Macen JL et al., 1991, Myxoma virus expresses a secreted protein with homology to the tumor necrosis factor recepter gene family that contributes to viral virulence, *Virology,* **184:** 370–82.

Usherwood EJ, Nash AA, 1995, Lymphocyte recognition of picornaviruses, *J Gen Virol,* **76:** 499–508.

Usherwood EJ, Ross AJ et al., 1996, Murine gammaherpesvirus-induced splenomegaly: a critical role for CD4 T cells, *J Gen Virol,* **77:** 627–30.

del Val M, Hengel H et al., 1992, Cytomegalovirus prevents antigen presentation by blocking in transport of peptide-loaded major histocompatibility complex class I molecules into the medial-Golgi-compartment, *J Exp Med,* **176:** 729–38.

Vicari AP, Zlotnik A, 1996, Mouse NK11 T cells: a new family of T cells, *Immunol Today,* **17:** 71–5.

Vilcek J, Sen GC, 1996, Interferons and other cytokines, *Fields' Virology,* 3rd edn, eds Fields BN, Knipe DM et al., Raven-Lippincott, New York, 375–400.

Vitiello A, Ishioka G et al., 1994, Development of a specific immunostimulant to treat chronic HBV infection: demonstration of de novo induction of HBV specific CTL in man, *J Clin Invest,* **95:** 341–9.

Vrijsen R, Mosser A, Boeye A, 1993, Postadsorption neutralization of poliovirus, *J Virol,* **67:** 3126–33.

Wabl M, Steinberg C, 1996, Affinity maturation and class switching, *Curr Opin Immunol,* **8:** 89–92.

Webster RG, Bean WJ et al., 1992, Evolution and ecology of influenza A viruses, *Microbiol Rev,* **56:** 152–79.

Wei X, Ghosh S et al., 1995, Viral dynamics in human immunodeficiency virus type 1 infection, *Nature (London),* **373:** 117–22.

Wharton S, Calder I et al., 1995, Electron microscopy of antibody complexes of influenza virus haemagglutinin in the fused pH conformation, *EMBO J,* **14:** 240–6.

Wiertz EJHJ, Jones TR et al., 1996, The human cytomegalovirus US11 gene product dislocates MHC class I heavy chains from the endoplasmic reticulum to the cytosol, *Cell,* **84:** 769–79.

Wohlfart C, 1988, Neutralization of adenoviruses: kinetics, stoichiometry and mechanisms, *J Virol,* **62:** 2321–8.

Wong GH, Goeddel DV, 1986, Tumour necrosis factors alpha and beta inhibit virus replication and synergize with interferons, *Nature (London),* **323:** 819–22.

Yao Z, Fanslow WC et al., 1995, *Herpesvirus saimiri* encodes a new cytokine, IL-17, which binds to a novel cytokine receptor, *Immunity,* **3:** 811–21.

Yasukawa M, Zarling JM, 1984, Human cytotoxic T cell clones directed against herpes simplex virus-infected cells. Lysis restricted by HLA class II MB and DR antigens, *J Immunol,* **133:** 422–7.

York IA, Roop C et al., 1994, A cytosolic herpes simplex virus protein inhibits antigen presentation to CD8 T lymphocytes, *Cell,* **77:** 523–35.

Zinkernagel RM, 1995, Immunology taught by viruses, *Science,* **271:** 173–8.

THE ROLE OF CYTOKINES IN VIRAL INFECTIONS

M S Künzi and P M Pitha

1   INTRODUCTION

The pathological manifestation of viral disease is the result of complex interactions between the direct cytopathic effect of viral infection and the local and systemic immune responses to infection. Cytokine production is responsible for common manifestations of viral diseases such as fevers, chills and myalgia, and the cytokine response has been associated with complications secondary to some viral infections such as immunosuppression and dementia. It is also clear now that cytokines produced either directly in infected cells or indirectly by lymphocytes and macrophages activated by the immune response to viral proteins play an important role both in the outcome of the viral infection and in its virulence. These proteins can inhibit viral replication either directly by inducing the antiviral state in the host cells or indirectly by increasing the expression of major histocompatibility antigens, initiating inflammatory responses and stimulating the development of cytotoxic T cells as well as the differentiation of B cells into antibody-producing plasma cells. Cytokines also play a crucial role in the activation of macrophages and natural killer (NK) cells.

Recently, a new dimension of complexity has been added to the virus-mediated immune response by the finding that certain viruses have evolved mechanisms that allow them to overcome some of the components of the host-induced cytokine response by producing proteins that mimic cytokines or their receptors. Other viruses have developed defence mechanisms that enable them to interfere with the transcriptional activation of cytokine genes or with their mechanisms of action. Thus, many of the viral genes that are not required directly for viral replication may be essential for pathogenicity of the virus in vivo. These aspects of viral escape from immune surveillance are discussed elsewhere in this volume (Chapter 10).

Local immune responses seem to be especially important in the development of cell-mediated immunity and antibody production. The cytokine expression profile defined as Th1, associated with the production of interferon (IFN)-γ, interleukin (IL)-2 and IL-12, leads predominantly to cell-mediated immunity. The Th2 profile of cytokine expression, in which IL-4, IL-5, IL-6 and IL-10 are produced, results in the production of virus-specific antibodies. Depending on the type of infection, the Th1 or Th2 response can be local or systemic, as has been suggested for human immunodeficiency virus type 1 (HIV-1) infection. This chapter deals with the role of cytokines in viral infection and reviews the main cytokines elicited by different viral infections. Particular emphasis is given to the viral infections of the central nervous system (CNS), HIV-1, herpesvirus and hepatitis virus infections, where there is clear evidence of a close relationship between cytokine production, viral replication and pathogenicity. The use of recombinant viruses to examine the effect of a selected cytokine is also discussed.

2   CYTOKINES INDUCED DURING VIRAL INFECTIONS

2.1   Interferons

IFNs have a broad antiviral action against many

viruses. They are the earliest defence mounted by the host during viral infection, until immune mechanisms can be fully engaged. An important element of the extensive cytokine network, IFNs also play a crucial role in the modulation of the immune system (de Maeyer and de Maeyer-Guignard 1991). Functionally, IFNs can be divided into 2 groups: type I IFNs, IFN-α, IFN-β and IFN-ω, and type II IFN, IFN-γ (Table 11.1).

Normally silent, IFN genes are rapidly induced in response to viral infection. A deficiency in the IFN system can lead to fulminant viral disease (Levin and Hahn 1985). Human type I IFN genes lack introns and map to the short arm of chromosome 9. There are more than 20 IFN-α genes and pseudogenes, 5 IFN-ω genes, but only one IFN-β gene (Diaz 1995). The single IFN-γ gene contains 3 introns and maps to the long arm of chromosome 12. Whereas IFN-α is a family of non-glycosylated monomeric proteins (Allan and Fantes 1980), IFN-β, IFN-ω and IFN-γ are N-glycosylated. Functionally, IFN-β is a dimer, whereas IFN-γ is a tetramer. Synthesis of IFN-α takes place mainly in cells of lymphoid origin. IFN-β is synthesized in fibroblasts, epithelial cells and macrophages and IFN-ω in leucocytes and trophoblasts. Production of IFN-γ is a specialized function of T lymphocytes although NK cells and macrophages can produce IFN-γ as well. Competitive binding studies (Merlin, Falkoff and Auget 1985) indicate that a common receptor for IFN-α β and ω, as well as the receptor for IFN-γ, are encoded by genes mapping to chromosome 21.

Upon binding to their respective receptors, IFNs exert their multiple effects through receptor-mediated transduction pathways resulting in the induction of IFN-stimulated genes (Darnell, Kerr and Stark 1994). The pathway involves the activation of several JAK kinases that are associated with IFN receptors and the consequent tyrosine phosphorylation of pre-existing transcriptional factors called STAT (signal transducers and activators of transcription). STAT proteins, upon phosphorylation, assemble into multimeric complexes and are transported to the nucleus, where they interact with interferon-responsive elements present in the 5′ flanking region of interferon-stimulated genes (ISGs) (Levy 1995). IFNs activate an array of genes encoding proteins with antiviral properties and others participating in viral recognition (Samuel 1991). Type I and type II IFNs are essential for antiviral defence and they are not functionally redundant (Muller et al. 1994). Both types of IFNs modulate the expression of major histocompatibility complex (MHC) antigens. It is via that mechanism that IFN-α/β increases the susceptibility of fibroblasts infected with vaccinia virus or lymphocytic choriomeningitis virus (LCMV) to cytotoxic T lymphocyte (CTL) lysis (Bukowski and Welsh 1985). Although both type I and type II IFNs modulate MHC II antigen expression, IFN-γ and tumour necrosis factor (TNF)-α are the most powerful inducers of MHC II antigens. IFN-γ enhances expression of MHC II antigens on accessory cells, stimulates the interaction of these cells with T cells and promotes CTL development. Murine IFN-α and IFN-β can block IFN-γ-mediated class II antigen up-regulation (de Maeyer and de Maeyer-Guignard 1991).

IFNs act via a paracrine loop. Virus-induced IFNs are secreted by the cell and activate neighbouring cells into an antiviral state characterized by the expression of a number of ISGs. Several of the proteins encoded by ISGs have direct antiviral activities (Samuel 1991). The antiviral activities of 2′,5′-oligoadenylate synthetase (2′,5′-OAS), PKR protein kinase and Mx proteins have been well characterized (Fig. 11.1).The 2′,5′-OAS pathway comprises 3 enzymes. 2′,5′-OAS, upon activation by dsRNA, polymerizes ATP into pppA(2′p5′A)n, (2′,5′A) (Kerr and Brown 1978). 2′,5′A in turn activates a cellular endonuclease, 2′,5′-OAS-dependent RNaseL (Williams and Silverman 1985, Zhou, Hassel and Silverman 1993). RNaseL is present in the cells in an inactive form. When activated by 2′,5′A, it degrades both cellular and viral RNAs at UU or AU nucleotides. 2′,5′-phosphodiester-

Table 11.1 Human interferons

Name	Genes	Proteins	Producer cells	Effect
IFN-α	>20 No introns Chromosome 9	Non-glycosylated 166 aa Monomer	Lymphoid cells Macrophages	Antiviral state ISG induction MHC I induction
IFN-β	1 No introns Chromosome 9	N-glycosylated 166 aa Dimer	Fibroblasts Epithelial cells Macrophages	Antiviral state ISG induction MHC I induction
IFN-ω	5 No introns Chromosome 9	N-glycosylated 172 aa ...	Leucocytes Trophoblasts	Presumably similar to IFN-α
IFN-γ	1 3 introns Chromosome 12	N-glycosylated 146 aa Tetramer	T cells Macrophages NK cells	2′,5′-OAS induction IL-1 enhancement MHC I induction MHC II induction

IFN, interferon; aa, amino acid; ISG, interferon-stimulated gene; MHC, major histocompatibility complex; 2′,5′-OAS, 2′,5′-oligoadenylate synthetase.

ase (Lengyel 1982) catalyses the degradation of 2',5'A. Expression of 2',5'-OAS (40 kDa) in cells leads to the establishment of an antiviral state which results in the selective inhibition of the replication of picornaviruses such as mengo- and encephalomyocarditis viruses (Chebath et al. 1987). The antiviral effect of the 2',5'-OAS system is specific for picornaviruses and no inhibition of VSV or HSV-1 has been observed.

Activation of the IFN-induced kinase, PKR, depends on the presence of dsRNA. The phosphorylation of the α subunit of protein synthesis initiation factor eF-2 (Samuel 1979, Berry et al. 1985) by PKR has been implicated in the inhibition of viral protein synthesis (Pathak, Schindler and Hershey 1988). The crucial role of PKR in the antiviral effect of IFN is further indicated by the observation that a number of viruses have developed mechanisms to negate the function of PKR. Adenovirus encodes small RNAs, VA-RNA, which are synthesized in the late stages of the replication cycle and interfere with the activation of PKR and phosphorylation of eF-2a (Davies et al. 1989). Vaccinia virus encodes a specific PKR inhibitory factor (SKIF) which appears to prevent the activation of PKR (Akkaraju et al. 1989).The reovirus encoded protein G3 binds dsRNA and inhibits the activation of PKR by

competing for dsRNA (Imani and Jacobs 1988). Poliovirus, on the other hand, inactivates PKR by inducing the autophosphorylation of PKR and its subsequent degradation. In cells infected with influenza virus, PKR is also inactivated; the inhibitor in this case is a cellular protein (Lee et al. 1990). Inhibition of PKR activity by HIV-1 has also been suggested (Roy et al. 1991).

The antiviral activity of Mx proteins is virus-selective. The specific antiviral properties of Mx1 protein are directed primarily against influenza virus (Haller et al. 1979, Samuel 1991). It has recently been shown that the Mx protein is also involved in the inhibition of hantavirus replication (Frese et al. 1995). However, the mechanism of action of Mx proteins remains to be elucidated.

These and possibly other IFN-regulated proteins confer on IFN its broad antiviral spectrum. IFN induces inhibition of viral translation in many viruses, such as vaccinia virus, reovirus, vesicular stomatitis virus (VSV), influenza virus and mengovirus (Johnston and Torrence 1984). IFN has been shown, however, to block other steps of the viral life cycle. IFN-α inhibits cytomegalovirus (CMV) at the level of transcription of viral immediate-early (IE) genes, in particular that of

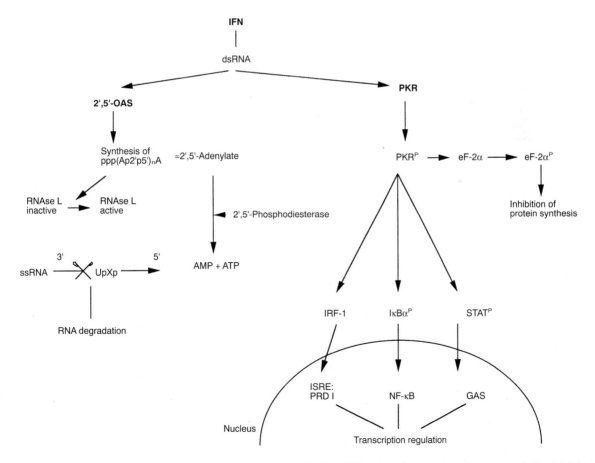

Fig. 11.1 dsRNA-dependent interferon-stimulated antiviral activities. GAS, γ-interferon-activated sequence; IκBα, inhibitor protein binding NF-κB transcription factors; IRF-1, interferon responsive factor 1; ISRE/PRD 1, interferon-sensitive response element/positive regulatory domain 1; p, phosphorylated; STAT, signal transduction activator transducer; UpXp, (by convention) a short RNA sequence in which the phosphorylated base uridine is followed by any other phosphorylated base (A, C or G).

the major genes *IE1*, *IE2* and *IE3*; consequently, steady-state levels of late transcripts are reduced, while early gene expression is only partially affected (Martinotti and Gribaudo 1992). Whereas both IFN-α and IFN-γ inhibit adenovirus early gene expression, only IFN-γ inhibits late transcription (Mistchenko, Diez and Falcoff 1989). IFN-α inhibits HIV-1 at many steps of its life cycle, but predominantly at the level of reverse transcription in acutely infected T cells and monocytes (Shirazi and Pitha 1992, 1993) and at the level of virus assembly in chronically infected cells (Pitha 1991). Inhibition of virus assembly and maturation is the major mechanism by which IFN blocks the replication of murine retroviruses (Pitha 1980). IFN-α, IFN-β and IFN-γ, alone or in combination, inhibit integration of human T cell leukaemia virus I (HTLV-I) provirus in MT-2 cells, but a combination of IFN-α and IFN-β or IFN-γ and IFN-α is necessary to inhibit its transcription (D'Onofrio et al. 1992).The transient nature of hantavirus infection in vascular endothelial cells is due to the induction of IFN-β (Pensiero et al. 1992). IFN-α protects against influenza A virus infection either directly by inducing the expression of the Mx protein or indirectly by promoting neutrophil respiratory burst responses (Little, White and Hartshorn 1994). Stimulation of HLA class 1 expression on measles virus infection is mediated by IFN-β.

The availability of purified and recombinant IFN preparations has made possible the clinical use of IFN-α for the treatment of papilloma virus infections of the larynx, the anogenital regions and the skin (Fingerote et al. 1995). IFN-α has also become the treatment of choice for chronic hepatitis B and hepatitis C virus infections. Hepatitis virus replication is inhibited by IFN-induced 2′,5′-OAS in mouse peritoneal macrophages. The antiviral effect of 2′,5′-OAS is not sufficient, however, to prevent the hepatocellular injury associated with hepatitis virus infection (Fingerote et al. 1995). Intranasal use of IFN-α for rhinovirus infections causes substantial damage to the nasal mucosa (Finter et al. 1991, Gutterman 1994). The major role of IFN-γ in antiviral defence is to modulate the immune response to viral infection. IFN-γ has, however, a direct antiviral effect, possibly through the induction of 2′,5′-OAS (de Maeyer and de Maeyer-Guignard 1991). In mice, IFN-γ controls T-cell-mediated viral clearance in acute cutaneous and ocular infection with herpes simplex (HSV-1) and in poxvirus infection. In macrophages, IFN-γ inhibits HSV-1 and vaccinia virus replication by inducing the production of nitric oxide in the infected cells (Karupiah et al. 1993). The growth of hepatitis virus is restricted in mice by IFN-γ-activated macrophages (Vassao, Mello and Pereira 1994). IFN-γ is also necessary for a normal antigen-specific immunoglobulin G2a response, as demonstrated in mice lacking the IFN-γ receptor (Huang et al. 1993). Intraperitoneal infection with mouse cytomegalovirus (CMV) or herpes simplex virus (HSV) results in inflammatory infiltrates, consisting mainly of macrophages with increased expression of IFN-γ and TNF-α. CMV titres

are increased in IFN-γ-depleted mice and in mice with severe combined immunodeficiency (SCID) (Heise and Virgin 1995). The antiviral effect of IFN-γ has also been demonstrated by the observation that the replication of recombinant vaccinia virus expressing IFN-γ is markedly inhibited, compared to that of wild type virus (Ramshaw et al. 1992). The virulence of poxvirus infection is increased in mice lacking IFN-γ, and one of the myxoma virus genes implicated in the growth of the virus in vivo encodes the IFN-γ receptor (Upton, DeLange and MacFadden 1987).

Viruses have, however, evolved mechanisms to evade the antiviral effects of IFN. As discussed earlier (p. 195), many viruses have developed mechanisms by which they negate the function of RNA-activated protein kinase (PKR) (Reich et al. 1988). By contrast, flaviviruses (e.g. West Nile and Kunjin viruses) induce expression of intercellular adhesion molecule-1 (ICAM-1) by 2 distinct mechanisms. First, induction is mediated by type I IFN and occurs only in quiescent fibroblasts in G0 phase; the second induction is cytokine-independent and occurs within hours of viral challenge. The induction of cell–cell contact via ICAM-1 expression early in infection may significantly enhance the ability of the virus to spread before the immune response is triggered (Shen, Devery and King 1995).

2.2   Tumour necrosis factor

Tumour necrosis factor (TNF)-α (cachectin) and β (lymphotoxin) are 2 related peptides encoded by linked genes mapping within the major histocompatibility complex (MHC) (Spies et al. 1986). Although TNF-α is secreted mainly by macrophages/monocytes and TNF-β by T cells, they compete for a common receptor. TNF-α, like IFN, can establish an antiviral state, and TNF-α-mediated induction of 2′,5′-OAS has been demonstrated in a number of cell lines (Mestan et al. 1988). IFN-γ and IFN-β synergize with TNF-α to increase levels of 2′,5′-OAS and viral inhibition (Mestan et al. 1988). Studies in vivo, with mice as a model for encephalomyocarditis (EMCV) infection, have shown that TNF-α alone is not sufficient to inhibit viral replication, but requires combined treatment with IFN-γ (Czarniecki 1993). The same requirement has been observed with murine CMV (Anderson et al. 1993). The direct antiviral effect of TNF-α has been well documented with recombinant vaccinia virus expressing TNF-α (Ramshaw et al. 1992). In contrast, the replication of retroviruses, such as simian immunodeficiency virus (SIV) and HIV, is activated by TNF-α (Lairmore et al. 1991). Although IL-6 mRNA levels are increased in response to TNF-α, IL-6 alone does not seem to contribute to the TNF-α-induced antiviral state (Jacobsen et al. 1989).

Both RNA and DNA viruses can induce TNF-α expression in peripheral blood mononuclear cells (PBMCs) and macrophages. Influenza virus increases TNF-α mRNA levels in monocytes (Nain et al. 1990), respiratory syncytial virus (RSV) stimulates TNF-α secretion in macrophages (Franke-Ullman et al. 1995) and human herpesvirus-6 (HHV-6) triggers TNF-α secretion in PBMCs (Flamand et al. 1991). TNF-α secretion by PBMCs from patients with chronic hepatitis B virus infection correlates with the level of virus replication. TNF-α inhibits replication of stomatitis virus (VSV) in WISH cells and replication of EMCV in HeLa cells. Another mechanism by which TNF-α limits viral spread is by enhancing viral cytotoxicity. TNF-α induces cytolysis of HSV-1 and HSV-2-infected rat embryo cells (Koff and Fann 1986). Cytolysis is also observed with either TNF-α or TNF-β in VSV or adenovirus-2-infected A549 cells. In vivo, however, adenovirus *E1A* gene encodes a 14.7 kDa protein which suppresses TNF-α-mediated cytolysis and thereby allows escape from the antiviral effects of TNF-α (Laster, Wold and Gooding 1994). Furthermore, co-expression of the adenovirus 14.7 kDa protein in a recombinant vaccinia virus expressing TNF-α inhibits the TNF-α-mediated attenuation of vaccinia virus virulence (Tufariello, Cho and Horwitz 1994). Also, one of the genes in the terminal repeat of myxoma virus involved in modulating the replication of the virus in vivo encodes a soluble TNF-α receptor. Because induction of TNF-α is an essential part of the cellular defence against myxoma virus infection, the virus is able to neutralize the effect of TNF-α. Induction of TNF-α as well as IFN-γ and IL-1 during dengue virus infection in macrophages may result in permeability of vascular endothelial cells and plasma leakage, which are characteristic of the haemorrhagic fever secondary to dengue virus infection. Not all viruses, however, can induce TNF-α. HSV-1, for instance, is a strong inducer, whereas Epstein–Barr virus (EBV) down-regulates the levels of TNF-α mRNA and protein in PBMCs (Gosselin et al. 1992).

2.3 Interleukin-1

The interleukin-1 (IL-1) family is composed of 2 cytokines, IL-1α and IL-1β, and one inhibitor, IL-1 receptor antagonist (IL-1ra). Although IL genes are highly conserved across species, they share little homology with one another and their regulation is different. Both IL-1α and IL-1β are synthesized as membrane bound precursors of 270 aa, cleaved by proteases to yield circulating soluble proteins. IL-1 is produced mainly by macrophages, but T and B cells, dendritic cells, fibroblasts, epithelial cells and astrocytes can synthesize IL-1 as well. IL-1 has no direct antiviral activity but, together with IL-2, induces IFN-γ synthesis and thus contributes indirectly to the antiviral immune response. IFN-α has been reported to down-regulate IL-1β in bone marrow stromal cells while stimulating expression of the IL-1 receptor, thereby contributing to the myelosuppression associated with viral infections (Arman et al. 1994). Not all viral infections result in the induction of IL-1. Whereas influenza virus induces substantial IL-1 activity in macrophages, RSV induces IL-1 inhibitor activity (Roberts, Prill and Mann 1986). In situ hybridization studies have shown that HIV-1, herpesviruses, EBV and CMV, adenovirus and chronic hepatitis B virus (HBV) infection induce

IL-1β and IL-6 genes; not, however, in the infected cells themselves but in macrophages and epithelial cells adjacent to the infected cells (Devergne et al. 1991). IL-1, together with TNF-α and IL-6, is a key cytokine expressed during inflammation. In mice, cerebral expression of IL-1α and 1β and TNF-α correlates with the onset of neurodegenerative processes secondary to scrapie infection (Campbell et al. 1994). Although both adult T cell leukaemia (ATL) and HTLV-associated myelopathy/tropical spastic paraparesis (HAM/TSP) are associated with HTLV-I infection, the difference in virus-induced cytokine expression may underlie the differences in pathogenesis between the 2 diseases: IFN-γ, TNF-α and IL-1β expression is induced in HAM/TSP, whereas elevated levels of transforming growth factor β (TGF-β') are secreted by leukaemic cells in ATL (Tendler et al. 1991).

2.4 Interleukin-6

IL-6 is produced by T and B cells, macrophages, fibroblasts and endothelial cells. During viral infection, IL-6 seems to play an essential role in antibody production, since it induces B cells to differentiate into antibody-producing cells. Mice with targeted disruption of the IL-6 gene have a reduced number of IgA-producing cells. Expression of IL-6 enhances systemic and mucosal antibody responses in mice infected with a recombinant fowlpox virus expressing influenza virus haemagglutinin and IL-6 (Ramsay et al. 1994). In contrast, IFN-γ expression in those animals inhibits antibody responses but not cell-mediated immunity (Leong et al. 1994). Both RNA and DNA viruses induce IL-6 expression. Thus, HTLV-I transactivator protein Tax induces IL-6 expression through the direct activation of the IL-6 NF-κB site (Mori et al. 1994). Chronic virus-producing, but not chronic latent, hepatitis B infection increases serum IL-6 activity, and IL-6 levels are further enhanced during acute exacerbation of the disease (Kakumu et al. 1991). Dengue virus, which is transmitted through mosquito bites, induces a rapid expression of IL-6 in fibroblasts, as well as granulocyte/macrophage colony stimulation factor (GM-CSF) and IFN-β; IFN protects uninfected cells from infection and limits virus spread (Kurane, Janus and Ennis 1992). Elevated serum levels of IL-6, IL-1 and TNF-α are also found in patients with dengue haemorrhagic fever (Hober et al. 1993). HIV-1 transactivating protein tat can induce IL-6 production in uninfected PBMCs in vitro and IL-6-dependent IgG and IgA synthesis (Rautonen et al. 1994). In the presence of IL-4, HIV-1 infection induces an autocrine IL-6 loop in B cells. AIDS-associated Kaposi's sarcoma cells express the IL-6 receptor and use IL-6 as an autocrine growth factor (Masood et al. 1994). Macaque monkeys infected with a lethal variant of SIV (SIVsmm/PBj-14) show a marked increase in both IL-6 mRNA in inflamed tissues and IL-6 protein in serum (Birx et al. 1993).

Virally induced IL-6 participates in inflammatory reactions together with IL-1 and TNF-α. Live or inactivated RSV induces increased levels of IL-6 as well as

TNF-α mRNA in alveolar macrophages. The combination of these 2 cytokines (IL-6 and TNF-α) does not seem, however, to have a direct antiviral effect but modulates the inflammatory response to RSV infection (Becker, Quay and Soukup 1991). In a similar manner, live or UV-irradiated Coxsackie virus B3 (CVB3) stimulates the release of IL-6, IL-1 and TNF-α in infected human monocytes, and supernatants from CVB3-infected monocytes are cytotoxic to heart cells, suggesting that these cytokines induced by viral infection may contribute to the pathology of CVB3-induced myocarditis. In patients with cerebrospinal inflammation, however, it is acute bacterial meningitis and not viral meningitis (such as is caused by mumps virus) that is associated with increased IL-6 activity (Torre et al. 1992).

2.5 Interleukin-7, 8 and 10

IL-7 is a 177 aa protein secreted by thymic stroma cells and acts as a T cell growth and differentiation factor and a macrophage activation factor. IL-7 also augments an *env*-specific CTL response in HIV-1 infected individuals in a dose- and time-dependent manner and promotes the maturation of precursor CTLs independently of IL-2. IL-8 is a member of a large family of factors secreted by macrophages and endothelial cells which act as mediators in inflammation. Constitutive expression of IL-8 and IL-6 by tracheobronchial and nasal epithelial cells is significantly increased upon viral infection (Adler et al. 1994). RSV in particular induces the release of IL-8 and IL-6 in the human epithelial cell line A549 in a time- and viral load-dependent manner. In addition, pro-inflammatory cytokines such as TNF-α and IL-1 synergistically enhance IL-8 secretion in RSV-infected A549 cells (Arnold et al. 1994). IL-10, appropriately termed cytokine synthesis inhibitory factor, inhibits the production of IFN-γ, and secretion of IL-1, IL-6 and TNF-α by macrophages. An open reading frame from EBV, *BCRF1*, shows extensive homology with IL-10, and it has been suggested that viral IL-10 expression enables infected cells to escape from immune surveillance (Moore et al. 1990) (Table 11.2).

2.6 Interleukin-4 and 12

IL-4 is a 20 kDa glycoprotein, B cell growth and differentiation factor which is secreted by Th2 cells and plays an essential role in the initiation of humoral immunity. IL-12, also known as NK cell stimulatory factor (Kobayashi et al. 1989), is a heterodimer which stimulates IFN-γ production. It has become clear now that IL-12 and IL-4 play pivotal roles in the differentiation of naive T cells into Th1 and Th2 subsets. Although viruses tend to trigger cell-mediated immunity, not all do so. CNS infection with live measles virus induces IL-4 expression and Th2 cell activation (Ward and Griffith 1993). Sindbis virus, which causes acute encephalomyelitis in mice, also triggers a Th2 response in the brain, characterized by increased expression of IL-4, IL-16, IL-10 and TGF-β in the brain (Wesselingh et al. 1994). IL-4 and IL-12 also seem to have an enhancing effect on HIV-1 replication, as is described in detail later (section 4, p. 199). The role of IL-4 and IL-12 in the Th1 and Th2 immune responses is explored more fully later in this chapter (section 3.1, below).

3 MODULATION OF THE IMMUNE RESPONSE

3.1 Th1–Th2 shift

As mentioned earlier (p. 193), T lymphocytes are required for cell-mediated immune responses and antibody production by B cells. This dual role is controlled by 2 distinct T-helper (Th) cell subsets. Th1 cells produce IL-2 and IFN-γ and direct cell-mediated immunity, whereas Th2 cells produce IL-4, IL-6 and IL-10 and promote antibody production for humoral immunity. IL-12, secreted by macrophages and B cells, stimulates the production of IFN-γ in T cells and NK cells. IL-12 has been shown to act directly on CD4+ naive T cells derived from T receptor transgenic mice to induce IFN-γ production and T cell differentiation towards Th1 development (Seder et al. 1993). In contrast, IL-4 has been shown, in the same system, to drive Th2 cell development and Th2-specific cytokine

Table 11.2 Virus-induced modulation of cytokine effects

Virus	Viral gene	Cellular homologue	Effect
Poxviruses	MGF	EGF/TGFα	Cell growth
	T2	TNF receptor	TNF inhibition
	T7	IFN-γ receptor	IFN-γ inhibition
	Unmapped	IL-1 receptor	IL-1 inhibition
EBV	BCRF1 = vIL-10	IL-10	Escape from immune surveillance
Adenovirus	E1A = 14·7 kDa protein	...	Suppresses TNF lysis
	E1B = 19 kDa protein		Counteracts TNF effects
	VA RNA		Inhibits IFN-α/β

EBV, Epstein–Barr virus; EGF, epidermal growth factor; IFN, interferon; IL, interleukin; TGF, transforming growth factor; TNF, tumour necrosis factor.

expression. Moreover, Th2-specific cytokines, IL-4 and IL-10 inhibit IL-12 production in human macrophages and, thereby, the Th1 response. As both IL-12 and IL-10 are produced by macrophages, these can either promote or inhibit Th1 cell development, depending on the relative production of either cytokine by these cells. IFN-α stimulates production of Th1 cells and IFN-γ blocks Th2 development (Sher et al. 1992). Th1 and Th2 responses play important roles in viral clearance. In mice, Th1 clones are protective against lethal challenges with influenza virus, whereas Th2 clones are not protective and delay viral clearance (Graham, Braciale and Braciale 1994). A switch from Th1 to Th2 responses has been suggested as playing a role in HIV infection and progression to AIDS. According to this model, HIV-specific T cell responses of the Th1 type would keep the infection under control. An increased viraemia would result in a Th2 response, antibody production and progression to AIDS. In this model, any stimulus or pathogen that could promote a switch from Th1 to Th2 would act as a cofactor in the progression to AIDS. If this model holds true, treatment with exogenous IL-12 might support and maintain Th1 cell function and thus delay the progression of the disease. This question is being explored in a number of clinical trials.

4 ROLE OF CYTOKINES IN SPECIFIC VIRAL INFECTIONS

4.1 HIV replication and pathogenicity

Human immunodeficiency virus (HIV-1) (Chapter 38) is recognized as the aetiological agent of the slowly progressing immune deficiency in humans that culminates in the development of acquired immune deficiency syndrome (AIDS) (Barré-Sinoussi et al. 1983). The rate of progression of this lentiviral infection and the onset of the disease seem to depend on viral determinants (multiplicity of infection, virus strain or isolate), the interaction of HIV-1 with the host immune system and a number of co-factors, such as secondary viral and bacterial infections, cytokines or stress factors. The primary targets of HIV-1 infection are CD4+, especially T cells and the cells of the myeloid lineage, monocytes and macrophages.

Initial infection with HIV-1 is followed within 3–5 weeks by an acute phase characterized by influenza-like symptoms, lymphadenopathy, plasma viraemia and a significant decrease in circulating CD4+ cells. During the acute phase, HIV-1 disseminates to other tissues, particularly to the lymph nodes. The generation of an immune response at those sites results in the suppression of HIV-1 levels in the blood and restoration of the CD4+ cells. Infection then enters a state of clinical latency, when little virus can be detected in plasma. However, viral replication takes place in lymph nodes, where it continues to infect the CD4+ cells (Pantaleo et al. 1993). Recent studies from several laboratories have shown that, during these seemingly asymptomatic stages, virus-infected T cells are

rapidly cleared from the circulation by the vigorous immune response (Coffin 1995, Ho et al. 1995). The high replication rate of HIV-1 results in the death of lymphocytes that are continuously being replenished by the immune system. This leads to the gradual decrease in CD4+ T cells and the deterioration of the immune response. In the final stages of infection, HIV-1 reappears in the blood as a consequence of a breakdown of lymph node ultrastructure; the paucity of CD4+ cells and the lack of appropriate immune response facilitate numerous opportunistic infections and the development of neoplasia.

EFFECT OF HIV INFECTION ON CYTOKINE GENE EXPRESSION

The production of cytokines by macrophages and T cells is part of the inflammatory response to viral infection, which is essential for lymphocyte activation, generation of cytotoxic cellular responses and antibody production.

Increased levels of TNF-α, IL-1, IL-6, transforming growth factor β, (TGFβ) and IFN-α and IFN-β have been found in the sera of AIDS patients (Birx et al. 1990, Breen et al. 1990). However, in vitro, the spontaneous and LPS-stimulated production of TNF-α, IL-1, and IL-6 does not seem to be significantly different in peripheral blood lymphocytes (PBLs) isolated from AIDS and uninfected donors (D'Addario et al. 1990, Molina et al. 1990, Yamato et al. 1990). In another set of reports, an increase in TNF-α production in PBLs has been observed with the progression of HIV-1 infection (Rossol et al. 1992). An increase in the relative levels of TNF-α, IL-1 and IL-6 mRNAs has also been observed in LPS-stimulated alveolar macrophages isolated from individuals with AIDS, compared with the levels of mRNAs present in macrophages isolated during the early stages of HIV infection. Polyclonal activation of B cells (Reickmann et al. 1991) and increased levels of IL-6 may be associated with the higher frequency of B cell malignancies seen in AIDS patients.

Increased levels of IFN-α and IFN-γ (acid-labile IFN-α) were found both in pre-AIDS and in AIDS patients, but the frequencies and levels were higher in AIDS patients (Künzi and Pitha 1995). Elevated levels of IFN-α serum have been associated with a poor prognosis (Voth et al. 1990). It is not clear, however, what type of cell is responsible for IFN-α production in people infected with HIV-1 because, in vitro, HIV-1 infection of PBLs does not result in the induction of IFN gene expression; PBMCs isolated from individuals infected with HIV-1 or from AIDS patients has impaired IFN production upon stimulation with dsRNA, NDV or HSV-1 (Fitzgerald-Bocarsky et al. 1989). This impairment in IFN production seems to occur at the transcriptional level (Gendelman et al. 1990).

In contrast, HIV-1 infection of wild type in vitro seems to induce cytokine expression. Thus, stimulation of HIV-1-infected wild type with bacterial antigens from *Pneumocystis carinii* or *Mycobacterium avium* results in enhanced expression of TNF-α, IL-1, IL-6 and IL-8 mRNAs, compared to those present in stimulated but uninfected controls (Newman et al. 1993, Kandil et al. 1994). Both enhanced and unaltered cytokine expression have, however, been reported in HIV-1-infected wild type stimulated with LPS, and no difference in cytokine production between HIV-1-infected and uninfected wild type has been observed after stimulation with endotoxin or dsRNA (Gendelman et al. 1990, Molina et al. 1990). A large variability in reported results suggests that inducible expression of cytokine genes in wild type may depend both on genetic determinants and on the nature of the inducer.

The molecular mechanism by which HIV-1 infection alters spontaneous and inducible cytokine gene expression is not clear. However, as most of the cytokines (whose expression is up-regulated by HIV-1 infection) contain an NF-κB enhancer in their promoter and NF-κB-specific binding is essential for transcription activation, it is likely that the binding of the HIV-1 or gp120 to the CD4 receptor induces change in the signalling pathways, such as those leading to the activation of NF-κB heterodimers, that alter both the constitutive and the inducible expression of the cytokine genes.

EFFECT OF CYTOKINES ON HIV-1 REPLICATION

Transcription of HIV-1 is controlled by cellular and viral transactivators that bind to regulatory sequences present both in the long terminal repeat (LTR) of HIV-1 provirus and in the untranslated leader sequence of viral RNAs. Activation of viral transcription occurs upon binding of virally encoded tat protein to the tat-binding region present in all viral mRNAs (Rosen, Sodroski and Haseltine 1985, Cullen and Green 1989). In contrast, DNA elements present in the HIV-1 LTR, such as NF-κB enhancer (Nabel and Baltimore 1987), play a major role in the activation of the promoter by cellular and extracellular factors. Additional regulation of the inducible response is mediated through specific interaction between nuclear transactivators and the AP-1, NFAT, LBP-1, HLP-1 and TCF-1 DNA binding sequences (Jones, Luciw and Duchange 1988).

Many inflammatory cytokines stimulate HIV-1 transcription from the LTR and affect HIV-1 replication (Butera 1993, Poli and Fauci 1993). This observation is of biological importance, because cytokines are released during the immune response to HIV-1 infection and increased cytokine expression can be detected in lymph nodes in the vicinity of the focus of infection (Emille et al. 1991). The local environment in the infected lymph nodes allows for extensive interactions between activated B cells and T cells, resulting in the production of a variety of cytokines secreted in both an autocrine and a paracrine fashion. The profile of cytokines induced at the site of infection can then not only determine the nature of the immune response (cellular immunity mediated by cytotoxic T cell lymphocyte (CTL) response vs antibody response) but also directly affects HIV-1 repli-

cation and thus positively or negatively enhances the progression of disease.

Cytokine-mediated up-regulation of HIV-1 replication

Of the stimulatory cytokines, TNF-α probably has the most significant effect on HIV-1 replication and a direct role in the pathogenicity of HIV-1 infection has been attributed to it. In vitro, TNF-α can up-regulate the transcriptional activity of HIV-1 LTR and the effect is mediated by the induction of NF-κB binding in the nucleus (Duh et al. 1989, Osborn, Kunkel and Nabel 1989). It has been shown that the TNF-α-mediated signal transduction pathway begins with the binding of TNF-α to one of the membrane receptors TNF-Rβ (55 kDa) and proceeds through sphingomyelinase and ceramide (Schutze et al. 1992). The TNF-α-mediated activation is not limited to the HIV-1 LTR; TNF-α can also effectively induce the expression of poorly expressed (latent) HIV-1 provirus in both T cells and monocytes. An interesting feature of TNF-α activation from the point of view of HIV-1 replication is that it is independent of tat-mediated transactivation. TNF-α can effectively rescue transcription and viral replication of a mutant HIV-1 provirus in which the tat region is deleted and therefore transcriptionally inactive (Popik and Pitha 1993). These results point to the existence of an alternative pathway in HIV-1 transcription regulation that is independent of the virus-encoded transactivator, tat. Because elevated levels of TNF-α can be detected in the serum in the later stages of HIV-1 infection, it is assumed that TNF-α is one of the factors that contribute to the progression of the disease and to some of the clinical signs, such as AIDS-associated weight loss (Serwadda et al. 1985). The ability of TNF-α to activate HIV-1 replication in a tat-independent manner has important implications for the antiviral strategies aimed at eliminating tat transactivation. Effective inhibition of HIV-1 replication requires both tat and NF-κB inhibition, and, in the presence of TNF-α, the drug RO5 that blocks tat transactivation is not effective (Popik and Pitha 1994). Thus, the presence of TNF-α in the serum and the ability of TNF-α to transactivate HIV-1 replication in a tat-independent fashion may be one of the reasons why the drug RO5 was ineffective in clinical trials.

Several other cytokines up-regulate HIV-1 transcription and HIV-1 provirus in vitro. In vitro IL-1 stimulates transcription of a latent HIV-1 provirus in both T cells and monocyte lines (Poli et al. 1994); the induction was associated with the stimulation of NF-κB activities. IL-3 and the proteins of the colony stimulating factor (CSF) family, GM-CSF and M-CSF, up-regulate HIV-1 replication in primary macrophages and in monocyte and myeloid cell lines (Gendelman et al. 1990). It is interesting that CSF-mediated stimulation does not seem to be mediated entirely through NF-κB binding, as the region upstream of the NF-κB enhancer is also required for activation (Zack, Arrigo and Chen 1990). IL-6 is another cytokine that has been implicated in the up-regulation of HIV-1 replication (Poli, Kinter and Fauci 1994). In contrast to the other cytokines, IL-6-mediated enhancement does not seem to take place at the transcriptional level, but occurs at the post-transcriptional level. The exact mechanism of this enhancement is not known. Of importance from a biological point of view is the synergy between IL-6 and TNF-α or IL-1 which leads to a significant enhancement of HIV-1 replication (Poli et al. 1990, Poli, Kinter and Fauci 1994).

Cytokine-mediated down-regulation of HIV-1 infection

Recent data indicate that progression to AIDS is accompanied by a shift from a Th1 cytokine response and production of IL-2 and IFN-γ to a Th2 cytokine response, with production of IL-4, IL-6 and IL-10. In vivo, production of IFN-γ during the Th1 response may play a role in the down-regulation of HIV-1 infection. Although in vitro HIV-1 infection in wild type or primary macrophages does not induce IFN-α or IFN-β production, IFN-α can be detected in serum during the later stages of HIV-1 infection. The biological role in vivo of this IFN is not known, but IFN-α, IFN-β and IFN-γ can effectively inhibit HIV-1 replication in vitro.

In vitro, IFNs inhibit HIV-1 replication both in primary cells (wild type and macrophages) and in established T cells and monocytic cell lines (Yamamoto 1986, Kornbluth et al. 1989, Poli et al. 1989, Gendelman et al. 1990). In a single cycle infection in T cells (Shirazi and Pitha 1992) or in IFN-producing cells (Bednarik et al. 1989), IFN inhibits early steps in HIV-1 replication and HIV-1 transcripts cannot be detected in these cells (Shirazi and Pitha 1993). Furthermore, in primary macrophages, IFN decreases the levels of integrated provirus (Kornbluth et al. 1990). Hence, in multiple infection cycles or in chronic infection, IFN inhibited HIV-1 replication at the post-translational level and decreased the levels of virus released into the culture medium, but did not substantially affect the synthesis of viral RNA and proteins in infected cells. The mechanism by which IFN inhibits HIV-1 replication at the pre-integrational step is not clear. Inhibition of the early replication steps has been observed in cells constitutively producing low levels of IFN-β, and it has been suggested that inhibition occurs at the level of viral uptake.

IFN also inhibits the activation of HIV-1 provirus by external stimuli in vitro. Poli et al. (1989) have shown that TNF-α-mediated stimulation of HIV-1 provirus is inhibited by IFN-α, and it has been suggested that the IFN-mediated block is at the level of virus maturation and assembly. Activation of a *tat*-defective provirus by 12-*O*-tetradecanylphorbol 13-acetate (TPA) or by HSV-1 is also inhibited in the presence of IFN. However, the inability of these inducers to activate HIV-1 provirus in the presence of IFN occurs at the transcriptional level, and is associated with the alteration of NF-κB-specific binding (Popik and Pitha 1991, 1992).

Several studies have shown that, although HIV-1 infection does not induce IFN type I synthesis in vitro, it can modulate the levels of at least 2 dsRNA-dependent enzymes, 2',5'-OAS and RNaseL, and induce expression of Mx protein. It has also been shown that the activation of PKR by tat-binding region (Edery, Petryshyn and Sonenberg 1989) inhibits the translation of HIV-1 mRNAs and that inhibition of protein synthesis correlates with phosphorylation of eF-2. Yet none of these IFN-induced proteins seems to play a significant role in the IFN-mediated inhibition of HIV-1 replication. Neither small nor large 2',5'-OAS can be detected in HIV-1-infected cells (Popik and Pitha, unpublished). Productive HIV-1 infection leads to a decrease, not an increase, in cellular PKR activity. It has been suggested that the binding of the cellular protein TRBP to the tat-binding region interferes with recognition of the dsRNA structure and prevents induction of PKR (Park et al. 1994) in HIV-1-infected cells. Together, these results indicate that IFN can inhibit many steps of the HIV-1 replication cycle with differing efficiency and they suggest that, in vivo, IFN may have a broad spectrum of action (Fig. 11.2).

Cytokines with both stimulatory and inhibitory effects on HIV-1 replication

The wide range of biological properties of certain cytokines is often manifested by their bifunctional effects. This is also true of their effects on HIV-1 replication. TGFβ pretreatment can stimulate HIV-1 replication in primary T cells and in myeloid and monocytic cell lines (Lazdins et al. 1991, Poli et al. 1991). However, when TGFβ is applied to infected cultures, it inhibits PMA, TNF and IL-6-mediated stimulation of HIV-1 replication (Poli et al. 1991). IL-4 is another cytokine with a bifunctional effect on HIV-1 replication: it can either induce or inhibit HIV-1 replication in myeloid cells. In undifferentiated monocytes, IL-4 stimulates HIV-1 replication as well as the proliferation of the cells (Kazazi et al. 1992, Foli et al. 1995) whereas, in differentiated macrophages, IL-4 suppresses HIV-1 replication (Novak et al. 1990). In T cells, however, IL-4 does not affect HIV transcription. This indicates that differences in host cells and types of infection, as well as the timing of exposure to cytokines, may determine the outcome of the cytokine effects.

4.2 Herpesvirus infections

Herpesviruses selectively regulate pro-inflammatory cytokine synthesis. Human herpesvirus 6 (HHV-6) infection induces high levels of IL-1β and TNF-β in wild type cultures but inhibits the induction of IL-6. In the same cells, EBV inhibits TNF-α secretion (Gosselin et al. 1992). The pattern of cytokine expression during herpes simplex virus (HSV)-induced keratitis (HSK) has been well studied in the mouse and human cornea. HSV-1 infection in murine keratinocytes induces transient expression of TNF-α, IL-6 and IL-1, a cytokine profile that is characteristic of a transient inflammatory response (Sprecher and Becker 1992). Exogenous IL-10, a cytokine with inflammatory suppressive activity, also significantly decreases IL-6 levels in HSV-1-infected murine cornea and sharply reduces the incidence of blindness sec-

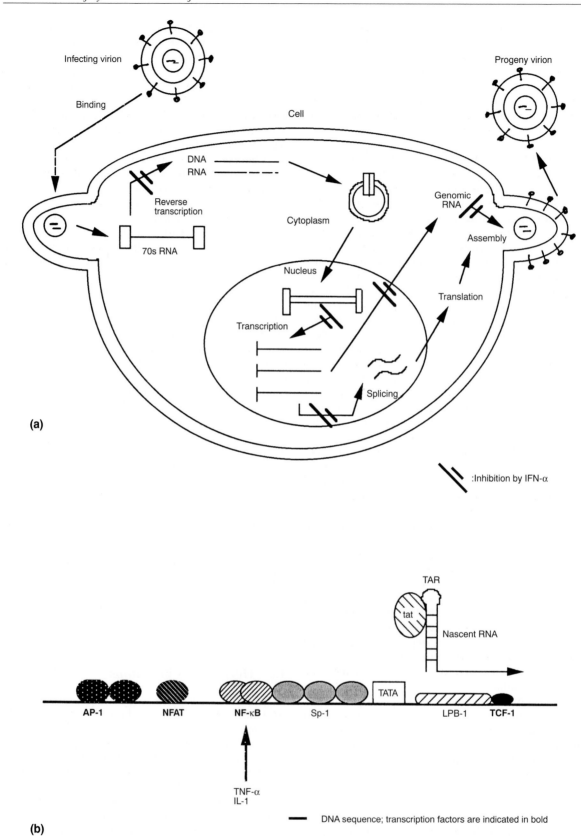

Fig. 11.2 (a) IFN-α inhibition of the HIV-1 life cycle. (b) Cytokine activation of HIV long terminal repeats.

ondary to the HSV-1-induced inflammatory response, even though IL-1α levels are not decreased (Tumpey et al. 1994). At low concentrations, IFN-γ and TNF-α induce a synergistic antiviral effect against HSV-1 in human corneal cells (Chen, Oakes and Lausch 1994). Cells isolated from eyes in the active phase of HSK have been found to be of the CD4+ Th1 subset, secreting IL-2, IFN-γ and TNF-α but not IL-4 or IL-10 (Niemialtowski and Rouse 1992). Treatment with monoclonal antibodies specific for IFN-γ or IL-2 reduces the severity of HSV-1-induced corneal inflammation in mice, and inhibition of IFN-γ production by UV-irradiation enhances IL-4 production as well as zosteriform skin lesions (Hendricks, Tumpey and Finnegan 1992, Yasumoto et al. 1994). These findings indicate that Th1 and Th2 responses define the pathogenicity of HSV-1 in the cornea and the skin. HSV-1 and HSV-2 activate macrophages and induce IFN-α/β production, which synergizes with TNF-α in an autocrine manner to protect macrophages from herpetic infection (Ellerman-Eriksen, Christensen and Morgensen 1994).

EBV infection is associated with acute, self-limiting, infectious mononucleosis, chronic infectious mononucleosis and lymphoproliferative disease (LPD). In all acute forms of EBV infection, IFN-γ, TNF-α, IL-2 and IL-6 are elevated (Linde et al. 1992). EBV-associated LPDs are a common complication of primary immunodeficiency and are associated with elevated serum levels of IL-4 and, to a lesser extent, IL-5, IL-10 and IFN-γ (Mathur et al. 1994). Cyclosporin A, used in immunosuppressive therapy, increases EBV-associated lymphoproliferative disorders by inducing IL-6 expression in T cells and by increasing the number of EBV-immortalized B cells expressing viral lytic antigens. Exposure to EBV stimulates IL-6 expression in B cells and in monocytes (Tanner and Menezes 1994).

EBV-infected B cells express IL-10 and B cell regulatory factor (BCRF) 1, the viral homologue of IL-10, and expression of both viral and cellular cytokines is maintained during transformation. Inhibition of viral IL-10 (vIL-10) expression with antisense oligonucleotides at the time of viral challenge prevents EBV B cell transformation; conversely, transformation is rescued by exogenous cellular IL-10. These observations indicate that EBV-encoded IL-10 is a latency gene involved in B cell transformation (Miyazaki, Cheung and Dosh 1993). EBV has been implicated in the aetiology of Sjögren's syndrome, a disease characterized by lymphocytic infiltration, squamous cell metaplasia and a decrease in goblet cell numbers in the conjunctival epithelium of the eye. Although the marker for latent EBV infection, EBNA-1 or EBV IL-10 is not expressed at a higher frequency than in the normal eye, HLA-DR, ICAM-1 and IL-6 expression is significantly increased in Sjögren's syndrome (Jones et al. 1994).

4.3   Infections with hepatitis viruses

Hepatitis virus clearance and persistence hinge upon the intricate, and as yet not fully understood, modulation of virus-induced cytokines. Monocytic production of IL-6, the mediator of acute-phase protein synthesis in hepatocytes, is decreased in chronic hepatitis B virus (HBV) infection, whereas it is normal in chronic hepatitis C virus (HCV) and in acute hepatitis A virus (HAV), HBV and HCV infections. Exacerbation of chronic HBV induces expression of IL-6 and TNF-α which correlates with an increase in HBV DNA levels in serum (Kakumu et al. 1991, Sheran et al. 1991). Moreover, IL-6 contains recognition sites for the segment of the HBV envelope protein through which the virus binds to cell surfaces (Neurath, Strick and Sproul 1992).

HBV is not cytopathic, but it evokes a strong lymphomononuclear inflammatory response in the liver during acute and chronic infections. Transgenic mice whose hepatocytes do not secrete HBV but retain the antigen in the endoplasmic reticulum, are highly susceptible to liver damage induced by bacterial lipopolysaccharide, a potent inducer of inflammatory cytokines. The effect seems to be mediated by both IFN-γ and TNF-α. Hepatocellular injury and induction of inflammatory cytokines coincide with a reduction in HBV steady-state mRNA content (Gilles et al. 1992). TNF-α induces 2 other proinflammatory cytokines, IL-8 and IL-6, in patients with chronic HBV. Inflammatory cytokines appear to down-regulate HBV expression by both TNF-α-dependent and TNF-α-independent pathways. Administration of exogenous recombinant TNF-α, IL-2, IFN-α and IFN-β has been shown to reduce steady-state levels of HBV RNA in transgenic mice. TNF-α antibodies block the effect of TNF-α and IL-2 but not that of IFNs. Administration of exogenous IFN-γ, IL-1, IL-3, IL-6 or TNF-α has no effect on the HBV RNA levels (Guidotti, Guilhot and Chisari 1994). Deregulation of the inflammatory cascade can have disastrous effects, as illustrated by fulminant hepatic failure, characterized by a striking elevation of IL-6, TNF-α, IL-1Rα and IL-1β levels (Sekiyama, Yoshiba and Thomson 1994). IFN-γ and HBV X protein increase the rate of transcription of intercellular adhesion molecule 1 (ICAM 1), a molecule critically important to adhesion-dependent leucocyte functions, such as antigen presentation and target cell lysis (Hu, Yu and Vierling 1992). IFN-γ initially also activates HBV-specific class I restricted CTL, suppressing expression of the HBV gene.

Chronic hepatitis B, C or D may lead to cirrhosis, hepatocellular failure or hepatocellular carcinoma. IFN-α has recently become the treatment of choice for chronic hepatitis, because HBV and HCV infections respond well to treatment with it. Sustained loss of HBV DNA and HBV nucleocapsid and surface antigens leads to the restoration of normal liver function. However, the relatively high prevalence of resistance of HBV to IFN is of concern. It was shown that the terminal domain of HBV polymerase is responsible for the resistance of the virus to IFN-α and IFN-γ. Individuals infected with several HCV quasi-species seem to be less responsive to IFN therapy than are those with a single major species (Gutterman 1994, Dusheiko 1995).

5 CYTOKINE RESPONSES TO VIRAL INFECTIONS OF THE CENTRAL NERVOUS SYSTEM

There is increasing evidence that local cytokine production induced as a response to viral infection of cells of the CNS or infiltrating lymphoid cells plays a crucial role in the pathogenicity and outcome of viral infection in this location (Benveniste 1992).

Local synthesis of TNF-α within the CNS seems to be especially damaging. TNF-α damages glial cells and has a direct toxic effect on neurons. In vitro, TNF-α induces demyelination of oligodendrocytes, whereas the closely related TNF-β kills oligodendrocytes by inducing apoptosis. Production of both TNF-α and TNF-β in the CNS results in the death of myelin-producing oligodendrocytes. TNF-α can also act indirectly by stimulating microglia and astrocytes to produce nitric oxide and the neurotoxic metabolites of arachidonic acid (Benveniste 1995). TNF-α also stimulates synthesis of other cytokines such as GM-CSF, G-CSF and M-CSF, which enhance inflammatory responses as well as the synthesis of IL-6 (Doherty, Allan and Clark 1989, Moskophidis et al. 1991, Campbell et al. 1994). IL-6 enhances inflammation in the CNS as well as stimulating the proliferation of B cells and their differentiation into antibody-producing cells.

The local immune responses in the CNS and the outcome of the infection are affected by the cytokines induced in situ, whether directly in infected cells (Sebire et al. 1993, Wesselingh et al. 1994), as a response to viral infection (e.g. IFNs, TNF-α or IL-6 in astrocytes or microglia) or by infiltrating T cells and macrophages during local inflammation (Shankar et al. 1992, Gillespie et al. 1993).

It is interesting that the profile of cytokines synthesized in the CNS seems to be determined by the type of the infecting virus rather than by the type of the host cells. Thus, infection of neurons with lymphocytic choriomeningitis virus (LCMV) leads to synthesis of TNF-α, IL-1, IL-6 and IFN-γ, generating a strong CTL response (Campbell et al. 1994).The strong Th1 cytokine response and induction of cytotoxic T cells leads ultimately to death, whereas viral replication alone is regulated by the presence of IFNs. The association of LCMV pathogenicity with the immune response provided the first clear evidence that viral pathogenicity may be mediated by the immune response of the host (Rowe 1954). In contrast, the infection of neurons with the Sindbis virus (an alphavirus closely related to Western equine encephalitis virus), which causes acute encephalomyelitis in mice, results in generation of the Th2 cytokine response (Wesselingh et al. 1994). Increases in mRNAs and IL-1, IL-4, IL-6, IL-10 and TNF-α proteins have been observed during the early stages of acute infection in mice, followed by the appearance of antiviral antibodies and clearance of virus from the CNS (Tyor et al. 1989, Levine et al. 1991). Although it has been suggested that the CNS may provide an environment that favours B cell antibody response, it is difficult at present to generalize

this finding. Thus, recovery from acute HSV infection depends on a T cell response, whereby the MHC class I-restricted CD8+ cytotoxic T lymphocytes control HSV infection in the brain (Schmidt and Rouse 1992, Nash and Cambouropoulos 1993). Secretion of IFN-γ from activated T cells is critical for clearing of herpes virus infection (Raniero et al. 1990, Lucin et al. 1992). Recently, it has been shown that the T cell inflammatory response and production of IFN-γ persist in trigeminal ganglia long after HSV-1 has established the latent phase of infection (Cantin et al. 1995). This observation may indicate that the prolonged production of IFN-γ and possibly also of other cytokines (e.g. TNF-α) (Schmidt and Rouse 1992) may block or suppress HSV-1 replication after reactivation from latency (Cunningham and Merigan 1983, Torseth and Merigan 1986).

Deregulated local production of cytokines in the brain has also been observed in patients with AIDS dementia complex (ADC), which afflicts 30–50% of all people infected with HIV-1 (Johnson, McArthur and Narayan 1988). In the CNS, HIV-1 can be found primarily in infiltrating monocytes and macrophages as well as in resident microglia (Koenig et al. 1986, Wiley et al. 1986), but there is evidence for major damage to neurons (Ketzler et al. 1990). There is no explanation at present for the cause of this extensive neurological impairment. It has been suggested that cytokines produced in macrophages and glial cells in response to HIV-1 infection (Gelbard et al. 1994) may either directly damage the neurons or alter the function of astrocytes and, consequently, neuronal function (Benveniste 1992, 1995).

Analysis of the cerebrospinal fluid from ADC patients has shown elevated levels of IL-1, TNF-α, IL-6 and neopterin, an indicator of the presence of IFN-γ (Grimaldi et al. 1991). With the exception of IFN-γ, all these substances are the products of activated macrophages and microglia; IFN-γ is most likely to be produced by infiltrating CD8+ cells (Tyor et al. 1992). The expression of cytokine mRNA in the brain has been analysed (Wesselingh et al. 1993). The results reveal a strong association between increased levels of TNF-α mRNA and ADC. As discussed above, TNF-α induces many abnormalities in the CNS and so its overproduction may be one of the causes of the neuron dysfunction in ADC. It is interesting that an increased number of TNF-α-producing cells was also observed in patients with other neurological disease such as multiple sclerosis (Benveniste 1995). These data suggest that TNF-α may play a major role in inflammatory disorders of the CNS.

6 DIRECTED CYTOKINE EXPRESSION WITH RECOMBINANT VIRUSES

(See also Chapter 40, section 1.3) The role of individual cytokines in response to viral infection has been studied by using recombinant cytokines administered systematically. This approach does not mimic well conditions in vivo, in which cytokines are acting locally and presumably in much higher concentrations (Biron, Young and Kasaian 1990). Results from experiments with transgenic animals expressing IL-2 (Ishida et al. 1989), IL-4 (Tepper et al. 1990), IL-5 (Tominaga et al. 1991) or GM-CSF (Lang et al. 1987) have often been difficult to interpret, because of the widely spread expression. More clear-cut results have been obtained with experiments in which animals with a homozygous deletion of a given cytokine or its receptor are used (e.g. IFN-γR nu/nu mice (Huang et al. 1993), IL-6 nu/nu mice) or when production of cytokines is suppressed by monoclonal antibodies (Leist, Eppler and Zinkernagel 1989).

Recently, a new technique has been used, whereby a cytokine gene inserted in a non-essential part of a recombinant virus is able to target cytokine production directly to the focus of infection. This makes it possible to determine the effect of local cytokine production on viral replication and the immunological consequences of cytokine overproduction. The most common type of virus for cytokine delivery has been vaccinia virus (Ramshaw et al. 1992), although HSV-1 (Mester, Pitha and Glorioso 1995) and mouse CMV (Burnes 1995, personal communication) have also been used.

Vaccinia virus is a complex DNA virus that replicates in the cytoplasm. Foreign DNA can easily be inserted into the virus under the control of a viral promoter (Davidson and Moss 1989), and foreign proteins are processed and transported with fidelity (Moss and Flexner 1987). Furthermore, a large region of this virus DNA genome is not essential for replication. Insertion of the IL-2 gene into vaccinia virus enhances neither T cell-mediated immunity nor the immune response, but it decreases the virulence of the virus and enables immune-suppressed mice to resolve infection (Ramshaw et al. 1992). Enhancement of NK cytotoxic activity is an important factor in the clearance of infection in nude mice, and it has been found that IFN-γ plays an essential role in IL-2-mediated recovery. Since no host response was demonstrated that explained the rapid clearance of IFN-γ-expressing virus, these authors concluded that the observed inhibition in viral replication is caused by the direct antiviral effect of IFN. Similarly, the recombinant virus expressing TNF-α was rapidly cleared without any detectable involvement of the host immune system. Furthermore, local production of TNF-α was not toxic and no pathogenicity induced by TNF-α could be detected. Thus, TNF-α, like IFN-γ, seems to inhibit viral replication by the direct antiviral effect (Sambhi, Kohonen-Corish and Ramshaw 1991). These results indicate that overproduction of Th1 cytokines inhibits viral replication. Inhibition of viral replication is localized and limited to the recombinant virus and does not affect the co-inoculated control virus (Ramshaw et al. 1992).

To determine the effect of Th2 cytokines on the course of viral infection, recombinant viruses expressing Th2 cytokines have been constructed. In normal mice, recombinant virus encoding IL-4 replicates more efficiently than control virus, whereas expression of IL-5 or IL-6 has no apparent antiviral effect. However, vectors encoding IL-5 and IL-6 significantly increase terminal differentiation of IgA-committed B cells and mucosal IgA antibody response in vivo (Ramsey and Kohonen-Corish 1993, Ramsey et al. 1994). Expression of IL-6 augments both the primary systemic antibody and the mucosal antibody responses. In contrast, expression of IFN-γ significantly inhibits antibody responses without affecting the general cell-mediated immune response (Leong et al. 1994). Furthermore, the vectors expressing IL-6 are able to reconstitute the IgA and IgG responses in IL-6-deficient mice (Ramsey et al. 1994). These results indicate that IL-6 plays a critical role in the induction of mucosal immunity.

Herpes simplex virus type 1 (HSV-1) has also been used for targeted delivery of cytokine genes. Weir and Elkins (1993) inserted a human IFNA gene into a replication-incompetent herpesvirus and showed that IFN expressed in infected monocytes is able to inhibit HIV-1 replication. Murine IFNA has been inserted in both replication-competent and incompetent HSV-1. HSV-1-derived IFNA gene expression did not inhibit HSV-1 replication in vitro; however, preinfection of the cells with the non-replicating HSV–IFN vector provided complete protection against a subsequent viral challenge (Mester et al. 1995). Replication-defective vectors derived from HSV-1 have also been used for delivering genes to neurons (Fink et al. 1992), suggesting their usefulness for analysing cytokine effects within the nervous system. In summary, these approaches suggest a novel and highly effective approach to the study of local cytokine effects in viral infections and to the effectiveness of virus-derived vectors in vaccine development and cytokine gene therapy.

7 CONCLUSION

It is evident that viral infection induces a complex host response mediated by the induction of genes encoding various cytokines and lymphokines, as well as stress proteins. This response can be induced directly in the infected cells or indirectly in cells of lymphoid origin tethered to the focus of infection during the immune response. The primary function of these cytokines is either to inhibit viral replication or to activate the cells mediating the cellular and humoral immune responses. However, inflammatory cytokines, produced during the immune response, are not always beneficial to the host and can contribute to the pathogenicity and side effects of viral infections. The detrimental effect of cytokines can be most clearly demonstrated in conditions in which infection is localized to a specific organ or system such as the CNS. Then, production of even relatively low levels of cytokines, such as TNF-α, can have profoundly toxic effects and result in the death of neurons or the dysfunction of oligodendrocytes.

Several viruses have developed ways to eliminate or

overcome the effect of cytokines. This again demonstrates the great plasticity of some viral genomes and their ability to adapt. Thus, HIV-1 has modified its regulatory region to resemble the promoter of some of the inflammatory cytokines, and can therefore use several of the inflammatory cytokines to stimulate its own replication. Other viruses, such as the poxviruses, carry several genes that encode soluble cytokine receptors; others, such as adenovirus, have developed a specific mechanism that can allow them to inhibit the effects of cytokines. Some of the HIV-1-encoded accessory proteins may carry similar functions. Expression of viral genes that inhibit cytokine functions seems to be essential for the replication of many of these viruses in vivo, because the replication and pathogenicity of mutants with 'mimicry' functions deleted are usually considerably diminished. One of the main objects of future research should, therefore, be to characterize these cytokine-inhibiting viral functions; this would help not only to understand the role that a given cytokine plays in a particular viral infection but also to generate attenuated, non-pathogenic viruses that could be used for vaccine development. However, the real challenge will be to use the mechanisms that viruses have developed to avoid the immune response as selective tools to eliminate viral infections.

REFERENCES

Adler KB, Fischer BM et al., 1994, Interactions between respiratory epithelial cell and cytokines: relationship to lung inflammation, *Ann N Y Acad Sci*, **725:** 128–45.

Akkaraju GR, Whitaker-Dowling P et al., 1989, Vaccinia specific kinase inhibitory factor prevents translational inhibition by double-stranded RNA in rabbit reticulocyte lysate, *J Biol Chem*, **264:** 10321–5.

Allan G, Fantes K, 1980, A family of structural genes for human lymphoblastoid (leukocyte-type) interferon, *Nature (London)*, **287:** 408–11.

Anderson KP, Lie YS et al., 1993, Effects of tumor necrosis factor-alpha treatment on mortality in murine cytomegalovirus-infected mice, *Antiviral Res*, **21:** 343–55.

Arman MJ, Keller U et al., 1994, Regulation of cytokine expression by interferon-alpha in human bone marrow structural cells: inhibition of hematopoietic growth factors and induction of interleukin-1 receptor antagonist, *Blood*, **84:** 4142–50.

Arnold R, Humbert B et al., 1994, Interleukin-8, interleukin-6 and soluble tumor necrosis factor receptor type I release from a human pulmonary epithelial cell line (A549) exposed to respiratory syncytial virus, *Immunology*, **82:** 126–33.

Barré-Sinoussi F, Chermann J-C et al., 1983, Isolation of a T-lymphotropic retrovirus from a patient at risk for acquired immune deficiency syndrome (AIDS), *Science*, **220:** 868–71.

Becker S, Quay J, Soukup S, 1991, Cytokine (tumor necrosis factor, IL-6 and IL-8) production by respiratory syncytial virus-infected human alveolar macrophages, *J Immunol*, **147:** 4307–12.

Bednarik DP, Mosca JD et al., 1989, Inhibition of human immunodeficiency virus (HIV) replication by HIV-*trans*-activated α2-interferon, *Proc Natl Acad Sci USA*, **86:** 4958–62.

Benveniste EN, 1992, Inflammatory cytokines within the central nervous system: sources, function and mechanism of action, *Am J Physiol*, **263:** C1–16.

Benveniste EN, 1995, Role of cytokines in multiple sclerosis, autoimmune encephalitis and other neurological disorders, *Human Cytokines: their role in research and therapy*, eds Aagarwal BB, Puri RK, Blackwell Science, Cambridge MA, 195–216.

Berry MJ, Knutson GS et al., 1985, Purification and substrate specificities of the double-stranded RNA-dependent protein kinase from untreated and interferon-treated mouse fibroblasts, *J Biochem*, **260:** 11240–7.

Biron CA, Young HA, Kasaian MT, 1990, Interleukin 2-induced proliferation of murine natural killer cells *in vivo*, *J Exp Med*, **171:** 173–88.

Birx DL, Redfield RR et al., 1990, Induction of interleukin-6 during human immunodeficiency virus infection, *Blood*, **76:** 2303–10.

Birx DL, Lewis MG et al., 1993, Association of IL-6 in the pathogenesis of acutely fatal SIVsmm-PBj-14 in pigtailed macaques, *AIDS Res Hum Retroviruses*, **9:** 1123–9.

Breen E, Rezal A et al., 1990, Infection with HIV is associated with elevated IL-6 levels and production, *J Immunol*, **144:** 480–4.

Bukowski JF, Welsh RM, 1985, Interferon enhances the susceptibility of virus-infected fibroblasts to cytotoxic T cells, *J Exp Med*, **161:** 257–62.

Butera S, 1993, Cytokine involvement in viral permissiveness and the progression of HIV disease, *J Cell Biochem*, **53:** 336–42.

Campbell IL, Hobbs MV et al., 1994, Cerebral expression of multiple cytokine genes in mice with lymphocytic choriomeningitis, *J Immunol*, **152:** 716–23.

Cantin EM, Hinton DR et al., 1995, Gamma interferon expression during acute and latent nervous system infection by herpes simplex virus type 1, *J Virol*, **69:** 4898–905.

Chebath J, Benech P et al., 1987, Constitutive expression of (2'-5') oligo A synthetase confers resistance to picornavirus infection, *Nature (London)*, **330:** 587–8.

Chen SH, Oakes JE, Lausch RN, 1994, Synergistic anti-herpes effect of TNF-alpha and IFN-gamma in human corneal epithelial cells compared with that in corneal fibroblasts, *Antiviral Res*, **25:** 201–13.

Coffin JM, 1995, HIV population dynamics *in vivo*: implications for genetic variation, pathogenesis, and therapy, *Science*, **267:** 483–9.

Cullen BR, Greene WC, 1989, Regulatory pathways governing HIV-1 replication, *Cell*, **58:** 423–6.

Cunningham AL, Merigan TC, 1983, γ-Interferon production appears to predict time of recurrence of herpes labialis, *J Immunol*, **130:** 2397–400.

Czarniecki CW, 1993, The role of tumor necrosis factor in viral disease, *Antiviral Res*, **22:** 223–58.

D'Addario M, Roulston A et al., 1990, Coordinate enhancement of cytokine gene expression in human immunodeficiency virus type 1-infected promonocytic cells, *J Virol*, **64:** 6080–9.

Darnell JE, Kerr IM, Stark GR, 1994, Jak-STAT pathways and transcriptional activation in response to IFNs and other extracellular signaling proteins, *Science*, **264:** 1415–20.

Davidson AJ, Moss B, 1989, Structure of vaccinia virus early promoters, *J Mol Biol*, **210:** 771–84.

Davies MV, Furtado M et al., 1989, Complementation of adenovirus virus-associated RNA I gene deletion by expression of a mutant eukaryotic translation initiation factor, *Proc Natl Acad Sci USA*, **86:** 9163–7.

Devergne O, Peuchmaur M et al., 1991, In vivo expression of IL-1 beta and IL-6 genes during viral infection in humans, *Eur Cytokine Netw*, **2:** 183–94.

Diaz MO, 1995, The human type 1 interferon gene cluster, *Semin Virol*, **6:** 143–9.

Doherty PC, Allan JE, Clark IA, 1989, Tumor necrosis factor inhibits the development of viral meningitis or induces rapid death depending on the severity of inflammation at time of administration, *J Immunol*, **142:** 3576–80.

D'Onofrio C, Franzese O et al., 1992, Antiviral activity of individual versus combined treatments with interferon alpha, beta and gamma on early infection with HTLV-I in vitro, *Int J Immunopharmacol*, **14:** 1069–79.

Duh EJ, Maury WJ et al., 1989, Tumor necrosis factor α activates human immunodeficiency virus-1 through induction of a nuclear factor binding to the NF-κB sites in the long terminal repeat, *Proc Natl Acad Sci USA*, **86:** 5974–8.

Dusheiko GM, 1995, Treatment and prevention of chronic viral hepatitis, *Pharmacol Ther*, **65:** 47–73.

Edery I, Petryshyn R, Sonenberg N, 1989, Activation of double-stranded RNA-dependent kinase (dsl) by the TAR region of HIV-1 mRNA: a novel translational control mechanism, *Cell*, **56:** 303–12.

Ellerman-Eriksen S, Christensen MM, Mogensen SC, 1994, Effect of mercuric chloride on macrophage-mediated resistance mechanisms against infection with herpes simplex virus type 2, *Toxicology*, **93:** 269–87.

Emille D, Peuchmaur M et al., 1991, Production of interleukins in human immunodeficiency virus 1-replicating lymph nodes, *J Clin Invest*, **86:** 148–59.

Fingerote RJ, Cruz BM et al., 1995, A 2′,5′-oligoadenylate analogue inhibits murine hepatitis virus strain 3 (MHV-3) replication in vitro but does not reduce MHV-3-related mortality or induction of procoagulant activity in susceptible mice, *J Gen Virol*, **76:** 373–80.

Fink DJ, Sternberg LR et al., 1992, *In vivo* expression of β-galactosidase in hippocampal neurons by HSV-mediated gene transfer, *Hum Gene Ther*, **3:** 11–19.

Finter NB, Chapman S et al., 1991, The use of interferon-alpha in virus infections, *Drugs*, **42:** 749–65.

Fitzgerald-Bocarsky P, Feldman M et al., 1989, Deficient interferon-gamma production and natural NK activity in AIDS patients with HIV-2 infection, *J Infect Dis*, **160:** 1084–5.

Flamand L, Gosselin J et al., 1991, Human herpesvirus 6 induces interleukin-1b and tumor necrosis factor alpha, but not interleukin-6 in peripheral blood mononuclear cell cultures, *J Virol*, **65:** 5105–10.

Foli A, Saville MW et al., 1995, Effects of the Th1 and Th2 stimulatory cytokines interleukin-12 and interleukin-4 on human immunodeficiency virus replication, *Blood*, **86:** 2114–23.

Franke-Ullman G, Pfortner C et al., 1995, Alteration of pulmonary macrophage function by respiratory syncytial virus infection in vitro, *J Immunol*, **154:** 268–80.

Frese M, Kochs G et al., 1995, MxA protein mediates resistance to hantavirus, *J Interferon Cytok Res*, **15, suppl 1:** S231.

Gelbard HA, Nottet HSLM et al., 1994, Platelet-activating factor: a candidate human immunodeficiency virus type 1-induced neurotoxin, *J Virol*, **68:** 4628–35.

Gendelman HE, Baca LM et al., 1990, Regulation of HIV replication in infected monocytes by IFN-α: mechanisms for viral restriction, *J Immunol*, **145:** 2669–76.

Gilles PN, Guerrette DL et al., 1992, HBsAg retention sensitizes the hepatocyte to injury by physiological concentrations of interferon-gamma, *Hepatology*, **16:** 655–63.

Gillespie JS, Cavanagh MA et al., 1993, Increased transcription of interleukin-6 in the brains of mice with chronic enterovirus infection, *J Gen Virol*, **74:** 741–3.

Gosselin S, Flamand L et al., 1992, Infection of peripheral blood mononuclear cells by herpes simplex and Epstein–Barr viruses: differential induction of interleukin-6 and tumor necrosis factor-α, *J Clin Invest*, **89:** 1849–56.

Graham MB, Braciale VL, Braciale TJ, 1994, Influenza virus-specific CD4+ T helper type 2 T lymphocytes do not promote recovery from experimental virus infection, *J Exp Med*, **180:** 1273–82.

Grimaldi LME, Martion GV et al., 1991, Elevated alpha-tumor necrosis factor levels in spinal fluid from HIV-1-infected patients with central nervous system involvement, *Ann Neurol*, **29:** 21–5.

Guidotti LG, Guilhot S, Chisari FV, 1994, Interleukin-2 and alpha/beta interferon down-regulate hepatitis B virus gene expression in vivo by tumor necrosis factor-dependent and -independent pathways, *J Virol*, **68:** 1265–70.

Gutterman JU, 1994, Cytokine therapeutics: lessons from interferon α, *Proc Natl Acad Sci USA*, **91:** 1198–205.

Haller O, Arnheiter H et al., 1979, Genetically determined, interferon-dependent resistance to influenza virus in mice, *J Exp Med*, **149:** 601–12.

Heise MT, Virgin HW, 1995, The T-cell-independent role of gamma interferon and tumor necrosis factor alpha in macrophage activation during murine cytomegalovirus and herpes simplex virus infection, *J Virol*, **69:** 904–9.

Hendricks RL, Tumpey TM, Finnegan A, 1992, IFN-gamma and IL-2 are protective in the skin but pathologic in the corneas of HSV-1 infected mice, *J Immunol*, **149:** 3023–8.

Ho DD, Neumann AU et al., 1995, Rapid turnover of plasma virions and CD4 lymphocytes in HIV-1 infection, *Nature (London)*, **373:** 123–6.

Hober D, Poli L et al., 1993, Serum levels of tumor necrosis factor-alpha (TNF-alpha), interleukin-6 (IL-6), and IL-1 beta in dengue infected patients, *Am J Trop Med Hyg*, **48:** 324–31.

Hu KQ, Yu CH, Vierling JM, 1992, Up-regulation of intercellular adhesion molecule 1 transcription by hepatitis B virus X protein, *Proc Natl Acad Sci USA*, **89:** 11441–5.

Huang S, Hendriks W et al., 1993, Immune response in mice that lack the interferon-γ receptor, *Science*, **259:** 1742–5.

Imani F, Jacobs BL, 1988, Inhibitory activity for the interferon-induced protein kinase is associated with the reovirus serotype 1 sigma 3 protein, *Proc Natl Acad Sci USA*, **80:** 7887–91.

Ishida I, Nishi M et al., 1989, Effects of deregulated expression of human interleukin-2 in transgenic mice, *Int Immunol*, **1:** 113–19.

Jacobsen M, Mestan J et al., 1989, Beta-interferon subtype induction by tumor necrosis factor, *Mol Cell Biol*, **9:** 3037–42.

Johnson RT, McArthur JC, Narayan O, 1988, The neurobiology of human immunodeficiency virus infections, *FASEB J*, **2:** 2970–81.

Johnston MI, Torrence PF, 1984, The role of interferon-induced proteins, double-stranded RNA and 2′,5′-oligoadenylate in the interferon-mediated inhibition of viral translation, *Interferon*, vol 3, *Mechanisms of Production and Action*, ed Friedman RM, Elsevier, Amsterdam, New York, Oxford, 189–298.

Jones DT, Monroy D et al., 1994, Sjögren's syndrome: cytokine and Epstein–Barr viral gene expression within the conjunctival epithelium, *Invest Ophthalmol Vis Sci*, **35:** 3493–504.

Jones KA, Luciw PA, Duchange N, 1988, Structural arrangements of transcription control domains within the 5′-untranslated leader regions of the HIV-1 and HIV-1 promoters, *Genes Dev*, **2:** 1101–14.

Kakumu S, Shinagawa T et al., 1991, Serum interleukin-6 levels in patients with chronic hepatitis B, *Am J Gastroenterol*, **86:** 1804–8.

Kandil O, Fishman JA et al., 1994, Human immunodeficiency virus type 1 infection of human macrophages modulates the cytokine response to *Pneumocystis carinii*, *Infect Immun*, **62:** 644–50.

Karupiah G, Fredrickson et al., 1993, Importance of interferons in recovery from mousepox, *J Virol*, **67:** 4214–26.

Kazazi F, Mathijs JM et al., 1992, Recombinant interleukin 4 stimulates human immunodeficiency virus production by infected monocytes and macrophages, *J Gen Virol*, **73:** 941–9.

Kerr IM, Brown RE, 1978, pppA2′p5′A: an inhibitor of protein synthesis synthesized with an enzyme fraction from interferon treated cells, *Proc Natl Acad Sci USA*, **75:** 256–60.

Ketzler S, Weis S et al., 1990, Loss of neurons in the frontal cortex in AIDS brains, *Acta Neuropathol*, **80:** 92–4.

Kobayashi M, Fitz I et al., 1989, Identification and purification of natural killer cell stimulatory factor (NKSF), a cytokine with multiple biological effects on human lymphocytes, *J Exp Med*, **170:** 827–45.

Koenig S, Gendelman HE et al., 1986, Detection of AIDS virus in macrophages in brain tissue from AIDS patients with encephalopathy, *Science*, **233:** 1089–93.

Koff WC, Fann AV, 1986, Human tumor necrosis factor-α kills herpes virus infected but not normal cells, *Lymphokine Res*, **5:** 215–21.

Kornbluth RS, Oh PS et al., 1989, Interferons and bacterial lipopolysaccharides protect macrophages from productive infection by human immunodeficiency virus in vitro, *AIDS*, **3:** 301–13.

Kornbluth RS, Oh PS et al., 1990, The role of interferons in the control of HIV replication in macrophages, *Clin Immunol Immunopathol*, **54:** 200–19.

Künzi MS, Pitha PM, 1995, Identification of human immunodeficiency virus primary isolates resistant to interferon-α and correlation of prevalence to disease progression, *J Infect Dis*, **171:** 822–8.

Kurane I, Janus J, Ennis FA, 1992, Dengue virus infection of human skin fibroblasts in vitro production of IFN-beta, IL-6 and GMCSF, *Arch Virol*, **124:** 21–30.

Lairmore MD, Post AA et al., 1991, Cytokine enhancement of simian immunodeficiency virus (SIV/mac) from a chronically infected T-cell line (HuT-78), *Arch Virol*, **121:** 43–53.

Lang RA, Metcalf D et al., 1987, Transgenic mice expressing a haemopoietic growth factor gene (GM-CSF) develop accumulations of macrophages, blindness and a fatal syndrome of tissue damage, *Cell*, **51:** 675–86.

Laster SM, Wold WSM, Gooding LR, 1994, Adenovirus proteins that regulate susceptibility to TNF also regulate the activity of PLA$_2$, *Semin Virol*, **5:** 431–42.

Lazdins JK, Klimkait T et al., 1991, *In vitro* effect of transforming growth factor-β on progression of HIV-1 infection in primary mononuclear phagocytes, *J Immunol*, **147:** 1201–7.

Lee TG, Tomita J et al., 1990, Purification and partial characterization of a cellular inhibitor of the interferon-induced protein kinase of Mr 68,000 from influenza virus-infected cells, *Proc Natl Acad Sci USA*, **87:** 6208–12.

Leist TP, Eppler M, Zinkernagel RM, 1989, Enhanced virus replication and inhibition of lymphocytic choriomeningitis virus disease in anti-γ interferon-treated mice, *J Virol*, **63:** 2813–19.

Lengyel P, 1982, Biochemistry of interferons and their actions, *Annu Rev Biochem*, **51:** 251–82.

Leong KH, Ramsay AJ et al., 1994, Selective induction of immune responses by cytokines coexpressed in recombinant fowlpox virus, *J Virol*, **68:** 8125–30.

Levin S, Hahn T, 1985, Interferon deficiency syndrome, *Clin Exp Immunol*, **60:** 267–73.

Levine B, Hardwick JM et al., 1991, Antibody-mediated clearance of alphavirus infection from neurons, *Science*, **254:** 856–60.

Levy DE, 1995, Interferon induction of gene expression through the JAK-Stat pathway, *Semin Virol*, **6:** 81–9.

Linde A, Andersson B et al., 1992, Serum levels of lymphokines and soluble cellular receptors in primary Epstein–Barr virus infection and in patients with chronic fatigue syndrome, *J Infect Dis*, **165:** 994–1000.

Little R, White MR, Hartshorn KL, 1994, Interferon-alpha enhances neutrophil respiratory burst responses to stimulation with influenza A virus and FMLP, *J Infect Dis*, **170:** 802–10.

Lucin P, Pavic I et al., 1992, Gamma interferon-dependent clearance of cytomegalovirus infection in salivary glands, *J Virol*, **66:** 1977–84.

de Maeyer E, de Maeyer-Guignard J, 1991, Interferons, *The Cytokine Handbook*, ed Thomson AW, Harcourt, Brace, Jovanovich, London, 215–39.

Martinotti MG, Gribaudo G, 1992, Effects of interferon alpha on murine cytomegalovirus replication, *Microbiologia*, **15:** 183–6.

Masood R, Lunardi-Iskandar Y et al., 1994, Inhibition of AIDS-associated Kaposi's sarcoma cell growth by DAB389-interleukin-6, *AIDS Res Hum Retroviruses*, **10:** 969–75.

Mathur A, Kamat DM et al., 1994, Immunoregulatory abnormalities in patients with Epstein–Barr virus-associated B cell lymphoproliferative disorders, *Transplantation*, **57:** 1042–5.

Merlin G, Falcoff E, Aguet M, 1985, ^{125}I-labelled human interferons alpha, beta and gamma: comparative receptor-binding data, *J Gen Virol*, **66:** 1149–52.

Mestan J, Brockhaus M et al., 1988, Antiviral activity of tumor necrosis factor. Synergism with interferons and induction of (2′,5′)A$_n$-synthetase, *J Gen Virol*, **69:** 3113–20.

Mester JC, Pitha PM, Glorioso JC, 1995, Antiviral activity of herpes simplex virus vectors expressing murine α1-interferon, *Gene Therapy*, **2:** 187–96.

Mistchenko AS, Diez RA, Falcoff E, 1989, Inhibitory effect of interferon-gamma on adenovirus replication and late transcription, *Biochem Pharmacol*, **38:** 1971–8.

Miyazaki I, Cheung RK, Dosh HM, 1993, Viral interleukin-10 is critical for the induction of B cell growth transformation by Epstein–Barr virus, *J Exp Med*, **178:** 439–47.

Molina J-M, Scadden DT et al., 1990, Human immunodeficiency virus does not induce interleukin-1, interleukin-6, or tumor necrosis factor in mononuclear cells, *J Virol*, **64:** 2901–6.

Moore KW, Vieira P et al., 1990, Homology of cytokine synthesis inhibitory factor (IL-10) to the Epstein–Barr virus gene BCRFI, *Science*, **248:** 1230–4.

Mori N, Shirakawa F et al., 1994, Transcriptional regulation of the human interleukin-6 gene promoter in human T-cell leukemia virus type 1-infected T-cell lines: evidence for the involvement of NF-κB, *Blood*, **84:** 2904–11.

Moskophidis D, Frei K et al., 1991, Production of random classes of immunoglobulins in brain tissue during persistent viral infection paralleled by secretion of interleukin-6 (IL-6) but not IL-4, IL-5, and gamma interferon, *J Virol*, **65:** 1365–9.

Moss B, Flexner C, 1987, Vaccinia virus expression vectors, *Annu Rev Immunol*, **5:** 305–24.

Muller U, Steinhoff U et al., 1994, Functional role of type I and type II interferons in antiviral defense, *Science*, **264:** 1918–21.

Nabel G, Baltimore D, 1987, An inducible transcription factor activates expression of human immunodeficiency virus in T-cells, *Nature (London)*, **326:** 711–13.

Nain M, Hinder F et al., 1990, Tumor necrosis factor-α production in influenza A virus-infected macrophages and potentiating effect of lipopolysaccharide, *J Immunol*, **147:** 1921–8.

Nash AA, Cambouropoulos P, 1993, The immune response to herpes simplex virus, *Semin Virol*, **4:** 181–6.

Neurath AR, Strick N, Sproul P, 1992, Search for hepatitis B virus cell receptors reveals binding sites for interleukin-6 on the virus envelope, *J Exp Med*, **175:** 461–9.

Newman GW, Kelley TG et al., 1993, Concurrent infection of human macrophages with HIV-1 and *Mycobacterium avium* results in decreased cell viability, increased *M. avium* multiplication and altered cytokine production, *J Immunol*, **151:** 2261–72.

Niemialtowski MG, Rouse BT, 1992, Predominance of Th1 cells in ocular tissues during herpetic stromal keratitis, *J Immunol*, **149:** 3035–9.

Novak RM, Holzer TJ et al., 1990, The effect of interleukin 4 (BSF-1) on infection of peripheral blood monocyte-derived macrophages with HIV-1, *AIDS Res Hum Retroviruses*, **6:** 973–6.

Osborn L, Kunkel S, Nabel GJ, 1989, Tumor necrosis factor α and interleukin 1 stimulate the human immunodeficiency virus enhancer by activation of the nuclear factor κB, *Proc Natl Acad Sci USA*, **86:** 2336–40.

Pantaleo G, Grailosi C, Fauci AS, 1993, The role of lymphoid organs in the pathogenesis of HIV infection, *Semin Immunol*, **5:** 157–63.

Park H, Davis MV et al., 1994, TAR RNA-binding protein is an inhibitor of the interferon-induced protein kinase, PKR, *Proc Natl Acad Sci USA*, **91:** 4713–17.

Pathak VK, Schindler D, Hershey JWB, 1988, Generation of a mutant form of protein synthesis initiation factor eIF-2 lacking the site of phosphorylation of eIF-2 kinase, *Mol Cell Biol*, **8:** 993–5.

Pensiero MN, Sharefkin JM et al., 1992, Hantaan virus infection of human endothelial cells, *J Virol*, **66:** 5929–36.

Pitha PM, 1980, The effect of interferon in mouse cells infected with MuLV, *Ann N Y Acad Sci*, **350:** 301–13.

Pitha PM, 1991, Multiple effects of interferon on HIV-1 replication, *J Interferon Res*, **11:** 313–18.

Poli G, Fauci AS, 1993, Cytokine modulation of HIV expression, *Semin Immunol*, **5:** 165–73.

Poli G, Kinter AL, Fauci AS, 1994, Interleukin 1 induces expression of the human immunodeficiency virus alone and in synergy with interleukin 6 in chronically infected U1 cells; inhibition of inductive effects by the interleukin 1 receptor antagonist, *Proc Natl Acad Sci USA*, **91:** 108–12.

Poli G, Orenstein JM et al., 1989, Interferon-α but not AZT suppresses HIV expression in chronically infected cell lines, *Science*, **244:** 575–7.

Poli G, Bressler P et al., 1990, Interleukin 6 induces human immunodeficiency virus expression in infected monocytic cells alone and in synergy with tumor necrosis factor α by transcriptional and post-transcriptional mechanisms, *J Exp Med*, **172:** 151–8.

Poli G, Kinter AL et al., 1991, Transforming growth factor β suppresses human immunodeficiency virus expression and replication in infected cells of the monocyte/macrophage lineage, *J Exp Med*, **173:** 589–97.

Popik W, Pitha PM, 1991, Inhibition by interferon of herpes simplex virus type 1-activated transcription of tat-defective provirus, *Proc Natl Acad Sci USA*, **88:** 9573–7.

Popik W, Pitha PM, 1992, Transcriptional activation of the Tat-defective human immunodeficiency virus type-1 provirus: effect of interferon, *Virology*, **189:** 435–47.

Popik W, Pitha PM, 1993, Role of tumor necrosis factor alpha in activation and replication of the *tat*-defective human immunodeficiency virus type 1, *J Virol*, **67:** 1094–9.

Popik W, Pitha PM, 1994, The presence of Tat protein or tumor necrosis factor alpha is critical for herpes simplex virus type 1-induced expression of human immunodeficiency virus type 1, *J Virol*, **68:** 1324–33.

Ramshaw I, Ruby J et al., 1992, Expression of cytokines by recombinant vaccinia viruses: a model for studying cytokines in virus infection in vivo, *Immunol Rev*, **127:** 157–82.

Ramsay AJ, Kohonen-Corish M, 1993, Interleukin-5 expressed by a recombinant virus vector enhances specific soluble IgA response in vivo, *Eur J Immunol*, **23:** 3141–5.

Ramsay AJ, Husband AJ et al., 1994, The role of interleukin-6 in mucosal IgA antibody responses in vivo, *Science*, **264:** 561–3.

Raniero DE, Stasio P, Taylor MW, 1990, Specific effect of interferon on the herpes simplex virus type 1 transactivation event, *J Virol*, **64:** 2588–93.

Rautonen J, Rautonen R et al., 1994, HIV type 1 Tat protein induces immunoglobulin and interleukin 6 synthesis by uninfected peripheral blood mononuclear cells, *AIDS Res Hum Retroviruses*, **10:** 781–5.

Reich NC, Pine R et al., 1988, Transcription of interferon-stimulated genes is induced by adenovirus particles, but suppressed by E1A gene products, *J Virol*, **62:** 114–19.

Reickmann P, Poli G et al., 1991, Activated B lymphocytes from human immunodeficiency virus-infected individuals induce virus expression in infected T cells and a promonocytic cell line, U1, *J Exp Med*, **173:** 1–5.

Roberts NF Jr, Prill AM, Mann TN, 1986, Interleukin 1 and interleukin 1 inhibitor production by human macrophages exposed to influenza virus or respiratory syncytial virus: respiratory syncytial virus is a potent inducer of inhibitor activity, *J Exp Med*, **163:** 511–19.

Rosen CA, Sodroski JG, Haseltine WA, 1985, The location of *cis*-acting regulatory sequences in the human T cell lymphotropic virus type III (HTLV-III/LAV) long terminal repeat, *Cell*, **41:** 813–23.

Rossol S, Glanni G et al., 1992, Cytokine-mediated regulation of monocyte/macrophage cytotoxity in human immunodeficiency virus-1 infection, *Med Microbiol Immunol*, **181:** 267–81.

Rowe WP, 1954, Studies on pathogenesis and immunity in lymphocytic choriomeningitis infection of the mouse, *Naval Med Res Inst Rep*, **005-048.14.01**.

Roy S, Agy M et al., 1991, The integrity of the stem structure of human immunodeficiency virus type I Tat-responsive sequence RNA is required for interaction with the interferon-induced protein kinase, *J Virol*, **65:** 632–40.

Sambhi SK, Kohonen-Corish M, Ramshaw IA, 1991, Local production of tumour necrosis factor encoded by recombinant vaccinia virus is effective in controlling viral replication *in vivo*, *Proc Natl Acad Sci USA*, **88:** 4025–9.

Samuel CE, 1979, Mechanism of interferon action. Phosphorylation of protein synthesis initiation factor eIF-2 in interferon-treated human cells by a ribosome-associated kinase possessing site specificity similar to hemin-required rabbit reticulocyte kinase, *Proc Natl Acad Sci USA*, **76:** 600–4.

Samuel CE, 1991, Antiviral actions of interferon. Interferon-regulated cellular proteins and their surprising selective antiviral activities, *Virology*, **183:** 1–11.

Schmidt DS, Rouse BT, 1992, The role of T cell immunity in control of herpes simplex virus, *Curr Top Microbiol Immunol*, **179:** 57–74.

Schutze S, Potthoff K et al., 1992, TNF activates NF-κB by phosphatidylcholine-specific phospholipase C-induced 'acidic' sphingomyelin breakdown, *Cell*, **71:** 765–76.

Sebire G, Emilie D et al., 1993, In vitro production of IL-6, IL-1-beta, and tumor necrosis factor-alpha by human embryonic microglial and neural cells, *J Immunol*, **150:** 1517–23.

Seder RA, Gazzinell R et al., 1993, Interleukin 12 acts directly on CD4+ T cells to enhance priming for interferon-γ production and diminishes interleukin 4 inhibition of such priming, *Proc Natl Acad Sci USA*, **90:** 10188–92.

Sekiyama KD, Yoshiba M, Thomson AW, 1994, Circulating proinflammatory cytokines (IL-1 beta, TNF-alpha, and IL-6) and IL-1 receptor antagonist (IL-1Ra) in fulminant hepatic failure and acute hepatitis, *Clin Exp Immunol*, **98:** 71–7.

Serwadda D, Sewankambo NK et al., 1985, Slim disease: a new disease in Uganda and its association with HTLV-III infection, *Lancet*, **2:** 849–52.

Shankar V, Kao M et al., 1992, Kinetics of virus spread and changes in levels of several cytokine mRNAs in the brain after intranasal infection of rats with Borna disease virus, *J Virol*, **66:** 992–8.

Shen J, Devery JM, King NJ, 1995, Early induction of interferon-independent virus-specific ICAM-1 (CD45) expression by flavivirus in quiescent but not proliferating fibroblasts: implications for virus–host interactions, *Virology*, **208:** 437–49.

Sher A, Gazzinelli RT et al., 1992, Role of T-cell derived cytokines in the downregulation of immune responses in parasitic and retroviral infection, *Immunol Rev*, **127:** 183–204.

Sheran N, Lau S et al., 1991, Increased production of tumor necrosis factor alpha in chronic hepatitis B virus infection, *J Hepatol*, **2:** 241–5.

Shirazi Y, Pitha PM, 1992, Alpha interferon inhibits early stages of the human immunodeficiency virus type 1 replication cycle, *J Virol*, **66:** 1321–8.

Shirazi Y, Pitha PM, 1993, Interferon α-mediated inhibition of human immunodeficiency virus type 1 provirus synthesis in T-cells, *Virology*, **193:** 303–12.

Spies T, Morton CC et al., 1986, Genes for the tumor necrosis factors α and β are linked to the major histocompatibility complex, *Proc Natl Acad Sci USA*, **83:** 8699–702.

Sprecher E, Becker Y, 1992, Detection of IL-1 beta, TNF-alpha and IL-6 gene transcription by the polymerase chain reaction in keratinocytes, Langerhans cells and peritoneal exudate cells during infection with herpes simplex virus-1, *Arch Virol*, **126:** 253–69.

Tanner JE, Menezes J, 1994, Interleukin-6 and Epstein–Barr

virus induction by cyclosporin A: potential role in lymphoproliferative disease, *Blood*, **84**: 3956–64.

Tendler CJ, Greenberg SJ et al., 1991, Cytokine induction in HTLV-1 associated myelopathy and adult T cell leukemia: alternate molecular mechanisms underlying retroviral pathogenesis, *J Cell Biochem*, **46**: 302–11.

Tepper RI, Levinson DA et al., 1990, IL-4 induces allergic-like inflammatory disease and alters T cell development in transgenic mice, *Cell*, **62**: 457–67.

Tominaga A, Takaki S et al., 1991, Transgenic mice expressing a B cell growth and differentiation factor gene (interleukin-5) develop eosinophilia and autoantibody production, *J Exp Med*, **173**: 429–36.

Torre D, Zeroli C et al., 1992, Cerebrospinal fluid levels of IL-6 in patients with acute infections of the central nervous system, *Scand J Infect Dis*, **24**: 787–91.

Torseth JW, Merigan CT, 1986, Tumor necrosis factor α and β inhibit virus replication and synergize with interferons, *Nature (London)*, **323**: 819–22.

Tufariello J, Cho S, Horwitz MS, 1994, The adenovirus E3 14.7 kilodalton protein which inhibits cytolysis by tumor necrosis factor increases the virulence of vaccinia virus in a murine pneumonia model, *J Virol*, **68**: 453–62.

Tumpey TM, Elner VM et al., 1994, Interleukin-10 treatment can suppress stromal keratitis induced by herpes simplex virus type 1, *J Immunol*, **153**: 2258–65.

Tyor WR, Moench TR, Griffin DE, 1989, Characterization of the local and systemic B cell response of normal and athymic nude mice with Sindbis virus encephalitis, *J Neuroimmunol*, **24**: 207–15.

Tyor WR, Glass JD et al., 1992, Cytokine expression in the brain during AIDS, *Ann Neurol*, **31**: 349–60.

Upton C, DeLange EM, MacFadden G, 1987, Tumorigenic poxviruses genomic organization and DNA sequence of the telomeric region of Shope fibroma virus genome, *Virology*, **160**: 20–30.

Vassao RC, Mello IG, Pereira CA, 1994, Role of macrophages, interferon-gamma and procoagulant activity in the resistance of genetic heterogeneous mouse populations to mouse hepatitis virus infection, *Arch Virol*, **137**: 277–88.

Voth R, Rossol S et al., 1990, Differential gene expression of IFNα and tumor necrosis factor-α in peripheral blood mononuclear cells from patients with AIDS related complex and AIDS, *J Immunol*, **144**: 970–5.

Ward BJ, Griffin DE, 1993, Changes in cytokine production after measles virus vaccination: predominant production of IL-4 suggests induction of a Th2 response, *Clin Immunol Immunopathol*, **67**: 171–7.

Weir JP, Elkins KL, 1993, Replication-incompetent herpesvirus vector delivery of an interferon α gene inhibits human immunodeficiency virus replication in human monocytes, *Proc Natl Acad Sci USA*, **90**: 9140–4.

Wesselingh SL, Power C et al., 1993, Intracerebral cytokine messenger RNA expression in acquired immunodeficiency syndrome dementia, *Ann Neurol*, **33**: 576–82.

Wesselingh SL, Levine B et al., 1994, Intracerebral cytokine mRNA expression during fatal and nonfatal alphavirus encephalitis suggests a predominant type 2 T cell response, *J Immunol*, **152**: 1289–97.

Wiley CA, Schrier RD et al., 1986, Cellular localization of human immunodeficiency virus infection within the brains of acquired immune deficiency syndrome patients, *Proc Natl Acad Sci USA*, **83**: 7089–93.

Williams BRG, Silverman RH, 1985, *The 2-5A System*, Alan R Liss, New York.

Yamamoto JK, Barre-Sinoussi F et al., 1986, Human alpha- and beta-interferon but not gamma suppress the in vitro replication of LAV, HTLV-III, and ARV-2, *J Interferon Res*, **6**: 143–52.

Yamato K, El-Hajjaoul Z et al., 1990, Modulation of interleukin 1β RNA in monocytoid cells infected with human immunodeficiency virus 1, *J Clin Invest*, **86**: 1109–16.

Yasumoto S, Mori Y et al., 1994, Ultraviolet-B irradiation alters cytokine production by immune lymphocytes in herpes simplex virus-infected mice, *J Dermatol Sci*, **8**: 218–23.

Zack JA, Arrigo SJ, Chen ISY, 1990, Control of expression and cell tropism of human immunodeficiency virus type 1, *Adv Virus Res*, **38**: 125–46.

Zhou A, Hassel BA, Silverman RH, 1993, Expression cloning of 2-5A-dependent RNAase: a uniquely regulated mediator of interferon action, *Cell*, **72**: 753–65.

C h a p t e r **1 2**

VIRAL ONCOGENICITY

James C Neil and John A Wyke

1 **Introduction**	4 **Principles of the management of virus-associated cancer**
2 **The pathogenesis of tumour viruses**	
3 **Implication of viruses in the aetiology of cancer**	5 **Conclusions**

1   INTRODUCTION

1.1   A brief history of tumour virology

The incidence of tumours in animals and humans often shows geographical variation. This clustering sometimes reflects genetic differences in the populations at risk but more often results from environmental factors that vary between populations. Features of the environment that enhance the risk of tumour development (i.e. carcinogens) comprise physical factors (such as ultraviolet and other irradiation that impinges on and penetrates the body), chemical factors (ingested or contaminating the body surface) and infectious agents. Of the last, the most important are viruses. Viruses that produce tumours in animals have been known since the early 1900s, but it is only in recent decades that they have excited great interest. The reasons for this are two-fold.

First, as diverse viruses were increasingly implicated as causes of cancer in animals of all vertebrate classes, it was hoped that they might also be important in the aetiology of human neoplasia. This concept was attractive, not least because it suggested that, if the causative organisms could be identified and characterized, the incidence of cancer might be reduced by the prophylactic measures so successful against other infectious agents. The development of a tumour is usually a rare outcome of virus infection but it has nevertheless been estimated that up to 20% of human tumours have a viral risk factor (zur Hausen 1991a) (Fig. 12.1). Only one family of RNA-containing viruses, the retroviruses, has well established oncogenic members (Table 12.1), but representatives of all the major subdivisions of DNA-containing viruses (except the parvoviruses) in vertebrates have been implicated in neoplasia. Examples are given in Tables 12.2 and 12.3 but, because all these agents receive

attention elsewhere in this volume, this chapter will concentrate on general principles rather than specific details.

The second reason for an interest in viruses was their promise as tools for studying the basic mechanisms underlying neoplastic change. This idea rested on several earlier developments in laboratory research. Inbreeding of laboratory animals produced some strains with high incidence of various virus-associated neoplasms. In addition, inbred strains permitted transplantation studies, which demonstrated that a single donor cell could produce a tumour in the recipient animal. This finding focused attention on changes that occurred at a subcellular level and provided the rationale for studying oncogenesis in vitro rather than in the whole animal. This switch in emphasis was facilitated by new tissue culture techniques and, at the same time, it was found that tissue culture was an ideal way to measure the cytopathic effects of viruses, so that animal virologists could adopt the quantitative approach developed in studies on bacteriophages.

A correlation soon emerged between the ability of viruses readily to cause solid mesenchymal tumours in animals and their induction of morphological transformation of cultured cells (Fig. 12.2). This finding had important implications, not widely appreciated at the time. Following Theodore Boveri's proposals in 1914, the notion that tumours were clones of cells whose altered properties result from accumulated mutations was accepted by many scientists. However, before molecular genetic technology was developed, they could not conceive ways of identifying, among the thousands of genes in every somatic cell, the putative subsets that were mutated. Tumour viruses seemed to offer a way round this impasse. Some of them possessed only a few genes among which, it was argued, were those that transformed cells in vitro and induced

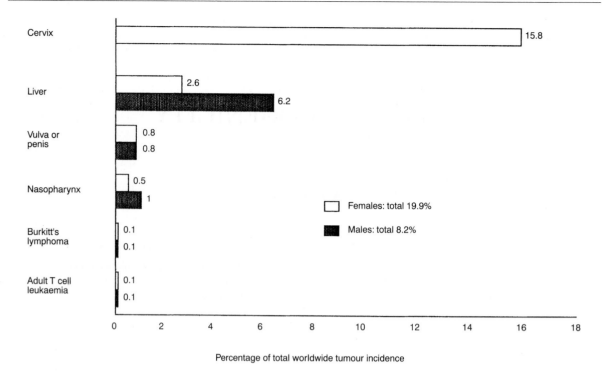

Percentage of total worldwide tumour incidence

Fig. 12.1   Incidence of human tumours in which virus infection is a risk factor. The viruses most strongly implicated are papillomaviruses – tumours of cervix and external genitalia (Chapter 16); hepatitis B virus – primary liver tumours (Chapter 36); Epstein–Barr virus – Burkitt's lymphoma and nasopharyngeal carcinoma (Chapter 20); and human T cell leukaemia viruses – adult T cell leukaemia (Chapter 38). (Modified, with permission, from zur Hausen 1986.) Note that these estimates do not include recent changes in cancer incidence due to HIV infection (Chapters 38 and 42).

tumours in vivo. Identification of these viral cancer genes (oncogenes) should help define the molecular basis of cancer, because they might have functional analogues among the cellular genes required for neoplasia. Although naive in hindsight, this concept proved correct for the retroviruses used widely by laboratory workers. Indeed, for the retroviruses its significance exceeded expectations, for in many cases the viral oncogenes were descended from cellular cognates, the proto-oncogenes. These, in turn, have been convincingly implicated in the genesis of a range of animal and human tumours of both viral and non-viral aetiology. The DNA tumour viruses have also provided vital insights into the cancer process because their oncogenes encode proteins that interact with and inactivate pivotal tumour suppressor proteins.

These concepts gave rise to a large amount of work, reviewed elsewhere (Bishop 1991; Vogelstein and Kinzler 1992). This chapter will summarize in turn the 2 broad divisions of tumour virology: (1) studies on the molecular mechanisms of virus-induced neoplasia, and (2) attempts to implicate viruses in the aetiology of cancer. These divisions, however, share concepts and techniques, and are increasingly considered together (Minson et al. 1994). Such a unitary approach is particularly important when attempting to combat virus-associated cancer, as outlined in the third part of this chapter.

1.2   Cancer – a disorder of cellular controls

The development of a fertilized egg into a multicellular organism and the subsequent maintenance of its form and function require complex controls over cell proliferation and cell death, and the expression of differentiated cell functions. These attributes of cells result from an interplay between stimuli from outside the cell and its current programme of activity. Many of these stimuli are mediated by chemical signals classified according to their origin; endocrine signals originate from distant cells, paracrine signals from cells in the neighbourhood of the recipient and autocrine signals from the recipient cell itself. Whatever their origin and consequence, these signals have an effect only if the recipient cell has appropriate cell surface or internal receptors for the signal, an appropriate machinery of second messengers to process it and the metabolic capacity to respond.

Perturbations in these controls can lead to local increases in tissue mass. These may be the response of a normal cell to abnormal stimuli, leading to cell hypertrophy or, if the cells can multiply, to hyperplasia. On the other hand, the cells themselves may be altered, so their growth and behaviour are no longer controlled in the same way as their normal counterparts and they become neoplastic. We might expect

Table 12.1 Some RNA viruses implicated in cancers of animals and humans

Virus classification	Virus	Associated tumours	Other risk factors
Retroviridae			
B type retroviruses	Mouse mammary tumour virus	Mammary adenocarcinomas T cell lymphoma	Pregnancy (altered hormone levels)
Avian leucosis–sarcoma viruses	Avian leucosis viruses Rous sarcoma virus	Various sarcomas, some carcinomas, lymphomas and leukaemias	Genetic susceptibility affecting virus penetration replication and spread
Avian reticuloendotheliosis virus complex	Reticuloendotheliosis virus	Lymphomas and leukaemias	
Mammalian C type viruses	Murine leukaemia and sarcoma viruses	Lymphomas, leukaemias and sarcomas	Genetic susceptibility to viral infection and spread
	Feline leukaemia and sarcoma viruses	Lymphosarcomas (mainly T cell) Myeloid leukaemias, fibrosarcomas	Age at exposure Immunosuppression
HTLV–BLV group	Human T cell leukaemia virus (HTLV-I, II) Bovine leukaemia virus	Adult T cell leukaemia Lymphosarcoma (B cell)	
D type viruses	Mason–Pfizer monkey virus	Fibrosarcomas	
Lentiviruses	Human immunodeficiency virus	B lymphomas, Kaposi's sarcoma	EBV, Kaposi's sarcoma herpesvirus (KSHV)
	Simian immunodeficiency virus	B lymphomas	Simian herpesvirus
	Feline immunodeficiency virus	B lymphomas	Feline leukaemia virus
Flaviviridae	Hepatitis C virus	Hepatocellular carcinoma	

neoplasia to result from a change in any of the components of the system by which the cell responds to external signals, and there is now considerable evidence that in neoplastic cells mutations exist that change the function of various components in the signalling pathway controlling cell proliferation. As we shall see, viral oncogenes frequently act to stimulate growth in this way.

However, the oncogenes represent only one facet of the genetic basis of cancer. The requirement for recessive mutations in cancer was long suspected, both from the occurrence of inherited cancer syndromes (Knudson 1993) and from classic in vitro cell fusion studies where the transformed phenotype was often found to be extinguished in hybrid cells (Harris 1985). It was suspected that the genes underlying these phenomena might play a role in commitment to terminal differentiation, with loss of function leading to a block at an immature, highly proliferative stage. Although this notion may be correct in some instances, the tumour suppressor genes are proving to be a diverse set, and the best characterized gene of this class is actually dispensable for normal development. Mice lacking functional p53 are ostensibly normal, but are prone to develop tumours, particularly lymphomas (Donehower et al. 1992). The normal physiological role of p53 is as a component of a response pathway to DNA damage; induction of p53 leads to cell cycle arrest and allows repair synthesis to occur. Whilst this phenomenon is a partial explanation for the protective role of p53, there is another important facet to the story. Cells in which p53 is induced may also undergo programmed cell death or **apoptosis** as a consequence (Yonish-Rouach et al. 1991). Although the importance of this cell suicide pathway in normal development was recognized some years ago, its relevance to cancer has only recently come to prominence. For cancer to develop, it seems that cells must acquire mutations which block cell death as well as those which drive cellular proliferation (Liebermann, Hoffman and Steinman 1995).

As shown in Fig. 12.3, the oncogenes are defined as those which act to drive proliferation or to block the processes of cell death or differentiation. Their action is genetically dominant, a single active oncogene overriding the effects of any endogenous counterpart. In contrast, the tumour suppressors are recessive genes and their functions must be lost for tumours to develop. Representatives of this class have been found which act as checks to unscheduled cell proliferation or as mediators of apoptosis or terminal differentiation. Paradoxically, certain oncogenes (e.g. c-*myc*) have been shown to induce cell death instead of proliferation when overexpressed in serum-starved cells,

Table 12.2   Some oncogenic small DNA viruses of animals and humans

Virus family	Virus	Host of origin	Associated tumours	Other risk factors
Hepadnaviridae	Hepatitis B group	Humans, apes, rodents, ducks	Primary hepatocellular carcinoma	In humans: alcohol, smoking, fungal toxins, other viruses
Papovaviridae	Polyoma	Mouse	Various carcinomas and sarcomas	...
	SV40	Monkey	Sarcomas (in rodents)	...
	BK and JC	Human	None in humans; neural tumours in rodents and monkeys	...
	Papilloma	Human	Genital, laryngeal and skin warts; may progress to:	
			Cervical carcinoma	Smoking, herpes simplex viruses, immunosuppression
			Laryngeal carcinoma	X-irradiation, smoking
			Skin carcinoma	Sunlight, genetic disorders
		Cattle	Genital, alimentary, skin warts; may progress to:	
			Alimentary carcinoma	Carcinogens and immunosuppressants in bracken fern
			Skin carcinoma	Sunlight, genetic predisposition (lack of pigmentation)
		Other mammals	Papillomas; may progress to carcinomas	Experimentally, carcinogens such as methylcholanthrene

suggesting that apoptosis may be an important physiological defence against mutations which might otherwise initiate cancer (Evan et al. 1992). As viruses appear to have evolved subtle ways of interfering with the cell death process to establish persistent infection, their ability to act as weak initiators of tumour development becomes more understandable.

2   THE PATHOGENESIS OF TUMOUR VIRUSES

Reasoning from first principles, we can envisage many ways by which features of virus infection might favour the development of tumours. The interactions between viruses and their hosts are such that it is clear that most of these mechanisms exist in naturally occurring cancers. Indeed, the genesis of a given neoplasm may be influenced by more than one mechanism, because they are not mutually exclusive.

2.1   Direct oncogenic mechanisms

A first major category of pathogenic mechanism is direct or intrinsic, in which the tumour cells, or at least their ancestral lineage, are infected by the causative virus. Although this mechanism was presumed to be involved in studies of tumour viruses in vitro, only one aspect of it was useful to the experimenter – that in which all or part of the virus genome persisted in the tumour lineage. Genome persistence provides a marker that pinpoints crucial events in tumorigenesis, either because a specific portion of the virus is always present or because the genome is inserted in a specific region of the host chromosome DNA.

The consistent presence of a viral gene, either free in the cell or integrated randomly in host DNA, suggests that it directly contributes to the neoplastic phenotype. These viral oncogene functions can supersede those of the cell and invariably mediate either oncogenicity by the virus or its presumed counterpart in vitro, cell transformation (see Fig 12.2).

THE RETROVIRAL ONCOGENES

The oncogenes of most retroviruses play no part in virus replication. Indeed, many replace portions of viral replicative genes in the virus genome. These oncogenes (v-*onc*) are related to sequences in normal host cells from which they are believed to evolve after capture (transduction) of the cellular gene, known as a proto-oncogene (c-*onc*), during some ancestral infection (Table 12.4). Such transduction is observed in certain naturally occurring tumours; however, because it is sporadic, and because oncogene transduction

Table 12.3 Some oncogenic large DNA viruses of animals and humans

Virus family	Virus	Host of origin	Associated tumours	Other risk factors
Adenoviridae	Types 2, 5, 12	Human	None in humans; sarcomas in hamsters	...
Herpesviridae	Frog herpesvirus	Leopard frog	Adenocarcinomas	Ambient temperature
	Marek's disease	Fowl	Neurolymphomatosis (T cell)	Genetic predisposition of unknown basis
	Herpesvirus ateles and saimiri	Monkeys	Lymphoma, leukaemia	...
	Epstein–Barr virus (EBV)	Human	Burkitt's lymphoma	Malaria, HIV
			Hodgkin's disease	...
			Immunoblastic lymphoma	Immunodeficiency
			Nasopharyngeal carcinoma	Salted fish in infancy, HLA type
	Herpes simplex (types 1 and 2)	Human	Cervical neoplasia	Papillomaviruses, smoking, immunodeficiency
	Cytomegalovirus	Human	Cervical neoplasia	Immunodeficiency, HLA type
	Kaposi's sarcoma herpesvirus (KSHV/HHV8)	Human Human	... Kaposi's sarcoma	... HIV
Poxviridae	Shope fibroma	Rabbit	Fibroma	...
	Yaba virus	Monkey	Nodular fibromatous hyperplasia	Not relevant; progressive tumours never develop
	Molluscum contagiosum	Human	Nodular epidermal hyperplasia	...

confers no conceivable advantage on the virus, it is often considered to be a relatively unimportant mode of pathogenesis. However, the onset of tumours in domestic cats infected with feline leukaemia virus (FeLV) is often associated with *de novo* transduction of cellular genes (Neil et al. 1991). This may be a more accurate representation of C-type retrovirus pathogenesis under natural conditions, because there is no other evidence to suggest that FeLV is a particularly recombinogenic virus. Transduction has major implications for understanding the mechanism of neoplasia because, if cell proto-oncogenes can mediate neoplasia when incorporated within a virus genome, they might also be able to do so in other circumstances. A considerable body of evidence now suggests that this is the case, some of the earliest data coming from work on the mode of tumour virus pathogenesis is described next.

Since the first glimpses of oncogenes in rapidly transforming retroviruses, it has been apparent that their products can be demonstrated in many different cellular sites; their functions, where elucidated (Table 12.4), identify them as components in the chain of information reception, transfer and response depicted in Fig. 12.4. Thus they can be altered forms of growth factors (e.g. v-*sis*), transmembrane growth factor receptors (some of which are protein tyrosine kinases such as v-*erb*-B) or 'G proteins' that couple ligand–receptor interactions to intracellular signalling events (e.g. the *ras* gene family). Others are second messengers, such as the intracellular protein tyrosine kinases and serine–threonine kinases. The oncogenes whose products are located in the nucleus can affect DNA synthesis or, more probably, gene expression; it is known that at least 2 of these, v-*jun* and v-*fos*, encode nuclear proteins that assemble as heterodimers to form a well characterized transcription factor complex (AP-1). It is easy to appreciate that mutations altering the expression of one of these genes, or their products, might short-circuit normal cell controls and lead to unregulated growth and behaviour. However, it remains a major challenge to understand the detailed mechanism of many of these perturbations. For a comprehensive listing of the known oncogenes and their properties, the reader is referred to a recently published compendium (Hesketh 1995).

The leukaemogenic retroviruses, bovine leukaemia virus (BLV), human T cell leukaemia viruses (HTLV-I and II) and simian T cell leukaemia virus (STLV-I) form a discrete subgroup where a normal constituent

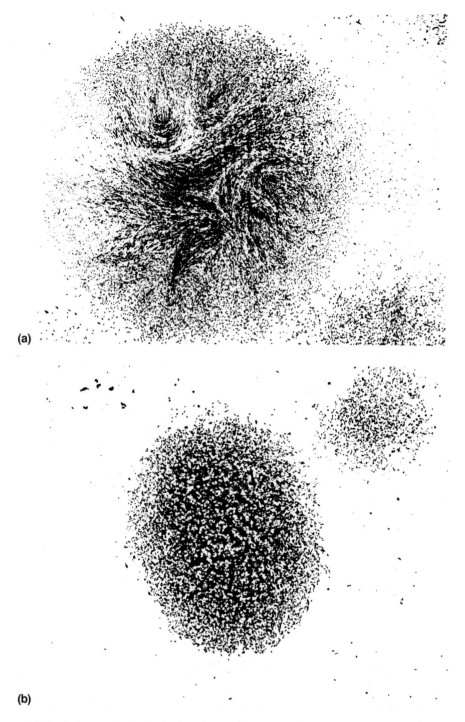

Fig. 12.2   The morphological appearance of colonies of normal and transformed cells in tissue culture (× 20). (a) A colony of BHK-21/C13, a cell line derived from Syrian hamster kidney. Note that the colony is flat and the cells are lined in parallel array. (b) The same cell line after transformation by polyomavirus. The cells are piled on one another and lack orientation.

of the viral genome is implicated in transformation. They contain a region, called pX, which encodes Tax and Rex, and a series of minor products.. The Tax protein is the most clearly implicated in in vitro transformation by these viruses. It acts on the long terminal repeat (LTR) of the integrated provirus, usually to increase viral transcription, through interaction with cellular transcription factors (Fig. 12.5); as a result of this activity it can also activate the transcription of

some crucial cellular genes (see Chapter 38). However, it should be noted that tumours are rare and a very late consequence of HTLV infection, and that the requirement for viral gene expression in maintaining the tumour phenotype remains uncertain.

THE ONCOGENES OF DNA TUMOUR VIRUSES

The transforming genes of the oncogenic DNA viruses bear no close relationship to cellular gene products;

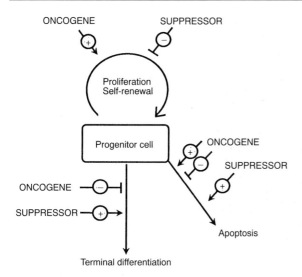

Fig. 12.3 Cell fate and the effect of oncogenes and tumour suppressor genes. Normal stem cells respond to regulatory signals which control self-renewal by proliferation or drive cells towards terminal differentiation. Oncogenes may promote unscheduled proliferation and self-renewal or block terminal differentiation, or both. In contrast, the tumour suppressor genes may act either to check proliferation or as essential mediators of differentiation pathways. Apoptosis, or programmed cell death, is a normal physiological process which acts to restrict normal or abnormal cell growth. Some oncogenes (e.g. members of the *bcl-2* family) are potent inhibitors of cell death pathways and hence act synergistically with others (e.g. *myc*) which induce proliferation but concomitantly trigger cell death. Some tumour suppressor genes act through apoptotic pathways.

they are integral components of the viral genome and provide important functions early in the replicative cycle. If the viral replication cycle fails to proceed past the expression of these early gene products, the result is a persistently infected, transformed cell. In this abortive mode of replication, the host cell is induced to multiply abnormally and will present few viral antigens to the host immune system, with obvious advantages to the virus in establishing latent or persistent infection.

The observation that SV40 T antigen binds tightly to a cellular protein, p53 (Lane and Crawford 1979, Linzer and Levine 1979), was the first step towards the elucidation of a transformation mechanism common to many of the DNA tumour viruses. For the adenoviruses (Sarnow et al. 1982) and papillomaviruses (Werness, Levine and Howley 1990), viral oncogene products also exert their effects by binding to 2 tumour suppressor proteins, p53 and pRb. Binding results in the inactivation or degradation of the cellular target proteins, removing the normal barriers to cell cycle progression. The viral effectors involved are listed in Table 12.5.

There are other mechanisms by which DNA tumour viruses can interfere with cell growth regulation, as shown by polyomavirus middle T antigen which interacts in subtle ways to activate non-receptor tyrosine kinases at the plasma membrane (Kiefer, Courtneidge

and Wagner 1994). For Epstein–Barr virus, a subset of 6 viral gene products has been implicated in the efficient immortalization of B cells, including a series of nuclear proteins (EBNAs) and 2 membrane proteins (LMP 1 and 2), and the same gene products are expressed in EBV-positive immunoblastic lymphomas which arise in immunosuppressed transplant recipients and AIDS patients (Rickinson 1994). A more limited subset of EBV proteins (EBNA-1, LMP-1 and 2) is expressed in nasopharyngeal carcinoma cells, while Burkitt's lymphoma cells express only EBNA-1. The functions encoded by these genes are mostly unknown but EBNA-5 has been reported to interact with p53 and pRB (Szekely et al. 1993), LMP-1 induces the expression of *bcl-2*, a cellular oncogene whose product inhibits apoptosis (Henderson et al. 1991), and EBNA-1 is a nuclear protein with a possible role in transactivation of host cell genes (see Chapter 20).

For hepatitis B virus, analysis of viral oncogenic functions has been hampered by the lack of tractable in vitro systems. However, both HBx and the large envelope protein preS can transactivate cellular genes (Rossner 1992), and there have been recent reports that HBx protein can bind p53.

Despite their potency in various in vitro transformation assays, most DNA tumour viruses are very weakly oncogenic, particularly in their natural hosts. This may be explained in part by the efficiency of the host immune response in controlling virus replication and destroying potential tumour cells that express virus-coded cell surface antigens or T cell epitopes.

INSERTIONAL MUTAGENESIS

Many retroviruses lack an oncogene but induce clonal tumours in which their genome is integrated as a DNA provirus in a specific region of the host chromosome (Fig. 12.6). This insertion is mutagenic, so it changes the sequence of DNA in that region, and can have either of 2 results: activation of a gene or its ablation. In most cases proviral insertion activates a nearby gene, either by qualitative alteration or by augmentation of its expression (Peters 1990, Kung, Boerkel and Carter 1991). In some cases the activated gene proves to be the cellular counterpart of a known retrovirus oncogene. Thus, B cell lymphomas induced by avian leucosis virus (ALV) and T cell lymphosarcoma induced by feline leukaemia virus (FeLV) often contain a c-*myc* gene activated by insertional mutagenesis. In ALV-induced erythroleukaemia, on the other hand, it is the c-*erb*-B proto-oncogene that is activated. These findings support a role for proto-oncogenes in neoplasia, and in the latter case also suggest the means by which viral oncogenes may be transduced (Nilsen et al. 1985).

By extrapolation from the observed activation of known proto-oncogenes by proviral insertion, it can be argued that, when an inserted virus consistently activates an adjacent limited region of the host genome in a tumour, the activated region is a putative oncogene. In this way a large number of loci have been identified, of which the activation is characteristic of certain virus-induced tumours; the available

Table 12.4 Examples of genes transduced by retroviruses

Viral oncogene	Location, structural features of gene product	Normal function of host cell gene	Transducing virus	Associated tumours
v-*sis*	Secreted growth factor	B chain PDGF	GaLV/FeLV	Sarcoma
v-*erb*-B		EGF receptor	ALV	Erythroblastosis
v-*kit*		SCF receptor	FeLV	Fibrosarcoma
v-*fms*		CSF-1 receptor	FeLV	Fibrosarcoma
v-*ros*	Transmembrane	...	ALV	...
v-*mpl*	receptors	Thrombopoietin receptor	MLV	Myeloproliferative disease
v-*sea*				
v-*tcr*		...	ALV	Erythroblastosis
		β chain T cell receptor	FeLV	T cell lymphoma
v-*abl*		...	MLV/FeLV	B cell leukaemia, fibrosarcoma
v-*fes*/v-*fps*		...	FeLV/ALV	Fibrosarcoma
v-*fgr*	Plasma membrane	...	FeLV	Fibrosarcoma
v-*ryk*	tyrosine kinases	...	ALV	...
v-*src*		...	ALV	Fibrosarcoma
v-*yes*		...	ALV	Fibrosarcoma
v-Ha-*ras*	Plasma membrane	...	MLV	Sarcoma
v-Ki-*ras*	G proteins	...	MLV	Sarcoma
v-mos	Cytoplasmic	...	MLV	Sarcoma
v-*raf*/v-*mil*	serine/threonine kinase	...	MLV/ALV	Sarcoma, carcinoma
v-*crk*	Cytoplasmic adapter	...	ALV	Sarcoma
v-*erb*-A	Cytoplasm/nucleus	Thyroid hormone receptor	ALV	Erythroblastosis
v-*maf*		...	...	...
v-*ski*		...	ALV	...
v-*myb*		...	ALV	Myeloblastosis
v-*myc*	Nuclear transcription factors	...	ALV, FeLV	Myelocytomatosis, lymphoma
v-*rel*		NFκB transcription factor	REV	Reticuloendotheliosis
v-*fos*		AP-1 transcription factor	MLV	Sarcoma
v-*jun*		AP-1 transcription factor	ALV	Sarcoma

ALV, avian leucosis virus; FeLV, feline leukaemia virus; GaLV, gibbon ape leukaemia virus; MLV, murine leukaemia virus; REV, reticuloendotheliosis virus.

evidence as to the nature of these loci strongly supports the concept that their activation is relevant to neoplasia.

Although the first example of insertional mutagenesis came from avian lymphomas (Neel et al. 1981), most recent work to identify new oncogenes by retroviral 'gene tagging' has been in the laboratory mouse. This trend is accounted for by the parallel development of techniques for the manipulation of the mouse genome. Thus, the introduction of mutant proto-oncogenes into the mouse germ-line has confirmed their oncogenic potential, whilst their inactivation by homologous recombination has provided valuable insights into their normal functions (Berns et al. 1989).

Insertional mutagenesis is also a prominent oncog-

enic mechanism for at least one representative of the hepadnaviruses; woodchuck hepatitis virus (WHV) often activates the c-*myc* or N-*myc* genes in the genesis of liver tumours that arise without the extensive cirrhosis that precedes HBV-associated cancers (Buendia 1994). In contrast, there is only fragmentary evidence for insertional mutagenesis in HBV-associated tumours. The reasons for the marked difference in mode of action between 2 similar viral agents are unknown.

So far we have focused on the capacity of integrated viruses to activate genes. The converse of this process, gene disruption by retroviral insertion, underlies some developmental mutations in laboratory mice (Lock, Jenkins and Copeland 1991). In such cases it is possible to reveal the disruptive effects of a single insertion

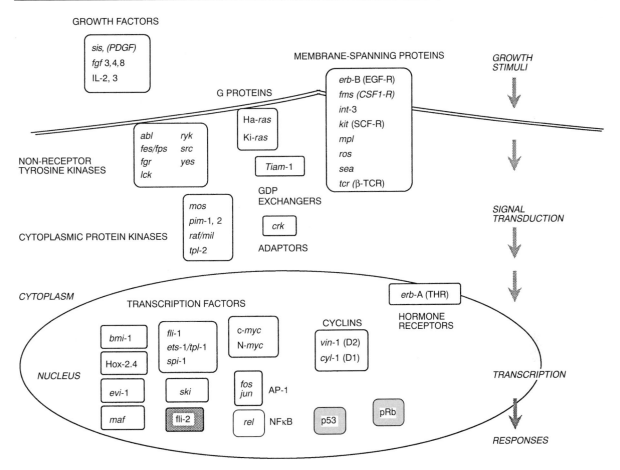

Fig. 12.4 Location and function of oncogene and tumour suppressor gene products implicated in viral carcinogenesis. Oncogenes are indicated by open boxes, tumour suppressors by shaded boxes. As can be seen, many levels of signal transduction and response pathways are represented. The complexity of this picture would be multiplied by the potential interactions between these oncogene and suppressor gene mutations and the differentiated cell environments in which they may occur.

by back-crossing to generate a homozygous mutation. In somatic cells, gene ablation is an improbable outcome because it requires inactivating insertions at both alleles. Nevertheless, there are at least 2 instances in which retroviral insertions have been shown to ablate gene function in tumour cells. Both examples come from Friend murine leukaemia virus-induced erythroleukaemias. The first to be identified was at the prototype tumour suppressor gene, p53, which can be inactivated by proviral insertion at both alleles or by a combination of one insertion event with loss of the other allele by deletion or other mutations. The second case is the *fli-2* locus, where the target is a transcription factor gene, NF-E2, which is necessary for globin gene expression (Lu et al. 1994). The effect of the loss of NF-E2 function seems most likely to be a block to differentiation.

At first sight, mutagenic ablation might be thought to be more likely because it is less specific than activation, and so insertion anywhere within the coding region would destroy the integrity of the gene. However, mutational activation seems to operate by such a variety of mechanisms that it, too, can result from insertion at many locations near the activated gene (Fig. 12.6). In the classic example of avian B cell lym-

phomas, c-*myc* transcription is driven by the viral promoter in an LTR situated 5′ to the gene (Fig. 12.6b). However, the subsequent discovery of enhancers in retroviral LTRs, their non-polar action over long distances and their effects predominantly on the nearest promoters now indicate that, in different circumstances, a viral LTR can augment activity of a gene either 5′ or 3′ to itself in either orientation (Fig. 12.6e–g). Moreover, it is theoretically possible that an inserted provirus may activate a gene by simply separating it from *cis*-acting cellular repressors.

A significant minority of common insertion sites remains unaccounted for in terms of gene activation (Table 12.6). Whilst some of these loci may simply require further close characterization, it is possible that some of the target genes have escaped detection because they involve long-range *cis*-activation of a target gene. Evidence in favour of this mechanism comes from the *evi*-1 and the c-*myc* loci where insertions in one of several distinct clustered sites appear to activate the genes at a considerable distance (up to 300 kb).

Although the focus of most current research is type C retroviruses in the laboratory mouse, the mechanism of insertional mutagenesis is relevant in tumours induced by other members of the type C and

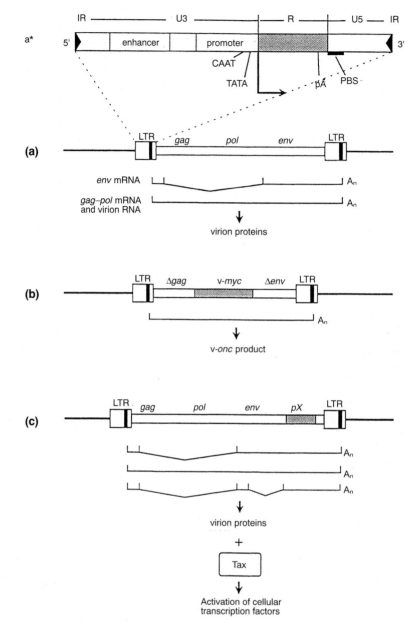

Fig. 12.5 Chapter 38 considers retroviruses at length. This Figure and Fig. 12.6 give only enough detail to appreciate their pathogenesis. (a*) Detail of a typical retroviral long terminal repeat (LTR). Each LTR resembles an insertion sequence, having an inverted repeat (IR) at its extremities. A direct repeat (R) derives from either end of the virion RNA, with a cap site at its 5′ end (large arrow) and a polyadenylation signal (pA) close to its 3′ end. The 3′ boundary is marked by a primer binding site (PBS) to which is bound the tRNA primer for reverse transcription of virion RNA. The remainder of the LTR comprises U3 and U5 regions, derived respectively from the 3′ and 5′ ends of viral RNA. U3 contains a promoter region, with characteristic 'CAAT' and 'TATA' boxes that regulate proviral transcription. Upstream (5′) to the promoter is an enhancer with a non-polar stimulatory effect on gene expression. (a) A retroviral provirus (boxes) integrated in cell DNA (thick line). LTRs flank and control the expression of coding regions that comprise, in replication-competent retroviruses, at least 3 genes, *gag*, *pol* and *env*, expressed through unspliced or spliced polyadenylated mRNAs. (b) A retroviral provirus bearing a viral oncogene (v-*onc*), in this case the v-*myc* in the avian myelocytomatosis virus MC29. In transducing v-*myc* the virus has lost the *pol* gene and portions of *gag* and *env*, so it can be propagated only if these missing functions are provided in *trans* in the same cell by a 'helper' virus of the sort shown in (a). (c) A simplified diagram of the human T cell leukaemia virus. The oncogene region of this virus (pX) encodes Tax, Rex and a series of other minor products (p30, p12), which have no known cellular counterparts. Tax interacts with cellular transcription factors to transactivate a range of cellular genes, including IL-2 and its receptor.

Table 12.5 Interaction of DNA tumour virus gene products with tumour suppressor proteins

Target	Virus	Effector
p53	SV40	T antigen
	Adenovirus	E1B protein
	Human papillomavirus	E6 protein
	Epstein–Barr virus	EBNA-5*
	Hepatitis B virus	pX*
Rb	SV40	T antigen
	Adenovirus	E1A protein
	Human papillomavirus	E7 protein
	Epstein–Barr virus	EBNA-5*

*The biological significance of these reported interactions is not yet clear.

type B retrovirus families. Other agents and the relevant target loci are listed in Table 12.7.

OTHER EVIDENCE IMPLICATING PROTO-ONCOGENES IN NEOPLASIA

A detailed consideration of the molecular and cell biology of neoplasia is outside the scope of this chapter, but the following brief survey is intended to provide some understanding of the basis of viral oncogenicity. Readers are referred to recent reviews on this subject (Bishop 1991, Knudson 1993).

Two major lines of investigation have further incriminated proto-oncogenes in cancer.

1 DNA from certain tumour cells, but not DNA from their normal counterparts, can induce morphological transformation of, or confer tumorigenicity upon, appropriate recipient cells in culture. The genes responsible are often mutant members of the *ras* oncogene family, first encountered as the v-*onc* genes of certain murine sarcoma viruses. However, as with insertional mutagenesis by viruses, DNA 'transfection' has revealed further novel putative oncogenes whose properties, where known, are compatible with a role in neoplasia (Bishop 1995).

2 Many cancers display characteristic karyological abnormalities, typically deletions, translocations or amplification of identifiable regions of chromosomes. In some cases the genes affected by translocation and amplification are the cellular relatives of known v-*onc* genes; again a number of novel loci are deemed guilty by association (Rabbitts 1994).

In short, proto-oncogenes have been incriminated in neoplasia by a variety of phenomena, and some genes have been implicated in several ways. The mutations suffered by proto-oncogenes in tumour cells – be they single base changes, transduction or gross disruption by viruses or massive, microscopically visible aberrations in karyotype – have one (or both) of 2 effects: they change either the expression of the gene or the nature of its product.

'HIT AND RUN' MECHANISMS

The pattern of virus persistence in a tumour may be complex but is amenable to study. The same cannot be said for those instances in which a virus is implicated in tumour formation in vivo or cell transformation in vitro but in which it is impossible to demonstrate either persistence of a specific portion of the viral genome or integration in a limited region of host DNA. The virus in such cases is presumed to act transiently. It may operate by one of the mechanisms detailed above but the genes involved are required only in the early stages of tumour evolution and unknown selective pressures against the virus eliminate it during tumour progression.

The absence of bovine papillomavirus type 4 from the alimentary carcinomas that it causes may reflect such a mechanism, because at least some papillomaviruses are known to carry transforming genes. On the other hand, this virus, as proposed for herpes simplex viruses and cytomegalovirus in cervical cancer, may act as a mutagen, through an ephemeral association of its genome with cell DNA or, possibly, through the action of viral enzymes (Minson 1984, Macnab 1987). The mechanisms in either case are hard to study and investigators have invoked this 'hit and run' explanation only after eliminating other possibilities.

2.2 Indirect mechanisms

The second major category of pathogenic mechanism is also frustrating for the student of in vitro systems but is clinically significant, whether operating alone or in concert with mechanisms outlined above. In these indirect, or extrinsic, mechanisms neither the cells of the tumour nor their ancestral lineage need ever have been infected by the causative virus; instead, tumours arise in response to virus infection of other cells, the nature of the response taking several forms.

Cell death or impaired function as a direct or indirect effect of virus infection can have different consequences depending on the type of cell affected. If the immune system is compromised the outgrowth of cells might be permitted from many tissues that had acquired neoplastic potential by various means; in practice, however, immunosuppression leads to increases in the incidences of a relatively small spectrum of tumours, a significant proportion of which are associated with viral risk factors (Fig. 12.1). Cell death, or untoward cell proliferation, among haemopoietic tissues can also upset delicate homoeostatic cellular interrelations, and compensatory proliferation in other lineages may favour independent neoplastic alterations in these reactive cells.

A number of tumour viruses cause immune impairment (Table 12.8), probably by a variety of mechanisms. Immunosuppression by some viruses may be due to cytotoxicity, reflecting, in the case of avian reticuloendotheliosis viruses, the burden of intracellular unintegrated viral DNA. The immunosuppressive effect of human immunodeficiency virus (HIV) could also result simply from cytopathic effects on CD4+ T cells, but the extent of infection does not seem suf-

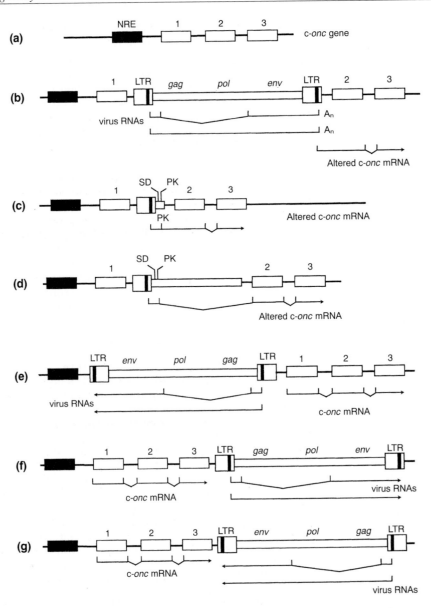

Fig. 12.6 Modes of insertional mutagenesis. The examples given show insertional mutagenesis by a retroviral provirus, but woodchuck hepatitis virus (Buendia et al. 1994) and others may have comparable effects. (a) Diagram of a proto-oncogene (c-*onc*) comprising 3 exons (open boxes), the first of which is largely non-coding, and an upstream negative regulatory element (NRE; closed box), which helps to ensure that the gene is often poorly transcribed. (b) Insertion of a provirus between exons 1 and 2 of the c-*onc* gene. Expression of c-*onc* is elevated by 'promoter insertion', regulatory elements in the 3′ LTR driving transcription of a viral c-*onc* hybrid message. (c) Insertion of a truncated provirus, with c-*onc* transcription initiating in the 5′ LTR. In this instance the transcript is not spliced at the donor site (SD) for generating subgenomic viral mRNA, so it includes the sequence (PK) 3′ to SD that permits packaging of the RNA into virions. This altered c-*onc* mRNA may thus be incorporated in an infectious virion, and infection leading to reverse transcription and genetic recombination with another viral RNA could generate a virus containing a transduced *onc* gene. (d) Another example of promoter insertion by a truncated provirus. In this case the packaging signal is spliced out of the mRNA so, like subgenomic viral mRNA, it is unlikely to be incorporated into virions. (e) Proviral insertion 5′ to c-*onc*, but in the opposite transcriptional orientation, precluding enhancement of *onc* expression by the viral promoter. The virus thus acts either through the effect of its enhancer alone or by distancing c-*onc* from the 'upstream' NRE. (f and g) Proviral insertion 3′ to c-*onc* in either transcriptional orientation. In these instances it appears that the virus can augment proto-oncogene expression only by virtue of its enhancer.

ficient to account for the degree of immune impairment. Moreover, feline immunodeficiency virus (FIV) also causes immunosuppression and a similar depletion of CD4+ cells despite its broader tropism and apparent use of a non-CD4 entry pathway (Willett and Hosie 1994). Various theories of HIV immunosuppression have been elaborated, including virus-induced autoimmune attack, T cell apoptosis following non-specific immunosuppression, cytokine dysregulation, and cell destruction due to chronic antiviral

Table 12.6 MLV insertions in tumours with unknown effects on gene expression

Locus	Chrom. location	Tumour	Virus	Other remarks
ahi-1	10	T lymphoma	Abelson helper	Between c-*myb*, *mis*-2[a]
bla-1	?	B lymphoma	Moloney	bmi-1/pal-1 complementation
dsi-1	4	T lymphoma (rat)	Moloney	
evi-3	18	Myeloid leukaemia	AKXD	
evi-5	5	T lymphoma	AKXD	Close to *gfi*-1/*pal*-1
fim-1	13	Myeloid leukaemia	Friend	
fis-1	7	Myeloid leukaemia, lymphoma	Friend	c. 75 kb *int*-2, 300 kb cyclin D1[b]
gin-1	19	T lymphoma	Gross passage A	Closely linked to *his*-2
his-1	2	Myeloid leukaemia	Cas-Br-M	
his-2	19	Myeloid leukaemia	Cas-Br-M	Closely linked to *gin*-1
mis-2	10	T lymphoma	Moloney	c. 160 kb from c-*myb*[c]
pal-1	5	B, T lymphoma	Moloney	Close to *gfi*-1/*evi*-5
tic-1[a]	17	T lymphoma	Moloney	

[a]Previously known as *pim*-2.
[b]Suggested long-range activation of cyclin D1.
[c]No evidence for long-range activation of *myb*.

Table 12.7 Insertional mutagenesis by retroviruses other than murine leukaemia virus

Virus	Locus	Gene product	Tumour
Avian leucosis virus	c-*erb*-B	RK	Erythroleukaemia
	c-*myc*	N	B lymphoma
	c-*bic*	…	…
	c-*brav*-o	…	…
	c-Ki-*ras*	GP	Nephroblastoma
	c-*fos*	N	…
RE virus	c-*myc*	N	T lymphoma
Feline leukaemia virus	c-*myc*	N	T lymphoma
	pim-1	PK	…
	flvi-2 (=*bmi*-1)	N	…
	fit-1	…	…
	flvi-1	…	Splenic lymphoma
Gibbon ape leukaemia virus	IL-2	GF	T cell leukaemia (cell line)
Mouse mammary tumour virus	*wnt*-1(*int*-1)	GF	Mammary carcinoma
	int-2[*fgf*3,4]	GF	…
	int-3	RK	…
	wnt-3(*int*-4)	GF	…
	int-5	P450	…
	int-6	?	…
	fgf-8	GF	…

GF, growth factor (-like); GP, G protein; PK, cytoplasmic protein kinase; N, nuclear protein/transcription factor; P450, cytochrome P450-like; RK, receptor kinase.

immune responses (Zinkernagel and Hengartner 1994). Two points should be noted at this juncture: (1) with the possible exception of HIV and its relatives, the tumour viruses that are immunosuppressive also seem to have efficient and direct means of inducing neoplasia; (2) immunosuppression is the only indirect mode of viral carcinogenesis that does not necessarily involve cell proliferation as an early stage.

Death or damage to non-haemopoietic cells may likewise favour neoplastic change, but in uninfected cells of the same lineage that are dividing in an attempt at tissue regeneration. This is one way in which chronic hepatitis B or hepatitis C infections may increase the risk of primary liver cancer (Slagle, Becker and Butel 1994).

Virus infection may also stimulate cells to produce growth factors of various types. In some cases, the viruses themselves carry growth factor-like genes, such as the Epstein–Barr virus BCRF1 gene which has homology with IL-10 (Morein and Merza 1991). When the producing cell itself possesses receptors for these factors, their effects can be autocrine with the virus acting directly, as described above. Examples include

Table 12.8 Viral functions implicated in cancer

Function	Virus group (and representatives)							
	Retroviruses							
	Type C MLV ALV FeLV	Type B MMTV	HTLV BLV	Lenti HIV SIV	Hepadna HBV WHV	Papova SV40 Polyoma	Papilloma HPV BPV	Herpes EBV HVS
Viral gene product stimulates proliferation	+/−	+	++	+/−	+	++	++	++
Insertional mutagenesis	++	++	−	+/−	+ (WHV)	−	+/−	−
Non-specific induction of proliferation (cell regeneration, immune stimulation, inflammation)	+	−	−	+	+ (HBV)	−	−	−
Immunosuppression	+	−	−	++	−	−	−	−

ALV, avian leucosis virus; BLV, bovine leukaemia virus; BPV, bovine papillomavirus; EBV, Epstein–Barr virus; FeLV, feline leukaemia virus; HBV, hepatitis B virus; HIV, human immunodeficiency virus; HPV, human papilloma virus; HTLV, human T cell leukaemia virus; HVS, herpesvirus saimiri; MLV, murine leukaemia virus; MMTV, mouse mammary tumour virus; SIV, simian immunodeficiency virus; WHV, woodchuck hepatitis virus.

the stimulation of IL-2 and its receptor by HTLV-I in infected T cells (Ruben et al. 1988), and the induction of IL-9 by certain murine leukaemia viruses which can also activate the IL-9 receptor by insertional mutagenesis (Flubacher, Bear and Tsichlis 1994).

A second type of cell stimulation may be operative in those chronic retroviral infections that lead to lymphoma. It is suggested that lymphoma cells bear immunoglobulin receptors for viral envelope glycoproteins, the cellular precursors having been propelled into hyperplasia by chronic antigenic stimulation (McGrath and Weissman 1979). In the case of T cell lymphomas induced by murine leukaemia virus (MuLV) this mechanism is direct because the lymphoma cells are also infected by the viruses to which they are responding (and the viruses also act as insertional mutagens) (Table 12.9). However, there seems to be no reason *a priori* why stimulation of uninfected cells should not favour their neoplastic conversion. This may be the mechanism of oncogenesis in B cell leukaemias associated with infection by the T cell tropic HTLV-I, since the tumour cells seem committed to produce immunoglobulins that recognize HTLV-I antigens (Mann, Desantis and Mark 1987). A comparable phenomenon is seen in HIV-1-associated B cell lymphomas.

A further example of viral interplay with host immunoregulatory systems is provided by the mouse mammary tumour viruses (MMTV) which encode superantigens. Endogenous MMTVs in the mouse genome express these polymorphic proteins which stimulate developing T cells via the Vβ of the αβTCR, leading to clonal deletion of reactive cells and a consequent bias in the Vβ repertoire of mature T cells. This phenomenon may be regarded as an aberrant outcome of viral sequestration in the mouse germ-line. However, it seems that the expression of these ligands on B cells is an important early event in establishment of infection by MMTV, because this may stimulate mature T cells to release growth factors that drive proliferation of the infected cell. Along the way, the virus usurps the host immune response to favour its own dissemination (Hesketh 1995).

The potential stimulatory effects of viral antigens may also be due to their mimicry of ligands for receptors on a range of cell types. If these receptors modulate normal cell growth and behaviour, chronic unscheduled binding of ligand analogues may lead to hyperplasia and then neoplasia. Such effects probably are widespread, and the oncogene of the spleen focus-forming component of mouse Friend leukaemia retrovirus is perhaps the best characterized example. This oncogene has no cell counterpart, being derived entirely from virus envelope gene sequences, but it appears to interact with the erythropoietin receptor, replacing the requirement for exogenous growth factors (Li et al. 1990).

3 IMPLICATION OF VIRUSES IN THE AETIOLOGY OF CANCER

The pathogenic strategies just discussed are clearly crucial to the concepts of the genesis of virus-associated tumours but are only part of this complex process. Experimental, clinical and epidemiological observations all suggest that malignancy results from a step-by-step accumulation of stable cellular alterations whose occurrence reflects, and is greatly accelerated by, exposure to multiple risk factors. The age of the animal and the duration, intensity and frequency of exposure to risk factors are important elements in tumour evolution, and these variables tend to obscure any causal relationship between virus infection and the eventual development of malignancy. We must take account of these other components if we are to understand the aetiological significance of viruses.

Table 12.9 Common insertion sites for murine leukaemia viruses in tumours where genes have been identified

Locus	Chrom. location	Gene function	Tumour	MLV strain
bmi-1	2	Transcription factor	B lymphoma	Moloney
evi/CB1/*fim*-3	3	Transcription factor	Myeloid leukaemia	AKXD
			Non-B non-T leukaemia	Friend, Cas-Br-M
evi-2[a]	11	Transmembrane protein NF1 tumour suppressor	Myeloid leukaemia	BXH
fim-2	18	c-*fms* (CSF-1 receptor)	Myeloid leukaemia	Friend
fli-1 (*sic*-1)	9	Transcription factor	Erythroleukaemia	Friend
			Non-B, non-T leukaemia	Cas-Br-E
fli-2[a]	15	Transcription factor NF-E2	Erythroleukaemia	Friend
lck	4	Non-receptor protein tyrosine kinase	T lymphoma	Moloney
myb	10	Transcription factor	Myelomonocytic	Moloney
myc/*mlvi*-1 (*mis*-1)/*mlvi*-4[b]	15	Transcription factor	T lymphoma	Moloney
N-*myc*	12	Transcription factor	T lymphoma	Moloney
Notch1	2	Transmembrane receptor	T lymphoma	Moloney
p53[a]	11	Transcription factor tumour suppressor	Erythroleukaemia Non-B, non-T	Friend Cas-Br-E
pim-1	17	Ser/thr protein kinase	T, B lymphomas	Moloney
pim-2	X	Ser/thr protein kinase	T, B lymphomas	Moloney
Prlr	15	Prolactin receptor	T lymphoma (rat)	Moloney
spi-1	2	Transcription factor	Erythroleukaemia	Friend SFFV
Tiam-1	16	GDP exchange protein	T lymphoma	Moloney
til-1	17	Transcription factor	T lymphoma	Moloney
tpl-1 (*ets*-1)	9	Transcription factor	T lymphoma	Moloney
tpl-2	18	Ser/thr protein kinase	T lymphoma (rat)	Moloney
vin-1	6	Cyclin D2	T lymphoma	BL/VL3 RadLV

[a]Insertion ablates gene expression.
[b]Insertions at *mlvi*-4 may have additional effects.

The influence of risk factors on viral carcinogenesis can be considered by dividing them into 3 major, but overlapping, categories: (1) factors associated with the virus infection and its effect on host cells; (2) factors that determine the evolution and properties of neoplastic cells; and (3) factors that affect the host response to both virus and tumour. We can consider in turn the interplay of these factors during 3 arbitrary stages of tumour development: (1) the successful infection of the organism by a virus and, when the virus acts by a direct means, its infection of the tumour cell lineage; (2) the conversion within the tumour cell lineage of a normal cell to neoplastic growth and behaviour; and (3) the survival and growth of its descendants to form a detectable tumour. An assessment of the relative importance of the different risk factors at each stage of tumour development is shown in the histogram in Fig. 12.7. In this diagram the 3 stages of development are shown on the abscissa, which is thus a time scale axis; it is, however, impossible to draw this to scale. Stage 2 is probably the longest period; important stage 2 events probably often precede those in stage 1.

3.1 Virus infection/transmission

An animal becomes infected with an oncogenic virus by one of 3 routes (Weiss 1984). The first is genetic transmission, by which most individuals, of many species, have acquired endogenous retroviruses during evolution. These viruses seem to be non-essential but innocuous passengers in the genomes of their hosts and they are often xenotropic (i.e. capable of replication only in other species). A clear exception to this harmlessness is that certain strains of mice harbour endogenous viruses that are ecotropic (i.e. they can infect mouse cells). Moreover, these viruses evolve by recombination with other defective endogenous proviruses, generating variants with enhanced leukaemogenicity (Stoye, Moroni and Coffin 1991). Comparable variants of altered, if not augmented, pathogenicity can also arise by recombination of FeLV with endogenous cat retroviruses (Neil et al. 1991). In both mice and cats the recombinant viruses reveal altered viral envelope glycoproteins, some of which have an increased propensity to bind to and stimulate proliferation of immune-responsive and other cells.

RISK FACTORS AFFECTING

1 The characteristics of virus infection

    (a) Exposure to virus

    (b) Genetic susceptibility to virus

    (c) Non-cytolytic virus–host interaction

2 The inherent nature of the neoplastic cell

    (a) Exposure to other initiating agents or
        complete carcinogens

    (b) Exposure to promoting agents

3 The host response to virus and neoplasia

    (a) Lack of passive immunity

    (b) Impaired active specific and non-specific
        immunity to virus and neoplastic cell

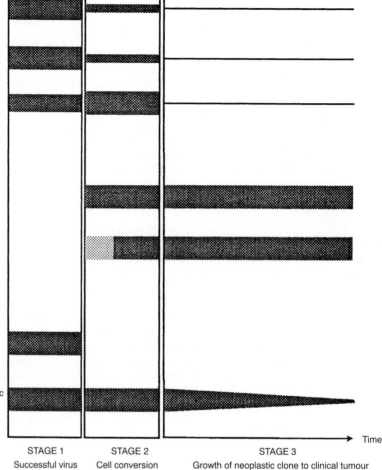

STAGE 1 — Successful virus infection

STAGE 2 — Cell conversion to neoplasia

STAGE 3 — Growth of neoplastic clone to clinical tumour

Time

Fig. 12.7 Risk factors in viral carcinogenesis; the relationship between the arbitrary stages of virus-associated neoplasia, the features of the neoplastic process and the risk factors that influence each feature. The stages of neoplasia are shown on the abscissa. The breaks in the time axis indicate that these stages vary in length and they are not shown to scale (in general, stage 1 is likely to be relatively short and stage 2 is usually the longest period). The risk factors affecting either of the 3 features characterizing virus-associated neoplasia are shown on the ordinate and they may operate at different, and often more than one, stages of the disease process. The thickness of the bars indicates the relative importance of each risk factor at each stage of neoplasia, broken lines indicating periods at which the risk factors are of no or uncertain significance. (Modified, with permission, from Wyke and Weiss 1984.)

The second route, congenital transmission of exogenous viruses across the placenta or oviduct, is important in the case of leukaemogenic avian, feline and bovine retroviruses. However, for these and many others the third route, horizontal transmission peri- and postnatally is also significant. Whereas the papovaviruses are hardy, the enveloped herpesviruses and retroviruses are far more labile; their horizontal spread is therefore more efficient when animals are grouped together and make close contact with carriers. Moreover, such conditions increase the risk of repeated exposure to high doses of virus early in life, a pattern which, in turn, appears to encourage the eventual appearance of neoplasia.

With regard to the routes of transmission, the pat-

tern of virus spread is also greatly influenced by its site of replication in the animal. Thus, for FeLV and EBV, free virus is shed in the buccal cavity and transmitted in saliva. Marek's disease virus of fowls, on the other hand, replicates in feather follicle epithelium and is spread in dander, whereas BLV and HTLV remain cell-associated and require the transmission of whole cells. In the case of the last 2 viruses, iatrogenic transfer and 'flying pin' arthropod vectors might be expected to be significant routes of infection, and epidemiological data support this notion.

3.2 Genetic susceptibility to viruses

All viruses require the means to enter a cell, express their genomes and assemble progeny for spread to other cells; exposure to virus will have no untoward effects unless the host genotype permits at least some stages of this process. Interspecies variation in the susceptibility of cells to viruses – often associated with severe constraints on the virus life cycle – are taken for granted but there can also be pronounced variation within a species. In cases of virus-associated neoplasia, such variation is indicated by clustering of tumour incidence. Clusters are often due to variation in the other risk factors discussed here, but difference in virus susceptibility is a likely cause when clustering is demonstrably familial. In domestic animals, where breeding is often controlled and one male can sire many dispersed offspring, it is easier to discern familial clusters. The clusters of, for example, bovine leucosis, reflect genetic factors that are not well defined, but in other instances the basis for the underlying enhanced susceptibility is better understood. The species in which this has been studied most comprehensively is, of course, the laboratory mouse (Tsichlis and Lazo 1991).

The need for entry of virus into cells provides a crucial barrier to infection; in many cases, efficient penetration is highly specific, not only for the whole animal but also for particular types of cell within the host. Retroviruses enter cells whose surfaces bear receptors to which the viral envelope glycoprotein can bind. In chickens, receptors are found on a wide range of cell types but their specificity (and hence host susceptibility to virus) reveals genetically determined polymorphisms between individual birds (Payne 1992). Other receptors are of limited distribution within the host: human CD4 lymphocyte antigen is an important component of the HIV-1 receptor, this stringency explaining in part the tropism of HIV-1 for a particular T cell subset (Dalgleish et al. 1984). These receptors do not of course exist merely to facilitate virus penetration and, indeed, not all binding sites serve this role. They clearly have structural or other functional purposes on the cell surface. For the mammalian type C retroviruses, related families of transmembrane transporter proteins for basic amino acids and phosphate have been identified as mediators of viral entry (Cunningham and Kim 1994). However, the relevance of these to oncogenesis seems to be slight, as there is little evidence of effects on cell growth and viability emanating from virus binding to these receptors.

Epstein–Barr virus gains entry to B cells via binding to the complement receptor molecule CR2 (Nemerow et al. 1987). Other oncogenic DNA virus receptors have yet to be identified.

Once inside cells, viruses may do some damage, which will, however, be greatly limited by any further restrictions on their replication and spread. For instance, retroviruses are subject to both physiological and genetic constraints after penetration. For the type C retroviruses, stable integration of a complete DNA

transcript of the virion RNA genome can occur only in cells that synthesize DNA; on the other hand, the early gene functions of polyomaviruses can themselves stimulate DNA synthesis. The host range restrictions of ectropic mouse leukaemia virus mediated by the mouse Fv-1 locus also operate during this early part of the infectious cycle. Recently, the retroviral LTR (see Fig. 12.5) has attracted considerable attention and there is a wealth of evidence to suggest that its potency varies with cell type. Cellular factors interact in *trans* with the LTR enhancer to modulate the level of transcripts mediated by this element in a given cell and hence the extent of viral replication, the oncogenic potential of the virus and its cell tropism (Tsichlis and Lazo 1991). Thus, the pathogenesis of, for example, retrovirus-induced mouse leukaemia is a very complex process in which both the virus and the tumour cell evolve. When virus infection of an appropriate host results in proviral insertion at a specific site, the expression is stimulated of one or more of a range of cell genes (see Table 12.9). The amplitude of this expression may depend on the potency of the viral LTR in that cell (Morrison, Soni and Lenz 1995).

3.3 Non-cytolytic virus–host interactions

Virus diseases result from the release of progeny from infected cells and their dissemination within the host. Some tumour-associated viruses, such as hepatitis B and many retroviruses, can be released by living cells but for many others cytolysis is necessary for escape of virus. Cytolysis is, of course, incompatible with direct mechanisms of virus oncogenesis, so neoplasia is likely to be a rare and aberrant consequence of infection by these viruses. In such cases, either the host restricts the later stages of virus replication or the virus is defective in directing these events, but, in both instances, viral functions needed to induce neoplasia are retained.

Two other properties of tumour viruses are worth mentioning here: virus integration and latent virus infection. The viruses of all families that include directly oncogenic members can exist as DNA within the cell, inserted in the host chromosome. This may be a rare outcome of infection or, as with retroviruses, an essential part of the virus life cycle. Virus integration is obligatory for oncogenesis by insertional mutagenesis but there seems to be no reason why it should be required for other forms of oncogenesis. Indeed, as virus genomes are absent from some tumours for which viruses are considered risk factors, integration is presumably not essential – at least in the later stages of tumour evolution. Poxviruses, although not true tumour viruses, need special consideration because they can induce proliferating lesions, probably through the action of viral genes that encode molecules resembling cell growth factors (Stroobant, Rice and Gullick 1985) but the nodules produced never progress to full-blown cancer. It is possible that poxviruses fail to induce tumours because they replicate in the cytoplasm, never integrate and so do not achieve a sufficiently stable association with the host cell. A number of RNA viruses also achieve persistent infections, yet they rarely, if ever, integrate and only one representative (hepatitis C virus) has so far been incriminated in neoplasia. Integration is clearly important in achieving a stable infection but may have additional undefined significance.

Latency is a characteristic of 2 families of oncogenic viruses: the retroviruses and the herpesviruses. Prolonged latent infection is a common sequel of primary FeLV infection in cats. It is associated with a humoral and cellular immune response and can be abolished by treatment with immunosuppressive agents (Rojko et al. 1982). Without such insults, however, this form of latent infection tends to resolve in recovery with subsequent immunity (Pacitti and Jarrett 1985). Latent infection with BLV has also been described but in this case a non-immunoglobulin plasma protein seems to be involved in virus suppression (Gupta and Ferrer 1982). Like those of many endogenous retroviruses, latent exogenous genomes may be in the configuration of inactive chromatin, which is highly methylated. This has practical significance because tumour cells do not usually express their resident viral genomes unless the animals are immunosuppressed or the cells are cultured, with or without agents intended to activate silent genomes. At the mechanistic level, the role of latency in neoplasia is not obvious, but, like integration, it may serve primarily to ensure persistence of the viral genome, thus facilitating its interactions with the other risk factors germane to neoplasia.

In the case of EBV, the capacity for latent infection seems to be critical to virus persistence and central to its involvement in tumours. EBV-positive tumour cells display one of 3 patterns of gene expression with increasingly complex expression patterns (latency I, II and III) typified by Burkitt's lymphoma, nasopharyngeal carcinoma and immunoblastic lymphomas, respectively. It is notable that latency III tumours, where at least 6 EBV proteins are expressed, are associated with immunosuppressed states in which immune surveillance of viral antigens is ineffective (Rickinson 1994).

3.4 Viruses and the multi-step development of neoplasia

Many of the viruses that transform cells in vitro carry oncogenes of which the activity is under the control of powerful viral regulatory elements (see Fig. 12.5). Oncogenes – perhaps aided by a spreading virus infection – are very potent carcinogens that rapidly induce tumours in host animals. In some circumstances, however, oncogene-mediated viral carcinogenesis is far less efficient and the appearance of a neoplastic cell phenotype requires other genetic or epigenetic events such as the loss of tumour suppressor genes or the acquisition of additional, activated oncogenes. There is abundant evidence for this. Some tumour viruses carry more than one oncogene, each of which contributes to their tumour-inducing capacity. In the example of the retrovirus avian erythroblastosis virus,

erb-B encodes a transmembrane protein (EGF receptor) and *erb*-A a nuclear protein (thyroid hormone receptor) (see Table 12.4). Other examples are the presence of the c-*myc* nuclear oncogene and the protein kinase oncogene *mil/raf* in avian carcinoma virus MH2, and the presence of 2 nuclear oncogenes, *myb* and *ets* in avian myeloblastosis virus.

Further evidence of the co-operative action of multiple genes in lymphoma development comes from murine leukaemia virus infection, in which several different insertional mutagenic events can be observed in a single tumour (Tsichlis, Gunter-Strauss and Lohse 1985). Furthermore, mice carrying one oncogene as a transgene may show greatly accelerated tumour onset when infected with the virus, and activation of co-operating genes by insertional mutagenesis occurs at high frequency (van Lohuizen et al. 1991). Thus, infection of *pim*-1 transgenic mice with Moloney murine leukaemia virus leads to rapid tumour onset, and in these tumours viral insertion invariably occurs at c-*myc* or N-*myc* but never at both genes (van Lohuizen et al. 1989). Further evidence of the co-operative action of these genes is given by the strongly synergistic effect on tumour development of crossing mice carrying different activated oncogenes (e.g. c-*myc* and *pim*-1). In this way, a complementation map of oncogenesis is gradually emerging, with genes from distinct groups supplying co-operating functions. In a similar way, MMTV has been used in conjunction with transgenics to demonstrate the synergistic relationship between insertions at *wnt*-1 and *int*-2 (*fgf*-3) in the development of mammary tumours and to identify further related genes (*wnt*-3, *fgf*-8) as alternative targets for the virus (Lee et al. 1995, MacArthur, Shankar and Shackleford 1995).

In naturally occurring cancer the requirement for multiple cellular changes is mirrored in the time- and risk factor-dependent pattern of tumour development. Many clinically important tumour viruses, particularly those of humans, need the operation of additional chemical, physical or infectious risk factors to initiate or promote neoplasia (see Tables 12.1, 12.2 and 12.3). Because these viruses are incomplete carcinogens, it is not certain whether they act as initiators or promoters of oncogenesis.

Viruses have often been considered initiators, for a number of reasons. Initiation in experimental systems is a dose-dependent, irreversible event with many hallmarks of mutation (Montesano and Slaga 1983), and direct models of virus oncogenesis either induce or introduce mutant genes. Moreover, virus infection is often observed early in life in the susceptible individual, perhaps before exposure to other likely risk factors. However, aside from instances of possible transient effects (see p. 221), virus-induced cancer is often associated with persistent infections, virus integration and possibly latency. Infection early in life may simply be a prerequisite for achieving persistence, a prolonged exposure to virus that can be significant in 2 ways. First, it may increase the chance of crucial, if rare, virus–cell interactions. Second, and this seems particularly relevant to viruses that act indirectly, it may enhance the possibility that other environmental risk factors that may be encountered can be influenced by a chronic viral tumour-promoting activity. Some instances, however, are not clear-cut. Consider, for example, tumour induction by EBV and HTLV-I: both seem to stimulate a proliferation of lymphoid cells that is strictly neoplastic (in that it is driven from within the cell and results from a 'mutation') but which resembles hyperplasia in being polyclonal. These viruses seem to behave as tumour promoters, and subsequent clonal events such as c-*myc* translocation in EBV-associated Burkitt's lymphoma are more likely to be the result of initiation. It seems that the concepts of initiation and promotion that have been so fruitful in studying experimental carcinogenesis are not so readily applicable to viral cancer. The consequences of virus infection are, however, clearly capable of contributing to several stages of neoplasia.

3.5 The host response

The ability of the infected animal to limit both virus infection and the multiplication of neoplastic cells is of great importance in virus-associated neoplasia, particularly the leukaemias in which the tumours themselves are prone to perturb both specific and non-specific immune regulation. Establishment of virus persistence increases the chance of viral pathogenic mechanisms coming into play; persistence can often be achieved by exposing a young animal, with waning maternal immunity, to large and repeated doses of virus, resulting in impaired ability to limit the extent of the infection. Episodes of immune impairment later in life, due to nutritional or hormonal factors, disease or other physiological stresses, can reinforce this effect or even favour infection of a previously virus-free animal. When the viral risk factor is itself an immunosuppressant (see Fig. 12.7) the problem is exacerbated, and, once a tumour burden develops, it may reinforce the predisposing impairment.

An intimate association with compromised immunity is often seen in the natural history of virus carcinogenesis. Examples from avian, feline and human haemopoietic neoplasms, in which the virus infection contributes wholly or partially to the immunosuppression, have been given above. In other instances, another risk factor is responsible. Thus, an immunosuppressant in bracken fern seems to be important in the aetiology of papillomavirus-associated alimentary carcinomas in cattle (Jarrett 1985). In humans, iatrogenic immunosuppression is associated with an increased incidence of certain tumours, many of which had prior association with a virus risk factor. Indeed, so striking is this that Kinlen (1992) has suggested that all human tumours of which the incidence increases in immunosuppressed patients may have a viral component in their cause. In short, the host response seems to be more important in controlling virus infection than other aspects of cell neoplasia.

3.6 The search for new viruses

There are 3 important motifs in naturally occurring viral cancers in animals and humans: (1) virus, (2) immune impairment and (3) co-carcinogen. The first 2 components appear to be particularly important in most animal tumours, whereas the third is of greater importance in humans. These must all be considered in assessing the roles of other potential tumour viruses.

The most profitable tumours for study are those showing clustering that can be familial, geographic or social/occupational, implying important genetic or environmental risk factors, both of which can point to viruses. Another important clue is any evidence of increased tumour prevalence in immunosuppressed individuals.

Both intact animals and tumours must be examined for characteristics of virus infection. Virus isolation from tumour material may require culture of tumour cells to demonstrate any latent virus, perhaps with addition of hormones, or of chemicals such as bromo- or iododeoxyuridine or activate endogenous viruses, or 5'-azacytidine which inhibits cytosine methylation. Virus can sometimes also be detected by electron microscopy or immunological techniques. It is important to try to discover an appropriate cell type for virus propagation in vitro because the tumour itself is often an unsuitable host. The complexity of the mammalian genome was a barrier to solving this problem by subtractive hybridization methods, but innovative PCR-based techniques have recently been devised to identify small amounts of foreign DNA in tumour cells (representational difference analysis). This approach has borne fruit with the discovery of a new human herpesvirus (KSHV) in Kaposi's sarcoma cases (Chang et al. 1994).

Isolation of a candidate virus provides the opportunity for a more detailed study of its association with the tumour. If, however, isolation fails, much can be learned by comparison with known tumour viruses together with the screening of tumour cells for molecular evidence of viral infection and examination of intact animals for epidemiological clues. If infection with a virus is common in a population, features of the infection peculiar to the tumour-bearing hosts should be sought. Is the infection unusually persistent? Is the serological response abnormal? Is the virus in the tumour defective? Are unusual viral antigens expressed? Even when a virus cannot be identified, a specific tumour antigen may be an important clue to a viral aetiology.

Epidemiological evidence is crucial in humans, in whom it is impossible to test a causal role for the agent by virus inoculation. Case–control studies can associate the virus with the tumour, and laboratory investigations will establish the features of high- and low-risk groups. Retrospective and, ideally, prospective studies of high-risk groups can establish a temporal relationship between virus infection, other risk factors and tumour development. This knowledge can then serve as a basis for the management of the tumour.

4 PRINCIPLES OF THE MANAGEMENT OF VIRUS-ASSOCIATED CANCER

Although little is known of many aspects of the pathogenesis of virus-associated tumours, the knowledge that a virus is implicated can be used to try to manage the disease at any of 3 arbitrary stages of virus neoplasia described earlier (Fig. 12.7). Two points should be remembered. First, a wider range of prophylactic measures can be applied in veterinary medicine (where the health of the herd can override the survival of the individual) than in human practice. Secondly, for all tumours in which a virus is implicated, the detection of virus infection at any stage of the disease might be of diagnostic or prognostic use. This is clearly the case in the few diseases in which infection often leads to tumour formation. However, even when neoplasia is rare, detailed knowledge of the role played by the virus might identify features of the infection that are characteristic of hosts at high risk.

4.1 Prevention of virus infection

Before infection, steps can be taken to: (1) decrease the concentration of virus in the hosts' environment; (2) increase the natural (genetic) resistance of host populations; and (3) increase the resistance of the hosts by active or passive immunization.

THE SOURCE OF VIRUS

This is determined by the density of symptomatic or asymptomatic carriers in the population, the ability of the virus to survive outside its host and whether other animals act as natural reservoirs for the virus. Many tumour viruses are species-specific and in practice only the first 2 factors are amenable to prophylactic measures.

The identification of carriers often requires specialized techniques to detect virus infection. It is thus costly and further action is effective only when the carrier can be killed, cured or isolated from the susceptible population. For these reasons, identification of human carriers poses ethical problems but can be important for several groups of patients. The first are those whose habits place them at particular risk, for example intravenous drug abusers in the case of HIV and hepatitis B infections and the sexually promiscuous in the case of papillomavirus and herpesvirus infections. The second are those who have acquired iatrogenic infections, such as HIV and hepatitis B virus from contaminated blood products. The third are mothers infected with HTLV, where breast milk can be a very important but avoidable means of transmission.

Identification of carriers can be useful in the control of avian, feline and bovine lymphoid leukaemias. A small proportion of cats infected with FeLV do not develop immunity and remain viraemic. Such animals can either be removed from colonies or identified before introduction into virus-free groups. Eradication of enzootic bovine leucosis is greatly assisted by tests for virus carriers, whose lineage can be maintained free of virus by the transfer of well washed embryos (with the zona pellucida intact) to virus-negative recipients (see reviews in Onions and Jarrett 1987).

Improved hygiene to reduce the source of the virus is probably of little significance within susceptible host populations but, in combination with appropriate husbandry, can reduce the dissemination of disease between local concentrations of animals such as the spread of ALV from one poultry farm to another. Many tumour viruses are highly susceptible to chemical disinfectants, drying and other inactivating agents, but horizontal and congenital spread depend on such intimate contact between hosts that disinfection is impracticable. Papillomas and enzootic bovine leucosis are exceptions to this because the causal viruses can be spread on the instruments of stockmen and veterinarians. Another possible measure, applicable to BLV and HTLV-I, is the control of insects that may spread infection. The social and hygiene practices in many Western countries delay some EBV infections until puberty or later, but these increase the incidence of infectious mononucleosis. A delay in the age of acquisition of EBV infection in Africa and Asia might reduce the incidence of Burkitt's lymphoma or nasopharyngeal carcinoma, but this has not yet been demonstrated. However, one virus-associated human neoplasm for which a change in habits should reduce incidence is carcinoma of the uterine cervix. As with other venereally transmitted infections, the spread of papillomavirus and HSV type 2 has been favoured by promiscuity and changes in contraceptive practices.

THE GENETIC SUSCEPTIBILITY OF HOST ANIMALS

The selective breeding of genetically resistant stock is possible only in animals, and particularly in those that have a short generation time. It has been successful in reducing the incidence of avian lymphoid leucosis; the causal virus exists in the field as 2 major subtypes, characterized by the presence of particular glycoproteins on the viral envelope. These glycoproteins interact with specific cell surface receptors to allow the viruses to penetrate the host cells. Strains of domestic chicken have been bred that lack the surface receptors for the field strains of avian leucosis virus and these birds are resistant to infection (Crittenden and Motta 1969). Some strains partly resistant to lymphoid leucosis apparently permit infection but not tumour development. A similar genetic resistance is seen in the production of Marek's disease lymphomas.

IMMUNITY TO VIRUS INFECTION

Although a number of commercial vaccines exist for oncogenic viruses of animals, proposals to produce vaccines against human oncogenic viruses are controversial, for several reasons.

1   In many instances the role of the virus in the tumour is uncertain; indeed, proof of a causal role may rely on the prophylactic effect of vaccination. This leads to the dilemma of whether to embark

on such measures before they can be shown to be necessary.

2 Tumour production may be a rare outcome of infection by a widespread and not very pathogenic virus.

3 The presence of many latently infected carriers and the frequent acquisition of infection early in life (e.g. with human herpesviruses) will limit vaccine efficacy.

4 Because tumours can result from an aberrant virus–cell interaction, a traditional type of vaccine, based on inactivated or attenuated virus, may itself pose a risk of oncogenicity. This last objection might be overcome by the use of purified immunogens either produced by genetically manipulated portions of viral genomes or synthesized in the laboratory.

However, the first 2 considerations suggest that the returns (in terms of improved health of the human population) may justify the outlay only if 3 conditions are fulfilled: (1) the virus causes significant disease in addition to its oncogenic potential (as is the case with HIV and hepatitis B virus); (2) the populations concerned are clearly defined, small and at high risk; (3) the virus is the only clearly defined risk factor in the genesis of a common tumour (as with EBV-associated nasopharyngeal carcinoma).

The first successful commercial vaccines against a neoplasm were produced for Marek's disease and have proved of great value to the poultry industry. Avirulent strains of the virus, either natural or artificially attenuated, have been used as vaccine, as has a related herpesvirus of turkeys; continual modification of the vaccine, however, has been necessary to try to keep up with the emergence of highly virulent strains (Schat 1987). The vaccine virus strains establish a latent infection and induce tumour-associated surface antigens in lymphoid cells, sometimes with minor cytopathic effects and neuritis. There is, however, no immunosuppression and vaccinated birds resist challenge with oncogenic virus (Calnek et al. 1979), apparently by an immunity directed against both viral and tumour antigens.

Approaches to vaccination against human herpesviruses have been more conservative, most efforts being directed to the testing of recombinant subunit vaccines in animal models. Using recombinant subunit vaccines based on viral surface glycoproteins, protection against infectious virus challenge has been achieved against EBV in a cottontop tamarin model, and against HSV in mice (reviewed in Morein and Merza 1991). While it would be desirable to eradicate both of these viruses from the human population, the case for large scale vaccination is not clear-cut.

Recombinant subunit vaccines based on hepatitis B virus surface antigen have been available since 1982 and have proved effective in reducing the incidence of infection in selected at-risk groups. However, these measures have had little impact on the overall incidence of infection in the population, leading to calls for mass vaccination to be considered (Margolis, Alter and Hadler 1991).

Vaccines made from ground-up wart tissue have long been used for prophylaxis and therapy of papillomas in animals. This empirical approach illustrates the potential for vaccination against papillomavirus infection, but is clearly incompatible with modern quality-control standards for human medicine. More recently, recombinant gene products of bovine papillomavirus, both early and late genes, have been efficacious in preventing warts and in accelerating rejection (Campo 1995). Translation of these results to human vaccination is complicated by the multiplicity of HPV types and our limited knowledge of the natural history of HPV infections (Galloway 1994).

A number of commercial vaccines have been developed for feline leukaemia, including inactivated virus, infected cell extracts and recombinant subunit *env* vaccines (Jarrett 1994), and attempts to produce a bovine leucosis vaccine are also under way.

Although prophylactic vaccination is also considered highly desirable as a means of containing the HIV epidemic, only small scale safety trials have been mounted at this time, and there is uncertainty over the likely efficacy of existing subunit vaccines. Experiments with animal lentivirus models such as simian and feline immunodeficiency viruses have shown only weak protection or short-term suppression of virus replication with conventional subunit or inactivated virus vaccines, and the problem of vaccine escape due to strain variation is significant (Schild and Stott 1993). Although more robust protection has been achieved with attenuated virus vaccines, these have serious safety drawbacks and are unlikely to be tested in the human population in the near future (Baba et al. 1995).

ANTIVIRAL THERAPY

Another approach to the control of oncogenic viruses (one popular with the pharmaceutical industry) is to try to limit the infection – usually after it is clinically evident – with antiviral chemotherapy. This, too, poses problems inherent in the close symbiosis between viruses and their host cells, because drugs must be devised that are selectively toxic for the virus. One approach is to direct research to the development of inhibitors of processes essential to the virus but dispensable by the cell, such as reverse transcriptase by RNA-dependent DNA polymerase. Within these constraints, some widely used and moderately effective drugs have been developed against, for instance, herpesviruses and retroviruses. These drugs may assist in the control of virus replication but in their current modes of use have shown no beneficial effect on tumour development or on established cancers. For example, the most widely used anti-retroviral agent, azidothymidine, was first tested as a potential anticancer agent but its long-term use in AIDS patients does not appear to reduce, and might conceivably increase, the incidence of non-Hodgkin's lymphoma (Pluda et al. 1990).

The use of interferons to control virus-associated

cancers was considered an exciting prospect in the last decade but clinical trials have, in general, been disappointing. Striking exceptions have been the effects of interferon-α in virus-associated laryngeal and genital papillomas and in hairy cell leukaemias. However, effects other than antiviral activity may be involved in the former examples (Gangemi et al. 1994) while in the latter case the ability of interferon to induce cell differentiation seems to be the most likely mechanism (Vedantham et al. 1992).

4.2 Prevention of cell conversion to neoplasia

The problems of tackling viral infection suggest that other potentially avoidable risk factors (see Tables 12.1, 12.2 and 12.3), which tend to operate in association, might provide easier targets for preventive measures. Such hopes, however, seem largely misplaced. In humans these risk factors include habits (notably smoking), dietary factors (which may be even harder to eliminate than smoking unless, like aflatoxin contamination, their deleterious effects are obvious) and other diseases. The most striking example of the last is malaria, a risk factor in Burkitt's lymphoma in certain tropical areas but also a major disease problem in its own right in many parts of the world. Indeed, the reduction or elimination of some of these risk factors would have benefits far beyond the postulated decrease in cancer incidence. This is so self-evident that there must be doubt as to whether the incentive of cancer prevention *per se* will succeed where other imperatives have failed.

4.3 Therapy of virus-associated cancers

Once a virus-infected cell has become neoplastic the prevention of further tumour growth depends on therapy rather than prophylaxis. But with virus-associated tumours, the detection of infection at any stage of the disease might itself influence prognosis. In cases in which neoplasia is a rare outcome of virus infection, knowledge of the role played by the virus might identify features characteristic of hosts at high risk. Such knowledge has been used, for instance, in attempts at early diagnosis of nasopharyngeal carcinoma by screening populations at risk in China for EBV-specific salivary IgA (Zeng, Zhang and Li 1982).

When viral aetiology is established, immunotherapy might be considered as a means of achieving regression. Indeed, early experimentation demonstrated that most virally induced tumours were quite readily rejected, unlike those without obvious viral aetiology (Klein and Klein 1977). However, these experiments involved the inoculation of immunocompetent animals with tumours expressing readily detectable viral antigens. In contrast, the human malignancies most tightly linked to virus infection are seen in the context of obviously impaired immunity (e.g. AIDS or transplant patients) or express very little if any viral antigens (e.g. HTLV-I associated adult T cell leukaemia (ATL), Burkitt's lymphoma). Moreover, the latter tumours may have arisen in individuals with specific deficits in their immunological repertoire, as suggested by associations with specific types of major histocompatibility complex. In these contexts, immunotherapy seems much less promising and it may be necessary instead to consider the means of repairing the defective response. One way to achieve this may be to create tumour cell vaccines by transfection with co-receptor or cytokine genes. Ironically, the retroviruses have recently found a role as vectors to mediate this type of gene therapy for cancer (Vieweg and Gilboa 1995).

Papillomavirus-associated neoplasms have long been treated with extracts of tumours. For example, treatment of bovine ocular squamous cell carcinoma (a common neoplasm in light-skinned cattle in areas of high sunlight) with an allogeneic tumour extract resulted in remissions (Hoffmann, Jennings and Spradbrow 1981). However, it is not clear whether viral antigens were targets in the regression of this malignancy. As discussed earlier (p. 231), the possibility that vaccines against HPV-16 and 18 might be able to cause regression of cervical carcinoma should be considered.

Finally, if viral genes can be shown to play a role in the maintenance of the tumour state, then direct inhibition of their expression or even their downstream effectors may be a route to therapy. For example, antisense inhibition of NF-κB was found to limit the growth of HTLV Tax-transformed cells in a mouse tumour model, while antisense to Tax itself was ineffective (Kitajima et al. 1992).

5 CONCLUSIONS

In recent years, research on tumour viruses has identified some of the genetic lesions that underly neoplasia and has led to some remarkable advances in basic cancer research. These studies are now influencing areas of cell biology and biochemistry that seem far removed from their virological origins. At the same time, however, tumour viruses have become more important to the virologist. We now appreciate that viruses are often one of a complex of risk factors that predisposes to a significant proportion of human disease. Although the part they play often results from an insidious and intractable pathogenic process, they are, in theory, avoidable risk factors. As such, they may provide the key to the management of many cancers.

REFERENCES

Baba TW, Jeong YS et al., 1995, Pathogenicity of live attenuated SIV after mucosal infection of neonatal macaques, *Science*, **267:** 1820–5.

Berns A, Breuer M et al., 1989, Transgenic mice as a means to study synergism between oncogenes, *Int J Cancer*, **S4:** 22–5.

Bishop JM, 1991, Molecular themes in oncogenesis, *Cell*, **64:** 235–48.

Bishop JM, 1995, The rise of the genetic paradigm, *Genes Dev*, **9:** 1309–15.

Buendia MA, 1994, Hepatitis B viruses and liver cancer: the woodchuck model, *Viruses and Cancer*, eds Minson A, Neil J, McCrae M, Cambridge University Press, Cambridge, 174–87.

Calnek BW, Carlisle JC et al., 1979, Comparative pathogenesis studies with oncogenic and nononcogenic Marek's disease viruses and turkey herpesvirus, *Am J Vet Res*, **40:** 541–8.

Campo MS, 1995, Infection by BPV and prospects for vaccination, *Trends Microbiol Sci*, **3:** 92–7.

Chang Y, Cesarman E et al., 1994, Identification of herpesvirus-like DNA sequences in AIDS-associated Kaposi's sarcoma, *Science*, **266:** 1865–9.

Crittenden LB, Motta JV, 1969, A survey of genetic resistance to leukosis-sarcoma viruses in commercial stocks of chickens, *Poultry Sci*, **48:** 1751–7.

Cunningham JM, Kim JW, 1994, Cellular receptors for type C retroviruses, *Cellular Receptors for Animal Viruses*, ed Wimmer E, Cold Spring Harbor Press, Cold Spring Harbor NY, 49–59.

Dalgleish AG, Beverley PC et al., 1984, The CD4 (T4) antigen is an essential component of the receptor for the AIDS retrovirus, *Nature (London)*, **312:** 763–7.

Donehower LA, Harvey M et al., 1992, Mice deficient for p53 are developmentally normal but susceptible to spontaneous tumours, *Nature (London)*, **356:** 215–21.

Evan GI, Wyllie AH et al., 1992, Induction of apoptosis in fibroblasts by c-myc protein, *Cell*, **69:** 119–28.

Flubacher MM, Bear SE, Tsichlis PN, 1994, Replacement of interleukin-2 (IL-2)-generated mitogenic signals by a mink cell focus-forming (MCF) or xenotropic virus-induced IL-9-dependent autocrine loop – implications for MVCF virus-induced leukemogenesis, *J Virol*, **68:** 7709–16.

Galloway DA, 1994, Human papillomaviruses: a warty problem, *Infect Agents Dis*, **3:** 187–93.

Gangemi JD, Piris L et al., 1994, HPV replication in experimental models: effects of interferon, *Antiviral Res*, **24:** 175–90.

Gupta P, Ferrer JF, 1982, Expression of bovine leukemia virus genome is blocked by a nonimmunoglobulin protein in plasma from infected cattle, *Science*, **215:** 405–7.

Harris H, 1985, Suppression of malignancy in hybrid cells: the mechanism, *J Cell Sci*, **79:** 83–94.

zur Hausen H, 1986, Intracellular surveillance of persistent viral infections: human genital cancer results from deficient cellular control of papilloma viral gene expression, *Lancet*, **2:** 489–91.

zur Hausen H, 1991, Viruses in human cancers, *Science*, **254:** 1167–73.

Henderson S, Rowe M et al., 1991, Induction of bcl-2 expression by Epstein–Barr virus latent membrane protein 1 protects infected B cells from programmed cell death, *Cell*, **65:** 1107–15.

Hesketh R, 1995, *The Oncogene Factsbook*, Academic Press, London.

Hoffmann D, Jennings PA, Spradbrow PB, 1981, Autografting and allografting of bovine ocular squamous carcinoma, *Res Vet Sci*, **31:** 48–53.

Jarrett O, 1994, Transmission and control of feline leukaemia virus, *Viruses and Cancer*, eds Minson A, Neil J, McCrae M, Cambridge University Press, Cambridge, 235–46.

Jarrett WFH, 1985, The natural history of bovine papillomavirus infection, *Adv Viral Oncology*, **5:** 83–102.

Kiefer F, Courtneidge SA, Wagner EF, 1994, Oncogenic properties of the middle T antigens of polyomaviruses, *Adv Cancer Res*, **64:** 125–57.

Kinlen LJ, 1992, Immunosuppressive therapy and acquired immunological disorders, *Cancer Res*, **52:** 5474–6.

Kitajima I, Shinohara T et al. 1992, Ablation of transplanted HTLV-I Tax-transformed tumors in mice by antisense inhibition of NF-kappa-B, *Science*, **258:** 1792–5.

Klein G, Klein E, 1977, Rejectability of virus-induced tumors and nonrejectability of spontaneous tumors: a lesson in contrasts, *Transplant Proc*, **9:** 1095–104.

Knudson AG, 1993, Antioncogenes and human cancer, *Proc Natl Acad Sci USA*, **90:** 10914–21.

Kung H-J, Boerkel C, Carter TH, 1991, Retroviral mutagenesis of cellular oncogenes: a review with insights into the mechanisms of insertional activation, *Curr Top Microbiol Immunol*, **171:** 1–25.

Lane DP, Crawford LV, 1979, T antigen is bound to a host protein in SV40-transformed cells, *Nature (London)*, **278:** 261–3.

Lee FS, Lane TF et al., 1995, Insertional mutagenesis identifies a member of the *Wnt* gene family as a candidate oncogene in the mammary epithelium of int2/fgf3 transgenic mice, *Proc Natl Acad Sci USA*, **92:** 2268–72.

Li JP, Andrea AD et al., 1990, Activation of cell growth by binding of Friend Spleen Focus-Forming Virus gp55 glycoprotein to the erythropoietin receptor, *Nature (London)*, **343:** 762–4.

Liebermann DA, Hoffman B, Steinman RA, 1995, Molecular controls of growth arrest and apoptosis: p53-dependent and independent pathways, *Oncogene*, **11:** 199–210.

Linzer DIH, Levine AJ, 1979, Characterization of a 54Kdalton cellular SV40 tumour antigen in SV40-transformed cells and uninfected embryonal carcinoma cells, *Cell*, **17:** 43–52.

Lock LF, Jenkins NA, Copeland NG, 1991, Mutagenesis of the mouse germline using retroviral insertion, *Curr Top Microbiol Immunol*, **171:** 27–41.

Lu S-J, Rowan S et al., 1994, Retroviral integration within the *Fli*-2 locus results in inactivation of the erythroid transcription factor NF-E2 in Friend erythroleukemias: evidence that NF-E2 is essential for globin expression, *Proc Natl Acad Sci USA*, **91:** 8398–402.

Macarthur CA, Shankar DB, Shackleford GM, 1995, *Fgf-8*, activated by proviral insertion, cooperates with the *Wnt-1* transgene in murine mammary tumorigenesis, *J Virol*, **69:** 2501–7.

McGrath MS, Weissman IL, 1979, AKR leukemogenesis: identification and biological significance of thymic lymphoma receptors for AKR retroviruses, *Cell*, **17:** 65–75.

Macnab JCM, 1987, Herpes simplex virus and human cytomegalovirus: their role in morphological transformation and genital cancers, *J Gen Virol*, **68:** 2525–50.

Mann DL, Desantis P, Mark G, 1987, HTLV-I-associated B-cell CLL: indirect role for retroviruses in leukemogenesis, *Science*, **236:** 1103–6.

Margolis HS, Alter MJ, Hadler SC, 1991, Hepatitis B: evolving epidemiology and implications for control, *Semin Liver Dis*, **11:** 84–92.

Minson A, Neil J, McCrae M, eds, 1994, *Viruses and Cancer*, Cambridge University Press, Cambridge.

Minson AC, 1984, Cell transformation and oncogenesis by herpes simplex virus and human cytomegalovirus, *Cancer Surv*, **3:** 91–111.

Montesano R, Slaga TJ, 1983, Initiation and promotion in carcinogenesis: an appraisal, *Cancer Surv*, **2:** 613–21.

Morein B, Merza M, 1991, Vaccination against herpesviruses: fiction or reality?, *Scand J Infect Dis*, **23:** 110–18.

Morrison HL, Soni B, Lenz J, 1995, Long terminal repeat enhancer core sequences in proviruses adjacent to c-myc in T-cell lymphomas induced by a murine retrovirus, *J Virol*, **69:** 446–55.

Neel B, Hayward WS et al., 1981, Avian leukosis virus-induced tumors have common proviral integration sites and synthesize discrete new RNAs: oncogenesis by promoter insertion, *Cell*, **23**: 323–34.

Neil JC, Fulton R et al., 1991, Feline leukaemia virus: generation of pathogenic and oncogenic variants, *Curr Top Microbiol Immunol*, **171**: 67–93.

Nemerow GR, Mold C et al., 1987, Identification of gp350 as the viral glycoprotein mediating attachment of Epstein–Barr virus (EBV) to the EBV/C3d receptor of B cells: sequence homology of gp350 and C3 complement fragment C3d, *J Virol*, **61**: 1416–20.

Nilsen T, Maroney PA et al., 1985, c-*erb*B activation in ALV-induced erythroblastosis: novel RNA processing and promoter insertion results in expression of an amino-truncated EGF receptor, *Cell*, **41**: 719–26.

Onions DE, Jarrett O, 1987, Viral oncogenesis: lessons from naturally occurring animal viruses, *Cancer Surv*, **6**: 161–80.

Pacitti AM, Jarrett O, 1985, Duration of the latent state in feline leukaemia virus infections, *Vet Rec*, **117**: 472–4.

Payne LN, 1992, Biology of avian retroviruses, *The Retroviridae*, ed Levy JA, Plenum Press, New York, 299–404.

Peters G, 1990, Oncogenes at viral integration sites, *Cell Growth Differentiation*, **1**: 503–10.

Pluda JM, Yarchoan R et al., 1990, Development of non-Hodgkins' lymphoma in a cohort of patients with severe human immunodeficiency virus infection on long-term antiretroviral therapy, *Ann Intern Med*, **113**: 276–82.

Rabbitts TH, 1994, Chromosomal translocations in human cancer, *Nature (London)*, **372**: 143–9.

Rickinson AB, 1994, EBV infection and EBV-associated tumours, *Viruses and Cancer*, eds Minson A, Neil J, McCrae M, Cambridge University Press, Cambridge, 81–100.

Rojko JL, Hoover EA et al., 1982, Reactivation of latent feline leukemia virus infection, *Nature (London)*, **298**: 385–8.

Rossner MT, 1992, Review: hepatitis B virus X-gene product: a promiscuous transcriptional activator, *J Med Virol*, **36**: 101–17.

Ruben S, Poteat H et al., 1988, Cellular transcription factors and regulation of IL-2 receptor gene expression by HTLV-I Tax gene product, *Science*, **241**: 89–92.

Sarnow P, Ho YS et al., 1982, Adenovirus E1B-58kd tumour antigen and SV40 large T antigen are physically associated with the same 54kd cellular protein in transformed cells, *Cell*, **28**: 387–94.

Schat KA, 1987, Marek's disease: a model for protection against herpesvirus-induced tumours, *Cancer Surv*, **6**: 1–37.

Schild GC, Stott EJ, 1993, Where are we now with vaccines against AIDS?, *Br Med J*, **306**: 947–8.

Slagle BL, Becker SA, Butel JS, 1994, Hepatitis viruses and liver cancer, *Viruses and Cancer*, eds Minson A, Neil J, McCrae M, Cambridge University Press, Cambridge, 149–71.

Stoye JP, Moroni C, Coffin JM, 1991, Virological events leading to spontaneous AKR thymomas, *J Virol*, **65**: 1273–85.

Stroobant P, Rice AP, Gullick W, 1985, Purification and characterisation of vaccinia virus growth factor, *Cell*, **42**: 383–93.

Szekely L, Selivanova G et al., 1993, EBNA-5 an EBV encoded nuclear antigen, binds to the RB and p53 proteins, *Proc Natl Acad Sci USA*, **90**: 5455–59.

Tsichlis PN, Gunter-Strauss P, Lohse MA, 1985, Concerted DNA rearrangements in Moloney leukemia virus-induced thymomas: a potential synergistic relationship in oncogenesis, *J Virol*, **56**: 258–67.

Tsichlis PN, Lazo PA, 1991, Virus–host interactions and the pathogenesis of murine and human oncogenic retroviruses, *Curr Top Microbiol Immunol*, **171**: 95–172.

Van Lohuizen M, Verbeek S et al., 1989, Predisposition to lymphomagenesis in pim-1 transgenic mice: cooperation with c-*myc* and N-*myc* in murine leukemia virus-induced tumors, *Cell*, **56**: 673–82.

Van Lohuizen, M, Verbeek S et al., 1991, Identification of cooperating oncogenes in E-mu-*myc* transgenic mice by provirus tagging, *Cell*, **65**: 737–52.

Vedantham S, Gamliel H, Golomb HM, 1992, Mechanism of interferon action in hairy cell leukemia: a model of effective cancer biotherapy, *Cancer Res*, **52**: 1056–66.

Vieweg J, Gilboa E, 1995, Considerations for the use of cytokine-secreting tumor cell preparations for cancer treatment, *Cancer Invest*, **13**: 193–201.

Vogelstein B, Kinzler KW, 1992, p53 function and dysfunction, *Cell*, **70**: 523–6.

Weiss R, 1984, Experimental biology and assay of RNA tumor viruses, *RNA Tumor Viruses*, eds Weiss R, Teich N et al., Cold Spring Harbor Laboratory, Cold Spring Harbor NY, 209–60.

Werness BA, Levine AJ, Howley PM, 1990, Association of human papillomavirus types 16 and 18 E6 proteins with p53, *Science*, **248**: 76–9.

Willett BJ, Hosie, M J, 1994, FIV and cell tropism, *Feline Immunology and Immunodeficiency*, eds Willett BJ, Jarrett O, Oxford University Press, Oxford, 205–19.

Wyke JA, Weiss RA, 1984, The contribution of tumour viruses to human and experimental oncology, *Cancer Surv*, **3**: 1–24.

Yonish-Rouach E, Resnitsky D et al., 1991, Wild type p53 induces apoptosis of myeloid leukaemic cells that is inhibited by IL-6, *Nature (London)*, **352**: 345–7.

Zeng Y, Zhang LG, Li HY, 1982, Serological mass survey for early detection of nasopharyngeal carcinoma in Wuzhou City, China, *Int J Cancer*, **29**: 139–41.

Zinkernagel RM, Hengartner H, 1994, T-cell-mediated immunopathology versus direct cytolysis by virus: implications for HIV and AIDS, *Immunol Today*, **15**: 262–7.

Chapter 13

THE EPIDEMIOLOGY OF VIRAL INFECTIONS

A S Monto

1 INTRODUCTION

Epidemiology describes the occurrence of illness in populations and, by means of specific study designs, facilitates analysis of the risk factors that determine its distribution. Such investigations are often observational and do not involve experimentation or intervention but, rather, they gather and interpret events as they occur in nature. In the process, the occurrence of diseases is quantified according to their characteristics. Hypotheses concerning aetiology and other variables are generated and are tested using statistical techniques. Epidemiology also provides experimental approaches for evaluating the efficacy of interventions such as vaccines to prevent or drugs to treat disease. Infectious diseases were the primary concern of epidemiologists for many years, and concepts were developed to evaluate the infectious process in populations. Now, most epidemiologists work on non-communicable diseases, and methods originally developed to study acute infections are being used to evaluate aetiology and risk factors for conditions such as coronary heart disease and cancer.

Whilst similar methods are now employed to study both communicable and non-communicable diseases, the unique nature of replicating agents makes certain techniques more relevant to infectious illnesses, especially in examining questions of aetiology. Debate has raged about the appropriateness of separating causes of diseases into 'necessary' and 'contributing' (Susser 1973). For example, it is impossible to produce a case of polio without the poliovirus, although contributing factors may be involved in determining the consequences of the infection, i.e. whether disease develops and how severe it is. Epidemiological approaches may also be required to evaluate some of the basic characteristics of infectious agents in humans, such as the infectious dose, which is important in terms of both the amount of pathogen required to initiate infection and the ease and likelihood of transmission. When animal models are available, many of these variables can be estimated. Results may or may not be applicable to humans, so epidemiological studies are needed for confirmation. They are essential when no animal model is available.

When dealing with viral infections (as opposed to those caused by other infectious agents), epidemiological principles are modified only because of characteristics of the pathogens. Most reflect differences in the ability of the agents to persist in the environment (typically more limited with viruses) and the comparative lack of the intermediate hosts that exist with animal parasites. Features such as the possibility of persistent infection and induction of chronic disease and malignancies are not unique to viruses, but are certainly more characteristic of infection with some of them than with other types of agents. In this chapter, the examination of the epidemiology of viral infections emphasizes the elements that are unique to viruses, but the discussion is not limited to them. More general issues are also covered and viral infections serve as illustrations of the principles and methods discussed.

2 CLASSIFYING MECHANISMS OF VIRAL TRANSMISSION

2.1 Direct transmission

In the cycle of infection, the period during transmission of the agent from one host to the next is when the virus is exposed to the environment and therefore most vulnerable. Systems have been developed to divide the transmission mechanisms of infectious agents into different categories and subcategories. There are classification systems based on portals of entry and exit of the agent to and from the host (Fox, Hall and Elveback 1970). That shown in Table 13.1 is based on duration and route in transit from one host to the next, but some categories are limited to specific portals such as the skin or the respiratory tract (American Public Health Association 1985). The major division is between **direct** transmission, which is essentially immediate, and **indirect** transmission, which is delayed. Direct contact generally implies no exposure of the agent to the environment. This type of transmission occurs during sexual intercourse, as with human immunodeficiency virus (HIV) or hepatitis B, or during direct skin contact, as with herpes gladiatorum, a herpes simplex infection of wrestlers transmitted as they rub their skin against that of an opponent (Belongia et al. 1991). In most cases, virus-containing fluids are involved and the viruses are often cell-associated. Direct contact includes, by extension, **vertical** transmission which may take place transplacentally, during the birth process or in breast milk. All these extended mechanisms are documented for HIV, which can be transmitted directly but is not well transmitted when the agent comes in contact with the environment (Friedland and Klein 1987).

Droplets of various sizes are expelled as part of respiratory discharges; the larger droplets, greater than 5 μm in diameter, settle out rapidly and do not spread further than about 1 m, rendering this form of transmission essentially immediate. Thus, even though the previously and the newly infected hosts are not in contact with each other, this is also considered to be a form of direct transmission, because of the limited transit time of this class of infected droplets which do not stay in the air for long periods. Agents potentially destroyed by longer exposure to the environment can still be transmitted by this mechanism. Rhinoviruses are spread by large droplets. As a result, rhinovirus disease transmission, which generally peaks in the autumn when schools reopen, is in fact a summation of

Table 13.1 Principal mechanisms of transmission

Direct (essentially immediate)
Contact (touching, kissing, sexual intercourse etc.)
Large droplet – limited distance
Indirect
Vehicle-borne
Indirect contact – fomites
Other inanimate objects and biological
substances (water, milk, urine, stool etc.)
Vector-borne
Mechanical – without multiplication
Biological – with multiplication
Dusts and air-borne droplet nuclei (aerosols)

mini-outbreaks produced by concurrent dissemination of many different serotypes (Monto, Bryan and Ohmit 1987). Some large droplets evaporate to become aerosols that may stay suspended and remain infectious for long periods. Influenza is spread by both large droplet and aerosol; a single viral subtype is generally responsible for outbreaks (Couch et al. 1966), in contrast to the relatively limited nature of transmission via large droplets alone. The childhood exanthemata, measles, mumps and chickenpox, are transmitted mainly by large droplets, which explains why outbreaks may take months to run their course in a partially immune population.

2.2 Indirect transmission

Indirect transmission covers many diverse mechanisms which have in common only the fact that there can be a delay, often prolonged, in the infectious agent reaching a new host. Indirect transmission is divided into 3 categories (Table 13.1). Vehicles are varied non-living entities, ranging from inanimate objects to water and biological products such as milk, urine or human tissue on or in which the infectious agent remains in transit to a new host. Personal inanimate objects, such as combs, blankets and writing materials serving as vehicles for transmission of infective agents, are termed fomites. Many important viruses can be transmitted by fomites, including the agents of measles, chickenpox and smallpox, but the period in transit cannot be long. Again, the issue is one of survival during exposure to environmental extremes. Because infections known to be transmitted from person to person can also be spread via freshly contaminated fomites, the definition of a contagious disease was extended to include this route, which is sometimes termed 'indirect contact'. Thus, a contagious disease is one transmitted by direct or indirect contact. In reality, contagious agents are transmitted mainly directly, especially by large droplets. Only infrequently are fomites involved, because this route is a relatively inefficient means of transmission.

Whereas some viruses transmitted by vehicle are spread in water, urine and milk, this kind of transmission is more common with bacteria that can survive in the environment for prolonged periods. The spread of picornaviruses (Chapter 25), other enteric viruses (Chapter 26) and hepatitis A and E viruses (Chapter 34) has been related to exposure to infected water. These viruses, known to be associated with faecal contamination, may be spread not only by drinking water itself but also by ingesting shellfish which filter and concentrate the virus (Hedstrom and Lycke 1964, Portnoy et al. 1975). Transmission from infected urine occurs with a number of the viruses whose primary hosts are sylvatic, such as the arenavirus Machupo (Chapter 31). Likewise, hantaviruses such as the agents of Korean haemorrhagic fever and the hantavirus pulmonary syndrome (Chapter 30), recently described in southwestern USA may be transmitted from infected urine or faeces (Johnson et al. 1966, Childs et al. 1994). For these, and for other agents similarly transmitted, rodents are the reservoir of infection. They often live close to or in human dwellings and infect humans via their excreta.

Vector transmission is divided into mechanical and biological categories. Mechanical transmission implies that the vector, typically an arthropod, is involved only in providing transport for the agent, i.e. moving it from one site to another without multiplication taking place. This occurs with certain enteric bacteria, in which the pathogen may adhere to the surface of the vector. It rarely takes place with viruses because the agents would be inactivated by the environmental exposure. No multiplication of the agent occurs, so it is not an efficient form of transmission. In contrast, biological transmission is highly efficient. Most of the large group of viruses transmitted by this mechanism were formerly termed the arthropod-borne or arboviruses (Chapter 29). They are now divided into different families, such as the flaviviruses and the togaviruses (Westaway et al. 1985a, 1985b). By definition, arboviruses are transmitted by mosquitoes, ticks or other arthropods, and, in the process, the quantity of virus increases, thus enhancing the probability of infection. Multiplication takes place in the body of the arthropod, and, for example, is released from the salivary glands during a mosquito bite. There has been speculation that non-arboviruses such as hepatitis B might be mosquito-transmitted, because epidemiological data suggested that distribution was related to mosquito density (Papaevangelou and Kourea-Kremastinou 1974). However, multiplication has never been demonstrated, so the likelihood of a bite producing transmission is low even if infected blood has been taken up (Berquist et al. 1976).

Infected dusts are rarely involved in transmitting viral infections by the air-borne route, because desiccation usually inactivates them if they stay exposed to the environment for prolonged periods. Certain respiratory viral infections such as influenza and coxsackie virus A21 are commonly transmitted by small droplets or droplet nuclei (Couch et al. 1966). The droplet nuclei are formed from large droplets as they evaporate while suspended in the air around a spicule of dust. In most cases it has not been possible to demonstrate by air sampling the presence of virus in aerosols, but this mechanism is assumed to operate because of the ability of a virus to infect large numbers. These are the true viral aerosols: the small droplets are able to stay in the air and remain suspended long enough to infect occupants of an entire naval vessel or aircraft with influenza, or to transmit smallpox from one infected person to another through the air-conditioning system of a hospital (Wehrle et al. 1970, Moser et al. 1979). The small droplets also have the ability to reach into the lower respiratory tract, which influences the character of illness that results.

3 QUANTIFICATION OF CHARACTERISTICS OF VIRAL INFECTION

3.1 Infectious dose and secondary attack rate

Epidemiology provides definitions that help to quantify the occurrence of infection and disease in a population. Experimental infection of laboratory animals is always accompanied by quantification; similarly, for work in human infection and disease, quantification is needed. However, because the situation is typically observational and not experimental, different terms and definitions are used. For example, to calculate the infectious dose required to initiate infection in animals, a 50% infectious dose (ID50) is determined by inoculation of serial dilutions. Except for certain self-limited infections such as those caused by the rhinoviruses, such experimental studies cannot be carried out in humans (Tyrrell et al. 1960). Even when experimental infection of humans is ethically possible, there are always questions concerning their comparability with those that occur naturally. Such questions apply to experimental studies of influenza, where large droplet inoculation in the nose does not mimic the aerosol spread of natural infection in which the lower respiratory tract is exposed.

The epidemiological measure historically used to approximate indirectly the infectivity of an agent in humans is the so-called secondary attack rate (SAR). It is more than a measure of infectivity: it describes numerically the communicability of a contagious disease, which is in part related to the ID50 of the virus but is also affected by loss of viability during transmission and the susceptibility of the recipient. An index or primary case is identified in a family or other similar semi-closed group. Cases that subsequently occur in the group during the incubation period (the time between inoculation and development of illness) are regarded as secondary; those that occur before are considered co-primary, i.e. a separate introduction into the group. The denominator for the calculation is based on the total number in the group less the index or co-primary cases. Other variations are possible, especially when using laboratory data to identify those truly at risk of infection or illness – i.e. those without prior evidence of infection such as antibody and therefore susceptible to infection. The classic calculation of the SAR is most appropriate for diseases with relatively long incubation periods, such as rubella and mumps. A problem arises with diseases of shorter incubation period (c. 2–4 days), such as influenza and the common cold, in which it is difficult to distinguish between co-primary and secondary cases because they are only days apart or may overlap. It is possible mathematically to model transmission: if infection rates are known for sufficient numbers of families to be representative of the community, statistical methods can be used to adjust the observed, or so-called apparent, SAR by the probability of acquiring from the community a new infection that had seemed to be a secondary case (Longini et al. 1982). Among infections of high SAR are measles and chickenpox. Rubella is less contagious, thus leaving residual susceptibles among young women entering childbearing age (Sever, Schiff and Huebner 1964).

3.2 Pathogenicity and virulence

'Pathogenicity' sometimes compares the capacity of different organisms to cause disease, whereas 'virulence' compares the severity of disease caused by different strains of the same organism (see Chapter 9, section 3: p. 237). Here, these terms are specified somewhat differently. In the epidemiological sense, 'pathogenicity' is the proportion of total infections that produce overt disease, which varies from virus to virus and may be affected by host factors (e.g. prior infection with the agent). 'Virulence' here indicates the capacity of a pathogen to produce severe disease. The likelihood of a fatal outcome is calculated as the case-fatality rate or ratio. It is not a true rate, which should cover a specific period, but is in fact a proportion, the denominator being represented by all recognized cases and the numerator by all deaths included in the denominator. Case fatality is high in many hantavirus and filovirus infections; it still is 100% in clinical cases of rabies, with rare and often questionable exceptions (Hattwick et al. 1972, Peters et al. 1994). There have been attempts to quantify virulence other than as case fatality, which has the disadvantage of not being a fixed quantity but one that can be reduced in most situations by appropriate treatment. Also, many diseases with the capacity to produce severe illness infrequently cause death; thus the measure is not a good indication of virulence. A persistent problem in quantifying severity is defining exactly what is meant by this term. In contrast, death as an endpoint is unambiguous. Polio is an illustration of the relative independence of pathogenicity and virulence; the disease is potentially very severe or virulent if it occurs, but only 0.1–1% of infections are symptomatic. Therefore the virus would be considered of relatively low pathogenicity but of relatively high virulence (Melnick and Ledinko 1951).

4 OBSERVATIONAL EPIDEMIOLOGY

4.1 Viral infections in person, place and time

Many epidemiological studies of infections involve description of the occurrence of disease and identification of factors that appear to be related to their distribution. **Description** is the first phase of an epidemiological investigation. It accepts that there is in fact an infection problem and permits development of hypotheses concerning aetiology, risk factors and other variables determining distribution. These relationships may be investigated further in analytical studies. Occurrence of the infectious disease can be described on the basis of a number of criteria. For some conditions, a **case definition** may be used: a list of signs and symptoms that are required before a case is recognized. Laboratory confirmation may or may not be included in this definition. Sometimes the aim is to identify inapparent infections as well as cases of disease. Here the criteria may be based on laboratory data only, such as virus identification or significant change in antibody titre.

PERSONAL FACTORS

Descriptions of infections or diseases are made in terms of their occurrence in person, place and time. Whilst temporal, geographical and personal factors are interrelated, it is useful to examine each separately as a systematic way of describing the occurrence of an infectious disease. Age is the most important personal determinant of disease because of development and ageing of the immune system, accumulation of exposures over time, and behavioural changes that affect the likelihood of exposure to infectious agents. It is impossible to generalize how age affects pathogenicity or virulence. Hepatitis A and polio are typically mild in young children and become increasingly virulent as children become young adults. Polio emerged as a recognized problem in northern and western Europe only at the end of the nineteenth century. It was called infantile paralysis because it infected mainly the very young, but as time passed it also caused disease in older children. In developing countries the process is being repeated; polio infections often occur in the first 6 months of life, modified by the universal presence of maternal antibody, but the disease is now present also in older children (Nathanson and Martin 1979). Hepatitis A has had a similar progression as the age at the time of infection has changed. In contrast, respiratory viruses such as respiratory syncytial virus (RSV) and parainfluenza produce the most severe disease in young children. In the USA the median age of infants hospitalized because of RSV is 3 months (Parrot et al. 1973).

The proportion of those infected who develop overt disease also falls with increasing age, in part as the result of repeated exposure to those agents that have the capacity to reinfect with regularity (Monto and Lim 1971). Previous exposures result in a spectrum of outcomes ranging from asymptomatic infection to disease of diminished severity. Other personal factors affecting outcomes of infection are listed in Table 13.2.

Position in the family affects the occurrence of infections best transmitted in that setting (e.g. the respiratory viruses and enteric agents such as the rotaviruses). An only child in a family will experience lower rates of respiratory infection until other siblings are born (Monto and Ross 1977). Other exposures, such as in day care, may increase the probability of the youngest child acquiring an agent which can then be introduced into and spread within the family (Bartlett et al. 1985). There is evidence that this pattern of occurrence is common with hepatitis A; in fact, community-wide outbreaks of hepatitis A have frequently been traced to day care transmission (Matson et al. 1989). Occupational exposure plays a role in the acquisition of, for example, sylvatic or jungle yellow fever by people working in the forest. The risk from rabies among veterinarians is another type of occupational exposure, but such infections do not result in further dissemination.

FACTORS RELATED TO PLACE

Place of occurrence of viral infection may be related to purely local biological or physical factors. Regional characteristics such as climate and resident flora and fauna determine whether transmission can take place. Most arboviruses are found in specific locations, determined by the distribution of the appropriate vectors or animal hosts. Sometimes the range of a particular agent is quite limited, minor ecological variation producing a niche where transmission can take place. Similarly, agents that are transmitted mainly among animals are limited to the range of that particular animal. Humans are often infected only incidentally, having been in the area where transmission is occurring to the animal hosts or vectors. Infections of animals in which humans are not involved in the major cycle of transmission but are occasionally infected are termed zoonoses.

Other physical or biological environmental factors determine whether common source outbreaks, such as those produced by hepatitis A or E from contaminated water, can occur at a particular location. Generally, special situations in the area, such as sewage outflows or substandard wells are responsible. The presence of an individual in certain locations such as a hospital could result in transmission of hepatitis B in those parts of the world where nosocomial transmission still occurs. In certain areas of Africa where the Ebola virus is present, being in a hospital adds greatly to risk (Baron, McCormick and Zubeir 1981). Events seemingly associated with place are often equally related to person or to time. **Clusters** of illnesses are sometimes detected, indicating that transmission of infection is taking place in a particular location. For a cluster to be recognized the transmission must occur over a limited period of time. Such a cluster may involve everyone in that location or may be limited to certain individuals. Reports of clusters are an

Table 13.2 Examples of personal factors important in viral illness

Age and gender
Position in family – birth order
Income
Education
Crowding
Socioeconomic status
Occupation – exposures
Genetic and related factors
Immunity
Nutrition

important alert that unusual transmission is taking place. The first cases of AIDS were detected as simultaneous clusters, in several cities, of a disease producing Kaposi's sarcoma or opportunistic infections in young homosexual men (Gottlieb et al. 1981, Friedman-Kien et al. 1982). The existence of these clusters focused attention on an infectious aetiology of the disease, which at the time was thought by some to have other causes such as exposure to environmental toxins or to drugs. HIV transmission was later found to be the explanation.

TEMPORAL FACTORS: CLASSIFICATION OF OUTBREAKS

Time of occurrence may be the most systematically evaluated of the 3 factors. Much of the terminology used in epidemiology has a temporal component. The terms **epidemic**, **endemic** and **sporadic** do not have any statistical definitions but simply mean, respectively, occurrence of an infection at a higher than expected frequency, at the expected frequency, or only rarely and in seemingly unconnected fashion. Another term frequently used, also without statistical definition, is **pandemic**, meaning an epidemic appearing in many geographic locations at about the same time. The term has been used for influenza outbreaks occurring on a global scale following appearance of variants with a new haemagglutinin or a new haemagglutinin and new neuraminidase. It is now appropriately applied to HIV/AIDS which has involved all continents in its inexorable spread (World Health Organization/Global Program on AIDS 1994). The years this has taken contrasts with the months needed for an influenza pandemic to involve the whole world. This contrasting pattern is related to differences in transmission characteristics between HIV, spread by direct contact, and influenza, transmitted by droplet and air-borne routes.

The characteristics of outbreaks are described according to the occurrence of cases over time. These characteristics are generally studied by creating an epidemic curve, with cases on the ordinate and time (in days or hours, depending on the speed of development) on the abscissa. Figure 13.1 shows the pattern of a point source outbreak of Norwalk virus infection in which all individuals were exposed at the same time and either became infected and ill with diarrhoeal disease or remained well (Warner et al. 1991). The group exposed was large (3000 people) and the attack rate, at 48%, was high. The times of onset were divided into 4-hour intervals. The suspect meal in question was consumed at noon on Monday; illnesses reported earlier are viewed as baseline cases of diarrhoea unrelated to the exposure. Such cases are typical in investigations of a common illness such as gastroenteritis, which can be produced by many agents. The time from the exposure to the peak of the outbreak is the mean incubation period of the pathogen, in this case 40 hours. The peak occurred during the 4-hour period beginning at 5 a.m., Wednesday.

If the source remains infectious for a time, the outbreak may continue. The new cases are still being

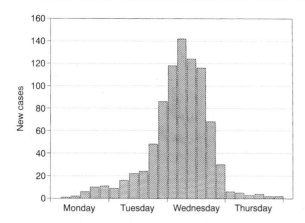

Fig. 13.1 A point source outbreak of enteritis attributed to Norwalk virus after a meal eaten at noon, Monday. Onset of illness (moving means) shown in intervals of 4 h. (From Warner et al. 1991.)

infected from the source and the outbreak may now be better termed common rather than point source. A contaminated well is an example of a common source. With viruses such as hepatitis A or Norwalk-like agents cases may arise in lower numbers even when the source is no longer infectious. Such continued occurrence is possible only for viruses that can also spread from person to person, a different type of transmission. Pure point source outbreaks assume exposure from one site or at one point in time, the time from exposure to peak being the median incubation period. In contrast, in propagated source outbreaks the infectious agents spread exclusively from person to person. Spread may be by different transmission mechanisms, often large droplet. Even with influenza, which may be transmitted by the more efficient air-borne route, one person can infect only 2 or 3 individuals, and the outbreak takes 6–10 weeks (or more) to move through a community. It should be remembered that the incubation period of the infection is only 2–4 days, so many generations of spread occur until the outbreak has run its course (Monto and Kioumehr 1975).

Many infectious diseases such as hepatitis A and rubella do not occur at uniform levels in populations but undergo predictable changes in frequency. Certain terms are used to describe these changes. **Seasonal variation** describes the phenomenon, well recognized with the respiratory viruses, of much higher frequency in colder than in warmer months. Other seasonal variations are less obvious, with rubella generally increasing (before vaccine control) in the spring and hepatitis A in the autumn. In temperate zones, transmission of rotavirus takes place almost exclusively during cold weather. Figure 13.2 shows 5 years of data from the study of young children hospitalized for diarrhoea in Washington DC (Brandt et al. 1983). Hospitalizations over all are most common in colder months. **Cyclical variation** refers to changes of frequency over periods of years, with gradual increases in intensity of transmission. Hepatitis A, for example, has a cycle of 5–7 years. This means that, when inten-

sity of transmission is increasing, illness in the autumn is more frequent than in the previous autumn. The term 'cycle' also implies that there is not only a waxing but also a waning period. In contrast, the term 'secular' is used to indicate long-term trends, which can be unidirectional in nature. The time periods involved must be long, generally more than 10 years.

4.2 Incidence and prevalence

INCIDENCE

Two critical terms used in epidemiology that have temporal definitions are **incidence** and **prevalence**. 'Incidence' is the number of new cases of a disease arising during a fixed period in a population of given size; for example, 1000 or 10 000 individuals. Incidence is sometimes further specified as either a cumulative incidence which expresses incidence as a risk or probability, or as an incidence density which does so as a rate.

These terms, whilst often used interchangeably, provide 2 types of information (Kleinbaum, Kupper and Morgenstein 1982). **Risk** is the probability of a disease-free person developing the disease of interest over a defined time and not dying from any other disease during that period. As a probability, risk can have values between zero and one. Risk is measured as cumulative incidence, the proportion of the study population becoming ill in a given period: for example, 'the risk of becoming ill with influenza-like illness in the study population was 12.8/1000 persons per year'. The need to specify a period can be appreciated by looking at the extreme case of mortality from all causes. If a cohort of 1000 subjects is followed for 120 years, the risk of dying during this period will be 1000/1000 per 120 years. However, during any one year of this period, the risk of dying will be much smaller. Thus, when applied to a vector-borne infection, risk of acquiring dengue over a 4-month mosquito season in an endemic area might be 10/100, but only 1.2/100 for a given week. The term **attack rate** is a cumulative incidence measure used to describe the number in a defined population who become infected or ill during the period of transmission of an agent; for example, the number of children infected with measles in the course of a school outbreak, using the number of susceptible children as the denominator of the proportion. This is more properly termed a risk, and is an example of cumulative incidence. The secondary attack rate, described above, is also an example of such a risk.

In contrast to risk, the **incidence rate**, sometimes called incidence density, describes the occurrence of new cases in the population per unit of time. Incidence density is most useful for testing epidemiological hypotheses when a long time is needed to follow a cohort to estimate risk, as in most chronic conditions and in some population-based studies of infection. The rate over a period of time is typically estimated using person-time as the denominator of the rate calculation. Person-time is the amount of time each study subject contributes to a study before becoming ill or

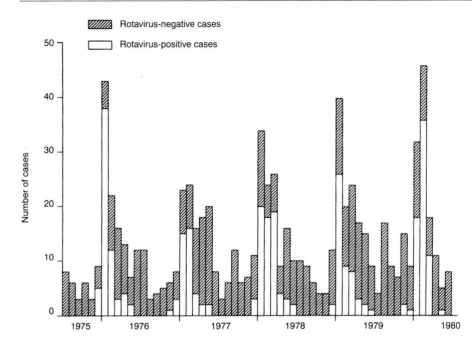

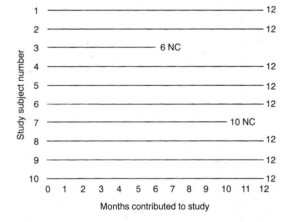

Fig. 13.2 Distribution by month over a 5-year period of children hospitalized for gastroenteritis and the proportions rotavirus-positive. Children's Hospital National Medical Center, Washington DC. (From Brandt et al. 1983.)

leaving the study for some reason. Sometimes new individuals may be added to the study population. Figure 13.3 illustrates the calculation of person-time. Among 10 people who were followed over differing periods of time, 2 cases of disease developed. In the incidence density calculation, 8 subjects completed the study, each contributing 12 person-months or a total of 96 person-months. Subjects 3 and 7 contributed 6 and 10 person-months respectively before becoming ill. The number of new cases (2) divided by the total number of person-months (112) yields a rate of 2/112 or 1.78/100 person-months. Dividing person-months by 12 would give person-years. Thus, the above translates to a rate of 1.78/8.33 person-months or 21/100 person-years. The same data could be used for an incidence density calculation for 10 subjects at risk. The data would give a rate of 2 new cases per 10 persons at risk, or 20/100 per year. The differences between the risk and rate calculations, while small, would have been greater with more cases developing or if the study had been carried out for a longer period.

PREVALENCE

The other important term, prevalence, is used less often when dealing with acute illnesses. Most often, the concept is defined as point prevalence, the point here being an arbitrary point in time. In prevalence, it is not new but existing cases that are identified, thus the ideal would be to enumerate them as a simultaneous count. Again the denominator is the population at risk from which the cases are drawn. Enumeration of all cases of AIDS existing in the population of interest at one time, whatever their date of onset, would provide a prevalence rate (Elandt-Johnson 1975).

Prevalence is often used in viral epidemiology when doing serological surveys based on collecting one

Fig. 13.3 Hypothetical one year study of 10 individuals. Two new cases (NC) of disease developed during this period, giving a risk calculation of 2/10 per year and a rate calculation of 2.1/10 person-years.

specimen per person. Serum banks have been established to reflect past experience with infectious diseases in a population. Ideally, the specimens should be representative of the population from which they have been drawn. Antibody present at a specific titre in a population sample collected to represent all age groups will indicate the pattern of past infection. For certain agents, such as arboviruses present intermittently in a geographical area, and for other more common agents such as measles in isolated populations, age-specific prevalence will indicate when infection was last present in that population, the years of birth of the youngest cohort with antibody indicating the last period of spread of the agent (Black 1989). Documenting the occurrence of influenza A subtypes over the last century is another example of use of antibody prevalence. Antibody present in sera, collected before the appearance of a new subtype of type A, has been taken as evidence for the spread of that subtype many years before (Masurel and Marine 1973). When sero-epidemiology is carried out with paired sera, change in antibody titre can be sought between 2 specimens collected from the same individual. The results are the equivalent to incidence, not prevalence, because they indicate that a new infection has occurred in the interval. This is also the case when examining IgM antibody in a single specimen for agents such as hepatitis A, known to produce that antibody for only a short time and thus indicating recent infection.

4.3   Monitoring and surveillance

The descriptive variables time, place and person are employed in monitoring and surveillance of viral disease. For infections that occur regularly the intention is to detect unusual increases. The expected frequency of these conditions, identified either by laboratory tests or on the basis of standard case definitions of illness, can be calculated. An example of the latter involves the use in the USA of reported deaths from pneumonia and influenza (P & I) from 121 cities. The reports are based on a list of specific causes of death, not on the laboratory detection of influenza infection, and are calculated weekly as a proportion of total deaths. Results of the method are shown in Fig. 13.4, with distribution of isolates by type in each of the influenza seasons. The P & I mortality curve has 3 components: the expected value, the threshold value (1.65 *SD* above the expected) and the actual values observed in the various cities. The expected values are a mathematical expression of past observed values derived from observations of periods without influenza transmission (Serfling 1963). They are higher in winter months than in summer, because of other non-influenza causes of pneumonia deaths that increase at the same time, such as those caused by primary bacterial infections. As can be seen in Fig. 13.4, in some years the observed mortality considerably exceeds the threshold level for several weeks. Typically, these are years in which there is considerable transmission of type A(H3N2) virus (Eickhoff, Sherman and Serfling 1961). In some years (not shown in the Figure), excess mortality has also occurred with type B transmission but this is observed less frequently (Nolan et al. 1980). When examining the data in Fig. 13.4, it is important to realize that the mortality data are the result of clinical diagnoses at the time of death, i.e. without laboratory evidence that the death was related to influenza. Thus the data for laboratory surveillance on which the annual distribution of isolates is based can be viewed as an independent determination. Only influenza produces this characteristic increase in mortality. The phenomenon is remarkable because the data are collected nationally in a country as large as the USA, in which outbreaks do not necessarily occur synchronously in different regions (Glezen et al. 1982). Similar systems are in use in other parts of the world, the data on virus circulation being based on collection of specimens in standard surveillance systems based in physicians' practices (Johnson et al. 1991).

Other diseases only rarely increase in frequency sufficiently to become noticeable in data collected nationally. Most infections are likely to be more localized, and the detection of outbreaks is based on the recognition of the unusual occurrence of cases in time, place or person. Outbreaks are variously defined according to expected occurrence; for some entities a single case may be so unusual as to produce an outbreak investigation. Rabies cases in areas of developed countries where this disease is unusual will be investigated on the basis of a single event. The virus causing hantavirus pulmonary syndrome was recognized and identified as a newly emerging pathogen in southeastern USA on the basis of deaths and severe illnesses clustered in time, place and, in part, person (Centers for Disease Control 1994). The regional nature of the outbreak contributed to its recognition; had the same number of cases occurred in a wider area, they would have gone unnoticed. As with other similar situations, prospective surveillance initiated after identification of the 'new' virus suggested that it had occurred at low frequency in the past and that recognition was due to an unusual natural event that produced a cluster of cases; in the case of the hantavirus pulmonary syndrome, the increase in food available for the rodent hosts resulted in their proliferation and an increased likelihood of interfacing with humans.

4.4   Primary analytical methods

CASE–CONTROL STUDIES

The descriptive phases of epidemiological investigations generate hypotheses about factors influencing the occurrence of a disease. Analytical studies then follow, and may involve formal outbreak investigations or more elaborate longitudinal studies. The investigations have in common the use of specific study designs. These designs are divided into **case–control** and **cohort** studies. In the first, cases of the disease or outcome being studied are identified and controls without the particular outcome are selected by matching or similar methods to be comparable to the cases in age and other characteristics. Past exposures or risk factors are then examined to determine if they are associated with the disease (Schlesselman 1982). In contrast, in the cohort design individuals are selected according to characteristics other than presence of the disease or infection of interest. They are followed over time and cases of the disease outcome are observed (Breslow and Day 1987).

Case–control studies can be relatively straightforward in their design and produce results quickly because all the exposures and outcomes have already occurred. The investigation of an outbreak of an infectious disease is generally case–control in nature, one group having the disease and the comparison group not having it. For example, an outbreak of vomiting and diarrhoea occurred in a group outing on an American lake where food was served in common and where many had gone swimming (Koopman et al. 1982). Individuals who developed disease according to a case definition were compared with those who did not. The food intake and other exposures of the cases

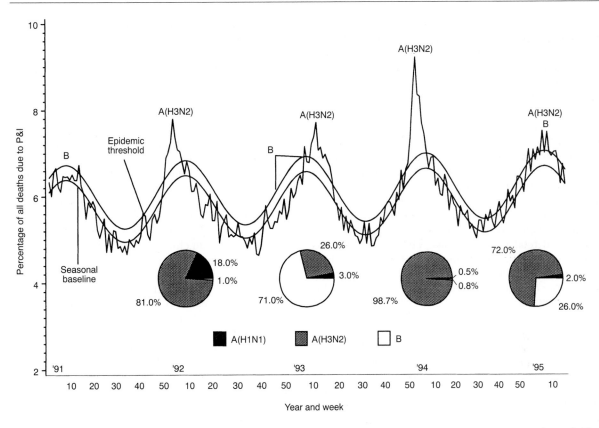

Fig. 13.4 Data on pneumonia and influenza mortality for 121 US cities, collected by the Centers for Disease Control. The curve indicates the observed mortality data, superimposed on the seasonal baseline and epidemic threshold. Also shown are the distributions of influenza isolates from specimens collected independently during the 4 seasons.

and the controls were then compared. There was no significant difference between cases and controls in terms of foods consumed or other relevant characteristics. However, swimming in the lake, especially with the head submerged, was the risk factor that was more common in those who developed diarrhoea compared to those who did not, and the differences were statistically significant. Furthermore, some samples, when available, showed rises in titre for the Norwalk virus, suggesting that it was the agent responsible. In this sort of outbreak investigation, the group studied is small. However, it is very important that the cases and controls have similar possibilities of exposure; in this case, people not at the lake would be ineligible.

Larger and more elaborate case–control studies were used to confirm the role of rubella as a cause of congenital anomalies. The original description of clusters of congenital anomalies involving the eyes, and then the heart, ears and other organs occurring in children whose mothers had experienced rubella in pregnancy allowed development of an aetiological hypothesis (Gregg 1941, Swan, Tostevin and Black 1946). The clusters seemed to be related to the epidemic behaviour of rubella, since frequency of the abnormality increased cyclically when rubella was widespread (Sever, Nelson and Gilkeson 1965). Many of the initial studies were simply a series of cases. For the analytical studies, cases were children with certain types of abnormalities identified at birth or shortly

thereafter and controls were children without abnormalities born in the same locations. Pregnancy histories of mothers of both case and control children were obtained; because rubella and other conditions of interest do not generally result either in a doctor being consulted or in hospitalization, data are generally obtained by interviewing the mothers. This has a disadvantage of introducing potential recall bias: mothers know whether their children had birth defects or were normal and, if the former, are more likely to remember every event that might possibly have been related to the defect (Klemetti and Saxen 1967). Methods can sometimes be developed to try to validate these reported events. If possible, medical or other records collected before the birth are used. By their very nature, case–control studies are nearly always retrospective: cases and controls are identified on the basis of the outcome, and the prior factors determining the development or non-development of the disease are compared. Table 13.3 lists some of the advantages and disadvantages of the basic study designs. Accurate recall of previous events is an inherent problem with case–control studies because of knowledge of the outcome, but the design has other attractive features. It is highly cost efficient, especially for outcomes that are relatively rare. Cases can be gathered easily and, because they have already occurred, the study can be carried out quite quickly. Another inherent problem of the design, however, is the selection of controls. Controls should be similar to the cases in all characteristics except the disease in question. This is often difficult to achieve and questions are always raised about this point. Typically there are 2 choices of populations from which to draw controls: hospital databases or the community. Each has its own advantages and disadvantages. In the study of infectious diseases, controls must have similar probabilities of exposure to the infections as the cases. In terms of, for example, rubella, cases and controls must have the same opportunity to be exposed and to experience rubella, which varies by both time and place in intensity of transmission. The case–control studies concluded that there was a high level of association between rubella in the first trimester of pregnancy and fetal malformations. That association was very strong and suggested that the risk of fetal malformation was greater than 50% in some studies, in one case 80% (Pitt 1957, Ingalls et al. 1960) (see also Chapter 28).

COHORT STUDIES

Cohort studies are generally undertaken after case–control studies indicate the likelihood of an association between a particular exposure and disease outcome. With rubella, these studies began relatively early, because of recognition of biases associated with obtaining histories on the cases. Such investigations are typically prospective in nature, and allow collection of data as new events occur, thus minimizing the possibility of recall bias. However, they must generally be larger with enough participants to allow for reasonable numbers of dropouts, and must last long enough to achieve the necessary numbers of events. As a precondition, the outcome of interest must be so frequent that the group followed does not need to be too large or followed for too long. For all these reasons, cohort studies are carried out less frequently than case–control studies because they are more

Table 13.3 Advantages and disadvantages of study designs

Advantages	Disadvantages
Case–control	
Efficiency – results rapidly available	Selection of comparable controls
Superior for rare outcome	Recall problems
Relatively inexpensive	Validity of recorded data
Cohort studies	
Reduction in potential bias	Duration – may be long
Greater ability to generalize results	Greater expense
No necessity to select healthy comparable controls	Uncertainty of adequate numbers and loss to follow-up
	Rare diseases require large numbers

expensive and problematic in terms of producing the required number of observations. However, when feasible, they are powerful evidence for confirming results of case–control studies, as many sources of bias can be avoided and there is not the problem of selecting comparable controls.

In this design the cohort is the population unit selected for study. The only requirement is that the selection cannot be on the basis of disease outcome or anything that might be closely related to the disease. Typically the unit may be individuals in an occupational group, such as nurses or physicians or people living in a certain area. In the case of rubella, 2 kinds of cohort studies have been carried out (Manson, Logan and Loy 1960, Sever et al. 1969). In the most powerful design, all children born during specific periods in particular hospitals were studied. Because all children born at the appropriate time were eligible, there was no need to identify controls, and all adverse outcomes of pregnancy could be followed in the cohort. Some mothers would have been exposed to rubella and might therefore give birth to children born with malformations. Most would not.

Another cohort design attempts to minimize the number of non-exposed women who would have to be included. This method identifies an exposure cohort (mother exposed to rubella) and a comparison cohort of mothers not exposed. Note that the selection here is based not on the outcome, congenital abnormalities, as would be the situation in a case–control study, but on exposures, so this remains a cohort study. There is no issue of recall bias because the comparison group is selected on documented lack of exposure. However, it has the potential problem of not being as representative as if all individuals, rather than a selected subgroup, were followed up. Estimates of the risk of maternal rubella in the first trimester in producing malformations was as low as 7–17% in some cohort studies, although others felt that, depending on length of follow-up and definitions used it might actually be higher (Jackson and Fisch 1958, Lundstrom 1962). This reduction in risk estimation had public health implications before the vaccine era, because pregnancies were often terminated after maternal rubella. From an epidemiological standpoint, cohort studies are better than case–control studies in providing data and results that can be generalized to the population of interest so that appropriate decisions can be made.

OTHER USES OF ANALYTICAL STUDIES

Although vaccines are usually evaluated by randomized controlled trials, an experimental study design involving an intervention, observational designs can also be employed successfully to evaluate the effectiveness of vaccines. The term 'efficacy' is generally employed for results of randomized trials; 'effectiveness' is used to indicate the results of observations when the intervention is in general use, especially when the outcome is not a laboratory-confirmed infection but a clinical diagnosis. The latter sort of study is the only type possible when, as is the case in North America for influenza vaccine for the elderly, ethical considerations preclude use of a placebo and questions still exist as to the value of the preparation. The observational design does not require that vaccine be denied to part of the group, as would be the case if a placebo were employed. The purpose of using inactivated influenza vaccine in older people is to prevent serious complications of the disease, especially those requiring hospitalization. However, unless a large population can be followed, these hospitalizations do not occur sufficiently often to allow the use of the cohort design. For this reason, 2 multi-year case–control studies were carried out, one in the USA and the other in Canada (Foster et al. 1992, Fedson et al. 1993, Ohmit and Monto 1995). The exact designs varied, but in both cases the influenza season was identified and possible influenza complications were defined from hospital records. Recognizing the need for generalization of results, both studies were designed to select their controls not from hospitals but from comparable community residents. In both, the vaccine was found to be significantly effective in preventing hospitalization, and, in the Canadian study, in preventing deaths in the influenza seasons coded as being related to respiratory diseases. Another study used a cohort design to confirm these findings (Nichol et al. 1994). As expected, many people needed to be followed up. The effectiveness of the vaccine was comparable with that in the previous case–control investigations. That several differently designed non-experimental studies came to similar conclusions is convincing evidence that the results in a single investigation were not simply a chance occurrence.

4.5 Observational studies to confirm aetiology

Koch's postulates in their various forms were the first systematic approach for determining that a pathogen caused a disease (Rivers 1937). They were formulated after early observations that simply isolating an agent from an individual with a particular disease did not necessarily mean that the agent caused that disease. The postulates were based on experiments, provided that disease could be reproduced in laboratory animals. They did not allow for asymptomatic infection because they stated that the agent should always produce disease. They also assumed that the potential pathogen had a unique role in producing a disease: only one hepatitis virus could produce hepatitis. We now know that clinical syndromes can frequently be caused by a variety of agents and that clinical manifestations of infection vary greatly in terms of age and other factors, so it might not seem that the same pathogen was involved. In addition, many viruses may not infect experimental animals at all or, if they do, will not produce diseases comparable to those in humans. For this reason, Koch's postulates have been complemented (or modified) by epidemiological studies, usually observational, to confirm aetiology. Typically, case–control designs are used, because they are easy to carry out and require smaller numbers of observations. Studies of this sort are particularly necessary when dealing with agents that produce chronic infections.

Another problem occurs when a potential pathogen is shed for prolonged periods from people who have had an illness in the past, or after an asymptomatic infection. Agents may be isolated from individuals who develop another illness, and thought, incorrectly, to cause the current instead

of the preceding illness. This misconception can occur with the herpesviruses. At the very least, an agent must be identified significantly more frequently in cases with the disease than in comparable controls. This analytical design assumes that asymptomatic or chronic infection will occur and that some controls will be virus positive, but not as frequently as cases. Aetiological association of infectious mononucleosis with Epstein–Barr virus (EBV) was difficult to accomplish, because of continuing shedding of the virus (Hallee et al. 1974). Even more difficult has been the demonstration of the association of hepatitis B virus with primary hepatocellular carcinoma, because of the long period between infection and development of the disease (Beasley 1982).

When observational approaches, rather than experimentation, are used to demonstrate aetiology, additional standards are generally applied to assist in deciding that there is a statistically significant aetiological relationship between a disease and an agent or other potential precipitation factor. These standards were developed to evaluate the relationship between environmental exposure and chronic diseases, specifically cigarette smoking and lung cancer; they apply equally to viral infection (Hill 1965). There must always be a proper temporal relationship: the putative aetiological factor is present before the disease occurs. This point is not particularly difficult to understand; in fact, there is often a tendency to assume an aetiological role on the basis of a simple temporal relationship. It is further required that the aetiological agent must have a scientifically logical role in the disease it is thought to cause. In other words, hepatitis B virus has a logical role in producing chronic liver disease, whereas it would be difficult to hypothesize such a role for the influenza virus. Strength of the association is also critical; i.e. if the associations are strongly statistically significant, an aetiological role is more likely. Most critical, as illustrated by the examples given above, is reproducibility of results. Consistent results from different study designs are strong evidence of an aetiological association.

The road to demonstrating aetiology involves an initial hypotheses and a series of studies. Such a road can be followed in the demonstration in North America of the role of aspirin in the production of Reye's syndrome. The syndrome is a combination of encephalopathy and acute liver abnormalities involving mitochondrial damage. It was recognized for many years to be an unusual complication of various infections, mainly influenza and chickenpox, occurring a few days after the acute illness. Why it happened in a small proportion of infected children was unknown. Descriptive studies suggested that aspirin ingestion might be involved, but this notion was rejected by many investigators because of lack of a clear dose–response relationship (Starko et al. 1982). However, the characteristics of aspirin intoxication provided a credible scientific basis for the relationship. A series of independent case–control studies demonstrated such a statistically strong and consistent role for aspirin that the last study was suspended in the pilot phase and an educational programme was begun (Halpin et al. 1982, Waldman et al. 1982, Hurwitz et al. 1985). Cohort studies were not carried out because Reye's syndrome was too rare to allow use of that design and the associations in the case–control studies were so strong.

5 EXPERIMENTAL EPIDEMIOLOGY

5.1 Simulations

Although most contributions of epidemiology to our understanding of viral infections are observational, experimental approaches are often useful in understanding relationships not defined by other methods. Two will be considered: one involving actual interventions and the other involving simulations. The latter method has mainly been applied to modelling transmission and epidemics mathematically and identifying the effects of various interventions that might be used to prevent or interrupt the outbreaks of infection. Mathematical models have evolved from rather simple approaches ranging from the use of balls to simulate individuals (Monte Carlo models) to elaborate computer structures designed to resemble a community with families and schools that mix with each other. The 2 basic types are deterministic models, which use differential equations, and stochastic models, which use random number generation to approximate the manner in which events take place naturally (Abbey 1952, Bailey 1957).The latter type of simulation is now easier with use of powerful computers so that many replications can be carried out. One of the first infections to be studied with these methods was influenza. Simulations were performed to determine the effects of, for example, vaccinating school age children with influenza vaccine (Elveback et al. 1976, Longini, Ackerman and Elveback 1977). As demonstrated in one experiment, vaccination of school age children increased immunity, sometimes termed herd immunity, in the segment of the population most responsible for introducing the virus into families and spreading it in the community (Monto et al. 1970). The result was not only protection of the vaccinated children but also interruption of transmission, which indirectly protected the rest of the community. Simulation modelling has also been applied to HIV transmission and AIDS forecasting, and has been particularly valuable, given the long-term nature of the infection and the difficulty in predicting spread (Hethcote, Van Ark and Longini 1991). Most recently, it has been especially useful in assessing the effects that vaccination could have on the future occurrence of the disease.

5.2 Controlled trials

The most accepted intervention study in infectious disease epidemiology is the **randomized controlled trial**. Traditionally, the intervention has been vaccination, although more recently antivirals have frequently been studied. Methods for randomized clinical trials have been the subject of a number of reviews and comments, and the many issues and approaches will not be discussed here (Spilker 1991). The endpoint for acute illnesses is generally prevention of the disease.

The efficacy of hepatitis B vaccine was evaluated by antibody production and prevention of acute disease in populations of homosexual males (Szmuness et al. 1975). The design was a randomized, controlled trial. The group chosen for study was at high risk of infection and the study could be concluded in a short period of time. Potentially eligible participants were screened and only those without antibody were included. The frequencies of infection and disease at various periods after vaccination were compared in those who received the active preparation and those who received placebo. The results demonstrated the value of this vaccine in primary prevention. In addition to protecting against acute infection in adults living in developed countries, the vaccine is now used in developing countries, not only to prevent the acute illness but mainly to prevent primary hepatocellular carcinoma. If this tumour decreases in frequency as a result of vaccination, it will be ultimate proof of aetiology. Similarly, with Reye's syndrome, education about the role of aspirin in the disease resulted in decreased use. Reye's syndrome has nearly disappeared in areas where it was previously common, adding further evidence for an aetiological connection (Remington et al. 1986). Certain potential aetiological relationships have bedevilled investigators for many years. It is thought that certain viral infections trigger attacks of asthma in sensitive children. The data are better for children than for adults, and, in both, rhinoviruses seem to be the virus most frequently involved (Mcintosh et al. 1973, Minor et al. 1974). A similar situation applies to triggering exacerbations of chronic respiratory disease in the elderly, although the relationship here is more tenuous. If use of an antiviral to prevent or treat rhinoviral infection also reduces episodes of the chronic condition, it would be the final demonstration of an aetiological relationship.

6 EPIDEMIOLOGICAL CHARACTERISTICS OF RESPIRATORY VIRUSES

6.1 Causes of common respiratory illnesses

Many viruses are responsible for the bulk of respiratory infections. Although the agents are very different from a virological standpoint, they do share epidemiological characteristics. Being surface infections, they do not produce long-lasting immunity. Instead they have the capacity to reinfect, even without antigenic change (Glezen et al. 1986). Other than influenza (Chapter 22), which can produce severe disease in older children and adults, some viruses such as parainfluenza and RSV (see Chapter 23), may cause severe disease in infants and young children on initial infection and mild or inapparent infection indistinguishable from the common cold in older people. Thus, older siblings who introduce a particular infection to the family may contract a mild illness, while the younger child may experience bronchiolitis or pneumonia. RSV is the principal cause of severe lower respiratory illness in young children. The mean age for hospitalization, which occurs in a small proportion of infected children, is 3 months (Parrott et al. 1973). This early age of onset prompted the hypothesis, later proven to be incorrect, that maternal antibody, which is always present to this ubiquitous virus, is responsible for the pathogenesis of the disease. It has now been shown that children born with the highest titres of maternal antibody are those least likely to develop severe disease (Glezen et al. 1981). As a result, maternal immunization is being examined as a way of modifying the initial infantile infection and the use of immune globulin is being examined for prophylaxis and treatment. Parainfluenza virus types 1 and 2 are the major agents of laryngotracheobronchitis (croup). The peak age for these initial, recognizable infections is later than that for RSV, and the protective effect of maternal antibody was never in doubt (Monto 1973).

Rhinoviruses (Chapter 25) and coronaviruses (Chapter 24), in contrast to RSV and parainfluenzaviruses, produce only cold-like symptoms regardless of whether they infect children or adults. Rhinoviruses, as the principal agents of the common cold, infect individuals many times throughout life. Even in the first years of age, when attention is usually directed to the other agents that may produce lower respiratory infection, the rhinoviruses are more commonly isolated (Monto, Koopman and Bryan 1986). Data on the annual incidence of respiratory infections due to all causes were collected from residents of the small community of Tecumseh, Michigan (Monto and Sullivan 1993). These data are shown as curves in Fig. 13.5, with results arranged by gender. As can be seen, there is a suggestion of sparing of infants aged <1 year, because of the presence of maternal antibody. Thereafter the frequencies fall off with increasing age, rising again in young adulthood when individuals start their families and are exposed to young children. The higher frequency of illnesses in females as compared to males is well recognized. In women who work outside the home, the frequency of illness in those aged 20–34 years is higher than in those who do not. Thus continual exposure to children must be a major factor. The age-specific frequency of rhinoviruses roughly parallels these curves. This similarity is a result of the major role of rhinoviruses in the aetiology of the common cold and other frequent respiratory illnesses (Monto, Bryan and Ohmit 1987). Coronaviruses are responsible for illnesses similar to those caused by rhinoviruses. Because they are difficult to isolate and occur much less frequently than the rhinoviruses, much less information is available on their occurrence in populations. Newer tests involving antigen detection may increase our knowledge of their behaviour and distribution (MacNaughton 1982).

Respiratory virus infections differ in their seasonality (Monto and Sullivan 1993). Although, over all, viral respiratory infections increase in frequency in cold weather in many geographic areas, isolation of rhinoviruses peaks in the period after schools reopen: children come into contact with each other for long periods and can spread these viruses that require relatively close contact for transmission. Rhinoviruses account for most of the respiratory illnesses in the community at that time. In other geographic areas, although the autumn peak is prominent, another peak of infection in the spring is also recognized (Hendley, Gwaltney and Jordan 1969). Other respiratory viruses have different periods of spread in different regions. In many areas, RSV transmission peaks in winter or early spring and parainfluenza virus in spring and late autumn, the exact occurrence varying by place and by year. Outside the temperate zones, periods of activity are different and must be defined locally. Because person to person transmission is always involved, the agents take weeks to move through even a small community.

6.2 Influenza

Influenza (Chapter 22) is potentially serious in all individuals who develop disease. Infection rates are highest in children and adults who are sufficiently ill to seek medical advice (Monto, Koopman and Longine 1985). However, the elderly and those with chronic illnesses experience the most severe disease, often with complications such as pneumonia (Chin et al. 1960). Reasons for the susceptibility of older individuals are varied, and probably related to depressed cell-mediated immunity (Phair et al. 1978). Because of the danger of illness in older people and those with chronic conditions, vaccination programmes in many countries are not intended to prevent infection in the young. Rather, older people are vaccinated as a means of preventing hospitalization or death. As result, disease in the young, who sustain the major burden of a complicated infection, is not affected, and outbreaks continue. An exception is Japan, where a former policy was designed to limit spread by vaccinating school-age children (Dowdle et al. 1980).

Influenza, like other respiratory agents, is seasonal, no obvious transmission taking place in warmer months of the year in the temperate zones, although asymptomatic infections have been detected serologically, particularly with type A viruses. Outbreaks of influenza in cold seasons can be recognized by various indicators, including increased visits to physicians or school absenteeism. These indicators can be found during major outbreaks of all types and subtypes of influenza; they are a reflection of the high infection frequency in the general population. Transmission of influenza types A(H3N2) and B can also be detected by the ability of these viruses to be fatal in older people and those with high risk conditions. Such deaths, as complications of the primary viral infection, generally occur 2 weeks after the initial episode, so excess mortality is a delayed indication of transmission.

Although seasonal outbreaks of influenza may be caused by one viral type or subtype, mixed or sequential outbreaks of different types may also occur. The viruses appear at various other times in tropical cli-

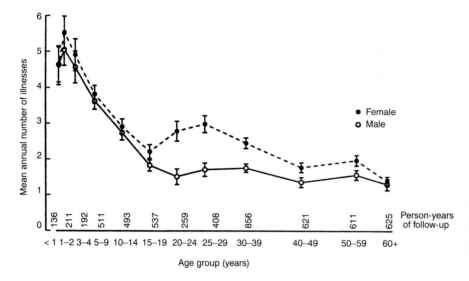

Fig. 13.5 Mean number of respiratory illnesses per person-year (95% confidence intervals) in males and females living in Tecumseh, Michigan. (From Monto and Sullivan 1993.)

mates, either throughout the year or during the rainy season, and such regions are likely to be the source of new strains. Pandemics of type A influenza take place at irregular intervals following sudden changes in the viral haemagglutinin or the neuraminidase, or both ('antigenic shift'). For a time, it was thought that new viruses with pandemic potential emerged at regular intervals, approximately every 10 years. In retrospect, these conclusions were based on confusion concerning whether a shift in surface antigens had occurred during the period 1918–1956, and observations during only a limited period thereafter. It had always been assumed that, when a type A strain with new surface antigen or antigens emerged, it would totally replace the previous A subtype. In 1977, the A(H1N1) subtype reappeared 20 years after it had been completely replaced in 1957 by type A(H2N2). The type A(H3N2) viruses have been circulating since 1968 and, instead of replacing these viruses, both subtypes have co-circulated since that time. Type A(H1N1) has largely been restricted to the younger segment of the population and type A(H3N2) has occurred in all age groups (Masurel 1976, Kendal et al. 1977).

When pandemics of influenza have followed a shift in type A antigens, the same age-specific morbidity and mortality patterns have been observed as in the annual epidemics of influenza but at much higher frequency. However, in 1918, the pandemic viruses thought, on the basis of serological epidemiology, to be related to swine influenza, produced unusually high mortality in young adults, a group usually experiencing significant morbidity but little mortality. A total of 20 million people died world-wide during this pandemic, which is still a unique and unexplained event, possibly related to unusual bacterial superinfections (Shope 1936). Recent pandemic strains of influenza first caused outbreaks of disease in humans in southern China. There, the combination of high population density and animals, especially domestic ducks and pigs, living in close contact with humans, often in the same dwellings, might have been responsible

(Kawaoka et al. 1993). Many domestic animals have their own type A influenza viruses, but such infections are not true zoonoses because these viruses are not pathogenic for humans.

New pandemic viruses seem to result from reassortment made possible by the segmented genome of the influenza virus. The gene segments coding for the surface antigens of the animal strains replace the comparable segments of the strains pathogenic for humans. The result is a new virus with internal components from the old pathogenic virus but with new haemagglutinin and sometimes a new neuraminidase from the animal strain. Type B influenza viruses do not infect animals, and pandemics of type B do not occur, strengthening the hypothesis of the animal origin of pandemic type A variants. Thus, the only changes seen with type B viruses are gradual year-to-year variations, referred to as 'antigenic drift'. The same drift also occurs with type A strains over the years, in addition to the episodic shift associated with pandemics. This regular drift makes it necessary to incorporate fresh strains in the vaccine, because efficacy drops if there is not a good match between circulating variants and in the vaccine strains. Updating is usually done annually with type A(H3N2) and not as often with type A(H1N1) and type B viruses, reflecting more rapid changes in type A(H3N2).

7 VIRUSES INFECTING THE GASTROINTESTINAL TRACT

7.1 Agents of diarrhoeal disease

Diarrhoeal disease in industrialized countries is of varied aetiology. Unlike respiratory illnesses, in which viruses are the principal pathogens, enteric illnesses are sometimes of bacterial or parasitic origin, especially when they occur as outbreaks. Much of the disease that occurs more regularly in families is of viral origin and its frequency increases in the cold season, reflecting greater opportunities for transmission (Monto and Koopman 1980). Rotaviruses are the main cause of dehydrating diarrhoeal disease in young children throughout the world (see Chapter 27). Although infants and young children in developing countries may die of these infections if they are not rehydrated with salt-containing solutions (orally or sometimes intravenously), the disease is rarely so severe in the developed world, mainly because of such factors as better nutrition (Black et al. 1981). These are surface infections that recur throughout life. Whilst initial infections in infants may be severe, reinfections usually produce mild illness or asymptomatic infection. As with the respiratory viruses, this has implications for spread within families.

Paradoxically, the pattern of occurrence of rotavirus infection is more like that of the respiratory viruses than of other enteric agents, although transmission clearly takes place by the faecal–oral route; whereas large amounts of virus are shed in the stools, none has been detected in the upper respiratory tract. As with respiratory viruses it is possible to examine the role of the family and the community in determining the occurrence of infection. All rotavirus types are seasonal in the temperate zones, most illness occurring in the colder months (Brandt et al. 1982, Vesikari et al. 1992). Rotavirus vaccines, prepared from live attenuated strains, are being developed for use in infants (see Chapter 27). Because of the need for multiple types, there has been at least a potential problem with interference, a phenomenon common to live attenuated vaccines, with difficulty in producing immunity simultaneously to several types. The purpose of vaccination is not necessarily to prevent infection or illness completely but to render it more like reinfection, thus preventing severe dehydration.

Rotaviruses are responsible for only some of the enteric illnesses experienced in the community during the cold season. Identifying the aetiological agents of other common illnesses has been complicated by the difficulty or impossibility of growing many of them in cell culture. Norwalk virus, now recognized to be a calicivirus, is one of a group of viruses causing water-related outbreaks (see Chapter 26). A variety of exposures are involved, including drinking and swimming in water containing the virus, especially when the head is submerged; contaminated seafood has also been implicated (Gunn et al. 1980, Kaplan et al. 1982). Person-to-person transmission also occurs, increasing the potential for spread in families and the community.

Immune electron microscopy was the basic method for identifying rise in antibody titre and reagents had to be prepared by inoculating human volunteers (Herrmann et al. 1985). The recent cloning of the Norwalk agent will allow better understanding of its epidemiology as reagents become available for testing sera. Similarly the enteric adenoviruses, types 40 and 41, originally detected only by electron microscopy can now be identified by enzyme immunoassay (EIA) (Johansson et al. 1985). The association of these viruses with enteric disease in infants is an example of use of the case–control design. The respiratory adenoviruses, which could at that time be easily cultivated in cell culture, were isolated in equal numbers from the stools of cases (children hospitalized with diarrhoea) and controls (children hospitalized with other conditions). However, adenoviruses that could not be cultivated in routine cell cultures were significantly more commonly detected in children with disease than in controls (Brandt et al. 1985). It has been suggested that an autumnal increase in enteric illness is related to these adenoviruses but such seasonality could not be demonstrated in hospital-based studies.

7.2 Polio and enteric hepatitis viruses

The enteroviruses are generally transmitted by the faecal–oral route. Some exceptions exist, however, such as coxsackie virus A21, an unusual cause of respiratory infection which can spread by aerosol. The dynamics and characteristics of this infection were well studied in the military, in whom it had presented an occasional problem. Polio is the best known of the enteroviruses, producing a potentially serious disease in a small proportion of those infected. Global elimination of polio is underway, by use of the live attenuated vaccine administered universally and repeatedly to young children. The method is based on the known transmission pattern of the vaccine virus, which resembles that of the wild virus in being shed in large quantities and for long periods in the stool of inoculated children (Hull et al. 1994). The shed virus can be transmitted to contacts, especially other children, and to adults in the family. By inoculating children regularly (annually or more frequently) as part of a mass vaccination programme, it is possible to spread the vaccine viruses in the environment so that children who are missed by the vaccine programme are indirectly exposed to them. This approach, which combines herd immunity, or increasing the level of antibody in a population so that susceptibles are rare and transmission is interrupted, together with the special characteristics of transmissibility of the live polio vaccine, has resulted in the elimination of transmission of wild polio virus in the Americas. The procedure is now being applied in other parts of the developing world (Centers for Disease Control 1995).

Hepatitis A is classified as an enterovirus; it shares epidemiological characteristics with other enteroviruses but is unusual in having a relatively long incubation period (median 28 days) (Lemon 1985). Spread in the developed countries typically occurs from person to person in the family or in settings such as day care centres for children, especially when they are not toilet trained. Much of the infection in North America has been traced to these day care outbreaks, from which spread continues in families and older individuals (Hadler and McFarland 1986). In developing countries and in special situations in the industrialized world, spread can often occur through contaminated water or by consuming uncooked shellfish from contaminated waters. Other food transmission is possible whenever there is faecal contamination. In the developing world, infection occurs at an early age and is often asymptomatic. In the industrialized countries, infection is delayed and often will not occur at all, rendering much of the population susceptible if exposed. Travellers to developing countries generally do not have protective antibodies from past exposure, and are thus at increased risk. One solution, before vaccine became available, was use of immune globulin, which gives temporary protection. There are now vaccines that can protect individuals from developed countries who will be exposed in the developing world. Such infection has been a major risk, especially for people exposed for long periods in areas with poor standards of hygiene (Wagner et al. 1993). Hepatitis E appears to have epidemiological characteristics similar to those of hepatitis A, and increasing availability of reagents will allow better understanding of its behaviour in populations. Some outbreaks of disease thought to be due to hepatitis A are now recognized to have been, in all probability, caused by hepatitis E (Wong et al. 1980).

8   VIRAL INFECTIONS WITH BLOOD-BORNE TRANSMISSION

8.1   Hepatitis B and related viruses

Hepatitis B was, before the discovery of HIV, the most extensively studied blood-borne pathogen. During the course of many viral infections, there is often a phase of viraemia; however, blood-borne transmission is unlikely when viraemia lasts for only a period of hours. The probability of such transmission is increased when viraemia persists for days or, as is the case with some infected with hepatitis B, for years. The likelihood that infection will persist decreases with increasing age at time of exposure. Thus, perinatal infection is most likely to result in chronic viraemia. The transmission of hepatitis B by blood or blood products was documented well before the virus or its antigens were identified (Sawyer et al. 1944). During the second world war, yellow fever vaccine used by the US military was stabilized by the addition of human albumin. Those who received the vaccine developed hepatitis and, by epidemiological evidence, it became clear that it was contaminated by what is now known to be hepatitis B virus. On initial study, the cases of hepatitis that were detected did not seem to bear any temporal relationship to an exposure to persons with infection or to a common event. Then it was realized that vaccination might be the common source. Because vaccinations had been administered over a long period, cases were occurring in an apparently unrelated fashion. Plotting of duration since vaccination resulted in a typical epidemic curve, with cases distributed around the long median incubation period of c. 120 days from exposure.

Hepatitis B is transmissible not only through blood and blood products but also through sexual contact. Simply living in a family with an infected person slightly increases the probability of transmission. It is not clear exactly how this occurs. The virus is present in various body fluids, in addition to blood and semen (Irwin et al. 1975). Transmission requires only very small amounts of blood, so leakage through minor abrasions and tears may be responsible. Hepatitis B was known to be more common in certain professional groups such as dentists, almost certainly because of exposure to small amounts of infected blood commonly lost in dental procedures rather than through virus present in saliva (Mosley et al. 1975). It

was especially common among homosexual men, especially those with multiple partners. In fact, the trial of hepatitis B vaccine was conducted in uninfected sexually active homosexual men, because exposure was predictable. The transmission was clearly sexual, but how much of it involved transfer of small quantities of highly infectious blood and how much other infected bodily fluids was difficult to quantify. Various specific sexual practices such as anal intercourse were identified as risk factors even before the study of HIV transmission (Szmuness et al. 1975).

A particular problem with hepatitis B, especially in eastern Asia (including China) and in sub-Saharan Africa, is that transmission is mainly vertical and children become infected at birth from transplacental and direct exposure to maternal blood (Stevens et al. 1975). When infection occurs at this age, it is likely to persist, and thus may be carried to the next generation. Hepatitis C shares many features with hepatitis B, including its transmission by blood and blood products. Risk groups differ somewhat; as newly developed reagents are used, these differences can be defined more precisely (Alter et al. 1989).

8.2   Human immunodeficiency virus

When human immunodeficiency virus (HIV) was first described, its epidemiology was found to be remarkably similar to that of hepatitis B (see Chapter 38). Differences are related to the natural history of the disease and to the far lower transmissibility of HIV under most conditions. A persistently high level of viraemia allows hepatitis B virus transmission to occur with relative ease for long periods. In contrast, transmission of HIV is most likely early in the infectious process when there is viraemia of high titre, or later in the development of AIDS itself when the level of viraemia increases again. The early period is probably the most important for transmission, because at that time individuals may not know they are infected and remain sexually active (Jacquez et al. 1994). Because of its importance, the epidemiology of HIV has been studied intensively over the short period since the virus was identified and many characteristics of its distribution are now well established. Much attention has been given to the role that various behaviours play in transmission, since, in the developed countries, antibody tests have ensured that blood and blood products are safe and transmission by that route of infection no longer occurs. Among homosexual men, receptive anal intercourse is the prime risk factor, but other sexual practices are possibly to blame, if not nearly as risky. Heterosexual intercourse also can transmit the virus efficiently, but male-to-female transmission is accomplished more easily than the reverse (Padian, Shiboski and Jewell 1991). As with hepatitis B, injecting drug use appears to be an independent risk factor for transmission. Transmission also occurs through breast milk and artificial insemination. In one controversial case, the argument for transmission of virus to the patients of an HIV-infected dentist was strengthened by the similarity of the viral nucleic acids in the various cases, a technique sometimes referred to as molecular epidemiology (Crandall 1995).

In the developed countries, the disease has predominantly been one of males, both homosexual and bisexual men and injecting drug users. Heterosexual transmission has often involved sexual partners of these individuals. In the USA, African-Americans and other minority groups are increasingly involved. In developing countries, the male to female ratio often is 1 : 1, and the prevalence of infection in the general population, especially in certain countries of Africa, is high. The infection has entered south and southeast Asia, where transmission has been rapid. Mathematical epidemiology has been used to study the relative probability of different transmission mechanisms when several may be involved, and to predict the course of the pandemic. Simulations have been particularly valuable in trying to understand how altering transmission by vaccination or behaviour modification will affect the course of the epidemic in different regions.

9 ZOONOSES AND VECTOR-BORNE INFECTION

9.1 Zoonoses not involving arthropods

Many, but not all, of the vector-borne viral infections are also zoonoses and are discussed together. The zoonoses are human infections in which the principal reservoirs of the viral agent are wild and domestic mammals, birds and possibly other species such as reptiles. Cycles of infection can be maintained in these reservoirs without the involvement of humans, in whom infection occurs incidentally. Zoonoses not involving arthropod-vector transmission are listed in Table 13.4, with animal reservoir and route transmission. Rabies (see Chapter 33) is an example of a zoonosis not involving vectors. In most of the world, rabies is widely distributed in a variety of mammals, the predominant species varying from region to region. In North America, foxes, skunks and raccoons are mainly involved (Anderson et al. 1984). Of these, only raccoons frequently invade human habitations but in most cases transmission remains within the particular species. Transmission sometimes involves domestic animals such as dogs or cats, who, because of their activities outside the home, will occasionally come in contact with the wildlife hosts. Insectivorous bats also maintain rabies in their own colonies but, because they often live in human dwellings, direct transmission to humans occasionally occurs. Vaccination of domestic pets is used to create a barrier between wildlife rabies and humans; it is highly effective, with the possible exception of preventing direct bat transmission. There have been several years in the USA without a single case of human rabies, even though extensive transmission in animals still occurs. In other parts of the developed world, the species involved in maintaining wildlife rabies differ. In Europe foxes are often involved, and attempts are now being made to control transmission in these hosts by drops of baited food containing vaccine (Brochier et al. 1991). This is possible only when the geographic areas are relatively limited. In remote areas, many more species are involved and control is impractical.

Some parts of the world, typically islands such as Great Britain and Hawaii, are rabies-free; because potential hosts are present in the wild, exclusion of animals who might be responsible for importation is a critical part of control activity. In many developing countries, rabies of domestic animals is common, especially of dogs which are barely domesticated and often form feral packs. Transmission from dog to dog does occur, as well as from dog to humans. This is in contrast to the typical situation in the developed world, where the dog, as well as humans who become infected, are 'dead-end hosts'; that is, they are generally not responsible for any further transmission. The few human cases that occur in industrialized countries are often imports from developing countries, where exposure of travellers to infected domestic animals is more likely. Molecular techniques, based on differences in viral nucleic acid structure in rabies viruses transmitted in different parts of the world, are often used to determine the source of exposure (Smith et al. 1992). The few cases and intensive study of those that do occur have allowed recognition of unusual sources of infection, such as a transplanted cornea obtained from a cadaver whose death was caused by undetected rabies (Houff et al. 1979).

Zoonoses not involving arthropods are typical of infections produced by arenaviruses and hantaviruses. With both, rodents and other wildlife hosts are responsible for transmission and maintenance of infection. Sometimes the rodents become diseased, but in most cases the infections are inapparent. Humans become involved incidentally and have no further role in maintenance of the chain of transmission. Viruses such as the arenaviruses (Machupo, the cause of Bolivian haemorrhagic fever, and Junin, the cause of Argentine haemorrhagic fever), as well as the hantaviruses (producing Korean haemorrhagic fever and the newly recognized hantavirus pulmonary syndrome in North America) are limited geographically by the area ranged by the rodents primarily infected. Human-to-human transmission is rare; most human infection appears to result from exposure to rodent urine heavily contaminated with virus, and possibly other animal products such as faeces or saliva (Peters et al. 1974, Mercado 1975). The rodents often live in or near dwellings, and humans may be exposed via aerosol or through abraded skin. Increases in frequency of the disease, which, for example, led to the recognition of the hantavirus pulmonary syndrome in southwestern USA, are related to changes in the environment affecting numbers and activities of the rodent host (Hjelle et al. 1994). It is suggested that an overproduction of pine nuts, the rodents' principal food, led to the emergence of the disease in the 'Sin Nombre' area of the USA.

9.2 Yellow fever and dengue

The term 'arbovirus' was used for many years to describe a large group of enveloped, lipid-containing

Table 13.4 Zoonotic viral infections without arthropod transmission

Virus and disease	Animal reservoir	Mode of transfer
Rhabdoviruses		
Rabies	Foxes, skunks, bats, raccoons, mongooses, dogs, cats etc.	Bite. Possibly saliva through abraded skin or air-borne
Arenaviruses		
Lymphocytic choriomeningitis	*Mus musculus*	Contact with urine, faeces or other infected fluids
Junin-Argentine haemorrhagic fever	*Calomys musculinus*	
Machupo-Bolivian haemorrhagic fever	*Calomys callosus*	
Guanarito virus disease– Venezuelan haemorrhagic fever	*Sigmodon hispidus*	Rarely person to person or nosocomial spread. Possible air-borne distribution
Lassa fever	*Mastomys natalensis*	
Bunyaviruses/hantaviruses		
Hantaan virus		Contact with urine, faeces, and saliva
Korean haemorrhagic fever	Field mice	
Seoul virus	Urban rats	
Sin Nombre virus		May be aerosolized or enter through abraded skin
Hantavirus pulmonary syndrome	Deer mice and other rodents	
Puumulavirus Nephropathia epidemica	Voles	
Filoviruses		
Marburg	Reservoir not clear	Contact with infected monkeys
Ebola	Reservoir not clear	Blood and other personal contact after infection in humans
Poxviruses		
Cowpox, monkeypox	Cows, monkeys, sheep	Animal skin lesion to abraded human skin
Contagious pustular dermatitis (orf)		
Herpesvirus		
Herpesvirus B	Rhesus monkeys	Saliva by bite or contact
Orthomyxovirus		
Swine influenza virus	Pigs	Close contact
Picornavirus		
Encephalomyocarditis	Rodents and monkeys	Possible contamination by urine and faeces

viruses that had in common transmission by arthropods (Theiler 1957). This diverse group of viruses has many epidemiological features in common (see Chapters 29 and 30. The principal vector is the mosquito, although there are important infections involving ticks and other arthropods. Many are also zoonoses, in which the infection is maintained in wild or domestic animals (the reservoirs), humans being involved only occasionally as dead-end hosts. Because of the nature of the vectors and the reservoirs, particular arboviruses are often geographically limited in distribution. Certain mosquitoes cannot exist outside the tropical or subtropical areas, so climate becomes a major determi-

nant, as does other vector behaviour, including preferences in multiplication sites, sources of blood meals and flight distances.

A list of some important arthropod-borne viral infections, according to geographical area of their occurrence is given in Table 13.5. Two important infections, both transmitted preferentially by the mosquito *Aedes aegypti*, which can be spread from human to human by the vector, are yellow fever and dengue. Thus, unlike many other arboviruses, dengue and (in this context) yellow fever are not zoonoses. The mosquito is closely associated with human dwellings in urban areas of the tropics and subtropics, but does not persist in areas with cold winter seasons. Urban outbreaks are typical, because infected humans are ready sources for the transmission of viruses to others. In certain regions, outbreaks of the infections are a regular seasonal occurrence. Control of yellow fever was accomplished in many cities of the Americas before availability of insecticides by eradicating the vector from urban areas. Early control of yellow fever transmission made possible the construction of the Panama Canal. With no urban yellow fever, sylvatic or jungle yellow fever was detected in areas without the usual vectors. The same virus caused the disease, which was found to have a zoonotic host, i.e. sub-human primates. It could be transmitted to humans, especially to people working or living in the forests, by haemagogus mosquitoes. *Aedes aegypti* has recently returned to many cities from which it had been eliminated, and, with it, urban outbreaks of yellow fever.

Several vaccines have been developed to control outbreaks of yellow fever and for primary prevention in endemic areas. The most successful, the 17-D vaccine, is a live attenuated preparation that confers long-term protection.

Dengue is currently the most important arthropod-borne virus because of its widespread distribution in large parts of the tropics and subtropics and the potential there for extensive outbreaks of life-threatening disease. Urbanization in these regions has led to an increase in the probability of dengue infection because the virus is transmitted by the vector mosquito

from one human host to another without the involvement of a zoonotic reservoir. The high concentration of susceptibles in the sprawling cities results in large-scale outbreaks. The vector *A. aegypti* is well adapted to multiplying in the small pools of water that are frequently found in these areas, especially in seasons with heavy rainfall. In its acute form, dengue is debilitating with high fever and deep pain; and infection can result in dengue haemorrhagic fever/dengue shock syndrome (DHF/DDS). These are life-threatening conditions, which affect mainly children. There are 4 types of dengue virus, and infection with one type produces only partial immunity to another type. The principal hypothesis to explain the pathogenesis of dengue haemorrhagic fever is based on epidemiological observations (Halstead 1970). The disease is widespread when a second outbreak of infection, typically caused by type 2, follows shortly after another outbreak caused by a different type. Reinfection appears to be the common factor; this occurs mainly in children, and maternal antibody may play a role in infants. A number of immunological characteristics of the disease support this hypothesis, although there is some evidence that the syndrome can be produced on initial infection in individuals without maternal antibody (Barnes and Rosen 1974). In recent years, dengue has been spreading, especially in the Americas. This is of particular concern in the USA because *A. aegypti* is present in the southern states.

Table 13.5 Arthropod-borne viruses of global importance and their vectors

Diseases	Family/Genus	Vector
Tropics and subtropics		
Yellow fever	*Flaviviridae/Flavivirus*	*Aedes* and haemagogus mosquitoes
Dengue	*Flaviviridae/Flavivirus*	*Aedes aegypti* and *A. albopictus*
Sandfly fever	*Bunyaviridae/Phlebovirus*	Phlebotomine sandflies
American		
Eastern, western, Venezuelan equine encephalitis	*Togaviridae/Alphaviruses*	*Aedes* and *Culex* mosquitoes
St Louis encephalitis	*Flaviviridae/Flavivirus*	*Culex* mosquitoes
California encephalitis	*Bunyaviridae/Bunyavirus*	*Aedes* mosquitoes
California tick fever	*Reoviridae/Orbivirus*	*Dermacentor* ticks
Eurasian		
Tick-borne encephalitis (Russian spring–summer/central European)	*Flaviviridae/flavivirus*	Ixodid ticks
Crimean haemorrhagic fever (Crimean–Congo)	*Bunyaviridae/Nairovirus*	*Hyalomma* ticks
Omsk haemorrhagic fever	*Flaviviridae/Flavivirus*	*Dermacentor* ticks
Japanese B encephalitis	*Flaviviridae/Flavivirus*	*Culex* mosquitoes
African		
Rift Valley fever	*Bunyaviridae/Phlebovirus*	*Culex* and *Aedes* mosquito
Chikungunya fever	*Togaviridae/Alphavirus*	*Aedes aegypti* and others
West Nile fever	*Flaviviridae/Flavivirus*	*Culex* mosquitoes
Australasian		
Murray Valley encephalitis	*Flaviviridae/Flavivirus*	*Culex* mosquitoes
Ross River fever	*Togaviridae/Alphavirus*	*Aedes* and *Culex* mosquitoes

9.3   Other arboviruses

For arboviruses that are principally zoonoses, disease in humans is generally sporadic or occasional. In North America, eastern equine encephalitis (EEE) is an example of an agent that occurs sporadically, during the summer. Many of the infections are inapparent. Symptomatic infection occurs only occasionally, but may manifest as severe encephalitis with residual mental retardation. The reservoir is wild and domestic birds; maintenance of infection does not require either humans or horses, both of which are dead-end hosts. With arboviruses in the temperate zones there is always the question of persistence through the winter (overwintering) during the period when there is no vector activity. Migrating birds infected by the virus winter in areas where mosquitoes are present and are responsible for the continued transmission of the agent. They return, some being infected, in the spring (Lord and Calisher 1970). With other arboviruses there is some evidence that animals in hibernation may serve to overwinter the virus (Reeves 1974).

In the Eurasian land mass, tick-borne encephalitis (TBE), also called Russian spring–summer encephalitis, is an important, though uncommon, sporadic disease associated with forested areas. The reservoir is small mammals and, to a lesser extent, birds; humans moving into sites where transmission is occurring become infected incidentally. Transovarian transmission can take place in ticks in which the virus is passed to the next generation, further maintaining the infection. In contrast, the most important arbovirus of eastern and southeast Asia, Japanese encephalitis, may be responsible for large numbers of cases of relatively severe encephalitis in humans. This disease is mosquito-transmitted and occurs in rice-growing regions which generally have a high mosquito density. The principal reservoir is pigs, also common in the region. Because vector control in these areas has been difficult, emphasis has been placed on vaccination.

10   VIRUSES AND CHRONIC DISEASES

Persistent infection is well documented for many DNA viruses and some RNA viruses. The herpesvirus group is well known for producing persistent infections, for example recurrent cold sores or genital ulcers caused by herpes simplex virus and herpes zoster due to varicella-zoster virus. The retroviruses, including HIV, are also characterized by long-term chronic infection. It is difficult to establish the role of various viruses to late, seemingly unrelated, events such as the development of cirrhosis and primary hepatocellular carcinoma (PHC) or carcinoma of the cervix. Relating these conditions to viral infections requires the application of epidemiological study designs. For hepatitis B and the production of primary hepatocellular carcinoma, the studies were mainly conducted in Taiwan, where there is a combination of high prevalence of chronic infec-

tion and a health care system that allowed a longitudinal study of health care workers. A problem in any of these evaluations is the long time between the infection, which may have been acquired perinatally, and development of the tumour, which can occur many decades later. Demonstration of viral antigen in the tumour is of help, but is not conclusive proof of aetiology where the population has a history of widespread infection with the agent. The major epidemiological evidence for aetiology has come from a series of case–control and cohort studies that noted a strong association between the persistent infection and primary hepatocellular carcinoma even after controlling for potential confounding variables (Beasley 1988). Similar work is now underway to investigate the link between hepatitis C and PHC.

Epidemiological approaches have also provided evidence of involvement of certain types of papilloma virus in carcinoma of the cervix (Chapter 16). Descriptive epidemiological studies have long suggested that an infectious entity, probably sexually transmitted, was involved in aetiology. Attention was first focused on behavioural differences and on herpes simplex virus. Case–control studies revealed that herpes antibody titres were higher in people with tumours than in those without (Rawls et al. 1970). It was possible to identify viral components in excised tumour, and other factors seemed to confirm the relationship. However, the link was not well sustained in studies controlling for confounding factors, such as sexual activity. When it became easier to work with papillomaviruses, epidemiological studies confirmed the specificity of the association with certain types. Moreover, it was possible to replicate the relationship in different studies in different parts of the world and to demonstrate the strength of the association with the specific papilloma types in question (Reeves et al. 1987). This again illustrated the importance of comparative studies.

Research into the long-term consequences of viral infection is very important, because it brings together acute and chronic outcomes affecting the health of populations. Examples include the relationship of EB virus to the later development of nasopharyngeal carcinoma and Burkitt's lymphoma. Work in this area is diverse, and ranges from efforts to relate acute respiratory infection to later chronic bronchitis and emphysema to studies attempting to relate infectious agents to the pathogenesis of atherosclerosis. All these investigations must use appropriate epidemiological methods, especially as these techniques are a recognized component of other investigations of risk factors for chronic disease.

REFERENCES

Abbey H, 1952, An examination of the Reed Frost theory of epidemics, *Hum Biol*, **24**: 201–33.

Alter HJ, Purcell RH et al., 1989, Detection of antibody to hepatitis C virus in prospectively followed transfusion recipients with acute and chronic non-A, non-B hepatitis, *N Engl J Med*, **321**: 1494–500.

American Public Health Association, 1985, *Control of Communi-*

cable Diseases of Man, 14th edn, ed Beneson AS, APHA, Washington DC, 457–9.

Anderson LJ, Nicholson KG et al., 1984, Human rabies in the United States, 1960 to 1979: epidemiology, diagnosis, and prevention, *Ann Intern Med*, **100**: 728–35.

Bailey NTJ, 1957, *The Mathematical Theory of Epidemics*, Griffin, London.

Barnes WJS, Rosen L, 1974, Fatal hemorrhagic disease and shock associated with primary dengue infection on a Pacific island, *Am J Trop Med Hyg*, **23**: 495–506.

Baron RC, McCormick JB, Zubeir OA, 1981, Ebola virus disease in southern Sudan: hospital dissemination and intrafamilial spread, *Bull W H O*, **61**: 997–1003.

Bartlett AV, Moore M et al., 1985, Diarrheal illness among infants and toddlers in day care centers. II. Comparison with day care homes and households, *J Pediatr*, **107**: 503–9.

Beasley RP, 1982, Hepatitis B virus as the etiologic agent in hepatocellular carcinoma – epidemiologic considerations, *Hepatology*, **2**: 215–65.

Beasley RP, 1988, Hepatitis B virus. The major etiology of hepatocellular carcinoma cancer, *Cancer*, **61**: 1942–56.

Belongia EA, Goodman JL et al., 1991, An outbreak of herpes gladiatorum at a high school wrestling competition, *N Engl J Med*, **325**: 906–10.

Berquist KR, Maynard JE et al., 1976, Experimental studies on the transmission of hepatitis B by mosquitoes, *Am J Trop Med Hyg*, **25**: 730–2.

Black FL, 1989, *Measles in Viral Infections of Humans: epidemiology and control*, 3rd edn, ed Evans AS, Plenum Medical, New York and London, 457.

Black RE, Merson MH et al., 1981, Incidence and severity of rotavirus and *Escherichia coli* diarrhea in rural Bangladesh. Implications for vaccine development, *Lancet*, **1**: 141–3.

Brandt CD, Kim HW et al., 1982, Rotavirus gastroenteritis and weather, *J Clin Microbiol*, **16**: 478–82.

Brandt CD, Kim HW et al., 1983, Pediatric viral gastroenteritis during eight years of study, *J Clin Microbiol*, **18**: 71–8.

Brandt CD, Kim HW et al., 1985, Adenoviruses and pediatric gastroenteritis, *J Infect Dis*, **151**: 437–43.

Breslow NE, Day NE, 1987, *Statistical Methods in Cancer Research. Vol II. The Design and Analysis of Cohort Studies*, International Agency for Research on Cancer, Lyon.

Brochier B, Kieny MP et al., 1991, Large-scale eradication of rabies using recombinant vaccinia–rabies vaccine, *Nature (London)*, **354**: 520–2.

Centers for Disease Control, 1994, Hantavirus pulmonary syndrome – United States, 1993, *Morbid Mortal Weekly Rep*, **43**: 45–8.

Centers for Disease Control, 1995, Progress toward poliomyelitis eradication – South East Asia region, 1988–1994, *Morbid Mortal Weekly Rep*, **44**: 791–801.

Childs JE, Ksiazek TG et al., 1994, Serologic and genetic identification of *Peromyscus maniculatus* as the primary rodent reservior for a new hantavirus in the southwestern United States, *J Infect Dis*, **169**: 1271–80.

Chin TDY, Foley JF et al., 1960, Morbidity and mortality characteristics of Asian strain influenza, *Public Health Rep*, **75**: 149–58.

Couch RB, Cate TR et al., 1966, Effect of route of inoculation on experimental respiratory viral disease in volunteers and evidence for airborne transmission, *Bacteriol Rev*, **30**: 517–531.

Crandall KA, 1995, Intraspecific phylogenetics: support for dental transmission of human immunodeficiency virus, *J Virol*, **69**: 2351–6.

Dowdle WR, Millar JO et al., 1980, Influenza immunization policies and practices in Japan, *J Infect Dis*, **141**: 258–64.

Eickhoff TC, Sherman IL, Serfling RE, 1961, Observations on excess mortality associated with epidemic influenza, *JAMA*, **176**: 104–10.

Elandt-Johnson RC, 1975, Definition of rates: some remarks on their use and misuse, *Am J Epidemiol*, **102**: 261–71.

Elveback LR, Fox JP et al., 1976, An influenza simulation model for immunization studies, *Am J Epidemiol*, **103**: 152–65.

Fedson DS, Wajda A et al., 1993, Clinical effectiveness of influenza vaccine in Manitoba, *JAMA*, **270**: 1956–61.

Foster DA, Talsma A et al., 1992, Influenza vaccine effectiveness in preventing hospitalization for pneumonia in the elderly, *Am J Epidemiol*, **136**: 296–307.

Fox JP, Hall CE, Elveback LR, 1970, *Epidemiology, Man and Disease*, Macmillan, London.

Friedland GH, Klein RS, 1987, Transmission of the human immunodeficiency virus, *N Engl J Med*, **317**: 1125–35.

Friedman-Kien AE, Laubenstein LJ et al., 1982, Disseminated Kaposi's sarcoma in homosexual men, *Ann Intern Med*, **96**: 693–700.

Glezen WP, Paredes A et al., 1981, Risk of respiratory syncytial virus infection for infants from low-income families in relationship to age, sex, ethnic group, and maternal antibody level, *J Pediatr*, **98**: 708–15.

Glezen WP, Payne AA et al., 1982, Mortality and influenza, *J Infect Dis*, **146**: 313–21.

Glezen WP, Taber LH et al., 1986, Risk of primary infection and reinfection with respiratory syncytial virus, *Am J Dis Child*, **140**: 543–6.

Gottlieb MS, Schroff R et al., 1981, *Pneumocystis carinii* pneumonia and mucosal candidiasis in previously healthy homosexual men: evidence of a new acquired cellular immunodeficiency, *N Engl J Med*, **305**: 1425–31.

Gregg NM, 1941, Congenital cataract following German measles in the mother, *Trans Ophthal Soc Aust*, **3**: 35–46.

Gunn RA, Terranova WA et al., 1980, Norwalk virus gastroenteritis aboard a cruise ship: an outbreak on five consecutive cruises, *Am J Epidemiol*, **112**: 820–7.

Hadler SC, McFarland L, 1986, Hepatitis in day care centers. Epidemiology and prevention, *Rev Infect Dis*, **154**: 231–7.

Hallee TJ, Evans AS et al., 1974, Infectious mononucleosis at the US military academy: a prospective study of a single class over four years, *Yale J Biol Med*, **47**: 182–95.

Halpin TJ, Holtzhauer FJ et al., 1982, Reye's syndrome and medication use, *JAMA*, **248**: 687–91.

Halstead SB, 1970, Observations relating to pathogenesis of dengue hemorrhagic fever. VI. Hypotheses and discussion, *Yale J Biol Med*, **42**: 350–62.

Hattwick MAW, Weis TT et al., 1972, Recovery from rabies: a case report, *Ann Intern Med*, **76**: 931–42.

Hedstrom C, Lycke E, 1964, An experimental study on oysters as virus carriers, *Am J Hyg*, **79**: 134–42.

Hendley JO, Gwaltney JM Jr, Jordan WS Jr, 1969, Rhinovirus infections in an industrial population. IV. Infections within families of employees during two fall peaks of respiratory illness, *Am J Epidemiol*, **89**: 184–96.

Herrmann JE, Nowak NA et al., 1985, Detection of Norwalk virus in stools by enzyme immunoassay, *J Med Virol*, **17**: 127–33.

Hethcote HW, Van Ark JW, Longini I Jr, 1991, A simulation model for AIDS in San Francisco. I. Model formulation and parameter estimation, *Math Biosci*, **106**: 203–22.

Hill AB, 1965, The environment and disease: association or causation?, *Proc R Soc Med*, **58**: 295.

Hjelle B, Jenison S et al., 1994, A novel hantavirus associated with an outbreak of fatal respiratory disease in the southwestern United States: evolutionary relationships to known hantaviruses, *J Virol*, **68**: 592–6.

Houff SA, Burton RC et al., 1979, Human-to-human transmission of rabies virus by corneal transplant, *N Engl J Med*, **30**: 603–4.

Hull HF, Ward NA et al., 1994, Paralytic poliomyelitis: seasoned strategies, disappearing disease, *Lancet*, **343**: 1331–7.

Hurwitz ES, Barrett MJ et al., 1985, Public health service study on Reye's syndrome and medications, *N Engl J Med*, **313**: 849–57.

Ingalls TH, Babbott FL Jr et al., 1960, Rubella: its epidemiology and teratology, *Am J Med Sci*, **239**: 363–83.

Irwin GR, Allen AM et al., 1975, Hepatitis B antigen in saliva, urine, and stool, *Infect Immun*, **11**: 142–5.

Jackson ADM, Fisch L, 1958, Deafness following maternal rubella: results of a prospective investigation, *Lancet*, **2**: 1241–4.

Jacquez J, Koopman JS et al., 1994, Role of the primary infection in epidemic HIV of gay cohorts, *J Acquired Immune Defic Syndr*, **7**: 1169–84.

Johansson ME, Uhnoo I et al., 1985, Enzyme-linked immunosorbent assay for detection of enteric adenovirus 41, *J Med Virol*, **17**: 19–27.

Johnson KM, Kuns ML et al., 1966, Isolation of Machupo virus from wild rodent *Calomys callosus*, *Am J Trop Med Hyg*, **15**: 103–6.

Johnson N, Mant D et al., 1991, Use of computerised general practice data for population surveillance: comparative study of influenza data, *Br Med J*, **302**: 763–5.

Kaplan JE, Gary GW et al., 1982, Epidemiology of Norwalk gastroenteritis and the role of Norwalk virus in outbreaks of acute nonbacterial gastroenteritis, *Ann Intern Med*, **96**: 756–61.

Kawaoka Y, Bean WJ et al., 1993, The roles of birds and pigs in the generation of pandemic strains of human influenza, *Options for the Control of Influenza II*, eds Hannoun C, Kendal AP et al., Elsevier Science, Amsterdam, 187–91.

Kendal AP, Joseph JM et al., 1977, Laboratory-based surveillance of influenza virus in the United States of 1977–1978. I. Periods of prevalence of H1N1 and H3N2 influenza A strains; their relative rates of isolation, *Am J Epidemiol*, **110**: 449–61.

Kleinbaum DG, Kupper LL, Morgenstein LL, 1982, *Epidemiologic Research: principles and quantitative methods*, Lifetime Learning Publications, Belmont CA.

Klemetti A, Saxen L, 1967, Prospective versus retrospective approach in the search for environmental causes for malformations, *Am J Public Health*, **57**: 2071–5.

Koopman JS, Eckert EA et al., 1982, Norwalk virus enteric illness acquired by swimming exposure, *Am J Epidemiol*, **115**: 173–7.

Lemon SM, 1985, Type A viral hepatitis: new developments in an old disease, *N Engl J Med*, **313**: 1059–67.

Longini IM, Ackerman E, Elveback LR, 1977, An optimization model for influenza A epidemics, *Math Biosci*, **38**: 141–57.

Longini IM Jr, Koopman JS et al., 1982, Estimating household and community transmission parameters for influenza, *Am J Epidemiol*, **115**: 736–51.

Lord RD, Calisher CH, 1970, Further evidence of southward transport of arboviruses by migratory birds, *Am J Epidemiol*, **92**: 73–8.

Lundstrom R, 1962, Rubella during pregnancy. A follow-up study of children born after an epidemic of rubella in Sweden, 1951, with additional investigations on prophylaxis and treatment of maternal rubella, *Acta Paediat*, **133**: 1–110.

Mcintosh K, Ellis EF et al., 1973, The association of viral and bacterial respiratory infections with exacerbations of wheezing in young asthmatic children, *J Pediatr*, **82**: 578–90.

MacNaughton MR, 1982, Occurrence and frequency of coronavirus infections in humans as determined by enzyme-linked immunosorbent assay, *Infect Immun*, **38**: 419–23.

Manson MM, Logan WPD, Loy RM, 1960, *Rubella and Other Virus Infections during Pregnancy*, Reports on public health and medical subjects, No 101, Ministry of Health/Her Majesty's Stationery Office, London.

Masurel N, 1976, Swine influenza virus and the recycling of influenza A viruses in man, *Lancet*, **2**: 244–7.

Masurel N, Marine WM, 1973, Recycling of Asian and Hong Kong influenza A virus hemagglutinins in man, *Am J Epidemiol*, **97**: 44–9.

Matson DO, Estes MK et al., 1989, Human calicivirus-associated diarrhea in children attending day care centers, *J Infect Dis*, **159**: 71–8.

Melnick JL, Ledinko N, 1951, Social serology: antibody levels in a normal young population during an epidemic of poliomyelitis, *Am J Hyg*, **54**: 354–82.

Mercado R, 1975, Rodent control programmes in areas affected by Bolivian hemorrhagic fever, *Bull W H O*, **52**: 691–6.

Minor TE, Dick EC et al., 1974, Viruses as precipitants of asthmatic attacks in children, *JAMA*, **227**: 292–8.

Monto AS, 1973, The Tecumseh study of respiratory illness. V. Patterns of infection with the parainfluenzaviruses, *Am J Epidemiol*, **97**: 338–48.

Monto AS, Kioumehr F, 1975, The Tecumseh study of respir-

atory illness. IX. Occurrence of influenza in the community, 1966–1971, *Am J Epidemiol*, **102**: 553–63.

Monto AS, Koopman JS, 1980, The Tecumseh Study. XI. Occurrence of acute enteric illness in the community, *Am J Epidemiol*, **112**: 323–33.

Monto AS, Lim SK, 1971, The Tecumseh study of respiratory illness. III. Incidence and periodicity of respiratory syncytial virus and *Mycoplasma pneumoniae* infections, *Am J Epidemiol*, **94**: 290–301.

Monto AS, Ross H, 1977, Acute respiratory illness in the community: effect of family composition, smoking, and chronic symptoms, *Br J Prev Soc Med*, **31**: 101–8.

Monto AS, Sullivan KM, 1993, Acute respiratory illness in the community: frequency of illness and the agents involved, *Epidemiol Infect*, **110**: 145–60.

Monto AS, Bryan ER, Ohmit S, 1987, Rhinovirus infections in Tecumseh, Michigan: frequency of illness and numbers of serotypes, *J Infect Dis*, **156**: 43–9.

Monto AS, Koopman JS, Bryan ER, 1986, The Tecumseh study of illness. XIV. Occurrence of respiratory viruses, 1976–1981, *Am J Epidemiol*, **124**: 359–67.

Monto AS, Koopman JS, Longini IM Jr, 1985, The Tecumseh study of illness. XIII. Influenza infection and disease, 1976–1981, *Am J Epidemiol*, **121**: 811–22.

Monto AS, Davenport FM et al., 1970, Modification of an outbreak of influenza in Tecumseh, Michigan, by vaccination of schoolchildren, *J Infect Dis*, **122**: 16–25.

Moser MR, Bender TR et al., 1979, An outbreak of influenza aboard a commercial airliner, *Am J Epidemiol*, **110**: 1–7.

Mosley JW, Edwards VM et al., 1975, Hepatitis B virus infection in dentists, *N Engl J Med*, **293**: 729–34.

Nathanson N, Martin JR, 1979, The epidemiology of poliomyelitis: enigmas surrounding its appearance, epidemicity, and disappearance, *Am J Epidemiol*, **110**: 672–92.

Nichol KL, Margolis KL et al., 1994, The efficacy and cost effectiveness of vaccination against influenza among elderly persons living in the community, *N Engl J Med*, **331**: 778–84.

Nolan TF Jr, Goodman RA et al., 1980, Morbidity and mortality associated with influenza B in the United States 1978–1980. A report from the Centers for Disease Control, *J Infect Dis*, **142**: 360–2.

Ohmit SE, Monto AS, 1995, Influenza vaccine effectiveness in preventing hospitalization among the elderly during influenza type A and B seasons, *Int J Epidemiol*, **24**: 1240–8.

Padian NS, Shiboski SC, Jewell NP, 1991, Female-to-male transmission of human immunodeficiency virus, *JAMA*, **266**: 1664–7.

Papaevangelou G, Kourea-Kremastinou T, 1974, Role of mosquitoes in transmission of hepatitis B virus infection, *J Infect Dis*, **130**: 78–80.

Parrott RH, Kim HW et al., 1973, Epidemiology of respiratory syncytial virus infection in Washington, DC, *Am J Epidemiol*, **98**: 289–300.

Peters CJ, Kuehne RW et al., 1974, Hemorrhagic fever in Cochabamba, Bolivia, 1971, *Am J Epidemiol*, **99**: 425–33.

Peters CJ, Sanchez A et al., 1994, Filoviruses as emerging pathogens, *Semin Virol*, **5**: 147–54.

Phair J, Kauffman CA et al., 1978, Failure to respond to influenza vaccine in the aged: correlation with B-cell number and function, *J Lab Clin Med*, **92**: 822–8.

Pitt DB, 1957, Congenital malformations and maternal rubella, *Med J Aust*, **1**: 233–9.

Portnoy BL, Mackowiak PA et al., 1975, Oyster-associated hepatitis: failure of shellfish certification program to prevent outbreaks, *JAMA*, **233**: 1065–8.

Rawls WE, Iwamoto K et al., 1970, Herpesvirus type 2 antibodies and carcinoma of the cervix, *Lancet*, **2**: 1142–3.

Reeves WC, 1974, Overwintering of arboviruses, *Prog Med Virol*, **17**: 193–220.

Reeves WC, Caussy D et al., 1987, Case–control study of human papillomaviruses and cervical cancer in Latin America, *Int J Cancer*, **40**: 450–4.

Remington PL, Rowley D et al., 1986, Decreasing trends in Reye's syndrome and aspirin use in Michigan 1979–1984, *Pediatrics*, **77**: 93–8.

Rivers T, 1937, Viruses and Koch's postulates, *J Bacteriol*, **33**: 1–12.

Sawyer WA, Meyer KF et al., 1944, Jaundice in army personnel in the western region of the United States and its relation to vaccination against yellow fever, *Am J Hyg*, **39**; **40**: 337–430; 35–107.

Schlesselman JJ, 1982, *Case–Control Studies: design, conduct, analysis*, Oxford University Press, New York.

Serfling RE, 1963, Methods for current statistical analysis of excess pneumonia–influenza deaths, *Pub Health Rep*, **78**: 494–506.

Sever JL, Hardy JB et al., 1969, Rubella in the collaborative perinatal research study. II. Clinical and laboratory findings in children through 3 years of age, *Am J Dis Child*, **118**: 123–32.

Sever JL, Nelson KB, Gilkeson MR, 1965, Rubella epidemic, 1964: effect on 6,000 pregnancies. I. Preliminary clinical and laboratory findings through the neonatal period: a report from the collaborative study on cerebral palsy, *Am J Dis Child*, **110**: 395–407.

Sever JL, Schiff GM, Huebner RJ, 1964, Frequency of rubella antibody among pregnant women and other human and animal populations, *Obstet Gynecol*, **23**: 153–9.

Shope RE, 1936, The incidence of neutralizing antibodies for swine influenza virus on the sera of human beings of different ages, *J Exp Med*, **63**: 669–84.

Smith JS, Orciari LA et al., 1992, Epidemiologic and historical relationships among 87 rabies virus isolates as determined by limited sequence analysis, *J Infect Dis*, **166**: 296–307.

Spilker B, 1991, *Guide to Clinical Trials*, Raven Press, New York.

Starko KM, Ray CG et al., 1982, Reye's syndrome and salicylate use, *Pediatrics*, **66**: 859–64.

Stevens CE, Beasley RP et al., 1975, Vertical transmission of hepatitis B antigen in Taiwan, *N Engl J Med*, **292**: 771–4.

Susser M, 1973, *Causal Thinking in the Health Sciences*, Oxford University Press, New York.

Swan G, Tostevin AL, Black GHB, 1946, Final observations on congenital defects in infants following infectious diseases during pregnancy with special reference to rubella, *Med J Aust*, **2**: 889–908.

Szmuness W, Much MI et al., 1975, On the role of sexual behavior in the spread of hepatitis B infection, *Ann Intern Med*, **83**: 489–95.

Szmuness W, Stevens CE et al., 1980, Hepatitis B vaccine: demonstration of efficacy in a controlled clinical trial in a high-risk population in the United States, *N Engl J Med*, **303**: 833–41.

Theiler M, 1957, Action of sodium deoxycholate on arthropodborne viruses, *Proc Soc Exp Biol Med*, **96**: 380–2.

Tyrrell DA, Bynoe ML et al., 1960, Some virus isolations from common colds. I. Experiments employing human volunteers, *Lancet*, **1**: 235–7.

Vesikari T, Ruuska T et al., 1992, Protective efficacy against serotype 1 rotavirus diarrhea by live oral rhesus–human reassortant rotavirus vaccines with human rotavirus VP7 serotype 1 or 2 specificity, *Pediatr Infect Dis J*, **11**: 535–42.

Wagner G, Lavanchy D et al., 1993, Simultaneous active and passive immunization against hepatitis A studied in a population of travellers, *Vaccine*, **11**: 1027–32.

Waldman RJ, Hall WN et al., 1982, Aspirin as a risk factor in Reye's syndrome, *JAMA*, **247**: 3089–94.

Warner RD, Carr RW et al., 1991, A large nontypical outbreak of Norwalk virus: gastroenteritis associated with exposing celery to nonpotable water and with *Citrobacter freundii*, *Arch Intern Med*, **151**: 2419–24.

Wehrle PF, Posch J et al., 1970, An airborne outbreak of smallpox in a German hospital and its significance with respect to other recent outbreaks in Europe, *Bull. W H O*, **43**: 669–79.

Westaway EG, Brinton MA et al., 1985a, *Flaviviridae*, *Intervirology*, **24**: 183–92.

Westaway EG, Brinton MA et al., 1985b, *Togaviridae*, *Intervirology*, **24**: 125–39.

Wong DC, Purcell RH et al., 1980, Epidemic and enteric hepatitis in India: evidence for a non-A, non-B hepatitis virus aetiology, *Lancet*, **2**: 876–8.

World Health Organization/Global Programme on AIDS, 1994, *The Current Global Situation of the HIV/AIDS Pandemic*, WHO, Geneva.

PARVOVIRUSES

G Siegl and P Cassinotti

| 1   Characteristics of the viruses | 2   Clinical and pathological aspects |

1 CHARACTERISTICS OF THE VIRUSES

1.1 Introduction

Parvoviruses comprise a group of small spherical viruses with a genome of linear single-stranded DNA. They infect a variety of hosts, including invertebrates, birds and mammals. Many of the viruses were isolated by chance in the early 1960s from tumour-bearing animals, experimentally transplanted tumours or cell cultures derived from them. Experimental injection of such isolates into laboratory rodents produced a broad spectrum of syndromes ranging from fetal and neonatal death to congenital malformations, hepatitis, enteritis, myocarditis and cerebellar dysfunction. Because such syndromes are also well known to occur under natural conditions in animals and humans, much time was spent in the following years to link them to infection with specific parvoviruses. In most instances, however, discovery of the causative agents of distinct syndromes occurred by chance rather than as the result of planned attempts. This situation is well illustrated by the discovery of the human parvovirus B19. The agent was first recognized as a new antigen in a serum sample labelled B19 when, in 1975, blood from healthy donors was screened for hepatitis B surface antigen (HBsAg) by counter-current electrophoresis (Cossart et al. 1975). Five years later, the virus was observed again in sera of patients suffering from febrile illness (Shneerson, Mortimer and Vandervelde 1980). A first, regular, association of the agent with a distinct human disease was established in 1981, when B19 virus was detected in the blood of patients with sickle-cell anaemia presenting with aplastic crisis (Pattison et al. 1981, Serjeant et al. 1981). It took another 2 years to prove the causative role of the virus in erythema infectiosum ('fifth disease'), a well known infection of childhood.

So far, B19 virus is known to be responsible for a continually enlarging spectrum of clinical manifestations in humans, and a growing number of parvoviruses are found to be associated with various economically important diseases of animals. It is most interesting that all clinical manifestations resulting from infection with these viruses, irrespective of whether they concern congenital malformations, dwarfism, myocarditis, encephalopathy, panleucopenia or aplastic anaemia, seem to result from a single, seemingly simple pathogenic principle, i.e. the dependence of the replication of these viruses on host cell functions displayed in actively proliferating cells in a specific state of differentiation. Characterization of factors involved in that dependence at the levels of the virus, the infected cell, and the infected organism has become the main theme of today's parvovirus research.

1.2 Classification

All viruses grouped in the family *Parvoviridae* are non-enveloped, isometric particles, 18–26 nm in diameter (Fig. 14.1). Their genome is a linear molecule of single-stranded DNA (ssDNA), 4–6 kb in size. Some members of the family preferentially encapsidate ssDNA of negative polarity, whereas others encapsidate ssDNA of either polarity in equivalent or varying proportions. These basic properties, distinct differences in genome organization, and specific aspects of viral replication and host range have recently been used to reclassify parvoviruses in one family, 2 subfamilies and 6 genera (Table 14.1). All parvoviruses within the subfamily Parvovirinae infect vertebrates. Members of the genus *Parvovirus* are capable of autonomous replication, which is independent of helper virus. This characteristic applies also to the genus *Erythrovirus*, of which B19 virus is so far the only accepted member. In contrast, efficient replication of dependoviruses depends on co-infection with helper adenoviruses or herpesviruses. There are only a few, very specific conditions (e.g. presence of mutagens) that allow replication of dependoviruses to proceed in the absence of helper viruses. Finally, the subfamily Densovirinae comprises autonomous viruses infecting only invertebrate species. These viruses are further subgrouped into 3 genera according to differences in the organization and coding strategy of their genomes.

1.3 Morphology and structure

The capsids of parvoviruses are composed of 60 copies of capsid protein arranged according to the symmetrical requirements of an icosahedral structure. In those viruses that have been studied in greater detail (i.e. canine parvovirus, feline panleucopenia virus, B19 virus), c. 95% of protein mass is made up of VP2 (for molecular details, see below, p. 263). The few molecules of VP1 also present in the capsid seem to be necessary for the virus to assume its mature conformation and for its ability to induce neutralizing antibodies. X-ray crystallographic analysis revealed a protrusion ('spike') on the 3-fold axes, a canyon encircling the 5-fold axes and a depression at the 2-fold axes. Two dominant neutralizing antigenic determinants were found on the 3-fold spike of the CPV capsid (Strassheim et al. 1994). It is assumed that, by analogy with the rhinoviruses, the canyon is the site of receptor attachment (Tsao et al. 1991).

Capsid proteins account for 63–81% of virion mass which, including viral DNA as a second component, amounts to a mol. wt of 5500–6200 kDa.

Mature infectious parvovirus virions have sedimentation coefficients (S) of 110–122 and band at a density (ρ) of 1.42 g/cm³ during equilibrium centrifugation in caesium chloride gradients. Viral harvests from both infected cell cultures and tissues contain additional structures such as empty capsids (70S, ρ = 1.32 g/cm³), particles containing defective genomes (ρ = 1.33–1.39 g/cm³) and immature infectious particles (ρ = 1.44–1.47 g/cm³).

Parvoviruses are extraordinarily stable. They resist treatment with lipid solvents, heating to 60°C for 60 minutes, pH ranges of 3–9 and high salt concentrations. This outstanding resistance makes it difficult

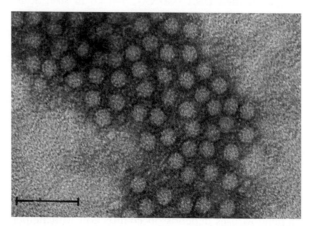

Fig. 14.1 Immunoelectron micrograph of human parvovirus B19, from plasma of an asymptomatic blood donor. Bar = 100 nm.

to eliminate their infectivity from biological materials such as blood and blood products. Laurian and colleagues (Laurian et al. 1994) have shown that current methods for pasteurization of such products are not sufficient to guarantee freedom from parvovirus infectivity.

1.4 Genome structure and function

The parvovirus genome consists of a single copy of a linear, non-permuted DNA molecule 4–6 kb in size and with a mol. wt of 1500–2000 kDa. For parvoviruses infecting vertebrates, sequences coding for the structural (or capsid) proteins and those coding for non-structural proteins (i.e. proteins concerned with transcription, synthesis of viral DNA and modulation of viral replication) are both exclusively confined to the negative strand of the viral DNA. They comprise the central 90% of the molecule. The remaining terminal regions consist of palindromic sequences that fold into hairpin structures. In the genome of members of the genus *Parvovirus* the respective sequences differ at the 3′ and the 5′ end. In contrast, genomes of B19 virus (genus *Erythrovirus*) and of the dependoviruses have identical palindromes at each end.

In invertebrate parvoviruses, coding sequences are found both on the negative and on the complementary positive strand of viral DNA. However, whereas members of the genera *Iteravirus* and *Contravirus* encode both structural and most of the non-structural proteins on the negative strand and carry only a minor open reading frame (so far of unknown significance) on the positive strand, the coat proteins and the proteins functional in viral replication of densoviruses are encoded separately on complementary DNA strands.

Figure 14.2 illustrates the overall organization and the principal transcriptional strategy of the genomes of 3 representative members of parvovirus genera infecting animals and humans. It shows that, although the organization of the genomes is very similar, with the non-structural (NS or Rep) proteins confined to the left (3′) half, and the structural (Cap) proteins to the right (5′) half, the viruses have different means of generating varying numbers of proteins. Thus, in the case of parvovirus MMV, transcription from 2 promoters and splicing in 2 different regions of the genome gives rise to 3 messenger RNA (mRNA) molecules. AAV (genus *Dependovirus*) relies on 3 promoters together with splicing in a distinct genome region to generate 6 different mRNAs. Finally, multiple, extensive splicing of transcripts originating from a single promoter allows the human parvovirus B19 (genus *Erythrovirus*) to produce a total of 9 distinct messenger RNAs. All mRNA species are capped and polyadenylated.

The palindromic sequences at the termini of the single-stranded parvovirus genome are required for DNA replication. They are capable of forming hairpin structures and, from the 3′-hydroxyl group, are able to induce self-primed synthesis of the complementary DNA strand. The various steps in the complex replication process of parvovirus DNA as well as the different intermediate molecules generated thereby are described in detail by Berns (1990).

Table 14.1 Taxonomic structure of the Family *Parvoviridae*

Genus	Species	Abbreviation
Subfamily Parvovirinae		
Parvovirus	Aleutian mink disease virus	AMDV
	Bovine parvovirus	BPV
	Canine parvovirus	CPV
	Chicken parvovirus	ChPV
	Feline panleucopenia virus	
	Feline parvovirus	FPV
	Goose parvovirus	GPV
	HB virus	HBPV
	H-1 virus	H-1PV
	Kilham rat virus	KRV
	Lapine parvovirus	LPV
	LuIII virus	LuIIIV
	Mink enteritis virus	MEV
	Mice minute virus	MMV
	Canine minute virus	CMV
	Porcine parvovirus	PPV
	Raccoon parvovirus	RPV
	RT parvovirus	RTPV
	Tumour virus X	TVX
Erythrovirus	B19 virus	B19V
Dependovirus	Adeno-associated virus 1	AAV-1
	Adeno-associated virus 2	AAV-2
	Adeno-associated virus 3	AAV-3
	Adeno-associated virus 4	AAV-4
	Adeno-associated virus 5	AAV-5
	Avian adeno-associated virus	AAAV
	Bovine adeno-associated virus	BAAV
	Canine adeno-associated virus	CAAV
	Equine adeno-associated virus	EAAV
	Ovine adeno-associated virus	OAAV
Subfamily Densovirinae		
Densovirus	*Galleria mellonella* densovirus	GmDNV
	Junonia coenia densovirus	JcDNV
Iteravirus	*Bombyx mori* densovirus	BmDNV
Contravirus	*Aedes aegypti* densovirus	AaDNV
	Aedes albopictus densovirus	AlDNV

1.5 Polypeptides

Two to 3 **structural proteins** are found in the capsids of the various parvoviruses infecting vertebrates and 4 in the capsids of the parvoviruses of invertebrates. Depending on the virus, VP1, the largest structural polypeptide, has a molecular weight of 80–96 kDa. The molecular weight of VP2 is in the range 64–85 kDa; of VP3, 60–75 kDa; and of VP4, 49–52 kDa. In all particles of the vertebrate parvoviruses, the principal protein is either VP2 or VP3. The major polypeptide in virions of members of the genus *Densovirus* is VP4. As determined by tryptic digestion, and in good agreement with the transcriptional strategy of parvovirus genomes, the structural proteins of a parvovirus contain overlapping amino acid sequences derived from the same coding sequence. The 2 larger proteins are usually translated from alternatively spliced transcripts. For the autonomous rodent parvoviruses (see Fig. 14.2) the smallest capsid protein VP3 is then produced by proteolytic cleavage of VP2. In the case of the dependoviruses, VP2 and VP3 are translated from the same transcript; but translation starts from different, distinct ACG and AUG codons within the mRNA molecule.

Parvovirus **non-structural (NS) proteins** are usually translated from unspliced or, alternatively, spliced transcripts originating from a common promoter or from 2 distinct promoters located close to the 3′ end of the parvovirus genome (see Fig. 14.2). The number of NS proteins detected thus far in cells infected with the various vertebrate parvoviruses varies from 1 to 4. For MMV, the best studied member of the autonomously replicating parvoviruses, there is good evidence that at least 4 closely related NS proteins are encoded. However, only NS1 (at 83 kDa the largest NS protein) seems to be essential for productive infection of all susceptible cells (Cater and Pintel 1992, Legendre and Rommelaere 1992). The human parvovirus B19, so far the only member of the

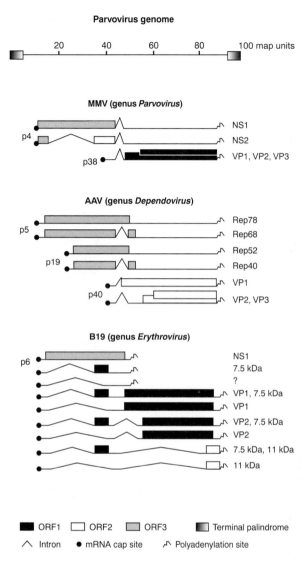

Fig. 14.2 Genome organization of 3 representative parvoviruses. 100 map units correspond to c. 5 kb. The size of the elements shown is approximate.

genus *Erythrovirus*, possesses one major non-structural protein of similar size. In addition, the existence of 2 proteins, 11 and 7.5 kDa in size and derived from small genomic transcripts, has been demonstrated (Luo and Astell 1993). Dependoviruses specify 4 non-structural proteins termed Rep78, Rep68, Rep52 and Rep40 (Mendelson, Trempe and Carter 1986).

Both NS and Rep proteins are multifunctional and play an essential role in parvovirus replication. NS1, Rep78 and Rep68 are sequence-specific DNA-binding proteins that have ATPase, helicase and site-specific endonuclease activities. The respective functions are required at various intermediate steps in the replication of parvoviral DNA and especially during the generation of the single-stranded progeny genome. Moreover, Rep78 and Rep68 seem to be involved in targeted integration of dependovirus DNA into a small defined region of human chromosome 19 in cultured cells, and thus in an essential step in the induction of dependovirus latency (Berns and Linden 1995).

An additional important property of NS1 and Rep78/68 proteins is their regulatory role in viral replication by trans-activating or down-regulating endogenous promoters under

both permissive and non-permissive conditions of viral replication. This ability can evidently also be extended to modulation of various heterologous viral as well as cellular promoters (Sol et al. 1993, Hermonat 1994). It may serve the infecting virus by facilitating takeover of the host cell's synthetic machinery. The cytotoxic effect of NS proteins as well as their inhibition of cell proliferation, observed in several experimental studies, may also be closely related to the modulating function of this group of parvoviral proteins.

The functions of the small non-structural proteins are not well documented. In one instance Reps 52/40 have been implicated in the packaging of progeny viral genomes.

1.6 Antigens

As we have seen, parvoviruses are rather simple particles made up of, at most, 4 structural proteins. Moreover, these proteins share overlapping peptide sequences, so one would expect little variation in their antigenic reactivity. The great majority of parvoviruses of vertebrates possess the ability to agglutinate red blood cells of various species. Whenever demonstrable, this ability is associated with all particle forms (i.e. empty capsids, defective particles, mature virions and 'heavy', immature, infectious virions). The receptor to which these particulate structures bind at the surface of the agglutinated red blood cell is probably a glycoprotein structure (Mochizuki, Konishi and Ogata 1978). None of the densoviruses has so far been shown to haemagglutinate.

If used under sufficiently standardized conditions, inhibition of haemagglutination (HI) with specific antisera is the most convenient means for the serological identification of parvoviruses. Neutralization of infectivity is only slightly more sensitive. The results obtained by HI and neutralization are thus generally comparable. Fifteen antigenically distinct groups of isolates or, in other words, distinct serotypes have so far been identified among members of the genus *Parvovirus*, and 10 serotypes make up the genus *Dependovirus*. If polyclonal antisera raised against purified virus particles are used in the tests, no common group antigen can be detected; and the antigenicity of an individual serotype seems to be extraordinarily stable. The host range variants of the feline panleucopenia virus serotype (i.e. FPV, MEV, CPV and RPV) are also not easily distinguished by standard HI or neutralization tests. However, individual viruses of this serotype can be readily identified by use of specific monoclonal antibodies, which also reveal minor variations in antigenicity among several other parvoviruses. Such changes involve both neutralizing and non-neutralizing surface epitopes. Under the selective pressure exerted by monoclonal antibodies present in the medium of infected cell cultures, viruses with new epitopes appeared at frequencies between 10^{-4} and 10^{-7}. The continuous evolution at the surface of the parvovirus particle is also illustrated by repeated reports of the appearance of non-haemagglutinating variants of well known haemagglutinating parvoviruses (Siegl 1990).

Immunofluorescent (IF) staining is a standard technique for detecting parvovirus antigens in tissues of infected animals and in infected cell cultures. Cross-staining of cells infected with different parvoviruses with antisera raised against highly purified virus preparations usually yields results broadly comparable with those of HI and neutralization tests. However, tests with sera of animals recovering from active parvovirus infection pointed to the existence of one or more group antigens in members of the individual genera of vertebrate parvoviruses. These group antigens are evidently closely related to the NS or Rep proteins. Serological cross-reactivity among these proteins has its basis in a common, widely conserved central part of the NS1/Rep78 molecule. Cross-reactivity of NS1 proteins has also been demonstrated between B19 virus (genus *Erythrovirus*) and various members of the genus *Parvovirus*.

1.7 Replication

PRODUCTIVE INFECTION

Productive infection of all parvoviruses in fully susceptible cells seems to follow a more or less identical scheme. In a first step, virus adsorbs to a specific host cell receptor. For most parvoviruses the exact nature of this receptor is unknown, but *N*-acetylneuraminic acid residues seem to play an essential role in binding of rodent parvoviruses. The cellular receptor for B19 virus was found to be identical with globoside or erythrocyte P antigen (Brown, Anderson and Young 1993). Experiments with purified virus showed that susceptible cells may be able to bind up to 10^5 particles. The process of virus internalization most probably occurs via coated pits. In electron micrographs of infected cells the internalized virus is seen in vesicular structures within the cytoplasm. Uncoating or release of the viral genome takes place either in the nucleus or in cytoplasm in close vicinity to it; research on this aspect of parvovirus replication has so far failed to yield conclusive results. However, no free ssDNA can be found in the cytoplasm early in infection; and capsid proteins of the infecting virus seem to be essential for inducing an early, intranuclear step in the replication of autonomous parvoviruses. Uncoating is thus most probably confined to the nucleus.

Subsequent steps in parvovirus replication such as formation of double-stranded replicative form (dsRF) DNA, generation of progeny single-stranded genomes, transcription of mRNA and translation of these molecules into viral non-structural as well as structural proteins are only partly controlled by the viral genome. These events depend to a large extent on helper functions. In the case of the so-called autonomous parvoviruses, such helper functions are provided by the host cell which, to make at least some of them available, has to pass actively through the phase of DNA synthesis (S-phase) in its life cycle. Consequently, autonomous parvoviruses replicate in vitro most efficiently in cell cultures exhibiting a high degree of mitotic activity, and in vivo, in rapidly proliferating tissues or in organs that are still differentiating. The nature of the host cell-specified helper function(s) as well as their temporal location early or late in the S-phase are still matters of dispute. Moreover, the specific event in virus replication on which the cellular functions are centred is not yet clear. Tattersall and Gardiner (1990) suggested it to be the synthesis of a complementary DNA strand on the infecting ssDNA genome. This creates a duplex DNA template for viral transcription and a parental dsRF DNA molecule as the basis for subsequent amplification of the viral genome. However, synthesis of the primary dsDNA structure in the replication of parvoviral DNA is not sufficient to ensure full viral gene expression. There is good evidence both from circumstantial observations and from many experiments with cell type-specific, so-called allotropic viral variants that, at this stage, productive parvovirus infection is also controlled by interaction of a strain-specific viral locus ('allotropic determinant') with a differentiation-dependent ('developmentally regulated') host cell factor. For MMV the viral locus has been mapped to a sequence of about 200 nucleotides around map position 70 in the part of the viral genome specifying capsid proteins VP1 and VP2. A few singular mutations in that region proved sufficient to alter host cell specificity and apparently also to affect the host range of parvoviruses (Parrish, Aquadro and Carmichael 1988). If the viral and host cell determinants are incompatible, initiation of viral transcription decreases dramatically and parvovirus replication is severely restricted.

For replication of the dependovirus AAV, the necessary helper functions are most efficiently supplied by a co-infecting adenovirus or herpesvirus. The helper functions involve exclusively early gene products of these viruses. In a co-infection with adenovirus, the E1a gene product evidently transactivates AAV transcription. E1b and E4 products seem to allow accumulation of AAV mRNA and E2a is assumed to be involved in transport of mRNA to the cytoplasm. Finally, adenovirus virus-associated RNAs are thought to work at the level of translation. Under exceptional environmental conditions (e.g. presence of mutagens, synchronization of cell growth by treatment with hydroxyurea), certain specific susceptible cells have also been reported to support AAV replication even in the absence of a known helper virus.

Although a few reports suggest that the non-structural proteins have to be synthesized before the structural proteins can be expressed in the course of parvovirus replication, these viruses seem to have no true 'early' and 'late' gene products. A considerable number of the large NS and Rep proteins (see section 1.5, p. 263) are, however, essential for replication of dsRF DNA and for generation of progeny single-stranded viral genomes. The latter processes are complex and are best described by the so-called rolling hairpin model of parvovirus DNA replication, developed first by Tattersall and Ward (1976). Since then the model has been continually modified to accommodate new information on intermediate nucleic acid structures as well as on differences between the replication of the genomes of autonomous parvoviruses and of the dependoviruses. A concise description would exceed the scope of this chapter and the interested reader is therefore referred to the excellent article on this subject by Tattersall and Cotmore (1990).

There is also good evidence that the final step in parvovirus DNA replication (i.e. accumulation of progeny viral ssDNA) requires the presence of capsid proteins, most probably in the form of empty capsids, to sequester the newly synthesized genomes. Overall, parvovirus replication seems to be very efficient in a fully competent parvovirus/cell system. Carter (1990) calculated that a single AAV-infected cell can produce more than 10^7 virus capsids. One-tenth, or about 10^6 capsids, package the viral genome and become mature, infectious virions. Because the particle : infectivity ratio for mature AAV particles is in the range of 50–100 : 1, the final yield in progeny infectious virus from a single infected cell amounts to c. 10^4 cell culture infectious units.

The massive production of viral components in an infected cell evidently results in formation of the intranuclear inclusion bodies found so frequently in parvovirus-infected cells and tissues. Moreover, under permissive conditions, replication of all parvoviruses generally leads to lysis of the infected cell and release of progeny virus capable of starting a new cycle of infection.

PERSISTENT AND LATENT INFECTION

Autonomous parvoviruses have frequently been isolated from both primary and continuous cell cultures after multiple passages in vitro. The viruses evidently can persist in such cells over a prolonged period without inducing a lytic replication cycle despite repeated provision of S-phase-dependent helper functions. However, such infected cultures can suddenly show signs of massive virus replication associated with destruction of all but a few of the cells. An explanation can be derived from the behaviour of experimentally established carrier cultures and from our understanding of the interaction of viral and cellular determinants in the modulation of parvoviral replication. Apparently, only a small fraction of cells in a carrier culture express determinants allowing for permissive replication of the predominant viral genotype. Mutational changes within the structural gene of the virus may then give rise to the appearance of a variant virus fully adapted to replication in the majority of available cells. Variant cells lacking expression of an appropriate cellular determinant will be resistant to the attack of the new virus and hence will survive and form the starting point of a new culture.

It can be imagined that such a continuous interplay between virus and cells is also the basis for the well known persistence of parvoviruses in their animal hosts, even in the presence of a high degree of humoral immunity. An additional factor possibly operative in this context may be the ability of parvoviruses to infect and subsequently persist in mitotically quiescent cells over a prolonged period without losing their ability to start replication as soon as the infected cell enters S-phase. The ability of autonomous parvoviruses to integrate into the genome of the host cell is also a matter for speculation. So far, however, attempts to demonstrate such an integration in the course of productive infection or in persistently infected cultures have failed.

By contrast, integration of the genome of the dependoviruses into host cell DNA is well established. In the absence of helper virus co-infection, the dependovirus genome is uncoated within the nucleus and supports at least minimal translation of the *rep* gene. In human cells the *rep* function is evidently essential for efficient integration of the viral genome at a specific site, which has been mapped to the q arm of chromosome 19 (Kotin, Linden and Berns 1992). The *rep* gene product does not seem to contain integrase activity. Homology between integrated dependovirus DNA and the flanking cellular sequences is limited to a 1–5 base overlap at the junctions. Integrated sequences are mostly present as a linear tandem of several copies of the viral genome. Co-infection with a helper adenovirus efficiently rescues the dependovirus genome from its integrated state and, provided a full set of viral genes is available, initiates productive and lytic replication.

2   CLINICAL AND PATHOLOGICAL ASPECTS

Over a period of almost 30 years of parvovirus research, no evidence could be found linking dependovirus infections with any specific pathological effect in either animals or humans. Together with the ability of dependoviruses to infect a wide variety of cell types, and of the dependovirus genome to integrate readily into host cell DNA, this apparent, well documented lack of pathogenicity seemed to make these viruses an ideal vector system for introducing foreign genetic information into a variety of cells and tissues (Flotte et al. 1993, Srivastava 1994). A few recent observations now point to a possible involvement of dependoviruses in fetal death and abortion early in pregnancy, both in experimentally infected mice and under natural conditions in humans. Consequently, the suitability of the dependovirus vector system for gene transfer and molecular therapeutics has to be re-evaluated (Berns and Linden 1995).

By contrast with the dependoviruses, autonomous parvoviruses have been recognized as potent pathogens both under experimental conditions and in the course of natural infection since their discovery at the end of the 1950s. A wealth of information has accumulated concerning the factors governing interaction between parvoviruses and their animal hosts, as well as the wide range of clinical syndromes resulting therefrom. These data provide a sound basis for evaluating and interpreting the broad spectrum of clinical disease observed in recent years in the human host, as the result of infection by parvovirus B19.

2.1 Parvovirus diseases in animals

Epidemiology

Serological screening revealed that the great majority of animal parvoviruses are highly endemic in populations of their natural host. This situation is clearly favoured by the tendency of the agents to establish latent, clinically inapparent infections; by the shedding of viruses by infected animals in faeces, urine, saliva and nasal secretions; and, last but not least, by the outstanding stability of the virus particle in the environment. The last characteristic guarantees survival of parvoviruses even under unfavourable conditions for up to 6 months and makes it almost impossible to prevent susceptible animals from contracting infection in a contaminated environment.

Because of the high prevalence of antibodies in populations of their natural host(s), most breeding females transmit immunity to their offspring. Under this protective shield, infection of the young animal with the ubiquitous virus leads to an active, long-lasting immune response rather than to overt disease. In consequence, clinically manifest infection is a rare event under such endemic conditions. It is usually observed only in an exceptionally predisposed susceptible organism, i.e. mostly under conditions negatively affecting the immune system. Overt and often fatal disease in epizootic and sometimes even panzootic form can nevertheless develop when the virus is introduced into an immunologically naive host population. Such fulminant epizootics in their natural hosts have been reported for goose parvovirus and feline panleucopenia virus. Panzootic spread of parvoviruses also occurred when variants of the feline parvovirus acquired the ability to cross species barriers and, as MEV and CPV, spread rapidly in previously unaffected populations of mink and dogs, respectively (Siegl 1990).

Pathogenesis

The spectrum of parvovirus disease ranges from acute, lethal affections to slowly progressing, sometimes chronic, illness. Whether the clinical picture of infection develops in one or the other way is determined by an interplay of factors such as the genetic composition of the virus, the genetic background of the host, the availability of appropriately differentiated cells in proliferating tissues, the ability of the organism to respond immunologically to infection and, last but not least, the epidemiological situation. Many of these factors are closely related to age or, in other words, to the state of development of the host organism. There is also increasing evidence that they are valid for every parvovirus/host system and that clinicopathological manifestations observed in one of these systems can be revealed, although sometimes only upon careful examination, in every other system. Small differences in clinical presentation from system to system are most probably due to variations in the complexity and the time course of differentiation of the host.

The 'age' of the infected host can be taken as synonymous with the availability of cells and tissues capable of supporting the replication of a parvovirus. However, age in terms of the state of development also determines the degree to which regeneration of tissues and organs can take place. In the case of parvovirus infections this means that cytolytic replication of the virus in tissues or organs capable of efficient regeneration (e.g. the liver in a young animal) leads to acute yet self-limiting disease with no permanent residue. By contrast, destruction of tissues lacking or limited in regenerative potential, such as the developing cerebellum, will leave permanent defects.

Fetal infection

The principles outlined above are clearly illustrated by the results of intrauterine parvovirus infections. Here, the extent to which a parvovirus is present in a host population determines the likelihood of immunity of the pregnant animal and, hence, the likelihood of transplacental infection. The regenerative potential of tissues and organs, and hence their susceptibility to viral infection, is determined by the developmental state of the embryo or fetus. Finally, the extent to which virus replicates and is spread within the fetus and especially within an infected newborn animal is modified by the ability of such an organism to mount an effective immune response.

The effects on the fetus are most severe if infection occurs in the first and the early part of the second trimester of gestation. At that time infections tend to be generalized and fatal. Hamster embryos infected with H-1 or LuIII virus, or bovine and porcine fetuses infected respectively with BPV or PPV, mostly die and are absorbed or aborted. After mid-gestation, especially in the third trimester and in the neonatal period, infection tends to become less overwhelming, probably because of the increasing ability of the fetuses to mount an immune response. With the changing pattern of susceptibility of cells in the differentiating fetus, infection also becomes more organ-specific and consequently gives rise to distinct syndromes. Thus, hamsters, rats, ferrets, kittens and, to some extent, even calves develop cerebellar ataxia when the dividing cells in the outer germinal layer of the cerebellum are infected. The degree of ensuing clinical disease depends on the stage of differentiation of the definitive granular cortex at the time of infection. Similarly, puppies infected with CPV between 8 days before and 5 days after birth can develop an interstitial myocarditis with loss of myofibres and multifocal myofibre necrosis. Early in life such animals often show acute respiratory distress and may die from congestive heart failure. Infection of the myocardium is not limited to CPV but has been observed with many other autonomous parvoviruses.

The most dramatic effect of parvovirus infection of rodents late in pregnancy or soon after birth results in the so-called osteolytic syndrome. Owing to cytolytic replication of parvoviruses in osteogenic tissues such as the costochondral junctions of long bones, the differentiating cranial sutures and the developing dentition, affected animals develop mongoloid features with small flat faces, microcephalic heads, protruding eyes and tongue, missing or abnormal teeth and fragile bones. In rodents, the whole of the developing skeleton may be affected, resulting in persistent dwarfism. In pigs, calves, goslings and chickens, stunted growth as a result of infection with the respective parvoviruses has also been observed, but this manifestation of infection is eventually overcome with increasing age.

POSTNATAL INFECTION

After birth, the final stages of differentiation are completed and this, together with concomitant maturation of the immune system, favours the development of various syndromes (e.g. ataxia, myocarditis) unless the pattern of disease characteristic for the adult animal develops. In spite of this evident trend, generalized disease with systemic involvement of almost all organs and tissues and a high rate of mortality is often observed following parvovirus infection of newborn rodents and of newly hatched goslings and chickens. In larger animals, however, generalized disease in the newborn seems to be rare.

The intestinal epithelium and the reticuloendothelial system retain their proliferative activity in the fully differentiated organism; it is therefore not surprising that parvoviruses often affect these organs. The extent to which the 2 systems are involved and react may vary with host and virus, so infections may manifest as enteritis, leucopenia or anaemia. In many instances, however, the involvement of other susceptible types of cells contributes to a complex clinicopathological picture.

Enteritis

Enteritis is probably the best known individual syndrome associated with parvovirus infection in animals. It can present in varying form from mere listlessness with borderline enteric signs to heavy discharge of watery, sometimes blood-stained, stools associated with severe dehydration and, not infrequently, death. Such infections have been observed in rodents, cats, dogs, mink, raccoons, calves, goslings and chickens. Signs usually appear within 4–7 days after infection in parallel with virus replication in cells of the crypt epithelium in the duodenum, the jejunum and, to a lesser extent, the ileum, colon and caecum. The severity of symptoms is directly related to necrosis of the crypt epithelium and this in turn to the mitotic activity of epithelial cells. Increased mitotic activity within the crypt epithelium is observed in the young animal in association with a dramatic alteration of the intestinal bacterial flora as a consequence of the change of diet during weaning. In the mature and old animal, proliferation of intestinal cells can also be stimulated by dietary stress but the factor most often aggravating intestinal parvovirus disease is co-infection with other viruses, bacteria or parasites.

Hepatitis

The extended period of mitotic activity of hepatocytes from an early intrauterine state to full maturation of the animal makes the liver an excellent target for replication of parvoviruses. In fact, infection of the liver occurs in many animals, but, because of the high regenerative potential of this organ, severe prolonged hepatitis or persisting defects as a result of parvovirus infection are rarely observed. The exception are goslings, in which hepatitis is a prominent symptom of infection with GPV.

Encephalopathy

Haemorrhages and necrosis in the brain and the spinal cord in association with acute fatal paralysis have been observed in rats during reactivation by immunosuppressive treatment of latent rat parvovirus infection (El Dadah et al. 1967). Encephalopathy could also be experimentally induced by infection with FPV in cats and ferrets. Furthermore, encephalomalacia and severe necrotizing vasculitis were reported in association with disseminated CPV infection in a dog (Johnson and Castro 1984).

Leucopenia and anaemia

Leucopenia is a very constant feature in animal parvovirus infections. It may be severe, and a hallmark of infection, as in cats in which it is a prominent specific syndrome (feline panleucopenia); a constant yet not specifically recognized manifestation, as in mink and dogs infected respectively with MEV and CPV; transient as in pigs; and a subclinical infection of rather brief duration in calves and rodents. Within 24–48 h of infection all animal parvoviruses involved in such infections replicate in the tonsils, thymus, regional lymph nodes, Peyer's patches and spleen. Towards the end of that period and in parallel with a pronounced viraemia, the bone marrow becomes infected and quantitative changes in the myeloid and megakaryocytic cell lines result in lymphopenia, panleucopenia and, not infrequently, in neutropenia. A clear-cut effect of animal parvoviruses on erythropoiesis has so far been reported only in infection with the newly discovered simian parvovirus in cynomolgus monkeys (O'Sullivan et al. 1994).

Aleutian mink disease

Aleutian mink disease is a persistent, slowly progressive, frequently fatal infection of mink by the Aleutian mink disease [parvo]virus (AMDV). Its course is determined with hyperglobulinaemia, plasmacytosis, glomerulonephritis, interstitial nephritis, polyarteritis, and splenomegaly is observed only in adult mink homozygous for the recessive gene of the Aleutian coat colour. Clinical disease may differ in severity both within and between genotypes. The predominant pathological changes and lesions are the result of an aberrant immune mechanism, as indicated by the presence of large quantities of immunoaggregates, rather than the direct effect of virus replication. In newborn mink, AMDV can cause a fatal acute interstitial pneumonitis with permissive virus replication in alveolar cells. The clinical signs and pathological lesions resemble those in preterm human infants with respiratory distress syndrome.

2.2 Parvovirus infections in humans

Parvoviruses of all 3 genera within the subfamily Parvovirinae infect humans. Of these agents, there is evidence that dependoviruses play a role in human disease. Moreover, B19 virus in the genus *Erythrovirus* gives rise to a broad spectrum of clinical manifestations.

DEPENDOVIRUSES

Antibodies against serotypes AAV-1, AAV-2, AAV-3 and AAV-5 are found at prevalences of up to 80% in the human population. Most infections with these viruses seem to occur in childhood or early adulthood, evidently in parallel with the high rate of adenovirus infections in these age groups. In spite of the evidence of frequent infections, no specific clinical disease was found to be directly associated with AAV infection. On the contrary, AAV infection could be shown to inhibit transformation of cells by adenoviruses in vitro and to interfere with induction of tumours by group A adenoviruses in the Syrian hamster. The latter observations stimulated serological surveys to test the possibility of so-called cancer surveillance of dependoviruses in their human host. The data indicated that, whereas c. 80% of the study population proved seropositive for AAV-2 and AAV-3, the prevalence of positive sera from patients with either cervical carcinoma or carcinoma of the prostate was markedly lower at 14% (Sprecher-Goldberger et al. 1971). Moreover, control patients had considerably higher antibody titres against AAV-5 than cervical cancer patients. These data were interpreted to mean that, if present, latent AAV infection is activated by tumour formation, which in turn leads to destruction of the developing tumour.

Botquin and colleagues (1994) showed that AAV induces early abortion in pregnant mice. Stimulated by this observation Tobiasch and co-workers (1994) looked for the presence of AAV-2 in human genital tissues as well as in curettage material from spontaneous abortions. By amplification with the polymerase chain reaction (PCR) they found low concentrations of AAV-2 DNA (compatible with latent infection) in 19 of 30 biopsy specimens of the uterine mucosa. Large amounts of viral DNA as well as viral proteins were detected in abortion material from the first trimester, but not in material from the second or third trimesters. Compared to a control population, women with spontaneous abortion or cervical intraepithelial neoplasia had a significantly higher prevalence of anti-AAV-2 IgM. The authors speculated that, on the one hand, these data point to a widespread, latent presence of AAV in the uterine mucosa. On the other hand, latent AAV-infection seems to be reactivated during pregnancy by the concomitant hormonal changes, by the physiological decline of cellular immunity, or by helper viruses such as cytomegalovirus or herpes simplex virus, which, in turn, may become reactivated during pregnancy. The ensuing replication of AAV-2 might then interfere with development of the placenta and thus lead to abortion. Further studies are needed to show to what extent this

suggested role of dependoviruses in early miscarriage can be substantiated.

HUMAN PARVOVIRUS B19
Epidemiology

Parvovirus B19 has a worldwide distribution. The virus is usually endemic and infections can be observed throughout the year. Nevertheless, more or less extended outbreaks are not uncommon. In temperate climates they tend to occur in the late winter, spring and early summer months. These outbreaks are often centred on primary schools where up to 40% of children may be clinically infected. In such situations, adult immunologically naive contacts run a high risk of becoming infected.

In addition to seasonality, longer term cycles of virus activity have been recorded. In Europe there are peaks every 4–6 years. In contrast, the cycle seems to be only 3–4 years in Jamaica, where B19 was responsible for outbreaks of aplastic crisis among patients with chronic haemolytic anaemia.

Infection with parvovirus B19 virus is a common occurrence and the overall seroprevalence of anti-B19 IgG antibody found in blood donors of most countries is c. 60% (Cohen, Mortimer and Pereira 1983). However, prevalence is typically age-dependent (Cohen and Buckley 1988). Whereas the seroprevalence of anti-B19 IgG antibody is 5–15% in children 1–5 years old and 50–60% in people 16–40 years of age, it rises to >85% in people older than 70 years (Cohen and Buckley 1988). A low prevalence of anti-B19 IgG antibody (16%) has been reported from Singapore (Matsunaga et al. 1994). It is thought to indicate a low incidence of parvovirus B19 infection during the last 2 decades.

Parvovirus B19 is primarily transmitted via the respiratory route and can be detected in throat swabs over a period of about 5 days within the week following infection. In addition, B19 is infectious when inoculated intranasally in human volunteers (Anderson et al. 1985). There are some anecdotal reports that B19 is also shed in the faeces of infected patients. True faecal–oral transmission, however, has not yet been established. It is also not clear whether individuals persistently infected over periods of months or even years (see 'Persistent infection', p. 272) shed the virus continuously or intermittently and are thus a constant source of the virus within the population.

High-titre viraemia during which the virus is present at concentrations of up to 10^{12} particles/ml of blood forms a further important source of infection. It is the prerequisite for vertical transmission of B19 virus from mother to fetus (Public Health Laboratory Service Working Party on Fifth Disease 1990). Moreover, B19 virus is efficiently transmitted by blood and blood products (e.g. factor VIII). Although the incidence of virus in donated blood varies between 1 per 200 and 1 per 70 000 donations according to the epidemic conditions prevailing, infection via transfusion of individual blood units is of relatively little concern. Blood products prepared from large pools of donations, however, carry the virus quite frequently and the known stability of parvoviruses makes it difficult if not impossible to remove B19 infectivity from such products.

Clinical manifestations

The common manifestation of B19 infection is a mild febrile illness with a maculopapular rash of variable intensity. Especially in children, the first sign of illness is often an erythema of the cheeks ('slapped cheek' appearance); in adults this is less common, and the rash is frequently followed by joint involvement. These are the symptoms of erythema infectiosum, or 'fifth disease'. This syndrome has long been known to clinicians and regarded as infectious; yet it was only in 1983 that B19 virus was recognized as the cause (Anderson et al. 1983). Since then, the development and use of specific laboratory tests for diagnosing B19 infection has revealed a spectrum of disease in which erythema infectiosum still occupies a central position. However, a large proportion of patients suffer from B19 infection without ever developing an erythema and at least 20% of infections are completely asymptomatic (Woolf et al. 1989). All infections, whether manifesting in the classic way or proceeding without signs of erythema, can lead to a broad spectrum of complications which, without appropriate laboratory diagnosis, will not necessarily be associated with B19 virus.

Prodromal symptoms and influenza-like illness There is a conspicuous absence of reports of prodromal symptoms in erythema infectiosum. The results of studies in volunteers, however (Anderson et al. 1985), supported early findings of a febrile episode, with non-specific symptoms of headache, chills, myalgia and malaise accompanying the viraemic phase of B19 infection. During this illness, virus may be detected in the respiratory tract where its replication may be associated with sore throat. The ensuing clinical picture of an influenza-like illness is typical of the prodromal phase of erythema infectiosum; it may, however, also be the only clinically apparent manifestation of acute B19 infection. It is then often difficult to link complications (e.g. hydrops fetalis or arthropathies, which may occur with a delay of several weeks) to such an ill-defined febrile illness.

Erythema infectiosum Following the prodromal illness, infected individuals are symptom-free for about one week before the onset of the exanthematous phase or erythema infectiosum (EI) which in its classic form has 3 stages (Anderson et al. 1985). The first stage begins some 18 days after acquisition of infection, and is characterized by the appearance on the cheeks of a bright red rash, the edges of which may be slightly raised. The second stage of the exanthem begins 1–4 days after the onset of facial involvement, with the appearance of an erythematous, maculopapular rash on the trunk and limbs. The rash is initially discrete but spreads to involve large areas. Towards the end of this stage there is central clearing of the rash to give the characteristic lacy or reticular pattern

(Fig. 14.3; see also Plate 14.3). The third stage is highly variable in duration, lasting from 1 to 3 weeks, and consists of changes in the intensity of the rash with periodic complete evanescence and recrudescence. These fluctuations are related to environmental factors such as exposure to sunlight and to varying temperatures. EI is common in children of both genders and may also be observed with relative frequency in women. In contrast, influenza-like symptoms are often the unique manifestation of a B19 infection in men.

The rash in EI appears simultaneously with the rise in anti-B19-antibody. Therefore, it is probably related to the formation and deposition of immune complexes. Direct detection of B19 virus DNA by PCR in a skin biopsy specimen supports this concept (Schwarz, Wiersbitzky and Pambor 1994).

Arthropathy This is the most common complication of EI. If only patients with obvious EI are taken into account, arthralgias and arthritis are rare (c.10%) in children of both sexes; they occur in c. 35% of adult men and complicate B19 infection in up to 85% of affected women. Studies that included patients lacking the classic signs of EI but with laboratory indicators of acute B19 infection now suggest that the overall incidence of arthritis and arthralgias may be similar in all age groups and occur in >80% of infected individuals (Nocton et al. 1993).

The extent and course of joint affections has been studied best in adult women in whom the most common presentation is a sudden onset of symmetric arthritis affecting mainly the joints of the hand, wrists, ankles, knees or any combination of these. The severity of the arthropathy ranges from mild arthralgia to acute arthritis. In most cases the arthritis resolves within 2–4 weeks. In some cases, however, B19-associated arthritis takes a prolonged course over some months to several years and shows some similarities with rheumatoid arthritis (Saal et al. 1992, Foto et al. 1993, Nocton et al. 1993). In one study, persistent B19-associated arthritis fulfilling the criteria for the diagnosis of juvenile rheumatoid arthritis was observed in

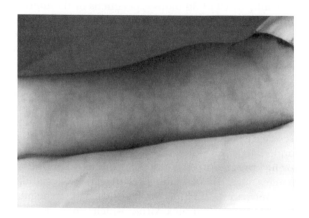

Fig. 14.3 Erythema infectiosum: rash on the arm of a patient infected with B19 virus. For colour, see Plate 14.3. (Courtesy of H Hochreutener, Ostschweizerisches Kinderspital, St Gall, Switzerland.)

6 of 22 children with arthritis or arthralgia (Nocton et al. 1993). In other studies, parvovirus B19 DNA was demonstrated by PCR in the synovial membrane of 15 of 20 patients with rheumatoid arthritis (Saal et al. 1992) and in bone marrow aspirates from 4 patients with chronic arthropathy (Foto et al. 1993). However, studies of 155 twins discordant for rheumatoid arthritis (Hajeer et al. 1994) and searches for parvovirus B19 DNA or anti-B19 antibodies in serum or synovial fluid samples from patients with rheumatoid arthritis (Nikkari et al. 1994, Cassinotti et al. 1995) were unable to confirm a direct role of human parvovirus B19 in inducing rheumatoid arthritis.

There is evidence that B19-associated arthropathy may closely resemble that observed in acute rubella (Smith, Woolf and Lenci 1987, Anderson 1988), in Lyme disease (Fatehnejad et al. 1992, Mayo and Vance 1991), Still's disease (Pouchot et al. 1993) or systemic lupus erythematosus (Kalish et al. 1992, 1993, Glickstein 1993).

Transient aplastic crisis (TAC) The predominant targets of B19 virus in the human organism are erythroid precursor cells. Lytic infection of these cells halts erythroid production. In the haematologically normal, immunocompetent individual, this cessation can be detected from the transient decrease in reticulocyte counts as well as from a transient fall in haemoglobin concentration. In these circumstances, the symptoms and signs, beginning with the appearance of viraemia, extend over 5–14 days and are readily compensated thereafter. However, in patients with underlying chronic haemolytic anaemia such as sickle-cell disease, hereditary spherocytosis, β-thalassaemia intermedia, pyruvate kinase deficiency or autoimmune haemolytic anaemia, who have in common a drastically shortened cell survival time, the profound reticulocytopenia of B19 virus infection results in complete red cell aplasia in the bone marrow and in severe haemoglobulinaemia in the peripheral blood (Fig. 14.4; see also Plate 14.4). Consequently, TAC often requires transfusion and can be fatal if not treated immediately.

Thrombocytopenia and leucopenia may also be observed in TAC. It is not yet clear, however, how these changes are brought about by B19 infection.

Parvovirus B19 infection in pregnancy The ability to infect the fetus transplacentally is a common feature of animal parvoviruses (Siegl 1984). Transplacental passage of the viruses usually happens in the course of acute maternal infection, when the fetus is not protected by passively acquired immunity. Viral replication then takes place in mitotically active, appropriately differentiated cells of the fetus. In general, the most severe effects are observed during the first or second trimester of gestation and comprise a wide spectrum of syndromes ranging from fetal death and abortion to very specific defects in individual organs (see 'Fetal infection', p. 267) (Siegl 1988).

A similar pattern is now emerging to some extent in human infections with B19 virus. During infection a high-titre viraemia develops, in the course of which B19 virus may cross the placenta and infect the fetus

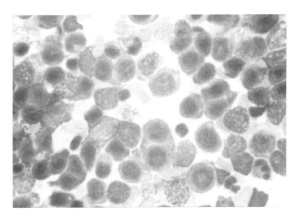

Fig. 14.4 Appearance of bone marrow in the course of B19 virus infection in a patient with β-thalassaemia and transient aplastic crisis. For colour, see Plate 14.4. (Courtesy of L Schmid, Institute for Clinical Chemistry and Haematology, St Gall, Switzerland.)

(Fig. 14.5; see also Plate 14.5). This can happen throughout the course of pregnancy and has been estimated to occur in about 30% of susceptible women showing clinical signs of B19 infection. Under these conditions, the risk of fetal death due to B19 virus infection has been calculated as c. 9% (Public Health Laboratory Service Working Party on Fifth Disease 1990). However, Smoleniec and co-workers (1994) observed that, in a group of pregnant women with serologically proven B19 infection, only 27% were symptomatic. There was also evidence for a higher rate of fetal affection following asymptomatic maternal infection than in women presenting with characteristic clinical symptoms. If these data can be substantiated, the number of fetal deaths due to B19 virus infection may be higher than estimated.

Most reported fetal deaths and spontaneous abortions secondary to parvovirus infection have occurred at 20–28 weeks of gestation but occasionally such losses also occur well outside this range (Centers for

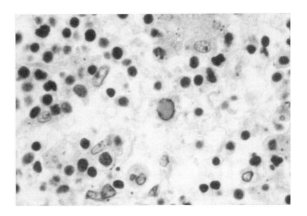

Fig. 14.5 Parvovirus B19-infected erythroblast with intranuclear alterations in fetal liver. The nucleus is eosinophilic, enlarged and ballooned, showing marginal inclusions (staining: haematoxylin and eosin). For colour, see Plate 14.5. (Courtesy of T Schwarz, Max v Pettenkofer-Institut, Munich, Germany.)

Disease Control 1989, Cassinotti et al. 1994, Sheikh and Ernest 1995). Nevertheless, despite recent observations concerning the impact of dependovirus infections on early human miscarriage, there is at present no indication that B19 virus is a significant cause of early spontaneous abortion (Rogers et al. 1993).

Infection with B19 virus in the second trimester is mostly associated with the development of non-immune hydrops fetalis. Although incompletely resolved, the mechanism leading to fetal hydrops is likely to be multifactorial (Morey et al. 1992, Sheikh and Ernest 1995). A major feature is the development of fetal anaemia, probably caused by the cytolytic replication of parvovirus B19 in erythroid precursor cells in the liver. The fetus is particularly at risk of infection owing to rapid erythroid progenitor cell proliferation, a shortened red blood cell life-span of 45–70 days and the lack of protective immunity. In this situation, the fetus is unable to eliminate the virus and chronic infection may be established, potentially leading to chronic anaemia and ultimately a fatal aplastic crisis. Additional factors frequently associated with the development of fetal hydrops are myocarditis, which is evidently due to replication of the virus in myocardial cells (Morey et al. 1992, Sheikh and Ernest 1995), congestive heart failure, and hypoalbuminaemia caused by hepatic dysfunction (Morey et al. 1992, Sheikh and Ernest 1995). The time between maternal infection and the manifestation of hydrops or fetal death is usually 4–6 weeks but may be as much as 12 weeks (Bond et al. 1986).

Fetal hydrops secondary to parvovirus B19 infection is not necessarily fatal. Spontaneous resolution of symptoms with delivery of healthy babies has been repeatedly described (Morey et al. 1991, Pryde et al. 1992, Zerbini et al. 1993).

The extent to which B19 infection of the developing human fetus leads to specific and permanent organic defects is still unresolved. So far, no controlled studies have been published on this subject, but a few reports seem to indicate that such an effect of B19 infection should be taken into account. In one case an aborted B19-infected fetus with eye anomalies and damage to several other tissues was reported (Weiland et al. 1987). A second fetus with proven B19 infection had multiple structural defects at prenatal ultrasound examination; at termination of pregnancy, a bilateral cleft lip and palate, micrognathia and webbed joints were found (Tiessen et al. 1994). Children born after intrauterine B19 infection and treatment with intrauterine blood transfusion were also found to have hypoglobulinaemia at birth and to develop chronic anaemia closely resembling congenital red cell aplasia or Diamond–Blackfan anaemia (Brown et al. 1994a). Finally, there has been a preliminary report describing 3 live-born infants with severe nervous system abnormalities following serologically confirmed B19 infection in utero. Neuroimaging studies revealed a wide range of pathological changes, for example cerebral atrophy, reduction in size of the brain stem and cerebellum, calcification of the basal ganglia and thalamus as well as periventricular calcification. One neonate

died and B19 virus was detected in brain tissue. The other 2 showed significant developmental delay and several neurological complications during follow-up (Török 1995).

For a more detailed account of parvovirus infections in pregnancy and in the foetus, see Chapter 41, section 4.

Persistent infection B19 infection in normal, immunocompetent individuals takes a self-limited brief course. Virus can be detected almost exclusively during the incubation period and, as suggested by the results of volunteer studies and by observations of naturally acquired infection, is rapidly cleared following the appearance of anti-B19 antibody (Fig. 14.6). This clear-cut picture may apply to a large proportion of all B19 infections, but is only one facet of the interaction of the virus with its human host. There is good evidence that, as with many other autonomous parvoviruses, B19 virus remains in the infected organism after resolution of clinical disease and in the presence of demonstrable antiviral immunity. The most likely place for persistence of this latent infection is the bone marrow. By sensitive means (PCR amplification) B19 has been repeatedly detected in samples of bone marrow months and even years after primary infection and in the absence of any clinical or laboratory diagnostic signs of a continuing, active infection. It is not yet known whether B19 virus, like the dependoviruses, can maintain such a latent infection via integration of its genome into cellular DNA or if there is a carrier state with low level virus replication in a few infected cells. Because persistent viraemia, with virus concentrations detectable only by the most sensitive amplification techniques (i.e. 10^2–10^3 genome copies/ml of serum), could be followed over periods of several months to almost 5 years in healthy individuals (Kerr et al. 1995a), a carrier state seems to be the more likely.

Latent (or low-level persistent) infection can be reactivated under conditions impairing the immune system of the host and providing a substrate of rapidly replicating, appropriately differentiated cells for replication of B19 virus. Such conditions include immunosuppression in the course of chemotherapy for cancer (e.g. acute lymphatic leukaemia), bone marrow or organ transplantation, and infection with the human immunodeficiency virus (HIV). These conditions, together with congenital immunodeficiencies, such as Nezelof's syndrome (combined T and B cell defect), also predispose to the development of chronic B19 disease following active primary virus infection (Kurtzman et al. 1988, Tang, Kemp and Moaven 1994). The patients then frequently present with unexplained chronic anaemia or have a history of pure red cell aplasia lasting several years. In general, their antibody response to B19 virus is absent or inadequate. Kurtzman and co-workers (1989) have presented evidence that antibodies produced in these immunodeficient individuals either lack the ability to neutralize B19 or block viral epitopes important for neutralization. The genome copy number in sera of chronically infected individuals is usually several orders of magnitude lower (10^5–10^{10} genome copies/ml serum) than in acute primary infection (10^{10}–10^{14} genome copies/ml of serum).

The range of clinical manifestations associated with persistent B19 infection in immunocompromised hosts is not limited to pure red cell aplasia. Other cellular components of the blood can apparently be affected either individually or in combination. Thus persistent or recurrent neutropenia, thrombocytopenia, pancytopenia and even agranulocytosis have been reported. In addition, there is evidence, albeit controversial, of long-term persistence of B19 virus in the synovial membranes of patients with rheumatoid arthritis (Saal et al. 1992). The latter type of persistence also appears to be associated with an absent or inappropriate immune response: c. 40% of patients with B19 DNA restricted to the synovial membrane lacked detectable anti-B19 antibody.

Finally, fetal B19 disease might also be regarded as a persistent infection. Transplacental passage of the virus in general takes place in the course of primary infection of a non-immune mother who, within a relatively short time, reacts to and overcomes infection by mounting an immune response. In spite of the resulting presence of anti-B19 IgG, which should be able to cross the placenta, B19 virus can persist and multiply for weeks in the blood-forming organs, as well as in many other tissues of the fetus, until fetal disease becomes manifest. As mentioned above under 'Parvovirus B19 infection in pregnancy' (see p. 271), persistent fetal infection may continue until after birth and may then present as congenital anaemia.

Neurological disease   Central nervous system involvement is a rare but well documented complication of parvovirus B19 infection in children and adults. Indeed, encephalitis and encephalopathy in patients with erythema infectiosum were described before B19 virus had been implicated in its aetiology (Balfour, Schiff and Bloom 1970, Hall and Horner 1977). Since then, the association between acute parvovirus B19 infection and neurological disease has been confirmed serologically by the demonstration of anti-B19 IgM antibody as well as by detection of parvovirus B19 DNA in blood and cerebrospinal fluid (CSF) of children with erythema and encephalopathy (Watanabe, Satoh and Oda 1994). Aseptic meningitis has been observed in a 35 year old man presenting with mild pancytopenia (Cassinotti et al. 1993) and in a 7 year old boy following EI (Okumura and Ichikawa 1993). In both patients acute parvovirus infection was serologically confirmed and B19 DNA was detected in CSF as well as in their blood during the course of the disease.

Neurological manifestations complicating parvovirus B19 infection usually resolve within one or 2 weeks without sequelae, but symptoms may persist (Hall and Horner 1977, Faden, Gary and Korman 1990).

Vasculitis and other clinical manifestations   Acute and chronic parvovirus B19 infections have been described in patients with polyarteritis nodosa (Corman and Dolson 1992, Finkel et al. 1994), Wegener's granulomatosis (Finkel et al. 1994), purpuric vasculitis (Shiraishi et al. 1989, Mortimer et al. 1985) and Henoch–Schönlein purpura (Lefrere et al. 1986). In addition, 2 reports linked B19 infection with Kawasaki disease (Nigro et al. 1994, Nigro, Pisano and Krzysztofiak 1993), an acute multisystem disease with vasculitic features, frequent in infancy and early childhood (Hicks and Melish 1986). However, since some laboratories failed to find convincing evidence for an association between B19 and Kawasaki disease (Cohen 1994, Yoto et al. 1994) or polyarteritis nodosa (Leruezville et al. 1994), it is possible that the presence of B19 virus in those patients was coincidental rather than causative.

The list of clinical manifestations ascribed to infection with B19 virus has grown rapidly during the past few years. It includes myocarditis and heart failure in both infants and adults (Saint-Martin et al. 1990, Tsuda et al. 1994), acute respiratory disease (Wiersbitzky et al. 1991), childhood idiopathic thrombocytopenic purpura (Murray et al. 1994), papular-purpuric or petechial 'gloves and socks' syndrome (Harms, Feldmann and Saurat 1990, Halasz, Cormier and Den 1992), systemic lupus erythematosus (Kalish et al. 1992), fibromyalgia (Leventhal, Naides and Freundlich 1991) and Still's disease (Pouchot et al. 1993). In most of these syndromes, a close association with an active or persistent B19 infection could be demonstrated; even so, as in the case of vasculitic diseases, the true role of parvovirus in the pathogenesis of these diseases remains to be elucidated.

Pathogenesis

Three main components are operative in B19 virus pathogenicity. The first and most important is the virus itself, with its ability to infect, to replicate and to lyse susceptible cells. The second component consists of cellular factors that restrict virus replication to actively proliferating cells in a particular state of development, and hence define the target tissues for B19 pathogenicity. The third factor is the immune response, which controls the extent of virus replication and determines whether disease is self-limiting or becomes chronic.

As has been mentioned (see 'Productive infection', p. 265), B19 virus is a typical autonomous parvovirus that can replicate productively without the presence of a helper virus in susceptible cells. There seem to be no specific types or strains of B19 virus responsible for the distinct clinical syndromes so far observed. Nevertheless, genetic variation among circulating virus strains has been reported (Kerr et al. 1995b). Genetic variant viruses also seem to appear readily in the course of persistent infection with B19 (Umene and Nunoue 1993). By analogy with many other viral infections, continual generation of such variants is very probably a prerequisite for the persistence of B19.

Lytic infection with B19 is similar to animal parvovirus infections, in which disease affects organs or tissues in which a large proportion of the cells are susceptible to infection and have a high mitotic rate. The most sensitive target organ in B19 infection is the erythropoietic cell series, which carry the P antigen that is the receptor for B19 virus. Moreover, although virus can be found in giant erythroid precursors in vitro, only late proliferating erythroid precursors (of the pronormoblast and normoblast phenotype) are fully permissive for B19 infection. Consequently, it must be assumed that they display the full spectrum of cell cycle-specific and differentiation-dependent factors required for fully productive B19 replication.

Productive infection in erythroid precursor cells leads to lysis of these cells and, hence, to arrest of erythrocyte production. The ultrastructural changes observed in infected cells in recent studies in vitro comprised nucleolar degeneration, extreme margination of the nuclear heterochromatin and cytoplasmic vacuolization, i.e. features typical of cells undergoing individual programmed cell death (apoptosis) (Morey, Ferguson and Fleming 1993). The possible triggering of this process in erythroid precursors by B19 would be compatible with the apparent lack of a strong inflammatory response to B19 infection, especially in the fetus.

In the haematologically normal individual, arrest of erythrocyte production is not clinically apparent, although bone marrow aspirates taken 10 days after inoculation from volunteers experimentally infected with B19 show a complete absence of erythroid cells of all developmental stages (Potter et al. 1987). In individuals with a shortened red cell survival time, this arrest results in transient, profound anaemia or aplastic crisis. In the fetus, immaturity of the immune response permits persistence of B19 infection and concomitant cessation of red cell production, leading to hydrops fetalis (Frickhofen and Young 1989).

Lytic infection and high-titre viraemia during the prodromal phase of B19 infection are accompanied by an influenza-like illness, including mild upper respiratory tract symptoms (Fig. 14.6). Their pathogenesis has not been fully defined, but the presence of virus in the respiratory tract secretions suggests that they are probably due to replication of the virus in cells of the respiratory tract.

The second phase of B19 disease is characterized by specific clinical manifestations such as erythema infectiosum or arthralgias and arthritis. At least 20% of parvovirus B19 infections are, however, asymptomatic (Woolf et al. 1989). Symptoms, when they occur, become apparent when virus disappears from the blood and a specific immune response in the form of anti-B19 IgM and, later, anti-B19 IgG can be detected (Fig. 14.6). Rash and arthralgias are likely to be mediated by this immune response, as it has been repeatedly observed that previously asymptomatic patients with chronic parvovirus B19 infection develop rashes and arthralgias following treatment with anti-B19 immunoglobulin (Kurtzman et al. 1988, Kurtzman et al. 1989, Ramage et al. 1994).

There is so far no explanation of why children and, to some extent, adult women (in contrast to adult men) are apparently predisposed to the development

of rash. Neither is it clear why some patients react with both rash and arthralgia and others only with one or the other. Some studies suggest that genetic factors, and specifically the major histocompatibility system, may play a role in this context. HLA-DR4 has been reported at increased frequency in patients with B19-related arthritis (Klouda et al. 1986) and the presence of HLA-B27 has been correlated with B19-associated arthritis persisting for >9 months (Jawad 1993). These findings, however, are still controversial.

Circumstantial evidence suggests that erythroid precursor cells are not the only targets for B19 virus replication. Intranuclear inclusions indicative of productive virus infection have been found in various fetal tissues and, with some regularity, in myocardial cells. Moreover, development of vascular disease may well be related to replication of the virus in endothelial cells, which carry the antigen equivalent to the B19 receptor on their surfaces (Brown et al. 1994b).

The importance of the immune system as a regulatory component in B19 disease is not limited to its role in the generation of rash and, possibly, arthralgias. It is more likely that a combination of humoral and cellular immune response is essential to make B19 infection self-limiting. Minor defects such as delayed switching from IgM to IgG isotype or failure of the antibodies to recognize distinctive viral epitopes predispose the patient to protracted or persistent B19 infection. Major defects in the immune system, whether congenital, pre-existing or acquired owing to immunosuppressive treatment, co-infection with immunosuppressive viruses or neoplastic disease, invariably lead either to persistence of virus and chronic disease following primary B19 infection or to reactivation of a pre-existing latent infection.

Immune response

The serological response to B19 infection in the controlled experimental infection of volunteers accords well with the data obtained in the investigation of natural infection. B19-specific IgM is first detectable as the viraemia wanes, 9–10 days after inoculation, and rises rapidly to reach peak concentrations within one week (Fig. 14.6). During the early part of the IgM response, much of the antibody circulates as virion–antibody complexes that do not fix complement. In the early studies, B19-specific IgG was not detectable until viraemia had cleared. However, with modern serological techniques for measuring the immune response and the ability to detect even small quantities of virus, B19 itself, anti-B19 IgM and anti-B19 IgG can frequently be demonstrated in parallel.

After an acute, self-limiting infection, anti-B19 IgM can usually be detected over a period of 2–3 months. Under conditions of persistent infection, as well as in cases in which reactivation of latent B19 infection was suspected, prolonged or fluctuating primary or short-lived secondary IgM responses have also been observed. Furthermore, it is assumed that an early switch from anti-B19 IgM to anti-B19 IgG is essential for efficient clearance of circulating virus.

Following transplacental infection, an anti-B19 IgM

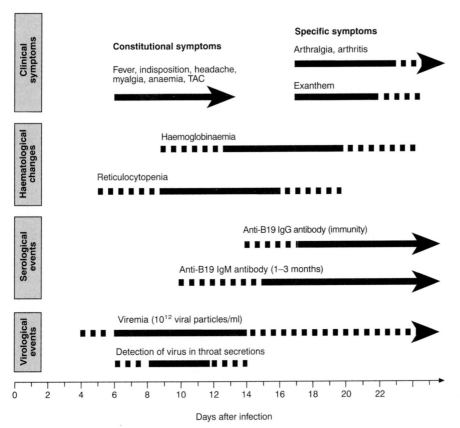

Fig. 14.6 Course of B19 infection in the human host.

response is not necessarily demonstrable, either in the mother or in the offspring infected in utero (see 'Laboratory diagnosis'). In some instances, no anti-B19 antibodies at all can be detected; in others, the only assessable immunological response to proved infection is the appearance of anti-B19 IgG.

Finally, the significance of anti-B19 IgG in antiviral immunity remains to be clarified. Epidemiological data give strong indications that this type of antibody confers life-long immunity to B19 infection. However, in some patients, their anti-B19 IgG either failed to neutralize the virus or, during pregnancy, could not prevent reinfection of the mother and subsequent infection of the fetus (Cassinotti et al. 1994). These findings might be explained at least in part by postulating that the antibodies present in these patients and detected by the available serological test were not directed against a major neutralizing epitope of B19 virus.

Laboratory diagnosis

Diagnostic tools Laboratory diagnosis of parvovirus B19 infection can be performed either by direct demonstration of the virus or by detection of anti-B19 antibodies.

Direct diagnosis of a parvovirus B19 infection by demonstration of the virus in clinical specimens is hindered by the lack of an appropriate, easily handled cell culture system. Although replication of parvovirus B19 has been reported in bone marrow cells (Ozawa, Kurtzman and Young 1986), cord blood, fetal liver cells and in various cell lines (Shimomura et al. 1992,

Munshi et al. 1993, Takahashi et al. 1993), these systems are not satisfactory for routine diagnostic purposes.

Haemagglutination assays have been used for detecting and quantifying most autonomous parvoviruses. B19 virus also agglutinates red blood cells of baboon and human origin (Brown and Cohen 1992). However, the presence of inhibitors in human serum makes this technique cumbersome and unreliable. B19 virus in clinical specimens can be demonstrated more easily by electron microscopy or detection of viral antigen by radioimmunoassay, enzyme immunoassay or counter-current immunoelectrophoresis. Furthermore, B19 DNA can be assayed by dot-blot hybridization. Because of their limited sensitivity, the usefulness of all these tests is restricted to detecting B19 virus in the acute phase of viraemia, i.e. during the prodromal phase of infection. This drawback can be partly overcome by amplification of the B19 genome with the PCR technique, which has a sensitivity several orders of magnitude higher and allows detection of even small amounts of virus (Koch and Adler 1990, Cassinotti, Weitz and Siegl 1993).

The most frequently used method for laboratory diagnosis of parvovirus B19 infection is the demonstration of anti-B19 antibodies of both IgM and IgG types. A broad range of test systems has been developed for this purpose. The standard was set by sensitive and specific radioimmunoassay (RIA) or enzyme-linked immunosorbent assay (ELISA) using native parvovirus B19 antigen (Cohen, Mortimer and Pereira 1983, Anderson et al. 1986). At present, however, this antigen can be obtained only from viraemic patients and is thus scarce. To overcome this problem, numerous tests based on the use of synthetic peptides (Fridell, Trojnar and Wahren 1989, Fridell, Cohen and Wahren 1991, Patou and Ayliffe 1991), recombinant VP1 or VP2 structural proteins (Sisk and Berman 1987, Brown et al. 1990) or empty capsids consisting of recombinant VP2 alone or in combination with VP1 have been developed (Kajigaya et al. 1991, Brown et al. 1991, Salimans et al. 1992). These tests vary greatly in sensitivity and specificity, and require careful validation by the diagnostic laboratory (see 'Parvovirus B19 infection in pregnancy', p. 271) to yield reliable results. For instance, anti-B19 IgM may be absent or undetectable by certain test systems in acute phase as well as in early convalescent sera following infection in pregnancy. It may then be necessary to apply more than one test. Attempts to overcome the resulting diagnostic ambiguity by assay of anti-B19 IgA failed, as this type of anti-B19 antibody obviously tends to persist for long periods after infection.

Little information is available concerning the antibody response to the non-structural protein NS1 of parvovirus B19. Von Poblotzki and co-workers (1995) used recombinant NS1 protein expressed in *Escherichia coli* to detect the corresponding antibodies. They showed that such antibodies were present in the sera of patients with arthritis, but not in those of patients with uncomplicated acute or previous B19 infection.

Erythema infectiosum and asymptomatic infection In patients presenting with erythema infectiosum or in those with an asymptomatic parvovirus B19 infection, the laboratory diagnosis, if necessary at all, is performed by demonstrating anti-B19 antibody in blood (see Fig. 14.6). In an acute infection, anti-B19 IgM antibody appears shortly before the onset of specific signs and can be detected for 2–3 months (Cohen, Mortimer and Pereira 1983, Anderson et al. 1986), or even longer. The presence of anti-B19 IgM antibody usually indicates an acute infection. The anti-B19 IgG response starts a few days after the IgM response and remains detectable for years. Its persistence is considered to confer immunity to reinfection (Anderson et al. 1985, Kurtzman et al. 1989) and is generally indicative of past infection. Anti-B19 IgA antibody is highly prevalent among healthy blood donors (Erdman et al. 1991), indicating prolonged persistence following acute infection and limiting its diagnostic use as an indicator of acute infection.

Chronic parvovirus infection Although parvovirus B19 infections are generally acute and easily diagnosed by demonstration of anti-B19 antibodies in serum, they may take a persistent course, often characterized by chronic anaemia. Immunocompromised patients with deficient humoral responses are particularly prone to develop persistent parvovirus infection. In such patients the diagnosis of a parvovirus B19 infection by serological means is not reliable and must be complemented by detection of parvovirus B19 DNA in blood. Because of its high sensitivity, PCR is the diagnostic procedure of choice in immunocompromised patients with low level viraemia.

Transient aplastic crisis Individuals experiencing transient aplastic crisis (TAC) against a background of chronic haemolytic anaemia are able to mount an effective immune response against B19 virus. Serological results are thus fully reliable in this situation. In the acute phase of TAC it is, however, advisable to seek B19 DNA, either by hybridization assay or by PCR. In patients with sickle-cell disease, persistence of anti-B19 IgM has been reported for up to 10 months (Rao, Miller and Cohen 1992).

Arthralgia and arthritis Arthralgia and arthritis associated with B19 infection usually resolve within 2–4 weeks. In these circumstances laboratory diagnosis based on demonstration of anti-B19 IgM and IgG antibodies is reliable. In some instances, however, these symptoms can persist for years and often only anti-B19 IgG is detectable. Persistent infection can then be verified by detection of viral DNA in blood or synovial fluid. Further studies are required to judge the usefulness of anti-B19 NS1 antibody in the diagnosis of B19-associated arthritis.

Parvovirus B19 infection in pregnancy The diagnosis of a B19 infection during pregnancy is not straightforward. The presence of anti-B19 IgM cannot be regularly demonstrated in the course of parvovirus B19 infection in pregnancy, either in maternal blood or in fetal blood obtained by cordocentesis, nor in the blood of the baby at birth. Hence, serology alone is unreliable and, in suspected acute B19 infection in pregnancy, it is essential to search directly for the virus, preferably by PCR. The appropriate samples are maternal blood, cord blood, amniotic fluid or ascites fluid. In the case of abortion, B19 can usually be readily detected in various fetal tissues and in the placenta. Once parvovirus B19 infection has been confirmed, ultrasound scans at regular intervals are helpful for monitoring the hydropic state of the fetus. Another possible method of closely following fetal parvovirus B19 infection is testing for elevated maternal serum α-fetoprotein (AFP) levels, which have been reported to indicate an increased risk of fetal death (Carrington et al. 1987, Bernstein and Capeless 1989, Soothill 1990). Recent observations suggest, however, that parvovirus B19 infection during pregnancy is not necessarily related to elevated levels of maternal AFP (Johnson et al. 1994, Pustilnik and Cohen 1994).

Prevention and treatment

There is as yet no vaccine for parvovirus B19 but such a vaccine based on recombinant virus particles is under development.

The virus is spread by the respiratory route, but most clinically apparent cases are no longer infectious. Therefore, isolation of patients with erythema infectiosum serves no useful purpose. Patients with aplastic crisis may be excreting virus at presentation and should therefore be isolated from seronegative patients. Caution must also be exercised with children with leukaemia or under immunosuppressive treatment. Finally, B19 is highly infectious, and handling of blood or serum samples containing the virus in high concentrations has repeatedly led to infections among laboratory personnel.

There is no specific antiviral treatment for B19 infection. Symptomatic therapy for erythema infectiosum is rarely necessary and treatment of arthralgias associated with B19 infection, if required, is by non-specific methods.

Cases of aplastic crisis require transfusion with erythrocytes until a satisfactory haemoglobin concentration is attained. In pure red cell aplasia, in chronic bone marrow failure and in all other instances of chronic B19 disease, treatment with immune serum globulin (ISG) over various periods has repeatedly proved successful. In immunologically normal patients, ISG evidently helps the organism to mount a protective immune response of its own; in patients with an underlying immune defect, repeated or even continuous treatment may be necessary.

Infections in utero respond favourably to intrauterine exchange transfusions. However, this procedure may be associated with considerable complications. Consequently, the use of intravenous ISG to protect mother and fetus has recently been suggested as an efficient alternative (Selbing et al. 1995). Because, on the one hand, B19-associated fetal hydrops may resolve spontaneously and, on the other, neonates transfused in utero may present with persisting anaemia, a decision to undertake intrauterine exchange transfusion has to be taken with great caution.

REFERENCES

Anderson MJ, 1988, Rash illness due to B19 virus, *Parvoviruses and Human Disease*, ed Pattison JR, CRC Press, Boca Raton FL, 93–104.

Anderson MJ, Jones SE et al., 1983, Human parvovirus: the cause of erythema infectiosum (fifth disease)?, *Lancet*, **2**: 1378.

Anderson MJ, Higgins PG et al., 1985, Experimental parvoviral infection in humans, *J Infect Dis*, **152**: 257–65.

Anderson LJ, Tsou C et al., 1986, Detection of antibodies and antigens of human parvovirus B19 by enzyme-linked immunosorbent assay, *J Clin Microbiol*, **24**: 522–6.

Balfour HH Jr, Schiff GM, Bloom JE, 1970, Encephalitis associated with erythema infectiosum, *J Pediatr*, **77**: 133–6.

Berns KI, 1990, Parvovirus replication, *Microbiol Rev*, **54**: 316–29.

Berns KI, Linden RM, 1995, The cryptic life style of adeno-associated virus, *Bioessays*, **17**: 237–45.

Bernstein IM, Capeless EL, 1989, Elevated maternal serum alpha-fetoprotein and hydrops fetalis in association with fetal parvovirus B19 infection, *Obstet Gynecol*, **74**: 456–7.

Bond PR, Caul EO et al., 1986, Intrauterine infection with human parvovirus, *Lancet*, **1**: 448–9.

Botquin V, Cidarregui A, Schlehofer JR, 1994, Adeno-associated virus type 2 interferes with early development of mouse embryos, *J Gen Virol*, **75**: 2655–62.

Brown CS, Salimans MM et al., 1990, Antigenic parvovirus B19 coat proteins VP1 and VP2 produced in large quantities in a baculovirus expression system, *Virus Res*, **15**: 197–211.

Brown CS, van Lent JWM et al., 1991, Assembly of empty capsids by using baculovirus recombinants expressing human parvovirus B19 structural proteins, *J Virol*, **65**: 2702–6.

Brown KE, Cohen BJ, 1992, Haemagglutination by parvovirus-B19, *J Gen Virol*, **73**: 2147–49.

Brown KE, Anderson SM, Young NS, 1993, Erythrocyte-P antigen – cellular receptor for B19 parvovirus, *Science*, **262**: 114–17.

Brown KE, Green SW et al., 1994a, Congenital anaemia after transplacental B19 parvovirus infection, *Lancet*, **343**: 895–6.

Brown KE, Hibbs JR et al., 1994b, Resistance to parvovirus B19 infection due to lack of virus receptor (erythrocyte P antigen), *N Engl J Med*, **330**: 1192–6.

Carrington D, Whittle MJ et al., 1987, Maternal serum α-fetoprotein: a marker of fetal aplastic crisis during intrauterine human parvovirus infection, *Lancet*, **1**: 433–5.

Carter BJ, 1990, The growth cycle of adeno-associated virus, *CRC Handbook of Parvoviruses*, vol 1, ed Tijssen P, CRC Press, Boca Raton FL, 155–68.

Cassinotti P, Weitz M, Siegl G, 1993, Human parvovirus-B19 infections – routine diagnosis by a new nested polymerase chain reaction assay, *J Med Virol*, **40**: 228–34.

Cassinotti P, Schultze D et al., 1993, Persistent human parvovirus B19 infection following an acute infection with meningitis in an immunocompetent patient, *Eur J Clin Microbiol Infect Dis*, **12**: 701–4.

Cassinotti P, Schultze D et al., 1994, Parvovirus B19 infection during pregnancy and development of hydrops fetalis despite the evidence for preexisting anti-B19 antibody: how reliable are serological results?, *Clin Diagn Virol*, **2**: 87–94.

Cassinotti P, Bas S et al., 1995, Association between human parvovirus B19 infection and arthritis, *Ann Rheum Dis*, **54**: 498–500.

Cater JE, Pintel DJ, 1992, The small non-structural protein-NS2 of the autonomous parvovirus minute virus of mice is required for virus growth in murine cells, *J Gen Virol*, **73**: 1839–43.

Centers for Disease Control, 1989, Risks associated with human parvovirus B19 infection, *Morbid Mortal Weekly Rep*, **38**: 81–97.

Cohen BJ, 1994, Human parvovirus B19 infection in Kawasaki disease, *Lancet*, **344**: 59.

Cohen BJ, Buckley MM, 1988, The prevalence of antibody to human parvovirus B19 in England and Wales, *J Med Microbiol*, **25**: 151–3.

Cohen BJ, Mortimer PP, Pereira MS, 1983, Diagnostic assays with monoclonal antibodies for the human serum parvovirus-like virus (SPLV), *J Hyg*, **91**: 113–30.

Corman LC, Dolson DJ, 1992, Polyarteritis nodosa and parvovirus B19 infection, *Lancet*, **339**: 491.

Cossart YE, Field AM et al., 1975, Parvovirus-like particles in human sera, *Lancet*, **1**: 72–3.

El Dadah AN, Nathanson N et al., 1967, Viral hemorrhagic encephalopathy of rats, *Science*, **156**: 392–4.

Erdman DD, Usher MJ et al., 1991, Human parvovirus B19 specific IgG, IgA, and IgM antibodies and DNA in serum specimens from persons with erythema infectiosum, *J Med Virol*, **35**: 110–15.

Faden H, Gary W Jr, Korman M, 1990, Numbness and tingling of fingers associated with parvovirus B19 infection, *J Infect Dis*, **161**: 354–5.

Fatehnejad S, Fikrig MK et al., 1992, Parvovirus arthritis mistaken for Lyme arthritis [letter], *J Rheumatol*, **19**: 1002–3.

Finkel TH, Török TJ et al., 1994, Chronic parvovirus B19 infection and systemic necrotising vasculitis: opportunist infection or aetiological agent? *Lancet*, **343**: 1255–8.

Flotte TR, Afione SA et al., 1993, Stable in vivo expression of the cystic fibrosis transmembrane conductance regulator with an adeno-associated virus vector, *Proc Natl Acad Sci USA*, **90**: 10613–17.

Foto F, Saag KG et al., 1993, Parvovirus B19 specific DNA in bone marrow from B19 arthropathy patients – evidence for B19 virus persistence, *J Infect Dis*, **167**: 744–8.

Frickhofen N, Young NS, 1989, Mini-review. Persistent parvovirus B19 infections in humans, *Microb Pathog*, **7**: 319–27.

Fridell E, Cohen BJ, Wahren B, 1991, Evaluation of a synthetic-peptide enzyme-linked immunosorbent assay for immunoglobulin M to human parvovirus B19, *J Clin Microbiol*, **29**: 1376–81.

Fridell E, Trojnar J, Wahren B, 1989, A new peptide for human parvovirus B19 antibody detection, *Scand J Infect Dis*, **21**: 597–603.

Glickstein SL, 1993, Lupus-like presentation of human parvovirus B19 infection, *J Rheumatol*, **20**: 1253.

Hajeer AH, Macgregor AJ et al., 1994, Influence of previous exposure to human parvovirus B19 infection in explaining susceptibility to rheumatoid arthritis: an analysis of disease discordant twin pairs, *Ann Rheum Dis*, **53**: 137–9.

Halasz CLG, Cormier D, Den M, 1992, Petechial glove and sock syndrome caused by parvovirus B19, *J Am Acad Dermatol*, **27**: 835–8.

Hall CB, Horner FA, 1977, Encephalopathy with erythema infectiosum, *Am J Dis Child*, **131**: 65–7.

Harms M, Feldmann R, Saurat JH, 1990, Papular-purpuric 'gloves and socks' syndrome, *J Am Acad Dermatol*, **23**: 850–4.

Hermonat PL, 1994, Down-regulation of the human c-*fos* and c-*myc* proto-oncogene promoters by adeno-associated virus Rep78, *Cancer Lett*, **81**: 129–36.

Hicks RV, Melish ME, 1986, Kawasaki syndrome, *Pediatr Clin North Am*, **33**: 1151–75.

Jawad ASM, 1993, Persistent arthritis after human parvovirus-B19 infection, *Lancet*, **341**: 494.

Johnson BJ, Castro AE, 1984, Isolation of canine parvovirus from a dog brain with severe necrotizing vasculitis and encephalomalacia, *J Am Vet Med Assoc*, **184**: 1398.

Johnson DR, Fisher RA et al., 1994, Screening maternal serum alpha-fetoprotein levels and human parvovirus antibodies, *Prenat Diagn*, **14**: 455–8.

Kajigaya S, Fujii H et al., 1991, Self-assembled B19 parvovirus capsids, produced in a baculovirus system, are antigenically and immunogenically similar to native virions, *Proc Natl Acad Sci USA*, **88**: 4646–50.

Kalish RA, Knopf AN et al., 1992, Lupus-like presentation of human parvovirus B19 infection, *J Rheumatol*, **19**: 169–71.

Kalish RA, Knopf AN et al., 1993, Lupus-like presentation of human parvovirus B19 infection. Reply, *J Rheumatol*, **20**: 1253.

Kerr JR, Curran MD et al., 1995a, Persistent parvovirus B19 infection, *Lancet*, **345**: 1118.

Kerr JR, Curran MD et al., 1995b, Genetic diversity in the nonstructural gene of parvovirus B19 detected by single-stranded conformational polymorphism assay (SSCP) and partial nucleotide sequencing, *J Virol Methods*, **53**: 213–22.

Klouda PT, Corbin SA et al., 1986, HLA and acute arthritis following human parvovirus infection, *Tissue Antigens*, **28**: 318–19.

Koch WC, Adler SP, 1990, Detection of human parvovirus B19 DNA by using the polymerase chain reaction, *J Clin Microbiol*, **28**: 65–9.

Kotin RM, Linden RM, Berns KI, 1992, Characterization of a preferred site on human chromosome 19q for integration of adeno-associated virus DNA by non-homologous recombination, *EMBO J*, **11**: 5071–8.

Kurtzman GJ, Cohen B et al., 1988, Persistent B19 parvovirus infection as a cause of severe chronic anaemia in children with acute lymphocytic leukaemia, *Lancet*, **2**: 1159–62.

Kurtzman GJ, Cohen BJ et al., 1989, Immune response to B19 parvovirus and an antibody defect in persistent viral infection, *J Clin Invest*, **84**: 1114–23.

Laurian Y, Dussaix E et al., 1994, Transmission of human parvovirus B19 by plasma derived factor VIII concentrates, *Nouv Rev Fr Hematol*, **36**: 449–53.

Lefrere JJ, Courouce AM et al., 1986, Henoch–Schönlein purpura and human parvovirus infection [letter], *Pediatrics*, **78**: 183–4.

Legendre D, Rommelaere J, 1992, Terminal regions of the NS1 protein of the parvovirus minute virus of mice are involved in cytotoxicity and promoter trans inhibition, *J Virol*, **66**: 5705–13.

Leruezville M, Lauge A et al., 1994, Polyarteritis nodosa and parvovirus B19, *Lancet*, **344**: 263–4.

Leventhal LJ, Naides SJ, Freundlich B, 1991, Fibromyalgia and parvovirus infection, *Arthritis Rheum*, **34**: 1319–24.

Luo WX, Astell CR, 1993, A novel protein encoded by small RNAs of parvovirus B19, *Virology*, **195**: 448–55.

Matsunaga Y, Goh KT et al., 1994, Low prevalence of antibody to human parvovirus B19 in Singapore, *Epidemiol Infect*, **113**: 537–40.

Mayo DR, Vance DW Jr, 1991, Parvovirus B19 as the cause of a syndrome resembling Lyme arthritis in adults [letter], *N Engl J Med*, **324**: 419–20.

Mendelson E, Trempe JP, Carter BJ, 1986, Identification of the trans-acting rep proteins of adeno-associated virus by antibodies to a synthetic oligopeptide, *J Virol*, **60**: 823–33.

Mochizuki M, Konishi S, Ogata M, 1978, Studies on feline panleukopenia. II. Antigenicities of the virus, *Nippon Juigaku Zasshi*, **40**: 375–83.

Morey AL, Ferguson DJP, Fleming KA, 1993, Ultrastructural features of fetal erythroid precursors infected with parvovirus-B19 in vitro – evidence of cell death by apoptosis, *J Pathol*, **169**: 213–20.

Morey AL, Nicolini U et al., 1991, Parvovirus B19 infection and transient fetal hydrops, *Lancet*, **337**: 496.

Morey AL, Keeling JW et al., 1992, Clinical and histopathological features of parvovirus-B19 infection in the human fetus, *Br J Obstet Gynaecol*, **99**: 566–74.

Mortimer PP, Cohen BJ et al., 1985, Human parvovirus and purpura [letter], *Lancet*, **2**: 730–1.

Munshi NC, Zhou SZ et al., 1993, Successful replication of parvovirus-B19 in the human megakaryocytic leukemia cell line MB-02, *J Virol*, **67**: 562–6.

Murray JC, Kelley PK et al., 1994, Childhood idiopathic thrombocytopenic purpura: association with human parvovirus B19 infection, *Am J Pediatr Hematol Oncol*, **16**: 314–19.

Nigro G, Pisano P, Krzysztofiak A, 1993, Recurrent Kawasaki disease associated with co-infection with parvovirus B19 and HIV-1, *AIDS*, **7**: 288–90.

Nigro G, Zerbini M et al., 1994, Active or recent parvovirus B19 infection in children with Kawasaki disease, *Lancet*, **343**: 1260–1.

Nikkari S, Luukkainen R et al., 1994, Does parvovirus B19 have a role in rheumatoid arthritis, *Ann Rheum Dis*, **53**: 106–11.

Nocton JJ, Miller LC et al., 1993, Human parvovirus B19-associated arthritis in children, *J Pediatr*, **122**: 186–90.

Okumura A, Ichikawa T, 1993, Aseptic meningitis caused by human parvovirus-B19, *Arch Dis Child*, **68**: 784–5.

O'Sullivan MG, Anderson DC et al., 1994, Identification of a novel simian parvovirus in cynomolgus monkeys with severe anemia. A paradigm of human B19 parvovirus infection, *J Clin Invest*, **93**: 1571–6.

Ozawa K, Kurtzman G, Young N, 1986, Replication of the B19 parvovirus in human bone marrow cell cultures, *Science*, **233**: 883–6.

Parrish CR, Aquadro CF, Carmichael LE, 1988, Canine host range and a specific epitope map along with variant sequences in the capsid protein gene of canine parvovirus and related feline, mink, and raccoon parvoviruses, *Virology*, **166**: 293–307.

Patou G, Ayliffe U, 1991, Evaluation of commercial enzyme linked immunosorbent assay for detection of B19 parvovirus IgM and IgG, *J Clin Pathol*, **44**: 831–4.

Pattison JR, Jones SE et al., 1981, Parvovirus infections and hypoplastic crisis in sickle-cell anaemia, *Lancet*, **1**: 664–5.

Potter CG, Potter AC et al., 1987, Variation of erythroid and myeloid precursors in the marrow and peripheral blood of volunteer subjects infected with human parvovirus (B19), *J Clin Invest*, **79**: 1486–92.

Pouchot J, Ouakil H et al., 1993, Adult Still's disease associated with acute human parvovirus-B19 infection, *Lancet*, **341**: 1280–1.

Pryde PG, Nugent CE et al., 1992, Spontaneous resolution of nonimmune hydrops fetalis secondary to human parvovirus B19 infection, *Obstet Gynecol*, **79**: 859–61.

Public Health Laboratory Service Working Party on Fifth Disease, 1990, Prospective study of human parvovirus (B19) infection in pregnancy, *Br Med J*, **300**: 1166–70.

Pustilnik TB, Cohen AW, 1994, Parvovirus B19 infection in a twin pregnancy, *Obstet Gynecol*, **83**: 834–6.

Ramage JK, Hale A et al., 1994, Parvovirus B19-induced red cell aplasia treated with plasmaphaeresis and immunoglobulin, *Lancet*, **343**: 667–8.

Rao SP, Miller ST, Cohen BJ, 1992, Transient aplastic crisis in patients with sickle cell disease – B19 parvovirus studies during a 7-year period, *Am J Dis Child*, **146**: 1328–30.

Rogers BB, Singer DB et al., 1993, Detection of human parvovirus-B19 in early spontaneous abortuses using serology, histology, electron microscopy, in situ hybridization, and the polymerase chain reaction, *Obstet Gynecol*, **81**: 402–8.

Saal JG, Steidle M et al., 1992, Persistence of B19 parvovirus in synovial membranes of patients with rheumatoid arthritis, *Rheumatol Int*, **12**: 147–51.

Saint-Martin J, Choulot JJ et al., 1990, Myocarditis caused by parvovirus [letter], *J Pediatr*, **116**: 1007–8.

Salimans MMM, Vanbussel MJAWM et al., 1992, Recombinant parvovirus B19 capsids as a new substrate for detection of B19-specific IgG and IgM antibodies by an enzyme-linked immunosorbent assay, *J Virol Methods*, **39**: 247–58.

Schwarz TF, Wiersbitzky S, Pambor M, 1994, Detection of parvovirus B19 in a skin biopsy of a patient with erythema infectiosum – case report, *J Med Virol*, **43**: 171–4.

Selbing A, Josefsson A et al., 1995, Parvovirus B19 infection during pregnancy treated with high-dose intravenous gammaglobulin, *Lancet*, **345**: 660–1.

Serjeant GR, Topley JM et al., 1981, Outbreak of aplastic crises in sickle cell anaemia associated with parvovirus-like agent, *Lancet*, **2**: 595–7.

Sheikh AU, Ernest JM, 1995, Clinical picture and consequences of fetal parvovirus B19 infection, *Ann Med*, **27**: 7–8.

Shimomura S, Komatsu N et al., 1992, First continuous propagation of B19 parvovirus in a cell line, *Blood*, **79**: 18–24.

Shiraishi H, Umetsu K et al., 1989, Human parvovirus (HPV/B19) infection with purpura, *Microbiol Immunol*, **33**: 369–72.

Shneerson JM, Mortimer PP, Vandervelde EM, 1980, Febrile illness due to a parvovirus, *Br Med J*, **2**: 1580.

Siegl G, 1984, Biology and pathogenicity of autonomous parvoviruses, *The Parvoviruses*, ed Berns KI, Plenum Press, New York & London, 297–362.

Siegl G, 1988, Patterns of parvovirus disease in animals, *Parvoviruses and Human Disease*, ed Pattison JR, CRC Press, Boca Raton FL, 43–67.

Siegl G, 1990, Variability, adaptability, and epidemiology of autonomous parvoviruses, *CRC Handbook of Parvoviruses*, vol 2, ed Tijssen P, CRC Press, Boca Raton FL, 59–74.

Sisk WP, Berman ML, 1987, Expression of human parvovirus B19 structural protein in *E. coli* and detection of antiviral antibodies in human serum, *Bio/Technology*, **5**: 1077–80.

Smith CA, Woolf AD, Lenci M, 1987, Parvoviruses: infections and arthropathies, *Rheum Dis Clin North Am*, **13**: 249–63.

Smoleniec JS, Pillai M et al., 1994, Subclinical transplacental parvovirus B19 infection – an increased fetal risk, *Lancet*, **343**: 1100–1.

Sol N, Morinet F et al., 1993, Trans-activation of the long terminal repeat of human immunodeficiency virus type 1 by the parvovirus B19 NS1 gene product, *J Gen Virol*, **74**: 2011–14.

Soothill P, 1990, Intrauterine blood transfusion for non-immune hydrops fetalis due to parvovirus B19 infection [letter], *Lancet*, **336**: 121–2.

Sprecher-Goldberger S, Thiry L et al., 1971, Complement-fixation antibodies to adenovirus-associated viruses, cytomegaloviruses and herpes simplex viruses in patients with tumors and in control individuals, *Am J Epidemiol*, **94**: 351–8.

Srivastava A, 1994, Parvovirus-based vectors for human gene therapy, *Blood Cells*, **20**: 531–8.

Strassheim ML, Gruenberg A et al., 1994, Two dominant neutralizing antigenic determinants of canine parvovirus are found on the threefold spike of the virus capsid, *Virology*, **198**: 175–84.

Takahashi T, Ozawa K et al., 1993, DNA replication of parvovirus-B-19 in a human erythroid leukemia cell line (JK-1) in vitro, *Arch Virol*, **131**: 201–8.

Tang ML, Kemp AS, Moaven LD, 1994, Parvovirus B19-associated red blood cell aplasia in combined immunodeficiency with normal immunoglobulins, *Pediatr Infect Dis J*, **13**: 539–42.

Tattersall P, Cotmore SF, 1990, Reproduction of autonomous parvovirus DNA, *CRC Handbook of Parvoviruses*, vol 1, ed Tijssen P, CRC Press, Boca Raton FL, 123–40.

Tattersall P, Gardiner EM, 1990, Autonomous parvovirus–host-cell interactions, *CRC Handbook of Parvoviruses*, vol 1, ed Tijssen P, CRC Press, Boca Raton FL, 111–21.

Tattersall P, Ward DC, 1976, Rolling hairpin model for replication of parvovirus and linear chromosomal DNA, *Nature (London)*, **263**: 105–8.

Tiessen RG, Vanelsackerniele AMW et al., 1994, A fetus with a parvovirus-B19 infection and congenital anomalies, *Prenat Diagn*, **14**: 173–6.

Tobiasch E, Rabreau M et al., 1994, Detection of adeno-associated virus DNA in human genital tissue and in material from spontaneous abortion, *J Med Virol*, **44**: 215–22.

Török T, 1995, Human parvovirus B19, *Infectious Diseases of the Fetus and Newborn Infant*, eds Remington JS, Klein JO, WB Saunders Co, Philadelphia, 668–702.

Tsao J, Chapman MS et al., 1991, The three-dimensional structure of canine parvovirus and its functional implications, *Science*, **251**: 1456–64.

Tsuda H, Maeda Y et al., 1994, Parvovirus B19-associated haemophagocytic syndrome with prominent neutrophilia, *Br J Haematol*, **86**: 413–14.

Umene K, Nunoue T, 1993, Partial nucleotide sequencing and characterization of human parvovirus-B19 genome DNAs from damaged human fetuses and from patients with leukemia, *J Med Virol*, **39**: 333–9.

Von Poblotzki A, Gigler A et al., 1995, Antibodies to parvovirus B19 NS-1 protein in infected individuals, *J Gen Virol*, **76**: 519–27.

Watanabe T, Satoh M, Oda Y, 1994, Human parvovirus B19 encephalopathy, *Arch Dis Child*, **70**: 71.

Weiland HT, Vermey-Keers C et al., 1987, Parvovirus B19 associated with fetal abnormality [letter], *Lancet*, **1**: 682–3.

Wiersbitzky S, Schwarz TF et al., 1991, Acute obstructive respiratory diseases in infants and children associated with parvovirus B19 infection [letter], *Infection*, **19**: 252.

Woolf AD, Campion GV et al., 1989, Clinical manifestations of human parvovirus B19 in adults, *Arch Intern Med*, **149**: 1153–6.

Yoto Y, Kudoh T et al., 1994, Human parvovirus B19 infection in Kawasaki disease, *Lancet*, **344**: 58–9.

Zerbini M, Musiani M et al., 1993, Symptomatic parvovirus-B19 infection of one fetus in a twin pregnancy, *Clin Infect Dis*, **17**: 262–3.

ADENOVIRUSES

W C Russell

1 Introduction	3 Clinical and pathological aspects
2 Properties of the viruses	

1   INTRODUCTION

The term adenoviruses was coined in 1956 (Enders et al.) to describe infectious agents that had been isolated from human adenoids (Rowe et al. 1953) and were similar to those associated with outbreaks of respiratory disease in military recruits (Hilleman and Werner 1954). The virus family was initially characterized in terms of cross-reactivity in serological tests and it soon became apparent that adenoviruses sharing this common antigen were to be found in a wide variety of species. Fundamental studies on adenoviruses and their interactions with their host cells were greatly stimulated by the discovery by Trentin and his colleagues (1962) that some human adenovirus serotypes could induce tumours in hamsters. However, later studies could not demonstrate any association with human tumours. This finding, coupled with the observations that adenoviruses did not appear to be associated with any serious morbidity and that they could readily be grown in a wide variety of cell lines, led to their being used extensively as model systems of the molecular basis of virus infection (for a review, see Horwitz 1990).

2   PROPERTIES OF THE VIRUSES

2.1   Classification

Adenoviruses are characterized on the basis of a common genus-specific antigen and a very characteristic morphology. Serotypes are classified by their ability to induce specific neutralizing antibodies. A serotype can therefore be defined as one that either exhibits no cross-reaction in neutralization with other animal typing antisera or shows a homologous : heterologous neutralization ratio of >16 (in both directions). For ratios of 8 or 16 a serotype assignment is made on the basis of other serological, biophysical or biochemical differences.

Two genera are now recognized on the basis of the presence of a genus-specific antigen: the mastadenoviruses covering 9 groups that infect mammals (bovine, canine, caprine, equine, human, murine, ovine, porcine, simian); and the aviadenoviruses with 5 groups infecting birds (duck, fowl, goose, pheasant, turkey), giving a total of at least 120 different viruses. The most intensively studied are the 47 serotypes isolated from humans (Mautner 1989, Russell et al. 1995).

2.2   Morphology and structure

The virions are non-enveloped, 80–110 nm in diameter and their capsids have icosahedral symmetry (Figs. 15.1 and 15.2). They have 240 non-vertex capsomeres (hexons) 8–10 nm in diameter and 12 vertex capsomeres (pentons). The pentons consist of penton bases and attached fibres, each in close association with a ring of 5 hexons; these are termed the peripentonal hexons. Each of the penton bases has one (or occasionally 2) fibres that protrude 9–30 mm from the capsid. Several other structural polypeptides (VI, VIII, IX, IIIa) are associated with the capsid and serve to cement the hexons and to link the capsid to the core (Stewart, Fuller and Burnett 1993). The latter consists of a double-stranded DNA genome with a covalently linked terminal protein (TP) (Rekosh et al. 1977) in tight association with three other polypeptides, V, VII and X(μ) (Fig. 15.1). The structure of this nucleoprotein core has not been established and the core polypeptides are shown in hypothetical locations in Fig. 15.1. The major capsid protein, the hexon, has been crystallized and its 3-dimensional structure shown to be based on a composite of 3 identical and interlocking polypeptide chains that form a triangular tower superimposed on a pseudohexagonal base (see Fig. 15.3). The virus is stable between pH 6.0 and 9.5, is resistant to chloroform, ether and fluorocarbons, and on heating to 56°C disintegrates, releasing core structures (Russell, Valentine and Pereira 1967).

On examination by electron microscopy some preparations of adenoviruses are seen to be contaminated by small round adeno-associated viruses (Fig. 15.2). These ssDNA parvoviruses belong to the genus Dependovirus (see Volume 1, Chapter 14) and require adenoviruses (or herpesviruses) for their replication (Porterfield 1989).

2.3 Genome structure and function

The mastadenovirus virion contains a single linear dsDNA genome of c. $(20–25) \times 10^3$ kDa; that of the aviadenoviruses is slightly larger, at c. 3×10^3 kDa. A virus-coded terminal protein is covalently linked to the 5' end of each DNA strand. The genome of the prototype human adenovirus type 2 has 35 937 bp and contains inverted terminal repetitions (ITRs) of 103 bp (Roberts et al. 1986). A number of other adenoviruses have been completely sequenced and all contain ITRs, but of variable length. Viruses replicate in the nuclei of a wide variety of cells of the species that they normally infect, giving a characteristic pattern of nuclear staining. Some adenoviruses can replicate in cells of other species; such infections are often abortive and, under suitable conditions, may give rise to morpho-

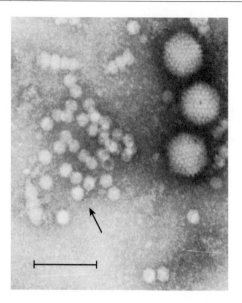

Fig. 15.2 Three adenovirus virions with dependoviruses (arrowed), negatively stained with phosphotungstic acid. Scale bar = 100 nm

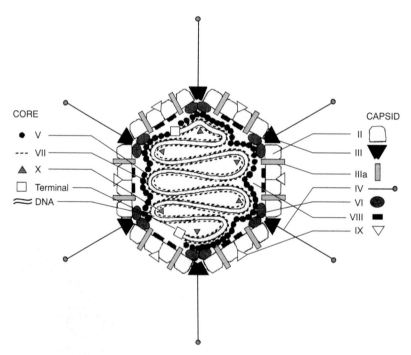

Fig. 15.1 Stylized cross-section of the adenovirus particle. The hexon bases are packed together to form a protein shell with 12 pentons at the apices of the icosahedral capsid. The positions of hexons (II), penton bases (III), fibres (IV) and protein (IX) are well established; 12 copies of polypeptides IX are found between 9 hexons in the centre of each facet. The positions of proteins IIIa, VI and VIII are tentatively assigned. Two monomers of IIIa appear to penetrate the hexon capsid at the edge of each facet. Multiple copies of VI form a ring underneath the peripentonal hexons. The 12 penton bases are formed by the interaction of 5 polypeptides (III) and are less tightly associated with the neighbouring (peripentonal) hexons. Each of the vertex pentons carries one or 2 fibres, each consisting of 3 polypeptides (IV) that interact to form a shaft of characteristic length and a distal knob. Polypeptide VIII has been assigned to the inner surface of the capsid. Other polypeptides (monomers of IIIa, trimers of IX and multimers of VI) seem to interact with hexons to stabilize the capsid. The 'core' consists of the DNA genome complexed with 4 polypeptides [V, VII, X(μ), terminal]. (Based on data supplied by P. Stewart and R. Burnett)

logical transformation (McDougall, Dunn and Galli-more 1975).

Entry of virus is by attachment of the fibre via its knob (Fig. 15.1) to ill-defined cellular receptors numbering $3–6 \times 10^3$ per cell (Defer et al. 1990). Adsorption is followed by an energy-dependent clustering of virus particles at the cell surface (Patterson and Russell 1983). Internalization of the virus particles then occurs via clathrin-coated vesicles into endosomes. At this stage the penton base appears to interact with cellular integrins (Wickham et al. 1993) facilitating the release of the engulfed virus particles into the cytoplasm. These steps may be modulated by other factors not yet defined (see Russell and Kemp 1995 for further details).

The events governing the onward passage of the virus and the eventual delivery of the virus genome to the nucleus are not at all clear but it seems likely that most of the capsid proteins are removed and the resulting core structure enters the nucleus through the nuclear pores, to become attached to the nuclear matrix via the viral terminal protein (Fredman and Engler 1993).

The adenovirus genome becomes available for transcription (Schaak et al. 1990) using cellular transcription factors that are abundant in the nuclear matrix. This process is well regulated and involves the synthesis of 4 major classes of 'early' transcripts (E1–E4), minor 'intermediate' transcripts and late transcripts (L1–L5). The last are initiated at the 'major late pro-

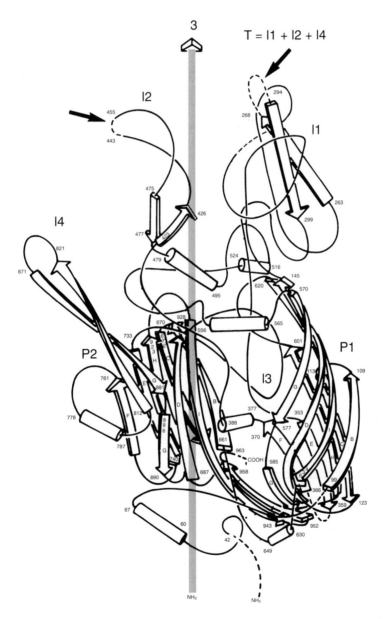

Fig. 15.3 Schematic diagram of the 3-dimensional structure of the Ad2 hexon monomer. P1 and P2 represent the two basal β barrel domains. T represents the surface tower domain comprising loops l1, l2 and l4. The dotted lines represent structures not resolved by x-ray crystallography. The arrows show the location of the regions presumed to be related to type specificity. Three of these monomers interweave in a complex manner to form the mature hexon. The 3-fold axes of symmetry of the hexon are indicated. (Based on Toogood, Crompton and Hay 1992 and Roberts et al. 1986)

moter', and, allied to a tripartite leader formed by a series of splicing events, drive the synthesis of most of the structural proteins; the 'early' transcripts are also subject to complex splicing mechanisms (Fig. 15.4). The mechanism of transcriptional regulation has not been elucidated but it has been suggested that the topology of the virus genome can be affected by the core proteins limiting template availability for transcription. After synthesis of the early transcripts and synthesis of 'early' proteins (e.g. virus DNA binding protein), further alterations in template topology and availability could permit virus DNA replication, thereby creating new progeny templates for late transcription. However, all these transcriptional events are subject to other regulatory controls of a quite complex nature (Wold and Gooding 1991).

2.4 Virus DNA replication

Adenovirus DNA synthesis is initiated at either end of the linear double-stranded DNA and at least 3 'early' viral proteins are required together with at least 3 cellular proteins. The initial event involves the interaction of one of the early proteins, the precursor of the terminal protein (pTP), with specific terminal DNA sequences followed by association with another early protein (polymerase) and then the formation of an ester bond between the phosphate of dCMP (C being the first nucleotide in the DNA sequence) and a serine residue in pTP. This can then function as a primer to extend a progeny DNA strand using one strand of the virus DNA as template; this process utilizes the viral polymerase and the co-operation of 3 other proteins,

2 of them cellular. The latter (NF1 and NF3) are also transcription factors and bind to specific sequences in the viral DNA, presumably facilitating the formation of the initiation complex. The other early virus protein, the DNA-binding protein (DBP), also plays a role in virus DNA initiation as well as facilitating strand separation during elongation and binding to the progeny DNA strands. A third cellular protein (NF2) seems to be required for complete elongation of the progeny strand and appears to be equivalent to cellular topoisomerase I. Synthesis of the second strands takes place after that of the first strands and the formation of a 'pan handle' structure formed by the interacting ITRs, thus allowing replication by a similar mechanism. The precise molecular mechanisms involved in these events have not yet been elucidated (for a review, see Hay and Russell 1989).

2.5 Polypeptides and maturation of the virion

The adenovirus genome has been completely sequenced (Roberts et al. 1986) and the dispositions of the polypeptide genes have been mapped. It became apparent that, by virtue of its splicing mechanisms, the genome makes efficient use of template information and synthesizes about 40 different polypeptides, 13 of these being incorporated into the mature virus particle (see Fig. 15.4 and Table 15.1). Three of the non-structural proteins synthesized early in infection are involved in virus DNA replication and are derived from the *E2* transcription region. The remainder of these 'early' non-structural proteins

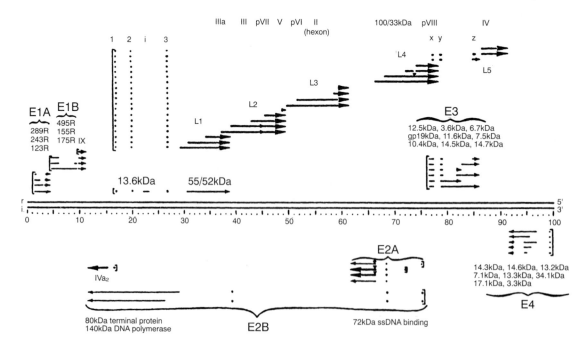

Fig. 15.4 Transcription map of the human Ad2 genome. The parallel lines indicate the linear duplex genome of 36 kbp; *r* and *l* refer to rightward and leftward transcription, 289R, 13.6 kDa, IIIa etc. refer to polypeptides. The split arrows indicate the spliced structures of the mRNAs. E1A, E4 etc. refer to early transcription units. Most of the late genes are in the 'major late transcription unit' which initiates at map position 16 (MLP) of the *r* strand and which includes the '1', '2' and '3' leaders as well as the L1, L2, L3, L4 and L5 families of mRNAs (see also Table 15.1). (Based on Wold and Gooding 1991)

seem to function as modulators of the host cell, so that virus transcription and replication are favoured, and to counteract the host immune response. A number of these polypeptides are phosphorylated and a few are glycosylated; the significance of these modifications is not, however, apparent in most cases.

The transcriptional units, in general, encode for products with related functions. Thus, regions *E1A* and *E1B* encode proteins that interact with cellular proteins and regulate the expression of other viral genes. These E1 proteins play a critical role in the initiation and maintenance of the transformed phenotype alluded to under section 2.3 (p. 282) (Shenk and Flint 1991). The *E2* region codes for proteins necessary for viral DNA replication, whereas the E3 gene products all appear to facilitate evasion of the host immune response (Wold and Gooding 1991) (see below). The E4 gene products are diverse and some at least are required for efficient tripartite splicing used in the transcription of the late genes (*L1–L5*). Not all the 'late' genes are structural (Table 15.1): a major product of c.100 kDa seems to function as a chaperone for other structural proteins but is not itself encapsidated, and the non-structural 52/55 kDa gene product appears to play a role as a scaffolding complex in assembling the virus particle. Two other

gene products, polypeptides IX and IV_{a2}, are regulated independently of the others and, whereas IX is clearly a structural component, the evidence that IV_{a2} is structural is not very strong.

The maturation of adenovirus is intimately linked to the functioning of the adenovirus gene-coded 23 kDa protease. This enzyme is synthesized late in infection and performs cleavages, leading to maturation, on 6 virus structural proteins: IIIa, pVI, pVII, pVIII, pTP and protein X (Webster et al. 1989). The enzyme is a cysteine protease of an as yet undetermined class and recognizes consensus sequences (M, L,I)XGX$\downarrow$G or (MLI)XGG$\downarrow$X (Webster et al. 1989). It also has the unusual characteristic of requiring for activation a disulphide-bonded dimer of an 11 residue peptide derived from the C terminus of polypeptide pVI (Webster, Hay and Kemp 1993). Recent investigations have also shown that, in an in vitro assay, pVI will bind to the principal capsid component, the hexon, but binding is very significantly enhanced whenever pVI is cleaved by the protease (Matthews and Russell 1994). This suggests that the primary maturation event is the interaction of adenovirus protease with pVI in a 'young' virion, i.e. that formed by the introduction of virus DNA and associated proteins into the precapsid. The protease is then activated, allowing cleavage of pVI to VI accompanied by tight binding to hexons, probably also with conformational changes leading to the proteolytic cascade that marks virion maturation.

Table 15.1 Polypeptides encoded by human adenovirus serotype 2 (prototype)

Mol. mass (kDa)	Transcription class	Description
13, 27, 32	E1A	NS
16, 21, 55	E1B	NS
59	E2A	NS; 72 kDa[a] DBP
120	E2B	NS; 140 kDa[a] DNA pol
75	E2B	S; Term[b], 80 kDa[a] pTP
4, 7, 8, 10, 12 13, 15, 15, 19	E3	NS
7, 13, 13, 14 15, 17	E4	NS
47	L1	NS[b]; maturation 52/55 kDa[a]
64	L1	S (IIIa)[b], p-protein
10	L2	S (X)[b]; and μ
22	L2	S (pVII); major core[b]
42	L2	S (V); minor core
63	L2	S (III); penton[a]
23	L3	S; protease
27	L3	S (pVI)[b]
109	L3	S (II); hexon
25	L4	NS; 33 kDa[a] p-protein
25	L4	S (pVIII)[b]
90	L4	NS; 100 kDa[a]
62	L5	S (IV); fibre
14	Intermediate	S (IX)
51	Intermediate	S (IVa2)

Polypeptide molecular weights deduced from sequence data. Mol. wts rounded to nearest kDa are presented as unmodified and uncleaved gene products.
The E1A gene products are also described in terms of the number of residues: E1A: 123R, 243R, 289R; E1B: 155R, 175R, 495R. E1B-175R is also called E1B-19K. DBP, DNA binding protein; DNA pol, DNA polymerase; NS, non-structural; p-protein, phosphoprotein; S, structural; Term, terminal protein.
[a]Mol. wts are significantly different from those obtained by SDS-PAGE.
[b]Cleaved by viral protease; other ORFs are not yet identified.

These events take place in the cell nucleus and many thousands of virions can be assembled, often in paracrystalline assays. In some cells the assembly process seems to be inefficient, so that many structural proteins (mostly capsomers) are made in excess and these can also form paracrystalline arrays (Wills et al. 1973). Release of the virus results from disintegration of the host cell. Abortive infections by adenovirus can occur whereby some of the early genes are expressed and, given the appropriate circumstances, can lead to morphogical transformation and tumour formation. There are also indications that adenoviruses can persist in vivo, engendering life-long immunity.

2.6 Antigens

As noted in section 2.1 (p. 281), the Adenoviridae are divided into two genera on the basis of their cross-reacting (or 'group') antigens and further subdivided into serotypes based on neutralization. Most adenoviruses can haemagglutinate rat or monkey cells and this characteristic has been used to subgroup the human adenoviruses and to confirm serospecificity (Table 15.2). These subgroups also correlate to some extent with clinical patterns (see section 3.1 and Table 15.3) and with the ability to induce tumours in hamsters. The utility of these serological assays has undoubtedly been enhanced by the relatively large amount of antigens (mostly associated with the capsomers) released during infection.

The serotype-specific antigens are located on the surface of the virions and are responsible for the formation of the neutralizing antibodies. Both hexons and fibres can induce neutralizing antibodies, whereas pentons and fibres appear to function in haemagglutination. The hexon serotype-specific antigens can be assigned to the tower regions of the structure (see Fig. 15.3) whereas the genus-specific antigens can be postulated to reside on the basal surfaces of the hexons at the region where they interact with each other and with polypeptide VI (Matthews and Russell 1994).

A range of hexon and fibre monoclonal antibodies has been prepared and has been instrumental in defining type and group specificities as well as antigenic relationships both within and between subgroups (Russell et al. 1981, Watson, Burdon and Russell 1988); they have also proved useful in diagnosis (see section 3.5, p. 289).

Classification of adenoviruses by serological procedures has been supplemented more recently by restriction enzyme analysis of virus DNA extracted from infected cells. By using a defined and limited range of restriction enzymes, patterns characteristic of adenovirus serotypes can be obtained; furthermore, this approach allows analysis into defined 'genotypes' (Kemp and Hierholzer 1986, Johansson et al. 1991).

3 CLINICAL AND PATHOLOGICAL ASPECTS

Adenoviruses are widespread in many species and can be isolated from both sick and healthy individuals. Antibodies can be detected in almost all humans, reflecting infection early in childhood and possibly lifelong persistence in adenoid and lung tissues. Mortality and morbidity associated with infection are relatively low and undoubtedly ensure that the virus retains its biological niche. Nevertheless, pneumonia and gastrointestinal disease can be serious.

3.1 Clinical manifestations

Adenovirus infections are mostly asymptomatic but may be associated with diseases of the respiratory, ocular and gastrointestinal systems (Table 15.3). Volunteers have been infected by rubbing virus into their conjunctivae or by administration of aerosols but, in general, it has been difficult to demonstrate unequivocally that the viruses cause disease, because they can be found in apparently normal tonsils and adenoids. Infections with human adenovirus serotypes 1, 2, 3, 5 and 6 usually take place in early childhood, giving mild respiratory infections. It has been suggested that

Table 15.2 Subgrouping of human adenoviruses: haemagglutination and oncogenicity

Subgroup	Serotypes	Species giving HA titres	Oncogenicity in hamsters
A	12, 18, 31	Rat (incomplete)	High
B	3, 7, 11, 14, 16, 21, 34, 35	Monkey	Weak
C	1, 2, 5, 6	Rat (incomplete)	No
D	8, 9, 37	Rat, mouse, human, guinea pig, dog	No
	10, 19, 26, 27, 36, 38, 39	Rat, mouse, human	
	13, 43	Rat, mouse, human, monkey	
	15, 22, 23, 30, 44–47	Rat, mouse, monkey	
	17, 24, 32, 33, 42	Rat, mouse	
	20, 25, 28, 29	Rat, monkey	
E	4	Rat (incomplete)	No
F	40, 41	Rat (atypical)	No

The subgrouping is based on a variety of criteria: differential haemagglutination, fibre length, oncogenic potential in rodents, percentage DNA homology, G + C content of viral DNAs and the ability to recombine with other members of the subgroup (see Horwitz 1990 for a more detailed explanation). Table derived from information presented by Hierholzer (1992) and Horwitz (1990).

Table 15.3 Subgrouping of human adenoviruses; association with disease

Syndrome	Principal serotypes involved in subgroups					
	A	B	C	D	E	F
Upper respiratory illness	...	All	...	...	...	...
Lower respiratory illness	...	3, 7, 21	...	...	4	...
Pertussis syndrome	...	...	5	...	...	...
Acute respiratory disease	...	7, 21	...	...	4	...
Pharyngoconjunctival fever	...	3, 7	...	...	4	...
Epidemic keratoconjunctivitis	...	...	...	8, 19, 37	...	...
Acute haemorrhagic conjunctivitis	...	11	...	...	...	...
Acute haemorrhagic cystitis	...	7, 11, 21, 35	...	...	...	...
Immunocompromised host disease	31	All	All	29, 30, 37, 43, 45	...	...
Infant gastroenteritis[a]	31	...	2	...	...	40, 41
Central nervous system disease	...	3, 7	...	...	...	...
Sexually transmitted disease[b]	...	...	2	19, 37	...	...

[a]Gastroenteritis is due predominantly to types 40 and 41 and to a lesser extent to types 2 and 31.
[b]Penile and labial ulcers and urethritis.
Table derived from information presented by Hierholzer (1992) and Horwitz (1990).

these infections may well induce sufficient immunological defences to modulate the progress of subsequent infections by related serotypes. The importance of adenoviruses in paediatric respiratory tract infection is not as great as that of respiratory syncytial and parainfluenza viruses, and it has been estimated that only about 5–10% of paediatric respiratory infection can be attributed to them. Nevertheless, acute respiratory infections in children (with some mortality) have been reported, particularly in association with type 7 (Kajon and Wadell 1992). Adenovirus respiratory infections may also be important in military recruits, of whom 30–80% may become infected, usually with types 4, 7, 14 or 21; up to 20% may require hospitalization. This morbidity has such an effect on training schedules that the US government invested heavily in the development of appropriate vaccines. Explosive outbreaks have also been reported in boarding schools and other institutions where young people live in close association.

Epidemic keratoconjunctivitis ('shipyard eye') was first associated with adenovirus type 8, but other serotypes (e.g. 3, 4, 7, 19 and 37) have also been incriminated in this syndrome. Adenovirus type 11 has been associated with haemorrhagic cystitis in school-age boys, and cases have been reported after renal and bone marrow transplantation. Adenoviruses are often a problem in patients undergoing immunosuppressive treatment and in AIDS patients. Indeed, a range of new serotypes was first isolated from patients with AIDS (Hierholzer 1992), suggesting that persistent long-term infection by adenoviruses kept under control by immune surveillance may be the usual situation.

The role of adenoviruses in gastrointestinal disease is, however, much more important; infection of the colon and the gut can cause severe diarrhoea and acute gastroenteritis, especially in developing countries. Serotypes 40 and 41 seem to be mainly responsible for these outbreaks and the viruses can be detected in large numbers in the faeces of infected children. Up to 15% of children hospitalized with acute gastroenteritis can be attributed to these enteric adenoviruses, second only to rotaviruses as the cause of infantile viral diarrhoea. It is interesting that faecal shedding of adenoviruses appears to be a characteristic of all serotypes, but types 40 and 41 are particularly associated with enteric disease. The tropisms of these serotypes differ from those of others in that they fail to infect standard tissue cell lines such as HeLa and Hep2 and require primary human kidney cells or the adenovirus-transformed human cell line 293 (Graham et al. 1977).

Adenovirus infections are common in many animal species. As in humans, they appear to be mostly asymptomatic and there is therefore a paucity of information on the mode and mechanics of virus transmission. There is some evidence that a virus that is asymptomatic in its natural host can produce disease in other species. Thus epidemics of reduced laying and production of soft shell or shell-less eggs in some chicken flocks have been attributed to a duck adenovirus (EDS'76). As in humans, most of the animal adenoviruses can be isolated from the tissues of healthy animals and there is very little evidence that they cause disease in wild populations. Nevertheless, two serotypes of canine adenovirus (CAV) do seem to cause different patterns of disease: CAV-1 is responsible for infectious canine hepatitis and, along with CAV-2, is among the viruses causing the 'kennel cough' syndrome. Epizoötic infections with CAV-1 in foxes, bears, wolves, coyotes and skunks have also been reported. CAV-2, on the other hand, seems to be confined to infections of the canine respiratory tract (reviewed by Russell 1994).

3.2 Epidemiology

Adenovirus infections are widespread and appear to be transmitted primarily by the faecal–oral rather than the respiratory route. The latter may, however, be more important for the lower numbered human serotypes. Seasonal variation of adenovirus epidemics is well recognized. Most outbreaks of pharyngoconjunctival fever in school-age children occur in summer; in contrast, epidemics in military recruits appear almost exclusively in the winter.

Infections with adenoviruses occur early in life: by 5 years of age almost all children have been infected by at least one, generally a low numbered serotype. The epidemiology of individual serotypes has been elucidated in more detail by using restriction enzyme analysis to distinguish between isolates of type-specific viruses. In this way, the provenance of particular genotypes within these serotypes (e.g. Ad8, Ad19, Ad37) can be traced in the population. Such studies suggest that some genotypes may be associated with increased morbidities (Kajon and Wadell 1992). They also indicate that multiple persistent infections probably provide opportunities for recombinational events.

3.3 Pathogenesis and pathology

In susceptible cells, adenoviruses cause early rounding and aggregation, followed by the appearance of characteristic basophilic nuclear inclusions. In organ cultures of human embryonic nasal mucosa and trachea, they infect and destroy the ciliated epithelium and it is likely that the same process occurs in vivo. Although organs outside the respiratory tract may be affected during severe adenovirus infection, replication rarely occurs unless the patient is immunologically compromised.

Considerable progress has been made in our understanding of adenovirus pathogenesis by studies in cotton rats (*Sigmodon hispidus*). These animals are susceptible to intranasal infection with human adenovirus type 5 (and other members of subgroup C), developing pulmonary histopathology very similar to that in human cases (Prince et al. 1993). The virus replicates in the bronchiolar epithelial cells, but in situ hybridization also shows early gene expression in macrophages/monocytes and in both alveoli and hilar lymph nodes. It is interesting that only early gene expression is needed to produce the pathology, of which there is an 'early' and a 'late' phase. The early (*E3*) region, which does not function in viral replication, plays an important role in the natural history of infection by at least the subgroup C viruses, which appear to produce latent infections in lymphocytes. The 19 kDa glycoprotein (see Table 15.1) markedly reduces transport of class I MHC components to the surface of infected cells and thereby thwarts attack by cytotoxic T cells. The E3 14.7 kDa protein reduces the presence of polymorphonuclear leucocytes in the early-phase pathological inflammatory exudate. The E1B 55 kDa polypeptide is essential to the late phase, which affects peribronchiolar and perivascular regions with an infiltrate consisting almost exclusively of lymphocytes. In both phases the predominant process is the response of the host to infection, rather than direct viral damage to cells. Only early genes seem to be

required to induce pathological changes in cotton rats and it was possible to demonstrate that tumour necrosis factor α (TNF-α), interleukin-1 (IL-1) and IL-6 are elaborated during the first 2–3 days of infection; but only TNF-α seems to play a major role in the early phase of pathogenesis. In nude mice this late inflammatory response does not appear, indicating that it derives primarily from T cells. Steroids too can almost eliminate the pneumonic inflammatory response to infection (Yang et al. 1995).

The importance in pathogenesis of proteins derived from early genes has been further emphasized by the observation that E1B products confer a survival function in adenovirus-infected cells and prevent premature cell death or apoptosis. It appears that the E1A proteins inactivate several cellular factors, thereby inducing apoptosis, whereas the E1B proteins effectively counteract this process (Subramanian et al. 1984, Sabbatini et al. 1995).

3.4 Immune response

Adenoviruses induce the full spectrum of responses from the immune system. The humoral response, which includes type-specific antibodies, plays a major role in protection and this observation led to the development of effective vaccines for military recruits. The finding that crystalline hexon could also confer protection indicated the importance of structural proteins in inducing immunity (unpublished observations).

The response to adenovirus infection by the immune system is efficient and well orchestrated and undoubtedly accounts for the generally low levels of morbidity. Cell-mediated responses are mounted but the virus can counteract most of these by means of products expressed from the *E3* gene cassette. One of these, gp19 kDa (of Ad2) is an abundant trans-membrane protein which binds class I MHC antigens and retains the complex in the endoplasmic reticulum. Since surface expression of class I antigens complexed with viral peptides is required for recognition and lysis by virus-specific cytotoxic T cells (CTLs), this strategy effectively thwarts the host T cell response. Although CTLs are one means by which the host eliminates virus-infected cells, there are others, involving secretion of cytokines such as TNF. It appears that E1A-derived proteins can induce susceptibility to TNF lysis, but this can be initiated by yet another *E3* gene product (14.7 kDa in Ad2) and by the E1B 19 kDa product (in human cells). Two other *E3* gene products, 10.4 kDa and 14.5 kDa, also participate in this protective response by co-operating to down-regulate the EGF receptor in infected cells, thus interfering with signal transduction (Yang et al. 1995). It is interesting that the *E3* promoter is unique among the adenoviral promoters in that it contains binding sites for E1A-independent transcription of *E3* in lymphoid cells and this may explain why adenoviruses (especially of subgroup C) appear to persist in lymphoid tissues (Williams et al. 1990).

The proliferative T cell responses in humans are mediated by CD4+ T cells, and structural proteins are important targets. In addition, proliferative responses to the uncommon adenovirus type 35 have been found in individuals without serological evidence of previous Ad35 infection (Flomenberg et al. 1995).

These findings suggest that CD4+ cells recognize conserved antigens and that this may play a role in modulating infections with a range of serotypes. Cellular and humoral immune responses have been of intense interest following the development of recombinant adenovirus vaccines as vehicles for gene therapy (Graham 1990, Wilson 1993) (see also Chapter 160). These techniques have appeared to be most promising in delivering the *CTFR* gene to the airways of cystic fibrosis patients. However, expression of the correct gene is only transient and is associated with the development of inflammation. Furthermore, the efficacy of the recombinant adenovirus becomes much less with repeated doses and this seems to be related to the accentuated induction of a multifactorial immune response (Yang et al. 1995).

3.5 Diagnosis

Adenovirus infections are ideally diagnosed by isolation of virus from appropriate clinical samples in a variety of sensitive indicator cell cultures such as HeLa, Hep2, KB or A549. The use of the 293 line of adenovirus-transformed cells also facilitates the isolation of the enteric adenoviruses 40 and 41. Rounding and aggregation of cells appear after incubation for 1–4 weeks. The culture fluids containing virus and soluble antigens can be used to characterize the virus further by neutralization and by haemagglutination inhibition (see Table 15.2).

More sensitive and rapid tests have been introduced over the last few years and have found a place in many diagnostic laboratories. They include, for example, enzyme immunoassays (Gleaves, Militoni and Ashley 1993), latex agglutination (Grandien et al. 1987), immunoelectron microscopy (Wood et al. 1988), and hybridization with synthetic nucleotide probes (Scott-

Taylor et al. 1993). Characterization of serotypes by restriction enzyme mapping is also of significant value.

The most sensitive technique for antigen recognition is the polymerase chain reaction (PCR). The use of primers based on the group-specific region of the hexon provides a rapid method of detecting all the human serotypes (Allard et al. 1990).

Other pairs of primers have been devised that successfully detected each of the two enteric adenoviruses Ad40 and 41 (Allard et al. 1990, Roussell et al. 1993). There seems little doubt that, as sequence information becomes available, it should be possible to devise appropriate primers for detecting and distinguishing all the serotypes of adenoviruses.

3.6 Control

Vaccination has been used with some success to control epidemics of adenovirus infection in military recruits and in bovines. Both inactivated and live adenovirus vaccines have been used in military recruits but live vaccines proved more effective in reducing the incidence of disease. Initial development concentrated on type 4; unattenuated virus was fed to volunteers in enteric-coated capsules to establish an asymptomatic infection in the lower alimentary tract. The virus induced moderate amounts of neutralizing antibody and, more important, did not spread to susceptible contacts. The type 4 vaccines grown in human diploid cells have been given to several hundred thousand military recruits with no untoward side effects and with a significant reduction in morbidity. A triple vaccine incorporating types 4, 7 and 21 was also successful (Takafuji et al. 1979). Vaccines have not, however, been released for use in the general population; the cost of development, production and control would be quite substantial and not commensurate with the risk of clinically significant infection.

REFERENCES

Allard A, Girones R et al., 1990, Polymerase chain reaction for detection of adenoviruses in stool samples, *J Clin Microbiol*, **28**: 2659–67.

Defer G, Berlin M-T et al., 1990, Human adenovirus–host cell interactions: comparative study with members of subgroups B and C, *J Virol*, **64**: 3661–73.

Enders JF, Bell JA et al., 1956, 'Adenovirus' – group name proposed for new respiratory tract viruses, *Science*, **124**: 119–20.

Flomenberg P, Piaskowski V et al., 1995, Characterisation of human T cell responses to adenovirus, *J Infect Dis*, **171**: 1090–6.

Fredman JN, Engler JA, 1993, Adenovirus precursor to terminal protein interacts with the nuclear matrix *in vivo* and *in vitro*, *J Virol*, **67**: 3384–95.

Gleaves CA, Militoni J, Ashley RL, 1993, An enzyme immunoassay for the detection of adenovirus in clinical specimens, *Diagn Microbiol Infect Dis*, **17**: 57–9.

Graham FL, 1990, Adenoviruses as expression vectors and recombinant vaccines, *Trends Biotechnol*, **8**: 85–7.

Graham FL, Smiley J et al., 1977, Characteristics of a human cell line transformed by DNA from human adenovirus type 5, *J Gen Virol*, **36**: 59–65.

Grandien M, Pettersson CA et al., 1987, Latex agglutination test for adenovirus diagnosis in diarrhoeal disease, *J Med Virol*, **23**: 311–16.

Hay RT, Russell WC, 1989, Recognition mechanisms in the synthesis of animal virus DNA, *Biochem J*, **258**: 3–16.

Hierholzer JC, 1992, Adenoviruses in the immunocompromised host, *Clin Microbiol Rev*, **5**: 262–74.

Hillemann MR, Werner JR, 1954, Recovery of a new agent from patients with acute respiratory illness, *Proc Soc Exp Biol Med*, **85**: 183–8.

Horwitz MS, 1990, Adenoviridae and their replication, *Virology*, 2nd edn, eds Fields BH, Krupe DM, Raven Press, New York, 1679–721.

Johansson ME, Brown M et al., 1991, Genome analysis of adenovirus type 31 strains from immunocompromised and immunocompetent patients, *J Infect Dis*, **163**: 293–9.

Kajon AE, Wadell G, 1992, Molecular epidemiology of adenoviruses associated with acute lower respiratory disease of children in Buenos Aires, Argentina (1984–1988), *J Med Virol*, **36**: 292–7.

Kemp M, Hierholzer JC, 1986, Three adenovirus type 8 genome types defined by restriction enzyme analyses: prototype stability in geographically separated populations, *J Clin Microbiol*, **23**: 469–74.

McDougall JK, Dunn AR, Gallimore PH, 1995, Recent studies on the characterization of adenovirus infected and transformed cells, *Cold Spring Harbor Symp Quant Biol*, **39**: 591–600.

Matthews DA, Russell WC, 1994, Adenovirus protein–protein interactions: hexon and protein VI, *J Gen Virol*, **75**: 3365–74.

Mautner V, 1989, Adenoviridae, *Andrewes' Viruses of Vertebrates*, 5th edn, ed Porterfield JS, Baillière Tindall, London, 249–82.

Patterson S, Russell WC, 1983, Ultrastructural and immunofluorescent studies of early events in adenovirus–HeLa cell interactions, *J Gen Virol*, **64**: 1091–9.

Porterfield JS, 1989, Parvoviridae, *Andrewes' Viruses of Vertebrates*, 5th edn, ed Porterfield JS, Baillière Tindall, London, 371–94.

Prince GA, Porter DD et al., 1993, Pathogenesis of adenovirus type 5 pneumonia in cotton rats (*Sigmodon hispidus*), *J Virol*, **67**: 101–11.

Rekosh DMK, Russell WC et al., 1977, Identification of a protein linked to the ends of adenovirus DNA, *Cell*, **11**: 283–95.

Roberts MM, White JL et al., 1986, Three-dimensional structure of the adenovirus major coat protein hexon, *Science*, **232**: 1148–51.

Roberts RJ, Akusjarvi G et al., 1986, A consensus sequence for the adenovirus 2 genome, *Dev Mol Virol*, **8**: 1–51.

Roussell J, Zajdel MEB et al., 1993, Rapid detection of enteric adenoviruses by means of the polymerase chain reaction, *J Infection*, **27**: 271–5.

Rowe WP, Huebner RJ et al., 1953, Isolation of a cytopathogenic agent from human adenoids undergoing spontaneous degeneration in tissue culture, *Proc Soc Exp Biol Med*, **84**: 570–3.

Russell WC, 1994, Animal adenoviruses, *Encyclopaedia of Virology*, Academic Press, New York, 14–17.

Russell WC, Kemp GD, 1995, Role of adenovirus structural components in the regulation of adenovirus infection, *The Molecular Repertoire of Adenovirus*, vol. 1, eds Doerfler W, Bohm P, Springer Verlag, Berlin, 81–98.

Russell WC, Valentine RA, Pereira HG, 1967, The effect of heat on the anatomy of adenovirus, *J Gen Virol*, **1**: 509–22.

Russell WC, Patel G et al., 1981, Monoclonal antibodies against adenovirus type 5: preparation and preliminary characterisation, *J Gen Virol*, **56**: 393–408.

Russell WC, Adrian T et al., 1995, Adenoviridae. In Virus Taxonomy, Classification and Nomenclature of Viruses, 6th Report, *Arch Virol*, **suppl.10**: 128–33.

Sabbatini P, Chou S-K et al., 1995, Modulation of p53-mediated transcriptional repression and apoptosis by the adenovirus E1B 19K protein, *Mol Cell Biol*, **15**: 1060–70.

Schaak J, Ho WY-W et al., 1990, Adenovirus terminal protein mediates both nuclear matrix association and efficient transcription of adenovirus DNA, *Genes Dev*, **4**: 1197–208.

Scott-Taylor T, Akluwalia G et al., 1993, Detection of enteric adenoviruses with synthetic oligonucleotide probes, *J Med Virol*, **41**: 328–37.

Shenk T, Flint SJ, 1991, Transcriptional and transforming activities of the adenovirus E1A proteins, *Adv Cancer Res*, **57**: 47–85.

Stewart PL, Fuller D, Burnett R, 1993, Difference imaging of adenovirus: bridging the restriction gap between x-ray crystallography and electron microscopy, *EMBO J*, **12**: 2589–99.

Subramanian T, Kuppuswamy M et al., 1984, 19 kDa tumor antigen coded by early region E1b of adenovirus 2 is required for efficient synthesis and for protection of viral DNA, *J Biol Chem*, **259**: 11777–83.

Takafuji ET, Gaydos JC et al., 1979, Simultaneous administration of live, enteric-coated adenovirus types 4, 7 and 21 vaccines: safety and immunogenicity, *J Infect Dis*, **140**: 48–53.

Toogood CIA, Crompton J, Hay RT, 1992, Antipeptide sera define neutralising epitopes on the adenovirus hexon, *J Gen Virol*, **73**: 1429–35.

Trentin JJ, Yabe Y, Taylor G, 1962, The quest for human cancer viruses, *Science*, **137**: 835–41.

Watson G, Burdon MG, Russell WC, 1988, An antigenic analysis of the adenovirus type 2 fibre polypeptide, *J Gen Virol*, **69**: 525–35.

Webster A, Hay RT, Kemp GD, 1993, The adenovirus proteases is activated by a virus-coded disulphide-linked peptide, *Cell*, **72**: 97–104.

Webster A, Russell S et al., 1989, Characterisation of the adenovirus proteinase: substrate specificity, *J Gen Virol*, **70**: 3224–34.

Wickham TJ, Mathias P et al., 1993, Integrins $\alpha_v\beta_3$ and $\alpha_v\beta_5$ promote adenovirus internalisation but not virus attachment, *Cell*, **73**: 309–19.

Williams JL, Garcia J et al., 1990, Lymphoid specific gene expression of the adenovirus early region 3 promoter is mediated by NF-κB binding motifs, *EMBO J*, **9**: 4435–42.

Wills EJ, Russell WC, Williams JF, 1973, Adenovirus-induced crystals: studies with temperature sensitive mutants, *J Gen Virol*, **20**: 407–11.

Wilson JM, 1993, Vehicles for gene therapy, *Nature (London)*, **365**: 691–2.

Wold WSM, Goding LR, 1991, Region E3 of adenovirus: a cassette of genes involved in host immunosurveillance and virus–cell interactions, *Virology*, **184**: 1–8.

Wood DJ, Longhurst R et al., 1988, One year prospective cross-sectional study to assess the importance of Group F adenovirus infections in children under 2 years admitted to hospital, *J Med Virol*, **26**: 429–35.

Yang Y, Hildegun CJE et al., 1995, Cellular and humoral immune responses to viral antigens create barriers to lung-directed gene therapy with recombinant adenoviruses, *J Virol*, **69**: 2004–11.

Chapter 16

PAPOVAVIRUSES

H zur Hausen

1 GENERAL DESCRIPTION

The family *Papovaviridae* contains 2 genera, *Polyomavirus* and *Papillomavirus*. They differ substantially in genomic organization and biological properties, although the morphology of the virions is similar.

Polyomaviruses frequently cause inapparent infections in susceptible hosts which may reactivate under immunosuppression and then result in overt disease. Representatives of this virus group infecting humans are the BK and JC viruses. Both are widespread in virtually all human populations; no recognizable disease is associated with the primary infection. Under prolonged immunosuppression, however, JC virus may cause a rare demyelinating disease, progressive multifocal leucoencephalopathy (PML), whereas reactivation of BK, and to a lesser extent JC, may result in haemorrhagic urinary tract infections. Polyomavirus infections are also found in a number of animal species: monkeys, cattle, mice, hamsters and even birds. Again, they usually cause inapparent persistent infections; the exceptions are murine K virus, which causes acute pneumonia in newborn mice, and the hamster polyomavirus, which gives rise to skin papillomas and lymphomas in its natural host. With the possible exception of avian polyomaviruses, all members of this group are oncogenic when injected into newborn rodents.

Papillomaviruses are characteristically epitheliotropic and cause proliferative lesions in infected epidermal or mucosal epithelia. They are commonly designated wart viruses, although many members of the group induce only discrete lesions that differ histologically from common warts. This virus group is remarkably heterogeneous and contains more than 75 human pathogenic genotypes (de Villiers 1994). Some of these types are causally involved in cancer of the cervix and other anogenital cancers and their precursor lesions (zur Hausen 1994a, 1994b); others have been linked to cancers in the rare hereditary condition, epidermodysplasia verruciformis (EV) (Orth et al. 1979). Non-melanoma skin cancers were also shown to contain novel human papillomavirus (HPV) genotypes (Shamanin et al. 1994, Berkhout et al. 1995). The relationship of members of this virus group to these widely distributed cancers has evoked intense interest in their molecular and biological properties, in their interaction with the infected cell and in host defence mechanisms engaged in the control of viral carcinogenesis.

The first part of this chapter characterizes the structure, biological properties and pathogenesis of polyomaviruses. The second deals primarily with human pathogenic papillomaviruses, with emphasis on genotypes known or suspected to be carcinogenic.

2 POLYOMAVIRUSES

2.1 Morphology and genome organization

Table 16.1 lists representative members of the polyomavirus group.

The diameter of polyomavirus particles is c. 45 nm. The virion contains 72 capsomers arranged with icosahedral symmetry. The particles contain a closed, double-stranded, circular DNA consisting of 4700–5300 nucleotide base pairs. Sequence analysis reveals a basically similar genome organization among members of the polyomavirus group. This is outlined schematically in Fig. 16.1.

The genome is almost equally divided into an 'early' and a 'late' region. With the exception of murine and hamster polyomaviruses, the early region codes for 2 proteins, **large T antigen** and **small t antigen**. Murine and hamster polyomaviruses code in addition for a third protein, **middle t antigen**. All these proteins play a role in stimulating the growth of infected cells. The late region codes for 3 structural proteins, VP1, VP2 and VP3, that form the structure of the viral particles and determine host range and infectivity.

Table 16.1 Polyomaviruses

Virus	Host
BK virus	Human
JC virus	Human
Simian virus 40 (SV40)	Rhesus monkey
B-lymphotropic papovavirus	African green monkey
Simian agent 12 (SA12)	Baboon
Bovine polyomavirus	Cattle
Rabbit kidney vacuolating agent	Rabbit
Polyomavirus	Mouse
K virus	Mouse
Hamster papovavirus	Hamster
Budgerigar fledgling disease virus	Budgerigar

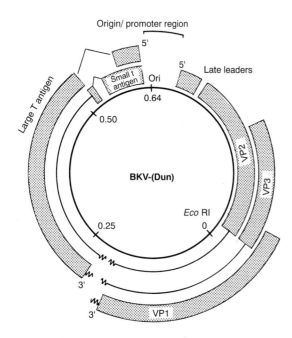

Fig. 16.1 The organization of the BKV-(Dun) genome. Transcription occurs bidirectionally, the early genes being transcribed in an anticlockwise, the late genes in a clockwise, direction. (Modified from McCance and Gardner 1987.)

2.2 Pathogenesis of animal polyomavirus infections

Exposure of the natural hosts to animal polyomaviruses regularly results in asymptomatic infections, with long-lasting persistence of the viruses and the development of neutralizing antibodies. Persistence has been demonstrated predominantly in neuronal tissue and within the kidneys. Primary infection with K virus in newborn mice causes interstitial pneumonia (Greenlee 1979). Pneumonia has also been observed as the consequence of primary infection of budgerigar fledglings with an avian polyomavirus.

2.3 Immortalization and transformation by polyomaviruses and oncogenicity

The early proteins of polyomaviruses are responsible not only for extending the lifespan of infected cells but also for the relatively rare induction of continued growth of cultured cells ('immortalization') and for malignant changes ('transformation'), shown by the induction of malignant tumours upon injection of transformed cells into immunocompromised animals or by inoculation of these viruses into newborn rodents. Such inoculations result in tumours arising after latency periods of several months or even >1 year. Although immortalization and induction of malignant tumours clearly depend on the expression of these viral oncogenes, their expression *per se* is not sufficient for these cellular changes and requires in addition the modification of specific host cell genes (Pereira-Smith and Smith 1981, zur Hausen 1991, Whitaker, Kidston and Reddel 1992).

Large T antigen binds the cellular tumour suppressor proteins p53 and Rb (Lane and Crawford 1979, Linzer and Levine 1979, DeCaprio et al. 1988), apparently inactivating their function. Besides stimulating their progression through the cell cycle (Oshima et al. 1993), binding of p53 also contributes to the observed chromosomal instability of latently SV40-infected cells (Drews, Chan and Schnipper 1992, Laurent, Frances and Bastin 1995). Presumably by the same mechanism, T antigens efficiently antagonize the induction of cell death by apoptosis (Zheng et al. 1994).

Transformation-specific functions of polyomavirus T antigens have been analysed in some detail in cells infected with SV40 and murine polyomavirus. Infection of non-permissive rodent cells by SV40 virus leads to an abortive infection with the expression of viral early gene products and no late protein synthesis. Immortalization or transformation of these cells results in a drastically altered phenotype with loss of contact inhibition, anchorage independence and reduced serum requirements. The need of viral early gene expression for the induction of these changes has been demonstrated repeatedly: immortalization and transformation can be achieved by transfection of the early viral region only, and conditional mutants of SV40 and murine polyomavirus T antigens are immortalized and transformed only under permissive conditions (DiMayorca et al. 1969, Eckardt 1969, Abrahams et al. 1975, Martin and Chou 1975, Freund et al. 1992).

With the exception of murine and hamster polyomaviruses, oncogenicity of known members of this group in their natural hosts either does not occur or is a very rare event. SV40, the best-studied polyoma type virus, is not oncogenic in the rhesus monkey, its natural host. Furthermore, inadvertent inoculation into humans as a contaminant of poliomyelitis vaccines did not result in detectable oncogenicity, although unconfirmed individual reports suggested a 2-fold increase in neurological malignancies in children whose mothers received the contaminated poliovaccine during pregnancy (Heinonen et al. 1973), and SV40-like DNA has been reported in ependymomas and choroid plexus tumours (Berdsagel et al. 1992). The mechanism of protection of the natural hosts against the oncogenic properties of these viruses, which, however, are relatively efficient carcinogens in newborn rodents, is not entirely understood.

Murine polyomavirus induces a wide variety of different tumours upon inoculation into its natural host (Stewart, Eddy and Borgese 1958), with a predominance of salivary gland tumours when injected into newborn animals (Gross 1953) and of benign skin appendage tumours after infection of these animals at later ages (Dawe 1963). Hamster polyomavirus induces skin papillomas and lymphomas in its natural host, the Syrian hamster (Graffi et al. 1969).

The potential oncogenicity of T antigens of these viruses is underlined by experiments in mice transgenic for T antigens of SV40, the lymphotropic papovavirus or the human pathogenic members BK and JC (Ornitz et al. 1987, Dalrymple and Beemon 1990, Levine et al. 1991, Held et al. 1994a, 1994b). The use of organ-specific promoters even permits targeting of the tumour development to specific sites.

Persistence of viral DNA in immortalized or transformed cells frequently occurs at a low genome copy number, usually not more than 10 copies per cell. This DNA may become integrated into the host cell genome but may also persist in an episomal state in experimental as well as in natural infections.

In SV40-infected cells both the large T and the small t antigens play a role in transformation, although the large T antigen is sufficient for transformation in certain circumstances (Topp, Lane and Pollack 1980). The middle t antigen of murine polyomavirus is the major transforming protein of this virus subgroup.

2.4 Human pathogenic polyomaviruses

ORIGINAL ISOLATION AND CELL CULTURE STUDIES

The human pathogenic members of the polyomavirus group, BK and JC virus, were both isolated in 1971. BK was initially isolated from the urine of a renal transplant recipient receiving immunosuppressive therapy (Gardner et al. 1971). Although serological studies indicated that BK virus infections are ubiquitous in human populations, virus was isolated mainly from the urine of patients under immunosuppression. JC virus was isolated by Padgett et al. (1971) from the brain of a patient with Hodgkin's disease and PML.

BK virus, and JC virus even more so, replicates slowly or not at all in cell cultures. BK virus can be propagated in human embryonic kidney cells, human fibroblast cultures and several cell lines of African green monkey origin (e.g. Vero and BSC-1). The infectious cycle seems to be longer than that of SV40 virus. JC virus grows predominantly in primary human glial cells and human vascular endothelial cells (Fareed, Takemoto and Gimbrone 1978). Certain strains have also been adapted to growth in other cell cultures. Heilbronn and co-workers (1993) have shown that human cytomegalovirus acts as an efficient helper for JC virus replication in human fibroblasts. Infections by members of the *Herpesviridae* (Schlehofer et al. 1983), and treatment by chemical and physical carcinogens (Lavi 1981, Matz et al. 1985), regularly result in a substantial amplification of latent polyomavirus genomes.

CLINICAL ASPECTS OF HUMAN POLYOMAVIRUS INFECTIONS

Primary infections are usually asymptomatic. Antibodies to BK and JC viruses can be detected in childhood; c. 70–80% of adults possess either neutralizing or haemagglutinating antibodies. Latent viral DNA can be detected by the polymerase chain reaction in human brain tissue and in peripheral blood leucocytes (Arthur, Dagostin and Shah 1989, Atwood et al. 1992, Elsner and Dörries 1992).

Virus has been isolated from immunologically compromised patients, including those receiving chemotherapy for malignant disease. In renal transplant recipients up to 40% have been reported to excrete BK virus (Hogan et al. 1988). This obviously results from reactivation of latent infection, and highlights the importance of immunological surveillance in these infections. Reactivation may lead to clinical disease, which may be life-threatening. In BK virus reactivation, haemorrhagic urinary tract infections, specifically those of the ureter and bladder, may represent serious post-transplant complications (Hogan et al. 1988). Similarly, reactivated BK virus can be recovered from the urine of c. 3% of women in the last trimester of pregnancy (Coleman et al. 1977).

Induction of disease as the consequence of JC virus reactivation under severe immunosuppression is documented in PML. This disease was first described in humans in 1958 (Astrom, Mancall and Richardson 1958). It develops in patients suffering from long-lasting immunosuppression caused by malignant conditions (e.g. Hodgkin's disease, lymphatic leukaemias, acquired immunodeficiency syndrome). Signs of neurological deterioration develop over a period of 3–6 months prior to death. Plaque-like foci of demyelination are widespread within the brains of PML patients; they contain oligodendroglial cells with basophilic nuclear inclusions and large astrocytic cells. Papovavirus-like particles were demonstrated within such lesions by electron microscopy (Silverman and Rubinstein 1965, Zu Rhein and Chou 1965). In 1971 Padgett and co-workers isolated JC virus from affected brain tissue in primary human fetal glial cells.

In PML, permissive infection of oligodendroglial cells by JC virus results in demyelinization. Astrocytes within these lesions show some characteristics of polyomavirus-transformed cells (Narayan 1976). Coexisting gliomas are occasionally found (Richardson 1965, Castaigne et al. 1974).

ONCOGENICITY OF HUMAN PATHOGENIC POLYOMAVIRUSES

Inoculation of newborn hamsters with BK virus induces ependymomas, choroid plexus tumours, insulinomas, osteosarcomas and fibrosarcomas (Costa et al. 1976, van der Noordaa 1976, Corallini et al. 1978, Uchida et al. 1979) and immortalizes and transforms various rodent and monkey cells in tissue culture (van der Noordaa 1976, Bradley and Dougherty 1978, Portolani et al. 1978). Abortive transformation of human cells (Portolani et al. 1978) and persistent infection of transformed human glial cells by BK virus have been reported (Takemoto et al. 1979).

JC virus is highly oncogenic in newborn hamsters (Walker et al. 1973) and produces cerebral tumours when injected into the brains of owl monkeys (London et al. 1978). Inoculation of this virus into hamster brains induces brain tumours of various histological types. Transformation of human amnion cells by BK virus has also been noted. The transformed cells contain a JC virus-specific T antigen. Animals transgenic for BK virus T antigens develop kidney carcinomas and thymoproliferative disorders (Dalrymple and Beemon 1990).

Neither BK nor JC virus has been found consistently in any human tumours. Their rare presence in brain tumours at copy numbers far lower than one per tumour cell seems to result from the harbouring by individual brain cells of latent DNA of these human papovaviruses (Pater et al. 1980). De Mattei and co-workers (1995) described the frequent occurrence of BK virus sequences not only in brain tumours, osteosarcomas and Ewing tumours but also in apparently normal brain tissue and peripheral blood samples. The significance of these findings, as well as that of the reported frequent occurrence of SV40 in human mesotheliomas (Carbone et al. 1994), remains to be assessed.

OTHER HUMAN PATHOGENIC POLYOMAVIRUSES

Whereas BK and JC viruses are widespread within all human populations tested, there are few reports of isolations of typical SV40 virus from PML cases and individual tumours (Weiner et al. 1972, Soriano, Shelbourne and Gokcen 1974). About 2–4% of the population of the USA possess neutralizing antibody to SV40 virus without known exposure to this agent (Shah 1972). A report of the presence of SV40 antigens in human mesotheliomas (Carbone et al. 1994) awaits confirmation.

A B-lymphotropic papovavirus (LPV) has been isolated from African green monkeys (zur Hausen and Gissmann 1979). This virus differs substantially in sequence composition from other known members of the polyomavirus group (Pawlita, Clad and zur Hausen 1985) and was found to infect human B lymphoma cells with high efficiency. Up to 20% of sera from adults contain antibodies to this virus that precipitate all structural proteins, some at high titre (Brade, Muller-Läntzsch and zur Hausen 1980),

suggesting infection by a closely related agent also present in the human population. Until now, however, attempts to isolate a human LPV have been unsuccessful.

2.5 Laboratory diagnosis of polyomavirus infections

It is important to do diagnostic tests for human polyomavirus in patients under prolonged immunosuppression who develop urinary tract infections, particularly haemorrhagic cystitis, and in those with suspected PML. Virus particles can be demonstrated in urine samples from such patients by electron microscopy after negative staining. They can also be found in oligodendrocytes in brain sections from PML patients. The type of the infecting virus can be identified by using type-specific primer combinations in the polymerase chain reaction.

Serological tests for BK and JC viruses are of limited value in view of the high prevalence of antibodies within the human adult population. Haemagglutination inhibition tests with human group O erythrocytes, ELISA tests and related assays are the most frequently used. In addition, immunofluorescence and in situ hybridization procedures can be used to study infected cells and tissues.

Isolation of these viruses from clinical specimens is usually difficult. This is particularly true of JC virus, because isolations depend on the availability of primary human embryonic glial cell cultures. BK virus grows in a number of primary human cells (e.g. human fibroblasts and kidney cells) and can be adapted to established cell cultures. However, cytopathic changes, consisting of gradual degeneration of the infected cell layer, often take weeks to develop after inoculation.

2.6 Treatment

There is no specific treatment for polyomavirus infections.

3 PAPILLOMAVIRUSES

3.1 Morphology and genome organization

The diameter of HPV particles (Fig. 16.2) is c. 55 nm. They contain a circular dsDNA molecule of 7.2–8.0 kbp. Their lack of an envelope renders these viruses relatively resistant to heating and to organic solvents (Bonnez et al. 1994).

Papillomaviruses cannot be grown in cell cultures. Virus-like particles containing the structural components of various types of HPV can, however, be obtained by the expression of these proteins in recombinant vectors (Kirnbauer et al. 1992, Hagensee, Yaegashi and Galloway 1993); obviously the L1 protein suffices for formation of these particles. This protein has a molecular weight of c. 55 kDa and is highly conserved among different papillomavirus types. The

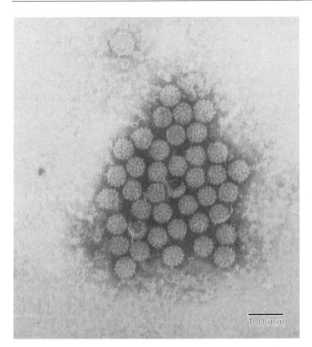

Fig. 16.2 Electron micrograph of a cluster of papillomavirus particles, negatively stained. Bar = 100 nm.

GENOME STRUCTURE AND GENE PROPERTIES

Papillomavirus genomes can be divided into 3 regions: a long control region (*LCR*) covering about 10% of the genome, an early (*E*) and a late (*L*) region. The *L* genes code for structural proteins, the *E* region mainly for regulatory functions concerned with genome persistence, DNA replication and activation of the lytic cycle. The structure of the genome is outlined schematically in Fig. 16.3.

The *E5*, *E6* and *E7* genes code for growth-stimulating proteins; in certain types, *E6* and *E7* are involved in progression to malignancy. The interaction of E6 of some HPV types with the cellular protein p53 (Werness, Levine and Howley 1990) results in rapid degradation of the latter (Scheffner et al. 1990). The E7 protein of the same types forms a complex with the cellular tumour suppressor protein RB (Dyson et al. 1989), thereby releasing the cellular transcription factor E2F from binding to RB and activating the cell cycle.

E1 codes for a polycistronic RNA and is involved in viral DNA replication. The same is true of *E2*, which in addition regulates the transcription of HPV genomes from the *LCR* by forming dimers at specific binding sites. E4 proteins seem to be incorrectly assigned as early gene products. They seem to be involved in virus maturation and particle release and form a cytoplasmic network co-localizing with cytokeratin filaments (Doorbar et al. 1991).

second structural protein, L2, is less conserved; its molecular weight is c. 75 kDa.

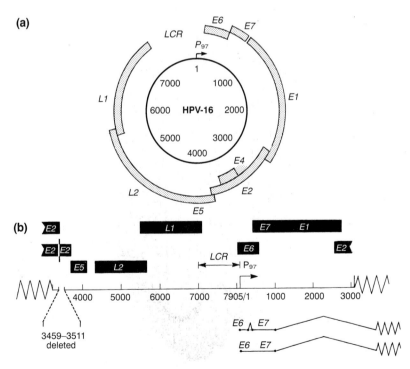

Fig. 16.3 (a) Circular map of the HPV-16 genome. Early (*E*) and late (*L*) open reading frames as well as the long control region are indicated. Transcription occurs from one strand only in a clockwise direction. (b) Structure of the integrated HPV-16 DNA in the human cervical cancer cell line SiHa. Integration occurred within the *E2* open reading frame. The structure of the transcripts is indicated. (Modified from Huibregtse and Scheffner 1994.)

The L1 and L2 proteins are components of the viral capsid, L1 being the major constituent.

The regulation of viral gene expression is complex and controlled by cellular and viral transcription factors. Most of these regulations occur within the *LCR* region, which varies substantially in nucleotide composition between individual HPV types. It can be subdivided into a promoter, an enhancer and a distal region, responsible for epithelium-specific transcription. The enhancer is modulated by steroid hormones and by intracellular signalling pathways activated via membrane-bound receptors.

TAXONOMY

Since 1976 (Gissmann and zur Hausen) the genetic heterogeneity of the human papillomavirus group has become more and more apparent. So far, 77 distinct HPV genotypes have been described and their genomic sequences analysed (Delius and Hoffmann 1994, de Villiers 1994). They are listed in Table 16.2. About 26 additional partial sequences of putative novel HPV types have been obtained, suggesting that the total number of HPV genotypes well exceeds 100. The rapid increase in the identification of novel types originates from technical advances, particularly PCR technology. The arbitrary definition of new types, a difference of more than 10% in the nucleotide sequences in the *E6, E7* and *L1* open reading frames, seems to define natural taxonomic units, since most recent isolates either represent novel types or are identical or nearly so with established prototypes (Ho et al. 1993). In spite of the great heterogeneity of these viruses, mutational changes seem to be rare, suggesting that

diversification had already taken place in prehistoric times.

The heterogeneity of the human papillomavirus group is not restricted to those infecting humans, the large number of which seems to reflect the intensity of investigation. Thus far 8 bovine papillomavirus types have been isolated. Four have been cloned from monkeys and apes and all these are more related to specific HPV types than several of the human types are to each other, indicating again the ancient origin of these viruses.

TARGET TISSUES

All HPV types isolated so far primarily infect epithelial cells. Most types can be subgrouped according to nucleotide homologies. Broadly speaking, these subgroups show tropisms for the infection of specific sites and tissues: more than 30 types, comprising one of the subgroups, infect the anogenital mucosa. Close to 20 types form another subgroup. They are found predominantly in skin infections of patients with EV, the rare hereditary condition characterized by extensive verrucosis. Two additional subgroups are also observed primarily in infections of the skin, one containing 5 members (HPV-4, 48, 50, 60, 65), the other 3 (HPV-1, 41, 63). They seem to have radiated from 4 ancestral prototypes early in the prehominid phase.

The molecular basis for the tissue tropisms is not fully understood. Virus-like particles obtained via recombinant plasmids attach to and even penetrate cells of various origin (Roden et al. 1994, Müller et al. 1995b). It is therefore likely that tissue-specific regulatory factors determine the tropisms of these infections.

Table 16.2 Characterized HPV types

HPV type	Predominant site
1	Plantar warts
2	Common warts
3	Flat warts
4	Common warts
5	Benign and malignant EV lesions
6	Genital warts, laryngeal papillomatosis
7	'Butchers' warts', oral papillomas of patients with HIV infections
8	Benign and malignant EV lesions
9	EV lesions
10	Flat warts
11	Laryngeal papillomas, genital warts
12	EV lesions
13	Oral focal epithelial hyperplasia
14	EV lesions
15	EV lesions
16	Anogenital intraepithelial neoplasias and cancers
17	EV lesions
18	Anogenital intraepithelial neoplasias and cancers
19	EV lesions
20	EV lesions
21	EV lesions
22	EV lesions

Table 16.2 Continued

HPV type	Predominant site
23	EV lesions
24	EV lesions
25	EV lesions
26	Common warts in immunosuppressed patients
27	Common warts
28	Flat warts
29	Common warts
30	Laryngeal carcinoma
31	Anogenital intraepithelial neoplasias and cancers
32	Oral focal epithelial hyperplasia, oral papillomas
33	Anogenital intraepithelial neoplasias and cancers
34	Anogenital intraepithelial neoplasias
35	Anogenital neoplasias and cancers
36	Actinic keratosis, EV lesions
37	Keratoacanthoma[a]
38	Melanoma[a]
39	Anogenital intraepithelial neoplasias and cancers
40	Anogenital intraepithelial neoplasias
41	Cutaneous squamous cell carcinomas
42	Anogenital intraepithelial neoplasias
43	Anogenital intraepithelial neoplasias
44	Anogenital intraepithelial neoplasias
45	Anogenital intraepithelial neoplasias and cancers
46[b]	EV lesions
47	EV lesions
48	Cutaneous squamous cell carcinoma
49	Flat warts under immunosuppression
50	EV lesions
51	Anogenital intraepithelial neoplasias and cancers
52	Anogenital intraepithelial neoplasias and cancers
53	Anogenital intraepithelial neoplasias
54	Anogenital intraepithelial neoplasias
55	Anogenital intraepithelial neoplasias
56	Anogenital intraepithelial neoplasias and cancers
57	Oral papillomas and inverted maxillary sinus papillomas
58	Anogenital intraepithelial neoplasias and cancers
59	Anogenital intraepithelial neoplasias
60	Epidermoid cysts
61	Anogenital intraepithelial neoplasias
62	Anogenital intraepithelial neoplasias
63	Myrmecia warts
64	Anogenital intraepithelial neoplasias
65	Pigmented warts
66	Cervical carcinoma
67	Anogenital intraepithelial neoplasias
68	Anogenital intraepithelial neoplasias
69	Anogenital intraepithelial neoplasias and cancers
70	Vulvar papilloma
71	Anogenital intraepithelial neoplasias
72	Oral papilloma (HIV patient)
73	Oral papilloma (HIV patient)
74	Anogenital intraepithelial neoplasias
75	Common wart in organ allograft recipient
76	Common wart in organ allograft recipient
77	Common wart in organ allograft recipient

From de Villiers, 1989, 1994, and unpublished data.
[a]Individual isolates only.
[b]Now designated HPV-20b.
EV, epidermodysplasia verruciformis; HIV, human immunodeficiency virus.

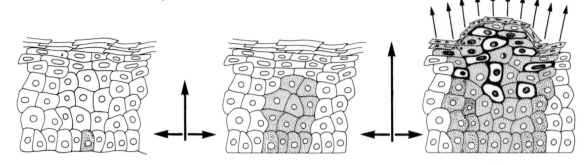

Fig. 16.4 Schematic representation of early events in HPV infection of keratinocytes. The primary infection occurs in a cell of the basal layer, accessible either through microlesions or at junctions of different epithelia. This results in an infected clone which spreads laterally, with a delay in differentiation. Eventually, differentiation takes place, permitting the replication of viral DNA, viral capsid protein synthesis and virion assembly within the differentiating cells. (Modified from zur Hausen and de Villiers 1994.)

DEVELOPMENT OF PAPILLOMAVIRUS LESIONS

Papillomaviruses infect epidermal cells still capable of proliferating, commonly basal layer cells, via microlesions or at sites where such cells are naturally exposed to the surface. This occurs regularly at the junctions of different epithelia, and seems to account for the preferential localization of cervical intraepithelial neoplasias (CINs) at the transformation zone, where c. 90% of all cervical lesions develop. The large transformation zone in young women seems particularly vulnerable to these infections. Similarly, laryngeal papillomas develop predominantly at junctions of the laryngeal epithelium with the respiratory tract.

The initial infection provides a growth stimulus for the infected cells, leading to their lateral expansion (zur Hausen and de Villiers 1994) and in most instances to a delay in differentiation, outlined schematically in Fig. 16.4. During the proliferative phase of the infected cells, viral gene expression is restricted. In HPV-16 and 18 infections, at most a low level of E6/E7 gene expression is detectable. Upon initiation of differentiation, however, this situation changes: early as well as late viral genes become abundantly expressed, viral capsid synthesis takes place within the stratum spinosum and stratum granulosum (Fig. 16.5) and virions can be visualized by electron microscopy in cell nuclei within the differentiating layers. Particle release occurs during desquamation from the surface of these lesions.

3.2 Clinical aspects of HPV infections

GENERAL FEATURES

Major manifestations of HPV infections are visible on the skin, the anogenital mucosa and the orolaryngeal mucosa. Skin warts can be classified according to appearance and histological criteria. Common warts, most frequently found on the soles of the feet, on hands (Fig. 16.6) and around knuckles, commonly contain HPV types 1, 2, 4, 7, 27 and 29. Flat warts (verruca plana) usually contain HPV type 3 or 10 (Fig. 16.7).

The high prevalence and long duration of HPV-7 infections in butchers is remarkable (Orth et al. 1981). The reason for the high prevalence of HPV-7 in this trade is not as yet clear.

Plantar warts often contain HPV-1 DNA. In a report relating only to Japanese patients, HPV-60 was regularly found in epidermoid cysts (Egawa et al. 1994). Filiform warts are often devoid of detectable HPV types. Some of them, however, have been reported to contain HPV-1, 2 or 7 (de Villiers et al. 1986, Melton and Rasmussen 1991).

Many cutaneous types have been described in EV (reviewed by Jablonska and Majewski 1994). This condition is found world-wide, although at very low prevalence. The skin lesions are polymorphic, consisting of red macules and brownish plaques, in addition to plane wart-like proliferations. Many of these papillomatous lesions contain more than one type of HPV. The EV-associated papillomaviruses form a separate subgroup of HPV. The same types of infections are also seen in organ allograft recipients and in some patients suffering from infections with the human immunodeficiency virus (Prose et al. 1990, Berger et al. 1991). It seems that, whereas infections with these HPV types must be very common in every population, the development of macroscopically visible lesions is well controlled by the immune systems of healthy individuals. Only under conditions of prolonged and severe immunosuppression do specific proliferative changes become apparent.

In the anogenital tract some papillomavirus infections cause genital warts (condylomata acuminata) and others intraepithelial neoplasias (Fig. 16.8). Genital warts typically contain HPV-6 in c. 60% of all lesions or HPV-11 in c. 30%. They develop into cauliflower-like tumours. Histologically they are characterized by acanthosis, papillomatosis and, within the superficial layers, by an extensive koilocytosis. The same virus types are also found in inverse frequency in tumours at an entirely different location, viz. laryngeal papillomas. Here HPV-11 prevails, being present in c. 60% of these lesions, whereas HPV-6 occurs in c. 30%.

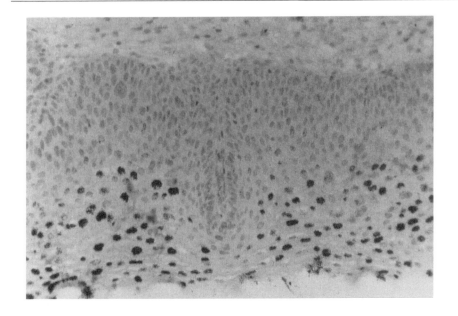

Fig. 16.5 Demonstration of viral DNA synthesis by in situ hybridization in HPV-16-positive cervical intraepithelial neoplasia. Viral DNA synthesis is restricted to the differentiating layer. (Courtesy of Professor Achim Schneider, Jena.)

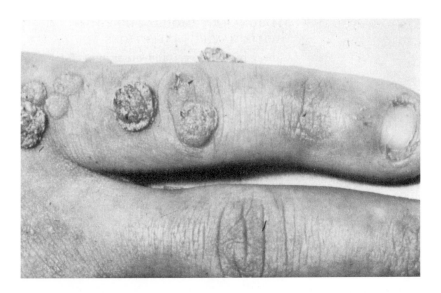

Fig. 16.6 Hand warts containing HPV-2 DNA. (Courtesy of Professor Wolfgang Meinhof, Aachen.)

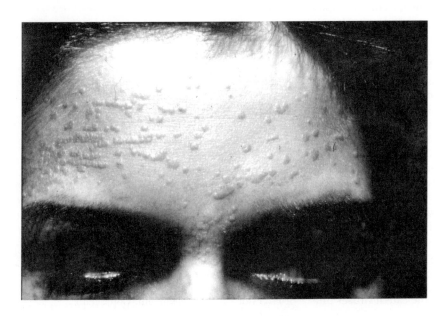

Fig. 16.7 Flat warts containing HPV-3. (Courtesy of Professor Wolfgang Meinhof, Aachen.)

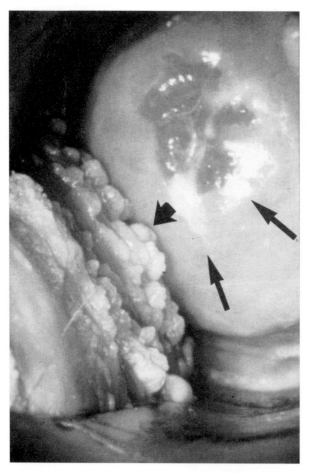

Fig. 16.8 Cervical intraepithelial lesions (small arrows) and vaginal condylomata acuminata (broad arrow) in the same patient. (Courtesy of Professor Achim Schneider, Jena.)

A rare anogenital form of condyloma acuminatum is represented by the Buschke–Löwenstein tumours. These are giant condylomata acuminata which grow invasively but metastasize only rarely. They can also be considered as a special variant of a verrucous carcinoma. All the tumours tested thus far contain either HPV-6 or HPV-11 DNA (Boshart and zur Hausen 1986).

The second major clinical manifestation of anogenital HPV infections are intraepithelial neoplasias of the cervix or other anogenital sites, often diagnosed as Bowen's disease or as bowenoid papulosis. CINs contain a spectrum of more than 30 different HPV types (Matsukura and Sugase 1995), some being found predominantly in low grade lesions, others more frequently in high grade intraepithelial neoplasias. The most frequent type observed in the latter is HPV-16, found in the majority of studies in more than 50% of these lesions, followed by HPV-18, and in southeast Asia by HPV-58. Infections with these virus types, which are also regularly found in anogenital cancer biopsies, are considered as high risk for malignant conversion. Consequently these types are considered as **high risk** viruses, by contrast with virus types commonly found in genital warts (zur Hausen 1986). The latter rarely become malignant, the causal viruses thus

being designated **low risk** HPV. A functional differentiation between these virus types has become possible: high risk viruses rapidly induce chromosomal instability and an aneuploid karyotype, whereas low risk viruses fail to do so (zur Hausen 1991).

In the oral cavity typical condylomata, verrucous hyperplasias and other types of papillomatous lesions have often been recorded (Fig. 16.9). Whereas condylomatous lesions usually contain HPV-11 or HPV-6, in other papillomatous proliferations HPV-13 or HPV-32 are most common. Papillomatous lesions in HIV-infected patients often contain HPV-7 DNA, otherwise mainly found in butchers' warts.

Laryngeal papillomatosis seems regularly to result from anogenital HPV infections, mainly by HPV-11 and HPV-6. The incidence rate of these lesions is low; they are acquired during early childhood, probably perinatally from mothers suffering from condyloma acuminatum or as early postnatal infections (see Chapter 41). They usually persist for long periods and recur regularly after surgical ablation.

MALIGNANT TUMOURS LINKED TO PAPILLOMAVIRUS INFECTIONS

Cancer of the cervix and other anogenital cancers

A role for papillomaviruses in cancer of the cervix (Fig. 16.10) was postulated over 20 years ago (zur Hausen 1976). In 1983 and 1984 HPV-16 and HPV-18 DNAs were isolated in my laboratory and demonstrated in c. 70% of all cervical biopsies tested (reviewed in zur Hausen 1994a). A number of

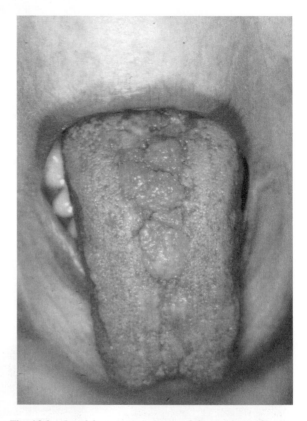

Fig. 16.9 Condylomata acuminata of the tongue. (Courtesy of Professor Christine Neumann, Göttingen.)

additional HPV types from biopsies of cancer of the cervix were subsequently characterized, most of them related to the 2 original prototypes. So far, more than 90% of biopsies from this type of cancer, obtained from various regions of the world, contain HPV DNA (Bosch et al. 1995).

Both experimental and epidemiological data support a causal role of high risk HPV types in the development of cervical cancer: specific viral genes (*E6/E7*) are transcribed in HPV-positive cancer biopsies. In approximately two-thirds of the biopsies viral DNA is integrated into the host cell genome, resulting in a prolonged lifespan of E6/E7 oncoproteins (Jeon and Lambert 1995). *E6/E7* genes immortalize human keratinocytes on transfection, permitting their unlimited growth in tissue culture. Their expression is apparently necessary for the initiation of permanent growth, for the maintenance of the immortalized cells and also for generating the malignant phenotype of cervical carcinoma cells. A switch-off of *E6/E7* gene activity results in cessation of growth and an inability to cause tumours. Besides their property of directly stimulating cell proliferation, probably by activating cyclin E and cyclin A, E6 and E7 proteins interfere with cellular factors, p53 and pRB, negatively regulating the mitotic cycle. The genes for both proteins have been defined as immunosuppressor genes. p53 is efficiently degraded by E6 and pRB is bound by the E7 protein, releasing it from a complex with the transcription factor E2F.

The degradation of p53 is apparently the main contributor to the induction of chromosomal instability and aneuploidy, regularly observed as a consequence of high risk HPV infection (White, Livanos and Tlsty 1994). Modifications in host cell DNA, apparently within genes regulating signalling pathways interfering with viral oncogene expression and transcription (zur Hausen 1994b), eventually result in the dysregulation of viral oncogene activity and progression to a malignant phenotype. The mutagenic properties of oncoproteins of these papillomaviruses are not shared by

low risk HPV, which probably explains their low carcinogenic potential.

The reported experimental data are supported by a rapidly increasing number of epidemiological case–control and cohort studies, pointing to high risk HPV as the main or even sole risk factor for the development of cancer of the cervix and its precursors (Muñoz et al. 1992, Schiffman et al. 1993). Thus cervical carcinoma, as the second most frequent malignancy in women world-wide, represents a major human cancer whose viral aetiology can be considered as proven.

High risk HPVs are also demonstrable in cancers of the vulva and penis, and in anal and vaginal cancers. Vulval intraepithelial neoplasias and vulval cancers contain these viruses in 40–60% of all biopsies tested; similar data were recorded for vaginal cancers. A review of the available literature indicates that the overall prevalence of HPV in penile cancers is 54% (International Agency for Research on Cancer 1995). A prevalence greater than 60% is recorded for anal and perianal cancers. It remains to be seen whether the tumours thus far negative for HPV DNA contain different types or have been caused by other factors.

Non-melanoma skin cancers

The involvement of papillomavirus infections in specific cancers of the skin was first demonstrated in patients suffering from EV. In this condition cancers develop in papillomatous lesions at sun-exposed sites after long persistence of these proliferations, usually for >10 years. Specific types of HPV have been discovered within the malignant lesions, predominantly types 5 and 8. The consistency of their presence, including the expression of viral oncogenes, points to a role of these infections in the development of such malignancies.

As mentioned under 'General features' (p. 298), EV-linked HPV types are also found in papillomas arising in immunocompromised patients following organ allograft treatment or in severe immunodeficiency as the consequence of HIV infections. A number of putatively novel HPV types have been isolated from squamous and basal cell carcinomas of such patients (Shamanin et al. 1994, Berkhout et al. 1995). The proportion of positive cancers is now well over 50% and by including positive signals – not as yet characterized – in the PCR reaction almost reaches 100% (Shamanin et al. 1996). Although it is still premature to conclude from these data that papillomaviruses are involved in the development of such malignancies, isolation of the novel types provides the tools for studying this question in detail.

HPV DNA has also been demonstrated in a small percentage of squamous cell carcinomas of the skin in immunocompetent patients. A detailed and systematic analysis (Shamanin et al. 1996) revealed HPV sequences, again including some novel types, in at least 30% of squamous and basal cell carcinomas derived from such patients. The spectrum of HPV types found in these cancers differed from that

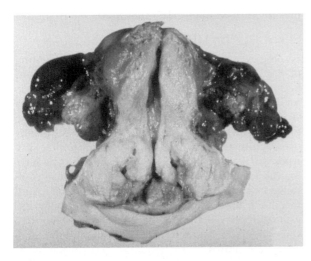

Fig. 16.10 Macroscopic appearance of cancer of the cervix after hysterectomy. (Courtesy of Dr Rolf Schmauz, Hamburg.)

observed in similar tumours in immunocompromised patients.

A specific skin malignancy, cancer of the nail beds, has been regularly linked to HPV-16 infections (Moy, Eliezri and Nuovo 1989, Eliezri, Silverstein and Nuovo 1990). This finding accords well with previous observations of the presence of HPV-16 DNA in a precursor syndrome, Bowen's disease (Ikenberg et al. 1983).

Basal and squamous cell carcinomas are the most frequent malignancies within the caucasian population. Future studies should clarify the role of HPV infections in the induction of these tumours. Their almost exclusive occurrence at sun-exposed sites may point to an interesting interaction between an environmental physical carcinogen (sunlight) and a virus infection.

Cancers of the oral cavity, the nasal sinuses and the oesophagus

HPV DNA has been demonstrated in a small number of cancers of the larynx and tongue, and in those at other oropharyngeal sites (reviewed by Snijders et al. 1994a). The high prevalence (>50%) of genital HPV types (16 and 33) in biopsies from cancer of the tonsils is particularly striking (Snijders et al. 1994b). Again, it is as yet impossible to assess the relevance of these findings. Additional systematic studies, including that of the spectrum of recently discovered HPV types, are needed to determine to what extent HPV infections contribute to these types of cancer.

Inverted papillomas of the nasal sinuses and malignant tumours of these sites have been reported to contain the DNA of a specific virus type, HPV-57, related to a virus commonly found in hand warts, HPV-2 (Hirsch-Behnam, Delius and de Villiers 1990). The number of tumours analysed is still very limited and the data do not permit firm conclusions.

It has been postulated that HPV is aetiologically related to cancer of the oesophagus; this supposition is based on the similarities of precursor lesions to CINs and the presence of koilocytes (Syrjänen 1982). Although there are claims of the presence of HPV antigens in the precursor lesions and of HPV DNA in some of the biopsies obtained from these tumours, further testing is required to substantiate them.

3.3 Epidemiology of HPV infections

Most epidemiological studies have been concerned with genital HPV infections; much less is known about non-genital HPV infections. Genital HPVs are transmitted primarily through sexual contacts. In sexually inexperienced women, HPV DNA or antibodies to anogenital HPV types are only rarely detected (Fairley et al. 1992, Andresson-Ellstrom et al. 1994, Rylander et al. 1994). In addition, there is a strong positive trend between increasing numbers of sexual partners and the prevalence of genital HPV infections. Isolated reports of periungual infections with HPV-16 and of anogenital warts in children without evidence of sexual abuse may point to occasional manual trans-

missions from one site to the other (Handley et al. 1993).

Transmission of non-genital HPV types occurs more efficiently on macerated or abraded epithelial surfaces. Concrete surfaces, such as the surrounds of swimming pools, seem to favour easy transmission of plantar warts. HPV-7-positive common warts, often found on the fingers of butchers and of fish and poultry handlers, may arise from accidental wounds from sharp implements.

The few available data on the incidence of genital warts indicate a dramatic rise between the 1950s and the late 1970s. In a study performed in Rochester, Minnesota, the age- and gender-adjusted incidence rose within this period from 13 per 100 000 to 105 per 100 000 (Chuang et al. 1984). Also within this period the rates of other sexually transmitted diseases (STDs) increased dramatically within Europe and the USA (Aral and Holmes 1994). Similar data have been obtained in Sweden for carcinomata in situ of the cervix, where the rate per 100 000 increased from <10 in 1958 to c. 100 in 1988 (Pontén et al. 1995).

Geographical differences in the prevalence of HPV infections are not readily apparent, although HPV-58 infections seem to occur with relatively high frequency in southeast Asia (Matsukura and Sugase 1995) and HPV-18 and 45 infections have been recorded more consistently in Africa and Indonesia than in Europe and the USA (ter Meulen et al. 1992, Bosch et al. 1995). Moreover, Bosch and co-workers (1995) detected HPV-39 and 59 almost exclusively in Central and South American cervical cancer biopsies.

A number of cohort studies have assessed the risk of genital cancer-linked HPV infections progressing to CIN and subsequently to invasive cancer (reviewed by Schiffman 1994). In these, and even more in case–control studies, the odds ratios of the relative risks were mostly >10. Well designed studies using reliable HPV test methods yielded the highest odds ratios. No negative results have been reported at the time of writing. From the epidemiological data alone it can be concluded that, world-wide, >90% of cervical cancers may be attributable to HPV infections.

Serology of HPV infections

Serological procedures permitting large scale testing of the humoral immune response to HPV infections became available with the expression of HPV structural proteins in recombinant baculo- or vaccinia virus-infected systems and the formation of virus-like particles (Kirnbauer et al. 1992). Studies have mainly been conducted with virus proteins of anogenital HPV types, particularly 6 and 11, and 16 and 18. The serological detection rate among HPV DNA-positive cases ranged in most studies between 50% and 70%, and was much lower in controls. The magnitudes of risk estimates derived from these studies are lower than those obtained from tests for DNA, although the tendencies are similar.

Besides reactivity to structural proteins, antibodies to high risk HPV E7 proteins are also elevated in cervical cancer patients, particularly at late stages of the disease, by comparison with controls, who rarely react with these antigens (Jochmus, Bouwes Bavinck and Gissmann 1992, Müller et al. 1995).

3.4 Immunological control of HPV infections

The highly increased frequency of warts and papillomas in immunosuppressed individuals strongly suggests an important role for the immune system in the control of HPV infections (Lutzner 1985). Generalized warts have been observed in patients with inherited immunodeficiencies (Lawlor et al. 1974), in organ allograft recipients (Benton, Shahidulah and Hunter 1992) and, with respect to anogenital neoplasia, in HIV-infected patients (Braun 1994). The available data suggest that the absolute deficit in CD4+ cells plays an important role in the emergence of HPV lesions. Disorders of the humoral immune system do not seem to lead to increased susceptibility.

The immunological control of papillomavirus-induced lesions is further emphasized by studies of regressing warts. They are characterized by a mononuclear cell infiltrate dominated by CD4+, CD45RO+ T cells and macrophages (Stanley, Coleman and Chambers 1994). Surveillance of HPV infections appears to depend on both MHC-restricted and non-restricted mechanisms. In cervical squamous cell carcinomas, MHC class I expression is consistently down-regulated (Connor and Stern 1990), a function that seems to be controlled post-transcriptionally (Cromme et al. 1993). This may lead to interference with T cell recognition of target antigens and block T cell effector mechanisms. Although normal cervical epithelium, with the exception of squamous metaplastic cells, does not express MHC class II antigens, a large percentage of high grade CINs and cervical cancers re-express these antigens.

An association between HLA haplotypes and the development of cervical carcinoma was first reported in 1991 (Wank and Thomssen) and finds strong experimental support in rabbits infected with cotton-tail rabbit papillomavirus, in which regression or progression of the papillomas is linked to the DR and DQ phenotypes of the animals (Han et al. 1992).

3.5 Diagnosis of HPV infections

Besides the macroscopic or colposcopic identification of HPV infections, the histological or cytological demonstration of koilocytes is considered a hallmark of HPV infections (Meisels and Fortin 1976, Purola and Savia 1977).

The demonstration of individual HPV genotypes is at present based exclusively on DNA technology. The most usual approach is based on the polymerase chain reaction, using different sets of degenerate consensus primers (Manos et al. 1989, Shamanin et al. 1994, 1996). This method has been applied successfully to the study of HPV infections in cancer of the cervix and in papillomavirus-linked skin cancers. The procedure permits amplification of a broad spectrum of HPV types in a single reaction. Conserved regions within the *L1* or *E1* open reading frames are usually used for the amplification protocol.

Besides the polymerase chain reaction, commercial kits can be used to detect a limited spectrum of HPV types. They are based on DNA–RNA hybrid capture assays and are useful for detecting the most common HPV types in anogenital lesions.

Southern blot techniques require the purification of cellular DNA, the availability of various HPV-type DNAs and good experience of hybridization techniques. They are relatively laborious and expensive procedures and are therefore not useful in large scale epidemiological investigations. On the other hand, this is the only method for the relatively quick identification of viral subtypes and for providing evidence of viral DNA integration.

In addition to these procedures, in situ hybridizations and filter in situ hybridizations are being used to detect HPV genomes. Both methods lack the specificity and sensitivity of the test systems already described. Histological in situ hybridizations, however, provide the basis for localization of HPV sequences in specific cell types and cellular compartments.

Serological techniques have so far not contributed to the diagnostic arsenal for HPV infections, but with the increasing availability of suitable reagents (e.g. virus-like particles) this situation may change.

3.6 Therapy of HPV infections

There is as yet no specific therapy for HPV infections. Surgical removal or ablation of the lesions by various local treatments (laser, electrodiathermy, cryotherapy etc.) are still the most reliable methods for treating papillomas and intraepithelial neoplasias.

Systemic and intralesional administration of interferon has been attempted in laryngeal papillomatosis and in recurrent condylomata acuminata. The evidence for success is so far not fully convincing. Retinoic acid may have some therapeutic potential, since this compound has been shown to suppress HPV transcriptional activity (Bartsch et al. 1992).

3.7 Vaccination

DNA-free virus-like particles, consisting exclusively of L1 and L2, or solely of L1 proteins, have been used to prevent the development of papillomas and cancers in rabbits inoculated with the cottontail rabbit papillomavirus (Breitburd et al. 1995). Similar methods are being applied to the development of a vaccine against human anogenital high risk HPV infections (reviewed by Tindle and Frazer 1994); there now seems to be a realistic chance of a preventive vaccine for cervical neoplasias and cancer of the cervix in the foreseeable future.

Therapeutic vaccines immunizing against viral oncoproteins may also have some potential. It is, however, difficult at present to assess the chances of these approaches, particularly in view of our limited knowledge of HLA restriction of viral antigenic epitopes. In general, papillomaviruses seem to represent good targets for immunoprevention, and possibly also for immunotherapy. A number of laboratories are now engaged in the development of suitable vaccines.

REFERENCES

Abrahams PJ, Malder C et al., 1975, Transformation of primary rat kidney cells by fragments of simian virus 40 DNA, *J Virol*, **16**: 818–23.

Andersson-Ellstroem A, Dillner J et al., 1994, No serological evidence for non-sexual spread of HPV 16, *Lancet*, **344**: 1435.

Aral SO, Holmes KK, 1994, Epidemiology of sexually transmitted disease, *Sexually Transmitted Diseases*, eds Holmes KK, Mardh PH et al., McGraw-Hill, New York, 126–41.

Arthur RR, Dagostin S, Shah KV, 1989, Detection of BK virus and JC virus in urine and brain tissue by the polymerase chain reaction, *J Clin Microbiol*, **27**: 1174–9.

Astrom KE, Mancall EL, Richardson EP Jr, 1958, Progressive multifocal leukencephalopathy: a hitherto unrecognized complication of chronic lymphatic leukemia and Hodgkin's disease, *Brain*, **81**: 93–111.

Atwood WJ, Amemiya K et al., 1992, Interaction of the human polyomavirus, JCV, with human B-lymphocytes, *Virology*, **190**: 716–23.

Bartsch D, Boye B et al., 1992, Retinoic acid-mediated repression of human papillomavirus 18 transcription and different ligand regulation of the retinoic acid receptor β gene in non-oncogenic and oncogenic HeLa hybrid cells, *EMBO J*, **11**: 2283–91.

Benton C, Shahidulah H, Hunter IAA, 1992, Human papillomaviruses in the immunosuppressed, *Papillomavirus Rep*, **3**: 23–6.

Berdsagel DJ, Finegold MJ et al., 1992, DNA sequences similar to those of simian virus 40 in ependymomas and choroid plexus tumors of childhood, *N Engl J Med*, **326**: 988–93.

Berger TG, Sawchunk WS et al., 1991, Epidermodysplasia verruciformis associated with human immunodeficiency disease, *Br J Dermatol*, **124**: 79–83.

Berkhout RJM, Tieben LM et al., 1995, Detection and typing of epidermodysplasia verruciformis-associated human papillomavirus types in cutaneous cancers from renal transplant recipients: a nested approach, *J Clin Microbiol*, **33**: 690–5.

Bonnez W, Elswick RK Jr et al., 1994, Efficacy and safety of 0.5% podofilox solution in the treatment and suppression of anogenital warts, *Am J Med*, **96**: 420–5.

Bosch FX, Manos MM et al., 1995, Int Biol Study Cervical Cancer (IBSSC) Study Group: Prevalence of human papillomavirus in cervical cancer: a worldwide perspective, *J Natl Cancer Inst*, **87**: 796–802.

Boshart M, zur Hausen H, 1986, Human papillomaviruses (HPV) in Buschke–Loewenstein tumours: physical state and identification of a tandem duplication in the non-coding region of a HPV 6-subtype, *J Virol*, **58**: 963–6.

Brade L, Müller-Lantzsch N, zur Hausen H, 1980, B-lymphotropic papovavirus and possibility of infections in humans, *J Med Virol*, **6**: 301–8.

Bradley MK, Dougherty RM, 1978, Transformation of African green monkey cells with the RF strain of human papovavirus BKV, *Virology*, **85**: 231–40.

Braun L, 1994, Role of immunodeficiency virus infection in the pathogenesis of human papillomavirus-associated cervical neoplasia, *Am J Pathol*, **144**: 209–14.

Breitburd F, Kirnbauer R et al., 1995, Immunization with virus-like particles from cottontail rabbit papillomavirus (CRPV) can protect against experimental CRPV infection, *J Virol*, **69**: 3959–63.

Carbone M, Pass HI et al., 1994, Simian virus 40-like DNA sequences in human pleural mesothelioma, *Oncogene*, **9**: 1781–90.

Castaigne P, Rondot P et al., 1974, Leucoencephalopathie multifocale progressive et gliomes multiples, *Rev Neurol*, **130**: 379–92.

Chuang TY, Perry HO et al., 1984, Condyloma acuminatum in Rochester, Minn, 1950–1978. I. Epidemiology and clinical features, *Arch Dermatol*, **120**: 469–75.

Coleman DV, Daniel RA et al., 1977, Polyomavirus in urine during pregnancy, *Lancet*, **2**: 709–10.

Connor ME, Stern PL, 1990, Loss of MHC class I expression in cervical carcinomas, *Int J Cancer*, **46**: 1029–34.

Corallini A, Altavilla G et al., 1978, Ependymomas, malignant tumours of pancreatic islets, and osteosarcomas induced in hamsters by BK virus, a human papovavirus, *J Natl Cancer Inst*, **61**: 875–83.

Costa J, Yee C et al., 1976, Hamster ependymomas produced by intracerebral inoculation of human papovavirus (MMV), *J Natl Cancer Inst*, **56**: 863–4.

Cromme FV, Snijders PJ et al., 1993, MHC class I expression in HPV 16 positive cervical carcinomas is post-transcriptionally controlled and independent from c-*myc* overexpression, *Oncogene*, **8**: 2969–75.

Dawe CJ, 1963, Skin-appendage tumours induced by polyoma virus in mice, *J Natl Cancer Inst Monogr*, **10**: 459–88.

Dalrymple SA, Beemon KL, 1990, BK virus T antigens induce kidney carcinomas and thymoproliferative disorders in transgenic mice, *J Virol*, **64**: 1182–91.

DeCaprio JA, Ludlow JW et al., 1988, SV40 large tumour antigen forms a specific complex with the product of the retinoblastoma susceptibility gene, *Cell*, **54**: 275–83.

De Mattei M, Martini F et al., 1995, High incidence of BK virus large-T-antigen-coding sequences in normal human tissues and tumours of different histiotypes, *Int J Cancer*, **61**: 756–60.

Delius H, Hofmann B, 1994, Primer-directed sequencing of human papillomavirus types, *Curr Top Microbiol Immunol*, **186**: 13–31.

Di Mayorca G, Callender J et al., 1969, Temperature sensitive mutants of polyoma virus, *Virology*, **38**: 126–33.

Doorbar J, Ely S et al., 1991, Specific interaction between HPV-16 E1–E4 and cytokeratins results in collapse of the epithelial cell intermediate filament network, *Nature (London)*, **352**: 824–7.

Drews RE, Chan VT-W, Schnipper LE, 1992, Oncogenes result in genomic alterations that activate a transcriptionally silent dominantly selectable reporter gene (neo), *Mol Cell Biol*, **12**: 198–206.

Dyson N, Howley PM et al., 1989, The human papillomavirus-16 E7 oncoprotein is able to bind to the retinoblastoma gene product, *Science*, **243**: 934–7.

Eckardt W, 1969, Complementation and transformation by temperature sensitive mutants of polyoma virus, *Virology*, **38**: 120–5.

Egawa K, Honda Y et al., 1994, Multiple plantar epidermoid cysts harboring carcinoembryonic antigen and human papillomavirus DNA sequences, *J Am Acad Dermatol*, **30**: 494–6.

Eliezri YD, Silverstein SJ, Nuovo GJ, 1990, Occurrence of human papillomavirus type 16 DNA in cutaneous squamous and basal cell neoplasms, *J Am Acad Dermatol*, **23**: 836–42.

Elsner C, Dörries K, 1992, Evidence of human polyomavirus BK and JC infection in normal brain tissue, *Virology*, **191**: 72–80.

Fairley CK, Chen S et al., 1992, The absence of genital human papillomavirus DNA in virginal women, *Int J STD AIDS*, **3**: 414–17.

Fareed GC, Takemoto KK, Gimbrone MA Jr, 1978, Interaction of simian virus 4 and human papovaviruses, BK and JC, with human vascular endothelial cells, *Microbiology*, ed Nester EW, Academic Press, New York, 427–31.

Freund R, Sotnikov A et al., 1992, Polyoma virus middle t is essential for virus replication and persistence as well as for tumor induction in mice, *Virology*, **191**: 716–23.

Gardner SD, Field AM et al., 1971, New human papovirus (BK) isolated from urine after renal transplantation, *Lancet*, **1**: 1253–7.

Gissmann L, zur Hausen H, 1976, Human papilloma viruses: physical mapping and genetic heterogeneity, *Proc Natl Acad Sci USA*, **73**: 1310–13.

Graffi A, Bender E et al., 1969, Induction of transmissible lymphoma in syrian hamster by application of DNA from viral hamster papovavirus induced tumors and by cell-free filtrates from human tumors, *Proc Natl Acad Sci USA*, **64**: 1172–5.

Greenlee JE, 1979, Pathogenesis of K virus infection in newborn mice, *Infect Immun*, **26**: 705–13.

Gross L, 1953, A filtrable agent, recovered from Ak leukemic extracts, causing salivary gland carcinomas in C3H mice, *Proc Soc Exp Biol Med*, **83**: 414–21.

Hagensee ME, Yaegashi N, Galloway DA, 1993, Self-assembly of human papillomavirus type 1 capsids by the expression of the L1 protein alone or by coexpression of the L1 and L2 capsid proteins, *J Virol*, **67**: 315–22.

Han R, Breitburd F et al., 1992, Linkage of regression and malignant conversion of rabbit viral papillomas to MHC class II genes, *Nature (London)*, **356**: 66–8.

Handley J, Dinsmore W et al., 1993, Anogenital warts in prepubertal children: sexual abuse or not?, *Int J STD AIDS*, **4**: 271–9.

zur Hausen H, 1976, Condylomata acuminata and human genital cancer, *Cancer Res*, **36**: 794.

zur Hausen H, 1986, Genital papillomavirus infections, *Viruses and Cancer*, eds Rigby PWJ, Wilkie NM, Cambridge University Press, Cambridge, 83–90.

zur Hausen H, 1991, Human papillomaviruses in the pathogenesis of anogenital cancer, *Virology*, **184**: 9–13.

zur Hausen H, 1994a, Molecular pathogenesis of cancer of the cervix and its causation by specific HPV types, *Curr Top Microbiol Immunol*, **86**: 131–56.

zur Hausen H, 1994b, Disrupted dichotomous intracellular control of human papillomavirus infection in cancer of the cervix, *Lancet*, **343**: 955–7.

zur Hausen H, Gissmann L, 1979, Lymphotropic papovavirus isolated from African green monkey and human cells, *Med Microbiol Immunol*, **167**: 137–53.

zur Hausen H, de Villiers E-M, 1994, Human papillomaviruses, *Annu Rev Microbiol*, **48**: 427–47.

Heilbronn R, Albrecht I et al., 1993, Human cytomegalovirus induces JC virus replication in human fibroblasts, *Proc Natl Acad Sci USA*, **90**: 11406–10.

Heinonen OP, Shapiro S et al., 1973, Immunization during pregnancy against poliomyelitis and influenza in relationship to childhood malignancy, *Int J Epidemiol*, **2**: 229–35.

Held WA, Pazik J et al., 1994a, Genetic analysis of liver oncogenesis in SV40 T antigen transgenic mice implies a role for imprinted genes, *Cancer Res*, **34**: 6489–95.

Held WA, O'Brian JG et al., 1994b, Chromosome 8 alterations accompany oncogenesis in renin-SV40 T antigen transgenic mice, *Cancer Res*, **34**: 6496–9.

Hirsch-Behnam A, Delius H, de Villiers E-M, 1990, A comparative sequence analysis of two human papillomavirus (HPV) types 2a and 57, *Virus Res*, **18**: 81–98.

Ho L, Chan SY et al., 1993, The genetic drift of human papillomavirus type 16 is a means of reconstructing prehistoric viral spread and the movement of ancient human populations, *J Virol*, **67**: 6413–24.

Hogan TF, Borden FC et al., 1988, Human polyomavirus infections with JC virus and BK virus in renal transplant patients, *Ann Intern Med*, **92**: 373–8.

Huibregtse JM, Scheffner M, 1994, Mechanisms of tumour suppressor protein inactivation by the human papillomavirus E6 and E7 oncoproteins, *Semin Virol*, **5**: 357–67.

Ikenberg H, Gissmann L et al., 1983, Human papillomavirus type 16 related DNA in genital Bowen's disease and in bowenoid papulosis, *Int J Cancer*, **32**: 563–4.

International Agency for Research on Cancer, 1995, *Monograph on Papillomaviruses and Cancer*, IARC, Lyon.

Jablonska S, Majewski S, 1994, Epidermodysplasia verruciformis: immunological and clinical aspects, *Curr Top Microbiol Immunol*, **186**: 157–75.

Jeon S, Lambert PF, 1995, Integration of human papillomavirus type 16 DNA into the human genome leads to increased stability of *E6/E7* mRNAs: implications for cervical carcinogenesis, *Proc Natl Acad Sci USA*, **92**: 1654–8.

Jochmus I, Bouwes Bavinck IN, Gissmann L, 1992, Detection of antibodies to the E4 or E7 proteins of human papillomaviruses (HPV) in human sera by western blot analysis: type-specific reaction of anti-HPV 16 antibodies, *Mol Cell Probes*, **6**: 319–25.

Kirnbauer R, Booy F et al., 1992, Papillomavirus L1 major capsid protein self-assembles into virus-like particles that are highly immunogenic, *Proc Natl Acad Sci USA*, **89**: 12180–4.

Lane DP, Crawford LV, 1979, T antigen is bound to a host protein in SV 40-transformed cells, *Nature (London)*, **278**: 261–3.

Laurent S, Frances V, Bastin M, 1995, Intrachromosomal recombination mediated by the polyomavirus large T antigen, *Virology*, **206**: 227–33.

Lavi S, 1981, Carcinogen-mediated amplification of viral DNA sequences in SV40-transformed Chinese hamster embryo cells, *Proc Natl Acad Sci USA*, **78**: 6144–8.

Lawlor GJ Jr, Ammann AJ et al., 1974, The syndrome of cellular immunodeficiency with immunoglobulins, *J Pediatr*, **84**: 183–92.

Levine DS, Sanchez CA et al., 1991, Formation of the tetraploid intermediate is associated with the development of cells with more than four centrioles in the elastase-simian virus 40 tumor antigen transgenic mouse model of pancreatic cancer, *Proc Natl Acad Sci USA*, **88**: 6427–31.

Linzer DIH, Levine AJ, 1979, Characterization of a 54 kdalton cellular SV40 tumour antigen present in SV40-transformed cells and uninfected embryonal carcinoma cells, *Cell*, **17**: 43–52.

London WT, Houff SA et al., 1978, Brain tumours in owl monkeys following inoculation with a human papovavirus (JC virus), *Science*, **201**: 1246–9.

Lutzner MA, 1985, Papillomavirus lesions in immunodepression and immunosuppression, *Clin Dermatol*, **3**: 165–9.

McCance DJ, Gardner SD, 1987, In *Principles and Practice of Clinical Virology*, eds Zuckerman AJ, Banatvala JE, Pattison JR, John Wiley, Chichester, 479.

Manos MM, Wright DK et al., 1989, The use of polymerase chain reaction amplification for the detection of genital human papillomaviruses, *Molecular Diagnostics of Human Cancer*, vol 7. *Cancer Cells*, eds Furth M, Greaves M, Cold Spring Harbor Laboratory Press, Cold Spring Harbor NY, 209–14.

Martin RG, Chou JY, 1975, Simian virus 40 functions required for the establishment and maintenance of malignant transformation, *J Virol*, **15**: 599–612.

Matsukura T, Sugase M, 1995, Identification of genital human papillomaviruses in cervical biopsy specimen: segregation of specific virus types in specific clinicopathologic lesions, *Int J Cancer*, **61**: 13–22.

Matz B, Schlehofer JR et al., 1985, HSV- and chemical carcinogenesis-induced amplification of SV40 DNA sequences in transformed cells is cell-line dependent, *Int J Cancer*, **35**: 521–5.

Meisels A, Fortin R, 1976, Condylomatous lesions of the cervix and vagina. I. Cytologic patterns, *Acta Cytol*, **20**: 505–9.

Melton JL, Rasmussen JE, 1991, Clinical manifestations of human papillomavirus infection in nongenital sites, *Dermatol Clin*, **9**: 219–33.

ter Meulen J, Eberhardt HC et al., 1992, Human papillomavirus (HPV) infection, HIV infection and cervical cancer in Tanzania, East Africa, *Int J Cancer*, **51**: 515–21.

Moy RL, Eliezri YD, Nuovo GJ, 1989, HPV DNA in periungual SSC, *JAMA*, **261**: 2669–73.

Müller M, Gissmann L et al., 1995a, Papillomavirus capsid binding and uptake by cells from different tissues and species, *J Virol*, **69**: 948–54.

Müller M, Viscidi RP et al., 1995b, Antibodies to the E4, E6, and E7 proteins of human papillomavirus (HPV) type 16 in patients with HPV-associated diseases and the normal population, *J Invest Dermatol*, **104**: 138–41.

Muñoz N, Bosch FX et al., 1992, The causal link between human papillomavirus and invasive cervical cancer: a population-based case–control study in Colombia and Spain, *Int J Cancer*, **52**: 743–9.

Narayan O, 1976, On the neoplastic viral transformation of astrocytes in cases of progressive multifocal leukencephalopathy, *J Neuropathol Exp Neurol*, **35**: 313.

van der Noordaa J, 1976, Infectivity, oncogenicity, and transforming ability of BK virus and BK virus DNA, *J Gen Virol*, **30**: 371–3.

Ornitz DM, Hammer RE et al., 1987, Pancreatic neoplasia induced by SV40 T antigen expression in acinar cells of transgenic mice, *Science*, **238**: 188–93.

Orth G, Jablonska S et al., 1979, Characteristics of the lesions and risk of malignant conversion as related to the type of the human papillomavirus involved in epidermodysplasia verruciformis, *Cancer Res*, **39**: 1074–82.

Orth G, Jablonska S et al., 1981, Identification of papillomaviruses in butchers' warts, *J Invest Dermatol*, **76**: 97-102.

Oshima J, Steinmann KE et al., 1993, Modulation of cell growth, p34^{cdc2} and cyclin A levels by SV-40 large T antigen, *Oncogene*, **8**: 2987–93.

Padgett BL, Walker DL et al., 1971, Cultivation of papova-like virus from human brain with progressive multifocal leucoencephalopathy, *Lancet*, **1**: 1257–60.

Pater MM, Pater A et al., 1980, BK viral sequences in human tumours and normal tissues and cell lines, *Viruses in Naturally Occurring Cancers*, eds Essex M, Todaro G, zur Hausen H, Cold Spring Harbor Laboratory Press, Cold Spring Harbor NY, 329–41.

Pawlita M, Clad A, zur Hausen H, 1985, Complete DNA sequence of lymphotropic papovavirus (LPV): prototype of a new species of the polyomavirus genus, *Virology*, **143**: 196–211.

Pereira-Smith OM, Smith JR, 1981, Expression of SV40 antigen in finite lifespan hybrids of normal and SV40-transformed fibroblasts, *Somatic Cell Genet*, **7**: 411–21.

Pontén J, Adami H-O et al., 1995, Strategies for global control of cervical cancer, *Int J Cancer*, **60**: 1–26.

Portolani M, Borgatti M et al., 1978, Stable transformation of mouse, rabbit, and monkey cells and abortive transformation of human cells by BK virus, a human papovavirus, *J Gen Virol*, **38**: 369–74.

Prose N, von Knebel-Doeberitz C et al., 1990, Widespread flat warts associated with human papillomavirus type 5: a cutaneous manifestation of human immunodeficiency virus infection, *J Am Acad Dermatol*, **23**: 978–81.

Purola E, Savia E, 1977, Cytology of gynaecologic condyloma acuminata, *Acta Cytol*, **21**: 26–31.

Richardson EP Jr, 1965, Progressive multifocal leukencephalopathy, *N Engl J Med*, **265**: 815–23.

Roden RB, Kirnbauer R et al., 1994, Interaction of papillomaviruses with the cell surface, *J Virol*, **68**: 7260–6.

Rylander E, Ruusuvaara L et al., 1994, The absence of vaginal human papillomavirus 16 DNA in women who have not experienced sexual intercourse, *Obstet Gynecol*, **83**: 735–7.

Scheffner M, Werness BA et al., 1990, The E6 oncoprotein encoded by human papillomavirus types 16 and 18 promotes the degradation of p53, *Cell*, **63**: 1129–36.

Schiffman MH, Bauer HM et al., 1993, Epidemiological evidence showing that human papillomavirus infection causes most cervical intraepithelial neoplasia, *J Natl Cancer Inst*, **85**: 958–64.

Schiffman MH, 1994, Epidemiology of cervical human papillomavirus infections, *Curr Top Microbiol Immunol*, **86**: 56–81.

Schlehofer JR, Gissmann L et al., 1983, Herpes simplex virus induced amplification of SV40 sequences in transformed Chinese hamster cells, *Int J Cancer*, **32**: 99–103.

Shah KV, 1972, Evidence for an SV40 related papovavirus infection in man, *Am J Epidemiol*, **95**: 199–206.

Shamanin V, Glover M et al., 1994, Specific types of HPV found in benign proliferations and in carcinomas of the skin in immunosuppressed patients, *Cancer Res*, **54**: 4610–13.

Shamanin V, zur Hausen H et al., 1996, HPV infections in non-melanoma skin cancers from renal transplant recipients and non-immunosuppressed patients, *J Natl Cancer Inst*, **88**: 802–81.

Silverman L, Rubinstein LJ, 1965, Electron microscopic observations on a case of progressive multifocal leukencephalopathy, *Acta Neuropathol*, **5**: 215–24.

Snijders PJF, van den Brule AJC et al., 1994a, Papillomaviruses and cancer of the upper digestive and respiratory tracts, *Curr Top Microbiol Immunol*, **86**: 177–98.

Snijders PJF, Steenbergen RD et al., 1994b, Analysis of p53 status in tonsillar carcinomas associated with human papillomavirus, *J Gen Virol*, **75**: 2769–75.

Soriano F, Shelbourne CE, Gokcen M, 1974, Simian virus 40 in human cancer, *Nature (London)*, **249**: 421–4.

Stanley M, Coleman N, Chambers M, 1994, The host response to lesions induced by human papillomavirus, *Vaccines against Virally Induced Cancers*, ed Frazer I, John Wiley, Chichester, 21–46.

Stewart SE, Eddy BE, Borgese N, 1958, Neoplasms in mice inoculated with a tumour agent carried in tissue culture, *J Natl Cancer Inst*, **20**: 1223–43.

Syrjänen K, 1982, Histological changes identical to those of condylomatous lesions found in esophageal squamous cell carcinomas, *Arch Geschwulstforsch*, **51**: 283–92.

Takemoto KK, Linke H et al., 1979, Persistent BK papovavirus infection of transformed human fetal brain cells, *J Virol*, **29**: 1177–85.

Tindle RW, Frazer IH, 1994, Immune response to human papillomaviruses and the prospects for human papillomavirus-specific immunization, *Curr Top Microbiol Immunol*, **86**: 218–52.

Topp WC, Lane C, Pollack R, 1980, Transformation by SV40 and polyomavirus, *DNA Tumor Viruses*, ed Tooze J, Cold Spring Harbor Laboratory Press, Cold Spring Harbor NY, 205–96.

Uchida S, Watanabe S et al., 1979, Polyoncogenicity and insulinoma-inducing ability of BK virus, a human papovavirus in Syrian golden hamsters, *J Natl Cancer Inst*, **63**: 119–26.

de Villiers E-M, 1989, Heterogeneity of the human papillomavirus group, *J Virol*, **63**: 4898–903.

de Villiers E-M, 1994, Human pathogenic papillomaviruses: an update, *Curr Top Microbiol Immunol*, **86**: 1–12.

de Villiers E-M, Neumann C et al., 1986, Butcher's wart virus (HPV 7) infections in non-butchers, *J Invest Dermatol*, **87**: 236–8.

Walker DL, Padgett BL et al., 1973, Human papovavirus (JC) induction of brain tumors in hamsters, *Science*, **181**: 674–6.

Wank R, Thomssen C, 1991, High risk of squamous cell carcinoma of the cervix for women with HLA-DQw3, *Nature (London)*, **352**: 723–5.

Weiner LP, Herndon RM et al., 1972, Further studies of a simian virus 40-like virus isolated from human brains, *J Virol*, **10**: 147–9.

Werness BA, Levine AJ, Howley PM, 1990, Association of human papillomavirus types 16 and 18 E6 proteins with p53, *Science*, **248**: 76–9.

Whitaker NJ, Kidston EL, Reddel RR, 1992, Finite lifespan of hybrids formed by fusion of different simian virus 40-immortalized human cell lines, *J Virol*, **66**: 1202–6.

White AE, Livanos EM, Tlsty TD, 1994, Differential disruption of genomic integrity and cell cycle regulation in normal human fibroblasts by the HPV oncoproteins, *Genes Dev*, **8**: 666–77.

Zheng DQ, Vayssière JL et al., 1994, Apoptosis is antagonized by large T antigens in the pathway to immortalization by polyomaviruses, *Oncogene*, **9**: 3345–51.

Zu Rhein GM, Chou S-M, 1965, Particles resembling papovaviruses in human cerebral demyelinating disease, *Science*, **148**: 1477–9.

Chapter 17

HERPESVIRUSES: GENERAL PROPERTIES

A J Davison and J B Clements

1 **Classification**	4 **Genome structure**
2 **Morphology and structure**	5 **Genetic content**
3 **Replication**	6 **Gene function**

The involvement of herpesviruses in a range of prominent medical or veterinary diseases makes them one of the most important virus families. Their ubiquitous occurrence, genetic complexity, evolutionary diversity and widely differing biological properties have motivated great research effort world-wide, so our understanding of these agents is now considerable. This is particularly apparent in the area of molecular genetics, and we can expect the knowledge gained to be applied increasingly to key questions about herpesvirus biology and to the development of effective therapies.

In this overview, we have focused on the best characterized member of the family, herpes simplex virus type 1 (HSV-1). Although a number of properties are shared by herpesviruses, many are not. For this reason, we have included pertinent information on the other human herpesviruses and, in a few cases, herpesviruses with non-human hosts. It is impossible in this review to develop a comprehensive bibliography for such a vast area of research. Moreover, selective referencing, even if applied liberally, can appear arbitrary and be of restricted value. Thus, we have chosen instead to refer to recent reviews and to a limited selection of research papers.

1 CLASSIFICATION

1.1 The family *Herpesviridae*

The family *Herpesviridae* comprises over 100 viruses that infect a wide range of vertebrates, including fish, amphibians, reptiles, birds, marsupials and mammals including humans (Minson 1989, Roizman et al. 1992). These viruses are ubiquitous and highly successful parasites, but each is usually restricted in natural infection to a single species and spreads from host to host by direct contact or by the respiratory route.

All herpesviruses have large enveloped virions containing double-stranded linear DNA genomes which exhibit considerable diversity of size and structure. Herpesviruses vary greatly in their pathology and biology, but one common feature is their ability, following primary infection, to establish lifelong latent infections which can recrudesce to cause a second round, or even recurrent rounds, of disease. Herpesviruses are well adapted to their hosts, and it is not uncommon for primary or recurring latent infections to be inapparent or trivial in the natural setting. Under certain conditions, however, particularly those resulting in a degree of immune suppression, herpesviruses can be life-threatening. Several herpesviruses have also been implicated in various types of cancer.

On the criteria of host range, duration of reproductive cycle, cytopathology and characteristics of latent infection, herpesviruses have been divided into 3 subfamilies: the *Alpha-*, *Beta-* and *Gammaherpesvirinae*. Each subfamily is subdivided: for example, the *Alphaherpesvirinae* comprise the *Simplexvirus* and *Varicellovirus* genera. In later sections of this chapter, however, we have employed a simplified terminology used widely in the literature; for example, using α-herpesvirus (subfamily) and α_1-herpesvirus (genus) instead of *Alphaherpesvirinae* and *Simplexvirus*. The herpesvirus nomenclature recommended by the International Committee on Taxonomy of Viruses uses the taxonomic unit to which the natural host belongs followed by a number. This rational scheme is used for many herpesviruses, but most human herpesviruses are generally known by their common names.

Alphaherpesvirinae have a variable host range in cell culture, have a short growth cycle, spread rapidly with efficient destruction of infected cells and are neurotropic in that they have the capacity to establish latent infections primarily in sensory ganglia. *Betaherpesvirinae* are typified by a narrow host range and a long reproductive cycle in cell culture with slow virus spread. Infected cells frequently become enlarged and carrier cultures may be established. Viruses may become latent in secretory glands and lymphoreticular cells. *Gammaherpesvirinae* are associated with lympho-proliferative diseases in their natural hosts, and infect lymphoblastoid cells in vitro. Some cause lytic infections in certain epithelial and fibroblastoid cell lines. Viruses are specific for B or T lymphocytes, in which infection is frequently arrested without production of infectious progeny, and latent virus may be found in lymphoid tissue. The term 'lymphotropic' has been used to describe these viruses, but this is arguably a misleading term as lymphocytes are at best semi-permissive.

This classification scheme, which is based predominantly on biological features, has been largely vindicated by studies of genetic relationships deduced from analyses of DNA sequence data, although there have been some notable examples of misclassification. Genetic data have superseded biological properties for classifying herpesviruses; their impact on herpesvirus phylogeny is described later (section 5.4, see p. 315).

1.2   Human herpesviruses

To date, 8 different herpesviruses have been identified whose natural host is humans (Table 17.1). The fact that 3 were discovered within the last decade leads one to anticipate that additional human herpesviruses will be isolated. HHV-6 was first isolated from patients with a variety of lymphoproliferative and immunosuppressive disorders (Salahuddin et al. 1986); it exists in two very closely related forms, one of which has been implicated as a causative agent of exanthem subitum (or roseola infantum), a common disease of infancy (Yamanishi et al. 1988). HHV-7 was first isolated from activated CD4+ cells from a healthy person (Frenkel et al. 1990), and has also been implicated in exanthem subitum (Tanaka et al. 1994). Both HHV-6 and HHV-7 are ubiquitous in human populations. The eighth human herpesvirus stems from the recent discovery that DNA sequences most closely related to γ_2-herpesviruses are present in Kaposi's sarcoma (KS) tissue from AIDS patients but not in normal tissue (Chang et al. 1994, Moore et al. 1996). These sequences were subsequently detected in KS tissue from patients displaying the classic or endemic African forms of the disease and, in association with Epstein–Barr virus (EBV), in AIDS-related lymphomas that occur in the body cavities. The new herpesvirus from which these sequences originated is understandably exciting interest as a possible causative agent of KS.

Entire DNA sequences for 4 human herpesvirus genomes are now available, and those for the others are not likely to lag far behind. Consequently, we know a great deal about how the genes are organized and what their functions are. Relating this type of information to general and particular aspects of herpesvirus pathogenesis presents an exciting challenge and has as objectives the control or prevention of infection in human populations.

2   MORPHOLOGY AND STRUCTURE

Herpesviruses have a characteristic morphology, which is the main factor in assigning viruses to this family. Virions are comprised of four distinct structural elements: envelope, tegument, capsid and core (Dargan 1986).

The lipid envelope is visible in negatively stained preparations as a pleomorphic structure with many short glycoprotein spikes. In thin sections it appears as a trilaminar, osmophilic ring with a diameter of about 120 nm. Contained within the envelope is the characteristic icosadeltahedral capsid 100 nm in diameter, which in negatively stained preparations appears as an orderly array of stain-penetrated capsomers. Forming the icosahedron are 12 pentavalent capsomers at the vertices, 60 hexavalent capsomers at the 20 faces and 90 hexavalent capsomers along the 30 edges – a total of 162 capsomers (Wildy, Russell and Horne 1962). Electron-dense material is clearly present between the envelope and capsid, and the term 'tegument' has been used to describe this poorly understood region which contains several proteins. Recently, electron cryomicroscopy has been used to study frozen, hydrated specimens of α-herpesviruses (Schrag et al. 1989). This approach allows direct examination of the 3-dimensional structure without the use of stain or fixative. When combined with computer-assisted image enhancement, considerable surface detail is visible (Fig. 17.1). Electron cryomicroscopic studies have also shown that the densely staining spherical core inside the capsid consists of the viral DNA packed at high density apparently without internal protein associations.

3   REPLICATION

The replication cycle has been studied most fully with HSV-1, and this is the basis of the brief account given here. Detailed accounts of specific aspects of this subject are given in subsequent sections. An outline of the events that occur during HSV-1 replication is shown in Fig. 17.2.

General aspects of the HSV-1 replication cycle are identical with HSV-2, but for other human herpesviruses less information is available, largely because of difficulties in propagating the viruses. No truly permissive cell culture system exists for EBV, and studies have been largely restricted to examination of latently infected cell lines. The diverse nature of human herpesviruses implies that details of their patterns of replication will vary. Nevertheless, replication cycles are all consistent with a sequential order of three major regulated phases of transcription and protein synthesis (Roizman and Sears 1990).

The external glycoproteins of the virion have important roles in adsorption of virus to cells and subsequent penetration (Spear 1993). It seems that fusion of the virus envelope with the plasma membrane occurs at the cell surface rather than in internalized vesicles. The capsid and at least some associated tegu-

Table 17.1 Human herpesviruses

Virus	Abbreviation	Genus	Designation	G + C content (mol%)	Genome (bp)
Herpes simplex virus type 1	HSV-1	α_1	Human herpesvirus 1	67	152259
Herpes simplex virus type 2	HSV-2	α_1	Human herpesvirus 2	69	~154000
Varicella-zoster virus	VZV	α_2	Human herpesvirus 3	46	124884
Epstein–Barr virus	EBV	γ_1	Human herpesvirus 4	60	172282
Human cytomegalovirus	HCMV	β_1	Human herpesvirus 5	57	229354
Human herpesvirus 6	HHV-6	β_2	Human herpesvirus 6	43	159321
Human herpesvirus 7	HHV-7	β_2	Human herpesvirus 7	40	~145000
Kaposi's sarcoma-associated herpesvirus	HHV-8 (KSHV)	γ_2	Human herpesvirus 8	?	?

?, not known

ment proteins then migrate to the nucleus where transcription, replication of viral DNA and capsid assembly take place.

Virus DNA is transcribed into mRNA throughout infection by host RNA polymerase II, various viral factors participating at all stages (Wagner 1985). Initially, a series of immediate-early (IE) or α genes is expressed whose transcription is independent of virus protein synthesis and is greatly enhanced by a tegument protein (O'Hare 1993). Certain IE proteins are *trans*-acting regulators of virus genes, and initiate a cascade of expression of early (or β) and late (or γ) genes (Honess and Roizman 1974). The products of early genes, defined as the subset expressed in the presence of functional IE products and before the onset of DNA replication, include several enzymes involved in DNA replication and nucleotide metabolism and a subset of glycoproteins. Late genes are dependent on functional IE proteins for expression, and in addition full levels of late protein synthesis require DNA replication. They encode mainly virion proteins.

A subset of virus genes is involved in DNA replication and packaging of DNA into capsids. DNA synthesis is initiated from one or more origins of DNA replication, generating head-to-tail concatemeric genomes apparently by a rolling circle mechanism. Concatemers are then cleaved and packaged into preformed capsids. The process by which virion maturation occurs is not fully understood, but several genes seem to have roles in envelopment and egress. Addition of tegument may occur at the nuclear envelope, but there is evidence from some herpesviruses that it may occur in a cytoplasmic compartment. Similarly, although enveloped particles are present in the cytoplasm, there is evidence that envelopment occurs at the cytoplasmic membranes. A plausible model involves a single envelopment event at the nuclear membrane, followed by glycoprotein maturation in the Golgi apparatus and release by reverse endocytosis.

The effects of these processes on host cells vary with the different viruses, and, for an individual virus,

depend on the cell type. The time taken for cytopathic effect to become evident may range from hours to days, and cells may lyse, round up or fuse. Also, the proportion of particles that are released from infected cells and the fraction that are enveloped are very variable.

Infection with HSV-1 leads to a rapid inhibition of host macromolecular synthesis. The initial phase of host shutoff is mediated by a virion component, and late in the cycle a second shutoff function may reduce host protein synthesis further. Reduction by the virion shutoff component of the functional half-lives of both infected cell and viral mRNAs could facilitate more rapid changes in viral gene expression in response to alterations at the level of transcription.

In addition to a lytic cycle of infection, all herpesviruses examined to date are able to undergo a latent cycle. Details of HSV-1 latency are described in Chapter 18.

4 GENOME STRUCTURE

4.1 Types of structure

Herpesvirus genomes range in size from 125 to 240 kbp and have nucleotide compositions ranging from 32 to 74% G + C (Honess 1984). The γ-herpesviruses exhibit a deficit in the CG dinucleotide, presumably as an evolutionary result of latency in dividing cells. The genome structures of many herpesviruses are known, but the majority of viruses in this family have not been examined at this level. Figure 17.3 illustrates the 6 types of genome arrangement that have been characterized thus far. A common characteristic is the presence of repeated regions at the ends of, or internally within, the genome.

The simplest genome arrangement is that of group 1, which consists of a unique sequence flanked by a direct repeat. It was first described for channel catfish virus (CCV), and has since been found for equine herpesvirus 2 (EHV-2; γ$_2$-herpesvirus) and HHV-6. The genome of murine cytomegalovirus (a β$_1$-herpesvirus)

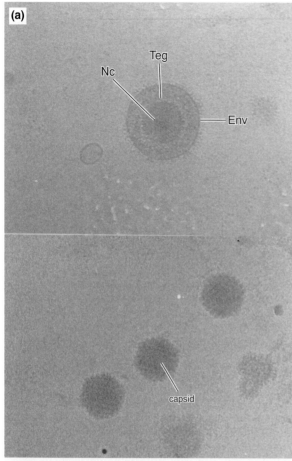

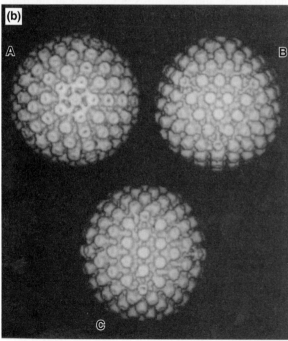

Fig. 17.1 (a) Electron cryomicrographs of HSV-1 virions and capsids. Visible in the enveloped particles are the capsid (Nc), tegument (Teg) and envelope (Env) with associated glycoprotein spikes. (b) Three-dimensional reconstructions of capsid surface structure as determined by computer analysis of electron cryomicrograph images of ice-embedded capsids. **A** shows the view along the 5-fold axis; **B** shows the view along the 2-fold axis; **C** shows the three-fold axis of symmetry. (By courtesy of Dr FJ Rixon and Dr W Chiu.)

also has this arrangement, but the direct repeats are much smaller. This distribution of the group 1 structure in different herpesvirus subfamilies illustrates the point that gross genome structure is not a reliable taxonomic tool.

Group 2 genomes contain a shorter sequence repeated a variable number of times at the termini instead of a single direct repeat, and are found among the γ_2-herpesviruses typified by the monkey virus herpesvirus saimiri (HVS). The addition of a variable number of the terminal repeats in inverse orientation internally results in the group 3 genome structure, which has been described for cottontail rabbit herpesvirus, also a γ_2-herpesvirus. This genome exists in 4 equimolar isomers in virion DNA, because inversion of the 2 unique regions can occur by recombination between inverted repeats. The group 4 structure results from the presence of an internal set of direct repeats unrelated to the terminal set and is typified by EBV. The 2 unique regions do not invert in such a structure because of lack of homology between internal and terminal repeats.

In the group 5 structure 2 unique regions (U_L and U_S) are each flanked by unrelated inverted repeats (TR_L/IR_L and TR_S/IR_S). The 2 orientations of U_S are present in equimolar amounts in virion DNA, but U_L is found completely or predominantly in a single orientation. Group 5 genomes have been described only for the α_2-herpesviruses, such as varicella-zoster virus (VZV).

The group 6 structure is the most complex, although it was the first type to be described, for HSV-1 (Sheldrick and Berthelot 1974). It is similar to that of group 5, except that TR_L/IR_L is much larger and the 2 orientations of U_L are present in equimolar amounts in virion DNA. HSV-2 and bovine herpesvirus 2, also an α_1-herpesvirus, and human cytomegalovirus (HCMV) share this structure. Unlike group 5 genomes, group 6 genomes are terminally redundant, possessing a short sequence (termed the *a* sequence, some 400 bp in HSV-1) which is repeated directly at the genome termini and inversely at the IR_L–IR_S junction (Wagner and Summers 1978).

4.2 Human herpesviruses

Figure 17.4 shows a scale representation of the genome structures of 7 human herpesviruses. Since the eighth virus, Kaposi's sarcoma-associated herpesvirus (KSHV), has not yet been isolated, the genome structure is unknown. The HSV-1 and HSV-2 genomes exhibit a group 6 structure and are essentially co-linear; the most striking difference is the presence of an additional 1500 bp in the coding sequence of HSV-2 gene US4. Preparations of virion DNA from both viruses contain equivalent amounts of 4 isomers which differ in the relative orientations of U_L and U_S (Hayward et al. 1975), a phenomenon termed genome isomerization. These isomers seem to be functionally equivalent, and one has been chosen arbitrarily to serve as a prototype for depicting restriction endonuclease sites and the gene arrangement. As the

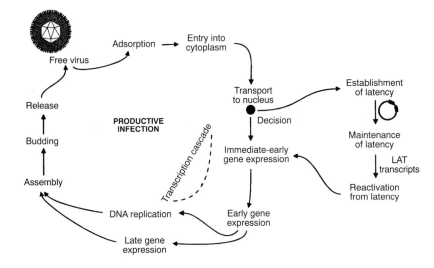

Fig. 17.2 The replication cycle of HSV-1.

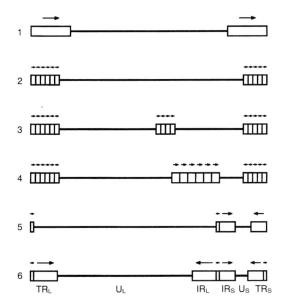

Fig. 17.3 Types of herpesvirus genome structure. The genomes are not drawn to scale. Unique and repeat regions are shown as horizontal lines and rectangles, respectively. The orientations of repeats are shown by arrows. The nomenclature used to designate regions of the HSV-1 genome is shown at the foot of the Figure. (From Davison and McGeoch 1995, by courtesy of Cambridge University Press.)

a sequence contains signals for cleavage and packaging concatemeric DNA generated during viral DNA replication, the presence of internal copies as alternative sites, in combination with homologous recombination events between TR_L and IR_L or TR_S and IR_S, provides a means for generating the 4 genome isomers.

The VZV genome, as an example of a group 5 structure, is not terminally redundant although sequences involved in cleavage and packaging of replicated DNA are present at the genome termini. U_L is flanked by a small inverted repeat of 88 bp which results in 5% of virions containing genomes with U_L inverted, and U_S is found equally in both orientations.

The general arrangement of the HCMV genomes resembles that of HSV-1, with a similar arrangement of unique and repeated elements and the presence of 4 equimolar genome isomers, although it is 50% larger. Phylogenetic studies indicate that the genome structures of HSV-1 and HCMV developed independently.

EBV DNA displays a linear, non-inverting structure. The terminal regions consist of up to 12 copies of a 500 bp tandem repeat, and the internal repeat region comprises 6–12 tandemly repeated copies of a 3072 bp sequence.

In addition to large scale repeat elements, each human herpesvirus genome contains several regions consisting of tandem reiterations of short sequence elements. The presence of the repeated elements in variable copy numbers results in genome size heterogeneity. These sequences may be coding or non-coding; in the former case, they exist as multiples of 3 bp and encode repeated amino acid sequences. A further type of genome heterogeneity is represented by the loss or gain of restriction endonuclease sites and is presumably due to differences in individual nucleotides. DNA cleavage patterns have demonstrated that epidemiologically unrelated HSV-1 and HSV-2 isolates are not identical, and the patterns are stable when viruses are passed in cell culture. This characteristic has an important diagnostic use and has been employed to examine modes of transmission and epidemiology of HSV-1 and HSV-2 in human populations (Sakaoka et al. 1994).

5 GENETIC CONTENT

5.1 Arrangement and expression

The complete DNA sequences of 9 herpesviruses have been published to date: HSV-1 (McGeoch et al. 1988), VZV (Davison and Scott 1986), equine herpesvirus 1 (EHV-1, an α_2-herpesvirus) (Telford et al. 1992), HCMV (Chee et al. 1990), HHV-6 (Gompels et al. 1995), EBV (Baer et al. 1984), HVS (Albrecht et al. 1992), EHV-2 (Telford et al. 1995) and CCV, which

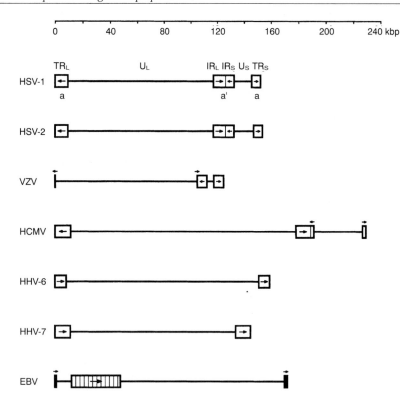

Fig. 17.4 Sizes and structures of human herpesvirus genome shown to scale. Unique and repeat regions are shown as horizontal lines and rectangles, respectively. The orientations of repeats are shown by arrows. The nomenclature used to designate regions of the HSV-1 genome is shown at the top of the Figure. The sequence that is directly repeated at the genome termini and also present internally in inverse orientation is shown as *a* and *a'*, respectively.

appears to be unrelated to α-, β- and γ-herpesviruses (Davison 1992). In addition, substantial parts of other herpesvirus genomes have been sequenced. Analyses of these sequences have given an overview of genetic content and usually form the starting point for experimental studies on particular genes.

The numbers of genes identified from sequence analyses range from about 70 in smaller genomes (e.g. HSV-1 and VZV) to 200 in the larger (e.g. HCMV). In general, the great majority of the DNA is protein-coding, and genes are arranged about equally between the 2 strands. Regions of overlap between genes in different reading frames on the same strand or on opposing strands are infrequent and usually not extensive. Certain small non-coding RNAs transcribed from γ-herpesvirus genomes are probably transcribed by RNA polymerase III. Most genes are expressed as single exons from their own promoters, but it is common for families of genes arranged tandemly on the same strand to share a polyadenylation site downstream from the most 3′ member (Wagner 1985). Few HSV-1 genes specify spliced mRNAs, but splicing is thought to be more common in HCMV and EBV. Most splicing in EBV specifically involves genes expressed during latency (Kieff and Liebowitz 1990), particularly a family of genes distributed over 100 kbp which is expressed by differential splicing of transcripts from a common promoter.

5.2 HSV-1

HSV-1 is the best characterized herpesvirus at the molecular level. At the present state of analysis, HSV-1 is considered to contain 74 different genes, 3 of them

present twice in the inverted repeats. The gene arrangement is shown in Fig. 17.5. Data continue to accumulate on the properties and functions of the proteins encoded by these genes, and the current state of knowledge is summarized in Table 17.2. Over all, more than 85% of the DNA is protein-coding, and genes are tightly packed with about equal numbers oriented rightwards and leftwards. Several examples of 2 or more genes specifying mRNAs that share a 3′ terminus are visible in Fig. 17.5. Larger mRNAs within these nested families contain more than one reading frame, and conventional wisdom suggests that translation initiates at the AUG codon proximal to the mRNA 5′ end. Owing to this nested arrangement, promoter sequences for certain internal mRNAs lie within the protein-coding sequences of overlapping mRNAs. HSV-1 has 4 genes that are expressed as spliced mRNAs, 2 (UL15 and RL2) with introns in protein-coding regions and 2 (US1 and US12) with a common spliced 5′ non-coding leader. In addition, the HSV-1 latency-associated transcripts (LATs), which probably do not encode protein, are also spliced. The LATs are the only transcripts expressed during latency (see Chapter 18 for more information).

Presumably, all the genes present in a herpesvirus genome are required for natural growth and transmission of the virus. Surprisingly, about half of the genes present in HSV-1 are 'non-essential', and each of these genes may be removed without eliminating viral growth in cell culture (Roizman and Sears 1990, McGeoch and Schaffer 1993). These genes are indicated in Table 17.2. Many of these mutants, however, are attenuated when assayed in animal models.

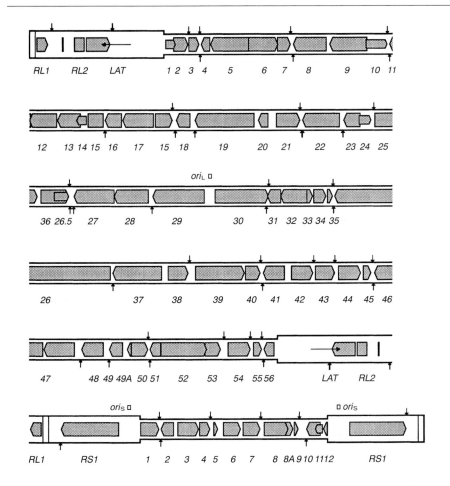

Fig. 17.5 Arrangement of genes in the HSV-1 genome. The genome is shown in 6 panels, each 25 kbp long. Inverted repeats are denoted by the thicker parts of the genome outline, and protein-coding regions are shown as shaded horizontal arrows. For the sake of clarity, the prefixes 'UL' (58 genes), 'US' (13 genes) have been omitted from the gene nomenclature given below the genome; see Fig. 17.4 for the locations of these regions. The major LAT RNA, presumed to be derived from a stable intron generated from a larger transcript, is also indicated by a horizontal arrow. Genes RL2 and UL15 contain 3 and 2 exons, respectively. Possible polyadenylation sites for mRNAs are indicated by vertical arrows above and below the genome for right and left orientated genes, respectively. The locations of ori_S and ori_L are shown by white rectangles above the genome. (Adapted from Davison 1992a, by courtesy of R & W Publications.)

5.3 Other herpesviruses

Comparisons of amino acid sequences predicted from DNA sequence data have shown that, despite substantial differences in nucleotide composition or genome structure, members of the same subfamily share the great majority of genes in a very similar layout. For example, all but 5 VZV genes have counterparts at equivalent locations in the HSV-1 genome. The utility of comparing a poorly understood genome (e.g. VZV) with a better characterized one (HSV-1) depends on this genetic correspondence. When viruses in the 3 subfamilies are compared, however, divergence is much greater, with a set of about 40 'core' genes conserved in blocks which have been rearranged during evolution. These genes are indicated in bold type in Table 17.2, and presumably function in processes that are central to growth and survival. A few genes are found in only 2 of the 3 subfamilies, and may reflect independent capture of a cellular gene or loss of a gene from one lineage. Examples are thymidine kinase and the small subunit of ribonucleotide reductase, which are not found in the β-herpesviruses. The remaining 'non-core' genes are characteristic of a single subfamily, and some are unique to one or a few specific viruses. Many of these genes are involved in

aspects of pathogenesis that contribute to survival of the virus in its particular ecological niche. Most genes involved in control processes and latency also fall into this category.

5.4 Herpesvirus evolution

Analyses of the genetic relationships between α-, β- and γ-herpesviruses indicate that they have evolved from a common ancestor by processes including substitution, deletion and insertion of nucleotides to modify genes or produce genes *de novo* and recombination processes resulting in gene duplication and divergence, capture of host genes and gene rearrangement (McGeoch 1992, Davison and McGeoch 1995). Results from recent phylogenetic studies are in general accord with the notion that herpesviruses have evolved with their vertebrate hosts, and this has allowed an evolutionary time-scale to be proposed (Fig. 17.6). These studies provide a firm basis for herpesvirus classification based on genetic relationships rather than on phenotypic properties.

The situation regarding fish herpesviruses is less clear, because CCV is not convincingly related at the genetic level to herpesviruses that infect mammals or birds (Davison 1992). However, evidence relating to

Table 17.2 Properties of HSV-1 proteins

Gene	Predicted mass	Status	Function or properties
RL1	26194	NE	Neurovirulence factor (ICP34.5)
RL2	78452	NE	IE protein (Vmw110); transcriptional regulator
UL1	24932	E	Glycoprotein L; complexes with glycoprotein H (UL22)
UL2	36326	NE	Uracil-DNA glycosylase
UL3	25607	NE	?
UL4	21516	NE	?
UL5	98710	E	Component of DNA helicase–primase complex; possesses helicase motifs
UL6	74087	E	Minor capsid protein
UL7	33057	E	?
UL8	79921	E	Component of DNA helicase–primase complex
UL9	94246	E	*Ori*-binding protein
UL10	51389	NE	Virion surface glycoprotein M
UL11	10486	NE	Myristylated tegument protein; role in virion envelopment
UL12	67503	(E)	Deoxyribonuclease; role in maturation/packaging of DNA
UL13	57193	NE	Tegument protein; probable protein kinase
UL14	23454	E	?
UL15	80918	E	Role in DNA packaging; putative terminase component
UL16	40440	NE	?
UL17	74577	E	?
UL18	34268	E	Capsid protein (VP23); component of intercapsomeric triplex
UL19	149075	E	Major capsid protein (VP5); forms hexons and pentons
UL20	24229	E/NE	Integral membrane protein; role in egress of nascent virions; host range phenotype; *syn* locus
UL21	57638	NE	Tegument protein
UL22	90361	E	Virion surface glycoprotein H; complexes with glycoprotein L (UL1); role in cell entry
UL23	40918	NE	Thymidine kinase
UL24	29474	NE	*Syn* locus
UL25	62664	E	Capsid-associated tegument protein
UL26	62466	E	Autocatalytically cleaved by N-terminal protease domain to give capsid protein (VP24) from N terminus and minor scaffold protein (VP21) of immature capsids
UL26.5	33758	(E)	Cleaved by UL26 protein to give major scaffold protein (VP22a) of immature capsids
UL27	100287	E	Virion surface glycoprotein B; role in cell entry; *syn* locus
UL28	85573	E	Role in DNA packaging
UL29	128342	E	Single-stranded DNA-binding protein
UL30	136413	E	Catalytic subunit of replicative DNA polymerase; complexes with UL42 protein
UL31	33951	E	?
UL32	63946	E?	?
UL33	14436	E	Role in DNA packaging
UL34	29788	E?	Membrane-associated phosphoprotein; substrate for US3 protein kinase
UL35	12095	E?	Capsid protein (VP26); located on tips of hexons
UL36	335841	E	Very large tegument protein
UL37	120549	E?	Tegument protein
UL38	50260	E	Capsid protein (VP19C); component of intercapsomeric triplex
UL39	124043	E/NE	Ribonucleotide reductase large subunit
UL40	38017	E/NE	Ribonucleotide reductase small subunit
UL41	54914	NE	Tegument protein; virion host shutoff factor
UL42	51156	E	Subunit of replicative DNA polymerase; increases processivity; complexes with UL30 protein
UL43	44905	NE	Probable integral membrane protein
UL44	54995	NE	Virion surface glycoprotein C; role in cell entry
UL45	18178	NE	Tegument/envelope protein

Table 17.2 Continued

Gene	Predicted mass	Status	Function or properties
UL46	78239	NE	Tegument protein; modulates IE gene transactivation by UL48 protein
UL47	73812	NE	Major tegument protein; modulates IE gene transactivation by UL48 protein
UL48	54342	E	Major tegument protein (Vmw65); transactivates IE genes
UL49	32252	NE?	Major tegument protein
UL49A	9201	NE?	Envelope protein disulphide-linked to tegument
UL50	39125	NE	Deoxyuridine triphosphatase
UL51	25468	(E)	?
UL52	114416	E	Component of DNA helicase–primase complex
UL53	37570	(E)	Glycoprotein K
UL54	55249	E	IE protein (Vmw63); post-translational regulator of gene expression
UL55	20491	NE	?
UL56	25319	NE	?
RS1	132835	E	IE protein (Vmw175); transcriptional regulator
US1	46521	E/NE	IE protein (Vmw68); host range phenotype; involved in modification of host RNA polymerase II
US2	32468	NE	?
US3	52831	NE	Protein kinase; phosphorylates UL34 protein
US4	25236	NE	Virion surface glycoprotein G
US5	9555	NE	Proposed glycoprotein J
US6	43344	E	Virion surface glycoprotein D; role in cell entry
US7	41366	NE	Virion surface glycoprotein I; complexed with glycoprotein E (US8) in Fc receptor
US8	59090	NE	Virion surface glycoprotein E; complexed with glycoprotein I (US7) in Fc receptor
US8A	16801	NE	?
US9	10026	NE	Major tegument protein
US10	34053	NE	Virion protein
US11	17756	NE	Virion protein; ribosome-associated in infected cell
US12	9792	NE	IE protein (Vmw12); interferes with maturation of MHC class I molecules

?, not known.
Developed from Davison (1986), McGeoch et al. (1988), McGeoch (1989), McGeoch and Schaffer (1993), McGeoch, Barnett and MacLean (1993), Davison (1993) and Ward and Roizman (1994).
Genes in bold type are conserved in the three herpesvirus subfamilies. The status of each gene in cell culture is indicated: E, essential; E?, probably essential; (E), a mutant is viable but very disabled; E/NE, non-essential under certain conditions; NE, non-essential; NE?, probably non-essential.

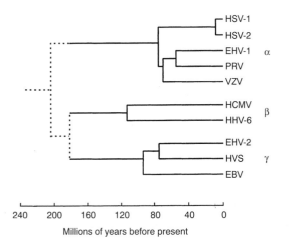

240 200 160 120 80 40 0

Millions of years before present

Fig. 17.6 A phylogenetic tree for the herpesviruses derived from sequence comparisons, with a time-scale based on the hypothesis that viruses co-speciate with their hosts (McGeoch et al. 1995). Broken lines indicate regions of lower confidence. (By courtesy of Academic Press Ltd.)

capsid structure and assembly indicates that all these herpesviruses have a common ancestor, presumably dating from the time when the lineages leading to fish and other vertebrates separated, but have diverged so far that their shared inheritance is no longer discernible by amino acid sequence comparisons.

6 GENE FUNCTION

6.1 Determination of function

Computer-aided comparisons of predicted amino acid sequences have facilitated the identification of some herpesvirus gene functions, but the majority of evidence has come from direct genetic and biochemical experimentation based on sequence information. Much of this information has been gained for HSV-1, and derived functions have been imputed to homologous genes in other herpesviruses. The major categories of gene functions are described below.

6.2 **Control**

Some proteins are involved in control processes, the most intensively studied acting directly or indirectly at the level of transcription to regulate gene expression during the infectious cycle. One such, the HSV-1 virion transactivator (Campbell, Palfreyman and Preston 1984), an essential structural component of the tegument termed Vmw65 (VP16 or α-TIF; gene UL48), acts to stimulate selective transcription of IE genes (O'Hare 1993). Although the transactivation function of Vmw65 is not essential for virus growth, mutants replicate poorly and are avirulent in some animal model systems. Induction of HSV-1 IE genes may determine aspects of cell tropism and could play a role in reactivation from latency. Transactivation by a related protein may also occur in other α-herpesviruses, but it is not clear that the mechanism is the same. An unrelated virion protein may transactivate in HCMV (Liu and Stinski 1992).

Coordinate induction of IE genes requires a consensus DNA signal (TAATGARAT) that is well conserved upstream of all 5 IE genes. This positive regulation of IE transcription acts through the cellular Oct-1 DNA-binding protein, and studies of Vmw65 function have shed light on the assembly of multicomponent transcriptional complexes (O'Hare 1993). Of the 5 HSV-1 IE proteins, 4 are involved in the regulation of early and late virus genes (Everett 1987). Two, Vmw175 (ICP4; gene RS1) and Vmw63 (ICP27; gene UL54), are essential for replication, but precisely how these 2 proteins function remains obscure. Vmw175 is required throughout productive infection (Watson and Clements 1980), and acts at the transcriptional level, exhibiting non-specific DNA-binding. Vmw63 acts post-transcriptionally (Sandri-Goldin and Mendoza 1992), also affecting virus transcription and DNA replication. Vmw110 (ICP0; gene RL2) is not absolutely required for HSV-1 replication but is required for reactivation from latency, and Vmw68 (ICP22; gene US1) affects phosphorylation of RNA polymerase II, probably to facilitate transcription of viral DNA (Rice et al. 1995).

Other virus proteins modulate replicative processes in the infected cell. Among the α-herpesviruses, 2 protein kinase families are likely to act in this way. For HSV-1, the protein kinase encoded by gene US3 phosphorylates a virion protein encoded by UL34, and the UL13 protein kinase phosphorylates Vmw68 and the tegument protein encoded by gene UL49. Mention should be made of the virion host shutoff function encoded by gene UL41, which reduces the cytoplasmic stability of both cellular and viral mRNAs and serves to switch off synthesis of host cell proteins. These effects may contribute to the down-regulation of early viral gene expression. Viruses in each subfamily also appear to have genetic mechanisms for suppressing the host's immune response.

Considerable information (largely from HCMV studies) is available on regulation of β-herpesvirus gene expression, particularly on gene functions that promote the regulated cascade of gene expression and on the viral *cis*-acting DNA sequences involved (Stinski 1990). Similarly, EBV has been well studied both in terms of gene expression during latent infection of B lymphocytes, and in terms of lytic gene expression occurring following treatment of latently infected cell lines with various inducers (Kieff and Leibowitz 1990). These studies have shown that all herpesviruses examined encode strong transcriptional regulators that are expressed in the IE replication phase. However, these activators exhibit considerable diversity at the primary sequence level, and seem to have developed separately in the herpesvirus lineages. This diversity is also shown by the DNA sequences that regulate synthesis of these proteins. Perhaps a similarity in tertiary structure enables these proteins to act in similar ways; alternatively, they may exert their effects by interaction with different host cell factors.

6.3 **Nucleotide metabolism**

Herpesviruses specify several enzymes involved in nucleotide metabolism or DNA repair (Morrison 1991). Virus-specified enzyme activities generally have biochemical properties that differ from their cellular counterparts, and they are an important feature for specific targeting of certain antiviral compounds (Coen 1992).

Two HSV-1 enzymes catalyse reactions in the biosynthesis of DNA precursors: thymidine kinase (TK) and ribonucleotide reductase (RR). HSV-1 TK appears to be evolutionarily derived from the cellular deoxycytidine kinase, and in being able to phosphorylate thymidine and deoxycytidine is more accurately described as a deoxypyrimidine kinase (dPyK). The HSV-1 TK activity is important for the inhibitory action of nucleoside analogues, such as acyclovir, which have to be phosphorylated to their monophosphate forms by the virus enzyme and subsequently to the di- and triphosphate forms by cellular enzymes. HSV-1 TK activity is not essential for virus replication in actively growing cells but is required for growth in serum-starved cells. The pathogenicity of TK-deficient viruses is reduced in animal models, presumably because TK activity is required to raise dTTP levels in target non-dividing cells. As might be expected, the enzymatic properties of TK enzymes specified by different herpesviruses differ, for example in their relative ability to phosphorylate thymidine and deoxycytidine. The TK gene is not ubiquitous: the α- and γ-herpesviruses (and even CCV) contain TK genes, but the β-herpesviruses such as HCMV and HHV-6 do not.

RR catalyses the reduction of nucleoside diphosphates to deoxynucleoside diphosphates, and comprises a large and a small subunit encoded by contiguous genes. It occupies a central role in metabolic routes for the supply of DNA precursors, and is required for efficient growth of virus in cell culture; RR-deficient viruses grow slowly and are non-pathogenic. Kinetic experiments have shown that this is one of the earliest HSV-1 gene functions to be expressed. The genes encoding both subunits of RR are present in α- and γ-herpesvirus genomes, but only that encoding the large subunit is present in the β-herpesviruses; presumably the β-herpesviruses use the small subunit of the cellular enzyme for viral RR activity. CCV lacks both genes. A feature peculiar to HSV-1 and HSV-2 is an additional domain of some 320 amino acid residues at the N terminus of the RR large subunit which may not be required for enzymatic activity. However, a protein kinase activity has been implicated for this domain. A synthetic oligopeptide corresponding to the C-terminal 9 residues of the RR small subunit specifically inhibits RR activity in vitro by disrupting a specific interaction between the 2 subunits (Cohen et al. 1986, Dutia et al. 1986). Interest has focused on this interaction as a target for antiviral compounds, and this has turned attention to essential interactions between other herpesvirus proteins, such as those involved in DNA replication, capsid assembly and DNA packaging (Marsden 1992).

HSV-1 also encodes a deoxyuridine triphosphatase (dUTPase) which is not essential for growth in cell culture. This enzyme catalyses conversion of dUTP to dUMP, which can then be methylated to dTMP by cellular thymidylate synthase. The important function of viral dUTPase in infected cells, however, may be to reduce misincorporation of uracil during DNA synthesis. A dUTPase gene is present in all herpesviruses studied to date, and appears to have developed in the α-, β- and γ-herpesviruses by capture of the gene, followed by gene duplication and fusion of the 2 protein-coding regions. An analysis of conserved motifs casts strong doubt, however, on whether the β-herpesvirus gene is a functional dUTPase.

HSV-2 encodes a uracil-DNA glycosylase, which is likely to function in removing spontaneously deaminated cytosine and misincorporated uracil residues from viral DNA and thus reduce mutations. The highly conserved uracil-DNA glycosylase gene is present in the α-, β- and γ-herpesviruses (but not CCV), but is not essential for growth of HSV-1 in cell culture.

Two other enzymes with roles in nucleotide supply have been characterized in certain herpesviruses, although neither is specified by HSV-1, HCMV or EBV. Thymidylate synthase (TS), which catalyses methylation of dUMP to dTMP, is encoded by VZV and HVS; dihydrofolate reductase, which catalyses reduction of dihydrofolate to tetrahydrofolate, an essential step in purine synthesis and in the action of TS, is specified by HVS. These genes may represent relatively recent capture of the cellular genes in certain virus lineages.

6.4 DNA replication

Seven HSV-1 proteins constitute essential components of the DNA synthesis machinery, including a replicative DNA polymerase comprising 2 subunits, a single-stranded DNA-binding protein, 3 constituents of a helicase–primase complex and a protein that recognizes the origins of viral DNA replication (Challberg 1991). There has been significant progress in understanding the roles of these proteins, and several interactions in the replication complex have been characterized. The possible involvement of cellular proteins, however, has not been investigated in any detail, and no origin-

dependent in vitro DNA replication system has been developed. The replicative machinery of α-, β- and γ-herpesviruses is, in broad outline, the same, since counterparts of 6 of the 7 proteins are present in all mammalian herpesviruses. However, each subfamily uses a different means of directing the replication complex to viral DNA, and this is reflected in the lack of conservation of the α-herpesvirus origin-binding protein in the other subfamilies and the observation that each subfamily uses a different type of origin of replication. These differences have presumably arisen as a result of evolutionary pressures exerted on each virus during the lytic and latent cycles of infection.

HSV-1 has an origin of replication (ori_S) which, being located in TR$_S$/IR$_S$, is present in 2 copies in the genome (Stow 1982) (see Fig. 17.4). In addition, a related origin (ori_L) is located near the centre of U$_L$. Other α-herpesviruses also possess ori_S at an equivalent location. Most have ori_L, in some cases at a different location in U$_L$, but VZV lacks this origin of replication. Both copies of ori_S or the single copy of ori_L may be deleted from the HSV-1 genome without affecting virus viability. Ori_S and ori_L are related in sequence and consist of an AT-rich palindrome flanked by short sequences that are recognized by the origin-binding protein, and both probably function during lytic replication. EBV also has 2 unrelated origins of DNA replication but, in contrast to HSV-1, these function at different stages of the life cycle (Hammerschmidt and Mankertz 1991). Ori_P is required for maintaining genome copy number in dividing cells, and is recognized by a protein specific to EBV. Ori_{Lyt}, which is required for lytic amplification of EBV genomes, consists of a much more extended region than HSV-1 ori_S or ori_L, and contains several important sequence elements. A lytic origin of replication has also been identified in the HCMV genome, but an origin equivalent in function to EBV ori_P has not yet been found.

DNA polymerase has been well characterized at the genetic and biochemical levels. The catalytic subunit (encoded by gene UL30) is the target of antiviral agents, such as phosphoformic and phosphoacetic acids, which mimic dNTPs, and is the site of genetic resistance to such compounds (Coen 1992). The associated, smaller subunit of DNA polymerase (encoded by gene UL42) seems to increase the processivity of the holoenzyme. Two of the components of the helicase–primase complex (encoded by genes UL5 and UL52) are essential for both enzymic activities; the UL5 protein contains a helicase domain. The third component (encoded by gene UL8) has an auxiliary function, and also interacts with the origin-binding protein. The origin-binding protein (encoded by gene UL9) consists of a homodimer, with each subunit comprising a domain that binds to the origin of replication and a helicase domain that may function in unwinding the origin to allow access to the replication complex. The single-stranded DNA-binding protein (encoded by gene UL29) also interacts with the origin-binding protein.

6.5 DNA packaging

The events that occur during packaging of viral DNA into immature capsids are not well understood. As with capsid assembly, this area is attracting increasing interest because of the possibility of antiviral intervention in essential herpesvirus-specific processes.

Seven HSV-1 genes have thus far been identified from their phenotypic effects on mutant viruses as having roles in DNA packaging (UL6, UL25, UL15, UL28, UL32, UL33 and UL12). It is unlikely that this list is complete, or that the products of the genes listed are all central to the DNA packaging mechanism. The UL6 and UL25 proteins are virion components, the former exclusively as part of the capsid and at least a proportion of the latter as a capsid-associated protein. The UL15 protein is of interest because it bears sequence similarity to ATPases and to the large subunit of the bacteriophage T4 terminase, which is responsible for energy-driven insertion of DNA into the capsid. This observation suggests that some aspects of HSV-1 DNA packaging might find parallels in bacteriophage T4. The UL15 gene is unusual in that it has highly conserved counterparts in all herpesviruses (even CCV) and is expressed as a spliced mRNA. UL12 encodes an alkaline exonuclease that may be responsible for resolving DNA structures produced during packaging.

6.6 Virion structure

DEGREE OF COMPLEXITY

About half of the total number of HSV-1 genes specify components of the viral particle. These proteins include 8 capsid constituents, at least 20 tegument components, and more than 10 proteins, most glycosylated, in the envelope. The proteins making up the capsid are much better characterized than those in the envelope or tegument (Rixon 1993). Capsid proteins can be envisaged as providing a robust, self-assembling container for the viral genome, tegument proteins as ancillary factors responsible for enhancing viral infection, and envelope proteins as molecules involved in allowing infecting virions to enter cells efficiently and facilitating mature virions to exit the infected cell successfully.

CAPSID

The proteins that make up HSV-1 capsids are conserved in other herpesviruses, and the capsid structures of widely diverged members (such as HSV-1 and CCV) are similar. Thus, it is likely that the same basic mechanism for capsid maturation is fundamental to all herpesviruses. The proteins that make up the HSV-1 capsid have undergone extensive characterization, and the structure of the capsid has been analysed in some detail by electron cryomicroscopy (Zhou et al. 1994). A single protein, VP5, makes up the hexameric and pentameric capsomers of the HSV-1 capsid, and the intercapsomeric regions are composed of a complex of 2 copies of VP23 plus a single copy of VP19C (known as a triplex). The external tips of hexameric capsomers are decorated with a small protein, VP26. The capsid also contains a protease, VP24. Recently, the protein encoded by the UL6 gene has been identified as a capsid constituent that is present in a small number of copies per capsid.

The steps that occur during capsid formation are reminiscent of those that take place during maturation of certain DNA-containing bacteriophages, such as T4, in that replicated DNA enters preformed immature capsids containing a core of scaffolding proteins, which are expelled in a process that involves specific proteolytic events. The HSV-1 scaffold proteins are encoded by the overlapping genes UL26 and UL26.5 (Liu and Roizman 1991) (see Fig. 17.4). The UL26.5 protein is identical to the C-terminal portion of the UL26 protein. Proteolytic action of the N-terminal domain of the UL26 protein on the UL26 protein itself at 2 locations, one central and one near the C terminus, and on the UL26.5 protein at the site near the C terminus generates VP24 (the protease) and VP21 (the minor scaffold protein) from the UL26 protein, and VP22a (the major scaffold protein) from the UL26.5 protein. During DNA packaging, VP21 and VP22a are expelled from the capsid interior, but VP24 is retained. The molecular events that occur during capsid maturation are now being unravelled with the aid of a system in which the HSV-1 proteins are expressed from baculovirus recombinants (Tatman et al. 1994, Thomsen, Roof and Homa 1994). Using this approach, VP5, VP23 and VP19C have been shown to be essential for capsid assembly, plus either the gene UL26.5 protein which gives rise to VP22a or, at a reduced efficiency, the gene UL26 protein which gives rise to VP21 and VP24. The proteolytic function of the UL26 protein is thus not essential in this system, but its requirement for virus production during HSV-1 infection indicates that it is involved in removal of the scaffold proteins during DNA packaging.

TEGUMENT

The tegument has a complex composition but its structure has not yet been defined in any herpesvirus. It is a feature of all members of the family but, in contrast to capsid proteins, most components of the tegument are specific to a particular subfamily or genus and are therefore likely to have important roles in modulating the virus–host interaction, rather than as passive structural components of the virion. Examples of such roles for HSV-1 tegument proteins are the virion host shutoff factor (encoded by UL41), Vmw65 (encoded by UL48) and the UL13 protein kinase. It is likely that additional functions for tegument proteins will emerge as this area of research develops.

ENVELOPE

At least 11 HSV-1 genes encode membrane-associated glycoproteins, and several of these are present in the virion envelope. A summary of the properties of HSV-1 glycoproteins is given in Table 17.3, and genetic information is give in Table 17.2. Most information is available for the major structural glycoproteins gB, gC and gD; less is known about the minor glycoproteins, particularly those that have been discovered only recently. In fact, gJ has not yet been identified, and presently has the status of a predicted glycoprotein based on its imputed amino acid sequence. The glycoproteins are located in membranes by virtue of one or several hydrophobic domains, and thus are exposed on the exterior of infected cells or virions. Also, they are functionally associated with initial virus–host interactions (Spear 1993) and are therefore likely to be of considerable importance for pathogenicity. For these reasons, glycoproteins have been the subject of intense scrutiny, particularly regarding their use as a route for vaccine development.

Many glycoproteins are specific to genera or subfamilies. For example, 3 HSV-1 glycoproteins lack counterparts in VZV (gD, gG, gJ). Only gB, gH, gL and gM have counterparts across the α-, β- and γ-herpesviruses. HCMV contains extensive families of related glycoprotein genes that appear to have been generated by gene duplication and divergence (Chee et al. 1990), and thus represent a striking evolutionary experiment in generating genetic diversity.

The primary interaction of HSV-1 with cells involves the binding of gC to heparan sulphate present on cell surface proteoglycans (WuDunn and Spear 1989). Viral mutants that lack gC are infectious but with very much reduced binding. Another HSV-1 glycoprotein, gB, exhibits heparin binding, and binding is dependent on gB when gC is absent; viruses lacking both gC and gB fail to bind to cells.

Herpesviruses enter cells by fusion with the plasma membrane. Three glycoproteins (gB, gD and gH) are required for cell penetration by HSV-1, and gK and gL are probably also required for this process. Like HSV, HCMV uses heparan sulphate as a cell surface receptor for the initial binding of virus. EBV, however, binds to cells in a different manner. The EBV virion glycoprotein gp350/220, which lacks sequence counterparts in the α- and β-herpesviruses, binds the cellular receptor CR2 (now CD21) which is found on B lymphocytes (Fingeroth et al. 1984); an unidentified cellular receptor for EBV is present on epithelial cells.

Of the HSV-1 glycoproteins that are not required for growth of virus in cell culture, 3 interact with key elements of the immune system: gC binds to the C3b component of the complement system, and gE and gI form a complex that can bind the Fc constant region of immunoglobulin G. Of the essential glycoproteins, gH and gL associate during maturation in endoplasmic reticulum and are present as a heterodimer in

virions. Also, HSV-1 is unusual in that gB in other herpesviruses is processed by a trypsin-like cleavage into a disulphide-linked dimer.

6.7 Pathogenesis

Although most viral proteins have some effect on pathogenicity, some are known to have or are suspected of having specific roles in disease processes, including latency. These proteins, because they help to fit a virus to an ecological niche, are usually specific to a subfamily or even to a genus. They may have little effect on the growth of virus in cell culture but may profoundly influence virus virulence in vivo. Some of the proteins in this group apparently modulate the immune response of the host; these seem to be more numerous in the β- and γ-herpesviruses (e.g. the MHC class I homologue of HCMV and the complement control proteins of HVS). In addition to gC, gE and gI which can interact with the immune system, a gene specific to HSV-1 and HSV-2 (gene US12) encodes an immediate-early protein (Vmw12; ICP47) which has recently been shown to interfere with maturation of MHC class I proteins in infected cells by interacting with the TAP peptide transporter complex (York et al. 1994). Other proteins also seem to affect the interaction between the virus and the infected cells in ways that are not yet fully defined. These include the G-coupled protein receptors of β- and γ2-herpesviruses, and the product of gene RL1 (ICP34.5) that is specific to HSV-1 and HSV-2 (gene RL1), which is related to proteins implicated in cell differentiation, and has a profound effect on neuropathogenicity (Chou et al. 1991). RL1 null mutant viruses are not neurovirulent in vivo, and exhibit limited replication at peripheral sites but fail to replicate in neurons of the peripheral nervous system. These viruses can, however, establish latent infections from which they can be reactivated.

Functional analyses of proteins such as that encoded by the RL1 gene which impart the capacity to invade and destroy central nervous system neurons, and of others which modulate the latent state, are fundamental to our understanding of herpesviruses as infectious agents. Information of this sort is crucial for the design of safe and efficient herpesvirus vectors for

Table 17.3 Properties of HSV-1 glycoproteins

Property	HSV-1 glycoproteins										
	gB	**gC**	**gD**	**gE**	**gG**	**gH**	**gI**	**gJ**	**gK**	**gL**	**gM**
Present in VZV	+	+	−	+	−	+	+	−	+	+	+
Present in α-, β- and γ-herpesviruses	+	−	−	−	−	+	−	−	−	+	+
Essential for replication in cell culture	+	−	+	−	−	+	−	−	+	+	−
Present in virions	+	+	+	+	+	+	+	?	−	+	+
Mediates absorption	+	+	−	−	?	−	−	?	−	−	?
Essential for penetration	+	−	+	−	−	+	−	−	?	+	−
Primary role in cell fusion (syncytia)	+	−	−	?	?	?	?	?	+	?	?
Neutralization	+	+	+	+	+	+	+	?	?	?	?
Cell-mediated immunity	+	+	+	+	+	?	?	?	?	?	?

?, not known

gene replacement and tumour therapy and for the development of live vaccines. Research in this area promises to be particularly exciting, and it is likely that

many different mechanisms used by herpesviruses to control the processes of natural infection will be elucidated in coming years.

REFERENCES

Albrecht J-C, Nicholas J et al., 1992, Primary structure of the herpesvirus saimiri genome, *Virology*, **66:** 5047–58.

Baer R, Bankier AT et al., 1984, DNA sequence and expression of the B95-8 Epstein–Barr virus genome, *Nature (London)*, **310:** 207–11.

Campbell MEM, Palfreyman JW, Preston CM, 1984, Identification of herpes simplex virus DNA sequences which encode a *trans*-acting polypeptide responsible for stimulation of immediate early transcription, *J Mol Biol*, **180:** 1–19.

Challberg MD, 1991, Herpes simplex virus DNA replication, *Semin Virol*, **2:** 247–56.

Chang Y, Cesarman E et al., 1994, Identification of herpesvirus-like DNA sequences in AIDS-associated Kaposi's sarcoma, *Science*, **266:** 1865–9.

Chee MS, Bankier AT et al., 1990, Analysis of the protein-coding content of the sequence of human cytomegalovirus strain AD169, *Curr Top Microbiol Immunol*, **154:** 125–69.

Chou J, Kern ER et al., 1990, Mapping of herpes simplex virus-1 neurovirulence to $\gamma_1 34.5$, a gene nonessential for growth in culture, *Science*, **250:** 1262–5.

Coen DM, 1992, Molecular aspects of anti-herpesvirus drugs, *Semin Virol*, **3:** 3–12.

Cohen EA, Gaudreau P et al., 1986, Specific inhibition of herpesvirus ribonucleotide reductase by a nonapeptide derived from the carboxy terminus of subunit 2, *Nature (London)*, **321:** 441–3.

Dargan DJ, 1986, The structure and assembly of herpesviruses, *Electron Microscopy of Proteins*, vol. 5, eds Harris JR, Horne RW, Academic Press, London, 359–436.

Davison AJ, 1992a, Genetic structure and content of herpesviruses, *Equine Infectious Diseases VI*, eds Plowright W, Rossdale PD, Wade JF, R & W Publications, Newmarket, 165–74.

Davison AJ, 1992b, Channel catfish virus: a new type of herpesvirus, *Virology*, **186:** 9–14.

Davison AJ, 1993, Herpesvirus genes, *Rev Med Virol*, **3:** 237–44.

Davison AJ, McGeoch DJ, 1995, *Herpesviridae, Molecular Basis of Viral Evolution*, eds Gibbs AJ, Calisher C, Garcia-Arenal F, Cambridge University Press, Cambridge, 290–309.

Davison AJ, Scott JE, 1986, The complete DNA sequence of varicella-zoster virus, *J Gen Virol*, **67:** 1759–816.

Dutia BM, Frame MC et al., 1986, Specific inhibition of herpesvirus ribonucleotide reductase by synthetic peptides, *Nature (London)*, **321:** 439–41.

Everett RD, 1987, The regulation of transcription of viral and cellular genes by herpesvirus immediate-early gene products, *Anticancer Res*, **7:** 589–604.

Fingeroth JD, Weis JJ et al., 1984, Epstein–Barr virus receptor of human B lymphocytes is the C3d receptor CR2, *Proc Natl Acad Sci USA*, **81:** 4510–16.

Frenkel N, Schirmer EC et al., 1990, Isolation of a new herpesvirus from human CD4+ T cells, *Proc Natl Acad Sci USA*, **87:** 748–52.

Gompels UA, Nicholas J et al., 1995, The DNA sequence of human herpesvirus 6: structure, coding content, and genome evolution, *Virology*, **209:** 29–51.

Hammerschmidt W, Mankertz J, 1991, Herpesviral DNA replication: between the known and unknown, *Semin Virol*, **2:** 257–69.

Hayward GS, Jacob RJ et al., 1975, Anatomy of herpes simplex virus DNA: evidence for four populations that differ in the relative orientations of their long and short components, *Proc Natl Acad Sci USA*, **72:** 4243–7.

Honess RW, 1984, Herpes simplex and 'The Herpes Complex':

diverse observations and a unifying hypothesis, *J Gen Virol*, **65:** 2077–107.

Honess RW, Roizman B, 1974, Regulation of herpesvirus macro-molecular synthesis. I. Cascade regulation of the synthesis of three groups of viral proteins, *J Virol*, **14:** 8–19.

Kieff E, Liebowitz D, 1990, Epstein–Barr virus and its replication, *Fields' Virology*, 2nd edn, eds Fields BN, Knipe DM, Raven Press, New York, 1889–920.

Liu F, Roizman B, 1991, The promoter, transcriptional unit, and coding sequence of the herpes simplex virus 1 family 35 proteins are contained within and in frame with the $U_L 26$ open reading frame, *J Virol*, **65:** 206–12.

Liu B, Stinski MF, 1992, Human cytomegalovirus contains a tegument protein that enhances transcription from promoters with upstream ATF and AP-1-*cis*-acting elements, *J Virol*, **66:** 4434–44.

McGeoch DJ, 1989, The genomes of the human herpesviruses: contents, relationships and evolution, *Annu Rev Microbiol*, **43:** 235–65.

McGeoch DJ, 1992, Molecular evolution of large DNA viruses of eukaryotes, *Semin Virol*, **3:** 399–408.

McGeoch DJ, Schaffer PA, 1993, Herpes simplex virus, *Genetic Maps*, 6th edn, vol 1, ed O'Brien S, Cold Spring Harbor Press, Cold Spring Harbor NY, 147–56.

McGeoch DJ, Barnett BC, MacLean CA, 1993, Emerging functions of alphaherpesvirus genes, *Semin Virol*, **4:** 125–44.

McGeoch DJ, Dalrymple MA et al., 1988, The complete DNA sequence of the long unique region in the genome of herpes simplex virus type 1, *J Gen Virol*, **69:** 1531–74.

McGeoch DJ, Cook S et al., 1995, Molecular phylogeny and evolutionary timescale for the family of mammalian herpesviruses, *J Mol Biol*, **247:** 443–58.

Marsden HS, 1992, Disruption of protein–subunit interactions, *Semin Virol*, **3:** 67–75.

Minson AC, 1989, *Herpesviridae, Andrewes' Viruses of Vertebrates*, 5th edn, ed Porterfield JS, Baillière Tindall, London, 293–332.

Moore PS, Gao SJ et al., 1996, Primary characterization of a herpesvirus agent associated with Kaposi's sarcoma, *J Virol*, **70:** 549–58.

Morrison JM, 1991, *Virus Induced Enzymes*, Wiley, Chichester.

O'Hare P, 1993, The virion transactivator of herpes simplex virus, *Semin Virol*, **4:** 145–55.

Rice SA, Long MC et al., 1995, Herpes simplex virus immediate early protein ICP22 is required for viral modification of host RNA polymerase II and establishment of the normal viral transcription program, *J Virol*, **69:** 5550–9.

Rixon FJ, 1993, Structure and assembly of herpesviruses, *Semin Virol*, **4:** 135–44.

Roizman B, Sears AE, 1990, Herpes simplex viruses and their replication, *Fields' Virology*, 2nd edn, eds Fields BN, Knipe DM, Raven Press, New York, 1795–841.

Roizman B, Desrosiers RC et al., 1992, The family *Herpesviridae*: an update, *Arch Virol*, **123:** 425–49.

Sakaoka H, Kurita K et al., 1994, Quantitative analysis of genomic polymorphism of herpes simplex virus type 1 strains from six countries: studies of molecular evolution and molecular epidemiology of the virus, *J Gen Virol*, **75:** 513–27.

Salahuddin SZ, Ablashi DV et al., 1986, Isolation of a new virus, HBLV, in patients with lymphoproliferative disorders, *Science*, **234:** 596–601.

Sandri-Goldin R, Mendoza GE, 1992, A herpesvirus regulatory protein appears to act post-transcriptionally by affecting mRNA processing, *Genes Dev*, **6:** 848–63.

Schrag JD, Prasad BVV et al., 1989, Three-dimensional structure of the HSV1 nucleocapsid, *Cell*, **56:** 651–60.

Sheldrick P, Berthelot N, 1974, Inverted repetitions in the chromosome of herpes simplex virus, *Cold Spring Harbor Symp Quant Biol*, **39:** 667–78.

Spear PG, 1993, Entry of alphaherpesviruses into cells, *Semin Virol*, **4:** 167–80.

Stinski MF, 1990, Cytomegalovirus and its replication, *Fields' Virology*, 2nd edn, eds Fields BN, Knipe DM, Raven Press, New York, 1959–80.

Stow ND, 1982, Localization of an origin of DNA replication within the TR$_S$/IR$_S$ region of the herpes simplex virus type 1 genome, *EMBO J*, **1:** 863–7.

Tanaka K, Kondo T et al., 1994, Human herpesvirus 7: another causal agent for roseola (exanthem subitum), *J Pediatr*, **125:** 1–5.

Tatman JD, Preston VG et al., 1994, Assembly of herpes simplex virus type 1 capsids using a panel of recombinant baculoviruses, *J Gen Virol*, **75:** 1101–13.

Telford EAR, Watson MS et al., 1992, The DNA sequence of equine herpesvirus-1, *Virology*, **189:** 304–16.

Telford EAR, Watson MS et al., 1995, The DNA sequence of equine herpesvirus 2, *J Mol Biol*, **249:** 520–8.

Thomsen DR, Roof LL, Homa FL, 1994, Assembly of herpes simplex virus (HSV) intermediate capsids in insect cells infected with recombinant baculoviruses expressing HSV capsid proteins, *J Virol*, **68:** 2442–57.

Wagner EK, 1985, Individual HSV transcripts, *The Herpesviruses*, eds Fields BN, Knipe DM, Plenum Press, New York, 45–104.

Wagner MJ, Summers WC, 1978, Structures of the joint region and the termini of the DNA of herpes simplex virus type 1, *J Virol*, **27:** 374–87.

Ward PL, Roizman B, 1994, Herpes simplex genes: the blueprint of a successful human pathogen, *Trends Genet*, **10:** 267–74.

Watson RJ, Clements JB, 1980, A herpes simplex virus type 1 function continuously required for early and late virus RNA synthesis, *Nature (London)*, **285:** 329–30.

Wildy P, Russell WC, Horne RW, 1960, The morphology of herpesvirus, *Virology*, **12:** 204–22.

WuDunn D, Spear PG, 1989, Initial interaction of herpes simplex virus with cells is binding to heparan sulphate, *J Virol*, **63:** 52–8.

Yamanishi K, Okuno T et al., 1988, Identification of human herpesvirus-6 as a causal agent for exanthem subitum, *Lancet*, **1:** 1065–7.

York IA, Roop C et al., 1994, A cytosolic herpes simplex protein inhibits antigen presentation to CD8+ T lymphocytes, *Cell*, **77:** 525–35.

Zhou ZH, Prasad BVV et al., 1994, Protein subunit structures in the herpes simplex virus A-capsid determined by 400 kV spotscan electron cryomicroscopy, *J Mol Biol*, **242:** 456–69.

ALPHAHERPESVIRUSES: HERPES SIMPLEX AND VARICELLA-ZOSTER

A C Minson

Herpes simplex virus	Varicella-zoster virus
1 Clinical manifestations	7 Clinical manifestations
2 Epidemiology	8 Epidemiology
3 Pathology and pathogenesis	9 Pathogenesis and pathology
4 Immune response	10 Immune response
5 Diagnosis	11 Diagnosis
6 Control	12 Control

Herpes simplex virus types 1 and 2 (HSV-1 and HSV-2) and varicella-zoster virus (VZV) are alphaherpesviruses that are related in their genetic and biological properties. Their genomes are composed of homologous sets of genes organized in a co-linear fashion; they cause productive cytolytic infection of epithelial cells and establish life-long latent infections in sensory nerve ganglia. There are, however, important biological differences. VZV infection has a viraemic phase whereas HSV infectivity is usually limited to the epithelium and sensory nerves at the infection site; HSV is transmitted only by contact whereas VZV is air-borne and contagious; VZV is highly species specific whereas HSV can infect, experimentally, a wide range of species. Indeed our knowledge of HSV pathogenesis and immunity derives largely from studies of the virus in rodents. HSV-1 and HSV-2 are closely related: they cross-react antigenically, exhibit extensive nucleotide sequence homology and their genes are functionally homologous because stable intertypic recombinants can be generated readily in tissue culture. However, despite the fact that HSV-1 and HSV-2 can infect similar sites in humans, recombination between these viruses does not appear to occur in vivo, and genetic comparison suggests that the 2 subtypes have evolved independently for more than 5 million years (McGeoch and Cook 1994).

HERPES SIMPLEX VIRUS

1 CLINICAL MANIFESTATIONS

Herpes simplex virus infects mucosal epithelium or damaged cutaneous epithelium, and infection can therefore occur at a variety of sites, but oral and genital infections are most common. HSV-2 is predominantly responsible for genital infection but HSV-1 contributes significantly, representing 30–50% of genital isolates in some studies (Buckmaster et al. 1984, Ross, Smith and Elton 1993). In contrast, HSV-2 is rarely isolated from oral lesions. The basis of this preference for different mucosal surfaces by the 2 virus types is unknown but the predominance of HSV-2 'below the waist' and HSV-1 'above the waist' extends to other sites. Thus anal lesions, cutaneous lesions of the thighs and buttocks, and infections of the neonate during birth are more frequently caused by HSV-2 whilst eye infections and cutaneous lesions of the head and neck are usually caused by HSV-1. Regardless of the site of infection or the virus type, HSV enters sensory nerve endings during primary infection and is transported to the neuronal cell body where latent infection is established. Since oral and genital infections are by far the most common, the trigeminal and sacral ganglia are the usual sites of latent infection by HSV-1 and HSV-2 respectively. The majority of the adult population is latently infected with HSV, but it is clear that infection rates greatly exceed clinical disease rates and many, perhaps most, individuals who are latently infected with HSV have no recollection of primary infection and do not suffer recurrent lesions.

Primary oral infection presents as an acute gingivostomatitis comprising painful ulcers in the mouth, which resolve within a few weeks, often accompanied by fever and enlargement of local lymph nodes. A significant proportion of sore throats is also thought to be caused by primary oral HSV, and this may be the most common manifestation of primary infection. During the course of primary infection the virus establishes a life-long latent infection in neurons of the trigeminal ganglia, and 'reactivation' results in the reseeding of virus into the oral epithelium and shedding in saliva. A minority of seropositive people suffer periodic clinical recurrences, the classic 'cold sores', crops of vesicles on the mucocutaneous junctions of the mouth and nose which ulcerate, crust and heal within 4–7 days (Fig. 18.1). These individuals recognize a prodromal tingling or burning sensation which heralds the development of the recurrent lesion. Recurrences are provoked by a variety of stimuli, including sunlight, physical trauma, stress, respiratory infections and hormonal change, but it is not known whether these stimuli act by a common pathway. The development of a cold sore requires reactivation of the latent virus in the ganglia followed by the establishment of a focus of epithelial infection; a provoking stimulus might operate either by triggering a reactivation in the ganglia or by modifying the susceptibility of the relevant epithelium such that a ganglionic reactivation, which would otherwise have been silent, results in a clinical recurrence.

Genital herpes consists of painful vesicles on the genitalia or anal region. Aseptic meningitis has been reported as a complication of primary infection, and proctitis has been reported in homosexual men. As with oral infection, many primary genital infections are inapparent and the first indication of infection may be a recurrence, an episode that has been termed 'initial infection' to distinguish it from the primary infection (Corey et al. 1983). Genital herpes infections

recur at a higher frequency than oral infections, and genital HSV-2 infections recur more frequently than genital HSV-1 infections (Lafferty et al. 1987). The frequency and severity of recurrent episodes usually decrease with time but recurrent genital herpes is a painful and distressing disease, and many patients suffer frequent recurrences for many years. Reactivation of latent virus and shedding in genital secretions occur at a much higher rate than clinical disease.

Infection of the skin, manifest as a crop of classic herpetic vesicles, can occur on any part of the body, most commonly the head or neck, and probably always results from the contamination of damaged skin by virus in saliva or genital secretions. Infection may result from intimacy or activities likely to cause abrasion, such as wrestling (herpes gladiatorum) or rugby (scrum pox). Lesions on the fingers (herpetic whitlows) are an occupational hazard for healthcare workers. A particularly severe disease results from infection of eczematous skin (eczema herpeticum), in which the virus spreads widely, causing large areas of ulceration.

Herpes infections of the eye are second only to oral and genital infections in frequency. Primary infections are associated with keratoconjunctivitis and are often bilateral whereas recurrences are usually unilateral and result in dendritic ulcers or stromal involvement. Repeated recurrences may lead to scarring and opacification of the cornea, and consequent sight impairment.

Invasion of the central nervous system (CNS) is manifest as herpes encephalitis, a cytolytic infection, primarily of neurons, with a propensity to focus in the temporal lobes (see Chapter 40). Untreated, the disease has a mortality of >70% and most survivors are neurologically impaired. All age groups are susceptible but the disease is rare; about one case per million population is reported each year in the UK and the USA. Symptoms generally begin with fever and headache, rapidly followed by disorientation and progressive deterioration in consciousness, but the symptoms are not diagnostic and can be confused with other syndromes. Predisposing factors are unknown. Herpes encephalitis can apparently result from primary or recurrent infection (Nahmias et al. 1982, Whitley et al. 1982), but the route to the CNS is uncertain. A focal encephalitis, similar to that observed in humans, results from infection of mice by the olfactory route (Anderson and Field 1983). Aciclovir (acyclovir) therapy has greatly reduced the morbidity and mortality of herpes encephalitis but effective treatment depends on prompt diagnosis.

The neonate is highly susceptible to HSV infection, and neonatal infection is frequently fatal. The disease presents classically as a generalized infection affecting multiple organs, including the lung, liver, adrenals, CNS and skin, but in some cases the infection is more limited, involving the skin or the CNS or both. The prognosis is very poor for those with disseminated or CNS infection. In the USA neonatal herpes is estimated to occur with an incidence of 1 per 2000–5000 deliveries and is perceived as a major public health

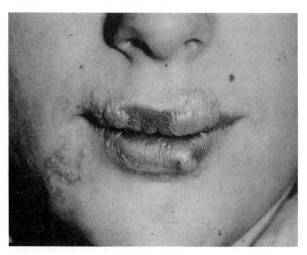

Fig. 18.1 Vesicular cold sores due to recurrent herpes simplex. (Photograph by kind permission of Professor J H Subak-Sharpe, Institute of Virology, Glasgow.)

problem, but in the UK the disease is rare (Sullivan-Bolyai et al. 1983, PHLS Report 1987), an unexplained discrepancy that cannot be accounted for by differences in the overall frequency of genital herpes in the 2 populations. The infection is most commonly acquired during birth from a genital infection of the mother but infections in utero and in the immediate postnatal period have also been documented and probably represent a significant proportion of the total. Primary infection in the mother close to term presents a much higher risk to the neonate than does recurrent infection (Prober et al. 1987), probably owing to the higher virus titres present during primary infection and perhaps to the protective effect of maternal antibody present in the neonate exposed to recurrent infection. Delivery by caesarean section is usually recommended when genital lesions are present at term. Superficial damage to the skin by fetal scalp monitors is thought to provide the virus with a route of entry, and the use of scalp monitors is contra-indicated if the mother has a history of recurrent genital infection.

Not surprisingly, the immunocompromised patient has an increased susceptibility to HSV infection. The most common manifestation is a reduced capacity to control recurrent oral lesions, which occur more frequently, spread more widely in the mouth and on the head and neck, and resolve more slowly, if at all, in the absence of therapy. Although these infections can be very severe, they are nevertheless limited to the skin and mucosa, even in profoundly immunosuppressed patients. Disseminated, generalized infection, as seen in the neonate, has been reported in adults very rarely.

2 EPIDEMIOLOGY

A wide range of mammalian species can be infected experimentally with HSV but there is no evidence that this occurs naturally. Humans are the only natural host, and latent virus in trigeminal and sacral ganglia is the reservoir. The source of transmitted virus is oral or genital secretions, and transmission requires contact. There is no seasonal variation in disease incidence. Because HSV-2 is primarily a sexually transmitted disease and occurs only rarely as an oral infection, evidence of HSV-2 infection is found almost exclusively in adolescents and adults, whereas HSV-1 is a common infection of childhood. Despite this straightforward picture, which emerges from a large number of seroepidemiological and virological studies, precise data on the incidence of HSV-1 and HSV-2 infections in different study populations have been difficult to obtain because of the high proportion of asymptomatic infections and problems in distinguishing antibodies to the 2 subtypes.

In many populations virtually all children are infected with HSV-1 during the first 5 years of life, but seroconversion rates vary greatly with geographic area and socioeconomic group. In higher socioeconomic groups in industrialized countries, seroconversion may be as low as 20% during the first 5 years, rising to 40–60% during adolescence and early adulthood. Young children secrete virus asymptomatically more frequently and for much more prolonged periods than seropositive adults; this, together with higher levels of contact activity, probably accounts for the high attack rates in this group. Seroepidemiological surveys emphasize the view that HSV-2 is transmitted primarily by the sexual route: antibodies specific for HSV-2 are virtually non-existent in nuns but are found in the majority of prostitutes, and the appearance of HSV-2 antibodies correlates with the onset of sexual activity. The reported overall incidence of HSV-2 antibodies in the adult population varies in different studies, and many historical surveys suffer from technical problems associated with the serological cross-reactivity of HSV-1 and HSV-2. More recent studies estimate that 15–25% of the adult US population is infected with HSV-2, and broadly similar data have been obtained in the UK (Ades et al. 1989), though prevalence rates vary significantly among different ethnic groups. As noted above, HSV-1 can also be transmitted by the sexual route, and in some studies nearly 50% of genital isolates were of this type (Ross, Smith and Elton 1993). It is supposed, though not proven, that the large number of HSV-1 genital infections and the occasional HSV-2 oral infection result from orogenital sex.

3 PATHOLOGY AND PATHOGENESIS

The portal of entry in primary infection is the damaged skin or mucosa and the classic lesion is a vesicle beneath the keratinized squamous epithelial cells (Fig. 18.2). The infection of epithelial cells is cytolytic; the cells lose adhesion, occasionally become multi-nucleate as a result of virus-induced cell fusion and contain Cowdry type A nuclear inclusions. The vesicle and surrounding tissue contain a dense infiltrate of inflammatory cells, mostly mononuclear. The vesicle drains and the lesion crusts before healing occurs, sometimes with residual scarring, and draining lymph nodes are commonly enlarged during this process. Recurrent lesions are morphologically and histologically similar but are usually less extensive, and lymph node swelling is inapparent. In the immune competent patient the lesion resolves within 7–10 days of its appearance.

3.1 Latency and reactivation

During primary infection of the skin or mucosa the virus enters sensory nerve endings and is transported by fast retrograde axonal flow to the neuronal bodies of the dorsal root ganglia innervating the site of infection. In animal models this is followed by a period of limited virus replication in the ganglia, during which virus antigen can be detected in a small number of neurons. Within about 10 days, no infectious virus can be detected in the ganglia or at the site of inoculation, but the presence of latent virus can be detected for

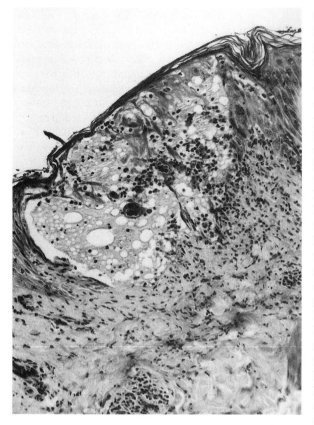

Fig. 18.2 Herpes simplex vesicle: the vesicle contains a serous exudate with inflammatory cells and large multinucleated cells; a light mixed inflammatory cell infiltrate is also present in the underlying dermis. The roof of the vesicle shows reticular degeneration – a result of progressive swelling and eventual rupture of the keratinocytes with only their cell walls remaining. Haematoxylin and eosin × 150. (Photograph by courtesy of Dr Morag Seywright, Pathology Department, Western Infirmary, Glasgow.)

the lifetime of the infected animal by dissection and in vitro culture of the relevant sensory ganglia (Stevens and Cook 1971, Hill, Field and Blyth 1975). Similarly, 'in vitro reactivation' of latent virus can be achieved by culture of trigeminal ganglia from cadavers of HSV-1 seropositive humans.

Many lines of evidence show that HSV establishes a true latent infection rather than a low level chronic infection. Mutant viruses that are incapable of replicating at the internal temperature of the mouse establish and maintain latency (McLennan and Darby 1980). Long-term treatment of infected mice or humans with aciclovir does not cure latency (Fife et al. 1994); the state of the viral genome in latent infection is unique. HSV DNA within virus particles is a linear molecule whereas viral DNA in latently infected ganglia is endless and is thought to be present as a circular episome (Mellerick and Fraser 1987). The latently infected ganglion contains a unique set of transcripts, the 'latency associated transcripts' (LATs) synthesized from a single promoter (the LAT promoter) situated in the repeat sequences flanking the unique long region of the viral genome (Stevens

et al. 1987). These transcripts are readily detected by in situ hybridization in latently infected human trigeminal ganglia or in ganglia from experimental animals, and they are found exclusively in neurons (Fig. 18.3) – consistent with other evidence that this cell type is the site of latent infection. The function of these molecules is, however, unknown. No translation product has been identified, and mutations that modify the transcripts or abolish their synthesis do not prevent the virus from establishing or maintaining latent infection (reviewed by Ho 1992) but appear to reduce the frequency of reactivation (Krause et al. 1995). Indeed, despite extensive study, no HSV gene has been identified that is essential for latent infection, and one view is that latency requires no gene function but occurs by default if the productive cycle fails. On this supposition the transcriptional machinery of the neuron is the key factor in latency and reactivation: if the neuron fails to transcribe the viral immediate early genes (see Chapter 17), the productive cycle cannot be initiated and the viral genome is latent by default, but at some later time perturbation of the sensory nerve may change the transcriptional programme of the neuron. The viral immediate early genes may then be expressed, the productive cycle is initiated and the latent virus reactivates. The evidence for this mechanism is largely negative but is consistent with the characteristics of an in vitro latency model in which the level of expression of one of the immediate early genes appears to be a key factor in determining whether the virus enters the lytic cycle or remains latent (Harris et al. 1989).

Perturbation of the sensory nerve can induce HSV reactivation, an observation first made by Cushing (1905), who noted the frequent appearance of cold sores after sectioning the posterior sensory root of the trigeminal ganglion, a result that has been confirmed in animal models. Furthermore, virus in latently infected rat sympathetic ganglia cultured in vitro reactivates after withdrawal of nerve growth factor (Wilcox et al. 1990). Nevertheless, the specific neuronal changes that lead to reactivation are unknown. A wide variety of stimuli provoke clinical recurrence but, as noted earlier (section 1, p. 325), many of these stimuli may act to enhance virus replication at the periphery rather than to induce reactivation in the ganglion. What is certain is that reactivation and virus shedding are much more common than clinical recurrence. The fate of the neuron in which reactivation occurs is also unknown. It is axiomatic of HSV infection that the productive cycle is cytolytic, yet reactivation and seeding of epithelium with infectious particles must require productive infection in the neuron. There is no evidence of sensory loss, even in patients who suffer frequent recurrences over a very long period, and it is uncertain whether reactivation results in the loss of the neuron or if, unlike other cell types, the neuron can survive virus replication.

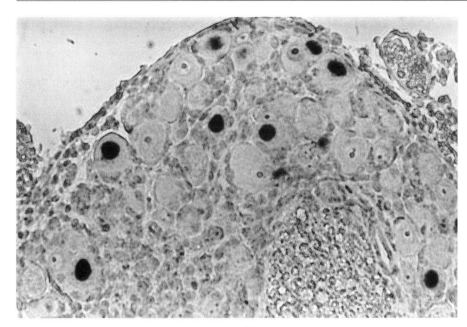

Fig. 18.3 Virus-specific transcripts in a sensory ganglion from a mouse latently infected with HSV-1. Latency-associated transcripts are detected by hybridization in situ within the nuclei of a minority of sensory neurons. No viral antigens, productive cycle transcripts or virus particles are detectable. Latent infection of the tissue can be demonstrated by explant culture. (Photograph by courtesy of Dr R Lachmann, Department of Pathology, University of Cambridge.)

4 IMMUNE RESPONSE

Herpes simplex virus infection in humans induces a vigorous humoral and cell-mediated response, but studies of the details are confounded by the very large number of antigens specified by the virus (>70) and by the technical problem of examining the response to primary infection. Most studies in humans have been of the response to latent infection or recurrent disease, whereas much information on the primary response derives from experiments in inbred mice.

Infection is followed within a few days by the appearance of IgM antibodies, closely followed by IgG and IgA. IgG persists indefinitely and antibodies against at least 30 different viral polypeptides have been identified. The surface glycoproteins of the virus (of which there are at least 10) are among the most immunogenic and these are also the targets for complement-dependent and complement-independent antibody-mediated neutralization. Glycoprotein D, delivered as a subunit protein or using live vectors, is probably the most potent inducer of neutralizing antibody and, in humans, anti-gD titres correlate with serum neutralizing titres. The role of antibody in infection is, however, uncertain. High levels of passive antibody protect mice from infection and modulate infection (Simmons and Nash 1985) but B cell deficient mice recover more or less normally from infection and agammaglobulinaemic patients do not suffer particularly severe HSV infections (Corey and Spear 1986, Simmons and Nash 1987). While antibody can protect against infection, at least in mice, the cell-mediated responses are of central importance in controlling an established infection since, in humans and in mice, T cell deficiencies result in severe disease and inefficient clearance of virus. The importance of different T cell subsets and of innate cellular defence mechanisms varies in mice, depending on the strain and infection route. Nevertheless, CD4+ T cells pre-

dominate in clearance of infection from the skin and mucosa (Nash and Gell 1983, Schmid 1988), whereas classic MHC class I restricted cytotoxic T cells are readily detected in mice but difficult to detect in humans. There is evidence that CD8+ T cells control HSV in the nervous system but by a cytokine-mediated mechanism rather than by direct cytotoxicity (Simmons and Tscharke 1992). Innate defences are also likely to be of central importance. HSV has a very broad cell tropism yet systemic generalized disease is found almost exclusively in the neonate and not in profoundly immunosuppressed children or adults. In mice interferon responses, NK cell activity and macrophage function have all been shown to control HSV infection, and deficiencies in these defences may contribute to the susceptibility of the neonate (Gesser et al. 1976, Cunningham and Merigan 1983, Lopez 1985, Wu and Morahan 1992). Severe HSV infection in a child with an NK cell deficiency has been reported (Biron, Byron and Sullivan 1989) but there are conflicting data on the importance of NK cells in controlling HSV (Bukowski and Welsh 1986).

It is worth reiterating that studies of the response to HSV in the mouse are almost exclusively concerned with primary infections. Recurrent infections do not occur in inbred mice, and in guinea-pigs and rabbits, which exhibit recurrent disease, the immune response is not amenable to detailed analysis. In humans, recurrent episodes are not usually accompanied by significant changes in antibody levels but changes in T cell proliferative responses have been reported. Comparisons of immune responses in seropositive patients with and without recurrent disease have given no indication of a consistent quantitative or qualitative difference in response in these 2 groups, and it may be that other factors, such as latent virus load, rather than the immune response, determine recurrence frequency. Nevertheless, the fact that recurrences usually decrease in frequency with time and that immunocompromised patients suffer more recurrent episodes suggests that recurrences can be suppressed by an acquired immune response. This is an issue of some consequence because the identification of the key elements of the response might allow the development of immunotherapeutic approaches to the prevention of recurrent disease.

HSV has evolved a number of mechanisms to evade the immune response. Glycoprotein C binds to the C3b complement component and inhibits the complement cascade (Fries et al. 1986). The glycoprotein E/glycoprotein I complex binds to Fc regions of IgG and inhibits Fc-mediated effector mechanisms (Frank and Friedman 1989, Bell et al. 1990). The US12 gene product binds the peptide transporter (TAP) and prevents antigen presentation on MHC class I molecules (York et al. 1994, Hill et al. 1995). None of these evasion mechanisms operates efficiently in mice, and there is good reason to doubt, therefore, whether immune control of HSV in mice precisely mimics events in humans. Immune responses to HSV infection have been reviewed in detail by Rouse (1992).

5 DIAGNOSIS

HSV infection is usually diagnosed by virus culture. The virus is labile and sensitive to desiccation, so swabs should be kept in transport medium and cultured as soon as possible. HSV grows rapidly in a variety of fibroblasts and epithelial cell types, causing a characteristic cell rounding or 'ballooning'' which develops within a few days and spreads rapidly. Unlike laboratory passaged strains, which are often syncytial, fresh isolates cause little, if any, cell fusion. In combination with clinical presentation, the development of characteristic cytopathic effect (CPE) in culture is usually sufficient for confident diagnosis, but if necessary this can be confirmed by a variety of immunocytochemical or antigen capture tests. The sensitivity of these tests allows diagnosis within 24 hours of culture, before extensive CPE develops, and also allows distinction between HSV-1 and HSV-2 isolates with type-specific reagents. Primary infections can also be diagnosed serologically by the detection of virus-specific IgM or by the rising IgG titre. A variety of tests are available but complement fixation and ELISA are the most widely used. The diagnosis of herpes encephalitis presents a special problem and rapid diagnosis is of importance because of the urgency of appropriate treatment. Diagnosis used to require the identification of virus or virus antigen in brain biopsies, but is now achieved by detection of viral DNA in the cerebrospinal fluid using the polymerase chain reaction (Lakeman et al. 1995). The sample must, however, be taken before aciclovir therapy is begun.

The distinction between of serum antibodies to HSV-1 and HSV-2 is rarely of clinical relevance but is crucial in seroepidemiological surveys of infection incidence. Sera against either virus react with both types in all assays, and historical methods of measuring type-specific antibody such as cross-adsorption and kinetic neutralization were time consuming and unreliable.

More recent methods are based on the observation that glycoprotein G of HSV-1 and HSV-2 is highly immunogenic and shows very little antigenic cross-reaction. Glycoprotein G, purified from infected cells or prepared as a recombinant protein, can therefore be used as a target for type-specific antibody detection using standard enzyme-linked assays (Lee et al. 1986, Sanchez-Martinez et al. 1991, Ho et al. 1992). Although these methods are clearly an improvement on previous approaches, discrepant results have been reported when compared with 'western blot' assays, which are generally regarded as well validated but relatively tedious (Ashley et al. 1988, Safrin et al. 1992).

6 CONTROL

Like other non-epidemic diseases transmitted by contact, HSV infection cannot be controlled by public health measures. Reduction in sexual transmission can be attempted by public education on the risks of unprotected sex. Despite recent education campaigns aimed at reducing the spread of HIV, the reported incidence of genital herpes has risen in the UK over the past 5 years (Barton 1995), though it is questionable whether this represents a real increase in transmission frequency.

6.1 Vaccination

No licensed vaccine is currently available for prophylaxis against HSV. Indeed, the fact that reinfection is possible and that restimulation of the response by a recurrence does not prevent further recurrences has been used to argue that the development of a successful vaccine is impossible. Two lines of evidence suggest that this is not so. First, infection by HSV-1 decreases the incidence and severity of subsequent HSV-2 genital infections (Mertz et al. 1992). Secondly, a variety of immunogens, including killed virus, glycoprotein subunits, viral antigens expressed by live vectors, and attenuated or disabled HSV, will all protect mice and guinea-pigs from challenge infection. As noted previously, the virus has evolved immune evasion mechanisms that do not operate efficiently in rodents, and data obtained from animal models must be treated with caution. Nevertheless, these results suggest that a protective response can be mounted, and the successful development of attenuated vaccines against other human and animal alphaherpesviruses gives some confidence in the principle of vaccination against HSV. A number of immunogenic preparations have been tested in humans but many of these trials were inadequately controlled and most tested therapeutic efficacy against established recurrent infection rather than prophylactic vaccine efficacy. A glycoprotein mixture prepared from HSV-2-infected cells and mixed with alum adjuvant showed no significant benefit against primary genital infection in a controlled trial but the vaccine was poorly immunogenic (Mertz et al.

1990). This study illustrated the difficulty of conducting a properly controlled prophylactic trial, in particular the need to monitor participants for subclinical primary infection. More recently, recombinant HSV-2 glycoproteins, in combination with more potent adjuvants, have elicited responses as great or greater than those found following natural infection. Preliminary therapeutic trials with glycoprotein D show promise (Straus et al. 1994), and phase I and phase II trials have been conducted using a mixture of glycoproteins B and D (Langenberg et al. 1995). Phase III trials are in progress.

6.2 Chemotherapy

Herpes simplex virus, together with other human herpesviruses, is among the most studied targets for antiviral chemotherapy, a subject covered in detail elsewhere (see Chapter 45). Nucleoside analogues such as iododeoxyuridine (idoxuridine), trifluorodeoxyuridine and adenine arabinoside were used for many years to inhibit viral DNA replication, but these analogues lacked selectivity and their cytotoxicity limited their use to topical treatment in all but the most life-threatening circumstances. The development of aciclovir (acycloguanosine) transformed the treatment of HSV infections. Aciclovir is a guanosine analogue in which the sugar is replaced by an acyclic ring lacking the 2′ and 3′ carbons. The analogue is converted to the 5′ monophosphate by the HSV-specific thymidine kinase and then to the triphosphate by cellular kinases. The viral DNA polymerase incorporates the triphosphate into the growing viral DNA where it acts as a chain terminator. The inability of host cell kinases to convert aciclovir into its monophosphate accounts primarily for its selective action against HSV-infected cells and its non-toxicity, although, in addition, the viral DNA polymerase has a higher affinity than its cellular counterpart for the triphosphate. Aciclovir is available in a number of formulations and can be administered topically, orally or intravenously. Its oral bioavailability is 15–30% and plasma half-life about 2–3 hours, so relatively frequent doses are required to maintain therapeutic concentration. The route of administration depends on the site and severity of infection: topical application is used for eye infections and oral lesions, oral administration for severe genital infections and intravenous administration for encephalitis and life-threatening infection of immunocompromised patients. A cream formulation is available without a prescription ('over the counter') in the UK for cold sore treatment, but not in the USA.

Mutants of HSV resistant to aciclovir arise readily in culture, almost invariably due to loss of a functional virus thymidine kinase gene. This gene function is irrelevant for virus growth in vitro but its loss results in severe attenuation in vivo. Alternative routes to resistance are point mutations in the thymidine kinase gene or DNA polymerase gene which reduce enzyme affinity for aciclovir and aciclovir triphosphate respectively (Furman et al. 1981, Larder et al. 1983, Larder

and Darby 1984). Resistance to therapy in vivo seems to be infrequent and has been observed most frequently in immunocompromised patients receiving long-term therapy. The mutants isolated from these patients include those with altered thymidine kinase or DNA polymerase enzymes, but the most frequent finding is of a heterogeneous population of viruses with a range of thymidine kinase activities from entirely deficient to almost normal. The basis of this form of resistance is uncertain, but it is known that thymidine kinase negative viruses can be complemented, in vivo, by a wild type virus (Efstathiou et al. 1989) and it appears that aciclovir selective pressure, particularly in the immunocompromised, can maintain a dynamic mixture of thymidine kinase positive and negative viruses.

During the past 10 years a second generation of anti-herpes drugs based on aciclovir has been developed (penciclovir, famciclovir, valaciclovir) with the same mechanism of action. It is unlikely that these will replace aciclovir as the treatment of choice for HSV infections, but their different pharmacokinetic properties may offer an advantage in specific instances. A second class of analogues with anti-HSV activity are pyrophosphate analogues which act as inhibitors of HSV DNA polymerase. Phosphonoformate (foscarnet) is the sole example in clinical use. Topical application is well tolerated but intravenous administration can cause nephrotoxicity and severe nausea. Foscarnet has no advantage over aciclovir but is of value in treating aciclovir-resistant infections.

Finally, anti-herpes chemotherapy suppresses virus growth but has no apparent effect on latent infection. Patients who have been treated with aciclovir continuously for as long as 6 years experience recurrences after drug withdrawal (Fife et al. 1994).

VARICELLA-ZOSTER VIRUS

It has been recognized for many years that varicella (chickenpox) and zoster (shingles) are caused by the same virus and that zoster results from the reactivation of an endogenous virus acquired during primary varicella. Our understanding of the pathogenesis of VZV derives almost entirely from clinical studies. The virus is highly species-specific in vivo, though it has been adapted to grow in guinea-pig cells and isolates thus adapted will cause a varicella-like disease in guinea-pigs (Pavan-Langston and Dunkel 1989). A closely related virus, simian varicella herpesvirus, has been isolated from Old World monkeys (Soike, Rangan and Gerone 1984, Padovan and Cantrell 1986).

7 CLINICAL MANIFESTATIONS

7.1 Varicella

Chickenpox is one of the common childhood exanthems, affecting most children during their early school years. The incubation period is about 2 weeks, after which the characteristic rash appears, composed of macules which rapidly develop into fluid-filled vesicles. These vesicles crust within a few days and heal, usually without scarring, within a few weeks. The lesions appear in crops, so any one area will contain macules, vesicles and crusted lesions. The rash tends to be centripetal and is variable in severity; a high density of vesicles is present on all parts of the skin and on mucosal membranes of the mouth and genitalia in some cases, while at the other extreme the number of vesicles may be very small or the infection inapparent. The accompanying fever is usually low grade, but reflects the severity of the rash and persists as long as new lesions continue to appear. The incidence of complications in normal children is low, the most common problem being secondary infection of lesions and consequent scarring, a problem that can usually be solved by antibiotic treatment. Central nervous system involvement is rare and may take the form of an invasive encephalitis or a transient ataxia, or may be a prelude to Reye's syndrome. Although primary varicella is usually a benign disease of the normal child, infection of malnourished children is much more severe (Salomon, Gordon and Scrimshaw 1966). The main groups in which complications occur are, however, the adult, the neonate and the immunocompromised.

Infection of adults (Fig. 18.4) is generally more severe than in children; the vesicles heal more slowly, secondary bacterial infection and scarring are more common, and the accompanying fever is higher and more prolonged. The most serious complication is varicella pneumonia (Fig. 18.5) which appears a few days after onset of the rash and usually resolves in the immunocompetent patient, though there may be residual nodular calcification. Pregnant women are thought to be particularly prone to varicella pneumonia, symptomatic pneumonia being reported in as many as 10% of primary varicella cases, with occasional mortality, though some studies report much lower frequencies of morbidity and mortality (Brunell 1992).

Primary varicella during pregnancy places the fetus at risk from 2 routes: infection in utero and neonatal infection. Infection in utero can result in congenital malformations which include limb hypoplasia, cicatrizing skin lesions, and sensory and motor deficiencies. Primary varicella in the mother close to term is associated with severe disease in the neonate (Fig. 18.6): symptoms appear in the infant about 7 days after birth and include pneumonia and visceral involvement, particularly of the liver. A full account of maternal, fetal and neonatal infections with VZV is given in Chapter 11.

Varicella is severe and often life-threatening in immunocompromised patients. Leukaemic children form a major risk group but patients undergoing chemotherapy or steroid treatment or who have any acquired or inborn immune deficiency are at risk. The most common complications are varicella pneumonia, visceral involvement and CNS infection, but also include haemorrhagic varicella ranging from bleeding

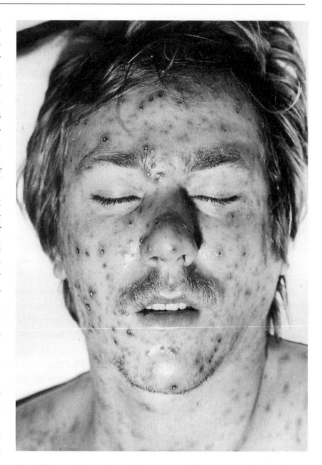

Fig. 18.4 Adult with chickenpox. (Photograph by courtesy of Dr A K R Chaudhuri and Mr R Milligan, Monklands Hospital, Airdrie.)

into lesions to purpura fulminans (Feldman, Hughes and Daniel 1975).

7.2 Herpes zoster

Like herpes simplex virus, varicella-zoster virus establishes a life-long latent infection of sensory dorsal root ganglia, but, because VZV is disseminated, latency is established in multiple ganglia. Reactivation and recurrences take the form of a unilateral rash, herpes zoster, limited to a single dermatome, the area of skin innervated by a single sensory ganglion. The rash appears most commonly in the thoracic dermatomes (Fig. 18.7), reflecting the high density of vesicles in this area during primary varicella, but also occurs (in about 10% of cases) as cranial zoster, often with eye involvement (Fig. 18.8) and may, in rare instances, appear on almost any part of the skin or mucosa. In healthy people zoster is relatively uncommon; many people never experience it and few have more than 1 or 2 episodes although it is common to suffer an episode in old age.

The rash of herpes zoster is usually preceded by pain in the involved dermatome, which begins a few days before the rash appears and remains during its development. The rash is composed of varicella-like vesicles but often so densely packed as to appear as a

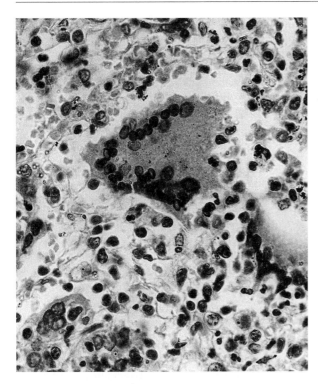

Fig. 18.5 Section of lung from patient dying of varicella pneumonia. Intense infiltration with lymphocytes and macrophages. The giant cell contains many nuclei, some with eosinophilic Cowdry type A inclusions. Haematoxylin and eosin stain. × 570 (Photograph by courtesy of L H Collier.)

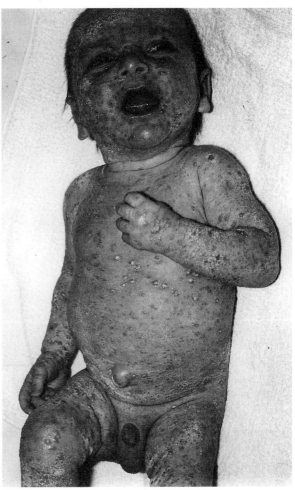

Fig. 18.6 Neonatal varicella. (Photograph by courtesy of Dr A K R Chaudhuri and Mr R Milligan, Monklands Hospital, Airdrie.)

continuous area of eruption. The rash develops over the course of about a week and usually crusts and heals in 2–3 weeks, but the course is variable, and particularly in the elderly the symptoms are often more severe and prolonged. Unlike oral HSV recurrences, no stimuli have been identified that provoke zoster. The susceptibility of the elderly to zoster has been interpreted to reflect a waning immunity, a view consistent with the increased frequency of zoster in the immunocompromised patient, but it is probable that the immune system controls reactivated virus rather than prevents reactivation. The detection of VZV DNA fragments in circulating mononuclear cells of healthy patients (Gilden et al. 1983) implies that reactivation of latent virus may be much more common than clinical zoster. *Zoster sine herpete* is the term applied to a syndrome in which a typical zoster prodrome is unaccompanied by the subsequent development of a zoster rash (Easton 1970, Gilden et al. 1992a).

Complications associated with zoster are uncommon in children and young adults but occur frequently in the elderly and the immunocompromised. Post-herpetic neuralgia is the most common complication and is defined as pain lasting longer than one month after lesions heal. It is rare in patients under 40 years of age but occurs in 50% of patients over 60 and, although the pain usually resolves in a few months, it can last for a year or more and is a major cause of morbidity in the elderly. It is most frequently associated with zoster of the ophthalmic branch of the trigeminal (cranial zoster), and cases of sufficient severity and protraction may require surgical ablation of the ganglion. In some instances, anaesthesia of the involved dermatome occurs and may result in residual palsy. The pathogenesis of post-herpetic neuralgia is unknown.

Other complications of zoster usually reflect underlying immunological defects. Zoster occurs with high frequency in immunocompromised patients and is unusually severe. Failure to control the recurrences is often illustrated by the spread of vesicles beyond the dermatome in which the initial rash occurs. The disease may become widely disseminated and correspond to severe varicella with involvement of the tissue, lungs or CNS. In these circumstances zoster may be fatal, most commonly as a result of pneumonia.

8 EPIDEMIOLOGY

VZV infects only humans. The reservoir is latent virus in sensory ganglia. Primary infection causes varicella, a common disease of childhood. Only a small minority

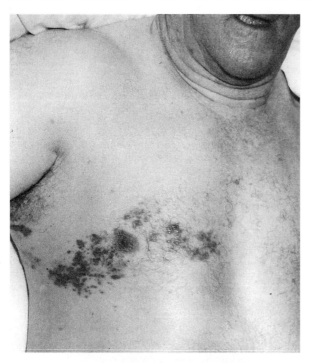

Fig. 18.7 Thoracic zoster. (Photograph by courtesy of Dr A K R Chaudhuri and Mr R Milligan, Monklands Hospital, Airdrie.)

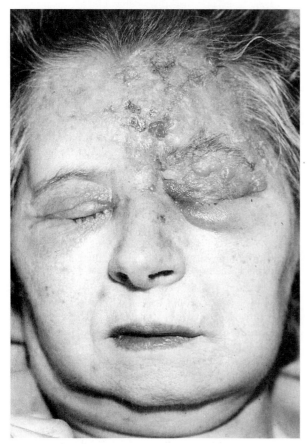

Fig. 18.8 Cranial zoster. (Photograph by courtesy of Dr A K R Chaudhuri and Mr R Milligan, Monklands Hospital, Airdrie.)

of young adults remain uninfected but by late middle age infection and immunity are virtually universal in industrial societies. Infection is usually accompanied by the characteristic syndrome; asymptomatic infection does occur, but the proportion of subclinical infections is difficult to estimate and is based largely on patient recall. The disease occurs in epidemics which, in temperate zones, usually appear in late winter every 2 or 3 years in young schoolchildren. Airborne spread has been demonstrated (Gustafson et al. 1982) and the attack rate is high: over 60% within households, and 20% in society as a whole (Yorke and London 1973), a rate lower than observed for measles. However, data collected before the advent of measles vaccination revealed that more young adults had been infected with VZV than with measles, a reflection of the fact that measles infection occurs almost exclusively during epidemics whereas varicella infection often occurs in unrecorded 'mini epidemics' or as isolated cases resulting from contact with zoster. The risk of varicella infection through contact with zoster within a household has been estimated to be about 3-fold lower than through contact with varicella (Hope-Simpson 1965).

Zoster exhibits no seasonal incidence, and is not correlated with outbreaks of varicella. Despite reports of 'outbreaks' of zoster, all evidence favours the view that zoster is the reactivation of latent virus rather than a transmissible syndrome and reports of 'outbreaks' almost certainly refer to statistical anomalies. In immunocompetent people the incidence of zoster correlates only with age, the disease incidence being approximately proportional to the age of the study group.

9 PATHOGENESIS AND PATHOLOGY

Like other benign diseases of humans, varicella pathogenesis cannot be studied in detail in the normal host. Our understanding of VZV pathogenesis derives, at least in part, from studies of severe or fatal disease and by analogy with other, better studied, exanthems. The route of entry is probably the upper respiratory tract or oropharynx where replication in epithelial cells occurs. During the incubation period of about 2 weeks cell-associated virus can be detected in the blood stream, primarily in mononuclear cells, and skin lesions are then initiated by infection of capillary endothelial cells. Whether the systemic amplification of virus is limited to circulating cells and capillary endothelium in the normal individual is unknown. In fatal varicella of the newborn or immunosuppressed, productive lesions can be found on all mucosal surfaces and in the parenchyma of almost every organ, and it is probable that limited replication at these sites contributes to the viraemia in normal benign infection. The cutaneous vesicles of varicella are histologically similar to those of herpes simplex (see section 1, p. 325). Vesicles on mucosal surfaces rapidly develop into shallow ulcers. The vesicle contains large numbers of free virus particles, suggesting that replication in epithelial cells results in secretion of free virus, whereas in most cell types VZV is strongly cell associated. The production of free virus in the oral cavity and upper respiratory tract is the probable major source of transmission. The patient is infectious for a few days before lesions appear until a few days after new lesions cease to appear.

The virus establishes latent infection in sensory ganglia. VZV DNA can be detected in the thoracic ganglia of seropositive cadavers, and similar results have been obtained with simian varicella virus (Gilden et al. 1983, Mahalingham et al. 1991). By analogy with herpes simplex virus, access to the ganglia is assumed to be from the skin via sensory nerve endings, but a haematogenous route cannot be excluded. VZV latency is poorly understood by comparison with HSV latency. The virus has not been reactivated from human ganglia by culture in vitro, the physical state of the viral genome has not been ascertained, and the pattern of transcription during latency, in contrast to herpes simplex virus, appears to involve the immediate early productive cycle genes (reviewed by Gilden et al. 1992b). Indeed there is some disagreement as to the cell type in which latent infection is established, and true latency, as opposed to chronic infection, is not proven (Gilden et al. 1987, Croen et al. 1988). Recurrent infection with herpes zoster, is, by analogy with HSV, assumed to result from reactivation of latent virus in a sensory ganglion and seeding of infectious virions into epithelium via sensory nerve endings, a view entirely consistent with the appearance of zoster within a single dermatome. The details of these events are uncertain. As noted earlier (section 7.2, p. 332), clinical zoster is an infrequent event and most triggering conditions, such as cytotoxic drug treatment, lymphoma or heavy metal poisoning, are immunosuppressive, suggesting a failure to control reactivated virus rather than stimulating reactivation. The frequency of reactivation rather than recurrence is unknown. The pain associated with zoster and the frequency and prolonged nature of post-herpetic neuralgia distinguish VZV recurrences from those of HSV, and it is proposed that these features reflect more widespread growth and consequent inflammation in sensory ganglia during VZV recurrence. This plausible explanation implies a quantitative difference between VZV and HSV recurrence but fundamental differences in the nature of latency, reactivation and recurrence of the 2 viruses cannot be excluded.

10 IMMUNE RESPONSE

Primary infection results in life-long immunity to exogenous reinfection. Humoral response, T cell proliferative responses and cytotoxic T cell responses are all detectable soon after symptoms appear, rise during convalescence and remain detectable throughout life. Recurrence is accompanied by a pronounced anamnestic response, an observation in contrast to HSV recurrence. Antibodies to at least 35 different VZV antigens have been identified in convalescent sera, including neutralizing antibodies directed against viral glycoproteins, but, despite the use of passive immunoglobulin in therapy, there is little evidence that humoral responses are important in controlling infection. No correlation has been found between titre or spectrum of VZV-specific antibodies and severity of varicella or the recurrence or severity of zoster (Brunell et al. 1987). Agammaglobulinaemic patients do not suffer from unusually severe varicella or from frequent or severe zoster. In contrast, many studies have demonstrated a correlation with deficiencies in cell-mediated immunity and the severity of varicella infection and the frequency and severity of zoster. T cell proliferative responses, cytotoxic T cell responses and interferon responses are all detected in human infection and in animal models (Arvin 1992, Rotbart, Levin and Hayward 1993). Responses to individual virus antigens, both structural and immediate early non-structural proteins, have been found, but the importance of particular responses to individual antigens has yet to be determined. The decline in cell-mediated responses to varicella-zoster virus in the elderly is thought to be responsible for the increased frequency of zoster in this group (Miller 1980, Berger, Luescher and Just 1981), and is consistent with the occurrence of zoster in immunocompromised patients. The maintenance of adequate levels of cell-mediated immunity to varicella in the population is therefore important but it is uncertain whether restimulation of the response occurs primarily through subclinical reactivation or results from re-exposure to varicella. Evidence exists for both mechanisms (Meyers, Flournoy and Thomas 1980, Arvin, Koropchak and Wittek 1983), but their relative contribution is of importance in predicting the possible consequences of mass vaccination and the need to vaccinate seropositive people carrying wild varicella-zoster virus.

11 DIAGNOSIS

Virus particles are present at high concentrations in vesicular fluid and can be cultured in a variety of human and primate cell lines. The cytopathic effect is focal and develops slowly with typical cell 'ballooning' and fusion. Immunofluorescence of infected cultures with specific antibody confirms the presence of VZV and allows more rapid diagnosis. The virus in culture is very strongly cell-associated and efficient storage of isolates requires freezing of viable infected cells. Electron microscopic examination of vesicular fluid reveals the presence of large numbers of herpesvirus particles, a method used historically to allow a rapid distinction between chickenpox and smallpox but which cannot distinguish VZV and HSV.

A wide range of serological tests for VZV-specific IgG have been described, including complement fixation, latex agglutination, radioimmune assay and ELISA. ELISAs for VZV-specific IgG and IgM are commercially available. A suspect rash can be confirmed as varicella by the presence of IgM or by a rising IgG titre. Zoster can be similarly confirmed because, in contrast to HSV, recurrence is usually associated with a significant rise in antibody titre. A skin test for cell-mediated immunity has been described (Kamiya et al. 1977, Takahashi et al. 1992) and is thought to provide a relevant measure of immunity to zoster.

12 CONTROL

12.1 Epidemiological control

No attempt is made to limit the spread of varicella in the general population because, as a rule, acquisition of the virus early in life is preferable to infection as an adult. Within hospitals, however, VZV infection has serious consequences for high risk groups such as premature babies, leukaemic children and transplant recipients, and patient isolation may be necessary to protect these groups. Healthcare staff can be monitored for immunity to VZV, and seronegative staff who suspect they have contracted varicella or staff suffering a zoster recurrence should avoid contact with high risk patients.

12.2 Vaccine

A live attenuated vaccine, the Oka strain, was developed in Japan by passage in guinea-pig cells and its efficacy first reported by Takahashi et al. (1974). Since then this vaccine has been used extensively in normal and immunocompromised children and in adults in Japan, and more recently in the USA where it is now licensed. American and Japanese experience with the vaccine is similar (reviewed by Gershon et al. 1992). A single vaccine dose to healthy children gives >90% seroconversion and c. 90% protection against subsequent varicella attacks, which, when they occur, are mild. Antibody persistence and protection in vaccinees are long lasting. Vaccination of leukaemic children provides similar levels of protection but vaccination of adults results in somewhat lower protection rates. There are few side effects of the vaccine in healthy children, some 5% suffering a mild rash occasionally accompanied by fever, but in leukaemic children side effects are more noticeable, about half the vaccinees developing a rash, in some cases resembling typical varicella. Nevertheless, the vaccine-related reactions in these patients are benign compared with the risk of varicella infection. Vaccination of seropositive adults results in an enhancement of cell-mediated immunity and may therefore be of value in protecting the elderly against zoster (Berger, Luescher and Just 1984, Takahashi et al. 1992).

It is not certain whether the vaccine establishes latent infection in all recipients. A few leukaemic vaccinees have experienced zoster due to recurrence of the vaccine strain but these individuals suffered a varicella rash following vaccination, consistent with the expectation that latency and recurrence are related to virus load in the skin during primary infection. Because most healthy vaccinees have no rash, it is reasonable to suppose that they will not suffer recurrence, and to date this is the case. In view of its safety and efficacy, the Oka strain has been proposed for universal vaccination of children. It has been used successfully in combination with measles, mumps and rubella vaccinations.

12.3 Passive antibody

Passive immunization with specific zoster immunoglobulin (ZIG – derived from donors with high anti-VZV titres) has been used to prevent or modify infection in high risk patients who are thought to have come into contact with varicella or zoster (Gershon, Stainberg and Brunell 1974, Zaia et al. 1983, Berger, Luescher and Just 1984, Takahashi et al. 1992). Examples include non-immune pregnant women, immunocompromised patients, premature babies in special care units and neonates born to mothers with varicella at term. This treatment is considered to be effective if administered within 2 days of contact with a disease case, though no strictly controlled trials have been conducted.

12.4 Chemotherapy

VZV, like HSV and other alphaherpesviruses, specifies a thymidine kinase (TK) and is sensitive to aciclovir. VZV is considerably less sensitive than HSV, however, and much higher doses are required to achieve therapeutic benefit. Nevertheless, aciclovir is now widely used in the treatment of varicella and zoster (Whitley 1992, reviewed by Griffiths 1995). Treatment of uncomplicated varicella in children with oral aciclovir within 24 hours of the onset of the rash resulted in fewer skin lesions and reduced fever but the benefit is relatively small. Similar treatment of adults, who suffer more severe varicella, achieved essentially similar results but the benefit was more pronounced. Oral aciclovir is used both prophylactically and therapeutically in immunocompromised patients at risk from or suffering from varicella. Because of the relatively poor oral bioavailability of the drug, hospitalized patients with severe varicella are treated intravenously.

Oral aciclovir reduces pain and duration of the rash in zoster patients but has little or no effect on post-herpetic neuralgia. Two pro-drug derivatives of aciclovir, famcyclovir and valacyclovir, with similar modes of action but different pharmacokinetic properties are now licensed for use against zoster. Their greater bioavailability offers advantages in some clinical settings (Carrington 1994, Murray 1995) (see also Chapter 46).

REFERENCES

Ades AE, Peckham CS et al., 1989, Prevalence of antibodies to herpes simplex virus type 1 and 2 in pregnant women and estimated rates of infection, *J Epidemiol Community Health*, **43**: 53–60.

Anderson JR, Field HJ, 1983, The distribution of herpes simplex type 1 antigen in the mouse central nervous system after different routes of inoculation, *J Neurol Sci*, **60**: 181–95.

Arvin AM, 1992, Cell mediated immunity to varicella zoster virus, *J Infect Dis*, **166, suppl 1:** 35–41.

Arvin AM, Koropchak CM, Wittek AE, 1983, Immunologic evidence of reinfection with varicella-zoster virus, *J Infect Dis*, **148:** 200–5.

Ashley R, Millitoni J et al., 1988, Comparison of western blot (immunoblot) and glycoprotein-G specific immunodot enzyme assays for detecting antibodies to herpes simplex virus types 1 and 2 in human sera, *J Clin Microbiol*, **26:** 662–7.

Barton SE, 1995, Current issues in the management of genital herpes, *Antiviral Chem Chemother*, **6, suppl 1:** 3–6.

Bell S, Cranage M et al., 1990, Induction of immunoglobulin G Fc receptors by recombinant vaccinia viruses expressing glycoproteins E and I of herpes simplex virus type 1, *J Virol*, **64:** 2181–6.

Berger R, Florent G, Just M, 1981, Decrease of the lymphoproliferative response to varicella zoster virus antigen in the aged, *Infect Immun*, **32:** 24–27.

Berger R, Luescher D, Just M, 1984, Enhancement of varicella-zoster specific immune responses in the elderly by boosting with varicella vaccine, *J Infect Dis*, **149:** 647.

Biron CA, Byron HS, Sullivan JL, 1989, Severe herpes virus infections in an adolescent without natural killer cells, *N Engl J Med*, **320:** 1731–5.

Brunell PA, 1992, Varicella in pregnancy, the fetus and the newborn: problems in management, *J Infect Dis*, **166, suppl 1:** 42–7.

Brunell PA, Novelli VM et al., 1987, Antibodies to the three major glycoproteins of varicella-zoster virus: search for the relevant host immune response, *J Infect Dis*, **156:** 430–5.

Buckmaster EA, Cranage MP et al., 1984, The use of monoclonal antibodies to differentiate isolates of herpes simplex virus types 1 and 2 by neutralisation and reverse passive haemagglutination tests, *J Med Virol*, **13:** 193–202.

Bukowski JF, Welsh RM, 1986, The role of natural killer cells and interferon in resistance to acute infection of mice with herpes simplex virus type 1, *J Immunol*, **136:** 3481–5.

Carrington D, 1994, Prospects for improved efficacy with antiviral prodrugs: will valaciclovir and famciclovir meet the clinical challenge?, *Int Antivir News*, **2:** 50–3.

Corey L, Spear PG, 1986, Infections with herpes simplex viruses, *N Engl J Med*, **314:** 686–91.

Corey L, Adams HG et al., 1983, Genital herpes simplex virus infections: clinical manifestations, course and complications, *Ann Intern Med*, **98:** 958–72.

Croen KD, Ostrove JM et al., 1988, Patterns of gene expression and sites of latency in human nerve ganglia are different for varicella zoster and herpes simplex viruses, *Proc Natl Acad Sci USA*, **85:** 9773–7.

Cunningham AL, Merigan TC, 1983, Gamma interferon production appears to predict time of recurrence of herpes labialis, *J Immunol*, **130:** 2397–400.

Cushing H, 1905, Surgical aspects of major neuralgia of the trigeminal nerve: report of 20 cases of operation upon the gasserian ganglion with anatomic and physiologic notes on the consequences of its removal, *JAMA*, **44:** 1002–8.

Easton HG, 1970, Zoster sine herpete causing acute trigeminal neuralgia, *Lancet*, **2:** 1065–6.

Efstathiou S, Kemp S et al., 1989, The role of herpes simplex virus type 1 thymidine kinase in pathogenesis, *J Gen Virol*, **70:** 869–79.

Enders G, Miller E et al., 1994, Consequences of varicella and herpes zoster in pregnancy: prospective study of 1739 cases, *Lancet*, **343:** 1548–51.

Feldman S, Hughes WT, Daniel CB, 1975, Varicella in children with cancer: seventy seven cases, *Pediatrics*, **56:** 388–97.

Fife KH, Crumpacker CS et al., 1994, Recurrence and resistance patterns of herpes simplex virus following cessation of >6 years of chronic suppression with acyclovir, *J Infect Dis*, **169:** 1338–41.

Frank I, Friedman HM, 1989, A novel function of the herpes simplex virus Fc receptor: participation in bi-polar bridging of antiviral immunoglobulin G, *J Virol*, **63:** 4479–88.

Fries LF, Friedman HM et al., 1986, Glycoprotein C of herpes simplex virus type 1 is an inhibitor of the complement cascade, *J Immunol*, **137:** 1636–42.

Furman PA, Coen DM et al., 1981, Acyclovir resistant mutants of herpes simplex virus type 1 express altered DNA polymerase or reduced acyclovir phosphorylating activity, *J Virol*, **40:** 936–41.

Gershon AA, Stainberg S, Brunell PA, 1974, Zoster immune globulin: a further assessment, *N Engl J Med*, **290:** 243–5.

Gershon A, La Russa P et al., 1992, Varicella vaccine: the American experience, *J Infect Dis*, **166, suppl 1:** 63–8.

Gesser I, Tovey MG et al., 1976, Role of interferon in the pathogenesis of virus diseases in mice as demonstrated by the use of anti interferon serum. II. Studies with herpes simplex, Moloney sarcoma, vesicular stomatitis, Newcastle disease and influenza virus, *J Exp Med*, **144:** 1316–23.

Gilden DH, Vafai A et al., 1983, Varicella-zoster virus DNA in human sensory ganglia, *Nature (London)*, **306:** 478–80.

Gilden DH, Rosemann Y et al., 1987, Detection of varicella zoster virus nucleic acid in neurons of normal human thoracic ganglia, *Ann Neurol*, **22:** 377–80.

Gilden DH, Dueland AN et al., 1992a, Varicella zoster virus reactivation without rash, *J Infect Dis*, **166, suppl 1:** 30–4.

Gilden DH, Mahalingham R et al., 1992b, Herpes zoster: pathogenesis and latency, *Progr Med Virol*, **39:** 19–75.

Griffiths PD, 1995, Progress in the clinical management of herpesvirus infections, *Antivir Chem Chemother*, **6:** 191–209.

Gustafson TL, Lavely GB et al., 1982, An outbreak of airborne nosocomial varicella, *Pediatrics*, **70:** 550–6.

Harris RA, Everett RD et al., 1989, Herpes simplex virus type 1 immediate early protein Vmw110 reactivates latent herpes simplex virus type 2 in an *in vitro* latency system, *J Virol*, **63:** 3513–15.

Hill A, Jugovic P et al., 1995, Herpes simplex virus turns off the TAP to evade host immunity, *Nature (London)*, **375:** 411–15.

Hill TJ, Field HJ, Blyth WA, 1975, Acute and recurrent infection with herpes simplex virus in the mouse: a model for studying latency and recurrent disease, *J Gen Virol*, **28:** 341–53.

Ho DWT, Field PR et al., 1992, Indirect ELISA for the detection of HSV-2 specific IgG and IgM antibodies with glycoprotein G (gG-2), *J Virol Methods*, **36:** 249–64.

Ho DY, 1992, Herpes simplex virus latency: molecular aspects, *Progr Med Virol*, **39:** 76–115.

Hope-Simpson RE, 1965, The nature of herpes zoster: a long-term study and a new hypothesis, *Proc Roy Soc Med*, **58:** 9–20.

Kamiya H, Ihara T et al., 1977, Diagnostic skin test reactions with varicella virus antigen and clinical applications of the test, *J Infect Dis*, **136:** 784–8.

Krause PR, Stanberry LR et al., 1995, Expression of the herpes simplex virus type 2 latency-associated transcript enhances spontaneous reactivation of genital herpes in latently infected guinea pigs, *J Exp Med*, **181:** 297–306.

Lafferty WE, Coombs RW et al., 1987, Recurrences after oral and genital herpes simplex virus infection. Influence of site of infection and viral type, *N Engl J Med*, **316:** 1444–9.

Lakeman FD, Whitley RJ et al., 1995, Diagnosis of herpes simplex encephalitis: application of polymerase chain reaction to cerebrospinal fluid from brain-biopsied patients and correlation with disease, *J Infect Dis*, **171**: 857–63.

Langenberg AGM, Burke RL et al., 1995, A recombinant glycoprotein vaccine for herpes simplex virus type 2: safety and efficacy, *Ann Intern Med*, **122**: 889–98.

Larder BA, Darby G, 1984, Virus drug resistance: mechanisms and consequences, *Antivir Res*, **4**: 1–42.

Larder BA, Derse D et al., 1983, Properties of purified enzymes induced by pathogenic drug resistant mutants of herpes simplex virus. Evidence for variants expressing normal DNA polymerase and altered thymidine kinase, *J Biol Chem*, **258**: 2027–33.

Lee FK, Pereira L et al., 1986, A novel glycoprotein for detection of herpes simplex virus type 1 specific antibodies, *J Virol Methods*, **14**: 111–18.

Lopez C, 1985, Natural resistance mechanisms in herpes simplex virus infections, *The Herpesviruses*, vol 4, eds Roizman B, Lopez C, Plenum Press, New York, 37–68.

McGeoch DJ, Cook S, 1994, Molecular phylogeny of the alphaherpesvirus subfamily and a proposed evolutionary timescale, *J Mol Biol*, **238**: 9–22.

McLennan JL, Darby G, 1980, Herpes simplex virus latency: the cellular location of virus in dorsal root ganglia and the fate of the infected cell following virus reactivation, *J Gen Virol*, **51**: 233–43.

Mahalingham R, Smith D et al., 1991, Simian varicella virus DNA in dorsal root ganglia, *Proc Natl Acad Sci USA*, **88**: 2750–2.

Mellerick DM, Fraser NW, 1987, Physical state of the latent herpes simplex virus genome in a mouse model system: evidence suggesting an episomal state, *Virology*, **158**: 265–75.

Mertz GJ, Ashley R et al., 1990, Double-blind placebo controlled trial of a herpes simplex virus type 2 glycoprotein vaccine in persons at high risk for genital herpes infection, *J Infect Dis*, **161**: 653–60.

Mertz GJ, Benedetti J et al., 1992, Risk factors for the sexual transmission of genital herpes, *Ann Intern Med*, **116**: 197–202.

Meyers JD, 1974, Congenital varicella in term infants: risks considered, *J Infect Dis*, **129**: 215–17.

Meyers JD, Flournoy N, Thomas ED, 1980, Cell mediated immunity to varicella zoster virus after allogenic marrow transplant, *J Infect Dis*, **141**: 479–87.

Miller AE, 1980, Selective decline in cellular immune response to varicella zoster in the elderly, *Neurology*, **30**: 582–7.

Miller E, Watson-Cradock JE et al., 1989, Outcome in newborn babies given anti-varicella zoster immunoglobulin after perinatal infection with varicella zoster virus, *Lancet*, **2**: 371–4.

Murray AB, 1995, Valaciclovir – an improvement over aciclovir for the treatment of zoster, *Antiviral Chem Chemother*, **6, suppl 1**: 34–8.

Nahmias AJ, Whitley RJ et al., 1982, Herpes simplex encephalitis: laboratory evaluations and their diagnostic significance, *J Infect Dis*, **145**: 829–6.

Nash AA, Gell PGH, 1983, Membrane phenotype of murine effector and suppressor T cells involved in delayed hypersensitivity and protective immunity to herpes simplex virus, *Cell Immunol*, **75**: 348–55.

Padovan D, Cantrell CA, 1986, Varicella-like herpesvirus infections of non-human primates, *Lab Anim Sci*, **36**: 7–13.

Pavan-Langston D, Dunkel EC, 1989, Ocular varicella zoster virus infection in the guinea pig, *Arch Ophthalmol*, **107**: 1068–72.

PHLS Report, 1987, Report from the PHLS Communicable Disease Surveillance Centre, *Br Med J*, **294**: 361–2.

Prober CG, Sullender WM et al., 1987, Low risk of herpes simplex virus infections in neonates exposed to the virus at the time of vaginal delivery to mothers with recurrent genital herpes simplex virus infection, *N Engl J Med*, **316**: 240–4.

Ross JDC, Smith IW, Elton RA, 1993, The epidemiology of herpes simplex types 1 and 2 infection of the genital tract in Edinburgh, 1978–1991, *Genitourin Med*, **69**: 381–3.

Rotbart HA, Levin MJ, Hayward AR, 1993, Immune responses to varicella zoster virus infections in healthy children, *J Infect Dis*, **167**: 195–9.

Rouse BT, ed, 1992, Herpes simplex virus: pathogenesis, immunobiology and control, *Curr Top Microbiol Immunol*, **179**.

Safrin S, Arvin A et al., 1992, Comparison of the western immunoblot assay and a glycoprotein G enzyme immunoassay for detection of serum antibodies to herpes simplex virus type 2 in patients with AIDS, *J Clin Microbiol*, **30**: 1312–14.

Salomon JB, Gordon JE, Scrimshaw NS, 1966, Studies of diarrheal disease in Central America. X. Associated chickenpox, diarrhea and kwashiorkor in a highland Guatemalan village, *Am J Trop Med Hyg*, **15**: 997–1002.

Sanchez-Martinez D, Schmid DS et al., 1991, Evaluation of a test based on baculovirus-expressed glycoprotein G for detection of herpes simplex virus type-specific antibodies, *J Infect Dis*, **164**: 1196–9.

Schmid DS, 1988, The human MHC-restricted cellular response to herpes simplex virus type 1 is mediated by CD4+, CD8– T cells and is restricted to the DR region of the MHC complex, *J Immunol*, **140**: 3610–16.

Simmons A, Nash AA, 1985, The role of antibody in primary and recurrent herpes simplex virus infection, *J Virol*, **53**: 944–8.

Simmons A, Nash AA, 1987, Effect of B cell suppression on primary and reinfection of mice with herpes simplex virus, *J Infect Dis*, **13**: 108–14.

Simmons A, Tscharke DC, 1992, Anti-CD8 impairs clearance of HSV from the nervous system: implications for the rate of virally infected neurones, *J Exp Med*, **175**: 1337–44.

Soike KF, Rangan SRS, Gerone PJ, 1984, Viral disease models in primates, *Adv Vet Sci Comp Med*, **28**: 151–99.

Stevens JG, Cook ML, 1971, Latent herpes simplex virus in sensory ganglia, *Science*, **173**: 843–5.

Stevens JG, Wagner EK et al., 1987, RNA complementary to a herpes alpha gene mRNA is prominent in latently infected neurones, *Science*, **235**: 1056–9.

Straus SE, Corey L et al., 1994, Placebo-controlled trial of vaccination with recombinant glycoprotein D of herpes simplex type 2 for immunotherapy of genital herpes, *Lancet*, **343**: 1460–3.

Sullivan-Bolyai J, Hull HF et al., 1983, Neonatal herpes simplex virus infection in King County, Washington: increasing incidence and epidemiological correlates, *JAMA*, **250**: 3059–62.

Takahashi M, Otsuka T et al., 1974, Live vaccine used to prevent the spread of varicella in children in hospital, *Lancet*, **2**: 1288–90.

Takahashi M, Ikatani T et al., 1992, Immunisation of the elderly and patients with collagen vascular disease with live varicella vaccine and use of varicella skin antigen, *J Infect Dis*, **166, suppl 1**: 58–62.

Whitley RJ, 1992, Therapeutic approaches to varicella-zoster virus infections, *J Infect Dis*, **166, suppl 1**: 51–7.

Whitley RJ, Lakeman AD et al., 1982, DNA restriction enzyme analysis of herpes simplex virus isolates obtained from patients with encephalitis, *N Engl J Med*, **307**: 1060–2.

Wilcox CL, Smith RL et al., 1990, Nerve growth factor dependence of herpes simplex virus latency in peripheral sympathetic and sensory neurones *in vitro*, *J Neurosci*, **10**: 1268–75.

Wu L, Morahan PS, 1992, Macrophages and other non-specific defenses: role in modulating resistance against herpes simplex virus, *Curr Top Microbiol Immunol*, **179**: 89–110.

York IA, Roop C et al., 1994, A cytosolic herpes simplex virus protein inhibits antigen presentation to CD8+ lymphocytes, *Cell*, **77**: 525–35.

Yorke JA, London WP, 1973, Recurrent outbreaks of measles, chickenpox and mumps. II. Systemic differences in contact rates and stochastic effects, *Am J Epidemiol*, **98**: 469–82.

Zaia JA, Levin MJ et al., 1983, Evaluation of varicella zoster immune globulin: protection of immunosuppressed children after household exposure to varicella, *J Infect Dis*, **147**: 737–43.

Chapter 19

BETAHERPESVIRUSES: CYTOMEGALOVIRUS, HUMAN HERPESVIRUSES 6 AND 7

W J Britt

Betaherpesviruses that infect humans include human cytomegalovirus (CMV), human herpesvirus 6 (HHV-6) and human herpesvirus 7 (HHV-7). These viruses have common biological characteristics that can be demonstrated both in vitro and in vivo. Restricted host cell tropisms are a hallmark of this group of viruses; in addition, they are characteristically highly cell associated and replicate slowly compared with alphaherpesviruses. This group of viruses also exhibits extensive genetic homology, especially in the organization of their genomic DNA (Lawrence et al. 1990, Inoue et al. 1993). There are antigenic cross-reactivities between conserved structural and nonstructural proteins encoded by these viruses (Adler et al. 1993, Loh et al. 1994). Finally, infections caused by betaherpesviruses are usually subclinical and acquired at an early age in most populations. Life- or organ-threatening disease following infection is limited to immunocompromised hosts.

CYTOMEGALOVIRUS

Infection with CMV is common in all populations and infrequently associated with symptomatic illness in normal hosts. In contrast, it is a major cause of multi-organ disease in immunocompromised patients, the severity of disease being related to the degree of immunosuppression. Although permissive infection in tissue culture is restricted to a very limited number of cell types, CMV infections in susceptible hosts are widespread with involvement of all organ systems. Although most investigators agree that CMV establishes a persistent infection, it remains unproven whether this represents a latent infection that can be reactivated.

1 CLINICAL MANIFESTATIONS

Although CMV rarely causes symptomatic infection in normal hosts, it is estimated to cause between 20% and 50% of cases of heterophile-negative infectious mononucleosis (Klemola et al. 1970). A characteristic syndrome of fever, hepatitis and atypical lymphocytosis following administration of blood products for cardiac surgery (post-perfusion syndrome) has been attributed to CMV and represents virus transmission from blood products (Perillie and Glenn 1962, Reyman 1966). A variety of other disease states including rheumatological diseases and genitourinary tract malignancies have been linked to CMV; however, the biological and epidemiological evidence of these associations is, at best, limited. More recent studies have renewed interest in a possible role of CMV in the development of atherosclerotic coronary artery disease (Speir et al. 1994).

Three groups of patients are at risk for invasive CMV disease: (1) newborn infants infected in utero, (2) immunocompromised allograft recipients and (3) patients with AIDS. Infants infected in utero may be born with subclinical infections or may have a constellation of clinical abnormalities characteristic of what was initially termed cytomegalic inclusion disease of the newborn (CID) (Jesionek and Kiolemenoglou 1904). Clinical findings include hepatosplenomegaly, jaundice, thrombocytopenia, purpura, microcephaly, chorioretinitis and, rarely, pneumonia (Table 19.1) (McCracken et al. 1969, Boppana et al. 1992). Mortality rates range from 11% to 20% in symptomatic infection, and long-term survivors frequently have deficits in perceptual and cognitive functions (McCracken et al. 1969, Alford 1984, Boppana et al. 1992). Infants with asymptomatic infections are also at risk of developmental abnormalities, hearing loss being the most common. Persistent infection with prolonged viral shedding is nearly universal in infants with either symptomatic or asymptomatic congenital infection (Stagno et al. 1975, Alford 1984).

Cytomegalovirus infections in the post-transplant period are a major cause of morbidity and mortality in allograft recipients. Infections can develop following reactivation of endogenous virus in the previously infected recipient or as the result of reinfection by virus present in the transplanted organ. The severity of infection depends on several characteristics but the 2 most consistently observed risk factors for severe infection are: (1) transplantation of an organ from a previously infected donor into a CMV non-immune host and (2) significant immunosuppression, including that caused by specific therapies directed at T lymphocyte function (Rubin et al. 1981, Singh et al. 1988, Weir et al. 1988). CMV infection in allograft recipients can range from asymptomatic excretion to fulminant multi-organ disease. The most common clinical syndrome associated with CMV infection in the post-transplant period is fever, leucopenia and mild to inapparent hepatic dysfunction (Table 19.1). Pneumonia attributed to CMV in the post-transplant population continues to carry a significant mortality rate. Infection of the central nervous system is rare in transplant patients.

In certain HIV-infected populations, the incidence of CMV infection is extraordinarily high with rates exceeding 95% (Drew et al. 1981, Collier et al. 1987).

It has been suggested that CMV may be the most common cause of clinically important opportunistic infection in long-lived AIDS patients in the USA (Gallant et al. 1992, Pertel et al. 1992). Although reports have documented CMV infection in every organ system in this patient population, the gastrointestinal tract, retina and brain represent the more commonly described sites of CMV disease (Jacobson and Mills 1988, Francis et al. 1989, Schmidbauer et al. 1989, Vinters et al. 1989, Pertel et al. 1992). Colitis, persistent diarrhoea with wasting, vision-threatening retinitis and encephalopathy are common manifestations of CMV infection in patients with end-stage HIV infections (Table 19.1) (Britt and Alford 1995).

2 EPIDEMIOLOGY

The epidemiology of CMV infections can be most readily understood by examining the sources of virus, identifying populations at risk for exposure to infectious virus and defining patients with deficits in immunity who are at risk of severe CMV infections. CMV can be cultured from most body fluids for extended periods following primary infection, significant amounts of infectious virus being found in urine, genital secretions (including semen), saliva and breast milk. Virus is also readily transmitted by cellular elements in blood products, especially leucocytes, and by solid organs during transplantation (Prince et al. 1971, Ho et al. 1975, Pass et al. 1978, Bowden et al. 1991). Periodic reactivation or persistent low level shedding from these sites is also a characteristic of CMV-infected hosts. Sources of infection in normal hosts include exposure to virus-infected body fluids, such as occurs in crowded living conditions in developing countries and in child-care centres in developed societies. In both situations there is frequent infection of children and of susceptible child carers (Pass et al. 1987, Adler 1989). An additional source of virus exposure in infancy is breast feeding, transmission occurring in 30–70% of infants breast fed by mothers with serological evidence of previous infection (Dworsky et al. 1983). After childhood, infection

Table 19.1 Clinical manifestations of CMV infection in different patient populations

Population	Clinical manifestation	
	Acute	Long term
Immuno-competent	Subclinical infection, mononucleosis syndrome	Prolonged virus shedding
Immunocompromised:		
Fetuses	Hepatitis, encephalitis, retinitis, thrombocytopenia microcephaly	Hearing loss, cognitive dysfunction, developmental delay, prolonged virus shedding
Allograft recipients	Fever, hepatitis, pneumonitis, haematological abnormalities	Graft dysfunction/loss, excessive long-term mortality
AIDS	Retinitis, encephalitis, colitis, oesophagitis	Vision loss, wasting syndrome, decreased survival time, encephalopathy

in non-hospitalized individuals is acquired commonly through sexual exposure (Chandler et al. 1985, Handsfield et al. 1985, Fowler and Pass 1991). Over all, it has been estimated that the rate of infection after childhood is c. 1% per year (Stagno et al. 1984).

Clinically significant infections develop in patients with deficits in immunity resulting from pharmacological immunosuppression, acquired deficits in immunity such as HIV infection or developmental immaturity of the immune system. The natural history of CMV infection in transplant recipients suggests that infection is nearly universal in those exposed, but that clinical disease is dependent on specific risk factors. In all but bone marrow allograft recipients, the single most important risk factor is the transplantation of an organ from a donor with previous infection into a CMV non-immune recipient (Rubin et al. 1985, Ho 1991). Disease rates as high as 70% in renal allograft recipients following CMV mismatched donor–recipient transplantation have been reported (Rubin and Colvin 1986). Mortality rates in excess of 50% in cardiac/lung transplants have limited mismatched donor–recipient transplantation in some centres (Smyth et al. 1991). As the severity of immunosuppression increases, so does the severity of the CMV infection, as illustrated by the often fatal CMV infections that occur in bone marrow allograft recipients (Meyers et al. 1982, Winston et al. 1990, Schmidt et al. 1991).

The natural history of CMV infections in AIDS patients has been most closely related to the depletion of CD4+ lymphocytes. Several prospective studies have documented high rates of CMV shedding in almost all AIDS patients, but invasive disease is significantly more common in patients with <50 CD4+ lymphocytes/mm^3 (Gallant et al. 1992). Reinfection is common and isolation of multiple strains of virus from one patient has been reported (Drew et al. 1984, Spector et al. 1984). Characteristics of CMV infection that lead to severe disease and specific organ involvement are not understood, but evidence has been presented that residual virus-specific immunity may modulate disease progression (Boppana et al. 1995).

Congenital CMV infection is the most common viral infection of the human fetus (Alford 1984). In the USA the incidence of congenital CMV infection is c. 1% in live births (Alford 1984, Fowler et al. 1993, Britt and Alford 1995). Of these, an estimated 10% have significant infections that result in long lasting central nervous system sequelae (Alford 1984, Fowler et al. 1993, Britt and Alford 1995). The characteristics of the maternal infection are of paramount importance to the outcome of fetal infection; pre-existing maternal immunity can limit damage to the fetus, a situation analogous to that in allograft patients (Fowler et al. 1993). Primary gestational infection with CMV results in a 35–50% fetal transmission rate, whereas gestational reactivation or reinfection in women with preconceptional immunity is associated with a fetal infection rate of <1% (Alford 1984, Britt and Alford 1995). Furthermore, it is estimated that fetal infection following primary maternal infection

during pregnancy results in damage 5–10 times more often than infection that follows reactivation or reinfection in women with preconceptional immunity (Fowler et al. 1993). Naturally acquired intrapartum or postnatal CMV infection in normal newborn infants has not been associated with severe infections and the permanent sequelae characteristic of infants infected in utero (see Table 19.1) (Alford 1984, Britt and Alford 1995).

3 PATHOGENESIS

In the context of currently available information, the pathogenesis of CMV infection must be viewed as a lytic viral infection resulting from a failure of host immunity to control effectively viral replication and spread. However, it is almost a certainty that CMV exerts its pathogenetic potential through non-lytic mechanisms as well. These may include modulation of normal host cell functions by limited expression of its genome, and perhaps by affecting neighbouring cellular functions through the induction of cytokine production. Other pathways of host cell damage may include the generation of host derived immunopathological responses that result in significant organ damage. Such a mechanism has been offered as an explanation of the severe pneumonia associated with CMV infection in bone allograft recipients (Grundy et al. 1987).

Pathological findings in CMV infection include evidence of viral infection in almost all organ systems (Britt and Alford 1995). Histological findings include large refractile cells (cytomegalic) with so-called owl's eye intranuclear inclusions. In some instances, organ dysfunction exceeds what would be expected from the number of infected cells detected by routine histopathological techniques. This discrepancy has been partially resolved by the use of more sensitive techniques for demonstration of CMV (Myerson et al. 1984).

4 IMMUNE RESPONSES

Protective immune responses against CMV have not been definitely identified, and may not be the same in different populations. Both cellular and antibody responses to CMV participate in the immune responses that resolve infection in normal hosts (Rasmussen 1990, Britt and Alford 1995). Most investigators who have suggested a dominant role for one arm of the immune system in protective immune responses against CMV have based these claims on findings from transplant populations (Pass et al. 1981, Quinnan et al. 1981, Reusser et al. 1991). In these patients, disease was associated with a decrease in either antibody or cellular responses to CMV as a result of immunosuppressive drug therapy. However, it must be noted that components of protective immunity in normal individuals have yet to be fully defined.

In both solid organ and bone marrow transplant

recipients, decreased cellular responses, especially CMV-specific CD8+, MHC-restricted T lymphocyte responses, have been associated with more severe CMV infections in the post-transplant period (Quinnan et al. 1981, Reusser et al. 1991). Reconstitution of these responses with in vitro expanded, CMV-specific cytotoxic T lymphocytes has been shown to reduce post-transplant mortality secondary to CMV (Riddell et al. 1993). Findings from pregnant women have also suggested a correlation of cellular responses to CMV and intrauterine transmission, but these studies remain controversial (Gehrz et al. 1981). In AIDS patients with invasive CMV disease, cellular responses are absent because of lymphocyte depletion. Cellular immune responses appear to be directed primarily at the protein components of virion tegument, the products of the UL83 open reading frame (ORF), phosphoprotein 65 (pp65), and the UL32 ORF, phosphoprotein 150 (pp150). Although other CMV-encoded proteins elicit cellular responses, responder cell frequency analysis has indicated that these 2 proteins represent dominant targets of cellular immunity. The role of cytokines in cellular responses against CMV is unknown. Finally, it has been reported that CMV infections are associated both with decreased cellular immune responses in normal individuals and with decreased CMV-specific responses in congenitally infected children (Gehrz et al. 1977, Pass et al. 1983). Depression in cellular immune responses may also contribute to superinfection with fungal pathogens in transplant recipients infected with CMV (Simmons et al. 1977).

5 ANTIBODY RESPONSES

Serological responses to CMV are complex because of the large number of virus proteins. Several studies have documented responses to a number of the more immunogenic proteins of CMV in both normal and immunocompromised hosts (Zaia et al. 1986, Hayes et al. 1987, Landini et al. 1988). These studies have provided important clues for identification of viral-encoded proteins that induce protective antibody responses as well as antibody responses which could be used in the diagnosis of acute and past CMV infections. The only well characterized in vitro assay of antibody activity that correlates with patient outcome is virus neutralizing antibody (Adler et al. 1995, Boppana and Britt 1995). Virus-neutralizing serological responses are limited to antibodies against virus-encoded glycoproteins, as these represent the only class of viral proteins that are surface exposed in a native form. The majority of virus-neutralizing antibodies are directed against the products of the UL55 (gB) and UL75 (gH) ORFs (Britt et al. 1990, Rasmussen et al. 1991). Studies have suggested that immunization with these proteins can induce neutralizing antibodies as well as antibodies reactive with the surface of virus-infected cells (Rasmussen 1990, Britt et al. 1995). The identification of intense and durable antibody responses to components of the viral

tegument, both pp65 and pp150, has provided a rationale for including these proteins in a recombinant protein based diagnostic assay for serological reactivity to CMV (Landini 1993). Conversely, the presence of significant IgM responses to a non-structural protein, pp50 (UL44), has led to its use as a serological target for detection of IgM and, therefore, recent infection (Landini 1993).

6 DIAGNOSIS

The diagnosis of CMV relies either on demonstration of the agent (virus, viral proteins, nucleic acids) in body fluids and/or tissue or on serological responses in a patient with clinical findings consistent with CMV infection. Because of the ubiquitous nature of CMV, it is important that a distinction be made between the detection of CMV and demonstration of CMV in the context of an infectious syndrome compatible with CMV. Multiple methods of recovering virus have been employed, including culture on permissive cells such as primary human fibroblasts and, more recently, centrifugation enhanced culture followed by early antigen detection with monoclonal antibodies. This latter technique is widely used and can provide positive results within 24 hours. In contrast, conventional tube culture may require up to 4 weeks to reveal cytopathology (Pass et al. 1995).

Techniques of viral antigen detection have been relatively limited with the exception of the antigen-aemia assay (Gerna et al. 1991, Miller et al. 1991), which uses the immunological detection of pp65 within polymorphonuclear leucocytes. Because this assay can be quantified relatively easily, it has been used to predict the likelihood of invasive disease in transplant patients and patients with AIDS (van der Bij et al. 1988, van den Berg et al. 1989). It is less sensitive than polymerase chain reaction (PCR) but this may offer some advantage, as the sensitivity of PCR has limited its predictive value in many circumstances.

Detection of viral nucleic acids has been used extensively to document CMV infections. Dot-blot hybridization, in situ hybridization and PCR have all been applied to clinical specimens. PCR is the most widely used assay and in certain clinical situations, such as screening newborn urine for CMV, is a highly sensitive method of diagnosis. PCR of plasma and peripheral blood buffy coat cells has been used to detect significant infection in transplant recipients and AIDS patients (Spector et al. 1992).

Serological assays of antibody reactivity to CMV include nearly every imaginable technology. Detection of IgG is straightforward and seropositivity is evidence of infection only, and relative titres are usually of little clinical value. Seropositivity does not indicate active virus shedding, but should be taken as evidence of the potential infectivity of blood or organs from the individual. The measurement of CMV-specific IgM responses offers the possibility of distinguishing between acute infection and past infection (Stagno et al. 1985, Landini 1993). Unfortunately, this assay is often associated with low sensitivity and, occasionally, low specificity (Stagno et al. 1985, Landini 1993). Furthermore, the presence of rheumatoid factors may lead to false positive IgM results (Griffiths et al. 1982). Lastly, IgM antibodies are not present in the absence of IgG reactivity, so competition for antigenic sites between IgG and IgM antibodies is possible.

7 CONTROL

7.1 Antiviral therapy

Two agents with activity against CMV are in current clinical use (Coen 1992). Both have significant toxicity, and resistant isolates have developed during treatment. Their use in AIDS patients is problematic since neither is virucidal and, when treatment is interrupted, virus replication resumes.

Ganciclovir is a nucleoside analogue that inhibits chain elongation both by its activity as a chain terminator and through direct inhibition of the viral DNA polymerase (Sullivan et al. 1992, 1993). It is inactive until phosphorylated by the phosphotransferase activity of the UL97 ORF (Sullivan et al. 1992). It has been used to treat invasive infections in transplant recipients, retinitis and colitis in AIDS patients, and as part of a protocol to examine its efficacy in limiting sequelae in infants with congenital CMV infections (Meyers 1991, Spector et al. 1993). It also has some value as an antiviral prophylaxis in bone marrow transplant recipients (Goodrich et al. 1993). Ganciclovir treatment causes primarily bone marrow toxicity with neutropenia as a major adverse effect.

Foscarnet is an inhibitor of CMV DNA polymerases (Snoeck et al. 1993). It is also active against a wide variety of viral polymerases. This agent has been used extensively in AIDS patients and has demonstrated efficacy in CMV retinitis (Palestine et al. 1991). It causes significant renal toxicity, thus limiting its use in transplant recipients.

Past and recent epidemiological studies have indicated that CMV is a vaccine-modifiable disease (Fowler et al. 1993). Previous efforts to develop vaccines have used replicating live viral vaccines. These were referred to as attenuated viruses; however, as CMV does not exhibit identifiable virulence markers, this claim was contentious. Vaccination of renal allograft recipients with one of these viruses, the Towne strain of CMV, provided some evidence that it could induce protective responses (Plotkin et al. 1991). In a recent study, this vaccine failed to protect normal women from reinfection following exposure to children in a group care setting (Adler et al. 1995). Thus, it is unclear whether this vaccine in its current formulation is sufficiently immunogenic to induce protective immunity. Clinical trials are currently underway using native glycoprotein B combined with an adjuvant as an alternative approach.

HUMAN HERPESVIRUSES 6 AND 7

Human herpesviruses 6 and 7 (HHV-6, HHV-7) are 2 newly described human viruses whose clinical importance continues to be defined. Isolation of HHV-6 from AIDS patients initially prompted speculation that it was an important co-factor in this disease (Salahuddin et al. 1986). This initial excitement was subsequently tempered by findings which demonstrated that HHV-6 infection was common and that persistent shedding was characteristic of the biology of this virus. A second lymphotrophic betaherpesvirus, HHV-7, was isolated from CD4+ T lymphocytes of normal individuals (Frenkel et al. 1990). Both viruses are acquired at an early age and seroprevalence is in excess of 60–80% by adulthood in most populations. Genetically, these viruses are closely related to CMV and exhibit genetic homology with CMV over an estimated two-thirds of their genomes (Lawrence et al. 1990, Inoue et al. 1993, Gompels et al. 1995). A single serotype of HHV-7 has been described, whereas HHV-6 can be divided into 2 groups, A and B, based on biology, serological reactivity and genetic composition (Ablashi et al. 1991, Schirmer et al. 1991).

8 CLINICAL MANIFESTATIONS

Recognizable clinical syndromes associated with HHV-6 and HHV-7 infection and confirmed by virological studies have been limited to primary infections in children. HHV-6 is the aetiological agent of exanthem subitum (roseola), a common febrile illness of early childhood (Yamanishi et al. 1988). The clinical findings of this illness include high fevers (>39°C) of 3–5 days' duration, non-specific findings such as pharyngeal injection and diarrhoea, and, perhaps most characteristically, rapid defervescence followed nearly coincidentally by the appearance of a generalized maculopapular rash (Okada et al. 1993, Asano et al. 1994, Hall et al. 1994). Symptoms including irritability, bulging anterior fontanelle and seizures in a significant percentage of infants with roseola have been suggested as evidence of central nervous system infection (Asano et al. 1994, Hall et al. 1994). HHV-6 and possibly HHV-7 are important causes of acute febrile illnesses in childhood, accounting for nearly 20% of hospital emergency room visits in the USA (Hall et al. 1994). Primary infection with HHV-7 is less well described but appears to cause a clinical syndrome very similar to that reported for HHV-6 (Tanaka et al. 1994, Asano et al. 1995). Clinically apparent infections in normal adults with either virus have been infrequently reported but, when diagnosed, resemble infectious mononucleosis (Steeper et al. 1990, Akashi et al. 1993). Reactivation of HHV-6 and possibly of HHV-7 often follows febrile illnesses, and reactivation of HHV-6 follows HHV-7 infection in vitro and in vivo (Kusuhara et al. 1991, Frenkel and Wyatt 1992, Asano et al. 1995). HHV-6 has also been associated with several rare disorders, including sinus histocytosis syndrome (Levine et al. 1992). There is currently little evidence to suggest that either HHV-6 or HHV-7 is an aetiological agent of chronic fatigue syndrome.

Infection with HHV-6 can result in severe organ involvement, especially in immunocompromised hosts. It has been associated with a variety of specific clinical entities, including encephalitis, pneumonitis, hepatitis and bone marrow dysfunction (Asano et al. 1990, Tajiri et al. 1990, Carrigan et al. 1991, Yoshikawa et al. 1992, Cone et al. 1993, Knox and Carrigan 1994). This latter disorder may result from HHV-6 infection of haematopoietic progenitor cells, contributing to graft dysfunction in bone marrow transplant recipients (Knox and Carrigan 1992, Carrigan and Knox 1994). Although numerous case reports have associated HHV-6 infection with specific organ damage in the post-transplant period, it remains to be determined whether HHV-6 is a major cause of morbidity in this patient population. Similarly, in patients with AIDS, HHV-6 and HHV-7 have been associated with a variety of clinical findings but their role, if any, in AIDS pathogenesis is unclear.

9 EPIDEMIOLOGY

The seroprevalence of HHV-6 increases rapidly through early childhood such that over 90% of infants in developed countries will be seropositive by the age of 2 years (Saxinger et al. 1988, Balachandra et al. 1989, Okuno et al. 1989). Serological reactivity in adults is also nearly universal. The vast majority of newborn infants are antibody positive, presumably because of transplacentally acquired maternal antibody, but become seronegative by 6 months of age (Balachandra et al. 1989, Yanagi et al. 1990). Because the rate of infection as measured by seroconversion increases rapidly during the interval between 6 and 12 months, it has been hypothesized that maternal antibody may provide protective immunity early in infancy. In contrast, the seroprevalence of HHV-7 increases steadily throughout childhood and by 10 years of age almost all individuals are seropositive (Wyatt et al. 1991). Furthermore, the prevalence of HHV-7 antibody reactivity in different geographical locations is more variable than that reported for HHV-6 (Wyatt et al. 1991, Yoshikawa et al. 1993, Ablashi et al. 1994). Serological reactivity for HHV-6 does not prevent infection with HHV-7. Intrauterine transmission of either virus seems to be exceedingly rare (Balachandra et al. 1989, Yanagi et al. 1990).

HHV-6 and HHV-7 can be readily isolated in the post-transplant period from both solid organ and bone marrow allograft recipients. Increases in serological responses and viraemia are commonly detected in up to 80% of transplant recipients in the first 3–4 weeks after transplantation (Okuno et al. 1990, Yoshikawa et al. 1991, Wilborn et al. 1994). However, as noted previously, the contribution of HHV-6 to post-transplant morbidity and mortality remains uncertain (Cone et al. 1994a).

Sources of virus include exposure to saliva, genital secretions and blood (Levy et al. 1990, Wyatt and Frenkel 1992, Black et al. 1993, Cone et al. 1994a, Leach et al. 1994). Although breast milk would seem to be a likely source of HHV-6 and HHV-7, current understanding of the natural history of these infections suggests that breast milk is not a common mode of transmission. Limited studies in families have suggested that exposure to respiratory secretions is the most likely mode of intrafamilial spread of HHV-6 (Mukai et al. 1994). HHV-6 and HHV-7 are persistently excreted in the saliva following primary infection and in individuals with past infections (Levy et al. 1990, Wyatt and Frenkel 1992). HHV-7 has been isolated from saliva in 60–80% of seropositive adults (Black et al. 1993, Hidaka et al. 1993). Both viruses can be detected in peripheral blood mononuclear cells (PBMC) from seropositive individuals using PCR, suggesting that blood may be an important source of virus transmission in hospitalized patients (Cone et al. 1994a).

The biological behaviour of the virus in tissue culture initially suggested the possibility of variants of HHV-6. Additional studies have documented the presence of 2 genetically and serologically distinct variants of HHV-6, type A and type B (Ablashi et al. 1991, Schirmer et al. 1991). These variants are associated with specific diseases as illustrated by the finding that over 95% of cases of roseola in the USA are caused by group B viruses (Dewhurst et al. 1993). Studies from 2 different transplant centres have also documented that the B variant is more frequently associated with infections in the post-transplant period (Frenkel et al. 1994, Wilborn et al. 1994a). The basis for the association between the B variant of HHV-6 and specific clinical syndromes remains unexplained. Recent comparisons of genomic sequences of B variants suggest that the B variant may be further divisible into 2 subtypes.

10 PATHOGENESIS

Little is known about the pathogenesis of HHV-6 and HHV-7 infections; however, it must be assumed that, as the majority of infections are subclinical, normal host responses can effectively limit virus-induced cellular damage. In addition, there are no consistent and specific histopathological changes in target organs that suggest direct virus mediated cytopathology (Kurata et al. 1990). Because the severity of roseola can be related to the level of HHV-6 viraemia, viral load may be an important determinant of this disease, and presumably of organ damage (Asano et al. 1991). The pathogenetic mechanism(s) leading to the clinical syndrome of roseola are unknown, but the lymphocyte tropism of the virus suggests that cytokines could contribute to the symptoms associated with this infection. HHV-6 infection of lymphocytes induces production of a variety of lymphokines, including TNF, IL-1β and interferons (Flamand et al. 1991). Using techniques that detect viral nucleic acids or viral antigens in the absence of histopathological changes, HHV-6 has been demonstrated in alveolar macrophages from transplant patients with pneumonitis, hepatocytes from patients with hepatitis, and brain tissue from patients with encephalitis (Asano et al. 1990, Carrigan et al. 1991, Carrigan and Knox 1994, Cone et al. 1994b). It has also been suggested that HHV-6 infection in bone marrow transplant recipients may contribute to more severe graft-versus-host disease (Wilborn et al. 1994a).

The association of HHV-6 infection with central nervous dysfunction, most commonly manifest as seizure activity, is particularly intriguing. As noted above (p. 343), roseola is frequently associated with irritability and a bulging anterior fontanelle, 2 non-specific findings of CNS involvement. Case reports have provided evidence of CNS infection by HHV-6 (Asano et al. 1990, Ishiguro et al. 1990, Yoshikawa et al. 1992). Other studies have also demonstrated, by PCR, viral nucleic acid in the CSF (Kondo et al. 1993, Suga et al. 1993, Achim et al. 1994, Caserta et al. 1994, Wilborn et al. 1994b). Because of the propensity of HHV-6 to reactivate after a febrile illness, including HHV-7 infection, the demonstration of viral nucleic acid in the CSF without additional evidence of tissue invasion or local replication of virus suggests only an association between HHV-6 and CNS dysfunction and not causality.

Since their discovery, HHV-6 and HHV-7 have been suspected to have a role in the pathogenesis of HIV infection. Several biological characteristics support this suspicion. These include: (1) growth in T lymphocytes in vivo and in vitro, (2) the use of CD4 as a cellular receptor by HHV-7, (3) induction of CD4 expression after infection of lymphocytes, and (4) transactivation of the HIV long terminal repeat (Ensoli et al. 1989, Takahashi et al. 1989, Ablashi et al. 1991, Lusso et al. 1991, Martin et al. 1991, Kashanchi et al. 1994, Lusso et al. 1994, Wang et al. 1994, Zhou et al. 1994, Lusso and Gallo 1995). However, epidemiological studies have provided little definitive evidence suggesting that HHV-6 plays an important role in the progression to AIDS in HIV-infected individuals (Fox et al. 1988, Spira et al. 1990). Furthermore, HHV-6 has been shown to inhibit the replication of HIV in vitro (Lusso et al. 1989). In contrast to this early finding, recent studies have suggested that co-infection of HIV-infected cells with lower inocula of HHV-6 may actually lead to enhanced HIV replication. Thus, it remains to be determined whether co-infection with HHV-6 contributes to the progression of HIV infections.

11 IMMUNITY

Immunological responses in normal hosts are sufficient to limit the replication and spread of HHV-6 and HHV-7 as evidenced by the infrequent development of symptomatic infection and the self-limited nature of the infection. The natural history of HHV-6 infection suggests that passively acquired immunity in early infancy is sufficient to prevent infection. Host immune responses that limit reactivation in normal hosts and curtail invasive infection in immunocompromised hosts are unknown, but, if analogous to other herpesvirus infections, are probably virus-specific cellular responses.

11.1 Cellular immune responses

As described above (p. 344), HHV-6 infection can induce the production of antiviral cytokines, including interferons. Natural killer cell activity has also been reported to be elevated in acute HHV-6 infection (Takahashi et al. 1992). Analysis of CD4+ lymphocyte clones derived from infected individuals has revealed that, although most were specific for HHV-6, about 10% responded to both HHV-6 and HHV-7 and an even smaller number were cross-reactive with HHV-6, HHV-7 and CMV (Yasukawa et al. 1993). Group A and B variants of HHV-6 could be distinguished by reactivity of 7% of the clones. MHC-restricted cytotoxic T cell clones specific for HHV-6 infected cells have also been isolated (Yakushijin et al. 1992). The antigen specificity of the cellular responses against HHV-6 and HHV-7 has not been elucidated.

11.2 Antibody responses

The serological responses to HHV-6 and HHV-7 are extraordinarily complex. A large number of virus-encoded proteins are recognized by convalescent sera, but to date the antibody components of protective immunity have not been defined. Immune precipitation of radiolabelled virus-infected cell proteins with convalescent serum revealed over 20 different proteins (Balachandran et al. 1991). At least 5 glycoproteins can be precipitated from infected cells by antibodies contained within convalescent sera (Balachandran et al. 1991). More recent studies have identified specific viral proteins that are targets of antibody responses including the gB and gH HHV-6 homologues (Ellinger et al. 1993, Liu et al. 1993, Qian et al. 1993). In addition, the major glycoprotein complex of the A variant of HHV-6, gp82-105, has been shown to be a target of neutralizing antibodies (Pfeiffer et al. 1993). A major antigenic protein of HHV-6, designated p100, is the homologue of CMV pp150 (UL32) and probably represents a dominant target of virus-specific antibodies (Neipel et al. 1992). Cross-reactivity exists between conserved structural proteins such as the major capsid protein and the non-structural protein CD41 (homologue of CMV pp50 (UL44)) (Loh and Britt 1993, unpublished, Loh et al. 1994). Interestingly, cross-reactivity has also been shown between the major envelope glycoprotein of CMV (gB) and HHV-6 (Adler et al. 1993). The serological response to HHV-7 is equally complex, with over 15 radiolabelled infected cell proteins demonstrable by immune precipitation (Foa-Tomasi et al. 1994). Antigenic cross-reactivity between HHV-6 and HHV-7 encoded proteins has also been demonstrated (Foa-Tomasi et al. 1994).

12   DIAGNOSIS

The diagnosis of HHV-6 and/or HHV-7 infection requires the detection of virus, viral antigens or viral nucleic acids in an appropriate specimen from a patient with a clinical syndrome compatible with infection by either of these viruses. Virus can be recovered from saliva or other body fluids by inoculation of umbilical cord lymphocytes. Other cells suitable for virus isolation include phytohaemagglutinin-stimulated PBMC. Cell lines such as HSB2, Sup T1 and Molt-3 have been used to propagate HHV-6, although tropism for specific cell lines may vary (Osman et al. 1993). Cell lines permissive for HHV-7 have not been described. Viral antigens within infected cells can be readily detected by immunological assays that incorporate HHV-6 or HHV-7 specific monoclonal antibodies (Yamamoto et al. 1990, Campadelli-Fiume et al. 1993, Parker and Weber 1993). Perhaps the most useful assays for HHV-6 and HHV-7 are PCR amplification of specific regions of the viruses. These can be carried out on a number different clinical specimens, including PBMC, saliva and plasma. The judicious selection of primers allows HHV-7 and the 2 variants of HHV-6 to be distinguished from one another (Aubin et al. 1994, Yamamoto et al. 1994, Secchiero et al. 1995).

Serological assays have yet to be rigorously standardized and, because of significant cross-reactivity between HHV-6 variants and HHV-7, confirmatory testing including absorption with heterologous viral antigens should be considered. With the identification of specific viral proteins and their corresponding ORFs, recombinant antigen-based serological assays will probably overcome issues of cross-reactivity and the high seroprevalence rates in the population.

13   CONTROL

Although ganciclovir and foscarnet are virustatic for both HHV-6 and HHV-7, current in vitro testing of antiviral susceptibility of these viruses is poorly standardized. Therefore, it is unclear whether adequate in vivo concentrations of drug can be achieved. The presence of the UL97 homologue in HHV-6 suggests that its sensitivity to ganciclovir will be similar to that of CMV. Consistent with this finding, some isolates have exhibited drug sensitivities comparable to those reported for CMV.

REFERENCES

Ablashi DV, Balachandran N et al., 1991, Genomic polymorphism, growth properties, and immunologic variations in human herpesvirus-6 isolates, *Virology*, **184:** 545–52.

Ablashi DV, Berneman ZN et al., 1994, Human herpesvirus-7 (HHV-7), *In Vivo*, **8:** 549–54.

Achim CL, Wang R et al., 1994, Brain viral burden in HIV infection, *J Neuropathol Exp Neurol*, **53:** 284–93.

Adler SP, 1989, Cytomegalovirus and child day care. Evidence for an increased infection rate among day-care workers, *N Engl J Med*, **321:** 1290–6.

Adler SP, McVoy M et al., 1993, Antibodies induced by a primary cytomegalovirus infection react with human herpes virus 6 proteins, *J Infect Dis*, **168:** 1119–26.

Adler SP, Starr SE et al., 1995, Immunity induced by primary human cytomegalovirus infection protects against secondary infection among women of childbearing age, *J Infect Dis*, **171:** 26–32.

Akashi K, Eizuru Y et al., 1993, Brief report: severe infectious mononucleosis-like syndrome and primary human herpesvirus 6 infection in an adult, *N Engl J Med*, **329:** 168–71.

Alford CA, 1984, Chronic intrauterine and perinatal infections, *Antiviral Agents and Viral Diseases of Man*, 2nd edn, eds Galasso GJ, Merigan JC, Buchanan RA, Raven Press, New York, 433–86.

Asano Y, Yoshikawa T et al., 1990, Fatal fulminant hepatitis in an infant with human herpesvirus 6 infection, *Lancet*, **335:** 862–3.

Asano Y, Nakashima T et al., 1991, Severity of human herpesvirus-6 viremia and clinical findings in infants with exanthem subitum, *J Pediatr*, **118:** 891–5.

Asano Y, Yoshikawa T et al., 1994, Clinical features of infants with primary human herpesvirus 6 infection (exanthem subitum, roseola infantum), *Pediatrics*, **93:** 104–8.

Asano Y, Suga S et al., 1995, Clinical features and viral excretion in an infant with primary human herpesvirus 7 infection, *Pediatrics*, **95:** 187.

Aubin JT, Poirel L et al., 1994, Identification of human herpesvirus 6 variants A and B by amplimer hybridization with variant-specific oligonucleotides and amplification with variant-specific primers, *J Clin Microbiol*, **32:** 2434–40.

Balachandra K, Ayuthaya PI et al., 1989, Prevalence of antibody to human herpesvirus 6 in women and children, *Microbiol Immunol*, **33:** 515–18.

Balachandran N, Tirawatnapong S et al., 1991, Electrophoretic analysis of human herpesvirus 6 polypeptides immunoprecipitated from infected cells with human sera, *J Infect Dis*, **163:** 29–34.

van den Berg AP, van der Bij W et al., 1989, Cytomegalovirus antigenemia as a useful marker of symptomatic cytomegalovirus infection after renal transplantation: a report of 130 consecutive patients, *Transplantation*, **48:** 991–5.

van der Bij W, Schirm J et al., 1988, Comparison between viremia and antigenemia for detection of cytomegalovirus in blood, *J Clin Microbiol*, **26:** 2531–5.

Black JB, Inoue N et al., 1993, Frequent isolation of human herpesvirus 7 from saliva, *Virus Res*, **29:** 91–8.

Boppana SB, Britt WJ, 1995, Antiviral antibody responses and intrauterine transmission after primary maternal cytomegalovirus infection, *J Infect Dis*, **171:** 1115–21.

Boppana SB, Pass RF et al., 1992, Symptomatic congenital cytomegalovirus infection: neonatal morbidity and mortality, *Pediatr Infect Dis J*, **11:** 93–9.

Boppana SB, Polis MA et al., 1995, Virus specific antibody responses to human cytomegalovirus (HCMV) in human immunodeficiency virus type 1-infected individuals with HCMV retinitis, *J Infect Dis*, **171:** 182–5.

Bowden RA, Slichter SJ et al., 1991, Use of leukocyte-depleted platelets and cytomegalovirus-seronegative red blood cells for prevention of primary cytomegalovirus infection after marrow transplant, *Blood*, **78:** 246–50.

Britt WJ, Alford CA, 1995, Cytomegalovirus, *Fields' Virology*, 3rd edn, eds Fields BN, Knipe DM et al., Raven Press, New York, 2493–523.

Britt WJ, Vugler L et al., 1990, Cell surface expression of human cytomegalovirus (HCMV) gp55-116 (gB): use of HCMV-vaccinia recombinant virus infected cells in analysis of the human neutralizing antibody response, *J Virol*, **64:** 1079–85.

Britt W, Fay J et al., 1995, Formulation of an immunogenic human cytomegalovirus vaccine: responses in experimental animals, *J Infect Dis*, **171:** 18–25.

Campadelli-Fiume G, Guerrini S et al., 1993, Monoclonal antibodies to glycoprotein B differentiate human herpesvirus 6 into two clusters, A and B, *J Gen Virol*, **74**: 2257–62.

Carrigan DR, Knox KK, 1994, Human herpesvirus 6 (HHV-6) isolation from bone marrow: HHV-6-associated bone marrow suppression in bone marrow transplant patients, *Blood*, **84**: 3307–10.

Carrigan DR, Drobyski WR et al., 1991, Interstitial pneumonitis associated with human herpesvirus-6 infection after marrow transplantation, *Lancet*, **338**: 147–9.

Caserta MT, Hall CB et al., 1994, Neuroinvasion and persistence of human herpesvirus 6 in children, *J Infect Dis*, **170**: 1586–9.

Chandler SH, Holmes KK et al., 1985, The epidemiology of cytomegaloviral infection in women attending a sexually transmitted disease clinic, *J Infect Dis*, **152**: 597–605.

Coen DM, 1992, Molecular aspects of anti-herpesvirus drugs, *Semin Virol*, **3**: 3–12.

Collier AC, Meyers JD et al., 1987, Cytomegalovirus infection in homosexual men. Relationship to sexual practices, antibody to human immunodeficiency virus, and cell-mediated immunity, *Am J Med*, **23**: 593–601.

Cone RW, Hackman RC et al., 1993, Human herpesvirus 6 in lung tissues from patients with pneumonitis after bone marrow transplantation, *N Engl J Med*, **329**: 156–61.

Cone RW, Huang ML et al., 1994a, Human herpesvirus 6 DNA in peripheral blood cells and saliva from immunocompetent individuals, *J Clin Microbiol*, **32**: 2633–7.

Cone RW, Huang ML et al., 1994b, Human herpesvirus 6 and pneumonia, *Leuk Lymphoma*, **15**: 235–41.

Dewhurst S, McIntyre K et al., 1993, Human herpesvirus 6 (HHV-6) variant B accounts for the majority of symptomatic primary HHV-6 infections in a population of US infants, *J Clin Microbiol*, **31**: 416–18.

Drew WL, Mintz L et al., 1981, Prevalence of cytomegalovirus infection in homosexual men, *J Infect Dis*, **143**: 188–92.

Drew WL, Sweet ES et al., 1984, Multiple infections by cytomegalovirus in patients with acquired immune deficiency syndrome: documentation by Southern blot hybridization, *J Infect Dis*, **150**: 952–3.

Dworsky M, Yow M et al., 1983, Cytomegalovirus infection of breast milk and transmission in infancy, *Pediatrics*, **72**: 295–9.

Ellinger K, Neipel F et al., 1993, The glycoprotein B homologue of human herpesvirus 6, *J Gen Virol*, **74**: 495–500.

Ensoli B, Lusso P et al., 1989, Human herpesvirus-6 increases HIV-1 expression in co-infected T cells via nuclear factors binding to the HIV-1 enhancer, *EMBO J*, **8**: 3019–27.

Flamand L, Gosselin J et al., 1991, Human herpesvirus 6 induces interleukin-1 beta and tumor necrosis factor alpha, but not interleukin-6, in peripheral blood mononuclear cell cultures, *J Virol*, **65**: 5105–10.

Foa-Tomasi L, Avitabile E et al., 1994, Polyvalent and monoclonal antibodies identify major immunogenic proteins specific for human herpesvirus 7-infected cells and have weak cross-reactivity with human herpesvirus 6, *J Gen Virol*, **75**: 2719–27.

Fowler KB, Pass RF, 1991, Sexually transmitted diseases in mothers of neonates with congenital cytomegalovirus infection, *J Infect Dis*, **164**: 259–64.

Fowler KB, Stagno S et al., 1993, Maternal age and congenital cytomegalovirus infection: screening of two diverse newborn populations, 1980–1990, *J Infect Dis*, **168**: 552–6.

Fox J, Briggs M et al., 1988, Antibody to human herpesvirus 6 in HIV-positive and negative homosexual men, *Lancet*, **2**: 396–7.

Francis ND, Boylston AW et al., 1989, Cytomegalovirus infection in gastrointestinal tracts of patients infected with HIV-1 or AIDS, *J Clin Pathol*, **42**: 1055–64.

Frenkel N, Wyatt LS, 1992, HHV-6 and HHV-7 as exogenous agents in human lymphocytes, *Dev Biol Standard*, **76**: 259–65.

Frenkel N, Schirmer EC et al., 1990, Isolation of a new herpesvirus from human CD4+ T cells, *Proc Natl Acad Sci USA*, **87**: 748–52.

Frenkel N, Katsafanas GC et al., 1994, Bone marrow transplant recipients harbor the B variant of human herpesvirus 6, *Bone Marrow Transplant*, **14**: 839–43.

Gallant JE, Moore RD et al., 1992, Incidence and natural history of cytomegalovirus disease in patients with advanced human immunodeficiency virus disease treated with zidovudine, *J Infect Dis*, **166**: 1223–7.

Gehrz RC, Markers SC et al., 1977, Specific cell-mediated immune defect in active cytomegalovirus infection of young children and their mothers, *Lancet*, **2**: 844–7.

Gehrz RC, Christianson WR et al., 1981, Cytomegalovirus specific humoral and cellular immune responses in human pregnancy, *J Infect Dis*, **143**: 391–5.

Gerna G, Zipeto D et al., 1991, Monitoring of human cytomegalovirus infections and ganciclovir treatment in heart transplant recipients by determination of viremia, antigenemia, and DNAemia, *J Infect Dis*, **164**: 488–98.

Gompels UA, Nicholas J et al., 1995, The DNA sequence of human herpesvirus-6: structure, coding content, and genome evolution, *Virology*, **209**: 29–51.

Goodrich JM, Bowden RA et al., 1993, Ganciclovir prophylaxis to prevent cytomegalovirus disease after allogeneic marrow transplant, *Ann Intern Med*, **118**: 173–8.

Griffiths PD, Stagno S et al., 1982, Infection with cytomegalovirus during pregnancy: specific IgM antibodies as a marker of recent primary infection, *J Infect Dis*, **145**: 647–53.

Grundy JE, Shanley JD et al., 1987, Is cytomegalovirus interstitial pneumonitis in transplant recipients an immunopathological condition?, *Lancet*, **2**: 996–9.

Hall CB, Long CE et al., 1994, Human herpesvirus-6 infection in children. A prospective study of complications and reactivation, *N Engl J Med*, **331**: 432–8.

Handsfield HH, Chandler SH et al., 1985, Cytomegalovirus infection in sex partners: evidence for sexual transmission, *J Infect Dis*, **151**: 344–8.

Hayes K, Alford CA et al., 1987, Antibody response to virus-encoded proteins after cytomegalovirus mononucleosis, *J Infect Dis*, **156**: 615–21.

Hidaka Y, Liu Y et al., 1993, Frequent isolation of human herpesvirus 7 from saliva samples, *J Med Virol*, **40**: 343–6.

Ho M, 1991, *Cytomegalovirus Biology and Infection*, Plenum Press, New York, 269.

Ho M, Suwansirikul S et al., 1975, The transplanted kidney as a source of cytomegalovirus infections, *N Engl J Med*, **293**: 1109–12.

Inoue N, Dambaugh TR et al., 1993, Molecular biology of human herpesvirus 6A and 6B, *Infect Agents Dis*, **2**: 343–60.

Ishiguro N, Yamada S et al., 1990, Meningo-encephalitis associated with HHV-6 related exanthem subitum, *Acta Paediatr Scand*, **79**: 987–9.

Jacobson MA, Mills J, 1988, Serious cytomegalovirus disease in the acquired immunodeficiency syndrome (AIDS), *Ann Intern Med*, **108**: 585–94.

Jesionek A, Kiolemenoglou B, 1904, Uber einen befund von protozoenartigen gebilden in den organen eines heriditarluetischen fotus, *Münch Med Wochenschr*, **51**: 1905–7.

Kashanchi F, Thompson J et al., 1994, Transcriptional activation of minimal HIV-1 promoter by ORF-1 protein expressed from the Sall-L fragment of human herpesvirus-6, *Virology*, **201**: 95–106.

Klemola E, von Essen R et al., 1970, Infectious-mononucleosis-like disease with negative heterophil agglutination test. Clinical features in relation to Epstein–Barr virus and cytomegalovirus antibodies, *J Infect Dis*, **121**: 608–14.

Knox KK, Carrigan DR, 1992, In vitro suppression of bone marrow progenitor cell differentiation by human herpesvirus 6 infection, *J Infect Dis*, **165**: 925–9.

Knox KK, Carrigan DR, 1994, Disseminated active HHV-6 infections in patients with AIDS, *Lancet*, **343**: 577–8.

Kondo K, Nagafuji H et al., 1993, Association of human herpesvirus 6 infection of the central nervous system with recurrence of febrile convulsions, *J Infect Dis*, **167**: 1197–200.

Kurata T, Kawasaki T et al., 1990, Viral pathology of human herpesvirus 6 infection, *Immunobiology and Prophylaxis of Human Herpesvirus Infections*, eds Lopez C, Mori R et al., Plenum Press, New York, 39–47.

Kusuhara K, Ueda K et al., 1991, Do second attacks of exanthema subitum result from human herpesvirus 6 reactivation or reinfection?, *Pediatr Infect Dis J*, **10**: 468–70.

Landini MP, 1993, New approaches and perspectives in cytomegalovirus diagnosis, *Prog Med Virol*, **40**: 157–77.

Landini MP, Rossier E et al., 1988, Antibodies to human cytomegalovirus structural polypeptides during primary infection, *J Virol Methods*, **22**: 309–17.

Lawrence GL, Chee M et al., 1990, Human herpesvirus 6 is closely related to human cytomegalovirus, *J Virol*, **64**: 287.

Leach CT, Newton ER et al., 1994, Human herpesvirus 6 infection of the female genital tract, *J Infect Dis*, **169**: 1281–3.

Levine PH, Jahan N et al., 1992, Detection of human herpesvirus 6 in tissues involved by sinus histiocytosis with massive lymphadenopathy (Rosai–Dorfman disease), *J Infect Dis*, **166**: 291–5.

Levy JA, Ferro F et al., 1990, Frequent isolation of HHV-6 from saliva and high seroprevalence of the virus in the population, *Lancet*, **335**: 1047–50.

Liu DX, Gompels UA et al., 1993, Identification and expression of the human herpesvirus 6 glycoprotein H and interaction with an accessory 40k glycoprotein, *J Gen Virol*, **74**: 1847–57.

Loh LC, Britt WJ et al., 1994, Sequence analysis and expression of the murine cytomegalovirus phosphoprotein pp50, a homolog of the human cytomegalovirus UL44 gene product, *Virology*, **200**: 413–27.

Lusso P, Gallo RC, 1995, Human herpesvirus 6 in AIDS, *Immunol Today*, **16**: 67–71.

Lusso P, Ensoli B et al., 1989, Productive dual infection of human CD4+ T lymphocytes by HIV-1 and HHV-6, *Nature (London)*, **337**: 370–3.

Lusso P, De Maria A et al., 1991, Induction of CD4 and susceptibility to HIV-1 infection in human CD8+ T lymphocytes by human herpesvirus 6, *Nature (London)*, **349**: 533–5.

Lusso P, Secchiero P et al., 1994, CD4 is a critical component of the receptor for human herpesvirus 7: interference with human immunodeficiency virus, *Proc Natl Acad Sci USA*, **91**: 3872–6.

McCracken GJ, Shinefield HR et al., 1969, Congenital cytomegalic inclusion disease. A longitudinal study of 20 patients, *Am J Dis Child*, **117**: 522–39.

Martin ME, Nicholas J et al., 1991, Identification of a transactivating function mapping to the putative immediate-early locus of human herpesvirus 6, *J Virol*, **65**: 5381–90.

Meyers JD, 1991, Critical evaluation of agents used in the treatment and prevention of cytomegalovirus infection in immunocompromised patients, *Transplant Proc*, **23**: 139–43.

Meyers JD, Flournoy N et al., 1982, Nonbacterial pneumonia after allogeneic marrow transplantation: a review of ten years' experience, *Rev Infect Dis*, **4**: 1119–32.

Miller H, Rossier E et al., 1991, Prospective study of cytomegalovirus antigenemia in allograft recipients, *J Clin Microbiol*, **29**: 1054–5.

Mukai T, Yamamoto T et al., 1994, Molecular epidemiological studies of human herpesvirus 6 in families, *J Med Virol*, **42**: 224–7.

Myerson D, Hackman RC et al., 1984, Widespread presence of histologically occult cytomegalovirus, *Hum Pathol*, **15**: 430–9.

Neipel F, Ellinger K et al., 1992, Gene for the major antigenic structural protein (p100) of human herpesvirus 6, *J Virol*, **66**: 3918–24.

Okada K, Ueda K et al., 1993, Exanthema subitum and human herpesvirus 6 infection: clinical observations in fifty-seven cases, *Pediatr Infect Dis J*, **12**: 204–8.

Okuno T, Takahashi K et al., 1989, Seroepidemiology of human herpesvirus 6 infection in normal children and adults, *J Clin Microbiol*, **27**: 651–3.

Okuno T, Higashi K et al., 1990, Human herpesvirus 6 infection in renal transplantation, *Transplantation*, **49**: 519–22.

Osman HK, Wells C et al., 1993, Growth characteristics of human herpesvirus-6: comparison of antigen production in two cell lines, *J Med Virol*, **39**: 303–11.

Palestine AG, Polis MA et al., 1991, A randomized, controlled trial of foscarnet in the treatment of cytomegalovirus retinitis in patients with AIDS, *Ann Intern Med*, **115**: 665–73.

Parker CA, Weber JM, 1993, An enzyme-linked immunosorbent assay for the detection of IgG and IgM antibodies to human herpesvirus type 6, *J Virol Methods*, **41**: 265–75.

Pass RF, Long WK et al., 1978, Productive infection with cytomegalovirus and herpes simplex virus in renal transplant recipients: role of source of kidney, *J Infect Dis*, **137**: 556–63.

Pass RF, Reynolds DW et al., 1981, Impaired lymphocyte transformation response to cytomegalovirus and phytohemagglutinin in recipients of renal transplants: association with antithymocyte globulin, *J Infect Dis*, **143**: 259–65.

Pass RF, Stagno S et al., 1983, Specific cell mediated immunity and the natural history of congenital infection with cytomegalovirus, *J Infect Dis*, **148**: 953–61.

Pass RF, Little EA et al., 1987, Young children as a probable source of maternal and congenital cytomegalovirus infection, *N Engl J Med*, **316**: 1366–70.

Pass RF, Britt WJ et al., 1995, Cytomegalovirus, *Diagnostic Procedures for Viral, Rickettsial and Chlamydial Infections*, 7th edn, eds Lennette EH, Lennette DA, Lennette ET, APHA, Washington DC, 253–71.

Perillie PE, Glenn WWL, 1962, Fever, splenomegaly and eosinophilia: a new postpericardiotomy syndrome, *Yale J Biol Med*, **34**: 625–8.

Pertel P, Hirschtick R et al., 1992, Risk of developing cytomegalovirus retinitis in persons infected with the human immunodeficiency virus, *J Acquired Immune Defic Syndr*, **5**: 1069–74.

Pfeiffer B, Berneman ZN et al., 1993, Identification and mapping of the gene encoding the glycoprotein complex gp82–gp105 of human herpesvirus 6 and mapping of the neutralizing epitope recognized by monoclonal antibodies, *J Virol*, **67**: 4611–20.

Plotkin SA, Starr SE et al., 1991, Effect of Towne live virus vaccine on cytomegalovirus disease after renal transplant. A controlled trial, *Ann Intern Med*, **114**: 525–31.

Prince AM, Szumuness W et al., 1971, A serologic study of cytomegalovirus infections associated with blood transfusions, *N Engl J Med*, **284**: 1125–31.

Qian G, Wood C et al., 1993, Identification and characterization of glycoprotein gH of human herpesvirus-6, *Virology*, **194**: 380–6.

Quinnan GV, Kirmani N et al., 1981, HLA-restricted cytotoxic T lymphocyte and nonthymic cytotoxic lymphocyte responses to cytomegalovirus infection of bone marrow transplant recipients, *J Immunol*, **126**: 2036–41.

Rasmussen L, 1990, Immune response to human cytomegalovirus infection, *Curr Top Microbiol Immunol*, **154**: 222–54.

Rasmussen L, Matkin C et al., 1991, Antibody response to human cytomegalovirus glycoproteins gB and gH after natural infection in humans, *J Infect Dis*, **164**: 835–42.

Reusser P, Riddell SR et al., 1991, Cytotoxic T-lymphocyte response to cytomegalovirus after human allogeneic bone marrow transplantation: pattern of recovery and correlation with cytomegalovirus infection and disease, *Blood*, **78**: 1373–80.

Reyman TA, 1966, Postperfusion syndrome: a review and report of 21 cases, *Am Heart J*, **72**: 116–23.

Riddell SR, Gilbert MJ et al., 1993, Reconstitution of protective CD8+ cytotoxic T lymphocyte responses to human cytomegalovirus in immunodeficient humans by the adoptive transfer of T cell clones, *Multidisciplinary Approach to Understanding*

Cytomegalovirus Disease, eds Michelson S, Plotkin SA, Elsevier Science, Amsterdam, 155–64.

Rubin RH, Colvin RB, 1986, Cytomegalovirus infection in renal transplantation: clinical importance and control, *Kidney Transplant Rejection: diagnosis and treatment*, eds Williams GM, Burdick JF, Solez K, Marcel Dekker, New York, 283–304.

Rubin RH, Cosimi AB et al., 1981, Effects of antithymocyte globulin on cytomegalovirus infection in renal transplant recipients, *Transplantation*, **31**: 143–5.

Rubin RH, Tolkoff-Rubin NE et al., 1985, Multicenter seroepidemiologic study of the impact of cytomegalovirus infection on renal transplantation, *Transplantation*, **40**: 243–9.

Salahuddin SZ, Ablashi DV et al., 1986, Isolation of a new virus, HBLV, in patients with lymphoproliferative disorders, *Science*, **234**: 596–600.

Saxinger C, Polesky H et al., 1988, Antibody reactivity with HBLV (HHV-6) in US populations, *J Virol Methods*, **21**: 199–208.

Schirmer EC, Wyatt LS et al., 1991, Differentiation between two distinct classes of viruses now classified as human herpesvirus 6, *Proc Natl Acad Sci USA*, **88**: 5922–6.

Schmidbauer M, Budka H et al., 1989, Cytomegalovirus (CMV) disease of the brain in AIDS and connatal infection: a comparative study by histology, immunocytochemistry and in situ DNA hybridization, *Acta Neuropathol (Berl)*, **79**: 286–93.

Schmidt GM, Horak DA et al., 1991, A randomized, controlled trial of prophylactic ganciclovir for cytomegalovirus pulmonary infection in recipients of allogeneic bone marrow transplants, *N Engl J Med*, **324**: 1005–11.

Secchiero P, Carrigan DR et al., 1995, Detection of human herpesvirus 6 in plasma of children with primary infection and immunosuppressed patients by polymerase chain reaction, *J Infect Dis*, **171**: 273–80.

Simmons RL, Matas AJ et al., 1977, Clinical characteristics of the lethal cytomegalovirus infection following renal transplantation, *Surgery*, **82**: 537–46.

Singh N, Dummer JS et al., 1988, Infections with cytomegalovirus and other herpesviruses in 121 liver transplant recipients: transmission by donated organ and the effect of OKT3 antibodies, *J Infect Dis*, **158**: 124–31.

Smyth RL, Scott JP et al., 1991, Cytomegalovirus infection in heart–lung transplant recipients: risk factors, clinical associations, and response to treatment, *J Infect Dis*, **164**: 1045–50.

Snoeck R, Neyts J et al., 1993, Strategies for the treatment of cytomegalovirus infections, *Multidisciplinary Approach to Understanding Cytomegalovirus Disease*, eds Michelson S, Plotkin SA, Elsevier Science, Amsterdam, 269–78.

Spector SA, Hirata KK et al., 1984, Identification of multiple cytomegalovirus strains in homosexual men with acquired immunodeficiency syndrome, *J Infect Dis*, **150**: 953–6.

Spector SA, Merrill R et al., 1992, Detection of human cytomegalovirus in plasma of AIDS patients during acute visceral disease by DNA amplification, *J Clin Microbiol*, **30**: 2359–65.

Spector SA, Weingeist T et al., 1993, A randomized, controlled study of intravenous ganciclovir therapy for cytomegalovirus peripheral retinitis in patients with AIDS. AIDS Clinical Trials Group and Cytomegalovirus Cooperative Study Group, *J Infect Dis*, **168**: 557–63.

Speir E, Modali R et al., 1994, Potential role of human cytomegalovirus and p53 interaction in coronary restenosis, *Science*, **265**: 391–4.

Spira TJ, Bozeman LH et al., 1990, Lack of correlation between human herpesvirus-6 infection and the course of human immunodeficiency virus infection, *J Infect Dis*, **161**: 567–70.

Stagno S, Reynolds DW et al., 1975, Comparative, serial virologic and serologic studies of symptomatic and subclinical congenital and natally acquired cytomegalovirus infection, *J Infect Dis*, **132**: 568–77.

Stagno S, Cloud G et al., 1984, Factors associated with primary cytomegalovirus infection during pregnancy, *J Med Virol*, **13**: 347–53.

Stagno S, Tinker MK et al., 1985, Immunoglobulin M antibodies

detected by enzyme-linked immunosorbent assay and radioimmunoassay in the diagnosis of cytomegalovirus infections in pregnant women and newborn infants, *J Clin Microbiol*, **21**: 930–5.

Steeper TA, Horwitz CA et al., 1990, The spectrum of clinical and laboratory findings resulting from human herpesvirus-6 in patients with mononucleosis-like illnesses not resulting from Epstein–Barr virus or cytomegalovirus, *Am J Clin Pathol*, **93**: 776–83.

Suga S, Yoshikawa T et al., 1993, Clinical and virological analyses of 21 infants with exanthem subitum and central nervous system complications, *Ann Neurol*, **33**: 597–603.

Sullivan V, Talarico CL et al., 1992, A protein kinase homologue controls phosphorylation of ganciclovir in human cytomegalovirus-infected cells, *Nature (London)*, **358**: 162–4.

Sullivan V, Biron KK et al., 1993, A point mutation in the human cytomegalovirus DNA polymerase gene confers resistance to ganciclovir and phosphonylmethoxyalkyl derivatives, *Antimicrob Agents Chemother*, **37**: 19–25.

Tajiri H, Nose O et al., 1990, Human herpesvirus-6 infection with liver injury in neonatal hepatitis, *Lancet*, **335**: 863.

Takahashi K, Sonoda S et al., 1989, Predominant CD4 T-lymphocyte tropism of human herpesvirus 6-related virus, *J Virol*, **63**: 3161–3.

Takahashi K, Segal E et al., 1992, Interferon and natural killer cell activity in patients with exanthem subitum, *Pediatr Infect Dis J*, **11**: 369–73.

Tanaka K, Kondo T et al., 1994, Human herpesvirus 7: another causal agent for roseola, *J Pediatr*, **125**: 1–5.

Vinters HV, Kwok MK et al., 1989, Cytomegalovirus in the nervous system of patients with the acquired immune deficiency syndrome, *Brain*, **112**: 245–68.

Wang J, Jones C et al., 1994, Identification and characterization of a human herpesvirus 6 gene segment capable of transactivating the human immunodeficiency virus type 1 long terminal repeat in an Sp1 binding site-dependent manner, *J Virol*, **68**: 1706–13.

Weir MR, Henry ML et al., 1988, Incidence and morbidity of cytomegalovirus disease associated with a seronegative recipient receiving seropositive donor-specific transfusion and living related donor transplantation: a multicenter evaluation, *Transplantation*, **45**: 111–16.

Wilborn F, Brinkmann V et al., 1994a, Herpesvirus type 6 in patients undergoing bone marrow transplantation: serologic features and detection by polymerase chain reaction, *Blood*, **83**: 3052–8.

Wilborn F, Schmidt CA et al., 1994b, A potential role for human herpesvirus type 6 in nervous system disease, *J Neuroimmunol*, **49**: 213–14.

Winston DJ, Ho WG et al., 1990, Cytomegalovirus infections after bone marrow transplantation, *Rev Infect Dis*, **12**: S776–92.

Wyatt LS, Frenkel N, 1992, Human herpesvirus 7 is a constitutive inhabitant of adult human saliva, *J Virol*, **66**: 3206–9.

Wyatt LS, Rodriguez WJ et al., 1991, Human herpesvirus 7: antigenic properties and prevalence in children and adults, *J Virol*, **65**: 6260–5.

Yakushijin Y, Yasukawa M et al., 1992, Establishment and functional characterization of human herpesvirus 6-specific CD4+ human T-cell clones, *J Virol*, **66**: 2773–9.

Yamamoto M, Black JB et al., 1990, Identification of a nucleocapsid protein as a specific serological marker of human herpesvirus 6 infection, *J Clin Microbiol*, **28**: 1957–62.

Yamamoto T, Mukai T et al., 1994, Variation of DNA sequence in immediate-early gene of human herpesvirus 6 and variant identification by PCR, *J Clin Microbiol*, **32**: 473–6.

Yamanishi K, Okuno T et al., 1988, Identification of human herpesvirus 6 as causal agent for exanthem subitum, *Lancet*, **1**: 1065–7.

Yanagi K, Harada S et al., 1990, High prevalence of antibody to human herpesvirus 6 and decrease in titer in age in Japan, *J Infect Dis*, **161**: 153–4.

Yasukawa M, Yakushijin Y et al., 1993, Specificity analysis of human CD4+ T-cell clones directed against human herpesvirus 6 (HHV-6), HHV-7, and human cytomegalovirus, *J Virol*, **67:** 6259–64.

Yoshikawa T, Suga S et al., 1991, Human herpesvirus-6 infection in bone marrow transplantation, *Blood*, **78:** 1381–4.

Yoshikawa T, Nakashima T et al., 1992, Human herpesvirus-6 DNA in cerebrospinal fluid of a child with exanthem subitum and meningoencephalitis, *Pediatrics*, **89:** 888–90.

Yoshikawa T, Asano Y et al., 1993, Seroepidemiology of human herpesvirus 7 in healthy children and adults in Japan, *J Med Virol*, **41:** 319–23.

Zaia JA, Forman SJ et al., 1986, Polypeptide-specific antibody response to human cytomegalovirus after infection in bone marrow transplant recipients, *J Infect Dis*, **153:** 780–7.

Zhou Y, Chang CK et al., 1994, Transactivation of the HIV promoter by a cDNA and its genomic clones of human herpesvirus-6, *Virology*, **199:** 311–22.

GAMMAHERPESVIRUSES: EPSTEIN–BARR VIRUS

M A Epstein and D H Crawford

| 1 Properties of the virus | 2 Clinical and pathological aspects |

1 PROPERTIES OF THE VIRUS

1.1 Introduction

The Epstein–Barr virus (EBV) was discovered in 1964 (Epstein, Achong and Barr 1964) in the course of a sustained search (Epstein 1985) for a possible causative virus in tumour samples from cases of endemic (African) Burkitt lymphoma (BL). EBV has been in the human evolutionary tree for about 30–35 million years, since all Old World monkeys and great apes have closely related viruses (Deinhardt and Deinhardt 1979), whereas the New World monkeys that branched off the tree shortly before that time are free of these agents.

EBV infects almost all of the world's adult population and, like all human herpesviruses, establishes lifelong persistence. However, despite the trivial nature of the infection in most individuals, the virus is the most potent immortalizing agent for mammalian cells in vitro, is associated with a spectrum of human malignant proliferations in vivo, and causes rapidly fatal malignant tumours on experimental injection in cottontop tamarins.

EBV has a restricted host range with humans as its natural host, but certain non-human primates can be infected experimentally. The virus infects B lymphocytes in vitro (Pattengale, Smith and Gerber 1973), resulting in B cell immortalization and the generation of continuously proliferating lymphoblastoid cell lines (LCL) (Pope, Horne and Scott 1968). The virus also infects squamous epithelial cells in vitro which can support full viral replication with the release of virus particles and cell death (Sixbey et al. 1983). However, epithelial cell infection is very inefficient, so no fully permissive systems are available for the study of individual replicative gene functions by the generation of mutants. In contrast, latent infection has been studied in great detail because of the ease with which immortalization can be brought about.

1.2 Classification

EBV is a member of the *Herpesviridae* and is in gammaherpesvirus subfamily. This classification is based on DNA homology between the EBV genome and that of other gammaherpesviruses, the G + C content of the genome and the lymphotropism of the virus.

1.3 Morphology and particle structure

Like other herpesviruses, EBV has a protein core containing DNA, a nucleocapsid composed of 162 capsomers which forms an icosahedral protein shell, and an outer envelope derived from cellular membranes and containing virus-coded glycoprotein spikes.

1.4 Molecular biology

GENOME STRUCTURE AND FUNCTION

The EBV genome is a linear molecule of double-stranded DNA which contains 172 kb and has coding potential for 100–200 proteins. EBV DNA contains several internal repeats interspersed with unique sequences and flanked by 2 terminal repeat sequences (Fig. 20.1). EBV was the first herpesvirus to be cloned (Dambaugh et al. 1980) and sequenced (Baer et al. 1984). The nomenclature for the promoters and open reading frames within the viral genome has been assigned using the abbreviated name of the *Bam*HI restriction fragment; for example, BARF 1 is the first, rightward open reading frame in the *Bam*HI A fragment of the EBV genome.

Two types of EBV exist, A and B (also called 1 and 2) (Dambaugh et al. 1986), with an overall DNA

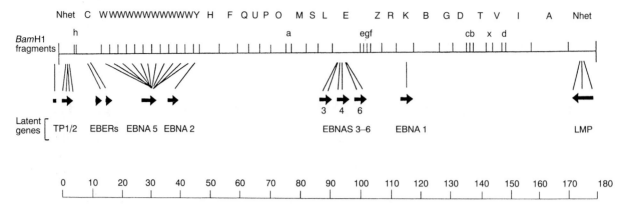

Fig. 20.1 Linear representation of the Epstein–Barr virus genome. *Bam*HI fragments are shown above and the location of the latent gene open reading frames is shown below. The arrows indicate the direction of transcription. The scale is in kilobases. EBERS, EB-coded small RNAs; EBNA, EB viral nuclear antigen; LMP, latent membrane protein; TP, terminal protein.

sequence homology of 70–85% (Sample et al. 1990). They differ mainly in the regions of the viral genome coding for the EBV nuclear antigens (EBNAs) 2, 3, 4, 6 (Rowe et al. 1989) and the EBV-encoded small RNAs (Arrand, Young and Tugwood 1989). These differences are reflected in biological diversity, A type viruses being more efficient than B type viruses at immortalization of B lymphocytes in vitro (Rickinson, Young and Rowe 1987). Type A EBV predominates world-wide. Type B is rare in Western societies but more common in African communities and in individuals with immunosuppression (Zimber et al. 1986, Sculley et al. 1990). However, no type-specific disease associations have been noted. In addition to EBV type variation, individual viral isolates differ in the number of tandem repeats in their internal DNA repeat sequences. This heterogeneity can be used to define individual EBV isolates (Falk et al. 1995).

Latent infection of a B lymphocyte is associated with circularization of the EBV genome to form an episome (Lindahl et al. 1976), which later amplifies to give multiple copies. Genome circularization is achieved by covalent linkage of the terminal repeat elements and the number of repeat sequences varies with different circularization events. Thus, when the viral episome is passed from one latently infected cell to a daughter cell (without linearizing) the number remains the same, indicating clonality. Estimation of the terminal repeats can therefore be used to determine whether virus infection of cells occurred before or after cell proliferation in tumour samples (Raab-Traub and Flynn 1986).

VIRUS-CODED PROTEINS

On infection of B lymphocytes in vitro, EBV establishes a latent type of infection with the expression of a restricted number of viral genes (latent genes) and continued cell survival and division without viral genome replication or production of viral progeny. The characteristics of these latent genes and their products are described below and listed with their alternative names in Table 20.1; the locations of their open reading frames are shown in Fig. 20.1. This type of infec-

tion can be switched to a lytic infection with new virus production and cell death by certain stimuli that induce B cell activation/differentiation and thereby cause the cell to become permissive for viral replication (Crawford and Ando 1986).

Latent proteins

The latent gene products include 6 EBNAs (1–6), 3 membrane proteins (latent membrane protein: LMP; terminal protein: TP1 and TP2). In addition, 2 small EBV-encoded RNAs (EBERs 1 and 2) are transcribed but not translated. EBNAs 1–6 initiate from promoters in either the W or C fragments of the genome as long polycistronic messages which are subsequently spliced to give individual mRNAs. In contrast, the latent membrane proteins each initiate from their own promoters. EBNAs 2, 3, 6 and LMP have been shown by analysis of recombinant mutant viruses to be essential for immortalization (see 'Immortalization', p. 356) whereas EBNA 4 and 5, TP1 and 2, and EBERs 1 and 2 are not. In addition to these proteins, complex transcripts arising from the *Bam*HI A open reading frame have been demonstrated in latently infected B cells but no protein products have yet been identified and their significance is unclear (Liebowitz and Kieff 1993).

EBNA 1

EBNA 1 is a phosphoprotein that is coded for by the BKRF1 open reading frame. It has a molecular weight ranging from 65 to 85 kDa, the variation being due to the different lengths of the repeat sequences in the molecule. EBNA 1 protein consists of c. 641 amino acids, is proline-rich and contains a glycine–alanine repeat sequence; it binds to a specific DNA sequence by the carboxy terminus domain which is rich in acidic and basic residues. Multiple EBNA 1 binding sites occur in the latent viral origin of replication (*oriP*) domain where the binding of EBNA 1 is the only viral factor required for maintenance of the viral episome (Yates, Warren and Sugden 1985). This binding also enhances transcription of EBNA 1 and other latent viral genes because it activates the *oriP* enhancer which

Table 20.1 EBV latent genes

Open reading frame*	Gene product	Alternative nomenclature	Mol. wt (kDa)	Cellular location	Required for immortalization	Suggested function/property
BKRF1	EBNA 1	...	65–85	Nucleus	Yes	Plasmid maintenance
BYRF1	EBNA 2	...	86	Nucleus	Yes	Viral oncogene, transactivator
BLRF3–BERF1	EBNA 3	EBNA 3A	140–157	Nucleus	Yes	NK
BERF2a–BERF2b	EBNA 4	EBNA 3B	148–180	Nucleus	No	NK
BWRF1	EBNA 5	ENBA leader protein	20–130	Nucleus	No	Binds Rb, p53
BERF3–BERF4	EBNA 6	ENBA 3c	160	Nucleus	Yes	Potential viral oncogene
BNLF1	LMP	LMP1	58–63	Membrane	Yes	Viral oncogene, cellular gene transactivator
BARF1/BNRF1	TP1	LMP2A	53	Membrane	No	Prevents Ca^{2+} mobilization
BNRF1	TP2	LMP2B	40	Membrane	No	NK
BCRF1	EBER1, 2	...	...	Cytoplasm/ nucleus	No	Regulation of PKR activity
BARFO	*Bam*HI A transcripts	...	...	Cytoplasm	NK	NK

*Abbreviated using the *Bam*HI(B) fragment (A–Z) LF or RF for left- or rightward open reading frame (ORF) followed by the number of the gene in a particular ORF.
EBNA, EB virus nuclear antigen; LMP, latent membrane protein; NK, not known; PKR, double-stranded RNA protein kinase; TP, terminal protein.

regulates the EBNA promoter, Cp, and the LMP promoter (Gahn and Sugden 1995).

EBNA 1 also binds non-specifically to DNA, a function that causes it to associate with metaphase chromosomes, thereby ensuring the equal partitioning of the viral episomes into the 2 daughter cells at mitosis. Thus EBNA 1 expression is a requirement not only for the maintenance of the viral episome in latently infected cells but also for the synchronization of virus genome replication with cell division.

EBNA 2

EBNA 2 is a phosphoprotein with a molecular weight of 86 kDa and is coded for by the BYRF1 open reading frame. The protein acts as a transcription factor which is essential for the immortalization of B lymphocytes in vitro (Cohen et al. 1989). It has an acidic activator domain near the carboxy terminus which interacts with the sequence-specific DNA binding proteins TFIIB, TAF40 and TFIIH, causing transcriptional activation (Johannessen et al. 1995). EBNA 2 does not bind directly to DNA but interacts with a variety of cellular factors, including the DNA binding proteins Jk (also called CBF1), which is ubiquitous, and PU1, which is expressed in a restricted number of haemopoietic cell types, including B cells (Ling et al. 1994, Johannessen et al. 1995). As a result of these interactions EBNA 2 transactivates the latent viral genes LMP and TP and a variety of cellular genes, including the oncogenes c-*fgr* and *bcl*-2 and the B cell activation molecules CD21 and CD23. EBNA 2 thereby plays a piv-

otal role in the immortalization of B cells in vitro. The EBNA 2 gene shows considerable DNA sequence diversity between type A and type B EBV, with an overall homology of c. 55%. The most conserved regions are at the amino and carboxy termini and include the regions that are essential for immortalization in vitro.

EBNA 3, 4, 6

These 3 proteins are coded for by the BERF open reading frames and clearly arise from a common origin. Their molecular weights range from 140 to 180 kDa owing to the variable repeat sequences present in each protein. Their functions are unknown although expression of EBNA 3 and 6 is required for immortalization (Tomkinson, Robertson and Kieff 1993). All 3 proteins show sequence divergence between EBV types A and B. EBNA 6 contains a leucine zipper motif, co-operates with EBNA 2 in the transactivation of LMP and also induces the cellular CD21 and vimentin genes, probably as a result of the up-regulation of LMP (Allday, Crawford and Thomas 1993).

EBNA 5

EBNA 5 is a phosphoprotein that is encoded by the BWRF1 open reading frame which forms either the leader sequence of the EBNA mRNAs or, by alternative splicing, EBNA 5 mRNA. Because of the DNA repeats in this part of the genome, EBNA 5 protein consists of multiple repeat sequences of 22 and 44 amino acids flanked by unique amino and carboxy termini. Because the DNA repeat sequences vary in number in different virus isolates, the size of EBNA 5 protein varies accordingly. Immunoblotting of EBNA 5 in electrophoretically separated proteins from EBV-infected B cells reveals a ladder of bands differing by 6–8 kDa and corresponding to products of 20–130 kDa, an effect probably due to differential splicing of the mRNA.

The function of EBNA 5 is unknown and it is not strictly essential for immortalization (Hammerschmidt and Sugden 1989). However, the protein has been reported to co-localize in the nucleus with the retinoblastoma gene product Rb (Jiang et al. 1991) and binds to both Rb and the tumour suppressor gene product p53 in vitro (Szekely et al. 1993). Coupled with the fact that B cells infected with EBNA 5 deletion mutants grow very poorly (Hammerschmidt and Sugden 1989), these findings suggest that EBNA 5 is involved in the control of cellular proliferation.

LMP

LMP is a cytoplasmic and membrane protein that is coded for by the BNLF1 open reading frame. It has a molecular weight of 58–63 kDa and is phosphorylated on serine residues. LMP mRNA is the most abundant viral transcript found in latently infected B cells. The predicted amino acid sequence of LMP suggests an integral membrane protein with a short cytoplasmic amino terminus, a large cytoplasmic carboxy terminus and 6 hydrophobic transmembrane segments forming 3 external loops. A smaller LMP mRNA also exists, coding for a protein that lacks the amino terminus of the full length protein, is expressed in lytically infected cells and is present in the virus particle.

Full length LMP is a classic viral oncoprotein that is essential for B cell immortalization (Kaye, Izumi and Kieff 1993). Transfection studies using the LMP gene under a heterologous promoter have shown that it induces loss of contact inhibition and anchorage dependence, altered cell morphology, and tumorigenic potential in rodent fibroblasts (Wang, Liebowitz and Kieff 1985). In human B cell lines, LMP causes increase in cell size and steady state calcium levels, up-regulation of cell activation and cell adhesion molecule (CAM) expression, as well as up-regulation of the cytoskeletal protein vimentin (Wang et al. 1988) and the oncogene *bcl*-2 which encodes an inhibitor of apoptosis (Henderson et al. 1991). The mechanism(s) by which LMP induces viral and cellular genes has not been elucidated but it is known that LMP can induce activation of the transcription factor NF-κB (Hammarskjold and Simurdo 1992).

The similarity between the structure of LMP and that of a growth factor receptor or ion channel has led to speculation on the mode of action of LMP. Recent studies showing the interaction of the LMP cytoplasmic C terminus with tumour necrosis factor (TNF) receptor-associated proteins link LMP to the signal transduction pathways used by TNF (Mosialos et al. 1995).

TP1 and 2

The sequences that make up the TP open reading frame are located at the 2 ends of the linear EBV genome in BARF1/BNRF1 and are completed only when the genome has circularized to form an episome (Laux, Perricaudet and Farrell 1988). TP1 and 2 are produced by alternative splicing of the mRNA, giving rise to proteins of 53 and 40 kDa respectively. Both are membrane proteins with 12 transmembrane segments and cytoplasmic amino and carboxy termini, but whereas TP1 has 119 amino acids in the amino terminus domain TP2 has only 3. Although little is known about the function of TP1 and 2 because of the lack of specific antibodies, TP1 associates with, and is phosphorylated by, the B lymphocyte *src* family of tyrosine kinases (Longnecker et al. 1991). This interaction inhibits calcium mobilization following stimulation of B lymphocytes latently infected with EBV and may thereby prevent fortuitous activation of the viral lytic cycle (Miller et al. 1994) which is known to be linked to B cell activation/differentiation processes (Crawford and Ando 1986).

EBERs 1 and 2

These 2 small, non-polyadenylated, RNA molecules are coded for by the BCRF1 open reading frame and are the most abundant RNAs in latently infected B cells. They are mainly localized in the nucleus where they bind to the La protein and the large ribosomal subunit protein L22 (Clemens 1994). Although the significance of this complex formation is not known, EBERs show sequence homology to the VA1 and the 2 RNAs of adenovirus which also bind La and are thought to be involved in RNA splicing. EBERs are not required for the in vitro immortalization process or for virus replication (Swaminathan, Tomkinson and Keiff 1991) but, like VA1, bind to and regulate the activity of the protein kinase PKR. This interaction may inhibit the antiviral and antiproliferative effects of interferon, because PKR is induced by, and mediates, interferon activity (Clemens 1994).

Lytic proteins

Genes expressed during the EBV lytic cycle have been characterized in LCL which have been induced by various agents (zur Hausen, O'Neill and Freese 1978, Luka, Kallin and Klein 1979, Tovey, Lenoir and Begon-Lours 1978); such genes have extensive homology with those of other herpesviruses. As with other herpesviruses, they follow an orderly sequence of expression, each set being activated by the previous set. Lytic genes can be divided into immediate early genes which are transcribed prior to viral protein synthesis, early genes which are transcribed in the absence of viral DNA synthesis, and late genes which represent the structural proteins and are expressed only after viral DNA synthesis. However, EBV is unique among herpesviruses in possessing a set of latent genes that are already transcribed in infected B cells and may therefore influence subsequent lytic gene expression although a viral transactivator of the immediate early genes has not been identified among them.

Immediate early genes

EBV possesses 2 genes that can be classified as immediate early genes: BZLF1 (Z) and BRLF1 (R). The products of these 2 genes are transactivators of the early genes and are derived from 3 mRNA species, one of which contains both R and Z sequences. Z is a DNA binding protein that shows homology to the DNA binding domain of the *c-jun* oncogene and binds to AP-1 sites (Farrell et al. 1989). The Z and R promoters (Zp, Rp) contain AP-1 sites and so Z transactivates its own activity as well as that of R. The early genes that Z and R have been shown to transactivate are BMRF1, BHRF1, BHLF1 and BRLF1.

Early genes

First identified by the staining pattern of sera containing antibodies to EBV when applied to the Raji cell line which lacks expression of the late genes, the early gene products (early antigens, EA) were characterized as diffuse (D) (nuclear and cytoplasmic staining) and restricted (R) (nuclear staining) (Henle, Henle and Klein 1971). It is now known that each of these complexes consists of c. 30 proteins, most of which have enzymic functions required for viral DNA replication. These include the D components BMLF1 and BMRF1 and the R components BHRF1 and BORF2 as well as others that are involved in viral DNA replication (Table 20.2).

Late genes

Viral capsid proteins   This antigen complex (VCA) consists of the viral structural proteins that have not yet been analysed in detail because of the lack of a fully lytic system in vitro. The major capsid protein p160 is coded for by the BALF4 open reading frame,

other components possibly arising from BNRF1 and BXRF1.

EBV glycoproteins   The EBV-coded glycoproteins are involved in viral infectivity and spread. Seven have been identified, most of which are inserted into the membranes of the infected cell and 3 of these become components of the viral envelope (membrane antigens, MA). Two (gp340/220 and gp85) have been studied in detail because they induce the production of neutralizing antibodies and are therefore potential vaccine candidates. Three show extensive homology to herpes simplex glycoproteins (Table 20.3).

The major envelope glycoprotein, gp340/220, is coded for by the BLLF1 open reading frame. The 2 forms of the protein are created by alternative splicing of the mRNA. It is found in the Golgi apparatus as well as the plasma membrane of infected cells. The mature protein is heavily *N*- and *O*-glycosylated, about 50% of the molecule being carbohydrate. Gp 340/220 mediates virus attachment to the B cell surface by binding to the EBV receptor CR2 (also called CD21) (Nemerow et al. 1987). Thus both naturally occurring and experimentally induced antibodies to gp340/220 prevent infection by blocking attachment.

Gp110 is coded for by the BALF4 open reading frame and has homology with the herpes simplex virus glycoprotein gB. It is *O*- and *N*-glycosylated and is localized to the nuclear and cytoplasmic membranes of infected cells but is not detected in the viral envelope.

Gp85 is coded for by the BXLF2 open reading frame and has homology to the herpes simplex virus glycoprotein gH. The protein is localized to the plasma membrane and viral envelope, where it induces fusion between the viral and cellular membranes.

Gp42 is coded for by the BZLF2 open reading frame

Table 20.2   Early proteins involved in EBV replication

Open reading frame	Mol. wt (kDa)	Cellular localization	Herpes simplex virus homology/putative function
BMLF5	...	...	DNA polymerase
BALF5	...	...	DNA polymerase
BXLF1	...	...	Thymidine kinase
BGLF5	...	...	Alkaline exonuclease
BORF1	140	...	Ribonucleotide reductase
BARF1	38	...	Ribonucleotide reductase
BMRF1	47	Nucleus	DNA polymerase-associated protein
BALF2	135	...	Single-strand DNA binding protein
BBLF4	...	...	Helicase/primase
BSLF1	...	...	Helicase/primase
BCRF2/3	...	...	Helicase/primase
BHRF1	18	Nuclear and cytoplasmic membrane	*bcl*-2 homologue
BKRF3	...	...	Uracil DNA glycosylase
BMLF1	...	Nucleus	Transactivator
BBLF2/3	...	...	Spliced primase–helicase complex component

Table 20.3 EBV glycoproteins

Open reading frame	Mol. wt (kDa)	Putative function	Present in viral envelope
BLLF1	350/220	Receptor (CR2) binding	Yes
BALF4	110	HSVgB homologue	No
BXLF2	85	Fusion of viral and cellular membranes HSV gH homologue	Yes
BZLF2	42	Binds MHC class II – viral penetration	Yes
BKRF2	25	HSV gL homologue	Yes
BILF2	78/55	...	Yes
BDLF3	150	...	Yes

HSV, herpes simplex virus.

and is involved in penetration of the virus through the cell membrane during infection

IMMORTALIZATION

Limiting dilution analysis reveals that c. 1–10% of B lymphocytes are immortalized after infection in vitro (Tosato, Blaese and Yarchoan 1985), indicating that EBV is the most potent known immortalizing agent for mammalian cells. The susceptible cell type is the small resting B cell expressing surface IgM (Steel et al. 1977).

Entry of the virus into B lymphocytes occurs through a ligand–receptor interaction between the major viral envelope glycoprotein gp340/220 and the cell surface complement receptor molecule CR2 (CD21) (Nemerow et al. 1987). CR2 is a member of the immunoglobulin superfamily and is expressed on all mature circulating B lymphocytes. It forms part of a signal transduction complex including CD19, TAPA1 and Leu-13 (Bradbury et al. 1992); it is postulated that the binding of EBV to CR2 induces initial activating signals, but these have not yet been clearly defined. Once bound, the viral envelope fuses with the cell membrane, releasing the capsid into the cytoplasm. The viral genome rapidly enters the cell nucleus where it circularizes to form an episome, which later amplifies to give multiple copies per cell.

EBNA 2 and 5, originating from the W promoter (Wp), are the first virus-coded proteins to be detected, at around 12 h post-infection. EBNA 2 protein then initiates a promoter switch from Wp to Cp (Woisetschlaeger et al. 1991) by complexing with Jk at the EBNA 2 response element upstream of Cp, thereby allowing expression of the full EBNA complex (EBNAs 1–6) by 24 h. EBNA 2 also induces LMP (Fåhraeus et al. 1990) so that, as a result of EBNA 2 transactivation, full latent viral gene expression is achieved by 48–72 h post-infection.

Cell enlargement and activation with the expression of the B cell activation marker CD23 occur at around 48 h post-infection and have been attributed to the action of LMP (Wang et al. 1990). By 72 h the cell has progressed through the G1, S and G2 phases of the cell cycle and is entering mitosis. The cells then continue to cycle indefinitely, giving rise to an immortalized LCL. The phenotype of cells in an LCL is similar to that of antigen-stimulated lymphoblasts with the expression of the B cell activation markers typical of this stage of B cell differentiation (e.g. CD23, CD39, CD30, CD70, ki24) as well as the CAMs, CD11a, CD54 and CD58.

A few cells in an LCL (0–5%) enter the lytic cycle, a switch that seems to be triggered by physiological stimuli such as differentiation of the cell (Crawford and Ando 1986), and that can be induced by B cell activating agents such as phorbol esters (zur Hausen, O'Neill and Freese 1978), sodium butyrate (Luka, Kallin and Klein 1979) and anti-immunoglobulin (Tovey, Lenoir and Begon-Lours 1978). Cells of LCLs are immortal but cytogenetically normal. They are not, by definition, transformed cells because they do not form colonies in soft agar or give rise to tumours in nude mice (Nilsson et al. 1971). These characteristics differ from those of EBV-carrying cell lines derived from BL biopsy material (see 'EBV gene expression').

EBV REPLICATION

The induction of the lytic cycle in B lymphocytes or squamous epithelial cells infected in vitro is associated with differentiation of the cell (Crawford and Ando 1986, Kirimi, Crawford and Nicholson 1995), suggesting that the availability of cellular transcription factors determines the outcome of infection. In addition, the lytic cycle can be activated by transfection of the BZLF1 gene or superinfection with the P3HR1 strain of virus, which contains defective virus in which BZLF1 is adjacent to Wp (Miller, Heston and Countryman 1984).

Replication of EBV DNA begins at the origin of lytic replication (*ori*lyt), which is 1.4 kb in length and contains many inverted repeat sequences (Hammerschmidt and Sugden 1988). *ori*lyt acts as an amplicon, giving rise to many linear concatemers of the genome by the rolling circle method, and EBV-coded DNA polymerase is required for this process. The terminal repeat elements are required for cleaving and packaging the newly formed virions.

EBV GENE EXPRESSION

Infection of B lymphocytes in vitro leads to initiation of transcription of the polycistronic EBNA mRNA from Wp with an EBNA 2-induced switch to Cp after

48–72 h (Woisetschlaeger et al. 1991). This results in expression of the whole EBNA complex (EBNAs 1–6) as well as expression of the latent membrane proteins (LMP, TP1 and 2) from their own promoters and is termed full latent gene expression or latency type III (Rowe et al. 1992). However, in vivo, other patterns of viral gene expression have been identified. The most restricted gene expression is seen in BL cells, which are small, non-activated cells expressing the cellular markers of a germinal centre B cell (CD10, CD77). Only EBNA 1 expression is detected in these cells (latency type I) (Rowe et al. 1986), and this EBNA 1 mRNA initiates from a promoter in the Q region of the genome (Qp). Wp and Cp are silent and have been shown to be methylated (Masucci et al. 1989). However, when BL cells are cultured, demethylation often occurs, associated with a drift to full latent viral gene expression and a lymphoblastoid phenotype (Rowe et al. 1987).

An alternative pattern of transcription (latency type II) is seen in Reed–Sternberg cells in EBV-positive Hodgkin's disease (Deacon et al. 1993) (see 'Hodgkin's disease', p. 361) and the malignant epithelial cells of nasopharyngeal carcinoma (Brooks et al. 1992) (see 'Other malignancies', p. 362). Here EBNA 1 is expressed from Qp, and LMP, TP1 and TP2 are also expressed in the absence of EBNAs 2–6 (Table 20.4). The significance of these different patterns of viral gene expression has not so far been elucidated.

2 CLINICAL AND PATHOLOGICAL ASPECTS

2.1 Introduction

As a very ancient parasite of humans, EBV has established a delicately balanced relationship with its host that is almost entirely benign under normal conditions. Natural primary infection is usually inapparent, and is always followed by a lifelong, silent, carrier state that becomes manifest as disease only if the virus–host balance is disturbed (Table 20.5).

2.2 Epidemiology

EBV is found in all human populations and, under natural conditions, primary infection occurs in early childhood; thus, in developing countries, 99.9% of all children are infected by 2–4 years of age, depending on geographical region. However, in industrialized countries with high standards of hygiene a considerable number of people do not become infected as young children, the percentage of each age group remaining free of infection as teenagers or young adults depending in Western societies on socio-economic status: the higher the standard of living, the greater the percentage (W Henle and Henle 1979). Among the very affluent as many as 50% of young adults may never have been infected. Today's lifestyle has affected the manner in which EBV spreads in the population.

Primary infection in early childhood is symptom-free and leads only to the generation of antibodies to the viral and virus-determined antigens (W Henle and Henle 1979) and to the development of specific cyto-toxic T lymphocytes (Murray et al. 1992). These humoral and cellular immunological responses are maintained continuously thereafter and are responsible for keeping the lifelong EBV infection in check; the virus persists as a latent infection in a few circulating B lymphocytes (Lewin et al. 1987) and as a productive infection somewhere in the mouth and pharynx, the urogenital tract and, perhaps, the salivary glands. EBV is shed into the buccal fluid in readily detectable amounts in c. 20% of those who have been infected and in small amounts from time to time in many of the remainder (Yao, Rickinson and Epstein 1985); the virus has also been detected in genital secretions (Sixbey, Lemon and Pagano 1986). There is currently controversy as to whether squamous epithelial cells or intraepithelial B lymphocytes at these various sites are the source of the infectious virus (Allday and Crawford 1988, Niedobitek and Young 1994). However, at the time of writing it appears that virus in the buccal fluid is the main source for transmission of the infection in the population, by droplets and casually contaminated objects in children and by direct salivary transfer during kissing among the sexually active.

Those who miss the clinically silent natural primary infection by the virus of childhood are likely, sooner or later, to undergo delayed primary infection. Although 50% of such delayed infections are symptom-free as in childhood, the other 50% are

Table 20.4 Latent viral gene expression in EBV-associated tumours

| Tumour | EBNA | | | | | | LMP | TP | | EBERs | Promoter usage |
	1	2	3	4	5	6		1	2		
Burkitt lymphoma	+	–	–	–	–	–	–	–	–	+	Qp
B lymphoproliferative disease	+	+	+	+	+	+	+	+	+	+	Cp/Wp
Nasopharyngeal carcinoma	+	–	–	–	–	–	+/–	+	+/–	+	Qp
Hodgkin's lymphoma	+	–	–	–	–	–	++	+	+	+	Qp

EBNA, EB viral nuclear antigen; EBERs, EB virus coded small RNAs; LMP, latent membrane protein; TP, terminal protein.

Table 20.5 Conditions associated with EBV infection in humans

1	Clinically silent childhood primary infection	Universal in developing countries Common in developed countries

2	Delayed primary infection (teenagers/young adults)	Seen in developed countries:
		  50% are clinically silent, as in childhood
		  50% have acute infectious mononucleosis –
		  usually resolves; may become chronic

3	Primary infection with fatal outcome	Very rare familial X-linked lymphoproliferative disease (Duncan syndrome)
4	Lymphomas in immunodepression	In organ graft recipients In AIDS patients
5	Oral hairy leucoplakia	In AIDS patients
6	Endemic Burkitt lymphoma	Common in children where falciparum malaria is hyperendemic
7	Nasopharyngeal carcinoma	Common in south Chinese and Inuit adults
8	Tumours with tenuous suspected links to EBV infection	Hodgkin's disease, some T cell lymphomas, leiomyosarcomas, salivary gland cancers, undifferentiated carcinoma of the stomach

accompanied by disease: classic infectious mononucleosis (IM) (Sawyer et al. 1971, Hallee et al. 1974).

2.3 Clinical manifestations

INFECTIOUS MONONUCLEOSIS

The fact that it is the teenagers and young adults in the upper classes of Western countries who tend to escape silent infection as children makes IM predominantly a disease of the most affluent groups and causes it to be exceptionally rare in developing countries. Although most cases of IM occur in adolescents and young adults, older children and the middle aged may occasionally develop the disease as a consequence of primary EBV infection, and rarely also the elderly. IM has long been known to be associated with kissing among young people (Hoagland 1955), and the pattern of acquisition results from a healthy carrier who is shedding virus in his or her saliva passing this during close buccal contact directly into the oropharynx of a partner who has not been primarily infected in the usual way as a child. This method of spread explains why case-to-case infection and epidemics are not seen with IM and why the incubation period, perhaps 30–50 days, is difficult to calculate. Primary EBV infection giving IM-like symptoms may also be transmitted by blood transfusion (Gerber et al. 1969) or organ grafting (Haque et al. 1996) from an infected donor to a previously uninfected recipient.

Symptoms and signs

There may be vague prodromal indisposition or an abrupt onset with sore throat, fever and sweating, anorexia, headache and marked malaise. Brief dysphagia and orbital oedema may be noticed. Severe oedema of the tonsils and pharynx can sometimes cause pharyngeal obstruction. Erythematous rashes occur in a small number of untreated patients but affect most of those who have been taking ampicillin. The pharynx, fauces, soft palate and uvula are red and

swollen, and may develop a greyish exudate. Generalized lymphadenopathy is almost invariable, most marked in the cervical region, with symmetrical, discrete, slightly tender glands; splenomegaly is seen in 60% of cases, an enlarged liver in 10% and actual jaundice in about 8%. Crops of palatal petechiae are found in about one-third of patients. If mild, IM may resolve in days, but usually continues for 1–2 weeks, and is often followed by a period of marked lethargy before complete recovery. The length of convalescence may be influenced by psychological factors, but about one case in 2000 continues in a truly chronic or recurrent form for several months or even years; exhaustive investigation of such patients has sometimes revealed minor immunological defects (Virelizier, Lenoir and Griscelli 1978).

In contrast, an extremely rare genetically determined, X-linked, lymphoproliferative condition (XLP disease or Duncan syndrome) (Bar et al. 1974) is due to a specific inability to respond normally to EBV during primary infection, and the affected young males of certain kindred die from IM owing to progressive destruction of vital organs and multisystem failure. Evidence suggests that an aberrant immune response to EBV in XLP disease gives rise to natural killer cell and cytotoxic T cell activity directed against the normal cells of organs instead of being concentrated on EBV-infected cells displaying virus-determined antigens (Weisenburger and Purtilo 1986).

Complications

Serious but rare complications include secondary bacterial throat infections, traumatic rupture of the enlarged spleen, asphyxia from pharyngeal oedema, massive hepatic necrosis, Guillain–Barré syndrome, and autoimmune manifestations such as thrombocytopenia and haemolytic anaemia (Finch 1969).

Pathogenesis

Children do not react with symptoms to primary EBV infection because, it seems, childhood is the appropriate time in evolutionary terms for this benign virus to establish its lifelong infection (W Henle and Henle 1979). When delayed primary infection occurs as a result of the high living standards of modern Western countries, young adults encounter the virus for the first time at an age when immunological reactions are more exuberant than those of children, reflecting clear physiological differences in responsiveness. Furthermore, the mode of infection and size of infecting dose are also different in the 2 groups: children come into contact with saliva from a shedder as air-borne droplets or contamination on some sucked object and thus receive a much smaller amount of virus than a young person taking in large quantities of virus-containing saliva from such a carrier during mouth-to-mouth kissing (Hoagland 1955). An exaggerated immunological response to a very large infecting dose of EBV fits well with the changes of IM: large numbers of activated CD8+ T cells stimulated by a mass of infected B cells (expressing all the known latent viral genes) (see 'Virus-coded proteins', p. 352) in the circulation, in lymph nodes, tonsils, lymphoid tissue of the mouth and pharynx, spleen, liver and elsewhere. These T cells, which kill EBV-infected target cells in a non-HLA restricted manner and secrete multiple lymphokines (Foss et al. 1994), are probably the cause, by recognizable immunopathological mechanisms, of the sore throat, fever, malaise, lymphadenopathy and hepatosplenomegaly.

Immune responses and diagnosis

During acute IM, serum IgM and IgG antibodies to VCA and IgG anti-EA antibodies appear early, whereas anti-EBNA 1 antibodies are not usually detectable until convalescence (W Henle and Henle 1979). On recovery, IgM anti-VCA and IgG anti-EA disappear but IgG antibodies to VCA and EBNA 1 are maintained for life (Fig. 20.2) (G Henle and Henle 1979).

Since it is not usually possible to document seroconversion, the presence of IgM antibodies to viral capsid antigen provides the most reliable diagnostic test. This may be corroborated by finding anti-EA antibodies (usually of D type) or the absence of antibodies to EBNA 1, or both (G Henle and Henle 1979). These tests depend on immunofluorescence staining of B cell lines expressing viral antigens, are time consuming and are usually carried out only in larger laboratories. A number of commercial ELISAs are appropriate for large scale screening but they lack sensitivity. The rapid screening Monospot test is more reliable: it has been adapted from the earlier Paul–Bunnell test for IgM heterophil antibodies which agglutinate red cells from non-human sources. Although the heterophil antibodies are not directed against viral-coded antigens they are present in up to 85% of IM sera, but it must be remembered that cases of Monospot-negative IM are frequent outside the classic 15–25 year age range, and false positives may occur in pregnancy and autoimmune disease (Okaro et al. 1988). An

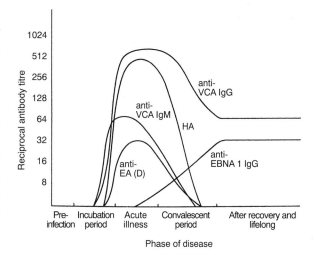

Fig. 20.2 Epstein–Barr virus-specific antibody response in infectious mononucleosis. Typical serum antibody titres as assessed by indirect immunofluorescence are indicated. EA (D), early antigen (diffuse); EBNA, EB viral nuclear antigen; HA, heterophile antibody; VCA, viral capsid antigen.

additional diagnostic feature of IM is the presence of a lymphocytosis of up to $15 \times 10^9/l$, most cells having an 'atypical' morphology. The clinical and haematological findings and a positive Monospot test give a reliable diagnosis, but, if the latter is negative, tests for IgM anti-VCA antibodies must be done. Retrospective diagnosis may be possible if suitable samples are available to allow seroconversion or a rising EBNA 1 IgG antibody titre to be detected.

ENDEMIC ('AFRICAN') BURKITT LYMPHOMA

Classic BL (Burkitt 1963) is a B cell tumour found in parts of Africa and Papua New Guinea, where the temperature does not fall below 16.5°C or the annual rainfall below 55 cm (Burkitt 1970a). BL is overwhelmingly a disease of children, and is extremely rare over the age of 14 years. In endemic areas, it is more common than all other childhood cancers added together. There is no evidence in the tumour belt for any tribal or racial susceptibility (Burkitt 1963). Endemic BL is distinct from the so-called Burkitt-like tumours (sometimes called 'American' or 'sporadic' BL) seen sporadically everywhere in the world, which have a different age incidence, anatomical distribution and response to therapy. The term 'Burkitt type' is sometimes also misguidedly applied to certain leukaemias because of morphological resemblances of the malignant cells.

Some 97% of endemic BL carries the EBV genome whereas only 12–25% of the sporadic tumours are EBV-positive (Ziegler et al. 1976); it would seem that the 3% of EBV-negative BLs occurring in endemic areas are in fact sporadic BLs that occur at low incidence world-wide.

The association between EBV and endemic BL is so close that it is now generally accepted that the virus is a necessary (albeit not solely sufficient) element in causation of the disease. It is an essential link, together with co-factors, in a complicated chain of events that leads to the malignant change (Epstein and Achong 1979). BL cells contain the EBV genome but only EBNA 1 is expressed (see 'EBV gene expression', p. 356). Hyperendemic falciparum malaria is an important co-factor, and its spread by anopheline mosquitoes requiring warmth and moisture explains the climate dependence of the tumour (Burkitt 1969).

Symptoms and signs

The tumour is usually multifocal, occurs in a variety of sites and the symptoms depend on the anatomical location of the lesions (Burkitt 1963). Tumours in the maxilla or mandible are present in 70% of patients and are the presenting feature of most of these (Fig. 20.3). They may be multiple in 2, 3 or even all 4 quadrants of the jaws, and are almost always accompanied by tumours elsewhere. A rapidly growing mass, loosening of teeth and exophthalmos from orbital spread are the main consequences. Abdominal tumours are also common, involving retroperitoneal nodes, liver, ovaries, intestine and kidneys. BL may present in the thyroid, the adolescent female breast, the testicles, the salivary glands and the skeleton. Extradural spinal tumours cause paraplegia of rapid onset. An unusual and characteristic feature of this lymphoma is its failure to involve the spleen and the peripheral lymph nodes.

Clinically, the tumours are firm, very rapidly growing and painless; even when large, they cause minimal constitutional disturbance. The clinical signs are determined by the tumour sites, but wherever these may be BL grows relentlessly and, in the absence of treatment, death ensues within a few months (Burkitt 1963).

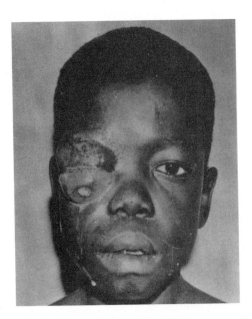

Fig. 20.3 A 9 year old girl with a typical Burkitt lymphoma of the right upper maxilla presenting through the orbit. The Epstein–Barr virus was first identified in cultured malignant lymphoblasts from this tumour.

Pathogenesis

Molecular biological investigations are successfully unravelling the sequence of EBV gene expression that enables the virus to immortalize normal human B lymphocytes in vitro into continuously growing cell lines (see 'Immortalization', p. 356). Explanations are also beginning to emerge as to how the viral genes, in combination with co-factors, can bring about the malignant change leading to BL. There are currently 2 possibilities:

1. EBV infection in the presence of the impaired immunological control brought about by hyperendemic malaria leads to a high level of EBV-driven B cell proliferation, perhaps by similar mechanisms to in vitro immortalization; this proliferation in turn increases the chances of one or another of 3 BL-specific chromosomal translocations (t8:14; t8:22; t2:8) occurring, each of which can deregulate the c-*myc* oncogene on chromosome 8 by bringing it under the influence of an immunoglobulin gene promoter on chromosome 14, 22 or 2. This deregulation causes malignant change in the affected cell and the rapid outgrowth of a clone of tumour cells (Klein 1987).

2. The chronic immunological stimulation of hyperendemic malaria generates a high turnover of pre-B cells in the bone marrow; one or more of these early lymphocytes acquires one of the 3 chromosomal translocations involving c-*myc* deregulation by an error occurring during immunoglobulin gene rearrangement, and this renders the affected cell responsive to growth signals; infection of such a cell by EBV finally provides viral functions conferring malignancy and a tumour clone grows out (Lenoir and Bornkamm 1987). In this connection, at least 2 EBV latent gene products are known to function as viral oncogenes (see Table 20.1).

But with either possibility the virus–host balance is disturbed by hyperendemic malaria.

Immune responses and diagnosis

In the appropriate geographical regions endemic BL can often be diagnosed on clinical grounds, but this should be confirmed by histological examination of a biopsy specimen. In addition, antibodies to EBV antigens have a unique pattern in BL; titres rise as the disease progresses and fall as tumours regress in response to treatment. These changes may be used to assess disease outcome. IgG antibodies to VCA are found at 8–10 times higher geometric mean titres than in healthy controls matched for age, gender and residence. IgG antibodies to EA-R and MA are also detectable (Henle et al. 1969) and likewise vary with disease progression; successful treatment causes a rise in anti-MA and a fall in anti-EA-R, whereas the reversal of this pattern usually heralds a recurrence of the tumour.

Therapy

Surgery and radiotherapy are not effective but excellent results are obtainable with moderate courses of chemotherapy (Burkitt 1970b). Cyclophosphamide is the drug of choice, and dramatic and sustained resolution is not uncommon when tumours are small.

LYMPHOMAS IN IMMUNOSUPPRESSED INDIVIDUALS

The lifelong EBV infection present in all normal seropositive individuals is controlled by cell-mediated immune mechanisms (Yao, Rickinson and Epstein 1985). In primary and secondary suppression of cellular immunity this control of persisting EBV infection is lost, leading to increased virus replication in the oral cavity, increased numbers of virus-carrying B lymphocytes in the circulation and increased levels of serum antibodies to lytic-cycle EBV antigens (VCA, EA). When this occurs it is sometimes described as a 'reactivated infection' although the condition is clinically silent. However, on occasions the loss of control results in EBV-associated lymphoproliferative disease. This type of disease also occurs when immunosuppressed individuals undergo primary infection and fail to mount the normal immunological response to the virus (Thomas, Allday and Crawford 1991).

Organ graft recipients

It has been known for many years that organ graft recipients who receive lifelong immunosuppressive drugs to prevent graft rejection have an increased risk of developing lymphoproliferative disease and lymphoma (28–100 times that of normal controls) (Penn 1983). Most of these conditions are of B cell origin, contain the EBV genome and express viral antigens in their cells. Lymphoproliferative disease has 2 forms of clinical presentation. In about 50% of cases it occurs within the first year after transplantation, in a young age group, has IM-like symptoms, and is associated with primary EBV infection in patients who were seronegative at the time of grafting. The second type of presentation occurs in older patients late after transplantation and takes the form of a localized mass, commonly in the gut, central nervous system or transplanted organ (Hanto et al. 1981, 1985). Biopsy of the lesion reveals large-cell lymphoma, which is usually monoclonal in origin, although progression from a polyclonal B cell proliferation probably occurs early in the disease (Frizzera et al. 1981, Frizzera 1987). The fact that all the EBV latent viral genes are expressed in these lymphoproliferative diseases, just as with lymphoblastoid cell lines immortalized by the virus in vitro, suggests that EBV is of prime importance in the aetiology of the lesions (Thomas et al. 1990), although other events, perhaps cytogenetic abnormalities, may be necessary to cause the monoclonal growth.

Reduction of immunosuppressive drugs, with or without aciclovir therapy, has caused complete and often sustained regression of the tumours in many cases (Starzl et al. 1984). This has therefore become the first line of treatment, cytotoxic drugs and/or radiotherapy being used only when there is no response or after recurrence. EBV-specific cytotoxic T cells grown in vitro have been given after bone marrow transplantation to protect against such EBV-driven lymphoproliferation prior to regeneration of the immune system (Rooney et al. 1995).

AIDS patients

Two types of lymphoma are seen with increasing frequency in AIDS patients: large-cell lymphoma and Burkitt lymphoma. Both of these may be associated with EBV (Kalter et al. 1985).

Large-cell lymphomas similar to those seen in organ graft recipients (see Chapter 38) occur in severely immunocompromised AIDS patients; their distribution is extranodal and involves many unusual sites, the most common being the central nervous system. These lymphomas have a strong association with EBV, which reaches 100% in cerebral tumours (Herndier, Kaplan and McGrath 1994). The clinical presentation depends on the site involved, but the progression is rapid, with a mean survival time from diagnosis of 3–4 months. The treatment of choice is radiotherapy, although the results are disappointing mainly because patients in the terminal stages of the underlying AIDS are in such poor general condition.

Burkitt lymphoma occurs earlier in the course of human immunodeficiency virus (HIV) disease, while the immune system is still relatively intact and is therefore more amenable to treatment. About 50% of these lymphomas contain EBV DNA.

HODGKIN'S DISEASE

There has long been a suspicion that EBV may play some part in the induction of Hodgkin's disease (HD) because of the similar socioeconomic epidemiology of HD and IM and because of the well established fact that within 5 years of IM there is a 4- to 6-fold increase in the likelihood of developing HD (Mueller et al. 1989). In recent years, evidence has been obtained that, in c. 60% of patients with HD, EBV DNA is carried and viral proteins expressed (latency II) see 'EBV gene expression', p. 356) in both Reed–Sternberg and the tumour reticulum cells (Weiss et al. 1989, Herbst and Niedobitek 1994). These intriguing findings are as yet insufficient to implicate EBV in the aetiology of HD, but point to the need for further investigation of a possible relationship.

T CELL LYMPHOMAS

EBV DNA has been detected with varying frequency in different types of T cell lymphoma. Detection rates have been recorded of up to 97% in angioimmunoblastic lymphadenopathy (Ott et al. 1992), 84% in nasal lymphoma (previously called midline granuloma) (Harabuchi et al. 1990) and in 46% of peripheral T cell lymphoma (Jones et al. 1988). In addition, sporadic cases of EBV-positive angiocentric T cell lymphoma and of T cell lymphoma related to immunosuppression and chronic EBV infection also occur. In these lesions the cell phenotype is usually that of clonal, mature T cells which more often express the CD4 than CD8 marker. The EBV gene expression is usually of the latency II type, but the latency III pattern has also been recorded.

Although it is now clear that EBV can infect T cells

under certain conditions, the involvement of the virus in the pathogenesis of T cell lymphoma remains to be elucidated.

VARIOUS OTHER MALIGNANCIES

Recent reports have linked EBV to various cancers, including some thymic epithelial tumours (Leyvraz et al. 1985, Wu and Kuo 1993), some undifferentiated salivary gland carcinomas (Hamilton-Dutoit et al. 1991) and, more regularly, to several types of gastric carcinoma (Tokunaga et al. 1993); surprisingly, smooth muscle tumours carrying EBV have also been reported in immunosuppressed children (Lee et al. 1995, McClain et al. 1995). Little is known about the EBV gene expression in any of these tumours and further work is required before a definite association can be established.

NASOPHARYNGEAL CARCINOMA

Nasopharyngeal carcinoma (NPC) arises from the squamous epithelial cells of the postnasal space; primary tumours are not found outside this well defined anatomical site. About 70% of NPC is undifferentiated in type; the remainder show squamous differentiation. The tumour occurs rarely throughout the world, but has a very high incidence in southern Chinese wherever they live and in the Inuit and related races of North America and Greenland. Among populations with a high incidence, NPC is the most common cancer of men and the second most common of women. There is also a high incidence of NPC in Malays, Dyaks, Indonesians, Filipinos and Vietnamese, and a moderately raised incidence in a belt across North Africa, down through the Sudan and into the Kenya Highlands. Comprehensive reviews have been given by Shanmugaratnam (1971, 1978). The tumour is usually a disease of middle or old age except that in medium-high incidence areas of Africa it has bimodal age peaks, the first involving children and young people under 20 years of age (Cammoun, Hoerner and Mourali 1974) and a second affecting much older people. The tumour cells of undifferentiated NPC always carry the EBV genome (Klein 1979, Niedobitek et al. 1991) and most authorities agree that the virus plays a role in causation as a necessary but not the sole element in the aetiological complex.

Symptoms and signs

About two-thirds of patients present with one or more symptoms caused by the local effects of the tumour: nasal obstruction, discharge or bleeding; deafness, tinnitus or earache; ocular paresis from tumour spread to affect cranial nerves. The remaining third of patients complain only of cervical lymph node enlargement due to metastatic spread from a primary tumour that is frequently occult. The signs result either from local tumour spread, causing soft tissue distortion around the postnasal space or cranial nerve palsies, or as a consequence of lymphatic spread to cervical and later supraclavicular lymph glands which become hard and fixed. Blood-borne metastases may be in any organ but are frequent in bones, liver and lungs, the signs

depending on the organ involved (Shanmugaratnam 1971).

Pathogenesis

Little is known of EBV gene function in normal infected epithelial cells but viral gene expression in the malignant cells of NPC is well characterized; although restricted, it is less so than in BL cells and LMP1 has been detected as well as EBNA 1 in every tumour cell of undifferentiated NPC (latency type II, see 'EBV gene expression', p. 356) (Young et al. 1988). In addition to the virus, racial predisposition plays a role, and, among southern Chinese, a modest genetic predisposition has also been demonstrated (Simons et al. 1974, Chan et al. 1983). Environmental co-factors associated with the Chinese way of life have emerged from studies on migrants (Buell 1974, Henderson 1974), and 2 likely candidates have been identified:

1 Traditional herbal remedies (taken as snuff) made from dried plants of the *Euphorbiaceae* and *Thymeliaceae* families, which contain tumour-promoting phorbol esters (Hirayama and Ito 1981).
2 Traditional salt fish dishes, which contain carcinogenic nitrosamines (Huang, Ho and Gough 1978).

Because EBV replicates in the nasopharynx of all carriers and southern Chinese always undergo primary infection as very young children (W Henle and Henle 1979), the taking of snuffs containing phorbol esters is significant because these chemicals are also powerful activators of EBV replication (zur Hausen et al. 1979) as well as having tumour-promoting effects. Thus, if virus production is greatly increased in people with a genetic predisposition to NPC, there will be an unusually large pool of EBV-infected cells that might progress to malignancy, perhaps through a combination of EBV LMP1 oncogene function with nitrosamine carcinogenicity and phorbol ester tumour-promoting effects.

Immune responses and diagnosis

The diagnosis of NPC is usually made histologically on a biopsy sample from the primary tumour or from an enlarged cervical lymph gland. In addition, serum antibody titres show a characteristic and specific pattern of reaction, regardless of geographical location, and can therefore be used for diagnosis; IgG and IgA antibodies to VCA and EA-D are raised, and IgA against these antigens can be found in the saliva (Klein 1979). In the high incidence areas of southern China, mass screening of susceptible populations for serum IgA antibodies to VCA has been successful in detecting very early cases of NPC (Zeng et al. 1982), an important achievement because such early lesions usually respond very well to treatment.

Therapy

The treatment of choice is radiotherapy, which gives 5 year survival rates of 60% or more in the earliest stages of the disease. Of those who survive, 70% remain permanently free of relapse (Ho et al. 1983).

More advanced stages have correspondingly worse prognoses.

ORAL HAIRY LEUCOPLAKIA

This unusual condition is seen fairly frequently in HIV-positive homosexual men, often before AIDS develops but sometimes heralding or accompanying the onset of clinical AIDS. Painless white patches occur on the tongue and/or the lateral buccal mucosa; the lesions are usually multiple, measure up to 3 cm in diameter, are slightly raised and have a 'hairy' or corrugated surface (Greenspan et al. 1985).

The squamous epithelial cells affected by this condition contain large amounts of actively replicating EBV (Greenspan et al. 1985). Aciclovir arrests the virus replication and the lesions regress, but only for the time that drug treatment is continued.

2.4 Vaccine prevention of infection

In the mid-1980s evidence linking EBV to some causative role in endemic BL and NPC was sufficiently strong to warrant the suggestion that vaccine prevention of the virus infection might be a way of decreasing the incidence of the associated cancers in high-risk populations (Epstein 1976). Although BL is of outstanding importance as a model for human viral carcinogenesis and is exceedingly common in endemic areas, in terms of world cancer it is insignificant; however, NPC is a major oncological problem for very large populations, justifying efforts to control it through the development of a vaccine against EBV. Vaccine protection against IM would also be useful.

A considerable body of early work demonstrated that the EBV MA component gp340 purified in various ways was able to induce neutralizing antibodies in experimental animals and protect immunized cottontop tamarins against a 100% carcinogenic challenge dose of the virus (Epstein 1984).

Subsequently, the gene for gp340 has been engineered into various mammalian cells that express gp340 in cultures from which the protein has been readily purified, and recombinant vaccinia viruses capable of expressing gp340 have also been made (Epstein 1993). Another approach is seeking to develop a vaccine based on synthetic peptide epitopes recognized by specific cytotoxic T cells, to be used in conjunction with appropriate adjuvant and CD4 T cell-mediated help (Moss and Suhrbier 1993).

Recent small scale trials in China with a recombinant vaccinia virus vaccine have given equivocal results (Gu et al. 1991), whilst in Australia volunteers are currently being recruited for a phase I trial of a prototype peptide epitope vaccine. If support were forthcoming from the international pharmaceutical industry, trials could also go forward using gp340 from genetically engineered mammalian cell cultures (Epstein 1994).

REFERENCES

Allday MJ, Crawford DH, 1988, Role of epithelium in EBV persistence and pathogenesis of B cell tumours, *Lancet*, **1**: 855–7.

Allday MJ, Crawford DH, Thomas JA, 1993, Epstein–Barr virus (EBV) nuclear antigen 6 induces expression of the EBV latent membrane protein and an activated phenotype in Raji cells, *J Gen Virol*, **74**: 361–9.

Arrand JR, Young LS, Tugwood JD, 1989, Two families of sequences in the small RNA-encoding region of Epstein–Barr virus (EBV) correlate with EBV types A and B, *J Virol*, **63**: 983–6.

Baer R, Bankier AT et al., 1984, DNA sequence and expression of the B95-8 Epstein–Barr virus genome, *Nature (London)*, **310**: 207–11.

Bar RS, Delor CJ et al., 1974, Fatal infectious mononucelosis in a family, *N Engl J Med*, **290**: 363–7.

Bradbury LE, Kansas GS et al., 1992, The CD19/CD21 signal transducing complex of human B lymphocytes includes the target of anti proliferative antibody-1 and Leu-13 molecules, *J Immunol*, **149**: 2841–50.

Brooks L, Yao QY et al., 1992, Epstein–Barr virus latent gene transcription in nasopharyngeal carcinoma cells: coexpression of EBNA1, LMP1, and LMP2 transcripts, *J Virol*, **66**: 2689–97.

Buell P, 1974, The effect of migration on the risk of nasopharyngeal carcinoma among Chinese, *Cancer Res*, **34**: 1189–91.

Burkitt D, 1963, A lymphoma syndrome in tropical Africa, *International Review of Experimental Pathology 2*, eds Richter GW, Epstein MA, Academic Press, New York, London, 67–138.

Burkitt DP, 1969, Etiology of Burkitt's lymphoma – an alternative hypothesis to a vectored virus, *J Natl Cancer Inst*, **42**: 19–28.

Burkitt DP, 1970a, Geographical distribution, *Burkitt's Lymphoma*, eds Burkitt DP, Wright DH, E & S Livingstone, Edinburgh, London, 186–97.

Burkitt DP, 1970b, Treatment: general features, *Burkitt's Lymphoma*, eds Burkitt DP, Wright DH, E & S Livingstone, Edinburgh, London, 43–51.

Cammoun M, Hoerner GV, Mourali N, 1974, Tumors of the nasopharynx in Tunisia: an anatomic and clinical study based on 143 cases, *Cancer*, **33**: 184–92.

Chan SH, Wee GB et al., 1983, HLA locus B and DR antigen associations in Chinese NPC patients and controls, *Nasopharyngeal carcinoma: current concepts*, eds Prasad U, Ablashi DV et al., University Malaya Press, Kuala Lumpur, 307–12.

Clemens MJ, 1994, Functional significance of the Epstein–Barr virus-encoded small RNAs, *Epstein–Barr Virus Rep*, **1**: 107–12.

Cohen JI, Wang F et al., 1989, Epstein–Barr virus nuclear protein 2 is a key determinant of lymphocyte transformation, *Proc Natl Acad Sci USA*, **86**: 9558–62.

Crawford DH, Ando I, 1986, EB virus induction is associated with B cell maturation, *Immunology*, **59**: 405–9.

Dambaugh T, Beisel C et al., 1980, EBV DNA. VII. Molecular cloning and detailed mapping of EBV (B95-8) DNA, *Proc Natl Acad Sci USA*, **77**: 2999–3003.

Dambaugh T, Wang F et al., 1986, Expression of the Epstein–Barr virus nuclear protein 2 in rodent cells, *J Virol*, **59**: 453–62.

Deacon EM, Pallesen G et al., 1993, Epstein–Barr virus and Hodgkin's disease: transcriptional analysis of virus latency in the malignant cells, *J Exp Med*, **177**: 339–49.

Deinhardt F, Deinhardt J, 1979, Comparative aspects: oncogenic animal herpesviruses, *The Epstein–Barr virus*, eds Epstein MA, Achong BG, Springer-Verlag, Berlin, Heidleberg, New York, 373–415.

Epstein MA, 1976, Epstein–Barr virus – is it time to develop a vaccine program?, *J Natl Cancer Inst*, **56**: 697–700.

Epstein MA, 1984, A prototype vaccine to prevent Epstein–Barr virus-associated tumours, *Proc Roy Soc London, B*, **221**: 1–20.

Epstein MA, 1985, Historical background: Burkitt's lymphoma and Epstein–Barr virus, *Burkitt's Lymphoma: a human cancer model*, eds Lenoir G, O'Conor G, Olweny CLM, International Agency for Research on Cancer, Lyon, 17–27.

Epstein MA, 1993, Epstein–Barr virus: retrospective reflections and future prospects, *Epstein–Barr Virus and Associated Diseases*, eds Tursz T, Pagano JS et al., INSERM/John Libbey Eurotext, London, **225**: 3–11.

Epstein MA, 1994, Le programme de vaccination pour la prevention des cancers associes au virus d'Epstein–Barr chez l'homme, *CR Acad Sci Ser G*, **11**: 11–18.

Epstein MA, Achong BG, 1979, The relationship of the virus to Burkitt's lymphoma, *The Epstein–Barr Virus*, eds Epstein MA, Achong BG, Springer-Verlag, Berlin, 321–37.

Epstein MA, Achong BG, Barr YM, 1964, Virus particles in cultured lymphoblasts from Burkitt's lymphoma, *Lancet*, **1**: 702–3.

Fåhraeus R, Jansson A et al., 1990, Epstein–Barr virus-encoded nuclear antigen 2 activates the viral latent membrane protein promoter by modulating the activity of a negative regulatory element, *Proc Natl Acad Sci USA*, **87**: 7390–4.

Falk K, Gratama JW et al., 1995, The role of repetitive DNA sequences in the size of Epstein–Barr virus (EBV) nuclear antigens and the identification of different EBV isolates using RFLP and PCR analysis, *J Gen Virol*, **76**: 779–90.

Farrell P, Rowe D et al., 1989, Epstein–Barr virus, BZLF-1 transactivator specifically binds to consensus AP-1 sites and is related to c-fos, *EMBO J*, **8**: 127–32.

Finch SC, 1969, Clinical symptoms and signs of infectious mononucleosis, *Infectious Mononucleosis*, eds Carter RL, Penman HG, Blackwell Scientific, Oxford, Edinburgh, 19–46.

Foss H-D, Herbst H et al., 1994, Patterns of cytokine gene expression in infectious mononucleosis, *Blood*, **83**: 707–12.

Frizzera G, 1987, The clinico-pathological expressions of Epstein–Barr virus infection in lymphoid tissues, *Virchows Arch B*, **53**: 1–12.

Frizzera G, Hanto DW et al., 1981, Polymorphic diffuse B-cell hyperplasias and lymphomas in renal transplant recipients, *Cancer Res*, **41**: 4262–79.

Gahn TA, Sugden B, 1995, An EBNA-1-dependent enhancer acts from a distance of 10 kilobase pairs to increase expression of the Epstein–Barr virus LMP gene, *J Virol*, **69**: 2633–6.

Gerber P, Walsh JH et al., 1969, Association of EB-virus infection with the post-perfusion syndrome, *Lancet*, **1**: 593–5.

Greenspan JS, Greenspan D et al., 1985, Replication of Epstein–Barr virus within the epithelial cells of oral 'hairy' leukoplakia, an AIDS-associated lesion, *N Engl J Med*, **313**: 1564–71.

Gu S, Huang T et al., 1991, A preliminary study on the immunogenicity in rabbits and in human volunteers of a recombinant vaccinia virus expressing Epstein–Barr virus membrane antigen, *Chinese Med Sci J*, **6**: 241–3.

Hallee TJ, Evans AS et al., 1974, Infectious mononucelosis at the United States Military Academy. A prospective study of a single class over four years, *Yale J Biol Med*, **47**: 182–95.

Hamilton-Dutoit SJ, Hamilton-Thirkildsen M et al., 1991, Undifferentiated carcinoma of the salivary gland in Greenland Eskimos: demonstration of Epstein–Barr virus DNA by in situ nucleic acid hybridization, *Hum Pathol*, **22**: 811–15.

Hammarskjold M-L, Simurdo MC, 1992, Epstein–Barr virus latent membrane protein trans-activates the human immunodeficiency virus type I long terminal repeat through induction of NF-κB activity, *J Virol*, **66**: 6496–501.

Hammerschmidt W, Sugden B, 1988, Identification and characterisation of oriLyt, a lytic orgin of DNA replication of Epstein–Barr virus, *Cell*, **55**: 427–33.

Hammerschmidt W, Sugden B, 1989, Genetic analysis of immortalising functions of Epstein–Barr virus in human B lymphocytes, *Nature (London)*, **340**: 393–7.

Hanto DW, Frizzera G et al., 1981, Clinical spectrum of lymphoproliferative disorders in renal transplant recipients and evidence for the role of Epstein–Barr virus, *Cancer Res*, **41**: 4253–61.

Hanto DW, Frizzera G et al., 1985, Epstein–Barr virus, immuno-

deficiency and B cell lymphoproliferation, *Transplantation*, **39**: 461–72.

Haque T, Thomas JA et al., 1996, Transmission of donor Epstein–Barr virus (EBV) in transplanted organs causes lymphoproliferative disease in recipients, *J Gen Virol*, **77**: 1169–72.

Harabuchi Y, Yamanaka N et al., 1990, Epstein–Barr virus in nasal T-cell lymphomas in patients with midline granuloma, *Lancet*, **1**: 128–30.

zur Hausen H, O'Neill FJ, Freese UK, 1978, Persisting oncogenic herpesvirus induced by the tumour promoter TPA, *Nature (London)*, **272**: 373–5.

zur Hausen H, Bornkamm GW et al., 1979, Tumor initiators and promoters in induction of Epstein–Barr virus virus, *Proc Natl Acad Sci USA*, **76**: 782–5.

Henderson BE, 1974, Nasopharyngeal carcinoma: present status of knowledge, *Cancer Res*, **34**: 1187–8.

Henderson S, Rowe M et al., 1991, Induction of *bcl*-2 expression by Epstein–Barr virus latent membrane protein 1 protects infected B cells from programmed cell death, *Cell*, **65**: 1107–15.

Henle G, Henle W, 1979, The virus as the etiologic agent of infectious mononucleosis, *The Epstein–Barr Virus*, eds Epstein MA, Achong BG, Springer-Verlag, Berlin, Heidelberg, New York, 279–320.

Henle G, Henle W, Klein G, 1971, Demonstration of two distinct components in the early antigen complex of Epstein–Barr virus-infected cells, *Int J Cancer*, **8**: 272–82.

Henle G, Henle W et al., 1969, Antibodies to EBV in BL and control groups, *J Natl Cancer Inst*, **43**: 1147–57.

Henle W, Henle G, 1979, Seroepidemiology of the virus, *The Epstein–Barr Virus*, eds Epstein MA, Achong BG, Springer-Verlag, Berlin, Heidelberg, New York, 61–78.

Herbst H, Niedobitek G, 1994, Epstein–Barr virus in Hodgkin's disease, *Epstein–Barr Virus Rep*, **1**: 31–5.

Herndier BG, Kaplan LD, McGrath MS, 1994, Pathogenesis of AIDS lymphoma, *AIDS*, **8**: 1025–49.

Hirayama T, Ito Y, 1981, A new view of the etiology of nasopharyngeal carcinoma, *Prev Med*, **10**: 614–22.

Ho JHC, Lau WH et al., 1983, Treatment of nasopharyngeal carcinoma: current status, *Nasopharyngeal Carcinoma – current concepts*, eds Prasad U, Ablashi DV et al., University of Malaya Press, Kuala Lumpur, 389–95.

Hoagland RJ, 1955, The transmission of infectious mononucleosis, *Am J Med Sci*, **229**: 262–72.

Huang DP, Ho JCH, Gough TA, 1978, Analysis for volatile nitrosomines in salt preserved foodstuffs traditionally consumed by southern Chinese, *Nasopharyngeal carcinoma: etiology and control*, eds de Thé G, Ito Y, International Agency for Research on Cancer, Lyon, 309–14.

Jiang W-Q, Szekely L et al., 1991, Colocalisation of the retinobastoma protein and the Epstein–Barr virus-encoded nuclear antigen EBNA-5, *Exp Cell Res*, **197**: 314–18.

Johannesen E, Koh E et al., 1995, Epstein–Barr virus nuclear protein 2 transactivation of the latent membrane protein 1 promotor is mediated by Jk and PU1, *J Virol*, **69**: 253–62.

Jones JF, Shurin S et al., 1988, T cell lymphomas containing Epstein–Barr viral DNA in patients with chronic Epstein–Barr virus infections, *N Engl Med J*, **318**: 733–41.

Kalter SP, Riggs SN et al., 1985, Aggressive non-Hodgkin's lymphoma in immunocompromised homosexual males, *Blood*, **66**: 655–9.

Kaye KM, Izumi KM, Kieff E, 1993, Epstein–Barr virus latent membrane protein 1 is essential for B lymphocyte growth transformation, *Proc Natl Acad Sci USA*, **90**: 9150–4.

Kirimi L, Crawford DH, Nicholson LJ, 1995, Identification of an epithelial cell differentiation responsive region within the BZLF1 promoter of the Epstein–Barr virus, *J Gen Virol*, **76**: 759–65.

Klein G, 1979, The relationship of the virus to nasopharyngeal carcinoma, *The Epstein–Barr Virus*, eds Epstein MA, Achong BG, Springer-Verlag, Berlin, Heidelberg, New York, 339–50.

Klein G, 1987, In defense of the 'old' Burkitt lymphoma scenario, *Advances in Viral Oncology 7*, ed Klein G, Raven Press, New York, 207–11.

Laux G, Perricaudet M, Farrell PJ, 1988, A spliced Epstein–Barr virus gene expressed in immortalized lymphocytes is created by circularization of the linear viral genome, *EMBO J*, **7**: 769–74.

Lee ES, Locker et al., 1995, The association of Epstein–Barr virus with smooth muscle tumors occurring after organ transplantation, *N Engl J Med*, **332**: 19–25.

Lenoir GM, Bornkamm GW, 1987, Burkitt's lymphoma, a human cancer model for the study of the multistep development of cancer; proposal for a new scenario, *Advances in Viral Oncology 7*, ed Klein G, Raven Press, New York, 173–206.

Lewin N, Åman P et al., 1987, Characterization of EBV-carrying B cell populations in healthy seropositive individuals with regard to density, release of transforming virus, and spontaneous outgrowth, *Int J Cancer*, **39**: 472–6.

Leyvraz S, Henle W et al., 1985, Association of Epstein–Barr virus with thymic carcinoma, *N Engl J Med*, **312**: 1296–9.

Liebowitz D, Kieff E, 1993, Epstein–Barr virus, *The Human Herpesvirus*, eds Roizman B, Whitley RJ, Lopes C, Raven Press, New York, 107–72.

Lindahl T, Adams A et al., 1976, Covalently closed circular duplex DNA of EBV in a human lymphoid cell line, *J Mol Biol*, **102**: 511–30.

Ling PD, Hsieh JJ-D et al., 1994, EBNA-2 upregulation of Epstein–Barr virus latency promoters and the cellular CD23 promoter utilize a common targeting intermediate, CBF1, *J Virol*, **68**: 5375–83.

Longnecker R, Druker B et al., 1991, An Epstein–Barr virus protein associated with cell growth transformation interacts with a tyrosine kinase, *J Virol*, **65**: 3681–92.

Luka J, Kallin B, Klein G, 1979, Induction of the Epstein–Barr virus (EBV) cycle in latently infected cells by *n*-butyrate, *Virology*, **94**: 228–31.

McClain KL, Leach CT et al., 1995, Association of Epstein–Barr virus with leiomyosarcomas in children with AIDS, *N Engl J Med*, **332**: 12–18.

Masucci MG, Contreras-Salazar B et al., 1989, 5-Azacytidine upregulates the expression of Epstein–Barr virus nuclear antigen 2 (EBNA2) through EBNA6 and latent membrane protein in the Burkitt's lymphoma line Rael, *J Virol*, **63**: 3135–41.

Miller G, Heston L, Countryman J, 1984, P3HR-1 EBV with heterogeneous DNA disrupts latency, *J Virol*, **50**: 174–82.

Miller CL, Lee JH et al., 1994, An integral membrane protein (LMP2) blocks reactivation of Epstein–Barr virus from latency following surface immunoglobulin crosslinking, *Proc Natl Acad Sci USA*, **91**: 772–6.

Mosialos G, Birkenbach M et al., 1995, The Epstein–Barr virus transforming protein LMP1 engages signalling proteins for the tumour necrosis factor receptor family, *Cell*, **80**: 389–99.

Moss DJ, Suhrbier A, 1993, Epstein–Barr virus vaccines: prospects and limitations, *Life Sci*, **5**: 30–4.

Mueller N, Evans A et al., 1989, Hodgkin's disease and Epstein–Barr virus, *N Engl J Med*, **320**: 689–95.

Murray RJ, Kurilla MG et al., 1992, Identification of target antigens for the human cytotoxic T cell response to Epstein–Barr virus (EBV): implication for the immune control of EBV-positive malignancies, *J Exp Med*, **176**: 157–68.

Nemerow GR, Mold C et al., 1987, Identification of gp350 as the viral glycoprotein mediating attachment of Epstein–Barr virus (EBV) to the EBV/C3d receptor of B cells: sequence homology of gp350 and C3 complement fragment C3d, *J Virol*, **61**: 1416–20.

Niedobitek G, Young LS, 1994, Epstein–Barr virus persistence and virus associated tumours, *Lancet*, **343**: 333–5.

Niedobitek G, Hansmann ML et al., 1991, Epstein–Barr virus and carcinomas: undifferentiated carcinomas but not squamous cell carcinomas of the nasopharynx are regularly associated with the virus, *J Pathol*, **165**: 17–24.

Nilsson K, Klein G et al., 1971, The establishment of lymphoblastoid lines from adult and foetal human lymphoid cells and its dependence on EBV, *Int J Cancer*, **8**: 443–50.

Okaro M, Thiele GM et al., 1988, Epstein–Barr virus and human diseases: recent advances in diagnosis, *Clin Microbiol Rev*, **1**: 300–12.

Ott G, Ott MM et al., 1992, Prevalence of Epstein–Barr virus DNA in different T-cell lymphoma entities in a European population, *Int J Cancer*, **51**: 562–7.

Pattengale PK, Smith RW, Gerber P, 1973, Selective transformation of B lymphocytes by EB virus, *Lancet*, **2**: 93–4.

Penn I, 1983, Lymphomas complicating organ transplantation, *Transplant Proc*, **15, suppl 1**: 2790–7.

Pope JH, Horne MK, Scott W, 1968, Transformation of foetal human leucocytes in vitro by filtrates of a human leukaemia cell line containing herpes-like virus, *Int J Cancer*, **3**: 857–66.

Raab-Traub N, Flynn K, 1986, The structure of the termini of the Epstein–Barr virus as a marker of clonal cellular proliferation, *Cell*, **47**: 883–9.

Rickinson AB, Young LS, Rowe M, 1987, Influence of the Epstein–Barr virus nuclear antigen EBNA2 on the growth phenotype of virus-transformed B cells, *J Virol*, **61**: 1310–7.

Rooney CM, Smith CA et al., 1995, Use of gene-modified virus-specific T lymphocytes to control Epstein–Barr virus-related lymphoproliferation, *Lancet*, **345**: 9–12.

Rowe DT, Rowe M et al., 1986, Restricted expression of EBV latent genes and T-lymphocyte-detected membrane antigen in Burkitt's lymphoma cells, *EMBO J*, **5**: 2599–2608.

Rowe M, Rowe DT et al., 1987, Differences in B cell growth phenotype reflect novel patterns of Epstein–Barr virus latent gene expression in Burkitt's lymphoma cells, *EMBO J*, **6**: 2743–51.

Rowe M, Young LS et al., 1989, Distinction between Epstein–Barr virus type A (EBNA 2A) and type B (EBNA 2B) isolates extends to the EBNA3 family of nuclear proteins, *J Virol*, **63**: 1031–9.

Rowe M, Lear AL et al., 1992, Three pathways of Epstein–Barr virus gene activation from EBNA1-positive latency in B lymphocytes, *J Virol*, **66**: 122–31.

Sample J, Young L et al., 1990, Epstein–Barr virus types 1 and 2 differ in their EBNA-3A, EBNA-3B, and EBNA-3C genes, *J Virol*, **64**: 4084–92.

Sawyer RN, Evans AS et al., 1971, Prospective studies of a group of Yale University freshman. I. Occurence of infectious mononucleosis, *J Infect Dis*, **123**: 263–70.

Sculley TB, Apolloni A et al., 1990, Coinfection with A- and B-type Epstein–Barr virus in human immunodeficiency virus-positive subjects, *J Infect Dis*, **162**: 643–8.

Shanmugaratnam K, 1971, Studies on the etiology of nasopharyngeal carcinoma, *International Review of Experimental Pathology 10*, eds Richter RW, Epstein MA, Academic Press, New York, London, 361–413.

Shanmugaratnam K, 1978, Histological typing of nasopharyngeal carcinoma, *Nasopharyngeal Carcinoma: etiology and control*, eds de Thé G, Ito Y, Davis W, International Agency for Research on Cancer, Lyon, 3–12.

Simons MJ, Wee GB et al., 1974, Immunogenetic aspects of nasopharyngeal carcinoma. I. Differences in HL-A antigen profiles between patients and control groups, *Int J Cancer*, **13**: 122–34.

Sixbey JW, Lemon SM, Pagano JS, 1986, A second site for Epstein–Barr virus shedding: the uterine cervix, *Lancet*, **2**: 1122–4.

Sixbey JW, Vesterinen EH et al., 1983, Replication of Epstein–Barr virus in human epithelial cells infected in vitro, *Nature (London)*, **306**: 480–3.

Starzl TE, Porter KA et al., 1984, Reversibility of lymphomas and lymphoproliferative lesions developing under cyclosporin-steroid therapy, *Lancet*, **1**: 583–7.

Steel CM, Philipson J et al., 1977, Possibility of EB virus preferentially transforming a subpopulation of human B lymphocytes, *Nature (London)*, **270**: 729–31.

Swaminathan S, Tomkinson B, Kieff E, 1991, Recombinant Epstein–Barr virus with small RNA (EBER) genes deleted transforms lymphocytes and replicates in vitro, *Proc Natl Acad Sci USA*, **88**: 1546–50.

Szekely L, Selivanova G et al., 1993, EBNA-5, an Epstein–Barr virus-encoded nuclear antigen, binds to the retinoblastoma and p53 proteins, *Proc Natl Acad Sci USA*, **90**: 5455–9.

Thomas JA, Allday MJ, Crawford DH, 1991, Epstein–Barr virus-associated lymphoproliferative disorders in immunocompromised individuals, *Adv Cancer Res*, **57**: 329–80.

Thomas JA, Hotchin N et al., 1990, Immunohistology of Epstein–Barr virus associated antigens in B cell disorders from immunocompromised individuals, *Transplantation*, **49**: 944–53.

Tokunaga M, Land CE et al., 1993, Epstein–Barr virus in gastric carcinoma, *Am J Pathol*, **143**: 1250–4.

Tomkinson B, Robertson E, Kieff E, 1993, Epstein–Barr virus nuclear proteins EBNA-3A and EBNA-3C are essential for B-lymphocyte growth transformation, *J Virol*, **67**: 2014–25.

Tosato G, Blaese MR, Yarchoan R, 1985, Relationship between immunoglobulin production and immortalization by Epstein–Barr virus, *J Immunol*, **135**: 959–64.

Tovey MG, Lenoir G, Begon-Lours J, 1978, Activation of latent Epstein–Barr virus by antibody to human IgM, *Nature (London)*, **276**: 270–2.

Virelizier JL, Lenoir G, Griscelli C, 1978, Persistent Epstein–Barr virus infection in a child with hypergammaglobulinaemia and immunoblastic proliferation associated with a selective defect in immune interferon secretion, *Lancet*, **2**: 231–4.

Wang D, Liebowitz D, Kieff E, 1985, An EBV membrane protein expressed in immortalized lymphocytes transforms established rodent cells, *Cell*, **43**: 831–40.

Wang D, Liebowitz D et al., 1988, Epstein–Barr virus latent infection membrane protein alters the human B-lymphocyte phenotype: deletion of the amino terminus abolishes activity, *J Virol*, **62**: 4137–84.

Wang F, Gregory C et al., 1990, Epstein–Barr virus latent membrane protein (LMP1) and nuclear proteins 2 and 3C are effectors of phenotypic changes in B lymphocytes: EBNA-2 and LMP1 cooperatively induce CD23, *J Virol*, **64**: 2309–18.

Weisenburger DD, Purtilo DT, 1986, Failure in immunological control of the virus infection: fatal infectious mononucleosis, *The Epstein–Barr Virus: recent advances*, eds Epstein MA, BG Achong BG, Heinemann Medical, London, 127–61.

Weiss LM, Movahed AM et al., 1989, Detection of Epstein–Barr viral genomes in Reed–Sternberg cells of Hodgkin's disease, *N Engl J Med*, **320**: 502–6.

Woisetschlaeger M, Jin XW et al., 1991, Role for the Epstein–Barr virus nuclear antigen 2 in viral promoter switching during initial stages of infection, *Proc Natl Acad Sci USA*, **88**: 3942–6.

Wu T-C, Kuo T-T, 1993, Study of Epstein–Barr virus early RNA1 (EBER1) expression by in situ hybridization in thymic epithelial tumours of Chinese patients in Taiwan, *Hum Pathol*, **24**: 235–8.

Yao QY, Rickinson AB, Epstein MA, 1985, A re-examination of the Epstein–Barr virus carrying state in healthy seropositive individuals, *Int J Cancer*, **35**: 35–42.

Yates JL, Warren N, Sugden B, 1985, Stable replication of plasmids derived from Epstein–Barr virus in mammalian cells, *Nature (London)*, **313**: 812–5.

Young LS, Dawson CW et al., 1988, Epstein–Barr virus gene expression in nasopharyngeal carcinoma, *J Gen Virol*, **69**: 1051–65.

Zeng Y, Zhang LG et al., 1982, Serological mass survey for early detection of nasopharyngeal carcinoma in Wuzhou City, China, *Int J Cancer*, **29**: 139–41.

Ziegler JL, Andersson M et al., 1976, Detection of Epstein–Barr virus DNA in American Burkitt's lymphoma, *Int J Cancer*, **17**: 701–6.

Zimber U, Adldinger HK et al., 1986, Geographical prevalence of two types of Epstein–Barr virus, *Virology*, **154**: 56–66.

Chapter 21

POXVIRUSES

Derrick Baxby

| 1 Properties of the viruses | 2 Clinical and pathological aspects |

1 PROPERTIES OF THE VIRUSES

1.1 Introduction

Ever since laboratory research on animal viruses started, considerable attention has been paid to vaccinia virus, largely because of the ease with which it can be handled, and so much of our knowledge of poxviruses in general and orthopoxviruses in particular has been derived from such studies. The large size of poxviruses made them ideal subjects for early electron microscopy, and fowlpox and vaccinia viruses were used in pioneering studies on growth of viruses in the chick embryo and cell culture. More recently, the complex nature of poxviruses, particularly their possession of virion-associated enzymes, has extended the concept of viruses beyond that of a simple nucleoprotein. Despite the eradication of smallpox (Fenner et al. 1988) interest in vaccinia virus has increased. Particular attention is focused on determining the role of individual gene products in pathogenesis (Smith 1994), and the development of attenuated strains that might be suitable vectors for recombinant vaccines (Baxby 1993a). Vaccinia virus also continues to be a model for similar studies on other poxviruses (Buller and Palumbo 1991, Binns and Smith 1992) and a general model for cytoplasmic DNA synthesis. The characteristics of poxviruses in general and orthopoxviruses in particular have been the subject of excellent reviews (Fenner, Wittek and Dumbell 1989, Dumbell 1989, Moss 1995).

1.2 Classification

Although poxviruses are not symmetrical and are somewhat pleomorphic, their appearance in negatively stained extracts or thin sections is sufficiently characteristic to enable a newly recognized virus to be regarded as a poxvirus. In this way poxviruses from hosts as diverse as primates, reptiles and insects have been recognized, although recognition of double-stranded DNA and replication in the cytoplasm are other important criteria.

The family *Poxviridae* is separated into 2 subfamilies. Insect poxviruses (*Entomopoxvirinae*) do not infect vertebrates and are not considered here (see reviews by Granados 1981, Moyer 1994). Table 21.1 shows that 8 genera of vertebrate poxviruses (*Chordopoxvirinae*) are recognized (Esposito et al. 1995). However, some viruses have yet to be allocated to genera and others, although assignable to a genus, have not had their relationship within it established. Traditionally, poxviruses have been named after their assumed reservoir host, but in some cases (e.g. 'cowpox', 'monkeypox') this has proved misleading.

There is cross-immunity and potential for genetic hybridization within but not between genera; the former property, and the apparently unique morphology of *Parapoxvirus* species, may be used to assign a virus to a particular genus. The importance of genome analysis for this purpose is, however, increasing.

IDENTIFICATION OF SPECIES

Because of the importance of smallpox and the ease with which orthopoxviruses can be grown, emphasis has usually been placed on the identification of these species by a suitable combination of biological tests. Details of such tests and their interpretation are available elsewhere (Tripathy, Hanson and Crandell 1981, Nakano and Esposito 1989). Increasing attention is, however, being paid to genome studies for separating species, in particular to analysis of the genome maps derived from digestion of virus DNA with various restriction endonucleases. For example, the enzyme *Hind*III is particularly useful for separation of *Orthopoxvirus* species (Esposito and Knight 1985). In general, the results have reinforced the earlier classification scheme based on biological characteristics, although 'buffalopox' virus is now regarded as a subspecies of vaccinia (Dumbell and Richardson 1993). Such studies have allowed volepox and raccoonpox viruses to be proposed as distinct *Orthopoxvirus* species

Table 21.1 Family *Poxviridae*[a]

Genus	Species[b]
Subfamily *Chordopoxvirinae* (poxviruses of vertebrates)	
Orthopoxvirus	**Vaccinia**,[c] smallpox,[d] cowpox,[e] camelpox, mousepox (infectious ectromelia), raccoonpox, volepox, Tatera (gerbil) pox viruses
Parapoxvirus	**Orf** (contagious pustular dermatitis), pseudocowpox (paravaccinia, milker's nodes), bovine papular stomatitis viruses. Probable members: parapoxvirus of New Zealand deer, Ausdyk (camel) virus
Capripoxvirus	**Sheeppox**, goatpox, lumpy skin disease viruses
Leporipoxvirus	**Myxoma**, rabbit (Shope) fibroma, hare fibroma, squirrel fibroma viruses, rabbit malignant fibroma virus
Suipoxvirus	**Swinepox** virus
Molluscipoxvirus	**Molluscum contagiosum** virus
Yatapoxvirus[f]	**Yaba** monkey tumour, tanapox viruses
Avipoxvirus	**Fowlpox**, canarypox, turkeypox, pigeonpox viruses (also isolates from starling, sparrow, quail etc.)
Subfamily *Entomopoxvirinae* (poxviruses of invertebrates)	
Three genera based on morphology, DNA characteristics and host range (see Granados 1981, Moyer 1994)	

[a]See also 'unclassified poxviruses' in text.
[b]Type species in bold.
[c]Includes buffalopox and rabbitpox as subspecies.
[d]Includes variola major and variola minor (alastrim).
[e]Includes isolates from felines and captive exotic species.
[f]From Yaba Tana.

(Knight et al. 1992), and viruses from 'unusual' hosts such as the domestic cat to be classified as cowpox virus (Naidoo et al. 1992). Similarly, use of the enzyme Kpnl has defined *Parapoxvirus* species (Robinson and Lyttle 1992). A greater range of enzymes can distinguish between individual isolates, which may be of epidemiological value (Naidoo et al. 1992). Orthopoxviruses can be identified by polymerase chain reaction amplification of species-specific sequences within the genes that code for the A-type inclusion protein (Meyer, Pfeffer and Rziha 1994), and the haemagglutinin antigen (Fig. 21.1) (Ropp et al. 1995). Such methods may be of value in situations where no virus is isolated. Molluscum contagiosum virus, the only *Molluscipoxvirus* species, has never been grown. Genome analysis has however, detected at least 3 major subgroups (Scholz et al. 1989, Porter and Archard 1994).

Genome analysis can also provide information about emerging viruses. Such evidence suggests that 'new' viruses may emerge naturally through genetic hybridization between leporipoxviruses, for example malignant rabbit fibroma (Upton et al. 1988), and between capripoxviruses (Gershon et al. 1989).

EVOLUTION

The separation of birds and mammals represents a major divergence of hosts, and the nucleotide sequence and genomic locations of the thymidine kinase (TK) of mammalian poxviruses are related more closely to each other than to the fowlpox TK (Schnitzlein and Tripathy 1991). Although apparent relationships may be explored in this way there are problems in relying too much on evidence from selected genes, and one cannot necessarily assume that hosts and parasites diverge at the same time.

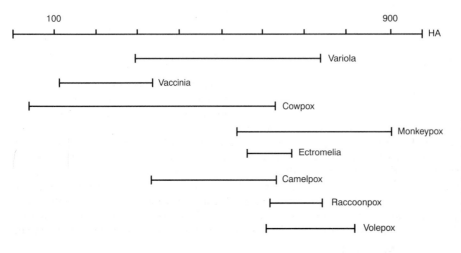

Fig. 21.1 Representation of the *Orthopoxvirus* haemagglutinin gene, showing sequences detectable by appropriate species-specific PCR primer pairs. Bars = 100 bp. (Modified from Ropp et al. 1995, with permission.)

The characteristic morphology and high G + C ratio (63%) of parapoxviruses may indicate early divergence from other genera, but the similar locations and nucleotide sequences of some parapoxvirus and orthopoxvirus genes probably indicate a common ancestor (Fleming et al. 1993). There is also similarity between the overall genome organization of capripoxviruses and orthopoxviruses (Gershon, Ansell and Black 1989). Within genera it is perhaps of interest that the genomes of New World orthopoxviruses (volepox and raccoonpox viruses) are related more closely to each other than to Old World orthopoxviruses (Knight et al. 1992).

There has for long been interest in the various origins of vaccinia viruses, which are regarded as laboratory strains with no natural reservoirs. Comparison of orthopoxvirus genomes indicates that vaccine strains are closely related and that vaccinia virus represents a distinct species (Esposito and Knight 1985). This finding supports historical analyses which indicate that it could not have been 'derived' from cowpox or smallpox viruses during the last 200 years (Baxby 1981).

Unclassified poxviruses

In addition to the viruses listed in Table 21.1, poxviruses, in some cases detected only by electron microscopy, have been reported from a variety of hosts. These include: viruses from 'molluscum contagiosum' in horses (Rahaley and Mueller 1983), kangaroos (Bagnall and Wilson 1974) and South American sea lions (Wilson and Poglayen-Neuwall, 1971); viruses with parapoxvirus and orthopoxvirus morphology isolated from grey seals (Osterhaus et al. 1990, 1994); 'Cotia' virus from South American rodents which seems to share properties with orthopoxviruses and leporipoxviruses (Ueda et al. 1978); and an orthopoxvirus related to ectromelia virus isolated from human epidemic erythromelalgia (Zheng et al. 1992). Poxviruses have also been detected in cold-blooded species, for example farmed Nile crocodiles (Horner 1988), lizards (Stauber and Gogolewski 1990), and chameleons (Jacobson and Telford 1990). A report of poxviruses in frogs (Cunningham et al. 1993) has not been confirmed (Cunningham, Bennett and Baxby 1995, unpublished).

1.3 Morphology and structure

Size and general organization

The virions are generally brick-shaped, but somewhat pleomorphic and variable in size. Parapoxviruses are c. 160 × 250 nm, and avipoxviruses c. 280 × 330 nm, but virions of most genera are c. 250 × 300 nm. In thin sections, mature virions have a dumb-bell-shaped core or nucleoid compressed by 2 lateral bodies and usually surrounded by one or more membranes (Fig. 21.2a–c). The configuration of the genome within the core is not known. Unduly stringent packaging is unlikely because infectious clones can be produced in which the genome has lost 47.6 kbp (Perkus et al. 1991) or had added to it 25 kbp (Smith and Moss 1983) of DNA. Cores, when released by detergent treatment, are usually larger than when within the virion (Fig. 21.2d).

Intracellular and extracellular virions

Studies on purified poxviruses were initially done on virus extracted artificially from cells by grinding, ultrasonic treatment, or both, and such virus is still often used. However, there are differences between such virions and those released naturally that have important implications for immunity and pathogenesis (Boulter and Appleyard 1973, Payne 1980, Smith 1993).

Intracellular naked virus

Also called intracellular mature virus, this is the infectious form found in artificial extracts and lacks an outer membrane or envelope (Fig. 21.2e). Although infectious, intracellular naked virus (INV) is in fact relatively immature and during the replication cycle is converted naturally to the forms described next.

Extracellular enveloped virus

This is infectious virus released naturally from infected cells and has an outer membrane or envelope not present in virus extracted artificially (Fig. 21.2f). In thin section it is best seen at the cytoplasmic membrane during or just after natural release where the envelope is most obvious (Fig. 21.2b). This important envelope (see below) is lost on manipulation and extracellular enveloped virus (EEV) is easily converted to INV.

Immature enveloped virus

This transient, presumably infectious, form, derived from INV during the replication cycle, has a double outer membrane or envelope (Fig. 21.2a). The outermost envelope is lost as this form converts naturally to EEV at the cytoplasmic membrane (Fig. 21.2b), and both envelopes are lost as it is converted to INV during artificial extraction. (See also section 1.5, p. 372, and Fig. 21.4.)

Mulberry and capsule forms

Two basic forms are seen when whole virions are negatively stained, the M ('mulberry') and C ('capsule') forms. M forms usually comprise 80–90% of the population but both are infectious and interconvertible; the differences are due to variation in the rates of drying and stain penetration (Harris and Westwood 1964). The surfaces of M forms of poxviruses other than *Parapoxvirus* are covered with randomly arranged tubules c. 10 nm wide. Those of *Molluscipoxvirus* are often more prominent and perhaps slightly longer than those of, for example vaccinia (Fig. 21.2e, f). The M form of parapoxviruses has one long surface tubule that winds round the virion (Fig. 21.2g). This gives a characteristic criss-cross appearance due to superimposition of the images of the top and bottom surfaces in electron micrographs (Nagington, Newton and Hall 1964). The C form is more uniformly electron dense and seems to be bounded by a 'capsule' 20–25 nm thick (Fig. 21.2h). This capsule is not the outer envelope of EEV described above, and M and C forms of EEV can be demonstrated. It has recently been sug-

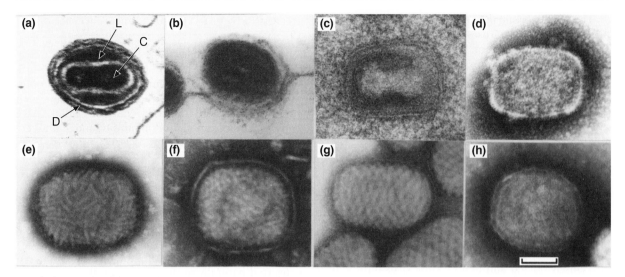

Fig. 21.2   (a) Thin section of intracellular virus showing double outer membrane (D), core (C) and lateral bodies (L). (b) Thin section of vaccinia virus showing loss of outer layer of double outer membrane during natural release. (c) Thin section of cowpox virus within A-type inclusion, showing multiple membranes. (d) Core of vaccinia virus. (e) Molluscum virion showing mulberry (M) form of intracellular naked virus (INV). (f) M form of vaccinia extracellular enveloped virus (EEV). (g) M form of parapox virus. (h) Capsule (C) form of vaccinia virus. (Whole core (d) and whole virions (e)–(h), negative stain. Bar = 100 nm).

gested that the M and C forms and the dumb-bell-shaped core are artefacts caused by inappropriate specimen preparation, and that the virus should more properly be represented as a more homogenous structure with a 30 nm coat similar to the C form (Dubochet et al. 1994). If this proves to be so, the surface structure of *Parapoxvirus* is difficult to interpret. The forms generally seen, artefacts or not, are remarkably consistent and a valuable aid to laboratory diagnosis.

1.4   Genome structure and function

General organization

Of all viruses, most information is available for orthopoxviruses in general and vaccinia virus in particular, and the entire genomes of strains of vaccinia and variola viruses have been sequenced (Goebel et al. 1990, Johnson, Goebel and Paoletti 1993, Shchelkunov, Massung and Esposito 1995). Individual genes and longer fragments from other viruses have been sequenced, and restriction maps of species from different genera are available, for example *Parapoxvirus* (Fleming et al. 1993), *Capripoxvirus* (Gershon and Black 1988), leporipoxviruses (Russell and Robbins 1989), *Molluscipoxvirus* (Scholz et al. 1989) and *Suipoxvirus* (Massung, Jayarama and Moyer 1993). The organization and function of the genome are best considered in relation to the *Hind*III restriction map of Copenhagen vaccinia, the first genome to be sequenced (Fig. 21.3).

The genome is a linear molecule of double-stranded DNA. There is some variation in length between genera, ranging from c. 130 kbp in *Parapoxvirus* to c. 260 kbp in *Avipoxivirus*. There is considerable difference in the genome lengths of *Orthopoxvirus* species, vaccinia being c. 190 kbp and cowpox

c. 220 kbp. The ends of the genome comprise inverted terminal repeat sequences (ITRs). At the extreme end these form short non-coding hairpin structures which cross-link the 2 DNA strands. The lengths of the ITRs vary from c. 700 bp in variola virus (Shchelkunov, Massung and Esposito 1995) to 12 kbp in Copenhagen vaccinia (Goebel et al. 1990). In the latter, and other viruses with sufficiently large ITRs, coding sequences are found in the ITR and the appropriate genes are transcribed at each end of the genome (Fig. 21.3). As discussed above ('Classification', p. 367) there is an overall similarity in the genomes of poxviruses. The general organization of the central region in particular is conserved, even between genera (see, e.g., Gershon, Ansell and Black 1989), although sequence homology is insufficient to permit genetic hybridization. Differences between species tend to occur at the ends (see, e.g., Esposito and Knight 1985, Robinson et al. 1987).

Genome function

The poxvirus genome is not infectious *per se* and other factors are needed to initiate replication (see section 1.5, p. 372). In general, the genome has been shown by direct analysis or sequence comparison to contain c. 200 major protein coding regions (Fig. 21.3) and the significance of some of them is discussed below (see sections 1.6, 2.4 and 2.5, p. 374, p. 378 and p. 379). Some are essential for virus replication, but of interest is the number of genes that are not essential for replication. These account for as much as 30% of the genome and include genes clustered at the termini (Fig. 21.3). As discussed in section 2.4 (p. 379) the role of such gene products in pathogenesis and virulence is of particular interest, as are the degrees of sequence and functional homology, not just between poxvirus genera but also in some cases between poxvirus and mammalian gene products (see, e.g., McFadden, Graham and Opgenorth 1994, Mossman, Barry and McFadden 1994, Smith 1994). Table 21.2

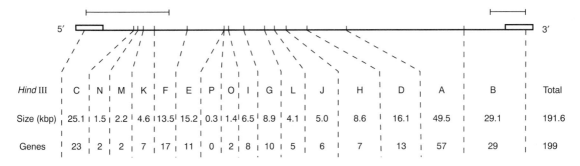

Hind III	C	N	M	K	F	E	P	O	I	G	L	J	H	D	A	B	Total
Size (kbp)	25.1	1.5	2.2	4.6	13.5	15.2	0.3	1.4	6.5	8.9	4.1	5.0	8.6	16.1	49.5	29.1	191.6
Genes	23	2	2	7	17	11	0	2	8	10	5	6	7	13	57	29	199

Fig. 21.3 Representation of genome of Copenhagen vaccinia showing *Hind*III restriction fragments labelled A–P according to decreasing size and arranged in order 5′–3′. Inverted terminal repeats (boxed) and 2 large non-essential regions (horizontal bars) are indicated. (Modified from Goebel et al. 1990 and Johnson, Goebel and Paoletti 1993, with permission.)

provides information on just some of the genes and gene products identified as important for virus replication and infection.

RECOMBINANT POXVIRUS VECTORS

Appreciation of the existence of non-essential coding regions, and of the relatively loose packaging of poxvirus DNA, has led to the development of infectious 'recombinant' poxviruses capable of expressing foreign genes inserted into the poxvirus genome (Binns and Smith 1992). The number of foreign genes studied, individually and in combination, is now very large, and the method has been used to study gene

expression and particularly to develop potential vaccines. Inevitably work has concentrated on vaccinia virus as a vector, and a vaccinia–rabies recombinant vaccine used for the control of wildlife rabies in Europe has been a considerable success (Pastoret et al. 1996). There are problems with the safety of vaccinia virus, partly solved by the development of attenuated strains (Tartaglia et al. 1992), but other vectors are being used. These include raccoonpox recombinant vaccines for the control of wildlife rabies in North America (Esposito et al. 1992), and species-specific capripox recombinant vaccines for the control of rinderpest (Romero et al. 1994). Of particular interest is

Table 21.2 Examples of gene products encoded by poxviruses

Gene[a]	Product[b]	Comment[c]
C22L	TNF receptor	Non-essential. Binds TNF, contributes to virulence. Disrupted in CopVac, present in other genera
C11L	Soluble EGF	Non-essential. Promotes cell proliferation, inactivation attenuates. Detected in all genera
C3L	C4b receptor	Non-essential. Binds C4b and inhibits C-dependent neutralization. Negative mutants attenuated
E9L	DNA polymerase	Essential early function of all poxviruses
J2R	TK	Thymidine kinase. Non-essential. Deletion may attenuate. Found in other genera
J6R/A24R	RNA polymerase	Major subunits of DNA-dependent enzyme. Essential component of all pox virions
A25/26R	ATI protein	Non-essential. Some protein, but not necessarily ATI, produced by all orthopoxviruses
A27L	Fusion protein	Surface antigen of INV. Required for EEV production. Antibody neutralizes all orthopoxviruses
A56R	Haemagglutinin	Non-essential antigen of EEV. Inhibits cell fusion, promotes virus attachment. Produced only by *Orthopoxvirus*
B5R	EEV antigen	Class 1 membrane glycoprotein. Important for *Orthopoxvirus* cross-immunity
B8R	IF-γ receptor	Non-essential. Binds IF-γ. Blocks host defences. Found in other genera
B13/14R	Serpin	Non-essential 38 kDa serpin. Non-functional in CopVac. Inhibits inflammatory response, particularly in cowpox
B16R	IL-1β receptor	Non-essential. Blocks IL-1β defence activity
(*CHO*)	Host range	Host range gene in cowpox, absent in CopVac, disrupted in WRVac (B4R). Non-expression causes apoptosis in CHO cells

[a]With reference to the genome of Copenhagen vaccinia. Initial letter denotes *Hind*III fragment, number indicates gene within that fragment, L and R indicate the direction of transcription. CHO, Chinese hamster ovary.
[b]ATI, A-type inclusion; C4b, complement component; EEV, extracellular enveloped virus; EGF, epidermal growth factor; IF, interferon; serpin, serine protease inhibitor; IL, interleukin; TK, thymidine kinase; TNF, tumour necrosis factor.
[c]CopVac, Copenhagen vaccinia, INV, intracellular naked virus; WRVac, Western Reserve vaccinia; other abbreviations as above.

the observation that avipoxvirus recombinants do not productively infect mammals but do immunize them against the appropriate disease (e.g. rabies) when the inserted gene is expressed via a poxvirus early promoter (Limbach and Paoletti 1996). Such vaccines could prove to be safe alternatives to vaccinia recombinants.

1.5 Replication

Vaccinia virus has been used as a model for poxvirus replication. It is cytocidal and its inhibition of host cell DNA and protein synthesis facilitates biochemical analysis of the replication cycle. The structural complexity of poxviruses permits analysis of replication by electron microscopy in a way not available to those who study simple viruses. Figure 21.4 provides a diagrammatic representation of the replication cycle. Detailed biochemical information can be found in the excellent, and extensively referenced, review by Moss (1995).

STRUCTURAL ANALYSIS

Virus adsorption is relatively non-specific, and inactivated virions are taken up almost as well as infective ones. Some enter by pinocytosis and are uncoated in cytoplasmic vesicles, but in most cases the outer viral membrane fuses with the cell membrane (Doms, Blu-

menthal and Moss 1990). Soon after infection the core is released and is then broken down. Replication takes place in so-called B-type inclusions, in which virions in various stages of assembly can usually be recognized. Concentrations of electron-dense material and crescent-shaped viral membranes are seen first. These progress to spherical or ovoid immature virions in which the developing core, often located excentrically, appears as a particularly electron-dense area. These forms mature to produce infectious virions (Fig. 21.5). The source of the membranes investing the intracellular forms is of interest. Recent cytoimmunological studies suggest that the transient forms described above (see Fig. 21.2a) derive their double membranes from the trans-Golgi network, a compartment between the rough endoplasmic reticulum and the Golgi complex (Schmelz et al. 1994). These forms then lose the outermost layer by fusion with the cytoplasmic membrane as they are released from the cells (see Fig. 21.2b, Fig. 21.4). In that sense, poxviruses may be said to exit by budding and to have an envelope.

Cowpox, ectromelia, raccoonpox, volepox and avipox viruses produce A-type inclusions (Fig. 21.5). These are large electron-dense bodies fringed with ribosomes. The inclusions of some virus isolates are devoid of virions, whereas those of others contain virions that are usually invested with multiple membranes (see Fig. 21.2c).

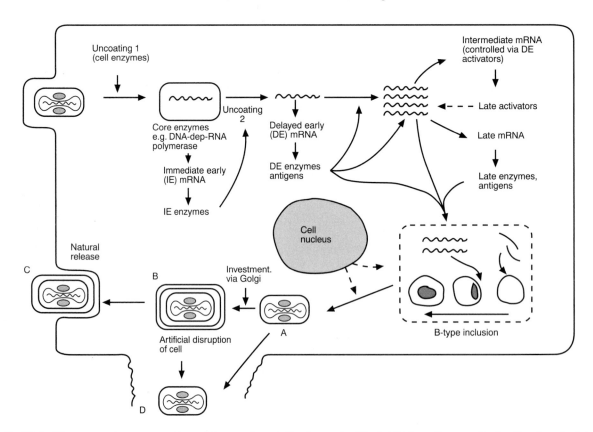

Fig. 21.4 Diagrammatic representation of the poxvirus replication cycle. The inhibition of pre-replicative functions by late gene products and the production of ATI by some orthopoxviruses are not shown. A = infectious INV which is detected when cells are extracted artificially (D), or converted naturally to a transient form with a double outer membrane (B). This may be converted to INV (D) as just described, or to EEV by natural loss of the outer element of the double envelope at the cell membrane (C).

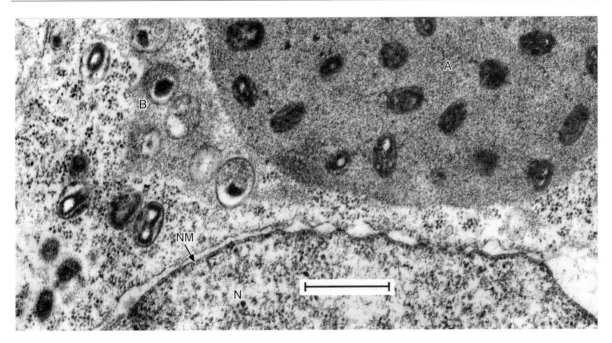

Fig. 21.5 Thin section of cell infected with cowpox virus. B = B-type inclusion showing virions in various stages of assembly. A = A-type inclusion (ATI) containing mature virions. N, nucleus, NM, nuclear membrane. Note that the ATI of some strains of virus do not contain virions. Bar = 500 nm.

BIOCHEMICAL ANALYSIS

Virus attachment to cells was thought to be relatively non-specific. A trypsin-sensitive cell surface epitope has, however, been detected which is involved in the attachment and penetration of poxviruses but not herpesviruses (Chang et al. 1995). Once inside the cell the core is released by constitutive cell enzymes and the DNA is released by 'immediate early' enzymes transcribed from the core. A number of enzymes and factors are present in the core (Moss 1995). These include a DNA-dependent RNA polymerase, transcription and termination factors, and RNA capping and methylating enzymes sufficient for the virus to transcribe at least part of the genome very early in the replication cycle. Such functions are essential for a DNA virus to replicate in the cytoplasm, and they explain why poxvirus DNA is not infectious. Further mRNAs are then transcribed from the genome of the inoculum. Such 'delayed early' gene products include the DNA polymerase, various structural proteins, and activators that regulate the transcription of 'intermediate' mRNA from progeny DNA (Baldick and Moss 1993). Late activators are then translated from intermediate mRNA and regulate production of 'late' mRNAs, enzymes and antigens (Wright, Keck and Moss 1991). These include the DNA-dependent RNA polymerase, which is incorporated into progeny virions to play its role in the next cells infected.

The DNA replicates via intermediates formed of pentameric concatemers, and the structure of the terminal hairpin loops is important for the resolution of the concatemers into linear molecules (Merchlinsky 1990, Moss 1995). Analysis of the transcriptional control of gene expression is facilitated by differences between early and late promoters and mRNAs.

Late promoters have a TAAATG recognition site and produce relatively large heterogeneous mRNAs. Early mRNAs tend to be shorter; their length is regulated by a TTTTTxT termination sequence (Yuen and Moss 1987). However, the distinction between pre- and post-replicative gene products is not always simple. Some early products are switched off by post-replicative control, others continue to be produced and the haemagglutinin (HA) is produced early and late from separate promoters (Brown, Turner and Moyer 1991). Poxvirus promoters lack TATA and CAAT, the usual consensus sequences, but genes from one poxvirus genus can be controlled by the promoters of another, and foreign genes inserted into recombinant poxviruses need to be controlled by poxvirus promoters.

Poxvirus gene products are subject to post-translational modification by, for example, glycosylation and proteolytic cleavage. The latter mechanism is mediated via an Ala–Gly–x motif conserved especially in core and late proteins (Whitehead and Hruby 1994). Although virus replication takes place in the cytoplasm, it does not take place in enucleated cells and there is evidence that components of the host cell RNA polymerase are transported from the nucleus and play some role in virus maturation (reviewed by Moyer 1987).

CULTIVATION

With the exception of molluscum contagiosum virus, which has not been cultivated (McFadden et al. 1979), poxviruses of warm-blooded hosts can usually be grown without difficulty. *Orthopoxvirus*, *Avipoxvirus* and *Leporipoxvirus* species can be grown on the chick chorioallantois, and the character of the pocks produced aids identification. Orthopoxviruses can also be grown, with the production of cytopathic effect, in a range of cell cultures usually wider than those from the host species. Other viruses tend to require, or grow better in, cells derived from the host species. The type of cytopathic effect is not particularly characteristic and the same virus isolate may produce a different effect in different cells. Host range genes have been studied, particularly *CHOhr* (see Table 21.2), the gene that permits growth of cowpox virus in Chinese hamster ovary cells. When not expressed, or absent as with vaccinia virus, the inoculated cells undergo apoptosis (Ink, Gilbert and Evan 1995).

1.6 Polypeptides: non-structural and structural

This topic is dealt with only briefly here. It is also discussed in section 2.5 (p. 379) in relation to important immunological differences between INV and EEV, and in section 2.4 (p. 378) regarding the pathogenic functions of soluble components. Over 100 polypeptides have been detected by 2-dimensional electrophoresis of disrupted virions (Essani and Dales 1979), and there is coding potential for twice this number (see Fig. 21.3). Virus-free extracts of infected cells contain structural polypeptides produced in excess, but more important is the variety of biologically active soluble proteins (e.g. cytokine receptors), which either interfere with host defence mechanisms or contribute to virulence, or both (see Table 21.2). The HA antigen, detectable in virus-free extracts, and long thought to be non-structural, is a component of the outer envelope of EEV.

Treatment of INV with non-ionic detergents separates surface proteins and the core. The latter can then be separated into the various enzymes etc. which initiate immediate transcription (see Moss 1995), and residual structural components. At least 4 core proteins have been recognized, including a major core protein VP8 (gene *L4R*) which binds to DNA (Yang and Bauer 1988, Moss 1995). A number of surface polypeptides have been characterized, including a fusion protein (mol. wt 14 kDa, gene *A27L*) (see Table 21.2), continued production of which is required to convert INV into EEV (Rodriguez and Smith 1990). The outer envelope of EEV contains 10 polypeptides not found in INV. Nine are glycoproteins, including the HA (Payne 1992). The predicted size of the HA (mol. wt 35 kDa, gene *A56R*) (Goebel et al. 1990) is less than is found in practice (89 kDa); the difference is due to extensive glycosylation.

1.7 Antigens

Cross-reactions between poxvirus genera are not easily detected and there is no cross-immunity. Nevertheless, early reports of an antigen common to all poxviruses and detectable in alkaline extracts of virions have been supported by workers using monoclonal antibodies (MAb) (Kitamoto et al. 1987). There is extensive antigenic cross-reaction between poxviruses of a particular genus. This can be detected by a variety of routine techniques, including cross-neutralization, and increasing use is being made of MAb.

Despite the importance of EEV in poxvirus immunity, work continues on INV. Differences found between this form in different species would certainly be of value in identification. INV is neutralized by antibody directed against a 35 kDa antigen (gene *H6L*), a 32 kDa antigen (gene *D8L*) and the 14 kDa fusion protein (gene *A27L*) (Rodriguez and Smith 1990, Demkowicz, Maa and Esteban 1992). More detailed analysis of different orthopoxviruses with a panel of MAb has emphasized the complex and close relationship within this genus (Czerny et al. 1994). These workers detected 21 distinct sites on the surface of INV, 9 of them neutralizing, distributed among 19 isolates of 4 species (vaccinia, cowpox, ectromelia, monkeypox). There was extensive cross-reaction but the possibility of detecting species-specific epitopes is suggested by such studies. Attempts are now being made to assign the epitopes to individual proteins; 6 sites, 4 responsible for neutralization, have been mapped onto the 14 kDa fusion protein (Czerny et al. 1994). The outer envelope of EEV has important antigenic sites through which it, but not INV, can be neutralized. The surface components of EEV have been characterized in some detail and the encoding genes identified. Even so, although antigenic sites have been recognized (Payne 1992) and some biological functions determined (Smith 1993), it is uncertain which particular epitopes elicit neutralizing antibody; the HA epitope is unlikely to be involved because antisera made against HA-negative viruses have neutralizing activity.

Because sites on EEV are important for cross-immunity between species, common neutralizing sites should be present on different species. It is of interest that the 42 kDa antigen encoded by gene *5BR* has been detected in different orthopoxviruses (Engelstad and Smith 1993), although the cross-neutralizing epitopes have not yet been identified.

2 CLINICAL AND PATHOLOGICAL ASPECTS

2.1 Introduction

Discussion of human poxvirus infections has always been dominated by the importance of smallpox. However, the last endemic case occurred in 1977 and in 1980 the WHO General Assembly accepted the conclusion of an independent international commission that smallpox had been eradicated. Smallpox virus is now restricted to 2 high security laboratories in the USA and Russia, and destruction of these stocks is debated regularly; in 1996, it was decided to destroy them in 1999. The importance of smallpox should not be forgotten. It had a marked impact on the development of civilization, was the first disease to be controlled by immunization, the first virus disease for which chemoprophylaxis was available, and the first to be eradicated. Smallpox is, however, mentioned here only to emphasize the importance of surveillance/containment rather than mass vaccination in the eradication programme. Those seeking authoritative information are directed to the excellent and detailed accounts by Hopkins (1983) and Fenner et al. (1988), which cover all aspects of smallpox including its history, its epidemiological and clinical features and the global eradication campaign.

Although conducted well before the use of properly controlled experiments, the investigations by Jenner and his contemporaries set historic precedents (Baxby 1981). In particular, attempts to evaluate the properties of 'true' and 'spurious' cowpox initiated important studies on the comparative epidemiological, clinical and immunological features of poxvirus zoonoses that still continue.

With smallpox eradicated, the remaining human poxvirus infections, with the exception of molluscum, are acquired directly or indirectly from infected animals. Although the clinical impact and incidence of these human infections are relatively low, they can cause considerable inconvenience, occasional serious infections and sometimes death.

Capripoxvirus infections are of considerable importance and, although parapox, fowlpox and camelpox infections are not perhaps as important as foot-and-mouth disease or rinderpest, they do cause considerable economic losses in communities dependent on the host species. Ectromelia can cause considerable disruption if accidentally introduced into laboratory mouse colonies, and the use of myxomatosis to control wild rabbits in Australia was an interesting failure with particular relevance to the evolution of host–parasite relations.

Although work continues on natural poxvirus infections in the field (Baxby 1988), laboratory studies are now increasingly focused on the role that particular gene products play in specific and non-specific immunity and pathogenesis. Some epidemiological and clinical information on poxvirus infections of human and veterinary importance is provided in Table 21.3; vaccinia is not listed but will be referred to where appropriate.

2.2   Clinical manifestations

Reservoir and indicator hosts

Although some poxviruses cause species-specific diseases (e.g. camelpox, swinepox), others, particularly cowpox virus, have a wide host range and the characteristics of the disease may depend on the host species infected. This perhaps reaches the extreme with ectromelia (mousepox), an infection of laboratory mice, in which exposure to virus can result in no infection, very mild but naturally transmissible infection, or severe lethal infection, depending on the genotype of the mice (Buller and Wallace 1988). In the case of cowpox, more is known about the disease in indicator (accidental) hosts than in the reservoir hosts in which the virus is maintained.

Nature of the lesions

Poxvirus infections are generally characterized by skin lesions. Nevertheless, despite the attention focused on smallpox and vaccinia, there is some variety in the nature of the lesions produced by members of the family,

and to regard those produced by any particular poxvirus as 'typical' is unrealistic.

Lesions produced by orthopoxviruses (particularly in humans) and by swinepox virus are seen first as macules and progress through papules, vesicles and pustules to crusts that separate leaving a scar (Kasza 1986, Fenner et al. 1988, Jezek and Fenner 1988). The bulk of the lesion is composed of some dermal proliferation, oedema and particularly leucocyte infiltration. Parapox, capripox, fowlpox and tanapox viruses tend to produce proliferative lesions with a granulomatous or nodular appearance, particularly obvious in lumpy skin disease (Davies 1991). In some instances parapoxviruses produce very large, long-lasting papillomatous lesions in human and animal patients. The term 'malignant' is sometimes used to describe capripox infections but in this context it indicates severity of infection rather than any particular pathological process. Molluscum and myxomatosis are characterized by the production of benign tumours. In the case of myxomatosis the lesions are larger and more obvious in *Oryctolagus*, originally an unnatural reservoir host, than in *Sylvilagus*, the natural reservoir (Fenner and Ratcliffe 1965).

Distribution of lesions

In most poxvirus infections, however acquired, multiple lesions are produced which tend to be distributed generally. In some (e.g. human tanapox), multiple lesions are uncommon (Jezek et al. 1985). In others, lesions may be concentrated in some areas, as with fowlpox in which lesions are often concentrated on the head and in the upper respiratory tract (Jordan 1982, Randall and Gafford 1994), and capripox in which they may be concentrated on the head and genitals (Kitching and Taylor 1985). Parapoxvirus infections and human cowpox are typically acquired by inoculation and, although multiple lesions may be produced by several inoculations, usually only one is produced (Johanneson et al. 1975, Baxby, Bennet and Getty 1994); in animal parapoxvirus infections they are typically found on the mouth, teats, or both (Robinson and Balassu 1981, Tripathy, Hanson and Crandell 1981). Although a primary lesion occurs in feline cowpox at the site of infection, generalized lesions develop subsequently (Bennett et al. 1990).

Severity of infection

Infections such as camelpox, capripox and human monkeypox are usually severe and have an appreciable mortality (Kriz 1982, Kitching and Taylor 1985, Fenner et al. 1988). These are generalized infections and internal organs, particularly the lungs, are affected. There is, however, not necessarily a correlation between the number of lesions and systemic **infection** on the one hand and the presence of such non-specific systemic **responses** as pyrexia, malaise and general debility on the other. Systemic infection occurs with swinepox and feline cowpox but systemic responses are relatively mild and recovery is the usual outcome. Although multiple and long-lasting lesions may occur in molluscum, the infection is rarely more

Table 21.3 Some characteristics of poxvirus infections of human and veterinary importance

Disease[a]	Natural hosts[b]	Distribution[c]	Transmission[d]	Comment[e]
Smallpox	Human	Eradicated	A, (F)	Severe generalized infection. Formerly world-wide, eradication certified 1980
Molluscum	Human	World-wide	C, F	Multiple skin lesions. Often sexually transmitted
Cowpox	Human (H), cats (Fe), cattle (B), rodents (R)	Europe, W CIS	H, B: C, F Fe, R: C, F, A	H: rare zoonosis, painful haemorrhagic ulcer. Fe: generalized infection. B: rare. R: presumed mild or asymptomatic
Monkeypox	Human, squirrel (R) monkey (?)	W Africa, esp. Zaire	H: A, C, F R: (A, C, F?)	H: rare zoonosis, generalized infection with 15% mortality. R: epidemiology, pathogenesis little studied, role of monkey uncertain
Buffalopox	Human, buffalo (R?)	India	H: C, F R: C, F	H: occupational hazard, painful skin lesion. R: epidemiology little studied, virus a subspecies of vaccinia
Orf/paravaccinia	Human, sheep (S, R), goats (G, R) cattle (B, R)	World-wide	H: C, F R: C, F, (Ap?)	H: common occupational hazard, relatively painless granulomatous lesions, reinfection occurs. S, G: scabby oral lesions in young interfere with feeding. B: 'ring-sore' on teats. Vaccine available
Tanapox	Human, monkeys (R)	E Africa	H, R: C, F	H: nodular, usually single, lesion with pyrexia
Capripox	Sheep (R), goat (R)	Africa, Asia	A, C, (Ap?)	R: serious generalized infection. Viruses probably represent host range variants of one species. Vaccine available
Lumpy skin disease	Cattle (B, R) goats (G), sheep (S)	Africa	C, F, Ap	B: multiple nodular skin lesions. Natural transmission to S, G rare. Vaccine available
Camelpox	Camel	M East, Africa	A, C, F	Severe generalized infection
Ectromelia	Laboratory mice	World-wide	C, F	Pathogen of laboratory mouse. Disease dependent on virus strain and host genotype
Myxomatosis	Rabbit	Americas, Europe, Australia	C, Ap, F	Benign tumours in original reservoir (*Sylvilagus*), fluctuating equilibrium but generally more severe in Australian and European reservoirs (*Oryctolagus*)
Swinepox	Pigs	World-wide	C, Ap, F	Generalized infection. Has also been caused by vaccinia virus
Fowlpox	Fowl (R), birds	World-wide	C, Ap, F, A	R: dermal infections and more severe respiratory disease. Vaccine available

[a]Arranged into human only, zoonotic, and non-human. See Table 21.1 for taxonomic position of viruses.
[b]R, reservoir. Other abbreviations used to identify hosts in other columns.
[c]CIS, Commonwealth of Independent States (former USSR); E, East, M, Middle; W, West. Zoonotic infections may occur anywhere in experimental animal handlers.
[d]A, close air-borne; Ap, mechanical transmission by arthropods: mosquito and rabbit flea (myxomatosis), lice (swinepox), various (others); C, contact (inoculation or infection via broken skin); F, fomites (utensils, bedding etc.).
[e]Abbreviations as in footnotes b and d.

than an inconvenience. A similar contrast can be seen in infections that produce single lesions. Human cowpox is a relatively severe infection with very painful lesions and considerable constitutional disturbance, whereas human parapox infection is surprisingly painless with little systemic reaction (Baxby, Bennett and Getty 1994).

Variation in the severity of myxomatosis in the European rabbit (*Oryctolagus*) is of interest. When the disease was first introduced into Australia it had a devastating effect, but within a few years less virulent strains of virus emerged naturally. At the same time, innate genetic resistance developed in the rabbit population. Thus a reasonably stable equilibrium has resulted which may temporarily favour the host, then the parasite. It is agreed that myxomatosis will not eradicate the rabbit but the exercise is a valuable experiment in evolution which still continues (Fenner 1983, Ross and Sanders 1987).

2.3 Epidemiology

GEOGRAPHICAL AND SEASONAL DISTRIBUTION

Although some poxviruses are geographically restricted, others are found world-wide (Table 21.3). This knowledge may be of value in diagnosis, but human infections may be acquired from experimentally infected animals wherever they are studied. The present-day distribution of viruses reflects the distribution of the reservoir hosts but is also affected by some of the early control programmes. For example, capripoxvirus infections no longer occur in Europe and parapoxvirus infections were presumably introduced into Australasia before adequate quarantine measures were implemented. The geographical restriction of cowpox and monkeypox is also related to the distribution of reservoir hosts and is discussed under 'Host range', below. Seasonal distribution of disease may be affected by differences in seasonal activity of the reservoir hosts and any arthropod vectors. Thus parapoxvirus infections tend to be more common during lambing and calving seasons. Similar effects occur with capripox infections, but may be obscured by poor animal husbandry that introduces infected animals into susceptible herds. Human and feline cowpox are most common in July–November (Baxby Bennett and Getty 1994) when the probable reservoir hosts are most active. Infections for which arthropod transmission is particularly important (e.g. myxomatosis and swinepox) occur most frequently when the vector is active.

HOST RANGE

Some poxviruses (e.g. molluscum, swinepox and camelpox viruses) are very host-specific; others have a wider host range (Table 21.3). The extreme is probably represented by cowpox virus, which infects a wide range of indicator hosts, including humans, cows, domestic and exotic captive cats, and captive elephants and rhinoceros (Pilaski 1988, Bennett et al. 1990, Baxby, Bennett and Getty 1994). When the reservoir hosts are closely related, cross-infection with related viruses may influence virus classification and nomenclature. Thus the early literature refers to sheeppox and goatpox, and sheeppox and goatpox viruses are listed as separate species. Nevertheless, the viruses cross-infect, producing very similar infections, and workers particularly interested in these viruses and the diseases they cause tend to regard them as host range variants of one virus type, capripoxvirus (Kitching and Taylor 1985, Kitching Hammond and Taylor, 1987). Early workers on cowpox and monkeypox viruses failed to appreciate the important difference between reservoir and indicator hosts, and these viruses were given inappropriate names. In the case of cowpox, bovine infection is very rare and the domestic cat is the most commonly detected victim. The likely reservoir hosts are rodents, and include susliks and gerbils in the former USSR (Marennikova, Shelukhina and Efremova 1984) and probably bank voles and woodmice in Britain (Crouch et al. 1995). Monkeypox virus was so named because it was isolated from captive Asiatic monkeys. Human monkeypox has, however, been detected only in Africa, particularly Zaire, and more recent studies suggest that squirrels are important reservoir hosts (Khodakevich et al. 1987, Richardson and Dumbell 1994). Although a subspecies of vaccinia has become established as the cause of buffalopox in India (Dumbell and Richardson 1993) it is not known whether wildlife reservoirs are involved.

TRANSMISSION

Poxvirus infections are transmitted naturally in a variety of ways and several routes may be involved in the transmission of one infection among one host species (Table 21.3). Air-borne transmission is relatively uncommon and occurs only over very short distances. Transmission by direct contact probably occurs to some extent in all poxvirus infections, but at least minor trauma that inoculates virus directly into the superficial layers of the skin is necessary to establish infection. Indirect transmission via fomites is also probably very common, but again virus must be implanted in order to infect. Such transmission may be over short distances, as would happen with contaminated bedding etc., but occasionally involves indirect spread as when parapox and cowpox infections are spread via utensils or veterinary surgeons' instruments. Molluscum may be transferred during contact sports or by sharing of contaminated towels but there is evidence that some cases are sexually transmitted (Postlethwaite 1970, Brown, Nalley and Kraus 1981).

In this context, arthropods are also fomites but they are treated separately in Table 21.3 because of their importance, particularly in the transmission of swinepox and myxomatosis. In the latter instance differences in the behaviour of rabbit fleas and mosquitoes explain the different rates of spread of myxomatosis in Europe and Australia (Fenner and Ratcliffe 1965). In distinguishing between arthropods and non-viable fomites it must be remembered that the virus does not replicate in the arthropod, which acts as a mechanical vector only. Under field conditions it may be extremely difficult to assess the relative importance of the various modes of transmission.

2.4   Pathogenesis

GENERAL CONSIDERATIONS

Poxviruses are dermatotropic, producing lesions in which epidermal proliferation, leucocyte infiltration or both are prominent features. In generalized infections a viraemia transfers virus to internal organs, particularly the lungs, and considerable damage is done during the incubation period and before the skin lesions develop. During the viraemic phase the virus is concentrated in the white cell fraction, but myxoma and malignant rabbit fibroma are probably unique among poxviruses in that the virus replicates in the lymphocytes. In localized infections the extent to which virus spreads to, and is controlled within, local and regional lymph nodes probably determines the extent of systemic reaction, and perhaps explains the relative severity of human cowpox and mild nature of human parapox infections. In molluscum the lesion is circumscribed and rarely penetrates the dermis; this again probably explains the relatively mild nature of the infection. In all cases it is important to note the overwhelming importance of EEV for the dissemination of individual virions both from cell to cell and by viraemia (Payne 1980).

GENE PRODUCTS AFFECTING PATHOGENESIS

Early attempts to investigate the virulence of vaccinia virus indicated that it was a complex multifactorial system. This has proved to be so, and there has been considerable progress in identifying the genes and gene products that contribute to virulence (see Table 21.2). Myxoma and vaccinia viruses have been particularly studied, but some effects have been extended by analysis or analogy to other poxviruses. This complex topic has been the subject of recent excellent reviews (Buller and Palumbo 1991, Smith 1993, Smith 1994, McFadden and Graham 1994, McFadden, Graham and Opgenorth 1994, Mossman, Barry and McFadden 1994, Smith and Goodwin 1994).

The term **viroceptor** refers to virus gene products that have functional homology with cellular receptors of cytokines and so inhibit cytokine-induced defence mechanisms. Poxviruses express soluble receptors for interleukin-1β (Alcami and Smith 1992), interferon-γ (IFN-γ) (Mossman, Barry and McFadden 1994) and tumour necrosis factor (Smith and Goodwin 1994) (see Table 21.2).

Recently, sequencing of several orthopoxvirus cognates of the cowpox virus Brighton tumour necrosis factor (TNF) receptor homologue, termed cytokine response modifier gene *crmB* (Pickup 1994), indicated that other cowpox strains and strains of monkeypox, camelpox, and variola virus contain *crmB* correlates that vary to about 80% identity, and that the gene is truncated or absent in various vaccinia and ectromelia strains (Loparev et al. 1996). The different genes encode a 348–360 amino acid secreted soluble glyco-

protein, CrmB, a cysteine-containing rich region that is 25% and 55% identical to parallel regions in human type-II TNF-receptor and the myxoma virus cognate, respectively. Selected virus cysteine-rich regions of CrmB expressed as *E. coli* fusion proteins formed multimers that bound human and murine TNF-α and lymphotoxin-α (LT-α) and blocked their ability to lyse mouse L cells in vitro. Interestingly, two other distinct TNF-binding homologues have been discovered: a 180-amino-acid protein of cowpox Brighton, termed CrmC (Smith et al. 1996), and a 320-residue protein of various ectromelia and cowpox strains termed CrmD (Loparev et al. 1996). A CrmC recombinant protein bound TNF-α but not LT-α and blocked TNF-α cytolysis in vitro. The CrmD protein, whether from virus-infected cells or synthesized *in vitro* as an *E. coli* fusion protein, bound both TNF-α and LT-α. The CrmD protein made in *E. coli* also inhibited the cytolytic activity of TNF-α and LT-α in an *in vitro* assay. Curiously, ectromelia virus CrmD appears to be produced 50-fold more abundantly than cowpox CrmD in cell cultures and antisera against a recombinant CrmD fusion protein partly blocked secondary plaque formation in ectromelia-infected cell monolayers, which suggests that CrmD might be on the surface of EEVs and might play a role in targeting virus to certain cells during infection in vivo.

The term **virokine** is used to describe virus gene products that have functional homology with cytokines and directly affect cellular functions in a similar way. Poxviruses express homologues of epidermal growth factor (EGF) (McFadden, Graham and Opnegorth 1994) and a vascular endothelial growth factor so far found only in orf virus (Lyttle et al. 1994). Other poxvirus gene products that have a relatively specific effect on host cell functions include a serine protease inhibitor (serpin) that inhibits cytokine activation and inflammation (Chua et al. 1990, Palumbo, Buller and Glasgow 1994), complement-binding proteins (Isaacs, Kotwal and Moss 1992) (see Table 21.2) and proteins that inhibit expression of MHC-I antigens at the cell surface (Boshkov, Macen and McFadden 1992). Although the above-mentioned are soluble proteins, structural proteins such as the 42 kDa envelope antigen also contribute to virulence (Engelstad and Smith 1993).

In general terms it is not difficult to envisage how the gene products mentioned above contribute to poxvirus pathogenesis by affecting specific and non-specific defence mechanisms. Their role has been demonstrated by showing that the virulence of strains not expressing a particular gene was diminished. Similarly, TK- and HA-negative strains also tend to be of diminished virulence in some circumstances. Nevertheless, it is difficult to assess the relative importance of the various gene products in different viruses. For example, most poxviruses produce a soluble EGF which probably contributes to virulence by promoting cell proliferation, and one might expect this factor to play a more important role in diseases such as myxomatosis in which cell proliferation is most marked (McFadden and Graham 1994). Despite the putative roles of individual gene products, co-operation is also essential with at least 3 gene products needed for inflammation (Palumbo, Buller and Glasgow 1994). The role of host species is also important, and much experimental work is done in hosts that are unnatural for the virus concerned. In that respect, studies on myxoma virus in rabbits are particularly important, and it is of interest that the IFN-γ and TNF receptors of myxoma virus act only on rabbit cells (Schreiber and McFadden 1994, Mossman, Upton and McFadden 1995). This is a fast moving area of research which is likely to produce much interesting information in the near future.

2.5 Immune responses

HUMORAL RESPONSES

Antigenic responses to poxvirus infection can be measured by several techniques, including the virus neutralization test, which has been used to measure immunity in vitro. Unfortunately, until the early 1970s the test virus was the artificially extracted INV form, whereas it is the additional antigens on the surface of naturally released EEV that are important (Boulter and Appleyard 1973, Payne 1980). The sera of animals inoculated with inactivated virus neutralize INV but not EEV, and such animals do not resist challenge. These observations explain the poor performance of inactivated poxvirus vaccines. INV is neutralized through 14, 32 and 35 kDa surface antigens (see section 1.7, p. 374) and EEV probably through the 42 kDa outer envelope antigen. It is interesting that mice inoculated with the 62 kDa (gene *A10L*) and 39 kDa (gene *A4L*) core antigens develop immunity (Demkowicz, Maa and Esteban 1992). Evidence that the humoral response is important comes from vaccination responses in individuals with B cell deficiencies, and therapeutic and experimental studies involving passive immunization (see, e.g., Cole and Blanden 1982). The humoral response tends to be related to the degree of lymphadenopathy, and localized infection may not stimulate sufficient response to prevent or even attenuate reinfection (see, e.g., Robinson and Balassu 1981, Baxby 1993b). Antibodies may be detected years after infection but, depending on the techniques used, may not reflect persistence of EEV neutralizing antibody (Nakano and Esposito 1989, Demkowicz, Maa and Esteban 1992).

CELL-MEDIATED RESPONSES

Virus antigens are expressed on the surface of infected cells and one would expect cell mediated immunity (CMI) to be important. However, antibody-dependent lysis of infected cells also plays an important role (Perrin, Zinkernagel and Oldstone 1977). Evidence for the importance of CMI comes from observations on immunodeficient vaccinees and experimental observations, particularly in mice. Although delayed hypersensitivity has generally been detected, the response of cytotoxic T lymphocytes (CTLs) would be expected to be more important. In mice with ectromelia, cytotoxic CMI plays the major role in recovery from infection (Cole and Blanden 1982, Buller and Wallace 1988), but results with other infections and host species are not easy to interpret. In lambs infected with orf there is relatively little CMI as measured by lymphoproliferative responses, whereas in human infection there is a vigorous proliferative response that quickly declines (Yirrell et al. 1989, Yirrell, Vestey and Norval 1994). These observations are consistent with the relatively poor immunity to reinfection observed in both host species. Although proliferative responses can be detected in smallpox vaccinees, limited attempts to detect CTLs in peripheral human blood after smallpox vaccination and revaccination proved unsuccessful. In the former case activity was thought to be due to non-specific 'killer' cells, and in the latter no CTL activity was detected; it is of course possible that CTLs are present in the spleen, lymph nodes or both (Perrin, Zinkernagel and Oldstone 1977, Graham et al. 1991). Experiments with vaccinia in mice indicated that the antigens that stimulate proliferative responses include the 32 kDa and 14 kDa fusion protein through which INV is neutralized (Demkowicz, Maa and Esteban 1992). Experiments with recombinant poxviruses suggest that antigens controlled by early promoters are important for induction of CMI (Coupar et al. 1986, Limbach and Paoletti 1996).

2.6 Diagnosis

CLINICAL DIAGNOSIS

The keys to the clinical diagnosis of poxvirus infections are appreciation of the importance of: the geographical distribution and host range of the viruses; epidemiological factors such as seasonal influence, contact with perhaps unusual animals, and possible transmission routes; clinical features such as nature, location and number of lesions and presence of any systemic reaction; and any factors (e.g. immunosuppression, eczema) that might exacerbate infection.

LABORATORY DIAGNOSIS

A satisfactory clinical diagnosis can often be made if adequate attention is paid to the information listed above. In other cases laboratory confirmation may be needed, and the importance of using electron microscopy (EM) sooner rather than later is emphasized; in some countries it may be used to distinguish poxvirus infection from foot-and-mouth disease or rinderpest. The characteristic morphology of parapoxviruses also permits a rapid differential diagnosis of capripox and parapox infections in sheep, goats and cattle and of camelpox and ausdyk in camels. In human infections EM allows rapid distinction between parapoxvirus and other virus infections; if putative orthopoxviruses are seen, clinical and epidemiological data would suggest whether the infection is cowpox, monkeypox, buffalopox or molluscum. In experienced hands and with suitable specimens, EM can be extremely sensitive; in a survey of human cowpox only 1 of 24 cases was missed when suitable material was available (Baxby, Bennett and Getty 1994). In one extreme case, clinical acumen and EM could have prevented unnecessary amputation (Johanneson et al. 1975). Laboratory diagnosis of parapox infection is usually made only by EM, and the distinction between human orf and pseudocowpox (paravaccinia) may be based on appropriate animal contact if known; in Great Britain, human cases are routinely reported as orf-paravaccinia.

Biological tests (see 'Identification of species', p. 367) may be used to identify poxviruses isolated in cell culture or on the chick chorioallantois, but increasing use is made of DNA analysis. If patients are seen too late to allow detection of virus, a variety of routine techniques can be used to detect antibody (Tripathy et al. 1981, Fenner et al. 1988, Nakano and Esposito 1989).

2.7   Control

EPIDEMIOLOGICAL CONTROL

A considerable measure of epidemiological control of poxvirus infections can be obtained, but the results will depend on the nature of the infection and the diligence with which such efforts are applied (Baxby 1988). The following measures may be used to control animal infections.

1   Segregation of infected and susceptible animals. This will prevent both the spread of capripox and camelpox infections between animals from different herds held on common grazing land, and the spread of these and parapox infections by not allowing infected adults to suckle young.
2   Not housing or grazing susceptible animals on areas contaminated by previous infection. This will apply where such animals as fowl, pigs, cattle and mice are reared intensively.
3   Careful attention to hygiene. Proper use of teat dips and utensil disinfectants will reduce the spread of parapox infections.

Molluscum may be controlled by avoiding contact with infected individuals and their contaminated belongings. Zoonotic infection may be prevented by using knowledge of the sources of infection and modes of transmission (see Table 21.3). Human monkeypox may be controlled by interposing a buffer zone between the forest and cultivated land. Human cowpox, buffalopox and parapox infections can never be completely eliminated. The last 2 are occupational hazards of farm and abattoir workers,and all 3 of veter-

inary surgeons; the domestic cat is a common source of human cowpox. Person-to-person spread of monkeypox and parapox infections is, however, uncommon, and rarely if ever occurs with cowpox. No case of human cowpox has been acquired from a cat after the feline infection had been recognized and obvious preventive measures taken.

VACCINATION

Vaccines are routinely available for capripox, lumpy skin disease (LSD), fowlpox and orf. Smallpox vaccine may still be available but is not advocated for the routine control of human monkeypox. Its use for those working with orthopoxviruses is debatable. Different countries have adopted different policies based on conflicting conclusions about the severity and effects of routine vaccination (Baxby 1993b). Any routine recombinant vaccines that use vaccinia as a vector will be based on attenuated strains (Tartaglia et al. 1992).

The use of vaccines for animal infections has not reflected the success of smallpox vaccination. In some cases immunity is relatively short lived, but the importance of this factor is diminished by the relatively short lifespan of animal populations. Orf vaccine is given to adult females before lambing and to lambs within 48 h of birth. This offers a measure of protection to lambs during their vulnerable early life. The orf vaccine contains fully virulent virus, but lambs are partly protected from the virulent effects of the vaccine by passive immunity. However, spread to unvaccinated animals and their handlers must be avoided.

A variety of capripoxvirus vaccines has been used in the past, including both inactivated and fully virulent sheep and goatpox viruses. Considerable success has been achieved with an attenuated vaccine that controls capripox in both sheep and goats (Kitching, Hammond and Taylor 1987). Various LSD vaccines have also been used , and an attenuated LSD recombinant rinderpest vaccine that offers dual protection is of particular interest (Romero et al. 1994). There is need for more work on animal virus vaccines in general; and the use of attenuated recombinant species-specific pathogens such as parapox, capripox, LSD and fowlpox viruses to provide immunity both to the species-specific pathogen and to the poxvirus vector is an interesting future prospect.

REFERENCES

Alcami A, Smith GL, 1992, A soluble receptor for interleukin-1β encoded by vaccinia virus, *Cell*, **71**: 153–67.

Bagnall BG, Wilson GR, 1974, Molluscum contagiosum in a red kangaroo, *Aust J Derm*, **15**: 115–20.

Baldick CJ, Moss B, 1993, Characterization and temporal regulation of mRNAs encoded by vaccinia virus intermediate stage genes, *J Virol*, **67**: 3515–27.

Baxby D, 1981, *Jenner's Smallpox Vaccine*, Heinemann Educational, London.

Baxby D, 1988, Poxvirus infections in domestic animals, *Virus Diseases in Laboratory and Captive Animals*, ed Darai G, Martinus Nijhoff, Boston MA, 12–35.

Baxby D, 1993a, Recombinant poxvirus vaccines, *Rev Med Microbiol*, **4**: 80–8.

Baxby D, 1993b, Indications for smallpox vaccination: policies still differ, *Vaccine*, **11**: 395–6.

Baxby D, Bennett M, Getty B, 1994, Human cowpox 1969–93: a review based on 54 cases, *Br J Dermatol*, **131**: 598–607.

Bennett M, Gaskell CJ et al., 1990, Feline cowpox virus infection: a review, *J Small Anim Pract*, **31**: 167–73.

Binns M, Smith GL, eds, 1992, *Recombinant Poxviruses*, CRC Press, Boca Raton FL.

Boshkov LK, Macen JL, McFadden G, 1992, Virus-induced loss of class I MHC antigens from the surface of cells infected with myxoma virus and malignant rabbit fibroma virus, *J Immunol*, **148**: 881–7.

Boulter EA, Appleyard G, 1973, Differences between extracellular and intracellular forms of poxviruses and their implications, *Prog Med Virol*, **16**: 86–108.

Brown ST, Nalley JF, Kraus SJ, 1981, Molluscum contagiosum, *Sex Transm Dis*, **8**: 227–34.

Brown CK, Turner PC, Moyer RW, 1991, Molecular characterization of the vaccinia virus haemagglutinin gene, *J Virol*, **65**: 3598–606.

Buller RML, Palumbo GJ, 1991, Poxvirus pathogenesis, *Microbiol Rev*, **55**: 80–122.

Buller RML, Wallace G, 1988, Ectromelia [mousepox] virus, *Virus Diseases in Laboratory and Captive Animals*, ed Darai G, Martinus Nijhoff, Boston MA, 63–82.

Chang W, Hsiao J-C et al., 1995, Isolation of a monoclonal antibody which blocks vaccinia virus infection, *J Virol*, **69**: 517–22.

Chua TP, Smith CE et al., 1990, Inflammatory responses and the generation of chemoattractant activity in cowpox virus-infected cells, *Immunology*, **69**: 202–8.

Cole GA, Blanden RV, 1982, Immunology of poxviruses, *Comprehensive Immunology*, vol 9, eds Nahmias AJ, O'Reilly RJ, Plenum Press, New York, 1–19.

Coupar BEH, Andrew ME et al., 1986, Temporal regulation of influenza haemagglutinin expression in vaccinia virus. recombinants and effect on the immune response, *Eur J Immunol*, **16**: 1476–87.

Crouch A, Baxby D et al., 1995, Serological evidence for the reservoir hosts of cowpox virus in British wildlife, *Epidemiol Infect*, **115**: 185–91.

Cunningham AA, Langton TES et al., 1993, Unusual mortality associated with poxvirus-like particles in frogs (*Rana temporaria*), *Vet Rec*, **133**: 141–2.

Czerny CP, Johann S et al., 1994, Epitope detection in the envelope of intracellular naked orthopox viruses and identification of encoding genes, *Virology*, **200**: 764–77.

Davies FG, 1991, Lumpy skin disease: an African capripoxvirus disease of cattle, *Br Vet J*, **147**: 489–503.

Demkowicz WE, Maa JS, Esteban M, 1992, Identification and characterization of vaccinia virus genes encoding proteins that are highly antigenic in animals and are immunodominant in vaccinated humans, *J Virol*, **66**: 386–98.

Doms RW, Blumenthal R, Moss B, 1990, Fusion of intra-and extracellular forms of vaccinia virus with the cell membrane, *J Virol*, **64**: 4884–92.

Dubochet J, Adrian M et al., 1994, Structure of intracellular mature vaccinia virus observed by cryoelectron microscopy, *J Virol*, **68**: 1935–41.

Dumbell KR, 1989, *Poxviridae, Andrewes' Viruses of Vertebrates*, 5th edn, ed Porterfield JS, Ballière Tindall, London, 395–427.

Dumbell KR, Richardson M, 1993, Virological investigations of specimens from buffaloes affected by buffalopox in Maharashtra State, India, between 1985 and 1987, *Arch Virol*, **128**: 257–67.

Engelstad M, Smith GL, 1993, The vaccinia virus 42kDa envelope protein is required for envelopment and egress of extracellular virus and for virulence, *Virology*, **194**: 627–37.

Esposito JJ, Baxby D et al., 1995, *Poxviridae, Arch Virol*, **suppl 10**: 79–91.

Esposito JJ, Knight JC, 1985, Orthopoxvirus DNA: a comparison of restriction profiles and maps, *Virology*, **135**: 230–51.

Esposito JJ, Summer JW et al., 1992, Raccoon poxvirus rabies glycoprotein recombinant for wildlife oral vaccine, *Vaccine 92: modern approaches to new vaccines including prevention of AIDS*, eds Brown F, Chanock RM et al., Cold Spring Harbor Press, Cold Spring Harbor NY, 321–30.

Essani K, Dales S, 1979, Biogenesis of vaccinia: evidence for more than 100 polypeptides in the virion, *Virology*, **95**: 385–94.

Fenner F, 1983, Biological control as exemplified by smallpox eradication and myxomatosis, *Proc Roy Soc London, B*, **218**: 259–85.

Fenner F, Henderson DA et al., 1988, *Smallpox and its Eradication*, World Health Organization, Geneva.

Fenner F, Ratcliffe FN, 1965, *Myxomatosis*, Cambridge University Press, Cambridge.

Fenner F, Wittek R, Dumbell KR, 1989, *The Orthopoxviruses*, Academic Press, Orlando FL.

Fleming SB, Blok J et al., 1993, Conservation of gene structure and arrangement between vaccinia virus and orf virus, *Virology*, **195**: 175–84.

Gershon PD, Ansell DM, Black DN, 1989, A comparison of the genome organization of capripoxvirus with that of orthopoxviruses, *J Virol*, **63**: 4703–8.

Gershon PD, Black DN, 1988, A comparison of the genomes of capripoxvirus isolates of sheep, goats, and cattle, *Virology*, **164**: 341–9.

Gershon PD, Kitching RP et al., 1989, Poxvirus genetic recombination during natural virus transmission, *J Gen Virol*, **70**: 485–9.

Goebel SJ, Johnson GP et al., 1990, The complete DNA sequence of vaccinia virus, *Virology*, **179**: 247–66.

Graham S, Green CP et al., 1991, Human cytotoxic T cell responses to vaccinia virus infection, *J Gen Virol*, **72**: 1183–6.

Granados RR, 1981, Entomopoxvirus infections in insects, *Pathogenesis of Invertebrate Microbial Disease*, ed Davidson I, Allenheld Osmu, Totowa NJ, 101–29.

Harris WJ, Westwood JCN, 1964, Phosphotungstate staining of vaccinia virus, *J Gen Virol*, **34**: 491–5.

Hopkins DR, 1983, *Princes and Peasants: Smallpox in History*, University of Chicago Press, Chicago.

Horner RF, 1988, Poxvirus in farmed Nile crocodiles, *Vet Rec*, **122**: 459–62.

Ink BS, Gilbert CS, Evan GI, 1995, Delay of vaccinia virus-induced apoptosis in non permissive Chinese hamster ovary cells by the cowpox virus *CHOhr* and adenovirus *EIB* 19K genes, *J Virol*, **69**: 661–8.

Isaacs SN, Kotwal GJ, Moss B, 1992, Vaccinia virus complement-control protein prevents antibody-dependent complement-enhanced neutralization of infectivity and contributes to virulence, *Proc Natl Acad Sci USA*, **89**: 628–32.

Jacobson ER, Telford SR, 1990, Chlamydial and poxvirus infections of circulating monocytes of a flap-necked chameleon (*Chamaeleo dilepsis*), *J Wildl Dis*, **26**: 572–7.

Jezek Z, Fenner F, 1988, Human monkeypox, *Monogr Virol*, **17**: 1–140.

Jezek Z, Arita I et al., 1985, Human tanapox in Zaire: clinical and epidemiological observations on cases confirmed by laboratory studies, *Bull W H O*, **63**: 1027–35.

Johanneson JV, Krogh H-K, 1975, Human orf, *J Cutan Path*, **204**: 265–83.

Johnson GP, Goebel SJ, Paoletti E, 1993, An update on the vaccinia virus genome, *Virology*, **196**: 381–401.

Jordan FTW, 1982, Viral diseases, *Poultry Diseases*, 2nd edn, eds Gordon RF, Jordan FTW, Ballière Tindall, London, 118–23.

Kasza L, 1986, Swine pox, *Diseases of Swine*, 6th edn, eds Leman AD, Straw B et al., Iowa State University Press, Ames, 315–21.

Khodakevich L, Szczeniowski M et al., 1987, The role of squirrels in sustaining monkeypox transmission, *Trop Geogr Med*, **39**: 115–22.

Kitamoto N, Tanimoto S et al., 1987, Monoclonal antibodies to cowpox virus: polypeptide analysis of several major antigens, *J Gen Virol*, **68**: 239–46.

Kitching RP, Hammond JM, Taylor WP, 1987, A single vaccine for the control of capripoxvirus infection in sheep and goats, *Res Vet Sci*, **42**: 53–60.

Kitching RP, Taylor RP, 1985, Clinical and antigenic relationship between isolates of sheep and goat pox viruses, *Trop Anim Health Prod*, **17**: 64–74.

Knight JC, Goldsmith CS et al., 1992, Further analysis of the orthopoxviruses volepox virus and raccoon poxvirus, *Virology*, **190**: 423–33.

Kriz B, 1982, A study of camelpox in Somalia, *J Comp Pathol*, **92**: 1–8.

Limbach P, Paoletti E, 1996, Non-replicating expression vectors: applications in vaccine development and gene therapy, *Epidemiol Infect*, **116**: 241–6.

Loparev VN, Esposito JJ et al., 1996, Orthopoxvirus TNF-receptor isologs, Abstract W33-1, 10th International Congress of Virology, Jerusalem.

Lyttle DJ, Fraser KM et al., 1994, Homologs of vascular endothelial growth factor are encoded by the poxvirus orf virus, *J Virol*, **68:** 84–92.

Marennikova SS, Shelukhina EA, Efremova EV, 1984, New outlook on the biology of cowpox, *Acta Virol*, **57:** 461–4.

Massung J, Jayarama V, Moyer RW, 1993, Sequence analysis of conserved and unique regions of swinepox virus: identification of genetic elements supporting phenotypic observations including a novel G protein-coupled receptor homologue, *Virology*, **197:** 511–28.

Merchlinsky M, 1990, Resolution of poxvirus telomeres: processing of vaccinia virus concatemer junctions by conservative strand exchange, *J Virol*, **64:** 3437–46.

Meyer H, Pfeffer M, Rziha H, 1994, Sequence alterations within and downstream of the A-type inclusion protein genes allow differentiation of orthopoxvirus species by polymerase chain reaction, *J Gen Virol*, **75:** 1975–81.

McFadden G, Graham K, 1994, Modulation of cytokine networks by poxvirus: the myxoma virus model, *Semin Virol*, **5:** 421–9.

McFadden G, Graham K, Opgenorth A, 1994, Poxvirus growth factors, *Viroceptors, Virokines and Related Immune Modulators encoded by DNA Viruses*, ed McFadden G, R G Landes, Austin TX, 1–15.

McFadden G, Pace WE et al., 1979, Biogenesis of poxviruses: transitory expression of molluscum contagiosum early functions, *Virology*, **94:** 297–313.

Moss B, 1995, Poxviridae: the viruses and their replication, *Fields' Virology*, 3rd edn, eds Fields BN, Knipe DM et al., Raven Press, New York, .

Mossman K, Barry M, McFadden G, 1994, Interferon γ receptors encoded by poxviruses, *Viroceptors, Virokines and Related Immune Modulators Encoded by DNA Viruses*, ed McFadden G, R G Landes, Austin TX, 41–54.

Mossman K, Upton C, McFadden G, 1995, The myxoma virus-soluble interferon-γ receptor homolog M-T7, inhibits interferon-γ in a species-specific manner, *J Biol Chem*, **270:** 3031–8.

Moyer RW, 1987, The role of the host cell nucleus in vaccinia virus morphogenesis, *Virus Res*, **8:** 173–91.

Moyer RW, 1994, Entomopoxviruses, *Encyclopedia of Virology*, eds Webster RG, Granoff A, Academic Press, Orlando FL, 392–8.

Nagington J, Newton AA, Horne RW, 1964, The structure of orf virus, *Virology*, **23:** 461–72.

Naidoo J, Baxby D et al., 1992, Characterization of orthopoxviruses isolated from feline infections in Britain, *Arch Virol*, **125:** 261-72.

Nakano JH, Esposito JJ, 1989, Poxviruses, *Diagnostic Procedures for Viral, Rickettsial and Chlamydial Infections*, 6th edn, eds Schmidt NJ, Emmons RW, American Public Health Association, Washington DC, 224–65.

Osterhaus ADME, Broeders HWJ et al., 1990, Isolation of an orthopoxvirus from pox-like lesions of a grey seal (*Halichoerus grypus*), *Vet Rec*, **127:** 91–2.

Osterhaus ADME, Broeders HWJ et al., 1994, Isolation of a parapoxvirus from pox-like lesions in grey seals, *Vet Rec*, **135:** 601–2.

Palumbo GJ, Buller RM, Glasgow WC, 1994, Multigenic evasion of inflammation by poxviruses, *J Virol*, **68:** 1737–49.

Pastoret P-P, Brochier B et al., 1996, The development and use of a vaccinia-recombinant oral vaccine for the control of wildlife rabies, *Epidemiol Infect*, **116:** 235–40.

Payne LG, 1980, Significance of extracellular enveloped virus in the in vitro and in vivo dissemination of vaccinia, *J Gen Virol*, **50:** 89–100.

Payne LG, 1992, Characterization of vaccinia virus glycoproteins by monoclonal antibody precipitation, *Virology*, **187:** 251–60.

Perkus ME, Goebel SJ et al., 1991, Deletion of 55 open reading frames from the termini of vaccinia virus, *Virology*, **180:** 406–10.

Perrin LH, Zinkernagel RM, Oldstone MB, 1977, Immune response in humans after vaccination with vaccinia virus: generation of a virus-specific cytotoxic activity by human peripheral lymphocytes, *J Exp Med*, **146:** 949–69.

Pickup DJ, 1994, Poxviral modifiers of cytokine responses to infection, *Infect. Agents and Disease* 3: 116–27.

Pilaski J, 1988, Poxvirus infection in zoo-kept mammals, *Virus Diseases in Laboratory and Captive Animals*, ed. Darai G, Martinus Nijhoff, Boston MA, 83–100.

Porter CD, Archard LC, 1994, Molluscum contagiosum virus, *Encyclopedia of Virology*, eds Webster RG, Granoff A, Academic Press, Orlando FL, 848–53.

Postlethwaite R, 1970, Molluscum contagiosum: a review, *Arch Environ Health*, 21: 432–52.

Rahaley RS, Mueller RE, 1983, Molluscum contagiosum in a horse, *Vet Pathol*, **20:** 247–50.

Randall CC, Gafford LG, 1994, Fowlpox virus, *Encyclopedia of Virology*, eds Webster RG, Granoff A, Academic Press, Orlando FL, 497–503.

Richardson M, Dumbell KR, 1994, Comparisons of monkeypox viruses from animal and human infections in Zaire, *Trop Geogr Med*, **46:** 327–9.

Robinson AJ, Balassu TC, 1981, Contagious pustular dermatitis [orf], *Vet Bull*, **51:** 771–82.

Robinson AJ, Barnes G et al., 1987, Conservation and variation in orf virus genomes, *Virology*, **157:** 13–23.

Robinson AJ, Lyttle DJ, 1992, Parapoxviruses: their biology and potential as recombinant vaccines, *Recombinant poxviruses*, eds Binns MM, Smith GL, CRC Press, Boca Raton FL, 285–327.

Rodriguez JF, Smith GL, 1990, IPTG-dependent vaccinia virus: identification of a virus protein enabling virion envelopment by Golgi membranes and egress, *Nucleic Acids Res*, **18:** 5347–51.

Romero CH, Barrett T et al., 1994, Protection of cattle against rinderpest and lumpy skin disease with a recombinant capripoxvirus expressing the fusion protein gene of rinderpest virus, *Vet Rec*, **135:** 152–4.

Ropp SL, Jin Q et al., 1995, Polymerase chain reaction strategy for identification and differentiation of smallpox and other orthopoxviruses, *J Clin Microbiol*, **33:** 2069–76.

Ross J, Sanders MF, 1987, Changes in the virulence of myxoma virus in Britain, *Epidemiol Infect*, **98:** 113–17.

Russell RJ, Robbins SJ, 1989, Cloning and molecular characterization of the myxoma virus genome, *Virology*, **170:** 147–59.

Schmelz M, Sodeik B et al., 1994, Assembly of vaccinia virus: the second wrapping cisterna is derived from the transGolgi network, *J Virol*, **68:** 130–47.

Schnitzlein WM, Tripathy DK, 1991, Identification and nucleotide sequence of the thymidine kinase gene of swinepox virus, *Virology*, **181:** 727–32.

Scholz J, Rosen-Wolff A et al., 1989, Epidemiology of molluscum contagiosum using genetic analysis of the viral DNA, *J Med Virol*, **27:** 87–90.

Schreiber M, McFadden G, 1994, The myxoma virus TNF-receptor homologue (T2) inhibits tumor necrosis factor α in a species-specific fashion, *Virology*, **204:** 692–705.

Shchelkunov SN, Massung RF, Esposito JJ, 1995, Comparison of the genome DNA sequences of Bangladesh-1975 and India-1967 variola viruses, *Virus Res*, **36:** 107–18.

Smith CA, Goodwin RG, 1994, TNF receptors in the poxvirus family, *Viroceptors, Virokines and Related Immune Modulators Encoded by DNA Viruses*, ed McFadden G, R G Landes, Austin TX, 29–40.

Smith CA, Pickup DJ et al., 1996, Cowpox virus genome encodes a second soluble homologue of cellular TNF receptors, distinct from CrmB, that binds TNF but not LTα, *Virology* 223: 132–47.

Smith GL, 1993, Vaccinia virus glycoproteins and immune evasion, *J Gen Virol*, **74:** 1725–40.

Smith GL, 1994, Virus strategies for evasion of the host response to infection, *Trends Microbiol*, **2:** 81–8.

Smith GL, Moss B, 1983, Infectious poxvirus vectors have capacity for at least 25,000 base pairs of foreign DNA, *Gene*, **25**: 21–8.

Stauber E, Gogolewski R, 1990, Poxvirus dermatitis in a tegu lizard (*Tupinambis teguixin*), *J Zoo Wildl Med*, **21**: 228–30.

Tartaglia J, Perkus ME et al., 1992, NYVAC: a highly attenuated strain of vaccinia virus, *Virology*, **188**: 217–32.

Tripathy DN, Hanson LE, Crandell RA, 1981, Poxviruses of veterinary importance: diagnosis of infections, *Comparative Diagnosis of Viral Diseases*, vol 3, eds Kurstak E, Kurstak C, Academic Press, Orlando FL, 267–346.

Ueda Y, Dumbell KR et al., 1978, Studies on Cotia virus, an unclassified poxvirus, *J Gen Virol*, **40**: 263–76.

Upton C, Macen JL et al., 1988, Tumorigenic poxviruses: fine analysis of the recombination junctions in malignant rabbit fibroma virus, a recombinant between Shope fibroma virus and myxoma virus, *Virology*, **166**: 229–39.

Whitehead SS, Hruby DE, 1994, Differential utilization of a conserved motif for the proteolytic maturation of vaccinia virus proteins, *Virology*, **200**: 154–61.

Wilson TM, Poglayen-Newall I, 1971, Pox in South American sea lions (*Otaria byronia*), *Can J Comp Med*, **35**: 174–7.

Wright CF, Keck JG, Moss B, 1991, Identification of factors specific for transcription of the late class of vaccinia virus genes, *J Virol*, **65**: 3715–20.

Yang WP, Bauer WR, 1988, Purification and characterization of vaccinia virus structural protein VP8, *Virology*, **167**: 578–84.

Yirrell DL, Reid HW et al., 1989, Immune response of lambs to experimental infection with orf virus, *Vet Immunol Immunopathol*, **22**: 321–32.

Yirrell DL, Vestey JP, Norval M, 1994, Immune response of patients to orf virus infection, *Br J Dermatol*, **130**: 438–43.

Yuen L, Moss B, 1987, Oligonucleotide sequence signalling transcriptional termination of vaccinia virus early genes, *Proc Natl Acad Sci USA*, **84**: 6417–21.

Zheng Z-M, Specter S et al., 1992, Further characterization of the biological and pathogenic properties of erythromelalgia-related poxviruses, *J Gen Virol*, **73**: 2011–19.

ORTHOMYXOVIRUSES: INFLUENZA

Nancy J Cox and Yoshihiro Kawaoka

1 INTRODUCTION

Influenza viruses are unique in their ability to cause recurrent epidemics and truly global pandemics during which acute febrile respiratory disease occurs explosively in all age groups. Excess hospitalization and death often accompany less serious but widespread morbidity during both influenza epidemics and pandemics.

Two features of influenza virus replication and evolution account for much of the epidemiological success of these viruses. First, there is the ability of novel influenza A viruses that have evolved and continue to circulate in avian or porcine reservoirs to emerge, either through genetic reassortment or through direct transmission, and spread in the human population at irregular intervals. Second, there is the relatively rapid and unpredictable antigenic change that accompanies the evolution of influenza viruses once they have become established in humans. Although influenza viruses have been studied intensively for more than 60 years and have often been used as a research model for other pathogens, much remains to be learned about influenza virus replication, pathogenicity, epidemiology and immunology.

1.1 Historical record

Influenza has probably existed from antiquity, although the lack of specific pathognomonic signs makes this assertion less definite than in the case of smallpox or cholera (Kilbourne 1987). Even so, historical records of rapidly spreading 'catarrhal fevers' in Great Britain (Table 22.1) suggest that major influenza epidemics affected human populations as early as the sixteenth century. Pandemic outbreaks are probably a more recent development, paralleling the increases in the world population and the growth of mass transportation systems. Animals may have played a leading role in past influenza epidemics. In the eighteenth and nineteenth centuries, for example, outbreaks of respiratory disease among horses were recorded concurrently with outbreaks in humans (Table 22.1). Although direct evidence for horse-to-human transmission of influenza viruses is lacking, the sizeable concentrations of these animals near previous centres of human population makes them attractive candidates as disease intermediaries (Hirsch 1883). In modern times, pigs have been accorded a prominent role in the generation of major influenza outbreaks (Goldfield et al. 1977, Scholtissek et al. 1985) (see 'Ecology of influenza', p. 414).

1.2 Seroarchaeology

Testing of sera from older adults for influenza virus antibodies (so-called seroarchaeology) suggests that the influenza in humans between 1889 and 1898 was caused by influenza A(H2N2) viruses (see section 2, p. 387), whereas epidemics or pandemics occurring in 1899–1917 and in 1918–1957 were the result of H3N8 and H1N1 viruses, respectively (Mulder and Masurel 1958, Masurel and Marine 1973, Noble 1982, Rekart et al. 1982, Masurel and Heijtink 1983) (Fig. 22.1). Recent pandemic strains share the haemagglutinin (HA) and neuraminidase (NA) subtypes of these earlier strains; however, they are probably not direct descendants, as they show a close relationship to avian viruses (Webster and Laver 1972, Scholtissek et al. 1978). Thus, the similarity of the HAs and NAs of recently circulating human viruses to those of the past may reflect certain properties of the surface molecules that favour viral replication in human hosts. Indeed, of the many HA and NA subtypes maintained in nature, only 3 have been identified in humans.

Table 22.1   Influenza: a summary of major epidemics affecting Great Britain and other regions of the world, 1510–1890

Epidemic year(s)	Season	Prevalence[a]	Temporally associated animal disease	Anomalous symptoms
1510	…	Pandemic	Murrain in cattle	'Gastrodynia'
1557	Autumn	Pandemic	…	Double tertian fever
1580	Autumn	European	Murrain in beasts (Kent)	Parotid swelling
1658	Spring	Britain, Europe	…	'Cephalic affection'
1675	Autumn	Britain, Europe	…	…
1688	…	Dublin	'Nasal defluxin' in horses	…
1693	Autumn	Britain, Europe	Antecedent nasal discharge in horses	…
1710	Spring	Britain, Europe	…	'Quick pulse'
1729	Winter	England, Europe	…	…
1732/3	Spring to winter	Pandemic	Cough in horses	Parotid swelling
1737/8	Autumn	England, Europe, North America	'Disease among horses'	…
1743	Spring	Britain, Europe	'Cough among horses'	…
1758	Autumn	North America, Europe, Britain	…	…
1762	Autumn	Britain, Europe	Antecedent 'horse colds' (1760)	Variable mortality
1767	Summer	Britain, Europe, North America	Dogs and horses, horse cold	…
1775	Autumn	Pandemic	Disease in dogs and horses	Prurigo, erysipelas, pustules
1782	Spring	Pandemic	…	…
1802/3	Spring	Britain, Europe	Cattle and domestic animals	'Interchanging with scarlatina'
1833	Spring	Pandemic	Concurrent disease in horses	…
1836/7	Winter	Pandemic	…	…
1847/8	Autumn	Pandemic	…	…
1889/90	Winter	Pandemic	…	Increased mortality age 20–60 (Jan. 1890)

From Kilbourne (1987).
[a]Pandemic implies historical evidence of involvement of more than two continents.

1.3   Virus isolation

The historical record of influenza viruses remained sparse until technological advances permitted their isolation. In 1901, a 'filterable agent' was isolated from chickens suffering from fowl plague (it was later classified by Schäfer (1955) as an influenza A virus). Smith, Andrewes and Laidlaw (1933) inoculated ferrets intranasally with human nasopharyngeal washes, which produced a form of influenza that spread to the animals' cage mates. The human virus [A/Wilson-Smith(WS)/33(H1N1)] was transmitted from an infected ferret to a junior investigator on the project (later Sir Charles Stuart-Harris), from whom it was subsequently re-isolated. An antigenically distinct virus, isolated by Francis (1940), was classified as a type B strain (B/Lee/40) to distinguish it from the 1933 isolate. The third major type of influenza virus, influenza C, was first isolated in 1947 by Taylor (1949).

1.4   Major research advances

Influenza research gained enormous momentum when it was shown that the virus could be isolated by

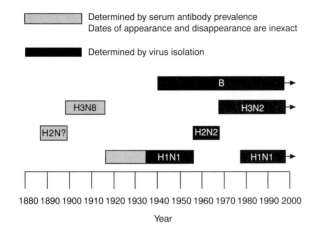

Determined by serum antibody prevalence
Dates of appearance and disappearance are inexact

Determined by virus isolation

Fig. 22.1 Eras of prevalence of influenza A and B viruses. The periods designated in black were defined by virus isolation while the periods designated in grey were approximated by determining serum antibody prevalence in retrospective serological studies.

inoculating samples into the chorioallantoic membrane of fertile hens' eggs (Francis and Magill 1937, Burnet 1940). Hirst (1941) and McClelland and Hare (1941) discovered that influenza virus particles agglutinate the erythrocytes of fowl as well as of other animal species. This advance established the concept of haemagglutinin inhibition in the detection of specific serum antibodies, making it possible to distinguish between viruses of the same type. Hirst (1950) further demonstrated the presence of a receptor-destroying enzyme, now known as neuraminidase. Later biochemical work (Gottschalk 1957) revealed that influenza viruses contain the HA and NA as major structural and antigenic components of the virus particle.

Subsequent advances included identification of the segmented nature of the RNA genome and assignment of corresponding protein products (McGeoch, Fellner and Newton 1976, Palese 1977); discovery of the antiviral compound amantadine (Davies et al. 1964); introduction of 'split' and subunit vaccines (Webster and Laver 1966); experimental work on cold-adapted vaccines (Maassab 1967); and elucidation of influenza gene replication (Inglis et al. 1979, Krug, Broni and Bouloy 1979, Lamb and Choppin 1979). More recently, the viral genome has been completely sequenced; the 3-dimensional structures of the HA (Wiley, Wilson and Skehel 1981) and the NA (Varghese, Laver and Colman 1983) have been resolved by x-ray crystallography; the ion channel activity of the M2 protein discovered (Sugrue et al. 1990, Pinto, Holsinger and Lamb 1992); and the reverse genetics technique established (Luytjes et al. 1989). Despite this progress, much remains to be learned about influenza viruses, particularly the molecular mechanism of influenza pathogenesis, interaction between viral and host gene products and the mechanisms giving rise to new pandemic strains.

2 CLASSIFICATION

The *Orthomyxoviridae* family consists of 4 genera: influenza virus A, influenza virus B, influenza virus C, and Thogotovirus which includes the Thogoto and Dhori viruses (Klenk et al. 1995, ICTV Executive Committee 1996). Orthomyxoviruses (Greek: *orthos*, straight or correct; *myxa*, mucus) contain segmented, linear and negative-sense (complementary to mRNA) single-stranded RNA. The number of RNA segments differs among the genuses: 8 for influenza A and B, 7 for influenza C, 6 for Thogoto virus, and probably 7 for Dhori virus. Accordingly, influenza A and B viruses contain HA and NA activities in different glycoproteins, whereas influenza C viruses lack NA, containing instead a haemagglutinin–esterase fusion protein (HEF). Thogoto and Dhori viruses possess a single glycoprotein (GP) that is not related to any known influenza virus protein but is related to the gp64 glycoprotein of baculoviruses (Morse, Marriott and Nuttall 1992). The virion has a molecular weight of 250 000 kDa and buoyant density in aqueous sucrose of 1.19 g/cm³. Virions are sensitive to heat, lipid solvents, non-ionic detergents, formaldehyde, irradiation and oxidizing agents.

Influenza A viruses are further classified into subtypes based on the antigenicity of their HA and NA molecules. Currently, there are 15 recognized HA subtypes (H1, H2, etc.) and 9 NA subtypes (N1, N2, etc.). The full nomenclature (WHO Memorandum 1980) for each new isolate includes the type of virus, the host of origin (except for human), geographical site of isolation, strain number and year of isolation. The antigenic description of the HA and NA is given in parentheses. For example, a type A virus isolated in Memphis, Tennessee, from a mallard duck in 1995 with a strain number of 123 and an H3N8 subtype would be designated A/mallard/Memphis/123/95 (H3N8). So far, no antigenic subtypes have been identified among the influenza B and C viruses. Thogoto and Dhori viruses do not cross-react antigenically.

3 MORPHOLOGY AND STRUCTURE

All influenza viruses have a segmented negative-sense RNA core surrounded by a lipid envelope (Fig. 22.2). The A and B types are distinguished by 2 integral membrane glycoproteins, HA and NA, that protrude from the virion surface. Influenza C virus, by contrast, contains only one type of membrane glycoprotein, HEF. Within the lipid envelope exists the matrix (M1) protein. The RNA segments are associated with nucleoprotein (NP) and 3 large polymerase proteins, designated PA, PB1 and PB2 on the basis of their overall acidic or basic amino acid composition, that are responsible for RNA replication and transcription (Krug et al. 1989).

Influenza virus particles are pleomorphic (Hoyle 1968) (Fig. 22.3). Among clinical isolates that have undergone a limited number of passages in eggs or tissue culture, there are more filamentous than spher-

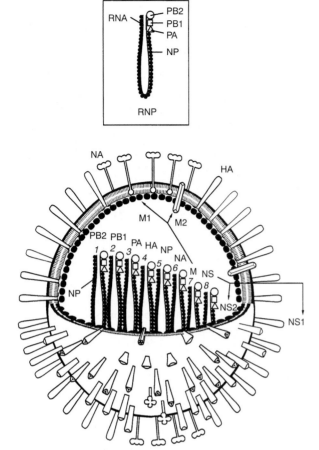

Fig. 22.2 Schematic diagram of an influenza A virion. The virion contains haemagglutinin (HA) and neuraminidase (NA) spikes in addition to a third membrane protein, M2. Within the viral envelope one finds ribonucleoprotein (RNP) consisting of RNA segments associated with nucleoprotein (NP), and the PA, PB1 and PB2 polymerase proteins. Three polymerase proteins are associated with RNP at its end (insert). The precise location of M1 in virions is unknown, although it is associated with virion envelope, RNP and NS2. (Courtesy of Dr R G Webster.)

ical particles, whereas extensively passaged laboratory strains consist almost exclusively of spherical virions (80–120 nm diam.). Despite their distinctive shape, the filamentous virions possess many of the serological, haemagglutinating and enzymatic characteristics of the spherical particles. The morphology of influenza virions seems to be determined by the M gene, although both the HA and the NP genes may contribute (Smirnov, Kuznetsova and Kaverin 1991).

The HA and NA molecules that stud the surface of influenza A and B viruses range from 10 to 12 nm in length (mean ratio of HA to NA spikes, c. 5:1). The HA spikes are rod-shaped, whereas the NA spikes resemble mushrooms with slender stalks (Fig. 22.4). They are not distinguishable by electron microscopy unless either the HA or the NA is removed from the virion surface with a protease or rosettes of the HA and NA are formed after virions are treated with detergent. The NA distribution on virions remains uncertain. If the HA is removed with trypsin, the NA

seems to be evenly distributed (Erickson and Kilbourne 1980); however, by immunoelectron microscopy with monoclonal antibodies, but not polyclonal antibodies, it seems to be clustered (Murti and Webster 1986, Amano et al. 1992). The HEF glycoproteins on influenza C viruses (8–10 nm long) are organized as hexagonal arrays of lattice-like structures on the virion surface (Flewett and Apostolov 1967, Hewat et al. 1984) (Fig. 22.5).

Within the lipid envelope, the viral RNA is associated with NP and 3 polymerase proteins, PA, PB1 and PB2. The organization of this ribonucleoprotein (RNP) complex within virions remains unclear. Electron microscopy has revealed helical structures in spontaneously lysed virions and in those partially disrupted with detergent (Fig. 22.6). Similar structures can be made only with use of purified M1 protein (Ruigrok, Calder and Wharton 1989), indicating a significant role for this component in the generation of the RNP complex, with which M1 is known to associate (Kawakami and Ishihama 1983). Isolated RNP forms rod-shaped, right-handed helices that vary in length from 50 to 150 nm (Compans, Content and Duesberg 1972). The 5′ and 3′ terminal ends of viral RNA, which are complementary to each other, form a panhandle-like structure (Hsu et al. 1987). All 3 polymerase proteins are associated with only one end of each RNP complex (Murti, Webster and Jones 1988).

The M1 protein is thought to add rigidity to the lipid bilayer, but direct evidence for this role is lacking. Immunogold labelling with monoclonal antibodies to M1 failed to decorate the protein in virions unless they were first treated with a protease or a detergent (Murti et al. 1992). Recent cryoelectron microscopic studies suggest that M1 can modify the lipid bilayer, causing thickening of the viral envelope (Fujiyoshi et al. 1994) (see Fig. 22.3d).

4 GENOME STRUCTURE AND FUNCTION

Influenza A and B viruses possess 8 single-stranded RNA segments, each encoding at least one protein, whereas influenza C viruses contain only 7 segments. Genome lengths differ widely among the 3 types of influenza viruses, some variations also being found among strains within the same type. Type B viruses have the longest genome (c. 14 600 nt) followed by A (c. 13 600 nt) and then C (c. 12 900 nt). Within each type the lengths of genes other than the HA and NA (for A and B viruses) and the HEF (for C viruses) are highly conserved. The viral genome constitutes 2% of the mass of the virion.

In each of the 8 RNA segments of all influenza A viruses, the first 12 nucleotides at the 3′ end and the last 13 at the 5′ end are highly conserved and form a panhandle that contains promoter activity (Parvin et al. 1989, Yamanaka et al. 1991, Li and Palese 1992, Seong and Brownlee 1992a, 1992b, Piccone, Fernandez-Sesma and Palese 1993, Fodor, Pritlove and Brownlee 1994, 1995, Neumann and Hobom 1995)

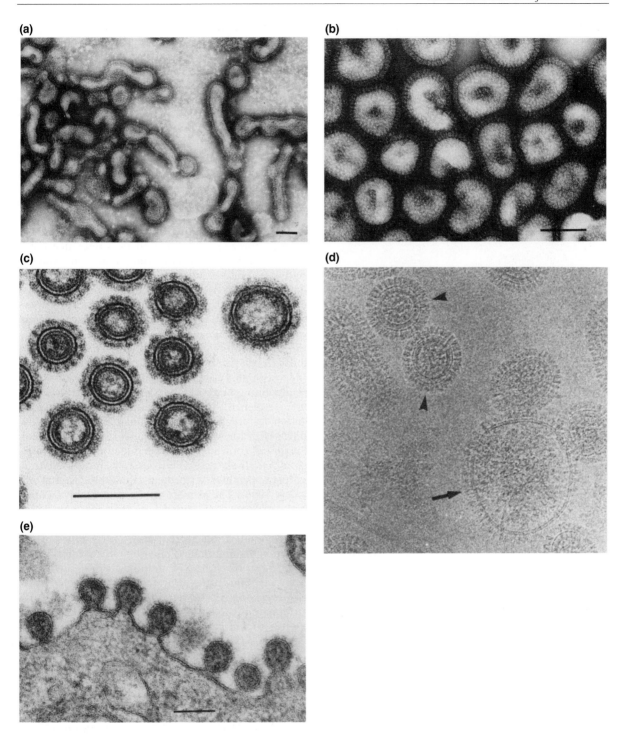

Fig. 22.3 Influenza A virus visualized by transmission electron microscopy. Two types of negatively stained virions are apparent: (**a**) filamentous and pleomorphic and (**b**) largely spherical. Bar = 100 nm. (Courtesy of Dr KG Murti.) (**c**) Sectioned virions with internal structures exposed. Bar = 100 nm. (**d**) High-resolution electron micrograph of influenza virus. Note the 2 distinct types of virions: those with thick membranes (arrowhead) and those with typical thin lipid bilayers (arrow). The former group possess more M1 proteins than do the latter. (Courtesy of Dr Y Fujiyoshi and Dr S Sato; from Fujiyoshi et al. 1994.) (**e**) Virus budding from plasma membrane. Bar = 100 nm.

(Fig. 22.7). Similar structures have been identified in the RNA segments of influenza B (conserved sequence: 5′ AGUAG(A/U)AACAA and 3′ UCGUCUUCGC) and C (conserved sequence: 5′ AGCAGUAGCAA and 3′ UCGU(U/C)UUCGUCC)

viruses as well. The panhandle regions of influenza A and B virus RNAs are interchangeable, although the chimaeric virus resulting from such modification is attenuated (Muster et al. 1991).

Most viral genes encode a single protein (Table

(a)

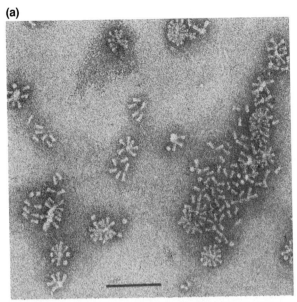

(b)

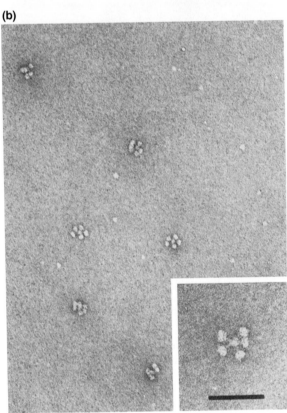

Fig. 22.4 (**a**) Haemagglutinin (HA) (bar = 100 nm) and (**b**) neuraminidase (NA) (bar = 50 nm) proteins isolated from detergent-disrupted virus. The molecules associate by hydrophobic C (HA) and N (NA) terminal sequences after the detergent has been removed. (by courtesy of Dr K G Murti.)

22.2); the exceptions are the M and NS genes of all influenza viruses and the NA gene of type B virus, which encode 2 proteins each (Lamb and Horvath 1991). The NS gene of type A virus encodes both a 26 kDa (NS1) protein translated from unspliced mRNA and a 14 kDa (NS2) protein translated from spliced mRNA (Inglis et al. 1979, Lamb and Choppin 1979) (Fig. 22.8a), which share the same AUG initiation codon and 9 subsequent amino acids. A similar protein-coding strategy is employed by the type B and C influenza viruses.

By contrast, each type of influenza virus possesses a different mechanism for expression of M gene products. The M gene of type A viruses generates an unspliced transcript encoding the M1 protein, as well as 2 other alternatively spliced RNAs, designated M2 and mRNA3, which differ in their use of 5′ splice sites (Inglis and Brown 1981, Lamb, Lai and Choppin 1981) (Fig. 22.8b). The leader sequence of the M2 mRNA contains the AUG initiation codon and codons for 8 subsequent residues that are shared with the M1 protein; this region is followed by a sequence encoding 88 residues in the +1 reading frame. The 9 amino acid peptide encoded by mRNA3 has not been detected in infected cells. By binding to the 5′ end of the viral M1 mRNA in a sequence-specific, cap-dependent manner, the viral polymerase complex promotes splicing at the M2 mRNA 5′ site over mRNA3 5′ site (Shih, Nemeroff and Krug 1995). The M gene of influenza B viruses also encodes 2 proteins, M1 and BM2, which are translated via a termination-reinitiation scheme of tandem cistrons; a pentanucleotide sequence, UAAUG, contains the termination codon for the M1 and the initiation codon for the BM2 (Horvath, Williams and Lamb 1990) (Fig. 22.8c). Finally, in contrast to the scheme employed by influenza A viruses, type C viruses rely on spliced transcripts to produce M1 protein (Yamashita, Krystal and Palese 1988). The primary transcript contains an open reading frame encoding 374 amino acids, from which M1 mRNA is spliced, such that a translational termination codon is introduced after 242 residues of the M1 open reading frame (Yamashita, Krystal and Palese 1988). The resulting 374 amino acid protein has not been identified unequivocally in virus-infected cells. However, one report describes a protein (CM2) with an apparent molecular weight of 18 kDa that corresponds to the carboxyl-terminal domain of the primary transcript (Hongo et al. 1994) (Fig. 22.8d).

Still another mechanism of viral protein expression is represented by the influenza B virus NA gene, which gives rise to a bicistronic mRNA containing 2 initiating AUG codons that are separated by 4 nucleotides (Fig. 22.8e). The 100 amino acid NB protein is translated from the 5′ AUG codon, while the 466 amino acid NA protein is translated from the second AUG codon. Even though the NA initiation codon is positioned downstream of the NB initiation site, greater amounts of NA protein (1:0.6) accumulate in cells (Williams and Lamb 1989).

4.1 Replication

The replication cycle of influenza viruses has been studied most extensively with type A strains; therefore, unless otherwise noted, the processes described below refer to viruses of that type (Fig. 22.9).

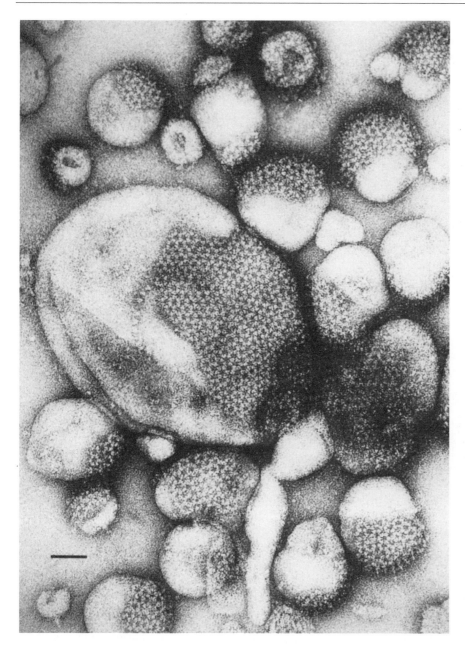

Fig. 22.5 Negatively stained influenza C virions with an array of extended glycoproteins. Bar = 50 nm. (Courtesy of Dr R W H Ruigrok.) (From Hewat et al. 1984.)

ATTACHMENT TO UNCOATING

An influenza virus infects cells through binding of its HA or HEF protein to the cell's sialyloligosaccharide receptor. After binding, the attached virion undergoes endocytosis (White, Kielian and Helenius 1983). The low pH of the late endocytotic vesicle triggers a conformational change in the cleavage-activated HA (Skehel et al. 1982), initiating fusion of the viral and vesicular membranes. Fusion releases the contents of the virion into the cytoplasm of the cell (uncoating). Before fusion, M2 proteins (possibly NB for type B viruses), by ion channelling, introduce protons into the inside of the virion, exposing the core to low pH (Sugrue et al. 1990, Hay 1992, Helenius 1992, Pinto, Holsinger and Lamb 1992) (Fig. 22.10). Such an event is thought to promote dissociation of the M1 from the RNP by disrupting their low pH-sensitive interaction between these molecules (Zhirnov 1990), allowing the

RNP to migrate to the nucleus through the nuclear pore in an ATP-dependent manner (Martin and Helenius 1991, Kemler, Whittaker and Helenius 1994). Exposure of the viral core to low pH, however, is not required for dissociation of M1 from RNP in type C viruses (Zhirnov and Grigoriev 1994).

TRANSCRIPTION AND TRANSLATION

Once the RNP migrates into the host cell nucleus, the associated polymerase complexes (PA, PB1 and PB2) begin primary transcription of mRNA (Krug, Broni and Bouloy 1979), which requires co-operation with ongoing transcription by cellular RNA polymerase II. The reason for this requirement is that initiation of influenza virus mRNA synthesis depends on $m^7GpppXm$-containing capped primers (10–13 nt long, containing 5′-GCA-3′ at their 3′ proximal ends) that are generated from host cell RNAs by an influ-

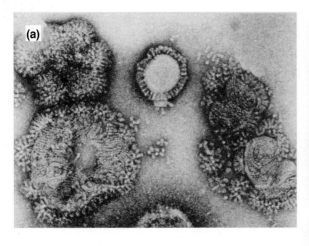

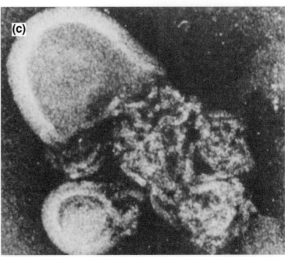

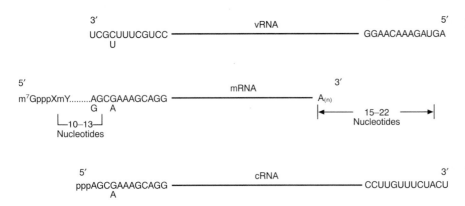

Fig. 22.6   Electron micrograph of the internal structure of an influenza virus. (**a**) Naturally disrupted virions. (**b**) Extended coil structures resulting from detergent treatment of virus. (c) M1 protein reconstituted into liposomes. (Courtesy of Dr. R.W.H. Ruigrok.) (From Ruigrok, Calder and Wharton 1989.)

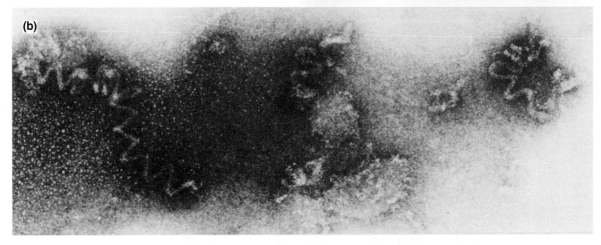

Fig. 22.7   Schematic diagram illustrating the differences between influenza virus virion RNA (vRNA) segments, mRNAs and full-length cRNA (template for vRNA). The conserved 12 nucleotides at the 3' end and 13 nucleotides at the 5' end of each of the influenza A virus vRNA segments are indicated. Similar conserved sequences are found at the 3' and 5' ends of the influenza B and C virus RNA segments.

enza virus-encoded, cap-dependent endonuclease (Plotch et al. 1981, Krug et al. 1989), whose activity requires both the 5' and the 3' ends of vRNA (Hagen et al. 1994).

mRNA synthesis begins with incorporation of a G residue complementary to the penultimate C residue on the vRNAs, and may involve not only the polymerase complex but also the NP (Bárcena et al. 1994). Transcription continues until it reaches the poly(A) addition site, located 15–25 nt from the 5' end of the vRNA. Newly synthesized NP promotes 'read-through' of the poly(A) site, allowing the synthesis of cRNA (Beaton and Krug 1986, Shapiro and Krug 1988). A

Table 22.2 Influenza A virus genome RNA and protein coding assignments

Segment	Length (nucleotides)[a]	Encoded polypeptide	Nascent polypeptide length (amino acids)	Experimentally determined mol. wt (kDa) of polypeptides	Carbohydrates	Approx. copy no. per virion	Remarks
1	2341	PB2	759	87	–	30–60	Component of RNA transcriptase complex. Host cell capped RNA recognition and possible endonuclease activity
2	2341	PB1	757	96	–	30–60	Component of RNA transcriptase complex. Initiation of RNA transcription
3	2233	PA	716	85	–	30–60	Component of RNA transcriptase complex. Precise function not known
4	1778	HA	566	63	+	500	Surface trimer glycoprotein. Cleaved into HA1 and HA2. Major antigenic determinant. Functions in virus binding to cell surface receptors and fusion
5	1565	NP	498	56	–	1000	Associated with RNA segments to form ribonucleoprotein
6	1413	NA	454	60	+	100	Surface tetramer glycoprotein, neuraminidase activity. Functions in virus release
7	1027	M1	252	27	–	3000	Major virion component involved in RNP transport out of nucleus
		M2	97	14	–	20–60	Coded from spliced mRNA, ion channel activity, target of amantadine
8	890	NS1	230	26	–	NA	Non-structural protein; inhibits mRNA transport from nucleus
		NS2	121	14	–	130–200	Coded from spliced mRNA, associated with M1

[a]The lengths of the HA and NA genes differ among the strains.
NA, not applicable.

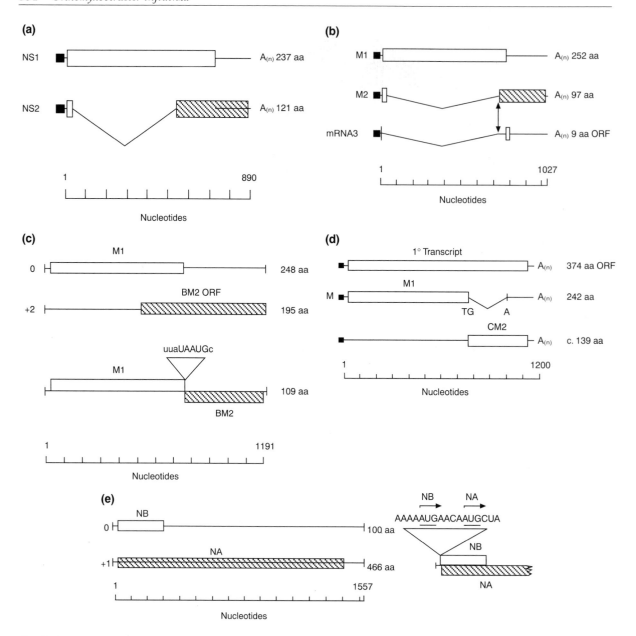

Fig. 22.8   Coding strategies of influenza virus genes. (**a**) Influenza A virus NS1 and NS2 mRNAs and their coding regions. NS1 and NS2 share 10 amino-terminal residues, including the initiating methionine. The reading frame of NS2 mRNA (nucleotide positions 529–861) differs from that of NS1. (**b**) Influenza A virus M1, M2 mRNAs and mRNA3 and their coding regions. M1 and M2 share 9 amino-terminal residues, including the initiating methionine; however, the reading frame of M2 mRNA (nucleotide positions 740–1004) differs from that of M1. A peptide that could be translated from mRNA3 has not been found in vivo. (**c**) Influenza B virus RNA segment 7 open reading frames (first 2 lines) and the organization of the open reading frames used to translate the M1 and BM2 proteins (third line). The stop–start pentanucleotide is also illustrated. (**d**) Influenza C virus mRNAs derived from RNA segment 6 and probable CM2 coding region (third line). The exact size of CM2 has not been determined. (**e**) Open reading frames in influenza B virus RNA segment 6, illustrating the overlapping reading frames of NB and neuraminidase (NA). Nucleotide sequence surrounding the 2 AUG initiation codons, in mRNA sense, is shown to the right. Thin lines at the 5′ and 3′ termini of the mRNAs represent untranslated regions. The shaded areas represent different coding regions. Introns in the mRNAs are shown by the V-shaped lines; filled rectangles at the 5′ ends of mRNAs represent heterogeneous nucleotides derived from cellular RNAs that are covalently linked to viral sequences. (From Lamb and Harvath 1991, with modification of part d).

stretch of uridines near the 5′ end of the virion RNA (optimal with 5–7 residues and 16 nt from the 5′ end (Li and Palese 1994)) serves as the poly(A) signal, and the RNA duplex of the panhandle structure is required for polyadenylation, suggesting that the viral RNA polymerase adds poly(A) by a slippage (stuttering) mechanism when it

reaches the double-stranded RNA barrier next to the uridine stretch (Luo et al. 1991). The primary transcripts are then used in the production of viral proteins by the cell's cytoplasmic translation machinery. Three polymerase proteins (PA, PB1 and PB2), as well as the NP and NS1 proteins, are transported to the nucleus. The negative-strand genomic segment

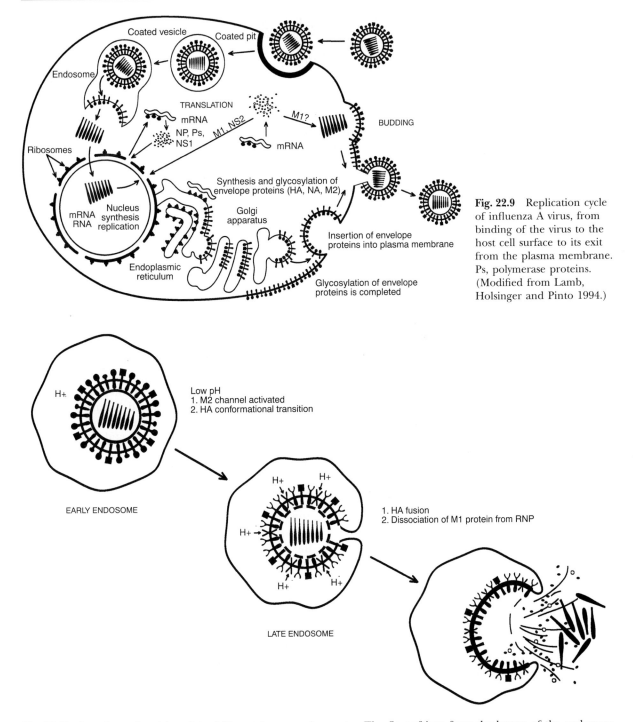

Fig. 22.9 Replication cycle of influenza A virus, from binding of the virus to the host cell surface to its exit from the plasma membrane. Ps, polymerase proteins. (Modified from Lamb, Holsinger and Pinto 1994.)

Fig. 22.10 Ion channel activity of the M2 protein upon virus entry. The flow of ions from the lumen of the endosome through the M2 channel into the virion interior allows the dissociation of protein–protein interactions between M1 and RNP, facilitating RNP transport to the nucleus. (From Lamb, Holsinger and Pinto 1994; © Mary K. Bryson.)

and the positive-strand antigenomic segments, but not viral mRNA, are coated with NP. NS1 inhibits the transport of cellular mRNA to the cytoplasm by binding to the poly(A) region (Qiu and Krug 1994) and maximizing the availability of capped primers for viral mRNA synthesis. The products of viral mRNA synthesis change as infection proceeds, indicating a temporal form of regulation (Hay et al. 1977, Hatada et al. 1989). Early in infection, the synthesis of mRNAs encoding NP and NS1 dominates; later the production of mRNAs for HA, NA and M1 increases, while tran-

scripts for the polymerase proteins are relatively low throughout the infection cycle, except at the earliest time. The relative amounts of mRNAs correlate with the amounts of their corresponding proteins, indicating that viral gene expression is regulated at the transcriptional level, in addition to the temporal control mechanisms governing the translational efficiency of viral mRNA (Yamanaka, Ishihama and Nagata 1988, Yamanaka, Nagata and Ishihama 1991). Full-length viral complementary RNA (cRNA) is not produced until viral protein has been synthesized. The same transcription complex responsible for mRNA synthesis also participates in cRNA synthesis. Equimolar quantities of cRNA are synthesized throughout infection (Hay et al. 1977), indicating a lack of regulation of this process.

After their translation in the endoplasmic reticulum (ER), viral membrane proteins – HA, NA and M2 for the type A viruses, NB for type B and HEF for type C – are translocated into the lumen of the ER, where they undergo oligomerization prior to their transport to the Golgi apparatus (Doms et al. 1993) and subsequent transport to the plasma membrane. The proteins are glycosylated in the ER (high mannose type), and then processed further in the Golgi to contain oligosaccharide of the complex type.

VIRION MORPHOGENESIS AND BUDDING

RNP transport from the nucleus to the cytoplasm cannot take place unless it is preceded by transport of M1 protein from the cytoplasm to the nucleus (Martin and Helenius 1991). Whether this requirement includes M1 transport from the nucleus back to the cytoplasm is controversial (Rey and Nayak 1992, Enami et al. 1993, Whittaker, Kemler and Helenius 1995). Electron microscopy of influenza virus-infected cells has not identified viral core structures, nor has an association of RNP with the plasma membrane been found; rather RNP seems to associate with viral membrane proteins only when the virion is beginning to assume its shape (Patterson, Gross and Oxford 1988). Few details of the final assembly process are known. Presumably, RNP buds outward through the cell membrane. Substantial amounts of M1 are found in the cytoplasm throughout the infection period, presumably interacting with cellular membranes (Hay 1974), in addition to those found in the nucleus. However, the role of cytoplasmic M1 is unknown. Because at least a fraction of M1 is associated with RNP in the virion (Rees and Dimmock 1981, Kawakami and Ishihama 1983), this protein possibly serves as a molecular 'glue', interacting with RNP on the one hand and with HA, NA or M2 on the other. Such interactions may function as a budding signal.

4.2 Polypeptides: non-structural and structural

Influenza A virus comprises 9 structural and 1 non-structural protein (see Table 22.2), compared with 9 structural and 2 non-structural proteins in influenza B virus, and 6 structural and 3 non-structural proteins in influenza C virus.

POLYMERASE PROTEINS

An acidic (PA) and 2 basic (PB1 and PB2) proteins, encoded by the 3 largest RNA segments, form a complex of either PB1–PB2 or PA–PB1–PB2 (St Angelo et al. 1987, Digard, Blok and Inglis 1989), which possess RNA-dependent RNA polymerase activity. The complex specifically recognizes RNA panhandle structures (Tiley et al. 1994) and is associated with the RNP at or near its end (Murti, Webster and Jones 1988). Each

of these is highly conserved in type A viruses (Kawaoka, Krauss and Webster 1989, Okazaki, Kawaoka and Webster 1989, Gorman et al. 1990a, 1990b).

PB1

This protein is required for the initiation and elongation of newly synthesized viral RNA (Braam, Ulmanen and Krug 1983). Conserved PB1 residues Ser444–Asp445–Asp446 of type A viruses (443–445 for type B and 445–447 for type C), which resemble the signature sequences of other viral RNA polymerases, may form the core of the transcriptase/replicase activity (Biswas and Nayak 1994). This protein contains 2 discontinuous regions, both essential for nuclear localization (Nath and Nayak 1990).

PB2

Apparently involved in the recognition and cleavage of type I cap structures of cellular mRNAs (Plotch et al. 1981, Blaas, Patzelt and Kuechler 1982, Ulmanen, Broni and Krug 1983), PB2 is essential for viral mRNA but not vRNA synthesis (Nakagawa et al. 1995). Two signals mediate nuclear localization of influenza A PB2 protein, one of which is involved in PB2 perinuclear binding (Mukaigawa and Nayak 1991). This protein also plays a role in host range restriction (Almond 1977, Subbarao, London and Murphy 1993).

PA

The function of the PA is not fully understood, but it may be involved in viral RNA replication (Krug et al. 1989). Expression of the PA by itself does not result in the accumulation of all the PA in the nucleus, and the PB1 and NS1 may be involved in the nuclear targeting or nuclear retention of the PA (Nieto et al. 1992).

HAEMAGGLUTININ

Encoded by the fourth largest RNA segment, the HA accounts for about 25% of viral protein and is distributed evenly on the surface of virions. It is responsible for the attachment and subsequent penetration of viruses into cells. The HA spikes, approximately 14×4 nm, protrude from the virion surface (Laver and Valentine 1969) (Fig. 22.11, and see Fig. 22.2). The HA homotrimer (Wiley, Skehel and Waterfield 1977) is synthesized as a single polypeptide chain (HA0) that undergoes post-translational cleavage by cellular proteases (Klenk et al. 1975, Lazarowitz and Choppin 1975). The resulting HA1 and HA2 subunits (36 and 27 kDa) are covalently attached by a disulphide bond, while the 'tow-chain' monomers are associated noncovalently to form trimers. An N terminal signal sequence is removed. HA cleavage is required for infectivity (Klenk et al. 1975, Lazarowitz and Choppin 1975) because of the hydrophobic amino terminus of HA2, which mediates fusion between the viral envelope and the endosomal membrane (White 1992).

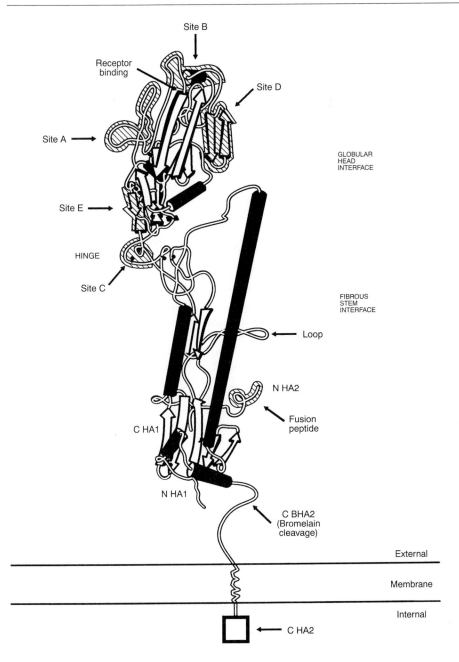

Site B

Receptor binding

Site D

Site A →

GLOBULAR HEAD INTERFACE

Site E →

HINGE

Site C

FIBROUS STEM INTERFACE

← Loop

N HA2

C HA1

Fusion peptide

N HA1

C BHA2 (Bromelain cleavage)

External

Membrane

Internal

← C HA2

Fig. 22.11 Schematic diagram of the Hong Kong haemagglutinin (HA) monomer, showing folding of the HA1 and HA2 polypeptides. The shaded areas show where 5 independent antigenic areas (sites A–E) may be located. Note that the fusion peptide is also buried in the intact molecule and is exposed only after a conformational change at low pH (Bullough et al. 1994). (From Wilson, Skehel and Wiley 1981.)

Three-dimensional structure

Bromelain-cleaved soluble HA (BHA) of A/Aichi/2/68(H3N2), which remains in trimeric form, has been crystallized and its 3-dimensional structure determined (Wiley, Wilson and Skehel 1981, Wiley and Skehel 1987, Wilson and Cox 1990). The BHA is 13.5 nm long and 1.4–4 nm in triangular cross-section, and contains all of the HA1 and the first 175 of the 221 amino acids of the HA2 subunit; it lacks only the hydrophobic membrane-anchoring peptide (Brand and Skehel 1972). The HA is folded into 2 structurally distinct domains, a globular head and a fibrous stalk. The globular head is entirely composed of HA1 residues and contains an 8-stranded antiparallel β-sheet. This framework supports the receptor-binding site, which is surrounded by highly variable antigenic loop structures. The fibrous stalk region, more proximal to the viral membrane, consists of residues from both HA1 and HA2. The cleavage site between HA1 and HA2 is located in the middle of the stalk. The C terminus of HA1 is exposed on the trimer surface, c. 2.2 nm from the terminus of HA2, indicating significant rearrangement and conformational change after cleavage of the HA0. The hydrophobic amino terminus of the HA2 (fusion peptide) is buried in the trimeric structure. The conformational states of the HA after exposure to low pH may differ among different subtypes of the molecules (e.g. H2 vs H3) (Puri et al. 1990). The trimeric structure is principally stabilized by the fibrous stem regions with a rather loose association of the globular heads. The variable antigenic determinants are located on the top of the stalk.

Folding, assembly and intracellular transport

During its synthesis in the ER, the HA interacts transiently with the BiP/GRP78 protein (Gething, McCammon and Sambrook 1986, Hurtley et al. 1989) and calnexin (Hammond, Braakman and Helenius 1994, Chen et al. 1995) before acquiring high mannose-type oligosaccharide and forming trimers, a prerequisite for its transport out of the ER (Doms et al. 1993). Cysteine residues in the ectodomain are essential both for efficient folding and for stabilization of the folded molecule (Segal et al. 1992). Disulphide bond formation occurs co-translationally (Cheng et al. 1995). In the Golgi apparatus, the oligosaccharide of the HA is further processed to the complex type. The HAs of virulent avian H5 and H7 viruses are cleaved in the trans-Golgi or trans-Golgi network by ubiquitous proteases (see below). In polarized cells, the final step of HA maturation is transport to the apical cell surface (Roth et al. 1983); its transport from the trans-Golgi network is energy-dependent (Gravotta, Adesnik and Sabatini 1990). A signal responsible for apical transport resides in the ectodomain, although a mutation in the cytoplasmic tail alters the polarized delivery (McQueen et al. 1986, Brewer and Roth 1991). The transmembrane and cytoplasmic domains contained signals for specific incorporation of the HA into virions in studies with a complementation assay (Naim and Roth 1993), although the HA tail-less mutant replicated almost as well as its parent (Jin, Leser and Lamb 1994).

HA cleavage

A link between HA cleavability and virulence is well established in avian influenza A viruses (Webster and Rott 1987, Klenk and Rott 1988). In virulent H5 and H7 avian viruses, the HAs contain multiple basic amino acids at the cleavage site, which are cleaved intracellularly by endogenous proteases. By contrast, in avirulent avian viruses as well as non-avian influenza A viruses, with the exception of H7N7 equine viruses (Dale et al. 1988, Kawaoka 1991), the HAs lack a series of basic residues and are not subject to cleavage by such proteases (Bosch et al. 1979, 1981). Thus, the tissue tropism of viruses may be determined by the availability of proteases responsible for the cleavage of different HAs, leading to differences in virulence.

Two groups of proteases seem to be responsible for HA cleavage. One includes enzymes recognizing a single arginine and able to cleave 'avirulent'-type HAs, such as plasmin (Lazarowitz, Goldberg and Choppin 1973), blood-clotting factor X-like protease (Gotoh et al. 1990), tryptase Clara (Kido et al. 1992) and bacterial proteases (Tashiro et al. 1987). The second group, which remains to be identified in vivo, comprises ubiquitous intracellular subtilisin-related proteases, furin and PC6, which cleave virulent-type HAs with multiple basic residues at the cleavage site (Stieneke-Grober et al. 1992, Horimoto et al. 1994). Studies with HA cleavage mutants have demonstrated that the number of basic amino acids at the cleavage site and the presence or absence of a nearby carbohydrate affect HA cleavability by intracellular proteases in an interrelated manner (Kawaoka, Naeve and Webster 1984, Kawaoka and Webster 1988, 1989, Ohuchi et

al. 1989, Vey et al. 1992). The proposed sequence requirement for HA cleavage by intracellular proteases, in the absence of a nearby carbohydrate (at residue 11 in H5 numbering) is Q–R/K–X–R/K–R (X = non-basic residue). If the carbohydrate moiety is present, virulence is maintained only if 2 amino acids are inserted (Q–X–X–R/K–X–R/K–R), or if the conserved glutamine at position –5 or the proline at position –6 is altered [i.e. B(X)–X(B)–R/K–X–R/K–R (B = basic residue)]. In addition, the amino acid immediately downstream of the cleavage site (the amino terminal residue of the HA2) affects HA cleavage by intracellular proteases (Horimoto and Kawaoka 1995). The HA cleavage enzyme seems to be located in either the trans-Golgi or the trans-Golgi network, to be calcium-dependent, and to have an acidic pH optimum (Klenk et al. 1974, Klenk, Garten and Rott 1984, Walker et al. 1992). Although the most HAs in influenza A and B viruses contain Arg at the C terminus of the HA1, H14 and some human H1s contain Lys at this position (Kawaoka et al. 1990, Günther et al. 1993).

Oligosaccharide side-chains

The location and number of glycosylation sites are not conserved among HAs of different strains and subtypes (Nobusawa et al. 1991). Rather, these sites are scattered throughout the HA, although they tend to cluster around the antigenic sites on the globular heads. The HAs of individual virus strains contain from 5 to 11 sites, with the glycosylation sequence around residues 20–22 conserved in type A strains, except in some virulent avian strains in which the HA is cleaved by intracellular proteases (corresponding to residue 11 in the H5 numbering system; see 'HA cleavage'). Some 17–20% of the total protein surface of the H3 HA could be covered by carbohydrate. The presence or absence of oligosaccharide side-chains in the HA affects antibody (Skehel et al. 1984) and CD4+ T cell (Jackson et al. 1994) recognition of the molecule, receptor specificity (Günther et al. 1993) and virulence (Kawaoka, Naeve and Webster 1984). Moreover, in H3 (Gallagher et al. 1992) and H7 (Roberts, Garten and Klenk 1993) HAs, no particular oligosaccharide side-chain is required for folding, intracellular transport or function of the molecule; however, at least 2 or 3 oligosaccharide chains (depending on the source of the HA) must be present to ensure transport of the molecule to the cell surface.

Acylation

The 3 cysteine residues in the carboxyl-terminal region of the HA2 are acylated with palmitic acid (Schmidt 1982) by a thioester linkage (Veit et al. 1990). The lack of HA acylation affects HAs differently depending on the subtype. For instance, loss of palmitic acid does not impede the fusion activity of the H3 (Steinhauer et al. 1991) or H7 HA (Veit et al. 1991, Philipp et al. 1995). In fact, an H3 virus with deletion of the HA cytoplasmic tail, which contains the acylation site, is generated by reverse genetics and replicates almost as well as its parent (Jin, Leser and Lamb 1994). On the other hand, a virus with a substitution at the C terminal cysteine of the HA (Cys563 in WSN HA numbering) was not generated by reverse genetics, possibly because of structural constraints rather than the altered palmitylation (Zurcher, Luo and Palese 1994). Results for the H2 HAs are more controversial. One report stresses the importance of each of the cysteine residues for fusion activity (Naeve and Williams 1990), while another indicates the absence of such an effect (Naim et al. 1992).

Receptor binding

Influenza A and B virus HAs bind to oligosaccharide-containing terminal sialic acids, including (α2,6)sialyllactose, *N*-acetylneuraminic acid-α2,6-galactose (NeuAcα2,6Galβ1),4Glc and (α2,3)sialyllactose, NeuAcα2,3Galβ1,4Glc. Topologically, the binding site is a depression. The amino acid residues that contact the terminal sialic acids (Weis et al. 1988, 1990a) are highly conserved among the different HA subtypes (Nobusawa et al. 1991). The hydroxy groups at C7 and C8 of the glycerol side-chain and the *N*-acetyl group, but not the hydroxy group of C9, are important for recognition by the HA (Kelm et al. 1992, Matrosovich, Gambaryan and Chumakov 1992). A second ligand-binding site, for which the affinity of sialyllactose is 4 times weaker than that for the primary site, has been identified in the HA (Sauter et al. 1992). The biological significance of the secondary ligand binding site is unknown.

The receptor specificity of the HA differs among influenza A viruses: most avian and equine influenza viruses bind preferentially the NeuAcα2,3Gal linkage, whereas human and classic H1N1 swine influenza viruses preferentially bind the NeuAcα2,6Gal linkage on the cell surface sialyloligosaccharides (Rogers and Paulson 1983, Rogers et al. 1983b, Rogers and D'Souza 1989). Epithelial cells in human trachea contain SA (sialic acid) α2,6Gal but not SAα2,3Gal sialyloligosaccharides on the cell surface (Baum and Paulson 1990), whereas those in duck intestine (the replication site of avian influenza viruses) and those in horse trachea contain SAα2,3Gal but not SAα2,6Gal sialyloligosaccharides (T Ito and Y Kawaoka, unpublished data from experiments with SA–Gal linkage-specific lectins; the types of SA were not determined, although normal human cells contain only NeuAc). In agreement with these findings, the virus with NeuAcα2,6Gal specificity binds epithelial cells lining human trachea, whereas that with NeuAcα2,3Gal specificity does not (Couceiro, Paulson and Baum 1993). It is interesting that epithelial cells in pig trachea contain both types of sialyloligosaccharides, which explains why both human and avian viruses replicate efficiently in pigs (Kida et al. 1994). Thus, the receptor specificities of the viruses correspond to the presence of the receptor at the replication site of the virus. The HAs of influenza B viruses also preferentially recognize NeuAcα2,6Gal linkages (Xu et al. 1994). Additionally, the H3 HAs with Leu at position 226 recognize 4-*O*-acetyl sialic acid, but non-H3 and B HAs with Gln at the position equivalent to 226 of the H3 HA do not (Matrosovich, Gambaryan and Chumakov 1992). Finally, the H1 HA binds NeuAcα2,6Galβ1,4GlcNAc with an affinity an order of magnitude higher than NeuAcα2,6Galβ1,4Glc, indicating

the importance of the asialic portion of the receptor (Matrosovich et al. 1993).

An amino acid at residue 226 of the H3 influenza A virus HA is involved in receptor specificity; that is, an alteration of this residue in human (Rogers et al. 1983a) and avian (Rogers et al. 1985) influenza A viruses shifts the receptor specificities from NeuAcα2,6Gal to NeuAcα2,3Gal and from NeuAcα2,3Gal to NeuAcα2,6, respectively. The mutant HA of A/Udorn/305/72(H3N2), which contains avian-like amino acids at residues 226 (Gln) and 228 (Gly), supports the replication of the virus in ducks when reassorted with other avian genes, whereas another mutant HA of A/Udorn/305/72, which contains only one avian-like amino acid at residue 226 (Gln) does not, establishing the importance of these residues for host range restriction (Hinshaw et al. 1983a, Naeve, Webster and Hinshaw 1983, Naeve, Hinshaw and Webster 1984). The molecular basis of the importance of the 228 mutation remains unknown.

Host cell-mediated selection of antigenic variants

The HA antigenicity of human influenza A and B viruses grown in embryonated hens' eggs differs from that of viruses isolated and passaged in a variety of cell cultures, including chicken embryo fibroblasts (Schild et al. 1983, Katz, Naeve and Webster 1987, Robertson et al. 1987, Katz and Webster 1992); even so, minor egg isolates contain the same antigenic phenotype as the tissue culture-grown viruses (Oxford et al. 1991). A similar phenomenon was discovered by Burnet (Burnet and Clarke 1942) as 'O (as **o**riginal)–D (as **d**erived)' variation during passages of human viruses in eggs; O form virus agglutinated human or guinea-pig erythrocytes in preference to fowl erythrocytes, while D form viruses agglutinated them equally. Because tissue culture-grown viruses contain the same amino acid sequences of the HA as those replicating in humans, mutants are selected during replication in eggs (Katz, Wang and Webster 1990, Rajakumar, Swierkosz and Schulze 1990, Robertson et al. 1990). This finding is supported by the greater efficiency of primary isolation of human virus in cell culture than in eggs (Dumitrescu et al. 1981, Monto, Maassab and Bryan 1981). Comparison of the HA sequence among viruses recently isolated in eggs or cell culture revealed mutations around the receptor binding pocket. This fact notwithstanding, differences in receptor specificity have not been demonstrated between egg- and tissue culture-grown viruses. However, the variability of erythrocyte agglutination by currently circulating human viruses, depending on the media used for isolation, suggests that such differences do exist. Egg variants can be selected by growing viruses isolated in tissue culture in cells lining the chorioallantoic membrane without allantoic fluid (Hardy et al. 1995); however, the variants selected do not represent all the viruses found during replication in embryonated eggs, suggesting the presence of other selective pressures (e.g. inhibitors in allantoic fluid). Inactivated vaccines prepared from tissue culture-grown viruses induce better protective immunity than do those from egg-grown viruses in animal models (Katz and Webster 1989, Wood et al. 1989, Newman et al. 1993) as well as in humans (Newman et al. 1993), although differences were not found when animals were immunized with vaccinia viruses that expressed the HAs of viruses grown in eggs or tissue culture (Rota, Shaw and Kendal 1987, 1989).

Fusion

The fusion of influenza viruses to the plasma membrane is mediated through the HA (Fig. 22.12) (White, 1992). Under conditions of neutral pH, the fusion peptide, which forms a small part of the amino terminus of the HA2, is located in the fibrous stem of the molecule (c. 3.5 nm away from the viral membrane and, hence, 10 nm from the target endosomal membrane), and is well integrated into the subunit interface by a network of hydrogen bonds. The importance of the peptide in HA-mediated fusion is evident from the ability of mutations in this region to alter (Daniels et al. 1985) or abolish (Gething et al. 1986) fusion activity. When the pH is c. 5 (late endosomal pH), the tertiary structure of the HA is altered (Skehel et al. 1982). Soon after, fusion peptides and other sequences buried in the stem become exposed (White and Wilson 1987), followed by a series of changes at the distal tips of the head domains, leading to dissociation of the globular heads from one another, as revealed by both epitope exposure (White and Wilson 1987) and electron microscopy (Ruigrok, Hewat and Wade 1992). Although this event is an essential step in membrane fusion (Godley et al. 1992, Kemble et al. 1992), complete dissociation of the head domains may not be required (Stegmann, Booy and Wilschut 1987, White and Wilson 1987). The binding of fusion peptides to the target membrane (Stegmann et al. 1991) is followed by a lag phase (Morris et al. 1989) whose length depends on HA surface density, pH and temperature, and whether a receptor is present in the target membrane (Stegmann, White and Helenius 1990). During the lag phase, rotational and lateral motions of HA trimers probably occur in the plane of the viral membrane (Junankar and Cherry 1986), leading to the aggregation of several of the trimers (Ellens et al. 1990, Stegmann, White and Helenius 1990) and to formation of a fusion pore within the interior of the aggregate, as indicated by electrophysiological (Spruce, Iwata and Almers 1991) and electron microscopic (Burger, Knoll and Verkleji 1988) studies. The transmembrane regions of the HA seem to have an important though still undefined role in the fusion process, as glycosylphosphatidylinositol-anchored HAs promote only hemifusion (a state in which lipids, but not the contents of the fusion compartments, mix) (Kemble, Danieli and White 1994).

How, then, do such peptides initiate fusion between viral and endosomal membranes? Biophysical analysis of an HA2 peptide corresponding to residues 54–89 (Carr and Kim 1993) and x-ray crystallographic analysis of a proteolytic fragment of BHA at the pH of membrane fusion (Bullough et al. 1994), obtained by trypsin/thermolysin treatment, revealed major refold-

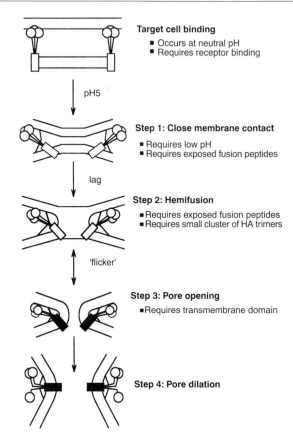

Target cell binding
- Occurs at neutral pH
- Requires receptor binding

pH5

Step 1: Close membrane contact
- Requires low pH
- Requires exposed fusion peptides

lag

Step 2: Hemifusion
- Requires exposed fusion peptides
- Requires small cluster of HA trimers

'flicker'

Step 3: Pore opening
- Requires transmembrane domain

Step 4: Pore dilation

Fig. 22.12 Steps in HA-mediated membrane fusion. Processes described in the diagram occur after a virus becomes attached to cell membrane. (From White 1994.)

ing of the secondary and tertiary structures of the molecule (Fig. 22.13). The loop preceding the buttressing helix of the neutral pH form becomes part of the coiled coil, extending the amino terminus of HA2. Such alteration could be expected to transport the fusion peptide 15 nm or more, bringing it in close contact with the endosomal membrane (Yu, King and Shin 1994). The carboxyl-terminal portion of the HA2 subunit also undergoes a major structural change. This alteration of the HA at the pH of membrane fusion would explain elevated pH optima for the fusion of mutants (Daniels et al. 1985, 1987) with alterations that destabilize structures in the stalk region (Daniels et al. 1985, Weis et al. 1990b).

NP

The NP, the most abundant component of RNP, is a type-specific antigen associated with viral RNA. It covers every 20 nucleotides (Duesberg 1969, Compans, Content and Duesberg 1972, Jennings et al. 1983), exposing the bases to the outside and inducing melting of the secondary structure (Baudin et al. 1994). By electron microscopy, purified NP has a rod-like shape with dimensions of 6.2 × 3.5 nm; most of these proteins exist in polymeric forms, ranging from trimers to large structures that are morphologically indistinguishable from the intact viral RNP (Ruigrok and Baudin 1995) (Fig. 22.14). Thus, vRNA may be

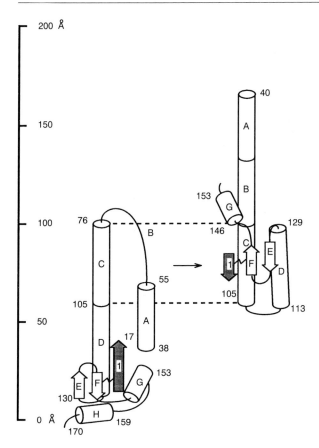

Fig. 22.13 Structural difference between equivalent regions of subunits of native haemagglutinin (HA) (left) and HA in the fusion pH conformation (right). The fusion pH structure was obtained by analysis of a fragment prepared by thermolytic digestion of HA at the fusion pH. The equivalent native structure is a partial diagram of the complete native structure. Consecutive regions of the HA2 chain are labelled A–H. The 2 structures are aligned on the C region, which is unaffected by the conformational change. The protease-treated, fusion-pH-exposed BHA (bromelain-cleaved soluble HA) lacks 39 amino-terminal residues. (From Bullough et al. 1994.)

wrapped around the NP scaffold, which by itself forms the same structure as RNP. The RNA-binding region of the NP of influenza A virus has been mapped between residues 91 and 188 (Kobayashi et al. 1994, Albo, Valencia and Portela 1995).

The NP possesses karyophilic signals (Davey, Dimmock and Colman 1985) and accumulates in the nucleus; later in infection it migrates back to the cytoplasm, presumably as a component of RNP (Martin and Helenius 1991, Rey and Nayak 1992). Free NP is needed for vRNA synthesis (Beaton and Krug 1986). It is also thought to play a role in host range restriction, as indicated by successful, host-dependent rescue of the *ts* phenotype (Scholtissek et al. 1985) and restriction of the replication of avian–human influenza A virus reassortants in primates (Snyder et al. 1987). This evidence notwithstanding, direct support for this role of the NP is lacking.

NA

The tetrameric NA protein of influenza A viruses (Fig. 22.15), a class II glycoprotein with its amino terminus inside the cell and its carboxyl terminus outside (Air and Laver 1989, Colman 1994), is one of 2 major glycoproteins on the virus surface. It has an uncleaved amino-terminal signal/anchor domain and a 6 amino-acid tail (Fields, Winter and Brownlee 1981, Blok et al. 1982). Although the precise location of the amino-terminal 6 polar residues is unknown, they are presumed to be exposed to the cytoplasm. The NA has a box-shaped head ($10 \times 10 \times 6$ nm) comprising 4 co-planar and roughly spherical subunits and contains the enzyme-active centre and major antigenic sites (Colman, Varghese and Laver 1983, Varghese, Laver and Colman 1983) (Fig. 22.16). The stalk is centrally attached to the head with a hydrophobic region by which the stalk is embedded in the viral membrane (Fields, Winter and Brownlee 1981, Blok et al. 1982). As demonstrated by studies with natural isolates (Blok and Air 1982a, 1982b), the stalk region is flexible in length and sequence and can be deleted almost completely or be extended by 58 amino acids to accommodate a variety of foreign sequences (Castrucci and Kawaoka 1993, Luo, Chung and Palese 1993, Castrucci et al. 1994). In contrast to the remainder of the NA, the 6 amino-acid cytoplasmic tail is highly conserved among all NA subtypes of influenza A virus (Blok and Air 1982a, 1982b). This region is important for incorporation of the NA into virions but is not essential for virus replication (Bilsel, Castrucci and Kawaoka 1993, García-Sastre and Palese 1995). Although deletion of 5 of these residues (leaving the initiating methionine) does not affect the viability of viruses, it causes attenuation because of the reduction in virion NA molecules. The mutant lacking the tail contains more filamentous than spherical parent virions, suggesting its interaction with other viral or cellular proteins during virion formation (L Mitnaul, M Castrucci and Y Kawaoka, unpublished data). The NA of influenza B viruses may be needed for assembly or budding of the virus (Yamamoto-Goshima et al. 1994).

An NA-deficient virus, generated by repeated passage in the presence of a bacterial NA and antibodies to viral NA, replicates in cell culture when a bacterial NA is added exogenously, as well as in immuno-deficient animals (Liu and Air 1993, Liu et al. 1995). The virus possesses an internal deletion of 800–900 nt, leaving regions encoding the cytoplasmic and trans-membrane domains and part of the stalk. Whether the truncated NA molecule exists in infected cell remains unknown.

The NA plays a role in host range restriction (Hinshaw et al. 1983a). It is also important for plaque formation by A/WSN/33(H1N1) in Madin–Darby bovine kidney (MDBK) cells and for the neurovirulence of this virus (Schulman and Palese 1977, Nakajima and Sugiura 1980, Sugiura and Ueda 1980), a phenotype characterized by loss of the oligosaccharide side-chain from the WSN NA, which is conserved among

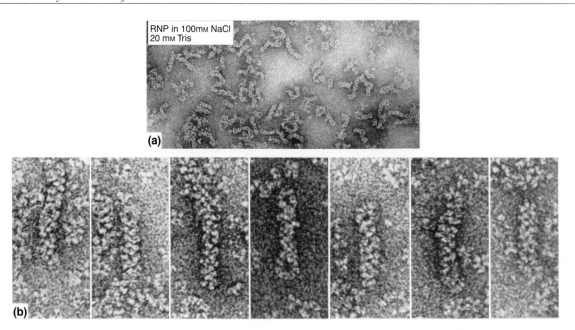

Fig. 22.14 Morphological features of RNP (**a**) and NP (**b**). (Courtesy of Dr Rob W H Ruigrok.) (From Ruigrok and Baudin 1995.)

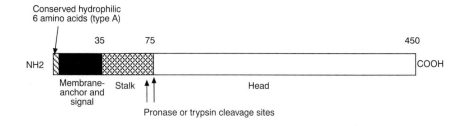

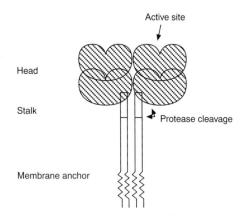

Fig. 22.15 Schematic diagram of the neuraminidase molecule. (Courtesy of Dr R G Webster.)

the NAs of all other influenza A viruses (Li et al. 1993b).

Three-dimensional structure

The NA 3-dimensional structure has been solved in both type A and B viruses. Despite the 28% homology between these 2 types of viruses, the overall folding patterns of their NAs are almost identical (Colman, Varghese and Laver 1983, Varghese, Laver and Colman 1983, Burmeister, Ruigrok and Cusack 1992, Janakiraman et al. 1994). The tetrameric NA protein

has circular 4-fold symmetry stabilized by calcium. The polypeptide chain folds into 6 topologically identical 4-stranded antiparallel β-sheets arranged like propeller blades (Fig. 22.16). The product of catalysis, sialic acid, is bound in a large pocket on the distal surface, flanked and surrounded by 9 acidic residues, 6 basic residues and 3 hydrophobic residues – each of which is strictly conserved in all known influenza viral NA sequences. Alteration of more than half of these residues results in molecules deficient in enzyme activity (Lentz, Webster and Air 1987). The 3-dimensional

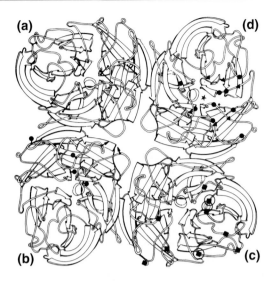

Fig. 22.16 Schematic illustration of the neuraminidase tetramer viewed from above down the symmetry axis. The 4 subunits highlight different features of the structure: (**a**) disulphide bonds; (**b**) carbohydrate attachment sites at positions 86, 146, 200 and 234 (circle) and metal ligands Asp 113 and Asp 114 (arrows); (**c**) residues that change in N2 (squares) and N9 (black circles) variants selected with monoclonal antibodies; (**d**) conserved acidic (circles) and basic (triangles) residues in influenza A and B neuraminidase and the sialic acid binding site (star). (Courtesy of Dr GM Air.) (From Air and Laver 1989.)

structure of the NA led to the synthesis of a potent sialidase inhibitor, 4-guanidino-2,4-dideoxy-2,3-dehydro-*N*-acetylneuraminic acid (Von Itzstein et al. 1993), which inhibits the NA activity of both type A and B viruses (inhibition constants, 10^{-9}–10^{-10} M).

Sialidase activity

The NA catalyses the cleavage of the α-ketosidic linkage between a terminal sialic acid and an adjacent sugar residue (Gottschalk 1957). The pH optimum of the enzyme ranges from 5.8 to 6.6, with an apparent K_m of 0.4 mM with use of *N*-acetylneuraminyllactose (Drzeniek 1972, Mountford et al. 1982). Removal of sialic acid residues by the NA promotes both entry and release of virus from infected cells (Palese et al. 1974). The majority of NAs of type A and B viruses cleave NeuAcα2,3Gal in preference to NeuAcα2,6Gal. The NA has little activity against 4–0–Ac–Neu (Pritchett and Paulson 1989), although some type A NA can hydrolyse NeuGc linked to Gal (Y Kawaoka, unpublished data). The preference of the linkage specificity of the human influenza A NA has shifted over the years, from NeuAcα2,3Gal to NeuAcα2,6Gal linkages, presumably corresponding to the preferential recognition of the latter linkages by the HA molecule (Baum and Paulson 1991).

Folding, assembly and intracellular transport

Synthesized as a monomer in the ER and translocated into the lumen of that structure, the NA rapidly forms a disulphide-linked dimer, which then non-covalently associates to form a tetramer ($t_{1/2}$ c. 1.5–2 min). After transiently associating with the BiP/GRP78 ($t_{1/2}$ c. 5 min), the NA is transported through the Golgi apparatus, where it acquires complex carbohydrates, rendering it resistant to endo H ($t_{1/2}$ c. 25 min), and finally to the cell surface (Hogue and Nayak 1992, Saito et al. 1994). The mature NA contains 2 apical sorting signals, one in the cytoplasmic (or transmembrane) domain and the other within the ectodomain, both of which are independently able to transport the protein to the apical plasma membrane (Kundu and Nayak 1994).

HA activity

The N1 and N9 NAs are different from the others in that they possess HA activity (Laver et al. 1984, Hausmann et al. 1995). The N9 HA activity can be transferred to the NAs of other NA subtypes by altering amino acid residues that are located apart from the NA active site (Nuss and Air 1991), indicating discrete HA- and NA-active sites in the N1 and N9 molecules. The biological significance of the HA activity in the N1 and N9 NAs remains unknown.

NB

The dimeric, integral membrane protein NB, unique to type B viruses and containing polygalactosaminoglycan (Williams and Lamb 1988), has an amino terminus portion that is exposed on the cell surface (Williams and Lamb 1986). Although it has not been found in virions, NB contains structural features similar to those of the M2 protein, suggesting that it may function as an ion channel.

M1

The most abundant virion protein and a type-specific antigen of influenza viruses, the M1 has long been thought to be located underneath and to add rigidity to the lipid bilayer, although direct evidence for such a role is lacking. Immunogold labelling with anti-M1 monoclonal antibodies failed to decorate the M1 in virions unless they were first treated with a protease or a detergent (Murti et al. 1992). Recent cryoelectron microscopic studies suggested that the M1 can modify the lipid bilayer, causing the viral envelope to thicken (Fujiyoshi et al. 1994) (see Fig. 22.3d). Located in both the nucleus and the cytoplasm (Smith et al. 1987, Patterson, Gross and Oxford 1988), this protein contains a karyophilic signal (residues 101–RKLKR–105) (Ye, Robinson and Wagner 1995) and multiple lipid-binding regions (Bucher et al. 1980, Gregoriades and Frangione 1981) (Fig. 22.17). In the cytoplasm it is associated with the membrane fraction (Hay 1974). The M1 proteins of influenza A and B viruses have a 'zinc finger' motif (Wakefield and Brownlee 1989), and purified virions contain zinc (Elster et al. 1994); however, the amount of zinc is not correlated with the RNA-binding activity of the protein, suggesting that zinc binding is independent of this activity. Although serine residues between amino acids 108 and 126 of A/WSN/33(H1N1) M1 are phosphorylated (Gregoriades, Guzman and Paoletti 1990), the role of this property in viral replication is unknown; it may be important for viral replication involving intracellular movement of the protein (Whittaker, Kemler and Helenius 1995). The influenza B M1 protein is also phosphorylated. M1 also inhibits RNP transcription activity (Zvonarjev and Ghendon 1980, Ye, Baylor and Wagner 1989), and thus is considered to serve as a molecular switch that initiates the final step of virus assembly. Although it is associated with RNP in virions, the molecules with which the protein interacts (e.g. vRNA, NP or polymerase proteins), remain unknown. M1 does contain RNA-binding domains (Ye, Baylor and Wagner 1989), which have been mapped between residues 90–109 and 129–164.

One of the M gene products (most likely M1) contributes to the dominance phenotype shown by cold-adapted A/Ann Arbor/6/60(H2N2) in co-infection studies with other strains, both in vitro and in vivo (Whitaker-Dowling, Lucas and Youngner 1990, Whitaker-Dowling, Maassab and Youngner 1991, Youngner et al. 1994). The M1 protein has also been linked to rapid virus growth (Baez, Palese and Kilbourne 1980, Yasuda, Bucher and Ishihama 1994).

M2

The integral homotetrameric M2 membrane protein (Lamb, Zebedee and Richardson 1985, Holsinger and Lamb 1991, Sugrue and Hay 1991, Panayotov and Schlesinger 1992), abundantly expressed at the surface of virus-infected cells, is nevertheless a relatively minor component of virions (Zebedee and Lamb 1988). Sharing 8 amino-terminal residues with M1, the M2 protein comprises 97 amino acids: 24 as the ecto-, 19 as the transmembrane, and 54 as the cytoplasmic domain. M2 proteins are palmitylated at Cys-50 with the exception of those in H3N8 equine viruses, but are not essential for virus replication (Sugrue, Belshe and Hay 1990, Veit et al. 1991). The protein is also phosphorylated, mainly at Ser-64 (85%), but also at Ser-82, 89 and 93 (Holsinger et al. 1995). M2 proteins are thought to function as a pH-activated ion channel that permits protons to enter the virion during uncoating (Sugrue et al. 1990, Pinto, Holsinger and Lamb 1992) and that modulates the pH of intracellular compartments, an essential function for the prevention of acid-induced conformational changes of intracellularly cleaved HAs (H5 and H7 HA subtypes

of virulent avian influenza A virus) in the trans-Golgi network (Sugrue et al. 1990, Ohuchi et al. 1994, Takeuchi and Lamb 1994). The activity of the M2 ion channel is blocked by the anti-influenza drug amantadine hydrochloride (see 'Chemotherapy', p. 420). The M2-associated ion channel activity resides in the transmembrane region (Duff and Ashley 1992), the primary site of mutations (residues 27, 30, 31 and 34) in amantadine-resistant mutants (Hay et al. 1985). Amantadine presumably blocks the ion channel activity of M2 by steric hindrance, resulting from insertion of the active drug between Val-27 and Ser-31 of the M2 molecule (Duff et al. 1994). The functional role of the M2 cytoplasmic region, the longest among the influenza viral membrane proteins, is unknown but is important for virus replication (Castrucci and Kawaoka 1995). M2 co-precipitates with the RNP core prepared from purified virus (Bron et al. 1993), indicating its high affinity for this protein, a property that presumably involves the M2 cytoplasmic tail. The M2 protein forms a homotetramer by non-covalent association of M2 dimers disulphide-linked at Cys-17 or 19, or both (Holsinger and Lamb 1991, Sugrue and Hay 1991, Panayotov and Schlesinger 1992). None of the cysteine residues in the M2 is essential for viral replication (M Castrucci and Y Kawaoka, unpublished data), although disulphide bond formation stabilizes the M2 tetramer (Holsinger and Lamb 1991). Post-translational modifications of the M2 do not affect its ion channel activity and may be involved in virion morphogenesis (Holsinger et al. 1995).

OTHER M GENE PRODUCTS OF TYPE B AND C VIRUSES

BM2, an M gene product of type B virus found in infected cells, has no obvious structural similarities with type A M2 protein (Briedis, Lamb and Choppin 1982), and its functional role remains unknown. CM2, which resides in infected cells (Hongo et al. 1994), is translated from unspliced transcripts of the M gene, from which a spliced mRNA for M1 is made. The coding region of CM2 corresponds to the 3' half of the transcript, but its exact length is unknown (132–139 amino acids), owing to the presence of multiple in-frame initiation codons at the anticipated initiation site. Although CM2 possesses a potential membrane-

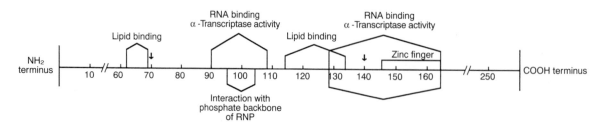

Fig. 22.17 Functional map of the M1 protein. Transcriptase inhibition sites and RNA binding sites were identified at amino acids 128–164 and 90–108 by Ye, Baylor and Wagner (1989). Hankins et al. (1989) placed the critical antitranscriptase sites at amino acids 70 and 140 (arrows). The lipid-binding sites have been placed at amino acids 62–68 and 114–133 by Gregoriades and Frangione (1981). Wakefield and Brownlee (1989) identified a zinc-finger motif at amino acids 146–160. Amino acid residues 101–105 serve as a karyophilic signal (Ye, Robinson and Wagner 1995.) (Modified from Herlocher, Bucher and Webster 1992.)

spanning region, its function and presence in virions remain unknown.

NS1

The only non-structural protein of influenza A virus, NS1 is made in abundance during early infection. It is encoded by a co-linear mRNA, consists of 124–237 amino acids depending on the virus strain, is phosphorylated (Privalsky and Penhoet 1978) and contains 2 karyophilic signals (Greenspan, Palese and Krystal 1988). It inhibits mRNA splicing and the nuclear export of cellular and viral mRNA (Alonso-Caplen et al. 1992, Lu, Qian and Krug 1994, Qiu and Krug 1994), maximizing the availability of substrate for capped primers, and thereby promoting viral mRNA synthesis. Two NS1 functional domains inhibit mRNA transport activity: the domain near the amino terminal end (amino acids 19–38), a region also containing a nuclear localization signal (Greenspan, Palese and Krystal 1988), binds to the poly(A) sequence; whereas the 'effector' domain, which resides in the carboxyl half of the molecule (residues 134–161), presumably interacts with host nuclear factors (Qian, Alonso-Caplen and Krug 1994). Nevertheless, the NS1 of A/Turkey/Oregon/71(H7N5) virus, which is not defective in growth in either embryonated eggs or tissue culture, is only 124 amino acids long (Norton et al. 1987), having a termination codon upstream of the effector domain. A temperature-sensitive mutant containing a 36 nt deletion in the NS1 gene shows host range restriction; the virus replicates in chicken kidney cells but not in MDCK cells (Maassab and DeBorde 1983, Buonagurio et al. 1984). An NS1 truncation mutant (90 instead of 281 total amino acids) has also been isolated from influenza B viruses (Tobita et al. 1990).

NS2

Encoded by a spliced mRNA (Inglis et al. 1979, Lamb and Choppin 1979), the NS2 protein comprises 121 amino acids (Lamb and Lai 1980), is phosphorylated, is located in the nucleus and cytoplasm of infected cells, and is found in virions, associating with RNP by interacting with the C terminal portion of M1 protein (Richardson and Akkina 1991, Yasuda et al. 1993). The function of this protein is unknown. The NS2 proteins of type A viruses are more conserved than the NS1 protein (76.9% vs 64.3%); however, neither product is conserved to the extent of other internal proteins (at least 90% for the PA (Okazaki, Kawaoka and Webster 1989), PB1 (Kawaoka, Krauss and Webster 1989) and PB2 (Gorman et al. 1990b)).

HEF

The HEF protein of influenza C virus, which is synthesized as a single polypeptide with subsequent trimer formation and then cleaved into 2 disulphide-linked subunits, HEF1 and HEF2 (Herrler, Compans and Meier-Ewert 1979, Hewat et al. 1984, Formanowski and Meier-Ewert 1988, Herrler and Klenk 1991), exists on the virion surface as projections and has a reticular structure consisting mainly of hexagons (Flewett and

Apostolov 1967) (see Fig. 22.5). Calcium ion is essential for maintenance of the HEF structure. The HEF facilitates binding of influenza C virus to its cell surface receptor, an oligosaccharide containing a terminal 9-O-acetyl-N-acetylneuraminic acid (Herrler et al. 1985a, Rogers et al. 1986).

The 9-O-acetyl group is critical for the binding of HEF, which does not recognize N-acetyl or N-glycolyl sialic acid (Rogers et al. 1986, Suzuki et al. 1992). The receptor-destroying enzyme (esterase) of influenza C virus resides in the HEF protein. Unlike the NA of type A and B viruses, HEF does not catalyse the cleavage of the α-ketosidic linkage between terminal sialic acid and an adjacent sugar residue, but instead catalyses the cleavage of the 9-O-acetyl group of 9-O-acetyl-N-acetylneuraminic acid (Herrler et al. 1985b, Vlasak et al. 1987). The active site of the esterase and the receptor-binding site differ, as di-isopropyl fluorophosphate inhibits only the esterase activity (Muchmore and Varki 1987). The protein also possesses fusion activity, which requires a low pH optimum (between 5.0 and 5.7) (Ohuchi, Ohuchi and Mifune 1982, Herrler et al. 1988). The acetylesterase activity may be required for entry of the C virus into target cells (Strobl and Vlasak 1993), but not for haemolysis (Herrler et al. 1992). The host cell-dependent variant selection also occurs in influenza C viruses with mutations in the HEF protein (Umetsu et al. 1992). HEF is also acylated, but with stearic acid instead of palmitic acid, as in type A and B HAs (Veit et al. 1990).

4.3 Reverse genetics

A major research advance occurred when Palese and colleagues established the reverse genetics system, which allows one to generate influenza viruses containing genes derived from cloned cDNA (Luytjes et al. 1989, Enami et al. 1990, García-Sastre and Palese 1993). Several research groups have established reverse genetics for other negative-strand RNA viruses (Pattnaik and Wertz 1990, Collins, Mink and Stec 1991, Park et al. 1991, Pattnaik et al. 1992, De and Banerjee 1993, Schnell, Mebatsion and Conzelmann 1994, Lawson et al. 1995). Using this technique, Palese and colleagues generated influenza A and B viruses (designated as transfectant viruses) with genes derived from cloned cDNA (Enami et al. 1990, Enami and Palese 1991, Barclay and Palese 1995). Although some modifications have been made from experiment to experiment (Kimura et al. 1992, Martin et al. 1992, Seong and Brownlee 1992a, de la Luna et al. 1993, Mena et al. 1994), the basic method (García-Sastre and Palese 1993) involves (1) preparation of RNA, containing exactly the same 5′ and 3′ sequences as viral RNA, from cloned influenza virus genes with RNA polymerase, (2) encapsidation of the RNA with influenza virus NP and polymerase proteins, (3) transfection of the encapsidated RNA, and (4) infection with a helper influenza virus to rescue the transfected RNA (Fig. 22.18). To generate transfectant viruses, selection of a virus containing transfected RNA is included as the last step. Reverse genetics has permitted novel investigations of the structure–function relationships of the HA (Jin, Leser and Lamb 1994, Zurcher, Luo and Palese 1994), the NA (Bilsel,

Castrucci and Kawaoka 1993, Castrucci and Kawaoka 1993, Luo, Chung and Palese 1993), the M1 (Yasuda, Bucher and Ishihama 1994) and the M2 (Castrucci and Kawaoka 1995). It also has allowed the generation of attenuated viruses for use in vaccine preparation (Muster et al. 1991, Subbarao, Kawaoka and Murphy 1993) and has opened the way for studies of influenza virus as a vaccine vector (Li et al. 1993, Castrucci et al. 1994, García-Sastre et al. 1994, Percy et al. 1994), genomic functions (Parvin et al. 1989, Luo et al. 1991, Yamanaka et al. 1991, Bergmann, García-Sastre and Palese 1992, Li and Palese 1992, 1994, Kimura et al. 1993, Piccone, Fernandez-Sesma and Palese 1993, Neumann and Hobom 1995), genomic replication (Nakagawa et al. 1995) and gene packaging (Enami et al. 1991).

5 ANTIGENS

5.1 Polymerase proteins

Cytotoxic T lymphocytes can recognize each of the 3

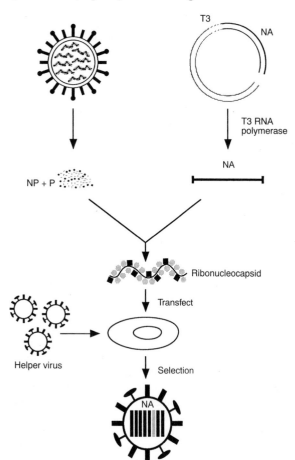

Fig. 22.18 Reverse genetics procedure. The diagram outlines the generation of an influenza virus containing the neuraminidase (NA) gene derived from cloned cDNA. NA vRNA is transcribed in the presence of NP and polymerase proteins to make artificial RNP, which is then transfected into cells that have been infected with a helper virus. With appropriate selection, one can generate a virus containing the transfected vRNA.

polymerase proteins (Bennink et al. 1984, 1987, Bastin, Townsend and McMichael 1987, Reay et al. 1989). These proteins have not been examined extensively for antigenic variants, although monoclonal antibodies to PA and PB2 are now available (Bárcena et al. 1994).

5.2 HA

The HA antigen is the major inducer of protective immunity to influenza viruses. Influenza A virus HAs show subtype specificity and are thought to possess 5 antigenic sites in the 3-dimensional structure (Wiley, Wilson and Skehel 1981, Wiley and Skehel 1987), although some subdivision and overlap of these areas have been noted (Caton et al. 1982, Daniels et al. 1983). For H3 virus strains (Wiley, Wilson and Skehel 1981, Wiley and Skehel 1987), the sites are A, B, C, D and E (see Fig. 22.11), and for the H1 strains they are Ca1, Ca2, Cb, Sa and Sb (Caton et al. 1982). Each of these sites was derived from amino acid sequence changes in antigenic variants selected with monoclonal antibodies, as well as in natural variants. Monoclonal antibodies to each of the 5 sites neutralize the infectivity of the virus (Wiley and Skehel 1987).

Helper T lymphocytes recognize several distinct regions of the HA1 and HA2 subunits located either on the surface or the interior of the intact molecule, as well as conformational determinants on the HA (Yewdell and Hackett 1989). Helper T lymphocyte recognition includes specificity for determinants on the variable regions of the molecule to which antibodies are also directed (Hackett et al. 1983, Mills et al. 1988). The immunodominant peptide most readily recognized by both subtype-specific and cross-reactive helper T lymphocyte clones is HA1 306–328 (H3 numbering system). Most memory T cell clones recognize sites B, C and E (HA1 56–76; H3 numbering) (Barnett et al. 1989, Graham et al. 1989). Residues important in antibody recognition affect T cell recognition (Barnett et al. 1989, Graham et al. 1989), indicating that both B and T cells may recognize similar sites on the HA and hence that both systems may provide selective immune pressure. Cytotoxic T cells recognize both the HA1 and HA2 subunits (Wabuke-Bunoti and Fan 1983, Wabuke-Bunoti et al. 1984).

5.3 NP

Although a type-specific protein, the NP of influenza A viruses shows antigenic variation (Herlocher, Bucher and Webster 1992). It contains at least 3 non-overlapping antigenic areas (Van Wyke et al. 1980), one of which is highly conserved. Monoclonal antibody binding to this site inhibits transcription of viral RNA in vitro (Van Wyke, Bean and Webster 1981). The NP epitopes recognized by dominant helper T lymphocytes in humans are located in residues 206–229, whereas those of mice are found in residues 260–283, with the distinct specificity of these regions depending on haplotypes. As a major antigen recognized by cytotoxic T lymphocytes, the NP possesses several T cell-specific epitopes that are conserved among human influenza A viruses (Bastin et al. 1987, Bodmer et al. 1988, Yewdell and Hackett 1989). Transfer of cytotoxic T lymphocytes specific to NP protects mice from lethal influenza challenge (Taylor and Askonas 1986).

5.4 NA

The subtype-specific influenza A virus NA has 4 antigenic sites, each consisting of multiple epitopes (Webster, Brown and Laver 1984). These antigenic sites differ in that antibodies to some but not other sites inhibit enzyme activity. Amino acids that change during antigenic drift cluster mainly in the distal surface loops connecting the various strands of β-sheets (Air et al. 1985).

Antigenic structures of the N9 NA have been extensively studied. Analysis of the crystal structure of a complex of N9 NA from A/tern/Australia/G75 with the Fab fragment of monoclonal antibody NC41 (Colman et al. 1987, Tulip et al. 1992) shows that the antibody contacts the NA over a surface area of 900 Å², comprising 19 amino acid residues localized on 5 polypeptide loops surrounding the enzyme active site. Site-specific mutagenesis indicates that, of the 19 amino acids in this epitope, only a few provide the critical contacts required for antibody recognition (Nuss, Whitaker and Air 1993). These findings support the observation of limited sites of sequence changes and local changes to the structure in escape mutants (Webster et al. 1987, Varghese et al. 1988, Tulip et al. 1991), implying (1) that antibody escape mutants are selected only when they contain changes at critical sites, or changes that introduce bulky side-chains capable of sterically preventing antibody attachment, and (2) that the other contact residues are providing 'passive surface complementarity' (Nuss, Whitaker and Air 1993). Antibodies to NA are inefficient in neutralizing the virus, but reduce plaque sizes in cell culture (Jahiel and Kilbourne 1966, Kilbourne et al. 1968, Rott, Becht and Orlich 1974). In agreement with these findings, immunity to NA in natural infection has only a small role in influenza protection as exemplified by the 1968 pandemic, whose causative agent possessed the NA from a previously circulating human virus; the immunity to the NA that existed in the human population did not protect humans from pandemic influenza (Cockburn, Delon and Ferreira 1969). However, in experimental infections in animal models, passive transfer of monoclonal antibodies to NA or immunization with the vaccinia virus expressing the NA protected animals against lethal challenge (Webster, Reay and Laver 1988) or reduced virus titres (Schulman, Khakpour and Kilbourne 1968, Rott, Becht and Orlich 1974). Helper and cytotoxic T lymphocyte responses to NA were found in influenza virus-infected mice, but were limited compared with responses to the HA, NP and M1 (Hurwitz et al. 1985, Reay et al. 1989, Wysocka and Hackett 1990, Caton and Gerhard 1992).

5.5 M1

Even though this protein is considered a highly conserved type-specific antigen, some variations have been found among influenza A strains studied with a panel of monoclonal antibodies (Van Wyke et al. 1984, Herlocher, Bucher and Webster 1992). Helper

T lymphocytes specific for the M1 protein are cross-reactive between viruses of different subtypes (Hurwitz et al. 1985). M1 is also recognized by cytotoxic T lymphocytes (Gotch et al. 1987).

5.6 M2

Antibodies to the M2 protein have been found in humans infected with influenza A virus (Black et al. 1993). Passively transferred monoclonal antibodies reduced virus replication in mice (Treanor et al. 1990), and it has recently been shown that M2 protein plays a role in recovery from infection in mice (Slepushkin et al. 1995). Some antigenic variation can be found among the M2s as a result of amino acid changes in the ectodomain (Zebedee and Lamb 1988). No helper or cytotoxic T lymphocytes specific for M2 have been isolated.

5.7 NS1

The influenza A virus NS1 proteins from different animal species cross-react with polyclonal antibodies. Although a panel of monoclonal antibodies distinguishes avian virus NS1 from those of human, swine and equine strains, there is no evidence of antigenic variations among the latter group of proteins (Brown, Hinshaw and Webster 1983). Cytotoxic T lymphocytes recognizing NS1 are highly cross-reactive (Bennink and Yewdell 1988).

5.8 NS2

The antigenic properties of NS2 are poorly understood; however, mouse cytotoxic T lymphocytes specific for this protein have been found (Yewdell and Hackett 1989).

6 CLINICAL MANIFESTATIONS AND PATHOGENESIS

The spectrum of symptoms occurring during influenza virus infections is highly variable, ranging from mild respiratory disease with rhinitis or pharyngitis to primary viral pneumonia with fatal outcome. Rates of asymptomatic infection may be nearly as high as those for symptomatic infection during some epidemics (Hayslett et al. 1962, Foy, Cooney and Allan 1976, Noble 1982). Often a physician's diagnosis is based on the patient's symptoms and the knowledge that influenza activity is occurring in the community. The presence of fever and cough along with sudden onset help distinguish influenza from other respiratory infections such as the common cold; however, the physical signs and symptoms of influenza are not distinct enough from those of other respiratory infections to make a firm clinical diagnosis without laboratory confirmation. In addition, symptoms in certain populations, notably elderly people, may be atypical.

ADULTS

Early symptoms in adults typically include fever, chills, headache, sore throat, dry cough, myalgias, anorexia and malaise. A fever of 38–40°C that peaks within 24 hours of onset is common, but peaks as high as 41°C can also occur. Pyrexia typically lasts 3 days but may last from 1 to 5 days. Other symptoms that occur less frequently include substernal soreness, photophobia and other ocular symptoms, nausea, abdominal pain and diarrhoea (Douglas 1975, Nicholson 1992, Betts 1995). Although most symptoms typically resolve within a week, cough and malaise may persist for 1 or more weeks after fever has subsided. Type A influenza viruses of the H1N1, H2N2 and H3N2 subtypes as well as type B influenza viruses cause a similar spectrum of illness (Frank, Taber and Wells 1985, Spelman and McHardy 1985, Nicholson 1992). However, in general, the frequency of severe infections requiring hospital admission or causing death is lower for influenza B than for influenza A. Elderly, debilitated people may have signs and symptoms that are not immediately recognized as influenza. Symptoms in uncomplicated disease in this group include lassitude, anorexia, cough, rhinitis, unexplained fever, general malaise and confusion.

INFANTS AND CHILDREN

Influenza A and B viruses are significant causes of both upper and lower respiratory tract illness in children (Kim et al. 1979, Glezen, Paredes and Taber 1980, Glezen et al. 1980). In children, symptoms are similar to those in adults, but gastrointestinal symptoms such as vomiting, abdominal pain and diarrhoea are seen more frequently. Maximum temperatures also tend to be higher in children than in adults, and febrile convulsions can occur. In addition, myositis, croup and otitis media occur more frequently in children. Influenza infection of neonates can be life-threatening and may be manifest only as an unexplained febrile illness (Meibalane et al. 1977). Hospitalization rates for infants and young children may increase during influenza outbreaks (Kim et al. 1979, Glezen 1980).

COMPLICATIONS

Complications of the upper respiratory tract after influenza infection include bacterial sinusitis and otitis media. Lower respiratory tract complications include exacerbation of chronic obstructive pulmonary disease and chronic congestive heart failure, croup, bronchitis, bronchiolitis, wheezing attacks in asthmatics and pneumonia (primary viral pneumonia, secondary bacterial pneumonia or combined bacterial and viral pneumonia) (Nicholson 1992, Betts 1995).

Primary influenza pneumonia, which often develops abruptly and progresses rapidly, was described in detail during the 1957/8 Asian influenza pandemic (Hers et al. 1957, Louria et al. 1959). This type of pneumonia is uncommon, and occurs mainly among those at increased risk for complications of influenza. Rapid respiration rate, tachycardia, cyanosis, high fever and hypotension are frequent symptoms. Diffuse pulmonary infiltrates and acute respiratory failure with a high mortality rate are also features of this disease. Combined viral and bacterial pneumonia is more common than primary viral pneumonia and may be clinically indistinguishable from it.

Secondary bacterial infections typically occur 5–10 days after initial onset of influenza symptoms and are responsible for most pneumonias during influenza epidemics. Productive cough, pleuritic chest pain and chills are common symptoms of this type of pneumonia. *Streptococcus pneumoniae*, *Staphylococcus aureus* and *Haemophilus influenzae* are the organisms most commonly involved (Schwarzmann et al. 1971). These illnesses respond to appropriate antimicrobial agents and have a lower case fatality rate than primary viral pneumonia.

Other reported but less frequent complications of influenza include myositis, myocarditis and pericarditis, acute renal failure, encephalopathy, encephalitis, transverse myelitis, Guillain–Barré syndrome and a range of other neurological complications, Reye's syndrome and toxic shock syndrome (Noble 1982, Betts 1995).

Higher rates of spontaneous abortion, stillbirths and premature births were reported among pregnant women during the major pandemics of 1918/19 and 1957/8 (Woolston and Conley 1918, Bland 1919, Hardy et al. 1961); increased maternal risk for death following influenza infection was also documented (Greenberg et al. 1958, Eickhoff, Sherman and Serfling 1961). In addition, case reports and limited studies suggest that women in the third trimester of pregnancy, including women without underlying risk factors, may be at increased risk for serious complications following influenza infection (Centers for Disease Control and Prevention 1996).

Serious complications of influenza most often occur in people 65 years of age and older, in the very young, and in those of any age with underlying chronic cardiac, pulmonary or metabolic disease (Barker and Mullooly 1980). Complications in elderly people, particularly among those with pulmonary, cardiovascular or other chronic diseases, account for most of the mortality in influenza epidemics (Eickhoff, Sherman and Serfling 1961). The highest rates of hospitalization and death following influenza infection occur in those at opposite ends of the age spectrum, i.e. less than a year old or 65 years and older. In general, hospital admissions are 10–20 times higher than the mortality rate (Barker and Mullooly 1980, Glezen Decker and Perrotta 1987).

PATHOGENESIS

Much remains to be learned about the pathogenesis of influenza virus replication and its relationship to the clinical manifestations and complications of the infection. Many studies to investigate the pathogenesis of influenza infections were conducted during the 1957/8 pandemic of Asian influenza (Hers and Mulder 1961, Walsh et al. 1961). These studies demonstrated that the principal site of replication is the columnar epithelial cells, but histological studies indicate that viral replication can occur throughout the respiratory tract. Infected ciliated columnar cells become vacuolated and lose their cilia, and infected mucosal and ciliated epithelial cells become necrotic and desquamate. In studies in which bronchoscopy was conducted on, or nasal and bronchial biopsy specimens were taken from, individuals with uncomplicated acute influenza infections, inflammation of the larynx, trachea and bronchi and desquamation of ciliated columnar epithelium into the lumen of the bronchus were observed. Regeneration of the respiratory epithelial cells takes c. 3–4 weeks, during which time pulmonary function abnormalities may persist (Hall et al. 1976). In these typical cases of influenza in which infection is confined to the respiratory tract, prostration, fever and myalgia often seem to be disproportionate to objective clinical signs or observed pathological changes.

Lungs from fatal cases of primary viral pneumonia most notably show hyaline membrane coverage of alveolar walls together with extensive intra-alveolar oedema and haemorrhage. Tracheitis and bronchitis are also observed. (Hers and Mulder 1961, Martin et al. 1959). Patients with secondary bacterial pneumonia have changes characteristic of bacterial pneumonia in addition to the tracheobronchial findings of influenza.

The occurrence of systemic illness and fever suggests dissemination of virus via the blood stream, but systematic studies (Kilbourne 1959, Minuse et al. 1962) and limited case reports (Naficy 1963, Lehmann and Gust 1971) suggest that viraemia is detected only rarely.

Apoptosis

Influenza A and B viruses induce apoptosis in both permissive (MDCK) and non-permissive cells (Takizawa et al. 1993, Hinshaw et al. 1994), which can be blocked by the *bcl*-2 product (Hinshaw et al. 1994). Apoptosis induced by influenza virus infection seems to involve activation of the Fas antigen-encoding gene (Takizawa et al. 1995). The role of apoptosis in the clinical signs and symptoms of influenza is unknown.

Mx protein

The pathogenesis of influenza virus infection is influenced by parameters specified by both the virus and the host. Relatively little is known about the role of host genes that control infection. One exception is the Mx family of proteins, which mediate inhibition of orthomyxovirus replication (Staeheli 1990). This family of proteins is induced by interferon and may act either in the cytoplasm, as in the case of the human MxA protein, or in the nucleus, as in the case of the mouse Mx1 protein (Pavlovic, Haller and Staeheli 1992). The Mx proteins bind GTP and exhibit GTPase activity required for antiviral activity (Horisberger 1992).

Host range restriction

Multiple genetic factors affect host range restriction for influenza viruses. Changes in host range can parallel changes in pathogenicity. At present, more is known about how particular amino acid changes at positions in or near the receptor-binding pocket of the haemagglutinin confer different receptor specificities and thus different host ranges. These receptor-binding specificities correspond to the composition of the receptor at the replication site in the host (see 'Receptor binding', p. 399).

There is also indirect evidence that other genes, particularly the *NP* and *NA* genes, play a role in host range restriction. For example, replacement of the *NP* gene of an avian virus with the *NP* gene of a human virus alters host range (Scholtissek, Koennecke and Rott 1978), and phylogenetic analyses of *NP* gene sequences have shown that there are 5 distinct host-specific lineages (Gammelin et al. 1990, Gorman et al. 1990a). Other internal genes of influenza A viruses also apparently play a role in host range and virulence (Klenk and Rott 1988).

6.1 Epidemiology

Although human type A and B influenza viruses were not isolated until 1933 and 1940, respectively, descriptions of epidemics and pandemics of respiratory disease with characteristics suggestive of influenza have been recorded for over 4 centuries (see 'Historical record', p. 385). Certain well documented epidemiological features of modern epidemics of influenza also emerge from the early accounts. Epidemics of varying severity occurred at irregular intervals, caused the highest mortality in elderly people and were thought to have spread from Asia. These records detail epidemics of cough, fever, chills and muscle aches that affected many people of different ages within a short time.

An epidemic of influenza is an outbreak of disease in a circumscribed location, which may affect a town, a city or an entire country. Localized epidemics within a community often have a characteristic pattern in which the epidemic begins abruptly, peaks within 2–3 weeks and has a total duration of 5–8 weeks (Glezen and Couch 1978). The spread of influenza virus through a community typically causes large increases in medical visits for febrile respiratory disease (Glezen 1982). Absence from school due to influenza often occurs early in the epidemic, and school children are believed to be important in disseminating the virus in the community. Although reports of increased numbers of children with febrile respiratory illness are often the first indication that influenza is circulating in a community, it is not uncommon for a laboratory-confirmed outbreak in a nursing home to be the first report that influenza is present. Absence from work, hospitalization for pneumonia and other complications of influenza, and death due to pneumonia and influenza and its complications all tend to peak later in the epidemic.

The size of epidemics that occur during the interpandemic intervals is quite variable, but almost always smaller than those that occur following the introduction of a new virus subtype. The size of epidemics and their impact reflect the interplay between the extent of antigenic variation of the virus, the extent of immunity in the population and the population groups that are most affected in a given year.

A pandemic of influenza is an epidemic of disease that involves most if not all age groups on several continents. Influenza experts agree that at least 3 true pandemics of influenza have occurred during the past century: Spanish influenza in 1918, Asian influenza A(H2N2) in 1957 and Hong Kong influenza A(H3N2) in 1968.

CURRENT EPIDEMIOLOGY

The simultaneous circulation of 2 subtypes of influenza A together with influenza B viruses since 1977 has made the current epidemiology of influenza unusually complex. Influenza B viruses have circulated continuously in humans since their first isolation in 1940, whereas influenza A(H3N2) viruses have been present since their emergence in pandemic form in 1968. Unlike the situation in 1957 and again in 1968 when new pandemic strains totally replaced the previously circulating influenza A strains, the influenza A(H1N1) viruses that emerged in 1977 were unable to supplant viruses of the A(H3N2) subtype. Instead, 2 distinct subtypes of influenza A viruses have co-circulated world-wide since then (see Fig. 22.1).

Prevalence of these 3 groups of viruses may vary temporally and geographically within a country (Chapman et al. 1993) and between countries and continents during a given influenza season (World Health Organization 1996). In the USA the circulation of influenza A(H3N2) viruses has, in recent years, been associated most often with excess pneumonia and influenza (P and I) mortality. Major peaks of excess P and I mortality were documented by the US 121 Cities Mortality Reporting System during the 1989/90 and 1993/4 influenza seasons, during which influenza A(H3N2) viruses accounted for over 98% of the viruses reported (see also Chapter 13).

TRANSMISSION AND SEASONALITY

It is generally accepted that influenza viruses are spread primarily by small particle aerosols of virus-laden respiratory secretions that are expelled into the air during coughing, sneezing or talking by an infected person (Moser et al. 1979, Betts 1995). Spread by direct contact is, however, also possible. The incubation period for influenza is relatively short (1–4 days), and the explosive nature of influenza epidemics and pandemics and simultaneous onset in many people suggest that a single infected person can transmit virus to a large number of susceptible individuals.

It is also generally accepted that influenza viruses are maintained in humans only by direct person-to-person spread, as there is no firm evidence for reintroduction from latently or persistently infected individuals. This is supported by evidence from local and global surveillance of influenza viruses, which has shown that antigenic variation and the consequent epidemiological behaviour of influenza viruses follow a relatively uniform pattern, each successive antigenic variant replacing the previously circulating one in such a way that the co-circulation of distinct antigenic variants of a given subtype occurs for relatively short periods (Stuart-Harris, Schild and Oxford 1985). These data have shown that consecutive epidemics in a community are caused by reintroduction of antigenically drifted or genetically distinct influenza viruses, or both. Intensive community-wide surveillance in large population centres has shown that influenza activity can often be detected during the summer months (Monto and Kioumehr 1975, Fox et al. 1982). Global influenza surveillance also indicates that influenza viruses are generally isolated every month from humans somewhere in the world (Noble 1982, World Health Organization 1996).

The seasonality of influenza activity has been well documented in many countries with temperate climates in Europe, North America and Asia. In these countries, influenza epidemics generally occur from December to March. Evidence that survival of influenza viruses in an aerosol is favoured by low relative humidity and low temperature (Hemmes, Winkler and Kool 1960, Schaffer, Soergel and Straube 1976) is often cited as an explanation for winter seasonality of influenza in temperate climates. Seasonality in tropical or subtropical climates is less well studied; however, influenza viruses may be isolated throughout the year, peaks of activity often occurring in the summer months (Reichelderfer et al. 1981). Other reports have suggested that peak influenza activity in tropical and subtropical areas may follow changes in weather such as onset of the rainy season (Rao et al. 1982). The environmental and epidemiological factors responsible for these observations remain to be elucidated.

ANTIGENIC DRIFT AND ITS IMPACT

The epidemiological success of influenza viruses is largely due to the 2 types of antigenic variation that occur in the HA and the NA. Antigenic variation renders an individual susceptible to new strains – despite previous experience with other influenza viruses. The first kind of variation, called antigenic drift, occurs with both influenza A and B viruses, and is the gradual alteration by point mutation of the HA and NA within type B influenza viruses or within a given subtype of influenza A viruses. This kind of variation results in the inability of antibody to previous strains to neutralize the mutant virus. Variations in the amino acid sequences of the HA and NA occur at a rate of <1% per year during antigenic drift.

Antigenic drift variants are responsible for periodic epidemics that occur between pandemics. Thus, influenza among humans is caused by distinguishable antigenic variant strains of influenza A and B viruses that emerge and become predominant over a period of 2–5 years, only to be replaced by the subsequently successful antigenic variant.

Phylogenetic analyses have revealed that HA genes of human influenza A and B viruses have a regular relationship between isolation date and their position on the evolutionary tree. When evolutionary rates are estimated by regression of the year of isolation against the number of nucleotide or amino acid substitutions from a common ancestor [A/Puerto Rico/8/34, A/USSR/90/77, A/Aichi/2/68 and B/Lee/40 for the old A(H1N1), contemporary A(H1N1), A(H3N2) and

B viruses, respectively], it is apparent that the HA genes of human influenza A viruses of the H1N1 and H3N2 subtypes evolve at about the same rates, whereas HA genes of influenza B viruses evolve more slowly (Table 22.3). Recent phylogenetic analyses have also shown that, although co-circulating lineages of HA genes of influenza B viruses can coexist longer than for influenza A HA genes, the overall patterns and the rates of evolution of the HA genes of these 2 types of influenza viruses are more similar than was previously believed (Cox and Bender 1995).

When amino acid changes in the HAs of field strains of influenza A(H3N2) viruses are plotted on the 3-dimensional structure of the HA, it is apparent that much of the surface of the molecule has been altered by amino acid substitutions during the circulation of these viruses since 1968 (Fig. 22.19; see also Plate 21.19). At least 4 changes that can be assigned to at least 2 antigenic sites have been observed between major epidemic strains of human influenza A viruses (Wilson and Cox 1990). Thus, the HA molecule seems to have a vast potential for antigenic change within a subtype as well as between subtypes without jeopardizing its function. This feature along with the apparent extensive nature of the antigenic regions in the HA molecule (Caton et al. 1982, Wilson and Cox 1990) make it unlikely that we will be able to predict future antigenic variants of influenza before they arise.

Morbidity

Quantifying morbidity due to influenza is difficult. The spectrum of symptoms occurring during influenza virus infections is quite variable. In addition, many other respiratory pathogens cause influenza-like illness, so parallel laboratory studies are essential to define influenza-related morbidity. Many methods have been used for estimating the impact of influenza illnesses in a community or country, including prospective surveillance of illnesses and influenza infections in all members of a defined population. Regular interviews of a randomly selected population to detect all symptomatic respiratory illnesses, coupled with laboratory studies to detect symptomatic and asymptomatic influenza infections, provide the most precise measurement of age-specific influenza morbidity and rates of asymptomatic infection. A number of these community- and family-based studies have been carried out during pandemic and interpandemic influenza outbreaks (Jordan, Badger and Dingle 1958, Philip et al. 1961, Hall et al. 1971, Hall, Cooney and Fox 1973, Monto and Ullman 1974, Foy, Cooney and Allan

1976, Jennings and Miles 1978). These studies have shown that influenza epidemics disrupt school attendance and work productivity, place heavy demands on health care systems, and result in morbidity and mortality among high-risk populations almost every year.

During average epidemics overall attack rates are estimated to be 10–20%, but in selected populations or age groups, attack rates of 40–50% are not unusual. It is apparent from studies conducted during both pandemic years and interpandemic periods that age-specific attack rates are highest in school children (Glezen 1996). This correlates well with the observation that school absenteeism is followed by employee absenteeism during influenza epidemics. Elderly people are often admitted to hospital during the latter part of the epidemic. Both type A and B influenza viruses are important causes of respiratory infection within nursing homes and other long-term care facilities.

Mortality

One of the hallmarks of influenza is the increase in mortality during pandemics and many epidemics. William Farr (1885) is credited with developing the concept of 'excess mortality', i.e. the number of deaths observed during an epidemic of influenza-like illness in excess of the number expected. Estimating influenza-associated excess mortality provides one of the most objective measures of the severity of influenza epidemics and pandemics. Methods for determining the baseline or expected number of deaths for the winter season in the absence of an influenza epidemic have changed over the years. Various statistical approaches, ranging from a moving average to cyclical regression models and ARIMA (autoregressive integrated moving average) time series analyses have been used to calculate the baseline and threshold values (Collins and Lehmann 1951, Choi and Thacker 1982, Lui and Kendal 1987, Simonsen et al. 1997).

Increased influenza mortality results not only from P and I but also from cardiopulmonary and other chronic diseases that can be exacerbated by influenza (Collins and Lehman 1951, Eickhoff, Sherman and Serfling 1961). Quantification of deaths caused by influenza is complicated by the fact that information recorded on death certificates may fail to indicate that influenza was a cause of death because a laboratory diagnosis was not made or because influenza was not listed as a primary underlying or contributory cause of death. Therefore, calculations of influenza-associated

Table 22.3 Evolutionary rates for the HA1 portion of the HA gene and protein

Virus	Period	Number	Nucleotide changes per nucleotide site per year	Amino acid changes per amino acid site per year
H1N1	1934–1957	24	3.9×10^{-3}	5.3×10^{-3}
H1N1	1977–1996	146	2.7×10^{-3}	4.2×10^{-3}
H3N2	1968–1996	340	3.7×10^{-3}	4.1×10^{-3}
B	1940–1996	168	1.2×10^{-3}	1.1×10^{-3}

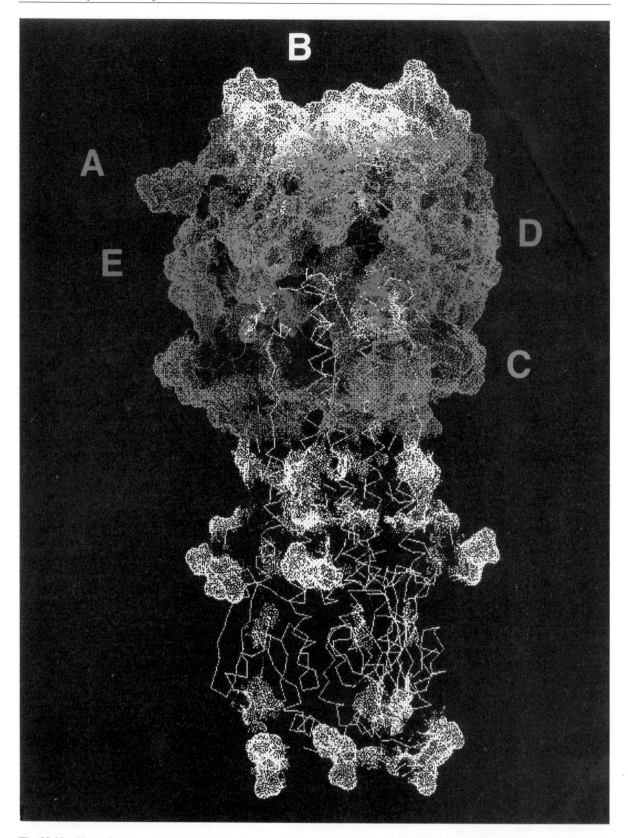

Fig. 22.19 Natural antigenic variation in the haemagglutinin (HA) of the H3 subtype of influenza A viruses circulating between 1968 and 1996. The HA trimer is depicted with the HA polypeptide backbone represented by an α-carbon trace in violet for the HA1 domain and in yellow for the HA2 domain. The solvent-accessible surface of residues that have changed during this period are represented by a dot surface. Antigenic regions are colour coded and designated A (red), B (yellow), C (magenta), D (blue) and E (green). Amino acid residues shown in white are surface accessible but not assigned to antibody-combining sites. This graphic representation demonstrates that most of the surface-accessible amino acids in the globular head region of the HA have changed during this 28-year period of circulation in humans of influenza A(H3N2) viruses. For colour, see Plate 22.19.

excess mortality are based both on excess deaths from P and I as well as from all causes. Although excess mortality occurs primarily in elderly people, it can occur in all age groups, particularly among individuals who are at increased risk for complications of influenza. Excess mortality has been documented during circulation of both type A and B influenza viruses, but has been associated most often with circulation of influenza A subtypes H2N2 and H3N2. Since 1986, excess mortality in the USA has been associated most frequently with the circulation of influenza A(H3N2) viruses (see Chapter 13); c. 90% of these influenza-associated excess deaths have occurred in individuals 65 or more years of age (Centers for Disease Control and Prevention 1996).

It is estimated that >20 000 influenza-associated excess deaths occurred in the USA during each of 9 different epidemics between 1972 and 1991; >40 000 influenza-associated deaths occurred during each of 3 of these epidemics (Simonsen et al. 1997) (Table 22.4).

ANTIGENIC SHIFT AND ITS IMPACT

Only influenza A viruses exhibit the second, more dramatic, kind of antigenic variation, called antigenic shift. Antigenic shift is the appearance in the human population of a new subtype of influenza A viruses containing a novel HA or a novel HA and NA immunologically distinct from isolates circulating previously. When antigenic shift occurs, the HA of the new strain would be expected to vary at the amino acid level 20–50% from the corresponding protein of previously circulating strains. Antigenic shift is responsible for worldwide pandemics, which occur at irregular and unpredictable intervals.

Although 15 subtypes of influenza HA have been identified in avian species, epidemics and pandemics of influenza among humans during this century seem to have been caused by viruses with HAs of only 3 different subtypes: H1, H2 and H3 (see Fig. 22.1). The most severe recorded pandemic of influenza was that of Spanish influenza in 1918–1919.

Retrospective serological evidence suggests that this pandemic was caused by viruses closely related to classic swine influenza A(H1N1) virus, but its origin is unknown. Outbreaks of disease occurred almost simultaneously in North America, Europe and Africa during the spring and early sum-

Table 22.4 Influenza excess mortality

Period	Excess deaths
'Spanish' influenza September 1918 to April 1919	500 000
'Asian' influenza September 1957 to March 1969	69 800
'Hong Kong' influenza September 1968 to March 1969	33 800
total	603 600
Interpandemic years 1957–1990	600 800

mer of 1918 (Crosby 1989). During the autumn of 1918 a second, more serious, wave of disease occurred. This wave peaked by the end of October but was followed by yet another wave of disease in mid-winter. Illness rates of nearly 40% occurred among school children during the autumn wave in the USA (Frost 1920). The differentiating features of this pandemic are the large numbers of cases with pneumonia and the unusually high case fatality rates, particularly in young healthy adults between the ages of 20 and 40 (Frost 1919). The social and medical consequences of the Spanish influenza pandemic are difficult to imagine today. About half of the 2 billion people living at that time were infected and at least 20 million of them died (Noble 1982). Hospitals were overflowing and there was a general shortage of medical services and vast disruption of community life.

Records indicate that the 1957/8 pandemic of Asian influenza A(H2N2) began in February in the southern Chinese province of Guizhou, spreading during March to Yunan province and during April to Singapore and Hong Kong (Stuart-Harris, Schild and Oxford 1985). The first virus isolates were obtained in Japan during May. This pandemic strain possessed completely different HA and NA antigens from the formerly circulating H1N1 viruses and spread rapidly world-wide by November 1957. Although H2N2 viruses were first isolated in the UK and the USA in June or July of 1957, peak incidence of the disease did not occur until October. This first wave of disease in both countries was followed by a second in January 1958; both waves were accompanied by excess mortality, primarily in the elderly. The timetable of key events for the pandemic of Asian influenza shown in Table 22.5 illustrates the short time frame for response to this pandemic and the missed opportunities for immunization after the first wave of disease. The highest attack rates during this pandemic were >50% in children aged 5–19 (Glezen 1996). Total influenza-associated excess mortality during this pandemic was estimated to be 69 800 (Noble 1982).

Viruses causing the Hong Kong H3N2 pandemic were first isolated in Hong Kong in July 1968. These viruses had a different HA antigen but shared the N2 NA antigen with the previously circulating Asian viruses. Widespread disease with increased excess mortality was observed in the USA during the winter of 1968/9, but in many other countries, including the UK, this did not happen until the winter of 1969/70 (Stuart-Harris, Schild and Oxford 1985). Total influenza-associated excess mortality for this pandemic was estimated to be 33 800 (Noble 1982).

In May 1977 the first outbreaks of disease caused by re-emerging influenza A(H1N1) viruses were observed in Tientsin, China (Kung et al. 1978). The H1N1 virus spread to other parts of Asia and reached Russia by November. Spread to Europe, North America and the southern hemisphere followed. Illness occurred almost exclusively among people less than 20 years of age and the highest attack rates of >50% were among school children. These viruses were antigenically and genetically similar to H1N1 viruses that had circulated widely during the early 1950s (Kendal et al. 1978, Nakajima, Desselberger and Palese 1978). The

Table 22.5 Timetable of events for the Asian influenza pandemic of 1957/58

February 1957	Outbreaks of influenza-like illness in Guizhou Province, China
Early March 1957	Outbreaks of influenza-like illness in Yunan Province, China
Mid March 1957	Outbreaks widespread in China
April 1957	Outbreaks in Hong Kong, Singapore and Taiwan
Mid May 1957	Virus isolated in Japan
June/July 1957	Virus first isolated in the USA. Outbreaks reported
September 1957	Widespread occurrence of influenza begun in the USA
October 1957	Peak incidence of disease occurred in the USA Attack rates were highest among school children and young adults
November 1957	Incidence of disease declined in the USA. First peak of pneumonia and influenza-related deaths observed
Early December 1957	Cumulative total of 60 million doses of vaccine released in the USA; much of the vaccine was unused
January/February 1958	Second peak of pneumonia and influenza-related mortality observed with a higher proportion than usual of deaths in the elderly. It was recognized retrospectively that a second wave of disease occurred in older adults and the elderly

absence of morbidity in people over 20 years of age has been explained by the fact that they were infected with similar viruses during the 1950s. Some workers have suggested that these H1N1 viruses may have been 'genetically frozen' in nature, while others have speculated that these viruses may have accidentally escaped from a laboratory; the source remains unknown.

Although antigenic shift seems to have been a requirement for the appearance of true pandemic influenza, the emergence of influenza A viruses of a new subtype in humans does not necessarily result in a pandemic (Dowdle and Millar 1978).

ECOLOGY OF INFLUENZA

The term influenza was used to describe a variety of acute respiratory and other diseases of a number of animal species, especially horses (see 'Historical record', p. 385), for many years. However, influenza A viruses have been isolated only from humans, swine, horses, a variety of sea mammals, and a wide variety of both domestic and wild birds, including ducks, geese, terns, shearwaters, gulls, turkeys, chickens, quail and pheasants (Easterday 1975, Hinshaw, Webster and Turner 1980, Webster et al. 1992).

Studies in Asia, Australia, Europe and North America have revealed that viruses with all 15 subtypes of HA and 9 subtypes of NA have been isolated from ducks and other feral water birds (Easterday 1975, Webster et al. 1992, Rohm et al. 1996) (Table 22.6), an observation suggesting that avian species serve as the primary reservoir for the emergence of new pandemic strains (Webster et al. 1992). These studies have also suggested that aquatic birds are likely to be the only source for influenza viruses in other species. Infections in avian species by most influenza viruses are asymptomatic, virus replicating preferentially in cells lining the intestinal tract (Webster et al. 1978). High titres of these viruses are excreted into their water habitat by asymptomatic birds. Avirulent influenza infections in birds may be the result of influenza viruses adapting to the host over many centuries. How-

ever, a few members of the H5 and H7 subtypes can cause a lethal systemic infection owing to the susceptibility of the HAs of these viruses to cleavage in many host tissues. The large reservoir for the 15 subtypes of influenza A viruses ensures their perpetuation in nature. The avian origin of strains of influenza in seals, whales, pigs, horses and domestic poultry has been documented (Webster et al. 1992, Webster and Kawaoka 1994).

Phylogenetic studies have revealed clues that have changed our thinking about the ecology and origins of influenza A viruses of different subtypes. There are species-specific lineages of viral genes (Kawaoka, Kraus and Webster 1989, Gorman et al. 1990a, 1990b, Ito et al. 1991, Bean et al. 1992), and it may be that all mammalian influenza viruses originate from the avian reservoir (Shortridge 1992, Webster and Kawaoka 1994).

Swine influenza

Koen (1919) reported the occurrence of an epizootic of respiratory disease among swine in Iowa, which seemed to be a new clinical entity and which coincided with the start of the 1918 pandemic of influenza in the Midwest of the USA. Because the clinical symptoms of the disease were similar to those occurring in humans, the disease was called swine influenza. Shope (1931) demonstrated the viral cause of swine influenza in 1930, 3 years before it was shown that influenza is a viral infection in people. Retrospective serological studies in humans (Davenport, Hennessy and Francis 1953) and subsequent investigations (reviewed by Stuart-Harris, Schild and Oxford 1985) provided strong circumstantial evidence that the Shope strain was antigenically close to the virus responsible for the 1918 pandemic of Spanish influenza.

Swine influenza A(H1N1) viruses have remained in the pig populations in many parts of the world to the present time and have also infected turkeys in the USA (Hinshaw et

Table 22.6 Influenza A viruses isolated from avian species, examples of HA and NA subtypes

HA subtype designation	NA subtype designation	Avian influenza A viruses
H1	N1	A/duck/Alberta/35/76(H1N1)[a]
	N8	A/duck/Alberta/97/77(H1N8)
H2	N9	A/duck/Germany/1/72(H2N9)[a]
	N9	A/duck/Germany/1/72(H2N9)
H3	N8	A/duck/Ukraine/1/63(H3N8)[a]
	N8	A/duck/England/62(H3N8)
	N2	A/turkey/England/69(H3N2)
H4	N6	A/duck/Czechoslovakia/56(H4N6)[a]
	N3	A/duck/Alberta/300/77(H4N3)
H5	N3	A/tern/South Africa/61(H5N3)[a]
	N9	A/turkey/Ontario/7732/66(H5N9)
	N1	A/chick/Scotland/59(H5N1)
H6	N2	A/turkey/Massachusetts/3740/65(H6N2)[a]
	N8	A/turkey/Canada/63(H6N8)
	N5	A/shearwater/Australia/72(H6N5)
	N1	A/duck/Germany/1868/68(H6N1)
H7	N7	A/fowl plague virus/Dutch/27(H7N7)[a]
	N1	A/chick/Brescia/1902(H7N1)
	N3	A/turkey/England/63(H7N3)
	N1	A/fowl plague virus/Rostock/34(H7N1)
H8	N4	A/turkey/Ontario/6118/68(H8N4)[a]
H9	N2	A/turkey/Wisconsin/1/66(H9N2)[a]
	N6	A/duck/Hong Kong/147/77(H9N6)
H10	N7	A/chick/Germany/N/49(H10N7)[a]
	N8	A/quail/Italy/1117/65(H10N8)
H11	N6	A/duck/England/56(H11N6)[a]
	N9	A/duck/Memphis/546/74(H11N9)
H12	N5	A/duck/Alberta/60/76(H12N5)[a]
H13	N6	A/gull/Maryland/704/77(H13N6)[a]
H14	N4	A/duck/Gurjev/263/83(H14N4)[a]
H15	N8	A/duck/Australia/341/83(H15N8)[a]
	N9	A/shearwater/Australia/2576/83(H15N9)

[a]Reference strains

al. 1983b). A number of cases or outbreaks attributable to swine H1N1 virus transmission from ill swine to people have been documented, and each is connected with concern stemming from the association of swine disease and antibodies to swine influenza viruses with the 1918 Spanish influenza pandemic. This concern is best exemplified by the swine influenza immunization campaign that was begun in the USA after a swine influenza virus (A/New Jersey/8/76) was isolated from a young military recruit who died of pneumonia (Goldfield et al. 1977). Serological evidence suggested that this virus was antigenically similar to the viruses believed to have caused the 1918 pandemic and that the virus had spread to other recruits (Dowdle and Millar 1978). Since that time additional fatal cases of swine H1N1 influenza in humans have been documented, but these viruses have so far shown a limited capacity to spread in humans.

Swine influenza virus is one of the most common causes of respiratory disease in swine, and serological surveys in the USA have indicated that nearly half of the herds have antibody against this virus. Clinical evidence indicates that influenza A strains vary in the severity of disease that they cause in infected swine. The relative prevalence of different influenza A viruses in swine varies throughout the world, but it is clear that a large reservoir of influenza A viruses exists in pigs world-wide.

Critical to the hypothesis that pigs may play a crucial role in the emergence of new pandemic strains of influenza is the observation that swine are susceptible to infection by swine, avian and human influenza viruses (see 'Receptor binding', p. 399). This susceptibility to a variety of subtypes of influenza viruses provides the opportunity for genetic reassortment in swine. These findings underscore the possible role of swine as a 'mixing vessel' for the emergence of novel influenza strains (Scholtissek et al. 1985). Furthermore, classic A(H1N1) swine viruses, avian A(H1N1) viruses and human A(H1N1) (H3N2) and type C influenza viruses have all been isolated from naturally infected swine. Experimental infection with avian viruses representing 13 of the 15 HA subtypes has also been reported (Kida et al. 1994).

6.2 Immune response

Infection with influenza viruses leads to induction of both virus-specific B and T cell immune responses. Antibodies are made against the viral external glycoproteins HA and NA as well as the internal type-specific proteins NP and M1 (see section 5, p. 406).

Neutralizing antibody directed against the HA is the primary immune mediator of protection from infection and clinical illness due to influenza viruses. Both mucosal and systemic immunity contribute to resistance to infection and disease (Clements et al. 1983, 1986). Influenza-specific lymphocytes have been detected in blood and lower respiratory tract secretions of infected subjects (Jurgensen et al. 1973, Yewdell and Hackett 1989). The primary cytotoxic T cell response is detectable in blood after 1–2 weeks but is relatively short lived (Ennis et al. 1981).

ANTIBODY TO HA AND NA

Antibody to HA is important in neutralization of virus, complement fixation, prevention of virus attachment and mediation of antibody-dependent cellular cytotoxicity. Resistance to infection is correlated with serum anti-HA antibody levels (Hobson et al. 1972, Dowdle et al. 1973) and by the demonstration of protection against challenge after passive transfer of immune serum in a mouse model (Virelizier 1975). More recent studies have shown that protection from live virus challenge is associated with local neutralizing antibody and secretory IgA as well as serum anti-HA antibody (Clements et al. 1986, Johnson et al. 1986). Although antibodies to NA are inefficient in neutralizing influenza viruses, they restrict virus release from infected cells, reduce the intensity of infection and enhance recovery (see section 5.4, p. 407).

Serum antibody to HA can persist for decades, and retrospective serosurveys suggest that a limited number of influenza subtypes have recycled (Masurel and Marine 1973). Decade-long persistence of immunity was demonstrated dramatically when influenza A(H1N1) strains, similar to viruses that had circulated in 1950, spread throughout the world during 1977/8. Little disease occurred in individuals born before 1950, indicating that substantial immunity remained after almost 30 years. Disease occurred in people ≤20 years old, however, irrespective of whether they were infected by influenza viruses of the H3N2 subtype. This and numerous observations during the pandemics of 1957 and 1968 suggest that intersubtypic immunity is weak in humans. In contrast, intrasubtypic immunity to influenza A(H3N2) viruses in adults can last for 4–7 years and include 2 or more variants of the same subtype, depending on the extent of antigenic drift (Couch and Kasel 1983).

The fact that a repeat infection with an antigenically related strain boosts the antibody response to the first virus encountered was originally described in 1953 by Davenport and colleagues. This phenomenon, known as 'original antigenic sin', is believed to be a selective anamnestic response orientated toward both the HA and the NA antigens experienced during the original infection. Thus, cross-reactive epitopes will stimulate a predominant secondary antibody response whereas new epitopes in the reinfecting variant induce a primary response. The precise importance of this phenomenon to immunity induced by infection or vaccination is unknown, but observations on original antigenic sin suggest that induced immunity during sequential infections may be biased toward older, less relevant strains rather than the current infecting strain.

Sequence analysis of the HA genes of monoclonal antibody escape variants, along with field isolates and location of amino acid changes on the 3-dimensional structure of the HA, have defined 5 antibody-combining sites (see section 5.2, p. 406). The relationship of these sites to antibodies produced via natural infection has yet to be determined precisely, but the specificity of the antibody response to HA seems to be limited in humans and may vary from individual to individual (Natali, Oxford and Schild 1981, Wang, Skehel and Wiley 1986). A limited range of specificities of anti-HA antibodies in individual mice and rabbits has also been demonstrated (Lambkin et al. 1994, Lambkin and Dimmock 1995). These findings may have implications for antigenic drift and the epidemiological success of influenza viruses in humans.

Among children with no previous exposure to influenza viruses, vaccination with live attenuated influenza viruses results in the appearance of serum anti-HA IgM, IgG and IgA antibodies within 2 weeks. IgM and IgA antibodies decline after this time, but the IgG response peaks after c. 6 weeks, declines over the next 6 months or so and then remains relatively stable for 2–3 years (Murphy et al. 1982, Murphy and Webster 1996). Antiviral IgA, IgG and IgM responses can be detected in nasal secretions in most individuals and persist for several months (Wright et al. 1983, Murphy and Clements 1989). A secondary response to infection in primed young adults results in serum IgG and IgA and mucosal IgA in most cases. Serum haemagglutination inhibition (HAI) responses decline initially after infection, but may then remain quite stable for years (Ada and Jones 1986). Serum antibodies to NA are rarely induced in primary infection and generally occur after re-exposure to NA of the same subtype. Antibodies to type-specific NP and M1 proteins are boosted via reinfection and may help diagnose a recent exposure to virus.

T CELL RESPONSES

CD4+ and CD8+ T cell responses to influenza are type-specific and are largely cross-reactive among influenza A viruses of different subtypes. T cell recognition of antigen is restricted by the MHC antigens, and the ability to respond to a given viral epitope depends on the HLA phenotype of an individual, a fact that complicates various approaches to vaccination against influenza. In naturally infected humans the CD4+ cell response seems to recognize epitopes on the internal proteins NP and M1 as well as the surface proteins NA and HA. CD8+ cytotoxic T lymphocytes seem to recognize epitopes within the HA, NP, M1 and PB2 proteins (Yewdell and Hackett 1989). Recent animal model studies have shown that both CD4+ and CD8+ T cells can contribute to immunity to influenza viruses. Animals that are deficient in both CD4+ and CD8+ T cells do not survive influenza infection, but animals deficient in only CD4+ or CD8+ T cells are able to clear virus (Lightman et al. 1987, Eichelberger et al. 1991a, 1991b).

6.3 Diagnosis

A number of techniques have been developed for the diagnosis of influenza virus infections. Virus isolation in cultured cells or in fertilized hens' eggs or demonstration of a 4-fold or greater rise in specific antibodies between acute and convalescent sera are techniques that have been used for many years. More recently, detection of viral antigens directly in clinical specimens by immunological methods and detection of viral nucleic acids by hybridization or using polymerase chain reaction (PCR) has greatly increased the speed of laboratory diagnosis.

Virus isolation and propagation

Embryonated hens' eggs, a number of primary tissue culture systems and continuous cell lines such as Madin–Darby canine kidney (MDCK; American Type Culture Collection, Rockville MD) cells can be used to isolate and grow influenza viruses for identification or research purposes. Recognition that proteolytic cleavage of the HA is necessary for viral infectivity and that inclusion of trypsin in the tissue culture fluid cleaves the HA expanded the culture systems available for influenza isolation and propagation. Replication of influenza viruses in all of its laboratory hosts is often detected by agglutination of erythrocytes added to culture fluid or by haemadsorption of erythrocytes to infected cells. On initial passage in eggs or tissue culture, some influenza viruses preferentially agglutinate guinea-pig over chicken erythrocytes, but on continued passage the viruses may preferentially agglutinate erythrocytes from chickens (Burnet and Bull 1943).

Isolation in embryonated eggs

Soon after the first identification of human influenza A viruses, Burnet (1936) reported that embryonated hens' eggs could serve as a host system for their propagation. This host system is still used for vaccine production and for generating large quantities of influenza virus that are occasionally necessary for research. To isolate both type A and type B influenza viruses, clinical samples are inoculated into the amniotic and allantoic cavities of 10–11 day old embryonated hens' eggs. The eggs are usually incubated at 33–34°C for 2–3 days before the virus is harvested. Most type A and B influenza viruses that are originally isolated in eggs will grow well in the allantoic cavity after one or 2 passages. Type C influenza viruses, on the other hand, grow only in the amniotic cavity and are best propagated in 7–8 day old embryonated hens' eggs after 5 days' incubation.

Isolation in tissue culture

Primary cynomolgus or rhesus monkey kidney cells (PMKC) are susceptible to a variety of respiratory viruses, including influenza viruses. Disadvantages with these cells include their cost and the presence of spumaviruses. Influenza A, B and C viruses can also be isolated in the MDCK cell line in the presence of trypsin. Primary monkey kidney and MDCK cells are most often used for the primary isolation of influenza viruses from humans.

Influenza virus isolation is still used in many laboratories world-wide. When performed correctly with properly collected specimens along with good quality laboratory cells and reagents, this method is highly sensitive. The shell vial tissue culture isolation method combines rapid detection of virus in the inoculated cells after 48–72 hours, increased sensitivity being obtained by centrifugation of specimens onto the cells. Monoclonal antibodies are often used for immunofluorescent detection of viral antigens in the inoculated cells (Kalin and Grandien 1993). Obtaining isolates for further antigenic and genetic characterization is an essential part of worldwide surveillance for the emergence of significant antigenic variants of influenza. Detection of these new variants may signal the need to revise the formulation of the influenza vaccine or to recommend other measures for public health control.

Serology

Serology may establish that infection by influenza viruses has occurred when the virus is not detected by any other method. Serological tests include complement fixation (CF), haemagglutination inhibition (HAI), neutralization and enzyme immunoassays (EIAs). These techniques are the fundamental tools in epidemiological and immunological studies as well as in the evaluation of the immunogenic properties of the vaccine.

The CF test measures antibodies against the NP and thus allows type-specific detection of antibodies to type A and B influenza viruses rather than a subtype- or strain-specific diagnosis. This test is relatively insensitive in detecting rises in pairs of serum titres from individuals with a recent infection, but can be used when more specific reagents are not available. HAI and neutralization are more sensitive and measure antibodies against subtype- and strain-specific antigens. EIA tests can be configured according to the nature of the antigens and the isotype of immunoglobulin chosen for the assay (Ziegler and Cox 1995).

The HAI test is the serological test most often applied to influenza viruses (Fig. 22.20). Because of the instability of HA, the dilution of antigen used must be precisely determined by HA titration each time the HAI test is performed. The test is also complicated by the presence in sera of several species of non-specific inhibitors of haemagglutination. These inhibitors interact with the HA molecule and prevent the agglutination of erythrocytes, even in the absence of specific antibodies. The non-specific inhibitors fall into 3 classes: α inhibitors, which are present in human serum and are heat-stable sialylated glycoproteins that inhibit haemagglutination but do not neutralize viral infectivity; β inhibitors, which are also present in human serum and but are heat-labile and have neutralizing activity; and γ inhibitors, which are present in horse serum and are heat-stable sialylated sialoproteins with neutralizing activity. The α and γ inhibitors function as receptor analogues by competing with red cell receptors for binding to HA. Removal of non-specific inhibitors from sera by using receptor-destroying enzyme or periodate is an essential step in the HAI test (Kendal, Skehel and Pereira 1982). In addition, interference by antineuraminidase antibody and variability of viruses in avidity for red cells and antibody can influence the test results.

RAPID VIRUS DIAGNOSIS

Virus antigens or nucleic acids can be detected in clinical specimens without prior virus growth in cell culture or hens' eggs if methods are sensitive enough. Rapid diagnosis of influenza viruses in respiratory secretions has been in use since the 1970s. Immunofluorescence (IF) techniques for direct detection were first developed followed by EIA and time-resolved fluoroimmunoassay. The most rapid method for diagnosing type A influenza virus infections is a commercially available EIA: it can be completed within 15 minutes, and the sensitivity and specificity of the test are quite high (Waner et al. 1991). Nucleic acid detection has also been developed, but specific amplification of nucleic acid present in respiratory specimens by PCR is more sensitive (Ziegler and Cox 1995).

The detection of virus antigens in exfoliated epi-

thelial cells in nasopharyngeal specimens by direct or indirect IF is a very sensitive and rapid method for the diagnosis of influenza and other respiratory virus infections. Monoclonal antibodies against virus types A and B are available commercially. The sensitivity of this method is greatly influenced by the quality, transport and processing of the specimen, as well as by the features of the fluorescence microscope and experience of laboratory staff with this method.

Several laboratories have used the reverse transcriptase PCR assay to detect influenza virus RNA in clinical specimens (Claas et al. 1993, Cherian et al. 1994). It seems that the overall sensitivity of PCR is comparable to that of standard virus isolation for influenza viruses. However, influenza virus RNA could sometimes be detected by PCR from experimentally infected volunteers even when infectious virus could no longer be isolated (Claas et al. 1993).

6.4   Control

The morbidity and mortality caused by influenza virus infections and the disruptive effects of epidemics and pandemics on the community justify strenuous efforts to prevent this disease. Two measures are currently available to reduce the impact of influenza: immunoprophylaxis with inactivated (killed virus) vaccine and chemoprophylaxis or therapy with the antiviral drugs

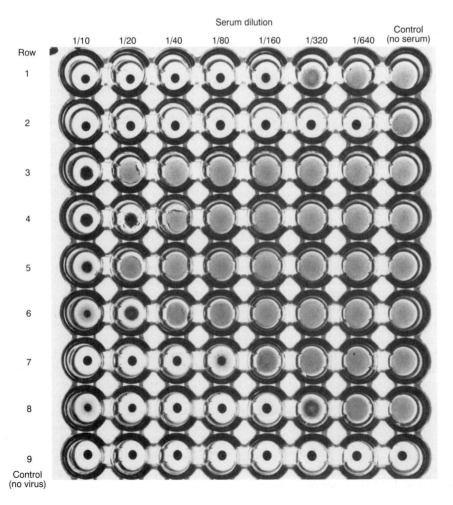

Fig. 22.20 Haemagglutination inhibition (HAI) test for influenza antibodies. The HAI is a competitive test in which antibodies present in an immune serum compete with red blood cells to bind the viral haemagglutinin. Row 1 shows results when antibodies are present and virus-induced haemagglutination of erythrocytes is inhibited with a consequent formation of erythrocyte 'buttons'. Row 3 shows results obtained when antibody is not present to inhibit viral haemagglutination.

amantadine or rimantadine. Research to develop additional influenza vaccines and antiviral agents is progressing rapidly, and it is likely that additional products for the prevention and control of influenza will become available.

IMMUNIZATION

Vaccination is currently the most effective measure for reducing the impact of influenza. Immunization is focused mainly on individuals at increased risk of complications of influenza infection and on individuals who might transmit influenza to such people (Fedson et al. 1995, Nicholson, Snacken and Palache 1995, Centers for Disease Control and Prevention 1996). For example, influenza vaccine is currently strongly recommended in the USA for anyone ≥6 months of age who, because of age or an underlying medical condition, is at increased risk for complications of influenza. They include people ≥65 years of age; people in residential or nursing homes; those with chronic disorders of the pulmonary or cardiovascular systems, including children with asthma; anyone who has required regular medical follow-up or hospitalization during the preceding year because of chronic metabolic diseases (including diabetes mellitus), renal dysfunction, haemoglobinopathies or immunosuppression (including immunosuppression caused by medications); and children and teenagers (6 months to 18 years of age) who are taking aspirin in the long term and may be at risk of developing Reye syndrome after influenza. People who should receive vaccination to reduce the likelihood of transmission to high-risk groups include: physicians, nurses and other personnel in both hospital and outpatient care settings; staff, visitors and volunteers in residential and nursing homes; providers of home care to individuals at high risk and household members (including children) of such people.

Vaccination is generally considered safe for anyone who can eat foods containing egg. Hypersensitivity to hens' eggs, the substrate for vaccine production, is the only contraindication. Desensitization to eggs followed by vaccination can be considered for individuals in high-risk groups.

Vaccine formulation

Each February the World Health Organization makes recommendations concerning the antigenic properties of the strains of influenza that are to be used in vaccines during the following influenza season. These recommendations are based on data gathered by the three WHO centres (Atlanta, USA, London, UK, and Melbourne, Australia) together with data gathered by many national WHO collaborating laboratories. The objective is to match the antigenic properties of the HA and NA of the recommended vaccine strains as closely as possible with those of strains that are emerging and are likely to circulate the following winter.

Three types of data are used to make the WHO influenza vaccine strain recommendations each year. First, data are obtained from reference antigenic and genetic analyses of influenza viruses isolated through WHO's global influenza surveillance network. These data are used to detect new antigenic variants that might have emerged since the previous recommendations were issued and to determine how these variants are genetically and antigenically related to other circulating strains. Second, epidemiological and virological data are combined to determine whether newly identified variants are detected in association with outbreaks of disease in multiple locations or are associated only with a single case or a few sporadic cases. Third, the ability of the existing vaccine strains to induce an antibody response in humans to the newly detected variants is examined. These 3 types of data are combined to determine what new antigenic variants are circulating, whether these variants are associated with significant disease, and whether immunization with the existing vaccine could protect against disease caused by the new variants.

Influenza vaccines in recent years have been trivalent, containing strains of the 2 influenza A subtypes that are circulating along with a representative type B strain (Table 22.7). Viruses used by vaccine manufacturers for the type B component of the vaccine are naturally occurring virus strains that replicate to relatively high titres in the allantoic cavity of embryonated hens' eggs. The strains most often used for the type A components are high-growth reassortant viruses that contain internal genes that specify the property of high growth in eggs derived from the A/PR/8/34(H1N1) laboratory adapted strain together with the surface glycoproteins, HA and NA, from the recommended field strain. Vaccine strains are grown individually in the allantoic cavity of embryonated hens' eggs and then purified and concentrated by zonal centrifugation or column chromatography and finally inactivated with formalin or other chemicals. Vaccines are routinely standardized by means of single radial diffusion tests (Wood et al. 1981) to contain 15 μg HA per virus strain per dose; the quantity of NA is not standardized and may vary between vaccines.

Influenza vaccines currently in use are inactivated whole-virus (WV), subvirion (SV) or surface antigen vaccines. WV vaccines contain intact, inactivated virus; SV vaccine contains detergent-disrupted inactivated virus; surface antigen vaccines contain isolated HA and NA proteins. Although current viruses are still produced by growing viruses in the allantoic sac of embryonated hens' eggs, numerous refinements have improved the immunogenicity and reactogenicity of current vaccines; they include the use of zonal centrifugation, the use of ether or other lipid solvents to disrupt the virus, the introduction of high-yield reassortants to improve yields, and the development of better methods to quantify the amount of viral antigens present in the vaccines. Thus modern influenza vaccines are associated with minimal side effects. Up to one third of vaccine recipients may feel some discomfort at the vaccination site for up to 2 days after vaccination; only about 1–2% have fever, malaise, myalgia or other systemic reaction, which may begin 6–12 hours after vaccination and persists for 1–2 days (Betts 1995, Centers for Disease Control and Prevention 1996).

Table 22.7 Influenza vaccine strains recommended by WHO, 1987/8 to 1996/7

Year	H1N1	H3N2	B
1987/8	A/Singapore/06/86-like[a]	A/Leningrad/360/86-like	B/Ann Arbor/1/86-like
1988/9	A/Singapore/06/86-like[a]	A/Sichuan/02/87-like	B/Beijing/1/87-like
1989/90	A/Singapore/06/86-like[a]	A/Shanghai/11/87-like	B/Yamagata/16/88-like
1990/1	A/Singapore/06/86-like[a]	A/Guizhou/54/89-like[c]	B/Yamagata/16/88-like
1991/2	A/Singapore/06/86-like[a]	A/Beijing/353/89-like	Either B/Yamagata/16/88-like or B/Panama/45/90-like
1992/3	A/Singapore/06/86-like[a]	A/Beijing/353/89-like	Either B/Yamagata/16/88-like or B/Panama/45/90-like
1993/4	A/Singapore/06/86-like[a]	A/Beijing/32/92-like	B/Panama/45/90-like
1994/5	A/Singapore/06/86-like[b]	A/Shangdong/09/93-like	B/Panama/45/90-like
1995/6	A/Singapore/06/86-like[b]	A/Johannesburg/33/94-like	B/Beijing/184/93-like[e]
1996/7	A/Singapore/06/86-like[b]	A/Wuhan/359/95-like[d]	B/Beijing/184/93-like[e]

[a]Most countries used the antigenically equivalent A/Taiwan/1/86 virus.
[b]Most countries used the antigenically equivalent A/Texas/36/91 virus.
[c]Most countries used the antigenically equivalent A/Shanghai/16/89 virus.
[d]Most countries used the antigenically equivalent A/Nanchang/33/95 virus.
[e]Most countries used the antigenically equivalent B/Harbin/7/94 virus.

Effectiveness of inactivated influenza vaccines

Inactivated parenterally administered influenza vaccines have been in use since the 1940s. A large number of trials in both military and civilian populations have demonstrated the efficacy of inactivated vaccines in the prevention of naturally occurring outbreaks of influenza A(H1H1), (H2N2) and (H3N2) viruses (for reviews, see Dowdle 1981, Couch et al. 1986, Ada et al. 1987, Monto and Terpenning 1996). The large variations in vaccine efficacy and clinical effectiveness reported in the literature are due to differences in the ages and immunocompetence of the vaccine recipients, the degree of antigenic similarity between the vaccine and circulating virus strains, the vaccine potency, the extent and intensity of transmission of influenza and other respiratory viruses circulating during the study period, as well as the surveillance and laboratory methods used for the studies. Current inactivated vaccines protect 70–90% of normal healthy adult recipients against naturally occurring disease when the antigens of the vaccine and those of the circulating influenza viruses are closely related. In people ≥65 years of age (a group that is a primary target of vaccination programmes in a number of countries), the antibody response to HA is reduced and clinical effectiveness of vaccine is lower. This is probably a reflection of reduced immunocompetence (Ershler 1984). For older people living in the community, the effectiveness of influenza vaccine in preventing hospitalization for P and I ranges from 30% to 70%. Among elderly people living in nursing homes, inactivated vaccines confer less protection against illness than in younger healthy individuals; they are more effective in preventing severe illness or secondary complications requiring hospitalization (50–60%) and death (80%) than in protecting against disease (30–40%). (Centers for Disease Control and Prevention 1996).

CHEMOTHERAPY

The chemically related drugs amantadine and rimantadine hydrochloride interfere with the replication cycle of all subtypes of type A but not type B influenza viruses (Van Voris and Newell 1992, Hayden 1996). Amantadine and rimantadine, its α-methyl derivative, share mechanisms of action, antiviral spectrums, oral bioavailability, prolonged plasma half-life and clinical efficacy. Both drugs inhibit the replication of influenza A viruses at low, clinically achievable concentrations of <1 μg/ml (Tominack and Hayden 1987), but concerns about side effects involving the central nervous system have limited the use of amantadine.

Amantadine and rimantadine are 70–90% effective in preventing illness caused by naturally occurring strains of type A influenza viruses when administered prophylactically to healthy adults or children when influenza viruses are circulating. These drugs can also reduce the severity and duration of illness caused by influenza A viruses when administered within 48 hours of onset of symptoms.

The antiviral activity of both of these compounds is exerted through interference with 2 different ion channel functions of the viral M2 protein (see 'M2', p. 404). The first involves inhibition of the acid-mediated dissociation of the matrix protein from the RNP complex within endosomes early in replication; this dissociation is essential for initiating viral replication (Sugrue et al. 1990, Pinto, Holsinger and Lamb 1992). A second effect on virus maturation relating to a low pH-mediated alteration of the HA protein during its transport to the cell surface occurs during the replication of certain avian influenza viruses (Sugrue et al. 1990, Ohuchi et al. 1994, Takeuchi and Lamb 1994).

Influenza A viruses are cross-susceptible and cross-resistant to amantadine and rimantadine. Viral strains responsible for pandemics and epidemics in recent years have all been drug-sensitive (Hayden 1996), but resistance to these compounds is readily selected by growth in the presence of these drugs either in vivo or in vitro. Resistance is associated with single nucleotide changes in RNA segment 7 and corresponding amino acid substitutions at one of 4 sites (amino acids 26, 27, 30 and 31 for human influenza A viruses) in the transmembrane region of the M2 protein (Hay 1992). Resistant viruses can emerge when either of these drugs is administered for treatment in adults or children. Although the frequency of the emergence of resistance is not firmly established, resistant variants have been recovered from c. 30% of treated children or adults (Hall et al. 1987, Hayden et al. 1989). Nevertheless, treated individuals who shed resistant viruses recover rapidly and the duration of shedding is relatively short, so the clinical significance of the emergence of resistance in an individual is unclear. Apparent transmission of resistant virus associated with failure of drug prophylaxis has been documented in nursing home residents receiving amantadine and in household contacts of rimantadine-treated individuals (Hayden et al. 1989, Mast et al. 1991, Degelau et al. 1992, Houck et al. 1995). Resistant viruses seem to be pathogenic and can cause typical influenza, but resistant viruses are no more transmissible or virulent than strains sensitive to amantadine and rimantadine (Hayden 1996).

NEW VACCINES AND ANTIVIRALS

Although the inactivated influenza vaccines currently in use achieve a reasonable degree of protection (70–90%) in normal healthy adults when the antigens of the vaccine and those of the circulating viruses are closely related, they are limited both in their ability to elicit mucosal antibody and cell-mediated immunity and in their reduced immunogenicity in unprimed individuals. People who are immunosuppressed may also fail to mount a protective antibody response after vaccination. In particular, these vaccines offer less protection to those who need it most, such as elderly debilitated individuals living in nursing homes whose immune response to the vaccine is often less than optimal. Although the antivirals amantadine and rimantadine are also 70–90% effective in preventing influenza when used prophylactically, associated side effects and the emergence of viruses resistant to these compounds are often viewed as impediments to their widespread use. Alternative vaccine and antiviral strategies are being explored because of these limitations.

Since the mid-1970s, extensive resources have been devoted to the development of intranasally administered live attenuated influenza virus vaccines that might induce local, systemic and cell-mediated immunity that is more complete and longer lasting than that induced by inactivated vaccines. Live

attenuated influenza vaccines are or have been under clinical investigation in a number of countries, but they have been used widely in Russia and China. At present the most promising are prepared by reassortment of a cold-adapted (ca) attenuated donor virus and a contemporary epidemic strain (Maassab 1967, Kendal et al. 1981, Wright, Johnson and Karzon 1986, Zhdanov 1986, Murphy 1993).

Considerable research has focused on the development of more potent adjuvants and alternative routes of vaccination to augment the immune response to inactivated influenza vaccines. Moderate improvements in immunogenicity in elderly people have recently been reported with a virosome influenza vaccine (Glück et al. 1994) and with the proprietary adjuvant MF59 (Martin 1996).

Both practical and theoretical problems associated with the use of embryonated eggs in inactivated influenza vaccines have led to efforts to develop alternative substrates for vaccine production. So far, successful human trials have been conducted with vaccines prepared from virus cultured in MDCK cells, a continuous cell line of canine kidney cells (Brands, Palache and van Scharrenburg 1996). In addition, recent safety and immunogenicity human trials with rDNA HA from the A/Beijing/32/9(H3N2) virus expressed in insect cells have indicated that this is a viable approach for producing inactivated influenza vaccine that can be updated annually as recommended (Treanor et al. 1996).

The development of 'naked DNA' vaccines has received a great deal of attention. Although NP DNA from influenza A virus was initially used only as a model for DNA vaccine development, positive results (Ulmer et al. 1993, Donnelly et al. 1995) have led to continuing DNA vaccine development for influenza. Both antibody and cell-mediated immune responses have been demonstrated in infected animals and, provided that safety of these vaccines can be achieved, this approach shows great promise.

It is noteworthy that the novel NA inhibitor GG167 has recently shown considerable promise as an antiviral drug against influenza. Phase I studies indicate that this compound is safe in healthy human subjects when administered intravenously, by nebulizer or by inhalation of dry powder (Hayden et al. 1994). Initial phase II studies have established that the compound is effective prophylactically and when used early in experimentally induced infection by influenza A/Texas/91 (H1N1) (Hayden et al. 1996).

REFERENCES

Ada GL, Jones PD, 1986, The immune response to influenza infection, *Curr Top Microbiol Immunol*, **128:** 1–54.

Ada G, Alexandrova G et al., 1987, Progress in the development of influenza vaccines: memorandum from a WHO meeting, *Bull W H O*, **65:** 289–93.

Ahmed AH, Nicholson KG, Nguyen-Van-Tam JS, 1995, Reduction in mortality associated with influenza vaccine during 1989–90 epidemic, *Lancet*, **346:** 591–5.

Air GM, Laver WG, 1989, The neuraminidase of influenza virus proteins: structure, function, and genetics, *Proteins*, **6:** 341–56.

Air GM, Els MC et al., 1985, Location of antigenic sites on the three-dimensional structure of the influenza N2 virus neuraminidase, *Virology*, **145:** 237–8.

Albo C, Valencia A, Portela A, 1995, Identification of an RNA binding region within the N-terminal third of the influenza A virus nucleoprotein, *J Virol*, **69:** 3799–806.

Almond JW, 1977, A single gene determines the host range of influenza virus, *Nature (London)*, **270:** 617–18.

Alonso-Caplen FV, Nemeroff ME et al., 1992, Nucleocytoplasmic transport: the influenza virus NS1 protein regulates the transport of spliced NS2 mRNA and its precursor NS1 mRNA, *Genes Dev*, **6**: 255–67.

Amano H, Uemoto H et al., 1992, Immunoelectron microscopy of influenza A virus neuraminidase glycoprotein topography, *J Gen Virol*, **73**: 1969–75.

Baez M, Palese P, Kilbourne ED, 1980, Gene composition of high-yielding influenza vaccine strains obtained by recombination, *J Infect Dis*, **141**: 362–9.

Bárcena J, Ochoa M et al., 1994, Monoclonal antibodies against influenza virus PB2 and NP polypeptides interfere with the initiation step of viral mRNA synthesis in vitro, *J Virol*, **68**: 6900–9.

Barclay WS, Palese P, 1995, Influenza B viruses with site-specific mutations introduced into the HA gene, *J Virol*, **69**: 1275–9.

Barker WH, Mullooly JP, 1980, Impact of epidemic type A influenza in a defined adult population, *Am J Epidemiol*, **112**: 798–813.

Barnett BC, Graham CM et al., 1989, The immune response of Balb/c mice to influenza hemagglutinin: commonality of the B cell and T cell repertoires and their relevance to antigenic drift, *Eur J Immunol*, **19**: 515–21.

Bastin JM, Townsend ARM, McMichael AJ, 1987, Specific recognition of influenza virus polymerase protein (PB1) by a murine cytotoxic T-cell clone, *Virology*, **160**: 278–80.

Bastin J, Rothbard J et al., 1987, Use of synthetic peptides of influenza nucleoprotein to define epitopes recognized by class I-restricted cytotoxic T lymphocytes, *J Exp Med*, **165**: 1508–23.

Baudin F, Bach C et al., 1994, Structure of influenza virus RNP. I. Influenza virus nucleoprotein melts secondary structure in panhandle RNA and exposes the bases to the solvent, *EMBO J*, **13**: 3158–65.

Baum LG, Paulson JC, 1990, Sialyloligosaccharides of the respiratory epithelium in the selection of human influenza virus receptor specificity, *Acta Histochemica Suppl*, **40**: 35–8.

Baum LG, Paulson JC, 1991, The N2 neuraminidase of human influenza virus has acquired a substrate specificity complementary to the hemagglutinin receptor specificity, *Virology*, **180**: 10–15.

Bean W, Schell J et al., 1992, Evolution of the H3 influenzavirus hemagglutinin from human and nonhuman hosts, *J Virol*, **66**: 1129–38.

Beaton AR, Krug RM, 1986, Transcription antitermination during influenza viral template RNA synthesis requires the nucleocapsid protein and the absence of a 5′ capped end, *Proc Natl Acad Sci USA*, **83**: 6282–6.

Bennink JR, Yewdell JW, 1988, Murine cytotoxic T lymphocyte recognition of individual influenza virus proteins. High frequency of nonresponder MHC class I alleles, *J Exp Med*, **168**: 1935–9.

Bennink JR, Yewdell JW et al., 1984, Recombinant vaccinia virus primes and stimulates influenza haemagglutinin-specific cytotoxic T cells, *Nature (London)*, **311**: 578–9.

Bennink JR, Yewdell JW et al., 1987, Anti-influenza virus cytotoxic T lymphocytes recognize the three viral polymerases and a nonstructural protein: responsiveness to individual viral antigens is major histocompatibility complex controlled, *J Virol*, **61**: 1098–102.

Bergmann M, García-Sastre A, Palese P, 1992, Transfection-mediated recombination of influenza A virus, *J Virol*, **66**: 7576–80.

Betts RF, 1995, Influenza virus, *Mandell, Douglas, and Bennett's Principles and Practice of Infectious Diseases*, 4th edn, eds Mandell GL, Bennett JE, Dolin R, Churchill Livingstone, New York, 1546–67.

Bilsel P, Castrucci MR, Kawaoka Y, 1993, Mutations in the cytoplasmic tail of influenza A virus neuraminidase affect incorporation into virions, *J Virol*, **67**: 6762–7.

Biswas SK, Nayak DP, 1994, Mutational analysis of the conserved motifs of influenza A virus polymerase basic protein 1, *J Virol*, **68**: 1819–26.

Blaas D, Patzelt E, Kuechler E, 1982, Identification of the cap binding protein of influenza virus, *Nucleic Acids Res*, **10**: 4803–12.

Black RA, Rota PA et al., 1993, Antibody response to the M2 protein of influenza A virus expressed in insect cells, *J Gen Virol*, **74**: 143–6.

Bland PB, 1919, Influenza in its relation to pregnancy and labor, *Am J Obstet Gynecol*, **79**: 184.

Blok J, Air GM, 1982a, Sequence variation at the 3′ end of the neuraminidase gene from 39 influenza type A viruses, *Virology*, **121**: 211–29.

Blok J, Air GM, 1982b, Variation in the membrane-insertion and 'stalk' sequences in eight subtypes of influenza type A virus neuraminidase, *Biochemistry*, **21**: 4001–7.

Blok J, Air GM et al., 1982, Studies on the size, chemical composition and partial sequence of the neuraminidase (NA) from type A influenza viruses show that the N-terminal region of the NA is not processed and serves to anchor the NA in the viral membrane, *Virology*, **119**: 109–21.

Bodmer HC, Pemberton RM et al., 1988, Enhanced recognition of a modified peptide antigen by cytotoxic T cells specific for influenza nucleoprotein, *Cell*, **52**: 253–8.

Bosch FX, Orlich M et al., 1979, The structure of the hemagglutinin, a determinant for the pathogenicity of influenza viruses, *Virology*, **95**: 197–207.

Bosch FX, Garten W et al., 1981, Proteolytic cleavage of influenza virus hemagglutinins: primary structure of the connecting peptide between HA1 and HA2 determines proteolytic cleavability and pathogenicity of avian influenza viruses, *Virology*, **113**: 725–35.

Braam J, Ulmanen I, Krug RM, 1983, Molecular model of eukaryotic transcription complex: function and movements of influenza P proteins during capped RNA-primed transcription, *Cell*, **34**: 609–18.

Brand CM, Skehel JJ, 1972, Crystalline antigen from the influenza virus envelope, *Nature (London)*, **238**: 145–7.

Brands R, Palache AM, van Scharrenburg GJM, 1996, Madin–Darby canine kidney (MDCK) cells for the production of inactivated influenza subunit vaccine. Safety characteristics and clinical results in the elderly, *Options for the Control of Influenza III*, eds Brown LE, Hampson AW, Webster RG, Elsevier Science, Amsterdam, 683–93.

Brewer CB, Roth MG, 1991, A single amino acid change in the cytoplasmic domain alters the polarized delivery of influenza virus hemagglutinin, *J Cell Biol*, **114**: 413–21.

Briedis DJ, Lamb RA, Choppin PW, 1982, Sequence of RNA segment 7 of the influenza B virus genome: partial amino acid homology between the membrane proteins (M_1) of influenza A and B viruses and conservation of a second open reading frame, *Virology*, **116**: 581–8.

Bron R, Kendal AP et al., 1993, Role of the M2 protein in influenza virus membrane fusion: effects of amantadine and monensin on fusion kinetics, *Virology*, **195**: 808–11.

Brown LE, Hinshaw VS, Webster RG, 1983, Antigenic variation in the influenza A virus nonstructural protein, NS1, *Virology*, **130**: 134–43.

Bucher DJ, Kharitonenkov IG et al., 1980, Incorporation of influenza virus M-protein into liposomes, *J Virol*, **36**: 586–90.

Bullough PA, Hughson FM et al., 1994, Structure of influenza haemagglutinin at the pH of membrane fusion, *Nature (London)*, **371**: 37–43.

Buonagurio DA, Krystal M et al., 1984, Analysis of an influenza A virus mutant with a deletion in the NS segment, *J Virol*, **49**: 418–25.

Burger KNJ, Knoll G, Verkleij AJ, 1988, Influenza virus-model membrane interaction. A morphological approach using modern cryotechniques, *Biochim Biophys Acta*, **939**: 89–101.

Burmeister WP, Ruigrok RWH, Cusack S, 1992, The 2.2 Å resolution crystal structure of influenza B neuraminidase and its complex with sialic acid, *EMBO J*, **11**: 49–56.

Burnet FM, 1936, Influenza virus on the developing egg. I.

Changes associated with the development of an egg-passage strain of virus, *Br J Exp Pathol*, **17**: 282–93.

Burnet FM, 1940, Influenza virus infections of the chick embryo lung, *Br J Exp Path*, **21**: 147–53.

Burnet FM, Bull RD, 1943, Changes in influenza virus associated with adaption to passage in chick embryos, *Aust J Exp Biol Med Sci*, **21**: 55–69.

Burnet FM, Clarke E, 1942, Influenza: a survey of the last 50 years in the light of modern work on the virus of epidemic influenza, *Monogr Res Med*, **4**: 1–118.

Carr CM, Kim PS, 1993, A spring-loaded mechanism for the conformational change of influenza hemagglutinin, *Cell*, **73**: 823–32.

Castrucci MR, Kawaoka Y, 1993, Biologic importance of neuraminidase stalk length in influenza A virus, *J Virol*, **67**: 759–64.

Castrucci MR, Kawaoka Y, 1995, Reverse genetics system for generation of an influenza A virus mutant containing a deletion of the carboxyl-terminal residue of M2 protein, *J Virol*, **69**: 2725–8.

Castrucci MR, Hou S et al., 1994, Protection against lethal lymphocytic choriomeningitis virus (LCMV) infection by immunization of mice with an influenza virus containing an LCMV epitope recognized by cytotoxic T lymphocytes, *J Virol*, **68**: 3486–90.

Caton AJ, Gerhard W, 1992, The diversity of the CD4+ T cell response in influenza, *Semin Immunol*, **4**: 85–90.

Caton AJ, Brownlee GG et al., 1982, The antigenic structure of the influenza virus A/PR/8/34 hemagglutinin (H1 subtype), *Cell*, **31**: 417–27.

Centers for Disease Control and Prevention, 1996, Prevention and control of influenza, *Morbid Mortal Weekly Rep*, **45(RR-5)**: 1–24.

Chapman LE, Tipple MA et al., 1993, Influenza – United States, 1988–89, *Morbid Mortal Weekly Rep*, **42(SS1)**: 9–22.

Chen W, Helenius J et al., 1995, Cotranslational folding and calnexin binding during glycoprotein synthesis, *Proc Natl Acad Sci USA*, **92**: 6229–33.

Cherian T, Bobo L, et al, 1994, Use of PCR–enzyme immunoassay for identification of influenza A virus matrix RNA in clinical samples negative for cultivable virus, *J Clin Microbiol*, **32**: 623–8.

Choi K, Thacker SB, 1982, Mortality during influenza epidemics in the United States, 1967–1978, *Am J Public Health*, **72**: 1280–3.

Claas EC, van Milaan AJ et al., 1993, Prospective application of reverse transcriptase polymerase chain reaction for diagnosing influenza infections in respiratory samples from a children's hospital, *J Clin Microbiol*, **31**: 2218–21.

Clements ML, O'Donnell SO et al., 1983, Dose response of A/Alaska/6/77 (H3N2) cold-adapted reassortant vaccine virus in adult volunteers: role of local antibody in resistance to infection with vaccine virus, *Infect Immun*, **40**: 1044–51.

Clements ML, Betts RL et al., 1986, Serum and nasal wash antibodies associated with resistance to experimental challenge with influenza A wild-type virus, *J Clin Microbiol*, **22**: 157–60.

Cockburn WC, Delon PJ, Ferreira W, 1969, Origin and progress of the 1968–69 Hong Kong influenza epidemic, *Bull W H O*, **41**: 345–8.

Collins SD, Lehmann J, 1951, Trends and epidemics of influenza and pneumonia, 1918–1951, *Public Health Rep*, **66**: 1487–516.

Collins PL, Mink MA, Stec DS, 1991, Rescue of synthetic analogs of respiratory syncytial virus genomic RNA and effect of truncations and mutations on the expression of a foreign reporter gene, *Proc Natl Acad Sci USA*, **88**: 9663–7.

Colman PM, 1994, Influenza virus neuraminidase: structure, antibodies, and inhibitors, *Protein Sci*, **3**: 1687–96.

Colman PM, Varghese JN, Laver WG, 1983, Structure of the catalytic and antigenic sites in influenza virus neuraminidase, *Nature (London)*, **303**: 41–4.

Colman PM, Laver WG et al., 1987, The three-dimensional

structure of a complex of influenza virus neuraminidase and an antibody, *Nature (London)*, **326**: 358–63.

Compans RW, Content J, Duesberg PH, 1972, Structure of the ribonucleoprotein of influenza virus, *J Virol*, **10**: 795–800.

Couceiro JNSS, Paulson JC, Baum LG, 1993, Influenza virus strains selectively recognize sialyloligosaccharides on human respiratory epithelium: the role of the host cell in selection of hemagglutinin receptor specificity, *Virus Res*, **29**: 155–65.

Couch RB, Kasel JA, 1983, Immunity to influenza in man, *Annu Rev Microbiol*, **37**: 529–49.

Couch RB, Kasel JA et al., 1986, Influenza: its control in persons and populations, *J Infect Dis*, **153**: 431–40.

Cox NJ, Bender CA, 1995, The molecular epidemiology of influenza viruses, *Semin Virol*, **6**: 359–70.

Crosby AW, 1989, *America's Forgotten Pandemic: the influenza of 1919*, Cambridge University Press, Cambridge.

Dale B, Brown R et al., 1988, Generation of vaccinia virus – equine influenza A virus recombinants and their use as immunogens in horses, *Equine Infectious Diseases V*, ed Powell DG, University Press of Kentucky, Lexington, 80–7.

Daniels RS, Douglas AR et al., 1983, Analysis of the antigenicity of influenza virus haemagglutinin at the pH optimum for virus-mediated membrane fusion, *J Gen Virol*, **64**: 1657–62.

Daniels RS, Downie JC et al., 1985, Fusion mutants of the influenza virus hemagglutinin glycoprotein, *Cell*, **40**: 431–9.

Daniels RS, Jeffries S et al., 1987, The receptor-binding and membrane-fusion properties of influenza virus variants selected using anti-haemagglutinin monoclonal antibodies, *EMBO J*, **6**: 1459–65.

Davenport FM, Hennessy AV, Francis T, 1953, Epidemiologic and immunologic significance of age distribution of antibody to antigenic variants of influenza virus, *J Exp Med*, **98**: 641–56.

Davey J, Dimmock NJ, Colman A, 1985, Identification of the sequence responsible for the nuclear accumulation of the influenza virus nucleoprotein in *Xenopus* oocytes, *Cell*, **40**: 667–75.

Davies WL, Grunert RR et al., 1964, Antiviral activity of 1-adamantanamine (amantadine), *Science*, **144**: 862–3.

Davis LE, Caldwell GG et al., 1970, Hong Kong influenza: the epidemiologic features of a high school family study analyzed and compared with a similar study during the 1957 Asian influenza epidemic, *Am J Epidemiol*, **92**: 240–7.

De BP, Banerjee AK, 1993, Rescue of synthetic analogs of genome RNA of human parainfluenza virus type 3, *Virology*, **196**: 344–8.

Degelau J, Somani SK et al., 1992, Amantadine-resistant influenza A in a nursing facility, *Arch Intern Med*, **152**: 390–2.

Digard P, Blok VC, Inglis SC, 1989, Complex formation between influenza virus polymerase proteins expressed in *Xenopus* oocytes, *Virology*, **171**: 162–9.

Doms RW, Lamb RA et al., 1993, Folding and assembly of viral membrane proteins, *Virology*, **193**: 545–62.

Donnelly JJ, Friedman A et al., 1995, Preclinical efficacy of a prototype DNA vaccine: enhanced protection against antigenic drift in influenza virus, *Nature Med*, **1**: 583–7.

Douglas RG Jr, 1975, Influenza in man, *Influenza Viruses and Influenza*, ed Kilbourne ED, Academic Press, New York, 395–447.

Dowdle WR, 1981, Influenza immunoprophylaxis after 30 years' experience, *Genetic Variation Among Influenza Viruses*, ICN–UCLA Symposia on Molecular and Cellular Biology, vol XXI, eds Nayak DP, Fox CF, Academic Press, New York, 525–34.

Dowdle WR, Millar JD, 1978, Swine influenza: lessons learned, *NY State J Med*, **62**: 1047–57.

Dowdle WR, Coleman MT et al., 1973, Inactivated influenza vaccines. 2. Laboratory indices of protection, *Postgrad Med J*, **49**: 159–63.

Drzeniek R, 1972, Viral and bacterial neuraminidases, *Curr Top Microbiol Immunol*, **59**: 35–74.

Duesberg PH, 1969, Distinct subunits of the ribonucleoprotein of influenza virus, *J Mol Biol*, **42**: 485–99.

Duff KC, Ashley RH, 1992, The transmembrane domain of influenza A M2 protein forms amantadine-sensitive proton channels in planar lipid bilayers, *Virology*, **190**: 485–9.

Duff KC, Gilchrist PJ et al., 1994, Neutron diffraction reveals the site of amantadine blockade in the influenza A M2 ion channel, *Virology*, **202**: 287–93.

Dumitrescu MR, Grobnicu M et al., 1981, A three years experience in using MDCK cell line for influenza virus isolation (1979–1981), *Arch Roum Pathol Exp Microbiol*, **40**: 313–16.

Easterday BC, 1975, Animal influenza, *Influenza Viruses and Influenza*, ed Kilbourne ED, Academic Press, New York, 449–81.

Edwards KM, Dupont WD et al., 1994, A randomized controlled trial of cold-adapted and inactivated vaccines for the prevention of influenza A disease, *J Infect Dis*, **169**: 68–76.

Eichelberger M, Allan W et al., 1991a, Clearance of influenza virus respiratory infection in mice lacking class I major histocompatibility complex-restricted CD8+ T cells, *J Exp Med*, **174**: 875–80.

Eichelberger MC, Wang M et al., 1991b, Influenza virus RNA in the lung and lymphoid tissue of immunologically intact and CD4-depleted mice, *J Gen Virol*, **72**: 1695–8.

Eickhoff TC, Sherman IL, Serfling RE, 1961, Observations on excess mortality associated with epidemic influenza, *JAMA*, **176**: 776–82.

Ellens H, Bentz J et al., 1990, Fusion of influenza hemagglutinin-expressing fibroblasts with glycophorin-bearing liposomes: role of hemagglutinin surface density, *Biochemistry*, **29**: 9697–707.

Elster C, Fourest E et al., 1994, A small percentage of influenza virus M1 protein contains zinc but zinc does not influence in vitro M1–RNA interaction, *J Gen Virol*, **75**: 37–42.

Enami M, Palese P, 1991, High-efficiency formation of influenza virus transfectants, *J Virol*, **65**: 2711–13.

Enami M, Luytjes W et al., 1990, Introduction of site-specific mutations into the genome of influenza virus, *Proc Natl Acad Sci USA*, **87**: 3802–5.

Enami M, Sharma G et al., 1991, An influenza virus containing nine different RNA segments, *Virology*, **185**: 291–8.

Enami K, Qiao Y et al., 1993, An influenza virus temperature-sensitive mutant defective in the nuclear-cytoplasmic transport of the negative-sense viral RNAs, *Virology*, **194**: 822–7.

Ennis FA, Rook A et al., 1981, HLA-restricted virus-specific cytotoxic T-lymphocyte responses to live and inactivated influenza vaccines, *Lancet*, **2**: 887–91.

Erickson AH, Kilbourne ED, 1980, Mutation in the hemagglutinin of A/N-WS/33 influenza virus recombinants influencing sensitivity to trypsin and antigenic reactivity, *Virology*, **107**: 320–30.

Ershler WB, Moore AAL, Socinski MA, 1984, Influenza and aging: age-related changes and the effects of thymosin on the antibody response to influenza vaccine, *J Clin Immunol*, **4**: 445–54.

Farr W, 1885, *Vital Statistics: Memorial Volume of Selections from the Writings of William Farr*, part IV, ed Humphrey N, Sanitary Institute of Great Britain, London, 330.

Fedson DS, Wajda A et al., 1993, Clinical effectiveness of influenza vaccination in Manitoba, *JAMA*, **270**: 1956–61.

Fedson DS, Hannoun C et al., 1995, Influenza vaccination in 18 developed countries, 1980–1992, *Vaccine*, **13**: 623–7.

Fields S, Winter G, Brownlee GG, 1981, Structure of the neuraminidase in human influenza virus A/PR/8/34, *Nature (London)*, **290**: 213–17.

Flewett TH, Apostolov K, 1967, A reticular structure in the wall of influenza C virus, *J Gen Virol*, **1**: 297–304.

Fodor E, Pritlove DC, Brownlee GG, 1994, The influenza virus panhandle is involved in the initiation of transcription, *J Virol*, **68**: 4092–6.

Fodor E, Pritlove DC, Brownlee GG, 1995, Characterization of the RNA-fork model of virion RNA in the initiation of transcription in influenza A virus, *J Virol*, **69**: 4012–19.

Formanowski F, Meier-Ewert H, 1988, Isolation of the influenza C virus glycoprotein in a soluble form by bromelain digestion, *Virus Res*, **10**: 177–91.

Fox JP, Hall CE et al., 1982, Influenzavirus infections in Seattle families, 1975–1979. I. Study design, methods and the occurrence of infections by time and age, *Am J Epidemiol*, **116**: 212–27.

Foy HM, Cooney MK, Allan I, 1976, Longitudinal studies of types A and B influenza among Seattle schoolchildren and families, 1968–1974, *J Infect Dis*, **134**: 362–9.

Francis T, 1940, A new type of virus from epidemic influenza, *Science*, **91**: 405–8.

Francis T, Magill TP, 1937, Direct isolation of human influenza virus in tissue cultures and in egg membranes, *Proc Soc Exp Biol (NY)*, **36**: 134–5.

Frank AL, Taber LH, Wells JM, 1985, Comparison of infection rates and severity of illness for influenza subtypes H1N1 and H3N2, *J Infect Dis*, **151**: 73–80.

Frost WH, 1919, The epidemiology of influenza, *JAMA*, **73**: 313–18.

Frost WH, 1920, Statistics of influenza morbidity: with special reference to certain factors in case incidence, *Public Health Rep*, **35**: 584–97.

Fujiyoshi Y, Kume NP et al., 1994, Fine structure of influenza A virus observed by electron cryo-microscopy, *EMBO J*, **13**: 318–26.

Gallagher PJ, Henneberry JM et al., 1992, Glycosylation requirements for intracellular transport and function of the hemagglutinin of influenza virus, *J Virol*, **66**: 7136–45.

Gammelin M, Altmuller A et al., 1990, Phylogenetics analysis of nucleoproteins suggests that human influenza A viruses emerged from a 19th-century avian ancestor, *Mol Biol Evol*, **7**: 194–200.

García-Sastre A, Palese P, 1993, Genetic manipulation of negative-strand RNA virus genomes, *Annu Rev Microbiol*, **47**: 765–90.

García-Sastre A, Palese P, 1995, The cytoplasmic tail of the neuraminidase protein of influenza A virus does not play an important role in the packaging of this protein into viral envelopes, *Virus Res*, **37**: 37–47.

García-Sastre A, Muster T et al., 1994, Use of a mammalian internal ribosomal entry site element for expression of a foreign protein by a transfectant influenza virus, *J Virol*, **68**: 6254–61.

Gething MJ, McCammon K, Sambrook J, 1986, Expression of wild-type and mutant forms of influenza hemagglutinin: the role of folding in intracellular transport, *Cell*, **46**: 939–50.

Gething MJ, Doms RW et al., 1986, Studies on the mechanism of membrane fusion: site specific mutagenesis of the hemagglutinin of influenza virus, *J Cell Biol*, **102**: 11–23.

Glezen WP, 1980, Consideration of the risk of influenza in children and indications for prophylaxis, *Rev Infect Dis*, **2**: 408–20.

Glezen WP, 1982, Serious morbidity and mortality associated with influenza epidemics, *Epidemiol Rev*, **4**: 25–43.

Glezen WP, 1996, Emerging infections: pandemic influenza, *Epidemiol Rev*, **18**: 64–76.

Glezen WP, Couch RB, 1978, Interpandemic influenza in the Houston area, 1974–76, *N Engl J Med*, **298**: 587–92.

Glezen WP, Decker M, Perrotta DM, 1987, Survey of underlying conditions of persons hospitalized with acute respiratory disease during influenza epidemics in Houston, *Am Rev Respir Dis*, **136**: 550–5.

Glezen WP, Paredes A, Taber LH, 1980, Influenza in children. Relationship to other respiratory agents, *JAMA*, **243**: 1345–9.

Glezen WP, Couch RB et al., 1980, Epidemiologic observations of influenza B virus in the Houston, Texas, 1976–77, *Am J Epidemiol*, **111**: 13–22.

Glück R, Mischier R et al., 1994, Immunogenicity of new virosome influenza vaccine in elderly people, *Lancet*, **344**: 160–3.

Godley L, Pfeifer J et al., 1992, Introduction of intersubunit disulfide bonds in the membrane-distal region of the influenza hemagglutinin abolishes membrane fusion activity, *Cell*, **68:** 635–45.

Goldfield M, Bartley JD et al., 1977, Influenza in New Jersey in 1976: isolations of influenza A/New Jersey/76 virus at Fort Dix, *J Infect Dis*, **136:** S347–55.

Gorman OT, Bean WJ et al., 1990a, Evolution of the nucleoprotein gene of influenza A virus, *J Virol*, **64:** 1487–97.

Gorman OT, Donis RO et al., 1990b, Evolution of influenza A virus PB2 genes: implications for evolution of the ribonucleoprotein complex and origin of human influenza A virus, *J Virol*, **64:** 4893–902.

Gotch F, McMichael A et al., 1987, Identification of viral molecules recognized by influenza-specific human cytotoxic T lymphocytes, *J Exp Med*, **165:** 408–16.

Gotoh B, Ogasawara T et al., 1990, An endoprotease homologous to the blood clotting factor X as a determinant of viral tropism in chick embryo, *EMBO J*, **9:** 4189–95.

Gottschalk A, 1957, The specific enzyme of influenza virus and *Vibrio cholerae*, *Biochim Biophys Acta*, **23:** 645–6.

Govaert, ME, Thijs CT et al., 1994, The efficacy of influenza vaccination in elderly individuals, *JAMA*, **272:** 1661–5.

Graham CM, Barnett BC et al., 1989, The structural requirements for class II (I-d)-restricted T cell recognition of influenza hemagglutinin: B cell epitopes define T cell epitopes, *Eur J Immunol*, **19:** 523–8.

Gravotta D, Adesnik M, Sabatini DD, 1990, Transport of influenza HA from the trans-Golgi network to the apical surface of MDCK cells permeabilized in their basolateral plasma membranes: energy dependence and involvement of GTP-binding proteins, *J Cell Biol*, **111:** 2893–908.

Greenberg M, Jacobziner H et al., 1958, Maternal mortality in the epidemic of Asian influenza, New York City, 1957, *Am J Obstet Gynecol*, **76:** 897–902.

Greenspan D, Palese P, Krystal M, 1988, Two nuclear location signals in the influenza virus NS1 nonstructural protein, *J Virol*, **62:** 3020–6.

Gregoriades A, Frangione B, 1981, Insertion of influenza M protein into the viral lipid bilayer and localization of site of insertion, *J Virol*, **40:** 323–8.

Gregoriades A, Guzman GG, Paoletti E, 1990, The phosphorylation of the integral membrane (M1) protein of influenza virus, *Virus Res*, **16:** 27–42.

Günther I, Glatthaar B et al., 1993, A H1 hemagglutinin of a human influenza A virus with a carbohydrate-modulated receptor binding site and an unusual cleavage site, *Virus Res*, **27:** 147–60.

Hackett CJ, Dietzschold B et al., 1983, Influenza virus site recognized by a murine helper T cell specific for H1 strains. Localization to a nine amino acid sequence in the hemagglutinin molecule, *J Exp Med*, **158:** 294–302.

Hagen M, Chung TD et al., 1994, Recombinant influenza virus polymerase: requirement of both 5' and 3' viral ends for endonuclease activity, *J Virol*, **68:** 1509–15.

Hall CB, Dolin R et al., 1987, Children with influenza A infection: treatment with rimantadine, *Pediatrics*, **80:** 275–82.

Hall CE, Cooney MK, Fox JP, 1973, The Seattle virus watch. IV. Comparative epidemiologic observations of infections with influenza A and B viruses, 1965–1969, in families with young children, *Am J Epidemiol*, **98:** 365–80.

Hall CE, Brandt MK et al., 1971, The virus watch program: a continuing surveillance of viral infections in metropolitan New York families. IX. A comparison of infections with several respiratory pathogens in New York and New Orleans families, *Am J Epidemiol*, **94:** 367–85.

Hall WJ, Douglas RG Jr et al., 1976, Pulmonary mechanics after uncomplicated influenza A infection, *Am Rev Respir Dis*, **113:** 141–7.

Hammond C, Braakman I, Helenius A, 1994, Role of N-linked oligosaccharide recognition, glucose trimming, and calnexin in glycoprotein folding and quality control, *Proc Natl Acad Sci USA*, **91:** 913–17.

Hankins RW, Nagata K et al., 1989, Monoclonal antibody analysis of influenza virus matrix protein epitopes involved in transcription inhibition, *Virus Genes*, **3:** 111–26.

Hardy JMB, Azarowicz EN et al., 1961, The effect of Asian influenza on the outcome of pregnancy, Baltimore 1957–1958, *Am J Public Health*, **51:** 1182–8.

Hardy TC, Young SA et al., 1995, Egg fluids and cells of the chorioallantoic membrane of embryonated chicken eggs can select different variants of influenza A (H3N2) viruses, *Virology*, **211:** 302–6.

Hatada E, Hasegawa M et al., 1989, Control of influenza virus gene expression: quantitative analysis of each viral RNA species in infected cells, *J Biochem (Tokyo)*, **105:** 537–46.

Hausmann J, Kretzschmar E et al., 1995, N1 neuraminidase of influenza virus A/FPV/Rostock/3 has haemadsorbing activity, *J Gen Virol*, **76:** 1719–28.

Hay A, 1974, Studies on the formation of influenza virus envelope, *Virology*, **60:** 394–418.

Hay AJ, 1992, The action of adamantanamines against influenza A viruses: inhibition of the M2 ion channel protein, *Semin Virol*, **3:** 21–30.

Hay AJ, Lomniczi B et al., 1977, Transcription of the influenza virus genome, *Virology*, **83:** 337–55.

Hay AJ, Wolstenholme AJ et al., 1985, The molecular basis of the specific anti-influenza action of amantadine, *EMBO J*, **4:** 3021–4.

Hayden FG, 1996, Amantadine and rimantadine – clinical aspects, *Antiviral Drug Resistance*, ed Richman DD, John Wiley, New York, 59–77.

Hayden FG, Belshe RB et al., 1989, Emergence and apparent transmission of rimantadine-resistant influenza A virus in families, *N Engl J Med*, **321:** 1696–702.

Hayden FG, Tunkel AR et al., 1994, Oral LY217896 for prevention of experimental influenza A virus infection and illness in humans, *Antimicrob Agents Chemother*, **38:** 1178–81.

Hayden FG, Treanor JJ et al., 1996, Safety and efficacy of the neuraminidase inhibitor GG167 in experimental human influenza, *JAMA*, **275:** 295–9.

Hayslett J, McCarroll J et al., 1962, Endemic influenza. I. Serologic evidence of continuing and subclinical infection in disparate populations in the post-pandemic period, *Am Rev Respir Dis*, **85:** 1–8.

Helenius A, 1992, Unpacking the incoming influenza virus, *Cell*, **69:** 577–8.

Hemmes JH, Winkler KC, Kool SM, 1960, Virus survival as a seasonal factor in influenza and poliomyelitis, *Nature (London)*, **188:** 430–1.

Herlocher ML, Bucher D, Webster RG, 1992, Host range determination and functional mapping of the nucleoprotein and matrix genes of influenza viruses using monoclonal antibodies, *Virus Res*, **22:** 281–93.

Herrler G, Compans RW, Meier-Ewert H, 1979, A precursor glycoprotein in influenza C virus, *Virology*, **99:** 49–56.

Herrler G, Klenk H-D, 1991, Structure and function of the HEF glycoprotein of influenza C virus, *Adv Virus Res*, **40:** 213–34.

Herrler G, Geyer R et al., 1985a, Rat alpha₁ macroglobulin inhibits hemagglutination by influenza C virus, *Virus Res*, **2:** 183–92.

Herrler G, Rott R et al., 1985b, The receptor-destroying enzyme of influenza C virus is neuraminate-O-acetylesterase, *EMBO J*, **4:** 1503–6.

Herrler G, Durkop I et al., 1988, The glycoprotein of influenza C virus is the haemagglutinin, esterase and fusion factor, *J Gen Virol*, **69:** 839–46.

Herrler G, Gross H-J et al., 1992, A synthetic sialic acid analogue is recognized by influenza C virus as a receptor determinant but is resistant to the receptor-destroying enzyme, *J Biol Chem*, **267:** 12501–5.

Hers JF, Mulder J, 1961, Broad aspects of the pathology and pathogenesis of human influenza, *Am Rev Respir Dis*, **83, suppl:** 54–67, 84–97.

Hers JFP, Goslings WRO et al., 1957, Deaths from Asiatic influenza in the Netherlands, *Lancet*, **2**: 1164–5.

Hewat EA, Cusack S et al., 1984, Low resolution structure of the influenza C glycoprotein determined by electron microscopy, *J Mol Biol*, **175**: 175–93.

Hinshaw VS, Webster RG, Turner B, 1980, The perpetuation of orthomyxoviruses and paramyxovirus in Canadian waterfowl, *Can J Microbiol*, **26**: 622–9.

Hinshaw VS, Webster RG et al., 1983a, Altered tissue tropism of human–avian reassortant influenza viruses, *Virology*, **128**: 260–3.

Hinshaw VS, Webster RG et al., 1983b, Swine influenza-like viruses in turkeys: potential source of virus for humans?, *Science*, **220**: 206–8.

Hinshaw VS, Olsen CW et al., 1994, Apoptosis: a mechanism of cell killing by influenza A and B viruses, *J Virol*, **68**: 3667–73.

Hirsch A, 1883, *Handbook of Geographical and Historical Pathology*, vol I, New Sydenham Society, London.

Hirst GK, 1941, Agglutination of red cells by allantoic fluid of chick embryos infected with influenza virus, *Science*, **94**: 22–3.

Hirst GK, 1950, Receptor destruction by viruses of the mumps–NDV–influenza group, *J Exp Med*, **91**: 161–75.

Hobson D, Curry RL et al., 1972, The role of serum hemagglutinin-inhibitory antibody in protection against challenge infection with A2 and B viruses, *J Hyg*, **70**: 767–77.

Hogue BG, Nayak DP, 1992, Synthesis and processing of the influenza virus neuraminidase, a type II transmembrane glycoprotein, *Virology*, **188**: 510–17.

Holsinger LJ, Lamb RA, 1991, Influenza virus M_2 integral membrane protein is a homotetramer stabilized by formation of disulfide bonds, *Virology*, **183**: 32–43.

Holsinger LJ, Shaughnessy MA et al., 1995, Analysis of the post-translational modifications of the influenza virus M_2 protein, *J Virol*, **69**: 1219–25.

Hongo S, Sugawara K et al., 1994, Identification of a second protein encoded by influenza C virus RNA segment 6, *J Gen Virol*, **75**: 3503–10.

Horimoto T, Kawaoka Y, 1995, The hemagglunitin cleavability of a virulent avian influenza virus by subtilisin-like endoproteases is influenced by the amino acid immediately downstream of the cleavage site, *Virology*, **210**: 466–70.

Horimoto T, Nakayama K et al., 1994, Proprotein-processing endoproteases PC6 and furin both activate hemagglutinin of virulent avian influenza viruses, *J Virol*, **68**: 6074–8.

Horisberger MA, 1992, Interferon-induced human protein MxA is a GTP-ase which binds transiently to cellular protein, *J Virol*, **66**: 4705–9.

Horvath CM, Williams MA, Lamb RA, 1990, Eukaryotic coupled translation of tandem cistrons: identification of the influenza B virus BM2 polypeptide, *EMBO J*, **9**: 2639–47.

Houck P, Hemphill M et al., 1995, Amantadine-resistant influenza A in nursing homes: identification of a resistant virus prior to drug use, *Arch Intern Med*, **155**: 533–7.

Hoyle L, 1968, Morphology and physical structure, *The Influenza Viruses*, Springer-Verlag, New York, 49–68.

Hsu MT, Parvin JD et al., 1987, Genomic RNAs of influenza viruses are held in a circular conformation in virions and in infected cells by a terminal panhandle, *Proc Natl Acad Sci USA*, **84**: 8140–4.

Hurtley SM, Bole DG et al., 1989, Interactions of misfolded influenza virus hemagglutinin with binding proteins (BiP), *J Cell Biol*, **108**: 2117–26.

Hurwitz JL, Hackett CJ et al., 1985, Murint T_H response to influenza virus: recognition of hemagglutinin, neuraminidase, matrix, and nucleoproteins, *J Immunol*, **134**: 1994–8.

ICTV Executive Committee, 1966, Meeting of the Executive Committee, 10–11 August 1996, Jerusalem, Israel.

Inglis SC, Brown CM, 1981, Spliced and unspliced RNAs encoded by virion RNA segment 7 of influenza virus, *Nucleic Acids Res*, **9**: 2727–41.

Inglis SC, Barrett T et al., 1979, The smallest genome RNA segment of influenza virus contains two genes that may overlap, *Proc Natl Acad Sci USA*, **76**: 3790–4.

Ito T, Gorman OT et al., 1991, Evolutionary analysis of the influenza A virus M gene with comparison of the M1 and M2 proteins, *J Virol*, **65**: 5491–8.

Jackson DC, Drummer HE et al., 1994, Glycosylation of a synthetic peptide representing a T-cell determinant of influenza virus hemagglutinin results in loss of recognition by CD4+ T-cell clones, *Virology*, **199**: 422–30.

Jahiel RI, Kilbourne ED, 1966, Reduction in plaque size and reduction in plaque number as differing indices of influenza virus-antibody reactions, *J Bacteriol*, **92**: 1521–34.

Janakiraman MN, White CL et al., 1994, Structure of influenza virus neuraminidase of B/Lee/40 complexed with sialic acid and a dehydro analog at 1.8-Å resolution: implications for the catalytic mechanism, *Biochemistry*, **33**: 8172–9.

Jennings LC, Miles JAR, 1978, A study of acute respiratory disease in the community of Port Chalmers. II. Influenza A/Port Chalmers/1/73: intrafamilial spread and the effect of antibodies to the surface antigens, *J Hyg*, **81**: 67–75.

Jennings PA, Finch JT et al., 1983, Does the higher order structure of the influenza virus ribonucleoprotein guide sequence rearrangements in influenza viral RNA?, *Cell*, **34**: 619–27.

Jin H, Leser GP, Lamb RA, 1994, The influenza virus hemagglutinin cytoplasmic tail is not essential for virus assembly or infectivity, *EMBO J*, **13**: 5504–15.

Johnson PR, Feldman S et al., 1986, Immunity to influenza A virus infection in young children: a comparison of natural infection, live cold-adapted vaccine, and inactivated vaccine, *J Infect Dis*, **154**: 121–7.

Jordan WS, Badger GF, Dingle JH, 1958, A study of illness in a group of Cleveland families. XVI. The epidemiology of influenza, 1948–1953, *Am J Hyg*, **68**: 169–89.

Junankar PR, Cherry RJ, 1986, Temperature and pH dependence of the haemolytic activity of influenza virus and of the rotational mobility of the spike glycoproteins, *Biochim Biophys Acta*, **854**: 198–206.

Jurgensen PF, Olsen GN et al., 1973, Immune response of the human respiratory tract. II. Cell-mediated immunity in the lower respiratory tract to tuberculin and mumps and influenza viruses, *J Infect Dis*, **128**: 730–5.

Kalin M, Grandien M, 1993, Rapid diagnostic methods in respiratory infections, *Curr Opin Infect Dis*, **6**: 150–7.

Katz JM, Naeve CW, Webster RG, 1987, Host cell-mediated variation in H3N2 influenza viruses, *Virology*, **156**: 386–95.

Katz JM, Wang M, Webster RG, 1990, Direct sequencing of the HA gene of influenza (H3N2) virus in original clinical samples reveals sequence identity with mammalian cell-grown virus, *J Virol*, **64**: 1808–11.

Katz JM, Webster RG, 1989, Efficacy of inactivated influenza A virus (H3N2) vaccines grown in mammalian cells or embryonated eggs, *J Infect Dis*, **160**: 191–8.

Katz JM, Webster RG, 1992, Amino acid sequence identity between the HA1 of influenza A (H3N2) viruses grown in mammalian and primary chick kidney cells, *J Gen Virol*, **73**: 1159–65.

Kawakami K, Ishihama A, 1983, RNA polymerase of influenza virus. III. Isolation of RNA polymerase–RNA complexes from influenza virus PR8, *J Biochem (Tokyo)*, **93**: 989–96.

Kawaoka Y, 1991, Equine H7N7 influenza A viruses are highly pathogenic in mice without adaptation: potential use as an animal model, *J Virol*, **65**: 3891–4.

Kawaoka Y, Krauss S, Webster RG, 1989, Avian-to-human transmission of the PB1 gene of influenza A virus in the 1957 and 1968 pandemics, *J Virol*, **63**: 4603–8.

Kawaoka Y, Naeve CW, Webster RG, 1984, Is virulence of H5N2 influenza viruses in chickens associated with loss of carbohydrate from the hemagglutinin?, *Virology*, **139**: 303–16.

Kawaoka Y, Webster RG, 1988, Sequence requirements for cleavage activation of influenza virus hemagglutinin expressed in mammalian cells, *Proc Natl Acad Sci USA*, **85**: 324–8.

Kawaoka Y, Webster RG, 1989, Interplay between carbohydrate in the stalk and the length of the connecting peptide determines the cleavability of influenza virus hemagglutinin, *J Virol*, **63**: 3296–300.

Kawaoka Y, Yamnikova S et al., 1990, Molecular characterization of a new hemagglutinin, subtype H14, of influenza A virus, *Virology*, **179**: 759–67.

Kelm S, Paulson JC et al., 1992, Use of sialic acid analogues to define functional groups involved in binding to the influenza virus hemagglutinin, *Eur J Biochem*, **205**: 147–53.

Kemble GW, Danieli T, White JM, 1994, Lipid-anchored influenza hemagglutinin promotes hemifusion, not complete fusion, *Cell*, **76**: 383–91.

Kemble GW, Bodian DL et al., 1992, Intermonomer disulfide bonds impair the fusion activity of influenza virus hemagglutinin, *J Virol*, **66**: 4940–50.

Kemler I, Whittaker G, Helenius A, 1994, Nuclear import of microinjected influenza virus ribonucleoproteins, *Virology*, **202**: 1028–33.

Kendal AP, Skehel JJ, Pereira MS, 1982, *Concepts and Procedures for Laboratory-based Influenza Surveillance*, US Department of Health and Human Services, Centers for Disease Control, Atlanta.

Kendal AP, Noble GR et al., 1978, Antigenic similarity of influenza A(H1N1) viruses from epidemics in 1977–1978 to 'Scandinavian' strains isolated in epidemics of 1950–1951, *Virology*, **89**: 632–6.

Kendal AP, Maassab HA et al., 1981, Development of cold-adapted recombinant live, attenuated influenza A vaccines in the USA and USSR, *Antiviral Res*, **1**: 339–65.

Kido H, Yokogoshi Y et al., 1992, Isolation and characterization of a novel trypsin-like protease found in rat bronchiolar epithelial Clara cells. A possible activator of the viral fusion glycoprotein, *J Biol Chem*, **267**: 13573–9.

Kida H, Ito T et al., 1994, Potential for transmission of avian influenza viruses to pigs, *J Gen Virol*, **75**: 2183–8.

Kilbourne ED, 1959, Studies on influenza in the pandemic of 1957–1958. III. Isolation of influenza A (Asian strain) viruses from influenza patients with pulmonary complications. Details of virus isolation and characterization of isolates, with quantitative comparison of isolation methods, *J Clin Invest*, **38**: 213–65.

Kilbourne ED (ed), 1987, History of influenza, *Influenza*, Plenum Press, New York, 3–22.

Kilbourne ED, Laver WG et al., 1968, Antiviral activity of antiserum specific for an influenza virus neuraminidase, *J Virol*, **2**: 281–8.

Kim HW, Brandt CD et al., 1979, Influenza A and B virus infection in infants and young children during the years 1957–1976, *Am J Epidemiol*, **109**: 464–79.

Kimura N, Nishida M et al., 1992, Transcription of a recombinant influenza virus RNA in cells that can express the influenza virus RNA polymerase and nucleoprotein genes, *J Gen Virol*, **73**: 1321–8.

Kimura N, Fukushima A et al., 1993, An in vivo study of the replication origin in the influenza virus complementary RNA, *J Biochem (Tokyo)*, **113**: 88–92.

Klenk HD, Garten W, Rott R, 1984, Inhibition of proteolytic cleavage of the hemagglutinin of influenza virus by the calcium-specific ionophore A23187, *EMBO J*, **3**: 2911–15.

Klenk HD, Rott R, 1988, The molecular biology of influenza virus pathogenicity, *Adv Virus Res*, **34**: 247–81.

Klenk HD, Wollert W et al., 1974, Association of influenza virus proteins with cytoplasmic fractions, *Virology*, **57**: 28–41.

Klenk HD, Rott R et al., 1975, Activation of influenza A viruses by trypsin treatment, *Virology*, **68**: 426–39.

Klenk HD, Cox NJ et al., 1995, *Orthomyxoviridae, Virus Taxonomy*, eds Murphy FA, Fauquet CM et al., Springer-Verlag, Vienna, 293–9.

Kobayashi M, Toyoda T et al., 1994, Molecular dissection of influenza virus nucleoprotein: deletion mapping of the RNA binding domain, *J Virol*, **68**: 8433–6.

Koen JS, 1919, A practical method for field diagnosis of swine diseases, *J Vet Med*, **14**: 468–70.

Krug RM, Broni BA, Bouloy M, 1979, Are the 5′ ends of influenza viral mRNAs synthesized in vivo donated by host mRNAs?, *Cell*, **18**: 329–34.

Krug RM, Alonso-Caplen FV et al., 1989, Expression and replication of the influenza virus genome, *The Influenza Viruses*, ed Krug RM, Plenum Press, New York, 89–152.

Kundu A, Nayak DP, 1994, Analysis of the signals for polarized transport of influenza virus (A/WSN/33) neuraminidase and human transferrin receptor, type II transmembrane proteins, *J Virol*, **68**: 1812–18.

Kung HC, Jen KF et al., 1978, Influenza in China in 1977. Recurrence of influenza virus A subtype H1N1, *Bull W H O*, **56**: 913–18.

Lamb RA, Choppin PW, 1979, Segment 8 of the influenza virus genome is unique in coding for two polypeptides, *Proc Natl Acad Sci USA*, **76**: 4908–12.

Lamb RA, Holsinger LJ, Pinto LH, 1994, The influenza virus M2 ion channel protein and its role in the influenza virus life cycle, *Cellular Receptors of Animal Viruses*, ed Wimmer E, Dr Cox: Cold Spring Harbour Laboratory Press, Cold Spring Harbour NY, 303–21.

Lamb RA, Horvath CM, 1991, Diversity of coding strategies in influenza viruses, *Trends Genet*, **7**: 261–6.

Lamb RA, Lai CJ, 1980, Sequence of interrupted and uninterrupted mRNAs and cloned DNA coding for the two overlapping nonstructural proteins of influenza virus, *Cell*, **21**: 475–85.

Lamb RA, Lai CJ, Choppin PW, 1981, Sequences of mRNAs derived from genome RNA segment 7 of influenza virus: co-linear and interrupted mRNAs code for overlapping proteins, *Proc Natl Acad Sci USA*, **78**: 4170–4.

Lamb RA, Zebedee SL, Richardson CD, 1985, Influenza virus M2 protein is an integral membrane protein expressed on the infected-cell surface, *Cell*, **40**: 627–33.

Lambkin R, Dimmock NJ, 1995, All rabbits immunized with type A influenza virions have a serum haemagglutination-inhibition antibody response biased to a single epitope in antigenic site B, *J Gen Virol*, **76**: 889–97.

Lambkin R, McLain L et al., 1994, Neutralization escape mutants of type A influenza virus are readily selected by antisera from mice immunized with whole virus: a possible mechanism for antigenic drift, *J Gen Virol*, **75**: 3493–502.

Laver WG, Valentine RC, 1969, Morphology of the isolated hemagglutinin and neuraminidase subunits of influenza virus, *Virology*, **38**: 105–19.

Lawson ND, Stillman EA et al., 1995, Recombinant vesicular stomatitis viruses from DNA, *Proc Natl Acad Sci USA*, **92**: 4477–81.

Lazarowitz SG, Choppin PW, 1975, Enhancement of the infectivity of influenza A and B viruses by proteolytic cleavage of the hemagglutinin polypeptide, *Virology*, **68**: 440–54.

Lazarowitz SG, Goldberg AR, Choppin PW, 1973, Proteolytic cleavage by plasmin of the HA polypeptide of influenza virus: host cell activation of serum plasminogen, *Virology*, **56**: 172–80.

Lehmann NI, Gust ID, 1971, Viraemia in influenza. A report of two cases, *Med J Aust*, **2**: 1166–9.

Lentz MR, Webster RG, Air GM, 1987, Site-directed mutation of the active site of influenza neuraminidase and implications for the catalytic mechanism, *Biochemistry*, **26**: 5351–8.

Li S, Rodrigues M et al., 1993a, Priming with recombinant influenza virus followed by administration of recombinant vaccinia virus induces CD8+ T-cell-mediated protective immunity against malaria, *Proc Natl Acad Sci USA*, **90**: 5214–18.

Li S, Schulman J et al., 1993b, Glycosylation of neuraminidase determines the neurovirulence of influenza A/WSN/33 virus, *J Virol*, **67**: 6667–73.

Li X, Palese P, 1992, Mutational analysis of the promoter

required for influenza virus virion RNA synthesis, *J Virol*, **66:** 4331–8.

Li X, Palese P, 1994, Characterization of the polyadenylation signal of influenza virus RNA, *J Virol*, **68:** 1245–9.

Lightman S, Cobbold S et al., 1987, Do L3T4⁺ T cells act as effector cells in protection against influenza virus infection? *Immunology*, **62:** 139–44.

Liu C, Air GM, 1993, Selection and characterization of a neuraminidase-minus mutant of influenza virus and its rescue by cloned neuraminidase genes, *Virology*, **194:** 403–7.

Liu C, Eichelberger MC et al., 1995, Influenza type A virus neuraminidase does not play a role in viral entry, replication, assembly, or budding, *J Virol*, **69:** 1099–106.

Louria DB, Blumenfeld HL et al., 1959, Studies on influenza in the pandemic of 1957–1958. II. Pulmonary complications of influenza, *J Clin Invest*, **38:** 213–65.

Lu Y, Qian X-Y, Krug RM, 1994, The influenza virus NS1 protein: a novel inhibitor of pre-mRNA splicing, *Genes Dev*, **8:** 1817–28.

Lui K-J, Kendal AP, 1987, Impact of influenza epidemics on mortality in the United States from October 1972 to May 1985, *Am J Public Health*, **77:** 712–16.

de la Luna S, Martin J et al., 1993, Influenza virus naked RNA can be expressed upon transfection into cells co-expressing the three subunits of the polymerase and the nucleoprotein from simian virus 40 recombinant viruses, *J Gen Virol*, **74:** 535–9.

Luo G, Chung J, Palese P, 1993, Alterations of the stalk of the influenza virus neuraminidase:deletions and insertions, *Virus Res*, **29:** 141–53.

Luo G, Luytjes W et al., 1991, The polyadenylation signal of influenza virus RNA involves a stretch of uridines followed by the RNA duplex of the panhandle structure, *J Virol*, **65:** 2861–7.

Luytjes W, Krystal M et al., 1989, Amplification, expression, and packaging of a foreign gene by influenza virus, *Cell*, **59:** 1107–13.

McClelland L, Hare R, 1941, The adsorption of influenza virus by red cells and a new in vitro method of measuring antibodies for influenza virus, *Can J Public Health*, **32:** 530–8.

McGeoch D, Fellner P, Newton C, 1976, Influenza virus genome consists of eight distinct RNA species, *Proc Natl Acad Sci USA*, **73:** 3045–9.

McQueen N, Nayak DP et al., 1986, Polarized expression of a chimeric protein in which the transmembrane and cytoplasmic domains of the influenza virus hemagglutinin have been replaced by those of the vesicular stomatitis virus G protein, *Proc Natl Acad Sci USA*, **83:** 9318–22.

Maassab HF, 1967, Adaptation in growth characteristics of influenza virus at 25°C, *Nature (London)*, **213:** 612–14.

Maassab HF, DeBorde DC, 1983, Characterization of an influenza A host range mutant, *Virology*, **130:** 342–50.

Martin C, Kunin CM et al., 1959, Asian influenza A in Boston, 1957–1958, *Arch Intern Med*, **103:** 516–31.

Martin JT, 1996, Enhanced immunogenicity of Chiron Biocine adjuvanted influenza vaccine in the elderly, *Options for the Control of Influenza III*, eds Brown LE, Hampson AW, Webster RG, Elsevier Science, Amsterdam, 647–52.

Martin J, Albo C et al., 1992, In vitro reconstitution of active influenza virus ribonucleoprotein complexes using viral proteins purified from infected cells, *J Gen Virol*, **73:** 1855–9.

Mast EE, Harmon MW et al., 1991, Emergence and possible transmission of amantadine-resistant viruses during nursing home outbreaks of influenza A(H3N2), *Am J Epidemiol*, **134:** 988–97.

Masurel N, Heijtink RA, 1983, Recycling of H1N1 influenza A virus in man – a haemagglutinin antibody study, *J Hyg (Lond)*, **90:** 397–402.

Masurel N, Marine WM, 1973, Recycling of Asian and Hong Kong influenza A virus hemagglutinins in man, *Am J Epidemiol*, **97:** 44–9.

Matrosovich MN, Gambaryan AS, Chumakov MP, 1992, Influ-

enza viruses differ in recognition of 4-*O*-acetyl substitution of sialic acid receptor determinant, *Virology*, **188:** 854–8.

Matrosovich MN, Gambaryan AS et al., 1993, Probing of the receptor-binding sites of the H1 and H3 influenza A and influenza B virus hemagglutinins by synthetic and natural sialosides, *Virology*, **196:** 111–21.

Meibalane R, Sedmak P et al., 1977, Outbreak of influenza in a neonatal intensive care unit, *J Infect Dis*, **91:** 974–6.

Mena I, de la Luna S et al., 1994, Synthesis of biologically active influenza virus core proteins using a vaccinia virus-T7 RNA polymerase expression system, *J Gen Virol*, **75:** 2109–14.

Mills KHG, Burt DS et al., 1988, Fine specificity of murine class II-restricted T cell clones for synthetic peptides of influenza virus hemagglutinin, *J Immunol*, **140:** 4083–90.

Minuse E, Willis PW III et al., 1962, An attempt to demonstrate viremia in cases of Asian influenza, *J Lab Clin Med*, **59:** 1016–19.

Monto AS, Kioumehr F, 1975, The Tecumseh study of respiratory illness. IX. Occurrence of influenza in the community, 1966–1971, *Am J Epidemiol*, **102:** 553–63.

Monto AS, Maassab HF, Bryan ER, 1981, Relative efficacy of embryonated eggs and cell culture for isolation of contemporary influenza viruses, *J Clin Microbiol*, **13:** 233–5.

Monto AS, Terpenning MS, 1996, The value of influenza and pneumococcal vaccine in the elderly, *Drugs Aging*, **8:** 445–51.

Monto AS, Ullman BM, 1974, Acute respiratory illness in an American community, *JAMA*, **227:** 164–9.

Morris SJ, Sarkar DP et al., 1989, Kinetics of pH-dependent fusion between 3T3 fibroblasts expressing influenza hemagglutinin and red blood cells, *J Biol Chem*, **264:** 3972–8.

Morse MA, Marriott AC, Nuttall PA, 1992, The glycoprotein of Thogoto virus (a tick-borne orthomyxo-like virus) is related to the baculovirus glycoprotein GP64, *Virology*, **186:** 640–6.

Moser MR, Bender TR et al., 1979, An outbreak of influenza aboard a commercial airliner, *J Epidemiol*, **110:** 1–6.

Mountford CE, Grossman G et al., 1982, Effect of monoclonal antineuraminidase antibodies on the kinetic behavior of influenza virus neuraminidase, *Mol Immunol*, **19:** 811–16.

Muchmore EA, Varki A, 1987, Selective inactivation of influenza C esterase: a probe for detecting 9-*O*-acetylated sialic acids, *Science*, **236:** 1293–5.

Mukaigawa J, Nayak DP, 1991, Two signals mediate nuclear localization of influenza virus (A/WSN/33) polymerase basic protein 2, *J Virol*, **65:** 245–53.

Mulder J, Masurel N, 1958, Pre-epidemic antibody against 1957 strain of Asiatic influenza in serum of older people living in the Netherlands, *Lancet*, **1:** 810–14.

Mullooly JP, Bennett MJ et al., 1994, Influenza vaccination programs for elderly persons: cost-effectiveness in a health maintenance organization, *Ann Intern Med*, **121:** 947–52.

Murphy B, 1993, Use of live attenuated cold-adapted influenza A reassortant virus vaccines in infants, children, young adults, and elderly adults, *Infect Dis Clin Pract*, **2:** 174–81.

Murphy BR, Clements ML, 1989, The systemic and mucosal response of humans to influenza A virus, *Curr Top Microbiol Immunol*, **146:** 107–16.

Murphy B, Webster RG, 1990, Orthomyxoviruses, *Fields' Virology*, 2nd edn, eds Fields BN, Knipe DM, Raven Press, New York, 1091–152.

Murphy B, Webster RG, 1996, Orthomyxoviruses, *Fields' Virology*, 3rd edn, eds Fields BN, Knipe DM et al., Lippincott-Raven, Philadelphia, 1397–445.

Murphy BR, Nelson DL et al., 1982, Secretory and systemic immunological response in children infected with live attenuated influenza A virus vaccines, *Infect Immun*, **36:** 1102–8.

Murti KG, Webster RG, 1986, Distribution of hemagglutinin and neuraminidase on influenza virions as revealed by immunoelectron microscopy, *Virology*, **149:** 36–43.

Murti KG, Webster RG, Jones IM, 1988, Localization of RNA polymerases on influenza viral ribonucleoproteins by immunogold labeling, *Virology*, **164:** 562–6.

Murti KG, Brown PS et al., 1992, Composition of the helical internal components of influenza virus as revealed by immunogold labeling/electron microscopy, *Virology*, **186**: 294–9.

Muster T, Subbarao EK et al., 1991, An influenza A virus containing influenza B virus 5′ and 3′ noncoding regions on the neuraminidase gene is attenuated in mice, *Proc Natl Acad Sci USA*, **88**: 5177–81.

Naeve CW, Hinshaw VS, Webster RG, 1984, Mutations in the hemagglutinin receptor-binding site can change the biological properties of an influenza virus, *J Virol*, **51**: 567–9.

Naeve CW, Webster RG, Hinshaw VS, 1983, Phenotypic variation in influenza virus reassortants with identical gene constellations, *Virology*, **128**: 331–40.

Naeve CW, Williams D, 1990, Fatty acids on the A/Japan/305/57 influenza virus hemagglutinin have a role in membrane fusion, *EMBO J*, **9**: 3857–66.

Naficy K, 1963, Human influenza infection with proved viremia, *N Engl J Med*, **269**: 964–6.

Naim HY, Roth MG, 1993, Basis for selective incorporation of glycoproteins into the influenza virus envelope, *J Virol*, **67**: 4831–41.

Naim HY, Amarneh B et al., 1992, Effects of altering palmitylation sites on biosynthesis and function of the influenza virus hemagglutinin, *J Virol*, **66**: 7585–8.

Nakagawa Y, Kimura N et al., 1995, The RNA polymerase PB2 subunit is not required for replication of the influenza virus genome but is involved in capped mRNA synthesis, *J Virol*, **69**: 728–33.

Nakajima K, Desselberger U, Palese P, 1978, Recent human influenza A (H1N1) viruses are closely related genetically to strains isolated in 1950, *Nature (London)*, **274**: 334–9.

Nakajima S, Sugiura A, 1980, Neurovirulence of influenza virus in mice. II. Mechanism of virulence as studied in a neuroblastoma cell line, *Virology*, **101**: 450–7.

Natali A, Oxford JS, Schild GC, 1981, Frequency of naturally occurring antibody to influenza virus antigenic variants selected in vitro with monoclonal antibody, *J Hyg Camb*, **87**: 185–90.

Nath ST, Nayak DP, 1990, Function of two discrete regions is required for nuclear localization of polymerase basic protein 1 of A/WSN/33 influenza virus (H1N1), *Mol Cell Biol*, **10**: 4139–45.

Neumann G, Hobom G, 1995, Mutational analysis of influenza virus promoter elements in vivo, *J Gen Virol*, **76**: 1709–17.

Newman RW, Jennings R et al., 1993, Immune response of human volunteers and animals to vaccination with egg-grown influenza A (H1N1) virus is influenced by three amino acid substitutions in the haemagglutinin molecule, *Vaccine*, **11**: 400–6.

Nichol KL, Margolis KL et al., 1994, The efficacy and cost effectiveness of vaccination against influenza among elderly persons living in the community, *N Engl J Med*, **331**: 778–84.

Nichol KL, Lind A et al., 1995, The effectiveness of vaccination against influenza in healthy, working adults, *N Engl J Med*, **333**: 889–93.

Nicholson KG, 1992, Clinical features of influenza, *Semin Respir Infect*, **7**: 26–37.

Nicholson KG, Snacken R, Palache AM, 1995, Influenza immunization policies in Europe and the United States, *Vaccine*, **13**: 365–9.

Nieto A, de la Luna S et al., 1992, Nuclear transport of influenza virus polymerase PA protein, *Virus Res*, **24**: 65–75.

Noble GR, 1982, Epidemiological and clinical aspects of influenza, *Basic and Applied Influenza Research*, ed Beare AS, CRC Press, Boca Raton FL, 11–50.

Nobusawa E, Aoyama T et al., 1991, Comparison of complete amino acid sequences and receptor-binding properties among 13 serotypes of hemagglutinins of influenza A viruses, *Virology*, **182**: 475–85.

Norton GP, Tanaka T et al., 1987, Infectious influenza A and B

virus variants with long carboxyl terminal deletions in the NS1 polypeptides, *Virology*, **156**: 204–13.

Nuss JM, Air GM, 1991, Transfer of the hemagglutinin activity of influenza virus neuraminidase subtype N9 into an N2 neuraminidase background, *Virology*, **183**: 496–504.

Nuss JM, Whitaker PB, Air GM, 1993, Identification of critical contact residues in the NC41 epitope of a subtype N9 influenza virus neuraminidase, *Proteins*, **15**: 121–32.

Ohuchi M, Ohuchi R, Mifune K, 1982, Demonstration of hemolytic and fusion activities of influenza C virus, *J Virol*, **42**: 1076–9.

Ohuchi M, Orlich M et al., 1989, Mutations at the cleavage site of the hemagglutinin alter the pathogenicity of influenza virus A/chick/Penn/83 (H5N2), *Virology*, **168**: 274–80.

Ohuchi M, Cramer A et al., 1994, Rescue of vector-expressed fowl plague virus hemagglutinin in biologically active form by acidotropic agents and coexpressed M2 protein, *J Virol*, **68**: 920–6.

Okazaki K, Kawaoka Y, Webster RG, 1989, Evolutionary pathways of the PA genes of influenza A viruses, *Virology*, **172**: 601–8.

Oxford JS, Newman R et al., 1991, Direct isolation in eggs of influenza A (H1N1) and B viruses with haemagglutinins of different antigenic and amino acid composition, *J Gen Virol*, **72**: 185–9.

Palese P, 1977, The genes of influenza virus, *Cell*, **10**: 1–10.

Palese P, Tobita K et al., 1974, Characterization of temperature-sensitive influenza virus mutants defective in neuraminidase, *Virology*, **61**: 397–410.

Panayotov PP, Schlesinger RW, 1992, Oligomeric organization and strain-specific proteolytic modification of the virion M2 protein of influenza A H1N1 viruses, *Virology*, **186**: 352–5.

Park KH, Huang T et al., 1991, Rescue of a foreign gene by Sendai virus, *Proc Natl Acad Sci USA*, **88**: 5537–41.

Parvin JD, Palese P et al., 1989, Promoter analysis of influenza virus RNA polymerase, *J Virol*, **63**: 5142–52.

Patterson S, Gross J, Oxford JS, 1988, The intracellular distribution of influenza virus matrix protein and nucleoprotein in infected cells and their relationship to haemagglutinin in the plasma membrane, *J Gen Virol*, **69**: 1859–72.

Pattnaik AK, Wertz GW, 1990, Replication and amplification of defective interfering particle RNAs of vesicular stomatitis virus in cells expressing viral proteins from vectors containing cloned cDNAs, *J Virol*, **64**: 2948–57.

Pattnaik AK, Ball LA et al., 1992, Infectious defective interfering particles of VSV from transcripts of a cDNA clone, *Cell*, **69**: 1011–20.

Pavlovic J, Haller O, Staeheli P, 1992, Human and mouse Mx protein inhibit different steps of the influenza virus multiplication cycle, *J Virol*, **66**: 2564–9.

Percy N, Barclay WS et al., 1994, Expression of a foreign protein by influenza A virus, *J Virol*, **68**: 4486–92.

Philip RN, Bell JA et al., 1961, Epidemiologic studies on influenza in familial and general population groups, 1951–1956, *Am J Hyg*, **73**: 148–63.

Philipp HC, Schroth B et al., 1995, Assessment of fusogenic properties of influenza virus hemagglutinin deacylated by site-directed mutagenesis and hydroxylamine treatment, *Virology*, **210**: 20–8.

Piccone ME, Fernandez-Sesma A, Palese P, 1993, Mutational analysis of the influenza virus vRNA promoter, *Virus Res*, **28**: 99–112.

Pinto LH, Holsinger LJ, Lamb RA, 1992, Influenza virus M_2 protein has ion channel activity, *Cell*, **69**: 517–28.

Plotch SJ, Bouloy M et al., 1981, A unique cap (m7GpppXm)-dependent influenza virion endonuclease cleaves capped RNAs to generate the primers that initiate viral RNA transcription, *Cell*, **23**: 847–58.

Pritchett TJ, Paulson JC, 1989, Basis for the potent inhibition of influenza virus infection by equine and guinea pig α_2-macroglobulin, *J Biol Chem*, **264**: 9850–8.

Privalsky ML, Penhoet EE, 1978, Influenza virus proteins: identity, synthesis, and modification analyzed by two-dimensional gel electrophoresis, *Proc Natl Acad Sci USA*, **75**: 3625–9.

Puri A, Booy FP et al., 1990, Conformational changes and fusion activity of influenza virus hemagglutinin of the H2 and H3 subtypes: effects of acid pretreatment, *J Virol*, **64**: 3824–32.

Qian X-Y, Alonso-Caplen F, Krug RM, 1994, Two functional domains of the influenza virus NS1 protein are required for regulation of nuclear export of mRNA, *J Virol*, **68**: 2433–41.

Qiu Y, Krug RM, 1994, The influenza virus NS1 protein is a poly(A)-binding protein that inhibits nuclear export of mRNAs containing poly(A), *J Virol*, **68**: 2425–32.

Rajakumar A, Swierkosz EM, Schulze IT, 1990, Sequence of an influenza virus hemagglutinin determined directly from a clinical sample, *Proc Natl Acad Sci USA*, **87**: 4154–8.

Rao L, Kadam SS et al., 1982, Epidemiological, clinical, and virological features of influenza outbreaks in Pune, India, 1980, *Bull W H O*, **60**: 639–42.

Reay PA, Jones IM et al., 1989, Recognition of the PB1, neuraminidase, and matrix proteins of influenza virus A/NT/60/68 by cytotoxic T lymphocytes, *Virology*, **170**: 477–85.

Rees PJ, Dimmock NJ, 1981, Electrophoretic separation of influenza virus ribonucleoprotein, *J Gen Virol*, **53**: 125–32.

Reichelderfer PS, Kendal AP et al., 1981, Influenza surveillance in the Pacific Basin, *Current Topics in Medical Mycology*, eds Chan YC, Doraisingham S, Ling AE, World Scientific, Singapore, 412–44.

Rekart M, Rupnik K et al., 1982, Prevalence of hemagglutination inhibition antibody to current strains of the H3N2 and H1N1 subtypes of influenza A virus in sera collected from the elderly in 1976, *Am J Epidemiol*, **115**: 587–97.

Rey O, Nayak DP, 1992, Nuclear retention of M1 protein in a temperature-sensitive mutant of influenza (A/WSN/33) virus does not affect nuclear export of viral ribonucleoproteins, *J Virol*, **66**: 5815–24.

Richardson JC, Akkina RK, 1991, NS2 protein of influenza virus is found in purified virus and phosphorylated in infected cells, *Arch Virol*, **116**: 69–80.

Roberts PC, Garten W, Klenk H-D, 1993, Role of conserved glycosylation sites in maturation and transport of influenza A virus hemagglutinin, *J Virol*, **67**: 3048–60.

Robertson JS, Bootman JS et al., 1987, Structural changes in the haemagglutinin which accompany egg adaptation of an influenza A (H1N1) virus, *Virology*, **160**: 31–7.

Robertson JS, Bootman JS et al., 1990, The hemagglutinin of influenza B virus present in clinical material is a single species identical to that of mammalian cell-grown virus, *Virology*, **179**: 35–40.

Rogers GN, D'Souza BL, 1989, Receptor binding properties of human and animal H1 influenza virus isolates, *Virology*, **173**: 317–22.

Rogers GN, Paulson JC, 1983, Receptor determinants of human and animal influenza virus isolates: differences in receptor specificity of the H3 hemagglutinin based on species of origin, *Virology*, **127**: 361–73.

Rogers GN, Paulson JC et al., 1983a, Single amino acid substitutions in influenza haemagglutinin change receptor binding specificity, *Nature (London)*, **304**: 76–8.

Rogers GN, Pritchett TJ et al., 1983b, Differential sensitivity of human, avian, and equine influenza A viruses to a glycoprotein inhibitor of infection: selection of receptor specific variants, *Virology*, **131**: 394–408.

Rogers GN, Daniels RS et al., 1985, Host-mediated selection of influenza receptor variants. Sialic acid alpha2,6Gal specific clones of A/duck/Ukraine/1/63 revert to sialic acid alpha2,3Gal-specific wildtype in ovo, *J Biol Chem*, **260**: 7362–7.

Rogers GN, Herrler G et al., 1986, Influenza C virus uses 9-*O*-acetyl-*N*-acetylneuraminic acid as a high affinity receptor determinant for attachment to cells, *J Biol Chem*, **261**: 5947–51.

Rohm C, Zhou N et al., 1996, Characterization of a novel influ-

enza hemagglutinin, H15: criteria for determination of influenza A subtypes, *Virology*, **217**: 508–16.

Rota PA, Shaw MW, Kendal AP, 1987, Comparison of the immune response to variant influenza type B hemagglutinins expressed in vaccinia virus, *Virology*, **161**: 269–75.

Rota PA, Shaw MW, Kendal AP, 1989, Cross-protection against microvariants of influenza virus type B by vaccinia viruses expressing haemagglutinins from egg- or MDCK cell-derived subpopulations of influenza virus type B/England/222/82, *J Gen Virol*, **70**: 1533–7.

Roth MG, Compans RW et al., 1983, Influenza virus hemagglutinin expression is polarized in cells infected with recombinant SV40 viruses carrying cloned hemagglutinin DNA, *Cell*, **33**: 435–43.

Rott R, Becht H, Orlich M, 1974, The significance of influenza virus neuraminidase in immunity, *J Gen Virol*, **22**: 35–41.

Ruigrok RWH, Baudin F, 1995, Structure of influenza virus ribonucleoprotein particles. II. Purified RNA-free influenza virus ribonucleoprotein forms structures that are indistinguishable from the intact influenza virus ribonucleoprotein particles, *J Gen Virol*, **76**: 1009–14.

Ruigrok RWH, Calder LJ, Wharton SA, 1989, Electron microscopy of the influenza virus submembranal structure, *Virology*, **173**: 311–16.

Ruigrok RWH, Hewat EA, Wade RH, 1992, Low pH deforms the influenza virus envelope, *J Gen Virol*, **73**: 995–8.

Saito T, Taylor G et al., 1994, Antigenicity of the N8 influenza A virus neuraminidase: existence of an epitope at the subunit interface of the neuraminidase, *J Virol*, **68**: 1790–6.

Sauter NK, Glick GD et al., 1992, Crystallographic detection of a second ligand binding site in influenza virus hemagglutinin, *Proc Natl Acad Sci USA*, **89**: 324–8.

Schäfer W, 1955, Sero-immunologic studies on incomplete forms of the virus of classical fowl plague [German], *Arch Exp Vet Med*, **9**: 218–30.

Schaffer FL, Soergel ME, Straube DC, 1976, Survival of airborne influenza virus: effects of propagating host, relative humidity, and composition of spray fluids, *Arch Virol*, **54**: 263–73.

Schild GC, Oxford JS et al., 1983, Evidence for host-cell selection of influenza virus antigenic variants, *Nature (London)*, **303**: 706–9.

Schmidt MF, 1982, Acylation of viral spike glycoproteins: a feature of enveloped RNA viruses, *Virology*, **116**: 327–38.

Schnell MJ, Mebatsion T, Conzelmann KK, 1994, Infectious rabies viruses from cloned cDNA, *EMBO J*, **13**: 4195–203.

Scholtissek C, Koennecke I, Rott R, 1978, Host range recombinants of fowl plague (influenza A) virus, *Virology*, **91**: 79–85.

Scholtissek C, Rohde W et al., 1978, On the origin of the human influenza virus subtype H2N2 and H3N2, *Virology*, **87**: 13–20.

Scholtissek C, Burger H et al., 1985, The nucleoprotein as a possible major factor in determining host specificity of influenza H3N2 viruses, *Virology*, **147**: 287–94.

Schulman JL, Khakpour M, Kilbourne ED, 1968, Protective effects of specific immunity to viral neuraminidase on influenza virus infection of mice, *J Virol*, **2**: 778–86.

Schulman JL, Palese P, 1977, Virulence factors of influenza A viruses: WSN virus neuraminidase required for plaque production in MDBK cells, *J Virol*, **24**: 170–6.

Schwarzmann SW, Adler JL et al., 1971, Bacterial pneumonia during the Hong Kong influenza epidemic of 1968–1969, *Arch Intern Med*, **127**: 1037–41.

Segal MS, Bye JM et al., 1992, Disulfide bond formation during the folding of influenza virus hemagglutinin, *J Cell Biol*, **118**: 227–44.

Seong BL, Brownlee GG, 1992a, A new method for reconstituting influenza polymerase and RNA in vitro: a study of the promoter elements for cRNA and vRNA synthesis in vitro and viral rescue in vivo, *Virology*, **186**: 247–60.

Seong BL, Brownlee GG, 1992b, Nucleotides 9 to 11 of the influenza A virion RNA promoter are crucial for activity in vitro, *J Gen Virol*, **73**: 3115–24.

Shapiro GI, Krug RM, 1988, Influenza virus RNA replication in vitro: synthesis of viral template RNAs and virion RNAs in the absence of an added primer, *J Virol*, **62**: 2285–90.

Shih S-R, Nemeroff ME, Krug RM, 1995, The choice of alternative 5′ splice sites in influenza M1 mRNA is regulated by the viral polymerase complex, *Proc Natl Acad Sci USA*, **92**: 6324–8.

Shope RE, 1931, Swine influenza; experimental transmission and pathology, *J Exp Med*, **54**: 349–59.

Shortridge KF, 1992, Pandemic influenza: a zoonosis?, *Semin Respir Infect*, **7**: 11–25.

Simonsen L, Clarke MJ et al., 1997, The impact of influenza epidemics on mortality: introducing a severity index, *Am J Public Health*, in press.

Skehel JJ, Baley PM et al., 1982, Changes in the conformation of the influenza virus hemagglutinin at the pH optimum of virus-mediated membrane fusion, *Proc Natl Acad Sci USA*, **79**: 968–72.

Skehel JJ, Stevens DJ et al., 1984, A carbohydrate side chain on hemagglutinins of Hong Kong influenza viruses inhibits recognition by a monoclonal antibody, *Proc Natl Acad Sci USA*, **81**: 1779–83.

Slepushkin VA, Katz JM et al., 1995, Protection of mice against influenza A virus challenge by vaccination with baculovirus-expressed M2 protein, *Vaccine*, **13**: 1399–402.

Smirnov YA, Kuznetsova MA, Kaverin NV, 1991, The genetic aspects of influenza virus filamentous particle formation, *Arch Virol*, **118**: 279–84.

Smith GL, Levin JZ et al., 1987, Synthesis and cellular location of the ten influenza polypeptides individually expressed by recombinant vaccinia viruses, *Virology*, **160**: 336–45.

Smith W, Andrewes CH, Laidlaw PP, 1933, A virus obtained from influenza patients, *Lancet*, **1**: 66–8.

Snyder MH, Buckler-White AJ et al., 1987, The avian influenza virus nucleoprotein gene and a specific constellation of avian and human virus polymerase genes each specify attenuation of avian/human influenza A/Pintail/79 reassortant viruses from monkeys, *J Virol*, **61**: 2857–63.

Spelman DW, McHardy CJ, 1985, Concurrent outbreak of influenza A and influenza B, *J Hyg Camb*, **94**: 331–9.

Spruce AE, Iwata A, Almers W, 1991, The first milliseconds of the pore formed by a fusogenic viral envelope protein during membrane fusion, *Proc Natl Acad Sci USA*, **88**: 3623–7.

St Angelo C, Smith GE et al., 1987, Two of the three influenza viral polymerase proteins expressed by using baculovirus vectors form a complex in insect cells, *J Virol*, **61**: 361–5.

Staeheli P, 1990, Interferon-induced proteins and the antiviral state, *Adv Virus Res*, **38**: 147–200.

Stegmann T, Booy FP, Wilschut J, 1987, Effects of low pH on influenza virus. Activation and inactivation of the membrane fusion capacity of the hemagglutinin, *J Biol Chem*, **262**: 17744–9.

Stegmann T, White JM, Helenius A, 1990, Intermediates in influenza induced membrane fusion, *EMBO J*, **9**: 4231–41.

Stegmann T, Delfino JM et al., 1991, The HA2 subunit of influenza hemagglutinin inserts into the target membrane prior to fusion, *J Biol Chem*, **266**: 18404–10.

Steinhauer DA, Wharton SA et al., 1991, Deacylation of the hemagglutinin of influenza A/Aichi/2/68 has no effect on membrane fusion properties, *Virology*, **184**: 445–8.

Stieneke-Grober A, Vey M et al., 1992, Influenza virus hemagglutinin with multibasic cleavage site is activated by furin, a subtilisin-like endoprotease, *EMBO J*, **11**: 2407–14.

Strobl B, Vlasak R, 1993, The receptor-destroying enzyme of influenza C virus is required for entry into target cells, *Virology*, **192**: 679–82.

Stuart-Harris CH, Schild G, Oxford JS, 1985, The epidemiology of influenza, *Influenza, the Viruses and the Disease*, 2nd edn, Edward Arnold, London, 118–30.

Subbarao EK, Kawaoka Y, Murphy BR, 1993, Rescue of an influenza A virus wild-type PB2 gene and a mutant derivative bearing a site-specific temperature-sensitive and attenuating mutation, *J Virol*, **67**: 7223–8.

Subbarao EK, London W, Murphy BR, 1993, A single amino acid in the PB2 gene of influenza A virus is a determinant of host range, *J Virol*, **67**: 1761–4.

Sugiura A, Ueda M, 1980, Neurovirulence of influenza virus in mice. I. Neurovirulence of recombinants between virulent and avirulent virus strains, *Virology*, **101**: 440–9.

Sugrue RJ, Belshe RB, Hay AJ, 1990, Palmitoylation of the influenza A virus M2 protein, *Virology*, **179**: 51–6.

Sugrue RJ, Hay AJ, 1991, Structural characteristics of the M2 protein of influenza A viruses: evidence that it forms a tetrameric channel, *Virology*, **180**: 617–24.

Sugrue RJ, Bahadur G et al., 1990, Specific structural alteration of the influenza haemagglutinin by amantadine, *EMBO J*, **9**: 3469–76.

Suzuki Y, Nakao T et al., 1992, Structural determination of gangliosides that bind to influenza A, B, and C viruses by an improved binding assay: strain-specific receptor epitopes in sialo-sugar chains, *Virology*, **189**: 121–31.

Taber LH, Paredes A et al., 1981, Infection with influenza A/Victoria virus in Houston families, 1976, *J Hyg (Lond)*, **86**: 303–13.

Takeuchi K, Lamb RA, 1994, Influenza virus M2 protein ion channel activity stabilizes the native form of fowl plague virus hemagglutinin during intracellular transport, *J Virol*, **68**: 911–19.

Takizawa T, Matsukawa S et al., 1993, Induction of programmed cell death (apoptosis) by influenza virus infection in tissue culture cells, *J Gen Virol*, **74**: 2347–55.

Takizawa T, Fukuda R et al., 1995, Activation of the apoptotic Fas antigen-encoding gene upon influenza virus infection involving spontaneously produced beta-interferon, *Virology*, **209**: 288–96.

Tashiro M, Ciborowski P et al., 1987, Role of staphylococcus protease in the development of influenza pneumonia, *Nature (London)*, **325**: 536–7.

Taylor PM, Askonas BA, 1986, Influenza nucleoprotein-specific cytotoxic T-cell clones are protective in vivo, *Immunology*, **58**: 417–20.

Taylor RM, 1949, Studies on survival of influenza virus between epidemics and antigenic variations of the virus, *Am J Public Health*, **39**: 171–8.

Tiley LS, Hagen M et al., 1994, Sequence-specific binding of the influenza virus RNA polymerase to sequences located at the 5′ ends of the viral RNAs, *J Virol*, **68**: 5108–16.

Tobita K, Tanaka T et al., 1990, Nucleotide sequence and some biological properties of the NS gene of a newly isolated influenza B virus mutant which has a long carboxyl terminal deletion in the NS$_1$ protein, *Virology*, **174**: 314–19.

Tominack RL, Hayden FG, 1987, Rimantadine hydrochloride and amantadine hydrochloride use in influenza A virus infections, *Infectious Disease Clinics of North America*, eds Knight V, Gilbert B, WB Saunders, Philadelphia, 459–78.

Treanor JJ, Tierney EL et al., 1990, Passively transferred monoclonal antibody to the M2 protein inhibits influenza A virus replication in mice, *J Virol*, **64**: 1375–7.

Treanor JJ, Betts RF et al., 1996, Evaluation of a recombinant hemagglutinin expressed in insect cells as an influenza vaccine in young and elderly adults, *J Infect Dis*, **173**: 1467–70.

Tulip WR, Varghese JN et al., 1991, Refined atomic structures of N9 subtype influenza virus neuraminidase and escape mutants, *J Mol Biol*, **221**: 487–97.

Tulip WR, Varghese JN et al., 1992, Refined crystal structure of the influenza virus N9 neuraminidase–NC41 Fab complex, *J Mol Biol*, **227**: 122–48.

Ulmanen I, Broni B, Krug RM, 1983, Influenza virus temperature-sensitive cap (m7GpppNm)-dependent endonuclease, *J Virol*, **45**: 27–35.

Ulmer JB, Donnelly JJ et al., 1993, Heterologous protection

against influenza by injection of DNA encoding a viral protein, *Science*, **259**: 1745–9.

Umetsu Y, Sugawara K et al., 1992, Selection of antigenically distinct variants of influenza C viruses by the host cell, *Virology*, **189**: 740–4.

Van Voris LP, Newell PM, 1992, Antivirals for the chemoprophylaxis and treatment of influenza, *Semin Respir Infect*, **7**: 61–70.

Van Wyke KL, Bean WJ, Webster RG, 1981, Monoclonal antibodies to the influenza A virus nucleoprotein affecting RNA transcription, *J Virol*, **39**: 313–17.

Van Wyke KL, Hinshaw VS et al., 1980, Antigenic variation of influenza A virus nucleoprotein detected with monoclonal antibodies, *J Virol*, **35**: 24–30.

Van Wyke KL, Yewdell JW et al., 1984, Antigenic characterization of influenza A matrix protein with monoclonal antibodies, *J Virol*, **49**: 248–52.

Varghese JN, Laver WG, Colman PM, 1983, Structure of the influenza virus glycoprotein antigen neuraminidase at 2.9 Å resolution, *Nature (London)*, **303**: 35–40.

Varghese JN, Webster RG et al., 1988, Structure of an escape mutant of glycoprotein N2 neuraminidase of influenza virus A/Tokyo/3/67 at 3 Å, *J Mol Biol*, **200**: 201–3.

Veit M, Herrler G et al., 1990, The hemagglutinating glycoproteins of influenza B and C viruses are acylated with different fatty acids, *Virology*, **177**: 807–11.

Veit M, Kretzschmar E et al., 1991, Site-specific mutagenesis identifies three cysteine residues in the cytoplasmic tail as acylation sites of influenza virus hemagglutinin, *J Virol*, **65**: 2491–500.

Vey M, Orlich M et al., 1992, Hemagglutinin activation of pathogenic avian influenza viruses of serotype H7 requires the protease recognition motif R–X–K/R–R, *Virology*, **188**: 408–13.

Virelizier JL, 1975, Host defenses against influenza: the role of anti-hemagglutinin antibody, *J Immunol*, **115**: 434–9.

Vlasak R, Krystal M et al., 1987, The influenza C virus glycoprotein (HE) exhibits receptor-binding (hemagglutinin) and receptor-destroying (esterase) activities, *Virology*, **160**: 410–25.

Von Itzstein M, Wu W-Y et al., 1993, Rational design of potent sialidase-based inhibitors of influenza virus replication, *Nature (London)*, **363**: 418–23.

Wabuke-Bunoti MA, Fan DP, 1983, Isolation and characterization of a CNBr cleavage peptide of influenza viral hemagglutinin stimulatory for mouse cytolytic T lymphocytes, *J Immunol*, **130**: 2386–91.

Wabuke-Bunoti MA, Taku A et al., 1984, Cytolytic T lymphocyte and antibody responses to synthetic peptides of influenza virus hemagglutinin, *J Immunol*, **133**: 2194–201.

Wakefield L, Brownlee GG, 1989, RNA-binding properties of influenza A virus matrix protein M1, *Nucleic Acids Res*, **17**: 8569–80.

Walker JA, Sakaguchi T et al., 1992, Location and character of the cellular enzyme that cleaves the hemagglutinin of a virulent avian influenza virus, *Virology*, **190**: 278–87.

Walsh JJ, Dietlein LF et al., 1961, Bronchotracheal response in human influenza, *Arch Intern Med*, **108**: 376–88.

Waner JL, Todd SJ et al., 1991, Comparison of Directigen Flu-A with viral isolation and direct immunofluorescence for the rapid detection and identification of influenza A virus, *J Clin Microbiol*, **29**: 479–82.

Wang M-L, Skehel JJ, Wiley DC, 1986, Comparative analyses of the specificities of anti-influenza hemagglutinin antibodies in human sera, *J Virol*, **57**: 124–8.

Webster RG, Brown LE, Laver WG, 1984, Antigenic and biological characterization of influenza virus neuraminidase (N2) with monoclonal antibodies, *Virology*, **135**: 30–42.

Webster RG, Kawaoka Y, 1994, Influenza – an emerging and re-emerging disease, *Semin Virol*, **5**: 103–11.

Webster RG, Laver WG, 1966, Influenza virus subunit vaccines. Immunogenicity and lack of toxicity for rabbits of ether and detergent-disrupted virus, *J Immunol*, **96**: 596–605.

Webster RG, Laver WG, 1972, Studies on the origin of pandemic influenza. I. Antigenic analysis of A₂ influenza viruses isolated before and after the appearance of Hong Kong influenza using antisera to the isolated hemagglutinin subunits, *Virology*, **48**: 433–44.

Webster RG, Reay PA, Laver WG, 1988, Protection against lethal influenza with neuraminidase, *Virology*, **164**: 230–7.

Webster RG, Rott R, 1987, Influenza virus A pathogenicity: the pivotal role of hemagglutinin, *Cell*, **50**: 665–6.

Webster RG, Yakhmo MA et al., 1978, Intestinal influenza: replication and characterization of influenza viruses in ducks, *Virology*, **84**: 268–78.

Webster RG, Air GM et al., 1987, Antigenic structure and variation in an influenza virus N9 neuraminidase, *J Virol*, **61**: 2910–16.

Webster RG, Bean WJ et al., 1992, Evolution and ecology of influenza A viruses, *Microbiol Rev*, **56**: 152–79.

Weis W, Brown JH et al., 1988, Structure of the influenza virus haemagglutinin complexed with its receptor, sialic acid, *Nature (London)*, **333**: 426–31.

Weis WI, Brünger AT et al., 1990a, Refinement of the influenza virus hemagglutinin by simulated annealing, *J Mol Biol*, **212**: 737–61.

Weis WI, Cusack SC et al., 1990b, The structure of a membrane fusion mutant of the influenza virus haemagglutinin, *EMBO J*, **9**: 17–24.

Whitaker-Dowling P, Lucas W, Youngner JS, 1990, Cold-adapted vaccine strains of influenza A virus act as dominant negative mutants in mixed infections with wild-type influenza A virus, *Virology*, **175**: 358–64.

Whitaker-Dowling P, Maassab HF, Youngner JS, 1991, Dominant-negative mutants as antiviral agents: simultaneous infection with the cold-adapted live-virus vaccine for influenza A protects ferrets from disease produced by wild-type influenza A, *J Infect Dis*, **164**: 1200–2.

White JM, 1992, Membrane fusion, *Science*, **258**: 917–24.

White JM, 1994, Fusion of influenza virus in endosomes: role of the hemagglutinin, *Cellular Receptors for Animal Viruses*, ed Wimmer E, Cold Spring Harbor Laboratory Press, Cold Spring Harbor NY, 281–301.

White J, Kielian M, Helenius A, 1983, Membrane fusion proteins of enveloped animal viruses, *Q Rev Biophys*, **16**: 151–95.

White JM, Wilson IA, 1987, Anti-peptide antibodies detect steps in a protein conformational change: low-pH activation of the influenza virus hemagglutinin, *J Cell Biol*, **105**: 2887–96.

Whittaker G, Kemler I, Helenius A, 1995, Hyperphosphorylation of mutant influenza virus matrix protein, M1, causes its retention in the nucleus, *J Virol*, **69**: 439–45.

WHO Memorandum, 1980, A revision of the system of nomenclature for influenza viruses: a WHO memorandum, *Bull W H O*, **58**: 585–91.

WHO Memorandum, 1995, Cell culture as a substrate for the production of influenza vaccines: memorandum from a WHO meeting, *Bull W H O*, **73**: 431–5.

Wiley DC, Skehel JJ, 1987, The structure and function of the hemagglutinin membrane glycoprotein of influenza virus, *Annu Rev Biochem*, **56**: 365–94.

Wiley DC, Skehel JJ, Waterfield M, 1977, Evidence from studies with a cross-linking reagent that the haemaglutinin of influenza virus is a trimer, *Virology*, **79**: 446–8.

Wiley DC, Wilson IA, Skehel JJ, 1981, Structural identification of the antibody-binding sites of Hong Kong influenza haemagglutinin and their involvement in antigenic variation, *Nature (London)*, **289**: 373–8.

Williams MA, Lamb RA, 1986, Determination of the orientation of an integral membrane protein and sites of glycosylation by oligonucleotide-directed mutagenesis: influenza B virus NB glycoprotein lacks a cleavable signal sequence and has an extracellular NH2-terminal region, *Mol Cell Biol*, **6**: 4317–28.

Williams MA, Lamb RA, 1988, Polylactosaminoglycan modification of a small integral membrane glycoprotein, influenza B virus NB, *Mol Cell Biol*, **8**: 1186–96.

Williams MA, Lamb RA, 1989, Effect of mutations and deletions in a bicistronic mRNA on the synthesis of influenza B virus NB and NA glycoproteins, *J Virol*, **63**: 28–35.

Wilson IA, Cox NJ, 1990, Structural basis of immune recognition of influenza virus hemagglutinin, *Annu Rev Immunol*, **8**: 737–71.

Wilson IA, Skehel JJ, Wiley DC, 1981, Structure of the haemagglutinin membrane glycoprotein of influenza virus at 3Å resolution, *Nature (London)*, **289**: 366–73.

Wood JM, Seagroatt V et al., 1981, International collaborative study of single-radial-diffusion and immunoelectrophoresis techniques for the assay of haemagglutin antigen of influenza virus, *J Biol Stand*, **9**: 317–30.

Wood JM, Oxford JS et al., 1989, Influenza A (H1N1) vaccine efficacy in animal models is influenced by two amino acid substitutions in the hemagglutinin molecule, *Virology*, **171**: 214–21.

Woolston WJ, Conley DO, 1918, Epidemic pneumonia (Spanish influenza) in pregnancy, *JAMA*, **71**: 1898.

World Health Organization, 1996, Influenza in the world, *Weekly Epidemiol Rec*, **71**: 1–7.

Wright PF, Johnson PR, Karzon DT, 1986, Clinical experience with live attenuated vaccines in children, *Options for the Control of Influenza*, eds Kendal AP, Patriarca PA, Alan R Liss, New York, 243–53.

Wright PF, Murphy BR et al., 1983, Secretory immunological response after intranasal inactivated influenza A virus vaccinations: evidence for immunoglobulin A memory, *Infect Immun*, **40**: 1092–5.

Wysocka M, Hackett CJ, 1990, Class I *H-2^d*-restricted cytotoxic T lymphocytes recognize the neuraminidase glycoprotein of influenza virus subtype N1, *J Virol*, **64**: 1028–32.

Xu G, Suzuki T et al., 1994, Specificity of sialyl-sugar chain mediated recognition by the hemagglutinin of human influenza B virus isolates, *J Biochem (Tokyo)*, **115**: 202–7.

Yamamoto-Goshima F, Maeno K et al., 1994, Role of neuraminidase in the morphogenesis of influenza B virus, *J Virol*, **68**: 1250–4.

Yamanaka K, Ishihama A, Nagata K, 1988, Translational regulation of influenza virus mRNAs, *Virus Genes*, **2**: 19–30.

Yamanaka K, Nagata K, Ishihama A, 1991, Temporal control for translation of influenza virus mRNAs, *Arch Virol*, **120**: 33–42.

Yamanaka K, Ogasawara N et al., 1991, In vivo analysis of the promoter structure of the influenza virus RNA genome using a transfection system with an engineered RNA, *Proc Natl Acad Sci USA*, **88**: 5369–73.

Yamashita M, Krystal M, Palese P, 1988, Evidence that the matrix protein of influenza C virus is coded for by a spliced mRNA, *J Virol*, **62**: 3348–55.

Yasuda J, Bucher DJ, Ishihama A, 1994, Growth control of influenza A virus by M1 protein: analysis of transfectant viruses carrying the chimeric M gene, *J Virol*, **68**: 8141–6.

Yasuda J, Nakada S et al., 1993, Molecular assembly of influenza virus: association of the NS2 protein with virion matrix, *Virology*, **196**: 249–55.

Ye ZP, Baylor NW, Wagner RR, 1989, Transcription-inhibition and RNA-binding domains of influenza A virus matrix protein mapped with anti-idiotypic antibodies and synthetic peptides, *J Virol*, **63**: 3586–94.

Ye Z, Robinson D, Wagner RR, 1995, Nucleus-targeting domain of the matrix protein (M_1) of influenza virus, *J Virol*, **69**: 1964–70.

Yewdell JW, Hackett CJ, 1989, Specificity and function of T lymphocytes induced by influenza viruses, *The Influenza Viruses*, ed Krug R, Plenum Press, New York, 361–429.

Youngner JS, Treanor JJ et al., 1994, Effect of simultaneous administration of cold-adapted and wild-type influenza A viruses on experimental wild-type influenza infection in humans, *J Clin Microbiol*, **32**: 750–4.

Yu YG, King DS, Shin Y-K, 1994, Insertion of a coiled-coil peptide from influenza virus hemagglutinin into membranes, *Science*, **266**: 274–6.

Zebedee SL, Lamb RA, 1988, Influenza A virus M2 protein: monoclonal antibody restriction of virus growth and detection of M2 in virions, *J Virol*, **62**: 2762–72.

Zhdanov VM, 1986, Live influenza vaccines in the USSR: development of studies and practical application, *Options for the Control of Influenza*, eds Kendal AP, Patriarca PA, Alan R Liss, New York, 193–205.

Zhirnov OP, 1990, Solubilization of matrix protein M1/M from virions occurs at different pH for orthomyxo- and paramyxoviruses, *Virology*, **176**: 274–9.

Zhirnov OP, Grigoriev VB, 1994, Disassembly of influenza C viruses, distinct from that of influenza A and B viruses, requires neutral-alkaline pH, *Virology*, **200**: 284–91.

Ziegler T, Hall HE et al., 1995, Type- and subtype-specific detection of influenza viruses in clinical specimens by rapid culture assay, *J Clin Microbiol*, **33**: 318–21.

Zurcher T, Luo G, Palese P, 1994, Mutations at palmitylation sites of the influenza virus hemagglutinin affect virus formation, *J Virol*, **68**: 5748–54.

Zvonarjev AY, Ghendon YZ, 1980, Influence of membrane (M) protein on influenza A virus virion transcriptase activity in vitro and its susceptibility to rimantadine, *J Virol*, **33**: 583–6.

Chapter 23

PARAMYXOVIRUSES

W J Bellini, P A Rota and L J Anderson

1 Properties of the viruses	3 Clinical and pathological aspects:
2 Clinical and pathological aspects: infections	paramyxovirus infections of birds and
of humans	animals

1   PROPERTIES OF THE VIRUSES

1.1   Classification

The parainfluenza viruses include several important human respiratory tract pathogens, as well as viruses affecting various species of mammals, birds and reptiles. Since the last edition of this book, the International Committee on Taxonomy of Viruses (Murphy et al. 1995) has reclassified the *Paramyxoviridae* family into 2 subfamilies: the *Paramyxovirinae* and the *Pneumovirinae*. Three genera comprise the *Paramyxovirinae* subfamily: *Paramyxovirus, Rubulavirus* and *Morbillivirus*. The subfamily *Pneumovirinae* contains the single genus *Pneumovirus*. In addition to morphology and genome organization, the new classification is based on the recent availability of genetic sequences for each of the viruses and the biological activities associated with the viral proteins. Viruses representative of each of the subfamilies and genera are listed in Table 23.1.

1.2   General properties

The paramyxoviruses are genetically stable viruses, primarily because they are composed of a single strand of unsegmented, negative-sense ribonucleic acid (RNA) that apparently does not undergo recombination. Thus, the only mechanism that permits some degree of variation is mutation. Members of this family of viruses infect humans and many species of animals, including terrestrial and aquatic mammals, birds and even reptiles (Richter et al. 1996). Paramyxoviruses that infect plants have not been described.

Paramyxoviruses are transmitted via close contact or the air-borne (droplet or aerosol) route. They infect their host cells by a primary interaction of cell surface receptors with virus-encoded glycoproteins, haemagglutinin/neuraminidase (HN), haemagglutinin (H) or G protein. This binding is followed by

Table 23.1   Representative members of each of the 4 genera comprising the family *Paramyxoviridae*

Subfamily *Paramyxovirinae*
Genus *Paramyxovirus*
Human parainfluenza viruses, types 1 and 3
Sendai virus
Bovine parainfluenza virus, type 3
Genus *Rubulavirus*
Human parainfluenza viruses, types 2, 4a and 4b
Mumps virus
Newcastle disease virus
Simian virus 5
Genus *Morbillivirus*
Measles virus
Canine distemper virus
Rinderpest virus
Peste des petits ruminants virus
Phocine distemper virus
Dolphin distemper virus
Equine morbillivirus (?)
Subfamily *Pneumovirinae*
Genus *Pneumovirus*
Human respiratory syncytial virus
Bovine respiratory syncytial virus
Pneumonia virus of mice
Turkey rhinotracheitis virus

fusion of host cell membrane and virus envelope. All paramyxoviruses possess a fusion (F) protein, but the fusion process is believed to require both glycoproteins. Syncytia formation, cell lysis or both are the common outcomes of infection by the paramyxoviruses. Table 23. 2 lists the general properties of the members of the family.

Table 23.2 General properties of the genera of the family *Paramyxoviridae*

Characteristic	Genus			
	Paramyxovirus	*Morbillivirus*	*Rubulavirus*	*Pneumovirus*
Genome	Single-stranded negative-sense RNA of c. 16 000 nucleotides			
Morphology	Quasispherical and filamentous particles			
Nucleocapsid:				
Symmetry	Helical	Helical	Helical	Helical
Diameter	18 nm	18 nm	18 nm	13–14 nm
Pitch	5.5 nm	5.5 nm	5.5 nm	6.7–7.0 nm
Virion characteristics:				
RNA polymerase	+	+	+	+
Haemagglutination	+	+	+	–
Neuraminidase	+	–	+	–
Spike length	8 nm	8 nm	8 nm	10–12 nm
Spike spacing	8–10 nm	8–10 nm	8–10 nm	7–10 nm
Multiplication	Cytoplasm	Cytoplasm	Cytoplasm	Cytoplasm
Structural proteins:				
Large polymerase	L (>160 kDa)	L (160–200 kDa)	L (>160 kDa)	L (160–200 kDa)
Attachment	HN (65–74 kDa)	H (76–85 kDa)	HN (65–74 kDa)	G (84–90 kDa)
Fusion	F0 (60–68 kDa)	F0 (60–62 kDa)	F0 (60–68 kDa)	F0 (66–70 kDa)
	F1 (48–59 kDa)	F1 (40–41 kDa)	F1 (48–59 kDa)	F1 (43–50 kDa)
	F2 (10–15 kDa)	F2 (20–25 kDa)	F2 (10–15 kDa)	F2 (19–24 kDa)
Nucleocapsid	N (56–61 kDa)	N (60 kDa)	N (56–61 kDa)	N (44 kDa)
Matrix	M (34–41 kDa)	M (34–38 kDa)	M (34–41 kDa)	M (27–33 kDa)
Phosphoprotein	P (44–84 kDa)	P (70–73 kDa)	P (44–84 kDa)	P (31–34 kDa)
Other transmembrane			SH (5 kDa)[a]	SH (13–40 kDa)
Nonstructural/other	C,C',V,Y1,Y2,D,W,I,X	C,V	C,V,W,I	NS1,NS2,M2

[a]Identified in some members of the genus only.

1.3 Morphology

Virus particles are generally spherical, with lipid envelopes derived from the plasma membrane of the host cell (Klenk and Choppin 1969, 1970). The lipid envelope surrounds the viral RNA genome, which is in the form of a protein–RNA nucleocapsid. Virus particles range from 150 to 400 nm in diameter and are generally round, but both pleomorphic and filamentous forms are frequently observed. The size and shape of the viral nucleocapsids are major morphological features that are used to distinguish the subfamily *Paramyxovirinae* from the *Pneumovirinae*. *Paramyxovirinae* nucleocapsids measure 18 nm in diameter, with a pitch of about 5.5 nm and a length of 1 μm. *Pneumovirinae* nucleocapsids are more slender, 13–14 nm in diameter with a pitch of 6.5–7.0 nm (Compans and Choppin 1967a, 1967b, Finch and Gibbs 1970). Paramyxoviruses contain 2 transmembrane glycoproteins that appear as spikes measuring 8–15 nm protruding from the viral envelope.

1.4 Chemical properties

The genomes of all paramyxoviruses are composed of single-stranded RNA with a density of c. 1.3 g/cm³. Protein comprises most of the virion composition by weight (69–74%). Paramyxoviruses are bounded by a lipid membrane derived from the host cell plasma membranes from which the viruses bud. Lipid makes up 20–25% of the weight of the viruses. The density of the virus particles is 1.18–1.20 g/cm³. Carbohydrate comprises 5–6% of the virion weight and is also host cell-dependent. Fusion activity is ubiquitous among the paramyxoviruses, whereas neuraminidase activity is associated with the *Paramyxovirus* and *Rubulavirus* genera. The infectious nature of the viruses is destroyed by reagents that disrupt lipids, such as organic solvents and detergents, as well as formaldehyde and oxidizing agents. The viruses are also inactivated by ultraviolet light, heating and drying.

1.5 Genome structure and function

The superfamily *Mononegavirales* is composed of the families *Paramyxoviridae*, *Rhabdoviridae* and *Filoviridae*. All members have a common genome structure that consists of a single strand of non-segmented, negative-sense RNA contained within a helical nucleocapsid formed by a head-to-tail assemblage of nucleoprotein. Viruses within the family *Paramyxoviridae* possess genomes of c. 15 000–16 000 nucleotides (nt) in length. Galinski and Wechsler (1991) listed the complete nucleotide sequences of a number of members of the family, including human parainfluenza virus 3 (HPIV-3), Sendai virus, mumps and SV5 viruses, measles and canine distemper morbilliviruses, and respiratory syncytial virus (RSV). The gene order of 3′ *NP–P–M–F–(SH)–HN–L* 5′ is highly conserved among the *Paramyxo-, Rubula-* and *Morbillivirus* genera (Fig. 23.1). The viral genomes contain 6 or 7 genes, with a phosphoprotein (*P*) gene encoding at least 2, and in some cases more than 6, different proteins. The newest addition to the *Morbillivirus* genus is equine morbillivirus (EMV) (Hyatt and Selleck 1996). EMV, unlike other morbilliviruses, has an unusual trailer sequence between the *P* and *M* genes with a short open reading frame (ORF). In addition, the long trailer at the 3′ end of *M* and the leader region at the 5′ end of *F* observed in some morbilliviruses is absent in the EMV genome (Gould 1996). Future studies will determine whether EMV will remain classified as a morbillivirus.

In contrast, the prototype of the pneumoviruses, RSV, contains 10 genes with distinguishing features relative to the other 3 genera (Fig. 23.1). The *L* gene overlaps the *M2* gene by 68 nt, i.e. transcripts of *L* message begin within the *M2* gene (formerly 22K), 68 nt upstream of the end of the *M2* gene (Elango et al. 1989). Although this overlap has also been described for bovine RSV, neither pneumonia virus of mice (PVM) (Compans and Choppin 1967a) nor turkey rhinotracheitis virus (TRTV) contains the overlapping sequences (Ling, Easton and Pringle 1992, Yu et al. 1992). Two genes encoding the non-structural proteins NS1 and NS2 precede the *N* gene, and a third (*NS3* or *1A* or *SH*) occurs between the *M* and *G* genes. The *M2* gene follows the *F* gene. Note that the order of the RSV glycoprotein genes, *G* and *F*, is switched with respect to the other genera. Whereas PVM has the same gene order as RSV, the gene order of TRTV differs in that the *SH–G* and *F–M2* gene pairs are inverted (Ling, Easton and Pringle 1992).

The genomes of member viruses of all 4 genera contain a 3′ leader region 40–50 nt in length that includes the promoter for the transcription of positive-sense mRNA. Within this region, the 3′ terminal 12–13 nt are highly conserved. The 5′ end of the genome contains an extragenic trailer region that includes the complement of the promoter for synthesis of the negative strand. There is complementarity between the 3′ and 5′ terminal sequences. It is speculated that base pairing of the termini may form a 'panhandle' structure that is recognized by the polymerase.

The genomes of members of the subfamilies *Paramyxovirinae* and *Pneumovirinae* contain nucleotide sequences at the start and end of each gene as well as between each gene (intergenic) that are more or less conserved. Depicted in Table 23.3 are examples of these transcriptional regulatory or 'punctuation' sequences for each of the 4 genera. In general, gene start regions are more guanosine- and cytosine-rich than the gene termination regions. The latter regions are very rich in adenosine and uridine and, without fail, end in a variable number of U residues. These regions are involved in transcript termination and in initiating the addition of the poly(A) tails that are present at the ends of all viral transcripts. The intergenic boundaries or junctions of the rubulaviruses and pneumoviruses are extremely variable in length and nucleotide sequence. In contrast, the morbilliviruses and paramyxoviruses have intergenic regions precisely 3 nt in length, made up predominantly of purine residues, and highly conserved in nucleotide sequence (Table 23.3). In general, the morbilliviruses contain long stretches of nucleotides between the termination of the matrix gene ORFs and the translational start of the fusion proteins. The function, if any, of these non-translated regions remains unknown.

1.6 Replication

ATTACHMENT AND PENETRATION

Attachment of virus particles to the host cell membranes occurs through the HN, H or glycoprotein (GP) depending on which genus is considered. Viruses in the *Paramyxovirus* and *Rubulavirus* genera bind sialic acid containing proteins or lipids, or both, on the cell surface. In contrast, the protein nature of the measles virus receptor has been known for some time (Krah 1991). A membrane co-factor protein, CD46, has been identified as a receptor for measles by several groups (Dorig et al. 1993, Naniche et al. 1993). Similar protein receptors have not been identified for any of the other morbilliviruses, and the nature of the pneumovirus receptor also remains unknown.

Following attachment to the cell surface, the F protein mediates fusion of the viral envelope with the plasma membrane. In all paramyxoviruses, F protein is synthesized as an F0 precursor molecule. The precursor protein is proteolytically cleaved to a large F1 subunit, yielding a new hydrophobic amino terminus (fusion peptide) and a smaller F2 subunit that remains linked to the F1 subunit by disulphide bonds. The fusion process occurs at neutral pH and is potentiated by the HN or H proteins. It is now widely

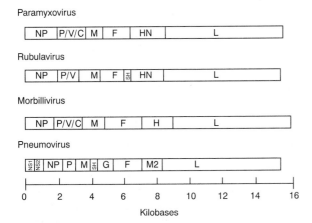

Fig. 23.1 Schematic diagrams of the respective gene orders of the 4 genera comprising the family *Paramyxoviridae*. All genomes are displayed 3′ to 5′ negative sense from left to right.

Table 23.3 Intergenic junction sequences and transcription signals (3′ to 5′ negative sense)

Virus	Gene	Gene start	Junction	Gene end
Paramyxovirus (Sendai)	NP	UCCCAGUUUC	GAA	CAUUCUUUUU
	P	UCCCACUUUC	GAA	AAUUCUUUUU
	M	UCCCACUUUC	GAA	UAUUCUUUUU
	F	UCCCUAUUUC	GAA	UAUUCUUUUU
	HN	UCCA-CUUUC	GGG	AAUUCUUUUU
	L	UCCCACUUAC	GAA	CAUUCUUUUU
Rubulavirus (mumps)	NP	UUCGGUCCUUCACC		UCAGAAAUUCUUUUUU
	P	UCCGGGCCUUUCUU	AA	GGAUAAUUUAUUUUUU
	M	UUCGUGCUUGUGUU	A	CUUUAAUAUCUUUUUU
	F	UUCGGAUCUUCCUA	A	UUUCUAAAUCUUUUUUU
	SH	UUCUUACUUAGAGG	GAUUUUA	UCUGUAUUUCUUUUUU
	HN	UUCGGUCUUGUCUG	CG	CUAAUAAUUCUUUUUU
	L	UCCGGUCUUACCGC	G	AAAAUUCUUUUUU
Morbillivirus (measles)	N	UCCUAAGUUCU	GAA	AAUAUUUUU
	P	UCCUUGGUCCA	GAA	AAUAUUUUU
	M	UCCUCGUUUCA	GAA	UUUGUUUU
	F	UCCCGGUUCC	GAA	UUAAUUUU
	H	UCCCACGUUCU	GAA	AUUCUUUUU
	L	UCCCAGGUUCA	GCA	UUUCUUU
Pneumovirus (RSV)	NS1	CCCCGUUUA		UC(A/C)(A/U)UNNNUUUU
	NS2	CCCCGUUUA	19N	UC(A/C)(A/U)UNNNUUUU
	N	CCCCGUUUA	26N	UC(A/C)(A/U)UNNNUUUU
	P	CCCCGUUUA	1N	UC(A/C)(A/U)UNNNUUUU
	M	CCCCGUUUA	9N	UC(A/C)(A/U)UNNNUUUU
	SH	CCCCGUUUA	9N	UC(A/C)(A/U)UNNNUUUU
	G	CCCCGUUUA	44N	UC(A/C)(A/U)UNNNUUUU
	F	CCCCGUUUA	52N	UC(A/C)(A/U)UNNNUUUU
	M2	CCCCGUUUA	46N	UCAAUAAAUUUU[a]
	L	CCCUGUUUA	[a]	UCAAUAAUUUU

[a] 5′ end of L mRNA overlaps 3′ end of M2 mRNA by 68 nucleotides.
N, any nucleotide.

accepted that, for cell membrane and viral membrane fusion to occur, the *Paramyxovirinae*, with the exception of SV5, require the co-expression of HN (H) and the F protein. It is postulated that a conformational change in the HN (H) molecule occurs after receptor interaction. This change triggers a conformational alteration in F, leading to exposure or release of the fusion peptide. Concomitant with membrane fusion, virus nucleocapsids are released into the cytoplasm (Lamb 1993).

PRIMARY TRANSCRIPTION AND REPLICATION

Replication of the paramyxoviruses seems to occur exclusively in the cytoplasm of infected cells. Primary transcription begins immediately after release of the viral nucleocapsids into the cytoplasm. The required polymerase complex decorates the newly introduced nucleocapsid, and the polymerase molecules, made up of the L and P proteins, enter from the 3′ end of the genomic RNA to produce one positive-sense mRNA (complementary to virion RNA) for each gene (with the exception of the *P* gene; see 'Phosphoproteins', p. 440). The single promoter region contained within the 3′ leader RNA sequence provides the initial entry point to the genome for the RNA-dependent RNA

polymerase. Transcriptional control regions dictate the start and end of each gene, and the resultant monocistronic mRNAs are capped at the 5′ end and polyadenylated at the 3′ end by the polymerase complex. As noted in section 1.5 (p. 436), the genes of all paramyxoviruses are arranged in a single linear sequence. Transcription proceeds with the polymerase stopping and reinitiating mRNA synthesis at each gene junction as it moves down the entire length of the genome; reinitiation process is that the abundance of each mRNA is proportional to its proximity to the 3′ end of the genome. Reinitiation at each subsequent gene junction is less efficient than the previous. Thus, regulation of viral gene expression is achieved by the establishment of this message gradient. The translation of primary transcripts leads to an accumulation of viral proteins, and a switch from transcription to antigenome synthesis. To serve as the template for more negative-sense viral RNA, the full-length antigenomes must be encapsidated in their entirety with the nucleoprotein (NP). In the presence of sufficient NP, the polymerase initiates at the same place as when performing transcription, but now it ignores all transcriptional regulatory signals and synthesizes a precise complementary copy of the negative-strand viral genome. Subsequent synthesis of antigenome and genome depends on the continued availability of the N protein. Synthesis of genomic RNA is initiated from a promoter located on the 3′ untranslated region of the antigenome. Nearly equivalent amounts of encapsidated genomic and antigenomic RNA can be found in infected cells and varying amounts of antigenomic RNA are packaged in virions. The phosphoproteins (P) form non-covalently linked complexes with the N proteins. On the basis of studies of VSV, these complexes are thought to keep the N protein soluble at high concentrations and accessible for assembly into nucleocapsids (Blumberg, Leppert and Kolakofsky 1981).

The replication of representative viruses from 2 different genera, Sendai virus and measles virus, is governed by the 'rule of six'. This surprising finding was discovered when studying defective interfering (DI) genome replication using expressed L, P and NP proteins. Calain and Roux (1993) had achieved the synthesis in vitro of a naturally occurring DI genome of Sendai virus. The system used cDNA copies of the genome, and attempts to manipulate the template led to shortening or lengthening of the genome by a few nucleotides. These genomes replicated very inefficiently, but were encapsidated. It was found that, when the total length of the genome was modified to a perfect multiple of 6, efficient replication returned. It is postulated that the NP protein covers precisely 6 nt when binding to the RNA (Egelman et al. 1989). Thus, beginning at the 5′ end of the genome the NP protein would bind in usual fashion, but if the rule of six were violated, binding of NP at the 3′ end would be disturbed. It is further postulated that the RNA polymerase might have difficulty recognizing the promoter at that imperfect 3′ end, adversely influencing the efficiency of replication. Similar results have been reported for measles genomes as well. In contrast, RSV does not seem to be governed by this rule (Samal and Collins 1996).

Virus assembly

The assembly of virus particles requires cessation of genome replication and preparation of completed nucleocapsids for packaging, and preparation of regions of the plasma membrane to accept nucleocapsids for budding. In the latter stages of genome replication, complete ribonucleoprotein (RNP) structures are formed from the pool of NP protein. These structures must also have polymerase complexes (L-P proteins) associated with them to initiate the next round of infection (Kingsbury, Hsu and Murti 1978). The M protein of vesicular stomatitis virus (VSV) inhibits RNP transcription (Carroll and Wagner 1979). Although never demonstrated, the M proteins of the paramyxoviruses are assumed to have similar functions.

Regions of plasma membrane that accept nucleocapsids and become sites for virus budding contain the fully processed and glycosylated HN (H or G) and activated F protein. For some time now, it has been assumed that the matrix (M) proteins of the *Para-*

myxoviridae associate with the cytoplasmic portions of the glycoproteins. In turn, other regions of the M protein are believed to interact with the nucleocapsids, forming the preferred budding site. This region somehow becomes devoid of cellular membrane proteins. The final assembly process of packaging and bud formation remains poorly understood. Paramyxovirus particles are pleomorphic and the sizes range from 150 to 200 nm. The helical nucleocapsid structure is surrounded by a membrane of host cell origin. The viral glycoproteins extend from the surface of the membrane, forming spikes that are visible by electron microscopy. Virions have haemagglutinating, haemolytic and neuraminidase activities.

Polypeptides: non-structural and structural

Nucleoproteins

The gene coding for the NP is nearest to the 3′ end of the genomes of the *Paramyxovirinae*. The complete nucleotide sequences and predicted amino acid sequences of many of the paramyxoviruses have been described (Collins et al. 1985, Rozenblatt et al. 1985, Galinski et al. 1986b, Ishida et al. 1986, Jambou et al. 1986, Sanchez et al. 1986, Sakai et al. 1987, Elango 1989b, Kondo et al. 1990, Yuasa et al. 1990, J Barr et al. 1991, Kamata et al. 1991, Lyn et al. 1991, Matsuoka and Ray 1991, Neubert, Eckerskom and Homann 1991, Tsurudome et al. 1991, Parks, Ward and Lamb 1992). The NP plays a pivotal role in several aspects of virus replication and assembly. Both genome and antigenome must be encapsidated by NP to serve as template for transcription or replication. The association with NP makes the encapsidated RNA resistant to treatment with RNAse. Of note is the fact that protease treatment of the nucleocapsids of measles, SV5 and Sendai viruses did not alter this resistance (Kingsbury and Darlington 1968). Trypsin treatment removes the carboxyl terminal 15–20 kDa, leaving the 45–48 kDa fragment associated with RNA. The C terminal regions of most of the *Paramyxovirinae* are the most poorly conserved; however, most are highly negatively charged (Hsu and Kingsbury 1982, Curran et al. 1993) and are highly phosphorylated (Mountcastle et al. 1974, Ryan, Portner and Murti 1993). Despite the non-essential nature of the C termini of NP in encapsidation, nucleocapsids assembled from C terminal-deleted NP do not serve as templates for replication (Dreyfuss et al. 1993). The NP interacts in some way with the polymerase complex, as well as with the matrix protein during virion assembly. Finally, the relative rates of transcription and replication, and perhaps the switch between transcription and replication, may be governed by the concentration of unassociated NP in the cytoplasm.

NP proteins range in size from about 391 to 557 amino acids (43.5–61 kDa; see Table 23.2), and these are the most abundant viral proteins in infected cells and virions. Within each genus there is 30–60% amino acid sequence conservation, but only 17–21% homology among the genera. Despite the close association of NP with RNA, classic RNA-binding motifs are absent from the predicted amino acid sequences examined (Dreyfuss et al. 1993).

Members of the subfamily *Pneumovirinae* contain the smallest of the NPs. Whereas PMV and RSV NPs cross-react antigenically, the amino acid sequences of this group have little similarity with the *Paramyxovirinae*. Several semi-conserved regions between the subfamilies have been described (J Barr et al. 1991).

Phosphoproteins

Members of the subfamily *Paramyxovirinae* have evolved unique mechanisms to maximize the available nucleotide sequences in these genes without expanding the overall genome size. This diversity includes translational choice that involves ribosomes initiating in separate places in the same reading frame or in several different reading frames, or at codons not usually associated with protein starts. Secondly, transcriptional diversity is generated by a mechanism first described as RNA editing but also referred to as pseudotemplated addition of nucleotides. By this mechanism, non-templated nucleotides (G residues) are placed precisely into mRNAs co-transcriptionally, thus diversifying transcripts and their products. The functions of the myriad proteins produced are mostly unknown at present. In contrast, members of the subfamily *Pneumovirinae* encode only a P protein from the cognate gene, thus defining a major difference between the subfamilies.

All encode a phosphoprotein (P), although the strategy for expression of this protein varies among the genera. Viruses belonging to the subfamily *Paramyxovirinae* (with the exception of HPIV1) express the P/C gene through RNA 'editing' in which non-templated G residues are inserted into the mRNA transcript by the viral polymerase (Paterson and Lamb 1990, Park and Krystal 1992). This insertion of one or more bases changes the reading frame of the mRNA, allowing the expression of alternate, downstream ORFs as chimaeric proteins. The editing site is highly conserved among all of the viruses in the *Morbillivirus*, *Paramyxovirus* and *Rubulavirus* genera. The paramyxoviruses, morbilliviruses, pneumoviruses and the rubulavirus Newcastle disease virus express the P protein from an unedited mRNA, whereas the chimaeric protein, V, which contains the amino terminal region of the P protein joined to the cysteine-rich V ORF, is coded for on a transcript containing a single G insertion. In the other rubulaviruses, the unedited transcript codes for the V protein, and P protein is expressed from an edited message containing a 2 G insertion.

The P proteins vary in size, pneumoviruses being the smallest (241 amino acids in length). Those of the rubulaviruses vary from 245 to 397 amino acid residues, and those of the paramyxoviruses and morbilliviruses range from 507 to 603 amino acid residues. The P proteins play a central role in RNA synthesis: P proteins are components of viral polymerase complexes, and are believed to serve as scaffolding or chaperone proteins binding both the NP and the L proteins. The P protein genes are the most variable

of the paramyxovirus genes, only 22–40% amino acid homology being observed between each genus. The predicted amino acid sequences of a great number of P proteins have been reported (Giorgi, Blumberg and Kolakofsky 1983, Barrett, Shrimpton and Russell 1985, Bellini et al. 1985, Galinski et al. 1986a, Shioda, Iwasaki and Shibuta 1986, Spriggs and Collins 1986, Spriggs et al. 1986, Varsanyi et al. 1987, McGinnes, McQuain and Morrison 1988, Thomas, Lamb and Paterson 1988, Cattaneo et al. 1989, Elango, Kovamees and Norrby 1989, Matsuoka et al. 1991, Berg et al. 1992, Takeuchi et al. 1988).

The P proteins seem to possess 2 distinct domains based on sequence conservation. The N termini seem to contain most of the sites for phosphorylation (threonine and serine) and regions of acidic residues (Deshpande and Portner 1985, Vidal et al. 1988). The first 78 amino acids of Sendai virus P protein contain domains that are required for RNA synthesis and encapsidation (Curran, Pelet and Kolakofsky 1994). Domains that interact with the L protein and provide the binding with NP have been localized to the C terminus of Sendai virus (Ryan and Portner 1990, Curran, Boeck and Kolakofsky 1991, Ryan, Morgan and Portner 1991, Boeck et al. 1992).

C proteins

Only the paramyxoviruses and morbilliviruses express C or C-related proteins, or both. The 180–204 amino acid residue C proteins carry a net positive charge and are expressed from a second ORF (+1 with respect to P) which overlaps the P gene (Giorgi, Blumberg and Kolakofsky 1983, Bellini et al. 1985). The protein termination signal of the C protein mRNA occurs upstream of the editing site, and therefore the expression of C is unaffected by editing. The C-related proteins, C', Y1 and Y2, are predicted to be generated via alternative protein start sites on the C ORF in some members of the paramyxoviruses (Sendai and HPIV1 viruses) (Curran, Pelet and Kolakofsky 1994). It is interesting that several of the start sites identified vary from the usual AUG initiator methionine codons. For example, ACG and GUG have been identified as initiating codons for C-related proteins (Curran and Kolakofsky 1988, Gupta and Patwardhan 1988, Boeck et al. 1992). Sendai virus C protein is found in small amounts in virions, associated with nucleocapsids (Lamb and Paterson 1991). RNA transcription and genome replication do not require the C protein, but the C protein inhibits transcription of Sendai virus in vitro (Curran, Marq and Kolakofsky 1992).

V proteins and other P gene-encoded proteins

Most rubulaviruses express the V protein from unedited transcripts (Thomas, Lamb and Paterson 1988). The V proteins of the paramyxo- and morbilliviruses require the pseudotemplated addition of a single G residue to switch from the N terminal P to C terminal V ORF. Thus, V proteins of the latter 2 genera are fusion proteins containing a negatively charged and phosphorylated N terminus (P protein N terminus) and a relatively short, cysteine-rich C terminus. In contrast, rubulavirus V proteins generally have a basic N terminus. This difference might be involved in the localization of rubulavirus V protein in virions, as opposed to localization in the cytoplasm (Thomas, Lamb and Paterson 1988, Takeuchi et al. 1990). In contrast to the relatively non-conserved nature of P protein sequences, the V-specific regions are among the most highly conserved. V proteins contain zinc-binding domains, and somehow inhibit genome replication in a dose-dependent fashion (Curran, Boeck and Kolakofsky 1991). This function, however, is independent of the cysteine-rich domain, because the W protein demonstrated similar activity.

Editing has also been predicted to generate the mRNA coding for the D protein in HPIV and BPIV and the W and I proteins in Sendai and rubulaviruses. The predicted D, W and I proteins have not always been found in infected cells, and their functions are unknown.

Matrix (M) proteins

Every member of the family *Paramyxoviridae* encodes a matrix or membrane protein. As noted earlier, the matrix (M) proteins are the most likely candidates for proteins that might interact with lipids, the cytoplasmic tails of the glycoproteins (Sanderson, Wu and Nayak 1993) and the newly formed nucleocapsids (Stricker, Mottet and Roux 1994, Yoshida et al. 1991) in preparation for budding (Peeples 1991). The M proteins vary between 341 and 375 amino acid residues in length, are non-glycosylated, and almost exclusively are basic proteins having net positive charges of +14 to +17 at neutral pH (Blumberg et al. 1984, Hidaka et al. 1984, Satake and Venkatesan 1984, Bellini et al. 1986, Galinski et al. 1987, Sakai et al. 1987, Elango 1989a, Kawano et al. 1990a, Limo and Yilma 1990, Sheshberadaran and Lamb 1990, Sharma et al. 1992). Although M proteins are hydrophobic in nature, none contains sufficient consecutive stretches of hydrophobic amino acids to span the plasma membrane. Thus, it is believed that these proteins interact with the inner surfaces of the virion lipid envelope and plasma membrane.

Persistent infections with Sendai virus (Roux and Waldvogel 1982) and in the measles-associated neurological disease subacute sclerosing panencephalitis (SSPE) (Cattaneo et al. 1987a, 1987b 1988a, 1988b) have been ascribed to the failure of M proteins to interact with one or more of the previously mentioned components. These findings underscore the central role of the M protein in virus budding.

A second M protein is encoded by the pneumovirus genome. The M2 protein (22K) is smaller than the M protein and lacks any sequence identity with the M proteins of members of the *Paramyxovirinae*. The RSV M2 protein is 194 amino acids in length, lacks a sufficient stretch of hydrophobic amino acids to span the plasma membrane, and is unglycosylated. Both the M and the M2 proteins remain virion-associated when the lipid envelope of the virus is removed with non-ionic detergents. Both are removed by high concentrations of salt. Co-localization studies indicate that the

M2 associates with the P and N proteins of RSV, and forms complexes with the N protein in immunoprecipitation studies (Huang, Collins and Wertz 1985). Similar results have been reported for bovine respiratory syncytial virus (Rima et al. 1995).

Recently, the M2 protein of RSV has been assigned a role in transcription elongation. During attempts to replicate a 'minigenome' of RSV, co-expression of N, P and L proteins was found to be required. The greater part of mRNA synthesis under these conditions resulted in premature mRNA termination. Co-expression of small quantities of the M2 protein with the N, P and L proteins was associated with successful mRNA elongation and correct termination (Collins et al. 1995).

Glycoproteins

Haemagglutinin/neuraminidase (HN)

The HN glycoproteins of the paramyxoviruses and rubulaviruses employ sialic acid-containing cell surface molecules as receptors. As is the case with all attachment proteins of paramyxoviruses, the HN proteins possess a type II transmembrane glycoprotein orientation in the plasma membrane. Such proteins have their NH_2 termini extending into the cytoplasm from the inner surface of the plasma membrane and the C termini extending from the outer surface of the plasma membrane into the extracellular milieu. The general structure is illustrated in Fig. 23.2a. The predicted amino acid sequences of many HN proteins have been reported, the proteins ranging in size from 565 to 582 amino acids in length (Markwell and Fox 1980, Blumberg et al. 1985b, Hiebert, Paterson and Lamb 1985, Millar, Chambers and Emmerson 1986, Suzu et al. 1987, Waxham et al. 1988, Kovamees, Norrby and Elango 1989, Kawano et al. 1990b, Sundqvist, Berg and Moreno 1992). These integral membrane proteins have between 3 and 6 potential sites for addition of *N*-linked carbohydrate residues.

The HN is also responsible for the ability of the viruses to bind erythrocytes. The neuraminidase activity cleaves sialic acid residues from budding virion to prevent self-aggregation. The HN of paramyxoviruses contains conserved cysteine, proline and glycine residues, suggesting that the protein structure must be conserved. The general structure of the HN contains a cytoplasmic domain, a membrane-spanning region, a stalk region and a globular head. The membrane distal globular head region contains the sialic acid-binding site. The functional HNs seem to be composed of disulphide-linked homodimers that interact to form a non-covalently associated tetramer (Markwell and Fox 1980, Thompson et al. 1988, Ng, Randall and Lamb 1989, Morrison et al. 1990, Russell, Paterson and Lamb 1994).

Paramyxoviruses contain a conserved amino acid sequence (Asn–Arg–Lys–Ser–Lys–Ser), similar to the sialic acid-binding site of influenza virus neuraminidase (Morrison and Portner 1991). Although it would seem logical that the sialic acid-binding site would also be responsible for agglutination activity, *ts* mutant and

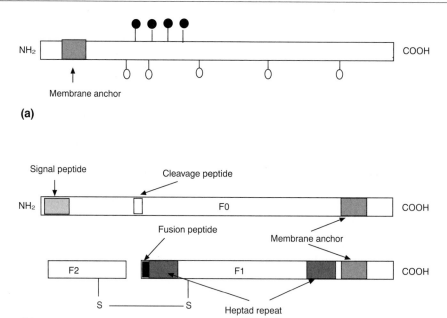

(a)

(b)

Fig. 23.2 Schematic diagrams depicting the most salient features of the attachment protein and fusion protein of the family *Paramyxoviridae*. (**a**) Idealized HN or H attachment type II glycoprotein. The stop transfer or membrane anchor sequences are shown near the amino-terminal end of the molecule. The lollipop structures in black along the top of the diagram display the clustering of *N*-linked glycosylation sites observed in the H genes of many morbilliviruses, and the open structures display the more general distribution observed for the HN proteins. The G proteins (not shown) share the same orientation in membrane, contain both *N*-linked and *O*-linked glycosylation sites, and are about one-half the size of either HN or H. (**b**) The fusion (F) type I glycoprotein. The uncleaved form of F, F0, is shown with a signal peptide at the NH₂ terminus, which permits entry into the Golgi endoplasmic reticular lumen for membrane-associated protein synthesis. The cleavage peptide, made up of one or more basic residues, is indicated by the open box. Finally, the membrane anchor sequence at the COOH terminus is depicted. Also shown is the cleaved form of F0. composed of F1 and F2 peptides. Note creation of a new NH₂ terminus on F1 containing the fusion peptide. Regions of F1 containing heptad repeats for the *Paramyxovirinae* subfamily are also clearly labelled. The F protein contains *N*-linked sugar residues primarily on the F2 molecule, but often on the F1 as well. The F1 and F2 subunits are covalently linked via a single disulphide bond.

monoclonal antibody studies suggest 2 separate sites for these activities (Portner et al. 1975, Portner 1981).

Recent studies have shown that the HN protein participates in fusion, as the ability of the F protein to fuse membranes is greatly enhanced in the presence of the homologous HN. It is believed that HN positions the membrane in the optimal place for access by the fusion peptide and/or causes a conformational change in F that allows fusion to occur.

Haemagglutinin

The receptor-binding molecule of the morbilliviruses is the haemagglutinin (H) protein. This surface glycoprotein is orientated in plasma membranes in the same way as the HN glycoproteins, but lacks neuraminidase activity. Although bacterial and viral sialidases destroyed the receptors of the HN proteins, the morbillivirus receptor(s) were resistant to this treatment (Howe and Lee 1972). Measles is the only morbillivirus for which a cell surface protein receptor (CD46) has been identified (Dorig et al. 1993, Naniche et al. 1993). This protein has been found on virtually every tissue in humans with the exception of erythrocytes, whereas primates have a CD46 homologue that is present on erythrocytes. These findings are consistent with the ability to use primate red cells for measles haemagglutinin assays, whereas human red cells do not agglutinate with measles virus.

The predicted amino acid sequence of most H proteins of the morbilliviruses has been determined from nucleic acid sequences (Curran, Clarke and Rima 1991, Alkhatib and Briedis 1986, Gerald et al. 1986, Tsukiyama et al. 1987, Kovamees, Blixenkrone-Møller and Norrby 1991, Curran et al. 1992, Blixenkrone-Møller et al. 1996). The H proteins of the morbilliviruses are larger than the HN proteins of parainfluenza virus and are 604–617 amino acids in length. The molecules are glycosylated with *N*-linked oligosaccharides only. The H proteins of vaccine strains of measles virus contain 5 potential glycosylation sites, but only the first 4 seem to be used (Hu et al. 1994). The glycosylation sites are more or less confined to the amino-terminal half of the protein (except for phocid and canine distemper viruses), that portion closest to the plasma membrane. There is conservation in the relative positions of 11–13 cysteine residues among the morbilliviruses. Like the HN proteins, H protein is believed to be a disulphide-linked homodimer. The H protein is highly antigenic, and antibody raised to the H protein neutralizes virus infection (Albrecht, Hermann and Bums 1981).

G proteins

The pneumovirus G proteins have little in common with HN or H proteins, apart from their type II glycoprotein configuration and attachment property. G proteins are about half the size of HN and H proteins, and have several other distinguishing features. The pneumovirus G proteins lack neuraminidase activity, and RSV G lacks haemagglutinating activity as well. In contrast, PVM has haemagglutinating activity (Harter and Choppin 1967). The major distinguishing feature of the pneumovirus G proteins is the abundance of *O*-linked sugar residues. *O*-linked glycosylation occurs at serine or threonine residues, which comprise 30% of the amino acid residues on RSV G protein (Wertz, Kreiger and Ball 1989, Collins and Mottet 1992). In addition, there are a variable number of potential sites for *N*-linked glycosylation. The predicted amino acid sequence of the RSV G protein is 298 amino acids with a predicted molecular mass of 32.587 kDa (Wertz et al. 1985, Satake et al. 1995). Thus, the apparent molecular weight in sodium dodecylsulphate-polyacrylamide gel electrophoresis (SDS-PAGE) of 90 kDa is due to carbohydrate addition. There are sufficient antigenic differences in RSV G proteins such that 2 groups, A and B, have been defined (Anderson et al. 1985).

N-linked glycosylation seems to occur co-translationally and is a requirement for the proper folding of the G proteins, as with HN and H. *O*-linked oligosaccharides are added after the folding is completed. In contrast, G proteins are not disulphide-linked dimers, but probably exist as non-covalently linked trimers or tetramers (Wertz, Kreiger and Ball 1989, Collins and Mottet 1992). Finally, about 15% of the total RSV G protein synthesized in the infected cell is secreted as a soluble form (Hendricks, McIntosh and Patterson 1988). It is interesting that the truncations occur post-translationally at the NH$_2$ termini and thus the molecules lack the cytoplasmic and membrane-spanning domains. It is speculated that the soluble G might interfere with the immune response to RSV infection, because antibody to the G protein is neutralizing and soluble G may bind the antibody first, allowing infection to go unchecked.

Fusion (F) proteins

All the paramyxoviruses contain a fusion (F) protein. F proteins are much more highly conserved than the attachment proteins. All are type I integral membrane glycoproteins that are initially synthesized in an inactive, F0, form (Fig. 23.2b). They all contain a signal sequence at the NH$_2$ terminus that is cleaved when the molecule is delivered to the endoplasmic reticular membrane for completion of synthesis. Likewise, all F proteins contain a hydrophobic domain (known as a stop transfer signal) at the C terminus that anchors the protein in the membrane (von Heijne 1981). A short cytoplasmic tail of between 20 and 40 amino acid residues in length extends into the cytoplasm. Among members of the *Paramyxovirinae*, F proteins contain 2 heptad repeats. Heptad repeat A occurs adjacent to the fusion peptide and may be involved in the confor-

mational alteration of this peptide that enhances fusion (Chambers, Pringle and Easton 1990). Heptad repeat B is located adjacent to an amino terminal of the transmembrane region. As such repeats can form triple-stranded coiled structures, this region might be important in supporting the F protein structure as a homotrimer (Pauling and Corey 1953, Buckland et al. 1992, Russell, Paterson and Lamb 1994).

Cleavage of F0 by intracellular or secreted host endoproteases creates 2 disulphide-linked subunits, F1 and F2. The efficiency of cleavage affects the host range and tissue tropism of the virus with greater cleavage efficiency generally associated with disseminated infections and increased virulence. The F1 subunit contains the amino-terminal fusion peptide and the carboxyl-terminal membrane anchor and cytoplasmic domain. The fusion peptide, which is highly conserved among the *Paramyxovirinae*, mediates the fusion of the viral envelope to the plasma membrane of the host cell. There is less conservation in the fusion peptide among the members of the subfamily *Pneumovirinae*, but hardly any exists between the member viruses of these 2 subfamilies (Table 23.4). Of note, however, is the consistent placement of glycine residues at position 3, 7 and 12 in the fusion peptide of the *Paramyxovirinae*, and 3 and 7 in the *Pneumovirinae*. These residues are known to greatly influence the fusion potential of the F1 peptide (Server et al. 1985, Horvath and Lamb 1992). Predicted amino acid sequences for the F protein have been deduced from nucleotide sequences for many of the paramyxoviruses (Paterson, Harris and Lamb 1984, Blumberg et al. 1985a, Elango et al. 1985, Chambers, Millar and Emmerson 1986, McGinnes and Morrison 1986, Richardson et al. 1986, Shioda, Iwasaki and Shibuta 1986, Spriggs et al. 1986, Suzu et al. 1987, Waxham et al. 1987, Kawano et al. 1990c, Visser et al. 1993).

The F protein cleavage sites contain either a single or multiple basic amino acids (Table 23.4). Viruses that contain a multibasic sequence are cleaved in the trans-Golgi network by a protease with the sequence specificity of R–X–K/R–R. An endoprotease, furin, has been identified as one protease having such properties (PJ Barr 1991, Hosaka et al. 1991, Ortmann et al. 1994). Cleavage sites containing a single basic residue are believed to be cleaved by proteases expressed at the cell surface. Several candidate proteases have been identified (Scheid and Choppin 1974, Gotoh et al. 1992). Of relevance to the tentative placement of EMV in the *Morbillivirus* genus (Gould 1996, Hyatt and Selleck 1996), the EMV cleavage site is most consistent with that of the paramyxoviruses, and its F1 fusion protein is the only one that begins with leucine instead of phenylalanine (Table 23.4).

Although regions of extensive amino acid homology are not obvious among the genera, there is similarity in the number and location of cysteine residues and the placement of glycine and proline residues, suggesting similar folded structures (Morrison and Portner 1991). Morbillivirus F proteins contain sites for the addition of *N*-linked sugars on the F2 peptide

Table 23.4 Fusion (F) protein cleavage sites and F1 termini of members of the family *Paramyxoviridae*

Paramyxoviruses		
HIPV-1	D–N–P–Q–S–R	F–F–G–A–V–I–G–T–I–A–L–G–V–A–T–A–A–Q–I–T
HPIV-3	D–P–R–T–K–R	F–F–G–G–V–I–G–T–I–A–L–G–V–A–T–S–A–Q–I–T
Sendai	G–V–P–Q–S–R	F–F–G–A–V–I–G–T–I–A–L–G–V–A–T–S–A–Q–I–T
Rubulaviruses		
Mumps	S–R–R–H–K–R	F–A–G–I–A–I–G–I–A–A–L–G–V–A–T–A–A–Q–V–T
SV5	T–R–R–R–R–R	F–A–G–V–V–I–G–L–A–A–L–G–V–A–T–A–A–Q–V–T
Morbilliviruses		
Measles	S–R–R–H–K–R	F–A–G–V–V–L–A–G–A–A–L–G–V–A–T–A–A–Q–I–T
CDV	S–R–R–K–K–R	F–A–G–V–V–L–A–G–A–A–L–G–V–A–T–A–A–Q–I–T
RPV	S–R–R–H–K–R	F–A–G–V–A–L–A–G–A–A–L–G–V–A–T–A–A–Q–I–T
EMV	L–V–G–D–V–K	L–A–G–V–V–M–A–G–I–A–I–G–I–A–T–A–A–Q–I–T
Pneumoviruses		
RSV	K–K–R–K–R–R	F–L–G–F–L–L–G–V–G–S–A–I–A–S–G–V–A–V–S–K
BRSV	K–K–R–K–R–R	F–L–G–F–L–L–G–I–G–S–A–I–A–S–G–V–A–G–S–K
PVM	K–R–K–K–R	F–L–G–L–I–L–G–L–G–A–A–V–T–A–G–V–A–L–A–K
	---------------	NH₂----3-----------7-------------12----------------
	Cleavage peptide	Fusion peptide

The amino acid sequence of the cleavage site for each virus group is underlined. The new amino-terminus is marked with NH$_2$ and glycines at positions 3, 7 and 12 are marked.

only. The other genera contain between 3 and 6 of these sites distributed between the F2 and F1 peptides.

L (polymerase component) protein

The gene closest to the 5′ end of the genome of members of *Paramyxoviridae* and the least abundant protein is the viral RNA-dependent RNA polymerase or large (L) nucleocapsid-associated protein. The large size of the protein (2200–2300 amino acids) is believed to be necessary for the many enzymatic and binding functions ascribed to this protein. The L protein or modified versions (L–P complexes) catalyse the synthesis of both positive- and negative-strand genome and mRNA. Thus, acceptor sites for all 4 nucleoside triphosphates, and P protein and nucleocapsids are necessary. Moreover, L catalyses the synthesis of capped and polyadenylated viral mRNA, as well as methylation. Whether L is involved in kinase and phosphorylating activities remains uncertain. The protein accounts for 40–50% of the coding capacity of the viral genome. Among the many L gene sequences available (Morgan and Rakestraw 1986, Yusoff et al. 1987, Blumberg et al. 1988, Galinski, Mink and Pons 1988, Kawano et al. 1991, Stec, Hill and Collins 1991, Higuchi et al. 1992, Okazaki et al. 1992, Parks, Ward and Lamb 1992, Sidhu et al. 1993), little information has been gleaned that would relate structure with function. As observed with other proteins, the greatest similarity lies within a genus, but significant similarities are shared among the genera. Four or 5 short regions of conserved amino acid sequence have been observed in the first half of the L protein. These regions range in size from 20 to 136 amino acids (Galinski and Wechsler 1991). Now that infectious clones of several of the *Paramyxoviridae* have been produced, progress toward understanding the structural and functional domains of the L proteins should be rapid.

Non-structural and other proteins

The gene encoding the SH proteins of SV5 and mumps virus lies between the F and HN genes. The SH protein is a small hydrophobic protein and seems to have no counterpart in the subfamily *Paramyxovirinae*. The SH protein of SV5 is 44 amino acids in length, and seems to be able to span the lipid membrane once. The hydrophilic NH$_2$ terminus is membrane associated whereas the carboxy-terminal end extends extracellularly from the plasma membrane by about 5 amino acids (Phillips 1954, Hiebert, Paterson and Lamb 1988).

The SH of mumps virus is somewhat larger, with a total of 57 amino acids. There is an analogous stretch of 25 hydrophobic amino acids, but on the mumps SH protein they reside within the N terminal portion of the protein (Elango et al. 1989). There is no sequence similarity between the 2 proteins and no known function has been described.

The SH gene of RSV is located between the M and G genes, and encodes a small integral membrane protein that is glycosylated, the SH protein (Collins, Chanock and McIntosh 1996). The protein contains 64 amino acid residues with an internal hydrophobic sequence capable of spanning the plasma membrane once. The membrane orientation of the SH protein is that of a type II integral membrane protein, consistent with the presence of a COOH terminal glycosylation site (Collins and Mottet 1993). At least 4 forms of the RSV SH protein have been identified. The predicted monomer is 7.5 kDa. Two other forms seem to be glycosylated: one of 13–15 kDa that contains one high mannose N-linked oligosaccharide chain, and a second of 21–30 kDa that is generated by the addition of polylactosaminoglycan to the N-linked carbohydrate chain. A smaller species of 4.8 kDa is believed to be the result of the initiation of protein synthesis at an internal AUG codon (Olmsted and Collins 1989, Anderson et al. 1992). The SH protein (or proteins) participates with the F protein in cell fusion but other functions have not been defined.

The RSV genome encodes 2 non-structural proteins, NS1 and NS2. The genes encoding these proteins lie just downstream of the leader sequence and upstream of the NP gene. This location necessarily leads to high copy numbers of both NS protein mRNAs and proteins. NS1 contains 139 amino acid residues and seems to decrease in molecular size during pulse-chase experiments (Huang, Collins and Wertz 1985). NS2 is 124 amino acid residues in length, has a short intracellular half-life, seems to increase in molecular size and is secreted (Collins, Chanock and McIntosh 1996). The function of these proteins is unknown, but they do not seem to be present in virions.

STRAIN VARIATION

Multiple strains of many paramyxoviruses and rubulaviruses have been compared using sequence analysis and monoclonal antibody binding patterns. Both HPIV-1 and HPIV-4 have been separated into 2 groups on the basis of reactivity with monoclonal antibodies. Sequence analysis of HPIV-1 and HPIV-3 has demonstrated the existence of multiple co-circulating lineages of virus. The lineages are stable over time and regionally distributed. There is no evidence for progressive evolution as seen with influenza A viruses. The number of nucleotide substitutions between wild type isolates of HPIV-1 or HPIV-3 is relatively low and the HN genes of these viruses differ by no more than 5.4%.

A similar evolutionary pattern has been observed on the basis of sequence analysis of the SH gene of mumps virus isolated in Europe and Japan. At least 6 co-circulating lineages have been identified, which also seem to be geographically restricted.

Multiple genotypes have been described for both group A and group B of RSV. The genotypes have a worldwide distribution. Viruses from the same genotype have been isolated from simultaneous outbreaks in various parts of the world. During seasonal outbreaks, multiple genotypes of both group A and B may co-circulate in the same area although the prevalence of each genotype varies from year to year (Cane and Pringle 1995).

Several distinct genotypes of measles virus have recently been identified (Rima et al. 1995, Rota, Rota and Bellini 1995, Rota et al. 1996). These genotypes seem to be stable for long periods. Although the degree of geographic restriction varies for each genotype, multiple genotypes of virus have been identified in many regions. Molecular epidemiological studies have been able to identify transmission pathways of measles virus and have recently documented the interruption of transmission of indigenous measles in the USA (Rota et al. 1996). Antigenic variation has been described for some wild type measles viruses, but all of these strains were neutralized by vaccine-induced antibody (Tamin et al. 1994).

2 CLINICAL AND PATHOLOGICAL ASPECTS: INFECTIONS OF HUMANS

This section discusses human parainfluenza, mumps, measles and respiratory syncytial viruses.

2.1 Human parainfluenza viruses

CLINICAL MANIFESTATIONS

Each of the human parainfluenza viruses – 1 (HPIV-1), 2 (HPIV-2), 3 (HPIV-3) and 4 (HPIV-4) – can cause various upper (URTI) and lower (LRTI) respiratory tract illnesses but the pattern of illness for each is different. HPIV-1 is most commonly associated with croup; HPIV-2 is also often associated with croup; HPIV-3 is second only to RSV as a cause of pneumonia and bronchiolitis in infants and young children (Glezen et al. 1971, Denny and Clyde 1986); and HPIV-4 has less often been detected in patients, presumably because it causes less severe illness (Rubin, Quennec and McDonald 1993). HPIV infection and illness is most commonly detected in infants and children, and illness associated with HPIV-3 occurs earlier than that associated with HPIV-1, 2 or 4 (Glezen et al. 1971, Centers for Disease Control 1978, Denny and Clyde 1986). Infections with HPIV have been associated with 2–10% of cases of URTI, 25–50% of cases of croup and 5–20% of cases of pneumonia and bronchiolitis (Glezen et al. 1971, Denny and Clyde 1986, Henrickson, Kuhn and Savatski 1994), but rarely with meningitis (Arisoy et al. 1993). Reinfection can occur throughout life, the elderly and the immunodeficient patient being at greatest risk of serious complications of infection in adults (Centers for Disease Control 1978, Glezen et al. 1984, Apalsch et al. 1995).

EPIDEMIOLOGY

Infections with HPIV usually occur during seasonal community outbreaks (Fig. 23.3) (Glezen et al. 1984, Knott, Long and Hall 1994). Outbreaks of HPIV-1 usually occur in the autumn every other year; in the USA over the last 20 years, they have occurred in odd-numbered years. Outbreaks of HPIV-2 infection have been detected in the autumn of every year in the USA, but in any given community can occur every other year. HPIV-3 is often detected throughout the year, with peaks in the spring. Patterns of HPIV-4 infections have not been well studied. Parainfluenza viruses spread efficiently and, by 5 years of age, virtually all children have serological evidence of past infection with HPIV-3, 75% with HPIV-1, 60% with HPIV-2 and 50% with HPIV-4 (Kilgore and Dowdle 1970, CE Hall et al. 1971). Infection and disease can recur throughout life despite the presence of neutralizing antibody. HPIV-1 and 3 can be important nosocomial pathogens in both children and adults (Centers for Disease Control 1978, Karron et al. 1993).

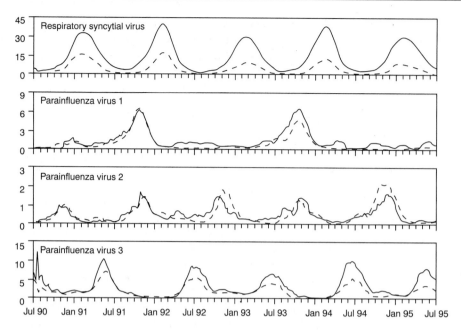

Fig. 23.3 Percentage of specimens that were positive (7-week running mean) by week and virus type, USA, July 1990 through June 1995. Solid lines indicate results of rapid antigen detection testing and dashed lines indicate isolations. (Data from the National Respiratory and Enteric Virus Surveillance System, CDC.)

PATHOLOGY AND PATHOGENESIS

Human PIVs are found in respiratory secretions and probably spread in a fashion similar to that of RSV (i.e. by large-particle aerosol, direct contact, fomites). They are stable for hours, but not days, in the environment (Brady, Evans and Cuartas 1990). Illness begins 1–7 days after infection and probably results from a combination of cytopathic effect of the virus and the immune or inflammatory response (or both) to infection (Chanock, Bell and Parrott 1961). Virus is usually shed for 3–10 days. With second infections, virus is shed for a shorter period, although in immunosuppressed patients it can be shed for prolonged periods.

IMMUNITY

Infection with HPIVs induces the production of IgA, IgG and IgM antibodies. The presence of serum neutralizing antibodies correlates with decreased risk of, but does not preclude, infection and disease (Chanock, Bell and Parrott 1961, Glezen et al. 1984). The cellular immune response to HPIV infections has not been well studied but is probably important in clearing infection. Both cytotoxic and lymphoproliferative responses have been detected in humans (Welliver, Sun and Rinaldo 1985, Slobod and Allan 1993).

DIAGNOSIS

Infection can be demonstrated by detection of the virus, viral antigens or genome, a diagnostic rise in virus-specific antibodies, or the presence of IgM antibodies. Critical to sensitivity of these assays is collection of well timed, appropriate specimens. For isolation and antigen detection, a nasopharyngeal aspirate or wash collected within 3–4 days after onset of illness is best (Downham, McQuillin and Gardner 1974). To detect a diagnostic rise in antibodies, the acute-phase serum specimen should be collected within a week of onset of illness and the convalescent-

phase specimen ≥2 weeks later. The paramyxoviruses have often been isolated in primary monkey kidney cells or human embryonic kidney cells. Several continuous cell lines supplemented with trypsin have also been used successfully; they include LLC-MK2 and, more recently, NCI-H292 cells (Castells, George and Hierholzer 1990). A number of enzyme-linked immunoassays (EIAs), immunofluorescent assays (IFAs), and reverse transcriptase polymerase chain reaction (RT-PCR) assays have been developed and give results similar to those for viral isolation (Downham, McQuillin and Gardner 1974, Sarkkinen, Halonen and Salmi 1981, Karron et al. 1994). Monoclonal antibodies are often used in IFAs and EIAs to detect HPIV antigens. Neutralization, complement fixation, haemagglutination inhibition and EIA-based assays have been used to detect antibodies. Infection with one HPIV can induce antibodies that cross-react with other HPIVs and mumps virus, and vice versa, especially with second infections.

PROPHYLAXIS AND TREATMENT

No antiviral chemotherapy is approved for use in the treatment of HPIV infections, and in most instances only supportive therapy is needed. Ribavirin has been used to treat immunodeficient patients with severe complications of infection. Live HPIV-3 vaccines are being developed and tested in clinical trials (Karron et al. 1995).

2.2 Mumps virus

CLINICAL MANIFESTATIONS

Before widespread vaccination, mumps was a common infection of childhood, peak incidence in the USA occurring in school-aged children. It is a systemic infection, the most characteristic clinical feature being parotitis. Onset of illness usually occurs 2–3 weeks after infection and begins with systemic symptoms, such as fever, myalgia and malaise, followed by parotitis. Parotitis is usually bilateral and diffuse, and resolves within 10 days after onset. About 30% of infections present with no symptoms of parotitis.

Some involvement of the meninges, as manifested by cerebrospinal fluid (CSF) pleocytosis, is common. Before large-scale vaccination programmes, mumps was the most commonly reported cause of viral encephalitis. Encephalitis, however, is an uncommon manifestation of infection and usually does not lead to significant sequelae (Pieper and Kurland 1958). Orchitis has been noted in as many as 25% of postpubertal males infected with the virus and oophoritis in 5% of females (Werner 1950). Testicular atrophy can occur but sterility is unusual. The high frequency with which virus can be isolated from urine suggests that renal involvement is common (Utz, Houk and Alling 1964). Some patients develop mild proteinuria and decreased glomerular filtration rates. Mumps has also been associated with ECG abnormalities indicating cardiac involvement (Bengtsson and Orndahl 1954), and in one study >4% of patients had some hearing loss after infection (Vuori, Lahikainen and Peltonen 1962).

EPIDEMIOLOGY

Before vaccination programmes, the epidemiology of mumps varied by population density. Large urban centres sustained endemic transmission and 80% or more of residents would be infected during childhood (Wesselhoeft and Walcott 1943). In remote areas, mumps would occur as periodic outbreaks every 2–7 years, and as few as 10–20% of the population might have serological evidence of past infection. In temperate climates in the northern hemisphere, the peak season for infection is winter and spring. Licensing of a safe and effective vaccine in 1967 and state immunization laws have effectively controlled mumps in the USA. Reported cases have decreased from over 150 000 cases in 1968 to a minimum of 1692 cases in 1993 (Centers for Disease Control and Prevention 1995). At present, in the USA, cases occur in both vaccinated and unvaccinated people, the cases in vaccinated people resulting from both primary and secondary vaccine failures (Briss et al. 1994, Centers for Disease Control and Prevention 1995). The institution of a second dose of measles, mumps and rubella vaccine in response to the resurgence of measles in 1989 probably contributed to the low number of mumps cases in 1993.

PATHOLOGY AND PATHOGENESIS

Mumps is a systemic virus infection and the associated disease reflects which tissues are infected. The virus is present in respiratory secretions and presumably spreads in a fashion similar to RSV (i.e. large-particle aerosol or droplet, direct contact, fomites). Illness usually begins 2–3 weeks after infection, with virus present in the respiratory tract 5–6 days before onset and 5–6 days after onset of illness (Henle et al. 1948). Virus can also be isolated from the blood and urine. A variety of other tissues can be infected, including the parotid gland, meninges, kidneys, pancreas and myocardium. Involved tissues manifest a local inflammatory response to the infection, and damage and disease presumably result from both the cytopathic effect of the virus and the inflammatory response to infection.

IMMUNITY

Infection with mumps virus, including live virus vaccines, induces IgA, IgG and IgM antibodies, cellular immunity and long-term protection from disease. Both cytotoxic T cells and lymphoproliferative responses (McFarland et al. 1980) have been detected after mumps infection. Reinfection can occur and is sometimes symptomatic (Briss et al. 1994, Gut et al. 1995).

DIAGNOSIS

Infection is usually demonstrated by isolating virus, demonstrating a diagnostic rise in specific antibodies or detecting specific IgM antibodies. Presumably, viral antigens could also be detected by IFA or EIA. Virus is most often isolated from respiratory secretions or the urine (5–6 days before and up to 12 days after onset of disease). Virus can also be isolated from CSF. A variety of cell lines, including primary monkey kidney cells, human embryonic kidney cells, HEp-2 cells, HeLa cells and human fibroblast cells, can be used to isolate mumps virus. Primary monkey kidney and human embryonic kidney cells give the best results. Because cytopathic effect is not consistently present, infection is most reliably detected by haemadsorption, using chicken, guinea-pig or human group O erythrocytes. A diagnostic rise in antibodies can be demonstrated in an acute-phase serum specimen collected at the onset of illness and a convalescent-phase serum specimen collected 2–3 weeks later. Various tests, including haemagglutination inhibition, complement fixation, neutralization and EIA, have been used to detect mumps antibodies. Cross-reacting antibodies induced by HPIVs can give false-positive results. IgM antibodies are usually present by 3 days after onset of illness and can persist for 3 or more months (Gut et al. 1985).

PROPHYLAXIS AND TREATMENT

Safe and effective live virus vaccines, such as that derived from Jeryl Lynn strain, have made it possible to prevent most mumps infections. Live virus vaccines induce an antibody response in over 90% of recipients that persists long term. As noted in the section 'Epidemiology' (see above), vaccination has proved very effective in controlling mumps in the USA (Centers for Disease Control and Prevention 1995). A killed virus vaccine developed in the 1960s was not effective. Although mumps can be a nosocomial pathogen, high rates of vaccination have markedly decreased the risk of nosocomial transmission.

2.3 Measles virus

CLINICAL MANIFESTATIONS

Measles has a very distinctive clinical presentation except when modified by actively or passively acquired prior immunity. Without prior immunity, people typically develop prodromal symptoms of fever, cough, coryza and conjunctivitis 10–14 days after exposure to measles. Adults sometimes have incubation periods as long as 21 days. Toward the end of the 2–3 day prodromal period, Koplik's spots (a white spot, 1–3 mm ($\pm$ 1 mm) on an erythematous base on the buccal mucosa) appear and are pathognomonic for measles. The end of the prodromal phase is heralded by the development of a maculopapular rash that typically begins on the neck and spreads to the rest of the body. The rash can become confluent, especially on the upper body, begins to fade 4 or more days later, and may desquamate. Common complications of infection include bronchitis, pneumonia, otitis media and diarrhoea. In one study, 50% of cases had X-ray evidence of a pulmonary infiltrate, and in another outbreak 1 in 150 patients with measles was hospitalized with pneumonia (Cherry et al. 1972). Measles-associated pneumonia can be caused by the virus or by bacterial superinfection. Otitis media has been reported in 5–15% of cases. Mortality in measles outbreaks has varied considerably from <0.5% to >25%, probable contributory factors including very young age, older age, lack of prior exposure to measles in the population and malnutrition. Measles during pregnancy, especially during the first trimester, often leads to fetal death. Patients with compromised immune systems can have difficulty controlling infection and are subject to serious complications, such as giant cell pneumonia.

Measles commonly involves the central nervous system (CNS), with as many as 50% of cases reported to have ECG abnormalities during the acute or convalescent phase of the illness (Gibbs et al. 1959). Clinical encephalitis manifested by convulsions, lethargy, irritability and possibly coma is reported in 0.5–1.0 cases, 5–30% progressing to death and 20–40% of survivors having residual deficits (LaBoccetta and Tornay 1964, Centers for Disease Control 1981). The encephalitis usually develops after the onset of rash (peak incidence at 6 days after onset of rash) and the risk may be greater when infection occurs after the age of 10 years (Greenberg, Pelliterri and Eisenstein 1955). The occurrence of encephalitis after the onset of rash and the difficulty in detecting virus in CSF or brain tissue raise the possibility that the patient's immune response contributes to the disease process.

SSPE is a late neurological complication that occurs in 0.6–2.2 per 100 000 measles cases and is uniformly fatal (Modlin et al. 1977). The risk is greater with measles infection at an earlier age. The average time from measles to SSPE is 7 years. SSPE begins insidiously with behaviour problems, decrease in motor and intellectual capabilities and convulsions. The disease progresses over 6–9 months to decorticate rigidity and death. Measles virus from brains of SSPE patients is defective in its ability to replicate (Katz and Koprowski 1973). The virus is difficult to recover, requiring cocultivation or brain explant techniques, yet measles proteins and RNA can readily be detected in brain tissue (Katz and Koprowski 1973, Liebert et al. 1986). Defective interfering particles and changes in M, F and H proteins have been identified, but it is not known which, if any, of these factors might be responsible for defective replication or for pathogenesis (WW Hall and Choppin 1979, Liebert et al. 1986, Cattaneo et al. 1988a, Sidhu et al. 1994). Changes in the M protein have generated considerable interest. The M protein often has extensive genetic changes, the amount of the M protein and antibodies against it are reduced, and the function of the M protein from some isolates in vitro is altered.

Infection can also occur in vaccinated people and result in classic measles, atypical measles, 'mild measles' or asymptomatic infection (Chen et al. 1990). Atypical measles occurred in recipients of a formalin-inactivated vaccine used in the 1960s (Brodsky 1972). In atypical measles, fever is often higher and prolonged, the rash often has vesicular or haemorrhagic features and starts peripherally rather than centrally, and pneumonitis is more common. Classic measles (generalized maculopapular rash lasting $\geq$3 days, fever $\geq$38.3°C, and cough, coryza or conjunctivitis) in recipients of live virus vaccines is thought to occur most often in people who fail to mount a primary response to vaccine, but sometimes from secondary vaccine failure, i.e. waning immunity (Atkinson and Orenstein 1992). Mild measles and asymptomatic infections may be common in outbreaks in vaccinated populations.

EPIDEMIOLOGY

In unvaccinated populations, measles causes periodic epidemics, with interepidemic periods varying between 2 and 5 years (Bartlett 1957, Griffiths 1973). The interval between epidemics decreases as the size and density of the population increases. In communities of less than 250 000–500 000 people, measles probably does not persist during interepidemic periods and is reintroduced to the local population for each outbreak. Measles is transmitted by aerosol very efficiently and can infect nearly all of a highly susceptible population over the course of an outbreak (Christensen et al. 1952). In communities that can support endemic measles, most members will have evidence of measles infection by the time they reach adulthood, the peak age at infection depending on types of contacts children have in the community. In communities where preschool children have limited contacts outside the household, most infections occur during the elementary school years. In communities where preschool children have more contacts outside the household, the peak age of cases may be <4 years. The infant <6 months of age is usually protected by maternal antibody.

In vaccinated populations, the interval between measles outbreaks increases and sufficiently high levels of vaccination can interrupt endemic transmission. With vaccination, the age distribution of cases is determined by which groups are likely to lack vaccine- or measles-induced immunity. In the USA, an extensive effort to achieve high levels of measles vaccination with a second dose of vaccine in school-aged children has resulted in a decrease in reported measles cases from 400 000–500 000 per year in the 1960s to a record minimum of 301 cases in 1995 (Centers for Disease Control 1989, Centers for Disease Control and Prevention 1996) (Fig. 23.4). During 1995, the greatest number of cases occurred in children <5 years of age (36%) and adults ≥20 years of age (32%). It is likely that endemic transmission of measles in the USA was interrupted in 1993, and subsequent cases have occurred via periodic introduction of measles from other countries, followed by limited spread (Cubie et al. 1995, JS Rota et al. 1996). Given widespread international travel, measles will continue to occur even in highly vaccinated populations until global eradication is achieved.

PATHOLOGY AND PATHOGENESIS

Measles virus infects via the respiratory tract, presumably by aerosol transmission, though close contact and fomites may also be involved. The virus establishes infection in the upper and lower respiratory tract and then spreads to local lymphoid tissue and disseminates throughout the body in a cell-associated viraemia (Esolen et al. 1993). A wide range of tissues are infected, including the skin, conjunctiva, kidney, lung, gastrointestinal tract, liver, vascular endothelium and brain. Infection in these tissues is not always clinically evident. During the prodromal period, virus is present in tears, respiratory secretions and urine. Endothelial cells, epithelial cells, monocytes and macrophages are the most common cell types infected (Kempe and Fulginiti 1965, Moench et al. 1988, Esolen et al. 1993). As discussed earlier (p. 442), CD46 or membrane co-factor protein has been identified as a cellular receptor for measles virus. Tissue infection is marked by giant cells with intranuclear and intracytoplasmic

inclusions. Histopathological studies of the rash and Koplik's spots show giant cells and a perivascular mononuclear cell infiltrate (Denton 1925).

IMMUNE RESPONSE

An IgM antibody response to natural measles becomes evident at the onset of rash or within 2–3 days thereafter. Measles-specific IgG and IgA antibodies can be detected a few days after the IgM antibodies. The IgM antibodies are short lived, whereas IgG antibodies persist long term, probably throughout life. IgA antibodies can be detected in as many as 25% of people with no evidence of recent infection. Antibodies to the N protein develop first and to the highest levels, followed by antibodies to H, F and M proteins (Graves et al. 1984). The fact that maternal antibody protects the newborn and passively administered antibody protects exposed people demonstrates that antibody can protect from acquisition of disease. Recovery from measles, on the other hand, seems to rely heavily on the cellular immune response. People with defects in cellular immunity often develop progressive disease, whereas those with selective hypogammaglobulinaemia recover (Burnet 1968). Both CD4 and CD8 T cells responsive to measles antigens are induced by infection. It seems that the early cellular response is associated with the production of cytokines suggestive of a type 1 response, whereas the cellular response after rash is associated with the production of cytokines suggestive of a type 2 response (Griffin and Ward 1993). Inactivated measles vaccines that were associated with atypical measles induced a delayed type hypersensitivity response to measles (suggestive of a type 1 T cell response) not seen with live virus infection and lower titres of antibody to the F protein (Griffin, Ward and Esolen 1994).

Natural measles and live measles vaccination are associated with transient defects of the immune response. During infection, delayed hypersensitivity responses, such as the tuberculin skin test and antibody and cellular responses to new antigens, are

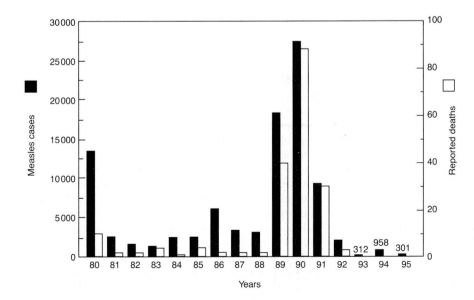

Fig. 23.4 Reported cases of measles and measles-associated deaths in the USA by year from 1980 to 1995.

impaired. The immunosuppression associated with measles probably increases the risk of secondary infections, which are important contributors to measles morbidity and mortality (Beckford, Kaschula and Stephen 1985).

DIAGNOSIS

The clinical presentation of 'classic measles', characterized by fever and rash with coryza, cough or conjunctivitis and Koplik's spots, has traditionally been sufficient to diagnose infection. However, in vaccinated populations, many healthcare providers will not have seen measles and are less likely to make the diagnosis. Moreover, infection in vaccinated people may be mild or asymptomatic. Consequently, good laboratory diagnostic tests are essential to identify measles in vaccinated populations.

A capture antibody assay for measles IgM antibodies has excellent sensitivity and specificity for diagnosing acute measles (Erdman et al. 1991) and usually requires collection of only one blood specimen. The IgM antibodies are present in c. 70% of people at rash onset, nearly 100% 3–4 days later, and begin to disappear 4–5 weeks after the onset of rash. IgM assays that do not use the antibody capture method may give false-positive or false-negative results. A variety of tests, including neutralizing, haemagglutination inhibiting, complement fixing and binding antibody assays, can be used to diagnose acute infection by detecting seroconversion or a significant rise in measles antibodies. The acute-phase serum specimen should be obtained as soon as possible after onset of rash (i.e. within 3–4 days) and the convalescent-phase serum specimen 3–4 weeks later.

Virus can also be isolated, or viral RNA, antigens or histological changes can be detected in respiratory tract secretions, urine, peripheral blood mononuclear cells or other affected tissues. An Epstein–Barr virus-transformed marmoset lymphocyte cell (B95-8) line has markedly improved isolation rates for measles virus (Kobune, Sakata and Suguira 1990). PCR assays have proved useful in detecting and sequencing virus from urine specimens (PA Rota et al. 1995). Measles-specific monoclonal antibodies have given good results in indirect immunofluorescence assays on respiratory tract specimens.

PREVENTION AND TREATMENT

The key to measles prevention is vaccination. Live measles virus vaccines are sufficiently safe and efficacious (90–95% efficacy after one dose and nearly 100% efficacy after 2 doses) to consider the possibility of global eradication (Hopkins et al. 1982). The fact that endemic transmission has been stopped in a number of countries, including the USA, Finland and several countries in Central and South America, suggests that global eradication of measles is possible (Peltola et al. 1994, de Quadros et al. 1996). The resurgence of measles in the USA in 1989–1991, however, demonstrated that 2 doses of vaccine are probably needed to achieve eradication (Centers for Disease Control 1989, Atkinson and Orenstein 1992).

Normal human immunoglobulin can be used to prevent disease in exposed people and, if indicated, it should be given as soon as possible after exposure (Centers for Disease Control 1989). There is no proven effective antiviral therapy, but ribavirin has been used to treat pneumonitis and subacute encephalitis (Mustafa et al. 1993, Forni, Schluger and Roberts 1994).

2.4   Respiratory syncytial virus

CLINICAL MANIFESTATIONS

RSV is the single most important cause of serious respiratory tract disease in infants and young children world-wide. The characteristic feature of RSV infection is bronchiolitis, but the most common manifestation of infection is a moderately severe URTI, with signs such as rhinorrhoea, cough and fever. In the infant and young child, asymptomatic infection is uncommon and 30–50% of infected children have physical signs of LRTI (wheezing, rales, rhonchi) (Kapikian et al. 1961, Glezen et al. 1986). Otitis media is also often present with RSV infections. Lower respiratory tract symptoms usually occur 1–3 days after onset of illness. About 1% of healthy children who become infected with RSV progress and develop tachypnoea, become hypoxaemic and require hospitalization with either bronchiolitis or pneumonia. The chest x-ray may show evidence of air trapping, interstitial pneumonitis or both. The very young or premature infant may present with lethargy and apnoeic spells and few respiratory tract symptoms (CB Hall et al. 1979). RSV has been detected in a few cases of sudden infant death.

RSV causes repeated infections throughout life which can result in LRTI and death even in adults (Henderson et al. 1979, Hall et al. 1991, Falsey et al. 1995). The risk of serious complications of infection is greatly increased in children with compromised cardiac or pulmonary function and in people of any age with compromised immune function (MacDonald et al. 1982, Hall et al. 1986, Groothuis, Gutierrez and Lauer 1988). Outbreaks of RSV disease in patients after bone marrow transplantation have been reported, with mortality rates >50% (Harrington et al. 1992).

EPIDEMIOLOGY

RSV is found in all parts of the world and causes yearly outbreaks in winter months in temperate climates. In the USA, outbreaks occur each year between November and April, the peak month varying between communities (see Fig. 23.3) (Gilchrist et al. 1994). Outbreaks in a community last for 2–7 months. The fact that during the same year many strains of RSV can circulate in the same community and different strains in other communities demonstrates that RSV outbreaks affect individual communities rather than whole regions or countries (LJ Anderson et al. 1991). RSV outbreaks are associated with an increase in hospitalization of children for bronchiolitis and pneumonia and in deaths from LRTI, the peak age for serious disease being 2–6 months (Brandt et al. 1973, LJ

Anderson, Parker and Strikas 1990). During outbreaks, RSV may be responsible for over 50% of the infants and young children to be admitted to hospital for LRTI. Rates of hospitalization seem to increase with male gender, urbanization and lower socioeconomic status.

The virus spreads efficiently and infects c. 50% of infants during their first year and nearly all by their second year of life. The risk of transmission is especially high in settings where close contact is common, such as households, hospitals and daycare centres. Nearly 50% of RSV-exposed family members, including adults, were found to be infected in one study, and rates of nosocomial transmission to patients and staff can be similarly high (Hall et al. 1975, 1976). Nosocomial transmission is of particular concern to patients who, because of an underlying disease, are at increased risk for serious complications of infection.

PATHOLOGY AND PATHOGENESIS

RSV establishes infection in the upper respiratory tract and probably progresses to the lower respiratory tract through cell-to-cell spread or aspirated secretions. Infection and disease seem to be limited to the respiratory tract, except in severely immunocompromised patients. Autopsy studies of children who died with RSV bronchiolitis show necrosis of bronchiolar epithelium and ciliated epithelial cells, peribronchiolar leucocytic infiltration and oedema, and cellular and mucus plugs blocking air passages (Aherne et al. 1970). These changes probably cause serious obstruction in the small airways of the young infant. Lungs of children who died of RSV pneumonia show changes in the bronchioles with necrosis of lung tissue, leucocytic infiltration of the alveolar walls, and cells, fibrin and fluid within alveoli. Many patients have an intermediate picture between pneumonia and bronchiolitis. Some strains are more virulent than others (Hall et al. 1990).

The pathogenesis of RSV bronchiolitis and its ability to cause severe disease in the presence of passively or actively acquired neutralizing antibodies is not understood. Some investigators have suggested that the virus or virus antigen–antibody complexes, possibly via virus-specific IgE, lead to the production of leukotrienes, histamine or other mediators of inflammation that cause bronchoconstriction.

The enhancement of RSV infection in children previously vaccinated with a formalin-inactivated vaccine clearly demonstrates the potential for the host immune response to contribute to disease (LJ Anderson and Heilman 1995). However, it is not known what, if any, aspects of vaccine-induced enhanced disease might be comparable to natural disease. Animal studies indicate that enhanced disease may be caused by induction of Th2-like memory T cells by the formalin-inactivated vaccine (Graham et al. 1993). In contrast, animal and human studies suggest that live RSV infection induces predominantly Th1-like memory T cells (Graham et al. 1993, LJ Anderson et al. 1994).

IMMUNE RESPONSE

RSV induces IgG, IgA and IgM antibodies. Humans mount an antibody response to several RSV proteins (Popow-Kraupp et al. 1989, Erdman and Anderson 1990). The F and G proteins induce neutralizing antibodies, the F protein inducing the highest titres of neutralizing antibodies and highest level of protection from challenge (Johnson et al. 1987). The F protein induces antibodies that react broadly against different strains, whereas the G protein induces antibodies that tend to be group or strain specific (Johnson et al. 1987, Cane et al. 1996). In humans and animals, passively administered neutralizing antibodies are protective when present in sufficiently high titre (Groothuis et al. 1993). Even high titres of neutralizing antibodies and natural infection, however, do not always protect. Cytotoxic T cells and antibody-dependent cellular cytotoxic and lymphoproliferative responses to RSV have been found in animals and humans. The cellular immune response seems to be particularly important for clearing infection, as illustrated by disease in humans and studies in animals (Graham et al. 1991, Harrington et al. 1992).

The fact that repeated naturally acquired infections do not prevent reinfection and only partially protect from disease underscores the difficulty in inducing a protective immune response to RSV.

DIAGNOSIS

Infection can be demonstrated by detection of the virus, viral antigens or genome, a diagnostic rise in specific antibodies, or presence of IgM antibodies. Critical to the sensitivity of these assays is the collection and correct handling of well timed, appropriate specimens. For isolation and antigen detection, nasopharyngeal aspirate or wash specimens provide much better sensitivity than swab specimens. These specimens should be collected within 3–4 days after onset of illness and, for isolation or RNA detection, handled with care to maintain the integrity of the virus. Infants may excrete virus for up to 3 weeks. In adults, the titre of virus is lower and detection more difficult. Several tissue culture systems, including HEp-2 cells, primary monkey kidney cells and human diploid fibroblast cells, have been used to isolate RSV. The ability to isolate RSV can vary between passages of the same cell line. Antigen detection is now commonly used to diagnose infection. A number of EIAs, IFAs and other assays have been developed that give results similar to those for isolation (Kellogg 1991). Most assays will detect RSV infection in 70–95% of isolation-positive patients as well as in some infected isolation-negative patients. PCR assays seem to be more sensitive than isolation or antigen detection (Freymuth et al. 1995). Antibodies against the virus and viral proteins have been measured effectively by a variety of assays, including complement fixation, neutralization and EIA. EIAs for IgG antibodies are the most sensitive. In older children and adults, 60–95% of isolation- or antigen-positive patients will develop a ≥4-fold rise in antibodies between acute- and convalescent-phase serum specimens. The infant <6 months old does not reliably mount a good antibody response to RSV. IgM and IgA antibodies can be detected, though IgA antibodies have not been helpful in diagnosing RSV infections (Erdman and Anderson 1990). Differences in antibody responses to the G protein can sometimes be used to distinguish between group A and B infections.

PREVENTION AND TREATMENT

Since RSV was discovered in the 1950s, a safe and effective vaccine has been sought, but so far unsuccessfully. The first attempt, a formalin-inactivated vaccine, caused enhanced disease and live attenuated candidate vaccine strains have been over- or under-attenuated (Anderson and Heilman 1995). Suitable attenuated strains are being sought. The recent development of an RSV infectious clone may provide the means to achieve this (Collins et al. 1995). Several groups are working on subunit vaccines, but progress has been hampered by concern over the possibility of enhanced disease.

Other measures are, however, effective in preventing RSV disease. RSV can be a serious nosocomial pathogen, and nosocomial transmission can, and should, be prevented. Compliance with contact isolation precautions, such as strict attention to good hand-washing practices, can prevent nosocomial transmission (Tablan et al. 1994). RSV intravenous immunoglobulin has been effective in decreasing both hospitalization and the days in intensive care among young children at risk for serious complications of infection (Groothuis et al. 1993). It was recently licensed in the USA for RSV prophylaxis in premature children and children with bronchopulmonary dysplasia. Ribavirin therapy may be indicated for some patients with, or at risk of, serious complications (American Academy of Pediatrics 1996).

3   CLINICAL AND PATHOLOGICAL ASPECTS: PARAMYXOVIRUS INFECTIONS OF BIRDS AND ANIMALS

This section includes discussion of Newcastle disease and other avian paramyxoviruses, bovine parainfluenza 3 and RSV, rinderpest, canine distemper and equine and aquatic morbillivirus infections.

3.1   Newcastle disease virus

CLINICAL MANIFESTATIONS OF INFECTION

Newcastle disease virus (NDV), also called avian paramyxovirus 1, causes epidemic disease in a wide range of domesticated and wild birds, most notably among poultry (Alexander 1995). It has been isolated from all orders of birds. The incubation period averages 5–6 days, with a range of 2–15 days. The type and severity of disease varies by infecting strain and age and with species of infected bird. For example, younger chickens are subject to more severe disease than older chickens. Although there is a continuum of clinical presentations, isolates have been separated arbitrarily into 4 groups based on the presence of enteric or neural disease and the speed with which they kill embryonating hens' eggs. All strains reduce egg production in chickens.

Lentogenic strains are associated with no or mild respiratory tract symptoms, and some have been developed into live virus vaccines. Young birds are most likely to develop illness when infected with these strains.

The **mesogenic form** is associated with an acute respiratory illness of moderate severity that is sometimes associated with life-threatening nervous system complications.

Neurotropic velogenic strains are associated with respiratory and neurological disease, such as paralysis of the legs. In outbreaks, death can occur in 5–10% or more of infected birds.

Viscerotropic-velogenic strains cause an acute, often lethal, infection with haemorrhagic gastrointestinal lesions. In outbreaks, mortality rates can be as high as 90%.

Both wild type and vaccine strains of NDV can infect humans (Chang 1981). After an incubation period of 1–4 days, the patient sometimes develops conjunctivitis, which is usually unilateral and, occasionally, systemic symptoms such as fever, myalgia and malaise. Symptoms usually resolve within a week.

MODE OF SPREAD

NDV can spread by inhalation or ingestion of infectious virus. Large amounts of infectious virus can be excreted in the faeces, which is likely to be the source of infectious virus in most instances. NDV can be introduced into new populations through natural movement of infected birds (e.g. migration, shipping infected birds from one location to another) or by fomites such as contaminated food, equipment or water. The virus can be transmitted quickly and efficiently in crowded populations, such as poultry houses. Humans presumably become infected by contamination of the hands and autoinoculation of the conjunctiva or inhalation of aerosolized virus. Most human infections have occurred after exposure to wild type virus in slaughterhouses or laboratories or to vaccine virus.

PATHOLOGY, PATHOGENESIS AND IMMUNE RESPONSE

The virus infects via the respiratory or gastrointestinal tract or the conjunctivae. With virulent strains, the virus first causes a local lytic infection and then becomes viraemic and infects multiple organs, including the brain, heart, kidneys and reticuloendothelial system. The speed and efficiency with which it infects different tissues seem to be key to its virulence and this, in turn, depends on the host species and strain of NDV. Efficient cleavage of the glycoproteins in a wide range of cell types seems to be characteristic of highly virulent strains (Rott and Klenk 1988). The titre of the inoculum can also alter the course of the infection. A low-titre inoculum can ameliorate disease caused by a virulent strain.

Infection by vaccine or naturally acquired infection confers resistance to later infection. Passively acquired antibody can also provide protection from disease. It has not yet been determined which components of the immune response are responsible for controlling and clearing established infection in the bird.

LABORATORY DIAGNOSIS

Diagnosis of NDV is often important in the context of control measures, and requires isolation and the characterization of the virus as virulent, avirulent or possibly vaccine-like. Respiratory, faecal or cloacal specimens from live birds or tissue specimens from affected organs from dead birds can be used to isolate the virus. Cell culture systems or embryonic chicken (or other fowl) eggs from flocks known to be pathogen or NDV free can be used to isolate the virus. The virus is then characterized by determining its virulence in embryonating hens' eggs, day-old chicks or 6 week old chickens. Molecular methods to characterize strains and track transmission are being developed and may provide alternative ways to determine virulence (Seal, King and Bennett 1995).

Antibodies against NDV can be detected by a variety of tests, including neutralization, haemagglutination inhibition and EIAs. Antibody tests have been used primarily to demonstrate past infection or response to vaccination.

PREVENTION

Vaccination and transmission control programmes have been used to prevent NDV infection. Live virus vaccines developed from B1 or Lasota lentogenic strains are most widely used. For poultry, the vaccines are administered orally in water, by intranasal or intraocular inoculation, or by aerosols. Quarantine of imported birds and quarantine and slaughter of infected flocks have been an integral part of NDV control in a number of countries.

3.2 Other avian paramyxoviruses

Eight other serotypes of avian paramyxoviruses have been isolated from a variety of birds. Although NDV is the most important pathogen, others have sometimes been associated with serious disease.

3.3 Bovine parainfluenza 3 (shipping fever)

Bovine parainfluenza virus 3 (BPIV-3) is a common infection of cattle, 60–90% of cattle in a herd often having serological evidence of past infection. Other animals, including buffalo, deer, horses and monkeys, also can have serological evidence of past infection with BPIV-3. Infection is not often associated with disease except when the cattle are stressed. Serious complications of infection are often related to secondary bacterial and mycoplasma infections. Pathological studies suggest that the upper and lower respiratory tracts are the primary targets of infection.

3.4 Bovine respiratory syncytial virus

CLINICAL MANIFESTATIONS

The clinical presentation of bovine respiratory syncytial virus (BRSV) is similar to that of human RSV, which is an acute upper and lower respiratory tract illness. Outbreaks of BRSV most often occur in weaned calves but can also occur in nursing calves and adult cattle. Illness is marked by upper respiratory symptoms, cough, hyperpnoea and, occasionally, respiratory distress and death. Bacterial secondary infection is not uncommon after infection. In some outbreaks, mortality has been as high as 20%.

EPIZOOTIOLOGY

Serological evidence of BRSV infection is detected in a high percentage of cattle in most herds. In temperate climates, outbreaks usually occur in the autumn and winter, often in animals that have been stressed.

3.5 Other animal RSVs

Isolates of RSV have also been made from goats (caprine RSV) and sheep (ovine RSV). These isolates are distinct from bovine and human RSV. Little is known about the clinical characteristics of naturally acquired infection in these species.

3.6 Other pneumonia virus infections of non-human species

Pneumonia virus of mice is present in many mouse colonies, but is not usually associated with disease. Some strains cause pneumonitis in mice. Turkey rhinotracheitis virus is a pathogen of turkeys and chickens (Naylor and Jones 1993). The virus causes an acute respiratory illness with sufficient mortality and morbidity that live attenuated vaccines have been developed.

3.7 Rinderpest

CLINICAL MANIFESTATIONS

Rinderpest can infect a variety of hoofed animals, including cattle, buffalo, sheep, goats and pigs, causing an acute febrile illness 3–15 days after infection. Typically, the animal then loses its appetite and develops nasal congestion, profuse lacrimal and nasal secretions, necrotic lesions on mucous membranes such as the mouth and tongue, profuse blood-streaked diarrhoea and dehydration. Mortality can be as high as 70–90%. There is considerable variation in the severity of symptoms, and even asymptomatic infections. This variability is probably in part related to differences in host susceptibility and virulence of the infecting strain.

EPIZOOTIOLOGY

Rinderpest has been eradicated from most of Europe, the Americas, Australia and New Zealand, but disease persists in parts of Asia, the Middle East, the Far East and Africa (Rweyemamu and Cheneau 1995). Endemic disease is commonly maintained in cattle and buffaloes, and the trade of cattle and movement of animals is responsible for the spread of disease.

PATHOLOGY, PATHOGENESIS AND IMMUNE RESPONSE

Virus can be detected in respiratory and lacrimal secretions, necrotic lesions, lymph nodes, blood and faeces. Respiratory secretions, and possibly urine and faeces, are probably the source of virus for transmission. Virus enters by the respiratory tract, becomes viraemic and spreads to lymph nodes, lungs, mucous membranes, and the gastrointestinal tract. Lytic infection of mucous membranes and the gastrointestinal tract is responsible for disease. Animals develop an antibody response to vaccine or naturally acquired infection that is associated with long-term protection from disease.

LABORATORY DIAGNOSIS

Diagnosis of rinderpest often has important implications for disease control programmes, such as quarantine or slaughter of affected animals, mass vaccination or restriction of animal movement. Classic rinderpest can be diagnosed clinically, but mild disease or disease in vaccinated populations must be diagnosed with the aid of laboratory testing (Diallo et al. 1995). Rinderpest virus can be detected by virus isolation, by antigen detection using various assays (e.g. agarose gel immunodiffusion, counterimmunoelectrophoresis, IFA or EIA) or by antibody detection in surviving animals by virus neutralization, EIA and other assays.

3.8 Canine distemper

CLINICAL MANIFESTATIONS

Canine distemper can infect a variety of carnivores, most notably the dog. Disease is most often seen in young animals but can cause disease in older animals as well. The animal develops fever, nasal and ocular discharge, vomiting, diarrhoea and pneumonia. Neurological disease such as seizures, incoordination or behavioural changes is often present and can develop acutely or weeks or months later. There can be considerable variation in the severity of disease. This variation is partly related to differences in the infecting strain and the infected species.

EPIZOOTIOLOGY

Canine distemper has been identified world-wide and has caused outbreaks, primarily in dogs but also in various other species, including lions in the Serengeti plains, javelinas in Arizona, mink, foxes and seals (Visser et al. 1993, Appel and Summers 1995, Roelke-Parker et al. 1996). Virus is usually maintained in dog populations by transmission to susceptible young via respiratory secretions. The virus is highly contagious.

PATHOLOGY AND PATHOGENESIS

Infection occurs in the upper respiratory tract and then spreads in a fashion similar to measles, i.e. via local spread or viraemia to various tissues, including the upper and lower respiratory tracts, gastrointestinal mucosa and brain. Many of the disease manifestations seem to result from the cytopathic effect of infection.

IMMUNE RESPONSE

Passively acquired maternal antibody and active immunity from vaccination or natural infection protect from disease. Specific IgM, IgA and IgG antibodies and cell-mediated immune responses can be detected with infection (Krakowka and Wallace 1979).

LABORATORY DIAGNOSIS

The virus can be isolated or specific antigens or RNA detected in infected secretions, blood or affected tissues. Dog kidney has been used, though not all strains grow well in this cell culture system. Viral antigens can be detected by EIA, IFA or immunohistological assays. Viral RNA has been detected by PCR assays.

PROPHYLAXIS

Modified live virus vaccines, Onderstepoort or Rockborn strains, are very successful in controlling disease. Maternal antibody decreases the effectiveness of the vaccine, so vaccine should be given after maternal antibody has disappeared, at 6–9 weeks of age (Chappuis 1995). Some workers recommend giving a second dose at 12–15 weeks of age to ensure an effective vaccination. Live virus vaccines have also been used in other species but can cause disease in some species and should be used only be if proven safe in that species. An inactivated vaccine in immunostimulating complexes (ISCOMs) has been used to vaccinate black-footed ferrets and seals (Visser et al. 1992).

3.9 Morbillivirus infections of aquatic mammals

Three distinct species of morbilliviruses – phocid distemper virus, dolphin morbillivirus and canine distemper virus – have caused deaths among seals, dolphins and porpoises (Barrett et al. 1995). Serological studies suggest that whales have also been infected with some of these viruses. Outbreaks of deaths probably result when interspecies transmission introduces or reintroduces the virus to a susceptible population. Pathological examination of animals from some outbreaks has revealed viral infection in the CNS, with evidence of encephalitis.

3.10 Equine morbillivirus

The recently described equine morbillivirus caused an outbreak of respiratory disease in horses and humans (Murray et al. 1995). The outbreak started in horses on a ranch in Australia with illness characterized by high fever and respiratory distress. Of 21 infected animals, 14 died or were killed with severe progressive illness. Two people working with the horses became ill; one survived, and one died with an interstitial pneumonia. In horses, the virus also causes a pneumonitis but infects a variety of other tissues, including the liver, kidney, lymphatic tissue and vascular endothelium. Experimentally, the virus can infect a wide range of animals. The source of virus for this outbreak is under investigation, but antibodies have been found in several fruit bats (*Pteropus* spp.) and the virus has been isolated from them.

REFERENCES

Aherne W, Bird T et al., 1970, Pathological changes in virus infections of the lower respiratory tract in children, *J Clin Pathol*, **23**: 7–18.

Albrecht P, Hermann K, Bums RG, 1981, Role of virus strain in conventional and enhanced measles plaque neutralization test, *J Virol Methods*, **3**: 251–60.

Alexander DJ, 1995, The epidemiology and control of avian influenza and Newcastle disease, *J Comp Pathol*, **112**: 105–26.

Alkhatib G, Briedis DJ, 1986, The predicted primary structure of the measles virus hemagglutinin, *Virology*, **150**: 479–90.

American Academy of Pediatrics, 1996, Reassessment of the indications for ribavirin therapy in respiratory syncytial virus infections, *Pediatrics*, **97**: 137–40.

Anderson K, King AM et al., 1992, Polylactosaminoglycan modification of the respiratory syncytial virus small hydrophobic (SH) protein: a conserved feature among human and bovine respiratory syncytial viruses, *Virology*, **191**: 417–30.

Anderson LJ, Heilman CA, 1995, Protective and disease-enhancing immune responses to respiratory syncytial virus, *J Infect Dis*, **171**: 1–7.

Anderson LJ, Parker RA, Strikas RL, 1990, Association between respiratory syncytial virus outbreaks and lower respiratory tract deaths of infants and young children, *J Infect Dis*, **161**: 640–6.

Anderson LJ, Hierholzer JC et al., 1985, Antigenic characterization of respiratory syncytial virus strains with monoclonal antibodies, *J Infect Dis*, **151**: 626–33.

Anderson LJ, Hendry RM et al., 1991, Multicenter study of strains of respiratory syncytial virus, *J Infect Dis*, **163**: 687–92.

Anderson LJ, Tsou C et al., 1994, Cytokine response to respiratory syncytial virus stimulation of human peripheral blood mononuclear cells, *J Infect Dis*, **170**: 1201–8.

Apalsch AM, Green M et al., 1995, Parainfluenza and influenza virus infections in pediatric transplant recipients, *Clin Infect Dis*, **20**: 394–9.

Appel MJG, Summers BA, 1995, Pathogenicity of morbilliviruses for terrestrial carnivores, *Vet Microbiol*, **44**: 187–91.

Arisoy ES, Demmler GJ et al., 1993, Meningitis due to parainfluenza virus type 3: report of two cases and review, *Clin Infect Dis*, **17**: 995–7.

Atkinson WL, Orenstein WA, 1992, The resurgence of measles in the United States, 1989–1990, *Annu Rev Med*, **43**: 451–63.

Barr J, Chambers P et al., 1991, Sequence of the major nucleocapsid protein gene of pneumonia virus of mice: sequence comparisons suggest structural homology between nucleocapsid proteins of pneumoviruses, paramyxoviruses, rhabdoviruses and filoviruses, *J Gen Virol*, **72**: 677–85.

Barr PJ, 1991, Mammalian subtilisins: the long-sought dibasic processing endoproteases, *Cell*, **66**: 1–3.

Barrett T, Shrimpton SB, Russell SE, 1985, Nucleotide sequence of the entire protein coding region of canine distemper virus polymerase-associated (P) protein mRNA, *Virus Res*, **3**: 367–72.

Barrett T, Blixenkrone-Møller M et al., 1995, Morbilliviruses in aquatic mammals: report on round table discussion, *Vet Microbiol*, **44**: 261–5.

Bartlett MS, 1957, Measles periodicity and community size, *J R Stat Soc*, **120**: 48–70.

Beckford AP, Kaschula ROC, Stephen C, 1985, Factors associated with fatal cases of measles: a retrospective autopsy study, *S Afr Med J*, **68**: 858–63.

Bellini WJ, Englund G et al., 1985, Measles virus P gene codes for two proteins, *J Virol*, **53**: 908–19.

Bellini WJ, Englund G et al., 1986, Matrix genes of measles virus and canine distemper virus: cloning, nucleotide sequences, and deduced amino acid sequences, *J Virol*, **58**: 408–16.

Bengtsson E, Orndahl G, 1954, Complications of mumps with special reference to the incidence of myocarditis, *Acta Med Scand*, **149**: 381–8.

Berg M, Hjertner B et al., 1992, The P gene of the porcine paramyxovirus LPMV encodes three possible polypeptides P, V and C: the P protein mRNA is edited, *J Gen Virol*, **73**: 1195–200.

Blixenkrone-Møller M, Bolt G et al., 1996, Comparative analysis of the attachment protein gene (H) of dolphin morbillivirus, *Virus Res*, **40**: 47–55.

Blumberg BM, Leppert M, Kolakofsky D, 1981, Interaction of VSV leader RNA and nucleocapsid protein may control VSV genome replication, *Cell*, **23**: 837–45.

Blumberg BM, Rose K et al., 1984, Analysis of the Sendai virus M gene and protein, *J Virol*, **52**: 656–63.

Blumberg BM, Giorgi C et al., 1985a, Sequence determination of the Sendai virus fusion protein gene, *J Gen Virol*, **166**: 317–31.

Blumberg B, Giorgi C et al., 1985b, Sequence determination of the Sendai virus IFN gene and its comparison to the influenza virus glycoproteins, *Cell*, **41**: 269–78.

Blumberg BM, Crowley JC et al., 1988, Measles virus L protein evidences elements of ancestral RNA polymerase, *Virology*, **164**: 487–97.

Boeck R, Curran J et al., 1992, The parainfluenza virus type 1 P/C gene uses a very efficient GUG codon to start its C′ protein, *J Virol*, **66**: 1765–8.

Brady MT, Evans J, Cuartas J, 1990, Survival and disinfection of parainfluenza viruses on environmental surfaces, *Am J Infect Control*, **18**: 18–23.

Brandt CD, Kim HW et al., 1973, Epidemiology of respiratory syncytial virus infection in Washington, DC. III. Composite analysis of eleven consecutive yearly epidemics, *Am J Epidemiol*, **98**: 355–64.

Briss PA, Fehrs JL et al., 1994, Sustained transmission of mumps in a highly vaccinated population: assessment of primary vaccine failure and waning vaccine-induced immunity, *J Infect Dis*, **169**: 77–82.

Brodsky AL, 1972, Atypical measles: severe illness in recipients of killed measles virus vaccine upon exposure to natural infection, *JAMA*, **222**: 1415–16.

Buckland R, Malvoisin E et al., 1992, A leucine zipper structure present in the measles virus fusion protein is not required for its tetramerization but is essential for fusion, *J Gen Virol*, **173**: 1703–7.

Burnet FM, 1968, Measles as an index of immunological function, *Lancet*, **2**: 610–13.

Calain P, Roux L, 1993, The rule of six, a basic feature for efficient replication of Sendai virus defective interfering RNA, *J Virol*, **67**: 4822–30.

Cane PA, Pringle CR, 1995, Molecular epidemiology of human respiratory syncytial virus, *Semin Virol*, **6**: 371–8.

Cane PA, Thomas HM et al., 1996, Analysis of the human serological immune response to a variable region of the attachment (G) protein of respiratory syncytial virus during primary infection, *J Med Virol*, **48**: 253–67.

Carroll AR, Wagner RR, 1979, Role of the membrane (M) protein in endogenous inhibition of in vitro transcription by vesicular stomatitis virus, *J Virol*, **29**: 134–42.

Castells E, George VG, Hierholzer JC, 1990, NCI-H292 as an alternative cell line for the isolation and propagation of the human paramyxoviruses, *Arch Virol*, **115**: 277–88.

Cattaneo R, Rebmann G et al., 1987a, Altered ratios of measles virus transcripts in diseased human brains, *Virology*, **160**: 523–6.

Cattaneo R, Rebmann G et al., 1987b, Altered transcription of a defective measles virus genome derived from a diseased human brain, *EMBO J*, **6**: 681–8.

Cattaneo R, Schmid A et al., 1988a, Biased hypermutation and other genetic changes in defective measles virus in human brain infections, *Cell*, **55**: 255–65.

Cattaneo R, Schmid A et al., 1988b, Multiple viral mutations rather than host factors cause defective measles virus gene expression in a subacute sclerosing panencephalitis cell line, *J Virol*, **62**: 1388–97.

Cattaneo R, Kaelin K et al., 1989, Measles virus editing provides an additional cysteine-rich protein, *Cell*, **56**: 759–64.

Centers for Disease Control, 1978, Parainfluenza outbreaks in extended-care facilities – United States, *Morbid Mortal Weekly Rep*, **27**: 475–6.

Centers for Disease Control, 1981, Measles encephalitis – United States, 1962–1979, *Morbid Mortal Weekly Rep*, **30**: 362–4.

Centers for Disease Control, 1989, Measles prevention: recommendations of the Immunization Practices Advisory Committee (ACIP), *Morbid Mortal Weekly Rep*, **38 (S-9)**: 1–18.

Centers for Disease Control and Prevention, 1995, Mumps surveillance – United States, 1988–1993, *Morbid Mortal Weekly Rep*, **44 (SS-3)**: 1–14.

Centers for Disease Control and Prevention, 1996, Measles – United States, 1995, *Morbid Mortal Weekly Rep*, **45**: 305–7.

Chambers P, Millar NS, Emmerson PT, 1986, Nucleotide sequence of the gene encoding the fusion glycoprotein of Newcastle disease virus, *J Gen Virol*, **67**: 2685–94.

Chambers P, Pringle CR, Easton AJ, 1990, Heptad repeat sequences are located adjacent to hydrophobic regions in several types of virus fusion glycoproteins, *J Gen Virol*, **71**: 3075–80.

Chang PW, 1981, Newcastle disease, *CRC Handbook Series in Zoonoses*, ed Beran GW, CRC Press, Boca Raton FL, 261.

Chanock RM, Bell JA, Parrott RH, 1961, Natural history of parainfluenza infection, *Perspect Virol*, **2**: 126–39.

Chappuis G, 1995, Control of canine distemper, *Vet Microbiol*, **44**: 351–8.

Chen RT, Markowitz LE et al., 1990, Measles antibody: reevaluation of protective titers, *J Infect Dis*, **162**: 1036–42.

Cherry JD, Feigin RD et al., 1972, Urban measles in the vaccine era: a clinical, epidemiologic, and serologic study, *J Pediatr*, **81**: 217–30.

Christensen PE, Henning S et al., 1952, An epidemic of measles in southern Greenland, 1951. Measles in virgin soil. II. The epidemic proper, *Acta Med Scand*, **144**: 430–49.

Collins PL, Chanock RM, McIntosh K, 1996, Parainfluenza viruses, *Fields' Virology*, 3rd edn, eds Fields BN, Knipe DM et al., Lippincott-Raven, Philadelphia, 1205–41.

Collins PL, Mottet G, 1992, Oligomerization and posttranslational processing of glycoprotein G of human respiratory syncytial virus: altered *O*-glycosylation in the presence of brefeldin A, *J Gen Virol*, **73**: 849–63.

Collins PL, Mottet G, 1993, Membrane orientation and oligomerization of the small hydrophobic protein of human respiratory syncytial virus, *J Gen Virol*, **74**: 1445–50.

Collins PL, Anderson K et al., 1985, Correct sequence for the major nucleocapsid protein mRNA of respiratory syncytial virus, *Virology*, **146**: 69–77.

Collins PL, Hill MG et al., 1995, Production of infectious human respiratory syncytial virus from cloned cDNA confirms an essential role for the transcription elongation factor from the 5′ proximal open reading frame of the M2 mRNA in gene

expression and provides a capability for vaccine development, *Proc Natl Acad Sci USA*, **92**: 11563–7.

Compans RW, Choppin PW, 1967a, Isolation and properties of the helical nucleocapsid of the parainfluenza virus SV5, *Proc Natl Acad Sci USA*, **57**: 949–56.

Compans RW, Choppin PW, 1967b, The length of the helical nucleocapsid of Newcastle disease virus, *Virology*, **33**: 344–6.

Cubie HA, Molyneaux PJ et al., 1995, Dot-blot hybridisation assay for detection of parvovirus B19 infections using synthetic obligonucleotides, *Mol Cell Probes*, **9**: 59–66.

Curran J, Boeck R, Kolakofsky D, 1991, The Sendai virus P gene expresses both an essential protein and an inhibitor of RNA synthesis by shuffling modules via mRNA editing, *EMBO J*, **10**: 3079–85.

Curran J, Kolakofsky D, 1988, Ribosomal initiation from an ACG codon in the Sendai virus P/C mRNA, *EMBO J*, **7**: 245–51.

Curran J, Marq JB, Kolakofsky D, 1992, The Sendai virus nonstructural C proteins specifically inhibit viral mRNA synthesis, *Virology*, **189**: 647–56.

Curran J, Pelet T, Kolakofsky D, 1994, An acidic activation-like domain of the Sendai virus P protein is required for RNA synthesis and encapsidation, *Virology*, **202**: 875–84.

Curran J, Homann H et al., 1993, The hypervariable C-terminal tail of the Sendai paramyxovirus nucleocapsid protein is required for template function but not for RNA encapsidation, *J Virol*, **67**: 4358–64.

Curran MD, Clarke DK, Rima BK, 1991, The nucleotide sequence of the gene encoding the attachment protein H of canine distemper virus, *J Gen Virol*, **72**: 443–7.

Curran MD, O'Loan D et al., 1992, Molecular characterization of phocine distemper virus: gene order and sequence of the gene encoding the attachment (H) protein, *J Gen Virol*, **73**: 1189–94.

Denny FW, Clyde WA Jr, 1986, Acute lower respiratory tract infections in nonhospitalized children, *J Pediatr*, **108**: 635–46.

Denton J, 1925, The pathology of fatal measles, *Am J Med Sci*, **169**: 531–43.

Deshpande KL, Portner A, 1985, Monoclonal antibodies to the P protein of Sendai virus define its structure and role in transcription, *Virology*, **140**: 125–34.

Diallo A, Libeau G et al., 1995, Recent developments in the diagnosis of rinderpest and peste des petits ruminants, *Vet Microbiol*, **44**: 307–17.

Dorig RE, Marcil A et al., 1993, The human CD46 molecule is a receptor for measles virus (Edmonston strain), *Cell*, **75**: 295–305.

Downham MAPS, McQuillin J, Gardner PS, 1974, Diagnosis and clinical significance of parainfluenza virus infections in children, *Arch Dis Child*, **49**: 8–15.

Dreyfuss G, Matunis MJ et al., 1993, hnRNP proteins and the biogenesis of mRNA, *Annu Rev Biochem*, **62**: 289–329.

Egelman EH, Wu SS et al., 1989, The Sendai virus nucleocapsid exists in at least four different helical states, *J Virol*, **63**: 2233–43.

Elango N, 1989a, Complete nucleotide sequence of the matrix protein MRNA of mumps virus, *Virology*, **168**: 426–8.

Elango N, 1989b, The mumps virus nucleocapsid mRNA sequence and homology among the *Paramyxoviridae* proteins, *Virus Res*, **12**: 77–86.

Elango N, Kovamees J, Norrby E, 1989, Sequence analysis of the mumps virus mRNA encoding the P protein, *Virology*, **169**: 62–7.

Elango N, Satake M et al., 1985, Respiratory syncytial virus fusion glycoprotein: nucleotide sequence of mRNA, identification of cleavage activation site and amino acid sequence of N-terminus of F1 subunit, *Nucleic Acids Res*, **13**: 1559–74.

Elango N, Kovamees J et al., 1989, mRNA sequence and deduced amino acid sequence of the mumps virus small hydrophobic protein gene, *J Virol*, **63**: 1413–15.

Erdman DD, Anderson LJ, 1990, Monoclonal antibody-based capture enzyme immunoassays for specific serum immunoglobulin G (IgG), IgA, and IgM antibodies to respiratory syncytial virus, *J Clin Microbiol*, **28**: 2744–9.

Erdman D, Anderson LJ et al., 1991, Evaluation of monoclonal antibody-based capture enzyme immunoassays for detection of specific antibodies to measles virus, *J Clin Microbiol*, **29**: 1466–71.

Esolen LM, Ward BJ et al., 1993, Infection of monocytes during measles, *J Infect Dis*, **168**: 47–52.

Falsey AR, Cunningham CK et al., 1995, Respiratory syncytial virus and influenza A infections in the hospitalized elderly, *J Infect Dis*, **172**: 389–94.

Finch JT, Gibbs AJ, 1970, Observations on the structure of the nucleocapsids of some paramyxoviruses, *J Gen Virol*, **6**: 141–50.

Forni AL, Schluger NW, Roberts RB, 1994, Severe measles pneumonitis in adults: evaluation of clinical characteristics and therapy with intravenous ribavirin, *Clin Infect Dis*, **19**: 454–62.

Freymuth F, Eugene G et al., 1995, Detection of respiratory syncytial virus by reverse transcription-PCR and hybridization with a DNA enzyme immunoassay, *J Clin Microbiol*, **33**: 3352–5.

Galinski MS, Mink MA, Pons MW, 1988, Molecular cloning and sequence analysis of the human parainfluenza 3 virus gene encoding the L protein, *Virology*, **165**: 499–510.

Galinski MS, Wechsler SL, 1991, The molecular biology of the *Paramyxovirus* genus, *The Paramyxoviruses*, ed Kingsbury DW, Plenum Press, New York, 41–82.

Galinski MS, Mink MA et al., 1986a, Molecular cloning and sequence analysis of the human parainfluenza 3 virus mRNA encoding the P and C proteins, *Virology*, **155**: 46–60.

Galinski MS, Mink MA et al., 1986b, Molecular cloning and sequence analysis of the human parainfluenza 3 virus RNA encoding the nucleocapsid protein, *Virology*, **149**: 139–51.

Galinski MS, Mink MA et al., 1987, Molecular cloning and sequence analysis of the human parainfluenza 3 virus gene encoding the matrix protein, *Virology*, **157**: 24–30.

Gerald C, Buckland R et al., 1986, Measles virus haemagglutinin gene: cloning, complete nucleotide sequence analysis and expression in COS cells, *J Gen Virol*, **67**: 2695–703.

Gibbs FA, Gibbs EL et al., 1959, Electroencephalographic abnormality to 'uncomplicated' childhood diseases, *JAMA*, **72**: 1050–5.

Gilchrist S, Torok TJ et al., 1994, National surveillance for respiratory syncytial virus, United States, 1985–1990, *J Infect Dis*, **170**: 986–90.

Giorgi C, Blumberg BM, Kolakofsky D, 1983, Sendai virus contains overlapping genes expressed from a single mRNA, *Cell*, **35**: 829–36.

Glezen WP, Loda FA et al., 1971, Epidemiologic patterns of acute lower respiratory disease of children in a pediatric group practice, *J Pediatr*, **78**: 397–406.

Glezen WP, Frank AL et al., 1984, Parainfluenza virus type 3: seasonality and risk of infection and reinfection in young children, *J Infect Dis*, **150**: 851–7.

Glezen WP, Taber LH et al., 1986, Risk of primary infection and reinfection with respiratory syncytial virus, *Am J Dis Child*, **140**: 543–6.

Gotoh B, Yamauchi F et al., 1992, Isolation of factor Xa from chick embryo as the amniotic endoprotease responsible for paramyxovirus activation, *FEBS Lett*, **296**: 274–8.

Gould AR, 1996, Comparison of the deduced matrix and fusion protein sequence of equine morbillivirus with cognate genes of the *Paramyxoviridae*, *Virus Res*, **43**: 17–31.

Graham BS, Bunton LA et al., 1991, Role of T lymphocyte subsets in the pathogenesis of primary infection and rechallenge with respiratory syncytial virus in mice, *J Clin Invest*, **88**: 1026–33.

Graham BS, Henderson GS et al., 1993, Priming immunization determines T helper cytokine mRNA expresssion patterns in lungs of mice challenged with respiratory syncytial virus, *J Immunol*, **151**: 2032–40.

Graves M, Griffin DE et al., 1984, Development of antibody to measles virus polypeptides during complicated and uncomplicated measles virus infections, *J Virol*, **49**: 409–12.

Greenberg M, Pelliterri O, Eisenstein DT, 1955, Measles encephalitis. I. Prophylactic effect of gamma globulin, *J Pediatr*, **46**: 642–7.

Griffin DE, Ward BJ, 1993, Differential CD4 T cell activation in measles, *J Infect Dis*, **168**: 275–81.

Griffin DE, Ward BJ, Esolen LM, 1994, Pathogenesis of measles virus infection: an hypothesis for altered immune responses, *J Infect Dis*, **170, suppl 1**: S24–31.

Griffiths DA, 1973, The effect of measles vaccination on the incidence of measles in the community, *J R Stat Soc*, **136**: 441–9.

Groothuis JR, Gutierrez KM, Lauer BA, 1988, Respiratory syncytial virus infection in children with bronchopulmonary dysplasia, *Pediatrics*, **82**: 199–203.

Groothuis JR, Simoes EAF et al., 1993, Prophylactic administration of respiratory syncytial virus immune globulin in high-risk infants and young children, *N Engl J Med*, **329**: 1524–30.

Gupta KC, Patwardhan S, 1988, ACG, the initiator codon for a Sendai virus protein, *J Biol Chem*, **263**: 8553–6.

Gut JP, Spiess C et al., 1985, Rapid diagnosis of acute mumps infection by a direct immunoglobulin M antibody capture enzyme immunoassay with labeled antigen, *J Clin Microbiol*, **21**: 346–52.

Gut JP, Lablache C et al., 1995, Symptomatic mumps virus reinfections, *J Med Virol*, **45**: 17–23.

Hall CB, Douglas RG Jr et al., 1975, Nosocomial respiratory syncytial virus infections, *N Engl J Med*, **293**: 1343–6.

Hall CB, Geiman JM et al., 1976, Respiratory syncytial virus infections within families, *N Engl J Med*, **294**: 414–19.

Hall CB, Kopelman AE et al., 1979, Neonatal respiratory syncytial virus infection, *N Engl J Med*, **300**: 393–6.

Hall CB, Powell KR et al., 1986, Respiratory syncytial viral infection in children with compromised immune function, *N Engl J Med*, **315**: 77–81.

Hall CB, Walsh EE et al., 1990, Occurrence of groups A and B of respiratory syncytial virus over 15 years: associated epidemiologic and clinical characteristics in hospitalized and ambulatory children, *J Infect Dis*, **162**: 1283–90.

Hall CB, Walsh EE et al., 1991, Immunity to and frequency of reinfection with respiratory syncytial virus, *J Infect Dis*, **163**: 693–8.

Hall CE, Brandt CD et al., 1971, The virus watch program: a continuing surveillance of viral infections in metropolitan New York families. IX. A comparison of infections with several respiratory pathogens in New York and New Orleans families, *Am J Epidemiol*, **94**: 367–85.

Hall WW, Choppin PW, 1979, Evidence for lack of synthesis of the M polypeptide of measles virus in brain cells in subacute sclerosing panencephalitis, *Virology*, **99**: 443–7.

Harrington RD, Hooton TM et al., 1992, An outbreak of respiratory syncytial virus in a bone marrow transplant center, *J Infect Dis*, **165**: 987–93.

Harter DH, Choppin PW, 1967, Studies on pneumonia virus of mice (PVM) in cell culture: replication in baby hamster kidney cells and properties of the virus, *J Exp Med*, **126**: 251–66.

von Heijne G, 1981, On the hydrophobic nature of signal sequences, *Eur J Biochem*, **116**: 419–22.

Henderson FW, Collier AM et al., 1979, Respiratory-syncytial-virus infections, reinfections and immunity: a prospective, longitudinal study in young children, *N Engl J Med*, **300**: 530–4.

Hendricks DA, McIntosh K, Patterson JL, 1988, Further characterization of the soluble form of the G glycoprotein of respiratory syncytial virus, *J Virol*, **62**: 2228–33.

Henle G, Henle W et al., 1948, Isolation of mumps virus from human beings with induced apparent or inapparent infections, *J Exp Med*, **88**: 223–32.

Henrickson KJ, Kuhn SM, Savatski LL, 1994, Epidemiology and cost of infection with human parainfluenza virus types 1 and 2 in young children, *Clin Infect Dis*, **18**: 770–9.

Hidaka Y, Kanda T et al., 1984, Nucleotide sequence of a Sendai virus genome region covering the entire M gene and the 3' proximal 1013 nucleotides of the F gene, *Nucleic Acids Res,* **12:** 7965–27.

Hiebert SW, Paterson RG, Lamb RA, 1985, Hemagglutinin–neuraminidase protein of the paramyxovirus simian virus 5; nucleotide sequence of the mRNA predicts an N-terminal membrane anchor, *J Virol,* **54:** 1–6.

Hiebert SW, Paterson RG, Lamb RA, 1988, Cell surface expression and orientation in membrane of the 44-amino-acid SH protein of simian virus 5, *J Virol Res,* **62:** 2347–57.

Higuchi Y, Miyahara Y et al., 1992, Sequence analysis of the large (L) protein of simian virus 5, *J Gen Virol,* **173:** 1005–10.

Hopkins DR, Koplan JP et al., 1982, The case for global measles eradication, *Lancet,* **1:** 1396–8.

Horvath CM, Lamb RA, 1992, Studies on the fusion peptide of a paramyxovirus fusion glycoprotein: roles of conserved residues in cell fusion, *J Virol,* **66:** 2443–55.

Hosaka M, Nagahama M et al., 1991, Arg–X–Lys/Arg–Arg motif as a signal for precursor cleavage catalyzed by furin within the constitutive secretory pathway, *J Biol Chem,* **266:** 12127–30.

Howe C, Lee LT, 1972, Virus–erythrocyte interactions, *Adv Virus Res,* **17:** 1–50.

Hsu C-H, Kingsbury DW, 1982, Topography of phosphate residues in Sendai virus proteins, *Virology,* **120:** 225–34.

Hu A, Cattaneo R et al., 1994, Role of N-linked oligosaccharide chains in the processing and antigenicity of measles virus hemagglutinin protein, *J Gen Virol,* **75:** 1043–52.

Huang YT, Collins PL, Wertz GW, 1985, Characterization of the 10 proteins of human respiratory syncytial virus: identification of a fourth envelope-associated protein, *Virus Res,* **2:** 157–73.

Hyatt AD, Selleck P, 1996, Ultrastructure of equine morbillivirus, *Virus Res,* **43:** 1–15.

Ishida N, Taira H et al., 1986, Sequence of 2617 nucleotides from the 3' end of Newcastle disease virus genome RNA and the predicted amino acid sequence of viral NP protein, *Nucleic Acids Res,* **14:** 6551–64.

Jambou RC, Elango N et al., 1986, Complete sequence of the major nucleocapsid protein gene of human parainfluenza type 3 virus: comparison with other negative strand viruses, *J Gen Virol,* **67:** 2543–8.

Johnson PR, Olmsted RA et al., 1987, Antigenic relatedness between glycoproteins of human respiratory syncytial virus subgroups A and B: evaluation of the contributions of F and G glycoproteins to immunity, *J Virol,* **61:** 3163–6.

Kamata H, Tsukiyama K et al., 1991, Nucleotide sequence of cDNA to the rinderpest virus mRNA encoding the nucleocapsid protein, *Virus Genes,* **5:** 5–15.

Kapikian AZ, Bell JA et al., 1961, An outbreak of febrile illness and pneumonia associated with respiratory syncytial virus infection, *Am J Hyg,* **74:** 234–48.

Karron RA, O'Brian KL et al., 1993, Molecular epidemiology of a parainfluenza type 3 virus outbreak on a pediatric ward, *J Infect Dis,* **167:** 1441–5.

Karron RA, Froehlich JL et al., 1994, Rapid detection of parainfluenza virus type 3 RNA in respiratory specimens: use of reverse transcription-PCR-enzyme immunoassay, *J Clin Microbiol,* **32:** 484–8.

Karron RA, Wright PF et al., 1995, A live attenuated bovine parainfluenza virus type 3 vaccine is safe, infectious, immunogenic, and phenotypically stable in infants and children, *J Infect Dis,* **171:** 1107–14.

Katz M, Koprowski H, 1973, The significance of failure to isolate infectious viruses in cases of subacute sclerosing panencephalitis, *Arch Gesamte Virusforsch,* **41:** 390–3.

Kawano M, Bando H et al., 1990a, Complete nucleotide sequence of the matrix genes of human parainfluenza type 2 virus and expression of the M protein in bacteria, *Virology,* **179:** 857–61.

Kawano M, Bando H et al., 1990b, Sequence determination of

the hemagglutinin–neuraminidase (HN) gene of human parainfluenza type 2 virus and the construction of a phylogenetic tree for HN proteins of all the paramyxoviruses that are infectious to humans, *Virology,* **174:** 308–13.

Kawano M, Bando H et al., 1990c, Sequence of the fusion protein gene of human parainfluenza type 2 virus and its 3' intergenic region: lack of small hydrophobic (SH) gene, *Virology,* **178:** 289–92.

Kawano M, Okamoto K et al., 1991, Characterizations of the human parainfluenza type 2 virus gene encoding the L protein and the intergenic sequences, *Nucleic Acids Res,* **19:** 2739–46.

Kellogg JA, 1991, Culture vs direct antigen assays for detection of microbial pathogens from lower respiratory tract specimens suspected of containing the respiratory syncytial virus, *Arch Pathol Lab Med,* **115:** 451–8.

Kempe CH, Fulginiti VA, 1965, The pathogenesis of measles virus infection, *Arch Gesamte Virusforsch,* **16:** 103–28.

Kilgore GE, Dowdle WR, 1970, Antigenic characterization of parainfluenza 4A and 4B by hemagglutination-inhibition test and distribution of HI antibody in human sera, *Am J Epidemiol,* **91:** 308–16.

Kingsbury DW, Darlington RW, 1968, Isolation and properties of Newcastle disease virus nucleocapsid, *J Virol,* **2:** 248–55.

Kingsbury DW, Hsu CH, Murti KG, 1978, Intracellular metabolism of Sendai virus nucleocapsids, *Virology,* **91:** 86–94.

Klenk HD, Choppin PW, 1969, Lipids of plasma membranes of monkey and hamster kidney cells and of parainfluenza virions grown in these cells, *Virology,* **38:** 255–68.

Klenk HD, Choppin PW, 1970, Plasma membrane lipids and parainfluenza virus assembly, *Virology,* **40:** 939–47.

Knott AM, Long CE, Hall CB, 1994, Parainfluenza viral infections in pediatric outpatients: seasonal patterns and clinical characteristics, *Pediatr Infect Dis J,* **13:** 269–73.

Kobune F, Sakata H, Suguira A, 1990, Marmoset lymphoblastoid cells as a sensitive host for isolation of measles virus, *J Virol,* **64:** 700–5.

Kondo K, Bando H et al., 1990, Sequencing analyses and comparison of parainfluenza virus type 4A and 4B NP protein genes, *Virology,* **174:** 1–8.

Kovamees J, Blixenkrone-Møller M, Norrby E, 1991, The nucleotide and predicted amino acid sequence of the attachment protein gene (H) of dolphin morbillivirus, *Virus Res,* **40:** 47–55.

Kovamees J, Norrby E, Elango N, 1989, Complete nucleotide sequence of the hemagglutinin–neuraminidase (HN) mRNA of mumps virus and comparison of paramyxovirus IFN proteins, *Virus Res,* **12:** 87–96.

Krah DL, 1991, Receptors for binding measles virus on host cells and erythrocytes, *Microb Pathog,* **11:** 221–8.

Krakowka S, Wallace AL, 1979, Lymphocyte-associated immune responses to canine distemper and measles virus in distemper-infected gnotobiotic dogs, *Am J Vet Res,* **40:** 669–72.

LaBoccetta AC, Tornay AS, 1964, Measles encephalitis. Report of 61 cases, *Am J Dis Child,* **107:** 247–55.

Lamb RA, 1993, Paramyxovirus fusion: a hypothesis for changes, *Virology,* **197:** 1–11.

Lamb RA, Paterson RG, 1991, The nonstructural proteins of paramyxoviruses, *The Paramyxoviruses,* ed Kingsbury DW, Plenum Press, New York, 181–214.

Liebert UG, Baczko K et al., 1986, Restricted expression of measles virus proteins in brains from cases of subacute sclerosing panencephalitis, *J Gen Virol,* **67:** 2435–44.

Limo M, Yilma T, 1990, Molecular cloning of the rinderpest virus matrix gene: comparative sequence analysis with other paramyxoviruses, *Virology,* **175:** 323–7.

Ling R, Easton AJ, Pringle CR, 1992, Sequence analysis of the 22K, SH, and G genes of turkey rhinotracheitis virus and their intergenic regions reveals a gene order different than that of other pneumoviruses, *J Gen Virol,* **73:** 1709–55.

Lyn D, Gill DS et al., 1991, The nucleoproteins of human parainfluenza virus type I and Sendai virus share amino acid sequences and antigenic and structural determinants, *J Gen Virol*, **72:** 983–7.

MacDonald NE, Hall CB et al., 1982, Respiratory syncytial viral infection in infants with congenital heart disease, *N Engl J Med*, **307:** 397–400.

McFarland NF, Pedone CA et al., 1980, The response of human lymphocyte subpopulations to measles, mumps, and vaccinia viral antigens, *J Immunol*, **125:** 221–5.

McGinnes L, McQuain C, Morrison T, 1988, The P protein and the non-structural 38K and 29K proteins of Newcastle disease virus are derived from the same open reading frame, *Virology*, **164:** 256–64.

McGinnes LW, Morrison TG, 1986, Nucleotide sequence of the gene encoding the Newcastle disease virus fusion protein and comparisons of paramyxovirus fusion protein sequence, *Virus Res*, **5:** 343–56.

Markwell MA, Fox CF, 1980, Protein–protein interactions within paramyxoviruses identified by native disulfide bonding or reversible chemical cross-linking, *Virology*, **33:** 152–66.

Matsuoka Y, Ray R, 1991, Sequence analysis and expression of the human parainfluenza type I virus nucleoprotein gene, *Virology*, **181:** 403–7.

Matsuoka Y, Curran J et al., 1991, The P gene of human parainfluenzavirus type I encodes P and C proteins but not a cysteine-rich V protein, *J Virol*, **65:** 3406–10.

Millar NS, Chambers P, Emmerson PT, 1986, Nucleotide sequence analysis of the haemagglutinin–neuraminidase gene of Newcastle disease virus, *J Gen Virol*, **67:** 1917–27.

Modlin JF, Jabbour JT et al., 1977, Epidemiologic studies of measles, measles vaccine, and subacute sclerosing panencephalitis, *Pediatrics*, **59:** 505–12.

Moench TR, Griffin DE et al., 1988, Acute measles in patients with and without neurological involvement: distribution of measles virus antigen and RNA, *J Infect Dis*, **158:** 433–42.

Morgan EM, Rakestraw KM, 1986, Sequence of the Sendai virus L gene: open reading frames upstream of the main coding region suggest that the gene may be polycistronic, *Virology*, **154:** 31–40.

Morrison T, Portner A, 1991, Structure, function, and intracellular processing of the glycoproteins of *Paramyxoviridae*, *The Paramyxoviruses*, ed Kingsbury DW, Plenum Press, New York, 347–82.

Morrison TG, McQuain C et al., 1990, Mature cell associated HN protein of Newcastle disease virus exists in two forms differentiated by posttransational modifications, *Virus Res*, **15:** 113–33.

Mountcastle WE, Compans RW et al., 1974, Proteolytic cleavage of subunits of the nucleocapsid of the paramyxovirus simian virus 5, *J Virol*, **114:** 1253–61.

Murphy FA, Fauquet CM et al., 1995, *Virus Taxonomy*, Springer-Verlag, Vienna.

Murray K, Selleck P et al., 1995, A morbillivirus that caused fatal disease in horses and humans, *Science*, **268:** 94–7.

Mustafa MM, Weitman SD et al., 1993, Subacute measles encephalitis in the young immunocompromised host: report of two cases diagnosed by polymerase chain reaction and treated with ribavirin and review of the literature, *Clin Infect Dis*, **16:** 654–60.

Naniche D, Varior-Krishnan G et al., 1993, Human membrane cofactor protein (CD46) acts as a cellular receptor for measles virus, *J Virol*, **67:** 6025–32.

Naylor CJ, Jones RC, 1993, Turkey rhinotracheitis: a review, *Vet Bull*, **63:** 439–49.

Neubert WJ, Eckerskom C, Homann HE, 1991, Sendai virus NP gene codes for a 524 amino acid NP protein, *Virus Genes*, **1:** 25–32.

Ng DTW, Randall RE, Lamb RA, 1989, Intracellular maturation and transport of the SV5 type II glycoprotein hemagglutinin–neuraminidase: specific and transient association with GPP78-Bip in the endoplasmic reticulum and extensive internalization from the cell surface, *J Cell Biol*, **109:** 3273–89.

Okazaki K, Tanabayshi K et al., 1992, Molecular cloning and sequence analysis of the mumps gene encoding the L protein and trailer sequence, *Virology*, **188:** 926–30.

Olmsted RA, Collins PL, 1989, The 1A protein of respiratory syncytial virus is an integral membrane protein present as multiple, structurally distinct species, *J Virol*, **63:** 2019–29.

Ortmann D, Ohuchi M et al., 1994, Proteolytic cleavage of wild type and mutants of the F protein of human parainfluenza virus type 3 by two subtilisin-like endoproteases, furin and Kex2, *J Virol*, **68:** 2772–6.

Park KE, Krystal M, 1992, In vivo model for pseudo-templated transcription in Sendai virus, *J Virol*, **66:** 7033–9.

Parks GD, Ward CD, Lamb RA, 1992, Molecular cloning of the NP and L genes of simian virus 5: identification of highly conserved domains in paramyxovirus NP and L proteins, *Virus Res*, **22:** 259–79.

Paterson RG, Harris TJR, Lamb RA, 1984, Fusion protein of the paramyxovirus simian virus 5: nucleotide sequence of mRNA predicts a highly hydrophobic glycoprotein, *Proc Natl Acad Sci USA*, **81:** 6706–10.

Paterson RG, Lamb RA, 1990, RNA editing by G-nucleotide insertion in mumps virus P-gene mRNA transcripts, *J Virol*, **64:** 4137–45.

Pauling L, Corey RB, 1953, Compound helical configurations of polypeptide chains: structure of protein of the α-keratin type, *Nature (London)*, **171:** 59–61.

Peeples ME, 1991, Paramyxovirus M proteins: pulling it all together and taking it on the road, *The Paramyxoviruses*, ed Kingsbury DW, Plenum Press, New York, 427–56.

Peltola H, Heinonen OP et al., 1994, The elimination of indigenous measles, mumps, and rubella from Finland by a 12-year, two-dose vaccination program, *N Engl J Med*, **331:** 1397–402.

Phillips IE, 1954, Erythema infectiosum: clinical and epidemiological observations, *South Med J*, **47:** 253–7.

Pieper SJL, Kurland LT, 1958, Sequelae of Japanese B and mumps encephalitis, *Am J Trop Med Hyg*, **7:** 481–90.

Popow-Kraupp T, Lakits E et al., 1989, Immunoglobulin-class-specific immune response to respiratory syncytial virus structural proteins in infants, children, and adults, *J Med Virol*, **27:** 215–23.

Portner A, 1981, The HN glycoprotein of Sendai virus analysis of site(s) involved in hemagglutinating and neuraminidase activities, *Virology*, **115:** 375–84.

Portner A, Scroggs RA et al., 1975, A temperature-sensitive mutant of Sendai virus with an altered hemagglutinin-neuraminidase polypeptide: consequences for virus assembly and cytopathology, *Virology*, **67:** 179–87.

de Quadros CA, Olive JM et al., 1996, Measles elimination in the Americas: evolving strategies, *JAMA*, **275:** 224–9.

Richardson C, Hull D et al., 1986, The nucleotide sequence of the mRNA encoding the fusion protein of measles virus (Edmonston strain): a comparison of fusion proteins from several different paramyxoviruses, *Virology*, **155:** 508–23.

Richter GA, Horner BL et al., 1996, Characterization of three paramyxoviruses isolated from three snakes, *Virus Res*, **43:** 77–83.

Rima BK, Earle JAP et al., 1995, Temporal and geographical distribution of measles virus genotypes, *J Gen Virol*, **76:** 1173–80.

Roelke-Parker ME, Munson L et al., 1996, A canine distemper virus epidemic in Serengeti lions (*Panthera leo*), *Nature (London)*, **379:** 441–5.

Rota PA, Rota JS, Bellini WJ, 1995, Molecular epidemiology of measles virus, *Semin Virol*, **6:** 379–86.

Rota PA, Khan AL et al., 1995, Detection of measles virus in RNA in urine specimens from vaccine recipients, *J Clin Microbiol*, **33:** 2485–8.

Rota JS, Heath JL et al., 1996, Molecular epidemiology of measles virus: identification of pathways of transmission and implications for measles elimination, *J Infect Dis*, **173:** 32–7.

Rott R, Klenk H-D, 1988, Molecular basis of infectivity and pathogenicity of Newcastle disease virus, *Developments in Veterinary*

Virology: Newcastle Disease, ed Alexander DJ, Kluwer Academic, Boston MA, 98–112.

Roux L, Waldvogel FA, 1982, Instability of the viral M protein in BHK-21 cells persistently infected with Sendai virus, *Cell*, **28:** 293–302.

Rozenblatt S, Eizenberg O et al., 1985, Sequence homology within the morbilliviruses, *J Virol*, **53:** 684–90.

Rubin EE, Quennec P, McDonald JC, 1993, Infections due to parainfluenza virus type 4 in children, *Clin Infect Dis*, **17:** 998–1002.

Russell R, Paterson RG, Lamb RA, 1994, Studies with cross-linking reagents on the oligomeric form of the paramyxovirus fusion protein, *Virology*, **199:** 160–8.

Rweyemamu MM, Cheneau Y, 1995, Strategy for the global rinderpest eradication programme, *Vet Microbiol*, **44:** 369–76.

Ryan KW, Morgan EM, Portner A, 1991, Two noncontiguous regions of Sendai virus P protein combine to form a single nucleocapsid binding domain, *Virology*, **180:** 126–34.

Ryan KW, Portner A, 1990, Separate domains of Sendai virus P protein are required for binding to viral nucleocapsids, *Virology*, **174:** 515–21.

Ryan KW, Portner A, Murti KG, 1993, Antibodies to paramyxovirus nucleoproteins define regions important for immunogenicity and nucleocapsid assembly, *Virology*, **193:** 376–84.

Sakai Y, Suzu S et al., 1987, Nucleotide sequence of the bovine parainfluenza 3 virus genome: its 3′ end and the genes of NP, P, C and M proteins, *Nucleic Acids Res*, **15:** 2927–44.

Samal SK, Collins PL, 1996, RNA replication by a respiratory syncytial virus RNA analog does not obey the rule of six, *J Virol*, **70:** 5075–82.

Sanchez A, Banerjee AK et al., 1986, Conserved structures among the nucleocapsid proteins of the *Paramyxoviridae*: complete nucleotide sequence of the human parainfluenza virus type 3 NP mRNA, *Virology*, **152:** 171–80.

Sanderson CM, Wu H-H, Nayak DP, 1993, Sendai virus M protein binds independently to either the F or the HN glycoprotein in vivo, *J Virol*, **68:** 69–76.

Sarkkinen HK, Halonen PE, Salmi AA, 1981, Type-specific detection of parainfluenzaviruses by enzyme-immunoassay and radioimmunoassay in nasopharyngeal specimens of patients with acute respiratory disease, *J Gen Virol*, **56:** 49–57.

Satake M, Venkatesan S, 1984, Nucleotide sequence of the gene encoding respiratory syncytial virus matrix protein, *J Virol*, **50:** 92–9.

Satake M, Coligan JE et al., 1995, Respiratory syncytial virus envelope glycoprotein (G) has a novel structure, *Nucleic Acids Res*, **113:** 7795–812.

Scheid A, Choppin PW, 1974, Identification of biological activities of paramyxovirus glycoproteins. Activation of cell fusion, hemolysis, and infectivity of proteolytic cleavage of an inactive precursor protein of Sendai virus, *Virology*, **57:** 475–90.

Seal BS, King DJ, Bennett JD, 1995, Characterization of Newcastle disease virus isolates by reverse transcription PCR coupled to direct nucleotide sequencing and development of sequence database for pathotype prediction and molecular epidemiologic analysis, *J Clin Microbiol*, **33:** 2624–30.

Server AC, Smith JA et al., 1985, Purification and amino-terminal protein sequence analysis of the mumps virus fusion protein, *Virology*, **144:** 373–83.

Sharma B, Norrby E et al., 1992, The nucleotide and deduced amino acid sequence of the M gene of phocid distemper virus (PDV). The most conserved protein of morbilliviruses shows a uniquely close relationship between PDV and canine distemper virus, *Virus Res*, **23:** 13–25.

Sheshberadaran H, Lamb RA, 1990, Sequence characterization of the membrane protein gene of paramyxovirus simian virus 5, *Virology*, **176:** 234–43.

Shioda T, Iwasaki K, Shibuta H, 1986, Determination of the complete nucleotide sequence of the Sendai virus genome RNA and the predicted amino acid sequences of the F, HN, and L proteins, *Nucleic Acids Res*, **14:** 1545–63.

Sidhu MS, Menonna JP et al., 1993, Canine distemper virus L gene: sequence and comparison with related viruses, *Virology*, **193:** 50–65.

Sidhu MS, Crowley J et al., 1994, Defective measles virus in human subacute sclerosing panencephalitis brain, *Virology*, **202:** 631–41.

Slobod KS, Allan JE, 1993, Parainfluenza type 1 virus-infected cells are killed by both CD8+ and CD4+ cytotoxic T cell precursors, *Clin Exp Immunol*, **93:** 363–9.

Spriggs MK, Collins PL, 1986, Sequence analysis of the protein genes of human parainfluenza virus type 3: patterns of amino acid sequence homology among paramyxovirus proteins, *J Gen Virol*, **12:** 2705–19.

Spriggs MK, Olmstead RA et al., 1986, Fusion glycoprotein of human parainfluenza virus type 3: nucleotide sequence of the gene, direct identification of the cleavage-activation site, and comparison with other paramyxoviruses, *Virology*, **152:** 241–51.

Stec DS, Hill MG, Collins PL, 1991, Sequence analysis of the polymerase L gene of human respiratory syncytial virus and predicted phylogeny of nonsegmented negative-strand viruses, *Virology*, **183:** 273–87.

Stricker R, Mottet G, Roux L, 1994, The Sendai virus matrix protein appears to be recruited in the cytoplasm by the viral nucleocapsid to function in viral assembly and budding, *J Gen Virol*, **75:** 1031–42.

Sundqvist A, Berg M, Moreno LI, 1992, The haemagglutinin–neuraminidase glycoprotein of the porcine paramyxovirus LPMV: comparison with other paramyxoviruses revealed the closest relationship to simian virus 5 and mumps virus, *Arch Virol*, **122:** 331–40.

Suzu S, Sakai Y et al., 1987, Nucleotide sequence of the bovine parainfluenza 3 virus genome: the genes of the F and HN glycoproteins, *Nucleic Acids Res*, **15:** 2945–58.

Tablan OC, Anderson LJ et al., 1994, Guideline for prevention of nosocomial pneumonia. The Hospital Infection Control Practices Advisory Committee, Centers for Disease Control and Prevention, *Infect Control Hosp Epidemiol*, **15:** 587–627.

Takeuchi K, Hishiyama M et al., 1988, Molecular cloning and sequence analysis of the mumps virus gene encoding the P protein: mumps virus P gene is monocistronic, *J Gen Virol*, **69:** 2043–9.

Takeuchi K, Tanabayashi K et al., 1990, Detection and characterization of mumps virus V protein, *Virology*, **178:** 247–53.

Tamin A, Rota PA et al., 1994, Antigenic analysis of current wild type and vaccine strains of measles virus, *J Infect Dis*, **170:** 795–801.

Thomas SM, Lamb RA, Paterson RG, 1988, Two mRNAs that differ from two nontemplated nucleotides encode the amino coterminal proteins P and V of the paramyxovirus SV5, *Cell*, **54:** 891–902.

Thompson SD, Laver WG et al., 1988, Isolation of a biologically active soluble form of the hemagglutinin–neuraminidase protein of Sendai virus, *J Virol*, **62:** 4653–60.

Tsukiyama K, Sugiyama M et al., 1987, Molecular cloning and sequence analysis of the rinderpest virus mRNA encoding the hemagglutinin protein, *Virology*, **160:** 49–54.

Tsurudome M, Naohiro O et al., 1991, Molecular relationships between human parainfluenza virus type 2 and simian viruses 41 and 5: determination of nucleoprotein gene sequences of simian viruses 41 and 5, *J Gen Virol*, **72:** 2289–92.

Utz JP, Houk VN, Alling DW, 1964, Clinical and laboratory studies of mumps, *N Engl J Med*, **270:** 1283.

Varsanyi TM, Jornvall H et al., 1987, F_1 polypeptides of two canine distemper virus strains: variation in the conserved N-terminal hydrophobic region, *Virology*, **157:** 241–4.

Vidal S, Curran J et al., 1988, Mapping of monoclonal antibodies to the Sendai virus P protein and the location of its phosphates, *J Virol*, **62:** 2200–3.

Visser IK, Vedder EJ et al., 1992, Canine distemper virus ISCOMs induce protection in harbour seals (*Phoca vitulina*) against phocid distemper but still allow subsequent infection with phocid distemper virus-1, *Vaccine*, **10:** 435–8.

Visser IKG, Van der Heijden RWJ et al., 1993, Fusion protein gene nucleotide sequence similarities, shared antigenic sites and phylogenetic analysis suggest that phocid distemper virus type 2 and canine distemper virus belong to the same virus entity, *J Gen Virol*, **74:** 1989–94.

Vuori M, Lahikainen EA, Peltonen T, 1962, Perceptive deafness in connection with mumps: a study of 298 servicemen suffering from mumps, *Acta Otolaryngol*, **55:** 231–6.

Waxham MN, Server AC et al., 1987, Cloning and sequencing of the mumps virus fusion protein gene, *Virology*, **159:** 381–8.

Waxham MN, Aronowski J et al., 1988, Sequence determination of the mumps virus HN gene, *Virology*, **164:** 318–25.

Welliver RC, Sun M, Rinaldo D, 1985, Defective regulation of immune responses in croup due to parainfluenza virus, *Pediatr Res*, **19:** 716–20.

Werner CA, 1950, Mumps orchitis and testicular atrophy. I. Occurrence, *Ann Intern Med*, **32:** 1066–74.

Wertz GW, Kreiger M, Ball LA, 1989, Structure and cell surface alteration of the attachment glycoprotein of human respiratory syncytial virus in a cell line deficient O-glycosylation, *J Virol*, **63:** 4767–76.

Wertz GW, Collins PL et al., 1985, Nucleotide sequence of the G protein gene of human respiratory syncytial virus reveals an unusual type of viral membrane protein, *Proc Natl Acad Sci USA*, **82:** 4075–9.

Wesselhoeft C, Walcott CF, 1943, Mumps as a military disease and its control, *War Med*, **2:** 213–22.

Yoshida T, Nakayama Y et al., 1986, Inhibition of the assembly of Newcastle disease virus by monensin, *Virus Res*, **4:** 179–195.

Yu Q, Davis PJ et al., 1992, Sequence and in vitro expression of the M2 gene of turkey rhinotracheitis virus pneumovirus, *J Gen Virol*, **73:** 1355–63.

Yuasa T, Bando H et al., 1990, Sequence analyses of the 3′ genome end and NP gene of human parainfluenza type 2 virus: sequence variation of the gene-starting signal and the conserved 3′ end, *Virology*, **179:** 777–84.

Yusoff K, Millar NS et al., 1987, Nucleotide sequence analysis of the L gene of Newcastle disease virus: homologies with Sendai and vesicular stomatitis viruses, *Nucleic Acids Res*, **15:** 3961–76.

CORONAVIRUSES, TOROVIRUSES AND ARTERIVIRUSES

S G Siddell and E J Snijder

1 Properties of the viruses	2 Clinical and pathological aspects

1 PROPERTIES OF THE VIRUSES

1.1 Introduction

Coronaviruses, toroviruses and arteriviruses are enveloped, positive-strand RNA viruses that infect vertebrates and can cause disease in their natural hosts. The genome organization and replication strategy are similar in all three groups of viruses but the differences in morphology and in genome size of the arteriviruses clearly set them apart. Coronaviruses and toroviruses are usually associated with respiratory or enteric disorders, although other organs (e.g. the central nervous system) can also be involved. The outcome of arterivirus infection can range from an asymptomatic, persistent carrier-state to lethal haemorrhagic fever.

The features that distinguish coronaviruses, toroviruses and arteriviruses from other positive-strand RNA viruses are primarily in the structure and function of the replicase gene:

1 The replicase gene comprises 2 overlapping open reading frames (ORFs), and expression of the downstream ORF is mediated by −1 ribosomal frameshifting.
2 Sequence analysis has identified common motifs, e.g. motifs characteristic of polymerase, proteinase or helicase functions, that are located at specific positions within the replicase gene.
3 In the infected cell, viral gene expression is mediated by a set of 4 or more 3′ co-terminal subgenomic mRNAs. Only the ORFs contained within the 5′ unique regions of each mRNA, i.e. the regions not found in the next smallest mRNA, are expressed as protein.

The features that distinguish coronaviruses, toroviruses and arteriviruses from each other are mainly in structure and function of the nucleoprotein gene:

1 The molecular weights of the nucleoprotein are 50–60 kDa for coronaviruses, c. 19 kDa for toroviruses and 12–14 kDa for arteriviruses.
2 The nucleocapsid structure has different morphologies: helical-extended for coronaviruses, helical-tubular for toroviruses and isometric for arteriviruses.

A number of other features help to define and distinguish these 3 groups of viruses. They include the organization of the virus genome, genome size, evidence of discontinuous transcription during subgenomic mRNA synthesis, the structure and function of the virus envelope (glyco)proteins and the intracellular budding of virus particles (Cavanagh et al. 1994, Holmes and Lai 1995, Plagemann 1995, Snijder and Spaan 1995).

1.2 Classification

At the present time the coronaviruses and the toroviruses represent 2 genera of the family *Coronaviridae*. The arteriviruses are designated as a separate, monogeneric family, the *Arteriviridae* (they were previously assigned to the family *Togaviridae*). It seems likely that a taxonomy recognizing the evolutionary relationships of the *Arteriviridae* and the *Coronaviridae* will be formulated in the near future. In this chapter, this relationship is acknowledged by referring to all 3 virus groups as the coronavirus-like (CV-like) superfamily. The viruses that currently comprise the CV-like superfamily are listed, with their abbreviations and natural hosts, in Table 24.1.

Fourteen viruses are classified as species in the *Coronaviridae* (Cavanagh et al. 1995a). The prototype of the *Coronavirus* genus is avian infectious bronchitis

Table 24.1   Coronaviruses, toroviruses and arteriviruses

Natural host	Virus	Abbreviation
Coronaviruses		
Chicken	Avian infectious bronchitis virus	IBV
Cattle	Bovine coronavirus	BCV
Dog	Canine coronavirus	CCV
Cat	Feline infectious peritonitis virus	FIPV
Humans	Human coronavirus 229E	HCV 229E
Humans	Human coronavirus OC43	HCV OC43
Mouse	Murine hepatitis virus	MHV
Rat	Rat coronavirus	RCV
Pig	Porcine epidemic diarrhoea virus	PEDV
Pig	Porcine transmissible gastroenteritis virus	TGEV
Pig	Porcine haemagglutinating encephalomyelitis virus	HEV
Turkey	Turkey coronavirus	TCV
Toroviruses		
Horse	Berne virus	BEV
Cattle	Breda virus	BRV
Arteriviruses		
Horse	Equine arteritis virus	EAV
Mouse	Lactate dehydrogenase-elevating virus	LDV
Monkey	Simian haemorrhagic fever virus	SHFV
Pig	Porcine reproductive and respiratory syndrome virus	PRRSV

virus. The name coronavirus is derived from the solar corona-like (Latin *corona*: crown) appearance of virus particles in negatively stained electron micrographs. The prototype of the *Torovirus* genus is Berne virus, the name torovirus being derived from the curved tubular (Latin *torus*: lowest convex moulding in the base of a column) morphology of the nucleocapsid structure. In addition to the viruses listed in Table 24.1, a further coronavirus, rabbit coronavirus (RbCV) is considered as a tentative species of the genus. Three more coronaviruses, feline enteric coronavirus (FECV), sialodacryoadenitis virus (SDAV) and porcine respiratory coronavirus (PRCV) are often discussed in the literature as coronavirus species but the available data suggest that they could equally well be considered as variants of FIPV, RCV and TGEV respectively. In relation to the *Torovirus* genus, there are reports of an enveloped virus in the stools of patients with gastro-enteritis that resembles Breda virus (Beards et al. 1986), and evidence for a porcine torovirus has been obtained by electron microscopy, polymerase chain reaction (PCR) amplification and sequencing of the nucleoprotein gene and seroconversion after infection (A Kroneman and M C Horzinek 1995, unpublished). However, neither virus is as yet recognized as a member of the genus. The antigenic and sequence relationships of coronaviruses and toroviruses have been analysed in a recent review (Siddell 1995a).

Four viruses are classified as species in the *Arteriviridae* (Cavanagh et al. 1995b). The prototype of the family is equine arteritis virus (EAV). The name arterivirus is derived from arteritis (inflammation of an artery), a disease caused by EAV. Porcine reproductive and respiratory syndrome virus (PRRSV) is also often referred to as swine infertility and respiratory syndrome virus (SIRSV) or Lelystad virus. Serological cross-reactions between arteriviruses have not been reported and, to date, there has been no extensive phylogenetic analysis of sequence relationships within the arterivirus genus. Godeny et al. (1993) have reported a phylogenetic analysis of sequence relationships within the CV-like superfamily based on a relatively limited region of the replicase gene. This analysis indicates that viruses of the CV-like superfamily comprise a distinct evolutionary lineage among positive-strand RNA viruses.

1.3   Morphology and structure

Coronaviruses are pleomorphic but roughly spherical enveloped particles, 120–160 nm in diameter with a characteristic 'fringe' of surface projections 20 nm long. An inner 'fringe' of short surface projections is sometimes seen on MHV, BCV, TCV and HCV OC43 particles. Toroviruses are also pleomorphic, enveloped particles, 120–140 nm in diameter; they are disc-, kidney- or rod-shaped and, like the coronaviruses, are decorated with 20 nm surface projections. The nucleocapsid of both coronaviruses and toroviruses is helical but differs in morphology. Coronavirus nucleocapsids are extended whereas those of toroviruses are tubular. Arteriviruses are c. 60 nm in diameter and consist of an isometric nucleocapsid of about 35 nm that is surrounded by a lipid envelope with ring-like surface structures of 12–15 nm. The morphological features and the assignment of structural proteins to the coronavirus, torovirus and arterivirus virions are illustrated in Fig. 24.1.

Coronaviruses have an estimated molecular mass of

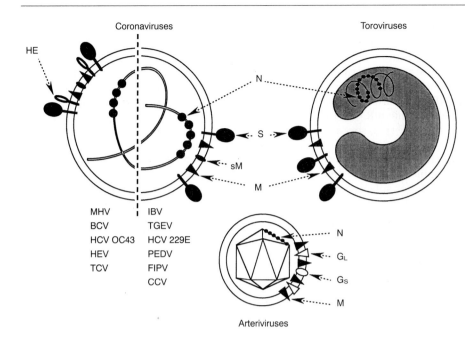

Coronaviruses

HE

MHV   IBV
BCV   TGEV
HCV OC43   HCV 229E
HEV   PEDV
TCV   FIPV
    CCV

Toroviruses

N — S — sM — M

Arteriviruses

N — G_L — G_S — M

Fig. 24.1 Schematic representation of coronavirus, torovirus and arterivirus virion structure, showing the locations of the structural proteins. The symmetries of the nucleocapsid structures and the division of coronaviruses into 'haemagglutinating' and 'non-haemagglutinating' subsets (see text, p. 473) are indicated. The stoichiometry of the virion components is shown arbitrarily. G_L, large glycoprotein; G_S, small glycoprotein; HE, haemagglutinin esterase; M, membrane; N, nucleoprotein; S, surface; sM, small membrane.

400×10^6 kDa and a buoyant density in sucrose of 1.15–1.19 g/cm^3. The buoyant density in CsCl is 1.23–1.24 g/cm^3 and the sedimentation coefficient $S_{20,w}$ is 300–500. Coronaviruses are sensitive to heat, lipid solvents, non-ionic detergents, formaldehyde and oxidizing agents. Toroviruses have a buoyant density of 1.16–1.17 g/cm^3 in sucrose and an estimated sedimentation coefficient ($S_{20,w}$) of 400–500. Virus infectivity is stable between pH 2.5 and 9.7 but rapidly inactivated by heat, organic solvents and irradiation. Arteriviruses have a buoyant density in sucrose of 1.13–1.17 g/cm^3 and 1.17–1.20 g/cm^3 in CsCl. The sedimentation coefficient is 200–230. The virions are highly unstable in solutions containing low concentrations of detergents.

1.4 Genome structure and function

The genome of coronaviruses and toroviruses is a positive-strand RNA molecule of c. 27 000–31 500 nucleotides (nt). This estimate of size is based on the nucleotide sequence of the IBV, MHV, HCV 229E and TGEV genomes (Boursnell et al. 1987, Lee et al. 1991, Herold et al. 1993, Eleouet et al. 1995) and the nucleotide sequence of a large part of the BEV genome (Snijder et al. 1988, 1990a, Snijder, Horzinek and Spaan 1990, den Boon et al. 1991b, Snijder et al. 1991a, 1991b). The coronavirus genomic RNA has a 5' cap structure, and coronavirus and torovirus genomic RNAs are polyadenylated at their 3' end. It is generally accepted that the genomic RNA of coronaviruses and toroviruses is infectious, a conclusion that is essentially based on the initiation of infection in susceptible cells with RNA extracted from purified virions (Brian, Dennis and Guy 1980, Snijder et al. 1988). In the light of the discovery of subgenomic RNAs in the virions of TGEV, BCV and IBV (Hofmann, Sethna and Brian 1990, Sethna, Hofmann and Brian 1991, Zhao, Shaw and Cavanagh 1993), it remains, however, to be shown that

the initiation of infection can be achieved with a cDNA clone corresponding to the full-length genomic RNA alone.

The positive-strand RNA genome of arteriviruses is significantly smaller than that of coronaviruses and toroviruses. Sequence analysis of the EAV, LDV and PRRSV genomes indicates a size of c. 13 000–15 000 nt (den Boon et al. 1991a, Godeny et al. 1993, Meulenberg et al. 1993). The genomic RNA of arteriviruses is polyadenylated at the 3' end. It has been reported that the genomic RNA of SHFV has a 5' cap structure but more recent data indicate that the LDV genome may, in fact, terminate with 5' phosphoryl-A (Chen, Faaberg and Plagemann 1994). Transfection experiments in vitro have shown that the genomic RNA of EAV and LDV is infectious (Brinton-Darnell and Plagemann 1975, van der Zeijst, Horzinek and Moennig et al. 1975). It has been shown, at least for LDV, that subgenomic mRNAs are not packaged into arterivirus virions (Chen, Faaberg and Plagemann 1994).

REGULATORY ELEMENTS

The genomes of coronaviruses and toroviruses contain a 5' non-translated region (NTR) of several hundred nucleotides. This region is almost devoid of AUG codons but a small ORF of 3–11 codons is conserved in the 5' NTR of viruses examined to date. It has been speculated that this 'mini-ORF' may play a role in regulating translation from the genomic RNA. The 5' NTR of arteriviruses is relatively short, about 150–220 nt, and does not contain a conserved 'mini-ORF'. By analogy with other positive-strand RNA viruses, it can be expected that secondary (or tertiary) structures in the 5' NTR, and possibly also elements located within coding regions of the genome (Kim, Jeong and Makino 1993, Kim and Makino 1995), will have a role in the replication and transcription of virus RNA.

As is described in the section 'Transcription' (p. 467), gene expression in the CV-like superfamily is mediated by the production of a set of subgenomic mRNAs in the infected cell. An element that plays an important role in this process is the so-called intergenic region. In coronaviruses and toroviruses, this motif is a species-specific AU-rich sequence of c. 10 nt, located upstream of the ORFs that are destined to become 5′ proximal in the subgenomic mRNAs. In the arteriviruses, the motif is also an AU-rich, species-specific sequence of 6 nt. However, in addition to its 'intergenic' locations, the arterivirus motif occurs many times in the genome, indicating that this element cannot be the only requisite for subgenomic mRNA synthesis.

It has been shown for the coronavirus MHV that the packaging of genomic RNA into virions is, at least partially, mediated by an RNA element located at the 3′ end of the replicase gene (Makino, Yokomori and Lai 1990, van der Most, Bredenbeek and Spaan 1991, Fosmire, Hwang and Makino 1992). This element, the so-called packaging signal, has been identified by the characterization of naturally occurring, packaged and non-packaged defective interfering (DI) RNA molecules and the analysis of packaging using in vitro synthesized, mutated DI RNA transfected into helper-virus-infected cells. It is surprising that the packaging of DI RNA in cells infected with the closely related coronavirus BCV does not seem to require the same element (Chang et al. 1994).

The 3′ NTR of viruses belonging to the CV-like superfamily comprises 60–150 nt (arteriviruses) or 200–500 nt (coronaviruses and toroviruses) following the last functional ORF and preceding the polyadenylate tract. It can be expected that secondary (or tertiary) structures in the 5′ NTR will have a role in replication and transcription (Yu and Leibowitz 1995b). In the coronaviruses, a common sequence, related to the motif $^G/_U GGAAGAGC^U/_C$, is found 70–80 nt from the 3′ end of all 3′ NTRs examined to date. The function of this conserved element is unknown. It is not present in the 3′ NTR of BEV or arteriviruses. The only significant nucleotide sequence conservation that has been found in the 3′ NTR of arteriviruses is located immediately upstream of the polyadenylate tract.

OPEN READING FRAMES

The available data suggest that the genomes of viruses belonging to the CV-like superfamily contain between 6 and 11 functional ORFs. The easiest to define are those located toward the 3′ end of the genome, encoding the structural proteins (Fig. 24.2). For coronaviruses and toroviruses, these are the surface (S), membrane (M) and nucleoprotein (N) ORFs and for the arteriviruses they are the large glycoprotein (G_L), small glycoprotein (G_S), membrane (M) and nucleoprotein (N) ORFs. The gene order, 5′-surface glycoprotein(s) ORF(s)/membrane protein ORF/nucleocapsid protein ORF-3′, is conserved in the genome of all CV-like viruses studied to date.

The genomes of coronaviruses contain a fourth structural protein ORF, encoding the sM (small membrane) protein, located 5′ proximal to the M pro-tein ORF. The genomes of toroviruses and a subset of coronaviruses (e.g. HCV OC43, MHV, BCV) also contain a fifth structural protein gene, the haemagglutinin esterase (HE) ORF. The location of this ORF in coronaviruses is 5′ proximal to the S protein gene, and in toroviruses it lies between the M and N protein genes. It seems that the HE gene is not essential and may be converted to a pseudogene; for example, during prolonged passage of virus in tissue culture.

In ORFs that encode non-structural proteins, the CV-like superfamily genome is dominated by the replicase (*rep*) gene (also referred to as the RNA polymerase gene or RNA polymerase locus). The replicase gene consists of 2 large ORFs encompassing c. 10 000 nt (arteriviruses) or 20 000 nt (coronaviruses and toroviruses) toward the 5′-end of the genome. These ORFs, *rep*1a and *rep*1b, overlap in the −1 reading frame. The extent of the overlap varies but invariably encompasses a specific sequence motif, UUUAAAC (or GUUAAAC in the case of EAV), which is referred to as the 'shifty' sequence. Immediately downstream of the shifty sequence is a characteristic RNA structure, the pseudoknot, which can be formed by base-pairing. Together, these 2 elements mediate −1 ribosomal frameshifting during expression of the replicase gene (Brierley, Digard and Inglis 1989).

In contrast to the replicase gene, the pattern and arrangement of the remaining non-structural protein ORFs in the genomes of CV-like viruses depend on the virus genus. In the toroviruses, there is no evidence for non-structural genes other than the replicase gene. In the arteriviruses, 2 putative genes, designated ORFs 3 and 4, are located between the large and small glycoprotein genes. The translation products of these ORFs have not yet been identified and they could, at least theoretically, be non-structural proteins. Based on the properties of the predicted proteins, however, it seems more likely that these ORFs encode structural proteins. Finally, in the coronaviruses there is a diverse and complex pattern of non-structural genes, even for viruses that are considered to be closely related. The reasons for this complexity are probably 2-fold. First, many coronavirus genes seem to encode proteins with accessory functions. Thus, under certain conditions (e.g. adaptation and propagation in cultured cells), mutations accumulate which lead to the inactivation and even deletion of these genes. Secondly, not only divergence from a common ancestor but also RNA recombination seem to have been a major driving force in the evolution of coronavirus (and torovirus) genomes (Lai et al. 1985, Keck et al. 1988, Luytjes et al. 1988, Kusters et al. 1990, Snijder et al. 1991b, Masters et al. 1994, Jia et al. 1995, Kottier, Cavanagh and Britton 1995).

1.5 Replication

A hallmark of the CV-like superfamily of viruses is the production of a set of multiple, subgenomic, 3′ co-terminal mRNAs in the infected cell. The subgenomic mRNAs are synthesized in non-equimolar amounts but in relatively constant proportions throughout the rep-

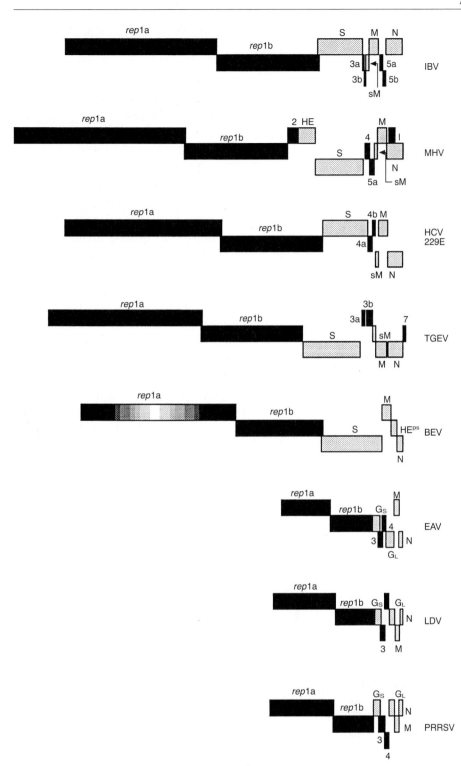

Fig. 24.2 Genomic structure of CV-like viruses. The genomic ORFs encoding structural proteins are lightly shaded; those encoding non-structural proteins are solid. The ORFs are drawn to scale in the correct relative reading frames. ORF *rep*1a is defined as reading frame zero. The ORF nomenclature is based on the recommendations of Cavanagh et al. (1990).

lication cycle. The structural relationship of these subgenomic mRNAs to the genomic RNA is illustrated for the murine coronavirus MHV in Fig. 24.3. The replication of MHV has been studied most intensively and it is assumed that MHV sets a paradigm for other CV-like viruses. However, it is already clear that the replication of coronaviruses, toroviruses and arteriviruses differs, at least in some details.

TRANSCRIPTION

The process by which viruses of the CV-like super-family generate multiple subgenomic mRNAs in the infected cell is complex and not fully understood. A detailed description of the extensive and sometimes conflicting literature in this area is beyond the scope of this chapter and only a summary of the most important aspects is presented here. For more information, the reader is referred to recent articles (den Boon, Spaan and Snijder 1995a, Holmes and Lai 1995, van der Most and Spaan 1995, Plagemann 1995).

1   The polycistronic genomic RNA of CV-like viruses is infectious.
2   Coronavirus and arterivirus subgenomic mRNAs are comprised of non-contiguous sequences. At their 5′ end they have a leader sequence of 65–100 nt (coronaviruses) or 150–210 nt (arteriviruses) that is derived from the 5′ end of the genome. Evidence for a common 5′ leader sequence in torovirus subgenomic mRNAs has not been obtained.
3   The site at which the leader and body of the mRNA are joined or, in the case of toroviruses, the 5′ end of the mRNA is defined by the position of a specific intergenic region preceding the mRNA body.

In the coronaviruses:

4   The bulk of the mRNA in the cell is produced from transcription intermediates that contain subgenomic, negative-strand RNA. There is one transcription intermediate per mRNA species.
5   The bulk of the subgenomic negative-strand RNAs have an anti-leader sequence at their 3′ end.
6   The subgenomic RNAs (positive or negative strand) are not able to initiate a transcription complex.

It has also recently been shown that EAV-infected cells contain a set of subgenomic transcription intermediates and it is likely that each intermediate contains a subgenomic minus-strand RNA with an anti-leader sequence (J A den Boon 1995, unpublished).

These observations can be interpreted using 2 dif-ferent models which essentially attempt to explain 3 basic questions. (1) How do subgenomic length templates arise? (2) How are the leader and body sequences in coronaviruses and arteriviruses joined? (3) What is the role of the intergenic sequence during the synthesis of mRNAs?

The first model (see Lai 1990) proposes that the genomic RNA enters the cell and is translated to produce RNA replicase that is used to synthesize a full-length negative-strand copy of the genome, the so-called antigenome. Transcription from the anti-genome is initiated at the 3′ end and a leader sequence is synthesized. This leader sequence is then used to prime transcription of the different mRNA bodies and a complete set of subgenomic mRNAs is synthesized. These mRNAs carry the RNA replicase into a transcription complex, negative-strand subgen-omic RNA is synthesized and serves as the template for the bulk of the mRNA synthesized in the cell. The essential features of this model are that discontinuous transcription takes place during positive-strand RNA synthesis and the complement of each intergenic sequence acts essentially as a promoter.

The second model (van Marle et al., 1995, Sawicki and Sawicki 1995) has a different 'scenario'. Again, the genomic RNA enters the cell and is translated to produce RNA replicase. The RNA replicase is then used, however, to produce not only antigenome but also a set of subgenomic negative-strand RNAs, the 3′ ends of which are defined by specific intergenic regions. These negative-strand RNAs then acquire an anti-leader sequence by a 3′ terminal extension process that involves discontinuous transcription. The 'full-length' negative-strand RNAs carry the RNA replicase into a transcription complex and act as templates for mRNA synthesis in the cell. In this model,

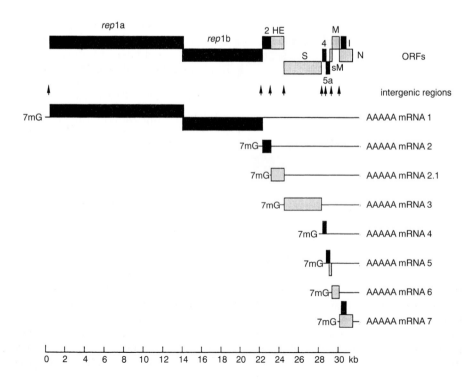

Fig. 24.3   Replication strategy of the murine coronavirus MHV, showing the genomic organization of MHV (as shown in Fig. 24.2), the structural relationship of the genomic and subgenomic mRNAs and the positions of intergenic regions. 7mG represents a 5′ cap structure and AAAA represents a 3′ polyadenylate tract. The ORF and mRNA nomenclature are based on the recommendations of Cavanagh et al. (1990).

discontinuous transcription takes place during negative-strand RNA synthesis and the intergenic sequences act essentially as attenuators of transcription.

In the torovirus mRNAs, which do not seem to have a 5′ leader sequence, both of the models described above can be easily modified to omit the element of discontinuous transcription (Snijder and Horzinek 1993). Also, as described above, it is implied that the intergenic regions play a pivotal role in the synthesis of mRNA, as promoters or attenuators of transcription. However, it has recently become evident that additional interactions, of RNA–RNA, RNA–protein or even protein–protein, may also be extremely important in this process (Yu and Leibowitz 1995a, Zhang and Lai 1995).

Translation

The production of a 3′ co-terminal set of subgenomic mRNAs in the infected cell allows for the expression of genes that are located internally on the non-segmented genome. By and large, the viral mRNAs are thought to be functionally monocistronic although usually, with the exception of the smallest mRNA, they are structurally polycistronic. This conclusion is based on the in vitro translation of coronavirus mRNAs (Rottier et al. 1981, Leibowitz et al. 1982, Siddell 1983, Stern and Sefton 1984, Jacobs, van der Zeijst and Horzinek 1986, de Groot et al. 1987) and conforms to the conventional 'ribosome scanning' model of translational initiation (Kozak 1989). Thus, taking MHV as an example (Fig. 24.3), the smallest mRNA, mRNA 7, encodes the nucleoprotein, mRNA 6 encodes the membrane protein, mRNA 3 encodes the surface protein and so on. If the genomic sequence is known and the position of the functional intergenic regions has been determined by sequence analysis of mRNAs, a 'translational model' can be deduced for each of the viruses belonging to the CV-like superfamily. It should be noted, however, that for arteriviruses, toroviruses and even the majority of coronaviruses this 'model' still needs to be confirmed by experiment.

The model outlined above describes the basic translational strategy of CV-like viruses. However, Fig. 24.3 indicates that there have to be exceptions. For example, MHV has no subgenomic mRNAs that could account for the expression of ORFs *rep*1b, sM or I in this manner. It is now clear that CV-like viruses also use a variety of alternative translation strategies to express some of their gene products.

In several coronaviruses (Brierley et al. 1987, Bredenbeek et al. 1990, Lee et al. 1991, Herold et al. 1993, Eleouet et al. 1995), BEV (Snijder et al. 1990a) and EAV (den Boon et al. 1991a) the region of RNA that encompasses the overlap of ORFs *rep*1a and *rep*1b is able to mediate a high frequency (20–30%) of –1 ribosomal frameshifting. Thus, ORF *rep*1b is expressed as a fusion protein with the ORF *rep*1a gene product. As described above, ribosomal frameshifting is mediated by a 'shifty' sequence, the actual position at which frameshifting takes place, and an RNA pseudoknot which is believed to slow or halt the ribosome as it translates this sequence (Somogyi et al. 1993). The most likely mechanism of frameshifting is simultaneous slippage of 2 ribosome-bound tRNAs present in the aminoacyl and peptidyl sites of the ribosome during decoding of the 'shifty' sequence (Jacks et al. 1988, Brierley 1995).

The subgenomic mRNAs encoding the sM proteins of MHV (mRNA 5) and IBV (mRNA 3) contain 2 and 3 ORFs, respectively, in their 5′ unique regions. The sM ORF is 3′-proximal in both cases and the mRNAs are functionally bi- and tricistronic, respectively (Budzilowicz and Weiss 1987, Liu et al. 1991). Therefore, the expression of the sM ORF has to involve the internal initiation of protein synthesis. The unique region of both mRNAs contains an element that is able to mediate the internal entry of ribosomes and initiate protein synthesis in a cap-independent manner (Liu and Inglis 1992, Thiel and Siddell 1994). This element has not yet been characterized but, by analogy with the picornavirus 'internal ribosome entry site' (IRES), it is likely to be comprised of a secondary (or tertiary) RNA structure.

Sequence analysis of the N protein gene of MHV and related coronaviruses (Lapps, Hogue and Brian 1987, Parker and Masters 1990, Kunita, Mori and Terada 1993) has revealed an internal ORF, the I ORF, which, in BCV, is expressed in infected cells and encodes a 23 kDa, membrane-associated protein (Senanayake et al. 1992). The I protein is translated from the same mRNA as the N protein, and it has been suggested, mainly on theoretical grounds, that the initiation of I protein synthesis conforms to the 'leaky ribosomal scanning' model proposed by Kozak (1989).

1.6 Non-structural polypeptides

Replicase

The replicase gene of viruses belonging to the CV-like superfamily encodes 2 polyproteins of extraordinary size and complexity. The translation of ORF *rep*1a theoretically produces a polyprotein of 450–500 kDa (coronaviruses) or 190–260 kDa (arteriviruses). Alternatively, as described above, –1 ribosomal frameshifting is used to express an ORF *rep*1a–1b fusion protein with a potential molecular weight of 750–800 kDa (coronaviruses) or 350–420 kDa (arteriviruses). Moreover, the polyproteins themselves are not the end-products of replicase gene expression. Instead, they are co- and post-translationally cleaved to produce a complex array of functional gene products. It is believed that, by and large, proteolytic processing of the replicase polyproteins is autocatalytic. The genetic analysis of MHV temperature-sensitive mutants with an RNA minus phenotype (Baric et al. 1990, Schaad et al. 1990, Fu and Baric 1994) supports this view.

Structural analysis of the predicted CV-like replicase polyproteins has revealed a number of putative functional domains that appear to have been conserved during evolution (Brown and Brierley 1995, Snijder and Spaan 1995). These domains and their approximate positions are illustrated in Fig. 24.4. In the predicted ORF *rep*1a polyprotein are found several domains characteristic of proteinase. These are of 2 types. First, domains indicative of papain-like cysteine proteinases (PCP) are located at the amino proximal end of the polyprotein. These may be single domains (e.g. IBV) or multiple domains (e.g. PRRSV). Secondly, towards the carboxyl end of the ORF *rep*1a polyprotein, a 3C-like cysteine protease domain (3CCP) is found in coronaviruses, with a counterpart in the form of a 3C-like serine proteinase domain (3CSP) in arteriviruses. The 3C-like proteinases are members of the superfamily of chymotrypsin-like proteolytic enzymes (Gorbalenya et al. 1989); despite the differences between the principal catalytic residues of the 3C-like proteinases of coronaviruses and arteriviruses, this domain is assumed to be part of the set of important domains that have been conserved during the evolution of the CV-like replicase gene (Snijder et al. 1996). This fact is reinforced by the similar substrate specificity of the 3CCP of coronaviruses (Liu and Brown. 1995, Lu, Lu and Denison 1995, Ziebuhr, Herold and Siddell 1995) and of the 3CSP of arteriviruses (Snijder et al. 1996). Thus, both enzymes cleave at sites that have a glutamine (coronaviruses) or glutamic acid (arteriviruses) at the P1 position and a small residue (glycine, alanine or serine) at the P1′ position.

In the *rep*1b gene product, which is expressed only in the *rep*1a–1b fusion protein, 4 domains have been conserved. First is a 'polymerase module' (POL) that is also found in a wide variety of putative RNA-dependent RNA polymerases. The alteration of the polymerase 'core' motif from glycine–aspartic acid–aspartic acid (GDD) to serine–aspartic acid–aspartic acid (SDD) is a feature that seems to be characteristic for the CV-like group of viruses. Second is a cysteine–

histidine-rich motif (C/H) that has been proposed to function as a zinc-finger, nucleic acid binding domain. Third is an NTP binding/helicase domain (HEL). The location of the helicase domain downstream of the polymerase module is unusual and characteristic of CV-like viruses. Fourth is a conserved domain at the carboxyl end of the ORF *rep*1b product, the so-called carboxy terminal domain (CTD), which also seems to be a feature of CV-like virus replicase polyproteins. As yet, no function has been suggested for this motif.

Compared with other positive-strand RNA viruses, the biochemical analysis of functions encoded in the CV-like replicase is still at an early stage. There have been occasional reports of RNA-dependent RNA polymerase activity in subcellular fractions of coronavirus-infected cells (Brayton et al. 1982, Dennis and Brian 1982, Mahy et al. 1983) or coronavirus-infected cells permeabilized with lysolecithin (Compton et al. 1987, Leibowitz and de Vries 1988). However, there is no evidence that these systems can initiate RNA synthesis and their application has been very limited. In contrast, there is an ever-increasing number of reports on the characterization of CV-like proteinases and the proteolytic processing of the replicase gene products (Weiss et al. 1994, den Boon et al. 1995b, Brown and Brierley 1995, Liu and Brown 1995, Lu et al. 1995, Snijder and Spaan 1995, Ziebuhr, Herold and Siddell 1995, Snijder et al. 1996). These analyses are, however, far from complete, and a detailed review of the subject is beyond the scope of this chapter. In summary, the papain-like proteinases seem to be largely responsible for the processing in *cis* of amino terminal and amino proximal products from the *rep*1a region of the replicase polyproteins, whilst the 3C-like proteinases are more likely to function in *trans* and are mainly responsible for self-excision and processing of the *rep*1a and

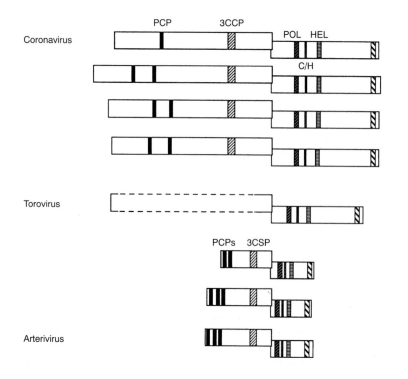

Fig. 24.4 Replicase gene organization of CV-like viruses. The replicase gene is shown as 2 ORFs that overlap at the site of ribosomal frame shifting (see text, p. 469). The ORFs are drawn to scale. Shaded boxes represent conserved domains. The relative positions of conserved domains are shown correctly but the extent of each domain cannot be defined precisely. The domains are usually defined in terms of their putative function. 3CCP, 3C-like cysteine proteinase; 3CSP, 3C-like serine proteinase; C/H, cysteine-histidine motif; CTD, carboxyl-terminal domain; HEL, helicase; PCP, papain-like cysteine proteinase; POL, polymerase.

*rep*1a–1b polyproteins downstream of the proteinase domain itself.

Other non-structural polypeptides

A variety of non-structural proteins (other than the RNA replicase) are encoded in the genomes of coronaviruses; little more is known about them than their predicted molecular weights and putative structural features deduced from computer-assisted analyses (Brown and Brierley 1995) (see Fig. 24.2). In some cases, the expression of non-structural proteins has been confirmed in coronavirus-infected tissue culture cells (Luytjes 1995) and evidence of post-translational modification (e.g. phosphorylation of the BCV ORF2 protein) (Cox, Parker and Babiuk 1991) has been obtained but the picture is very incomplete. Despite this lack of information, 2 interesting observations have been made. First, for some coronaviruses, variants have been obtained that are defective for the expression of one or more of these non-structural proteins but are able, nevertheless, to replicate normally in tissue culture. Thus, for example, MHV variants defective for the expression of the ORF2, ORF4 or ORF5a gene products have normal properties in vitro (Schwarz, Routledge and Siddell 1990, Yokomori and Lai 1991). This suggests that these proteins may be of functional significance only when the virus is replicating in vivo. Secondly, it seems that the functions carried by some non-structural proteins of the *Coronaviridae* may be looked upon as 'genetic cassettes'. Thus, for example, amino acid sequences that show significant homology to the ORF2 protein of MHV are encoded at the 3′ end of the BEV *rep*1a ORF (Snijder and Horzinek 1993). Another example of this concept are the proteins encoded by ORFs 4a and 4b of HCV 229E which seem to be equivalent to the single protein encoded by ORF3 of PEDV (Duarte et al. 1994).

1.7 Structural polypeptides

Whereas the RNA replicase provides clear evidence of an evolutionary link between viruses of the CV-like superfamily, the structural proteins indicate a complex phylogeny, probably involving both recombination and evolution from a common ancestor. For example, the nucleoproteins of CV-like viruses show no sign of any relationship (apart from the features common to almost all nucleoproteins) whilst the envelope proteins of coronaviruses and toroviruses are clearly related both structurally and functionally (for a discussion of the evolution of the CV-like superfamily, see Snijder and Spaan 1995). The structural proteins of coronaviruses, toroviruses and arteriviruses are listed in Table 24.2.

The nucleoprotein of CV-like viruses is a basic phosphoprotein that associates with the genomic RNA to form the nucleocapsid structure. However, the nature of this association must be very different for the 3 groups of virus. First, the sizes of the nucleoproteins differ markedly and, secondly, the nucleocapsid structures have very different morphologies. The coronaviruses and toroviruses have a helical nucleocapsid,

which is unique among positive-strand RNA enveloped viruses, whilst the arteriviruses have an isometric (cubical) nucleocapsid. The geometric parameters, the role of phosphorylation and the nature of the protein–RNA or protein–protein interactions that stabilize these structures have not yet been elucidated. On the basis of sequence analysis, Masters and colleagues have postulated a 3-domain structure for the coronavirus nucleoprotein and have shown that the central, hydrophilic basic domain is involved in RNA binding (Laude and Masters 1995).

CV-like viruses have a triple-membrane-spanning protein with a Nexo–Cendo configuration (den Boon et al 1991b, Faaberg and Plagemann 1995, Rottier 1995; see also Risco et al. 1995). For most M proteins, it is thought that one of the hydrophobic transmembrane domains functions as an internal signal sequence, although for the M proteins of TGEV, FIPV and CCV an amino terminal signal sequence is present. In the coronaviruses and toroviruses, transient expression studies have revealed that the M protein also carries a signal for retention in the Golgi apparatus (coronavirus) or endoplasmic reticulum (torovirus) of the cell. Only when it is associated with other components of the virion does the M protein proceed beyond these compartments. Despite the striking similarities in structure of CV-like M proteins, there are also significant differences. For example, only the M proteins of coronaviruses are glycosylated. In BCV, MHV and HCV OC43, *O*-glycosylation has been demonstrated; for the other coronaviruses, *N*-glycosylation is found (Rottier 1995).

There is good evidence that the coronavirus M protein is essential for virus budding. Throughout the infection there is a correlation between the intracellular sites at which progeny virions bud and the perinuclear location of the M protein. Also, in the presence of tunicamycin, spikeless, non-infectious coronavirions containing M protein are produced. However, it is probably incorrect to conclude that the M protein alone dictates the intracellular site of budding. Tooze and colleagues (Tooze, Tooze and Warren 1984) showed that the coronavirus 'budding compartment' actually lies between the rough endoplasmic reticulum and the *cis* side of the Golgi stack. Clearly other factors, for example interaction of the M protein with the nucleocapsid structure or other viral proteins (the S and sM proteins are likely candidates), may be required to 'organize' coronavirus budding in pre-Golgi membranes (Opstelten et al. 1994, Rottier 1995).

Very little is known about the functional role(s) of the arterivirus M protein. Recently, it has been shown that the EAV and LDV M and G_L proteins are associated in virus particles as disulphide-linked heterodimers and that covalent linkage is essential for virus infectivity (Faaberg et al. 1995, de Vries et al. 1995a).

The coronavirus and torovirus surface glycoproteins have a number of features in common: a large number (18–35) of potential *N*-glycosylation sites, an N terminal signal sequence, a C terminal transmembrane anchor domain, putative heptad repeat domains and,

Table 24.2   Structural proteins of CV-like viruses

Protein		Molecular weight (kDa)			Glycosylation	Abundance	Comments
		Corona-	Toro-	Arteri-			
Nucleoprotein	N	50–69	19	12–4	No	Major	Basic, phosphorylated
Membrane	M	30–35	27	18–9	Only coronavirus	Major	Triple-membrane-spanning protein
Surface	S	180–220	200	…*	Yes	Major	Peplomer structure with coiled-coil elements
Small membrane	sM	10–12	…	…	No	Minor	Acylated
Haemagglutinin esterase	HE	65	Pseudogene	…	Yes	Major	Subset of coronaviruses, disulphide-linked homodimer
Glycoprotein (small)	G_S	…	…	25	Yes	Minor	Disulphide-linked homodimer
Glycoprotein (large)	G_L	…	…	25–5	Yes	Major	Disulphide-linked heterodimers with M

*no such protein described

with the exception of some coronaviruses (e.g. TGEV, FIPV and HCV 229E), a centrally located, arginine-rich cleavage site for a 'trypsin-like' proteinase. When post-translational cleavage takes place (which varies according to the virus and the cell) the quaternary structure of the protein is an oligomer (dimer or trimer), each monomer being comprised of 2 sub-units, S1 (amino terminal) and S2 (carboxyl terminal), that are non-covalently linked. The S1 sub-unit is thought to be a globular protein that comprises the bulbous head of the peplomer. The heptad repeat domains, which are located in the S2 subunit, are thought to generate intrachain coiled coil secondary structure and provide the stalk of the peplomer with its rigid, elongated structure (Snijder et al. 1990b, Cavanagh 1995). The MHV S protein is acylated, and it has been speculated that fatty acid chains are associated with a cluster of cysteine residues located in the C terminal, hydrophilic tail of the protein (Schmidt 1982, van Berlo et al.1987).

The surface protein of coronaviruses has at least 2 major functions in virus replication. First, it binds to cellular receptors to initiate the infection process. The S protein-receptor interaction is complex and may involve the recognition of carbohydrates as well as protein (Schultze et al. 1991). However, the major class of protein receptor for MHV has been identified as isoforms of the Bgp glycoprotein, a group of murine, carcinoembryonic antigen (CEA)-related glycoproteins in the biliary glycoprotein subgroup (Dveksler et al. 1991, 1993). Similarly, the metalloprotease, aminopeptidase N (also called CD13) has been identified as the protein receptor for TGEV and HCV 229E (Delmas et al. 1992, Yeager et al. 1992). The second major function of the S protein is to mediate membrane fusion. This activity is necessary for the fusion of viral and cellular membranes at the cell surface during the initial stages of infection, and it may also occur later in infection by extensive formation of syncytium. In the coronaviruses, virus entry is thought to take place at the cell surface or within endosomes

prior to their acidification. However, mutants of MHV that depend on low pH for fusion activity have also been isolated (Gallagher, Escarmis and Buchmeier 1991). Cleavage of the S protein seems to enhance its fusion activity but it is not an absolute requirement for virus infectivity (Gombold, Hingley and Weiss 1993).

The arterivirus glycoprotein, G_L (also referred to as E or VP-3P), may be considered as 'equivalent' to the coronavirus S protein but its structure is completely different and quite unusual for a major viral envelope glycoprotein. Recent analyses suggest that it is a polytopic class I protein; after removal of the signal peptide, the processed protein consists of an N terminal ectodomain (about 30 amino acids for LDV and PRRSV, 95 amino acids for EAV) which is N-glycosylated, a segment that crosses the membrane 3 times and a C terminal endodomain of 50–75 amino acids (de Vries et al. 1992, Faaberg and Plagemann 1995, Meulenberg et al. 1995). The ectodomain of the EAV G_L protein carries a single polylactosaminoglycan, a very unusual modification for a viral glycoprotein. At the present time there is no information on receptor binding or fusion functions that are likely to be associated with this protein.

The second arterivirus glycoprotein, G_S (also referred to as VP-3M), seems to be a more conventional class I integral membrane glycoprotein with an N terminal signal peptide, a C terminal transmembrane segment and 1–4 potential N-glycosylation sites. The significant under-representation of G_S in EAV particles (at least in relation to its intracellular abundance) and the difficulty encountered in detecting the G_S protein in LDV and PRRSV virions raise the possibility that its incorporation into virus particles may be incidental. However, de Vries et al. (1995b) have shown that the G_S protein occurs in EAV-infected cells in 4 monomeric conformations and as disulphide-linked homodimers. Only the G_S dimers are specifically incorporated into virions, indicating that it may indeed have a functional role in particle morphogenesis.

The small membrane protein, sM, is unique to coronaviruses. All sM proteins are predicted to have a hydrophobic region, located in the amino terminal half of the polypeptide, which is flanked by charged residues. Adjacent to this hydrophobic domain is a cysteine-rich region, followed by an abundance of charged residues in the carboxy half of the polypeptide (Siddell 1995b). These features are indicative of an integral membrane protein, and a membrane location for the sM proteins of IBV, TGEV and MHV virions has been demonstrated (Liu and Inglis 1991, Godet et al. 1992, Yu et al. 1994). At present, the only post-translational modification attributed to the MHV sM protein is acylation (Yu et al. 1994). There are no published experimental data on the function of the coronavirus sM protein, although most authors have speculated on a possible role, namely in the assembly of virions. This is because small, integral membrane proteins have been described in several enveloped viruses and have often been implicated in the assembly process.

The haemagglutinin esterase glycoprotein is a structural protein that is restricted to a subset of the *Coronaviridae*. This subset is characterized by a strong haemagglutinating property and a second, shorter, fringe of peplomers on the virion surface. The subset of so-called haemagglutinating coronaviruses includes HEV, BCV, MHV, HCV OC43 and TCV (Brian, Hogue and Kienzle 1995). It should be noted that some other coronaviruses (e.g. TGEV and IBV) can also display strong haemagglutinating activity but this is a property of the surface glycoprotein S and is usually cryptic: treatment of the virus with, for example, neuraminidase is required to 'activate' haemagglutination. Finally, even for haemagglutinating coronaviruses, variants have been found that, for one reason or another, have lost the ability to express a functional HE protein. Thus, for example, the MHV strain A59 is defective in this respect (Luytjes et al. 1988). In the same way, it seems likely that the single isolate of BEV studied to date, which clearly carries the remnants of an HE protein gene but does not express an HE protein, is atypical. Further BEV isolates may, in fact, have a functional HE protein gene, as has been reported for BRV (Koopmans and Horzinek 1995).

The HE protein is a disulphide-linked homodimer. The monomer polypeptide (65–75 kDa) has a Nexo–Cendo configuration and is *N*-glycosylated in the ectodomain. Transient expression of the MHV and BCV HE proteins has shown that the protein has both haemagglutin and esterase activities (Parker, Yoo and Babiuk 1990, Pfleiderer et al. 1991, Yoo et al. 1992). The acetylesterase activity of BCV is specific for *N*-acetyl-9-*O*-neuraminic acid (Vlasak et al. 1988). Comparison of the coronavirus HE protein sequence and the sequence of the influenza C virus HEF protein reveals a remarkable degree of conservation, including, for example, many cysteine residues and the active site motif 'phenylalanine–glycine–aspartic acid–serine–arginine' (PGDSR) (Vlasak et al. 1988). It has been speculated that the HE gene of coronaviruses has been acquired by an RNA recombination event between ancestral coronaviruses and influenza C viruses (Luytjes et al. 1988).

The functional importance of the coronavirus HE protein is not yet clear. On the one hand, there is evidence for a functional role: for example, monoclonal antibodies specific for the BCV HE protein are able to neutralize virus infectivity (Derget and Babiuk 1987). On the other hand, MHV A59, which does not have an HE protein, is able to replicate quite normally in tissue culture. Moreover, it has been shown that, even for MHV strains that express high levels of HE, the HE-ligand interaction alone is not sufficient to mediate infection (Gagnetin et al. 1995). One possibility is that the interaction of HE with *N*-acetyl-9-*O*-neuraminic acid serves to concentrate virus on the cell membrane and thereby facilitates the interaction of the coronavirus S protein with its specific protein receptor molecule. As the levels of cell surface 9-*O*-acetylneuraminic acid can differ dramatically in vivo, this interaction may still be an important determinant of pathogenicity.

1.8 Immunogens

HUMORAL IMMUNITY

The surface glycoprotein, S (coronaviruses and toroviruses), and the large glycoprotein, G_L (arteriviruses), are the major inducers of neutralizing antibody during natural infection, although the degree to which this antibody affords protection varies from virus to virus (Coutelier et al. 1986, Horzinek et al. 1986, Balasuriya et al. 1995, Cavanagh 1995, Chirnside et al. 1995, Corapi et al. 1995). Only the antigenic structure of the coronavirus S protein has been studied in any detail and the picture that emerges is complex (Cavanagh 1995). Essentially, the majority of virus neutralization (VN) epitopes seem to be located on the S1 subunit (or the amino terminal half of the S protein if it is not cleaved) and they are 'conformational' in the sense that they are comprised of amino acids that are brought into close proximity by the folding of the protein. The VN epitopes are clustered into domains, one of which is usually immunodominant, although 2–3 domains may carry VN epitopes. Glycosylation seems to be an important component of VN epitope structure. Some studies have indicated that VN epitopes may be located on the S2 subunit (or carboxyl half of the protein) and that amino acids in the S2 subunit can modulate the recognition of VN epitopes located in the S1 subunit (Kusters et al. 1989, Luytjes et al. 1989, Grosse and Siddell 1994). It should be kept in mind that, although many VN epitopes have been defined, the mechanisms of virus neutralization remain essentially unknown.

Although the S and G_L proteins are the prime inducers of humoral immunity, antibody responses to other structural proteins of CV-like viruses may also have a role in protection. Some monoclonal antibodies specific for the MHV or TGEV M protein can neutralize virus infectivity in vitro (Woods, Wesley and Kapke 1988, Fleming et al. 1989, Risco et al. 1995) and, as already mentioned (see p. 473), HE-specific antibodies are able to neutralize BCV infectivity (Derget and Babuik 1987). It has been shown that sM specific antibodies are able to neutralize MHV infectivity in the presence of complement (Yu et al. 1994). The relevance of these observations to the situation in vivo is, however, unclear.

Cell-mediated immunity

As for most other viruses, the cell-mediated immune response to CV-like virus infection is less well characterized than the humoral immune response. Also, for technical reasons, most of the information we have relates to murine infections (MHV or LDV), often in an experimental setting. Nevertheless, there is good evidence that the coronavirus S, M and N proteins, as well as the arterivirus N protein, are targets for cellular immune recognition (Boots et al. 1992, Mobley et al. 1992, Bergmann, McMillan and Stohlman 1993, Ignjatovic and Galli 1993, Anton et al. 1995, Castro and Perlman 1995, Flory et al. 1995, Plagemann 1995, Stohlman et al. 1995, Xue, Jaszewski and Perlman 1995). In a few cases, specific T cell epitopes have been defined and helper or cytotoxic functions have been attributed to T cell subpopulations. There is some preliminary evidence that non-structural proteins may also represent T cell immunogens (Stohlman et al. 1993).

In addition to MHC-restricted immune responses, coronavirus infections elicit lymphokine responses. For example, MHV infection of 129/Sv mice triggers a transient increase in the level of IL-12 (p40) mRNA present in pooled spleen cells (Coutelier, van Broeck and Wolf 1995). Also, the M protein of TGEV can induce, directly or indirectly, the production of interferon-α in lymphocytes (Laude et al. 1992). The significance of these types of response for immunity has not yet been defined but there seems little doubt that they play an important role in particular situations.

2 Clinical and pathological aspects

2.1 Introduction

The spectrum of disease caused by CV-like viruses is summarized in Table 24.3. As is the case with many viruses, the majority of infections are asymptomatic, perhaps reflecting the pathogenic equilibrium reached during the co-evolution of host and pathogen. Many of the clinical diseases listed in Table 24.3 are, in fact, manifested only in immunodeficient animals (e.g. neonates or during pregnancy). In contrast, when a non-natural host is infected, or when the natural host is infected by an unusual route or virus variant, fulminant disease can also ensue. In the following review, only natural infections of major importance are discussed. For a discussion of less common and experimental infections with CV-like viruses the reader is referred to recent review articles (Plagemann and Moennig 1991, Plagemann et al. 1994, Dales and

Anderson 1995, Garwes 1995, de Groot and Horzinek 1995, Koopmans and Horzinek 1995).

2.2 Coronaviruses

Avian infectious bronchitis virus

Avian infectious bronchitis virus (IBV) is a pathogen of economic importance to the poultry industry worldwide. It causes a highly contagious disease affecting the respiratory, reproductive and renal systems of chickens. IBV infection results in a drop in egg production in adult birds and damages the developing reproductive system in young birds (Cook and Mockett 1995). Infection of the respiratory tract, most probably by aerosols, is the most important route of transmission. Young chickens are most susceptible to infection and the clinical signs include nasal discharge, sneezing, coughing and tracheal rales. IBV infection predisposes chickens to infection with secondary pathogens. Even young chickens will usually recover from an uncomplicated IBV infection, but the incidence of IBV-related nephritis, which can result in high mortality rates, seems to be increasing (Kinde et al. 1991).

Chickens respond to IBV infection by producing specific humoral antibodies of the IgM, IgG and IgA subclasses. The major viral antigens are the S and M proteins, and the S protein is a major immunogen. High concentrations of VN antibodies are thought to prevent the spread of virus from its primary replication site to the reproductive and renal organs. Local immune responses, in particular IgA, play a significant role in controlling the respiratory infection. Finally, cell-mediated immune responses also develop after IBV infection. Cell-mediated immune responses to the S, N and M proteins have been demonstrated (Ignjatovic and Galli 1993). At the moment, however, the relationship between cell-mediated immune responses and the degree of protective or long-term immunity has not been defined.

The diagnosis of IBV infection, in common with most other viruses, depends on 3 approaches: (1) isolation of the virus; (2) demonstration of a specific antibody response, usually by serological methods; and (3) demonstration of viral antigens or nucleic acid in clinical material.

Isolation   IBV can be isolated in tracheal organ cultures and embryonated eggs and propagated in tissue cultures. Infected allantoic fluid and tracheal organ culture supernatant fluid often contain enough virus particles to be visualized directly by electron microscopy. Alternatively, IBV isolates can be identified by immunofluorescence using polyclonal antisera or by antigen assays based on monoclonal antibodies. The existence of strain-specific monoclonal antibodies has also led to the development of serotype-specific ELISAs (Karaca and Naqi 1993).

Demonstration of antibody response   A range of serological tests are available to detect IBV antibodies. They include immunofluorescence, haemagglutinin inhibition, ELISA and virus neutralization. Probably

Table 24.3 CV-like virus infections in natural hosts

Virus	Host	Infection						Clinical disease
		Respiratory	Enteric	Reproductive	Neurological	MPS	Other	
Coronaviruses								
IBV	Chicken	++	..	+	..	..	+[a]	Infectious bronchitis
BCV	Cattle	..	++	..	..	..	..	Neonatal calf diarrhoea, winter dysentery
CCV	Dog	..	++	..	..	..	..	Enteritis
FIPV	Cat	+	++	..	+	..	+[b]	Enteritis, infectious peritonitis
HCV 229E	Human	++	?	..	..	..	..	Common cold
HCV OC43	Human	++	..	..	..	..	..	Common cold
MHV	Mouse	+	++	..	+	..	+[c]	Enteritis, rhinitis, hepatitis
RCV	Rat	++	..	..	..	..	+[d]	Pneumonitis
PEDV	Pig	..	++	..	..	..	..	Epidemic diarrhoea
TGEV	Pig	+	++	..	..	..	..	Transmissible gastroenteritis
HEV	Pig	+	++	..	++	..	..	Vomiting and wasting disease
TCV	Turkey	..	++	..	..	..	..	Transmissible enteritis
Toroviruses								
BEV	Horse	..	..	..	..	..	..	?
BRV	Cattle	+	++	..	..	..	..	Gastroenteritis
Arteriviruses								
EAV	Horse	+	..	..	..	++	+[e]	Rhinitis, abortion
LDV	Mouse	..	..	..	..	++	..	Asymptomatic
SHFV	Monkey	..	..	..	..	++	..	Asymptomatic
PRRSV	Pig	+	..	..	+	++	..	Pneumonia, abortion

MPS, mononuclear phagocyte system

++, main target for infection; +, secondary target for infection

?, circumstantial evidence of infection or disease

Other targets of infection are: a, kidney; b, serous membranes; c, liver; d, salivary, lacrimal glands; e, arteries the most sensitive tests are ELISAs using purified virus as antigen. In the future, it can be expected that these types of test will be significantly improved by the use of recombinant antigens.

Viral antigens   It is possible to detect IBV antigens or nucleic acids directly in clinical material. For antigens this can be done by using a monoclonal antibody-based immunoperoxidase procedure (Naqi 1990) or indirect immunofluorescence using antigen-specific monoclonal antibodies (Yagyu and Ohta 1990). For nucleic acids, PCR is a rapid and sensitive method to amplify and identify IBV RNA (Jackwood, Kwon and Hilt 1992, Kwon et al 1993). Combined with nucleotide sequencing, PCR will probably also become the preferred method for distinguishing between IBV serotypes.

At the present time, the control of IBV relies almost exclusively on vaccination and management. Both live attenuated and inactivated vaccines are available. It is generally believed that both vaccines can be used, usually in combination, to induce high levels of humoral antibody and that immunity represents protection against reproductive and renal disease rather than protection against respiratory infection (Cook and Mockett 1995). There are also 2 major problems associated with the use of vaccine. First, there are many serotypes of IBV and, although it is not necessary to develop a different vaccine for each serotype, occasionally serotypes emerge against which existing vaccines are not fully effective (Lambrechts, Pensaert and Ducatelle 1993, Pensaert and Lambrechts 1994). Secondly, although some serotypes probably emerge by antigenic drift (Cavanagh, Davis and Cook 1992a), there is at least circumstantial evidence to suggest that they may also emerge by recombination, possibly involving the live vaccine virus itself (Cavanagh et al. 1992, Jia et al. 1995).

HUMAN CORONAVIRUS

Human coronaviruses (HCVs) are now well accepted as a major cause of upper respiratory tract illness and, in particular, the common cold (McIntosh 1995). On the basis of serological cross-reactivity, it is possible to classify most HCV isolates into one of 2 main groups, of which HCV 229E and HCV OC43 are the prototypes. HCV 229E is related to the group of coronaviruses that include PEDV, TGEV, FIPV and CCV whilst HCV OC43 is related to the group of 'haemagglutinating' coronaviruses (Siddell 1995a). Infection with either HCV type results in essentially the same clinical picture. After an incubation period of about 3 days, the patient develops general malaise, headache, nasal discharge, sneezing and a mild sore throat. About one-tenth of patients also have a fever and one-fifth have a cough. The illness lasts about one week. Respiratory disease related to HCV infection is found world-wide, in all age groups and in both sexes (Myint 1995).

It is generally assumed that HCV infections are transmitted by aerosols. Epidemiological surveys of HCV 229E (Monto and Lim 1974) and HCV OC43

(Hamre and Beem 1972) infections indicate that the peak incidence of infection is in the winter and spring. Somewhere between 10% and 20% of individuals have serological responses indicative of HCV infection in any one year, although this figure may increase to 35% in some years. A high percentage of infections occur despite pre-existing antibody, and the frequency of infection gradually diminishes with age. Studies of coronaviruses as the cause of clinical illness indicate that human coronaviruses are responsible for c. 1–30% of all common colds, with a roughly equal number of subclinical infections (McIntosh et al. 1970, Wenzel et al. 1974). The possible association of coronavirus with more severe (lower) respiratory tract illness in children (Matsumoto and Kawana 1992), triggering exacerbation of asthma (Pattemore, Johnston and Bardin 1992) or as an enteric pathogen (Zhang et al. 1994), has also been discussed.

Little is known about the pathogenesis and immune response to HCV infection, mainly because there is no animal model available. Replication of the virus is optimal at 33–34°C and takes place in ciliated cells of the nasal epithelium (Afzelius 1994). Serum antibodies rise about one week after infection, peak at 2 weeks and decline to low levels after about 12–18 months. The serum antibody response is mainly directed toward the surface protein although membrane- and nucleoprotein-specific immunoglobulins are also synthesized (MacNaughton et al. 1981). It seems likely that the local immune response, perhaps including a cell-mediated immune component, is mainly responsible for controlling the primary infection (Tyrrell 1983). There is no evidence that HCV can spread from the nasal mucosa to other parts of the body, and the humoral immune response may be important for protection in this respect. Whatever the relative importance of local and humoral immune responses in controlling coronavirus infection, reinfections are nevertheless common and can occur within a year to the same serotype or within 2 months to a different serotype (Schmidt et al. 1986).

Human coronaviruses are notoriously difficult to isolate and, even after adaptation to tissue culture, propagation in vitro is very inefficient. Thus, the isolation of HCV in organ or tissue culture and the identification of HCV by electron microscopy or immunoelectron microscopy is possible only in specialized laboratories. Until a few years ago, the diagnosis of HCV infection relied mainly on serological methods, including, for example, ELISA, neutralization, immunofluorescence, Western-blotting and complement fixation (Myint 1995). These tests use purified viral antigen or, more recently, recombinant viral proteins (Pohl-Koppe et al 1995) and were generally employed for seroepidemiological studies rather than clinical diagnosis.

More recently, the detection of viral antigens and nucleic acids in clinical material has become a viable approach to the rapid diagnosis of HCV infection. HCV-specific monoclonal antibodies have been produced (Ziebuhr, Herold and Siddell 1995) and a 'nested' RT-PCR has been developed that is a sensitive and specific means of detecting both HCV 229E and HCV OC43 RNA in clinical material (Myint et al. 1994). Despite these advances, the detection of HCV infection is not generally done in routine diagnostic laboratories. This is undoubtedly due to the temporary and trivial nature of HCV infections and is unlikely to change unless an effective antiviral therapy becomes available. Even then, the diagnosis of HCV infection will probably be restricted to specific 'risk' groups.

PORCINE TRANSMISSIBLE GASTROENTERITIS VIRUS

The severity of disease caused by porcine transmissible gastroenteritis virus (TGEV) is related to the age of the animal. Infection of the piglet during the first 2 weeks of life causes vomiting followed by a profuse, watery diarrhoea that eventually results in dehydration and frequently death within 2–5 days. In older pigs, similar clinical signs are manifested but the mortality rate drops as the body weight of the animal at the time of infection increases. Transmission of TGEV is primarily from the ingestion of contaminated material, usually faeces or milk, and possibly via aerosols (Enjuanes and van der Zeijst 1995, Garwes 1995). TGEV has been reported in a large number of countries, but with different incidence and prevalence of disease. In countries where pig breeding has not been intensified, transmissible gastroenteritis is essentially epizootic with an incidence of disease every 2–3 years. In this situation, new outbreaks of disease are probably due to the cyclic reintroduction of virus. In countries with intensive pig breeding, transmissible gastroenteritis infection has become essentially enzootic. In this situation, the virus probably establishes a persistent infection in adult animals, in the gut or respiratory tract (Underdahl et al. 1974, Underdahl, Mebus and Torres-Medina 1975).

The pathogenesis and immune response to TGEV infection, especially in newborn animals, are quite well understood. The virus primarily infects and replicates in the apical tubovascular system of villous absorptive cells in the jejunum and ileum. Clinical signs seem to result from an increase in osmotic pressure in the lumen of the small intestine, caused by a failure to absorb milk lactose combined with an abnormal level of sodium secretion into the lumen (Garwes 1995). Because immunity requires the secretion of antibodies into the lumen of the gut, the rapid progression of the disease in the newborn animal probably provides insufficient time for immunity to develop, irrespective of whether the animals have reached a state of immune competence. The main source of immune protection for neonates, therefore, has to be antibodies provided by the mother in colostrum and milk (de Diego et al. 1992). Surprisingly, it has been shown that colostrum from non-immune sows can also provide some degree of protection (Enjuanes and van der Zeijst 1995).

Several techniques are available for the rapid diagnosis of TGEV infection, including immunofluorescence, reversed passive haemagglutination, ELISA, RIA and nucleic acid hybridization (Enjuanes and van der Zeijst 1995). Most important, a panel of type-, group- and interspecies-specific monoclonal antibodies have been developed to distinguish between viruses of the TGEV cluster, including PRCV (Sanchez et al. 1990). As described above, immune protection of piglets can be best achieved by natural lactogenic immunity provided by sows, or by artificial lactogenic immunity using serum or protective monoclonal antibodies. Virulent TGEV strains can be used to produce a solid immunity for both pregnant sows and their offspring (de Diego et al. 1992) but there is an obvious danger associated with this approach. Attenuated strains of TGEV and the PRCV variant have also been tested as vaccines but they have only limited efficacy (Saif and Wesley 1992). Efforts are being made to develop more effective vaccines. These may include non-infectious antigens that are targeted to the gut, and the use of live vectors with enteric tropism.

2.3 Toroviruses

BREDA VIRUS

There is clear evidence that torovirus infections are quite common in vertebrate species. For example, serological evidence of torovirus infection has been obtained in all ungulates that were tested using a BEV neutralization assay (horses, cattle, sheep, goats and pigs) and in rats, rabbits and some species of feral mice (Weiss et al. 1984). Torovirus-like particles have also been observed in stool specimens from horses, cattle, pigs, humans, cats and dogs (Koopmans and Horzinek 1995). It has been speculated that toroviruses may be associated with enteric disease in many species but, as yet, the only disease that can be definitely ascribed to a torovirus is Breda virus (BRV)-related gastroenteritis in cattle.

Seroepidemiological studies in a number of countries (Koopmans and Horzinek 1995) show that the infection of cattle with BRV (also known as bovine enteric torovirus) seems to be common throughout the world. In dairy cattle herds in the Netherlands, 85–95% of animals have antibodies to BRV by 1 year of age (Koopmans et al. 1989). Transmission probably takes place via the oral or the respiratory routes. BRV infections are usually limited to the gut, although there is some evidence for a possible respiratory involvement (Vanopdenbosch et al. 1992a, 1992b). The clinical signs of infection are watery diarrhoea with dehydration, weakness and depression. Predominantly affected are young animals 2–3 weeks of age; by the time they are 3–4 months old, they have only very mild or no diarrhoea, in association with virus shedding. There is some preliminary evidence that persistent BRV infection can be established in a herd (Koopmans et al. 1990).

The pathogenesis of BRV infection centres on the destruction of crypt and villus epithelial cells, particularly in the small intestine. Although the epithelial cells are rapidly replaced, the new cells lack a mature brush border and thus present insufficient absorptive surface and digestive enzymes. This decrease in absorptive and digestive capacity causes an accumulation of lactose in the gut lumen, which in turn results in water and electrolytic retention leading to diarrhoea. At least in young animals, the immune response following infection is probably of secondary importance, because protection depends mainly on maternal antibodies derived from colostrum and milk.

Attempts to isolate and propagate toroviruses have proved unsuccessful. BRV does not replicate in cell or tissue culture, and the isolation of BEV was a unique event that could be repeated only with the field sample of a single horse. The diagnosis of BRV infection has thus relied on immunological methods for the detection of BRV antigen or BRV-specific antibodies (Koopmans et al. 1989, 1990). However, there is evidence that BRV-infected animals shed ELISA-detectable amounts of virus for only 2–3 days (Woode et al. 1982), and the purification of BRV antigens from the faeces of experimentally infected gnotobiotic calves is a laborious and expensive procedure. More recently, nucleic acid hybridization and RT-PCR methods have been developed for the detection of BRV RNA in clinical material (Koopmans, Snijder and Horzinek 1991, Koopmans et al. 1993) and it is likely that this approach will be developed for diagnostic purposes and epidemiological studies. The control of torovirus-related disease currently depends on good management practices.

2.4 Arteriviruses

Equine arteritis virus

Equine arteritis virus (EAV) was first isolated in 1953 from an aborted equine fetus (Doll et al. 1957). Serological evidence suggests that EAV is widespread in the horse population (Timoney and McCollum 1988) but infections are generally subclinical and usually lead only to a mild, often unrecognized, infection of the respiratory tract. If the virus does cause overt disease, the clinical symptoms are acute anorexia and fever, usually accompanied by palpebral oedema, conjunctivitis, nasal catarrh and oedema of the legs, genitals and abdomen (Mumford 1985, Plagemann and Moennig 1991). The clinical symptoms of EAV infection vary widely, probably reflecting, at least in part, differences in virulence among EAV variants. Almost all naturally infected horses recover from EAV infection. Donkeys are the only other known host for the virus (Paweska et al. 1994).

The primary mode of EAV transmission is assumed to be via the respiratory route by contact with aerosol secretions from acutely infected animals (McCollum and Pricke 1971). The name 'equine arteritis virus' was derived from the characteristic necrosis of small muscular arteries following infection (Jones, Doll and Bryans 1957). Of greatest concern to the horse breeding industry, however, is the fact that the virus frequently causes abortion in pregnant mares (Doll, Knappenberger and Bryans 1957, Golnick, Moraillon and Colnik 1986). Furthermore, a carrier state exists in seropositive stallions in which EAV is produced in the semen (Timoney et al. 1986). These 'shedding

stallions' may thus infect brood mares by the venereal route.

Studies of experimentally infected horses have indicated that, as with other arteriviruses, the initial replication of EAV takes place in lung macrophages (McCollum et al. 1971). The virus infects the bronchial lymph nodes and then spreads throughout the body via the circulatory system. The cause of abortion in pregnant mares has not yet been elucidated. Neutralizing antibodies, mainly of the IgG class, are induced within a week of EAV infection, and this clears the virus from the circulation (McCollum 1969, Fukunaga et al. 1981). Clearly, however, this does not always prevent the virus from establishing a persistent infection, particularly in stallions. Neutralizing antibodies generally persist for years, and protective immunity is presumed to be lifelong (McCollum 1969, Mumford 1985). Only one EAV serotype has been recognized. As described above (see p. 473), the EAV G_L glycoprotein is the main inducer of neutralizing antibodies (Balasuriya et al. 1995, Chirnside et al. 1995).

Traditionally, the diagnosis of EAV infection has been based on the isolation and propagation of virus in tissue culture. The clinical materials most often used are nasopharyngeal, vaginal and rectal swabs or a buffy coat fraction from blood or semen. Rabbit kidney (RK-13), baby hamster kidney (BHK-21) and Vero cells are susceptible to infection and develop characteristic cytopathic effects.

Attempts to isolate virus from field cases have sometimes proved difficult. Several immunological assays for measuring EAV-specific antibodies in horse sera are available but the detection of neutralizing antibodies (TCID50 and plaque reduction assays) are used most commonly. The determination of the nucleotide sequence of the EAV genome has also allowed the development of assays based on RT-PCR (Chirnside and Spaan 1990, St Laurent, Morin and Archambault 1994). The control of EAV infection relies on a combination of vaccination and containment (Plagemann and Moennig 1991, Chirnside 1992). At present, a live attenuated and a killed virus vaccine are available. The live vaccine (McCollum 1969) induces long-lasting protection against clinical disease but does not prevent reinfection with wild type virus or temporary virus shedding (Mumford 1985, McCollum 1986). To avoid this problem, a formalin-inactivated vaccine (Fukunaga, Wada and Ka 1984) has been developed. Increased knowledge of the antigenic properties of the EAV G_L protein may provide the basis for the development of an EAV subunit vaccine (Chirnside et al. 1995).

2.6 Porcine reproductive and respiratory syndrome virus

Porcine reproductive and respiratory syndrome virus (PRRSV) is responsible for respiratory disease in pigs of all ages and for abortions and stillbirths in pregnant sows. The clinical signs of infection are transient fever, anorexia and respiratory distress. Mortality is generally

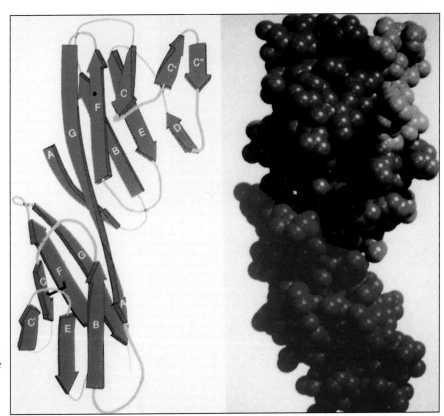

Plate 8.6 Backbone and solid representations of the 3-dimensional structure of CD4 (D1D2 domains). The D1 domain is in red, the D2 domain is in blue and the region of D1 implicated in the binding HIV gp120 is yellow. (From Bullough et al. 1994.)

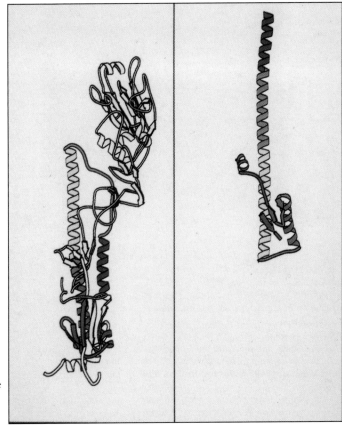

Plate 8.9 The conformational change induced by low pH in influenza virus HA. The neutral pH form of the HA1,2 monomer is shown on the left in the same orientation as in the HA trimer shown in Plate 8.3. The low pH form of the HA2 monomer is shown on the right. Corresponding regions are coloured identically. (From Bullough et al. 1994.)

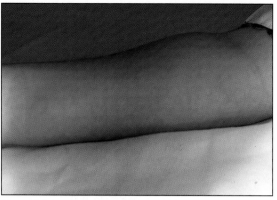

Plate 14.3 Erythema infectiosum: rash on the arm of a patient infected with B19 virus. (Courtesy of H Hochreutener, Ostschweizerisches Kinderspital, St Gall, Switzerland.)

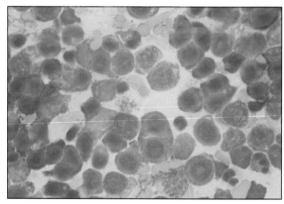

Plate 14.4 Appearance of bone marrow in the course of B19 virus infection in a patient with ß-thalassaemia and transient aplastic crisis. (Courtesy of L Schmid, Institute for Clinical Chemistry and Haematology, St Gall, Switzerland.)

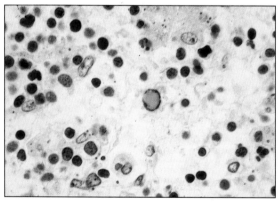

Plate 14.5 Parvovirus B19-infected erythroblast with intranuclear alterations in fetal liver. The nucleus is eosinophilic, enlarged and ballooned, showing marginal inclusions (staining: haematoxylin and eosin). (Courtesy of T Schwarz, Max v Pettenkofer-Institut, Munich, Germany.)

seen only in young piglets and is often associated with secondary infections (Meredith 1993, Plagemann 1995). Within the herd, PRRSV is thought to be transmitted mainly via aerosols. The virus is present in nasal secretions and swine can be readily infected by intranasal inoculation. Faecal–oral transmission may, however, also take place and infection between herds may involve the movement of infected animals or fomites. In pregnant sows PRRSV can be transmitted transplacentally, leading to reproductive failure in late gestation. The disease associated with PRRSV first appeared in the USA in the late 1980s. The first incidence of the disease in Europe was in northern Germany in 1991 and the virus is now common in the Netherlands and the UK (Drew et al. 1995). As with TGEV, the disease associated with PRRSV infection was originally epizootic but more recently the incidence of acute disease has decreased and mild, even inapparent, infections are becoming more commonplace.

Lung macrophages are the primary site of PRRSV infection and replication. Their destruction is probably the cause of the increased susceptibility of infected pigs to secondary bacterial infections. The virus may also spread to other organs. In addition to interstitial pneumonia, lymphocytic encephalitis is a common lesion found in PRRSV-infected animals. As with other arteriviruses, the initial phase of PRRSV infection is characterized by transient suppression of the cellular immune response coupled with an enhanced response to T cell dependent and T cell independent antigens (Murtaugh et al. 1993). PRRSV-specific humoral antibodies can be detected 1–2 weeks after infection and peak after 5–6 weeks. The neu-

tralizing antibody component reaches a maximum after 4–6 weeks and thereafter virus is generally cleared from the circulation. There is evidence that virus may persist in swine herds for periods of 2 years or longer but it is not clear whether this represents persistence in the individual animal, reinfection of animals or the infection of animals that have escaped earlier encounters with the virus.

The diagnosis and control of PRRSV infections still represents a significant problem. In tissue culture, PRRSV is most successfully isolated and propagated in primary pig lung macrophages. However, the costs involved preclude this as a routine diagnostic procedure. A number of continuous cell lines can be used for virus propagation but they do not seem to be equally susceptible to all isolates (Meredith 1993, Murtaugh et al. 1993). Serologically, PRRSV infections can be detected by virus neutralization, immunofluorescence and immunoperoxidase staining. However, it is clear that many isolates of PRRSV differ antigenically and it will be some time before the extent of this variation has been fully characterized (Drew et al. 1995). Finally, the detection of PRRSV RNA using RT-PCR is under development (Suarez et al. 1994, van Woensel, van der Wouw and Visser 1994) and promises to be the method of choice for the detection of low levels of viral RNA in the tissues of infected pigs. At present there are no vaccines or therapeutic measures available for the treatment or control of PRRSV. Control measures essentially consist of the eradication of infected herds and restrictions on the movement of pigs from enzootic areas. Both live and killed virus vaccines are under development.

REFERENCES

Afzelius BA, 1994, Ultrastructure of human nasal epithelium during an episode of coronavirus infection, *Virchows Arch*, **424**: 295–300.

Anton IM, Sune C et al., 1995, A transmissible gastroenteritis coronavirus nucleoprotein epitope elicits T helper cells that collaborate in the in vitro antibody response to the three major structural viral proteins, *Virology*, **212**: 746–51.

Balasuriya UB, Maclachlan NJ et al., 1995, Identification of a neutralization site in the major envelope glycoprotein (G$_L$) of equine arteritis virus, *Virology*, **207**: 518–27.

Baric RS, Fu K et al., 1990, Establishing a genetic recombination map for murine coronavirus strain A59 complementation groups, *Virology*, **177**: 646–56.

Beards GM, Brown DWG et al., 1986, Preliminary characterisation of torovirus-like particles of humans: comparison with Berne virus of horses and Breda viruses of calves, *J Med Virol*, **20**: 67–78.

Bergmann C, McMillan M, Stohlman S, 1993, Characterization of the Ld-restricted cytotoxic T-lymphocyte epitope in the mouse hepatitis virus nucleocapsid protein, *J Virol*, **67**: 7041–9.

van Berlo MF, van den Brink WJ et al., 1987, Fatty acid acylation of viral proteins in murine hepatitis virus-infected cells. Brief report, *Arch Virol*, **95**: 123–8.

den Boon JA, Snijder EJ et al., 1991a, Equine arteritis virus is not a togavirus but belongs to the coronaviruslike superfamily, *J Virol*, **65**: 2910–10.

den Boon JA, Snijder EJ et al., 1991b, Another triple-spanning envelope protein among intracellularly budding RNA viruses: the torovirus E protein, *Virology*, **182**: 655–63.

den Boon JA, Spaan WJM, Snijder EJ, 1995a, Equine arteritis virus subgenomic RNA transcription. UV inactivation and translation inhibition studies, *Virology*, **213**: 364–72.

den Boon JA, Faaberg KS et al., 1995b, Processing and evolution of the N-terminal region of the arterivirus replicase ORF1a protein: identification of two papainlike cysteine proteases, *J Virol*, **69**: 4500–5.

Boots AM, Benaissa TB et al., 1992, Induction of anti-viral immune responses by immunization with recombinant-DNA encoded avian coronavirus nucleocapsid protein, *Vaccine*, **10**: 119–24.

Boursnell ME, Brown TD et al., 1987, Completion of the sequence of the genome of the coronavirus avian infectious bronchitis virus, *J Gen Virol*, **68**: 57–77.

Brayton PR, Lai MMC et al., 1982, Characterization of two RNA polymerase activities induced by mouse hepatitis virus, *J Virol*, **42**: 847–53.

Bredenbeek PJ, Pachuk CJ et al., 1990, The primary structure and expression of the second open reading frame of the polymerase gene of the coronavirus MHV-A59; a highly conserved polymerase is expressed by an efficient ribosomal frameshifting mechanism, *Nucleic Acids Res*, **18**: 1825–32.

Brian DA, Dennis DE, Guy JS, 1980, Genome of porcine transmissible gastroenteritis virus, *J Virol*, **34**: 410–15.

Brian DA, Hogue BG, Kienzle TE, 1995, The coronavirus hemagglutinin esterase glycoprotein, *The* Coronaviridae, ed Siddell SG, Plenum Press, New York, 165–79.

Brierley I, 1995, Ribosomal frameshifting on viral RNAs, *J Gen Virol*, **76**: 1885–92.

Brierley I, Digard P, Inglis SC, 1989, Characterization of an efficient coronavirus ribosomal frameshifting signal: requirement for an RNA pseudoknot, *Cell*, **57**: 537–47.

Brierley I, Boursnell ME et al., 1987, An efficient ribosomal frame-shifting signal in the polymerase-encoding region of the coronavirus IBV, *EMBO J*, **6**: 3779–85.

Brinton-Darnell M, Plagemann PGW, 1975, Structure and chemical–physical characteristics of lactate dehydrogenase elevating virus, *J Virol*, **16**: 420–33.

Brown TDK, Brierley I, 1995, The coronavirus nonstructural proteins, *The* Coronaviridae, ed Siddell SG, Plenum Press, New York, 191–217.

Budzilowicz CJ, Weiss SR, 1987, In vitro synthesis of two polypeptides from a nonstructural gene of coronavirus mouse hepatitis virus strain A59, *Virology*, **157**: 509–15.

Castro RF, Perlman S, 1995, CD8+ T-cell epitopes within the surface glycoprotein of a neurotropic coronavirus and correlation with pathogenicity, *J Virol*, **69**: 8127–31.

Cavanagh D, 1995, The coronavirus surface glycoprotein, In *The Coronaviridae*, ed Siddell SG, Plenum Press, New York, 73–113.

Cavanagh D, Brian DA et al., 1990, Recommendations of the Coronavirus Study Group for the nomenclature of the structural proteins, mRNAs and genes of coronaviruses, *Virology*, **176**: 306–7.

Cavanagh D, Davis PJ, Cook JKA, 1992, Infectious bronchitis virus: evidence for recombination within the Massachusetts serotype, *Avian Pathol*, **21**: 401–8.

Cavanagh D, Davis PJ et al., 1992, Location of the amino acid differences in the S1 spike glycoprotein subunit of closely related serotypes of infectious bronchitis virus, *Avian Pathol*, **21**: 33–43.

Cavanagh D, Brian DA et al., 1994, Revision of the taxonomy of the *Coronavirus, Torovirus* and *Arterivirus* genera [news], *Arch Virol*, **135**: 227–37.

Cavanagh D, Brian DA et al., 1995a, Coronaviridae, *Virus Taxonomy*, eds Murphy FA, Fauquet CM et al., Springer-Verlag, Vienna, 407–11.

Cavanagh D, Brian DA et al., 1995b, Arterivirus, *Virus Taxonomy*, eds Murphy FA, Fauquet CM et al., Springer-Verlag, Vienna, 412–14.

Chang RY, Hofmann MA et al., 1994, A *cis*-acting function for the coronavirus leader in defective interfering RNA replication, *J Virol*, **68**: 8223–31.

Chen Z, Faaberg KS, Plagemann PG, 1994, Detection of negative-stranded subgenomic RNAs but not of free leader in LDV-infected macrophages, *Virus Res*, **34**: 167–77.

Chirnside ED, 1992, Equine arteritis virus: an overview, *Br Vet J*, **148**: 181–97.

Chirnside ED, Spaan WJM, 1990, Reverse transcription and cDNA amplification by the polymerase chain reaction of equine arteritis virus, *J Virol Methods*, **30**: 133–40.

Chirnside ED, de Vries AA et al., 1995, Equine arteritis virus-neutralizing antibody in the horse is induced by a determinant on the large envelope glycoprotein G_L, *J Gen Virol*, **76**: 1989–98.

Compton SR, Rogers DB et al., 1987, In vitro replication of mouse hepatitis virus strain A59, *J Virol*, **61**: 1814–20.

Cook JKA, Mockett APA, 1995, Epidemiology of infectious bronchitis virus, *The* Coronaviridae, ed Siddell SG, Plenum Press, New York, 317–35.

Corapi WV, Darteil RJ et al., 1995, Localization of antigenic sites of the S glycoprotein of feline infectious peritonitis virus involved in neutralization and antibody-dependent enhancement, *J Virol*, **69**: 2858–62.

Coutelier JP, Van-Broeck J, Wolf SF, 1995, Interleukin-12 gene expression after viral infection in the mouse, *J Virol*, **69**: 1955–8.

Coutelier J-P, van-Roost E et al., 1986, The murine antibody response to lactate dehydrogenase-elevating virus, *J Gen Virol*, **67**: 1099–108.

Cox GJ, Parker MD, Babiuk LA, 1991, Bovine coronavirus non-structural protein ns2 is a phosphoprotein, *Virology*, **185**: 509–12.

Dales S, Anderson R, 1995, Pathogenesis and diseases of the central nervous system caused by murine coronaviruses, *The* Coronaviridae, ed Siddell SG, Plenum Press, New York, 257–92.

Delmas B, Gelfi J et al., 1992, Aminopeptidase N is a major receptor for the entero-pathogenic coronavirus TGEV, *Nature (London)*, **357**: 417–20.

Dennis DE, Brian DA, 1982, RNA-dependent RNA polymerase activity in coronavirus-infected cells, *J Virol*, **43**: 153–64.

Deregt D, Babiuk LA, 1987, Monoclonal antibodies to bovine coronavirus: characteristics and topographical mapping of neutralizing epitopes on the E2 and E3 glycoproteins, *Virology*, **161**: 410–20.

de Diego M, Laviada MD et al., 1992, Epitope specificity of protective lactogenic immunity against swine transmissible gastroenteritis virus, *J Virol*, **66**: 6502–8.

Doll ER, Knappenberger RE, Bryans JT, 1957, An outbreak of abortion caused by the equine arteritis virus, *Cornell Vet*, **47**: 69–75.

Doll ER, Bryans JT et al., 1957, Isolation of a filterable agent causing arteritis of horses and abortion of mares. Its differentiation from equine (abortion) influenza virus, *Cornell Vet*, **47**: 3–41.

Drew TW, Meulenberg JJ et al., 1995, Production, characterization and reactivity of monoclonal antibodies to porcine reproductive and respiratory syndrome virus, *J Gen Virol*, **76**: 1361–9.

Duarte M, Tobler K et al., 1994, Sequence analysis of the porcine epidemic diarrhea virus genome between the nucleocapsid and spike protein genes reveals a polymorphic ORF, *Virology*, **198**: 466–76.

Dveksler GS, Pensiero MN et al., 1991, Cloning of the mouse hepatitis virus (MHV) receptor: expression in human and hamster cell lines confers susceptibility to MHV, *J Virol*, **65**: 6881–91.

Dveksler GS, Dieffenbach CW et al., 1993, Several members of the mouse carcinoembryonic antigen-related glycoprotein family are functional receptors for the coronavirus mouse hepatitis virus-A59, *J Virol*, **67**: 1–8.

Eleouet JF, Rasschaert D et al., 1995, Complete sequence (20 kilobases) of the polyprotein-encoding gene 1 of transmissible gastroenteritis virus, *Virology*, **206**: 817–22.

Enjuanes L, van der Zeijst BAM, 1995, Molecular basis of transmissible gastroenteritis virus epidemiology, *The* Coronaviridae, ed Siddell SG, Plenum Press, New York, 337–76.

Faaberg KS, Plagemann PGW, 1995, The envelope proteins of lactate dehydrogenase-elevating virus and their membrane topology, *Virology*, **212**: 512–25.

Faaberg KS, Even C et al., 1995, Disulfide bonds between two envelope proteins of lactate dehydrogenase-elevating virus are essential for viral infectivity, *J Virol*, **69**: 613–17.

Fleming JO, Shubin RA et al., 1989, Monoclonal antibodies to the matrix (E1) glycoprotein of mouse hepatitis virus protect mice from encephalitis, *Virology*, **168**: 162–7.

Flory E, Stühler A et al., 1995, Coronavirus-induced encephalomyelitis: balance between protection and immune pathology depends on the immunization schedule with spike protein S, *J Gen Virol*, **76**: 873–9.

Fosmire JA, Hwang K, Makino S, 1992, Identification and characterization of a coronavirus packaging signal, *J Virol*, **66**: 3522–30.

Fu K, Baric RS, 1994, Map locations of mouse hepatitis virus temperature-sensitive mutants: confirmation of variable rates of recombination, *J Virol*, **68**: 7458–66.

Fukunaga Y, Wada R, Ka M, 1984, Tentative preparation of an inactivated virus vaccine for equine viral arteritis, *Bull Eq Res Inst*, **21**: 56–64.

Fukunaga Y, Imagawa H et al., 1981, Clinical and virological findings on experimental equine viral arteritis in horses, *Bull Eq Res Inst*, **18**: 110–18.

Gagnetin S, Gout O et al., 1995, Interaction of mouse hepatitis virus (MHV) spike glycoprotein with receptor glycoprotein MHVR is required for infection with an MHV strain that expresses the hemagglutinin-esterase glycoprotein, *J Virol*, **69**: 889–95.

Gallagher TM, Escarmis C, Buchmeier MJ, 1991, Alteration of the pH dependence of coronavirus-induced cell fusion: effect of mutations in the spike glycoprotein, *J Virol*, **65**: 1916–28.

Garwes DJ, 1995, Pathogenesis of the porcine coronaviruses, *The* Coronaviridae, ed Siddell SG, Plenum Press, New York, 377–88.

Godeny EK, Chen L et al., 1993, Complete genomic sequence and phylogenetic analysis of the lactate dehydrogenase-elevating virus (LDV), *Virology*, **194**: 585–96.

Godet M, L'Haridon R et al., 1992, TGEV corona virus ORF4 encodes a membrane protein that is incorporated into virions, *Virology*, **188**: 666–75.

Golnik W, Moraillon A, Golnik J, 1986, Identification and antigenic comparison of equine arteritis virus isolated from an outbreak of epidemic abortion of mares, *J Vet Med*, **33**: 413–17.

Gombold JL, Hingley ST, Weiss SR, 1993, Fusion-defective mutants of mouse hepatitis virus A59 contain a mutation in the spike protein cleavage signal, *J Virol*, **67**: 4504–12.

Gorbalenya AE, Donchenko AP et al., 1989, Cysteine proteases of positive strand RNA viruses and chymotrypsin-like serine proteases: a distinct protein super-family with a common structural fold, *FEBS Lett*, **243**: 103–14.

de Groot RJ, Horzinek MC, 1995, Feline infectious peritonitis, *The* Coronaviridae, ed Siddell SG, Plenum Press, New York, 293–315.

de Groot R, ter Haar R et al., 1987, Intracellular RNAs of the feline infectious peritonitis coronavirus strain 79-1146, *J Gen Virol*, **68**: 995–1002.

Grosse B, Siddell SG, 1994, Single amino acid changes in the S2 subunit of the MHV surface glycoprotein confer resistance to neutralization by S1 subunit-specific monoclonal antibody, *Virology*, **202**: 814–24.

Hamre D, Beem M, 1972, Virologic studies of acute respiratory disease in young adults. V. Coronavirus 229E infections during six years of surveillance, *Am J Epidemiol*, **96**: 94–106.

Herold J, Raabe T et al., 1993, Nucleotide sequence of the human coronavirus 229E RNA polymerase locus, *Virology*, **195**: 680–91.

Hofmann MA, Sethna PB, Brian DA, 1990, Bovine coronavirus mRNA replication continues throughout persistent infection in cell culture, *J Virol*, **64**: 4108–14.

Holmes KV, Lai MMC, 1995, *Coronaviridae*: the viruses and their replication, *Fields' Virology*, 3rd edn, eds Fields BN, Knipe DM et al., Lippincott–Raven Publishers, Philadelphia, 1075–93.

Horzinek MC, Ederveen J et al., 1986, The peplomers of Berne virus, *J Gen Virol*, **67**: 2475–83.

Ignjatovic J, Galli N, 1993, Immune responses to structural proteins of avian bronchitis virus, *Avian Immunology in Progress*, Les Colloques No 62, ed Coudert F, Institut National de la Recherche Agronomique, Paris, 237–42.

Jacks T, Madhani HD et al., 1988, Signals for ribosomal frame-shifting in the Rous sarcoma virus gag–pol region, *Cell*, **55**: 447–58.

Jackwood MW, Kwon HM, Hilt DA, 1992, Infectious bronchitis virus detection in allantoic fluid using the polymerase chain reaction and a DNA probe, *Avian Dis*, **36**: 403–9.

Jacobs L, van der Zeijst B, Horzinek MC, 1986, Characterization and translation of transmissible gastroenteritis virus mRNAs, *J Virol*, **57**: 1010–15.

Jia W, Karaca K et al., 1995, A novel variant of avian infectious bronchitis virus resulting from recombination among three different strains, *Arch Virol*, **140**: 259–71.

Jones TC, Doll ER, Bryans JT, 1957, The lesions of equine viral arteritis, *Cornell Vet*, **47**: 52–68.

Karaca K, Naqi S, 1993, A monoclonal antibody blocking ELISA to detect serotype-specific infectious bronchitis virus antibodies, *Vet Microbiol*, **34**: 249–57.

Keck JG, Matsushima GK et al., 1988, In vivo RNA–RNA recombination of coronavirus in mouse brain, *J Virol*, **62**: 1810–13.

Kim YN, Jeong YS, Makino S, 1993, Analysis of *cis*-acting sequences essential for coronavirus defective interfering RNA replication, *Virology*, **197**: 53–63.

Kim YN, Makino S, 1995, Characterization of a murine coronavirus defective interfering RNA internal *cis*-acting replication signal, *J Virol*, **69**: 4963–71.

Kinde H, Daft BM et al., 1991, Viral pathogenesis of a nephrotropic infectious bronchitis virus isolated from commercial pullets, *Avian Dis*, **35**: 415–21.

Koopmans M, Horzinek MC, 1995, The pathogenesis of torovirus infections in animals and humans, *The* Coronaviridae, ed Siddell SG, Plenum Press, New York, 403–13.

Koopmans M, Snijder EJ, Horzinek MC, 1991, cDNA probes for the diagnosis of bovine torovirus (Breda virus) infection, *J Clin Microbiol*, **29**: 493–7.

Koopmans M, van den Boom U et al., 1989, Seroepidemiology of Breda virus in cattle using ELISA, *Vet Microbiol*, **19**: 233–43.

Koopmans M, Cremers H et al., 1990, Breda virus (*Toroviridae*) infection and systemic antibody response in sentinel calves, *Am J Vet Res*, **51**: 1443–8.

Koopmans M, Monroe SS et al., 1993, Optimization of extraction and PCR amplification of RNA from paraffin-embedded tissue in different fixatives, *J Virol Methods*, **43**: 189–204.

Kottier SA, Cavanagh D, Britton P, 1995, Experimental evidence of recombination in coronavirus infectious bronchitis virus, *Virology*, **213**: 569–80.

Kozak M, 1989, The scanning model for translation: an update, *J Cell Biol*, **108**: 229–41.

Kunita S, Mori M, Terada E, 1993, Sequence analysis of the nucleocapsid protein gene of rat coronavirus SDAV-681, *Virology*, **193**: 520–3.

Kusters JG, Jager EJ et al., 1989, Analysis of an immunodominant region of infectious bronchitis virus, *J Immunol*, **143**: 2692–8.

Kusters JG, Jager EJ et al., 1990, Sequence evidence for RNA recombination in field isolates of avian coronavirus infectious bronchitis virus, *Vaccine*, **8**: 605–8.

Kwoon HM, Jackwood MW et al., 1993, Polymerase chain reaction and a biotin-labelled DNA probe for detection of infectious bronchitis virus in chickens, *Avian Dis*, **37**: 149–56.

Lai MM, 1990, Coronavirus: organization, replication and expression of genome, *Annu Rev Microbiol*, **44**: 303–33.

Lai MM, Baric RS et al., 1985, Recombination between nonsegmented RNA genomes of murine coronaviruses, *J Virol*, **56**: 449–56.

Lambrechts C, Pensaert M, Ducatelle R, 1993, Challenge experiments to evaluate cross-protection induced at the trachea and kidney level by vaccine strains and Belgian nephropathogenic isolates of avian infectious bronchitis virus, *Avian Pathol*, **22**: 577–90.

Lapps W, Hogue BG, Brian DA, 1987, Sequence analysis of the bovine coronavirus nucleocapsid and matrix protein genes, *Virology*, **157**: 47–57.

Laude H, Masters PS, 1995, The coronavirus nucleocapsid protein, *The* Coronaviridae, ed Siddell SG, Plenum Press, New York, 141–63.

Laude H, Gelfi J et al., 1992, Single amino acid changes in the viral glycoprotein M affect induction of alpha interferon by the coronavirus transmissible gastroenteritis virus, *J Virol*, **66**: 743–9.

Lee HJ, Shieh CK et al., 1991, The complete sequence (22 kilobases) of murine coronavirus gene 1 encoding the putative proteases and RNA polymerase, *Virology*, **180**: 567–82.

Leibowitz JL, DeVries JR, 1988, Synthesis of virus-specific RNA in permeabilized murine coronavirus-infected cells, *Virology*, **166**: 66–75.

Leibowitz JL, Weiss SL et al., 1982, Cell-free translation of murine coronavirus RNA, *J Virol*, **43**: 905–13.

Liu DX, Brown TD, 1995, Characterisation and mutational analysis of an ORF 1a-encoding proteinase domain responsible for proteolytic processing of the infectious bronchitis virus 1a/1b polyprotein, *Virology*, **209**: 420–7.

Liu DX, Inglis SC, 1991, Association of the infectious bronchitis virus 3c protein with the virion envelope, *Virology*, **185**: 911–17.

Liu DX, Inglis SC, 1992, Internal entry of ribosomes on a tricistronic mRNA encoded by infectious bronchitis virus, *J Virol*, **66**: 6143–54.

Liu DX, Cavanagh D et al., 1991, A polycistronic mRNA specified by the coronavirus infectious bronchitis virus, *Virology*, **184**: 531–44.

Lu Y, Lu X, Denison MR, 1995, Identification and characterization of a serine-like proteinase of the murine coronavirus MHV-A59, *J Virol*, **69**: 3554–9.

Luytjes W, 1995, Coronavirus gene expression: genome organization and protein synthesis, *The* Coronaviridae, ed Siddell SG, Plenum Press, New York, 33–54.

Luytjes W, Bredenbeek PJ et al., 1988, Sequence of mouse hepatitis virus A59 mRNA 2: indications for RNA recombination between coronaviruses and influenza C virus, *Virology*, **166**: 415–22.

Luytjes W, Geerts D et al., 1989, Amino acid sequence of a conserved neutralizing epitope of murine coronaviruses, *J Virol*, **63**: 1408–12.

McCollum WH, 1969, Development of a modified viral strain and vaccine for equine viral arteritis, *J Am Vet Med Assoc*, **155**: 318–22.

McCollum WH, 1986, Responses of horses vaccinated with avirulent modified-live equine arteritis virus propagated in *E. derm* (NBL-6) cell line to nasal inoculations with virulent virus, *Am J Vet Res*, **47**: 1931–4.

McCollum WH, Pricke ME et al., 1971, Temporal distribution of EAV in respiratory mucosa, tissues and body fluids of horses infected by inhalation, *Res Vet Sci*, **2**: 459–64.

McIntosh K, 1995, Coronaviruses, *Fields' Virology*, 3rd edn, eds Fields BN, Knipe DM et al., Lippincott–Raven Publishers, Philadelphia PA, 1095–103.

McIntosh K, Kapikian AZ et al., 1970, Seroepidemiological studies of coronavirus infection in adults and children, *Am J Epidemiol*, **91**: 585–92.

MacNaughton MR, Hasony HJ et al., 1981, Antibody to virus components in volunteers experimentally infected with human coronavirus 229E group viruses, *Infect Immun*, **31**: 845–9.

Mahy BWJ, Siddell SG et al., 1983, RNA-dependent RNA polymerase activity in murine coronavirus-infected cells, *J Gen Virol*, **64**: 103–11.

Makino S, Yokomori K, Lai MM, 1990, Analysis of efficiently, packaged defective interfering RNAs of murine coronavirus: localization of a possible RNA-packaging signal, *J Virol*, **64**: 6045–53.

van Marle G, Luytjes W et al., 1995, Regulation of coronavirus mRNA transcription, *J Virol*, **69**: 7851–6.

Masters PS, Koetzner CA et al., 1994, Optimization of targeted RNA recombination and mapping of a novel nucleocapsid gene mutation in the coronavirus mouse hepatitis virus, *J Virol*, **68**: 328–37.

Matsumoto I, Kawana R, 1992, Virological surveillance of acute respiratory tract illnesses of children in Morioka, Japan. III. Human respiratory coronavirus, *Kansenshogaku Zasshi*, **66**: 319–26.

Meridith MJ, 1993, *Porcine Reproductive and Respiratory Syndrome*, Cambridge University Press, Cambridge.

Meulenberg JJ, Hulst MM et al., 1993, Lelystad virus, the causative agent of porcine epidemic abortion and respiratory syndrome (PEARS), is related to LDV and EAV, *Virology*, **192**: 62–72.

Meulenberg JJ, Petersen den Besten A et al., 1995, Characteriz-

ation of proteins encoded by ORFs 2 to 7 of Lelystad virus, *Virology*, **206**: 155–63.

Mobley J, Evans G et al., 1992, Immune response to a murine coronavirus: identification of a homing receptor-negative CD4+ T cell subset that responds to viral glycoproteins, *Virology*, **187**: 443–52.

Monto AS, Lim SK, 1974, The Tecumseh study of respiratory illness. VI. Frequency of and relationship between outbreaks of coronavirus infection, *J Infect Dis*, **129**: 271–6.

van der Most R, Bredenbeek PJ, Spaan WJ, 1991, A domain at the 3′ end of the polymerase gene is essential for encapsidation of coronavirus defective interfering RNAs, *J Virol*, **65**: 3219–26.

van der Most RG, Spann WJM, 1995, Coronavirus replication, transcription, and RNA recombination, *The* Coronaviridae, ed Siddell SG, Plenum Press, New York, 11–31.

Mumford JA, 1985, Preparing for equine arteritis, *Equine Vet J*, **17**: 6–11.

Murtaugh M, Collins JE, Rossow KD, 1993, Porcine respiratory and reproductive syndrome, *A D Leman Swine Conference*, University of Minnesota, Minneapolis MN, 43–53.

Myint SH, 1995, Human coronavirus infections, In *The* Coronaviridae, ed Siddell SG, Plenum Press, New York, 389–401.

Myint S, Johnston S et al., 1994, Evaluation of nested polymerase chain methods for the detection of human coronaviruses 229E and OC43, *Mol Cell Probes*, **8**: 357–64.

Naqi SA, 1990, A monoclonal antibody-based immunoperoxidase procedure for rapid detection of infectious bronchitis virus in infected tissues, *Avian Dis*, **34**: 893–8.

Opstelten DJ, de Groote P et al., 1994, Folding of the mouse hepatitis virus spike protein and its association with the membrane protein, *Arch Virol Suppl*, **9**: 319–28.

Parker MD, Yoo D, Babiuk LA, 1990, Expression and secretion of the bovine coronavirus hemagglutinin-esterase glycoprotein by insect cells infected with recombinant baculoviruses, *J Virol*, **64**: 1625–9.

Parker MM, Masters PS, 1990, Sequence comparison of the N genes of five strains of the coronavirus mouse hepatitis virus suggests a three domain structure for the nucleocapsid protein, *Virology*, **179**: 463–8.

Pattemore PK, Johnston SL, Bardin PG, 1992, Viruses as precipitants of asthma symptoms. I. Epidemiology, *Clin Exp Allergy*, **22**: 325–36.

Paweska JT, Volkmann DH et al., 1994, Sexual and in-contact transmission of asinine strain of equine arteritis virus among donkeys, *J Clin Microbiol*, **33**: 3296–9.

Pensaert M, Lambrechts C, 1994, Vaccination of chickens against a Belgian nephropathogenic strain of infectious bronchitis virus B1648 using attenuated homologous and heterologous strains, *Avian Pathol*, **23**: 631–41.

Pfleiderer M, Routledge E et al., 1991, High level transient expression of the murine coronavirus haemagglutinin-esterase, *J Gen Virol*, **72**: 1309–15.

Plagemann PWG, 1995, Lactate dehydrogenase-elevating virus and related viruses, *Fields' Virology*, 3rd edn, eds Fields BN, Knipe DM et al., Lippincott–Raven Publishers, Philadelphia PA, 1105–20.

Plagemann PGW, Moennig V, 1991, Lactate dehydrogenase-elevating virus, equine arteritis virus, and simian haemorrhagic fever virus: a new group of positive-stranded RNA viruses, *Adv Virus Res*, **41**: 99–192.

Plagemann PGW, Rowland RRR et al., 1994, Lactate dehydrogenase-elevating virus: an ideal persistent virus?, *Springer Semin Immunol*, **17**: 167–86.

Pohl-Koppe A, Raabe T et al., 1995, Detection of human coronavirus 229E-specific antibodies using recombinant fusion proteins, *J Virol Methods*, **55**: 175–83.

Risco C, Anton IM et al., 1995, Membrane protein molecules of transmissible gastroenteritis coronavirus also expose the carboxy-terminal region on the external surface of the virion, *J Virol*, **69**: 5269–77.

Rottier PJM, 1995, The coronavirus membrane glycoprotein, *The Coronaviridae*, ed Siddell SG, Plenum Press, New York, 115–39.

Rottier PJM, Spaan WJM et al., 1981, Translation of three mouse hepatitis virus strain A59 subgenomic RNAs in *Xenopus laevis* oocytes, *J Virol*, **38**: 20–6.

Saif LJ, Wesley RD, 1992, Transmissible gastroenteritis, *Diseases of Swine*, eds Leman AD, Straw B et al., Iowa State University Press, Ames, 362–86.

Sanchez CM, Jimenez G et al., 1990, Antigenic homology among coronaviruses related to transmissible gastroenteritis virus, *Virology*, **174**: 410–17.

Sawicki SG, Sawicki DL, 1995, Coronaviruses use discontinuous extension for synthesis of sub-genome length negative strands, *Corona- and Related Viruses*: Current Concepts in Molecular Biology and Pathogenesis, eds Talbot PJ, Levy GA, Plenum Press, New York, 499–506.

Schaad MC, Stohlman SA et al., 1990, Genetics of mouse hepatitis virus transcription: identification of cistrons which may function in positive and negative strand RNA synthesis, *Virology*, **177**: 634–45.

Schmidt MFG, 1982, Acylation of viral spike glycoproteins: a feature of enveloped RNA viruses, *Virology*, **116**: 327–38.

Schmidt OW, Allan ID et al., 1986, Rises in titers of antibody to human coronaviruses OC43 and 229E in Seattle families during 1975–1979, *Am J Epidemiol*, **123**: 862–8.

Schultze B, Gross HJ et al., 1991, The S protein of bovine coronavirus is a hemagglutinin recognizing 9-*O*-acetylated sialic acid as a receptor determinant, *J Virol*, **65**: 6232–7.

Schwarz B, Routledge E, Siddell SG, 1990, Murine coronavirus nonstructural protein ns2 is not essential for virus replication in transformed cells, *J Virol*, **64**: 4784–91.

Senanayake SD, Hofmann MA et al., 1992, The nucleocapsid protein gene of bovine coronavirus is bicistronic, *J Virol*, **66**: 5277–83.

Sethna PB, Hofmann MA, Brian DA, 1991, Minus-strand copies of replicating coronavirus mRNAs contain antileaders, *J Virol*, **65**: 320–5.

Siddell SG, 1983, Coronavirus JHM: coding assignments of subgenomic mRNAs, *J Gen Virol*, **64**: 113–25.

Siddell SG, 1995a, The *Coronaviridae*: an introduction, *The Coronaviridae*, ed Siddell SG, Plenum Press, New York, 1–10.

Siddell SG, 1995b, The small-membrane protein, *The* Coronaviridae, ed Siddell SG, Plenum Press, New York, 181–9.

Snijder EJ, Horzinek MC, 1993, Toroviruses: replication, evolution and comparison with other members of the coronavirus-like superfamily, *J Gen Virol*, **74**: 2305–16.

Snijder EJ, Horzinek MC, Spaan WJ, 1990b, A 3′-coterminal nested set of independently transcribed mRNAs is generated during Berne virus replication, *J Virol*, **64**: 331–8.

Snijder EJ, Spaan WJM, 1995, The coronaviruslike superfamily, *The* Coronaviridae, ed Siddell SG, Plenum Press, New York, 239–55.

Snijder EJ, Ederveen J et al., 1988, Characterization of Berne virus genomic and messenger RNAs, *J Gen Virol*, **69**: 2135–44.

Snijder EJ, den Boon JA et al., 1990a, The carboxyl-terminal part of the putative Berne virus polymerase is expressed by ribosomal frameshifting and contains sequence motifs which indicate that toro- and coronaviruses are evolutionarily related, *Nucleic Acids Res*, **18**: 4535–42.

Snijder EJ, den Boon JA et al., 1990b, Primary structure and posttranslational processing of the Berne virus peplomer protein, *Virology*, **178**: 355–63.

Snijder EJ, den Boon JA et al., 1991a, Characterization of defective interfering RNAs of Berne virus, *J Gen Virol*, **72**: 1635–43.

Snijder EJ, den Boon J et al., 1991b, Comparison of the genome organization of toro- and coronaviruses: evidence for two nonhomologous RNA recombination events during Berne virus evolution, *Virology*, **180**: 448–52.

Snijder EJ, Wassenaar ALM et al., 1996, The arterivirus nsp4 protease is the prototype of a novel group of chymotrypsin-like enzymes, the 3C-like serine proteases, *J Biol Chem*, **271**: 4864–71.

Somogyi P, Jenner AJ et al., 1993, Ribosomal pausing during translation of an RNA pseudoknot, *Mol Cell Biol*, **13**: 6931–40.

St Laurent G, Morin G, Archambault D, 1994, Detection of equine arteritis virus following amplification of structural and nonstructural viral genes by reverse transcription PCR, *J Clin Microbiol*, **32**: 658–65.

Stern DF, Sefton BM, 1984, Coronavirus multiplication: locations of genes for virion proteins on the avian infectious bronchitis virus genome, *J Virol*, **50**: 22–9.

Stohlman SA, Kyuwa S et al., 1993, Characterization of mouse hepatitis virus-specific cytotoxic T cells derived from the central nervous system of mice infected with the JHM strain, *J Virol*, **67**: 7050–9.

Stohlman SA, Bergmann CC et al., 1995, Mouse hepatitis virus-specific cytotoxic T lymphocytes protect from lethal infection without eliminating virus from the central nervous system, *J Virol*, **69**: 684–94.

Suarez P, Zardoya R et al., 1994, Direct detection of the porcine reproductive and respiratory syndrome (PRRS) virus by reverse polymerase chain reaction (RT-PCR), *Arch Virol*, **135**: 89–99.

Thiel V, Siddell SG, 1994, Internal ribosome entry in the coding region of murine hepatitis virus mRNA 5, *J Gen Virol*, **75**: 3041–6.

Timoney PJ, McCollum WH, 1988, Equine viral arteritis, epidemiology and control, *Equine Vet Sci*, **8**: 54–9.

Timoney PJ, McCollum WH et al., 1986, Demonstration of the carrier state in naturally acquired equine arteritis virus infection in the stallion, *Res Vet Sci*, **41**: 279–80.

Tooze J, Tooze S, Warren G, 1984, Replication of coronavirus MHV-A59 in sac- cells: determination of the first site of budding of progeny virions, *Eur J Cell Biol*, **33**: 281–93.

Tyrrell DA, 1983, Rhinoviruses and coronaviruses – virological aspects of their role in causing colds in man, *Eur J Respir Dis*, **64**: 332–5.

Underdahl NR, Mebus CA, Torres-Medina A, 1975, Recovery of transmissible gastroenteritis virus from chronically infected experimental pigs, *Am J Vet Res*, **36**: 1473–6.

Underdahl NR, Mebus CA et al., 1974, Isolation of transmissible gastroenteritis virus from lungs of market-weight swine, *Am J Vet Res*, **35**: 1209–16.

Vanopdenbosch E, Wellemans G et al., 1992a, Prevalence of torovirus infections in Belgian cattle and their role in respiratory, digestive and reproductive disorders, *Vlaams Diergeneesk Tijdschr*, **61**: 187–91.

Vanopdenbosch E, Wellemans G et al., 1992b, Bovine torovirus: cell culture propagation of a respiratory isolate and some epidemiological data, *Vlaams Diergeneesk Tijdschr*, **61**: 45–9.

Vlasak R, Luytjes W et al., 1988, The E3 protein of bovine coronavirus is a receptor-destroying enzyme with acetylesterase activity, *J Virol*, **62**: 4686–90.

de Vries AA, Chirnside ED et al., 1992, Structural proteins of equine arteritis virus, *J Virol*, **66**: 6294–303.

de Vries AA, Post SM et al., 1995a, The two major envelope proteins of equine arteritis virus associate into disulfide-linked heterodimers, *J Virol*, **69**: 4668–74.

de Vries AA, Raamsman MJ et al., 1995b, The small envelope glycoprotein (G$_S$) of equine arteritis virus folds into three distinct monomers and a disulfide-linked dimer, *J Virol*, **69**: 3441–8.

Weiss M, Steck F et al., 1984, Antibodies to Berne virus in horses and other animals, *Vet Microbiol*, **9**: 523–31.

Weiss SR, Hughes SA et al., 1994, Coronavirus polyprotein processing, *Arch Virol Suppl*, **9**: 349–58.

Wenzel RP, Hendley JO et al., 1974, Coronavirus infections in military recruits, *Am Rev Resp Dis*, **109**: 621–4.

van Woensel P, van der Wouw J, Visser N, 1994, Detection of porcine reproductive respiratory syndrome virus by the polymerase chain reaction, *J Virol Methods*, **47**: 273–8.

Woode GN, Reed DE et al., 1982, Studies with an unclassified virus isolated from diarrheic calves, *Vet Microbiol*, **7**: 221–40.

Woods RD, Wesley RD, Kapke PA, 1988, Neutralization of porcine transmissible gastroenteritis virus by complement-dependent monoclonal antibodies, *Am J Vet Res*, **49**: 300–4.

Xue S, Jaszewski A, Perlman S, 1995, Identification of a CD4+ T cell epitope within the M protein of a neurotropic coronavirus, *Virology*, **208**: 173–9.

Yagyu K, Ohta S, 1990, Detection of infectious bronchitis virus antigen from experimentally infected chickens by indirect immunofluorescent assay with monoclonal antibody, *Avian Dis*, **34**: 246–52.

Yeager CL, Ashmun RA et al., 1992, Human aminopeptidase N is a receptor for human coronavirus 229E, *Nature (London)*, **357**: 420–2.

Yokomori K, Lai MM, 1991, Mouse hepatitis virus S RNA sequence reveals that nonstructural proteins ns4 and ns5a are not essential for murine coronavirus replication, *J Virol*, **65**: 5605–8.

Yoo D, Graham FL et al., 1992, Synthesis and processing of the haemagglutinin-esterase glycoprotein of bovine coronavirus encoded in the E3 region of adenovirus, *J Gen Virol*, **73**: 2591–600.

Yu W, Leibowitz JL, 1995a, A conserved motif at the 3′ end of mouse hepatitis virus genomic RNA required for host protein binding and viral RNA replication, *Virology*, **214**: 128–38.

Yu W, Leibowitz JL, 1995b, Specific binding of host cellular proteins to multiple sites within the 3′ end of mouse hepatitis virus genomic RNA, *J Virol*, **69**: 2016–23.

Yu X, Bi W et al., 1994, Mouse hepatitis virus gene 5b protein is a new virion envelope protein, *Virology*, **202**: 1018–23.

van der Zeijst BAM, Horzinek MC, Moennig V, 1975, The genome of equine arteritis virus, *Virology*, **68**: 418–25.

Zhang X, Lai MM, 1995, Interactions between the cytoplasmic proteins and the intergenic (promoter) sequence of mouse hepatitis virus RNA: correlation with the amounts of subgenomic mRNA transcribed, *J Virol*, **69**: 1637–44.

Zhang XM, Herbst W et al., 1994, Biological and genetic characterization of a hemagglutinating coronavirus isolated from a diarrhoeic child, *J Med Virol*, **44**: 152–61.

Zhao X, Shaw K, Cavanagh D, 1993, Presence of subgenomic mRNAs in virions of coronavirus IBV, *Virology*, **196**: 172–8.

Ziebuhr J, Herold J, Siddell SG, 1995, Characterization of a human coronavirus (strain 229E) 3C-like proteinase activity, *J Virol*, **69**: 4331–8.

Chapter 25

PICORNAVIRUSES

P Minor

1 Introduction
2 Properties of the viruses
3 Clinical and pathological aspects
4 Epidemiology

5 Laboratory diagnosis
6 Control of enteroviral infections
7 Future prospects

1 INTRODUCTION

The earliest record of a disease believed to be caused by a virus is a New Kingdom Egyptian funerary stela of about 1300 BC depicting a priest with the typical withered limb and dropped foot deformity of poliomyelitis, caused by poliovirus, a picornavirus of the enterovirus genus. In 1909 the virus was transmitted from the spinal cord of a fatal case to monkeys by Landsteiner and Popper. Enders, Weller and Robbins (1949) showed that poliovirus could be grown in primate cells of non-neural origin, and the isolation of other enteroviruses followed. Coxsackie virus was isolated from 2 children with paralytic disease from the town of Coxsackie in New York State in 1948 by the inoculation of newborn mice with faecal extracts (Dalldorf and Sickles 1948). Robbins and co-workers isolated echoviruses (enterocytopathic human orphan viruses) from healthy children in 1951. The echo-, polio- and coxsackieviruses, with more recently discovered viruses identified by number, are classified as enteroviruses, as shown in Table 25.1.

The rhinovirus genus of the picornavirus family is one of the causative agents of the common cold. Kruse (1914) first demonstrated that a cold could be transmitted by bacteria-free filtrates. The Common Cold Research Unit at Salisbury (UK) was established in 1946 and investigation of transmission of the common cold to human volunteers eventually led to the cultivation of the virus in vitro. In the USA, 2 cytopathogenic agents, JH and 2060, were described (Price et al. 1959) and were originally classified as echovirus 28, later being reclassified as rhinovirus 1A, the type species of the genus (Kapikian et al. 1967). In 1960, Tyrrell and Parsons found that other viruses that caused common colds could be propagated in cultures of human embryonic kidney cells rolled at 33°C in medium with low pH. This observation and the introduction of

Table 25.1 Enterovirus serotypes

Group*	Major disease
Polioviruses 1–3	Paralytic poliomyelitis Aseptic meningitis
Coxsackieviruses A1–22, 24	Aseptic meningitis Herpangina Conjunctivitis (A24)
Coxsackieviruses B1–6	Aseptic meningitis Fatal neonatal disease Pleurodynia Myo- or pericarditis
Echoviruses 1–9, 11–27, 29–34	Aseptic meningitis Rashes Febrile illness
Enteroviruses 68–71	Conjunctivitis (enterovirus 70) Polio-like illness (enterovirus 71)

Echovirus 9 = coxsackievirus A23; echovirus 10 = reovirus; echovirus 28 = rhinovirus; echovirus 34 = coxsackievirus A24.
*In the current report of the International Committee on Taxonomy of Viruses these viruses are prefixed 'human' to distinguish them from animal viruses where relevant.

semi-continuous strains of diploid human embryonic lung fibroblasts (Hayflick and Moorhead 1961) led to a rapid increase in the number of viruses isolated. Rhinoviruses were also isolated from horses (Plummer 1963) and cattle (Bogel and Bohm 1962).

The Rhinovirus Collaborative Programme of the World Health Organization authenticated 100 serotypes of rhinovirus over the next 20 years (Hamparian et al. 1987).

2 PROPERTIES OF THE VIRUSES

The picornaviruses are small RNA-containing viruses. The complete sequences of the genomic RNA of many strains of picornaviruses have been determined, the first being that of the type 1 poliovirus strain Mahoney (Kitamura et al. 1981), and the atomic structures of representative viruses of each of the various genera have been resolved by x-ray crystallography (Hogle, Chow and Filman 1985, Rossmann et al. 1985, Ming Luo et al. 1987, Acharya et al. 1989). The discussion of the detailed molecular virology that follows refers to poliovirus except where stated otherwise.

2.1 Classification

The 6 genera that make up the *Picornaviridae* are (1) the enteroviruses (Table 25.1) (2) the rhinoviruses, (3) the aphthoviruses, which cause foot-and-mouth disease of cattle, (4) the cardioviruses of mice, which include mengovirus and encephalomyocarditis virus as well as Theiler's virus, (5) the hepatoviruses, which include only hepatitis A viruses (described in Chapter 34) and (6) a proposed new genus including echovirus 22 and 23, provisionally designated Orphanovirus. Comparisons of the sequences of the virus genomes play an increasing role in the classification scheme. In particular, Theiler's virus and hepatitis A virus were moved from the enteroviruses mainly because of the nature of their genomic organization and sequence, although they also have particular pathogenic features, whereas echovirus 22 and 23 appear to be typical enteroviruses in all except their sequences, which are very different.

The viruses of these genera share a number of characteristics (Palmenberg 1987), including size, icosahedral morphology, lack of a lipid envelope, a positive-sense RNA genome and the general arrangement of their structural proteins. The sedimentation coefficient is c. 155–160S.

2.2 Differences between genera

The picornavirus genera may be distinguished by a number of criteria. The enteroviruses, cardioviruses, hepatoviruses and orphanoviruses have a buoyant density in caesium chloride of 1.34 g/cm^3, the rhinoviruses of 1.40 g/cm^3 and the aphthoviruses of 1.43 g/cm^3. The enteroviruses, unlike rhinoviruses or aphthoviruses, are totally stable to pH 4 and resistant to pH 2, and this property formed the basis of early classification schemes for the picornaviruses.

The nucleotide sequences of the genomic RNAs of a number of picornavirus strains, including polioviruses, coxsackieviruses A and B, and hepatitis A virus, have been determined and indicate the relationships between the various genera (Palmenberg 1987). The enteroviruses are most closely related to the rhinoviruses, and more distantly to the aphtho- and cardioviruses. The genomes of both the aphtho- and the cardioviruses include a tract of cytidine residues not found in the other genera, and share a similar gen-omic structure distinct from that of the enteroviruses and rhinoviruses, as described below (p. 490). The properties of the picornavirus genera are summarized in Table 25.2.

2.3 Subgroups and species

The enteroviruses are divided into various subgroups, some of which are apparently serologically related. For example, poliovirus 1 and 2 share common antigens. Cross-relationships also exist between coxsackieviruses A3 and A8, A11 and A15, A13 and A18, echoviruses 1 and 8, 6 and 30, and 12 and 29.

In general, the echoviruses may be distinguished from the coxsackieviruses by their failure to cause pathological changes in newborn mice. However, most strains of echovirus 9 can produce flaccid paralysis in newborn mice, a finding that led to its early classification as coxsackievirus A23. Some strains of enterovirus 71 grow better in newborn mice than in cultures of primate cells. Conversely, coxsackievirus A9 is not pathogenic for mice unless passaged in cell culture, in which it grows readily, thus resembling the echoviruses.

The neutralization of rhinovirus infectivity by antisera is largely type specific, and is the basis of the numbering system by which rhinoviruses are classified into 100 serotypes (Hamparian et al. 1987). Minor serological variations may exist within a serotype. Within type 1 there are 2 subtypes, A and B: the low degree of cross-reaction between these subtypes may be reciprocal or one-way (Monto and Johnson 1966). 'Prime' strains of rhinovirus 22 that are antigenically broader than the prototype strain have been isolated (Schieble, Lennette and Fox 1970, Hamparian et al. 1987).

2.4 Resemblances to other viruses

A number of other viruses seem to be superficially similar to the picornaviruses. Astroviruses, which contain RNA and lack a lipid bilayer, are of similar size to picornaviruses, although with distinct morphology in electron micrographs. The caliciviruses are similar, but significantly larger, with a particle diameter of 30 nm, a characteristic morphology and a capsid consisting of a single protein species. Other small round viruses are found in the intestinal tract and may be confused with the true enteroviruses; their relationship, if any, with the enteric picornaviruses is not clear (see Chapter 26).

However, the picornaviruses are similar in many ways, including particle structure and genomic organization to the spherical plant viruses such as cowpea mosaic virus and to insect viruses such as cricket paralysis virus. Similarly, the picornaviruses and togaviruses share some features of genomic strategy and organization. These relationships, which have been revealed by detailed molecular biological characterization of the viruses, suggest intriguing possibilities for the evolutionary origin of picornaviruses (see, e.g., Rossmann 1987).

Table 25.2 Properties of the picornavirus genera

Property	Enterovirus	Hepatovirus	Rhinovirus	Cardiovirus	Aphthovirus	Orphanovirus[a]
Particle size	27 nm	27 nm	27 nm	27 nm	27 nm	27 nm
Sense or virion RNA	Messenger	Messenger	Messenger	Messenger	Messenger	Messenger
Sedimentation coefficient (S) of virion	156	156	149	156	142–146	156
RNA in virion (%)	31	31	31	34	38	31
Size of virion proteins (kDa):						
VP1	35	35	35	34	29	30.5
VP2	30	30	30	30	30	38
VP3	24	24	23	23	22	30
VP4	7	?[b]	7	7	8	…
Poly(A) tract	+	+	+	+	+	+
Size of genome:						
kb	7445	7450	7155	7832	8400	7340
kDa	2200	2200	2200	2300	2500	2200
Buoyant density in CsCl (g/cm³)	1.34	1.34	1.41	1.34	1.43	1.36
Acid stability	+	+	−	+	−	+
Poly(C) tract	−	−	−	+	+	−
Base composition:						
A (%)	30	29	32	26	26	32
U(%)	24	33	28	25	21	29
C (%)	23	16	20	26	28	19
G (%)	23	22	20	23	25	20

[a]Echoviruses 22 and 23 may be assigned to their own genus, provisionally entitled Orphanovirus, chiefly on the basis of their unique genomic sequences.
[b]It is not clear whether hepatoviruses contain VP4.

2.5 Morphology and structure

Picornaviruses usually appear in electron micrographs as roughly spherical particles not penetrated by negative staining methods. Figure 25.1 demonstrates some of the features of poliovirus, but similar results would be obtained with all picornaviruses. The viruses are 25–30 nm in diameter (Fig. 25.1a), and can occasionally present a hexagonal appearance (Fig. 25.1a) or form hexagonal arrays (Fig. 25.1b). Similarly, shadowed preparations can produce blunt-ended or pointed shadows, consistent with an icosahedral structure (Fig. 25.1c). In preparations positively stained after drying of the virus from ethanol where the RNA is extruded, the capsid may remain negatively stained and so the thickness of the virion wall can be seen to be c. 2.5 nm. A similar thickness has been determined for the empty capsids, which are in general penetrated by negative stain (Fig. 25.1d), although frequently there are regions from which the stain is excluded (Fig. 25.1e). When the particle is distorted during drying it may expand and break into circular or crescent-like portions (Fig. 25.1g). Similarly, heating (Fig. 25.1h, i) can give rise to 12 crescentic or circular structures, which are believed to correspond to the pentamers of the icosahedron.

Understanding of picornaviruses was extended immensely by the determination of the atomic structures of rhinovirus 14 (Rossmann et al. 1985), the type 1 poliovirus strain Mahoney (Hogle, Chow and Filman 1985), the cardiovirus mengovirus (Ming Luo et al. 1987) and foot-and-mouth disease virus (Acharya et al. 1989). The structure of the type 1 poliovirus strain Mahoney is shown in Fig. 25.2. Although all picornavirus structures solved to date are strikingly similar to each other, and to the spherical plant viruses such as southern bean mosaic virus and tomato bushy stunt virus, there are also clear differences between them.

The capsid of poliovirus is composed of 60 protomers, each being made up of one molecule of each of the 4 virion proteins VP1, VP2, VP3 and VP4. The protomers are arranged with icosahedral symmetry. Each of the 20 faces of the icosahedron is made up of 3 protomers, orientated so that the 12 apices of the icosahedron are occupied by 5 copies of VP1 while the centre of each face is occupied by 3 copies each of VP2 and VP3, alternating around the 3-fold axis of symmetry. The overall thickness of the shell is about 3 nm, extending 11–14 nm from the particle centre. However, the apices of the icosahedron extend to 16.5 nm, and the face at the 3-fold axis of symmetry extends 15 nm from the particle centre. These 2 elevated features are separated by a cleft or 'canyon' that circles the apex, and it has been suggested that, for

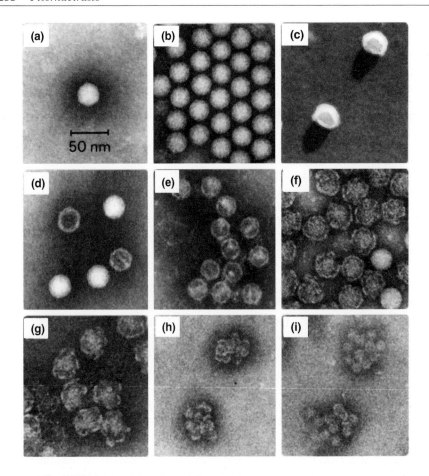

Fig. 25.1 Electron micrographs of poliovirus; all specimens (except c) stained with 4% sodium silicotungstate and all magnified × 200 000. (a) Whole virus particle (D antigen) c. 30 nm in diameter and displaying a hexagonal profile. (b) High concentration of virus in hexagonal array. (c) Freeze-dried virus with low angle platinum shadowing (print reversed to give black shadows); virus particles produce either pointed or blunt-ended shadows, which are consistent with an icosahedral particle. (d) Penetration of stain into empty particles reveals outer capsid. (e) Empty particles (C antigen) showing complete contents and outer capsid. (g) Flattened particles showing breakdown of capsid into angular or crescent-like portions. (h and i) Particles heated at 56°C for 2 min produce aggregates of c. 12 crescent-like or circular structures.

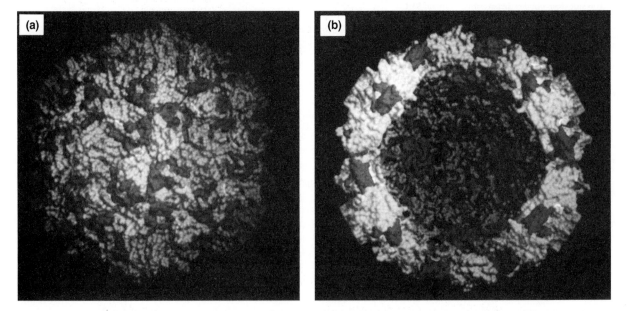

Fig. 25.2 Structure of the Mahoney strain of type 1 poliovirus showing (a) the complete capsid, and (b) the capsid with one pentamer removed to reveal the inside of the virion.

enteroviruses and rhinoviruses, the virus attaches to the specific receptor site on the cell by this feature.

The structural organization of the individual proteins that make up the virion is surprisingly similar, despite their differences in sequence (Fig. 25.3), if VP4 is regarded as an N-terminal extension of VP2 confined to the interior of the virus. Each protein has a wedge-shaped core structure composed of 8 strands of protein, shown as broad arrows in Fig. 25.3, arranged in an antiparallel β sheet array, the 8 strands collectively forming a barrel (termed the β barrel). The core structure of polioviruses, rhinoviruses and other spherical viruses, including plant viruses, are very similar in this respect. The features that are unique to the individual virus, including antigenic sites, arise from the loops that join the different β strands and the sequences at the N and C termini.

The narrow end of the β barrel of VP1 is located near the icosahedral apex of the virus while the corresponding regions of VP2 and VP3 alternate around the 3-fold axis of symmetry. The N-terminal portion of VP3 interacts with the VP1 β barrel, while the N-terminal portion of VP1 interacts with the β barrel of VP3, so the proteins interact extensively. VP4 forms a lattice around the inside of the pentameric apex, and the pentamer of 5 interleaved copies each of VP1, VP2, VP3 and VP4 forms an obviously stable structural unit. Interactions between adjacent pentamers include regions of secondary structure in the form of β sheets between the β barrels of VP2 and VP1.

In addition to the protein components of the virus

shell, the N terminus of each VP4 protein is covalently bound to a myristic acid residue (Chow et al. 1987). The myristate sequences penetrate the pentameric apex, possibly forming a framework for assembly.

The structures of poliovirus and rhinovirus are very similar but differ from that of the cardioviruses, typified by mengovirus (Ming Luo et al. 1987). A major loop found in VP1 of both poliovirus and rhinovirus, and which constitutes a principal antigenic site, is greatly truncated in mengovirus, and another loop is greatly extended. In VP2 a loop is deleted, and another in VP3 is displaced. Consequently the pentameric apex is surrounded by 5 distinct pores rather than a canyon. The 15 C-terminal residues of VP1 are disordered but exposed on the virus surface, whereas all C-terminal residues of VP1 are ordered in the poliovirus and rhinovirus.

The particle shell of foot-and-mouth disease virus is relatively smooth because of the truncation of certain loops, and there is no canyon or series of pits around the pentameric apex (Acharya et al. 1989). One loop

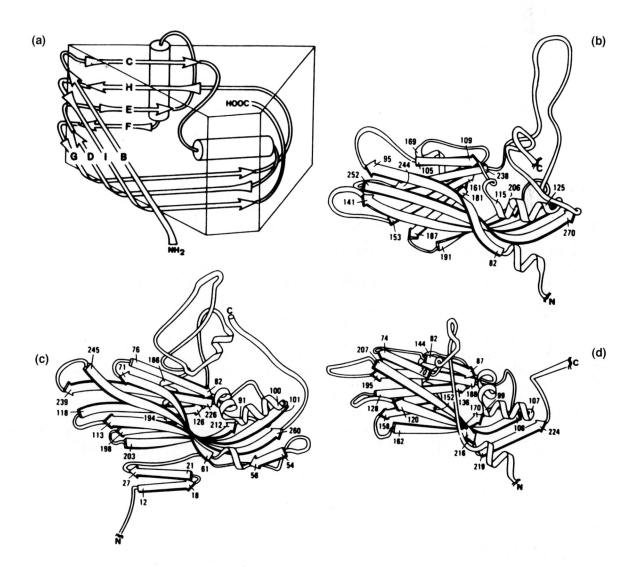

Fig. 25.3 Structure of the proteins making up the poliovirus capsid: (a) schematic diagram of β barrel structure (arrow) and connecting α helices (cylinders); (b) VP1; (c) VP2; (d) VP3.

in VP1 forms a disordered surface structure known to be a major antigenic site. The C terminus of VP1 is also a disordered surface feature lying in the region of the disordered loop. A residue in VP2 is covalently linked by a disulphide bridge to a residue in the disordered VP1 loop, and is therefore itself faint in the structure. It has been suggested that the highly exposed, disordered loop forms the site on the virus by which it attaches to the host cell, in contrast to the other picornaviruses which may attach to the cell via the canyon or pit regions.

2.6   Genome structure and function

The number of viral proteins identified in infected cells is too great to be encoded by the genomic RNA, which has a coding capacity of about 200 kDa (Putnak and Phillips 1981). The use of inhibitors demonstrated the existence of precursor proteins which are subsequently cleaved; very similar cleavages occur in vitro when polio RNA is translated in cell-free systems, suggesting that protease activity is virally encoded (Villa-Komaroff et al. 1974).

Sequences of the genomes of a number of picornaviruses representing strains from each genus have been determined. The genomic RNA, constituting about 33% of the mass of the virion, varies in size from about 7200 nucleotides for rhinovirus to 8500 nucleotides for foot-and-mouth disease virus (mol. wt 2000–3000 kDa). Virion RNA is infectious for cells, although less so than intact virus. The layout of the genome of poliovirus is presented in Fig. 25.4. The 5′ terminus of the RNA is covalently linked to a small protein (VPg) of 22 amino acids via the phenolic hydroxyl group of the tyrosine at residue 3 from the N terminus, a residue conserved in all picornaviral sequences of VPg to date. The following 740 nucleotides of the RNA constitute the 5′ non-coding region preceding the single open reading frame. The genome terminates in a short untranslated 3′ non-coding region of about 70 nucleotides, to which a sequence of 40–100 adenosine residues is attached, comparable to that found on many eukaryotic mRNAs. Sequence analysis of viral proteins has defined the genomic location and proteolytic cleavage sites used in processing. The structural proteins are encoded in the order VP4, VP2, VP3 and VP1, or 1A, 1B, 1C, 1D in the formal nomenclature (Rueckert and Wimmer 1984), from the 5′ end, making up the P1 region of the polyprotein which is excised as a single unit during replication. The non-structural proteins P2, consisting of proteins 2A, 2B and 2C, and P3, consisting of proteins 3A, 3B, 3C and 3D, are also considered to be single units. The rhinoviruses closely resemble the enteroviruses except that the 5′ non-coding region lacks the poorly conserved 100 nucleotide region immediately preceding the open reading frame.

The genomic organization of the cardioviruses and aphthoviruses differs from this general structure in that they encode a leader protein (L) before the P1 region and contain a polycytidylate tract in the 5′ non-coding region. In addition, protein 2A of foot-and-mouth disease virus is very small, and the genome includes 3 distinct copies of the protein VPg, any of which may be covalently linked to virus-derived RNA.

Complete cDNA copies of the genome of entero-, rhino- and hepatovirus can be generated and used either to recover infectious virus directly from the DNA (Racaniello and Baltimore 1981) or, after linking to transcription systems such as SP6 or T7, to generate infectious RNA. It is thus possible to study the effect of defined genetic manipulations on the phenotype of the virus. For technical reasons, complete infectious copies of aphtho- or cardiovirus genomes are more difficult to generate.

2.7   Antigens

Most studies of the antigenic properties of enteroviruses, and of poliovirus in particular, have been concerned with humoral immunity to structural proteins, which is believed to be the major factor in protection from disease, although some work has concerned sites involved in recognition by T cells (Mahon et al. 1995). In infection by foot-and-mouth disease, however, a major immune response is directed against the infection associated antigen (IAA) which has been shown to correspond to the non-structural RNA polymerase protein 3D.

Antigenic differences may occur between different isolates; for example isolates of type 3 polioviruses in Finland during 1984/85 differed from classic type 3 strains (Huovilainen et al. 1987) and UK strains of coxsackievirus B5 from 1973 were very different from the Faulkner strain isolated in 1952.

The infectious virus particles of polioviruses and other picornaviruses differ antigenically from the empty capsids. Mayer et al. (1957) resolved poliovirus preparations into distinct fractions by centrifugation on a sucrose step gradient; most of the infectious material appeared in the fourth layer (D) and reacted preferentially with convalescent sera, but viral antigens could also be detected in the lighter third layer (C) which reacted preferentially with acute phase sera. D antigenic material corresponds to infectious particles, and C to empty capsids. Others showed that the natural virus expressed one antigenic determinant (termed N antigen), whereas material heated at 56°C for 30 minutes expressed another (H antigen) (Hummeler and Tumilowicz 1960); in general, N and D antigens are equated, as are C and H antigens. Relatively mild treatments have a pronounced effect on antigenicity (Le Bouvier 1955). Whilst protective antibodies should be directed against the infectious virus or D antigen, antibodies raised against purified D antigenic material frequently react with C antigen and vice versa; it is therefore quite possible to raise a protective immune response with C antigenic material. Rhinoviruses also exhibit D and C antigen characteristics (Butterworth et al. 1976).

The development of monoclonal antibodies derived from mice immunized with poliovirus demonstrated that they could bind to the D or to the C antigenic forms of the virus

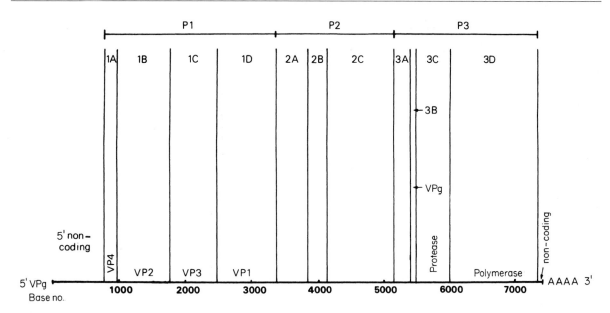

Fig. 25.4 Organization of the genome of enteroviruses showing the 5′ and 3′ non-coding regions and the location of the regions coding for the various proteins. Nomenclature is according to Rueckert and Wimmer (1984) and the common name where appropriate.

(Rombaut, Vrijsen and Boeye 1983), or to both (Ferguson et al. 1984). In addition, some D-specific antibodies bound to subunits that were precursors to virions in the assembly pathway, whereas others bound only to mature virus. The particular sites recognized by antibodies were identified by generating antigenic mutants resistant to neutralization by monoclonal antibodies (Minor et al. 1986a, Page et al. 1988). In many instances, C antigen generated from such antigenic mutants no longer reacts with particular C-specific monoclonal antibodies, implying that the D- and C-specific antibodies are recognizing the same amino acid sequences in different conformation on the 2 types of particle. This is consistent with the concept that relatively mild abuse of the virion can induce major conformational changes reflected in large alterations in antigenicity.

The specific amino acid substitutions found in antigenic mutants of poliovirus selected with murine antibodies have been identified, and examination of the atomic structure of the virus shows that they are clustered into several non-overlapping sites on the surface of the virion. The regions in which mutations have been identified are shown in Table 25.3, and each site is complex and conformational in nature. For poliovirus of both type 2 and type 3, site 1 seems to be the major target of the murine immune response, whereas antibodies against the corresponding region of type 1 have not been induced by immunization with native virus.

Antibodies directed against site 3 of poliovirus serotypes 1 and 3 tend to be highly strain specific, even to the extent that antigenic drift can be demonstrated during the period of excretion by vaccinees.

Site 1 contains a trypsin cleavage site (Minor et al. 1986c). Virus excreted by vaccinees is cleaved at this point and the antigenic properties of the site are destroyed or greatly altered as a result. Thus the virus growing in its natural ecological niche presents an

Table 25.3 Antigenic sites for the neutralization of poliovirus and rhinovirus by monoclonal antibodies

Poliovirus			Rhinovirus 14		
Site	Amino acids involved		Site	Amino acids involved	
1	VP1	89–100	Nim 1a	VP1	91, 95
	VP1	142	Nim 1b	VP1	83, 85, 138, 139
	VP1	166	...	...	
	VP1	253	...	...	
2	VP1	220–222	Nim II	VP1	210
	VP2	164–170	...	VP2	158, 159, 161, 162
	VP2	273	...	...	
3	VP1	286–290	Nim III	VP1	287
	VP3	58–60	...	VP3	72, 73, 75, 78, 203
	VP3	70–72	...	...	
4	VP3	77–80	...	...	
	VP2	72	...	...	

antigenic structure significantly different from that found in cell cultures or, presumably, in a viraemic state.

Neutralizing antibody is difficult to induce with isolated viral proteins or with short peptides based on sequences found within them. In this respect poliovirus contrasts with foot-and-mouth disease virus, for which such approaches have been very successful (Bittle et al. 1982), and with coxsackie B virus, against which high titres of neutralizing antibody have been induced with VP2 (Beatrice et al. 1980). The difference is attributable to the highly integrated and conformational nature of the antigenic sites. However, viruses can be constructed by genetic engineering, in which entire sites have been exchanged between different serotypes (Burke et al. 1988, Murray et al. 1988). Such constructs can have antigenic and immunogenic properties of both parents, although, even here, the inserted site is imperfectly expressed (Minor et al. 1990, 1991). The viruses usually grow poorly.

Similar antigenic studies have been performed for rhinovirus 14. Sherry and colleagues (1986) identified 4 antigenic sites recognized by monoclonal antibodies (Table 25.3). All are surface features. Under conditions in which 95% of infectious virus particles are neutralized, monoclonal antibodies to each of the 4 sites caused a shift in the isoelectric point of virions and inhibited virus attachment to cellular receptors (Colonno et al. 1989).

2.8 Replication

Entry into host cells

Viral RNA from poliovirus is able to induce a single round of replication in rabbit kidney cells, which are not normally susceptible to infection (Holland et al. 1959), indicating that the blockage is at the level of virus entry. Saturable receptors have been demonstrated (Lonberg-Holm, Crowell and Philipson 1976) and competition experiments showed that the 3 serotypes of poliovirus attach to the same site, distinct from that used by other enteroviruses. Monoclonal antibodies directed against cellular components have been raised that specifically block the binding of poliovirus (Minor et al. 1984) coxsackieviruses (Campbell and Cords 1983) and rhinovirus 14.

The gene coding for the poliovirus receptor was identified by Mendelsohn et al. (1986, 1989). It is a 3-domain protein of the immunoglobulin superfamily with an unglycosylated molecular weight of 42 kDa. The cellular receptor for most rhinoviruses is the cell adhesion protein ICAM-1, a 5-domain protein of the same superfamily (Greve et al. 1989, Staunton et al. 1989).

Other picornavirus receptors identified include decay accelerating factor (DAF), implicated in the complement pathway as the receptor for echovirus 7 among others (Ward et al. 1994) and integrin VLA2 for echovirus 1 (Bergelson et al. 1992). The possible need for additional molecules in attachment or penetration is suggested by the failure of mouse cells transfected with the genes for either ICAM-1 or DAF to support the growth of rhinovirus 14 or echovirus 7. Moreover, whereas mouse cells transfected with the poliovirus receptor are highly susceptible to poliovirus (Pipkin et al. 1993), it has been suggested that CD44 may also play a role (Shepley and Racaniello 1994). The poliovirus receptor and susceptibility to coxsackie B3 and echovirus 11 have been shown to be encoded on human chromosome 19 (Medrano and Green 1973, Miller et al. 1974). Transgenic mice carrying the gene for the human poliovirus receptor are susceptible to poliovirus infection by a variety of routes, developing paralysis similar to that seen in primates (Ren and Racaniello 1992). Penetration of the virus into the cell is presumed to be by receptor-mediated endocytosis.

Uncoating

When virus is allowed to bind to cells at room temperature and the cultures are then incubated at 37°C, up to 90% of the virus may be released into the medium. The released virus (A particles) has lost VP4, and has converted from D (N) antigenicity to C (H) antigenicity, although it retains the virion RNA (Joklik and Darnell 1961). Similar particles can be identified in the cells, and their production can be catalysed by soluble receptor in the case of poliovirus.

Protein synthesis

The genomic RNA is infectious and translated into virion proteins directly. The 5' terminus of many eukaryotic mRNA species is blocked by a 'cap' or 7-methylguanosine residue linked in the reverse orientation to the 5' terminal residue by phosphate groups. Ribosomes bind close to the free capped 5' end of the RNA and then 'scan' the sequence for the first suitable initiation codon (defined in part by the nucleotides that flank it) at which protein synthesis commences. Picornavirus RNAs are translated by another mechanism in which the 5' non-coding region acts as an internal initiation site for translation not requiring a free terminus (Pelletier and Sonenberg 1988). This mechanism had previously been thought extremely unlikely. Following the initiation of viral protein synthesis, host protein synthesis is rapidly shut off by mechanisms that are not fully understood but include the proteolytic cleavage of initiation factors required for the cap-dependent protein synthesis of the host cell by a mechanism involving the virus-coded protease 2A.

Post-translation processing

The proteases of polioviruses and other enteroviruses are extremely specific and have been proposed as possible targets for chemotherapeutic agents. In the case of poliovirus, the P1 protein comprising all the structural proteins is excised as a single unit by protease 2A, which cleaves between a tyrosine–glycine pair. This has the effect of removing the structural from the non-structural proteins before they are processed any further. The corresponding protease in coxsackie B3 virus is believed to cleave between a threonine–isoleucine pair. Later processing is carried out by protease 3C or the precursor molecule 3CD. It may be difficult to identify the active moiety, which may be an intermediate or a final product of the cleavage pathway. The processing protease in poliovirus cleaves between glutamine–glycine pairs, including those found in the P1 region between VP2 and VP3, and VP3 and VP1. The exposure and possibly the amino acid sequence surrounding the dipeptide govern whether cleavage occurs, as many such pairs are not cleaved. A similar sequence specificity seems to function in the coxsackie B viruses, but the situation is less clear in viruses such as hepatitis A, or other picornaviruses, such as EMC, in which cleavage does not seem to involve a specific dipeptide (Palmenberg 1987).

Two further proteolytic cleavages take place in the viral growth cycle. One occurs in protein 3D, at a tyrosine–glycine pair, and is thus probably performed by protein 2A. This may have the effect of reducing the amount of active polymerase in the cell, but the advantage of this is not understood, especially as at least the Sabin type 3 vaccine strain of poliovirus and viruses related to it do not carry out this step, although they grow to high titre in vivo and in vitro. The final cleavage involves the formation of VP2 and VP4 from the precursor VP0, which occurs as the last stage of maturation.

REPLICATION OF RNA

The synthesis of RNA requires an RNA template that is read from the 3′ to 5′ direction, whereas protein synthesis requires an RNA template read in the opposite direction. The 2 processes are therefore mutually exclusive, and the factors influencing the fate of a particular RNA molecule are not known.

The replication of poliovirus RNA requires the synthesis of both negative and positive strands of RNA (Kuhn and Wimmer 1987). Messenger-sense (positive-strand) RNA is synthesized in a great excess over the complementary-sense RNA. Infected cells contain complete double-stranded copies of one positive and one negative strand of viral RNA, termed replicative forms (RF) and partial double-stranded structures termed replicative intermediates (RI). All nascent strands of polio RNA of either sense are covalently linked to VPg at the 5′ terminus. This protein is absent from RNA associated with ribosomes. The association of VPg with nascent RNA presumably accounts for the fact that inhibitors of protein synthesis such as puromycin rapidly inhibit RNA synthesis.

Viral protein 3D is present in replication complexes isolated from infected cells (Lundquist, Ehrenfeld and Maizel 1974) and is able to synthesize poly(U) from a poly(A) template if primed with oligo(U) (Flanegan and Baltimore 1977). Protein 3B (VPg) is associated with nascent RNA strands and is also found as 3AB in membrane preparations that have RNA polymerase activity. This suggests a role for both 3A and 3B in RNA synthesis. Guanidine inhibits poliovirus RNA synthesis, and mutants that are either resistant to it or dependent on its presence for growth possess base changes in protein 2C, which is therefore also implicated in synthesis in some way. This protein may influence host range in polioviruses and in rhinoviruses. It is therefore likely that some host factor is involved, although this could, for example, involve structural factors contributed by the host, such as cell membranes.

The detailed mechanism of viral RNA synthesis is controversial, although it is accepted that it occurs in particulate or membranous regions of the infected cell. Replication of

virus in vitro has been reported in protein translation systems primed with polioviral RNA. Protein 3D is the main component of replicative complexes which may be prepared from infected cells by mild detergents. Such complexes synthesize both virion (+) and complementary (−) sense RNAs in vitro. Three models for RNA synthesis have been put forward.

1   Dasgupta, Zabel and Baltimore (1980) reported the presence of a 67 kDa protein able to initiate viral RNA synthesis in the absence of oligo(U). The protein has kinase activity, and the implication of host proteins in viral nucleic acid synthesis in other systems is well documented. However, this factor (host factor, or HF) leaves no clear role for VPg.
2   Flanegan and co-workers (Young, Tuschall and Flanegan 1985) have reported a host enzyme-terminal uridylate transferase (TUT) – which is able to add uridine residues to the 3′ termini of viral nucleic acid. Uridine bases added to the 3′ end of the virion RNA that carries a poly(A) tail would form a tail that could loop back and anneal to the poly(A) sequence as a primer for 3D. The 3′ terminus of the complementary RNA is UUUUAA, so there is a short sequence for such a hairpin structure to form and prime RNA synthesis on the negative-sense RNA. An analogous mechanism has been suggested in the replication of parvoviruses. The hairpin structure would be cleaved by VPg or a precursor, in the course of which VPg would be transferred to the 5′ end of the nascent strand.
3   There is a proposal that uridine residues are added to VPg to make VPg pUpU, which then functions as a primer. Such an intermediate has been reported.

Combinations of these models have been proposed and the reader is referred to Kuhn and Wimmer (1987) for further details and discussions of the experimental evidence available.

ASSEMBLY OF CAPSIDS

The structural proteins are synthesized and processed as a unit and assemble to form pentamers of VP0, VP1 and VP3 (Putnak and Phillips 1981). Isolated pentamers (or 14S particles) are able to assemble into procapsids, which are complete but empty viral shells, sedimenting at 75S. It is possible to prepare soluble fractions from infected cells containing 14S subunits able to assemble to give 75S empty shells. If the pH is allowed to fall, however, the 75S units become altered, adopting the C antigenic form, and are no longer dissociable.

The last step in the maturation of the infectious virion is the cleavage of VP0 to give VP2 and VP4. It has been proposed that this occurs autocatalytically by insertion of the nucleic acid as a proton donor in the presence of a serine residue at position 10 of VP2 close to the cleavage point (Rossmann et al. 1985). However, specific mutagenesis of residue 10 does not prevent cleavage of VP0. A possible model for virion assembly is that the empty 75S capsids act as a dissociable reservoir of structural proteins. As the units reassociate around the genomic RNA, the cleavage of VP0 to VP2 and VP4 occurs, making assembly essentially irreversible under the conditions pertaining in the infected cell. This scheme remains speculative but plausible.

2.9   Effects on host cells

Replication of enteroviruses is normally accompanied by lysis of the host cell by mechanisms that are unknown. Exceptions to this generalization have been reported for poliovirus (Sarnow, Bernstein and Baltimore 1986), hepatitis A virus, echovirus 6 and the coxsackie B viruses (Matteucci et al. 1985) which can give rise to persistent infections in appropriate cells. There is evidence for the persistent enterovirus infection in vivo of humans and rats (Bowles et al. 1986, Schnurr and Schmidt 1988, Yousef et al. 1988).

2.10   Resistance to physical and chemical agents

Enteroviruses can remain viable for years at −20°C and −70°C, and for weeks at 4°C, but lose infectivity slowly at room temperature and with increasing rapidity as the temperature is raised. Their inactivation at all environmental temperatures is inhibited by molar magnesium chloride; this property has led to the widespread use of magnesium chloride as a stabilizer of oral poliovaccine.

In the absence of organic matter, enteroviruses are rapidly inactivated by ultraviolet light and usually by drying.

Enteroviruses are insensitive to alcoholic and phenolic disinfectants, ether, chloroform and deoxycholate. Treatment with formaldehyde (0.3%), 0.1N HCl or free residual chlorine (0.3–0.5 ppm) causes rapid inactivation. The activity of chlorine is diminished by a high pH, low temperature and the presence of organic matter, and it may therefore be less effective when used under field conditions.

3   CLINICAL AND PATHOLOGICAL ASPECTS

3.1   Enteroviruses

The alimentary tract is the predominant site of replication of enteroviruses. Although infection is usually asymptomatic, enteroviruses are recognized causes of paralytic poliomylitis, encephalitis, aseptic meningitis, myocarditis, conjunctivitis and numerous other syndromes associated with target organs outside the alimentary tract. The serotypes comprising each group and the main disease caused by them are listed in Table 25.1.

HOST RANGE

The only natural host of polioviruses are humans, although most strains will infect Old World monkeys and chimpanzees. However, cotton rats, mice and hamsters and fertile hens' eggs may be infected by strains adapted in the laboratory. Other enteroviruses, notably the coxsackieviruses, will infect mice under laboratory conditions. Swine vesicular disease (SVD) is closely related to coxsackie B5.

PATHOGENESIS

Enteroviruses infect via the mouth or oropharynx. The incubation period is usually 7–14 days, with extremes of 2–35 days. Virus infects the mucosal tissues of the pharynx, gut or both, finally entering the blood stream and gaining access to cells of the reticuloendothelial system and specific target organs such as the meninges, myocardium and skin. Enteroviruses can generally be recovered from the pharynx during the first week of illness and from the faeces for 1–4 weeks after onset of illness; they have been isolated from CSF, spinal cord, brain, heart, conjunctivae and skin lesions.

Two or more enteroviruses may propagate simultaneously in the alimentary tract but usually multiplication of one virus interferes with the growth of the heterologous type.

Poliomyelitis

Poliomyelitis is the most serious disease caused by any of the enteroviruses. According to one view (Bodian 1955), the virus first multiplies in the tonsils and Peyer's patches of the small intestine before spreading to the more distant lymph nodes and thence by a viraemia to other sites, including the spinal cord. According to another view (Sabin 1955), the virus multiplies at mucosal surfaces and accumulates in the draining lymph nodes where some, but not all, strains may replicate. From there virus seeds peripheral sites, including peripheral nerves, and the virus generated at the distant sites is the source of the detectable viraemia. Antibodies appear early and are protective even when given as passive immunoglobulin (Hammon et al. 1953).

Virus may pass to the spinal cord along nerves under certain conditions; for example, in children with inapparent infection either at the time of tonsillectomy or at the time of injection with material causing local inflammation.

The anterior horn cells of the spinal cord are most readily infected by poliovirus, but in severe cases the intermediate grey ganglia and even the posterior horn and dorsal root ganglia may also be involved. In the brain, the reticular formation, the vestibular nuclei, the cerebellar vermis and the deep cerebellar nuclei are most often affected.

Other enteroviruses

The pathogenesis of non-polio enteroviruses is similar to that of poliovirus in the initial stages but the target organs vary. For example, echoviruses 6 and 9 may infect the CNS, causing meningitis. Coxsackievirus A7 and enterovirus 71 can cause paralysis, and others, such as coxsackie B viruses, may infect the heart or muscle.

Coxsackievirus A24 and enterovirus 70 resemble rhinoviruses, being spread by fomites and direct inoculation of the conjunctiva by contaminated fingers. The incubation period is very short (12–48 h); recovery is usually complete within 1–2 weeks.

Host factors

Age is an important determinant of the severity of enterovirus disease, the incidence of some syndromes being greatest in neonates (e.g. myo- or pericarditis).

Malnutrition may worsen disease. When marasmus was induced in normally resistant postweaning mice, challenge with coxsackie B3 virus gave more severe disease.

Physical exertion while incubating poliovirus infection is associated with a higher incidence or greater extent of paralysis. The severity of paralysis is increased in monkeys infected experimentally with poliovirus and made to swim until exhausted. Similarly, exercising mice infected with coxsackievirus A9 or B3 results in increased virus titres in their myocardium, in higher mortality rates, or both.

Pregnancy and parturition may be associated with a greater risk of paralysis with poliovirus infection or a greater risk of myocarditis with coxsackie B infection. Hypo- or agammaglobulinaemic individuals with impaired or absent B cell function but normal T cell function do not readily clear enterovirus infections, which may induce severe disease as well as persisting for abnormally long periods, even years. This provides further evidence for the importance of humoral immunity in the control of enteroviral infection. Maternal antibody may not protect from infection but will prevent disease.

Clinical syndromes

The description of clinical syndromes below is not exhaustive. Further details concerning enteroviral diseases may be found in reviews by Moore and Morens (1984), Melnick (1990) and Bendinelli and Friedman (1988).

Most enterovirus infections produce clinically inapparent or minor illness. The consequences of infection, when they do occur, range from specific clinical syndromes, such as fatal paralytic or cardiac illness, to minor undifferentiated febrile illnesses. Asymptomatic infection rates are reported as 90–95% for the polioviruses, 76% for the coxsackieviruses and 43% for the echoviruses.

Poliomyelitis

Exposure to poliovirus may have the following consequences.

1 **Inapparent infection** (90–95%).
2 **'Abortive'** or **'minor' illness** (4–8%) with symptoms of upper respiratory tract infection, gastrointestinal upset or influenza-like illness. The patient recovers within a few days.
3 **Non-paralytic poliomyelitis** (1–2%), an illness of about 2–10 days similar to 'aseptic' meningitis, often accompanied by back pain and muscle spasm. Recovery usually is rapid and complete.
4 **Paralytic poliomyelitis** (0.1–2%). The major illness, paralysis, usually follows a prodromal illness similar to the minor illness described above, especially in children. Thereafter the predominant feature is flaccid paralysis resulting from lower motor neuron damage. Paralytic poliomyelitis is termed **spinal** if the lower spine is involved or **bulbar** (from 'bulb' or medulla oblongata) if the upper spine and brain stem are involved. Bulbar poliomyelitis is the more serious because it affects the respiratory system.

A paralysed patient may recover completely or have varying degrees of residual deficit. A review of 203 cases between 1969 and 1981 in the USA (Moore et al. 1982) showed that residual paralysis was minor in 11% and significant or severe in 79%; 10% of the cases were fatal.

Post-polio syndrome has been described in which individuals who have survived an initial attack suffer a degeneration of function many years later. This may be anatomical in origin as advancing age results in the loss of nerve cells from an already damaged pathway. Sequences of enterovirus-related nucleic acid have been reported in the cerebrospinal fluid (CSF) of such cases, however, and some workers believe that the virus may persist.

'Aseptic' meningitis

Non-bacterial 'aseptic' meningitis (AM) is a common manifestation of enterovirus infection. Pleocytosis of the CSF is characteristically lymphocytic but may show transient predominance of polymorphonuclear leucocytes when cell counts are high in the early stage of illness, temporarily mimicking bacterial meningitis. Recovery is usually complete within a few weeks, although irritability and fatigue may persist for some weeks and there is a small risk of serious neurological damage in the first year of life (Wilfert et al. 1981). Second attacks of AM may occur from infection with other serotypes.

Paralytic disease

Polioviruses remain the dominant viral cause of paralysis in most of the world. Sporadic cases associated with coxsackievirus A7 continue to be reported (Gear 1984).

Paralysis has also been reported in association with coxsackieviruses B2–6 and echovirus types 3 (transverse myelitis), 4, 6, 9, 11 and 19.

Enterovirus 71 is capable of causing severe CNS disease with persisting flaccid paralysis, although it can also cause meningitis, encephalitis and hand-foot-and-mouth disease, depending on the outbreak (Melnick 1984).

Enterovirus 70, an agent of acute haemorrhagic conjunctivitis (AHC), has caused poliomyelitis-like illness (Kono et al. 1977).

Encephalitis

The dominant enterovirus associated with outbreaks of encephalitis is enterovirus 71, although poliovirus, coxsackieviruses A9, B3, B5 and B6 and echoviruses 6, 9, 17 and 19 have all been isolated from CSF or brain tissues.

Myalgic encephalomyelitis (post-viral fatigue syndrome)

Multiple symptoms are associated with this illness (Behan 1980), but always include extreme muscle fatigue following slight physical effort, muscle pain and psychological upset. The lack of objective physical signs, pronounced emotional lability and neuroticism and the unknown nature of the disorder have made it easy for some physicians to dismiss the illness as hysterical. Myalgic encephalomyelitis (ME) is not a fatal disease but recovery may take months or years; relapses during periods of physical or mental stress are common. Chronic infection with enteroviruses has been reported (Yousef et al. 1988).

Pleurodynia (Bornholm disease)

The group B coxsackieviruses are the main identified causes of pleurodynia, also known as Bornholm disease, epidemic myalgia or the devil's grippe. The chest pain is spasmodic, intensified by movement and may be severe. Abdominal pain resulting from involvement of the diaphragm occurs in approximately half the cases; in children this may be the chief complaint. The illness lasts for 2–14 days and is self-limited; recovery is complete although short relapses are common.

Sporadic cases of pleurodynia have also been associated with coxsackieviruses A4, A6 and A10; coxsackievirus A9 has been implicated in this syndrome and also in chronic diseases of the muscle and joints.

Congenital and neonatal infection

Prematurity, low birth weight, onset of illness within the first few days of life, occurrence during the 'enterovirus season' and recent antepartum or postpartum febrile illness in the mother are risk factors for the most severe, generalized and fatal neonatal enteroviral disease, most commonly associated with the coxsackie B virus, particularly B2 and B4. Neonatal illness has seldom been attributed to coxsackie A viruses but echoviruses (e.g. types 4, 9, 11, 17–20, 22 and 31) have been incriminated in both nursery outbreaks and sporadic infections. Fatal cases of echovirus infection generally present with progressive severe hepatitis and CNS involvement, whereas fulminant coxsackievirus B infections can be distinguished by the presence of severe myocarditis.

Cardiac disease

Severe myocarditis is usually a prominent feature of disseminated enterovirus infections of neonates; less severe myocarditis or pericarditis may follow infection of older children and adults. It has been estimated that c. 5% of all symptomatic coxsackievirus infections induce heart disease.

Nucleic acid hybridization has been used to detect enterovirus RNA in myocardial biopsies. Replicating enterovirus RNA was found in 19 of 81 patients with suspected myocarditis (Kandolf 1988) but in none of the controls. Endomyocardial biopsies from >100 patients with heart muscle disease were investigated by Archard et al. (1988). Enterovirus genomic RNA was detected in 60% with active myocarditis and 47% with healing myocarditis; tissue from cases of other specific heart muscle diseases was consistently negative. All patients who made a coxsackievirus B-specific IgM response also had detectable enterovirus RNA in biopsy tissue. Enterovirus-infected myocardial cells have also been detected by hybridization in situ in dilated myocardiomyopathy (Kandolf 1988). Persistence of enteroviral genomes may therefore be implicated in chronic heart disease.

Mucocutaneous syndromes

Herpangina is characterized by fever and a vesicular exanthem that typically involves the fauces and soft palate. It is chiefly associated with coxsackievirus A types 1–10, 16 and 22, and less commonly with coxsackieviruses B1–5 and some echoviruses. The disease occurs during the summer season and generally involves clusters of patients. Herpangina mainly affects young children but occasionally is seen in young adults. The illness is self-limited, with recovery in a few days.

Hand-foot-and-mouth disease (HFMD) is predominantly a childhood illness, usually associated with infection by coxsackievirus A16 or enterovirus 71. Occasionally, cases due to coxsackieviruses A5, A7, A9, A10, B2 and B5 have been reported. Typical cases of HFMD have vesicles and ulcers mainly in the front of the mouth, most frequently on the tongue, and a vesicular exanthem, mostly localized on the palms and soles; virus can be isolated readily from these sites. During outbreaks, c. 60–70% of cases show the complete clinical picture of HFMD. Recovery from HFMD is usually complete within 1–2 weeks.

Swine vesicular disease in humans Swine vesicular disease virus (SVDV) is a porcine enterovirus that is closely related to coxsackievirus B5 (Zhang et al. 1993). The disease in pigs was first recognized in Italy in 1966. Since then SVD has been seen throughout Europe as well as in Hong Kong and Japan. The lesions in pigs resemble those caused by foot-and-mouth disease and other vesicular diseases of pigs. No vesicles have been seen in workers with pigs affected with SVD although, in laboratories, inapparent human infection has occurred and antibodies have been detected. There are on record 4 human cases with presumptive evidence of infection with SVDV. One patient had a severe illness with fever, myalgia, weakness and abdominal pain, in 2 the disease was mild and the fourth had meningitis. In 3 of these patients infection occurred after exposure to pigs; the other was exposed to the virus in the laboratory.

Exanthems, usually transient and erythematous (rubelliform, maculopapular, rarely morbilliform or vesicular), have been reported in infections by enteroviruses, notably during outbreaks of infection with coxsackieviruses A9, A16 and B5 or echoviruses 4, 9 and 16. Rash is seldom the sole clinical feature in symptomatic enterovirus infections. Fever, malaise, cervical lymphadenopathy and aseptic meningitis may also occur in patients with rash. Rashes associated with coxsackievirus A9 and echovirus 9 can mimic rubella infection so closely as to merit diagnostic differentiation, particularly in pregnant women. Congenital abnormalities following maternal enterovirus infection have only rarely been reported.

Acute epidemic haemorrhagic conjunctivitis In 1970 there was a large epidemic of acute haemorrhagic conjunctivitis (AHC) in Singapore with more than 60 000 reported cases. The causal agent was identified as a variant of coxsackievirus A24. After an incubation period of 18–48 h, mild to severe conjunctivitis developed, with subconjunctival haemorrhage in a minority of cases; recovery was usually complete within 1–2 weeks. Epidemics of AHC recurred in southeast Asia in 1975 and again in 1985 and in the Americas.

Enterovirus 70 first emerged in an epidemic of AHC in Ghana in 1969, spread through the coastal areas of Africa, eventually reaching India, southeast Asia and Japan by 1970, ultimately involving hundreds of millions of people. Serological surveys in Ghana, Indonesia and Japan confirmed that the virus was not prevalent before the pandemic. The illness had a short incubation period (24 h), acute subconjunctival haemorrhage being the most characteristic sign; corneal involvement was usually transient and the prognosis good. The first outbreak in the western hemisphere was in Brazil in 1981 from where it then spread north, reaching Florida.

Rare cases of neurological complications accompanying or following enterovirus 70 conjunctivitis have been reported.

Respiratory disease

Respiratory illness caused by enteroviruses cannot be distinguished clinically from that caused by viruses such as rhinoviruses, parainfluenza viruses, respiratory syncytial virus and adenoviruses. However, these viruses predominate in the winter months, whereas respiratory infection by enteroviruses typically occurs during the summer and autumn.

Diabetes

A possible association of insulin-dependent diabetes mellitus (IDDM) with coxsackie B virus infection was first suggested by Gamble in 1969. Reviews by Gamble (1980), Barrett-Connor (1985) and Toniolo et al. (1988) provide comprehensive interpretations of the available data.

A long euglycogenic period, characterized by the presence of islet cell antibodies (ICAs) and T lymphocyte responses, precedes the appearance of hyperglycaemia following the near total disappearance of the β cells of the islets of Langerhans. There is some correlation of HLA haplotype (DR3 mainly in males, DR4 mainly in females) with this illness, suggesting that an autoimmune process is responsible for the chronic and irreversible loss of β cells. What triggers pancreatic autoimmunity in individuals is unknown.

Strains of coxsackievirus B4 and B5 shown to be diabetogenic in mice have been isolated from people developing diabetes (Toniolo et al. 1988). It has now been shown that most of the group B coxsackieviruses are potentially able to infect and damage pancreatic endocrine cells, causing hyperglycaemia. Serological studies have demonstrated that about one-third of the cases of IDDM in children are probably preceded by coxsackie B infection, although this may be a precipitating rather than causative factor.

Gastroenteritis

Although enteroviruses readily replicate within the gut, they are seldom the cause of gastroenteritis when this is the predominant feature.

Hepatitis

Hepatitis can accompany generalized coxsackievirus B and echovirus infections in neonates or occasionally in older children as well as following infection with hepatitis A virus (Chapter 34).

3.2 Rhinoviruses

Rhinoviruses are the major cause of common colds. In the US National Health Interview Survey for 1985, colds were associated with 161 million days of restricted activity and accounted for 26 million days of school absenteeism, 23 million days lost from work and 27 million visits to physicians. More than 800 oral cold remedies are available and the annual expenditure on such treatments exceeds $2 billion in the USA.

CLINICAL MANIFESTATIONS

About 30% of human volunteers inoculated intranasally with nasal secretions or tissue culture fluid containing rhinoviruses develop colds, whereas less than 5% of volunteers given uninfected material have symptoms (Tyrrell 1965). When virus is given to adults without antibody, up to 100% develop colds (D'Allessio et al. 1976). At least 15 different serotypes have been given to volunteers, with essentially the same results.

In studies of university students (Gwaltney and Jordan 1966, Hamre, Connelly and Procknow 1966, Phillips et al. 1968), industrial workers (Hamparian et al. 1964, Gwaltney et al. 1966), military personnel (Bloom et al. 1963) and civilian families (Elveback et al. 1966, Higgins, Ellis and Boston 1966, Hendley, Gwaltney and Jordan 1969, Monto and Cavallaro 1972, Fox, Cooney and Hall 1975, Fox et al. 1985), rhinoviruses were isolated from 7–40% of people (including children) with upper respiratory illness but from less than 2% of healthy people. These findings probably underestimate the importance of rhinoviruses, because virus can be isolated from only half of known infections. The same epidemiological studies also indicate that between 10% and 40% of rhinovirus infections are subclinical, with substantial differences in pathogenicity between serotypes.

Rhinovirus infections are more common and severe in young children than in adults (Fox, Cooney and Hall 1975). Rhinoviruses are also associated with lower respiratory disease in children or those with a history of chronic respiratory disease. However, in controlled studies, rhinoviruses were found in 3–8% of children in hospital either with lower respiratory illness or without respiratory symptoms (Chanock and Parrott 1965,

Holzel et al. 1965, Stott and Walker 1967, Mufson et al. 1970). Hence, the precise role of rhinoviruses in acute respiratory disease of children is unclear (Cherry 1973). In children with a history of wheezy bronchitis or asthma, rhinoviruses are associated with up to 33% of acute attacks, and virus was found more often in sputum than in the nose or throat, suggesting that virus multiplies in the lower respiratory tract (Horn, Reed and Taylor 1979).

Rhinoviruses can cause lower respiratory tract illness in adult volunteers infected with virus in a fine particle aerosol (Cate et al. 1965). Transient abnormal pulmonary function has also been found in a small proportion of healthy volunteers after intranasal instillation of rhinovirus and in a minority of natural infections. Although rhinoviruses have been isolated postmortem from the lungs of adults who died of pneumonia, they are not implicated as a significant cause of adult pneumonia. However, in people with chronic bronchitis, rhinovirus infections have been associated with 12–43% of exacerbations and virus frequently seems to invade the lower respiratory tract (Stott, Grist and Eadie 1968). Although Buscho and colleagues (1978) found that rhinoviruses could infect patients without exacerbating their chronic bronchitis, such patients are more susceptible to rhinovirus infection than are otherwise healthy people. Furthermore, Horn and Gregg (1973) found lower respiratory tract signs in 85–90% of rhinovirus infections in adults with a previous history of asthma or bronchitis but in only 5% of such infections in otherwise healthy adults.

Bovine rhinovirus types 1 and 3 have been isolated from cattle with respiratory disease but there is little evidence to show that they are clinically important (Stott et al. 1980, Yamashita, Akashi and Inaba 1985). There is one reported isolation of bovine type 2 virus (Reed et al. 1971). Similarly, although infection with equine rhinoviruses is widespread in horses, their precise contribution to the problem of respiratory disease is not yet clear (Powell et al. 1978).

PATHOGENESIS

Hand contact rather than aerosol is the prime mode of transmission of rhinoviruses (Gwaltney and Hendley 1978, Gwaltney, Moskalski and Hendley 1978). Virus has not been recovered from air in rooms occupied by infected people and it is not possible to transmit rhinovirus colds between volunteers separated by a double wire mesh allowing free flow of air but no direct contact. Under the same conditions coxsackievirus A21 was readily transmitted. Aerosols produced by talking, coughing and sneezing derive primarily from the saliva, which has a low titre of virus, and not from the nasal secretions in which titres are highest.

In contrast, rhinovirus can readily be isolated from the hands of people during the acute stage of a cold. Furthermore, the hand contacts the eye or nose, on average, once every 3 hours. Thus, in a comparison of routes of rhinovirus transmission, 11 or 15 hand contact exposures initiated infection but only 1 of 22 aerosol exposures was successful. Epidemiological findings indicate that colds spread poorly in workplaces where many people share the same air space but direct contact is minimal. In contrast, transmission occurs readily within families where direct contact is frequent.

Rhinoviruses replicate in and destroy the ciliated epithelium of both nasal and tracheal mucosae, but grow to highest titre in nasal epithelium (Hoorn and Tyrrell 1965). Ciliated cells are extruded from the epithelium, leaving a generally smooth surface (Reed and Boyde 1972). Mycoplasma replication is enhanced in such virus-damaged tissue (Reed 1972), which is also probably more susceptible to secondary invasion by bacteria and mycoplasmas. Although the target cell in the lower respiratory tract is not known, type II pneumocytes may be infected by rhinoviruses in vitro (Tyrrell et al. 1979). Rhinoviruses are rarely found outside the respiratory tract, partly because their growth is restricted by temperatures above 37°C.

Host responses to infection may cause the vascular engorgement, increased vascular permeability with transudation of serum proteins and increased mucus production that are characteristic of colds. Host responses include release of inflammatory mediators, such as kinins; influxes of inflammatory cells, including polymorphonuclear leucocytes; interferon; and probably neuroreflexes and associated cholinergic stimulation and neuropeptide release (Naclerio et al. 1988). Further evidence for the role of kinins is provided by the finding that intranasal instillation of bradykinin causes some of the symptoms and alterations in nasal mucus seen in rhinovirus colds.

IMMUNE RESPONSES

Rhinovirus infection stimulates an antibody response in 47–77% of cases (Fox, Cooney and Hall 1975). The response is greater in adults than in children. Severe lower respiratory infection induces higher antibody titres than mild upper respiratory infection. Furthermore, certain serotypes are more effective antigens than others. Specific antibody in the circulation is related to protection against reinfection of volunteers. In families in which exposure to known serotypes occurred, pre-existing serum antibody was 52–69% effective in preventing infection. Rhinovirus infections also stimulate local IgA production. Whether secretory IgA in the mucus of the upper respiratory tract or circulating antibody in the serum is the more important in protection remains contentious (Perkins et al. 1969, Douglas and Couch 1972).

3.3 Foot-and-mouth disease

Foot-and-mouth disease is a highly infectious disease of ungulates. There are a few reports of infection in humans and experimental infections of laboratory animals are readily initiated. Seven serotypes of foot-and-mouth disease virus are recognized – O, A, C, SAT1, SAT2, SAT3 and Asia 1 – and existing vaccines are based on inactivated preparations of the appropriate serotype. Synthetic peptides based on known antigenic sites are able to induce protective immune responses and are the most promising candidates for a chemically synthesized vaccine against any virus (Bittle et al. 1982, Clarke et al. 1987).

The first signs of disease in cattle are dullness, anorexia and rising temperature, followed by nasal discharge and the appearance of vesicles in the mouth and on the feet. Initially, the vesicles in the mouth are present on the tongue, hard palate and dental pad, lips and muzzle, and on the feet in the interdigital space or along the coronary band, giving rise to lameness. The incubation period varies from 1 to 14 days.

The main routes of infection are inhalation, ingestion or penetration of the epithelium. Virus may persist in the pharyngeal area for prolonged periods.

4 EPIDEMIOLOGY

Epidemiology is discussed in 2 sections: enteroviruses and rhinoviruses.

4.1 Enteroviruses

MODE OF TRANSMISSION

Humans are the only known reservoir for members of the human enterovirus group. Virus is generally shed for longer periods in faeces (1 month or more) than from the oropharynx, and faecal contamination is the usual source of infection although enterovirus 70, the agent of acute haemorrhagic conjunctivitis, has been found almost exclusively in conjunctival and throat specimens.

INFLUENCE OF CLIMATE

In temperate climates enteroviruses are more prevalent in the summer and autumn (i.e. when warmth and humidity are at their peak). In tropical climates they tend to circulate all the year round or are associated with the rainy season.

SPREAD WITHIN FAMILIES

Young children are the usual reservoir of enterovirus infection. The secondary attack rates in susceptible family members are reported as 92% for polioviruses, 76% for coxsackieviruses and 43% for echoviruses. The greater spread of polioviruses and coxsackieviruses may be related to their longer periods of excretion. Secondary coxsackievirus infections were more common in mothers (78%) than in fathers (47%). Coxsackieviruses spread to 75% of exposed susceptibles but to only 25% of exposed people who already had antibody to the infecting type; echoviruses infected 43% of susceptibles and only one person with homotypic antibody.

EPIDEMIOLOGICAL SURVEILLANCE

International data In 1963 the World Health Organization established a system for the collection and dissemination of information on viral infections. Although the level of reporting may be low and variable, the data are of interest in identifying viruses implicated in clinical syndromes. Examples from 1975 to 1983 are shown in Tables 25.4 and 25.5.

The commonest coxsackievirus reported was type A9, the serotype most readily detectable in cell cultures. Coxsackievirus A16 is the main cause of hand-

Table 25.5 Reports of echovirus infection by main clinical features, 1975–1983

Systems affected	Echovirus infections	
	Number	Predominant serotypes
Central nervous system:		
Total	16 668	E30, 11, 19, 9, 6
Paralytic	178	E11, 9
Cardiac	266	E11, 6, 22
Muscle/joint	223	E11, 6
Skin/mucosa	976	E9, 11
Respiratory	4 620	E11, 22
Gastrointestinal	7 763	E11, 22
Ophthalmic	72	E11
Others	4 106	…
No illness/data	3 497	…
Total	38 191	…

Data from the Global Surveillance Programme, World Health Organization, Geneva.

Table 25.4 Reports of coxsackievirus infections by main clinical features, 1975–1983

Systems affected	Coxsackievirus A infections		Coxsackievirus B infections	
	Number	Predominant serotypes	Number	Predominant aerotypes
Central nervous system:				
Total	1627	A9	4 364	B5, 4
Paralytic	68	A9, 1	112	B4, 5
Cardiac	57	A9	596	B4, 2
Muscle/joint	35	A9	302	B4
Skin/mucosa	1262	A16	360	B5, 4
Respiratory	741	A9	2 880	B4, 2
Gastrointestinal	996	A9	2 921	B4
Ophthalmic	30	A24	33	B4
Others	644	…	2 169	…
No illness/data	395	…	1 309	…
Totals	5787	…	14 934	…

Data from the Global Surveillance Programme, World Health Organization, Geneva.

foot-and-mouth disease. Over all, coxsackievirus B4 was the serotype associated with the widest range of syndromes; coxsackievirus B5 was the predominant serotype linked with non-paralytic CNS infections and rashes.

Almost half the reported echovirus infections were associated with CNS disease, especially aseptic meningitis (Table 25.5). Echoviruses 6, 9, 11, 19 and 30 are regularly encountered during outbreaks of aseptic meningitis, sometimes accompanied by a rash in echovirus 6 and 9 infections. Echovirus 22 is usually associated with a 'failure to thrive' syndrome in infants less than 1 year old and is seldom associated with CNS infection. The apparent role of coxsackieviruses A and B and, to a lesser extent, the echoviruses in paralytic disease should be interpreted with caution because most reports are based on virus isolation from faeces alone.

Infections due to enterovirus serotypes 68–71 reported to WHO during 1975–83 and the associated illnesses are listed in Table 25.6.

Illness due to enteroviruses 68 and 69 is uncommon. Although the figures clearly show the association of enterovirus 70 with eye infections, they fail to reveal the pandemic nature of this virus in acute haemorrhagic conjunctivitis; enterovirus 70 is difficult to isolate in cell culture and this alone might explain the discrepancy. Enterovirus 71 is more readily isolated from clinical specimens, and its associations with CNS infections and hand-foot-and-mouth disease (or both concurrently) are apparent from Table 25.6.

Peak virus activity was seen in July in the northern hemisphere, and during December to January in the southern hemisphere.

As shown in Table 25.7, enterovirus infections were more common in children, especially in those aged 1–4 years.

Table 25.6 Reports of enterovirus 68–71 infections in 217 cases by main clinical features, 1975–1983

Systems affected	Number of infections			
	Ev 68	Ev 69	Ev 70	Ev 71
Central nervous system:				
Total	1	0	1	93
Paralytic	0	0	1	3
Cardiac	0	0	0	0
Muscle/joint	0	0	0	0
Skin/mucosa	0	0	0	41
Respiratory	1	1	0	9
Gastrointestinal	0	4	0	10
Ophthalmic	0	0	33	0
Others	0	0	0	10
No illness/data	1	2	0	10
Totals	3	7	34	173

Data from the Global Surveillance Programme, World Health Organization, Geneva.

4.2 Rhinoviruses

Rhinovirus infections are seen throughout the year but are most prevalent in the spring and autumn when sudden changes in temperature are common. It has been suggested that rapid temperature changes are closely associated with the incidence of colds (Hope-Simpson 1958). Rhinoviruses are distributed throughout the world, and antibodies to them have been detected even in the remote communities of Alaskan Eskimos, Pacific Micronesians and Kalahari Hottentots.

The multiplicity of rhinovirus serotypes is a major factor in their epidemiology. Several serotypes circulate simultaneously within a community, and an individual may be infected with 2 serotypes at the same time (Cooney and Kenny 1977). Some serotypes persist continuously in a population for several years whereas others may appear transiently. The distribution of serotypes has changed over the years. Before 1967 most isolates belonged to the first 55 serotypes; in 1968 and 1969 fewer than half the isolates were serotypes 1–55 and an increasing number were types 56–89. Between 1970 and 1975, 50% of rhinoviruses isolated did not belong to the first 89 types (Fox 1976). However, more recent publications indicate that over 90% of rhinoviruses isolated can now be identified as known serotypes (Fox et al. 1985, Hamparian et al. 1987). Some serotypes, such as 1B, 12, 15 and 38, are isolated more often than others, possibly because they spread more effectively. Certainly, the more frequently isolated serotypes cause a higher secondary attack rate in family surveys (Fox, Cooney and Hall 1975). However, it must be remembered that frequency of isolation may just reflect the sensitivity of the cell cultures used rather than the distribution of viruses in a population.

5 LABORATORY DIAGNOSIS

5.1 Enteroviruses

Detailed descriptions of the principles and procedures for the diagnosis of enterovirus infections are published elsewhere (Grist et al. 1979).

COLLECTION OF SPECIMENS

The usual specimens for virus isolation are faeces (or rectal swabs) and throat swabs. **Faecal** excretion of virus commences within a few days of infection and may continue for weeks in children with poliovirus and coxsackievirus infections although it rarely exceeds 1 month with the echoviruses; in adults it is usually of shorter duration (1–2 weeks). Excretion in the faeces is often intermittent, so, ideally, more than one sample should be collected at least 1–2 days apart. Isolation of virus from **pharyngeal secretions** is possible up to 1 week after onset of symptoms. Culture of virus from the **CSF** is an essential part of the routine laboratory diagnosis of patients with aseptic meningitis.

Table 25.7 Global surveillance of enteroviral infections by age, 1975–1983

Viruses (no. of infections)	Percentage in each age group					
	<1 yr	1–4 yr	5–14 yr	15–24 yr	25+ yr	Unknown
Coxsackievirus A (5787)	18	41	20	5	11	5
Coxsackievirus B (14934)	25	34	18	5	14	4
Echovirus (38 191)	28	26	24	7	11	4
Enteroviruses 68–71* (217)	25	32	22	3	14	3

Data from the Global Surveillance Programme, World Health Organization, Geneva.
*Details available from only 217 of total of 864 infections reported to WHO.

VIRUS ISOLATION IN CELL CULTURES

Polioviruses, the coxsackie B group viruses and the echoviruses are readily isolated in kidney cell cultures prepared from rhesus or cynomolgus monkeys or baboons. Other susceptible cultures can be obtained from human amnion, diploid cells of human embryo lung and the RD cell line derived from a human rhabdomyosarcoma.

IDENTIFICATION OF SEROTYPES

Serotypes may be identified by reference antisera. These LBM pools (devised by Lim, Benyesh and Melnick) are issued in freeze-dried form to reference centres after formal requests to WHO, Geneva. There are 8 pools of antisera (A–H) against 42 enteroviruses that grow readily in cell culture and a further 7 pools (J–P) of antisera against 19 coxsackievirus A serotypes that grow readily only in newborn mice (Table 25.8) (Melnick and Wimberly 1985).

ANTIGENIC VARIATION

Antigenic variation in the enteroviruses can give rise to prime strains that may not be neutralized by sera

Table 25.8 Type-specific antisera included in each of eight 'intersecting' LBM pools A–H

Pool	Enteroviruses represented in each pool		
A	A7	B1, 4	E1, 4, 5, 7, 15, 29, 33 None
B	A7, 9	B2	E2, 3, 9, 19, 21, 26 P2
C	None	B1, 3, 5	E2, 6, 12, 24, 29, 30 P1
D	None	B2	E6, 13, 14, 16, 25, 26, 32, 33 P3
E	None	B4, 5	E5, 11, 13, 17, 18, 22, 30, 32 P2
F	None	B6	E7, 9, 14, 18–20, 26, 27, 29 P1
G	A9	B3	E4, 5, 16, 17, 20, 23, 30, 31 None
H	A16	B6	E1, 3, 9, 12, 22, 23, 32 P3

Antisera against 19 additional coxsackie A viruses are contained in pools J–P. Data from Melnick and Wimberly (1985).

to the prototype strain, but can induce antibodies that neutralize the homologous and prototype strains equally well. Intratypic variants have also been described for coxsackieviruses A24, B1–4, B6, echoviruses 4, 9 and 33 and enterovirus 70. Unlike prime strains, intratypic variants have a narrower antigenic spectrum than their corresponding prototype strains.

Aggregation of virions may also cause problems in the neutralization test. The Pesascek strain of echovirus 4 is poorly neutralized by homologous antisera, whereas the Du Toit strain is readily neutralizable. Virus in non-neutralizable aggregates was found to constitute up to 30% of untreated Pesascek stock virus preparations but only 0.1% of Du Toit stocks. Methods used to disaggregate enteroviruses include filtration or treatment with chloroform.

VIRUS ISOLATION IN NEWBORN MICE

Coxsackievirus A is not readily detected in cell cultures (Table 25.9). Isolation requires that specimens should be injected into litters of newborn mice (24–48 h old) by intracerebral, intraperitoneal and subcutaneous routes. The group A viruses induce general myositis of striated muscle, causing flaccid paralysis and death. The B group cause spastic paralysis and degenerative changes in the brain and necrosis of the brown fat.

TEST FOR ANTIBODIES

A few diseases – notably pleurodynia, hand-foot-and-mouth disease and acute haemorrhagic conjunctivitis – are so regularly associated with particular serotypes (viz. coxsackieviruses B1–5, coxsackievirus A16 and enterovirus 70 respectively) that their serological diagnosis is often feasible; in other situations virus isolation is the best approach. Antibody titres are compared in paired sera, the first sample being collected in the acute phase and the second 1–14 days later. ELISA or radioimmunoassay may be used as well as neutralization or, in some cases, haemagglutination inhibitor. Such methods can be used to assay for IgM specifically, and thus identify acute infections.

MOLECULAR BIOLOGICAL METHODS

The detection of virus-specific sequences by dot or slot blot, sandwich or nucleic acid hybridization in situ has led to the identification of viral sequences in postmortem and biopsy material and in isolates. The detection of coxsackievirus B2 RNA sequences in 9 of 17 patients with active or healed myocarditis or cardiopathy of

Table 25.9 Comparative sensitivity of enterovirus isolation systems

Virus group	Primary monkey[a]/baboon	Primary human ammion	Human embryo lung (semi-continuous)	RD[b]	Newborn mice
Poliovirus	++	+	+	++	−
Coxsackievirus A	±[c]	±	±[d]	+	++
Coxsackievirus B	++	±	±	−	+
Echovirus	++	+	+	++	±
Enterovirus	+	Variable	+	Variable	±

[a]Rhesus or cynomolgus
[b]RD = human rhabdomyosarcoma continuous cell line
[c]Coxsackie A7, A9, A10, A16
[d]Coxsackie A21
− = nil; ± = poor; + = good; ++ = very good

unknown origin (Bowles et al. 1986) illustrates the importance of this assay; until now, information on the role of enteroviruses in these diseases has depended largely on circumstantial evidence based on neutralization tests. The potential of these hybridization techniques, particularly in relation to chronic viral illness, is enormous (Kandolf 1988).

Polymerase chain reaction (PCR) is increasingly applied to clinical specimens and isolates, particularly using primers able to amplify a wide range of enterovirus sequences, which can then be studied further.

5.2 Rhinoviruses

Rhinovirus infections are normally diagnosed by isolation of virus from respiratory secretions. As for the enteroviruses, serological techniques have only limited value because of the large number of serotypes and the absence of a specific rhinovirus group antigen.

Rhinoviruses are most often isolated from nasal washings but throat or nasal swabs and sputa are suitable alternative samples. Virus is rarely isolated from blood.

Specimens should be transported to the laboratory in a buffered medium containing about 1 mg of protein (e.g. bovine plasma albumin) per millilitre and inoculated into cell cultures as soon as possible. Most rhinoviruses are strictly species-specific. Therefore, apart from the few strains that grow in monkey kidney cells, human rhinoviruses will grow only in cells of human origin. Semi-continuous cell strains from human embryonic lung are the most widely used for virus isolation, although certain virus strains are isolated more readily in diploid cells from human embryonic kidney or tonsils. Semi-continuous cell strains from different human embryos vary considerably in their sensitivity to rhinoviruses and these differences are not always revealed by titration of laboratory passaged viruses (Stott and Walker 1967, Fox, Cooney and Hall 1975). A continuous line of HeLa cells, sensitive to rhinoviruses, may also be used for primary isolation (Cooney and Kenny 1977). Bovine rhinoviruses are usually isolated in secondary calf kidney cells. All cell cultures inoculated with rhinoviruses should be rolled at 33°C in medium with pH below 7.6. Virus-infected cultures develop small areas of refractile cells, usually within 7 days. Such cytopathic agents are tentatively identified as rhinoviruses by demonstrating that they resist chloroform or ether,

pass through a 50 nm filter, grow in the presence of bromodeoxyuridine (a DNA inhibitor) and are destroyed at pH 5. Final identification of a rhinovirus serotype requires neutralization by specific antiserum but this procedure can be simplified by combining antisera into a scheme of pools (Kenny, Cooney and Thompson 1970).

Organ cultures of human embryonic trachea or nasal epithelium support the growth of some rhinoviruses that cannot be isolated in cell cultures. Although most of these viruses can subsequently be passaged in cell culture, some apparently replicate only in organ cultures.

When the infecting serotype is known, as in volunteer trials, virus antigen can be detected in nasal washings by ELISA, using specific polyclonal or monoclonal antibodies.

Molecular methods can also be applied. Deoxyoligonucleotides complementary to conserved sequence of the 5' noncoding region hybridize to the RNAs of all 57 rhinovirus serotypes so far tested and also detect virus in nasal washings specifically and efficiently (Bruce et al. 1988). This approach has the further advantage that cDNA to this region of viral RNA may be specifically amplified by the polymerase chain reaction, increasing the sensitivity of the technique.

Serological diagnosis of rhinovirus infection by demonstrating rising antibody titres is practicable only when the serotype of the infecting virus is known. The microneutralization test has been widely used for the detection of rhinovirus antibodies. The haemagglutination inhibition test is particularly useful for the rapid screening of volunteers for antibodies before inoculation (Reed and Hall 1973) but can, of course, be used only for serotypes that haemagglutinate. This restriction does not apply to ELISA or complement fixation tests.

6 CONTROL OF ENTEROVIRAL INFECTIONS

There are no antiviral agents for the prevention or treatment of enteroviral diseases. Quarantine of patients or contacts is of little use because most infections are inapparent and spread among close contacts is rapid. A degree of control can be achieved in special baby-care units (where enterovirus infections can often prove fatal), by 'barrier nursing', an increase in general hygiene of the staff and exclusion of staff and parents with even 'minor' illnesses. Similar precautions in eye clinics may help when acute haemorrhagic conjunctivitis is present in the community.

Use of immunoglobulin

Commercially prepared γ-globulin may be useful in preventing enteroviral disease, especially in nurseries threatened by serious outbreaks of group B coxsackieviruses. Its use halted an outbreak of echovirus 11 in a premature baby unit in England in 1983.

Prophylaxis: rhinoviruses

The use of formalin-inactivated rhinovirus 1A vaccine to induce antibody was first described in 1963 (Doggett et al. 1963, Mufson et al. 1963). Subsequently, similar inactivated vaccines made from rhinoviruses 2 and 13 have been administered by subcutaneous, intramuscular or intranasal routes and have protected volunteers against live virus challenge. The problem of numerous serotypes with little or no cross-protection remains.

Specific therapy

In a review of chemotherapy for rhinovirus infections, Sperber and Hayden (1988) have pointed out that treatment may be aimed at either the virus or the symptoms it induces.

Many compounds specifically inhibit rhinoviruses in vivo but few have beneficial effects against infection in vivo although some are used in symptom relief. Interferon, zinc salts, synthetic antiviral agents and monoclonal antibodies have been tested against rhinovirus colds in placebo-controlled trials.

Natural and recombinant human interferons have been tested clinically. Recombinant interferon-α_2 administered intranasally protects against natural and experimental rhinovirus infections. However, no therapeutic benefit is observed even if treatment is started within 30 hours of virus challenge.

Zinc salts inhibit the cleavage of viral polypeptides. This observation led to a clinical trial of zinc gluconate lozenges in which there seemed to be a major reduction in the duration of symptoms. Subsequently, 3 carefully conducted placebo-controlled trials failed to demonstrate any benefit from the lozenges against experimentally induced colds. Furthermore, field trials did not demonstrate any therapeutic benefit against naturally occurring colds. Finally, unpleasant side effects are often associated with oral administration of zinc salts.

A number of compounds are now available that specifically bind to rhinovirus capsids and block uncoating. The Sterling-Winthrop compound disoxaril and its derivations have powerful antiviral effects both in vitro and in animals inhibiting viral uncoating. It has been established by x-ray crystallography that this drug acts within the VP1 β barrel of the capsid. Two other compounds, dichloroflavan and R61837, also inhibit rhinovirus uncoating, and probably bind to a similar region of the capsid. In clinical trials, dichloroflavan is ineffective but R61837 has significant benefit when given intranasally before an experimental rhinovirus challenge. Enviroxime, a benzimidazole derivative, seems to inhibit the formation of the viral RNA polymerase replication complex. When given orally and intranasally before the challenge, enviroxime significantly reduces production of nasal mucus. However, no therapeutic benefit has yet been demonstrated.

Murine monoclonal antibodies directed against the major group cell receptor compete with rhinoviruses in vitro and displace previously bound virions from cells, thus inhibiting infection. One of these monoclonal antibodies, administered intransally and prophylactically to humans, modified experimental rhinovirus infection both clinically and virologically.

A major pharmacokinetic obstacle to effective therapy is the maintenance of an adequate concentration of drug in respiratory mucosae where rhinoviruses replicate. Furthermore, successful therapies must work rapidly and be free of any side effects.

Prophylaxis: the eradication of poliomyelitis

Polioviruses are believed to have been established throughout most of the population of the world from ancient times, surviving in an endemic form by infection of susceptible infants. Because of the universal presence of antibody to all 3 serotypes in women of child-bearing age, and the protective effect of maternal antibody on disease but not gut infection, most infants would be infected while still protected. Improvements in standards of hygiene in the late 19th century led to a delay in the exposure of infants to an age when maternal antibody had declined to non-protective levels. Patterns of disease then changed from the relatively uncommon and endemic kind to the occurrence of large epidemics, and poliomyelitis also became known as infantile paralysis. Safe and effective polio vaccines were developed and used in the 1950s and are among the most impressive public health achievements of the 20th century. The incidence of poliomyelitis in the USA between 1951 and 1979 is shown in Fig. 25.5, demonstrating the effect of vaccination.

Inactivated polio vaccine

The first of the currently used vaccines to be developed was the formalin-inactivated preparation of Salk (1960). Virus was treated with low concentrations of formalin under carefully controlled conditions to ensure that infectivity but not immunogenicity was lost. The resulting inactivated poliovaccine (IPV) is administered by injection; in the early days there were significant problems of production, particularly of the type 1 component which is the least immunogenic of the serotypes in IPV. Immediately after the licensure of the vaccine, batches were used that contained imperfectly inactivated virus, resulting in paralysis in recipients. This was the Cutter incident, and is attributed to the presence of aggregates in which the virus at the centre of a clump was protected from inactivation. Production was revised at once to introduce filter steps before and after treatment to remove aggregates, and no case of poliomyelitis attributable to IPV has been reported since. However, filtration removed viral antigen, making the supply problems more intense, and it was not until the 1980s with the development of improved high density cell culture systems that high potency IPV (enhanced potency IPV, EIPV) became available.

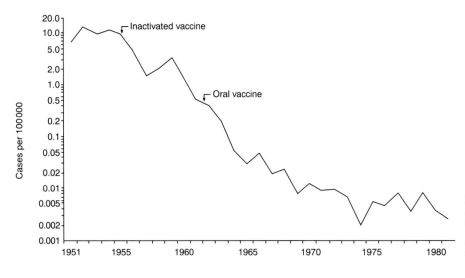

Fig. 25.5 Incidence of paralytic poliomyelitis in USA from 1951 to 1979, showing the effect of vaccination.

LIVE POLIO VACCINE

The relative merits of inactivated polio vaccine and live attenuated vaccines were a matter of heated debate. Both are highly effective and safe, but it was argued that the live, oral vaccine (OPV) developed by Sabin (Sabin and Boulger 1973), which imitated natural gut infection, also stimulated gut immunity, preventing reinfection and thus interrupting transmission. Whilst it can be shown that even recent OPV vaccinees can be reinfected by wild type strains, OPV is effective in breaking transmission in epidemics. This may be due in part to gut immunity or to simple competition. Where countries have used IPV alone, unimmunized subpopulations can suffer outbreaks. For example, a religious group in Holland experienced outbreaks of type 1 in 1976 and type 3 in 1993.

The Sabin vaccine strains were developed by passage in vivo or in vitro and selected for reduced neurotropism by tests in primates. The molecular basis of this attenuation for primates was studied intensively in the 1980s and 90s (Minor 1992).

The type 3 strain was studied in particular because it failed the primate safety test more often than types 1 and 2. Complete sequences of the genomes of the virulent precursor strain (Leon), the vaccine strain (Leon 12$_{a1b}$) and a virulent revertant isolated from a fatal case of vaccine-associated poliomyelitis were determined and compared to identify features common to the virulent strains that distinguished them from the vaccine strain. Recombinant viruses were made by genetic engineering, followed by recovery of virus from the infectious DNA, in which portions of the attenuated vaccine strain genome were exchanged for the equivalent region of the Leon genome to identify changes that would attenuate. Finally, a deattenuated version of the Sabin type 3 vaccine strain was made in which all bases thought to have an attenuating effect were reverted to the virulent form. The conclusion from these studies was that only 2 mutations were responsible for the great majority of the attenuation of the Sabin type 3 vaccine strain. They were a base change at residue 472 in the 5′ non-coding region, and a coding change leading to a substitution

of a phenylalanine residue for a serine residue at position 91 of the capsid protein VP3. The 5′ non-coding change leads to a loss of efficiency in the initiation of protein synthesis in in vitro translation systems (Svitkin, Maslova and Agol 1985), and the change in VP3 is responsible in large part for the fact that growth of the Sabin vaccine strain is greatly inhibited at high temperatures. Other changes may make some contribution to the attenuated phenotype, but these 2 cause the only effects readily detectable in the standard virulence tests.

Comparable recombinants were made between the type 1 Sabin and the virulent type 1 Mahoney strains. The relatively large number of differences between the strains made detailed analysis more difficult, but it was concluded that a major attenuating mutation was to be found at base 480 in the 5′ non-coding region, comparable to that found in type 3, and that other mutations were scattered through the genome. For type 2 there is evidence for a mutation in a similar location in the 5′ non-coding region at residue 481, and in structural protein VP1 at residue 143.

A striking feature of the mutations in the 5′ non-coding region is that, in studies of viruses excreted by vaccinees in the UK, they revert to the virulent form in all cases for type 2 and type 3 and in half the isolates for type 1. For type 3, the temperature-sensitive phenotype is also lost at a later stage. During the course of excretion, changes also occur in antigenic sites, at the extreme 3′ terminus, and by recombination. Such modifications are extremely common and rapid.

Despite these changes, the virus is antigenically stable in the sense that it is restricted to 3 serotypes, and the vaccine is very safe and effective. However, as shown in Fig. 25.5, the number of cases when OPV is used does not decline to zero, and many of the residual cases are attributable to a strain derived from the vaccine given. The incidence is currently calculated to be one per 2×10^6 vaccine recipients over all, or one per 530 000 in previously unimmunized infants. In practice, this frequency is so low as to be difficult to measure with confidence, but there is no doubt that there is a small risk of poliomyelitis associated with OPV in both recipient and contacts. The risk with types 2 and 3 is similar, and of the order of 5 times higher than for type 1.

THE ERADICATION OF WILD POLIOMYELITIS

In 1988 the World Health Organization declared the goal of eliminating all cases of poliomyelitis in the world due to wild type virus by the year 2000. This was to be done by the use of live attenuated vaccines, despite the belief that they are less effective in tropical countries because of interference by other enteric infections or for other reasons. Figure 25.6 shows that great progress has been made toward this goal. In the Americas no poliomyelitis has been recorded since 1992, the last case being in Peru. This has been achieved in large part by campaigns in which the aim is to immunize all children within a specified age range in a very short period of time. Thus children receive many doses of vaccine, susceptible individuals are colonized by vaccine rather than by wild type polio

strains, and transmission is interrupted. This contrasts with the strategy of immunizing children as they reach a certain age, which is also followed, and which focuses on protecting the individual rather than interrupting transmission.

One of the important factors in this exercise has been the demonstration that virus transmission has been interrupted. This has depended on the specific identification of virus strains, which has been accomplished by sequencing a relatively small part of the genome encoding the region around the VP1-2A gene (Rico-Hesse et al. 1987). Such sequences can be used to construct dendrograms of relatedness, and it has been possible to identify 'genotypes' of the different serotypes, defined as strains differing by 15% or less in sequence. The genotypes are found to be geographically clustered; thus an isolate from the Middle East made recently closely resembles other isolates from the Middle East, including those made some time ago. It is therefore possible to say whether a particular virus is indigenous to the country of origin or

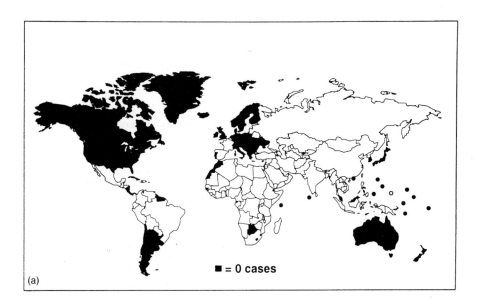

(a)

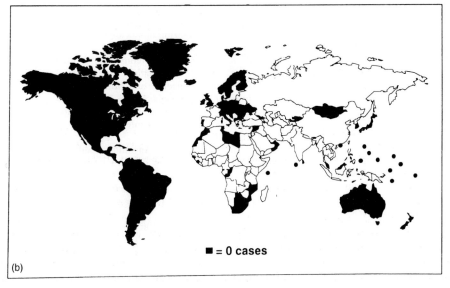

(b)

Fig. 25.6 Global distribution of poliomyelitis in (a) 1988 and (b) 1994. Shaded areas indicate countries with no reports of poliomyelitis due to wild type virus.

was imported, and if so from where. For example, in 1984 a small outbreak of type 3 poliomyelitis occurred in Finland in which there were 9 paralytic cases and one case of aseptic meningitis. Circulation of the strain was widespread despite the use of IPV in Finland, and there was some evidence that the strain was antigenically unusual. Genomic analysis revealed that the strain originated from the Middle East, possibly imported by soldiers serving with the UN.

The pattern of poliomyelitis cases in unimmunized populations is that 90% are caused by type 1, and most of the remainder by type 3. As eradication nears, the pattern changes to increase the role of type 3, which is the least effective of the live attenuated strains. The evidence suggests that infection by all 3 serotypes is equally common but that the type 1 serotype is intrinsically more virulent, exactly the reverse of the situation with the vaccines.

7 FUTURE PROSPECTS

It is possible that poliomyelitis due to wild type virus will be eliminated in the near future, although some areas such as Africa will be extremely difficult to deal with because of poor infrastructure and a deeper level of poverty than found in the Americas. At that point the only way of contracting poliomyelitis will be by vaccination, which will therefore presumably stop. The strategy for doing so has not yet been elaborated, but the risk is that the vaccine strains will occupy the niche occupied by wild poliovirus, and, in view of their ability to adapt, that they will become virulent. It will therefore be necessary to protect individuals for some time until it can be shown that the vaccine-derived strains are not circulating freely but have died out. It is likely that this will be done by changing to the use of IPV rather than OPV, accompanied by suitable environmental monitoring. In Finland after the 1984/85 outbreak, OPV was used extensively but was only detectable in sewage for a period of a few months. It is therefore possible that circulation will not be prolonged, and that poliomyelitis will become the second disease to be eliminated, after smallpox.

REFERENCES

Acharya R, Fry E et al., 1989, The three-dimensional structure of foot-and-mouth disease virus at 2.9 Å resolution, *Nature (London)*, **337:** 709–16.

Archard LC, Banner M et al., 1988, Persistence of enterovirus RNA in dilated myocardiopathy. A progression from myocarditis, *New Concepts in Viral Heart Disease*, ed Schultheib H-P, Springer-Verlag, New York, 349–62.

Barrett-Connor E, 1985, Is insulin-dependent diabetes mellitus caused by coxsackievirus B infection? A review of the epidemiologic evidence, *Rev Infect Dis*, **7:** 207–15.

Beatrice ST, Katze MG et al., 1980, Induction of neutralizing antibodies by the coxsackievirus B3 virion polypeptide, VP2, *Virology*, **104:** 426–38.

Behan PO, 1980, Epidemic myalgic encephalomyelitis, *Practitioner*, **224:** 805–7.

Bendinelli M, Friedman H, eds, 1988, *Coxsackieviruses: a general update*, Plenum Press, New York, London.

Bergelson JM, Shepley MP et al., 1992, Identification of the integrin VLA-2 as a receptor for echovirus 1, *Science*, **255:** 1718–20.

Bittle JL, Houghten RA et al., 1982, Protection against foot-and-mouth disease by immunization with a chemically synthesized peptide predicted from the viral nucleotide sequence, *Nature (London)*, **298:** 30–3.

Bloom HH, Forsyth BR et al., 1963, Relationship of rhinovirus infection to mild upper respiratory disease. 1. Results of a survey in young adults and children, *JAMA*, **186:** 38–45.

Bodian D, 1955, Emerging concept of poliomyelitis infection, *Science*, **122:** 105–8.

Bögel K, Böhm H, 1962, Ein rhinovirus des Rindes, *Zentralbl Bakteriol Orig Abt 1*, **187:** 2–14.

Bowles NE, Richardson PJ et al., 1986, Detection of Coxsackie B virus specific RNA sequences in myocardial biopsy samples from patients with myocarditis and dilated cardiomyopathy, *Lancet*, **1:** 1120–3.

Bruce CB, Al-Nakib W et al., 1988, Synthetic oligonucleotides as diagnostic probes for rhinoviruses [letter], *Lancet*, **2:** 53.

Burke KL, Dunn G, Ferguson M et al., 1988, Antigen chimaeras of poliovirus as potential new vaccines, *Nature (London)*, **332:** 81–2.

Buscho RO, Saxtan D et al., 1978, Infections with viruses and *Mycoplasma pneumoniae* during exacerbations of chronic bronchitis, *J Infect Dis*, **137:** 377–83.

Butterworth BE, Grunert RR et al., 1976, Replication of rhinoviruses, *Arch Virol*, **51:** 169–89.

Campbell BA, Cords CE, 1983, Monoclonal antibodies that inhibit attachment of group B coxsackieviruses, *J Virol*, **48:** 561–4.

Cate TR, Couch RB et al., 1965, Production of tracheobronchitis in volunteers with rhinovirus in a small particle aerosol, *Am J Epidemiol*, **81:** 95–105.

Channock RM, Parrott RH, 1965, Acute respiratory disease in infancy and childhood: present understanding and prospects for prevention, *Pediatrics*, **36:** 21–39.

Cherry JD, 1973, Newer respiratory viruses: their role in respiratory illness of children, *Adv Pediatr*, **20:** 225–90.

Chow M, Newman JFE et al., 1987, Myristylation of picornavirus capsid protein VP4 and its structural significance, *Nature (London)*, **327:** 482–4.

Clarke BE, Newton SE et al., 1987, Improved immunogenicity of a peptide epitope after fusion to hepatitis B core protein, *Nature (London)*, **330:** 381–4.

Colonno RJ, Callahan PL et al., 1989, Inhibition of rhinovirus attachment by neutralizing monoclonal antibodies and their Fab fragments, *J Virol*, **63:** 36–42.

Cooney MK, Kenny GE, 1977, Demonstration of dual rhinovirus infection in humans by isolation of different serotypes in human heteroploid (HeLa) and human diploid fibroblast cell cultures, *J Clin Microbiol*, **5:** 202–7.

D'Alessio DJ, Peterson JA et al., 1976, Transmission of experimental rhinovirus colds in volunteer married couples, *J Infect Dis*, **133:** 28–36.

Dalldorf G, Sickles GM, 1948, An unidentified, filtrable agent isolated from the faeces of children with paralysis, *Science*, **108:** 61–3.

Dasgupta A, Zabel P, Baltimore D, 1980, Dependence of the activity of the poliovirus replicase on the host cell protein, *Cell*, **19:** 423–9.

Doggett JE, Bynoe ML et al., 1963, Some attempts to produce an experimental vaccine with rhinoviruses, *Br Med J*, **1:** 34–6.

Douglas RG Jr, Couch RB, 1972, Parenteral inactivated rhinovirus vaccine: minimal protective effect, *Proc Soc Exp Biol Med*, **139:** 899–902.

Elveback LR, Fox JP et al., 1966, The virus watch program: a continuing surveillance of viral infections in metropolitan New York families. 3. Preliminary report on association of infections with disease, *Am J Epidemiol*, **83:** 436–54.

Enders JF, Weller TH, Robbins FC, 1949, Cultivation of the Lansing strain of poliomyelitis virus in cultures of various human embryonic tissues, *Science*, **109:** 85–7.

Ferguson M, Minor PD et al., 1984, Neutralization epitopes on poliovirus type 3 particles: an analysis using monoclonal antibodies, *J Gen Virol*, **65:** 197–201.

Flanegan JB, Baltimore D, 1977, Poliovirus specific primer dependent RNA polymerase able to copy poly(A), *Proc Natl Acad Sci USA*, **74:** 3677–80.

Fox JP, 1976, Is a rhinovirus vaccine possible?, *Am J Epidemiol*, **103:** 345–54.

Fox JP, Cooney MK, Hall CE, 1975, The Seattle virus watch. V. Epidemiologic observations of rhinovirus infections, 1965–1969, in families with young children, *Am J Epidemiol*, **101:** 122–43.

Fox JP, Cooney MK et al., 1985, Rhinoviruses in Seattle families, 1975–1979, *Am J Epidemiol*, **122:** 830–46.

Gamble DR, 1980, The epidemiology of insulin dependent diabetes with particular reference to the relationship of virus infection to its etiology, *Epidemiol Rev*, **2:** 49–70.

Gear JHS, 1984, Non polio causes of polio-like paralytic syndromes, *Rev Infect Dis*, **6, suppl 2:** S379–84.

Greve J, Davis G et al., 1989, The major human rhinovirus receptor is ICAM-1, *Cell*, **56:** 839–47.

Grist NR, Bell EJ et al., 1979, *Diagnostic Methods in Clinical Virology*, 3rd edn, Blackwell Scientific, Oxford, 129–145.

Gwaltney JM, Hendley JO, 1978, Rhinovirus transmission: one if by air; two if by hand, *Am J Epidemiol*, **107:** 357–61.

Gwaltney JM, Jordan WS, 1966, Rhinoviruses and respiratory illnesses in university students, *Am Rev Respir Dis*, **93:** 362–71.

Gwaltney JM, Moskalski PB, Hendley JO, 1978, Hand-to-hand transmission of rhinovirus colds, *Ann Intern Med*, **88:** 463–7.

Gwaltney JM, Hendley JO et al., 1966, Rhinovirus infections in an industrial population. 1. The occurrence of illness, *N Engl J Med*, **275:** 1261–8.

Hammon WM, Coriell LL et al., 1953, Evaluation of Red Cross gamma globulin as prophylactic agent for poliomyelitis; final report of results based on clinical diagnosis, *JAMA*, **151:** 1272–85.

Hamparian VV, Leagus MB et al., 1964, Epidemiologic investigations of rhinovirus infections, *Proc Soc Exp Biol Med*, **117:** 469–76.

Hamparian VV, Colonno RJ et al., 1987, A collaborative report: rhinoviruses – extension of the numbering system from 89 to 100, *Virology*, **159:** 191–2.

Hamre D, Connelly AP Jr, Procknow JJ, 1966, Virologic studies of acute respiratory disease in young adults. IV. Virus isolations during four years of surveillance, *Am J Epidemiol*, **83:** 238–49.

Hayflick L, Moorhead PS, 1961, The serial cultivation of human diploid cell strains, *Exp Cell Res*, **25:** 585–621.

Hendley JO, Gwaltney JM Jr, Jordan WS Jr, 1969, Rhinovirus infections in an industrial population. IV. Infections within families of employees during two fall peaks of respiratory illness, *Am J Epidemiol*, **89:** 184–96.

Higgins PG, Ellis EM, Boston DG, 1966, The isolation of viruses from acute respiratory infections. 3. Some factors influencing the isolation of viruses from cases studied during 1962–64, *Mon Bull Minist Health Public Health Lab Serv*, **25:** 5–17.

Hogle JM, Chow M, Filman DJ, 1985, Three dimensional structure of poliovirus at 2.9 Å resolution, *Science*, **229:** 1358–65.

Holland JJ, McLaren LC et al., 1959, The mammalian cell virus relationship. IV. Infection of naturally insusceptible cells with enterovirus ribonucleic acid, *J Exp Med*, **110:** 65–80.

Holzel A, Parker L et al., 1965, Virus isolations from throats of children admitted to hospital with respiratory and other diseases, Manchester 1962–4, *Br Med J*, **1:** 614–19.

Hoorn B, Tyrell DAJ, 1965, On the growth of certain 'newer' respiratory viruses in organ cultures, *Br J Exp Pathol*, **46:** 109–18.

Hope-Simpson RE, 1958, Discussion on the common cold, *Proc R Soc Med*, **51:** 267–74.

Horn ME, Gregg I, 1973, Role of viral infection and host factors in acute episodes of asthma and chronic bronchitis, *Chest*, **63, suppl:** 44S–8.

Horn ME, Reed SE, Taylor P, 1979, Role of viruses and bacteria in acute wheezy bronchitis in childhood: a study of sputum, *Arch Dis Child*, **54:** 587–92.

Hummeler K, Tumilowicz JS, 1960, Studies on the complement fixing antigens of poliomyelitis. II. Preparation of the type-specific anti-N and anti-H indicator sera, *J Immunol*, **84:** 630–4.

Huovilainen A, Hovi T et al., 1987, Evolution of poliovirus during an outbreak: sequential type 3 poliovirus isolates from several persons show shifts of neutralization determinants, *J Gen Virol*, **68:** 1373–8.

Joklik WL, Darnell JE, 1961, The adsorption and early fate of purified poliovirus in HeLa cells, *Virology*, **13:** 439–47.

Kandolf R, 1988, The impact of recombinant DNA techniques on the study of enterovirus heart disease, *Coxsackieviruses: a general update*, eds Bendinelli M, Friedman H, Plenum Press, New York, London, 293–318.

Kapikian AZ, Conant RM et al., 1967, Rhinoviruses: a numbering system, *Nature (London)*, **213:** 761–2.

Kenny GE, Cooney MK, Thompson DJ, 1970, Analysis of serum pooling schemes for identification of large numbers of viruses, *Am J Epidemiol*, **91:** 439–45.

Kitamura N, Semler BL et al., 1981, Primary structure, gene organization and polypeptide expression of poliovirus RNA, *Nature (London)*, **291:** 547–53.

Kono R, Miyamura K et al., 1977, Virological and serological studies of neurological complications of acute hemorrhagic conjunctivitis in Thailand, *J Infect Dis*, **135:** 706–13.

Kruse WV, 1914, Die Erreger von Husten und Schnupfen, *Münchener Med Wochenschr*, **61:** 1547.

Kuhn RJ, Wimmer E et al., 1987, The replication of picornaviruses, *The Molecular Biology of the Positive Strand RNA Viruses*, FEMS Symposium No 32, eds Rowlands DJ, Mayo MA, Mahy BWJ, Academic Press, London, 17–52.

Le Bouvier GL, 1955, The modification of poliovirus antigens by heat and ultraviolet light, *Lancet*, **2:** 1013–16.

Lonberg-Holm K, Crowell RL, Philipson L, 1976, Unrelated animal viruses share receptors, *Nature (London)*, **259:** 679–81.

Lundquist RE, Ehrenfeld E, Maizel JV Jr, 1974, Isolation of a viral polypeptide associated with poliovirus RNA polymerase, *Proc Natl Acad Sci USA*, **71:** 4773–7.

Mahon BP, Katrak K et al., 1995, Poliovirus-specific CD4+ Th1 clones with both cytotoxic and helper activity mediate protective humoral immunity against a lethal poliovirus infection in transgenic mic expressing the human poliovirus receptor, *J Exp Med*, **181:** 1285–92.

Matteucci D, Paglianti M et al., 1985, Group B coxsackieviruses readily establish persistent infections in human lymphoid cell lines, *J Virol*, **56:** 651–4.

Mayer MM, Rapp HJ et al., 1957, The purification of poliomyelitis virus as studied by complement fixation, *J Imunol*, **78:** 435–55.

Medrano L, Green H, 1973, Picornavirus receptors and picornavirus multiplication in human–mouse hybrid cell lines, *Virology*, **54:** 515–24.

Melnick JL, 1984, Enterovirus type 71 infections: a varied clinical pattern sometimes mimicking paralytic poliomyelitis, *Rev Infect Dis*, **6:** S387–90.

Melnick JL, 1990, Enteroviruses: polioviruses, coxsackieviruses, echoviruses and newer enteroviruses, *Fields' Virology*, 2nd edn, eds Fields BN, Knipe DM, Raven Press, New York, 549–605.

Melnick JL, Wimberly IL, 1985, Lyophilized combination pools of enterovirus equine antisera: new LBM pools prepared from reserves of antisera stored frozen for two decades, *Bull W H O*, **63:** 543–50.

Mendelsohn C, Johnson B et al., 1986, Transformation of a human poliovirus receptor gene into mouse cells, *Proc Natl Acad Sci USA*, **83:** 7845–9.

Mendelsohn C, Wimmer E et al., 1989, Cellular receptor for poliovirus: molecular cloning, nucleotide sequence, and expression of a new member of the immunoglobulin superfamily, *Cell*, **56:** 855–65.

Miller DA, Miller OJ et al., 1974, Human chromosome 19 carries a poliovirus receptor gene, *Cell*, **1:** 167–173.

Ming Luo, Vriend G et al., 1987, The atomic structure of Mengo virus at 3.0 Å resolution, *Science*, **235:** 182–91.

Minor PD, 1992, The molecular biology of poliovaccines, *J Gen Virol*, **73:** 3065–77.

Minor PD, Pipkin PA et al., 1984, Monoclonal antibodies which block cellular receptors of poliovirus, *Virus Res*, **1:** 203–12.

Minor PD, John A et al., 1986a, Antigenic and molecular evolution of the vaccine strain of type 3 poliovirus during the period of excretion by a primary vaccinee, *J Gen Virol*, **67:** 693–706.

Minor PD, Ferguson M et al., 1986b, Antigenic structure of polioviruses of serotypes 1, 2 and 3, *J Gen Virol*, **67:** 1283–91.

Minor PD, Ferguson M et al., 1986c, Conservation in vivo of protease cleavage sites in antigenic sites of poliovirus, *J Gen Virol*, **68:** 1857–65.

Minor PD, Ferguson M et al., 1990, Antigenic structure of chimeras of type 1 and type 3 poliovirus involving antigenic site 1, *J Gen Virol*, **71:** 2543–51.

Minor PD, Ferguson M et al., 1991, Antigenic structure of chimeras of type 1 and type 3 polioviruses involving antigenic sites 2, 3 and 4, *J Gen Virol*, **72:** 2475–81.

Monto AS, Cavallaro JJ, 1972, The Tecumseh study of respiratory illness. IV. Prevalence of rhinovirus serotypes, 1966–1969, *Am J Epidemiol*, **86:** 352–60.

Monto AS, Johnson KM, 1966, Serologic relationships of the B632 and ECHO-28 rhinovirus strains, *Proc Soc Exp Biol Med*, **121:** 615–19.

Moore M, Morens DM, 1984, Enteroviruses, including polioviruses, *Textbook of Human Virology*, ed Belshe RB, PSG Publishing, Littleton MA, 407–84.

Moore M, Katona P et al., 1982, Poliomyelitis in the United States, 1969–1981, *J Infect Dis*, **146:** 558–63.

Mufson MA, Ludwig WM et al., 1963, Effect of neutralizing antibody on experimental rhinovirus infection, *JAMA*, **186:** 578–84.

Mufson MA, Krause HE et al., 1970, The role of viruses, mycoplasmas and bacteria in acute pneumonia in civilian adults, *Am J Epidemiol*, **86:** 526–44.

Murray MG, Kuhn RJ et al., 1988, Poliovirus type 1/type 3 antigenic hybrid virus constructed in vitro elicits type 1 and type 3 neutralizing antibodies in rabbits and monkeys, *Proc Natl Acad Sci USA*, **85:** 3203–7.

Naclerio RM, Proud D et al., 1988, Kinins are generated during experimental rhinovirus colds, *J Infect Dis*, **157:** 133–42.

Page GS, Mosser AG et al., 1988, Three-dimensional structure of poliovirus serotype 1 neutralizing determinants, *J Virol*, **62:** 1781–94.

Palmenberg A, 1987, *The molecular biology of the positive strand RNA viruses*, FEMS Symposium No 32, eds Rowlands DJ, Mayo MA, Mahy BWJ, Academic Press, London, 1–16.

Pelletier J, Sonenberg N, 1988, Internal initiation of translation of eukaryotic mRNA directed by a sequence derived from poliovirus RNA, *Nature (London)*, **334:** 320–5.

Perkins JC, Tucker DN et al., 1969, Evidence for protective effect of an inactivated rhinovirus vaccine administered by the nasal route, *Am J Epidemiol*, **90:** 319–26.

Phillips CA, Melnick JL et al., 1968, Rhinovirus infections in a student population: isolation of five new serotypes, *Am J Epidemiol*, **87:** 447–56.

Pipkin PA, Wood DJ et al., 1993, Characterisation of L cells expressing the human poliovirus receptor for the specific detection of polioviruses in vitro, *J Virol Methods*, **41:** 333–40.

Plummer G, 1963, An equine respiratory enterovirus. Some biological and physical properties, *Archiv Gesamte Virusforsch*, **12:** 694–700.

Powell DG, Burrows R et al., 1978, A study of the infectious respiratory diseases among horses in Great Britain, 1971–1976, *Equine Infectious Diseases IV*, eds Bryans JT, Gerber H, Veterinary Publications, Princeton, 451–9.

Price WH, Emerson H et al., 1959, Studies of the JH and 2060 viruses and their relationship to mild upper respiratory disease in humans, *Am J Hyg*, **69:** 224–49.

Putnak JR, Phillips BA, 1981, Picornaviral structure and assembly, *Microbiol Rev*, **45:** 287–315.

Racaniello VR, Baltimore D, 1981, Cloned poliovirus complementary DNA is infectious in mammalian cells, *Science*, **214:** 916–19.

Reed SE, 1972, Viral enhancement of mycoplasma growth in tracheal organ cultures, *J Comp Pathol*, **82:** 267–.

Reed SE, Boyde A, 1972, Organ cultures of respiratory epithelium infected with rhinovirus or parainfluenza virus studied in a scanning electron microscope, *Infect Immun*, **6:** 68–76.

Reed SE, Hall TS, 1973, Hemagglutination-inhibition test in rhinovirus infections of volunteers, *Infect Immun*, **8:** 1–3.

Reed SE, Tyrell DA et al., 1971, Studies on a rhinovirus (EC11) derived from a calf. I. Isolation in calf tracheal organ cultures and characterization of the virus, *J Comp Pathol*, **81:** 33–40.

Ren R, Racaniello VR, 1992, Poliovirus spreads from muscle to the central nervous system by neural pathways, *J Infect Dis*, **166:** 747–52.

Rico-Hesse R, Pallansch MA et al., 1987, Geographic distribution of wild poliovirus type 1 genotypes, *Virology*, **160:** 311–22.

Robbins FC, Enders JF et al., 1951, Studies on the cultivation of poliomyelitis viruses in tissue culture. V, the direct isolation and serologic identification of virus strains in tissue culture from patients with paralytic and non-paralytic poliomyelitis, *Am J Hyg*, **54:** 286–293.

Rombaut B, Vrijsen R, Boeye A, 1983, Epitope evolution in poliovirus maturation, *Arch Virol*, **76:** 289–98.

Rossmann MG, 1987, The evolution of RNA viruses, *BioEssays*, **7:** 99–103.

Rossmann MG, Arnold E et al., 1985, Structure of a human common cold virus and functional relationship to other picornaviruses, *Nature (London)*, **317:** 145–53.

Rueckert RR, Wimmer E, 1984, Systematic nomenclature of picornavirus proteins, *J Virol*, **50:** 957–9.

Sabin AB, 1955, Pathogenesis of poliomyelitis: reappraisal in the light of new data, *Science*, **123:** 1151–7.

Sabin AB, Boulger LR, 1973, History of Sabin attenuated poliovirus oral live vaccine strains, *J Biol Standard*, **1:** 115–18.

Salk JE, 1960, Persistence of immunity after administration of formalin-treated poliovirus vaccine, *Lancet*, **2:** 715–23.

Sarnow P, Bernstein HD, Baltimore D, 1983, A poliovirus temperature-sensitive RNA synthesis mutant located in a noncoding region of the genome, *Proc Natl Acad Sci USA*, 571–5.

Schieble JH, Lennette EH, Fox VL, 1970, Antigenic variation of rhinovirus type 22, *Proc Soc Exp Biol Med*, **133:** 329–33.

Schnurr DP, Schmidt NJ, 1988, Persistent infections, *Coxsackieviruses: a general update*, eds Bendinelli M, Friedman H, Plenum Press, New York, London, 181–201.

Shepley MP, Racaniello VR, 1994, A monoclonal antibody that blocks poliovirus attachment recognizes the lymphocyte homing receptor CD44, *J Virol*, **68:** 1301–8.

Sherry B, Mosser AG et al., 1986, Use of monoclonal antibodies to identify four neutralization immunogens on a common cold picornavirus, human rhinovirus 14, *J Virol*, **57:** 246–57.

Sperber SJ, Hayden FG, 1988, Chemotherapy of rhinovirus colds, *Antimicrob Agents Chemother*, **32:** 409–19.

Staunton DE, Merluzzi VJ et al., 1989, A cell adhesion molecule, ICAM-1, is the major surface receptor for rhinoviruses, *Cell*, **56:** 849–53.

Stott EJ, Walker M, 1967, Human embryo kidney fibroblasts for the isolation and growth of rhinoviruses, *Br J Exp Pathol*, **48:** 544–51.

Stott EJ, Grist NR, Eadie MB, 1968, Rhinovirus infections in chronic bronchitis: isolation of eight possibly new rhinovirus serotypes, *J Med Microbiol*, **1:** 109–17.

Stott EJ, Thomas LH et al., 1980, A survey of virus infections of the respiratory tract of cattle and their association with disease, *J Hyg*, **85:** 257–70.

Svitkin YV, Maslova SV, Agol VI, 1985, The genomes of attenuated and virulent poliovirus strains differ in their in vitro translation efficiencies, *Virology*, **147:** 243–52.

Toniolo A, Federico G et al., 1988, Diabetes mellitus, *Coxsackieviruses: a general update*, eds Bendinelli M, Friedman H, Plenum Press, New York, London, 351–82.

Tyrrell DAJ, 1965, *Common Colds and Related Diseases*, Edward Arnold, London, 197.

Tyrrell DA, Mika-Johnson M et al., 1979, Infection of cultured human type II pneumonocytes with certain respiratory viruses, *Infect Immun*, **26:** 621–9.

Villa-Komaroff L, McDowell M et al., 1974, Translation of reovirus mRNA, poliovirus RNA and bacteriophage Qbeta RNA in cell-free extracts of mammalian cells, *Methods Enzymol*, **30:** 709–23.

Ward T, Pipkin PA et al., 1994, Decay-accelerating factor CD55 is identified as the receptor for echovirus 7 using CELICS, a rapid immuno-focal cloning method, *EMBO J*, **13:** 5070–4.

Wilfert CM, Thompson RJ Jr et al., 1981, Longitudinal assessment of children with enteroviral meningitis during the first three months of life, *Pediatrics*, **67:** 811–15.

Yamashita H, Akashi H, Inaba Y, 1985, Isolation of a new serotype of bovine rhinovirus from cattle. Brief report, *Arch Virol*, **83:** 113–16.

Young DC, Tuschall DM, Flanegan JB, 1985, Poliovirus RNA-dependent RNA polymerase and host cell protein synthesize product RNA twice the size of poliovirion RNA in vitro, *J Virol*, **54:** 256–64.

Yousef GE, Bell EJ et al., 1988, Chronic enterovirus infection in patients with postviral fatigue syndrome, *Lancet*, **1:** 146–50.

Zhang G, Wilsden G et al., 1993, Complete nucleotide sequence of a coxsackie B5 virus and its relationship to swine vesicular disease virus, *J Gen Virol*, **74:** 845–53.

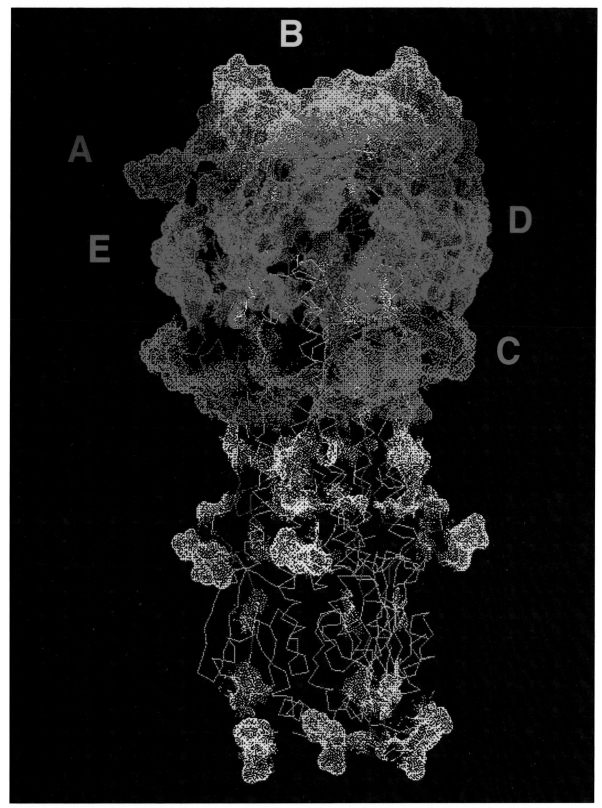

Plate 22.19 Natural antigenic variation in the haemagglutinin (HA) of the H3 subtype of influenza A viruses circulating between 1968 and 1996. The HA trimer is depicted with the HA polypeptide backbone represented by an α-carbon trace in violet for the HA1 domain and in yellow for the HA2 domain. The solvent-accessible surface of residues that have changed during this period is represented by a dot surface. Antigenic regions are colour coded and designated A (red), B (yellow), C (magenta), D (blue) and E (green). Amino acid residues shown in white are surface accessible but not assigned to antibody-combining sites. This graphic representation demonstrates that most of the surface-accessible amino acids in the globular head region of the HA have changed during this 28-year period of circulation in humans of influenza A(H3N2) viruses.

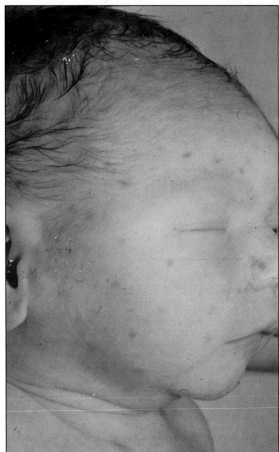

Plate 28.5 Purpuric rash in newborn infant with congenitally acquired rubella, who was subsequently found to have congenital heart disease and cataract.

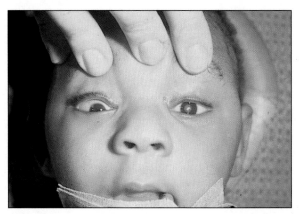

Plate 28.6 Congenital rubella cataract in a 9-month-old infant. Cataract present in the left eye was surgically removed.

HUMAN ENTERIC RNA VIRUSES: CALICIVIRUSES AND ASTROVIRUSES

I N Clarke, P R Lambden and E O Caul

---

1 **Historical perspectives**
2 **Enteric caliciviruses**

3 **Astroviruses**

---

1 HISTORICAL PERSPECTIVES

Diarrhoeal disease in humans, clinically distinct from bacterial gastroenteritis, was first reported in the southern USA. It was originally described as 'hyperemesis hiemis' or winter vomiting disease (Zahorsky 1929), a term that reflects its seasonality. The illness occurred in widespread epidemics with a high secondary attack rate, and was documented as a short, self-limiting episode of vomiting with some diarrhoea. Later, this syndrome was also recognized by clinicians in the UK (Miller and Raven 1936, Gray 1939, Bradley 1943). Its distinction from bacterial gastroenteritis was confirmed by investigations of institutional outbreaks in which stool cultures were consistently negative for pathogenic bacteria.

A variety of synonymous terms were used for this syndrome between the 1940s and early 1970s, including non-bacterial gastroenteritis, epidemic gastroenteritis, acute infectious non-bacterial gastroenteritis and epidemic vomiting disease. The transmissibility of an agent by oral inoculation of human volunteers with a faecal filtrate was repeatedly demonstrated (Reimann, Price and Hodges 1945, Gordan, Ingraham and Korns 1947, Jordan, Gordan and Dorrance 1953, Adler and Zickl 1969, Dolin et al. 1971, Clarke et al. 1972). This approach established the possibility of a viral aetiology and, although the natural history of this transmissible agent was comprehensively described, all attempts to isolate a bacterial pathogen or a viral agent failed.

Eventually, an outbreak of epidemic gastroenteritis in a primary school in Norwalk, Ohio, led to confirmation of its viral aetiology (Kapikian et al. 1972). Faecal filtrates from affected children were fed to volunteers, whose stools were examined by immunoelectron microscopy. A previously undescribed virus-like particle, 27 nm in diameter, was detected and subsequently named Norwalk virus. Further studies in volunteers established it as the agent responsible for the original outbreak. Seroconversions or rising IgG titres as well as virus excretion were demonstrated in infected volunteers, and the histopathology of jejunal biopsies from those with acute disease gave new insights into the cell tropism of Norwalk virus in the small intestine (Agus et al. 1973, Schreiber, Blacklow and Trier 1973). These studies heralded the discovery of other, taxonomically distinct, viruses associated with gastroenteritis.

Soon after the discovery of the Norwalk virus a small round 22 nm diameter virus (Wollan agent) was detected in stools from patients in Bristol, UK (Paver et al. 1973). Electron microscopy (EM) revealed fundamental differences in both size and morphology between the Norwalk and Wollan agents. Both the American and the British workers described their respective isolates as parvovirus-like on the basis of biophysical properties (Kapikian et al. 1973, Paver, Caul and Clarke 1974). It has since been shown that Norwalk virus is more correctly classified within the *Caliciviridae*. Subsequently, other parvo-like viruses morphologically indistinguishable from the Wollan agent were described in association with outbreaks of gastroenteritis and were termed the Ditchling agent (Appleton et al. 1977) and cockle agent (Appleton and Pereira 1977) respectively. The Wollan, Ditchling and cockle agents and many other morphologically similar small round viruses (SRVs) are likely to be classified within the family *Parvoviridae* and so far have no proven role in causing disease. Furthermore, SRVs indistinguishable from these 3 viruses are detectable in normal stool samples from the general population. The most likely explanation for the outbreaks with which these viruses were associated is that they were caused by Norwalk-like viruses that were not detected at the time. Further volunteer studies by American workers identified viruses morphologically similar to the Norwalk agent in 2 outbreaks of non-bacterial gastroenteritis. These viruses were termed Montgomery County and Hawaii respectively (Kapikian 1994), after the locations of the outbreaks. This mode of nomenclature became common (Caul 1988) and continues. These early EM studies demonstrated the difficulties of accurately establishing the taxonomic status and aetiological role of small round human faecal viruses and would give rise to considerable confusion in subsequent studies.

The widespread application of EM to the examination of diarrhoeal stool samples resulted in major advances in our knowledge of the aetiology of non-bacterial gastroenteritis. Rotaviruses were rapidly identified as major pathogens in endemic infantile gastroenteritis, and other viruses, including 'fastidious' adenoviruses, were added to the increasing list of enteric 'diarrhoea' viruses. There were many reports of an apparently wide range of SRVs varying in size and morphology. In many studies SRVs were identified by immunoelectron microscopy (IEM), which masks surface morphology, and often resulted in a confusing picture of the aetiology of non-bacterial gastroenteritis. Other SRVs were identified from their classic surface structure; and detailed descriptions of the morphology of the newly described astroviruses and 'classic' caliciviruses were published (Madeley 1979).

In an attempt to bring some order to the recognition of the many SRVs being reported, Caul and Appleton (1982) published an 'interim classification scheme' that was adopted to aid national surveillance within the UK and to establish which SRVs were causally related to viral gastroenteritis (Fig. 26.1). The scheme included comparative morphological criteria derived by EM examination of known animal and human SRVs. The authors concluded that SRVs could be readily subdivided into those viruses without any resolvable surface structure ('featureless') and those with an obvious surface morphology. The featureless group included both picornaviruses and parvovirus-like particles, the latter being represented by the Wollan, Ditchling, cockle and the Australian 'Parramatta' (Christopher et al. 1978) agents. All 4 agents had been previously implicated in outbreaks of non-bacterial gastroenteritis but conclusive evidence of their role in disease is so far lacking.

The second group of SRVs all possessed a surface morphology to which descriptive terms could be applied; they included the previously described astroviruses, 'classic' caliciviruses and viruses that shared the morphological features of an amorphous surface structure and 'ragged' edged virions. These viruses were represented by the prototype Norwalk virus; the Hawaii and Montgomery County viruses were added later. They were morphologically distinguishable from both astroviruses and the classic caliciviruses and were termed small round structured viruses (SRSVs). A prerequisite of this study was that all viruses were examined in the absence of antibody to ensure that any surface structure would not be obscured by antibody molecules.

The application of the interim classification scheme in the UK over many years has established important epidemiological information on the prevalence of astroviruses, caliciviruses and SRSVs as aetiological agents in non-bacterial gastroenteritis (Figs. 26.2 and 26.3). SRSVs emerged as the most important cause of epidemic non-bacterial gastroenteritis world-wide. All members of this group cause similar illnesses and are morphologically indistinguishable by EM.

This morphological classification scheme recognized fundamental differences between SRSVs and the classic caliciviruses, and was supported by epidemiological and immunological distinctions (Caul 1988, Blacklow and Greenberg 1991). The molecular characterization of SRSVs and the classic caliciviruses (Liu et al. 1995) also demonstrated significant differences despite the recent classification of SRSVs within the family *Caliciviridae* (Jiang et al. 1990, Jiang et al. 1993, Lambden et al. 1993, Lambden, Liu and Clarke 1995). The clinical, epidemiological and pathological aspects of SRSVs, caliciviruses and astroviruses (Table 26.1), as well as our current knowledge of their taxonomic status at the molecular level, will now be considered.

2   ENTERIC CALICIVIRUSES

2.1   Small round structured viruses

Norwalk virus particles were first visualized in 1972 by IEM with convalescent sera from a volunteer who became ill following ingestion of a faecal filtrate of the Norwalk virus (Kapikian et al. 1972). Morphologically indistinguishable agents have since been described in clinically similar outbreaks and were termed Hawaii (Wyatt et al. 1974, Thornhill et al. 1977), Snow Mountain (Morens et al. 1979, Dolin et al. 1982) and Taunton agents (Caul, Ashley and Pether 1979, Pether and Caul 1983).

The use of volunteers has considerably increased our knowledge of the transmissibility, pathogenesis and immunobiology of the Norwalk and Hawaii viruses (Schreiber, Blacklow and Trier 1973, Wyatt et al. 1974, Schreiber, Blacklow and Trier 1974, Parrino et al. 1977) and has established a previously undescribed and poorly characterized group of related viruses as important causes of epidemic gastroenteritis. Many other workers subsequently described morphologically similar viruses associated with an identical clinical syndrome, many of which have also been assigned a geographical nomenclature (Caul 1988). These viruses cause acute, explosive diarrhoea, vomiting or both, and are highly infective, with rapid secondary spread. Large outbreaks have been described in semi-closed communities throughout the world as a result of person-to-person spread (Kaplan et al. 1982, Pether and Caul 1983, Caul 1988, Christensen 1989). Point-source outbreaks resulting from

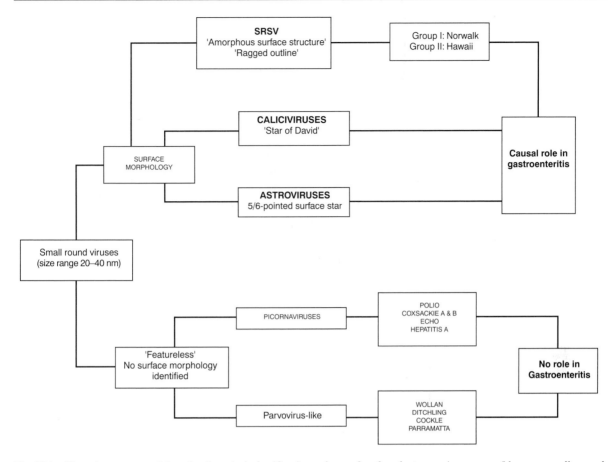

Fig. 26.1 Flow chart summarizing the 'interim' classification scheme for the electron microscopy of human small round viruses.

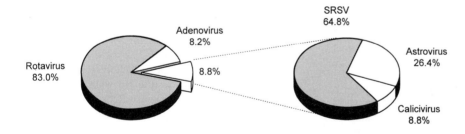

Fig. 26.2 Incidence of viruses causing acute non-bacterial gastroenteritis in England and Wales reported to the Communicable Disease Surveillance Centre (Colindale, England) between 1990 and 1994.

ingestion of sewage-contaminated water, contaminated shellfish or food (Morens et al. 1979, Murphy et al. 1982) emphasize the great public health importance of this group of viruses. There are major problems in controlling such outbreaks, and the economic implications, including those applicable to the food and shellfish industries, are being increasingly recognized.

The inability to propagate this group of viruses in vitro has severely hampered the development of reagents for laboratory assays, and EM remains the most widely used technique for identification and diagnosis. The introduction of the term 'small round structured virus' (SRSV) to describe and distinguish this group of viruses from other small round faecal viruses has facilitated recognition of their importance as major causes of epidemic gastroenteritis in the UK and elsewhere.

CLASSIFICATION AND MORPHOLOGY

These viruses were originally described as non-enveloped, round, 27 nm particles with a 'ragged' outer edge but lacking a definite surface structure (Kapikian et al. 1972). The paucity of virions found in stool samples together with their small size and amorphous structure has made them difficult to detect by direct EM. Many other small round structured viruses (Norwalk-like viruses) have been described which have in common a buoyant density of 1.33–1.41 g/cm^3, an inability to propagate in vitro and an RNA genome of positive polarity (Greenberg and Matsui 1992). Despite their amorphous structure, recent advances in the characterization of the genome have shown that the SRSVs are members of the family *Caliciviridae* (Jiang et al. 1993, Lambden et al. 1993, Dingle et al. 1995).

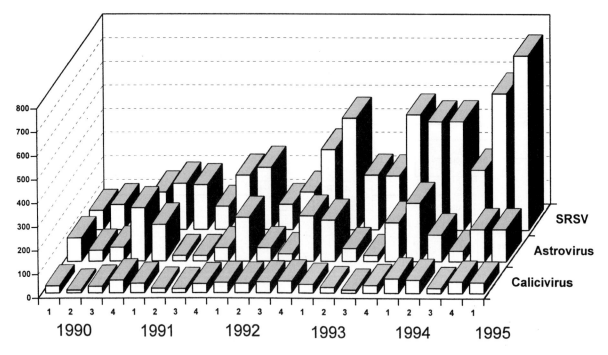

Fig. 26.3   Comparison of incidence rates of calicivirus, astrovirus and SRSV infections in England and Wales. The chart shows the relative incidence of cases attributable to the respective viruses reported to the Communicable Disease Surveillance Centre (Colindale, England) between 1990 and early 1995.

These viruses are characterized by a single capsid protein (Greenberg et al. 1981) but lack of a cell culture system has restricted production of capsid antigen to heterologous expression systems. Capsid proteins expressed in insect cells using baculovirus vectors spontaneously assemble to form virus-like particles and are released into the cell culture supernatant (Jiang et al. 1992, Dingle et al. 1995, Jiang et al. 1995). These virus-like particles are larger than SRSVs and have the appearance of empty virions (Fig. 26.4).

Cryoelectron microscopy and computer image processing techniques have determined the empty virion structure to a resolution of 2.2 nm (Prasad et al. 1994) (Fig. 26.5). The empty capsids are composed of 90 dimers of the capsid structural protein and are 38 nm in diameter with T = 3 icosahedral symmetry. Arch-like capsomers formed from dimers of the capsid structural protein and deep depressions at the 5- and 3-fold axes are distinctive features. Each virus-like particle has 32 surface hollows surrounded by the protruding arches. Twelve hollows are at the icosahedral 5-fold axis and have a small hump at the centre. The other 20 hollows at the 3-fold positions seem to be flat. This distinctive molecular architecture has also been described for a primate calicivirus (Prasad, Matson and Smith 1994) and it has been suggested that the primary sequence of the capsid protein may be organized into structural domains. The N terminal 250 residues may form an 8-strand β barrel in the lower shell, the remaining C terminal amino acids forming the protruding domains. Sequence comparisons indicate that the C terminal domain exhibits significant variation.

ORGANIZATION OF THE GENOME

Since the first reports of the molecular cloning of the Norwalk virus genome in 1990, rapid progress has been made in the genome analysis of SRSVs. Virus purified from faeces of volunteers infected with Norwalk virus was used to generate a library of cDNA clones representing most of the viral genome. Authentic clones were identified by hybridization to post- but not pre-infection stool nucleic acid. Sequence information indicated that the Norwalk virus genome is single-stranded, positive-sense RNA of about 7.5 kb and polyadenylated at the 3′ terminus (Jiang et al. 1990). In one of the viral clones a motif characteristic of viral RNA-dependent RNA polymerases was identified. Matsui and colleagues (1991) then cloned a region of the Norwalk virus genome that was immunoreactive when expressed in recombinant λ phage. Complete genome sequences (Jiang et al. 1993, Lambden et al. 1993, Dingle et al. 1995, Lambden, Liu and Clarke 1995) have since been determined, together with several partial sequences covering the RNA polymerase and capsid regions in the 3′ half of the genome (Green et al. 1994, Lew et al. 1994a, 1994b; 1994c, Wang et al. 1994, Green et al. 1995a).

Sequence comparisons of the RNA polymerase and capsid regions of the genome indicate that SRSVs may be divided into 2 genetic groups (Ando et al. 1994, Cubitt et al. 1994, Green et al. 1994, Wang et al. 1994). Two group I viruses (Norwalk and Southampton viruses) and one group II virus (Lordsdale virus) have been fully sequenced. The genome of group I viruses is slightly larger (7.7 kb) than the group II genome

Table 26.1 Properties of the human enteric caliciviruses and astroviruses

Virus	Appearance	Genome structure	Clinical features	Examples
SRSVs	Feathery, ragged outline No distinctive surface structure Some preparations resemble classic calicivirus No cell culture system	ssRNA, +ve polarity, polyadenylated, c. 7.7 kb group I and 7.5 kb group II ORF1 non-structural polyprotein ORF2 capsid ORF3 small basic protein Possible subgenomic RNA	'Winter vomiting disease' Epidemic nausea vomiting and diarrhoea Acquisition of antibodies is gradual, vomiters are more likely to seroconvert Peak illness in adults No immunity Clinical features identical for group I and group II viruses	**Group I:** Norwalk virus (school outbreak, USA 1969) Southampton virus (family outbreak, UK 1991) **Group II:** Hawaii virus (family outbreak, USA 1972) Lordsdale virus (hospital outbreak, UK 1993)
Calicivirus	Distinctive cup-shaped surface depressions, giving classic 'star of David' morphology No cell culture system	ssRNA, +ve polarity, polyadenylated, c.7.3 kb ORF1 non-structural polyprotein contiguous with and fused to capsid gene ORF2 small basic protein Additional small ORF overlapping capsid in alternative reading frame Subgenomic RNA and VPg present in animal virus	No seasonal variance Predominantly paediatric illness Antibodies acquired at young age Diarrhoeal illness is mild	HuCV/Sapporo isolated from an outbreak in an orphanage Sapporo, Japan (1982) HuCV/Manchester from a sporadic case of acute vomiting and diarrhoea in a 6 month old child (1993)
Astrovirus	Smooth surface outline with characteristic 5- or 6-pointed surface star Virus grows in cell culture and can be isolated directly from clinical samples	ssRNA, +ve polarity, polyadenylated, c. 6.8 kb ORF1a and b non-structural polyproteins in different reading frames produced by ribosome frame shifting ORF2 capsid precursor is cleaved Co-terminal subgenomic RNA 2.4 kb	No obvious seasonal variance Young children most susceptible Antibodies acquired at young age Diarrhoeal illness is mild Occasional outbreaks among elderly	7 recognized human serotypes (HAstV-1–7) Complete genome sequence available for serotypes 1 and 2 viruses grown and purified from CaCo2 cells

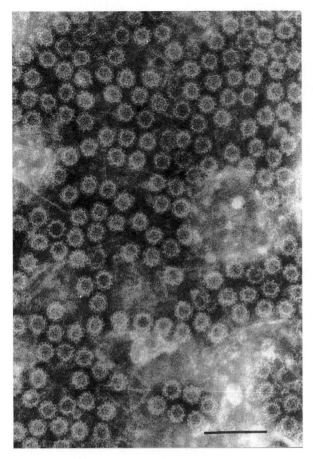

Fig. 26.4 Electron micrograph showing recombinant virus-like particles produced by expression of Southampton virus capsid protein from insect cells. Bar = 100 nm.

the capsid structural protein. At the 3′ end of the genome is a small ORF, predicted by computer analysis to encode a basic protein. The genome organization of SRSVs clearly distinguishes these viruses from other positive-stranded RNA viruses such as the picornaviruses.

The smaller size of the group II SRSV genome is attributable to its smaller ORF1. The nucleotide (nt) sequence in the 5′ region of ORF1 shows significant diversity between the 2 genetic groups although distal to this variable region both groups show the characteristic motifs of the helicase, cysteine protease and RNA polymerase in the same relative genomic positions. Sequence diversity at the 5′ end of the genome may reflect fundamental differences between the 2 groups of viruses in terms of secondary structures or regulatory signals.

The capsid coding region in the SRSV genome is similar to the arrangement in feline calicivirus (FCV) in which ORF2 is frame-shifted relative to ORF1 so that the N terminus of the capsid protein overlaps the C terminus of the putative RNA-dependent RNA polymerase. However, the extent of reading frame overlap differs between the 2 genetic groups of SRSVs: it is 17 nt in group I and 20 nt in group II. The small 3′ ORF is also in a different reading frame from the capsid. The first residue of the initiator codon of ORF3 overlaps the last base of the terminator codon of the capsid gene. A characteristic feature of the animal caliciviruses is the production of a 3′ co-terminal polyadenylated subgenomic RNA coding for the capsid and small 3′ ORF (Meyers, Wirblich and Thiel 1991). The subgenomic RNA is thought to provide an additional message for the production of capsid protein and in the case of rabbit haemorrhagic disease virus (RHDV) this additional RNA is packaged into mature virions (Meyers, Wirblich and Thiel 1991). It is not yet clear if SRSVs produce a subgenomic message although detection of RNA of over 2 kb by Northern blot analysis of total stool RNA from a volunteer infected with Norwalk virus suggested that this virus may also produce a subgenomic RNA (Jiang et al. 1993). A characteristic feature of the animal calicivirus genomic and

(7.5 kb), although computer analyses reveal that the reading frame usage of these 2 genetic groups is very similar and strikingly like that of the well characterized feline calicivirus (Carter et al. 1992). The genomes of both group I and group II SRSVs (Fig. 26.6) are characterized by a large 5′ open reading frame (ORF) encoding a non-structural polyprotein of c. 1700 amino acids followed by a smaller ORF encoding

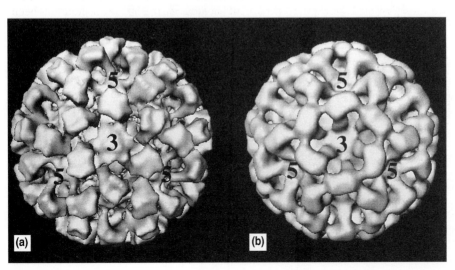

Fig. 26.5 Computer-generated images from cryoelectron microscopic preparations of (a) recombinant Norwalk virus capsids and (b) primate calicivirus. The images are viewed along the 3-fold axes. (Photograph by courtesy of Dr B V V Prasad, Baylor College of Medicine, Houston TX, USA.)

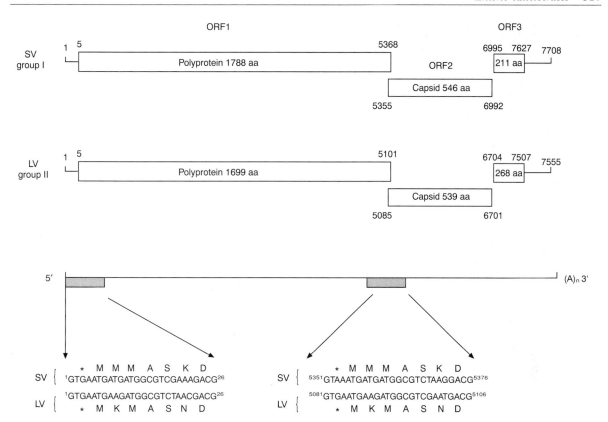

Fig. 26.6 Comparison of the genome structure of a group I and a group II SRSV. Open boxes represent computer-predicted open reading frames. Translation products and their sizes are indicated above the boxes. The conserved sequences at the 5′ genomic termini and the predicted 5′ termini of the subgenomic RNAs are aligned beneath the genome map. Shaded boxes represent the genomic position of these motifs. LV, Lordsdale virus (EMBL/GenBank Accession No X86557); SV, Southampton virus (EMBL/GenBank Accession No L07418).

subgenomic RNAs is that the 5′ termini are highly conserved (Lambden and Clarke 1995). The 5′ terminal sequence of ORF1 is repeated around the 5′ terminal region of ORF2. The first reported genome sequences did not reveal similar repeated motifs in the Norwalk and Southampton viruses, suggesting that the SRSVs may be fundamentally different from the animal caliciviruses (Jiang et al. 1993, Lambden et al. 1993). However, the use of alternative techniques for polymerase chain reaction (PCR) amplification of SRSV genome termini revealed similar highly conserved sequence motifs in both group I and group II SRSV genomes (Dingle et al. 1995, Lambden, Liu and Clarke 1995). These data strongly suggest that SRSVs, like their animal counterparts, also produce a subgenomic RNA.

VIRAL PROTEINS

Highly purified Norwalk virus (NV) recovered from CsCl equilibrium density gradients contains a single protein of 59 kDa (Greenberg et al. 1981). The single capsid protein was identified by radioimmunoprecipitation of purified virions with acute and convalescent sera from infected volunteers. Similar studies with the antigenically distinct Snow Mountain agent revealed a major structural polypeptide of 62 kDa (Madore, Treanor and Dolin 1986). In addition to the 59 kDa capsid protein of Norwalk virus, a soluble protein with

a molecular weight of 30 kDa was also detected in the supernatant of faecal suspensions. It has been estimated that up to 50% of the excreted antigen is present as soluble protein (Jiang et al. 1992). Until recently the source of the soluble protein remained uncertain and was suggested to be an immunogenic non-structural protein or a cleavage product derived from the capsid protein. However, by use of virus-like particles expressed from insect cells infected with recombinant baculovirus, the 30 kDa protein has been identified as a specific cleavage product of the viral capsid (Hardy et al. 1995). Recombinant Norwalk virus treated with trypsin released a 32 kDa protein and analysis of the N-terminal sequence of this product revealed that a trypsin-specific cleavage occurred at amino acid residue 227. The 30 kDa soluble protein reacted with rabbit polyclonal antisera raised against recombinant Norwalk virus capsids, and analysis of the N-terminal sequence of the 30 kDa soluble protein showed it to be identical with the 32 kDa trypsin cleavage product. In addition, it was shown that the 32 kDa proteolytic cleavage product is derived from soluble capsid protein and not intact assembled virions. These data suggest that the Norwalk virus capsid undergoes proteolytic cleavage during the course of infection. Japanese isolates antigenically related to the Hawaii virus also demonstrated immunoreactive structural proteins of 63 and 30 kDa by Western blot analysis (Hayashi et al. 1989, Oishi et al. 1992).

Several groups have described capsid gene sequences from a number of different SRSV isolates that encode proteins with predicted molecular weights of c. 60 kDa. Computer alignments of the capsid sequence data support the division of SRSVs into 2 major genetic groups. The capsid proteins have c. 68% amino acid sequence identity within a genetic group and 40% between groups. However, the SRSV capsids show only limited homology with the corresponding animal calicivirus protein. A dendrogram of the phylogenetic relatedness of the SRSVs and typical animal caliciviruses is given in Fig. 26.7. The prototype Norwalk virus and the antigenically distinct Southampton virus are both members of genetic group I together with the Desert Shield virus and a Japanese isolate, KY89. The recent UK isolate, Lordsdale virus, has been assigned to genetic group II along with Bristol virus, Snow Mountain agent, Hawaii virus, Toronto virus and another Japanese isolate, OTH-25.

The first major ORF encodes a polyprotein that is presumably processed by a proteolytic cascade analogous to that of picornaviruses. Computer analysis of the ORF1 sequence data has identified conserved amino acid motifs typical of the picornaviral 2C helicase, 3C protease and RNA-dependent RNA polymerase. Sequence comparisons of group I and II viruses reveal, apart from the short conserved sequence motifs, extreme sequence diversity at the 5′ proximal regions of the genomes. Thus it is not clear whether caliciviruses use the picornaviral internal ribosome entry site (IRES) mechanism of translation initiation or if the genome acts as a capped mRNA with translation by the conventional ribosome scan-

ning mechanism. In rabbit haemorrhagic disease virus (RHDV) the genomic and subgenomic RNAs are linked at their 5′ termini to a small protein analogous to picornaviral VPg although the caliciviral protein (c. 15 kDa) is considerably larger than the picornaviral equivalent (22 amino acids). The presence of a VPg-like protein, encoded by ORF1 in SRSVs, is strongly inferred by analogy with the animal caliciviruses.

At present no biological function has been assigned to the translation product of ORF3, although the fact that this ORF is present in all caliciviruses and SRSVs sequenced so far suggests an essential role for this protein. The ORF3 translation product shows considerable sequence variation both within and between genetic groups. This is surprising, if the predicted protein product has the same functional role in both groups of viruses.

ANTIGENIC VARIATION

Cross-challenge studies in volunteers have demonstrated that Norwalk and Hawaii viruses are antigenically distinct (Kapikian 1994) and further volunteer studies with the Montgomery County agent identified a one-way cross-protection with Hawaii virus. There was short-term homologous immunity after challenge of humans with all 3 viruses (Dolin et al. 1972, Wyatt et al. 1974). Long-term immunity to homologous challenge has also been demonstrated (Parrino et al. 1977), and this unusual aspect and the complexity of the immunobiology of SRSVs are under investigation (Kapikian 1994).

The antigenic relatedness of Norwalk, Hawaii and Snow Mountain viruses was studied by testing serological responses in volunteers. With an enzyme immunoassay (EIA), variable degrees of antigenic relatedness were observed with a 2-way cross-reaction between Snow Mountain and Hawaii virus and a one-way cross-reaction between Norwalk and Snow Mountain viruses (Madore et al. 1990). These results may reflect heterologous responses and contrast with the greater specificity of IEM or SPIEM (solid phase immunoelectron microscopy) which is based on the use of intact virions and capsid epitopes.

Four antigenic types of SRSV have been identified by IEM or SPIEM in the UK (Lewis 1990, 1991, Lambden et al. 1993), 6 in the USA (Lewis et al. 1995) and 9 in Japan (Okada et al. 1990). It has been suggested, on the basis of cross-reactions, that the 9 Japanese serotypes include similar viruses and may therefore be an overestimate of the actual number of serotypes. Definitive data on the antigenic relationship of SRSVs will have to await the development of specific monoclonal antibodies that are less broadly reactive than human convalescent or hyperimmune sera. This is a possibility now that some strains of SRSVs have been completely sequenced, allowing the production of expressed viral proteins and monoclonal antibodies. Despite the technical drawbacks, SPIEM has been useful in defining the changing prevalence of different SRSV antigenic types in the UK and for identifying appropriate isolates for molecular characterization.

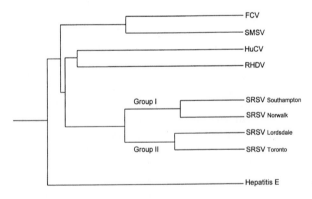

Fig. 26.7 Dendrogram of the phylogenetic relationship of the capsid proteins of members of the *Caliciviridae*. FCV (feline calicivirus, M86379); SMSV, (San Miguel sealion virus, M87481); HuCV (human enteric calicivirus, X86560); RHDV, (rabbit haemorrhagic disease virus, M67473); SRSV (small round structured virus: Southampton, L07418; Norwalk, M87661; Lordsdale, X86557; Toronto, U02030). The EMBL/GenBank accession numbers are shown in parentheses. Computer analyses were performed on the complete amino acid sequence of the capsid proteins. The length of the horizontal branches is proportional to the genetic distance between strains. The 2 genetic groups of SRSV are indicated on their respective branches.

CLINICAL MANIFESTATIONS

Detailed information on the clinical, immunological and pathological aspects of SRSVs have been established from investigations on volunteers (Kapikian 1994), in whom infections by Norwalk virus, Hawaii agent, Montgomery County agent and the Snow Mountain agent are clinically indistinguishable (Wyatt et al. 1974, Morens et al. 1979, Kapikian 1994). Following transmission by the faecal–oral route, volunteer and epidemiological studies have established an incubation period of c. 24 h (Kapikian 1994) with a dose-dependent range of 18–48 h (Blacklow and Herrmann 1988). Symptoms are sudden in onset and are accompanied by nausea and vomiting which can be projectile and severe. Low grade fever and diarrhoea usually occur, the latter being relatively mild. By contrast with bacterial gastroenteritis, diarrhoeal stools do not contain blood, mucus or white cells. Other symptoms include mild abdominal pain or cramps, malaise and headaches. Vomiting may arise from a decrease in gastric motility (Meeroff et al. 1980), giving rise to a reflux action into the stomach. Respiratory involvement has not been observed and nasopharyngeal washings from an acutely ill volunteer did not induce disease on passage to other volunteers (Dolin et al. 1972).

In general, SRSV infections are self-limiting and affected patients rarely need to be hospitalized. There have, however, been occasional reports of severe dehydration that required administration of intravenous fluids. Deaths associated with SRSV infections are exceptionally rare and have not been directly attributed to this group of viruses (Kaplan et al. 1982).

PATHOGENESIS

Volunteer studies show that as few as 10–100 infectious particles may be needed to initiate infection. Replication is considered to occur in the mucosal epithelium of the small intestine although direct evidence is lacking. Light microscopy of jejunal biopsies from volunteers infected with Norwalk virus showed partial flattening and broadening of the villi with disorganization of the mucosal epithelium (Agus et al. 1973, Schreiber, Blacklow and Trier 1973). The lamina propria was infiltrated with mononuclear cells and vacuolization of mucosal epithelium was noted. Crypt cell hyperplasia was common. At the ultrastructural level mucosal epithelial cells showed dilatation of the rough and smooth endoplasmic reticulum with an increase in multivesiculate bodies. Microvilli were significantly shortened and amorphous electron-dense material was present in the expanded intercellular spaces. The absence of SRSVs in damaged mucosal cells was noteworthy. The results of light and electron microscopy in volunteers infected with the Hawaii agent were similar, and, again, virus particles were not identified in biopsies (Schreiber, Blacklow and Trier 1974, Dolin et al. 1975). In general, SRSV infections seem to cause mild atrophy of the villi of the small intestine, assumed to arise from limited virus replication that damages the mucosal cells. The appearance of mucosal lesions was paralleled by a decrease in brush border enzymes, which returned to normal values in convalescence (Agus et al. 1973).

EPIDEMIOLOGY

SRSVs are now established as the most important cause of epidemic non-bacterial outbreaks of gastroenteritis throughout the world (Kaplan et al. 1982, Blacklow and Greenberg 1991, Kapikian 1994). Extensive seroepidemiological studies in the USA and the direct detection of SRSVs by EM in various countries, particularly in the UK and Japan, have reinforced the importance of these viruses in community-wide outbreaks, which often have significant economic importance. National surveillance and diagnosis by EM of outbreaks of non-bacterial gastroenteritis in the UK have recently shown that SRSVs are now a more common cause of infective gastroenteritis than salmonella (Evans et al. 1995). These data demonstrate an increasing prevalence of SRSVs in recent years with the suggestion of a winter seasonality (Fig. 26.8) and show that all age groups are affected. This epidemiology differs from that of astrovirus and calicivirus infections.

The diversity of settings associated with these economically important viruses is demonstrated by the early work in the USA. Norwalk virus caused a community-wide outbreak in Norwalk, Ohio; Hawaii and Montgomery County agents were responsible for small family outbreaks (Thornhill et al. 1977) whereas the Snow Mountain agent caused an outbreak at a holiday camp in Colorado (Morens et al. 1979). The Taunton agent caused considerable disruption in a hospital in southern England (Caul, Ashley and Pether 1979, Pether and Caul 1983). Subsequent surveillance and investigations of outbreaks in many parts of the world identified the potential of SRSVs for causing epidemic gastroenteritis in semi-closed or community-wide populations; for example, families, healthcare institutions, holiday locations including cruise ships, educational establishments and the catering industry (Cukor and Blacklow 1984, Caul 1988, Kapikian 1994). Outbreaks occur among children and adults but rarely among neonates or very young children (Blacklow and Greenberg 1991). By contrast, the 'classic' caliciviruses are rarely associated with epidemic gastroenteritis in adults. Although considerable data are available on the causal role of SRSVs in outbreaks, less is known about their role in endemic disease, perhaps because of the relative mildness of the illness. Hospitalization of individual cases is thus unusual and opportunities to investigate sporadic cases are scarce.

Despite the lack of secondary spread by the respiratory route, it is clear that many of the explosive outbreaks described cannot be due solely to faecal–oral transmission. SRSVs can be detected in vomitus (Greenberg, Wyatt and Kapikian 1979); the projectile vomiting associated with acute infections and consequent formation of aerosols offers an alternative mode of spread (Sawyer et al. 1988, Ho et al. 1989, Caul 1994a, Chadwick and McCann 1994). This in conjunction with the low infectious dose would explain the rapid, explosive outbreaks commonly observed in

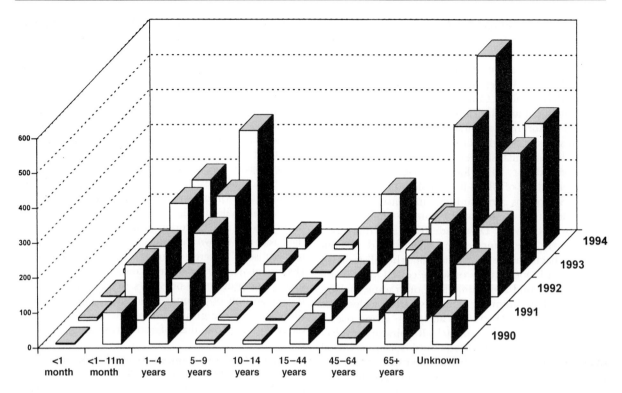

Fig. 26.8 SRSV incidence by age groups in England and Wales. The chart shows the numbers of cases reported to the Communicable Disease Surveillance Centre (Colindale, England) between 1990 and 1994. Reported cases occur across all the age groups.

semi-closed communities. The epidemiology of SRSV infections should thus include not only person-to-person spread but also mechanical transmission from hand to mouth. The likelihood of spread from inhalation of aerosol by contacts in close proximity to the index case has been suggested but not proved (Caul 1994a).

In addition to these modes of transmission, SRSVs are often associated with 'point-source' outbreaks (Okada et al. 1990, Caul et al. 1993, Kapikian 1994). In many cases a likely vehicle of transmission has been identified (Kapikian 1994). In the USA, contaminated water supplies – e.g. municipal water, drinking water on cruise ships, recreational swimming water (lake or pool) and commercially produced ice-cubes – have been incriminated (Greenberg et al. 1979, Cukor and Blacklow 1984, Blacklow and Greenberg 1991, Kapikian 1994). Food-borne outbreaks are well recognized, and food-specific attack rates have incriminated salads, bakery products, fresh fruit, cold foods, sandwiches and cooked meat (Griffin et al. 1982, Kuritsky et al. 1985, Caul 1994b, Kapikian 1994). The source of the contamination has often been identified as a symptomatic food handler (Pether and Caul 1983, Reid et al. 1988). The secondary attack rate of point-source outbreaks is often high. In the UK, 20–25% of SRSV outbreaks were associated with contaminated food (Caul 1994b) and 26 of 38 outbreaks in Japan were considered to be food-borne (Okada et al. 1990). The future application of molecular epidemiology should increase our knowledge of such outbreaks and the role of the food handler in transmission. The sec-

ondary attack rates in outbreaks in the USA reported by the Centers for Disease Control (CDC), Atlanta, ranged between 4% and 32% but attack rates of >50% have often been reported in semi-closed communities. Outbreaks have been prolonged by the introduction of susceptible individuals into an infected environment (e.g. aboard cruise ships and in hospitals).

Contaminated shellfish are major sources of epidemic gastroenteritis (Appleton and Pereira 1977, Christopher et al. 1978, Kaplan et al. 1982, Morse et al. 1986, Caul 1994b). The most commonly reported are the bivalve molluscs (oysters, cockles and mussels) which are filter-feeders and become infected from raw sewage. SRSVs are the major cause of viral gastroenteritis arising from eating shellfish in the UK, and both small and large outbreaks have been reported from a CDC study in the USA. In Australia, an outbreak of Norwalk virus gastroenteritis affecting more than 2000 people arose from a single batch of contaminated oysters (Murphy et al. 1979).

SEROEPIDEMIOLOGY

The inability to propagate SRSVs in cell culture and the lack of a suitable animal model severely limited seroprevalence studies in the past. American workers developed a number of serological assays, using faecal extracts containing Norwalk virus, to assess the acquisition of Norwalk antibody in different populations (Kapikian et al. 1978, Greenberg et al. 1979). It was acquired gradually during childhood, c. 20% of children <5 years old being positive. The prevalence of antibody rose rapidly to 45% in 18–35 year olds and to 55–60% in those aged 45–65 years. These findings accord with the prevalence of SRSV infections in older children and adults, and contrast with those of rotaviruses and classic caliciviruses. In developing countries, however, antibody is acquired very early in life. In Bangladesh 100% of children had acquired antibody by the age of 5 years whereas in Yugoslavia the seroprevalence rate was intermediate between that of the USA and those of less developed countries (Kapikian 1994); similar results have been reported from Taiwan and the Philippines. The prevalence of Norwalk virus antibody in blood donors in the USA, Belgium, Yugoslavia and Switzerland ranges from 54% to 77% and emphasizes the ubiquitous nature of this agent. Compelling evidence that Norwalk virus was responsible for many outbreaks throughout the world in the 1970s has been demonstrated by RIA tests (Kapikian 1994). All these studies were performed when Norwalk virus was circulating in the community.

The recent expression of recombinant Norwalk virus capsids in insect cells is a major advance (Jiang et al. 1992) and has allowed further seroepidemiological studies to be carried out using defined reagents in an ELISA format. Early results from the UK suggest that c. 25% of children aged 6–11 months had Norwalk antibody, a figure that increased to 90% in individuals over 60 years old (Gray et al. 1993). These high prevalences contrast with values obtained by molecular methods, which have not identified Norwalk virus as a circulating strain in recent years. The possibility that these assays detect heterologous SRSV responses rather than specific Norwalk virus antibody should be considered.

LABORATORY DIAGNOSIS

Virus isolation

At present there are no reports of the isolation of SRSVs in either cell or human intestinal organ cultures. Tests with a wide range of animals have also failed to identify a suitable model (Kapikian 1994). Some success has been achieved with the transmission of Norwalk virus in chimpanzees in which serological responses and excretion of Norwalk antigen in stools were described (Wyatt et al. 1978). Further investigations of this sort are clearly needed to study the cell tropism, cellular receptors and replication of these important viruses. It is, however, unlikely that isolation in cell cultures will ever be used for diagnosing individuals as in vitro methods are too slow and labour-intensive.

Serological methods

American workers have used reagents derived from human volunteers for both seroepidemiology and diagnostic serology in outbreaks of Norwalk virus infection. The development of RIA, EIA and immune adherence assay (IAHA) tests has greatly facilitated the understanding of the natural history of Norwalk virus infections. These assays provided compelling evidence of the aetiological role of Norwalk viruses in epidemic gastroenteritis in the 1970s (Kapikian 1994). Analysis of results with RIA and EIA suggested that they are more sensitive than EM methods for identifying Norwalk virus, as they detect both particulate (virion) and soluble antigens. The recent characterization of SRSV genomes will, however, supersede the use of reagents derived from humans and experimentally infected animals.

The preparation of hyperimmune antisera to recombinant Norwalk capsid antigens has facilitated development of an EIA for identifying naturally acquired or experimentally induced Norwalk virus antigen and antibody (Jiang et al. 1992, Treanor et al. 1993). Application of these improved assays to volunteer studies has provided new insights into Norwalk virus infection (Graham et al. 1994), showing that seroconversions were highest among volunteers who experienced vomiting. The assays for Norwalk virus are highly specific, revealing more subclinical infections, longer periods of virus excretion (up to 7 days) and higher infection rates than were previously recognized (Graham et al. 1994).

In summary, the development and application of reagents arising from the molecular characterization of SRSVs will considerably advance our epidemiological knowledge, as they will represent currently circulating strains of SRSV. It is, however, unlikely that serological methods will be useful in diagnostic laboratories in the future, in view of the need for rapid diagnosis both for managing patients and for the control of outbreaks.

Electron microscopy

EM is the most commonly used laboratory diagnostic method for direct detection of SRSV in stools. All SRSVs are indistinguishable in the EM when examined by routine negative staining methods (1.5% phosphotungstic acid at pH 6.5). Virions possess an amorphous surface structure, lacking a defined symmetry, with a ragged outline (Fig. 26.9) that probably explains the wide range of particle diameters (32–38 nm) reported. It is essential that preparations of SRSV are examined in the absence of antibody, which can mask the surface structure and lead to incorrect identification (Caul and Appleton 1982).

SRSVs are commonly excreted in faeces as small aggregates and in low numbers, close to the limit of sensitivity of the EM (10^6 viruses/g of stool), so careful examination of preparations is necessary. Contamination with other proteins in clinical samples often obscures SRSVs and can be overcome by applying SPIEM with human convalescent sera. Samples prepared in this way are far superior to conventional methods of virus concentration used in EM and increase the detection rate of SRSVs significantly. SPIEM is as sensitive as molecular methods for detecting SRSVs (Green et al. 1995b) and has the advantage of speed that is so important to the management of outbreaks. EM has the added value of being a 'catch-all' system whereby all viruses associated with gastroenteritis can be detected. EM will probably retain an important role in the investigation of future SRSV outbreaks for which rapid diagnosis is a prerequisite.

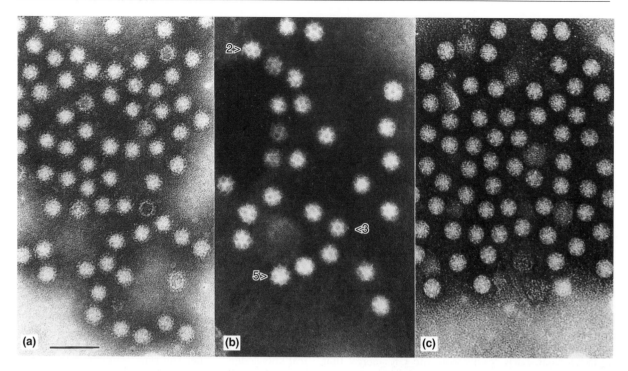

Fig. 26.9 Electron microscopic appearance of (a) SRSVs, (b) classic caliciviruses and (c) astroviruses. (a) SRSVs lack the distinctive surface morphology characteristic of classic caliciviruses and astroviruses although a ragged edge is clearly visible surrounding some of the particles. (b) The distinctive surface structures on a classic calicivirus viewed along the 2-, 3- and 5-fold (indicated) axes of symmetry. (c) Astroviruses occur in regular clusters, have a smooth surface outline and a characteristic 5- or 6-pointed star surface morphology. Bar = 100 nm for each panel.

Molecular diagnosis

The characterization of the SRSV genome has opened the prospect of applying molecular techniques to diagnosis. Although methods have now been described for applying PCR to the RNA polymerase region of the SRSV genome, continual refinement and design of new primers is necessary. It is surprising that the RNA polymerase and capsid regions of SRSVs show considerable heterogeneity, allowing division of isolates into 2 genetic groups (Green et al. 1994). Thus a continual assessment of SRSVs at the molecular level may be necessary, at least in the short term. Molecular epidemiology will be a powerful tool in future investigations of point-source outbreaks, particularly for examining shellfish (Atmar et al. 1993) and in monitoring spread of SRSVs between hospitals (Green et al. 1995b). These techniques are currently restricted to the research laboratory but will in the future play a major role in routine diagnosis, for which they will complement EM.

PREVENTION AND CONTROL

In volunteers, SRSVs induce both short- and long-term immunity but, until the mechanisms are fully understood, it is unlikely that a vaccine can be developed (Green et al. 1995b).

The high infectivity of SRSVs and the explosive outbreaks of gastroenteritis that often occur in semiclosed communities present a major challenge to control of infection and require aggressive intervention (Caul 1994a, Chadwick and McCann 1994). Measures

for interrupting the various modes of transmission (see 'Epidemiology', p. 519) must include 'enteric' precautions but these alone are ineffective and should be supplemented by measures to deal with patients who vomit.

Symptomatic healthcare workers should be excluded from contact with patients for at least 2 days after resolution of symptoms. Effective hand washing should be done routinely. People caring for patients should wear disposable gloves, gowns and masks when cleaning vomit, faecal material or contaminated clothing. Soiled linen and clothes should be handled carefully, to minimize generation of aerosols, and transported in plastic bags to the laundry. All potentially contaminated surfaces in toilets, bathrooms and rooms occupied by patients should be disinfected with a chlorine-based product and cleaned with a hot detergent solution. Contact with other patients should be avoided.

Common-source outbreaks are well documented. Symptomatic food handlers have often been incriminated and must be excluded from the workplace for at least 2 days after resolution of symptoms. Decontamination of all potentially infected surfaces within the kitchens and associated rest and toilet facilities is essential (Caul et al. 1993). Suspect water supplies may require shock chlorine treatments. Shellfish are a particular problem in the transmission of SRSVs and the most effective preventive measure is to grow them in clean waters. Depuration processes are not effective in eliminating SRSVs from shellfish, which futhermore are rendered unpalatable by effective heating.

2.2 Classic caliciviruses

CLASSIFICATION AND MORPHOLOGY

Distinctive virus particles 30 nm in diameter and differing from both astroviruses and the SRSVs were first recognized in faecal samples by negative staining techniques in 1976 (Madeley and Cosgrove 1976). These human enteric caliciviruses have a unique morphology: 'classic' particles viewed along their 3-fold axes of symmetry possess a central stain-filled cup (calyx) surrounded by 6 peripheral cups giving rise to the 'star of David' appearance. Viewed along their 2-fold axes of symmetry they have 4 cups (Fig. 26.9b). Particles viewed along their 5-fold axes present as 10-pointed spheres and may not be identified so readily as the classic particles described above. Unlike astroviruses, which possess a smooth, entire edge, caliciviruses have a ragged outline which makes accurate measurements difficult and explains the particle diameters of 31–38 nm quoted by most workers. Enteric human caliciviruses (HuCVs) have a buoyant density of 1.37–1.38 g/cm^3 (Terashima et al. 1983)

Detailed studies have been performed on a calicivirus isolated from lesions on the lip of a pygmy chimpanzee. The 3-dimensional structure of this primate calicivirus (see Fig. 26.5) was determined by cryo-electron microscopy and computer image-processing techniques (Prasad, Matson and Smith 1994). The virions are 40 nm in diameter and have a T = 3 icosahedral symmetry with 32 surface depressions at the 5-fold and 3-fold axes of symmetry. The surface depressions are surrounded by 90 arch-like capsomers, each of which is a capsid protein.

ORGANIZATION OF THE GENOME

Sequence analyses of isolates of classic HuCVs from the UK, USA and Japan indicate that they may be related more closely to the animal caliciviruses than to the SRSVs (Lambden et al. 1994, Liu et al. 1995, Matson et al. 1995).

Only one complete genome sequence of HuCV (UK/Manchester/93) has so far been described (Liu et al. 1995, Liu et al., 1997). The sequence and genome organization of this virus support the allocation of these viruses to a group separate from the SRSVs. The complete sequence of the Manchester isolate consists of 7431 nt with an overall G : C ratio of 51%. The 5′ terminus of the genome contains an untranslated leader sequence of 12 nt before the first predicted in-frame AUG codon at position 13. The 3′ end of the genome contains 84 untranslated nucleotide followed by a polyadenylate tail. Sequence analysis indicated 3 potential ORFs including a large 5′ ORF1 characteristic of SRSVs and other members of the *Caliciviridae*. The genome of HuCV (Fig. 26.10) is considerably smaller than those of group I SRSVs (Southampton virus, 7708 nt; Norwalk virus, 7642 nt) and smaller than the genome of a group II SRSV (Lordsdale virus, 7555 nt). The HuCV genome is very similar in size to RHDV (7437 nt).

A major difference between SRSVs and HuCVs is that the region of the HuCV genome predicted to encode the structural capsid protein is in the same frame as ORF1 and contiguous with the RNA polymerase, resulting in one large fused polyprotein. This genome organization is also found in the rabbit hepatotropic calicivirus, RHDV, and contrasts with those of all SRSVs so far sequenced. A second ORF of 495 nt coding for a small protein of 165 amino acids is predicted in frame –1 at the 3′ end of the genome and has a counterpart in all caliciviruses including the SRSVs. The translated product consists of 165 amino acids (17.8 kDa) and is larger than the equivalent animal virus proteins but smaller than the SRSV protein. The predicted protein is basic, hydrophilic and contains no cysteine residues. The AUG initiator codon of this 3′ ORF overlaps by one base the terminator codon of the polyprotein ORF1 and its position is similar to the arrangement in FCV and SRSVs.

Another surprising feature of the HuCV genome is a predicted second small ORF in a different frame that overlaps with the capsid region of the genome. Sequence analysis of 2 geographically separate isolates of HuCV in the UK revealed a third ORF of 483 nt coding for a small basic protein of 161 amino acids (17.5 kDa) in frame +1 and overlapping the N terminus of the putative capsid region of the polyprotein. The putative initiator codon of this second small ORF is 11 nt downstream of the predicted start codon of the capsid and is in the strongly favoured context, GCAAUGG, for translation initiation. This ORF is not seen in any of the animal caliciviruses or SRSVs but may be analogous to the small ORF3 of HEV (Bradley, 1992). The 2 HuCV isolates revealed extremely high sequence conservation in this region which strongly suggests that a biologically active translation product is produced from ORF3.

A major feature that distinguishes the caliciviruses from the picornaviruses is the production of one or more species of subgenomic RNAs during replication. In the case of RHDV, a subgenomic RNA is also encapsidated into mature virus particles. The 5′ terminal sequences of the subgenomic RNAs of FCV and RHDV are very similar to the 5′ genomic RNA terminus, suggesting an important regulatory role for this sequence. The existence of a subgenomic RNA has not been established for HuCV and only indirect evidence exists for Norwalk virus. The 5′ genomic terminus of HuCV was also defined by homopolymer tailing and PCR using cDNA generated from several specific primers. The consensus terminal sequence derived by this method was repeated in the capsid region of the genome although the level of sequence similarity was less than the analogous conserved motifs observed both for SRSVs and animal caliciviruses.

In summary, the arrangement of the 3 potential open reading frames of HuCV is distinct from that of the SRSVs but shares features with animal caliciviruses and the human HEV (Fig. 26.11). On the basis of genome organization alone it seems that the classic enteric caliciviruses are distinct from SRSVs.

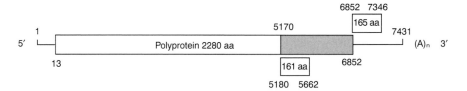

Fig. 26.10   Genome structure and organization of a classic human calicivirus (Manchester, EMBL/ GenBank Accession No X86560). Open boxes represent computer-predicted open reading frames. The shaded area at the 3′ terminus of ORF1 represents the capsid coding region which is fused to the ORF1 non-structural protein. An additional small ORF (161aa) is predicted within the capsid coding region in an alternative reading frame.

VIRAL PROTEINS

The lack of a productive cell culture system for HuCVs has severely impeded analysis of the viral polypeptides. During acute infection the viruses are, however, shed in relatively high concentrations. A single faecal specimen obtained during an outbreak of acute gastroenteritis in an orphanage in Sapporo, Japan, was used for the purification of HuCV virions (Terashima et al. 1983). This study showed that classic HuCV particles contain a single polypeptide of 62 kDa. This protein could be precipitated with convalescent (4 weeks) but not acute phase (2 days) serum from the same patient.

The large ORF1 has a coding potential of 2280 amino acids and includes conserved motifs typical of the 2C helicase, 3C protease and 3D RNA polymerase in relative genomic positions similar to those of other caliciviruses. Sequence comparisons of HuCV with other caliciviruses, including the SRSVs, show only 30–40% amino acid identity in the helicase, protease and RNA polymerase regions of the genome.

By analogy with RHDV, the capsid gene of HuCV is predicted to start at nt 5170 and code for 561 amino acids with a calculated molecular weight of 60 kDa, which agrees closely with that observed for the major structural polypeptide (62 kDa) of the HuCV Sapporo (Terashima et al. 1983). Capsid sequence comparisons with other caliciviruses demonstrated c. 30–40% identity in the conserved N-terminal B region but little homology in the C-terminal half of the protein. The predicted capsid amino acid sequence shows little similarity with those of either animal caliciviruses or the SRSVs.

CLINICAL MANIFESTATIONS

Symptomatic calicivirus infection occurs most often in infants and young children, in whom it seems indistinguishable from the milder forms of rotavirus infection (Suzuki et al. 1979, Cubitt and McSwiggan 1981, Cubitt 1987). Transmission is by person-to-person spread through the faecal–oral route and this is probably important in maintaining an endemic state in some semi-closed communities. Contaminated shellfish, cold foods and drinking water have also been implicated as vehicles of infection (Cubitt 1988).

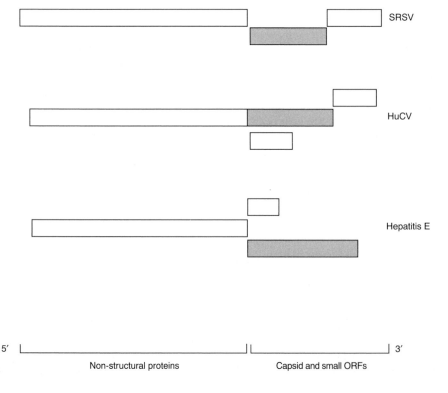

Fig. 26.11   Computer-predicted reading frames in SRSVs, HuCVs and the candidate calicivirus hepatitis E. Open boxes represent the viral non-structural proteins and the shaded boxes represent the viral structural capsid protein.

The incubation period is 1–3 days and symptoms persist for an average of 4 days. Diarrhoea and vomiting are common, whereas fever with upper respiratory symptoms is less so. There is no evidence that caliciviruses replicate in respiratory mucosal cells or that respiratory spread occurs. As respiratory symptoms have been described mainly in young children, they may arise from one of the concomitant respiratory viral infections common in this age group.

PATHOGENESIS

By contrast with SRSVs and astroviruses, there have been no reports of ultrastructural studies of human caliciviruses in the gut. Flewett and Davies (1976) demonstrated caliciviruses in the small intestinal lumen of a child dying of gastroenteritis. An aetiological role could not, however, be established as there were complicating factors and ultrastructural studies were not performed. Analogy with all the other 'diarrhoea viruses' suggests that caliciviruses replicate in mucosal cells lining the villi of the small intestine. Extensive studies on the pathology of a bovine calicivirus-like agent (Newbury) revealed damage to enterocytes at the bases of the villi (Hall et al. 1984); their relevance to the pathogenesis of the 'classic' human caliciviruses is unclear. In limited adult volunteer studies the virus was administered by the nasal/oral route (Cubitt 1994). Symptoms were inapparent or ranged from mild to moderately severe; the latter included nausea, vomiting, diarrhoea, pyrexia and abdominal pains. These clinical features resemble those in naturally acquired infections.

EPIDEMIOLOGY

In common with the other 'diarrhoea viruses' most of our data on the epidemiology of caliciviruses derives from EM observations and limited seroprevalence studies. The first report of a human enteric calicivirus was by Madeley and Cosgrove (1976), who detected classic calicivirus particles in both symptomatic and asymptomatic subjects in Glasgow, UK. They were unable, at that stage, to assign a causal role for caliciviruses in human disease, because 20% of children excreting them were asymptomatic. Subsequently, an outbreak of gastroenteritis in an infant and junior school in north London was investigated and a calicivirus was conclusively shown to be the causal agent (Cubitt, McSwiggan and Moore 1979). This outbreak was described as 'winter vomiting disease' although spread to others in the school and to home contacts was negligible, being perhaps limited by their immunity. These epidemiological and immunological features are not consistent with 'winter vomiting disease' caused by SRSVs. Caliciviruses have since been established as enteric pathogens (Christensen 1989, Cubitt 1994). In children hospitalized with sporadic diarrhoea, excretion rates of 0.9–6.6% have been reported (Suzuki et al. 1979, Cubitt and McSwiggan 1981, Monroe et al. 1991a). A similar excretion rate (2.9%) was reported in a day-care centre in the USA (Matson et al. 1989). All these studies suggest that, like astroviruses, caliciviruses are a minor cause of

clinically significant disease. By contrast with infection in older children, neonatal infection is often subclinical.

The clinical importance of HuCVs in the UK has been evaluated from national data reported by electron microscopists. Between 1985 and 1987 caliciviruses accounted for 0.9% of the total identifications of 'diarrhoea viruses' (Monroe et al. 1991a). Over 90% of these identifications were in children aged <5 years. More recent data (1990–1994) from England and Wales show that caliciviruses accounted for 0.8% of all positive 'diarrhoea virus' reports (see Fig. 26.2), a figure remarkably consistent with those in previous studies. Considering only SRSVs, classic caliciviruses and astroviruses associated with diarrhoea during this period, classic caliciviruses account for 8.8% of reports (see Fig. 26.2). Caliciviruses are thus a minor cause of clinically significant disease in the UK and infected children are rarely admitted to hospital.

HuCV is endemic in the UK, usually appearing sporadically in young children, although community and nosocomial outbreaks have also been recognized. Outbreaks have been reported in Japan (Chiba et al. 1979, Oishi et al. 1980), Australia (Grohmann et al. 1991), England (Cubitt, McSwiggan and Moore 1979, Cubitt, McSwiggan and Arstali 1980, Cubitt and McSwiggan 1981, Humphrey, Cruickshank and Cubitt 1984, Gray et al. 1987), Canada (Spratt et al. 1978) and Scandinavia (Kjeldsberg 1977), not only among children but also among elderly patients in nursing homes where the attack rates ranged from 50% to 70%. Outbreaks among adults and elderly patients are unusual and may represent infection in the face of waning immunity. A distinct seasonality has not been described for calicivirus infections (Fig. 26.12).

SEROEPIDEMIOLOGY

HuCVs with classic morphology have been grouped into 4 distinct antigenic types by IEM and share a common antigen detectable by RIA (Cubitt et al. 1987).

Caliciviruses are identified world-wide in faecal samples from young children with acute vomiting and diarrhoea. The high incidence of antibody in young children (>80%) suggests that subclinical infection in childhood is very common (Nakata, Estes and Chiba 1988). In contrast, SRSVs often cause epidemic gastroenteritis in all age groups. Furthermore, immunity to classic HuCV appears to be long-lived, whereas the short-term immunity to SRSVs allows symptomatic reinfections (Greenberg and Matsui 1992).

In Japan, antibody to calicivirus is rapidly acquired between 6 months and 2 years of age with a prevalence of 30%, rising to 65% in 2–5 year olds and c. 90% in older children and adults (Sakuma et al. 1981, Nakata et al. 1985a). Similar results have been reported from the USA (Nakata, Estes and Chiba 1988). Tests on pooled γ-globulin and serum samples in all continents confirm these findings (Christensen 1989). The high seroprevalence in early childhood agrees with the reported excretion rates of human caliciviruses in young children. The paucity of reports of calicivirus in hospitalized children with diarrhoea suggests that

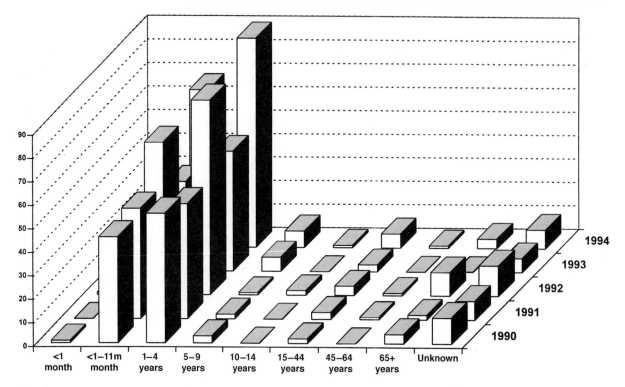

Fig. 26.12   Calicivirus incidence by age groups in England and Wales. The chart shows the numbers of cases reported to the Communicable Disease Surveillance Centre (Colindale, England) between 1990 and 1994. Peak incidence occurs in chldren under 4 years old.

asymptomatic or at least clinically insignificant disease in childhood is frequent. These clinical and epidemiological findings resemble those in astrovirus infections. In general, the rapid acquisition of both calicivirus and astrovirus antibodies in childhood is similar to that in rotavirus infections and markedly different from that reported for SRSVs.

LABORATORY DIAGNOSIS

Virus isolation

Unlike astroviruses, caliciviruses cannot be serially propagated in media containing trypsin. There is a single report of infections by HuCV in dolphin kidney and HEK cells in the presence of trypsin (Cubitt and Barrett 1984). Cytoplasmic replication was demonstrated only by immunofluorescence and by radiolabelling. This report has not been confirmed and many other workers have failed to propagate human caliciviruses in vitro.

Electron microscopy

The unique morphology (see section 2.2, p. 523) of HuCVs allows definitive identification by EM (Madeley 1979), and micrographs should always be checked to confirm direct observations with the EM. The characteristic morphology has been the main criterion for identifying human caliciviruses. If the morphology suggests a calicivirus but is not convincing, genetic analysis may confirm the diagnosis. EM is currently the only routine method available for laboratory diagnosis and requires skilled operators to achieve consistent results.

Immunoassays

The need for alternative methods of identifying caliciviruses in stool samples has been generally recognized. Nakata and co-workers (1983) found that a solid-phase RIA using a hyperimmune guinea-pig serum was more sensitive than EM. This assay was later modified to an EIA of similar sensitivity (Nakata, Estes and Chiba 1988). These tests are not yet available to the routine laboratory but will presumably become so.

Serology

Specific IgM, seroconversions or rising titres of specific IgG have been observed following infection (Chiba et al. 1979, Cubitt, McSwiggan and Moore 1979, Cubitt, McSwiggan and Arstali 1980, Cubitt, Pead and Saeed 1981, Nakata et al. 1985b). These techniques, although useful in epidemiological studies, are not ethically justified for diagnosing enteric 'diarrhoea virus' infections in young children because they involve taking blood samples.

PREVENTION AND CONTROL

The measures needed to prevent the spread of calicivirus infections are the same as those recommended in section 2.1 under 'Prevention and control' (p. 522).

3   ASTROVIRUSES

CLASSIFICATION AND MORPHOLOGY

Human astroviruses were discovered in the UK in 1975 by EM examination of faecal specimens (Appleton and Higgins 1975, Madeley and Cosgrove 1975). They were distinctive non-enveloped individual virus particles, 28–30 nm in diameter, that were often present in very large numbers and also appeared in clumps. Both reports concerned stool specimens from neonates who had developed acute non-bacterial gastroenteritis while in maternity wards. Direct negative contrast staining of stool specimens revealed that the virions have a smooth, round appearance with a clearly defined margin. Empty stain-penetrated particles are rarely observed. A characteristic surface structure is present in up to 10% of virions. In stool specimens, particles are often seen in orderly paracrystalline arrays, within which even spacing is thought to be maintained by surface projections beyond the resolution of the EM. The presence of projections has been confirmed from recent studies on astroviruses grown in cell culture, but the characteristic star shape was observed only after treatment with alkalized culture medium (Risco et al. 1995).

Under negative staining with potassium phosphotungstate the viruses are 28 nm in diameter with little variation and generally circular in outline. Virions with discernible surface structure have a star-shaped configuration of either 5 or 6 points which extends over the whole surface (see Fig. 26.9c). This stellate feature is not stain-penetrated and has a characteristic white displacing centre in electron micrographs, allowing clear differentiation from SRSVs and the classic caliciviruses. The distinctive stellate configuration suggested the name 'astrovirus' (Madeley and Cosgrove 1976). Later observations increased the range of diameters but these variations probably reflect differing staining and sample preparation techniques. Astroviruses have been isolated from both avian and mammalian species, including ducks, turkeys, sheep, pigs, cattle, cats, dogs and deer (Kurtz and Lee 1987).

The large number of astroviruses shed in acute phase infection has allowed purification directly from faecal specimens. Buoyant density gradient fractionation suggested a range of densities for isolates, especially those from animal species. Animal viruses have been reported to band at densities from 1.34 g/cm^3 for canine astrovirus (Williams 1980) to 1.39 g/cm^3 for ovine astrovirus (Herring, Gray and Snodgrass 1981). Buoyant density gradient fractionation of human astroviruses grown in cell culture show 2 bands, at 1.35 and 1.32 g/cm^3 respectively. The lower density band may comprise capsids devoid of RNA (Willcocks et al. 1990). CsCl gradient purified lamb astroviruses also gave 2 bands of buoyant densities, 1.365 and 1.39 g/cm^3, the denser of which was thought to be aggregated virus (Herring, Gray and Snodgrass 1981). Astroviruses are stable to lipid solvents, heat treatment and acid, and can survive heating to 60°C at pH 3.0 for up to 5 min (Kurtz and Lee 1987).

ORGANIZATION OF THE GENOME

Astroviruses contain a positive-sense single-stranded RNA genome of c. 7000 nt which is polyadenylated. In cells infected by human astrovirus, 2 infection-specific polyadenylated cytoplasmic RNA species of 7000 and 2500 nt (Monroe et al. 1991b) are detected. The smaller RNA species is a subgenomic mRNA that is 3′ co-terminal with the genomic RNA. This subgenomic RNA is synthesized in c. 5–10 times greater molar amounts than the genomic RNA during replication.

Complete nucleotide sequences are available for 2 of the 7 recognized human astrovirus serotypes (Jiang et al. 1993, Willcocks et al. 1994b). The overall organization and structure of both these astrovirus genomes are similar. Excluding the polyadenylate tail of 31 nt (Jiang et al. 1993), the complete genomic RNA sequence of the human astrovirus serotype 2 (HAstV-2), a UK isolate from Oxford, is 6797 nt in length. The 5′ terminus of this astrovirus genome contains an untranslated leader sequence of 82 nt before the first predicted in-frame AUG codon at position 83. The 3′ end of the genome also contains 82 untranslated nucleotides followed by the polyadenylate tail. Computer analysis predicts 3 large overlapping reading frames, termed ORFs 1a, 1b and 2 (Fig. 26.13). ORF2 is located at the 3′ terminus of the genome and encodes a capsid protein precursor of 796 amino acids. ORF1a encodes a polypeptide of 920 amino acids. ORF1b overlaps ORF1a by 70 nt and is in reading frame +1, although the first initiation codon is located 380 nt downstream from the termination codon for ORF1a and is in a weak context for translation initiation. No separate mRNA has been detected for ORF1b.

Detailed structural analysis of the 70 nt overlap region between ORFs 1a and 1b has suggested the presence of a potential ribosomal frame-shift signal (Jiang et al. 1993, Lewis et al. 1994, Willcocks et al. 1994b). This is thought to direct the synthesis of a large non-structural fusion polypeptide of >1400 amino acids derived from both ORF1a and ORF1b. An elegant study using reporter genes carrying the cloned ORF1a/ORF1b junctions of HAstV-1 translated in vitro using rabbit reticulocyte lysate has provided direct evidence for the operation of the frame-shifting mechanism (Marczinke et al. 1994). Frame-shifting efficiency in this in vitro system was 5%. The frameshift signal comprises 2 distinct components: a 7 nt 'slippery' sequence and a short 7 bp stem and 10 nt loop structure. Mutagenic analysis shows that these are the only structures involved in frame shifting. By analogy with other systems it is proposed that the −1 ribosome frame slippage site is the 7 nt sequence A$_6$C. The stem–loop feature is most similar to the *gag–pol* overlap region of the human type II T cell leukaemia virus in which a simple stem–loop structure is also required, giving a frame-shifting efficiency of 13% in rabbit reticulocyte lysates.

VIRAL PROTEINS
Early work

Before 1981 human astroviruses were available only from clinical specimens or from volunteer studies, so biochemical characterization was extremely limited. The first detailed biochemical characterization was

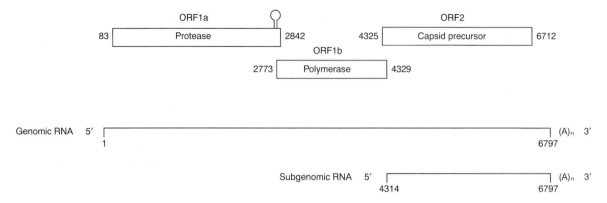

Fig. 26.13 Genome structure and organization of astrovirus (serotype 2, EMBL/GenBank Accession No L13745). Open boxes represent computer-predicted open reading frames. Location of the stem–loop structure predicted to cause ribosome frame shifting is indicated at the terminus of ORF1a. The nucleotide coordinates of the subgenomic RNA are indicated below the genome map. The genome structure and organization of human astrovirus serotype 1 (6813 nt, EMBL/GenBank Accession No Z25771) are similar.

performed on an animal astrovirus purified from infected epithelial cells extracted from the small intestines of infected gnotobiotic lambs (Herring, Gray and Snodgrass 1981). This seminal work showed that the astrovirus capsid is quite distinct from both those of picornaviruses and those of caliciviruses and comprises at least 2 structural proteins of molecular weights 30 and 32 kDa respectively.

Cell culture

In 1981 a major advance towards the molecular characterization of astroviruses was achieved by the adaptation of human astroviruses to growth in cell culture (Lee and Kurtz 1981). Using a faecal suspension from an infected volunteer, human embryo kidney (HEK) cells were infected with astrovirus in the presence of high concentrations of trypsin. Viral infectivity was monitored by immunofluorescent staining because the trypsin caused detachment of cells and obscured cytopathic effects. After 6 passages it was possible to propagate the virus both in a continuous line of rhesus kidney cells (LLCMK2) and in primary baboon kidney cells. Attempts to adapt the virus to other cell lines were unsuccessful.

Astroviruses grown in cell culture are morphologically identical to isolates from faecal specimens. Purification and sodium dodecyl sulphate–polyacrylamide gel electrophoresis (SDS-PAGE) of human astrovirus serotype 4 grown in cell culture indicated that the virus capsid is composed of 4 polypeptides of 36.5, 34, 33 and 32 kDa (Kurtz and Lee 1987). SDS-PAGE analysis of purified human astrovirus serotype 1 adapted to cell culture in HEK cells revealed 4 polypeptides of 34, 33, 26.5 and 5.2 kDa (Kurtz 1988). Other workers could not confirm the existence of the small polypeptide. The protein compositions of several animal and human astrovirus capsids have recently been thoroughly reviewed (Willcocks, Carter and Madeley 1992). The consensus is that astroviruses comprise 3 major protein species, 2 in the range 29–33 kDa and a smaller, more variable polypeptide in the range 13–26.5 kDa. Passage through primary HEK cells is clearly

impracticable for routine isolation of astroviruses and thus only a limited number of strains were adapted to cell culture in this way. In 1990 a continuous human colonic carcinoma cell line (CaCo2) was developed for isolating astroviruses directly from faeces (Willcocks et al. 1990). Reduction of the concentration of trypsin preserved the cell monolayer, which in turn allowed observation of a cytopathic effect. This technique was an important advance and is now used regularly for research purposes. Genome sequence analysis of isolates adapted to growth by initial passage through HEK cells revealed a 45 nt deletion in the ORF1a region of the genome that did not occur in isolates adapted to growth in CaCo2 cells (Willcocks et al. 1994a). This deletion is located approximately 300 nt upstream from the ribosomal frame-shifting signal and removes a partially repetitive amino acid sequence EQQVVK and KPQ. The biological function of this sequence is unknown.

Purified human astroviruses adapted to CaCo2 cells by direct infection from faeces contain 3 virus-specific structural polypeptides of 33.5, 31.5 and 24 kDa (Willcocks et al. 1990). There were no differences in the structural protein patterns between early and late passage virus in these cells. The 24 kDa protein was loosely associated with virions and could easily be removed by detergent treatment. Thus the 2 abundant structural proteins of 33.5 and 31.5 kDa in human astrovirus were thought to be very similar to the 2 found in purified ovine astrovirus (Herring, Gray and Snodgrass 1981).

In the absence of trypsin, astroviruses undergo a single cycle of replication in infected cells. The temporal synthesis of astrovirus proteins in LLCMK2 cells was followed in the absence of trypsin (Monroe et al. 1991b). Synthesis of the capsid proteins was analysed by precipitation with rabbit serum hyperimmune to purified astrovirus particles. In the absence of trypsin a 90 kDa astrovirus-specific polypeptide was synthesized. Treatment in vitro with trypsin caused specific cleavage of this large polypeptide to 3 fragments of

31, 29 and 20 kDa. Thus this study confirmed that the astrovirus capsid polypeptides are made from a 90 kDa precursor.

Molecular cloning of the capsid

The complete subgenomic RNAs of both human astrovirus serotype 1 (HAstV-1) and HAstV-2 have been cloned and sequenced (Monroe et al. 1993, Willcocks and Carter 1993). These RNA species, which are abundant in infected cells, comprise 2454 nt in HAstV-1 and 2484 nt in HAstV-2 excluding the polyadenylate tail. These subgenomic RNAs encode a single ORF of 786 and 796 amino acids respectively (ORF2) with predicted molecular weights in the region of 85–88 kDa. This is consistent with the estimated size of the capsid precursor previously observed in astrovirus-infected cells in the absence of trypsin (Monroe et al. 1991b). It was proposed that the subgenomic RNA encodes the capsid precursor polypeptide. A search of the databases revealed the amino acid sequence of the precursor polypeptide to be unique. It was thus proposed that astroviruses belong to a separate family of non-enveloped viruses, designated *Astroviridae*.

The ORF2 was also cloned and sequenced from another HAstV-1 strain (Lewis et al. 1994). ORF2 from this strain has 2361 nt encoding 787 amino acids that yield a predicted protein of 87 kDa. Radioimmune precipitation of ORF2 expressed in an in vitro coupled transcription/translation system with virion-specific monoclonal and polyclonal antisera provided formal proof that this ORF encodes the capsid precursor. In addition, an 87 kDa precursor was immunoprecipitated with these sera from astrovirus-infected cells. ORF2 has also been expressed as a c. 90 kDa product in baculovirus (Willcocks and Carter 1993, Lewis et al. 1994). In this heterologous expression system the large capsid precursor does not seem to undergo proteolytic cleavage.

The use of microsequencing and of monoclonal antibodies directed against conformation-dependent epitopes indicates that processing of the capsid precursor is complex, yielding several intermediate products (Sanchez-Fauquier et al. 1994). In HAstV-2 the 29 and 26 kDa polypeptides share primary sequences but originate from alternative processing of the precursor at residues 361 and 394 respectively. The C-terminal cleavage point of these products has not been determined.

Open reading frames

ORF1a and ORF1b encoded by the 5' half of the astrovirus genome are, by analogy with other single-stranded RNA virus genomes, considered to encode the viral non-structural polypeptides. Conclusive evidence for production of a single fused giant polyprotein in vivo has not been found. Sequence analysis of the ORF1a identified a region of similarity to the calicivirus (RHDV) 'cysteine' protease. It is interesting that the astrovirus protease has a serine instead of cysteine at the proposed catalytic site of the protease. In this respect astroviruses resemble the luteoviruses

of plants which also use a ribosomal frame-shifting mechanism for expressing their RNA polymerase.

Computer analysis of ORF1a also revealed 4 transmembrane α helical regions and a nuclear localization site (NLS), although their biological significance is unknown. The NLS is absolutely conserved between strains and fits the consensus bipartite motif for such sites, consisting of 2 clusters of basic amino acid residues separated by a 10-amino acid spacer. Bovine astrovirus proteins have been detected in the cell nucleus by immunofluorescence (Aroonprasert et al. 1989). Thus the NLS may have a role in transporting astrovirus proteins to this target site. The NLS is close to the region of the genome deleted during the adaptation of astroviruses to growth in LLCMK2 cells. Whether viruses deleted in this region target the cell nucleus is unknown. Actinomycin D, which inhibits DNA-dependent RNA polymerase, did not inhibit the replicative cycle of bovine astrovirus-infected cells (Aroonprasert et al. 1989). The role of the cell nucleus in astrovirus replication therefore remains to be determined.

ORF1b contains the classic RNA polymerase active site motif YGDD. Thus it appears that the expression of the RNA polymerase is modulated through the ribosomal frame-shifting mechanism during the replicative cycle of the virus. Extensive searching of sequence databases failed to reveal any significant similarities either to RNA helicase or to methyl transferase in the astrovirus genome. It has been speculated that astroviruses may have a VPg although at present there is no direct evidence for this hypothesis.

ANTIGENS

Human astroviruses are currently divided into 7 antigenic types on the basis of IEM and immunofluorescence of infected cells using polyclonal and monoclonal antisera (Lee and Kurtz 1982, Kurtz and Lee 1984, Lee and Kurtz 1994). The human astroviruses are also antigenically distinct from animal strains (Kurtz and Lee 1984). Complete capsid precursor sequences are available for human astrovirus serotypes 1, 2 and 4 (Monroe et al. 1993, Willcocks and Carter 1993, Lewis et al. 1994, Willcocks et al. 1995). Alignment of these complete capsid precursor sequences allowed identification of 3 distinct regions. The amino terminus of the capsid is highly conserved for the first 415 amino acids with 81–85% sequence identity. The central region of the capsid, residues 416–707, shows 38–42% identity and the carboxy terminus (residues 708 to terminus) is the most divergent, with only 16–24% identity (Willcocks et al. 1995). How these regions relate to the 3 defined capsid polypeptides is not yet clear. However, RT-PCR amplification and sequencing of a small segment of the capsid precursor has shown that the phylogenetic groupings are consistent with the original serotyping scheme (Noel et al. 1995).

CLINICAL MANIFESTATIONS

Astroviruses are transmitted from person to person by the faecal–oral route. Although this is the most common mode of transmission within semi-closed communities (families, hospital wards etc.), other, less often reported, routes are via fomites, food or water. There is an incubation period of 3–4 days preceding systemic signs and symptoms including fever, headache, nausea, malaise and (uncommonly) vomiting (Kurtz et al. 1979). These features resemble those caused by other gastroenteritis viruses and are not diagnostic.

Volunteers have been used to demonstrate that astroviruses are enteric pathogens: 17 were fed with a faecal filtrate containing astroviruses; one subsequently developed diarrhoea and a further 4 asymptomatic volunteers excreted astroviruses. The findings suggested that those with pre-existing antibody were protected from symptomatic reinfection (Kurtz et al. 1979). Although these researches are useful in assessing the potential of astroviruses as enteric pathogens and provide important clinical information, they are of limited value in assessing the overall burden of symptomatic primary infections in children, in whom most such infections occur.

PATHOGENESIS

Limited tests in humans showed that astroviruses infect the mucosal epithelium of the lower parts of the villi in the duodenum (Phillips, Rice and Walker-Smith 1982). Crystalline arrays of astrovirus particles within the cytoplasm have been noted. The results of the few ultrastructural studies of astrovirus infections in humans so far reported are compatible with the finding of transient villous atrophy in the small intestine of lambs (Snodgrass et al. 1979). In one investigation of human astrovirus infections short-term monosaccharide intolerance was reported (Nazer, Rice and Walker-Smith 1982) but was not a serious sequela.

Viral replication within mucosal epithelial cells presumably results in cell lysis and release of astrovirus particles into the gut lumen where they become detectable in faeces. Excretion of virus may be followed by diarrhoea which is sometimes watery, although asymptomatic excretion is common. Diarrhoea usually lasts for 2–3 days but may continue for a week or longer and virus excretion persists while symptoms last. During the acute stage 10^{10} particles/g of faeces can be detected. Symptomatic excretion may persist for months in immunocompromised patients (Kurtz and Lee 1987) and such cases may be an important source of nosocomial infections.

EPIDEMIOLOGY

Most of our knowledge of the epidemiology of astroviruses is based on the detection of morphologically typical particles by EM (Madeley 1979) and on limited seroprevalence studies. The virus has been reported in all 5 continents (Kurtz 1988) and is closely associated with childhood diarrhoea (Cukor and Blacklow 1984, Caul 1988, Christensen 1989, Blacklow and Greenberg 1991, Herrmann et al. 1991).

Investigations in Glasgow during the 1970s showed that 80% of babies excreting astroviruses were symptomatic, whereas 12% had no diarrhoea (Madeley 1979). Nosocomial spread is well documented, and many outbreaks in infants and young children in nurseries and paediatric wards have been described (Ashley, Caul and Paver 1978, Oshiro et al. 1981). In one large paediatric outbreak in Japan over 50% of children were symptomatic (Konno et al. 1982); in a children's ward in the UK, the infection spread to nursing staff (Kurtz, Lee and Pickering 1977), indicating that susceptibility is not restricted to neonates and children. In nurseries and paediatric wards astroviruses can become endemic as a result of the continual introduction of susceptible children. Asymptomatic excretion has been reported in 5–20% of both neonates and young children and represents a significant source of further spread in semi-closed communities.

Astroviruses seem to be a relatively minor cause of gastroenteritis in young children and are only occasionally incriminated in adult disease. Reports of longitudinal observations of astrovirus infections in the community are rare. Surveillance based on EM in England and Wales from 1985 to 1987 revealed that astroviruses are endemic, with distinct peaks in the winter (Monroe et al. 1991a). This seasonality seems to be constant in temperate climates. In one study there was a striking age-related prevalence, most reported symptomatic infections being in children aged <5 years. In a separate longitudinal investigation of infantile gastroenteritis in London, astrovirus infection was reported in 50 of 1802 (2.8%) children <6 years old, but none in those aged 6–12 years (Kurtz 1994). More recent national surveillance data in England and Wales confirmed that astroviruses seem to be a minor cause of viral gastroenteritis (see Fig. 26.2) in the UK and emphasize the age-related and seasonal distribution (Fig. 26.14).

Sporadic cases or outbreaks in adults are rarely reported. In one outbreak in a convalescent home for the elderly in Marin County, California, 51% of residents developed gastroenteritis and the outbreak persisted for 3 months (Oshiro et al. 1981). Although the virus was initially reported as a Norwalk-like agent the published micrographs suggested an astrovirus morphology (Caul 1988) and this has subsequently been confirmed (Gary et al. 1987). An unusually large outbreak of gastroenteritis affecting both students and teachers has been reported by Japanese workers (Oishi et al. 1994).

Food- or water-borne outbreaks seem to be rare but in one oyster-associated outbreak, involving 39 naval officers, one-third developed diarrhoea within 4 days of eating the oysters (Kurtz and Lee 1987).

In Oxford, SPIEM and immunofluorescence identified 6 antigenically distinct astroviruses over a 10 year period (Kurtz 1994). Of 165 strains, serotype 1 was the most prevalent (64%); the prevalence of the other serotypes varied from year to year. Since this report one additional serotype has been recognized. Hermann and colleagues (1988) developed a monoclonal antibody EIA with which they confirmed the antigenic

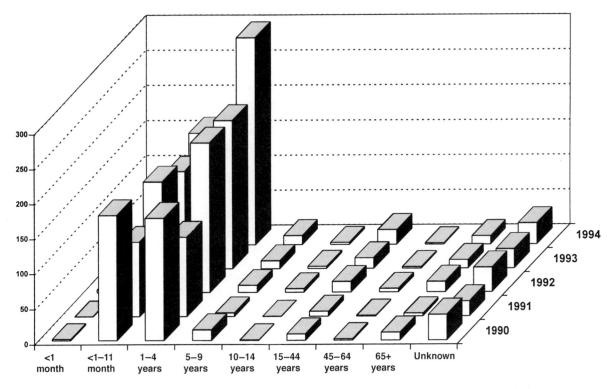

Fig. 26.14 Astrovirus incidence by age groups in England and Wales. The chart shows the number of cases reported to the Communicable Disease Surveillance Centre (Colindale, England) between 1990 and 1994. Peak incidence occurs in children under 4 years old.

variation described by Lee and Kurtz (1982, Kurtz and Lee 1984).

SEROEPIDEMIOLOGY

Limited antibody prevalence studies have confirmed that astroviruses are a minor cause of clinically significant disease in young children. One study in Oxfordshire showed that 64% of 3–4 year old children had been infected, and this prevalence rose to 87% in those aged 5–10 years (Kurtz and Lee 1978). These data are compatible with the finding that most clinical infections occur in young children (Fig. 26.14). The high prevalence of antibody in young children and the relatively few reports of astroviruses in symptomatic cases suggest that many infections are either subclinical or so mild that medical intervention is not required.

Some workers have suggested that the difficulties in identifying astroviruses by EM result in underestimates of their role in viral gastroenteritis (Oliver and Phillips 1988) and that the introduction of alternative methods has significantly improved their detection in clinical samples (Willcocks, Carter and Madeley 1992). Others have suggested that astroviruses are second in importance to rotaviruses as a cause of viral gastroenteritis in young children (Lew et al. 1990, Herrmann et al. 1991). These conclusions are not, however, sustainable without applying the newer techniques to all other enteric virus infections.

LABORATORY DIAGNOSIS

Isolation methods

Cell culture is well established for isolating viruses from clinical samples but is not the method of choice for diagnostic purposes because it is labour intensive, expensive and likely to be less sensitive than immunologically based assays.

Enzyme immunoassays

Herrmann and co-workers (1988) developed an EIA employing monoclonal antibodies to the group antigen that detected all astroviruses grown in cell culture. These workers later modified the test to detect astroviruses in stool samples (Herrmann et al. 1990) and compared this assay with IEM. The EIA has as high a sensitivity and specificity as IEM and will probably replace it in diagnostic laboratories.

Electron microscopy

The characteristic 5- or 6-pointed star morphology is enhanced in high contrast micrographs. Astroviruses are usually present in large numbers in faeces during the acute phase of the illness. Aggregates are quite common, probably resulting from the release of crystalline arrays from lysed cells. These features distinguish astrovirus infections from those due to caliciviruses. The possibility that aggregates of astrovirus result from antigen–coproantibody complexes is unlikely. The technique used for concentrating astroviruses from clinical samples for EM is important. Astroviruses are unstable if pelleted from CsCl gradients but can be purified and are stable in tartrate/glycerol gradients (Ashley and Caul 1982). IEM creates difficulties because aggregation of virions masks the characteristic surface morphology and leads to inaccurate identification, as demonstrated by the original classification of the Marin County agent as a Norwalk-like virus. In contrast, the capture of astrovirus particles on antibody-coated EM grids (SPIEM) is an elegant and highly sensitive method of identification and has allowed astrovirus capsids to be grouped into 7 serotypes (Kurtz 1994). Another major disadvantage of IEM is its high specificity compared with that of direct EM, which remains the only 'catch-all' technique available for all 'diarrhoea viruses'.

Molecular techniques

A sensitive dot-blot hybridization procedure for detecting astroviruses in faecal samples has also been described (Willcocks et al. 1991) but has not been validated in comprehensive field studies. The typing of human astroviruses by nucleotide sequencing (Noel et al. 1995) has an epidemiological rather than a diagnostic value.

PREVENTION AND CONTROL

Most astrovirus infections occur in childhood and although symptomatic infection has been described in adults it seems to be relatively uncommon, probably because immunity in childhood is long lasting. Volunteer studies suggest that humoral antibody is protective at least against symptomatic disease, so development of a vaccine is theoretically possible. The burden of clinically significant disease in children is, however, much less than that due to other enteric pathogens and the development of a vaccine cannot at present be justified.

Measures for controlling the spread of infection in semi-closed communities are similar to those described for SRSVs. Infections acquired from water and food, including shellfish, have been reported only occasionally. Unpublished reports of high numbers of astroviruses in sea-waters in the UK may indicate a public health problem but confirmation is urgently needed (Cook and Myint 1995).

REFERENCES

Adler I, Zickl R, 1969, Winter vomiting disease, *J Infect Dis*, **119:** 668–73.

Agus SG, Dolin R et al., 1973, Acute infectious nonbacterial gastroenteritis: intestinal histopathology. Histologic and enzymatic alterations during illness produced by the Norwalk agent in man, *Ann Intern Med*, **79:** 18–25.

Ando T, Mulders MN et al., 1994, Comparison of the polymerase region of small round structured virus strains previously classified in three antigenic types by solid-phase immune electron microscopy, *Arch Virol*, **135:** 217–26.

Appleton H, Higgins PG, 1975, Viruses and gastroenteritis in infants, *Lancet*, **1:** 1297.

Appleton H, Pereira MS, 1977, A possible virus aetiology in outbreaks of food-poisoning from cockles, *Lancet*, **1:** 780–1.

Appleton H, Buckley M et al., 1977, Virus-like particles in winter vomiting disease, *Lancet*, **1:** 409–11.

Aroonprasert D, Fagerland JA et al., 1989, Cultivation and partial characterization of bovine astrovirus, *Vet Microbiol*, **19:** 113–25.

Ashley CR, Caul EO, 1982, Potassium tartrate-glycerol as a density gradient substrate for separation of small, round viruses from human feces, *J Clin Microbiol*, **16:** 377–81.

Ashley CR, Caul EO, Paver WK, 1978, Astrovirus-associated gastroenteritis in children, *J Clin Pathol*, **31:** 939–43.

Atmar RL, Metcalf TG et al., 1993, Detection of enteric viruses in oysters by using the polymerase chain-reaction, *Appl Env Microbiol*, **59:** 631–5.

Blacklow NR, Greenberg HB, 1991, Medical progress – viral gastroenteritis, *N Engl J Med*, **325:** 252–64.

Blacklow NR, Herrmann JE, 1988, Norwalk virus, *Proceedings of the 9th BSG SK & F International Workshop*, 65–9.

Bradley DW, 1992, Hepatitis E: epidemiology, etiology and molecular biology, *Rev Med Virol*, **2:** 19–28.

Bradley WH, 1943, Epidemic nausea and vomiting, *Br Med J*, **1:** 309–12.

Carter MJ, Milton ID et al., 1992, The complete nucleotide sequence of a feline calicivirus, *Virology*, **190:** 443–8.

Caul EO, 1988, Small round human fecal viruses, *Parvoviruses and Human Disease*, CRC Press, Boca Raton FL, 139–63.

Caul EO, 1994a, Small round structured viruses – airborne transmission and hospital control, *Lancet*, **343:** 1240–2.

Caul EO, 1994b, Viruses in food, *Rapid Methods and Automation in Microbiology and Immunology*, eds Spencer RC, Wright EP, Newsom SWB, Intercept Ltd, Andover, Hampshire, 348–54.

Caul EO, Appleton H, 1982, The electron microscopical and physical characteristics of small round human fecal viruses: an interim scheme for classification., *J Med Virol*, **9:** 257–65.

Caul EO, Ashley CR, Pether JVS, 1979, 'Norwalk'-like particles in epidemic gastroenteritis in the UK, *Lancet*, **2:** 1292.

Caul EO, Sellwood NJ et al., 1993, Outbreaks of gastroenteritis associated with SRSVs, *PHLS Microbiol Digest*, **10:** 2–8.

Chadwick PR, McCann R, 1994, Transmission of a small round structured virus by vomiting during a hospital outbreak of gastroenteritis, *J Hosp Infect*, **26:** 251–9.

Chiba S, Sakuma Y et al., 1979, An outbreak of gastroenteritis associated with calicivirus in an infant home, *J Med Virol*, **4:** 249–54.

Christensen ML, 1989, Human viral gastroenteritis, *Clin Microbiol Rev*, **2:** 51–89.

Christopher PJ, Grohmann GS et al., 1978, Parvovirus gastroenteritis – a new entity for Australia, *Med J Aust*, **1:** 121–4.

Clarke SKR, Cook GT et al., 1972, A virus from epidemic vomiting disease, *Br Med J*, **3:** 86–9.

Cook N, Myint S, 1995, Astroviruses, *J Med Microbiol*, **42:** 1–2.

Cubitt WD, 1987, The candidate caliciviruses, *CIBA Found Symp*, **128:** 126–43.

Cubitt WD, 1988, Caliciviruses, *Proceedings of the 9th BSG SK & F International Workshop*, 82–4.

Cubitt WD, 1994, Caliciviruses, *Viral Infections of the Gastrointestinal Tract*, 2nd edn, ed Kapikian AZ, Marcel Dekker, New York, 549–68.

Cubitt WD, Barrett ADT, 1984, Propagation of human candidate calicivirus in cell culture, *J Gen Virol*, **65:** 1123–6.

Cubitt WD, McSwiggan DA, 1981, Calicivirus gastroenteritis in north west London, *Lancet*, **2:** 975–7.

Cubitt WD, McSwiggan DA, Arstali S, 1980, An outbreak of calicivirus infection in a mother and baby unit, *J Clin Pathol*, **33:** 1095–8.

Cubitt WD, McSwiggan DA, Moore W, 1979, Winter vomiting disease caused by calicivirus, *J Clin Pathol*, **32:** 786–93.

Cubitt WD, Pead PJ, Saeed AA, 1981, A new serotype of calicivirus associated with an outbreak of gastroenteritis in a residential home for the elderly, *J Clin Pathol*, **34:** 924–6.

Cubitt WD, Blacklow NR et al., 1987, Antigenic relationships between human caliciviruses and Norwalk virus, *J Infect Dis*, **156**: 806–14.

Cubitt WD, Jiang XJ et al., 1994, Sequence similarity of human caliciviruses and small round structured viruses, *J Med Virol*, **43**: 252–8.

Cukor G, Blacklow NR, 1984, Human viral gastroenteritis, *Microbiol Rev*, **48**: 157–79.

Dingle KE, Lambden PR et al., 1995, Human enteric *Caliciviridae*: the complete genome sequence and expression of virus-like particles from a genetic group II small round structured virus, *J Gen Virol*, **76**: 2349–55.

Dolin R, Blacklow NR et al., 1971, Transmission of acute infectious nonbacterial gastroenteritis to volunteers by oral administration of stool filtrates, *J Infect Dis*, **123**: 307–12.

Dolin R, Blacklow NR et al., 1972, Biological properties of Norwalk agent of acute infectious nonbacterial gastroenteritis, *Proc Soc Exp Biol Med*, **140**: 578–83.

Dolin R, Levy AG et al., 1975, Viral gastroenteritis induced by the Hawaii agent: jejunal histopathology and seroresponse, *Am J Med*, **59**: 761–9.

Dolin R, Reichmann RC et al., 1982, Detection by immune electron microscopy of the Snow Mountain agent of acute viral gastroenteritis, *J Infect Dis*, **146**: 184–9.

Evans H, Ross DP et al., 1995, A review of outbreaks of viral gastroenteritis in England and Wales 1992–1994, University of Warwick, 18–21 September, Unpublished.

Flewett TH, Davies H, 1976, Caliciviruses in man, *Lancet*, **1**: 311.

Gary GW, Anderson LJ et al., 1987, Norwalk virus-antigen and antibody-response in an adult volunteer study, *J Clin Microbiol*, **25**: 2001–3.

Gordan I, Ingraham HS, Korns RF, 1947, Transmission of epidemic gastroenteritis to human volunteers by oral administration of fecal filtrates, *J Exp Med*, **86**: 409–22.

Graham DY, Jiang X et al., 1994, Norwalk virus infection of volunteers: new insights based on improved assays, *J Infect Dis*, **170**: 34–43.

Gray JD, 1939, Epidemic nausea and vomiting, *Br Med J*, **1**: 209–11.

Gray JJ, Wreghitt TG et al., 1987, An outbreak of gastroenteritis in a home for the elderly associated with astrovirus type-1 and human calicivirus, *J Med Virol*, **23**: 377–81.

Gray JJ, Jiang X et al., 1993, Prevalence of antibodies to Norwalk virus in England: detection by enzyme-linked immunosorbent assay using baculovirus-expressed Norwalk virus capsid antigen, *J Clin Microbiol*, **31**: 1022–5.

Green SM, Dingle KE et al., 1994, Human enteric *Caliciviridae*: a new prevalent small round-structured virus group defined by RNA-dependent RNA polymerase and capsid diversity, *J Gen Virol*, **75**: 1883–8.

Green SM, Lambden PR et al., 1995a, Capsid diversity in small round-structured viruses: molecular characterisation of an antigenically distinct human enteric calicivirus, *Virus Res*, **37**: 271–83.

Green SM, Lambden PR et al., 1995b, Polymerase chain reaction detection of small round-structured viruses from two related hospital outbreaks of gastroenteritis using inosine-containing primers, *J Med Virol*, **45**: 197–202.

Greenberg HB, Matsui SM, 1992, Astroviruses and caliciviruses: emerging enteric pathogens, *Infect Agents Dis*, **1**: 71–91.

Greenberg HB, Wyatt RG, Kapikian AZ, 1979, Norwalk virus in vomitus, *Lancet*, **1**: 55.

Greenberg HB, Valdesuso J et al., 1979, Role of Norwalk virus in outbreaks of nonbacterial gastroenteritis, *J Infect Dis*, **139**: 564–8.

Greenberg HB, Valdesuso JR et al., 1981, Proteins of Norwalk virus, *J Virol*, **37**: 994–9.

Griffin MR, Surowiec JJ et al., 1982, Foodborne Norwalk virus, *Am J Epidemiol*, **115**: 178–84.

Grohmann G, Glass RI et al., 1991, Outbreak of human calici-virus gastroenteritis in a day-care center in Sydney, Australia, *J Clin Microbiol*, **29**: 544–50.

Hall GA, Bridger JC et al., 1984, Lesions of gnotobiotic calves experimentally infected with a calicivirus-like (Newbury) agent, *Vet Pathol*, **21**: 208–15.

Hardy ME, White LJ et al., 1995, Specific proteolytic cleavage of recombinant Norwalk virus capsid protein, *J Virol*, **69**: 1693–8.

Hayashi Y, Ando T et al., 1989, Western blot (immunoblot) assay of small, round-structured virus associated with an acute gastroenteritis outbreak in Tokyo, *J Clin Microbiol*, **27**: 1728–33.

Herring AJ, Gray EW, Snodgrass DR, 1981, Purification and characterization of ovine astrovirus, *J Gen Virol*, **53**: 47–55.

Herrmann JE, Hudson RW et al., 1988, Antigenic characterization of cell-cultivated astrovirus serotypes and development of astrovirus-specific monoclonal antibodies, *J Infect Dis*, **158**: 182–5.

Herrmann JE, Nowak NA et al., 1990, Diagnosis of astrovirus gastroenteritis by antigen detection with monoclonal antibodies, *J Infect Dis*, **161**: 226–9.

Herrmann JE, Taylor DN et al., 1991, Astroviruses as a cause of gastroenteritis in children, *N Engl J Med*, **324**: 1757–60.

Ho M, Glass RI et al., 1989, Viral gastroenteritis aboard a cruise ship, *Lancet*, **2**: 961–4.

Humphrey TJ, Cruickshank JG, Cubitt WD, 1984, An outbreak of calicivirus associated gastroenteritis in an elderly persons home – a possible zoonosis, *J Hyg*, **93**: 293–9.

Jiang B, Monroe SS et al., 1993, RNA sequence of astrovirus: distinctive genomic organization and a putative retrovirus-like ribosomal frameshifting signal that directs the viral replicase synthesis, *Proc Natl Acad Sci USA*, **90**: 10539–43.

Jiang X, Graham DY et al., 1990, Norwalk virus genome cloning and characterization, *Science*, **250**: 1580–3.

Jiang X, Wang M et al., 1992, Expression, self-assembly, and antigenicity of the Norwalk virus capsid protein, *J Virol*, **66**: 6527–32.

Jiang X, Wang M et al., 1993, Sequence and genomic organization of Norwalk virus, *Virology*, **195**: 51–61.

Jiang X, Matson DO et al., 1995, Expression, self-assembly, and antigenicity of a Snow Mountain agent-like calicivirus capsid protein, *J Clin Microbiol*, **33**: 1452–5.

Jordan WS, Gordan I, Dorrance WR, 1953, A study of illness in a group of Cleveland families. VII. Transmission of acute nonbacterial gastroenteritis to volunteers: evidence for two different etiologic agents, *J Exp Med*, **98**: 461–75.

Kapikian AZ, ed, 1994, Norwalk and Norwalk-like Viruses, *Viral Infections of the Gastrointestinal Tract*, 2nd edn, Marcel Dekker, New York, 471–518.

Kapikian AZ, Wyatt RG et al., 1972, Visualisation by immune electron microscopy of a 27-nm particle associated with infectious nonbacterial gastroenteritis., *J Virol*, **10**: 1075–81.

Kapikian AZ, Gerin JL et al., 1973, Density in cesium chloride of the 27nm '8FIIa' particle associated with acute infectious nonbacterial gastroenteritis: determination by ultracentrifugation and immune electron microscopy, *Proc Soc Exp Biol Med*, **142**: 874–7.

Kapikian AZ, Greenberg HB et al., 1978, Prevalence of antibody to the Norwalk agent by a newly developed immune adherence hemagglutination assay, *J Med Virol*, **2**: 281–94.

Kaplan JE, Gary GW et al., 1982, Epidemiology of Norwalk gastroenteritis and the role of Norwalk virus in outbreaks of acute nonbacterial gastroenteritis, *Ann Intern Med*, **96**: 756–61.

Kjeldsberg E, 1977, Small spherical viruses in faeces from gastroenteritis patients, *Acta Pathol Microbiol Scand*, **85**: 351–4.

Konno T, Suzuki H et al., 1982, Astrovirus-associated epidemic gastroenteritis in Japan, *J Med Virol*, **9**: 11–17.

Kuritsky JN, Osterholm MT et al., 1985, A statewide assessment of the role of Norwalk virus in outbreaks of foodborne gastroenteritis, *J Infect Dis*, **151**: 568.

Kurtz JB, 1988, Astroviruses, *Proceedings of the 9th BSG SK & F Workshop*, 84–7.

Kurtz JB, 1994, Astroviruses, *Viral Infections of the Gastrointestinal Tract*, 2nd edn, ed Kapikian AZ, Marcel Dekker, New York, 569–80.

Kurtz JB, Lee TW, 1978, Astrovirus gastroenteritis: age distribution of antibody, *Med Microbiol Immunol*, **166**: 227–30.

Kurtz JB, Lee TW, 1984, Human astrovirus serotypes, *Lancet*, **2**: 1405.

Kurtz JB, Lee TW, 1987, Astroviruses: human and animal, *CIBA Found Symp*, **128**: 92–107.

Kurtz JB, Lee TW, Pickering D, 1977, Astrovirus associated gastroenteritis in a children's ward, *J Clin Pathol*, **30**: 948–52.

Kurtz JB, Lee TW et al., 1979, Astrovirus infection in volunteers, *J Med Virol*, **3**: 221–30.

Lambden PR, Clarke IN, 1995, Genomic organization in the *Caliciviridae*, *Trends Microbiol*, **3**: 261–5.

Lambden PR, Liu BL, Clarke IN, 1995, A conserved sequence motif at the 5' terminus of the Southampton virus genome is characteristic of the *Caliciviridae*, *Virus Genes*, **10**: 149–52.

Lambden PR, Caul EO et al., 1993, Sequence and genome organization of a human small round-structured (Norwalk-like) virus, *Science*, **259**: 516–19.

Lambden PR, Caul EO et al., 1994, Human enteric caliciviruses are genetically distinct from small round structured viruses, *Lancet*, **343**: 666–7.

Lee TW, Kurtz JB, 1981, Serial propagation of astrovirus on tissue culture with the aid of trypsin, *J Gen Virol*, **57**: 421–4.

Lee TW, Kurtz JB, 1982, Human astrovirus serotypes, *J Hyg*, **89**: 539–40.

Lee TW, Kurtz JB, 1994, Prevalence of human astrovirus serotypes in the Oxford region 1976–92, with evidence for 2 new serotypes, *Epidemiol Infect*, **112**: 187–93.

Lew JF, Glass RI et al., 1990, Six year retrospective surveillance of gastroenteritis viruses identified at ten electron microscopy centers in the United States and Canada, *Pediatr Infect Dis J*, **9**: 709–14.

Lew JF, Kapikian AZ et al., 1994a, Molecular characterization and expression of the capsid protein of a Norwalk-like virus recovered from a Desert Shield troop with gastroenteritis, *Virology*, **200**: 319–25.

Lew JF, Kapikian AZ et al., 1994b, Molecular characterization of Hawaii virus and other Norwalk- like viruses: evidence for genetic polymorphism among human caliciviruses, *J Infect Dis*, **170**: 535–42.

Lew JF, Petric M et al., 1994c, Identification of minireovirus as a Norwalk-like virus in pediatric patients with gastroenteritis, *J Virol*, **68**: 3391–6.

Lewis DC, 1990, Three serotypes of Norwalk-like virus demonstrated by solid-phase immune electron microscopy, *J Med Virol*, **30**: 77–81.

Lewis D, 1991, Norwalk agent and other small-round structured viruses in the UK, *J Infect*, **23**: 220–2.

Lewis D, Ando T et al., 1995, Use of solid-phase immune electron-microscopy for classification of Norwalk-like viruses into 6 antigenic groups from 10 outbreaks of gastroenteritis in the United States, *J Clin Microbiol*, **33**: 501–4.

Lewis TL, Greenberg HB et al., 1994, Analysis of astrovirus serotype 1 RNA, identification of the viral RNA-dependent RNA polymerase motif, and expression of a viral structural protein, *J Virol*, **68**: 77–83.

Liu BL, Clarke IN et al., 1995, Human enteric caliciviruses have a unique genome structure and are distinct from the Norwalk-like viruses, *Arch Virol*, **140**: 1345–56.

Liu B, Clarke IN et al., 1997, The genomic 5' terminus of Manchester calicivirus, *Virus Genes*, **15**: in press.

Madeley CR, 1979, Comparison of the features of astroviruses and caliciviruses seen in samples of feces by electron microscopy, *J Infect Dis*, **139**: 519–23.

Madeley CR, Cosgrove BP, 1975, 28 nm particles in faeces in infantile gastroenteritis, *Lancet*, **2**: 451–2.

Madeley CR, Cosgrove BP, 1976, Caliciviruses in man, *Lancet*, **1**: 199–200.

Madore HP, Treanor JJ, Dolin R, 1986, Characterization of the Snow Mountain agent of viral gastroenteritis, *J Virol*, **58**: 487–92.

Madore HP, Treanor JJ et al., 1990, Antigenic relatedness among the Norwalk-like agents by serum antibody rises, *J Med Virol*, **32**: 96–101.

Marczinke B, Bloys AJ et al., 1994, The human astrovirus RNA-dependent RNA polymerase coding region is expressed by ribosomal frameshifting, *J Virol*, **68**: 5588–95.

Matson DO, Estes MK et al., 1989, Human calicivirus-associated diarrhea in children attending day care centers, *J Infect Dis*, **159**: 71–8.

Matson DO, Zhong W et al., 1995, Molecular characterization of a human calicivirus with sequence relationships closer to animal caliciviruses than other known human caliciviruses, *J Med Virol*, **45**: 215–22.

Matsui SM, Kim JP et al., 1991, The isolation and characterization of a Norwalk virus-specific cDNA, *J Clin Invest*, **87**: 1456–61.

Meeroff JC, Schreiber DS et al., 1980, Abnormal gastric motor functions in viral gastroenteritis, *Ann Intern Med*, **92**: 370–3.

Meyers G, Wirblich C, Thiel H, 1991, Genomic and subgenomic RNAs of rabbit hemorrhagic disease virus are both protein-linked and packaged into particles, *Virology*, **184**: 677–86.

Miller R, Raven H, 1936, Epidemic nausea and vomiting, *Br Med J*, **1**: 1242–4.

Monroe SS, Glass RI et al., 1991a, Electron microscopic reporting of gastrointestinal viruses in the United Kingdom, 1985–1987, *J Med Virol*, **33**: 193–8.

Monroe SS, Stine SE et al., 1991b, Temporal synthesis of proteins and RNAs during human astrovirus infection of cultured cells, *J Virol*, **65**: 641–8.

Monroe SS, Jiang B et al., 1993, Subgenomic RNA sequence of human astrovirus supports classification of Astroviridae as a new family of RNA viruses, *J Virol*, **67**: 3611–14.

Morens DM, Zweighaft RM et al., 1979, A waterborne outbreak of gastroenteritis with secondary person-to-person spread, *Lancet*, **1**: 964–6.

Morse DL, Guzewich JJ et al., 1986, Widespread outbreaks of clam- and oyster-associated gastroenteritis: role of Norwalk virus, *N Engl J Med*, **314**: 678–81.

Murphy AM, Grohmann GS et al., 1979, An Australia-wide outbreak of gastroenteritis from oysters caused by Norwalk virus, *Med J Aust*, **2**: 329–33.

Murphy AM, Grohmann GS et al., 1982, Norwalk virus gastroenteritis following raw oyster consumption, *Am J Epidemiol*, **115**: 348–51.

Nakata S, Estes MK, Chiba S, 1988, Detection of human calicivirus antigen and antibody by enzyme-linked immunosorbent assays, *J Clin Microbiol*, **26**: 2001–5.

Nakata S, Chiba S et al., 1983, Microtiter solid-phase radioimmunoassay for detection of human calicivirus in stools, *J Clin Microbiol*, **17**: 198–201.

Nakata S, Chiba S et al., 1985a, Prevalence of antibody to human calicivirus in Japan and southeast Asia determined by radioimmunoassay, *J Clin Microbiol*, **22**: 519–21.

Nakata S, Chiba S et al., 1985b, Humoral immunity in infants with gastroenteritis caused by human calicivirus, *J Infect Dis*, **152**: 274–9.

Nazer H, Rice S, Walker-Smith JA, 1982, Clinical associations of stool astrovirus in childhood, *J Pediatr Gastroenterol Nutr*, **1**: 555–8.

Noel JS, Lee TW et al., 1995, Typing of human astroviruses from clinical isolates by enzyme immunoassay and nucleotide sequencing, *J Clin Microbiol*, **33**: 797–801.

Oishi I, Maeda A et al., 1980, Calicivirus detected in outbreaks of acute gastroenteritis in school-children, *Biken J*, **23**: 163–8.

Oishi I, Yamazaki K et al., 1992, Demonstration of low molecular weight polypeptides associated with small, round-structured viruses by Western immunoblot analysis, *Microbiol Immunol*, **36:** 1105–12.

Oishi I, Yamazaki K et al., 1994, A large outbreak of acute gastroenteritis associated with astrovirus among students and teachers in Osaka, Japan, *J Infect Dis*, **170:** 439–43.

Okada S, Sekine S et al., 1990, Antigenic characterization of small, round-structured viruses by immune electronmicroscopy, *J Clin Microbiol*, **28:** 1244–8.

Oliver AR, Phillips AD, 1988, An electron microscopical investigation of faecal small round viruses, *J Med Virol*, **24:** 211–18.

Oshiro LS, Haley CE et al., 1981, A 27nm virus isolated during an outbreak of acute infectious nonbacterial gastroenteritis in a convalescent home: a possible new serotype, *J Infect Dis*, **143:** 791–5.

Parrino TA, Schreiber DS et al., 1977, Clinical immunity in acute gastroenteritis caused by Norwalk agent, *N Engl J Med*, **297:** 86–9.

Paver WK, Caul EO, Clarke SKR, 1974, Comparison of a 22 nm virus from human faeces with animal parvoviruses, *J Gen Virol*, **22:** 447–50.

Paver WK, Caul EO et al., 1973, A small virus in human faeces, *Lancet*, **1:** 237.

Pether JVS, Caul EO, 1983, An outbreak of foodborne gastroenteritis in 2 hospitals associated with a Norwalk-like virus, *J Hyg*, **91:** 343–50.

Phillips AD, Rice SJ, Walker-Smith JA, 1982, Astrovirus within human small intestinal mucosa, *Gut*, **23:** A923–4.

Prasad BVV, Matson DO, Smith AW, 1994, Three-dimensional structure of calicivirus, *J Mol Biol*, **240:** 256–64.

Prasad BVV, Rothnagel R et al., 1994, Three-dimensional structure of baculovirus-expressed Norwalk virus capsids, *J Virol*, **68:** 5117–25.

Reid JA, White DG et al., 1988, Role of infected food handler in hotel outbreak of Norwalk-like viral gastroenteritis: implications for control, *Lancet*, **2:** 321–3.

Reimann HA, Price AH, Hodges JA, 1945, The cause of epidemic diarrhea, nausea and vomiting (viral dysentery?), *Proc Soc Exp Biol Med*, **59:** 8–9.

Risco C, Carrascosa JL et al., 1995, Ultrastructure of human astrovirus serotype 2, *J Gen Virol*, **76:** 2075–80.

Sakuma Y, Chiba S et al., 1981, Prevalence of antibody to human calicivirus in general population of northern Japan, *J Med Virol*, **7:** 221–5.

Sanchez-Fauquier A, Carrascosa AL et al., 1994, Characterization of a human astrovirus serotype 2 structural protein (VP26) that contains an epitope involved in virus neutralization, *Virology*, **201:** 312–20.

Sawyer LA, Murphy JJ et al., 1988, 25- to 30-nm virus particle associated with a hospital outbreak of acute gastroenteritis with evidence for airborne transmission, *Am J Epidemiol*, **127:** 1261–71.

Schreiber DS, Blacklow NR, Trier S, 1973, The mucosal lesion of the proximal small intestine in acute infectious nonbacterial gastroenteritis, *N Engl J Med*, **288:** 1318–23.

Schreiber DS, Blacklow NR, Trier S, 1974, The small intestinal lesion induced by the Hawaii agent in infectious nonbacterial gastroenteritis, *J Infect Dis*, **142:** 705–8.

Snodgrass DR, Angus KW et al., 1979, Pathogenesis of diarrhoea caused by astrovirus infections in lambs, *Arch Virol*, **60:** 217–26.

Spratt HC, Marks I et al., 1978, Nosocomial infantile gastroenteritis associated with minirotavirus and calicivirus, *J Pediatr*, **93:** 922–6.

Suzuki H, Konno T et al., 1979, The occurrence of calicivirus in infants with acute gastroenteritis, *J Med Virol*, **4:** 321–6.

Terashima H, Chiba S et al., 1983, The polypeptide of a human calicivirus, *Arch Virol*, **78:** 1–7.

Thornhill TS, Wyatt RG et al., 1977, Detection by immune electron microscopy of 26- to 27-nm viruslike particles associated with two family outbreaks of gastroenteritis, *J Infect Dis*, **135:** 20–7.

Treanor JJ, Jiang X et al., 1993, Subclass-specific serum antibody responses to recombinant Norwalk virus capsid antigen (rNV) in adults infected with Norwalk, Snow mountain, or Hawaii virus, *J Clin Microbiol*, **31:** 1630–4.

Wang J, Jiang X et al., 1994, Sequence diversity of small, round-structured viruses in the Norwalk virus group, *J Virol*, **68:** 5982–90.

Willcocks MM, Carter MJ, 1993, Identification and sequence determination of the capsid protein gene of human astrovirus serotype-1, *FEMS Microbiol Lett*, **114:** 1–7.

Willcocks MM, Carter MJ, Madeley CR, 1992, Astroviruses, *Rev Med Virol*, **2:** 97–106.

Willcocks MM, Carter MJ et al., 1990, Growth and characterisation of human faecal astrovirus in a continuous cell line, *Arch Virol*, **113:** 73–81.

Willcocks MM, Carter MJ et al., 1991, A dot-blot hybridization procedure for the detection of astrovirus in stool samples, *Epidemiol Infect*, **107:** 405–10.

Willcocks MM, Ashton N et al., 1994a, Cell culture adaptation of astrovirus involves a deletion, *J Virol*, **68:** 6057–8.

Willcocks MM, Brown TDK et al., 1994b, The complete sequence of a human astrovirus, *J Gen Virol*, **75:** 1785–8.

Willcocks MM, Kurtz JB et al., 1995, Prevalence of human astrovirus serotype 4: capsid protein and comparison with other strains, *Epidemiol Infect*, **114:** 385–91.

Williams FP, 1980, Astrovirus-like, coronavirus-like and parvovirus-like particles detected in the diarrhoeal stools of beagle pups, *Arch Virol*, **66:** 215–26.

Wyatt RG, Dolin R et al., 1974, Comparison of three agents of acute infectious nonbacterial gastroenteritis by cross-challenge in volunteers, *J Infect Dis*, **129:** 709–14.

Wyatt RG, Greenberg HB et al., 1978, Experimental infection of chimpanzees with the Norwalk agent of epidemic viral gastroenteritis, *J Med Virol*, **2:** 89–96.

Zahorsky J, 1929, Hyperemesis hiemis or the winter vomiting disease, *Arch Pediatr*, **46:** 391–5.

Chapter 27

REOVIRUSES

U Desselberger

1 Introduction and general classification	4 Orbiviruses
2 Rotaviruses	5 Coltiviruses
3 Reoviruses	

1 INTRODUCTION AND GENERAL CLASSIFICATION

The *Reoviridae* family contains 9 genera: *Orthoreovirus*, *Rotavirus*, *Orbivirus*, all infecting animals and humans, *Coltivirus* infecting insects, rodents and humans, *Aquareovirus* infecting fish, *Cypovirus* infecting insects, and *Fijivirus*, *Phytoreovirus* and *Oryzavirus* infecting plants (Murphy et al. 1995). In this chapter *Orthoreovirus* is called *reovirus*, the term being an acronym derived from **r**espiratory, **e**nteric, **o**rphan viruses, and only the mammalian genera will be discussed.

Members of the *Reoviridae* have the following features in common:

1 They contain a genome of 10–12 segments of double-stranded RNA.
2 They are icosahedral, non-enveloped particles of c. 70–75 nm diameter with a double-shelled capsid.
3 They replicate in the cytoplasm of cells without complete uncoating, produce 5' end-capped, non-polyadenylated mRNAs and form intracytoplasmic inclusion bodies.

The *Reoviridae* are relatively heat stable, resistant to lipid solvents and resistant over a wide pH range (except orbiviruses which lose infectivity at low pH).

The genomes of several strains of reo-, rota- and orbiviruses have been fully sequenced and the gene protein assignments completed. The overall genome size in base pairs (bp; genomic molecular weight) is 23 540 bp (7770 kDa) for reoviruses (type 3 reovirus), 18 555 bp (6120 kDa) for rotaviruses (SA 11 rotavirus) and 19 218 bp (6340 kDa) for orbiviruses (bluetongue virus type 10) (Roy and Gorman 1991, Murphy et al. 1995).

Rotaviruses are the major cause of infantile gastroenteritis world-wide and the causative agent of acute diarrhoea in the young of many mammalian species (calves, piglets, lambs, chicks etc.). Reoviruses have been isolated from humans but have not been associated convincingly with a particular human disease. They cause systemic disease in rodents (mice). Orbiviruses mainly affect animals, producing severe disease (African horse sickness, epizootic haemorrhagic disease in cattle and deer, bluetongue disease in sheep). *Coltivirus* causes Colorado tick fever in humans. All mammalian reoviruses are ubiquitous, occurring in water supplies from which many infections may result. Whereas rotaviruses are most commonly spread by the faecal–oral route, orbiviruses are transmitted by a variety of ticks and mosquitoes.

2 ROTAVIRUSES

Rotaviruses are the major cause of gastroenteritis in infants and young children and in a wide range of animal species.

2.1 Genome, gene protein assignment and structure

Rotaviruses have a genome of 11 segments of double-stranded RNA which can be easily separated by polyacrylamide gel electrophoresis. The RNA segments code for 6 structural (VP1, VP2, VP3, VP4, VP6, VP7) and 5 non-structural proteins (NSP1–NSP5). The structural proteins are located in the core (VP1–VP3), inner shell (VP6) and outer shell (VP4, VP7) (Mattion, Cohen and Estes 1994). The wheel-like (Latin: *rota*) appearance of the double-shelled particles by electron microscopy is diagnostic (Fig. 27.1a). Figure 27.1b shows diagrammatically the gene coding capacity, how the structural proteins fit into the particles and their 3-dimensional (3D) structure as obtained by image processing techniques from cryoelectron micrographs.

Details of the 3D structure have been elucidated in

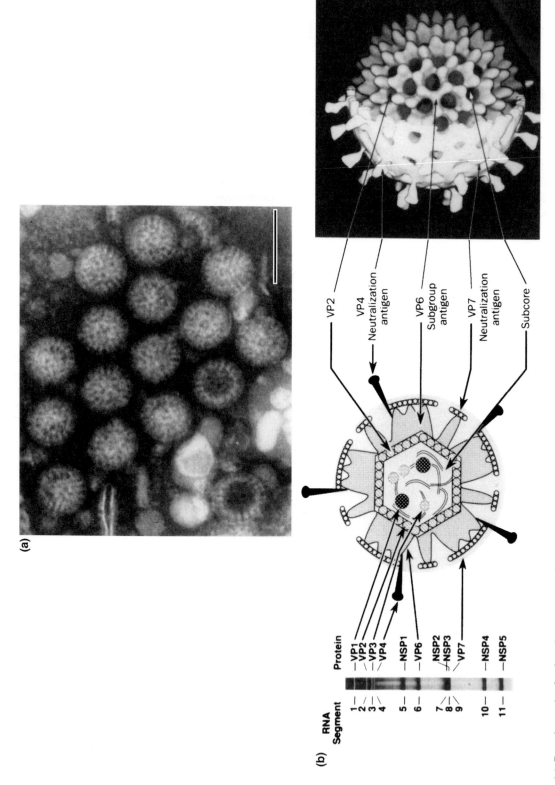

Fig. 27.1 (a) Rotaviruses in the faecal suspension of an infant suffering from acute gastroenteritis. Electron micrograph, PTA stain. (Courtesy of Dr E A C Follett, Regional Virus Laboratory, Ruchill Hospital, Glasgow. Bar = 100 nm) (b) RNA profile (10% SDS polyacrylamide gel, silver stain), protein products (gene protein assignment) and particle structure (diagram and reconstruction from a cryoelectron micrograph) of rotaviruses. (From Mattion, Cohen and Estes 1994, with permission of the authors and publisher.)

a number of excellent studies by the groups of Prasad and Chiu (Prasad et al. 1988, 1990, Shaw et al. 1993, Prasad and Chiu 1994) and Yeager (Yeager et al. 1990, 1994). According to their findings, the double-shelled capsid is ordered along 5-, 3- and 2-fold symmetry axes and is perforated by numerous channels. Table 27.1 lists the sizes of RNAs and their products, as well as post-translational modification and possible functions (see section 2.3; p. 540).

2.2 Classification into subgroups, serotypes and genotypes

A classification of rotaviruses has been derived from immunological reactivities of various components of the particles and from genomic composition. Groups A–E can be differentiated according to lack of serological cross-reactivities of the inner capsid protein VP6 with polyclonal and monoclonal antibodies. There may be 2 more groups, F and G (Bridger 1987). Within group A rotaviruses, subgroups (I; II; I+II; nonI,nonII) are defined according to exclusive reactivities of 2 VP6-specific monoclonal antibodies (Greenberg et al. 1982). Types within group A are

determined by cross-neutralization studies as **serotypes** or by sequence comparison as **genotypes**. (Typing in other rotavirus groups is rudimentary.) Because 2 surface proteins carry neutralization-specific antigens (VP4 and VP7), a double classification scheme similar to that developed for influenza viruses has been established, differentiating G types (for VP7 which is a **g**lycoprotein) and P types (for VP4 which is a **p**rotease-sensitive protein, being cleaved post-translationally into its subunits VP5* and VP8*). So far, 14 G types and more than 19 P types have been differentiated, indicating extensive genomic diversity within group A rotaviruses (Estes 1996). Because these proteins are coded for by different RNA segments and rotaviruses reassort readily in doubly infected cells both in vitro (Garbarg-Chenon, Bricout and Nicolas 1984, Graham et al. 1987) and in vivo (Gombold and Ramig 1986, Ward et al. 1990), the observed diversity resulting from various combinations of VP7 and VP4 types becomes very large. Table 27.2 shows the various combinations of VP4 and VP7 types detected so far in human and animal group A rotaviruses.

Table 27.1 Gene protein assignments of group A rotaviruses

RNA segment	Size (bp)	Protein product Designation	Deduced molecular weight (kDa)	Post-translational modification	Location and function
1	3302	VP1	125.0	…	Inner core protein; RNA polymerase
2	2690	VP2	102.7	Myristylation	Inner core protein; RNA binding; leucine zipper
3	2591	VP3	88.0	…	Inner core protein; guanylyl transferase
4	2362	VP4	86.7	Proteolytic cleavage (VP5* + VP8*)	Surface protein (dimer) Haemagglutinin Neutralization antigen Fusogenic protein Virulence Pathogenicity
5	1611	VP5 (NS53)	58.6	…	Non-structural (?) Zinc fingers; assembly
6	1356	VP6	44.8	Myristylation	Inner capsid protein (trimer); group and subgroup antigen
7[a]	1104	VP8 (NS35)	36.7	…	Non-structural RNA replication?
8[a]	1059	VP9 (NS34)	34.6	…	Non-structural RNA binding
9[a]	1062	VP7 (1)	37.4	Cleavage of signal sequence glycosylation	Surface glycoprotein
		VP7 (2)	33.9		Neutralization antigen (serotype specific); Ca^{2+} binding site?
10	751	VP10 (NS29)	20.3	Glycosylation	Non-structural; intracellular receptor Morphogenesis
11	667	VP11 (NS26)	21.7	Phosphorylation	Non-structural

[a]This gene protein assignment is for SA11 rotaviruses.
Slightly modified from Mattion et al. 1994, with permission of authors and publisher.

Table 27.2   Rotavirus G types (VP7 specific) and P types (VP4 specific) in the combinations found in animals (A) and humans (H)

P type	G type														
	1	2	3	4	5	6	7	8	9	10	11	12	13	14	NK
1			A			A									
2			A												
3			H/A												
4		H										H			
5						A		A		A					A
6	H	H			H/A										H
7			A		A						A				A
8	H		H	H					H						
9	H		H/A			H									
10								H							
11									H	H/A					A
12			A												
13			H/A												
14										H					
15			A												
16										A					
17							A								A
18			A												
19			A												
NK	A	H	A	A	A	A	A		H	H		H	A	A	

All G types are genotypes and serotypes; not all P types (genotypes) have yet been differentiated as serotypes.
NK, not known.
Data from Estes 1996.

2.3   Replication

Rotaviruses infect the small intestine after oral ingestion and spread via the faecal–oral route. Multiplication takes place in the mature epithelial cells at the tips of the villi of the small intestine.

Double-shelled particles attach to the host cell via the outer capsid protein VP4. For full infectivity this has to be cleaved into its components VP5* and VP8*. Replication occurs exclusively in the cytoplasm. After removal of the outer capsid the virion-associated RNA-dependent RNA polymerase is activated and synthesizes mRNAs, which leave the single-shelled particle via its aqueous pores and are translated into viral proteins. This process can readily be achieved in vitro (Cohen et al. 1979). Viral structural proteins (mainly VP2 and VP6) accumulate in the cytoplasm to form inclusion bodies (termed 'viroplasms') which are thought to be the site of assembly of subviral particles enclosing the 11 different segments of mRNA, which are then replicated to form dsRNA molecules. Single-shelled particles attach VP4 and bud through the endoplasmic reticulum where NS28 (VP10) acts as a receptor and VP7 is incorporated. Single-shelled particles thus become double-shelled and transiently enveloped. Virus release occurs by cell lysis when VP4 and VP7 form the ordered outer capsid structure and the envelope membrane is lost (Patton 1994). Co-expression of rotavirus capsid proteins VP2 and VP6 from baculovirus recombinants in insect cells has allowed the production of single-shelled (double-layered) particles, whereas co-expression of VP2, VP4, VP6 and VP7 leads to the formation of double-shelled (triple-layered) virus-like particles (VLPs) (Crawford et al. 1994).

2.4   Pathogenesis: animal models

Cell death and desquamation reduce digestion and adsorption of nutrients (primary malabsorption) and lead to villous atrophy (Greenberg et al. 1981). This is followed by a reactive crypt cell hyperplasia accompanied by increased secretion, which is thought to contribute to the severity of diarrhoea. The local pathogenesis is shown in Fig. 27.2.

The viral factors determining pathogenicity of rotaviruses have been investigated in several animal models (piglets, mice, rabbits). The product of RNA segment 4, VP4, is likely to be a major determinant (Offit et al. 1986, Gorziglia et al. 1988, Bridger et al. 1992, Burke, Bridger and Desselberger 1994, Burke, McCrae and Desselberger 1994), but products of other structural genes (RNA 3 coding for VP3 and RNAs 8 or 9 coding for VP7) and non-structural genes (RNA 5, coding for NSP1, RNA 8 coding for NSP2 and RNA 10 coding for NSP4) have also been associated with pathogenicity (Table 27.3) (Broome et al. 1993, Hoshino et al. 1993, 1995, Ball et al. 1996; review by Burke and Desselberger 1996).

2.5   Illness and treatment

After a short incubation period of 24–48 hours, the onset of illness is sudden with watery diarrhoea, vomit-

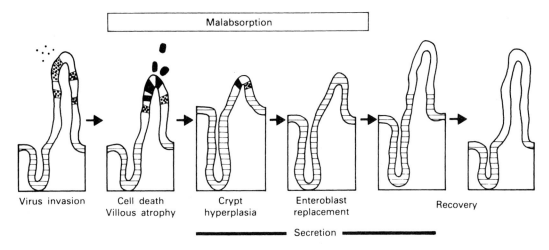

Fig. 27.2 Rotavirus pathogenesis. Development of damage to gut mucosa and ensuing diarrhoea. (From Phillips 1989, with permission of the author and publisher.)

Table 27.3 Rotavirus genes implicated in pathogenicity in different hosts

Gene segment	Gene product	Host	Reference
3	VP3	Pig	Hoshino et al. 1993, 1995
4	VP4	Mouse	Offit et al. 1986
		Human	Gorziglia et al. 1988
		Pig	Bridger et al. 1992
			Burger, Bridger and Desselberger 1994
			Burke, McCrae and Desselberger 1994
			Hoshino et al. 1993, 1995
5	NS53 (NSP1)	Mouse	Broome et al. 1993
7	NS35 (NSP2)	Mouse	Broome et al. 1993
8 or 9	VP7	Pig	Hoshino et al. 1993, 1995
10	NS28 (NSP4)	Pig	Hoshino et al. 1993, 1995
		Mouse, rat	Ball et al. 1995

ing and rapid dehydration. Untreated, rotavirus infection is a major cause of infant death in the developing world. It should be noted, though, that the clinical symptoms of rotavirus infection may vary widely, and asymptomatic infection of neonates with so-called nursery strains has been described (Hoshino et al. 1985).

Treatment is by oral, subcutaneous or intravenous rehydration. Table 27.4 gives the WHO approved formula of oral rehydration salts (ORS) to which glucose is added (Pierce and Hirshhorn 1977).

Table 27.4 Composition of oral rehydration solution for treatment of acute gastroenteritis in children

Compound	Concentration (mM/l)
Sodium	90
Potassium	20
Chloride	80
Bicarbonate or citrate	30
Glucose	110

2.6 Diagnosis

The number of virus particles in the gut at the peak of the diarrhoea can be as high at 10^{11}/ml of faeces. Diagnosis is therefore relatively easy by electron microscopy, ELISA or passive particle agglutination techniques.

Electron microscopy allows quick identification of the pathognomonic single- and double-shelled rotavirus particles. These particles differ grossly from other viruses causing acute gastroenteritis: enteroadenoviruses, small round structured viruses (SRSVs) such as calici-, Norwalk-like and astroviruses, and small round viruses (SRVs) (Doane 1994) (see Chapter 26).

Serological assays to detect rotaviruses are used widely, mostly applying direct or indirect enzyme-linked immunosorbent assays (ELISAs). The tests can be calibrated and quantified. If the detecting anti-rotavirus antibody is type-specific, the test can be used for G and P typing; this, however, depends on the presence of double-shelled virus particles in the clinical specimen. Another frequently used rapid technique is a passive particle agglutination test (Ruggeri et al. 1992). Details of procedures are described by Yolken and Wilde (1994).

The viral genome can be detected easily after phenol extraction of RNA from crude or semipurified rotavirus-containing specimens and separation by polyacrylamide gel electrophoresis (PAGE) followed by silver staining (e.g. Herring et al. 1982, Follett et al. 1984). The use of rotavirus-specific primers in a reverse transcription (RT) polymerase chain reaction (PCR) has allowed not only sensitive detection but also typing for both G and P types when the type-specifying sequence diversity is exploited (Gouvea et al. 1990a, Gentsch et al. 1992).

Human rotaviruses can be grown in vitro on monkey kidney cells in the presence of trypsin (Ward et al. 1984), but the procedure is not in routine use in most diagnostic laboratories. For diagnostic purposes the ELISA, which is much easier to perform, is usually preferred.

2.7   Immune response and correlates of protection

After neonatal or primary rotavirus infection a mainly serotype-specific humoral immune response is elicited, but there is also partial protection against subsequent heterotypic infections (Bishop et al. 1983, Chiba et al. 1986, Friedman et al. 1988, Linhares et al. 1989). The exact degrees of protection remain to be determined (Offit 1994), but the best are provided by coproantibodies of the IgA subclass (Corthier and Franz 1981, Coulson et al. 1992, Matson et al. 1993). The exact role of rotavirus-specific cytotoxic T cell (CTC) responses (Offit et al. 1993) is not known. There seems to be protection from **severe disease** after natural infection and vaccination (see section 2.9) even if the serotype of the challenging virus differs from that of the first infection or vaccination (Ward et al. 1992, Offit 1994, Velazquez et al. 1996). In the mouse model, homologous protection from infection depended on the level of mucosal IgA antibodies; heterologous protection could be achieved, but depended on dose and strain and also seemed to be correlated with the ability of the heterologous strain to stimulate detectable rotavirus-specific intestinal IgA antibody (Feng et al. 1994). In mice, rotavirus VP6-specific IgA monoclonal antibodies that lack direct neutralizing activity were found to protect from primary infection, possibly by intracellular viral inactivation during transcytosis (Burns et al. 1996). The extent to which heterotypic protection is efficient in humans remains unclear (Offit 1994).

2.8   Epidemiology

The epidemiology of rotavirus group A infections in humans is complex: at any one time and site there is co-circulation of rotaviruses of different G types, types G1–G4 representing 95% of co-circulating strains world-wide and type G1 c. 50% (Flores et al. 1988, Beards et al. 1989, Desselberger 1989, Gouvea et al. 1990b, Matson et al. 1990, Padilla-Noriega et al. 1990,

Noel, Beards and Cubitt 1991). Within one country different serotypes can show regional differences (Noel, Beards and Cubitt 1991, Bern et al. 1992, Bern and Glass 1994). Group B rotaviruses have caused widespread outbreaks in children and young adults in China (Hung 1988, Fang et al. 1989), but apparently not elsewhere.

2.9   Vaccine development

The development of a vaccine to protect against rotavirus infections has continued since the early 1980s and has been reviewed by Desselberger (1993), and more recently and comprehensively by Kapikian (1994) and Vesikari (1994). Owing to the enormous genomic and antigenic diversity of rotaviruses, results of vaccine trials have been varied. In most trials animal rotaviruses (of bovine or simian origin) have been used as live attenuated virus vaccines. Whereas protection from infection and mild disease was only modest, it was best when the vaccine serotype was related to that of the predominant circulating human wild type rotavirus strain. Partial protection preventing severe disease was achieved in most cases, possibly due to cross-reactive coproantibody (IgA) or CTL responses. The vaccine response is widened by applying a 'cocktail' of viruses, for example a native rhesus rotavirus (RRV) of G3 type and reassortants carrying the VP7 genes of human serotypes G1, G2 and G4 in the RRV genetic background. The outcome of a multicentre, placebo-controlled field trial in the USA has been published (Rennels et al. 1996). The trial involved 1278 children aged 5–25 weeks, who received 3 doses of 4 $\times 10^5$ pfu of monovalent RRV reassortant serotype G1 vaccine or tetravalent (TV) RRV 'cocktail' (G1–G4) at 2, 4 and 6 months of age. It was concluded that RRV-TV was safe and prevented 49% of rotavirus infections, 80% of severe disease episodes and 100% of cases of dehydration. RRV-TV induced better heterotypic protection than RRV-G1 (Rennels et al. 1996). A trial in Venezuela involving more than 2300 children yielded similar results (Kapikian et al. 1996). Rotavirus cocktail vaccines have now been submitted for FDA approval.

New approaches to immunization are under investigation; for example, applying inactivated virus or synthetic peptides (Conner et al. 1993), enhancing rotavirus immunogenicity by microencapsidation (Offit et al. 1994) or using VLPs obtained by co-expression of viral proteins (VP2, VP4, VP6 and VP7) from baculovirus recombinants in insect cells (Crawford et al. 1994). In view of the heterotypic immune responses observed after natural infection and immunization, it must be determined which of the epidemiologically important human P and G rotaviruses are mainly required for protection (Offit 1994).

3 REOVIRUSES

3.1 Genome, gene protein assignment and structure

Orthoreoviruses (reoviruses) are found world-wide in a wide range of vertebrates (mammals, including humans, birds and bats). They cause hepatic and neurological disease in mice, diarrhoea in cattle and sheep, and respiratory tract infections in dogs. In birds, reovirus infection is associated with hepatitis, arthritis and diarrhoea. Mammalian orthoreoviruses occur in 3 types: type 1 (strain Lang), type 2 (strain D5/Jones), and type 3 (strain Dearing).

The reovirus genome consists of 10 dsRNA segments that fall into 3 size classes, which for serotype 3 are: large (L), 3854–3916 bp; medium (M), 2203–2304 bp, and small (S) 1189–1416 bp. With the exception of RNA S1, they are monocistronic, but several protein products are modified post-translationally. Table 27.5 lists the genome segments, their coding capacity and some of the recognized functions of the protein products. The topography of reovirus proteins is shown in Fig. 27.3.

There are 8 structural (λ1, λ2, λ3, μ2, μ1C, σ1, σ2, σ3) and 2 non-structural (NS) proteins (μNSC, σNS). The inner core is made of λ1 and σ2 proteins into which are embedded 36 pentamers of λ2. Also within the core are λ3 and μ2 proteins. The λ3 protein is closely associated with the genomic RNA and has been identified as the RNA-dependent RNA polymerase. Trimers of σ1, the viral haemagglutinin, are located on top of the σ2 pentamers. The outer capsid comprises μ1C and σ3 proteins. Protein μ1 is myristylated at its amino terminus and is cleaved to μ1C when complexed with σ3.

3.2 Replication

Reoviruses adsorb to susceptible cells by interaction of the σ1 protein spikes with the cellular receptor, which is the β-adrenergic mammalian receptor. Penetration is by receptor-mediated endocytosis, but there is also direct penetration of so-called intermediate subviral particles (ISVPs) that have lost σ3 and possess an endoproteolytically cleaved μ1C (termed δ). The outer capsid is then completely removed in endocytic or lysosomal particles to yield subviral particles (SVPs) in which transcription starts. Outer uncoating is a prerequisite for transcription. Transcription is fully conservative, i.e. both strands of the parental genome remain in the SVPs. Only positive sense transcripts are made which are 'capped', the SVPs processing a full set of virus-coded capping enzymes (λ2 having guanylyltransferase and possibly also methyltransferase activity). Capped full length RNAs act as both mRNAs and templates for negative-strand RNA synthesis. There is transcriptional control in that the *L1*, *M3*, *S3* and *S4* genes are transcribed first and the other genes later. Replication occurs within nascent SVPs in which the plus strand RNA is packaged. The assembly of the correct number of RNA segments into SVPs is tightly controlled by as yet unknown mechanisms. At this late stage a second round of transcription can take place from the new SVPs, but this yields uncapped RNA. Both capped and uncapped RNAs undergo translation (the latter possibly supported by σ3). The relative rates of protein production are uneven: there is post-transcriptional control. The variability in translation might be due to differences in the structure of the individual mRNAs.

The morphogenesis is complex: the earliest SVPs still contain single-stranded RNA ('replicase particles'); once double-stranded RNA is made, they start secondary transcription ('transcription

Table 27.5 Gene protein assignment of mammalian reoviruses

RNA segment	Size (bp)	Proteins	Size (kDa)	Location and function
L1	3854	λ3	142	Core; RNA polymerase
L2	3916	λ2	144	Core spike; guanylyltransferase
L3	3896	λ1	137	Core
M1	2304	μ2	83	Core
M2	2203	μ1	76	Outer capsid
		μ1C	72	
M3	2235	μNS	80	Non-structural; ssRNA-binding; phosphoprotein
		μNSC	75	Unknown
S1	1416	σ1	49	Outer capsid; cell attachment protein; haemagglutinin; type-specific antigen
		σ1S	16	Unknown
S2	1331	σ2	47	Core
S3	1189	σNS	41	Non-structural; ssRNA-binding
S4	1196	σ3	41	Outer capsid; dsRNA-binding

Data obtained for reovirus type 3.
Slightly modified from Murphy et al. 1995, with permission of authors and publisher.

(a)

(b)

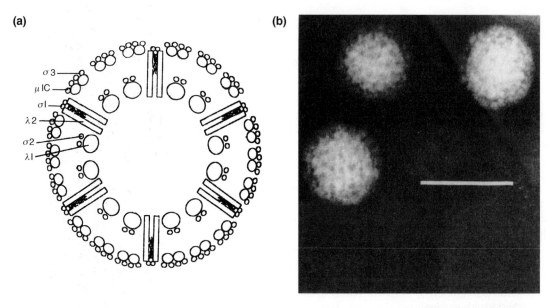

$\sigma 3$
$\mu 1C$
$\sigma 1$
$\lambda 2$
$\sigma 2$
$\lambda 1$

Fig. 27.3 (a) Schematic diagram showing the protein arrangements in capsid and (b) electron micrograph (uranyl formate stain; bar = 100 nm) of orthoreovirus. (From Murphy et al. 1995, with permission of the authors and publisher.)

particles'). The capsid and outer capsid proteins associate (NS proteins may be involved) around the SVPs. A peculiar feature is the occurrence of oligo-nucleotides (di- to nonanucleotides) in viral particles which seem to be synthesized at this late stage and represent 'aborted' 5′ ends of mRNAs. Virions are released from the cells by their lysis. Thus, viral replication is very similar though not identical to that of rotaviruses. (For details, see Joklik 1983, Schiff and Fields 1990.)

3.3 Pathogenesis: the mouse model

The elucidation of viral factors determining the pathogenesis of reoviruses is classic and is one of the major achievements of B N Fields' group. (For review, see Sharpe and Fields 1985, Tyler and Fields 1990.) The analysis is based on 2 observations:

1 Different reovirus types cause different diseases in mice (reovirus type 1: meningitis; reovirus type 3: encephalitis followed by hydrocephalus).
2 Different reovirus types have very different RNA profiles by PAGE (Fig. 27.4).

By doubly infecting cell cultures with reoviruses of types 1 and 3, numerous reassortants have been obtained for which the parental RNA segment derivation is established by co-electrophoresis of reassortant and parental RNA genomes. Careful observation of mice infected with various reassortants revealed the relative contributions of different genes or gene groups and their products to the pathogenic process.

The stages of viral pathogenesis are: (1) entry into host; (2) primary replication; (3) spread through the host; (4) specific cell and tissue tropism; and (5) host immune response. After oral inoculation in suckling mice, reovirus type 1 grows well in intestinal tissue but

type 3 does not. Studies with reassortants have shown that the capacity to grow in the gut is determined by the product of RNA segment *M2*: only viruses possessing the *M2* gene of type 1 grow in intestinal tissue. Type 3 lost its infectivity after chymotrypsin treatment in vitro; this characteristic was also traced to the *M2* product, suggesting that incoming and progeny virus carrying the *M2* gene of type 3 survive less well in the gut than do viruses carrying the *M2* gene of type 1.

Reovirus is taken up by Peyer's patches via the M cells, specialized gut epithelia overlying the lymphoid tissue of the Peyer's patches. From there virus spreads to mesenteric lymph nodes and spleen. The ability to spread from the site of entry is determined by the product of the *S1* gene, the viral haemagglutinin: only reoviruses carrying the *S1* gene of type 1 spread efficiently.

Reovirus types 1 and 3 can infect the central nervous system but each targets very different cells: type 1 reovirus infects ependymal cells, causing meningitis; type 3 infects neurons, causing encephalitis. Thus, type 3, which is avirulent when given orally, produces severe disease of the central nervous system when given parenterally; however, a reassortant type 3 virus carrying the *M2* gene of type 1 (or other reassortants of the *S1* type 3 *M2* type 1 gene combination) will cause encephalitis when given orally. Conversely, a type 1 reassortant carrying the *M2* gene of type 3 loses its ability to cause encephalitis when given orally.

By this and other genetic approaches, other factors determining pathogenicity of reoviruses have been elucidated; for example, infection of the pituitary (anterior, type 1; posterior, type 3, determined by the *S1* gene) or switching from acute lytic to persistent infection (mutations in *L2* and *S4* genes). (For review, see Sharpe and Fields 1985, Tyler and Fields 1990.)

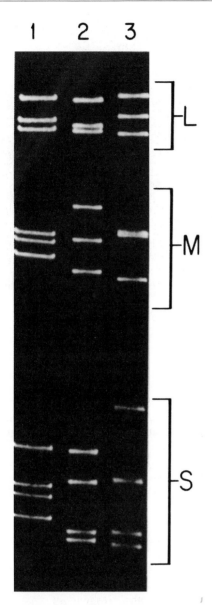

Fig. 27.4 RNA profiles of reoviruses type 2 (lane 1), type 1 (lane 2) and type 3 (lane 3), separated by electrophoresis on 10% SDS polyacrylamide gel and stained with ethidium bromide. (From Schiff and Fields 1990, with permission of the authors and publisher.)

3.5 Epidemiology

By 3 years of age, more than 70% of children have antibodies against all 3 types of reovirus. Antibodies to reoviruses are also found in most domestic animals. Reoviruses of all 3 types can be easily isolated from sewage and water supplies. Despite their ubiquity reoviruses have not been specifically shown to produce any human diseases (Tyler and Fields 1990).

4 ORBIVIRUSES

4.1 Genome, gene protein assignment and structure

The genome of orbiviruses consists of 10 segments of double-stranded RNA of 3 size classes termed *L1–L3*, *M4–M6* and *S7–S10*. The genome of bluetongue virus type 10 (BTV 10) has been fully sequenced (Roy 1989), and complete gene protein assignments have been made (Table 27.6) (Roy 1996a).

With the exception of RNA 10, all genes are monocistronic, coding for 7 structural and 4 non-structural proteins. The 5′ and 3′ termini of the RNA segments are conserved and have inverted complementarity (Roy 1996a), theoretically allowing 'panhandle' structure formation.

The inner core of the virion consists of the segmented genome with which 3 minor proteins, VP1, VP4 and VP6 (coded for by RNAs *L1*, *M4* and *S9*, respectively), are closely associated. These proteins represent the viral RNA polymerase, guanylyltransferase and RNA binding proteins, respectively. The inner core is surrounded by an inner capsid layer made up of VP3 trimers (inside; coded for by RNA *L3*) which forms a scaffold for VP7 trimers (outside; coded for by RNA *S7*). Genome and proteins VP1, VP4, VP6, VP3 and VP7 are also designated as core. This in turn is surrounded by the outer capsid consisting of VP5 (coded for by RNA *M5*), a glycoprotein, and VP2 (coded for by RNA *L2*). VP2 is the most variable of all BTV proteins and carries major epitopes determining serotype and neutralization specificity; it is a haemagglutinin and interacts with the cellular receptor (Roy 1996a). Specific antibody against VP2 protects animals but antibody directed against VP5 does not. There are 4 non-structural proteins NS1 (coded for by RNA *M6*), NS2 (coded for by RNA *S8*) and NS3/NS3A (coded for by RNA *S10* starting from 2 in-frame AUG triplets and differing in size by 1.5 kDa), the function of which is not fully elucidated (Roy 1992, 1996a).

It is interesting to compare the proteins of rota-, reo- and orbiviruses from a functional point of view. Although the 3 genera of the *Reoviridae* clearly have unique characteristics in structure, replication, pathogenesis and epidemiology, the parallels of functional equivalents are remarkable (Table 27.7). Thus, all viruses have a virion-associated RNA-dependent polymerase, have proteins of capping enzyme activity, have structural proteins that act as scaffolds at different levels and others that interact with receptors, haemagglutinate and determine neutralization (serotype) specificity. There is increasing evidence that the non-structural proteins have similar functions in morphogenesis, virion assembly and release.

3.4 Illness in humans

Reoviruses are recognized and well-studied pathogens in mice and other rodents, but it has been very difficult to link reovirus infections to any known disease in humans. Because adult humans have serological evidence of reovirus infections early in life, most of these infections must be asymptomatic. It has been suggested that there is an association of reovirus infections with enteritis in infants and children, upper respiratory tract infections and possibly neonatal biliary atresia, but confirmation is required (Tyler and Fields 1990).

Table 27.6   Gene protein assignments of orbivirus (bluetongue virus type 10)

RNA segment	Size (bp)	Protein Designation	Protein Deduced mol. wt (kDa)	Location in virion	Function (modification)
L1	3954	VP1	149.6	Inner core	RNA polymerase
L2	2926	VP2	111.1	Outer capsid	Haemagglutinin; cell attachment protein; type-specifying neutralization antigen
L3	2772	VP3	103.3	Core	Scaffold protein for VP7
M4	2011	VP4	76.4	Inner core	Guanylyltransferase
M5	1639	VP5	59.2	Outer capsid	Cross-reactive antigen (glycoprotein); not neutralization specific; positioning of VP2?
M6	1770	NS1	64.4	Non-structural	Tubule formation; translocation of virus particles?
S7	1156	VP7	38.5	Core surface	Group-specific antigen
S8	1123	NS2	41.0	Non-structural	Morphogenesis (phosphoprotein); binds ssRNA
S9	1046	VP6	35.8	Inner core	Binds ssRNA and dsRNA
S10	822	NS3	25.6	Non-structural	Virus release (glycoprotein)
		NS3A	24.0	Non-structural	?

Slightly modified from Roy 1996a, with permission of author and publisher.

Table 27.7   Functional similarities of proteins of rotavirus, bluetongue virus and reovirus

Topography	Function	Protein designation (and coding RNA segment) Rotavirus		Protein designation (and coding RNA segment) Bluetongue virus		Protein designation (and coding RNA segment) Reovirus	
Core (first layer)	RNA polymerase	VP1	(1)	VP1	(*L1*)	λ3	(*L1*)
	Guanylyltransferase	VP3	(3)	VP4	(*M4*)	λ2	(*L2*)
	RNA binding			VP6	(*S9*)		
	Scaffolding protein; RNA binding	VP2	(2)	VP3	(*L3*)	λ1 + σ2 (*L3 + S2*)	
Inner capsid (second layer)	Structural protein	VP6	(6)	VP7	(*S7*)	μ1/μ1C	(*M2*)
Outer capsid (third layer)	Structural protein	VP7	(7ᵃ)	VP5	(*M5*)	σ3	(*S4*)
	Haemagglutinin	VP4	(4)	VP2	(*L2*)	σ1	(*S1*)
Non-structural proteins	Diverse functions during replication (see text, p. 540, 543, 545)	NSP1	(5)	NS1	(*M6*)	μNS	(*M3*)
		NSP2	(8ᵃ)	NS2	(*S8*)	σNS	(*S3*)
		NSP3	(9ᵃ)				
		NSP4	(10)	NS3	(*S10*ᶜ)	σ1Sᵈ	(*S1*)
		NSP5	(11ᵇ)				

[a]Depending on the strain, VP7, NSP2 and NSP3 are coded for by RNA 7, 8 or 9.
[b]Also coding for NSP5A.
[c]Also coding for NS3A.
[d]ORF different from that of σ1.
Slightly modified from Mattion et al. 1994, with permission of authors and publisher.

4.2   Replication

Orbiviruses are special in that they replicate in both mammalian and insect cells at very different temperatures (37°C and 22–27°C, respectively).

Virions are adsorbed (via VP2) to sialic acid-containing receptors on the surface of mammalian cells; how-ever, the cellular receptor is not fully identified. It is remarkable that core particles (CPs) (lacking VP2 and VP5) adsorb well to and infect insect cells, suggesting that VP7 at the outside of the core may interact with insect cell receptor(s). Virus enters mammalian cells by endocytosis, after which the outer capsid (VP2 + VP5) is removed. The resulting core particle is active in transcription. The RNA polymerase has an optimum in vitro temperature of 28°C, but also works well at 37°C (Van Dijk and Huismans 1987), reflecting adaptation of viral replication to very different host cells. The transcription product is capped mRNA. There may be transcriptional control. Viral proteins are synthesized from 2–14 hours after infection and accumulate in the cytoplasm. NS1 protein forms extensive tubules throughout the cytoplasm but their function is unknown (Eaton, Hyatt and Brookes 1990).

Core-like and virus-like particles (CLPs, VLPs) largely self-assemble when combinations of viral proteins (CLPs: VP3 + VP7; VLPs: VP3 + VP7 + VP2 + VP5) are overexpressed simultaneously in insect cells from baculovirus recombinants (Fig. 27.5) (French, Marshall and Roy 1990).

Detailed morphological studies have been made of VLPs (Hewat, Booth and Roy 1994), and domains of the proteins required for self-interaction (e.g. trimer formation of VP3 and VP7) and interaction with each other or with nucleic acid have been identified (reviewed by Roy 1996a, 1996b). It is also possible to construct chimaeric VLPs. VP7 has been crystallized and its different domains have been described in detail (Grimes et al. 1995).

4.3 Pathogenesis

In animals BTV replicates mainly in the lymphoreticular system; it has a particular affinity with endothelial cells of capillaries, causing ischaemic lesions, inflammatory changes and oedema. There is an extensive viraemia that lasts for up to one month although neutralizing antibody appears 7–10 days after infection (Parsonson 1991). Like in vitro, different BTV serotypes reassort readily in their natural host (Samal et al. 1987).

4.4 Illness

The incubation period is 6–9 days. Illness starts with fever, followed by lesions developing mainly in the gastrointestinal but also in the respiratory tract, frequently associated with haemorrhages. Animals start to vomit and frequently die of bronchopneumonia. There is a wide range of host responses with many subclinical infections; morbidity ranges from 10% to 30%, and mortality is c. 5% (Parsonson 1991). Besides sheep, cattle are widely infected although mostly asymptomatic. Bluetongue virus can infect the fetus and is associated with abortions and fetal abnormalities in sheep and cattle (Parsonson 1991).

4.5 Epidemiology

Bluetongue viruses, which constitute one of at least 14 serogroups of orbiviruses (Murphy et al. 1995) and occur in 24 serotypes, infect sheep, cattle, goats and wild ungulates in many countries of the tropical and subtropical zones (Parsonson 1991). Their distribution is supported by a variety of insect vectors (*Culicoides* midges, ticks, mosquitoes etc.) in which the virus replicates (Mellor 1991). Other orbivirus serogroups, such as African horse sickness virus (AHSV) occurring in horses, donkeys and dogs, and epizootic haemorrhagic disease virus (EHDV), occurring in deer, have also diverged into various serotypes. Between BTV, AHSV and EHDV there is considerable conservation of the *VP3* gene products (55–79%), less of the *VP7* gene product (44–64%), the protein specifying the group antigen, and very little (17–23%) of

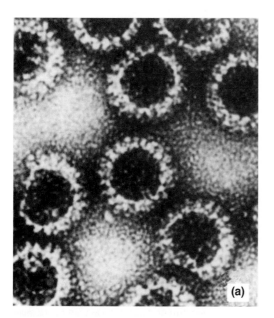 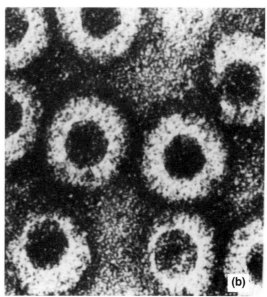

Fig. 27.5 (a) Core-like particles (CLPs) and (b) virus-like particles (VLPs) of bluetongue virus, obtained by co-expression of baculovirus recombinants in insect cells (CLPs: VP3 + VP7; VLPs: VP3 + VP7 + VP2 + VP5). (From French, Marshall and Roy 1990, with permission of the authors and publisher.)

the *VP2* gene product which specifies serotypes (Roy 1996a).

4.6 Vaccines

VP2 BTV-specific antibody is neutralizing and provides good homotypic protection (Huismans et al. 1987). The technology to make CLPs and VLPs by co-expression of viral genes in baculovirus recombinant-infected insect cells (e.g. French, Marshall and Roy 1990) has enabled the production of potent vaccine candidates (Roy, French and Erasmus 1992) which, either as mixtures derived from different serotypes or as particle chimaeras, have the potential to elicit broad protective immune responses.

5 COLTIVIRUSES

These viruses, which possess a genome of 12 segments of dsRNA, have recently been classified as a separate genus of the *Reoviridae* (Murphy et al. 1995). They are isolated from ticks, mosquitoes, rodents and humans. The Colorado tick fever virus (CTFV) can cause a fatal disease in humans. From RNA/RNA hybridization studies it became apparent that different isolates of CTFV differed mostly in their RNA segments 4 and 6, suggesting that their products are located on the outer capsid and carry neutralization specific epitopes (Bodkin and Knudson 1987).

CTFV is endemic in the Rocky Mountain region of the USA and Canada. In the insect vector (ticks of many species)

CTFV infects the midgut, from which it spreads to other organs, including salivary glands, allowing transmission to the next mammalian host by bite. As rodents have prolonged CTF viraemia they seem to be the main reservoir for tick infection in nature, but a variety of other mammals (marmots, deer, elk, sheep) can also become infected. Humans are infected by bite, but are a dead end of the transmission cycle (Monath and Guirakhoo 1996).

As is found with orbiviruses, CTFV can be isolated from red blood cells of humans up to 120 days after infection whereas it disappears from plasma very quickly (Bowen 1988). This cell-associated viraemia seems to originate from early infection of bone marrow stem cells; from there virus is continuously dispersed into the periphery in maturing erythrocytes. The viraemia persists in the presence of a strong neutralizing antibody response (Monath and Guirakhoo 1996).

After an incubation period of 4 (1–19) days, humans develop fever (possibly due to elevated interferon-α levels), leucopenia, gastrointestinal symptoms (20%), rash (10%) and meningitis/encephalitis (in 3–7% of cases). A severe haemorrhagic form of the disease (purpura, epistaxis, gastrointestinal bleeding) is rarely seen. The case-fatality rate is less than 0.1%.

Virus can be isolated from blood in continuous cell lines (Vero, BHK-21), and viral antigen can be detected in erythrocytes by IFT. Serological diagnosis is by IFT using infected Vero cells as antigen, or by ELISA.

Treatment is symptomatic; ribavirin has been used in cases of severe haemorrhagic disease.

REFERENCES

Ball JM, Tiang P et al., 1996, Age-dependent diarrhoea induced by a rotaviral nonstructural glycoprotein, *Science*, **272**: 101–4.

Beards GM, Desselberger U, Flewett TH, 1989, Temporal and geographical distributions of human rotavirus serotypes 1983–1988, *J Clin Microbiol*, **27**: 2827–33.

Bern C, Glass RI, 1994, Impact of diarrheal diseases worldwide, *Viral Infections of the Gastrointestinal Tract*, 2nd edn, ed Kapikian AZ, Marcel Dekker, New York, 1–26.

Bern C, Martines J et al., 1992, The magnitude of the global problem of diarrhoeic disease: a ten-year update, *Bull W H O*, **70**: 705–14.

Bishop RF, Barnes GL et al., 1983, Clinical immunity after neonatal rotavirus infection: a prospective longitudinal study in young children, *N Engl J Med*, **309**: 72–6.

Bodkin DK, Knudson DL, 1987, Genetic relatedness of Colorado tick fever virus isolates by RNA–RNA blot hybridization, *J Gen Virol*, **68**: 1199–204.

Bowen GS, 1988, Colorado tick fever, *The arboviruses: epidemiology and ecology*, CRC Press, Boca Raton FL, ed Monath TP, 159–76.

Bridger JC, 1987, Novel rotaviruses in animals and man, *Ciba Found Symp*, **128**: 5–23.

Bridger JC, Burke B et al., 1992, The pathogenicity of two porcine rotaviruses differing in their *in vitro* growth characteristics and genes 4, *J Gen Virol*, **73**: 3011–15.

Broome RL, Vo PT et al., 1993, Murine rotavirus genes encoding outer capsid proteins VP4 and VP7 are not major determinants of host range restriction and virulence, *J Virol*, **67**: 2448–55.

Burke B, Bridger JC, Desselberger U, 1994, Temporal correlation between a single amino acid change in the VP4 of a porcine rotavirus and a marked change in pathogenicity, *Virology*, **202**: 754–9.

Burke B, Desselberger U, 1996, Rotavirus pathogenicity, *Virology*, **218**: 299–305.

Burke B, McCrae MA, Desselberger U, 1994, Sequence analysis of two porcine rotaviruses differing in growth *in vitro* and in pathogenicity. Distinct VP4 sequences and conservation of NS53, VP6 and VP7 genes, *J Gen Virol*, **75**: 2205–12.

Burns JW, Siadet-Pajouh M et al., 1996, Protective effect of rotavirus VP6-specific IgA monoclonal antibodies that lack neutralizing activity, *Science*, **272**: 104–107.

Chiba S, Nakata S et al., 1986, Protective effect of naturally acquired homotypic and heterotypic rotavirus antibodies, *Lancet*, **ii**: 417–21.

Cohen J, Laporte J et al., 1979, Activation of rotavirus RNA polymerase by calcium chelation, *Arch Virol*, **60**: 177–86.

Conner ME, Crawford SE et al., 1993, Rotavirus vaccine administered parenterally induces protective immunity, *J Virol*, **67**: 6633–41.

Corthier G, Franz J, 1981, Detection of antirotavirus immunoglobulins A, G and M in swine colostrum, milk and faeces by ELISA, *Infect Immun*, **31**: 833–6.

Coulson B, Grimwood K et al., 1992, Role of coproantibody in clinical protection of children during reinfection with rotavirus, *J Clin Microbiol*, **30**: 1678–84.

Crawford SE, Labbé M et al., 1994, Characterization of viruslike particles produced by the expression of rotavirus capsid protein in insect cells, *J Virol*, **68**: 5945–52.

Desselberger U, 1989, Molecular epidemiology of rotaviruses, *Viruses and the Gut*, ed Farthing MJG, Swan Press, London, 55–65.

Desselberger U, 1993, Towards rotavirus vaccines, *Rev Med Virol*, **3**: 15–21.

Doane FW, 1994, Electron microscopy for the detection of gastroenteritis viruses, *Viral Infections of the Gastrointestinal Tract*, 2nd edn, ed Kapikian AZ, Marcel Dekker, New York, 101–30.

Eaton BT, Hyatt AD, Brookes SM, 1990, The replication of bluetongue virus, *Curr Topics Microbiol Immunol*, **162**: 89–118.

Estes MK, 1996, Rotaviruses and their replication, *Fields' Virology*, 3rd edn, eds Fields BN, Knipe DM et al., Lippincott-Raven Publ, Philadelphia, 1625–55.

Fang ZY, Ye Q et al., 1989, Investigation of an outbreak of adult diarrhoea rotavirus in China, *J Infect Dis*, **160:** 948–53.

Feng NG, Burns JW et al., 1994, Comparison of mucosal and systemic humoral immune responses and subsequent protection in mice orally inoculated with a homologous or a heterologous rotavirus, *J Virol*, **68:** 7766–73.

Flores J, Taniguchi K et al., 1988, Relative frequencies of rotavirus serotypes 1, 2, 3 and 4 in Venezuelan infants with gastroenteritis, *J Clin Microbiol*, **26:** 2092–5.

Follett EAC, Sanders RC et al., 1984, Molecular epidemiology of human rotaviruses. Analysis of outbreaks of acute gastroenteritis in Glasgow and the West of Scotland 1981/82 and 1982/83, *J Hyg (Camb)*, **92:** 209–22.

French TJ, Marshall JJA, Roy P, 1990, Assembly of double shelled virus particles of bluetongue virus by the simultaneous expression of four structural proteins, *J Virol*, **64:** 5695–700.

Friedman MG, Galil A et al., 1988, Two sequential outbreaks of rotavirus gastroenteritis: evidence of symptomatic and asymptomatic reinfections, *J Infect Dis*, **158:** 814–22.

Garbarg-Chenon A, Bricout F, Nicolas JC, 1984, Study of genetic reassortment between 2 human rotaviruses, *Virology*, **139:** 358–65.

Gentsch JR, Glass RI et al., 1992, Identification of group A rotavirus gene 4 types by polymerase chain reaction, *J Clin Microbiol*, **30:** 1365–73.

Gombold JL, Ramig RF, 1986, Analysis of reassortants of genome segments in mice mixedly infected with rotavirus SA11 and RRV, *J Virol*, **57:** 110–16.

Gorziglia M, Green K et al., 1988, Sequence of the fourth gene of human rotaviruses recovered from asymptomatic or symptomatic infections, *J Virol*, **64:** 2978–84.

Gouvea V, Glass RI et al., 1990a, Polymerase chain reaction amplification and typing of rotavirus nucleic acid from stool specimens, *J Clin Microbiol*, **28:** 276–82.

Gouvea V, Ho M et al., 1990b, Serotypes and electropherotypes of human rotavirus in the USA, 1987–1989, *J Infect Dis*, **162:** 362–7.

Graham A, Kudesia G et al., 1987, Reassortment of human rotavirus possessing genome rearrangements with bovine rotavirus: evidence for host cell selection, *J Gen Virol*, **68:** 115–22.

Greenberg HB, Wyatt RG et al., 1981, New insights in viral gastroenteritis, *Perspect Virol*, **11:** 163–87.

Greenberg HB, McAuliffe V et al., 1982, Serologic analysis of the subgroup protein of rotavirus using monoclonal antibody, *Infect Immun*, **39:** 91–9.

Grimes J, Basak AJ et al., 1995, The crystal structure of bluetongue virus VP7, *Nature (London)*, **373:** 167–70.

Herring AJ, Inglis NF et al., 1982, Rapid diagnosis of rotavirus infection by direct detection of viral nucleic acid in silver-stained polyacrylamide gels, *J Clin Microbiol*, **16:** 473–7.

Hewat EA, Booth TF, Roy P, 1994, Structure of the bluetongue virus-like particles by cryo-electron microscopy, *J Struct Biol*, **112:** 183–91.

Hoshino Y, Wyatt RG et al., 1985, Serotypic characterization of rotaviruses derived from asymptomatic human neonatal infections, *J Clin Microbiol*, **21:** 425–30.

Hoshino Y, Sereno M et al., 1993, Genetic determinants of rotavirus virulence studied in gnotobiotic piglets, *Vaccines*, eds Ginsberg HS, Brown F, Chanode RM, Lerner RA, Cold Spring Harbor Laboratory Press, Cold Spring Harbor NY, 277–82.

Hoshino Y, Saif LJ et al., 1995, Identification of group A rotavirus genes associated with virulence of a porcine rotavirus and host range restriction of a human rotavirus in the gnotobiotic piglet model, *Virology*, **209:** 274–80.

Huismans H, Van der Walt NT et al., 1987, Isolation of a capsid protein of bluetongue virus that induces a protective immune response in sheep, *Virology*, **157:** 172–9.

Hung T, 1988, Rotavirus and adult diarrhoea, *Adv Virus Res*, **35:** 193–218.

Joklik WK, 1983, The reovirus particle, *The Reoviridae*, ed Joklik WK, Plenum Press, New York, 9–78.

Kapikian AZ, ed, 1994, Rhesus rotavirus-based human rotavirus-vaccines and observations on selected non-Jennerian approaches to rotavirus vaccination, *Viral Infections of the Gastrointestinal Tract*, 2nd edn, ed Kapikian AZ, Marcel Dekker, New York, 443–70.

Kapikian AZ, Hoshino Y et al., 1996, Efficacy of the quadrivalent rhesus rotavirus (RRV), human RRV reassortant vaccine bearing VP7 specificity for each of the 4 epidemiologically important serotypes against rotavirus diarrhea of infants and young children, X International Congress of Virology, Jerusalem, August, abstracts, p. 12.

Linhares AC, Gabbag YB et al., 1989, Longitudinal study of rotavirus infections among children from Belém, Brazil, *Epidemiol Infect*, **102:** 129–45.

Matson DO, Estes MK et al., 1990, Serotype variation of group A rotaviruses in two regions of the USA, *J Infect Dis*, **162:** 605–14.

Matson D, O'Ryan M et al., 1993, Fecal antibody responses to symptomatic and asymptomatic rotavirus infections, *J Infect Dis*, **167:** 577–83.

Mattion NM, Cohen J, Estes MK, 1994, The rotavirus proteins, *Viral Infections of the Gastrointestinal Tract*, 2nd edn, ed Kapikian AZ, Marcel Dekker, New York, 169–249.

Mellor PS, 1991, The replication of bluetongue virus in *Culicoides* vectors, *Curr Topics Microbiol Immunol*, **162:** 143–61.

Monath TP, Guirakhoo F, 1996, Orbiviruses and coltiviruses, *Fields' Virology*, 3rd edn, eds Fields BN, Knipe DM et al., Lippincott-Raven Publ, Philadelphia, 1735–66.

Murphy FA, Fauquet CM et al., 1995, *Reoviridae, Virus Taxonomy. Classification and Nomenclature of Viruses*, 5th edn, eds Murphy FA, Fauquet CM et al., Springer Verlag, Vienna, New York, 208–39.

Noel JS, Beards GM, Cubitt WD, 1991, An epidemiological survey of human rotavirus serotypes and electropherotypes in young children admitted to two hospitals in north east London, *J Clin Microbiol*, **29:** 2213–19.

Offit PA, 1994, Rotaviruses: immunological determinants of protection against infection and disease, *Adv Virus Res*, **44:** 161–202.

Offit PA, Blavat G et al., 1986, Molecular basis for rotavirus virulence: role of rotavirus gene segment 4, *J Virol*, **57:** 46–9.

Offit PA, Hoffenberg EJ et al., 1993, Rotavirus-specific humoral and cellular immune response after primary symptomatic infection, *J Infect Dis*, **167:** 1436–40.

Offit PA, Khouri CA et al., 1994, Enhancement of rotavirus immunogenicity by microencapsidation, *Virology*, **203:** 134–43.

Padilla-Noriega L, Arias CF et al., 1990, Diversity of rotavirus serotypes in Mexican infants with gastroenteritis, *J Clin Microbiol*, **28:** 1114–19.

Parsonson TM, 1991, Pathology and pathogenesis of bluetongue virus infections, *Curr Top Microbiol Immunol*, **162:** 119–41.

Patton JT, 1994, Rotavirus replication, *Rotaviruses*, ed Ramig RF, Springer Verlag, Berlin, 107–27.

Phillips AD, 1989, Mechanisms of mucosal injury: human studies, *Viruses and the Gut*, ed Farthing MJG, Swan Press, London, 30–40.

Pierce NF, Hirshhorn J, 1977, Oral fluid is a single weapon against dehydration: how it works and how to use it, *W H O Chron*, **31:** 87–93.

Prasad BVV, Chiu W, 1994, Structure of rotaviruses, *Rotaviruses*, ed Ramig RF, Springer-Verlag, Berlin, 9–29.

Prasad BVV, Wang GY et al., 1988, Three-dimensional structure of rotavirus, *J Mol Biol*, **199:** 269–75.

Prasad BVV, Burns JW et al., 1990, Localization of VP4 neutralization sites in rotavirus by three-dimensional cryo-electron microscopy, *Nature (London)*, **343:** 476–9.

Rennels MB, Glass RI et al., 1996, Safety and efficacy of high-dose rhesus-human reassortant rotavirus vaccines. Report of the national multicenter trial, *Pediatrics*, **97:** 7–13.

Roy P, 1989, Bluetongue virus genetics and genome structure, *Virus Res*, **13:** 179–206.

Roy P, 1992, Bluetongue virus proteins, *J Gen Virol*, **73:** 3051–64.

Roy P, 1996a, Orbiviruses and their replication, *Fields' Virology*, 3rd edn, eds Fields BN, Knipe DM et al., Lippincott-Raven Publ, Philadelphia, 1709–34.

Roy P, 1996b, Orbivirus structure and assembly, *Virology*, **216:** 1–11.

Roy P, French TJ, Erasmus BJ, 1992, Protective efficacy of virus-like particles for bluetongue disease, *Vaccine*, **10:** 28–32.

Roy P, Gorman BM, 1991, Bluetongue viruses, *Curr Top Microbiol Immunol*, **162:** 1–200.

Ruggeri FM, Marziano ML et al., 1992, Laboratory diagnosis of rotavirus infection in diarrhoeal patients by immunoenzymatic and latex agglutination assays, *Microbiologica*, **15:** 249–57.

Samal SK, Livingstone CW et al., 1987, Analysis of mixed infection of sheep with bluetongue virus serotypes 10 and 17: evidence for genetic reassortment in the vertebrate host, *J Virol*, **61:** 1086–91.

Schiff LA, Fields BN, 1990, Reoviruses and their replication, *Fields' Virology*, 2nd edn, eds Fields BN, Knipe DM, Raven Press, New York, 1275–306.

Sharpe AH, Fields BN, 1985, Pathogenesis of viral infections. Basic concepts derived from the reovirus model, *N Engl J Med*, **312:** 486–97.

Shaw AL, Rothnagel R et al., 1993, Three-dimensional visualization of the rotavirus hemagglutinin structure, *Cell*, **74:** 693–701.

Tyler KL, Fields BN, 1990, Reoviruses, *Fields' Virology*, 2nd edn, eds Fields BN, Knipe DM, Raven Press, New York, 1307–28.

Van Dijk AA, Huismans H, 1987, The effect of temperature on the *in vitro* transcription reaction of bluetongue virus, epizootic haemorrhagic disease virus and African horse sickness virus, *Onderstepoort J Vet Res*, **54:** 629–33.

Velazquez FR, Matson DO et al., 1996, Rotavirus infection in infants as protection against subsequent infections, *N Engl J Med*, **335:** 1022–8.

Vesikari T, 1994, Bovine rotavirus-based rotavirus vaccines in humans, *Viral Infections of the Gastrointestinal Tract*, 2nd edn, ed Kapikian AZ, Marcel Dekker, New York, 419–42.

Ward RL, Knowlton DR, Pierce M, 1984, Efficiency of human rotavirus propagation in cell culture, *J Clin Microbiol*, **19:** 748–53.

Ward RL, Nakagomi O et al., 1990, Evidence for natural reassortants of human rotaviruses belonging to different genogroups, *J Virol*, **64:** 3219–25.

Ward R, Clemens J et al., 1992, Evidence that protection against rotavirus diarrhoea after natural infection is not dependent on serotype-specific neutralizing antibody, *J Infect Dis*, **166:** 1251–7.

Yeager M, Dryden KA et al., 1990, Three-dimensional structure of rhesus rotavirus by cryoelectron microscopy and image reconstruction, *J Cell Biol*, **110:** 2133–44.

Yeager M, Berriman JA et al., 1994, Three-dimensional structure of the rotavirus haemagglutinin VP4 by cryo-electron microscopy and difference map analysis, *EMBO J*, **13:** 1011–18.

Yolken RH, Wilde JA, 1994, Assays for detecting human rotavirus, *Viral Infections of the Gastrointestinal Tract*, 2nd edn, ed Kapikian AZ, Marcel Dekker, New York, 251–78.

Chapter 28

RUBELLA

J E Banatvala and Jennifer M Best

1 Properties of the virus	2 Clinical and pathological aspects

1   PROPERTIES OF THE VIRUS

1.1   Introduction

Rubella was first described by 2 German physicians, de Bergen and Orlow, in the mid eighteenth century. At that time it was frequently known by the German name 'Röteln', and it was due to the early interest of the German physicians and the general acceptance of a German name that the disease subsequently became known as 'german measles'. For many years german measles was frequently confused with measles and scarlet fever, other infectious diseases presenting with rash, and at one time was considered to be a cross between them. The clinical differences between these diseases were recognized in the nineteenth century and rubella was accepted as a distinct disease by an International Congress of Medicine in London in 1881 (Smith 1881). The disease received comparatively little attention, for infection was generally mild and severe complications were rare, until the 1940s when the association between maternal infection and such congenital defects as cataract, heart disease and hearing loss was first recognized (Gregg 1941). This report is discussed in more detail later (see p. 557).

Rubella virus (RV) was not isolated in cell culture until 1962, when Parkman, Buescher and Artenstein (1962) detected the presence of RV in primary vervet monkey kidney cell cultures by means of the interference technique and Weller and Neva (1962) reported unique cytopathic effects in primary amnion cell cultures. Tests for neutralizing and haemagglutination inhibition (HAI) antibodies were reported in 1962 (Parkman, Buescher and Artenstein 1962, Parkman et al. 1964) and 1967 (Stewart et al. 1967) respectively and these tests allowed seroepidemiological investigations to be conducted. The fine structure of RV was not determined until 1968 as it is difficult to obtain the high titres of virus required for electron microscopy (Best et al. 1967, Holmes et al. 1968). Much of the work on the molecular structure

and replication of RV was carried out in the late 1980s and early 1990s, some time after similar work on other viruses. This was probably because RV is slow to grow in cell culture, high levels of virus are difficult to produce consistently and the high G + C content of the genome has made sequencing difficult.

1.2   Classification

Rubella virus, an enveloped RNA virus, belongs to the family *Togaviridae* (Chapter 29) and is probably distantly related to the alphaviruses (Frey 1994). Unlike other togaviruses, RV has no known invertebrate host and has been placed by itself in the genus *Rubivirus*.

1.3   Morphology and structure

The virion has a mean diameter of 58 nm with a 30 nm core (Fig. 28.1) (Holmes et al. 1968, Murphy, Halonen and Harrison 1968). The core is surrounded by a lipoprotein envelope with surface spikes 5–8 nm in length. In thin sections of infected cells an electron-lucent zone is seen between the core and the envelope. The virion is pleomorphic, owing to the delicate non-rigid nature of the envelope. The symmetry of the nucleocapsid has been difficult to establish because of its instability, but rotational analysis of thin sections of rubella virions suggested that the core had a T = 3 icosahedral symmetry and 32 capsomers (Matsumoto and Higashi 1974).

Physical properties of RV are shown in Table 28.1 and were reviewed by Horzinek (1973, 1981). The stability of the virus is enhanced by the addition of proteins and $MgSO_4$ to the suspending medium. Because of the lipid content of the viral envelope, RV is inactivated by detergents and organic solvents. The effects of these and other chemicals have been reviewed (Parkman et al. 1964, Norrby 1969, Plotkin 1969, Horzinek 1973, 1981, Herrmann 1979).

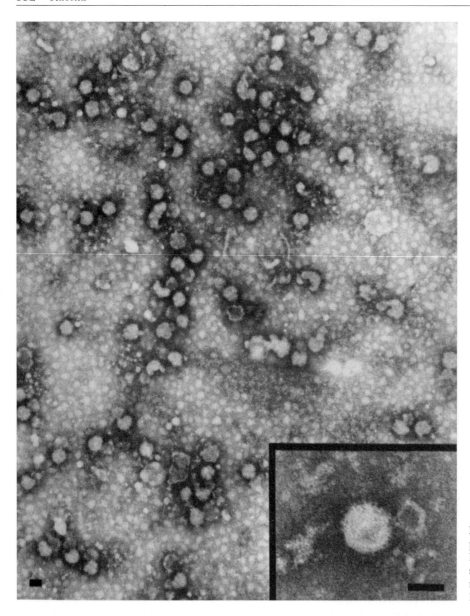

Fig. 28.1 Negatively stained preparation of rubella virus. Inset: an enlarged particle, showing spikes. Bar = 50 nm. (Kindly provided by Dr I Chrystie.)

1.4   Genome structure and function

The genome of RV is a single strand of RNA. This 40S genomic RNA is infectious, but the recovery of infectivity is poor (Hovi and Vaheri 1970b). The genome is 9759 nucleotides in length excluding the 3′ terminal poly(A) tail and is capped at the 5′ end (Dominguez, Wang and Frey 1990, Frey 1994). The cap is required for efficient translation as it serves as a ribosome recognition site. The base composition of the genome is A 14.9%, U 15.4%, G 30.8% and C 38.7%. The high G + C content (69.5%) of the genome has made sequence determination difficult and a number of sequencing errors are present in some of the original sequences reported (reviewed by Frey 1994). The genome is composed of 2 long open reading frames (ORFs) and has some features in common with the alphaviruses (Dominguez, Wang and Frey 1990). The 5′ proximal ORF is 6345 nucleotides (nuc) in length (nuc 41–6385) and codes for the non-struc-

tural proteins (NSP). The 3′ proximal ORF is 3189 nucleotides in length (nuc 6509–9697) and codes for the structural proteins (Fig. 28.2). The 2 ORFs are in the same translational frame and are separated by 123 nucleotides. The subgenomic RNA. which is capped, methylated and polyadenylated, is transcribed from the negative sense subgenomic RNA, for which the start site is nucleotide 6433 (U) (T Frey 1995, personal communication). Genome-length cDNA clones have been produced and used to synthesize infectious RNA transcripts (Wang, Dominguez and Frey 1994).

Sequences at the 5′ and 3′ ends of rubella virus RNA can form stable stem–loop structures. These structures are thought to be involved with virus replication and may be necessary for efficient translation (Pogue et al. 1993, Nakhasi et al. 1994). Recent work suggests that RV RNA interacts with host cell proteins. Cell proteins of 59 and 52 kDa bind to the 5′ stem–loop structure, these 2 proteins are related to the autoantigen La (Pogue et al. 1993, 1996). The host cell protein that

Table 28.1 Physical and morphological properties of rubella virus

Virus particle:		
Diameter	40–70 nm	Reviewed by Horzinek (1973)
Buoyant density:	in sucrose: 1.16–1.19 g/ml	
	in CsCl$_2$: 1.20–1.23 g/ml	Reviewed by Horzinek (1973)
Sedimentation	240S	Thomssen, Laufs and Müller (1968)
coefficient	342S	Russell, Selzer and Goetz (1967)
	350 ± 50S	Bardeletti, Kessler and Aymard-Henry (1975)
Nucleocapsid:		
Diameter	30–40 nm	Reviewed by Horzinek (1973)
Symmetry	Icosahedral	Reviewed by Horzinek (1973)
Buoyant density	in CsCl$_2$: 1.4 ± 0.4 g/ml	
Sedimentation	150S	Vaheri and Hovi (1972)
coefficient		
Molecular weight	2600–4000 kDa	Kenney et al. (1969)
Nucleic acid:	Single strand of RNA	
Buoyant density	1.634 g/ml	Hovi and Vaheri (1970a)
Sedimentation	38–40S	Sedwick and Sokol (1970)
coefficient		
Molecular weight	3200–3500 kDa	
Length of surface	5–6 nm	Holmes, Wark and Warburton (1969)
projections		Smith and Hobbins (1969)
		Voiland and Bardeletti (1980)
Chemical composition	RNA 2.4% Lipid 18.8%	
	Proteins 74.8% Carbohydrates 4.0%	
Major polypeptides	Envelope E1 58 kDa	Oker-Blom et al. (1983)
	E2 42–47 kDa	Waxham and Wolinsky (1985)
	Nucleocapsid C 33	
Thermal stability:		
4°C	Stable for ≥7 days	Fabiyi et al. (1966)
37°C	Inactivated at 0.1–0.4 log$_{10}$ TCID50/ml per h	Parkman (1965)
56°C	Inactivated at 1.5–3.5 log$_{10}$ TCID50/0.1 ml per h	Parkman (1965)
70°C	Inactivated at 5.5 log$_{10}$ TCID50/0.1 ml per ½ hour	Kistler and Sapatino (1972)
−70°C	Stable	Parkman et al. (1964)
Freeze drying	Stable	Parkman et al. (1964)
pH sensitivity	Stable at pH 6.0–8.1	Schell and Wong (1966), Norrby (1969)
	Unstable at more acid and alkaline pH	
UV sensitivity	Inactivated within 40 s	Fabiyi et al. (1966)
1350 W/cm^2	Inactivated at 7.0 log$_{10}$ TCID 50/0.1 ml per h	Kistler and Sapatino (1972)
Photosensitivity	Labile, K = 0.07/min in PBS	Booth and Stern (1972)
Sonication	Stable for ≥9min	Schell and Wong (1966)

TCID50 = 50% tissue culture infective dose.

binds to the 3′ stem–loop structure is autophosphorylated calreticulin, another putative autoantigen (Atreya, Singh and Nakhasi 1995). It has been suggested that these autoantigen–RV–RNA complexes may play a role in the replication and pathogenesis of RV, including arthropathy.

1.5 Replication

RV probably enters the cell by receptor-mediated endocytosis. The cellular receptor for the virus has not been identified, but membrane lipid molecules play an essential role (Mastromarino et al. 1990). The

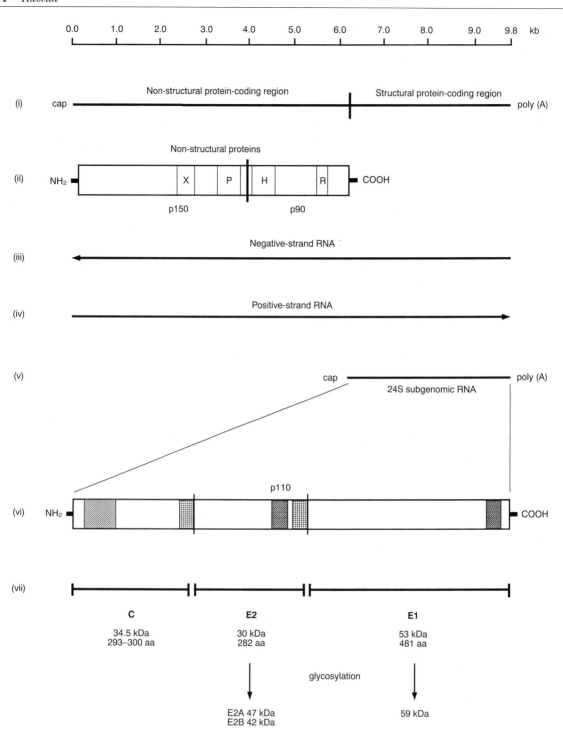

Fig. 28.2 Map of the rubella virus genome and strategy for the expression of rubella virus structural proteins. Translation of rubella RNA (i) results in production of non-structural proteins (ii), which initiate the synthesis of a full-length negative strand of RNA (iii), which acts as template for the synthesis of both full-length positive strand for new viral progeny (iv) and 24S subgenomic RNA (v). Translation of this 24S RNA results in the production of p110, a polyprotein (vi) which is proteolitially cleaved to produce the 3 structural proteins C, E2 and E1 (vii). Within the non-structural ORF the location of global amino acid motifs indicative of replicase (R), helicase (H) and cysteine protease (P) activity are indicated. X indicates a region of homology between rubella and alphaviruses.

▓ hydrophilic domain of C, putatively interacts with virion RNA
▦ hydrophobic signal sequences that precede the N terminal of E2 and E1
▨ the transmembrane sequences of E2 and E1

reproductive cycle takes place in the cytoplasm. It is probable that the process of penetration and uncoating resembles that of the alphaviruses (Chapter 29). The virion is internalized in a coated vesicle and transported to the endosomal compartment. At the low pH in the endosome the C protein becomes lipid soluble and this may allow association of the capsid with the viral membrane to uncoat the viral RNA within the viral envelope (Mauracher et al. 1991). The low pH also triggers a conformational change in the envelope glycoproteins and mediates fusion of the viral membrane and the endosomal membrane to allow release of viral RNA into the cytoplasm (Katow and Sugiura 1988).

The virion RNA is translated to produce the 2115 amino acid polyprotein encoded by the 5′ proximal ORF. This polyprotein is proteolytically cleaved to give the non-structural proteins (NSP) which may interact with host cell proteins to replicate a negative sense genome, which is then used as a template for the new positive sense RNA and subgenomic 24S RNA. The negative polarity RNA is present only in double-stranded form and functions solely as a template for positive polarity RNA synthesis. The subgenomic RNA that is transcribed from this negative template is translated to produce a polyprotein of 110 kDa, which is cleaved by host cell proteases to produce the 3 structural proteins: 2 glycoproteins, E1 and E2, and the capsid protein, C (Fig. 28.2) (Kalkkinen, Oker-Blom and Pettersson 1984, Oker-Blom 1984). Cleavage of the 110 kDa precursor is thought to occur at signal sequences that precede the amino termini of E2 and E1. The E2 and E1 signal sequences remain attached to the mature C and E2 respectively (Suomalainen et al. 1990, Marr et al. 1991, Baron, Ebel and Suomalainen 1992). The C protein of RV lacks the autoprotease activity found in the alphavirus C proteins. Cleavage is thought to be catalysed by signalase in the lumen of the endoplasmic reticulum (Oker-Blom, Jarvis and Summers 1990).

The C protein forms a non-covalently bonded dimer soon after translation in infected cells (Baron and Forsell 1991). RV capsid formation occurs in association with membranes for which the E2 signal sequence is required (Suomalainen et al. 1990). E1 and E2 form heterodimeric complexes and can be detected by immunoprecipitation within 30 min of synthesis (Baron and Forsell 1991). They are targeted to the Golgi apparatus. A *trans*-dominant Golgi retention signal has been identified within the C-terminal region of E2 (Hobman, Woodward and Farquhar 1995). Thus, all the structural proteins are transported to the Golgi complex.

The replication cycle of RV in vertebrate cell cultures is slow and less efficient than that of the alphaviruses. The high G + C content of RV RNA may contribute to the inefficiency (Frey 1994). Hemphill and colleagues (Hemphill et al. 1988) have shown that virus production reaches a peak at 48 hours after infection in Vero cells at high multiplicities of infection. Intracellular virus structural proteins were first detected by immunoprecipitation 16 hours after infection and all cells exhibited cytoplasmic immunofluorescence at 48 hours.

Viral genomic and subgenomic RNA was first detected 12 hours after infection and peaked at 26 hours. Hemphill et al. (1988) found no effect on total cell RNA synthesis but a modest inhibition of total cell protein synthesis; they suggested that the effect may vary in different cell types. Others have reported a stimulation of the metabolism of infected cells (Vaheri and Cristofalo 1967, Bardeletti 1977). Defective interfering (DI) RNAs have been detected (reviewed by Frey 1994) and were characterized by Derdyn and Frey (1993). More than 2 days after infection, membrane alterations and vacuolation are observed in infected cells. Membrane alterations include proliferation and distension and the appearance of crystalline inclusions and annulate lamellae (Kistler et al. 1967, Bardeletti et al. 1979, Pathak et al. 1994). Membrane-bound cytoplasmic vacuoles analogous to the replication complexes found in alphavirus-infected cells have been reported (Lee, Marshall and Bowden 1992).

There is limited information about the assembly of the RV particle. The 40S genomic RNA is encapsidated by the C protein. A 29 nucleotide RNA sequence (nucleotides 347–375) has been identified as essential for binding the RNA to the capsid protein, and a peptide domain (residues 28–56) with specific RNA binding activity has been located in the capsid protein (Liu et al. 1996). Virus is released from the cell by budding, probably at both the plasma membrane and the internal membranes. The nucleocapsid core buds from the modified cellular membrane and acquires host cell lipids and the viral proteins E1 and E2 to form the viral envelope. Bardeletti, Tektoff and Gautheron (1979) compared RV maturation and production in Vero and BHK-21 cells; Vero cells released more virus into the culture medium, because virus maturation occurred only at the plasma membrane. In Vero cells less intracellular virus is produced than in BHK-21 cells, in which maturation occurs at the plasma membrane and in the Golgi apparatus and vacuoles of the cytoplasm. Wolinsky (1996) suggests that the capacity to mature within intracellular vacuoles, avoiding the host's immune system, may enable the virus to establish persistent infections in humans. Pathak et al. (1994), using immunoelectron microscopy, reported spherules (pleomorphic membrane-bound structures containing a dense thread-like structure) as well as virions budding from the surface of infected Vero cells.

The structure and replication of RV has been reviewed by Frey (1994) and Wolinsky (1996).

1.6 Polypeptides

Forng and Frey (1995) used immunoprecipitation to identify the NSP in lysates of infected cells and confirmed that the order within the NSP-ORF is NH$_2$–P150–P90–COOH. They predicted that a motif of unknown function, described as X, and a protease domain reside in P150 and the helicase and replicase domains in P90. Using immunofluorescence, they showed that antibodies to P150 stained a perinuclear focus, the nuclear membrane and a thread-like network extending into the cytoplasm of infected cells. None of the antibodies to the NSP stained the nucleus.

The capsid protein C is 293–300 amino acids in length and is very basic, being rich in proline and arginine residues. It has a molecular weight of 33 kDa and is non-glycosylated and RNA-associated (see p. 555). In the virion it occurs as dimers. E2 and E1 are 282 and 481 amino acids in length respectively. However, carboxy-terminal sequencing has not been successful and it is possible that limited proteolytic tailoring occurs at these locations. E1 and E2 are membrane-bound glycoproteins exposed on the surface of the virus particle. E2 from most RV strains sequenced to date contains 4 potential N-linked glycosylation sites and a putative transmembrane domain near its C terminus. More than 2 forms of E2 occur (42–47 kDa) which differ in their degree of glycosylation (Bowden and Westaway 1985, Kalkkinen, Oker-Blom and Pettersson 1984, Pettersson et al. 1985, Waxham and Wolinsky 1985). The E1 protein has a molecular weight of 58 kDa and has 3 potential N-linked glycosylation sites. In the mature virion E1 and E2 exist as heterodimers, formed by multiple interchain disulphide bonds and project from the envelope as spikes (Baron and Forsell 1991, Waxham and Wolinsky 1983). E2 is relatively inaccessible to the action of enzymes and the immune response, suggesting that E2 is buried beneath E1 (Waxham and Wolinsky 1985).

The RV glycoproteins have been expressed in *Escherichia coli*, with vaccinia and baculovirus as vectors (Seppanen et al. 1991, Londesborough, Terry and Ho-Terry 1992, Oker-Blom et al. 1995). E1 and E2 have been expressed in soluble form (Hobman, Seto and Gillam 1994, Seto, Ou and Gillam 1995), and virus-like particles containing the 3 structural proteins have been produced in CHO and BHK cells (Hobman et al. 1994, Qiu et al. 1994).

1.7 Antigens

Early work on RV identified haemagglutinating, complement-fixing, precipitating (Le Bouvier 1969) and platelet-aggregating (Penttinen and Myllyla 1968) antigens. Kobayashi (1978) demonstrated that RV also has haemolytic activity.

The haemagglutinin (HA) is associated with the surface projections on the viral envelope. It can be obtained from the supernatant fluid of infected BHK-21 cell cultures if these are maintained on serum-free medium or if non-specific inhibitors of haemagglutination (serum lipoproteins) are first removed by kaolin treatment from the serum included in the maintenance medium (Stewart et al. 1967). Alternatively, treatment of the RV harvest with EDTA will separate HA from non-specific inhibitors by removing Ca^{2+} (Furukawa et al. 1967). Rubella HA can also be prepared by alkaline extraction of infected BHK-21 or Vero cell cultures (Halonen, Ryan and Stewart 1967). Although treatment of virus with ether destroys the HA activity, treatment with ether and Tween 80 retains this activity and increases the titre of the antigen, because of the formation of subunits. Ca^{2+} is required for the attachment of HA to erythrocytes. Optimum conditions for haemagglutination and further details of the non-specific inhibitors of HA and methods for their removal from test sera were reviewed by Herrmann (1979).

Three CF antigens have been described: (1) a large particle antigen with a density of 1.19–1.23 g/ml in sucrose gradients and associated with the infectivity and HA activity; (2) a small particle ('soluble') antigen, which is probably a subunit of the protein coat of the (Schmidt and Styk 1968); and (3) a 150S particle, which appears to be associated with the ribonucleoprotein core of the virus (Vesikari 1972). High-titre preparations of RV can be used as CF antigens. These are usually prepared either by concentration of infected cell culture fluids or by alkaline extraction of infected cells (Herrmann 1979). BHK-21 and Vero cells are used for the production of suitable high-titre virus.

During rubella infection, antibody responses are produced against all 3 structural proteins, but the E1 protein appears to be immunodominant (Cusi et al. 1989, Chaye et al. 1992a). Studies using murine monoclonal antibodies have identified several epitopes on E1; 3 of these which exhibit neutralizing or haemagglutinating activity have been mapped to residues 245–285 (Terry et al. 1988). A further well conserved neutralization domain has been identified within residues 211–239 (Chaye et al. 1992b, Mitchell et al. 1992, Wolinsky et al. 1993). Human sera react with synthetic peptides comprising residues 214–285 of the E1 protein, suggesting that this region may represent a major neutralization domain, and a recombinant protein containing these epitopes is recognized by most rubella antibody-positive human sera (Starkey et al. 1995). Murine and human antibody-binding domains also occur outside this region (Ilonen et al. 1992, Mitchell et al. 1993, Newcombe et al. 1994). A neutralization epitope has also been identified on the E2 glycoprotein (1–26) (Dorsett et al. 1985); other epitopes have been located between amino acids 51 and 105. At least 2 epitopes are present on the C protein (residues 9–29. 64–97) (reviewed by Frey 1994). The epitopes that confer protection are probably conformational (Wolinsky et al. 1991) and have not yet been identified.

All 3 structural proteins contain T cell epitopes. Immunoreactive regions have been identified within capsid protein residues 9–29, 14–29, 255–280, E2 residues 54–74 and E1 residues 273–284, 358–377 and 402–422 (Ou et al. 1993; reviewed by Frey 1994). The significance of these T cell epitopes in relation to protection is unclear.

BIOLOGICAL, ANTIGENIC AND NUCLEIC ACID SEQUENCE VARIATION

Differences in the biological activity of attenuated and wild type strains have been reported. The attenuated Cendehill strain has lower infectivity for rabbits and other laboratory animals than wild type strains (Zygraich, Peetermans and Huygelen 1971, Gill and Furesz 1973). Ohtawara and colleagues (Ohtawara et al. 1985) demonstrated that the growth of Japanese vaccine strains is restricted at 39°C, the body temperature of the rabbit. Chantler and colleagues (Chantler et al. 1993) have shown that the vaccine strains RA27/3 and Cendehill differ from wild type strains in growth characteristics, plaque morphology and temperature sensitivity. They have suggested that the processing in the Golgi of the viral glycoproteins from the attenuated strains was slower than for wild type strains, particularly in synovial cells (a human chondrocyte cell line and synovial membrane cells). The growth of the HPV77-DE5 vaccine strain was similar to the M33 strain from which it was derived.

Many studies in the late 1960s and 1970s failed to reveal any antigenic variation among RV strains and there was no reliable test to distinguish wild and attenuated strains. However, differences have been observed by cross-neutralization tests and neutralization kinetics (reviewed by Banatvala and Best 1990). More recent studies with monoclonal antibodies used in neutralization, HAI and enzyme immunoassay (EIA) revealed no significant differences between 9 RV strains tested, which included the vaccine strains Cendehill, RA27/3, HPV77-DE5 and TO336 (Best et al. 1992). However, Dorsett and colleagues (Dorsett et al. 1985) demonstrated strain specific epitopes within the E2 glycopolypeptide when disrupted virus was used.

RV is genetically stable when compared to other RNA viruses. Frey and Abernathy (1993) reported 0.7–3.6% interstrain nucleotide variation in the E1 coding region, but more recent studies have identified 8.77% interstrain nucleotide variation, mainly due to the variability of 2 RV isolates from India (Bosma et al. 1996). However, these nucleotide changes do not alter the deduced amino acid sequence. Nucleic acid sequencing has revealed that 5 characteristic nucleotide changes found within a 1300 nucleotide sequence of the E1 coding region of the RA27/3 vaccine strain distinguishes it from other isolates of RV (Frey and Abernathy 1993, Frey 1994). Despite this, deduced amino acid sequence of RV is remarkably stable (0.0–2.9%) (Frey and Abernathy 1993, Bosma et al. 1996).

2 CLINICAL AND PATHOLOGICAL ASPECTS

2.1 Introduction

In 1941, N McAlister Gregg, an Australian ophthalmologist, published his now famous retrospective study 'Congenital cataract following german measles in the mother', in which he showed that, if acquired in early pregnancy, rubella could cause congenital malformations. Seventy-eight babies, all with a similar type of congenital cataract, were born in New South Wales after an extensive rubella epidemic there in 1940 and many of the mothers gave a history of rubella, usually in the first or second month of pregnancy. Congenital defects of the heart were also noted in 66% of cases whose cardiac condition was recorded. These findings were soon confirmed in Australia, and deafness was also noted in many congenitally infected infants. Microcephaly, dental defects and low birth weight were also reported (Swan et al. 1943, Gregg 1944, Wesselhoeft 1947a, b).

Despite confirmation of Gregg's original observation, an annotation in the *Lancet* (Editorial 1944) suggested that additional studies were required, as it could not be proved that the illness with rash experienced by these mothers was in fact rubella; and that it was unlikely that such an association would have previously gone unnoticed. However, Hope-Simpson (1944) reported in the *Lancet* congenital cataract and heart defects in 2 babies in England after epidemic rubella. Similar defects had been noted before Gregg's original observation but their significance had not been appreciated. Additional retrospective studies reporting congenital defects induced by rubella in early pregnancy were subsequently carried out (reviewed by Hanshaw, Dudgeon and Marshall 1985).

Retrospective studies in which the starting point for investigations was an infant with one or more rubella-induced deformities suggested that a very high proportion of mothers who had rubella during pregnancy were delivered of infants with congenital malformations. The outcome of pregnancies in which maternal rubella was followed by the birth of unaffected infants was not recorded. Thus, in 1940, when rubella was at its peak incidence in New South Wales, Gregg and his colleagues (Gregg et al. 1945) reported that 96% of infants whose mothers had had rubella in early pregnancy suffered from congenital defects that were confined to cases in which maternal rubella had occurred before the 16th week of gestation.

In 1963/64, within a year of the first reports of RV isolation, the USA experienced one of the most extensive outbreaks of rubella ever recorded. During this epidemic it was shown that maternal rubella could result in a generalized and persistent fetal infection and that infants excreted virus not only at birth but also for many months after this, despite developing rubella-specific antibody responses. In addition, the spectrum of anomalies was much wider than had hitherto been described. The impact of this epidemic stimulated research into the development of rubella vaccines and, following this, attenuated vaccines were licensed for use, in the USA in 1969 and in Britain in 1970 (see p. 569). Congenitally acquired rubella therefore became a potentially preventable disease; national programmes, which achieved high uptake rates, have recently shown a marked reduction in both postnatally and congenitally acquired rubella.

2.2 Postnatally acquired infection

CLINICAL AND VIROLOGICAL FEATURES

After an incubation period of 14–21 days the characteristic features of rubella, rash and lymphadenopathy may appear. In young children the onset of illness is usually abrupt. Such constitutional symptoms as fever and malaise may be present for a day or two before onset of the rash but they usually subside rapidly after its appearance. Older children and adults may experience more pronounced constitutional symptoms 3–4 days before the rash appears, and during this prodromal phase an enanthem consisting of erythematous pinpoint lesions on the soft palate may be present. The exanthem is usually discrete, in the form of pinpoint maculopapular lesions. It appears first on the face and spreads rapidly to the rest of the body; lesions on the body may coalesce. The rash usually persists for about 3 days, occasionally longer, but may be fleeting. The mechanism by which rash is induced has not been established. Although immunopathological mechanisms may be responsible, RV has been isolated from skin biopsy specimens taken not only from areas with rash but also from parts of the skin without rash and from the skin of patients with subclinical infection (Heggie 1978). Furthermore, the development of rash may be prevented by the administration of pooled human immunoglobulin, although this does not prevent viraemia. Patients may complain of tender lymph nodes when or just before the rash appears. Follow-up studies of susceptible people exposed to rubella have revealed that lymphadenopathy may be present 7–10 days before the onset of rash, and sometimes for an even longer period after it has disappeared. Suboccipital, postauricular and cervical lymph nodes are most frequently affected. Rubella is rarely associated with severe complications. Encephalitis may occur in approximately one in 10 000 cases, but in general the prognosis is good (Krugman and Ward 1968). However, during an epidemic of rubella in Japan in 1987, when complications were reported rather more frequently than in previous epidemics, it was estimated that the incidence of encephalitis was much higher (1:1600 cases) (Moriuchi et al. 1990). Very occasionally, rubella is associated with thrombocytopenia, which may result in purpuric rash, epistaxis, haematuria and gastrointestinal bleeding. The commonest complication of postnatally acquired rubella is joint involvement; although this is rare among children and adult males, it may occur in up to 60% of postpubertal females. Symptoms generally develop as the rash subsides and vary in severity from mild stiffness of the small joints of the hands to a frank arthritis with severe pain, joint swelling and limitation of movement. The finger joints, wrists, knees and ankles are most frequently affected. The duration of these symptoms is usually about 3 days but occasionally they may persist for up to a month. Rubella-induced arthralgia is not associated with any sequelae.

Arthralgia occurs commonly in postpubertal females after administration of rubella vaccine. The mechanism by which naturally acquired and vaccine-induced infection causes arthralgia is probably complex. Thus, joint symptoms may result from direct infection of the synovial membrane by virus, for RV has been isolated from the joint aspirates of vaccinees with vaccine-induced arthritis (Weibel et al. 1969). Furthermore, studies in vitro have shown that attenuated virus strains will replicate in human synovial membrane cell cultures (Grayzel and Beck 1971). However, an immune mechanism is probably also involved, because, in addition to virus, joint aspirates have been shown to contain rubella-specific IgG (Ogra and Herd 1971, Mims, Stokes and Grahame 1985), which suggests that joint symptoms may be induced by immune complexes. It is therefore of interest that the presence of rubella antibody containing immune complexes in the serum has been associated with a high incidence of joint symptoms following rubella vaccination (Coyle et al. 1982). However, hormonal factors may also play a role, for, in addition to being common in postpubertal females, the development of joint symptoms appears to be related to the menstrual cycle; after rubella vaccination, they are most likely to occur within 7 days of the onset of the cycle (Harcourt, Best and Banatvala 1979).

RV has been suggested as a possible cause of chronic inflammatory joint disease, but studies on patients with that disease have yielded conflicting and unconfirmed results. It has been claimed that RV could be detected in synovial fluid or the synovium, as well as in lymphocytes from patients with both rheumatoid arthritis and seronegative arthritis (i.e. rheumatoid factor negative) (Grahame et al. 1981, Chantler et al. 1982, Chantler, Petty and Tingle 1985, Mims, Stokes and Grahame 1985). However, it is known that RV is able to establish persistent infection in vivo (p. 565) (Waxham and Wolinsky 1984) as well as in human synovial cell cultures and organ cultures (Cunningham and Fraser 1985, Miki and Chantler 1992) and that high levels of rubella antibody are found in joint fluid (Mims, Stokes and Grahame 1985). Although there is no doubt that RV may be isolated from synovial fluid after naturally acquired infection or vaccination and from occasional patients with chronic inflammatory joint disease, the incidence of vaccine-associated chronic complications has not been determined (Report 1994). Thus, there is no convincing evidence that RV plays a causal role in chronic inflammatory joint disease.

Rubella is often difficult to diagnose clinically because the illness may present atypically with minimal lymphadenopathy and an evanescent rash, and, conversely, typical rubelliform rashes may be induced by other viruses. Thus, such viruses as enteroviruses may occasionally induce rubella-like rashes. Chikungunya and Ross River viruses (Chapter 29) and parvovirus B 19 (Chapter 14) may induce not only a rubella-like rash but also arthralgia. Serological studies have shown that there is poor correlation between a past history of rubella and immune status, particularly among adults (Brown, Hambling and Ansari 1969). This is not surprising because not only may rubella present atypically, but disease without rash or subclinical infection may occur in up to 25% of children (Krugman and Ward 1954, Green et al. 1965).

The relation between clinical and virological features is shown in Fig. 28.3. The patient is potentially infectious for a prolonged period, as pharyngeal virus excretion may occur for up to a week before onset of rash and persist thereafter for 7–10 days. Virus may also be detected in the stools and urine, but excretion occurs over for a shorter time. These are not suitable specimens from which to isolate virus and do not play an important role in virus transmission. Viraemia is present for about a week before the onset of rash, but as this appears rubella antibodies develop and viraemia terminates.

EPIDEMIOLOGY

Rubella has a worldwide distribution. In temperate climates, before the introduction of rubella vaccination, epidemics usually happened in spring and early summer, rubella occurring less commonly among pre-

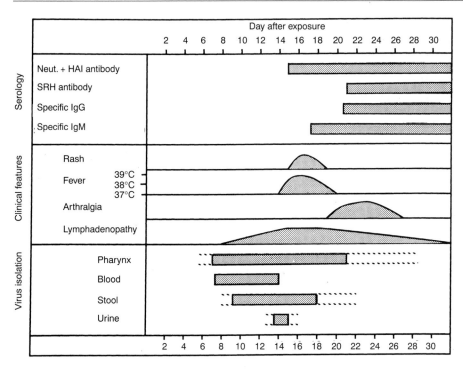

Fig. 28.3 Relation between clinical and virological features of postnatally acquired rubella. HAI, haem- agglutination inhibition; Neut., neutralizing; SRH, single radial haemolysis.

school children than among school children and young adults. Women of child-bearing age were often infected as a result of exposure to their own children or at work. Seroepidemiological studies showed that the proportion of seropositive people increased progressively with age, about 50% of 9- to 11-year-old children being immune. Among women of child-bearing age, the proportion increased to about 80–85% (Dowdle et al. 1970). In industrialized parts of the world (e.g. the UK, the USA and Scandinavia, which have achieved high uptake rates for rubella vaccine), postnatally and congenitally acquired rubella are now rare. In 1992, the lowest ever number of cases of rubella were reported in Britain (Miller et al. 1993). There is still, however, a large pool of rubella-susceptible 10- to 25-year-old males in the UK and such people were infected in localized outbreaks of rubella in 1993, transmitting infection to some susceptible pregnant women, most of them being young primigravidae and many of whom were immigrants (Miller et al. 1994). Despite the success of the rubella vaccination programme in the USA, a number of cases of congenitally acquired rubella were reported in California and among the Amish population in Pennsylvania in 1989/90, this resulting from infection of unvaccinated women (Lindegren et al. 1991). Figure 28.4 compares the epidemic periodicity of rubella and parvovirus B19, showing that in England and Wales in 1993 they occurred concurrently. In 1993–1996 many cases of rubella occurred in adolescent and adult males who had not been vaccinated (Miller et al. 1994).

Many developing countries have rubella susceptibility rates among women of child-bearing age similar to those reported in developed countries before to the introduction of rubella vaccine; in tropical countries the infection tends to occur at an earlier age than in temperate climates, although outbreaks of rubella are seldom reported. However, there is considerable regional variation (Table 28.2). High susceptibility rates may be found among island communities, owing to limited opportunities for the introduction of RV, as well as among some tribes in remote rural areas (de Freitas et al. 1990).

As yet, relatively few virological studies have assessed the impact of congenitally acquired rubella in developing countries. However, virological studies conducted in parts of South America and India among children who are deaf, blind, or both, suggest that the burden of congenitally acquired rubella may be considerable (Kishore, Broor and Seth 1990, de Azevedo Neto et al. 1994, Bosma et al. 1995a, Eckstein et al. 1996).

IMMUNE RESPONSES

Rubella-specific IgG, IgM and IgA responses develop rapidly after the onset of rash. Rubella-specific IgG persists for life, but may decline to low levels in old age. The IgG response is predominantly IgG1; IgG3 is detected in most sera from cases of recently acquired rubella and IgG4 occasionally in sera from cases of remote rubella (Stokes, Mims and Grahame 1986, Thomas and Morgan-Capner 1988). Rubella-specific IgM usually appears within 4 days of onset of rash and persists for 4–12 weeks but detection depends on the sensitivity of the technique employed. Specific IgM may sometimes persist for up to one year after both naturally acquired infection and rubella immunization (Pattison, Dane and Mace 1975, O'Shea et al. 1985). Serum and nasopharyngeal IgA responses are detectable for at least 5 years after infection. The specific serum IgA response is exclusively IgA1. Specific IgD and IgE responses develop rapidly after onset of infection and persist for at least 6 months. The results of

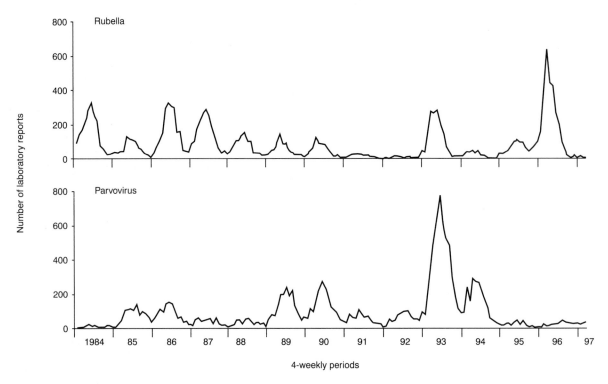

Rubella and Parvovirus - Laboratory reports
England and Wales 1984 - Mar 1997

Fig. 28.4 Epidemic periodicity of rubella and parvovirus B19 in England and Wales. Laboratory reports 1984 to March 1997 (Courtesy of Dr Elizabeth Miller).

Table 28.2 Immunity to rubella among women of child-bearing age in different countries

	Country		**%**
Africa	Angola		>73
	Ethiopia		>90
	Gambia		>93
	Ghana		>70
	Nigeria		75
	South Africa		>97
	Togo		33
	Uganda		>90
	Upper Volta		>90
Asia	Hong Kong	Caucasian	80
		Chinese	64
	India	Northern cities	80
		Calcutta	57
		Rural areas	72
	Japan	North	86–91
		South	75–86
	Korea		81
	Pakistan	Karachi	84
	China		>96*
South & Central America	Brazil		82
	Panama city		60
	Peru (urban)		67
	Barbados, Jamaica, Trinidad		28–52

*96 of 2399 persons aged 11–15 years tested (indicating a high level of immunity).

Mitchell, Zhang and Tingle (1992) suggest that males have a more rapid antibody response than females. Methods available for the detection and quantification of rubella antibodies are discussed under 'Laboratory Diagnosis' (see section 2.4, p. 566).

Immunoblotting for detection of polypeptide-specific antibodies is technically difficult. However, Zhang et al. (1992) demonstrated that antibodies to E1 and E2 were detected more effectively under non-reducing conditions than in the presence of 2-mercaptoethanol. The response to E1 is greater than to E2 and there is a strong response to C (Katow and Sugiura 1985, Zhang et al. 1992). Antibodies to E1 are essential for protection (Cusi et al. 1995). Avidity of IgG antibody to E1 matures during the 2 years after rubella infection, but IgG anti-E2 and anti-C show minimal avidity maturation (Mauracher, Mitchell and Tingle 1992).

A decrease in total leucocytes, neutrophils and T cells and a transient depression of lymphocyte responsiveness to mitogens and antigens such as purified protein derivative (PPD) is seen after rubella (Buimovici-Klein et al. 1976, Maller, Fryden and Soren 1978, Niwa and Kanoh 1979, Hyypiä et al. 1984). Cell-mediated immune responses, measured by lymphocyte proliferation assays, develop within a few days of onset of rash and persist for many years; lymphokine secretion has also been detected (Honeyman, Forrest and Dorman 1974, Buimovici-Klein, Lang and Ziring 1985). MHC class I-restricted CD8+ cytotoxic T lymphocytes have been demonstrated in rubella-immune individuals (Lovett et al. 1993).

Reinfection

Natural infection is followed by a high order of protection from reinfection. However, evidence of reinfection may be obtained by demonstrating a significant increase in antibody concentration following natural and experimental exposure to rubella. Such reinfection is generally asymptomatic (Horstmann et al. 1970, Vesikari 1972). Reinfection in pregnancy is hazardous only if viraemia occurs, and this has rarely been documented in experimental studies (O'Shea, Best and Banatvala 1983). Following maternal reinfection during the first 16 weeks in pregnancy, the risk of fetal infection has been estimated to be of the order of 8%, although fetal damage is rare (Best et al. 1989, Morgan-Capner et al. 1991). Although it is possible that, in such cases, transmission of virus to the fetus may be due to a specific defect in the maternal immune response, rubella reinfection is not associated with a lack of neutralizing antibodies or persistent impairment of rubella-specific lymphoproliferative responses (O'Shea et al. 1994). Sequence changes have not been identified in the E1 ORF of isolates from cases of reinfection (Bosma et al. 1996). Further studies are required to determine whether reinfection is due to a failure to produce an immune response to the protective epitopes of the virus. Reinfection in pregnancy will be eliminated if high rates of rubella vaccination are achieved and maintained among the target groups (p. 569). Rubella reinfection has been reviewed by Best (1993).

2.3 Congenitally acquired infection

CLINICAL MANIFESTATIONS

Although the early retrospective enquiries emphasized the frequency and importance of such defects as congenital anomalies of the heart and eyes, and deafness, it was not until follow-up studies had been carried out on infants whose mothers had had rubella during the extensive 1963/64 outbreak in the USA that it was fully appreciated that congenital rubella frequently caused widespread multisystem disease. However, follow-up studies showed that congenitally acquired rubella (CAR) was not a static disease and that prolonged careful evaluation of infants at risk was necessary before some or all of the features of CAR were apparent. The broader range of anomalies described after the US 1963/64 and subsequent outbreaks were probably due not to any change in viral virulence but rather to more careful and prolonged observation, since careful scrutiny of the records of infants with CAR who were born before these outbreaks revealed that such anomalies as thrombocytopenic purpura and osteitis, although not reported in the literature, occurred fairly frequently.

Cooper (1975) divided clinical features associated with rubella infection into those that were transient, developmental or permanent (Table 28.3). The pathogenesis of transient lesions is not understood, but they are usually present only during the first few weeks of life, do not recur and are not associated with the development of permanent sequelae. Intrauterine growth retardation resulting in low birth weight but at a normal gestational age ('small for dates' babies) is among the commonest of the transient features. Thus Cooper and his colleagues (Cooper et al. 1965) found that about 60% of infected infants fell below the 10th and 90% below the 50th percentile.

A petechial or purpuric rash is also common, particularly among infants whose mothers had had maternal rubella in early pregnancy (Fig. 28.5, Plate 28.5) (Cooper et al. 1965, Horstmann et al. 1965). However, low birth weight and a purpuric rash are seldom the sole manifestations of congenital rubella. These infants may have other anomalies such as congenital heart and eye defects, although they may not always be apparent at birth. Infants with thrombocytopenic purpura generally have a platelet count ranging from 3000 to 100 000/mm^3, this being associated with a decreased number of megakaryocytes, but of normal morphology, in the bone marrow. In general, the platelet count rises spontaneously during the first month of life, although (rarely) some infants die from such complications as intracranial haemorrhage.

Deafness

Of the permanent defects, the commonest is sensorineural deafness. This results from rubella-induced damage to the organ of Corti. However, central auditory impairment may also occur. Hearing loss, which may be unilateral or bilateral, mild or profound, may sometimes be the only rubella-induced congenital anomaly.

Table 28.3 Clinical features associated with congenitally acquired rubella

	Common	Uncommon
Transient	Low birth weight Thrombocytopenic purpura Hepatosplenomegaly Bone lesions Meningoencephalitis	Cloudy cornea Hepatitis Generalized lymphadenopathy Haemolytic anaemia Pneumonitis
Developmental	Sensorineural deafness Peripheral pulmonary stenosis Mental retardation Central language defects Diabetes mellitus	Severe myopia Thyroiditis Hypothyroidism Growth hormone deficiency 'Late onset disease'
Permanent	Sensorineural deafness Peripheral pulmonary stenosis Pulmonary valvular stenosis Patent ductus arteriosus Ventricular septal defect Retinopathy Cataract Microphthalmia Psychomotor retardation Microcephaly Cryptorchidism Inguinal hernia Diabetes mellitus	Severe myopia Thyroid disorders Dermatoglyptic abnormalities Glaucoma Myocardial abnormalities

Peckham (1972) followed up 218 children who were apparently normal at birth but who had been exposed to rubella in utero. When assessed for hearing loss at the age of 1–4 years, 50 (23%) were deaf; when 85 were re-examined between the ages of 6 and 8 years, further hearing defects were detected in another 9 children. Of the children with hearing defects, 90% were seropositive. Because rubella antibodies are uncommon before the age of 4 years, it is particularly important to follow up infants with persistent rubella antibody so that hearing defects can be recognized as early as possible. Delay in detecting deafness can be reduced by testing for auditory evoked responses (Wild et al. 1990).

Heart disease

Congenital anomalies of the cardiovascular system are responsible for much of the high perinatal mortality associated with CAR. Numerous studies have shown that the commonest lesions are persistence of a patent ductus arteriosus, proximal (valvular) or peripheral pulmonary artery stenosis, and a ventricular septal defect (Sperling and Verska 1966, Hastreiter et al. 1967, Cooper 1975).

Occasionally, neonatal myocarditis is found, often associated with other cardiac malformations (Korones et al. 1965). Rubella-induced damage to the intima of the arteries may result in obstructive lesions of the renal and pulmonary arteries (Rorke and Spiro 1967, Phelan and Campbell 1969).

Defects in the central nervous system

About 25% of infants who present at birth with clinical evidence of CAR have CNS involvement, usually in the form of a meningoencephalitis. Such infants are often lethargic at birth but may become irritable and often exhibit evidence of photophobia. They have a full anterior fontanelle, pleocytosis and an increased amount of protein in the CSF (Desmond et al. 1967). The outcome is variable and unpredictable. Although c. 25% of infants presenting with meningoencephalitis at birth may, by the age of 18 months, be severely retarded, suffering from communication problems, ataxia or spastic paresis, others appear to progress well neurologically despite poor development in the first 6 months of life.

Rubella panencephalitis is rare, about 20 cases having been reported as a sequel of congenital rubella infection and 2 following postnatally acquired disease. All but one of the patients were male, and clinical signs developed between the ages of 8 and 19 years (Lebon and Lyon 1974, Townsend et al. 1975, Weil, Itabashi and Creamer 1975, Wolinsky, Berg and Maitland 1976). RV has been recovered from the brain both with and without co-cultivation techniques; it has also been recovered from patients' lymphocytes (Cremer et al. 1975, Wolinsky et al. 1979). Elevated levels of rubella-specific IgG and occasionally IgM may be detected in the serum; the CSF may contain elevated concentrations of protein and immunoglobulin.

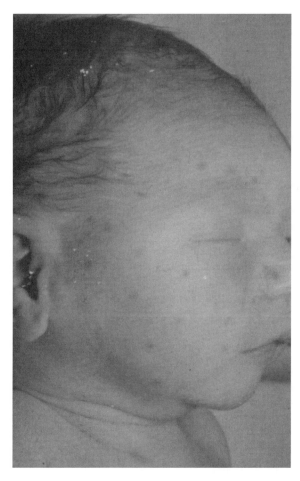

Fig. 28.5 Purpuric rash in newborn infant with congenitally acquired rubella, who was subsequently found to have congenital heart disease and cataract. For colour, see Plate 28.5.

Oligoclonal bands and a high CSF : serum rubella antibody ratio may be present (Wolinsky et al. 1982).

Histological studies show panencephalitis with a perivascular inflammatory response as well as a vasculitis. Rubella antigens have not been detected in brain sections by immunofluorescence. It has been postulated that post-rubella panencephalitis may be mediated by immune complexes (Waxham and Wolinsky 1984) or by virus-mediated autoreactivity to brain antigens (Martin et al. 1989).

Ocular defects

Many of the ocular defects characteristic of CAR were described by Gregg (1941), who drew particular attention to pigmented retinopathy and cataract. Pigmented retinopathy may be present in up to 50% of infants with CAR (Menser and Reye 1974) and may provide a useful aid in clinical diagnosis. The macular area of the retina is generally affected but the lesions rarely impair vision. Cataracts, although usually present at birth, may not be visible until several weeks later (Murphy et al. 1967). Lesions may be subtotal, consisting of a dense pearly-white central opacity (Fig. 28.6, Plate 28.6) or, total with a more uniform density throughout the lens. Microphthalmus is often associated with congenital cataract, but glaucoma, though

rare, is important to recognize because it may rapidly cause blindness. Microphthalmia and glaucoma result from disturbances in organogenesis, and retinopathy and cataract result from intrauterine tissue destruction. However, delayed manifestations of congenital infection have also been recorded including lens changes, chronic uveitis, glaucoma, choroidal neovascularization, corneal hydrops and keratoconus. Mechanisms postulated include virus persistence in the eye, resulting in RV-induced reduced growth rate and lifespan of cells, autoimmune phenomena or virally induced vascular damage and reactive hypervascularization (reviewed by Arnold et al. 1994).

Diabetes

Diabetes mellitus was originally believed to be a rare complication of CAR. However, follow-up studies of infants infected in utero during the Australian and US epidemics of 1940 and 1963/64 respectively have shown that 9 of 45 (20%) of Australian and 30 of 242 (12.4%) of US children eventually developed insulin-dependent diabetes mellitus (IDDM). A long latent period is characteristic, the mean age of children developing IDDM in the US study being 9 years; all the Australian patients were in their third decade (Menser et al. 1978, Ginsberg-Felner et al. 1985). Lymphocytic infiltration of the pancreas of an infant with CAR but without IDDM may suggest that RV can initiate the train of events that subsequently results in IDDM in later life (Bunnell and Monif 1972). It seems probably that autoimmune mechanisms are involved in the pathogenesis, because the HLA types in these patients are typical of those with autoimmune disease, there being a significant increase in prevalence of HLA-DR3, some increase in HLA-DR4 and a virtual absence of HLA-DR2. In addition, islet cell antibodies have been detected in 20% of these patients. These antibodies have a cytotoxic effect on cultured islet cells and predict the diabetic state. Although autoimmune responses may play an important role, the mechanism by which RV might trigger them remains to be established. Possible mechanisms have been reviewed by Banatvala (1987a).

Bone defects

Bone lesions may be detected by x-ray. Irregular areas of translucency are present in the metaphyseal portion of the long bones but without any evidence of periosteal reaction in over 20% of infants with congenital rubella (Cooper et al. 1965). These lesions generally resolve within 1–2 months. Cooper et al. (1965) detected these characteristic radiological changes in a fetus of 18 weeks' gestational age, suggesting that the process inducing such changes begins in early gestational life.

Late onset disease

Between the ages of about 3 and 12 months, some infants may present with such features as a chronic rubelliform rash, persistent diarrhoea and pneumonitis. Marshall (1973) referred to this syndrome as 'late onset disease'. Although mortality is high, some infants show a dramatic response to treatment with corticosteroids. This syndrome may reflect an immunopathological phenomenon; circulating immune complexes that appear to contain rubella antigen have been demonstrated in infants with late onset disease (Tardieu et al. 1980), and Coyle, Grospierre and Durandy (1982) demonstrated rubella antibody containing immune complexes in children with congenital rubella who developed new clinical problems some years after birth.

Some developmental defects may take many months or years to become apparent, but then persist permanently. Failure to recognize such defects in early infancy may not always be the result of difficulty in their detection. There is evidence which suggests that such defects as perceptive deafness, CNS anomalies and some ocular defects may actually develop or become increasingly noticeable some considerable time after birth. Thus Peckham (1972) showed that some 2-year-old children with apparently normal hearing had severe perceptive deafness when examined later. Menser and Forrest (1974) showed that it might be up to 4 years before the first rubella defects were recognized; further defects might continue to be recognized up to the age of 8 years. The progressive nature of congenitally acquired disease is emphasized by the finding that children with previously stable congenital rubella-induced defects developed a widespread subacute progressive panencephalitis with progressive motor retardation as late as the second decade in life (Townsend et al. 1975, Weil, Itabashi and Creamer 1975).

As a result of the extent and severity of rubella-induced congenital malformations, children who survive will need continuous specialized management, education and rehabilitation. However, a study carried out on 50 25-year-old patients with CAR born in Australia after the 1940/41 epidemic showed that, although many were deaf or had eye defects, they had developed far better than had been anticipated when assessed in early childhood. Many had married and produced normal children, and all but 4 were employed, most patients being of average intelligence

(Menser, Dods and Harley 1967). Follow-up studies so far reported on children with CAR following the 1963/64 US rubella epidemic suggest that it may have had a more catastrophic impact on the lives of affected children than did the 1940/41 Australian epidemic (Cooper 1975). This may be a reflection on the more modern methods of treatment available to the children born after this more recent epidemic; many might not have survived previously.

Although congenitally acquired rubella is now rare in countries that have adopted rubella vaccination programmes, a heavy burden from previous epidemics persists. A 20-year-old follow-up on 125 patients infected during the extensive 1963–1965 USA outbreak showed that, although many patients had multiple defects, ocular disease was the most commonly noticed disorder (78%) followed by sensorineural deafness (66%), psychomotor retardation (62%) and cardiac anomalies (58%). Ocular disease was frequently associated with hearing loss and cardiac anomalies (Givens et al. 1994).

PATHOGENESIS

The fetus is at risk during the period of maternal viraemia, because placental infection may occur at this time. The most likely source of virus is from the maternal viraemia. Virus may also be excreted via the cervix for up to 6 days after the onset of rash (Seppala and Vaheri 1974), and, because virus may exist in the genital tract for even longer, placental infection by direct contact or from ascending genital infection cannot be excluded.

After infection in early pregnancy, rubella induces a generalized and persistent virus infection in the fetus which may result in multisystem disease. Töndury and Smith (1966) conducted histopathological studies on the products of conception from mothers clinically diagnosed as infected with rubella: anomalies were present in 68% of 57 fetuses when maternal rubella was contracted in the first trimester; and when contracted in the first month of pregnancy, 80% were abnormal, sporadic foci or cellular damage being present in the heart, inner ear, lens, skeletal muscle and teeth. Those authors suggested that RV enters the fetus via the chorion, in which it induces necrotic changes in the epithelial cells as well as in the endothelial lining of the blood vessels; the damaged endothelial cells are desquamated into the lumen of the vessel and then transported as virus-infected 'emboli' into the fetal circulation to settle in and infect various fetal organs. Lesions in the chorion were present as early as the 10th day after the onset of maternal rash. Fetal endothelial damage was distributed widely and probably resulted from viral replication rather than from antibody-mediated damage, because the most extensive histopathological changes were present at a gestational period before the fetal immune defence mechanism was sufficiently mature to be activated. Indeed, a characteristic feature of rubella embryopathy following maternal rubella in early gestational life is the notable absence of an inflammatory cell response (Töndury and Smith 1966).

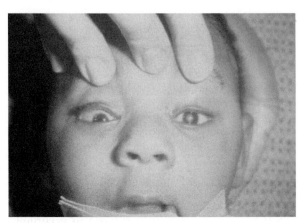

Fig. 28.6 Congenital rubella cataract in a 9-month-old infant. Cataract present in the left eye was surgically removed. For colour, see Plate 28.6.

At least 2 mechanisms have been suggested for inducing fetal damage: a virus-induced retardation in cell division, and tissue necrosis. Studies in vitro on embryonic cell cultures and rubella-infected fetuses suggest that RV may induce chromosomal damage and cause cells to divide more slowly than those that are uninfected (Plotkin et al. 1965). This may be due to a specific protein that reduces the mitotic rate of infected cells (Plotkin and Vaheri 1967). If retardation of cell division occurs during the critical phase of organogenesis, it is likely to result in congenital malformations. It has also been shown that the organs of rubella-infected infants are smaller and contain fewer cells than those of uninfected infants (Naeye and Blanc 1965). The fetal endothelial damage induced by rubella infection may cause haemorrhages in small blood vessels, leading to tissue necrosis and further damage of malformed organs over a longer period. Such organs as the liver, myocardium and organ of Corti may be affected. Studies on the products of conception obtained from virologically confirmed cases of rubella during the first trimester have shown that the fetus is almost invariably infected regardless of the time at which infection has occurred during this period (Rawls 1968, Thompson and Tobin 1970).

RV is isolated infrequently from neonates whose mothers developed infection after the first trimester, possibly because by then fetal immune mechanisms can effectively terminate infection. More mature fetal tissues do not have a reduced susceptibility to infection, for studies in vitro have shown that RV will replicate as well in organs derived from fetuses of 12–13 weeks' gestational age as in those of younger fetuses (Best et al. 1968). Nevertheless, even though severe congenital anomalies are rarely encountered following rubella after the first trimester, serological evidence of fetal infection has been shown to occur in 25–33% of infants whose mothers acquired maternal rubella between the 16th and 28th weeks of gestation (Cradock-Watson et al. 1980, Vejtorp and Mansa 1980).

Persistence of virus

Following intrauterine infection in early pregnancy, RV persists throughout gestation and can be isolated from most organs obtained at autopsy from infants who die in early infancy with severe and generalized infections. Virus may also be recovered from the nasopharyngeal secretions, urine, stools, CSF and tears of survivors. RV can be isolated from nasopharyngeal secretions of most neonates with severe congenitally acquired disease, but by the age of 3 months the proportion excreting virus has declined to 50–60% and by 9–12 months to 10% (Cooper and Krugman 1967). Particularly during the first few weeks after birth, those with severe disease may excrete high concentrations of virus and readily transmit infection to rubella-susceptible contacts. RV may persist in infants with congenitally acquired disease in secluded sites for even longer. Thus, RV has been recovered from a cataract removed from a 3-year-old child (Menser et al. 1967) and from the CSF of children with CNS involve-

ment up to the age of 18 months (Desmond et al. 1967). By immunofluorescence, rubella antigen was detected in the thyroid from a 5-year-old child with Hashimoto's disease (Ziring et al. 1977), and by cocultivation techniques RV was recovered from the brain of a child who developed rubella panencephalitis at the age of 12 years (Cremer et al. 1975, Weil, Itabashi and Creamer 1975). Experimental studies have shown that, within the CNS, the astrocyte is the main cell type in which virus replicates, high concentrations of virus being expressed. Intrauterine infection involving these cells may perhaps induce focal areas of necrosis resulting in the pattern of neurological deficit observed in congenitally acquired disease (Chantler, Smymis and Tai 1995).

The mechanism by which CAR may result in insulin-dependent diabetes mellitus (IDDM) has not been established. However, an experimental study employing human fetal islet cells showed that RV induced a depression of immunoreactive secreted insulin without being cytolytic (Numazaki et al. 1990). A further study suggested that autoimmune phenomena might be involved, because immunoreactive epitopes in the RV capsid shared antigenicity with islet β cell protein (molecular mimicry) (Karounos, Wolinsky and Thomas 1993).

How RV persists throughout gestation and for a limited period during the first year of life has not been clearly established. Possible mechanisms include defects in cell-mediated immunity (CMI), poor interferon synthesis and the possibility that a limited number of infected fetal cells give rise to infected clones which persist for a limited period (reviewed by Banatvala 1977). It has also been suggested that selective immune tolerance to the RV E1 protein may play a role (Mauracher, Mitchell and Tingle 1993). Studies in vitro show that RV replicates in T lymphocytes and macrophages and can also persist in B lymphocytes, causing inhibition of host-cell protein synthesis (Chantler and Tingle 1980, van der Logt, van Loon and van der Veen 1980). Infection of macrophages may interfere with their interactions with T cells. Postnatally acquired rubella causes a transient reduction in lymphocyte responses to phytohaemagglutinin (Buimovici-Klein et al. 1976, Maller, Fryden and Soren 1978, Vesikari 1980) as well as a decrease in the numbers of T cells (Niwa and Kanoh 1979). CAR might be expected to cause an even greater reduction in responsiveness. Indeed, significantly diminished lymphoproliferative responses to phytohaemagglutinin and rubella antigen, as well as diminished interferon synthesis, were demonstrated in 40 congenitally infected children aged 1–12 years (Buimovici-Klein et al. 1979). Impairment of CMI responses was related to the gestational age at which maternal infection occurred, and was greatest in infants whose mothers acquired rubella in the first 8 weeks of pregnancy. Hosking, Pyman and Wilkins (1983) suggested that children with nerve deafness due to CAR could be distinguished from those with immunity due to postnatally acquired rubella by their failure to produce lymphoproliferative responses to rubella antigen. We have also found that 10 of 13 (80%) children with CAR under the age of 3 years failed to mount a lymphoproliferative response (O'Shea, Best and Banatvala 1992). Congenitally infected infants also have impaired natural killer cell activity (Fuccillo et al. 1974) and persistent T cell abnormalities (Rabinowe et al. 1986). It is of interest that the defective CMI responses may persist into the second decade of life, well beyond the time when RV can be recovered from accessible sites.

RISKS TO THE FETUS

Whether maternal rubella induces fetal damage that causes intrauterine death or the birth of a malformed infant depends on the gestational age at which maternal rubella occurs, although other factors may also be involved. Maternal rubella may result in spontaneous abortion in up to 20% of cases (Siegel, Fuerst and Guinee 1971); this occurs most commonly when maternal infection is acquired during the first 8 weeks of pregnancy. To this must be added fetal wastage from therapeutic abortion following virologically confirmed rubella.

Maternal rubella in the first trimester

Many earlier prospective studies, the results of which are still quoted, underestimated the risks of congenital malformations, because maternal infections were included that were not rubella-induced and some rubella-infected infants were not followed up for sufficiently long. It is now known that 75–100% of infants born to mothers infected at this time will be congenitally infected and most of those infected will have associated defects (Enders 1982, Miller, Cradock-Watson and Pollock 1982, Grillner et al. 1983). Many infants, although apparently normal at birth, if followed up for periods ranging from a few months to some years, may eventually be shown to have such defects as perceptive deafness or minimal CNS anomalies. Figure 28.7 relates the gestational age of maternal rubella to the clinical manifestations of congenitally acquired disease among 376 infants infected in utero during the 1964 epidemic in the USA. When maternal infection is acquired during the first 8 weeks of pregnancy – the critical phase of organogenesis – cardiac and eye defects are likely to occur. Retinopathy, hearing and CNS defects are more evenly distributed throughout the first 16–20 weeks of gestational life.

Maternal rubella after the first trimester

RV is seldom isolated from infants whose mothers acquired rubella after the first trimester, although studies in vitro have shown that fetal tissues, regardless of gestational age, are susceptible to infection (Best, Banatvala and Moore 1968). Indeed, serological studies confirm that a high proportion of infants are infected as a result of maternal rubella contracted after the first trimester, rubella-specific IgM being detected in 25–33% of infants whose mothers had rubella between the 16th and 20th weeks of pregnancy (Cradock-Watson et al. 1980) However, because organogenesis is complete by 12 weeks and in more

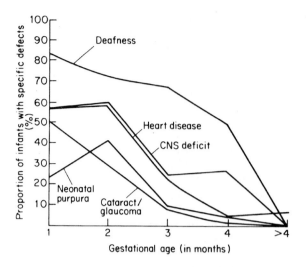

Fig. 28.7 Relation of clinical manifestations of congenital rubella to time of maternal infection, extrapolated from Cooper et al. (1969).

mature fetuses immune responses may limit or terminate infection, such infants rarely have severe or multiple anomalies. Deafness and retinopathy, which *per se* does not affect vision, are likely to be the only anomalies commonly associated with rubella after the first trimester. When the results of 4 studies conducted in different countries are combined it is seen that the risk is about 17% when infection occurs at 13–16 weeks and about 5.9% after infection at 17–20 weeks (Peckham 1972, Miller, Cradock-Watson and Pollock 1982, Grillner et al. 1983, Munro et al. 1987). Figure 28.7 shows that deafness is usually the sole clinical manifestation of fetal infection occurring between 13 and 16 weeks, and is relatively common, but that deafness or any other defects are only rarely encountered after this time.

Preconceptual rubella

Studies conducted in the Federal Republic of Germany and Britain indicate that preconceptual rubella does not result in transmission of RV to the fetus. Thus, Enders and colleagues (Enders et al. 1988) found no serological or clinical evidence of intrauterine infection in 38 infants whose mothers' rash appeared before or within 11 days after their last menstrual period (LMP). However, the fetus of a mother whose rash appeared 12 days after her LMP became infected, and all of 10 mothers who developed rash 3–6 weeks after their LMP transmitted infection to their fetuses.

2.4 Laboratory diagnosis

POSTNATALLY ACQUIRED INFECTION

A clinical diagnosis of rubella is unreliable and so laboratory confirmation is required, particularly for the diagnosis of rubella-like illness during pregnancy. Because the virus is slow to grow in cell cultures and a distinct cytopathic effect (CPE) is not produced (see p. 568), serological methods are employed. A significant rise in antibody concentration may be detected by a variety of methods, including HAI, enzyme immunoassay (EIA) or latex agglutination (LA) titration. Seroconversion can also be detected by single radial haemolysis (SRH). Although HAI antibodies develop within a day or 2 of onset of rash, antibodies detected by EIA, LA or SRH may be delayed until 7–8 days. Specific IgM antibodies may be detected by indirect and M-antibody capture assays, but capture assays are generally preferred. M-antibody capture radioimmunoassay (MACRIA) (Tedder et al. 1982) is used in the UK and a number of EIAs for rubella-specific IgM are available commercially. Care should be taken to ensure that the test chosen has a high degree of specificity and sensitivity (Hudson and Morgan-Capner 1996). Rubella-specific IgM usually appears within 4 days of onset of rash and persists for 4–12 weeks. More than 4 weeks after onset, detection will depend on the sensitivity of the technique employed.

Rubella-specific IgG and IgM antibodies may be detected in saliva using antibody capture radioimmunoassays; results correlate well with serum antibodies (Perry et al. 1993). The optimum time for detecting specific IgM is 1–5 weeks after onset of illness.

Reinfection is associated with a rise in antibody concentration, sometimes to very high levels. An IgM response may also be present, but is usually lower and more transient than that following primary infection. An accurate history of rubella contact, rubella vaccination and previous rubella antibody screening is required in order to interpret results. It may be particularly difficult to distinguish between a primary infection and reinfection, if blood is not obtained shortly after contact or if sera taken prior to contact (e.g. for screening purposes) are not available. However, reinfection may be distinguished from primary infection by examining the antigen-binding avidity of specific IgG, because the avidity of specific IgG from cases of recent primary rubella is low compared with that from people with remote infection or reinfection (Thomas and Morgan-Capner 1991).

Assessment of the risk to women exposed to or who develop rubella-like illness in pregnancy

Precise details on the date of onset of illness, presence and distribution of such clinical features as rash, lymphadenopathy and arthralgia should be obtained from pregnant women who present with rubella-like clinical features or the date, duration and type of contact (e.g. casual or more prolonged household contact), in order to interpret the results of virological investigations. In addition, enquiry should be made about results of previous screening tests for rubella antibodies and history of rubella vaccination.

Patients who have been exposed to rubella should be carefully followed up serologically because retrospective studies have shown that some women who delivered infants with CAR gave no history of a rubella-like illness during pregnancy (Sheppard et al. 1977). Blood should be collected from pregnant women with rubella-like features as soon as possible after the onset of symptoms. Provided that a blood sample is obtained within the first 3–4 days, it is usually possible to detect a significant rise in antibody concentration by such tests as HAI and EIA in a second blood sample taken a few days later. It is advisable to confirm the diagnosis by conducting tests for rubella-specific IgM.

Although most patients develop rubella antibodies within a few days of onset of symptoms, antibody responses may very occasionally be delayed for as long as 10 days. This underlines the importance of collecting further blood samples from patients who remain seronegative. Many patients present in the postacute phase of their illness, at which time antibody concentrations are likely to have reached maximum concentrations. It must be emphasized that there is no particular concentration of antibody ascertained by any test that can be regarded as indicative of recent or current infection. Because a virological diagnosis is usually required quickly for obstetric reasons, such patients should be tested for rubella-specific IgM with minimum delay.

Women who present within the incubation period and who have antibodies may be reassured, although it is often wise to obtain a second blood sample 7–10 days later to ensure that antibody concentrations are stable. The interpretation of results may depend on the accuracy of the history given by the patient. Sometimes an earlier blood sample is available (e.g. taken at the first antenatal visit) which can be tested in parallel with a sample taken after contact. If there is no change in antibody concentration the patient can be reassured with confidence that she was already immune.

Patients presenting after an interval greater than the incubation period and who are seropositive are more difficult to assess because antibodies may already have reached their maximum titre. The sera of such patients should therefore be tested for rubella-specific IgM.

Because rubella is unlikely to be acquired as a result of casual or brief contact (e.g. while shopping or in public transport), seronegative patients who experience this type of exposure should be reassured that the risks of acquiring rubella are small. Nevertheless, it is essential to follow up such people serologically. Those exposed more closely over a longer period are at greater risk, but even they may be reassured, particularly during non-epidemic times, by being told that the clinical diagnosis of rubella is often incorrect. Anxiety may be allayed by testing the index case, in order to confirm or refute the diagnosis. Patients who have been followed up but who remain seronegative should be offered rubella vaccination in the immediate postpartum period.

Rubella antibody screening

Tests for rubella antibodies are extensively used to identify susceptible women who should be offered rubella vaccination. In the UK, all antenatal patients are tested, as should women presenting to their general practitioners and 'well woman' clinics who have no history of vaccination or a previous positive antibody result. A number of tests are available commercially. EIA is used widely because it is readily automated and can easily be included in automated antenatal screening. LA has the advantage that a result is available in a few minutes. SRH is also widely used; the plates are usually prepared in the laboratory with commercially available reagents. Such techniques are preferred to HAI, which may sometimes give false-positive results owing to incomplete removal of β lipoprotein inhibitors of HA, and because it is more time consuming and labour intensive. Vaccination should be offered to women who are seronegative or have antibody concentrations <10–15 iu/ml. These techniques have been described in detail by Best and O'Shea (1995).

Rubella antibodies may be detected in saliva by IgG-capture RIA (GACRIA) (Parry et al. 1987). The use of saliva rather than serum has several benefits for screening and for seroepidemiological studies, especially those involving children and in developing countries (Eckstein et al. 1996).

Most rubella antibody tests use whole virus as antigen, but peptides and proteins produced by recombinant techniques have been evaluated (Mitchell et al. 1992, Hobman et al. 1994, Starkey et al. 1995) and some methods seem promising. One commercially available test employs virus-like particles produced by expression in BHK cells (Grangeot-Keros, Pustowoit and Hobman 1995).

Virus isolation and identification

RV may be detected in clinical samples by isolation in cell culture or by reverse transcription polymerase chain reaction (RT-PCR). Virus isolation techniques are rarely used for the diagnosis of postnatally acquired rubella because this may be established more reliably and rapidly by serological methods. However, virus isolation may be of value for determining the duration of excretion in congenitally infected infants (see p. 569), as they may transmit infection to susceptible contacts. RV isolates are also required to study the molecular epidemiology of the virus.

RV can be identified by the production of CPE in RK13, SIRC and certain sublines of Vero cells, by interference in primary VMK (Parkman, Buescher and Artenstein 1962) and other monkey kidney cultures, or by using immunofluorescence or immunoperoxidase for detection of antigen in such cells as RK13, BHK-21 and Vero. The most sensitive technique for isolation of RV is one or 2 passages in Vero cells, followed by passage in RK13 cells, in which the virus may be identified by immunofluorescence employing hyperimmune sera or monoclonal antibodies. These techniques have been described in detail by Best and O'Shea (1995). However, as virus isolation is labour intensive and a minimum of 3 weeks is required to obtain a result, this technique is available only in specialized laboratories.

A nested RT-PCR for the detection of RV RNA employing primers from the E1 region has been described by Bosma et al. (1995b). Results of this assay compared well with virus isolation. It has been applied to the pre- and postnatal diagnosis of congenital rubella (see p. 569).

LABORATORY DIAGNOSIS OF CONGENITAL RUBELLA

Postnatal tests

The National Congenital Surveillance Programme in the UK classifies suspected cases of congenital rubella according to the criteria listed in Table 28.4.

A diagnosis of CAR can be established by:

1 Detection of rubella-specific IgM in cord serum or serum samples obtained in early infancy. An IgM antibody capture assay is the method of choice for this purpose. Specific IgM has been detected in all symptomatic infants up to the age of 3 months, in 90% of infants aged 3–6 months, in fewer than 50% of infants aged 6–12 months and only occasionally in children over one year old (Chantler et al. 1982). The absence of specific IgM by IgM antibody capture assays in the neonatal period virtually excludes congenital rubella.

2 Detection of persistent rubella IgG antibody in serum or saliva at a time when maternal antibodies are no longer detectable (c. 8 months). This may be a useful technique when patients present too late for the detection of specific IgM.

3 Isolation of RV (see p. 568) or detection of RV RNA by RT-PCR (Bosma et al. 1995b) in specimens (such as pharyngeal swabs) taken from infants during early infancy. Facilities for RV isolation are not widely available, but RT-PCR can be applied to lens aspirates from cataracts in order to establish a diagnosis of CAR. Such lens aspirates can be transported from distant countries on dry ice or in physiological saline (Bosma et al. 1995a).

Table 28.4 Congenital rubella: case classification criteria (Miller et al. 1994)

Congenital rubella infection	
No rubella defects but congenital infection confirmed by isolation of virus, or detection of specific IgM or persistent IgG in infant	
Congenital rubella syndrome	
Confirmed	Typical rubella defect(s) plus virus-specific IgM or persistent IgG in infant; or 2 or more rubella defects plus confirmed maternal infection in pregnancy
Compatible	Two or more rubella defects with inconclusive laboratory data; or single rubella defect plus confirmed maternal infection in pregnancy
Possible	Compatible clinical findings with inconclusive laboratory data; e.g. single defect plus probable maternal infection in pregnancy
Unclassified	Insufficient information to confirm or exclude

RV can be isolated from the stools, urine, tears, CSF and nasopharyngeal secretions of infants with CAR. Cooper and Krugman (1967) isolated RV from the nasopharynx of almost all severely infected infants at birth, but by the age of 3 months the proportion declined to about 60% and, by 9–12 months, to c. 10%. However, RV may persist at other sites for even longer (see 'Persistence of virus', p. 565). There is a high perinatal mortality from CAR. RV can be isolated from most of the organs obtained at autopsy from severely infected infants who die in early infancy. Babies excreting virus may transmit infection to susceptible contacts; therefore, until virus is no longer being excreted, women of childbearing age, some of whom may be in the early stages of pregnancy, should be dissuaded from visiting such babies until serological tests confirm that they are immune.

Rubella-specific lymphoproliferative assays (O'Shea, Best and Banatvala 1992) and tests for low avidity specific IgG (Thomas et al. 1993) may be of value for retrospective diagnosis of CAR in children between the ages of one and 3 years.

Children with CAR may lose antibodies to the E1 glycoprotein (de Mazancourt et al. 1986, Mitchell et al. 1992, Mauracher, Mitchell and Tingle 1993) and consequently HAI antibodies may not be detected (Cooper et al. 1971, Ueda et al. 1975). In order to determine the immune status of such children in later life it may be necessary to use tests such as EIA and LA, which detect antibodies to all RV polypeptides.

Prenatal tests

Prenatal diagnosis of CAR may provide a more accurate estimate of risk when the mother is reluctant to have a therapeutic abortion following rubella in the first trimester (see p. 566), when maternal reinfection is confirmed or suspected and when serological results are equivocal, for example when patients present some time after a rubella-like illness. A prenatal diagnosis may be made by testing fetal blood samples obtained by fetoscopy for rubella-specific IgM (Daffos et al. 1984, Morgan-Capner et al. 1984), but, as IgM does not develop until about 20 weeks' gestation, this method should not be used until weeks 22–23 and even then false-negative results may be obtained (Enders and Jonatha 1987). This approach has the disadvantage that patients may have to wait for a long period, leaving little time for termination to be considered. RV may also be detected in chorionic villus samples or amniotic fluid by isolation in cell culture or RT-PCR (Bosma et al. 1995a). RT-PCR is preferred because results are available within 24–48 hours. However, the results of testing chorionic villus samples should be interpreted with caution, as the detection of RV in the placenta may not accurately reflect fetal infection (Bosma et al. 1995a). The detection of RV RNA in amniotic fluid and fetal blood seems more promising: sensitivities of 87.5% and positive predictive values of 100% were obtained when these specimens were tested by the RT-PCR of Bosma et al. (1995b) (G Enders and D Betzl 1996, personal communication).

2.5 Control

RUBELLA VACCINATION

Rubella and congenitally acquired rubella are preventable, and the marked reduction in CAR achieved in countries with well developed vaccination programmes results from the administration of attenuated rubella vaccines.

Rubella vaccines

The first attenuated strain of rubella was developed by the National Institutes of Health in the USA, this strain being isolated from a military recruit with acute rubella and attenuated by 77 passages in vervet monkey kidney cell cultures. Following preliminary trials in primates in which this vaccine was shown to be protective, controlled trials were conducted among institutionalized children, the vaccine strain having been passaged a further 5 times in duck embryo fibroblasts. Within a short time, further vaccine strains were prepared, being attenuated in primary rabbit kidney (Cendehill) and in human diploid cell cultures (RA27/3) (Proceedings 1969). The vaccine containing the RA27/3 strain, originally isolated from the fetal kidney of a rubella-infected conceptus, is the most widely used world-wide, although a number of vaccine strains developed in Japan are now used there (Perkins 1985). The accumulated data from trials employing rubella vaccines show that they are immunogenic, protective, and well tolerated. Vaccinees excrete virus via the nasopharynx but infection is not transmitted to susceptible contacts. The development and properties of different rubella vaccines have been reviewed by Banatvala and Best (1989) and Best (1991).

Vaccination programmes

Rubella vaccines were licensed in the USA in 1969 and in the UK in 1970. In the USA a policy of universal childhood immunization was adopted, this being aimed at interrupting transmission of virus by vaccinating pre-school children, thereby reducing the risk of pregnant women being exposed to rubella. Because high uptake rates were achieved, this policy markedly reduced the incidence of postnatally acquired and CAR (Fig. 28.8). However, in 1989/90 rubella occurred among unvaccinated women in some parts of the USA, resulting in cases of CAR (Lindegren et al. 1991). In contrast, a selective vaccination programme was initially adopted in the UK, this being directed first at pre-pubertal schoolgirls as well as women at particular risk of acquiring rubella (e.g. nurses and school teachers). Later it was recommended that all pregnant women be tested for rubella antibodies and those found seronegative offered rubella vaccine postpartum. Although a 90% uptake of vaccine was achieved among schoolgirls and the proportion of susceptible women of child-bearing age fell to only 2–3%, susceptible pregnant women were still infected when rubella was prevalent in the community. Because complete vaccination of the target population was an unrealistic goal, the vaccination

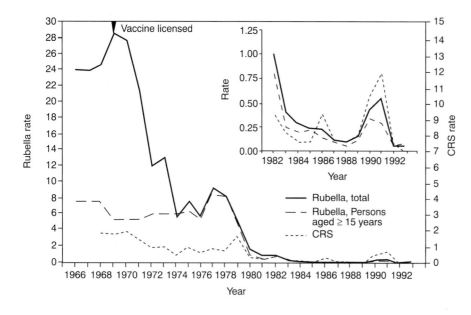

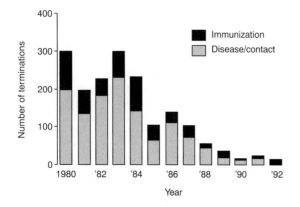

Fig. 28.8 Incidence rates of rubella and congenital rubella syndrome (CRS) in the USA, 1966–1993 Cases of rubella reported to the National Notifiable Disease Surveillance System per 100 000 population; cases of CRS reported to the National CRS Registry per 100 000 live births. (From Centers for Disease Control 1994.)

programme was augmented in 1988 by offering rubella vaccine to pre-school children of both sexes (Banatvala 1987b) and rubella is now given with measles and mumps (MMR) vaccine at about 15 months of age. This resulted in a fall in the number of reported cases of rubella and of terminations of pregnancy because of rubella (Fig. 28.9). Following the administration of MR vaccine to all 5- to 16-year-old school children in late 1994 to prevent a predicted measles epidemic, it was agreed to discontinue vaccination of schoolgirls, but to continue to ensure that susceptible pregnant women were vaccinated postpartum.

Although a significant proportion of young adult males remain susceptible, high rates of vaccine uptake among pre-school children together with the markedly reduced susceptibility among pregnant women have resulted in CAR being rare in the UK. Thus, in contrast to 1984 in which 52 cases were reported, in 1994 only 7 cases were notified to the National Congenital Rubella Surveillance Programme (P Tookey and CS Peckham 1995, personal communication).

Fig. 28.9 Terminations of pregnancy associated with rubella (England and Wales) 1980–1992. (From Miller et al. 1994.)

Most countries in Europe administer MMR vaccine between the first and second birthdays; although in some countries (e.g. Scandinavia) a second dose is given between 6 and 12 years (Galaska 1991).

Immune responses

About 95% of vaccinees develop an immune response. Serum antibodies develop between 10 and 28 days after vaccination and reach maximum levels about 6 months later. Occasionally, antibody responses may be delayed for up to 8 weeks. Failure to respond may result from concurrent infections, pre-existing low levels of antibody undetectable by less sensitive assays, or the presence of passively acquired antibody acquired maternally, via blood transfusion or administration of immunoglobulin. Failure to comply with the manufacturer's recommendations during storage or after reconstitution may result in virus inactivation and loss of potency of the vaccine.

Following vaccination, antibodies to the major structural proteins E1, E2 and C may be detected, and rubella-specific IgG, IgA and IgM responses are present. Specific IgM responses are detected in about 70% of vaccinees, persisting for about 6 months. Occasionally, rubella-specific IgM may persist at low levels for up to 4 years (O'Shea et al. 1985). Virus-specific IgA concentrations decline more rapidly than specific IgG. There is a transient oligomeric (10S) IgA response, is succeeded by a 7S response which may persist at low levels for 10–12 years after vaccination. The RA27/3 vaccine induces a secretory IgA response which persists for up to 5 years (O'Shea et al. 1985).

Although serum antibody levels detected by HAI and SRH persist for at least 21 years in most vaccinees, in c. 10% the levels decline to <15 iu/ml within 5–8 years; a small number may become completely seronegative (reviewed by Banatvala and Best 1989). However, when volunteers with low levels of antibody were challenged intranasally with high titre RA27/3 vaccine, most appeared to be protected although a transient low level of virus specific IgM was present in

4 of 19 and a transient viraemia was detected in one of 19 volunteers (O'Shea, Best and Banatvala 1983). A transient lymphoproliferative response has been detected following rubella vaccination (Buimovici-Klein and Cooper 1985).

Virus excretion

RV may be detected in nasopharyngeal secretions in most vaccinees 6–29 days after vaccination as well as in the breast milk of lactating women vaccinated postpartum. Although lack of transmission to susceptible contacts may result from low concentrations in nasopharyngeal secretions, it is possible that attenuation may alter the biological properties of the virus, resulting in poor replication in the respiratory tract. Very occasionally, virus has been transmitted to breast-fed infants but they do not develop any clinical features of infection.

Vaccine reactions

RV is well tolerated although lymphadenopathy, rash and arthropathy may occur between 10 and 30 days after vaccination. In general, such reactions are less severe than following naturally acquired infection. Indeed, vaccinees may fail to notice their lymphadenopathy and, if rash occurs, it is usually macular, faint and evanescent. Joint symptoms are related to age and gender, being rare in children of both sexes (2.5–10%) but occurring in up to 58% of postpubertal females. Most commonly the small joints of the hands are affected but the knees, wrists and ankles may also be involved. Symptoms rarely persist for longer than a week. However, a small proportion of vaccinees may develop an arthritis with pain and limitation of joint movement, which may occasionally recur intermittently. Joint symptoms rarely result in absence from work.

Contraindications

As with other live vaccines, immunocompromised patients should not be vaccinated. Such people include those with malignant disease and those being treated with cytotoxic drugs, radiotherapy or corticosteroids. Thrombocytopenic patients should not be vaccinated. HIV-positive people, with or without symptoms, are exceptions to these recommendations because they may be vaccinated with such live vaccines as MMR and polio. HIV-positive people do not react adversely to such live vaccines but, if unprotected, may experience serious complications, particularly if infected with measles.

Live vaccines may be administered concurrently, preferably at different sites (except in the case of MMR). If this is not possible, the 2 live vaccines should be separated by an interval of 3 weeks; a similar period should be allowed between the administration of rubella vaccine or MMR and BCG. If a vaccinee has a febrile illness, it is prudent to postpone rubella vaccination until the individual has recovered. The rubella vaccines may contain such antibiotics as neomycin, kanamycin or polymyxin, and anyone with established hypersensitivity to these antibiotics should not be vaccinated. As passively acquired antibodies may interfere with vaccine-induced responses, rubella vaccination should be delayed for 3 months after blood transfusion or administration of immunoglobulin. However, the administration of anti-D immunoglobulin does not suppress vaccine-induced immune responses although it may be prudent to confirm seroconversion 2–3 months after vaccination.

Vaccination during pregnancy

Although wild strains of rubella are teratogenic, the accumulated data from studies reported in different countries, in which over 500 rubella-susceptible women were vaccinated during pregnancy, a third during the high risk period between one week before and 4 weeks after conception, have shown that this has not resulted in rubella-induced fetal defects. Vaccine strains may, however, infect the conceptus because rubella vaccine strains have been isolated from the placenta, kidney and bone marrow for up to 94 days after vaccination. Furthermore, rubella-specific IgM responses or antibodies persisting for up to a year have been detected in about 3% of infants delivered of mothers inadvertently vaccinated during early pregnancy (reviewed by Best and Banatvala 1994).

The theoretical maximum risk of rubella vaccine-induced major malformations based on a 95% confidence limit of the binomial distribution has been calculated to be 1.2%, this being less than the 3% of major malformations occurring in 'normal' pregnancies (Bart et al. 1985, Enders 1985). These encouraging reports have resulted in a substantial reduction in terminations of pregnancy being carried out as a result of inadvertent vaccination in pregnancy in Britain. Nevertheless, it is still recommended that pregnant women should not be vaccinated against rubella and that pregnancy should be avoided for one month after vaccination (Department of Health 1992).

PASSIVE IMMUNIZATION

Normal human immunoglobulin does not confer any clear-cut protection (Report 1968, 1970). This preparation may reduce the incidence of clinically overt maternal infection, but subclinical infection may nevertheless occur, with a prolonged incubation period. Because inapparent infection is accompanied by viraemia, fetal damage is not prevented when it is used in pregnancy. However, it is possible that the administration of normal human globulin reduces the level of fetal infection or damage, or both (Peckham 1974, Hanshaw, Dudgeon and Marshall 1985).

High-titre rubella immunoglobulin has been used experimentally to determine whether infection induced by rubella vaccine can be prevented (Urquhart, Crawford and Wallace 1978). This preparation has not been properly evaluated in the field, but may be recommended for the few susceptible pregnant women who come into contact with clinical rubella and for whom therapeutic abortion is unacceptable.

REFERENCES

Arnold JJ, McIntosh ED FJ et al., 1994, A fifty-year follow-up of ocular defects in congenital rubella: late ocular manifestations, *Aust N Z J Ophthal*, **22:** 1–6.

Atreya CD, Singh NK, Nakhasi HL, 1995, The rubella virus RNA binding activity of human calreticulin is localised to the N-terminal domain, *J Virol*, **69:** 3848–51.

de Azevedo Neto RS, Silveira ASB et al., 1994, Rubella seroepidemiology in a non-immunized population of Sao Paulo State, Brazil, *Epidemiol Infect*, **113:** 161–73.

Banatvala JE, 1977, Health of mother, fetus and neonate following bacterial fungal and protozoal infections during pregnancy, *Infections and Pregnancy*, ed Coid CR, Academic Press, London, 437–88.

Banatvala JE, 1987a, Insulin-dependent and (juvenile-onset type 1) diabetes mellitus-coxsackie B virus revisited, *Prog Med Virol*, **34:** 33–54.

Banatvala JE, 1987b, Measles must go and with it rubella [editorial], *Br Med J*, **295:** 2–3.

Banatvala JE, Best JM, 1989, Rubella vaccines, ed Zuckerman AJ, Kluwer, Lancaster, 155–80.

Banatvala JE, Best JM, 1990, Rubella, *Topley and Wilson's Principles of Bacteriology, Virology and Immunity*, 8th edn, vol 4, eds Collier LH, Timbury M, Edward Arnold, London, 501–31.

Bardeletti G, 1977, Respiration and ATP level in BHK2Y135 cells during the earliest stages of rubella virus replication, *Intervirology*, **8:** 100–9.

Bardeletti G, Kessler N, Aymard-Henry M, 1975, Morphology, biochemical analysis and neuraminidase activity of rubella virus, *Arch Virol*, **49:** 175–86.

Bardeletti G, Tektoff J, Gautheron D, 1979, Rubella virus maturation and production in two host cell systems, *Intervirology*, **11:** 97–103.

Baron MD, Ebel T, Suomalainen M, 1992, Intracellular transport of rubella virus structural proteins expressed from cloned cDNA, *J Gen Virol*, **73:** 1073–86.

Baron MD, Forsell K, 1991, Oligomerization of the structural proteins of rubella virus, *Virology*, **185:** 811–19.

Bart SW, Stetler HC et al., 1985, Fetal risk associated with rubella vaccine: an update, *Rev Infect Dis*, **7, suppl 1:** S95–102.

Best JM, 1991, Rubella vaccines – past, present and future, *Epidemiol Infect*, **107:** 17–30.

Best JM, 1993, Rubella reinfection, *Curr Med Literature: Virology*, **2:** 35–40.

Best JM, Banatvala JE, 1994, Rubella, *Principles and Practice of Clinical Virology*, 3rd edn, eds Zuckerman AJ, Banatvala JE, Pattison JR, John Wiley, Chichester, 363–400.

Best JM, Banatvala JE, Moore BM, 1968, Growth of rubella virus in human embryonic organ cultures, *J Hyg*, **66:** 407–13.

Best JM, O'Shea S, 1995, Rubella, *Diagnostic Procedures for Viral, Rickettsial and Chlamydial Infections*, 7th edn, eds Lennette EH, Lennette DA, Lennette ET, American Public Health Association, Washington DC, 583–600.

Best JM, Banatvala JE et al., 1967, The morphological characteristics of rubella virus, *Lancet*, **2:** 237–9.

Best JM, Banatvala JE et al., 1989, Fetal infection after maternal reinfection with rubella: criteria for defining reinfection, *Br Med J*, **299:** 773–5.

Best JM, Thomson A et al., 1992, Rubella virus strains show no major antigenic differences, *Intervirology*, **34:** 164–8.

Booth JC, Stern H, 1972, Photodynamic inactivation of rubella virus, *J Med Microbiol*, **5:** 515–28.

Bosma TJ, Corbett KM et al., 1995a, Use of PCR for prenatal and postnatal diagnosis of congenital rubella, *J Clin Microbiol*, **33:** 2881–7.

Bosma TJ, Corbett KM et al., 1995b, Use of the polymerase chain reaction for the detection of rubella virus RNA in clinical samples, *J Clin Microbiol*, **33:** 1075–9.

Bosma TJ, Best JM et al., 1996, Nucleotide sequence analysis of a major antigenic domain of the E1 glycoprotein of 22 rubella virus isolates, *J Gen Virol*, **77:** 2523–30.

Bowden DS, Westaway EG, 1985, Changes in glycosylation of rubella virus envelope proteins during maturation, *J Gen Virol*, **66:** 201–6.

Brown T, Hambling MH, Ansari BM, 1969, Rubella-neutralising and haemagglutinin-inhibiting antibodies in children of different ages, *Br Med J*, **4:** 263–5.

Buimovici-Klein E, Cooper LZ, 1985, Cell-mediated immune response in rubella infections, *Rev Infect Dis*, **7, suppl 1:** S123–8.

Buimovici-Klein E, Weiss KE, Cooper LZ, 1977, Interferon production in lymphocyte cultures after rubella infection in humans, *J Infect Dis*, **135:** 380–5.

Buimovici-Klein E, Vesikari T et al., 1976, Study of the lymphocyte in vitro response to rubella antigen and phytohemagglutinin by a whole blood method, *Arch Virol*, **52:** 323–31.

Buimovici-Klein E, Lang PB et al., 1979, Impaired cell mediated immune response in patients with congenital rubella: correlation with gestational age at time of infection, *Pediatrics*, **64:** 620–6.

Bunnell CE, Monif GRG, 1972, Interstitial pancreatitis in the congenital rubella syndrome, *J Pediatr*, **80:** 465–6.

Centers for Disease Control and Prevention, 1994, Reported vaccine-preventable diseases – United States 1993, *Morbid Mortal Weekly Rep*, **43:** 57–60.

Chantler JK, Ford DK, Tingle AJ, 1982, Persistent rubella infections and rubella-associated arthritis, *Lancet*, **1:** 1323–5.

Chantler JK, Petty RE, Tingle AJ, 1985, Persistent rubella virus infections with chronic arthritis in children, *N Engl J Med*, **313:** 1117–23.

Chantler JK, Smymis L, Tai G, 1995, Selective infection of astrocytes in human glial cell cultures by rubella virus, *Lab Invest*, **72:** 334–40.

Chantler JK, Tingle AJ, 1980, Replication and expression of rubella virus in human lymphocyte populations, *J Gen Virol*, **50:** 317–28.

Chantler S, Evans CJ et al., 1982, A comparison of antibody capture radio- and enzyme immunoassays with immunofluorescence for detecting IgM antibody in infants with congenital rubella, *J Virol Methods*, **4:** 305–13.

Chantler JK, Lund KD et al., 1993, Characterisation of rubella virus strain differences associated with attenuation, *Intervirology*, **36:** 225–36.

Chaye HH, Mauracher CA et al., 1992a, Cellular and humoral immune responses to rubella virus structural proteins E1, E2, and C, *J Clin Microbiol*, **30:** 2323–9.

Chaye H, Chong P et al., 1992b, Localisation of the virus neutralising and hemagglutinin epitopes of E1 glycoprotein of rubella virus, *Virology*, **189:** 483–92.

Cooper LZ, 1975, Congenital rubella in the United States, *Progress in Clinical and Biological Research*, eds Krugman S, Gershon AA, Alan R Liss, New York, 1–22.

Cooper LZ, Krugman S, 1967, Clinical manifestations of postnatal and congenital rubella, *Arch Ophthalmol*, **77:** 434–9.

Cooper LZ, Green RH et al., 1965, Neonatal thrombocytopenic purpura and other manifestations of rubella contracted in utero, *Am J Dis Child*, **110:** 416–27.

Cooper LZ, Zirling PR et al., 1969, Rubella: clinical. manifestations and management, *Am J Dis Child*, **118:** 18–29.

Cooper LZ, Forman AL. et al., 1971, Loss of rubella hemagglutination inhibition antibody in congenital rubella. Failure of seronegative children with congenital rubella to respond to HPV-77 rubella vaccine, *Am J Dis Child*, **122:** 397–403.

Coyle PK, Wolinsky JS et al., 1982, Rubella-specific immune complexes after congenital. infection and vaccination, *Infect Immun*, **36:** 498–503.

Cradock-Watson JE, Ridehalgh MKS et al., 1980, Fetal. infection resulting from maternal rubella after the first trimester of pregnancy, *J Hyg*, **85:** 381–91.

Cremer NE, Oshiro LS et al., 1975, Isolation of rubella virus from brain in chronic progressive panencephalitis, *J Gen Virol*, **29:** 143–53.

Cunningham AL., Fraser JRE, 1985, Persistent rubella virus infection of human synovial cells cultured in vitro, *J Infect Dis*, **151:** 638–45.

Cusi MG, Metelli R et al., 1989, Immune responses to wild and vaccine rubella viruses after rubella vaccination, *Arch Virol*, **106:** 63–72.

Cusi MG, Valassina M et al., 1995, Evaluation of rubella virus E2 and C proteins in protection against rubella virus in a mouse model, *Virus Res*, **37:** 199–208.

Daffos F, Forestier F et al., 1984, Prenatal diagnosis of congenital rubella, *Lancet*, **2:** 1–3.

Department of Health, 1992, *Immunisation against Infectious Disease*, HMSO, London, 68–75.

Derdyn CA, Frey TK, 1993, Characterisations of defective-interfering RNAs of rubella virus generated during serial undiluted passage, *Virology*, **206:** 216–26.

Desmond MM, Wilson GS et al., 1967, Congenital. rubella encephalitis: course and early sequelae, *J Pediatr*, **71:** 311–31.

Dominguez G, Wang C-Y, Frey TK, 1990, Sequence of the genome of rubella virus. Evidence for genetic rearrangement during togavirus evolution, *Virology*, **177:** 225–38.

Dorsett PH, Miller DC et al., 1985, Structure and function of the rubella virus proteins, *Rev Infect Dis*, **7, suppl 1:** S150–6.

Dowdle WR, Ferreira W et al., 1970, Study on the sero-epidemiology of rubella in Caribbean and Middle and South American populations in 1968, *Bull W H O*, **42:** 419–22.

Eckstein MB, Brown DWG et al., 1996, Congenital rubella in south India: diagnosis using saliva from infants with cataract, *Br Med J*, **312:** 161.

Editorial, 1944, Rubella and congenital malformations, *Lancet*, **1:** 316.

Enders G, 1982, Röteln-Embryopathie noch heute?, *Geburtshilfe Frauenheilkd*, **42:** 403–13.

Enders G, 1985, Rubella antibody titres in vaccinated and non-vaccinated women and results of vaccination during pregnancy, *Rev Infect Dis*, **7, suppl 1:** S103–12.

Enders G, Jonatha W, 1987, Prenatal diagnosis of intrauterine rubella, *Infection*, **15:** 162–4.

Enders G, Nikerl-Pacher U et al., 1988, Outcome of confirmed periconceptional maternal rubella, *Lancet*, **1:** 1445–7.

Fabiyi A, Sever JL et al., 1966, Rubella virus: growth characteristics and stability of infectious virus and complement-fixing antigen, *Proc Soc Exp Biol Med*, **122:** 392–6.

Forng RY, Frey TK, 1995, Identification of the rubella virus non-structural proteins, *Virology*, **206:** 843–53.

de Freitas RB, Wong D et al., 1990, Prevalence of human parvovirus (B19) and rubella virus infections in urban and remote rural areas in northern Brazil, *J Med Virol*, **32:** 203–8.

Frey TK, 1994, Molecular biology of rubella virus, *Adv Virus Res*, **44:** 69–160.

Frey TK, Abernathy ES, 1993, Identification of strain-specific nucleotide sequences of the RA 27/3 rubella virus chain, *J Infect Dis*, **168:** 854–64.

Fuccillo DA, Steele RW et al., 1974, Impaired cellular immunity to rubella virus in congenital rubella, *Infect Immun*, **9:** 81–4.

Furukawa T, Plotkin SA et al., 1967, Studies on hemagglutination by rubella virus, *Proc Soc Exp Biol Med*, **126:** 745–50.

Galaska A, 1991, Rubella in Europe, *Epidemiol Infect*, **107:** 43–54.

Gill SD, Furesz J, 1973, Genetic stability in humans of the rabbit immunogenic marker of Cendehill rubella vaccine virus, *Archiv Gesamte Virusforsch*, **43:** 135–43.

Ginsberg-Fellner F, Witt ME et al., 1985, Diabetes mellitus and autoimmunity in patients with the congenital rubella syndrome, *Rev Infect Dis*, **7, suppl 1:** S170–6.

Givens KT, Lee DA et al., 1994, Congenital rubella syndrome:

ophthalmic manifestations and associated systemic disorders, *Br J Ophthalmol*, **78:** 79.

Grahame R, Armstrong R et al., 1981, Isolation of rubella virus from synovial fluid in five cases of seronegative arthritis, *Lancet*, **2:** 649–51.

Grangeot-Keros L, Pustowoit B, Hobman T, 1995, Evaluation of Cobas core rubella IgG EIA recomb, a new enzyme immunoassay based on recombinant rubella-like particles, *J Clin Microbiol*, **33:** 2392–4.

Grayzel AI, Beck C, 1971, The growth of vaccine strain of rubella virus in cultured human synovial cells, *Proc Soc Exp Biol Med*, **136:** 496–8.

Green RH, Balsamo MR et al., 1965, Studies of the natural history and prevention of rubella, *Am J Dis Child*, **110:** 348–65.

Gregg NMcA, 1941, Congenital cataract following german measles in the mother, *Trans Ophthalmol Soc Aust*, **3:** 35–46.

Gregg NMcA, 1944, Further observations on congenital defects in infants following maternal. rubella, *Trans Ophthalmol Soc Aust*, **4:** 119–31.

Gregg NMcA, Beavis WR et al., 1945, The occurrence of congenital defects in children following maternal rubella, *Med J Aust*, **2:** 122–6.

Grillner L, Forsgren M et al., 1983, Outcome of rubella during pregnancy with special reference to the 17th–24th weeks of gestation, *Scand J Infect Dis*, **15:** 321–5.

Halonen PE, Ryan IH, Stewart JA, 1967, Rubella hemagglutinin prepared with alkaline extraction of virus grown in suspension culture of BHK-21 cells, *Proc Soc Exp Biol Med*, **125:** 162–7.

Hanshaw JB, Dudgeon JA, Marshall WC, 1985, *Viral Diseases of the Fetus and New-born*, 2nd edn, WB Saunders, Philadelphia, London, Toronto.

Harcourt GC, Best JM, Banatvala JE, 1979, HLA antigens and responses to rubella vaccination, *J Hyg*, **83:** 405–12.

Harcourt GC, Best JM, Banatvala JE, 1980, Rubella–specific serum and nasopharngeal antibodies in volunteers with naturally acquired and vaccine-induced immunity after intranasal challenge, *J Infect Dis*, **142:** 145–55.

Hastreiter AR, Joorabchi B et al., 1967, Cardiovascular lesions associated with congenital rubella, *J Pediatr*, **71:** 59–65.

Heggie AD, 1978, Pathogenesis of the rubella exanthem: distribution of rubella virus in the skin during rubella with and without rash, *J Infect Dis*, **137:** 74–6.

Hemphill ML, Forng R-Y et al., 1988, Time course of virus-specific macromolecular synthesis during rubella virus infection in Vero cells, *Virology*, **162:** 65–75.

Herrmann KL, 1979, Rubella virus, *Diagnostic Procedures for Viral, Rickettsial and Chlamydial Infections*, 5th edn, eds Lennette EH, Schmidt NJ, American Public Health Association, Washington DC, 725.

Hobman TC, Seto NOL, Gillam S, 1994, Expression of soluble forms of rubella virus glycoproteins in mammalian cells, *Virus Res*, **31:** 277–89.

Hobman TC, Woodward L, Farquhar MG, 1995, Targeting of a heterodimeric membrane protein complex to the Golgi: rubella virus E2 glycoprotein contains a transmembrane Golgic retention signal, *Mol Cell Biol*, **6:** 7–20.

Hobman TC, Lundstrom ML et al., 1994, Assembly of rubella virus structural protein into virus particles in transfected cells, *Virology*, **202:** 574–85.

Holmes IH, Wark MC, Warburton MV, 1969, Is rubella an arbovirus? Ultrastructural morphology and development, *Virology*, **371:** 5–25.

Holmes IH, Wark MC et al., 1968, Identification of two possible types of virus particles in rubella infected cells, *J Gen Virol*, **2:** 37–42.

Honeyman MC, Forrest JM, Dorman DC, 1974, Cell-mediated immune response following natural rubella and rubella vaccination, *Clin Exp Immunol*, **17:** 665–71.

Hope-Simpson RE, 1944, Rubella and congenital malformations, *Lancet*, **1:** 483.

Horstmann DM, Banatvala JE et al., 1965, Maternal rubella and the rubella syndrome in infants: epidemiologic, clinical and virologic observations, *Am J Dis Child*, **110:** 408–15.

Horstmann DM, Liebhaber H et al., 1970, Rubella: reinfections of vaccinated and naturally immune persons exposed in an epidemic, *N Engl J Med*, **283:** 771–8.

Horzinek MC, 1973, The structure of togaviruses, *Prog Med Virol*, **16:** 109–56.

Horzinek MC, 1981, *Non-Arthropod-Borne Togaviruses*, Academic Press, London.

Hosking CS, Pyman C, Wilkins B, 1983, The nerve deaf child – intrauterine rubella or not?, *Arch Dis Child*, **58:** 327–9.

Hovi T, Vaheri A, 1970a, Rubella virus-specific ribonucleic acids in infected BHK21 cells, *J Gen Virol*, **6:** 77–83.

Hovi T, Vaheri A, 1970b, Infectivity and some physicochemical characteristics of rubella virus ribonucleic acid, *Virology*, **42:** 1–8.

Hudson P, Morgan-Capner P, 1996, Evaluation of 15 commercial enzyme immunoassays for the detection of rubella-specific IgM, *Clin Diagn Virol*, **5:** 21–6.

Hyypiä T, Eskola J et al., 1984, B-cell function in vitro during rubella infection, *Infect Immun*, **43:** 589–92.

Ilonen J, Seppanen H et al., 1992, Recognition of synthetic peptides with sequences of rubella virus E1 polypeptide by antibodies and T lymphocytes, *Viral Immunol*, **5:** 221–8.

Kalkkinen N, Oker-Blom C, Pettersson RF, 1984, Three genes code for rubella virus structural proteins E1, E2A, E2b and C, *J Gen Virol*, **65:** 1549–57.

Karounos DG, Wolinsky JS, Thomas JW, 1993, Monoclonal antibody to rubella virus capsid protein recognises a beta-cell antigen, *J Immunol*, **150:** 3080–5.

Katow S, Sugiura A, 1985, Antibody response to individual rubella virus proteins in congenital and other rubella virus infections, *J Clin Microbiol*, **21:** 449–51.

Katow S, Sugiura A, 1988, Low pH-induced conformational change of rubella virus envelope proteins, *J Gen Virol*, **69:** 2797–807.

Kenney MT, Albright MT et al., 1969, Inactivation of rubella virus by gamma radiation, *J Virol*, **4:** 807–10.

Kishore J, Broor S, Seth P, 1990, Acute rubella infection in pregnant women in Delhi, *Ind J Med Res*, **91:** 245–6.

Kistler GS, Sapatino V, 1972, Temperature and UV-light resistance of rubella virus infectivity, *Archiv Gesamte Virusforsch*, **38:** 11–16.

Kistler, Best JM et al., 1967, Elektronenmikroskopische Untersuchungen an rötelninfizierten menschlichen Organkulturen, *Schweiz Med Wochenschr*, **97:** 1377–82.

Kobayashi N, 1978, Hemolytic activity of rubella virus, *Virology*, **89:** 610–12.

Korones SB, Ainger LE et al., 1965, Congenital rubella syndrome: study of 22 infants. Myocardial damage and other new clinical aspects, *Am J Dis Child*, **110:** 434–40.

Krugman S, Ward R, 1954, The rubella problem, *J Pediatr*, **44:** 489–98.

Krugman S, Ward R, 1968, Rubella (german measles), *Infectious Diseases of Children*, 4th edn, CV Mosby, St Louis MO, 279–95.

Krugman S, Ward R, Jacobs KG, 1953, Studies on rubella immunization. 1. Demonstration of rubella without rash, *JAMA*, **151:** 285–8.

Lebon P, Lyon G, 1974, Non-congenital rubella encephalitis, *Lancet*, **2:** 468.

Le Bouvier GL, 1969, Precipitinogens of rubella virus-infected cells, *Proc Soc Exp Biol Med*, **130:** 51–4.

Lee J-Y, Marshall JA, Bowden DS, 1992, Replication complexes associated with the morphogenesis of rubella virus, *Arch Virol*, **122:** 95–106.

Lindegren M, Fehrs LJ et al., 1991, Update: rubella and congenital rubella syndrome, 1980–1990, *Epidemiol Rev*, **13:** 341–8.

Liu Z, Yang D et al., 1996, Identification of domains in rubella virus genomic RNA and capsid protein necessary for specific interaction, *J Virol*, **70:** 2184–90.

van der Logt JTM, van Loon AM, van der Veen J, 1980, Repli-

cation of rubella virus in human mono-nuclear blood cells, *Infect Immun*, **27:** 309–14.

Londesborough P, Terry G, Ho-Terry L, 1992, Reactivity of a recombinant rubella E1 antigen expressed in *E coli*, *Arch Virol*, **122:** 391–7.

Lovett AE, Chang SH et al., 1993, Rubella virus-specific cytotoxic T-lymphocyte responses: identification of the capsid as a target of major histocompatiblity complex class I – restricted lysis and definition of two epitopes, *J Virol*, **67:** 5849–58.

Maller R, Fryden A, Soren L, 1978, Mitogen stimulation and distribution of T- and B-lymphocytes during natural rubella infection, *Acta Pathol Microbiol Immunol Scand, Sect C, Immunology*, **86:** 93–8.

Marr LD, Wang C-Y, Frey TK, 1994, Expression of the rubella virus non-structural protein ORF and demonstration of the proteolytic processing, *Virology*, **198:** 586–92.

Marr LD, Sanchez A et al., 1991, Efficient *in vitro* translation and processing of the rubella virus structural proteins in the presence of microsomes, *Virology*, **180:** 400–5.

Marshall WC, 1973, *Intrauterine Infections*, Ciba Foundation Symposium No 10, Associated Scientific Publishers, Amsterdam.

Martin R, Marquardt P et al., 1989, Virus specific and autoreactive T cell lines isolated from cerebrospinal fluid of a patient with chronic rubella panencephalitis, *J Neuroimmunol*, **23:** 1–10.

Mastromarino P, Cioe L et al., 1990, Role of membrane phospholipids and glycolipids in the Vero cell surface receptor for rubella virus, *Med Microbiol Immunol*, **179:** 105–14.

Matsumoto A, Higashi M, 1974, Electron microscopic studies on the morphology and morphogenesis of togaviruses, *Annu Rep Inst Virus Res, Kyoto University*, **17:** 11–22.

Mauracher CA, Gillam S et al., 1991, pH independent solubility shift of rubella virus capsid protein, *Virology*, **181:** 773–7.

Mauracher CA, Mitchell LA, Tingle AJ, 1992, Differential IgG avidity to rubella virus structural proteins, *J Med Virol*, **36:** 202–8.

Mauracher CA, Mitchell LA, Tingle AJ, 1993, Selective tolerance to the E1 protein of rubella virus in congenital rubella syndrome, *J Immunol*, **151:** 2041–9.

de Mazancourt A, Waxham MN et al., 1986, Antibody responses to the rubella virus structural proteins in infants with the congenital rubella syndrome, *J Med Virol*, **19:** 111–22.

Menser MA, Dods L, Harley JD, 1967, A twenty-five year follow up of congenital rubella, *Lancet*, **2:** 1347–50.

Menser MA, Forrest JM, 1974, Rubella: high incidence of defects in children considered normal at birth, *Med J Aust*, **1:** 123–6.

Menser MA, Forrest JM, Bransby RD, 1978, Rubella infection and diabetes mellitus, *Lancet*, **1:** 57–60.

Menser MA, Harley JD et al., 1967, Persistence of virus in lens for three years after prenatal rubella, *Lancet*, **2:** 387–8.

Menser MA, Reye RDK, 1974, The pathology of congenital rubella: a review written by request, *Pathology*, **6:** 215–22.

Miki NPH, Chantler JK, 1992, Differential ability of wild-type and vaccine strains of rubella virus to replicate and persist in human joint tissue, *Clin Exp Rheumatol*, **10:** 3–12.

Miller E, Cradock-Watson JE, Pollock TM, 1982, Consequences of confirming maternal rubella at successive stages of pregnancy, *Lancet*, **2:** 781–4.

Miller E, Waight PA et al., 1993, Rubella surveillance to December 1992: second joint report of the PHLS and National Congenital Rubella Surveillance Programme, *Com Dis Rep Review*, **3:** R35–40.

Miller E, Tookey P et al., 1994, Rubella surveillance to June 1994: third joint report from the PHLS and the National Congenital Rubella Surveillance Programme, *Com Dis Rep*, **4:** R146–52.

Mims CA, Stokes A, Grahame R, 1985, Synthesis of antibodies including antiviral antibodies in the knee joints of patients with chronic arthritis, *Ann Rheum Dis*, **44:** 734–7.

Mitchell LA, Zhang T, Tingle AJ, 1992, Differential antibody responses to rubella virus infection in males and females, *J Infect Dis*, **166:** 128–65.

Mitchell LA, Zhang T et al., 1992, Characterisation of rubella virus specific antibody responses by using a new synthetic peptide based enzyme linked immunosorbent assay, *J Clin Microbiol*, **30**: 1841–7.

Mitchell LA, Décarie D et al., 1993, Identification of immunoreactive regions of rubella virus E1 and E2 envelope proteins by using synthetic peptides, *Virus Res*, **29**: 33–57.

Morgan-Capner P, Rodeck CH et al., 1984, Prenatal diagnosis of rubella, *Lancet*, **2**: 343.

Morgan-Capner P, Miller E et al., 1991, Outcome of pregnancy after maternal reinfection with rubella, *Com Dis Rep*, **1**: R56–9.

Moriuchi H, Yamasaki S et al., 1990, A rubella epidemic in Sasebo, Japan, in 1987, with various complications, *Acta Paediatr Jpn*, **32**: 67–75.

Munro ND, Sheppard S et al., 1987, Temporal relations between maternal rubella and congenital defects, *Lancet*, **2**: 201–4.

Murphy AM, Reid RR et al., 1967, Rubella cataracts. Further clinical and virologic observations, *Am J Ophthalmol*, **64**: 1109–19.

Murphy FA, 1980, Togavirus morphology and morphogenesis, *The Togaviruses*, ed Schlesinger RW, Academic Press, New York, 241–316.

Murphy FA, Halonen PE, Harrison AK, 1968, Electron microscopy of the development of rubella virus in BHK21 cells, *J Virol*, **2**: 1223–7.

Naeye RL, Blanc W, 1965, Pathogenesis of congenital rubella, *JAMA*, **194**: 1277–83.

Nakhasi H, Cao XQ et al., 1991, Specific binding of host cell proteins to the 3′ terminal stem loop structure of rubella virus, *J Virol*, **65**: 5961–7.

Nakhasi H, Singh NK et al., 1994, Identification and characterisation of host factor interactions with *cis*-acting elements of rubella virus RNA, *Arch Virol*, **9**: 255–67.

Newcombe J, Starkey W et al., 1994, Recombinant rubella E1 fusion protein for antibody screening and diagnosis, *Clin Diag Virol*, **2**: 149–63.

Niwa Y, Kanoh T, 1979, Immunological behaviour following rubella infection, *Clin Exp Immunol*, **37**: 470–6.

Norrby E, 1969, *Rubella Virus*, Virology Monographs, 7th edn, Springer-Verlag, Vienna, New York, 115–74.

Numazaki K, Goldman H et al., 1990, Infection by human cytomegalovirus and rubella of cultured human fetal islets of Langerhans, *In Vivo*, **4**: 49–54.

Ogra PL, Herd JL, 1971, Arthritis associated with induced rubella infection, *J Immunol*, **107**: 810–13.

Ohtawara M, Kobune F et al., 1985, Inability of Japanese rubella vaccines to induce antibody response in rabbits is due to growth restrictions at 39 degrees C, *Arch Virol*, **83**: 217–27.

Oker-Blom C, 1984, The gene order for rubella virus structural proteins is NH2–C–E2–E1–COOH, *J Virol*, **51**: 354–8.

Oker-Blom C, Jarvis DL, Summers MD, 1990, Translocation and cleavage of rubella virus envelope glycoproteins: identification and role of the E2 signal sequence, *J Gen Virol*, **71**: 3047–53.

Oker-Blom C, Kalkkinen N et al., 1983, Rubella virus contains one capsid protein and three envelope glyoproteins, E1, E2a and E2b, *J Virol*, **46**: 964–73.

Oker-Blom C, Blomster M et al., 1995, Synthesis and processing of the rubella virus p110 polyprotein in baculovirus-infected *Spodoptera frugiperda* cells, *Virus Res*, **35**: 71–9.

O'Shea S, Best JM, Banatvala JE, 1983, Viremia, virus excretion, and antibody responses after challenge in volunteers with low levels of antibody to rubella virus, *J Infect Dis*, **148**: 639–47.

O'Shea S, Best JM, Banatvala JE, 1992, A lymphocyte transformation assay for the diagnosis of congenital rubella, *J Virol Methods*, **37**: 139–48.

O'Shea S, Best JM et al., 1985, Development and persistence of class-specific serum and nasopharyngeal antibodies in rubella vaccinees, *J Infect Dis*, **151**: 89–98.

O'Shea S, Corbett KM et al., 1994, Rubella reinfection; role of

neutralising antibodies and cell-mediated immunity, *Clin Diag Virol*, **2**: 349–58.

Ou D, Chong P et al., 1993, Mapping T-cell epitopes of rubella virus structural proteins E1, E2 and C recognised by T-cell lines and clones derived from infected and immunised populations, *J Med Virol*, **40**: 175–83.

Parkman PD, 1965, Biological characteristics of rubella virus, *Arch Gesamte Virusforsch*, **16**: 401–11.

Parkman PD, Buescher EL, Artenstein MS, 1962, Recovery of the rubella virus from recruits, *Proc Soc Exp Biol*, **111**: 225–30.

Parkman PD, Buescher EL et al., 1964, Studies of rubella. 1. Properties of the virus, *J Immunol*, **93**: 595–607.

Parry JV, Perry KR, Mortimer PP, 1987, Sensitive assays for viral antibodies in saliva: an alternative to tests on serum, *Lancet*, **1**: 72–5.

Pathak S, Webb HE et al., 1994, Immunoelectron microscopical study of rubella virus grown in Vero cells with special reference to membrane bound spherules, *Electron microscopy 1994*, Proceedings of the 13th International Conference on Electron Microscopy, vol 3B, eds Jouffrey B, Colliex C, Editions de Physique, Les Ulis, France, 1381–2.

Pattison JR, Dane DS, Mace JE, 1975, Persistence of specific IgM after natural infection with rubella virus, *Lancet*, **1**: 185–7.

Peckham CS, 1972, Clinical laboratory study of children exposed in utero to maternal rubella, *Arch Dis Child*, **47**: 571–7.

Peckham CS, 1974, Clinical and serological assessment of children exposed in utero to confirmed maternal rubella, *Br Med J*, **2**: 259–61.

Penttinen K, Myllyla G, 1968, Interaction in human blood platelets, viruses and antibodies. 1. Platelet aggregation test with microequipment, *Ann Med Exp Biol Fenn*, **46**: 188–92.

Perkins FTC, 1985, Licensed vaccines, *Rev Infect Dis*, **7, suppl 1**: S73–8.

Perry KR, Brown WG et al., 1993, Detection of measles, mumps and rubella antibodies in saliva using antibody capture radioimunoassay, *J Med Virol*, **40**: 235–40.

Pettersson RF, Oker-Blom C et al., 1985, Molecular and antigenic characteristics and synthesis of rubella virus structural proteins, *Rev Infect Dis*, **7, suppl 1**: S140–6.

Phelan P, Campbell P, 1969, Pulmonary complications of rubella embryopathy, *J Pediatr*, **75**: 202–12.

Plotkin SA, 1969, Rubella virus, *Diagnostic Procedures in Viral and Rickettsial Diseases*, 4th edn, eds Lennette EH, Schmidt NJ, American Public Health Association, Washington DC, 364–413.

Plotkin SA, Vaheri A, 1967, Human fibroblasts infected with rubella virus produce a growth inhibitor, *Science*, **156**: 659–61.

Plotkin SA, Oski FA et al., 1965, Some recently recognized manifestations of the rubella syndrome, *J Pediatr*, **67**: 182–91.

Pogue GP, Cao X-Q et al., 1993, 5Δ Sequences of rubella virus RNA stimulate translation of chimeric RNAs and specifically interact with two host-encoded proteins, *J Virol*, **67**: 7106–17.

Pogue GP, Hoffmann J et al., 1996, Autoantigens interact with *cis*-acting elements of rubella virus RNA, *J Virol*, **70**: 6269–77.

Proceedings, 1969, Proceedings of the International Conference on Rubella Immunisation, *Am J Dis Child*, **118**: 2–399.

Qiu Z, Ou D et al., 1994, Expression and characterisation of virus like particles containing rubella virus structural proteins, *J Virol*, **68**: 4068–91.

Rabinowe SL, George KL et al., 1986, Congenital rubella: monoclonal antibody-defined T cell abnormalities in young adults, *Am J Med*, **81**: 779–82.

Rawls WE, 1968, Congenital rubella: the significance of virus persistence, *Prog Med Virol*, **10**: 238–85.

Report of the Public Health Laboratory Service Working Party on Rubella, 1968, Measurement of rubella antibody in immunoglobulin: its disappearance from the blood after infection, *Br Med J*, **3**: 206–8.

Report of the Public Health Laboratory Working Party on Rubella, 1970, Studies on the effect of immunoglobulin on rubella in pregnancy, *Br Med J*, **2**: 497.

Report, 1994, Report of an International Meeting on rubella vaccines and vaccination, 9 August 1993, Glasgow, United Kingdom, *J Infect Dis*, **170**: 507–9.

Rorke LB, Spiro AJ, 1967, Cerebral lesions in congenital rubella syndrome, *J Pediatr*, **70**: 243–55.

Russell B, Selzer G, Goetz H, 1967, The particle size of rubella virus, *J Gen Virol*, **1**: 305–10.

Schell K, Wong KT, 1966, Stability and stage of rubella complement fixing antigen, *Nature (London)*, **212**: 621–2.

Schmidt NJ, Styk B, 1968, Immunodiffusion reactions with rubella antigens, *J Immunol*, **101**: 210–16.

Sedwick WD, Sokol F, 1970, Nucleic acid of rubella virus and its replication in hamster kidney cells, *J Virol*, **5**: 478–87.

Seppala M, Vaheri A, 1974, Natural rubella infection of the female genital tract, *Lancet*, **1**: 46–7.

Seppanen H, Huhtala M et al., 1991, Diagnostic potential of baculovirus-expressed rubella virus envelope proteins, *J Clin Microbiol*, **29**: 1877–82.

Seto NO, Ou D, Gillam S, 1995, Expression and characterisations of secreted forms of rubella virus E2 glycoprotein in insect cells, *Virology*, **206**: 736–41.

Sheppard S, Smithells RW et al., 1977, National congenital rubella surveillance, *Health Trends*, **9**: 38–41.

Siegel M, Fuerst HT, Guinee VF, 1971, Rubella epidemicity and embryopathy. Results of a long term prospective study, *Am J Dis Child*, **121**: 469–73.

Smith JL, 1881, Contributions to the study of Rötheln, *Trans Int Med Congr Philadelphia*, **4**: 14.

Smith KO, Hobbins TE, 1969, Physical characteristics of rubella virus, *J Immunol*, **102**: 1016–23.

Sperling DR, Verska JJ, 1966, Rubella syndrome, *Calif Med*, **105**: 340–4.

Starkey WG, Newcombe J et al., 1995, Use of rubella E1 fusion proteins for the detection of rubella antibodies, *J Clin Microbiol*, **33**: 270–4.

Stewart GL, Parkman PD et al., 1967, Rubella-virus hemagglutination-inhibition test, *N Engl J Med*, **276**: 554–7.

Stokes A, Mims CA, Grahame R, 1986, Subclass distribution of IgG and IgA responses to rubella virus in man, *J Med Microbiol*, **21**: 283–5.

Suomalainen M, Garoff H et al., 1990, The E2 signal sequence of rubella virus remains part of the capsid protein and confers membrane association *in vitro*, *J Virol*, **64**: 5500–9.

Swan C, Tostevin AL et al., 1943, Congenital defects in infants following infectious diseases during pregnancy with special reference to relationship between german measles and cataract, deaf–mutism, heart disease and microcephaly, and to period of pregnancy in which occurrence of rubella is followed by congenital abnormalities, *Med J Aust*, **2**: 201–210.

Tardieu M, Grospierre B, Durandy A, 1980, Circulating immune complexes containing rubella antigens in late-onset rubella syndrome, *J Pediatr*, **97**: 370–3.

Tedder RS, Yao JL et al., 1982, The production of monoclonal antibodies to rubella haemagglutinin and their use in antibody capture assays for rubella-specific IgM, *J Hyg*, **88**: 335–50.

Terry GM, Ho-Terry LM et al., 1988, Localisation of the rubella E1 epitopes, *Arch Virol*, **98**: 189–97.

Thomas HIJ, Morgan-Capner P, 1988, Rubella-specific IgG subclass avidity: ELISA and its role in the differentiation between primary rubella and rubella reinfection, *Epidemiol Infect*, **101**: 591–8.

Thomas HIJ, Morgan-Capner P, 1991, The use of antibody avidity measurements for the diagnosis of rubella, *Rev Med Virol*, **1**: 41–50.

Thomas HIJ, Morgan-Capner P et al., 1993, Slow maturation of IgG1, avidity and persistence of specific IgM in congenital rubella: implications for diagnosis and immunopathology, *J Med Virol*, **41**: 196–200.

Thompson KM, Tobin JO'H, 1970, Isolation of rubella virus from abortion material, *Br Med J*, **2**: 264–6.

Thomssen R, Laufs R, Muller J, 1968, Physical properties and

particle size of rubella virus [in German], *Archiv Gesamte Virusforsch*, **23**: 332–45.

Töndury G, Smith DW, 1966, Fetal rubella pathology, *J Pediatr*, **68**: 867–79.

Townsend JJ, Baringer JR et al., 1975, Progressive rubella panencephalitis: late onset after congenital rubella, *N Engl J Med*, **292**: 990–3.

Ueda K, Nishida Y et al., 1975, Seven-year follow-up study of rubella syndrome in Ryuku with special reference to persistence of rubella hemagglutination inhibition antibodies, *Jpn J Microbiol*, **19**: 181–5.

Urquhart GED, Crawford RJ, Wallace J, 1978, Trial of high-titre human rubella immunoglobulin, *Br Med J*, **2**: 1331–2.

Vaheri A, Cristofalo VJ, 1967, Metabolism of rubella virus BHK21 cells, *Arch Gesamte Virusforsch*, **21**: 425–36.

Vaheri A, Hovi T, 1972, Structural proteins and subunits of rubella virus, *J Virol*, **9**: 10–16.

Vejtorp M, Mansa B, 1980, Rubella IgM antibodies in sera from infants born after maternal rubella, later than the 12th week of pregnancy, *Scand J Infect Dis*, **12**: 1–5.

Vesikari T, 1972, Antibody response in rubella reinfection, *J Infect Dis*, **4**: 11–16.

Vesikari T, 1980, Suppression of lymphocyte PHA – responsiveness after rubella vaccination with Cendehill and RA27/3 strains, *Scand J Infect Dis*, **12**: 7–11.

Voiland A, Bardeletti G, 1980, Fatty acid composition of rubella virus and BHK21/13 S infected cells, *Arch Virol*, **64**: 319–28.

Wang CY, Dominguez G, Frey TK, 1994, Construction of rubella virus genome–length cDNA clones and synthesis of infectious RNA transcripts, *J Virol*, **68**: 3550–7.

Waxham MN, Wolinsky JS, 1983, Immunochemical identification of rubella virus haemagglutinin, *Virology*, **126**: 194–203.

Waxham MN, Wolinsky JS, 1984, Rubella virus and its effect in the central nervous system, *Neurol Clin*, **2**: 367–85.

Waxham MN, Wolinsky JS, 1985, A model of the structural organisation of rubella virions, *Rev Infect Dis*, **7, suppl 1**: S133–9.

Weibel RE, Stokes J Jr et al., 1969, Live rubella vaccines in adults and children HPV-77 and Merck–Benoit strains, *Am J Dis Child*, **118**: 226–9.

Weil MJ, Itabashi H, Creamer NE, 1975, Chronic progressive panencephalitis due to rubella virus simulating subacute sclerosing panencephalitis, *N Engl J Med*, **292**: 994–8.

Weller TH, Neva FA, 1962, Propagation in tissue culture of cytopathic agents form patients with rubella-like illness, *Proc Soc Exp Biol Med*, **111**: 215–25.

Wesselhoeft C, 1947a, Rubella (german measles), *N Engl J Med*, **236**: 943–50.

Wesselhoeft C, 1947b, Rubella (german measles), *N Engl J Med*, **236**: 978–88.

Wild NJ, Sheppard S et al., 1990, Delayed detection of congenital hearing loss in high risk infants, *Br Med J*, **301**: 903–5.

Wolinsky JS, 1996, Rubella, *Fields' Virology*, 3rd edn, eds Fields BN, Knipe DM, Howley PM, Lippincott–Raven, Philadelphia PA, 899–929.

Wolinsky JS, Berg BO, Maitland CJ, 1976, Progressive rubella panencephalitis, *Arch Neurol*, **33**: 722–3.

Wolinsky JS, Dau PC et al., 1979, Progressive rubella panencephalitis: immunovirological studies and results of isoprinosine therapy, *Clin Exp Immunol*, **35**: 397–404.

Wolinsky JS, Waxham MN et al., 1982, Immunochemical features of a case of progressive rubella panencephalitis, *Clin Exp Immunol*, **48**: 359–66.

Wolinsky JS, McCarthy M et al., 1991, Monoclonal antibody defined epitope map of expressed rubella virus protein domains, *J Virol*, **65**: 3986–94.

Wolinsky JS, Sukholutsky E et al., 1993, An antibody- and synthetic peptide-defined rubella virus E1 glycoprotein neutralisation domain, *J Virol*, **67**: 961–8.

Zhang T, Mauracher CA et al., 1992, Detection of rubella virus-specific imunoglobulins G (IgG), IgM, and IgA antibodies by immunoblot assays, *J Clin Microbiol*, **30:** 824–30.

Ziring PR, Gallo G et al., 1977, Chronic lymphocytic thyroiditis: identification of rubella virus antigen in the thyroid of a child with congenital rubella, *J Pediatr*, **90:** 419–20.

Zygraich N, Peetermans J, Huygelen C, 1971, In vivo properties of attenuated rubella virus 'Cendehill strain', *Archiv Gesamte Virusforsch*, **33:** 225–33.

Chapter 29

ARBOVIRUSES (*TOGAVIRIDAE* AND *FLAVIVIRIDAE*)

Duane J Gubler and John T Roehrig

1 Basic concepts	3 *Flaviviridae*
2 *Togaviridae*	

1 BASIC CONCEPTS

Most of the viruses described in this chapter are **ar**thropod-**bo**rne, or arboviruses. Such viruses satisfy the criteria established by the World Health Organization (WHO 1967, 1985), which define arboviruses as viruses that are maintained in nature through biological transmission between susceptible vertebrate hosts by haematophagous arthropods. Arboviruses multiply and produce viraemia in the vertebrate, multiply in the tissues of arthropods and are passed on to new vertebrates when the arthropod takes a subsequent blood meal after a period of extrinsic incubation. The term 'arbovirus' has no taxonomic significance and encompasses a heterogeneous group of viruses in 7 taxonomic families, including the *Togaviridae* and *Flaviviridae* (Table 29.1). The International Catalogue of Arboviruses describes 535 viruses and gives their antigenic group, taxonomic status and rating as to whether they are considered arboviruses (Karabatsos 1985). Many of the viruses included in the book are zoonotic viruses that do not require an arthropod vector.

Almost all arbovirus infections are zoonoses. By definition, they have at least 2 hosts, one a vertebrate and the other a haematophagous arthropod species. The majority of arboviruses are maintained in complex life cycles involving a non-human primary vertebrate host and a primary arthropod vector (Fig. 29.1). These cycles remain undetected until humans encroach on the natural enzootic focus, or the virus escapes the primary cycle via a secondary vector or vertebrate host as the result of some ecological change. Humans and domestic animals generally become involved only after the virus is brought into the peridomestic environment by a bridge vector. These vertebrate hosts, which frequently develop clini-

cal illness, are considered 'dead-end' hosts because they do not produce significant viraemia and, therefore, do not contribute to the transmission cycle. Many arboviruses have several different vertebrate hosts and some are capable of transmission by more than one vector. A few arboviruses cause significant viraemia in humans and may be transmitted in a human–arthropod–human cycle (Fig. 29.2). This is generally an epidemic transmission cycle, but with some viruses, such as dengue, it may also be an endemic maintenance cycle. Occasionally, a secondary vector may transmit the virus to other vertebrates, which are usually dead-end hosts. In both types of transmission cycles, maintenance of the viruses in nature may be facilitated by transovarial transmission, in which the virus passes from the female through the eggs to the offspring. The significance of transovarial transmission or whether it occurs is not known for most arboviruses.

Arboviruses have a global distribution, but the majority are found in tropical developing countries. The greatest number of viruses has been described from Africa and South America, where the flora and fauna are diverse and extensive studies have been conducted. The smaller number of viruses described from Asia, which has ecological diversity comparable to Africa and tropical America, may simply reflect the lack of studies conducted in that region. The geographical distribution of each arbovirus is limited by the ecological parameters governing its transmission cycle. Important limiting factors include temperature, rainfall patterns, distribution of the arthropod vector and vertebrate reservoir host.

The majority of arbovirus infections in humans cause a febrile illness with no specific features. Onset is usually sudden with fever, headache, myalgias, malaise and occasionally prostration. Infection with some arboviruses may lead to more severe haemorrhagic dis-

Table 29.1 Relationship between antigenic groups and the taxonomic status of arboviruses

Family	Genus	Approximate number[a] of possible or definitive arboviruses
Bunyaviridae	*Bunyavirus*	137
	Phlebovirus	37
	Nairovirus	24
	Uukuvirus	6
	Hantavirus	2
	Unassigned (*Bunyavirus*-like)	42
Flaviviridae	*Flavivirus*	61
Reoviridae	*Orbivirus*	69
	Coltivirus	2
	Unassigned	6
Rhabdoviridae	*Vesiculovirus*	18
	Lyssavirus	15
	Unassigned	18
Togoviridae	*Alphavirus*	27
	Ungrouped	1
Arenaviridae	*Arenavirus*	4
Coronaviridae	?	1
Herpesviridae	?	1
Poxviridae	...	1
Orthomyxoviridae	...	2
Unclassified	?	10

[a]These figures exclude viruses that are known or suspected to have no arthropod vector.

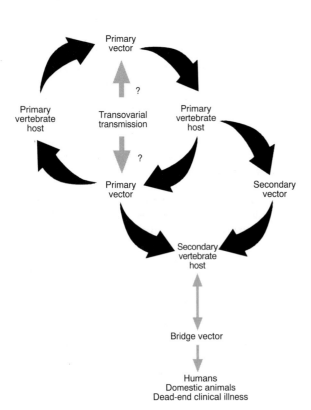

Fig. 29.1 Generalized arbovirus maintenance cycle.

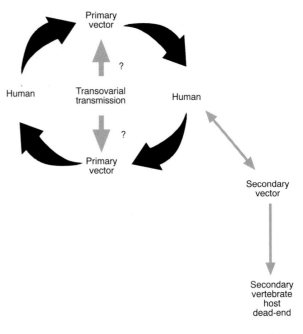

Fig. 29.2 Epidemic/maintenance arbovirus cycle involving humans as the primary vertebrate host.

ease or encephalitis, often with a fatal outcome or permanent neurological sequelae. The same virus may produce different syndromes in different subjects. The illnesses often follow a biphasic course. Mild fever, which is often unrecognized, occurs during the initial viraemic stage, and is followed by a much more serious illness during which viraemia may be masked by the host's immune response. Often only a small proportion of people infected with potentially encephalitic arboviruses progress to overt encephalitis; most patients develop only the first stage of the infection, which may even be asymptomatic.

Mosquitoes are the most important arbovirus vectors, followed by ticks, sandflies (phlebotomines) and midges *(Culicoides)*. Bedbugs *(Cimicidae)* are also involved in the transmission of some arboviruses. Although the great majority of arbovirus infections of humans follow exposure to the bite of an arthropod, infection may follow ingestion of infected cow's or goat's milk, inhalation of infected secretions, accidentally produced aerosols, or close contact with infected secretions or blood. Monath (1988) has edited a 5-volume compilation on arboviruses and their epidemiology and ecology. More recently, the major arboviral diseases have been reviewed in the second edition of the *Handbook of Zoonoses* (Beran et al. 1994).

2 *TOGAVIRIDAE*

2.1 Properties of the viruses

This family of enveloped, positive-stranded RNA viruses contains many agents responsible for important diseases in animals and humans. Members of the genus *Alphavirus* are arthropod-borne, principally by mosquitoes, whereas members of other genera (*Arterivirus, Rubivirus*) are not arboviruses but are transmitted both horizontally and vertically between vertebrate hosts, frequently causing congenital malformations after transplacental infection. Several alphaviruses are also capable of transovarial transmission in mosquitoes. The family name is derived from the Latin 'toga', a Roman mantle or cloak, a reference to the viral envelope.

CLASSIFICATION

The classification of the *Togaviridae* has changed substantially since the family was first defined, and further changes are expected in the near future. The family was initially established with 2 genera, *Alphavirus* (previously group A arboviruses) and *Flavivirus* (previously group B arboviruses) (Wildy 1971). Later, the genera *Pestivirus* and *Rubivirus* were added (Fenner 1976). When it was recognized that there are fundamental differences in the molecular biology of alphaviruses and flaviviruses, the latter were assigned to a new family, the *Flaviviridae* (Westaway et al. 1985a). At the same time, a new genus *Arterivirus* was added to the *Togaviridae*, restoring the number of genera to 4 (Westaway et al. 1985b). More recently, pestiviruses have been reclassified in the *Flaviviridae* (Horzinek and van Berlo 1987, Renard et al. 1987, Collett, Moennig and Horzinek 1989). Arterivirus classification is also in transition. Although they are positive single-stranded RNA viruses similar in size to alphaviruses and rubella virus, their replication strategy is more like that of coronaviruses. These viruses may soon be reclassified into their own family.

The genus *Rubivirus* contains only a single member, rubella virus, which is the subject of Chapter 28 and is not considered further here, except to note that its molecular biology is very like that of the alphaviruses.

All medically important vector-borne togaviruses are members of the *Alphavirus* genus. This genus has been serologically divided into at least 6 complexes, the prototypes of which are western equine encephalitis (WEE), eastern equine encephalitis (EEE), Venezuelan equine encephalitis (VEE), Semliki Forest (SF), Middelburg and Ndumu viruses. Recent gene sequencing studies have suggested, however, that WEE, Highlands J and Fort Morgan are recombinant New World alphaviruses whose glycoproteins were derived from a Sindbis-like virus, the rest of the genome being derived from an EEE-like virus (Hahn et al. 1988). These genetic studies suggest only 3 clearly defined virus groups: a VEE/EEE group, a SF group (including Middelburg virus), and a Sindbis (SIN) group. The genetic classification of the recombinant alphaviruses and Ndumu and Buggy Creek is less clear. An excellent review on the molecular biology of alphaviruses has recently been published (Strauss and Strauss 1994).

MORPHOLOGY AND VIRION STRUCTURE

Virions of all members have an external diameter of 50–70 nm, including the lipid envelope; lipid constitutes 26% of the weight of alphaviruses, and carbohydrate 6%. Sedimentation coefficients differ with different genera; densities are 1.17–1.19 g^{-1} ml^{-1} in sucrose for alphaviruses and rubivirus; arteriviruses occupy an intermediate position. Icosahedral symmetry is clearly defined only for alphaviruses, in which the envelope glycoproteins are arranged in trimers in a T = 4 icosahedral surface lattice (von Bonsdorff and Harrison 1978, Harrison 1986, Vogel et al. 1986).

GENOME STRUCTURE AND FUNCTION

Complete or partial genome sequences are available for many alphaviruses, including representatives from each major serological or genetic complex (Strauss and Strauss 1994). The genome of alphaviruses is a molecule of single-stranded positive-sense RNA almost 12 000 nucleotides in length, which is capped at the 5′ end and polyadenylated at the 3′ end. The naked RNA is infectious and has a sedimentation coefficient of 42–49S. The genome is organized into 2 distinct regions, the 5′ two-thirds encoding the non-structural proteins and the 3′ one-third encoding the structural proteins (Fig. 29). The structural proteins are translated from a 26S subgenomic messenger RNA. The base composition is: A, 28.3%; U, 20.8%; G, 24.8.%; and C, 26.1%.

The complete nucleotide sequence of the positive-sense, single-stranded genomic RNA has been derived for 2 strains of lactic dehydrogenase-elevating virus (Godney et al. 1993, Palmer et al. 1995), equine anaemia virus (den Boon et al. 1991), and porcine reproductive and respiratory syndrome virus (Meulenberg et al. 1993). The genomes range in size from 12.7 to 15.1 kb.

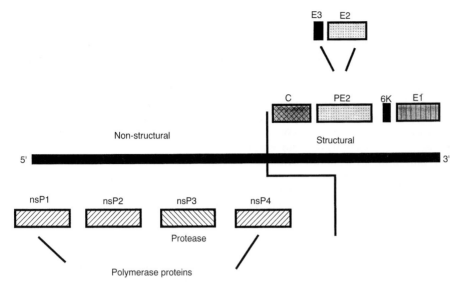

Fig. 29.3 *Alphavirus* genome organization.

POLYPEPTIDES: STRUCTURAL AND NON-STRUCTURAL

The 26S subgenomic RNA of alphaviruses is translated into a polyprotein, which is cleaved to form the structural proteins, namely the capsid protein C (30–34 kDa) and the envelope glycoproteins E1 and E2 (50–59 kDa). The 3-dimensional structure of a crystal of the SIN virus capsid protein has been solved at a 0.3 nm resolution (Choi et al. 1991, Tong et al. 1993). The C protein (260–270 amino acids in length) associates with the virion RNA to form the virus nucleocapsid. The diameter of the nucleocapsid is about 40 nm and contains 240 copies of the C protein in T = 4 triangulation. It is believed that the surface of the nucleocapsid interacts with the hydrophilic tail of the surface glycoprotein E2 during virus assembly. This association is further supported by the 1:1 ratio of C protein to envelope glycoproteins. The E1 (438–442 amino acids in length) and E2 (420–424 amino acids in length) associate as heterodimers. These heterodimers associate as trimers in the virion envelope. An additional envelope glycoprotein, E3 (10 kDa), which is derived from the cleavage of the precursor of the E2 glycoprotein (PE2), is associated with the SF virion. Recently the 6 kDa (6K) protein, which is derived from the E1 glycoprotein signal sequence, also has been associated with the SIN virus particle (Gaedigk-Nitschko and Schlesinger 1990).

The non-structural proteins are translated from a messenger RNA (that is indistinguishable from the genomic RNA) to yield polyproteins, which are cleaved to the final 4 non-structural proteins, nsP1, nsP2, nsP3 and nsP4. It is believed that the non-structural proteins are functional as both polyproteins and individual proteins during virus replication. All 4 non-structural proteins seem to be involved in RNA synthesis. The C terminal domain of the nsP2 seems also to be a virus-specific protease involved in the cleavage of the non-structural proteins.

Arteriviruses have 4 structural proteins, a nucleocapsid or core protein (VP1, or N, mol. wt 12–14 kDa) and 3 envelope proteins. The primary envelope glycoprotein, VP3, has a mol. wt of 30–42 kDa and is c. 255 amino acids long. There is also a non-glycosylated envelope protein (VP2, or M, mol. wt 18–19 kDa) and a minor envelope glycoprotein (Faaberg et al. 1995).

ANTIGENS

Because of their close association, the E1 and E2 share a number of biological functions and antigenic properties. The glycoprotein spike functions both in adsorption to cellular receptors and in fusion of cellular membranes. These proteins are primary in eliciting virus-neutralizing antibody and haemagglutination-inhibiting antibody. The E2 glycoprotein elicits high-titre, virus-specific, neutralizing antibody. Two domains capable of eliciting virus-neutralizing antibody have been identified in the E2 glycoprotein: amino acids 114–120, and amino acids 180–220 (or 230–250 for Ross River (RR) virus) using monoclonal antibody neutralization escape variants and rapid penetration variants (Johnson et al. 1990). Antibodies to the carboxyl-proximal domain neutralize virus infectivity by blocking virion attachment to susceptible cells (Roehrig and Hunt 1988). Antibodies to the E2 glycoprotein can also block virus haemagglutination, presumably because of its close association with E1. The amino terminal 25 amino acids of the VEE virus E2 glycoprotein protect mice from virus challenge (Hunt and Roehrig 1995). Mutations in the E2 glycoprotein have been associated with changes in virulence and ability to grow in mosquitoes (Woodward et al. 1991, Kinney et al. 1993).

The E1 glycoprotein contains a highly conserved amino acid sequence (amino acids 80–96), which has sequence and chemical similarities to regions responsible for cell membrane fusion in orthomyxoviruses and paramyxoviruses. Mutation of this region alters the fusion characteristics of the virus (Levy-Mintz and Kielian 1991). Because cell-membrane fusion seems, therefore, to be mediated by the E1 glycoprotein, it is not surprising that this glycoprotein elicits potent haemagglutination-inhibiting antibody. Virus-neutralizing anti-E1 antibodies have also been identified. Binding of these antibodies has been associated with E1 amino acid 132 using monoclonal antibody neutralization escape variants (Strauss et al. 1991). Anti-E1 antibodies are usually not serotype specific, and fix complement well.

Many of the biologically important epitopes on both the E1 and the E2 glycoproteins are conformational. This result makes mimicking these antigens in subunit or peptide vaccines difficult (Hunt et al. 1990). The C protein elicits broadly cross-reactive antibody and is also a major complement-fixing antigen.

The major glycoprotein, VP3, of arteriviruses elicits virus-neutralizing antibodies (Brinton-Darnell and Plagemann 1975).

REPLICATION

Studies on the replication strategy of alphaviruses have been facilitated by the derivation of full-length infectious cDNA clones for SIN, VEE, SF and RR viruses (Rice et al. 1987, Davis et al. 1989, Kuhn et al. 1991, Liljestrom et al. 1991, Kinney et al. 1993). Alphavirus infection is initiated by virion attachment to cellular receptors. Recent studies using a variety of techniques, including generation of anti-idiotypic antibodies, have identified the laminin receptor as a SIN virus receptor on baby hamster kidney (BHK-21) cells (Wang et al. 1992). Laminin receptor does not seem to be the major SIN virus receptor on chicken cells, however. After endocytosis, the capsid is apparently released into the cell cytoplasm by low-pH catalysed membrane fusion, presumably mediated by the E1 glycoprotein.

Two major RNA species are detectable in cells infected with alphaviruses. One, which sediments at 49S (SIN virus) or 42S (SF virus), is identical to genomic RNA; the other, at 26S, represents the subgenomic RNA identical with the 3' third of the genome. The parental RNA is first translated from the 5' end of the genome to yield the 4 non-structural proteins in the order 5'–nsP1–nsP2–nsP3–nsP4. The parental genome is copied to a full-length minus-strand with poly(U) at its 5' end. The minus strand serves as a template for the synthesis of 42–49S RNA in membrane-bound replicative intermediate structures. In addition to this full-length RNA, a 3' co-terminal subgenomic 26S mRNA, which encodes the structural proteins C–E3–E2–6K–E1–3', is synthesized by internal initiation (Strauss, Rice and Strauss 1984, Kääriäinen et al. 1987). Both positive-strand RNA forms are capped and methylated as they are synthesized. The non-structural proteins are translated as 2 precursor polyproteins, which are subsequently cleaved, one to form nsP1, nsP2 and nsP3, and the other nsP4.

The structural proteins are also formed by cleavage of a precursor polyprotein. The C protein is an autoprotease that releases itself from the nascent polypeptide chain. Insertion of the envelope glycoproteins into the cellular membrane is mediated by signal sequences (E3 for the E2 glycoprotein and 6K for the E1 glycoprotein). The E2 glycoprotein is synthesized as a precursor protein, PE2, which is presumably cleaved by a membrane-bound cellular serine protease related to bacterial subtilisins and similar or identical to the mammalian furin-like proteases (Barr 1991).

After the formation of the nucleocapsid, it is believed that the association of the virus core with the hydrophilic tail of the E2 glycoprotein drives the virus budding process. In mammalian cells, virus buds from the plasma membrane; however, in invertebrate cells virus buds into cytoplasmic vesicles. Alphaviruses rapidly produce cytopathic effects in virus-infected cells. The virus shuts down host cell macromolecular synthesis, and infected cells eventually die by a mechanism indistinguishable from apoptosis (Levine et al. 1993).

The replication of arteriviruses is poorly understood. Their genomic organization is most like that of the coronaviruses. The genome encodes 9 open reading frames (ORFs) and produces a nested set of 6 or 7 3' co-terminal subgenomic RNAs during infection. ORFs 1a and 1b encode the viral protease, replicase and helicase (den Boon et al. 1995). ORF5 encodes the major envelope glycoprotein VP3. ORF6 encodes VP2 (M), and ORF7 encodes the nucleocapsid protein, VP1 (N). ORF2 encodes a minor envelope protein. The coding assignments of ORFs 3 and 4 are unknown. As with the pestiviruses, the envelope proteins VP2 (M) and VP3 appear to associate by disulphide bridging that is required for virus infectivity (Faaberg et al. 1995).

2.2 Clinical and pathological aspects

Of the 27 currently described alphaviruses, at least 13 are known to cause disease in humans (Table 29.2), and Babanki virus has been isolated from human serum in the Cameroons, although without any association with disease. The pestiviruses cause hog cholera in pigs, mucosal disease and virus diarrhoea in bovine species, and border disease in sheep. Arteriviruses are responsible for disease in equine, murine and porcine species.

DISEASE CAUSED BY ALPHAVIRUSES: GENERAL FEATURES

Clinical manifestations

The syndromes associated with alphavirus infections in humans include undifferentiated febrile illness, fever with a rash, arthritis or arthralgia or encephalitis. The same virus can cause a variety of clinical syndromes. Some alphaviruses are responsible for disease in animals, notably *Equidae*.

Epizootiology and arthropod vectors

Every alphavirus has its own distinct epizootiology. For some, such as EEE and WEE viruses, birds are the principal natural reservoir host, but for many the maintenance host is not known with certainty. Several, including Chikungunya, EEE, WEE, VEE and SIN viruses, have been isolated from bats. All alphaviruses infecting humans are mosquito-borne. Middelburg virus has also been isolated from *Amblyomma variega-*

Table 29.2 List of alphaviruses

Virus	Geographical distribution	Other features
Aura	Brazil, Argentina	
Babanki	W & C Africa	
Barmah Forest[a]	Australia	Epidemics, Australia
Bebaru	Malaysia	
Bijou Bridge	USA	
Buggy Creek	Australia	
Cabassou	French Guiana	
Chikungunya[a]	Tropical Africa, S & SE Asia, Philippines	Epidemics, E Africa, Asia
Eastern encephalitis[a]	N & C America, Trinidad, Guyana, Brazil, Argentina	Epizootics, N America only
Everglades[a]	Florida	
Fort Morgan[b]	Western USA	
Getah	Malaysia, Japan, Australia, Cambodia, Philippines	One epizootic, Japan
Highlands J	Florida, eastern USA	
Igbo-Ora[a]	W & C Africa	
Kyzylagach	Azerbaijan SSR, former USSR	
Mayaro[a]	Trinidad, Brazil	
Middelburg	S, W & C Africa	
Mucambo	Brazil, Trinidad, Surinam	
Ndumu	S, W & C Africa	
Ockelbo[a]	Scandinavia, W (former) USSR	Epidemics, Sweden
O'nyong-nyong[a]	E & W Africa, Zimbabwe	Epidemics, E Africa, Zimbabwe
Pixuna	Brazil	
Ross River[a]	Australasia, South Pacific	Polyarthritis, epidemics Australia, S Pacific
Sagiyama	Japan, Okinawa	
Semliki Forest[a]	Africa	1 laboratory case Epidemic in Central African Republic
Sindbis[a]	Africa, E Mediterranean, S & SE Asia, Borneo, Philippines, Australia, Sicily	
Tonate	French Guiana, Surinam	
Una	Brazil, Colombia, Panama, Surinam, French Guiana, Trinidad	
Venezuelan encephalitis[a]	Venezuela, Colombia, S and C America	Mucambo also infects humans
Western encephalitis[a]	N America, Mexico, Guyana, Brazil, Argentina	Epizootics, N America only
Whataroa	New Zealand	
Zingilamo	Central African Republic	

[a]Known to cause human disease.
[b]This virus is carried by *Cimicidae*; the vectors for all others in this Table are mosquitoes.

tum ticks in South Africa. Chikungunya and SIN viruses have also been isolated from ticks. The principal arthropod vectors are discussed under individual viruses.

Pathogenesis

Experimental studies have shown that invasion of the central nervous system (CNS), when this occurs, generally follows initial virus replication in various peripheral sites and a period of viraemia. Entry to the CNS through the olfactory tract has been suggested, but the importance of this route is in question. RR and Chikungunya viruses are believed to replicate in striated muscle.

Immune response

Alphaviruses are highly immunogenic, and both cellular and humoral immune mechanisms contribute to recovery following natural or experimental infection.

Diagnosis

Alphavirus infections are diagnosed on the basis of both immunoglobulin M (IgM) and immunoglobulin G (IgG) serological responses. Isolation of virus from acute-phase serum is possible with some infections, but alphaviruses are seldom recovered from the CNS, including the cerebrospinal fluid (CSF), except from fatal cases. A large array of anti-alphavirus murine monoclonal antibodies are available for virus identification (Roehrig 1986).

Control

The interruption of transmission by mosquito control provides the only effective approach to the control of alphavirus infections. Equine vaccines are available for EEE, WEE and VEE, and under an investigational new drug permit for humans in high-risk jobs.

2.3 Encephalitis and other important *Alphavirus* diseases

EASTERN EQUINE ENCEPHALITIS

EEE virus occurs in focal locations along the eastern seaboard, the Gulf coast and some inland midwestern locations of the USA, and in Canada, some Caribbean Islands, and Central and South America (Morris 1988, Gibbs and Tsai 1994). Small outbreaks of human disease have occurred in the USA, the Dominican Republic, Cuba and Jamaica. Equine epizootics are common occurrences during the summer in coastal regions bordering the Atlantic and Gulf of Mexico, and in other eastern and midwestern states of the USA, and as far north as Quebec, Ontario and Alberta in Canada. Two distinct antigenic variants (North American and South American) of EEE virus have been isolated; however, North American strains of EEE virus are genetically quite stable (Roehrig et al. 1990).

EEE virus is maintained in nature in an enzootic cycle involving birds and *Culiseta melanura*, a mosquito that is found in swamp areas that support cedar, red maple and loblolly bay trees. The larval habitat of *C. melanura* is water collected at the base of trees in swampy, peat soils. The virus escapes from enzootic foci in swamp areas by bridge vectors such as *Coquilletidia perturbans* and *Aedes sollicitans*. These species feed on both birds and mammals and can transmit the virus to humans, horses and other hosts. Other species such as *Ae. vexans* in temperate regions and *Ae. taeniorhynchus*, *Culex taeniopus* and *Cx. nigripalpus* in the tropics are involved in transmission to humans and equines. A recent isolation of EEE virus from *Ae. albopictus* in Florida is of concern because this mosquito species has catholic blood-feeding habits, feeding aggressively on a variety of animals as well as humans, thus potentially increasing the risk of human infection if it becomes involved in the transmission cycle.

The incubation period for EEE in humans is 4–10 days. Onset of illness is sudden, with fever, malaise, headache, photophobia, nausea, vomiting, abdominal pain and myalgias followed by confusion, delirium, drowsiness and ultimately coma. Patients may have other neurological disorders such as abnormal reflexes, spasticity, paralysis and cranial nerve palsies. Infants may have convulsions and bulging fontanelles. The CSF is under pressure, has elevated protein and pleocytosis is common. Death may occur in 3–5 days after onset. Outcome and the occurrence of neurological sequelae are age-related. Sequelae are more common in children and include convulsions, paralysis and mental retardation. Older patients usually recover more completely. A fatal outcome occurs in 30–70% of cases, the fatality rates being highest in the elderly (c. 70%) and the lowest in young adults (c. 30%).

Vaccine is not available for general human use, although a formalin-inactivated vaccine prepared in chick embryos has been found to be effective in horses.

WESTERN EQUINE ENCEPHALITIS

WEE virus was first isolated in California in 1930 from the brain of a horse with encephalitis, and remains an important cause of encephalitis in *Equidae* and in humans in North America, mainly in western parts of the USA and Canada (Chamberlain 1987, Hardy 1987, Reeves 1987, Iversen 1994). Sporadic cases also occur in Central and South America. In the western United States, the enzootic cycle of WEE involves passerine birds, in which the infection is inapparent, and culicine mosquitoes, principally *Culex tarsalis*, a species that is associated with agriculture and irrigation systems. The virus has also been isolated from snakes (Gebhardt et al. 1964, Thomas et al. 1980) and from a variety of mammal species. Other important mosquito vector species include *Culiseta inornata, Ae. vexans* and *Ae. melanimon*. WEE virus was isolated from field-collected larvae of the last-named species, providing the first evidence that transovarial transmission may play an important role in the maintenance cycle of an alphavirus (Fulhorst et al. 1994).

Human cases are usually first seen in June or July in the northern hemisphere. Most WEE infections are asymptomatic or present as mild, non-specific illness. Patients with clinically apparent illness usually have a sudden onset with fever, headache, nausea, vomiting, anorexia and malaise, followed by altered mental status, weakness and signs of meningeal irritation. The CSF shows a pleocytosis. Children, especially those under 1 year old, are affected more severely than adults and may be left with permanent sequelae, which is seen in 5–10% of patients. The mortality is about 3%.

Strains of WEE virus seem to be relatively homogeneous by oligonucleotide fingerprinting and are clearly different from the serologically related Highlands J virus (Trent and Grant 1980, Hunt and Roehrig 1985).

VENEZUELAN EQUINE ENCEPHALITIS

VEE virus was first isolated in Venezuela in 1938 from the brain of a horse; like EEE and WEE viruses, it causes encephalitis in *Equidae* and humans. VEE is an important veterinary and public health problem in Central and South America. Focal outbreaks occur periodically, but, occasionally, there are large regional epizootics with thousands of equine cases and deaths. A large epizootic that began in Peru in 1969 reached Texas in 1971. It was estimated that over 200 000 horses died in that outbreak, which was controlled by a massive equine vaccination programme using the live attenuated TC-83 vaccine (Report 1972). There were several thousand human infections. A more recent VEE epidemic occurred in the fall of 1995 in Venezuela and Colombia, with an estimated 75 000 human infections.

Infection of humans is less severe than with EEE and WEE viruses, and fatalities are rare. Adults usually develop only an influenza-like illness; overt encephalitis is usually confined to children.

Six antigenic subtypes of VEE virus are now recognized. Subtype I is subdivided into 5 variants, IAB-IF (Calisher et al. 1980, 1985, Kinney, Trent and France 1983). Subtypes II–V include previously named viruses (II=Everglades, III= Mucambo, Tonate and Paramana, IV=Pixuna, V=Cabassou), and VI is an un-named isolate from Argentina (Ag80–663). Only subtypes I and II are associated with encephalitis in humans; Mucambo virus has been recognized as a cause of a febrile illness in humans, but the remaining subtypes are not known to be associated with human disease. VEE virus isolates have a common C protein, but show heterogeneity in the molecular weight of envelope glycoproteins (Wiebe and Scherer 1980, Kinney, Trent and France 1983) on which at least 7 epitopes have been defined (Mathews and Roehrig 1982, Roehrig and Mathews 1985).

Enzootic strains (subtypes ID, IE and IF) of VEE virus have a wide geographic distribution in the Americas. These viruses are maintained in cycles involving forest-dwelling rodents and mosquito vectors (probably *Culex* spp.). Occasional cases or small outbreaks of human disease are associated with these viruses. The most recent were outbreaks in Peru caused by subtype ID in 1994, and in Mexico (subtype IE) in 1993 and 1996. The epizootic IC strain, for which *Equidae* are the primary amplification hosts, was the aetiological agent of the 1995 epidemic in Venezuela and Colombia. The natural reservoir host for the epizootic strains is not known.

Chikungunya

Chikungunya virus was first isolated from patients and mosquitoes during an epidemic in the Newala district of Tanzania in 1952/53. The native name, which means 'doubled up', is derived from the main symptom of excruciating joint pains. Chikungunya virus has frequently been isolated from humans and mosquitoes during epidemics in India, southeast Asia, southeast Africa and sub-Saharan Africa. The largest epidemics in recent years have been in India and Indonesia.

After an incubation period of 2–4 days, there is a sudden onset of fever and crippling joint pains, which may incapacitate the patient, accompanied by chills, flushed face, headache, myalgias, backache, photophobia, and rash in c. 80% of patients. There may be conjunctival injection, and patients often have anorexia and constipation. The acute phase of illness lasts for 2–4 days with recovery in 5–7 days; the fever may be biphasic. Arthralgia is the most striking sign or symptom, occurring in c. 70% of cases. The areas affected include the metacarpophalangeal joints, wrists, elbows, shoulders, knees, ankles and metatarsal joints. Arthralgia may affect one or several joints. Reddening and swelling may occur, and arthralgias may persist for months in a small proportion of cases. The clinical picture resembles that of dengue fever, with which it is often confused (Carey 1971). Differential

diagnosis should include dengue, SIN and West Nile viruses.

In India and southeast Asia, Chikungunya virus has been implicated in outbreaks of haemorrhagic fever, often in association with dengue viruses. A careful review of the clinical presentation of Chikungunya virus infection in Asia, however, suggests that, although mild haemorrhagic manifestations may occur in a small proportion of cases, Chikungunya is not a cause of severe haemorrhagic disease. Haemorrhagic complications have not been reported in association with Chikungunya infections in Africa.

Chikungunya virus is transmitted in Africa by *Ae. africanus* and *Ae. aegypti*, whereas, *Ae. aegypti* transmits the disease in urban centres of India and southeast Asia. No vertebrate host other than humans has been discovered, although McIntosh et al. (1963) found evidence that monkeys might be maintenance hosts in Africa.

O'nyong-nyong

This virus caused a major epidemic that began in Uganda in 1959 and quickly spread to Kenya, Tanzania and Malawi, affecting an estimated 2 million people. The virus is closely related to Chikungunya virus, and the diseases produced by the 2 agents are very similar. However, O'nyong-nyong virus has a geographically limited distribution in East Africa and is transmitted by *Anopheles gambiae* and *An. funestus* mosquitoes, both of which also transmit malaria.

Ross River fever

Epidemics of benign polyarthritis have been recognized in Australia since 1927, but the causative agent, RR virus, was not isolated until 1963 (Nimmo 1928, Doherty, Carley and Best 1972). Epidemics of polyarthritis involving several thousand cases have occurred regularly in Australia, and currently the virus is endemic in most coastal regions of the country as well as inland, especially along waterways and rivers. Since the early 1980s, RR virus has expanded its geographic distribution into the Pacific, with outbreaks in New Guinea, Fiji, American Samoa, Raratonga, Tonga and New Caledonia. The natural maintenance cycle of RR virus is not known for sure. Serological surveys suggest that a diverse group of wild and domestic animals may be involved as reservoir hosts (Aaskov and Doherty 1994, Mackenzie et al. 1994). Humans have significant viraemia, and the virus in some epidemics has been maintained in a human–mosquito–human transmission cycle (Rosen, Gubler and Bennett 1981). In coastal regions, *Ae. vigilax* in the north and *Ae. camptorhynchus* in the south and west are important mosquito vectors. *Culex annulirostris* is also considered an important vector in Australia. In the Pacific islands, *Ae. polynesiensis*, *Ae. vigilax* and *Ae. aegypti* are important vectors (Gubler 1981, Rosen, Gubler and Bennett 1981, Mackenzie et al. 1994). The incubation period of RR virus is 2–21 days; the illness is generally mild. Patients with polyarthritis present with fever, arthralgia of the small joints of the hands and feet, maculopapular rash, paraesthesiae of the palms and the soles, myalgia, lethargy and headache. The painful arthritis frequently persists for several weeks, occasionally for a year or more, but recovery is complete and no fatalities have been reported. Women are affected more often than men, and children less commonly than adolescents or adults (Mudge and Aaskov 1983). There seems to be an association between clinical illness and the class II MHC antigen HLA-DR7 (Fraser et al. 1980).

No vaccine is available. Prevention and control measures are directed at the mosquito population, and at health education on how to protect against mosquito bites.

OTHER *ALPHAVIRUS* INFECTIONS

Barmah Forest virus

Isolated in Australia from *Cx. annulirostris* mosquitoes, this virus was initially placed in the family *Bunyaviridae*, but later tests established it as an *Alphavirus* (Dalgarno et al. 1984). It cross-reacts with other alphaviruses by haemaglutination-inhibition tests, but is distinct by complement-fixation and neutralization tests. Human infection with Barmah Forest virus was first reported in 1986, and the first epidemic of human disease occurred in 1992 in the Northern Territory (Mackenzie et al. 1994). Clinically, Barmah Forest virus causes a Ross River-like illness, but generally milder and with a higher frequency of rash and a lower frequency of arthralgias.

Little is known of the natural history of Barmah Forest virus but the virus has been isolated from several mosquito species; *Cx. annulirostris* appears to be the most widespread. It is interesting that Barmah Forest virus has also been isolated from *Culicoides marksi* in the Northern Territory (Standfast et al. 1984, Mackenzie et al. 1994).

Getah virus

This virus was originally isolated in Malaysia from *Cx. gelidus* mosquitoes and *Cx. tritaeniorhynchus*. It is closely related to Sagiyama, Bebaru and RR viruses, which are considered to be subtypes of Getah (Calisher et al. 1980). Getah virus is found throughout southeast Asia, including Japan, the Philippines and Australia, but serological cross-reaction with RR virus makes interpretation of serosurvey data difficult. Getah virus has not been associated with human disease, but has caused severe enzootic encephalitis in horses in Japan (Kamada et al. 1980).

Mayaro virus

Mayaro virus is closely related to Chikungunya and O'nyong-nyong viruses and causes a similar illness. Isolated first in Trinidad from human serum in 1954, it was subsequently isolated from humans in Brazil, Bolivia and Surinam. Serological surveys also suggest that it occurs in Guyana, Colombia, Peru, Panama and Costa Rica (Pinheiro and Travassos da Rosa 1994). Little is known about the natural history of Mayaro virus, but it has been isolated numerous times from *Haemagogus* spp. mosquitoes, suggesting a monkey–*Haemagogus* spp.–monkey maintenance cycle (Pinheiro and Travassos da Rosa 1994).

Igbo-Ora

This virus is also related to Chikungunya and O'nyong-nyong viruses and causes a similar clinical illness in humans in Nigeria, the Central African Republic and the Ivory Coast (Olaleye and Fagbami 1988).

Sindbis

Sindbis virus has been designated as the prototype *Alphavirus*. It was originally isolated in Egypt (Taylor et al. 1956) but has a wide distribution in Africa, India, tropical Asia, Australia and Europe. It rarely causes overt disease but has been associated with febrile illnesses in Africa (McIntosh et al. 1976) and India. SIN virus has a number of variants that have caused outbreaks of human illness in Sweden (Ockelbo disease), Finland (Pogosta disease), Russia (Karelian fever) and West and Central Africa (Babanki). A single case with haemorrhagic manifestations and joint pains has been reported from Australia (Guard et al. 1982). SIN virus is maintained in enzootic cycles involving a variety of birds and mosquito species of the genera *Culex*, *Aedes* and *Culiseta*.

Ockelbo   This SIN-related virus has been identified as the cause of a mosquito-borne fever characterized by rash. The disease is described under the names of Ockelbo disease in Scandinavia (Niklasson et al. 1984), Pogosta disease in Finland (Brummer-Korvenkontio and Kuusisto 1981) and Karelian fever in the USSR (Lvov et al. 1984).

Semliki Forest virus

Semliki Forest (SF) virus was isolated from *Aedes* mosquitoes collected in the course of yellow fever field studies in Uganda (Smithburn and Haddow 1944). The virus has been used widely in laboratory studies and was regarded as non-pathogenic until it caused a single, fatal infection in a laboratory worker (Willems et al. 1979). Antibodies to SF virus are commonly found in human serum collected from both East and West Africa, but no overt disease was recognized until 1987 when it caused a large outbreak of mild febrile illness in Bangui, Central African Republic. SF virus may be maintained in a monkey–*Ae. africanus*–monkey cycle (Jupp 1994).

2.4   Arterivirus infections

EQUINE ARTERITIS VIRUS

Equine arteritis virus causes disease in equine species. It multiplies in the smooth muscle cell of the small arteries, thus causing tissue necrosis; it also causes abortion in mares (Horzinek 1981).

LACTATE DEHYDROGENASE ELEVATING VIRUS

This virus infects both wild and domestic mice, *Mus musculus*, and also *Mus caroli*, but not other murine species. Macrophages are infected via Fc receptors by infectious antibody–virus complexes. Infection results in persistent, life-long viraemia. Serum titres of the enzyme lactate dehydrogenase are elevated 5–10-fold following infection, which gives the virus its name (Rowson and Mahy 1985). The rise in serum enzymes seems to be due to reduced clearance and may mean that primary sites of virus infection are the liver Kupffer cells.

SIMIAN HAEMORRHAGIC FEVER VIRUS

Simian haemorrhagic fever virus has caused major disease in at least 5 different primate centres, principally affecting Macaca monkeys. *Cercopithecus aethiops* and *Erythrocebus patas* monkeys and baboons (*Papio papio*) have silent infections and are probably the source of infection for rhesus monkeys held within the same colony (London 1977).

SWINE INFERTILITY AND RESPIRATORY SYNDROME VIRUS

This virus, first reported in the USA in 1987, has since been recognized in Europe, where it is most commonly known as Lelystad virus, the cause of porcine epidemic abortion and respiratory syndrome (Meulenberg et al. 1993). Swine are the only known host. Infection causes reproductive failure, pneumonia in piglets and increase preweaning mortality. At least 4 virus genotypes occur in the USA and Europe.

3 FLAVIVIRIDAE

3.1 Properties of the viruses

This family of enveloped, positive-strand RNA viruses contains over 70 members, of which about 50 are arthropod-borne; many are pathogenic for humans and other vertebrates. The family name is derived from that of the type species, yellow fever (YF) virus (Latin: *flavus* = yellow).

CLASSIFICATION

The family *Flaviviridae* contains 3 genera: *Flavivirus, Pestivirus* and hepatitis C viruses. All members of the *Flavivirus* genus are antigenically related. Cross-reactions are most evident by haemagglutination and haemagglutination-inhibition tests, and plaque reduction neutralization tests showing the greatest specificity. Seven subgroups or complexes were defined on the basis of cross-neutralization tests (de Madrid and Porterfield 1974), and this subdivision has recently been substantially confirmed and extended in a more comprehensive study (Calisher et al. 1989). Flaviviruses can also be divided into 3 biological subsets based on their mode of transmission, by mosquitoes or ticks, or by having no known arthropod vector. Table 29.3 shows the relationship between the subgroups determined by the plaque reduction neutralization test and the mode of transmission of currently named flaviviruses.

Three pathogens of farm animals – hog cholera virus or classic swine fever virus, bovine viral diarrhoea virus and border disease virus – constitute the *Pestivirus* genus. The *Ae. albopictus* cell-fusing virus is an additional member of the *Flaviviridae* but is outside the genus *Flavivirus*. Hepatitis C virus is the topic of another chapter (Chapter 35) and is not discussed further here.

MORPHOLOGY AND VIRION STRUCTURE

Flaviviruses possess an isometric core 30–35 nm in diameter, which contains a nucleocapsid or core (C) protein complexed with single-stranded positive-sense RNA. This core is surrounded by a lipid bilayer containing an envelope (E) protein and a matrix or membrane (M) protein, giving a total virion diameter of about 45 nm. Purified pestiviruses sometimes show a racquet type of morphology (Renard et al. 1985).

GENOME STRUCTURE AND FUNCTION

The genome of flaviviruses is a molecule of single-stranded, positive-sense RNA, c. 11 kb in length containing short untranslated regions at 3' and 5' ends, a 5' cap and a non-polyadenylated 3' terminus (Fig. 29.4). There is no subgenomic mRNA in flavivirus-infected cells. Complete genome sequences are known for yellow fever (Rice et al. 1985, Chambers, McCourt and Rice 1989), West Nile (Castle et al. 1985, Wengler et al. 1985, 1987, Nowak et al. 1989), all 4 serotypes of dengue (Mackow et al. 1987, Hahn et al. 1988, Osatomi and Sumiyoshi 1990, Fu et al. 1992), Japanese encephalitis (Sumiyoshi et al. 1987), Kunjin (Coia et al. 1988), Powassan (Mandl et al. 1993) and tick-borne encephalitis (Pletnev, Yamshikov and Blinov 1990) viruses. A number of partial genome sequences, primarily of the E glycoproteins, are also available. A single long open reading frame (10 223 nucleotides in the case of yellow fever) spans almost the entire length of the RNA.

The genome of pestiviruses has been reported to be 12.5 kb in length. The 3' end of the genomic RNA is not polyadenylated (Renard et al. 1987), and, unlike flaviviruses, the pestivirus RNA lacks a 5' cap structure (Brock, Deng and Riblet 1992). The base composition is: A, 32.2%; U, 22.1%; G, 25.7%; and C 20.0% (Collett et al. 1988a). The pestivirus genome encodes a single open reading frame with a theoretical coding capacity of about 4000 amino acids. Complete genome sequences have been determined for classic swine fever virus (Meyers, Rümenapf and Theil 1989, Moorman et al. 1990) and bovine viral diarrhoea virus (Collett et al. 1988b, Deng and Brock 1992). Partial gene sequences are available for border disease virus (Becher et al. 1994). As with the flaviviruses, the genes encoding the structural proteins are located at the 5' end of the genome.

POLYPEPTIDES: STRUCTURAL AND NON-STRUCTURAL

Cell-associated flaviviruses have a C protein of 13 kDa surrounded by a lipid bilayer containing the 2 membrane proteins E and pre-M (mol. wt 50 and 22 kDa, respectively). Extracellular virions contain the shorter M protein (mol. wt 8 kDa) instead of pre-M. At least 5, and up to 12, non-structural proteins have been described (see below, under 'Replication' p. 590). Because of the continued medical significance of the flaviviruses, the structure and function of the E glycoprotein (c. 500 amino acids) have been intensely investigated. Three antigenic domains (A, B and C) have been identified on the E glycoprotein (Mandl et al. 1989, Heinz and Roehrig 1990). The A domain (amino acids 50–130 and 185–300) is a linearly discontinuous domain that is divided by C domain (amino acids 130–185). The A domain structure is stabilized by 5 disulphide bridges and contains most of the conformationally dependent virus neutralizing epitopes. Much of the antigenicity of the B domain (amino acids 300–400) requires a disulphide bond between Cys 11 and Cys 12. The A, B and C domains constitute

Table 29.3 Relationship between *Flavivirus* subgroup and mode of transmission

Tick-borne viruses		No-vector viruses		Mosquito-borne viruses	
Virus	Subgroup	Virus	Subgroup	Virus	Subgroup
Karshi	1	Carey Island	1	Alfuy	(3)
Kyasanur Forest	1	Phnom Penh bat	1	Japanese encephalitis	3
Langat	1	...	...	Kedougou	3
Louping-ill	1	...	...	Kokobera	3(5?)
Negishi	1	Apoi	2A	Koutango	3
Omsk	1	Bukalassa bat	2A	Kunjin	3
Powassan	1	Dakar bat	2A	Murray Valley	3
Royal Farm	1	Entebbe bat	2A	St Louis	3
Tick-borne	1	Rio Bravo	2A	Stratford	3
encephalitis		Saboya	2A	Usutu	3
				West Nile	3
				Yaounde	(3ª)
Meaban	1A	Cowbone Ridge	2B	Spondweni	4
Saumarez Reef	1A	Jutiapa	2B	Zika	4
Tyuleniy	1A	Modoc	2B	...	...
		Sal Vieja	2B	Bagaza	5
		San Perlita	2B	Israel turkey	5
				Ntaya	5
				Tembusu	5
				Yokose	5
				Banzi	6
				Bouboui	6
				Edge Hill	6
				Potiskum	(6)ª
				Uganda S	6
				Dengue 1	7
				Dengue 2	...
				Dengue 3	7
				Dengue 4	7
Gadgets Gully	U	Aroa	U	Bussuquara	U
Kadam	U	Batu Cave	(U)ª	Ilheus	U
		Cacipacore	U	Jugra	U
		Montana ML	U	Naranjal	U
		Sokuluk	U	Rocio	U
		Tamana bat	U	Sepik	U
				Wesselbron	U
				Yellow fever	U
Totals	14		19		36=69

ªBatu Cave, Potiskum and Yaounde viruses were not examined in either series, but are included for completeness. Based on data from de Madrid and Porterfield (1974) and Calisher et al. (1989).
U, unrelated to any other virus.

the 'head' of the E glycoprotein. A 100 amino acid (c. amino acids 400–500) stalk that includes a 50 amino acid hydrophobic tail (amino acids 450–500) anchors the molecule in the virion envelope. The 2 Å molecular structure of the amino terminal 380 amino acids of the tick-borne encephalitis virus E glycoprotein homodimer has recently been solved (Rey et al. 1995). The protein folds into 3 distinct domains (I, II and III), which correlate well to the previously defined domains C, A and B. Because the locations of the E glycoprotein Cys residues are conserved among all flaviviruses, it is generally assumed that the overall structure is the same for all flaviviruses.

Three major non-structural proteins (NS1, NS3 and NS5) can be found in flavivirus-infected cells. The NS1 protein is a membrane-bound glycoprotein whose function has not been fully determined. It is possible that this protein is involved in virion morphogenesis. The NS2a and NS3 proteins seem to function in concert as a virus-specific protease. The NS5 protein is the virus polymerase.

The pestivirus proteins seem to be synthesized as a polyprotein. Four structural proteins – capsid (C, mol. wt 14 kDa) and 3 envelope proteins, E0 (44–48 kDa), E1 (33 kDa) and E2 (55 kDa) – have been identified. The envelope glycoproteins form dimers through disulphide bridging in both infected cells and virions. The E0 and E2 form homodimers, and the E1 and E2

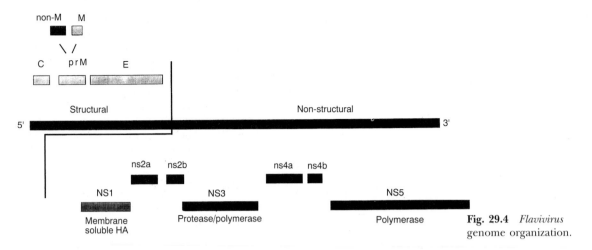

Fig. 29.4 *Flavivirus* genome organization.

form heterodimers (Thiel et al. 1991). A non-structural protein (23 kDa) that has autoproteolytic activity is located 5′ of the C protein. This protein has no analogue in the flaviviruses. Pestiviruses do not seem to have a protein analogue of the flavivirus NS1 protein. Another non-structural protein (80 kDa) is located 3′ of the envelope genes and apparently functions as a viral protease involved in polyprotein processing (Wiskerchen and Collett 1991). At least 3 other non-structural proteins have been identified (p54, p58 and p75). It is assumed that these non-structural proteins function in virus polymerase activity. The nomenclature for pestivirus proteins is currently under review.

ANTIGENS

The E protein represents the viral haemagglutinin, which also elicits neutralizing, enhancing and protective antibodies. The C protein contributes to the group reactivity detected by the complement fixation test. The NS1 protein is responsible for inducing the soluble complement-fixing antigen detected in cells infected with dengue and other flaviviruses. Monoclonal antibodies specific for the NS1 protein can protect animals from virus challenge.

The pestivirus E0 and E2 are primarily responsible for eliciting pestivirus neutralizing antibodies (Weiland et al. 1990, 1992). Because it is difficult to elicit virus-neutralizing antibody specific for the E1 protein, it is thought that most of this protein is buried in the virus envelope, similar to the flavivirus M protein.

REPLICATION

Although it has not been conclusively proven, it is assumed that flaviviruses infect cells by attaching to cellular receptors through the E protein. Flavivirus cellular receptor proteins have not been identified. After endocytosis, the nucleocapsid is released into the cytoplasm by membrane fusion catalysed by a low-pH dependent conformational change in the E protein. All flavivirus E proteins have a highly conserved sequence (amino acids 98–110) that has chemical similarities to regions responsible for cell membrane fusion in orthomyxoviruses and paramyxoviruses.

The gene order, using the nomenclature proposed by Rice et al. (1985) is 5′–C–prM–(M)–E–NS1–ns2a–ns2b–NS3–ns4a–ns4b–NS5–3′ (Fig. 129.4). Translation of viral mRNA yields a polyprotein, which undergoes extensive co-translational and post-translational proteolytic processing and cleavage by cellular signalase(s). Cleavage generates the primary amino acid sequence of the mature structural proteins, pre-M and E, and the amino terminus of the following non-structural protein, NS1. The amino-terminal portion of the polyprotein is released as a molecule, the anchored C protein, which is associated with membranes of the rough endoplasmic reticulum. The anchored C protein is converted to mature C protein by removal of the carboxyl-terminal hydrophobic segment. Cell-associated virions are constructed from the proteins C, pre-M and E. The pre-M protein is cleaved in the Golgi vesicles, resulting in loss of the amino-terminal fragment of this protein and release of mature virions from infected cells. It is currently believed that the pre-M protein functions as an E protein chaperone, protecting it from acid-catalysed denaturation during virus maturation. The cleavage sites generating the non-structural proteins NS2a, NS2b, NS4a and NS4b have been identified.

Flavivirus infection causes virus-specific cytopathic effects in mammalian cells. As with the alphaviruses, cytopathic effects in virus-infected arthropod cells are not as dramatic. The site of flavivirus budding is not fully defined. Nucleocapsids do not seem to accumulate at the plasma membranes, indicating that budding may be quite efficient.

Pestivirus-infected cells contain a single high molecular weight RNA, which is not polyadenylated. A preliminary map of the genome of bovine viral diarrhoea virus has been published, with the gene order 5′–p20–C–E0–E1–E2–p54–p80–p58–p75–3′, but precise identification of some of the virus-specific proteins is still lacking (Collett, Moennig and Horzinek 1989). The processing of the structural proteins has been recently described (Rümenapf et al. 1993). The envelope glycoproteins are produced as a precursor protein, E0123, which is rapidly cleaved to E01 and E2. The E01 precursor is then processed to E0 and E1. The E0 protein has no hydrophobic anchor sequence and can be found in infected cell supernatant. This cleavage pattern is like that seen with the flavivirus prM/E protein.

3.2 Clinical and pathological aspects

DISEASES CAUSED BY FLAVIVIRUSES: GENERAL FEATURES

The flaviviruses known to cause human disease are listed in Table 29.4, several of which may also cause disease in wild or domestic animals. For example, in South Africa, Wesselsbron causes disease in sheep and, to a lesser extent, goats and cattle (Coetzer and Theodoridis 1982); Kyasanur Forest disease has killed monkeys in India (Sreenivasan, Bhat and Bajagopalan 1979); and yellow fever virus can kill South American monkeys in nature and Asian monkeys in the laboratory, but not African monkeys. Israel turkey meningoencephalitis virus has caused economic losses in turkey farms in Israel and is also present in South Africa (Barnard et al. 1980).

Clinical manifestations

Flaviviruses cause a spectrum of clinical manifestations ranging from asymptomatic infections to undifferentiated febrile illnesses, fevers with rash or arthralgia or both, to haemorrhagic fevers, hepatitis and encephalitis, which may result in death. The same virus can cause a variety of syndromes.

Arthropod vectors

Much is known about the epidemiology of viruses such as dengue, yellow fever, Japanese encephalitis, St Louis encephalitis and Central European tick-borne encephalitis, but there are also many uncertainties about these and other flaviviruses. For example, there are substantial differences between the natural history of yellow fever in Africa and in the New World (Downs 1982). Yellow fever is the classic example of a mosquito-borne flavivirus, being transmitted in urban outbreaks by Ae. aegypti in both Africa and the Americas and by a variety of mosquito species in the forest cycle. It has also been recovered from ticks in West Africa (Germain et al. 1982), although it is not known whether these arthropods contribute to the maintenance of the virus in nature.

In general, mosquito-borne flaviviruses are more common in the tropics, whereas tick-borne flaviviruses tend to be prevalent in more temperate regions. The flaviviruses without a known vector are associated with rodents and bats, and are presumed to be transmitted by contact with infective secretions. Only one virus in this subset, Dakar bat virus, is known to infect humans naturally, but several other non-vector-borne flaviviruses have caused laboratory infections. Transovarial and trans-stadial transmission have been documented with several mosquito-borne and tick-borne flaviviruses (Rosen 1987).

Pathogenesis

Flavivirus infections in humans cause 3 main disease patterns – non-specific febrile illness (pantomorphic), encephalitis (neuromorphic) and haemorrhagic fever (visceromorphic) – which generally reflect the tropisms of the viruses for different target organs (Monath 1986). Symptoms in most flavivirus infections probably result from the direct effects of virus replication in the various target organs, which include the brain, liver, skin, lymphoid tissue and cells of the mononuclear phagocyte lineage. Most flaviviruses are pantomorphic, causing only a non-specific febrile illness in a large proportion of infections. Some, however, have virulence and evolutionary host characteristics that make them more neuromorphic or visceromorphic, thus causing encephalitis or haemorrhagic fever, respectively.

Both viral and host factors influence the pathogenesis of flaviviral infections of humans. Many flaviviruses vary naturally in virulence characteristics as a result of selection pressures associated with the arthropod vector or vertebrate host, or both. In addition, host factors such as age, immune status and genetic background may influence pathogenesis.

Immune response

Antigenically related flaviviruses may coexist within similar habitats. There is extensive cross-reactivity between flaviviruses in serological tests, and although there is no cross-protective immunity, heterologous flavivirus antibody may modulate clinical illness. This is especially important with dengue viruses, in that infection with a single serotype provides homotypic immunity, but may enhance infection with a heterologous dengue virus and increase the risk of dengue shock syndrome or dengue haemorrhagic fever.

Diagnosis

Isolation of virus, a process that has been facilitated by use of mosquitoes and mosquito cell lines, provides definitive evidence of flavivirus infection. In practice, however, most infections are diagnosed on the basis of serological tests, which include the classic neutralization, complement-fixation and haemagglutination-inhibition tests, and the enzyme-linked immunosorbent assay and radioimmunoassays for virus-specific IgM and IgG. A variety of flavivirus-derived murine monoclonal antibodies are available for virus identification (Roehrig 1986).

Control

Measures directed towards vector control provide the only practical means of limiting virus transmission for most flaviviruses. Vaccines are available for yellow fever, Japanese encephalitis and tick-borne encephalitis viruses.

3.3 Important mosquito-borne diseases

YELLOW FEVER

Although the yellow fever virus is believed to have originated in Africa, the first recorded outbreak was in Mexico in 1648. This was followed during the seventeenth, eighteenth and nineteenth centuries by

Table 29.4 Flaviviruses known to cause human disease

Virus	Geographical distribution	Other features
Mosquito-borne viruses		
Banzi	S & E Africa	2 cases only
Bussuquara	Brazil, Colombia, Panama	1 case only
Dengue types 1–4	World-wide in the tropics	Tropics and subtropics where the virus and a *Stegomyia* vector exist
Edge Hill	Australia	
Ilheus	C & S America	
Japanese encephalitis	E, SE & S Asia, W Pacific	
Kedougou	Africa	
Kokobera	Australia	
Kunjin	Australia, Sarawak	Laboratory infection
Murray Valley	Australia, New Guinea	
Rocio	Brazil	Epidemics of encephalitis
St Louis	N America, Panama, Jamaica, Trinidad, Brazil, Argentina	
Sepik	New Guinea	1 case only
Spondweni	E, W & S Africa	
Usutu	E, W & C Africa	
Wesselsbron	E, W & S Africa, Thailand	
West Nile	E, W & S Africa, S & SE Asia, India, Mediterranean area	Disease recognized mainly in Israel & France
Yellow fever	W & C Africa, S & C America	Periodical epidemics, e.g. Ethiopia, Nigeria
Zika	E & W Africa, Malayasia, Philippines	1 case in Uganda
Tick-borne viruses		
Absettarov	Europe	
Hanzalova	Europe	
Hypr	Europe	
Karshi	Asia	
Koutango	Africa	
Kumlinge	Europe	
Kyasanur-Forest	Mysore, India	
Langat	Malaysia	Only experiental cases proven
Louping-ill	British Isles	
Negishi	Asia	
Omsk	Central (former) USSR	
Powassan	Canada & USA	
Tick-borne encephalitis		
Western	Europe from Scandinavia to Balkans and from Germany to W (former) USSR	
Eastern	E (former) USSR, occasionally W (former) USSR & Czechoslovakia	
No known arthropod vector		
Apoi	Japan	Laboratory infection
Dakar bat	W, E & C Africa, Madagascar	2 cases only
Phnom-Penh bat	Cambodia, Malaysia	
Rio Bravo	USA, Mexico	

numerous epidemics in the West Indies, Central and South America and the eastern part of the USA as far north as New York. Epidemics in more temperate regions of the western hemisphere were the result of introductions through seaports and of transport of mosquito vectors and viruses along commercial ship-ping routes. The work of the US Army Commission in Cuba established that transmission of yellow fever virus from humans to humans was by infected *Ae. aegypti* mosquitoes (Reed 1902); subsequent control measures against this mosquito, along with immunization using a live attenuated virus vaccine (see below.

p. 593), effectively controlled urban yellow fever in the Americas. However, the disease persisted sporadically in rural areas of both Africa and South America as a consequence of sylvatic cycles involving monkeys and forest-dwelling mosquitoes, e.g. *Haemagogus* and *Sabethes* spp. in South America, *Ae. africanus* in East Africa, and a variety of *Aedes* spp. in West Africa (Strode 1951).

In rural areas, most yellow fever infections occur in people who visit or work in the forests of Africa and South America. Periodically the virus is introduced into urban areas where the highly domesticated mosquito *Ae. aegypti* occurs. This mosquito may become infected by feeding on a viraemic person who was infected in the forest, and secondary transmission can then ensue. Urban epidemics have historically been explosive with many cases because transmission is human to human via the *Ae. aegypti* mosquito, which feeds primarily on humans.

The disease varies from an inapparent infection to a fulminating disease terminating in death; 3 stages (infection, remission and intoxication) are commonly recognized. After an incubation period of 3–10 days, there is sudden onset of fever, rigors, headache and backache. The patient is usually intensely ill and restless, with flushed face, swollen lips, bright red tongue and congested conjunctivae; many patients suffer from nausea and vomiting. A bleeding tendency may be seen early on. This stage of active congestion is followed after 2–3 days by a brief remission and then a resumption of febrile illness. The facial oedema and flushing are replaced by a dusky pallor, the gums become swollen and bleed easily, and there is a pronounced haemorrhagic tendency with black vomit, melaena and ecchymoses. The pulse rate is slow, despite the high fever, and the blood pressure falls, resulting in albuminuria, oliguria and anuria. Death, when it occurs, is usually within 6–7 days of onset, and is rare after 10 days of illness. The jaundice, which gives the disease its name, is generally apparent only in convalescing patients. In patients with intoxication, mortality may occur in 20–50%. In a recent outbreak in Nigeria, mortality was over 50% (Nasidi et al. 1989). Most patients with severe disease have leucopenia, thrombocytopenia, elevated liver enzymes and coagulation defects. At autopsy the organs most affected are the liver, spleen, kidneys and heart. Typically, midzonal necrosis is apparent in the liver, affecting cells around the periphery of the lobule and sparing areas around the central vein. Hyaline necrosis is evident and Councilman inclusion bodies are usually present.

Treatment is supportive and confined to non-specific measures, including maintenance of fluid and electrolyte balances and replacement of any substantial amounts of blood lost through haemorrhage. One dose of live, attenuated 17D vaccine provides complete protection for 10 years and is notably free from reactions. A French vaccine prepared from a neurotropic strain of yellow fever virus has been widely used in Africa. It confers good protection and is cheaper than the 17D vaccine, but, because it has caused adverse reactions, including a number of cases of encephalitis, its use is limited.

DENGUE

There are 4 dengue virus serotypes (DEN-1, DEN-2, DEN-3 and DEN-4). These viruses are closely related to each other antigenically, and cross-reactivity occurs in serological tests. However, there is no lasting cross-protective immunity; Sabin (1952) showed that cross-protection between dengue virus serotypes lasted for only a few months. Thus, individuals can have as many as 4 dengue infections in their life, one with each serotype.

Major dengue epidemics have been caused by all 4 dengue serotypes. Generally one serotype predominates in an area until increased herd immunity decreases transmission. Then another serotype predominates. Dengue viruses change genetically during natural transmission, and significant biological differences have been shown between strains of the same serotype (Russell and McCown 1972, Gubler and Rosen 1977, Gubler et al. 1978).

The epidemiology of the 4 dengue virus serotypes is similar (Gubler 1988). All have a worldwide distribution in the tropics and are maintained in most tropical urban centres in a mosquito–human–mosquito cycle. In many urban centres, multiple virus serotypes co-circulate. The principal mosquito vector is *Ae. aegypti*, an African species that was spread around the world during the seventeenth, eighteenth and nineteenth centuries with the slave trade and shipping industry. This species became highly adapted to living in intimate association with humans and is a highly efficient epidemic vector in urban settings. Secondary vectors include other *Ae. stegomia* species such as *Ae. albopictus*, *Ae. polynesiensis* and *Ae. scutellaris*. These secondary vector species can transmit outbreaks, but are more important as maintenance vectors. Dengue viruses are also maintained in forest cycles in Asia and Africa. These involve monkeys and canopy-dwelling mosquitoes that rarely come in contact with humans. Current evidence suggests that these forest cycles are not important in contributing to urban epidemics.

Infection with dengue viruses causes a spectrum of clinical illness, ranging from inapparent infection to mild non-specific viral syndrome to classic dengue fever to severe and fatal haemorrhagic disease. The clinical picture of classic dengue fever in experimentally infected volunteers was described by Siler, Hall and Hitchens (1926) and Simmons et al. (1931). The classic form usually affects adults and older children. After an infective mosquito bite, there is an incubation period of 5–8 days (range 3–14 days), followed by the sudden onset of fever (which is often biphasic), severe headache, chills and generalized pains in the muscles and joints. A maculopapular rash generally appears on the trunk between days 3 and 5 of illness and spreads to the face and extremities. Lymphadenopathy, anorexia, constipation and altered taste sensation are common. Occasionally, petechiae are seen on the dorsum of the feet, legs, hands, axillae and palate late in the illness. In young children the illness is usually mild, but may be severe. The illness generally lasts for 5–7 days, after which recovery is usually complete, although convalescence may be prolonged. There is leucopenia with a relative lymphocytosis, and thrombocytopenia may occur. Liver enzymes may be elevated and haemorrhagic manifestations may occur.

Dengue haemorrhagic fever

Dengue haemorrhagic fever (DHF) is a severe form of dengue infection characterized by sudden onset of fever, usually of 2–7 days duration, and non-specific signs and symptoms (WHO 1986). The critical stage of DHF occurs 24 hours before to 24 hours after the temperature falls to or below normal. During this time, haemorrhagic manifestations usually occur, and signs of circulatory failure may appear. The patient may become restless or lethargic, experience acute abdominal pain, and have cold extremities, skin congestion and oliguria, usually on or after day 3 of illness. Clinical laboratory tests at this time show thrombocytopenia (platelet count $<100\,000\,\mathrm{mm}^3$) and evidence of a capillary leak syndrome, which may cause hypovolaemia, shock and death. The most common haemorrhagic manifestations are skin haemorrhages, but epistaxis, bleeding gums, gastrointestinal haemorrhage and haematuria may occur.

DHF is most commonly observed in children under the age of 15 years, but in recent epidemics in the Americas DHF was also observed in adults (Guzman et al. 1984a, 1984b, Schatzmayr, Noqueira and Travassos da Rosa 1986, CDC 1987). The pathogenesis of DHF is still not well understood. Classic DHF with a capillary leak syndrome seems to have a unique immunopathological basis mediated by heterologous dengue antibody-dependent enhancement of viral infection of cells of the mononuclear phagocyte lineage (Halstead 1980). Infection of these cells stimulates the release of a vasoactive mediator (or mediators) which apparently causes increased vascular permeability; if not promptly detected and corrected, this can lead to hypovolaemia, shock and death. Although the risk of DHF is higher in children experiencing a second dengue infection, DHF also occurs in patients experiencing primary infections with dengue viruses, suggesting that heterologous dengue antibody (previous infection) is not a necessary prerequisite for DHF. Furthermore, some strains of dengue viruses cannot be enhanced in vitro. Both field and laboratory evidence have been accumulating in recent years that support a more prominent role of viral factors in the pathogenesis of DHF and suggesting that virus strain and serotype are also important risk factors for severe disease (Rosen 1986b, 1989, Gubler 1988, Trent et al. 1989). Another complicating factor is that dengue infections with severe haemorrhage, but no evidence of a capillary leak syndrome, may have another pathogenetic mechanism (Gubler 1988). Because there is no good animal model for DHF, a full understanding of the pathogenetic mechanism of severe dengue disease will have to await careful field studies in dengue endemic areas.

There is no vaccine for dengue/DHF although significant progress has been made in developing one in recent years. Case-fatality rates can be reduced with early diagnosis and proper case management. Currently, prevention depends on mosquito control.

JAPANESE ENCEPHALITIS

Japanese encephalitis (JE) virus is widespread throughout Asia, from the maritime provinces of the former USSR to south India and Sri Lanka (Umenai et al. 1985, Rosen 1986a). It is the most important cause of arboviral encephalitis, with over 45 000 cases reported annually. In recent years, JE virus has expanded its geographic distribution with outbreaks in the Pacific (Paul et al. 1993, Hanna et al. 1995). Epidemics occur in late summer in temperate regions, but the infection is enzootic and occurs throughout the year in many tropical areas of Asia. The virus is maintained in a cycle involving culicine mosquitoes and water birds. The virus is transmitted to humans by *Culex* mosquitoes, primarily *Cx. tritaeniorhynchus*, which breed in rice fields. Pigs are the primary amplifying hosts of JE virus in the peridomestic environment.

The incubation period of JE is 5–14 days. Onset of symptoms is usually sudden, with fever, headache and vomiting. The illness resolves in 5–7 days if there is no CNS involvement. In patients with CNS involvement, lethargy is common, faces are expressionless and there are sensory and motor disturbances affecting speech, the eyes and limbs. There may be confusion and delirium progressing to coma, with convulsions in children as a presenting sign. Weakness and paralysis may affect any part of the body. The lesions are generally upper motor neuron in character. Neck rigidity and a positive Kernig sign are found, and reflexes are abnormal. Initial leucocytosis is followed by leucopenia. The mortality in most outbreaks of JE is less than 10%, but is higher in children and exceeded 30% in some outbreaks in India (Bu'Lock 1986) and in Korea (Umenai et al. 1985). Neurological sequelae in patients who recover are reported in up to 30% of cases.

A formalin-inactivated vaccine prepared in mice infected with the Nakayama strain of JE virus is used widely in Japan, Korea, Taiwan and Thailand; in China, inactivated vaccine prepared in hamster kidney cell cultures has been given to millions of children. A live attenuated vaccine prepared in primary hamster kidney cell culture has also given very promising results in children in China (Xin et al. 1988).

ST LOUIS ENCEPHALITIS

St Louis encephalitis (SLE) is one of the most important mosquito-borne encephalitides in the USA, causing periodic epidemics in the midwest and southeast. This virus is prevalent throughout the western hemisphere from Canada to Argentina, but epidemics are unknown in South and Central America (Monath and Tsai 1987). SLE virus is maintained in a culicine mosquito–bird–mosquito cycle, with periodic amplification by peridomestic birds and *Culex* mosquitoes. In Florida, the principal vector is *Cx. nigripalpus*; in the midwest; *Cx. pipiens pipiens* and *Cx. p. quinquefasciatus*; and in the western United States, *Cx. tarsalis.*

Only a small proportion of SLE infections lead to clinical illness. Onset of illness is usually insidious, with a non-specific prodrome. The disease is generally milder in children than in adults. In children who do have severe disease, however, there is a high rate of encephalitis. The elderly are at highest risk for severe disease and death. No vaccine is yet available, and prevention, therefore, is by mosquito control measures.

MURRAY VALLEY ENCEPHALITIS

Murray Valley encephalitis is endemic in New Guinea and in parts of Australia; it resembles JE. Inapparent infections are common, and the small number of fatalities have mostly been in children (Doherty 1987). Excellent reviews have recently been published (Aaskov and Doherty 1994, Mackenzie et al. 1994).

OTHER MOSQUITO-BORNE INFECTIONS

Kunjin

Kunjin virus is closely related to Murray Valley encephalitis and West Nile viruses, and is found only in Australia, where it normally causes mostly asymptomatic infections, but occasional cases of encephalitis have been reported (Muller et al. 1986).

Ilheus

Ilheus virus is active over wide areas of Central and South America, including Trinidad, and is probably maintained in a forest cycle involving birds and mosquitoes. Most human infections are asymptomatic, but occasional cases of encephalitis are recognized.

Rocio

Rocio virus is antigenically related to SLE virus and is known only from Brazil. Clinically it causes CNS disease like the encephalitis caused by other flaviviruses. It has been responsible for major epidemics in Brazil, principally in males 15–30 years of age (de Souza Lopes et al. 1981, Iversson 1988).

Spondweni

Spondweni virus is present in South Africa, and has produced overt human disease in a few expatriates in West Africa (Wolfe, Calisher and McGuire 1982).

Usutu

Usutu virus is present in East, West and Central Africa. A single case with fever and a rash has been reported.

Wesselsbron

Wesselsbron virus has wide distribution in Africa and causes epizootics in sheep, producing abortion and death in newborn lambs and ewes, and less severe disease in goats and cattle (Coetzer and Theodoridis 1982). The virus also infects humans in nature and in the laboratory (Justines and Shope 1969).

West Nile

West Nile virus is closely related to JE, Murray Valley encephalitis and SLE viruses, but produces a generally milder disease; it rarely causes overt encephalitis. A single case of hepatitis caused by West Nile virus has been reported from Africa (Georges et al. 1988). It has a wide geographical distribution in Africa and Asia.

3.4 Tick-borne infections of the central nervous system

TICK-BORNE ENCEPHALITIS

Tick-borne encephalitis (TBE) is caused by 2 closely related but biologically distinct viruses. The eastern subtype causes Russian spring–summer encephalitis and is transmitted by *Ixodes persulcatus*. The western subtype is transmitted by *I. ricinus* and causes Central European encephalitis. The latter name is somewhat misleading, because the condition occurs in foci extending from Scandinavia in the north to Greece and Yugoslavia in the south. Of the 2 subtypes, Russian spring–summer encephalitis is the more severe infection, having a mortality of up to 25% in some outbreaks, whereas mortality from Central European encephalitis seldom exceeds 5%.

The incubation period is 7–14 days. Infection usually presents as a mild, influenza-type illness or as benign, aseptic meningitis, but may result in fatal meningoencephalitis. Fever is often biphasic, and there may be severe headache and neck rigidity, with transient paresis of the limbs, shoulder girdle or, less commonly, of the respiratory musculature. A few patients are left with residual flaccid paralysis (Ackermann et al. 1986). Although the great majority of TBE infections follow exposure to ticks, infection has occurred through the ingestion of infected cow's or goat's milk.

Inactivated vaccines are available against both eastern and western subtypes of TBE. The vaccine against the western subtype is highly effective (Kunz, Heinz and Hoffman 1980).

LOUPING-ILL

Louping-ill is derived from an old Norse word meaning 'to leap'; louping-ill virus is a member of the TBE complex. It is known in the British Isles as a disease of sheep, characterized by CNS manifestations, in particular cerebellar ataxia, paralysis and death. It has never been a serious hazard to humans: most reported cases are the result of laboratory infections. A few natural infections do occur in people closely associated with sheep. The illness is generally biphasic with encephalitic involvement in the second stage. The vector is *I. ricinus* and the virus is maintained in rodents, deer and ground-living birds (Reid 1988).

POWASSAN VIRUS

Powassan virus is a member of the TBE complex. It is a rare cause of acute viral disease of the CNS in Canada and the USA, but is also present in the former USSR, where it has been recovered from mosquitoes, ticks and humans. It was first isolated from the brain of a 5-year-old child who died in Ontario in 1958, and has since caused a number of cases of encephalitis in Canada and the eastern USA (Artsob 1988). Patients who recover may have residual neurological sequelae. In addition to isolations from humans, the virus has been recovered from ticks (*I. marxi*, *I. cookei* and *Dermacentor andersoni*) and from the tissues of a skunk

(*Spiligale putorius*) (Johnson 1987). There is clinical and serological evidence that Powassan virus can cause fatal encephalitis in horses, which may be confused with rabies encephalitis (Little et al. 1985).

3.5   Tick-borne haemorrhagic fever

KYASANUR FOREST DISEASE

Since the Kyasanur Forest virus was first recognized in 1957 during a fatal epizootic affecting wild monkeys in Mysore State, India, thousands of infections have occurred in forest workers, with a mortality of up to 10%. The virus has been isolated from monkeys, humans and ticks. The principal tick vector appears to be *Haemaphysalis spinigera*; the vertebrate reservoir host is uncertain (Banerjee 1988). An inactivated vaccine is available.

An apparent subtype of Kyasanur Forest disease virus was recently isolated from a fatal human case of haemorrhagic disease in Jeddah, Saudi Arabia (A Zaki, DJ Gubler and J Chang, 1996, unpublished data). The virus was subsequently isolated from other patients with illness ranging from fatal haemorrhagic disease to viral syndrome. All known human infections to date have been associated with handling meat or drinking unpasteurized camels milk. The virus seems to be associated with sheep and camels, and to be transmitted by ticks.

OMSK HAEMORRHAGIC FEVER

This virus was first isolated in association with human disease in Siberia in 1945; illness was characterized by biphasic fever with lymphadenopathy and haemorrhages from mucous membranes. Omsk haemorrhagic fever virus is antigenically distinct from the eastern and western subtypes of TBE. Infection may be acquired from ticks, usually *D. pictus* or *D. marginatus*, or from exposure to infected water voles or muskrats (Lvov 1988).

OTHER TICK-BORNE INFECTIONS
Meaban, Saumarez Reef and Tyuleniy

These viruses are associated with sea-bird ticks in France, Australia and sub-arctic regions of the USA and Russian Federation (Clifford et al. 1971, Lvov et al. 1971, St George et al. 1977, Chastel et al. 1985).

Negishi virus

Negishi virus has caused at least 2 fatal cases of encephalitis in Japan (Okuno, Oya and Ho 1961). Although tick transmission has not been proven, this virus is closely related to other tick-borne flaviviruses (de Madrid and Porterfield 1974, Furuta et al. 1984, Calisher et al. 1989).

3.6   Pestivirus infections

BOVINE VIRUS DIARRHOEA

Infection with this virus occurs world-wide in many wild and domestic bovine species. Two clinical syndromes are recognized in cattle: bovine virus diarrhoea and mucosal disease. The former is a mild, transient infection with high morbidity but low mortality, which is followed by immunity. Viral infection during pregnancy can result in abortion or the birth of persistently infected offspring, some of which may have teratogenic defects. Two biotypes of virus have been recognized, only one of which is cytopathic. When persistently infected, antibody-negative animals carrying the non-cytopathic strain virus are reinfected with a serologically related cytopathic strain; they develop mucosal disease, which carries a high mortality (Baker 1987, Brownlie et al. 1987).

Antibodies reactive with pestivirus antigens have been detected in the serum of 2 children with microcephaly (Potts et al. 1987). With a monoclonal antibody prepared against bovine diarrhoea virus, Yolken et al. (1989) detected pestivirus antigens in the faeces of infants with gastroenteritis.

BORDER DISEASE

Border disease of sheep, originally recognized in the Scottish Border country, occurs also in New Zealand. The causative virus is closely related to that of bovine virus diarrhoea (Horzinek 1981, Nettleton 1987).

CLASSIC SWINE FEVER (HOG CHOLERA)

This important disease of pigs occurs world-wide and is associated with persistent infections, abortion and congenital malformations (Liess 1987).

REFERENCES

Aaskov JG, Doherty RL, 1994, Arboviral zoonoses of Australasia, *Handbook of Zoonoses*, section B: *Viral*, 2nd edn, eds Beran GW, Steele JH et al., CRC Press, Boca Raton FL, 289–304.

Ackermann R, Kruger et al., 1986, Spread of early-summer meningoencephalitis in the Federal Republic of Germany, *Dtsch Med Wochenschr*, **111**: 927–33.

Artsob H, 1988, Powassan encephalitis, *The Arboviruses: ecology and epidemiology*, vol IV, ed Monath TP, CRC Press, Boca Raton FL, 29–50.

Baker JC, 1987, Bovine viral diarrhea virus: a review, *J Am Vet Med Assoc*, **11**: 1449–58.

Banerjee K, 1988, Kyanasur Forest disease, *The Arboviruses: ecology and epidemiology*, vol III, ed Monath TP, CRC Press, Boca Raton FL, 93–116.

Barnard BJH, Buys SB et al., 1980, Turkey meningo-encephalitis in South Africa, *Onderstepoort J Vet Res*, **47**: 89–94.

Barr PJ, 1991, Mammalian subtilisins: the long-sought dibasic processing endoproteases, *Cell*, **66**: 1–3.

Becher P, Shannon AD et al., 1994, Molecular characterization of border disease virus, a pestivirus from sheep, *Virology*, **198**: 542–51.

Beran GW, Steele JH et al., eds, 1994, *Handbook of Zoonoses*, section B: *Viral*, 2nd edn, CRC Press, Boca Raton FL.

den Boon JA, Snijder EJ et al., 1991, Equine arteritis virus is not a togavirus but belongs to the coronavirus-like superfamily, *J Virol*, **65**: 2910–20.

den Boon JA, Faaberg KS et al., 1995, Processing and evolution of the N-terminal region of the arterivirus replicase ORF1a protein: identification of 2 papainlike cysteine proteases, *J Virol*, **69**: 4500–5.

Brinton-Darnell M, Plagemann P, 1975, Structure and chemical-physical characteristics of lactate dehydrogenase-elevating virus and its RNA, *J Virol*, **16**: 420–33.

Brock KV, Deng R, Riblet S, 1992, Nucleotide sequencing of 5′ and 3′ termini of bovine viral diarrhea virus by RNA ligation and PCR, *J Virol Methods*, **38**: 39–46.

Brownlie J, Clarke MC et al., 1987, Pathogenesis and epidemiology of bovine virus diarrhea infection of cattle, *Ann Rech Vet*, **18**: 157–66.

Brummer-Korvenkontio M, Kuusisto P, 1981, Has western Finland been spared the 'Pogosta'? [in Finnish], *Suomen Laakarilehti*, **32:** 2606.

Bu'Lock FA, 1986, Japanese B virus encephalitis in India – a growing problem, *Q J Med, NS 60*, **233:** 825–36.

Calisher CH, Monath TP et al., 1980, Arbovirus investigations in Argentina, 1977–1980. 3. Identification and characterization of viruses isolated, including new subtypes of western and Venezuelan equine encephalitis viruses and four new bunyaviruses (Las Maloyas, Resistencia, Barranqueras, and Antequera), *Am J Trop Med Hyg*, **34:** 956–65.

Calisher CH, Monath TP et al., 1985, Characterization of Fort Morgan virus, an alphavirus of the western equine encephalitis virus complex in an unusual ecosystem, *Am J Trop Med Hyg*, **29:** 1428–40.

Calisher CH, Karabatsos N et al., 1989, Antigenic relationships between flaviviruses as determined by cross-neutralization tests with polyclonal antisera, *J Gen Virol*, **70:** 37–43.

Carey DE, 1971, Chikungunya and dengue: a case of mistaken identity?, *J Hist Med Allied Sci*, **26:** 243–62.

Castle E, Nowak T et al., 1985, Sequence analysis of the viral core and the membrane associated proteins V1 and NV2 of the flavivirus West Nile virus and of the genome sequence of those proteins, *Virology*, **145:** 227.

CDC, 1987, Dengue hemorrhagic fever – Puerto Rico, *Morbid Mortal Weekly Rep*, **35:** 779–82.

Chamberlain RW, 1987, Historical perspectives on the epidemiology and ecology of mosquito-borne virus encephalitides in the United States, *Am J Trop Med Hyg*, **37:** 8–17S.

Chambers TJ, McCourt DW, Rice CM, 1989, Yellow fever virus proteins NS2A, NS2B, NS4B: identification and partial N-terminal amino acid sequence analysis, *Virology*, **169:** 100–9.

Chastel C, Main AJ et al., 1985, The isolation of Meaban virus, a new Flavivirus from the seabird tick *Ornithodoros* (*Alectorobius*) *maritimus* in France, *Arch Virol*, **83:** 129–40.

Choi H-K, Tong L et al., 1991, Structure of Sindbis virus core protein reveals a chymotrypsin-like serine proteinase and the organization of the virion, *Nature (London)*, **354:** 37–43.

Clifford CM, Yunker CE et al., 1971, Isolation of a group B arbovirus from *Ixodes uriae* collected on Three Arch Rocks National Wildlife Refuge, Oregon, *Am J Trop Med Hyg*, **20:** 461–8.

Coetzer JAW, Theodoridis A, 1982, Clinical and pathological studies in adult sheep and goats experimentally infected with Wesselsbron disease virus, *Onderstepoort J Vet Res*, **49:** 19–22.

Coia G, Parker MD et al., 1988, Nucleotide and complete amino acid sequences of Kunjin virus: definitive gene order and characteristics of the virus-specified proteins, *J Gen Virol*, **69:** 1–21.

Collett MS, Moennig V, Horzinek MC, 1989, Recent advances in pestivirus research, *J Gen Virol*, **70:** 253–66.

Collett MS, Larson R et al., 1988a, Molecular cloning and nucleotide sequence of the pestivirus bovine viral diarrhea virus, *Virology*, **165:** 191–9.

Collett MS, Larson R et al., 1988b, Proteins encoded by bovine viral diarrhea virus: the genomic organization of a pestivirus, *Virology*, **165:** 200–8.

Dalgarno L, Short NJ et al., 1984, Characterisation of Barmah Forest virus: an alphavirus with some unusual properties, *Virology*, **133:** 416–26.

Davis NL, Willis LV et al., 1989, *In vitro* synthesis of infectious Venezuelan equine encephalitis virus RNA from a cDNA clone: analysis of a viable deletion mutant, *Virology*, **171:** 189–204.

De Madrid AT, Porterfield JS, 1974, The flaviviruses (group B arboviruses): a cross-neutralization study, *J Gen Virol*, **23:** 91–6.

Deng R, Brock KV, 1992, Molecular cloning and nucleotide sequence of a pestivirus genome, noncytopathic bovine viral diarrhea virus strain SD-1, *Virology*, **191:** 867–79.

Doherty RL, 1987, William C Reeves and arbovirus research in Australia, *Am J Trop Med Hyg*, **37:** 87–93S.

Doherty RL, Carley JG, Best JC, 1972, Isolation of Ross River virus from man, *Med J Aust*, **1:** 1083–4.

Downs WG, 1982, The known and the unknown in yellow fever ecology and epidemiology, *Ecol Dis*, **1:** 103–10.

Faaberg KS, Even C et al., 1995, Disulfide bonds between 2 envelope proteins of lactate dehydrogenase-elevating virus are essential for viral infectivity, *J Virol*, **69:** 613–17.

Fenner F, 1976, Classification and nomenclature of viruses. Second report of the International Committee on Taxonomy of Viruses, *Intervirology*, **7:** 1–115.

Fraser JRE, Tait B et al., 1980, Possible genetic determinants in epidemic polyarthritis caused by Ross River virus infection, *Aust N Z J Med*, **10:** 597–603.

Fu J, Tan B-H et al., 1992, Full-length cDNA sequence of dengue type 1 virus (Singapore strain S275/90), *Virology*, **188:** 953–8.

Fulhorst CF, Hardy JL et al., 1994, Natural vertical transmission of western equine encephalomyelitis virus in mosquitoes, *Science*, **263:** 676–8.

Furuta I, Takashina I et al., 1984, Antigenic analysis of flaviviruses with monoclonal antibodies against Negishi virus, *Microbiol Immunol*, **28:** 1023–30.

Gaedigk-Nitschko K, Schlesinger MJ, 1990, The Sindbis virus 6K protein can be detected in virions and is acylated with fatty acid, *Virology*, **175:** 274–81.

Gebhardt LP, Stanton GJ et al., 1964, Natural overwintering hosts of the virus of western equine encephalitis, *N Engl J Med*, **271:** 172–7.

Georges AJ, Lesbordes JL et al., 1988, Fatal hepatitis from West Nile virus, *Ann Inst Pasteur (Paris): Virologie*, **138:** 237–44.

Germain M, Cornet M et al., 1982, Recent advances in research regarding sylvatic yellow fever in west and central Africa, *Bull Inst Pasteur*, **80:** 315–30.

Gibbs EPJ, Tsai TF, 1994, Eastern encephalitis, *Handbook of Zoonoses*, section B: *Viral*, 2nd edn, eds Beran GW, Steele JH et al., CRC Press, Boca Raton FL, 11–24.

Godney EK, Chen L et al., 1993, Complete genome sequence and phylogenetic analysis of the lactate dehydrogenase-elevating virus (LDV), *Virology*, **194:** 585–96.

Guard RW, McAuliffe MJ et al., 1982, Haemorrhagic manifestations with Sindbis infection, *Pathology*, **14:** 89–90.

Gubler DJ, 1981, Transmission of Ross River virus by *Aedes polynesiensis* and *Aedes aegytpi*, *Am J Trop Med Hyg*, **30:** 1303–6.

Gubler DJ, 1988, Dengue, *Epidemiology of Arthropod-Borne Viral Disease*, vol II, ed Monath TP, CRC Press, Boca Raton FL, 223–60.

Gubler DJ, Rosen L, 1977, Quantitative aspects of replication of dengue viruses in *Aedes albopictus* (Diptera: Culicidae) after oral and parenteral infection, *J Med Entomol*, **13:** 469–72.

Gubler DJ, Reed D et al., 1978, Epidemiologic, clinical and virologic observations on dengue in the Kingdom of Tonga, *Am J Trop Med Hyg*, **27:** 581–9.

Guzman MG, Kouri GP et al., 1984a, Dengue haemorrhagic fever in Cuba. 1. Serological confirmation of clinical diagnosis, *Trans R Soc Trop Med Hyg*, **78:** 235–8.

Guzman MG, Kouri GP et al., 1984b, Dengue haemorrhagic fever in Cuba. 2. Clinical investigations, *Trans R Soc Trop Med Hyg*, **78:** 239–41.

Hahn CS, Lustig S et al., 1988a, Western equine encephalitis virus is a recombinant virus, *Proc Natl Acad Sci USA*, **85:** 5997–6001.

Hahn YS, Galler R et al., 1988b, Nucleotide sequence of dengue 2 RNA and comparison of the encoded proteins with those of other flaviviruses, *Virology*, **162:** 167–80.

Halstead SB, 1980, Immunopathological parameters of togarvirus disease syndromes, *The Togaviruses: Biology, Structure, Replication*, ed Schleslinger RW, Academic Press, New York, 107–74.

Hanna J, Ritchie S et al., 1995, Probable Japanese encephalitis acquired in the Torres Strait, *Comm Dis Intell*, **19:** 206–8.

Hardy JL, 1987, The ecology of western equine encephalomyelitis virus in the central valley of California, 1945–1985, *Am J Trop Med Hyg*, **37:** 18–32S.

Harrison SC, 1986, Alphavirus structure, *The* Togaviridae *and* Flavirviridae, eds Schlesinger S, Schlesinger MJ, Plenum Press, New York, 21–34.

Heinz FX, Roehrig JT, 1990, Flavivirueses, *Immunochemistry of Viruses. II. The Basis for Serodiagnosis and Vaccines*, eds Van Regen mortel MHV, Neurath AR, Elsevier, Amsterdam, 289–305.

Horzinek MC, 1981, *Non-arthropod-borne Togaviruses*, Academic Press, New York.

Horzinek MC, van Berlo MF, 1987, The pestiviruses: where do they belong?, *Ann Rech Vet*, **18**: 115–19.

Hunt AR, Roehrig JT, 1985, Biochemical and biological characteristics of epitopes on the E1 glycoprotein of western equine encephalitis virus, *Virology*, **142**: 334–46.

Hunt AR, Roehrig JT, 1995, Localization of a protective epitope on a Venezuelan equine encephalomyelitis (VEE) virus peptide that protects mice from both epizootic and enzootic VEE virus challenge and is immunogenic in horses, *Vaccine*, **13**: 281–6.

Hunt AR, Johnson AJ et al., 1990, Synthetic peptides of Venezuelan equine encephalomyelitis virus E2 glycoprotein. I. Immunogenic analysis and identification of a protective peptide, *Virology*, **179**: 701–11.

Iversen JO, 1994, Western equine encephalomyelitis, *Handbook of Zoonoses*, section B: *Viral*, 2nd edn, eds Beran GW, Steele JH et al., CRC Press, Boca Raton FL, 25–31.

Iversson LB, 1988, *The Arboviruses: ecology and epidemiology*, vol. IV, ed Monath TP, CRC Press, Boca Raton FL, 77–92.

Johnson BJB, Brubaker JR et al., 1990, Variants of the Venezuelan equine encephalitis virus that resist neutralization define a domain of the E2 glycoprotein, *Virology*, **177**: 676–83.

Johnson HN, 1987, Isolation of Powassan virus from a spotted skunk in California, *J Wildlife Dis*, **23**: 152–3.

Jupp PG, 1994, Arboviral zoonoses of Africa, *Handbook of Zoonoses*, section B: *Viral*, 2nd edn, eds Beran GW, Steele JH et al., CRC Press, Boca Raton FL, 261–73.

Justines GA, Shope RE, 1969, Wesselsbron virus infection in a laboratory worker, with virus recovery from a throat washing, *Health Lab Sci*, **6**: 46–9.

Kääriäinen L, Takkinen K et al., 1987, Replication of the genome of alphaviruses, *J Cell Sci Suppl*, **7**: 231–50.

Kamada M, Ando Y et al., 1980, Equine Getah virus infection: isolation of the virus from racehorses during an enzootic in Japan, *Am J Trop Med Hyg*, **79**: 984–8.

Karabatsos N, 1985, *International Catalogue of Arboviruses, including certain other viruses of vertebrates*, American Society of Tropical Medicine and Hygiene, San Antonio TX.

Kinney RM, Trent DW, France JK, 1983, Comparative immunological and biological analyses of viruses in the Venezuelan equine encephalitis complex, *J Gen Virol*, **64**: 135–47.

Kinney RM, Chang G-J et al., 1993, Virulence of Venezuelan equine encephalitis (VEE) virus is encoded by the 5′ noncoding region and E2 envelope glycoprotein, *J Virol*, **67**: 1269–77.

Kuhn RJ, Niesters HGM et al., 1991, Infectious RNA transcripts from Ross River virus cDNA clones and the construction and characterization of defined chimeras with Sindbis virus, *Virology*, **182**: 430–1.

Kunz C, Heinz FX, Hoffmann H, 1980, Immunogenicity and reactigenicity of a highly purified vaccine against tick-borne encephalitis, *J Med Virol*, **6**: 103–9.

Levine B, Huang Q et al., 1993, Conversion of lytic to persistent alphavirus infection by the *bcl*-2 cellular oncogene, *Nature (London)*, **361**: 739–42.

Levy-Mintz P, Kielian M, 1991, Mutagenesis of the putative fusion active domain of Semliki Forest virus spike protein, *J Virol*, **65**: 4292–300.

Liess B, 1987, Pathogenesis and epidemiology of hog cholera, *Ann Rech Vet*, **18**: 139–45.

Liljestrom P, Lusa S et al., 1991, *In vitro* mutagenesis of a fulllength cDNA clone of Semliki Forest virus: the small 6000-

molecular-weight membrane protein modulates virus release, *J Virol*, **65**: 4107–13.

Little PB, Thorsen J et al., 1985, Powassan viral encephalitis: a review and experimental studies in the horse and rabbit, *Vet Pathol*, **22**: 500–7.

London WT, 1977, Epizootiology, transmission and approach to prevention of fatal simian haemorrhagic fever in rhesus monkeys, *Nature (London)*, **268**: 344–5.

Lvov DK, 1988, *Epidemiology of Arthropodborne Viral Disease*, vol 3, ed Monath TP, CRC Press, Boca Raton FL, 205–16.

Lvov DK, Timopheeva AA et al, 1971, Tuleniy virus. A new group B arbovirus isolated from *Ixodes (Ceratixodes) putus* Pick.-Camb. 1878 collected on Tuleniy Island, Sea of Okhotsk, *Am J Trop Med Hyg*, **20**: 456–60.

Lvov DK, Skortsova TM et al., 1984, Isolating of the Karelian fever agent from *Aedes communis* mosquitoes, *Lancet*, **2**: 399–400.

McIntosh BM, Harwin RM et al., 1963, An epidemic of chikungunya in south-eastern Southern Rhodesia, *Cent Afr J Med*, **9**: 351–59.

McIntosh BM, Jupp PC et al., 1976, Epidemics of West Nile and Sindbis viruses in South Africa with *Culex (Culex) univittatus*, *S Afr J Sci*, **72**: 295–300.

Mackenzie JS, Lindsay MD et al., 1994, Arboviruses causing human disease in the Australasian zoogeographic region, *Arch Virol*, **136**: 447–67.

Mackow E, Makino Y et al., 1987, The nucleotide sequence of dengue 4 virus: analysis of genes coding for non structural proteins, *Virology*, **158**: 217–28.

Mandl CW, Guirakhoo FG et al., 1989, Antigenic structure of the flavivirus envelope protein E at the molecular level, using tick-borne encephalitis virus as a model, *J Virol*, **63**: 564–71.

Mandl CW, Holzmann H et al., 1993, Complete genomic sequence of Powassan virus: evaluation of genetic elements in tick-borne versus mosquito-borne flaviviruses, *Virology*, **194**: 173–84.

Mathews JH, Roehrig JT, 1982, Determination of the protective epitopes on the glycoprotein of Venezuelan equine encephalomyelitis virus by passive transfer of monoclonal antibodies, *J Immunol*, **129**: 2763–7.

Meulenberg JJM, Hulst MM et al., 1993, Lelystad virus, the causative agent of porscine epidemic abortion and respiratory syndrome (PEARS) is related to LDV and EAV, *Virology*, **192**: 62–72.

Meyers G, Rümenapf T, Theil H-J, 1989, Molecular cloning and nucleotide sequence of the genome of hog cholera virus, *Virology*, **171**: 555–67.

Monath TP, 1986, Pathobiology of the flaviviruses, *The* Togaviridae *and* Flaviviridae, eds Schlesinger S, Schlesinger MJ, Plenum Press, New York, 375–440.

Monath TP, ed, 1988, *The Arboviruses: epidemiology and ecology*, vols 1–4, CRC Press, Boca Raton FL.

Monath TP, Tsai TF, 1987, St Louis encephalitis: lessons from the last decade, *Am J Trop Med Hyg*, **37**: 40–59S.

Moormann RJM, Warmerdam PAM et al., 1990, Molecular cloning and nucleotide sequence of hog cholera virus strain Brescia and mapping of the genomic region encoding envelope protein E1, *Virology*, **177**: 184–98.

Morris CD, 1988, Eastern equine encephalomyelitis, *The Arboviruses: epidemiology and ecology*, vol 3, ed Monath TP, CRC Press, Boca Raton FL, 1–20.

Mudge PR, Aaskov JG, 1983, Epidemic polyarthritis in Australia, 1980–1981, *Med J Aust*, **2**: 269–73.

Muller D, McDonald M et al., 1986, Kunjin virus encephalomyelitis, *Med J Aust*, **144**: 41–9.

Nasidi A, Monath TP et al., 1989, Urban yellow fever epidemic in western Nigeria, 1987, *Trans R Soc Trop Med Hyg*, **83**: 401–6.

Nettleton PF, 1987, Pathogenesis and epidemiology of border disease, *Ann Rech Vet*, **18**: 147–55.

Niklasson B, Espmark A et al., 1984, Association of a Sindbis-like virus with Ockelbo disease in Sweden, *Am J Trop Med Hyg*, **33:** 1212–17.

Nimmo JR, 1928, An unusual epidemic, *Med J Aust*, **1:** 549–50.

Nowak T, Farber P et al., 1989, Analyses of the terminal sequences of West Nile virus structural proteins and of the in vitro translation of these proteins allow the proposal of a complete scheme of the proteolytic cleavages involved in their synthesis, *Virology*, **169:** 365–76.

Okuno T, Oya A, Ho T, 1961, The identification of Negishi virus: a presumably new member of Russian spring–summer encephalitis virus family isolated in Japan, *Jpn J Med Sci Biol*, **14:** 51–9.

Olaleye OD, Fagbami AH, 1988, Igbo-ora virus (an alphavirus isolated in Nigeria): a serological survey for hemagglutination inhibiting antibody in humans and domestic animals, *Trans R Soc Trop Med Hyg*, **82:** 905–6.

Osatomi K, Sumiyoshi H, 1990, Complete nucleotide sequence of dengue type 3 virus genome RNA, *Virology*, **176:** 643–7.

Palmer GA, Kuo L et al., 1995, Sequence of the genome of lactate dehydrogenase-elevating virus heterogeneity between P and C, *Virology*, **209:** 637–42.

Paul WS, Moore PS et al., 1993, Outbreak of Japanese encephalitis on the island of Saipan, 1990, *J Infect Dis*, **167:** 1053–8.

Pinheiro FP, Travassos da Rosa APA, 1994, Arboviral zoonoses of Central and South America, *Handbook of Zoonoses,* section B*: Viral*, 2nd edn, eds Beran GW, Steele JH et al., CRC Press, Boca Raton FL, 201–25.

Pletnev AG, Yamshikov VF, Blinov VM, 1990, Nucleotide sequence of the genome and complete amino acid sequence of the polyprotein of tick-borne encephalitis virus, *Virology*, **174:** 250–63.

Potts BJ, Sever JL et al., 1987, Possible role of pestiviruses in microcephaly, *Lancet*, **1:** 972–3.

Reed W, 1902, Recent researches concerning etiology, propagation and prevention of yellow fever, by the United States Army Commission, *J Hyg*, **2:** 101–19.

Reeves WC, 1987, The discovery decade of arbovirus research in western North America, 1940–1949, *Am J Trop Med Hyg*, **37:** 94–100S.

Reid HW, 1988, Louping ill, *The Arboviruses: ecology and epidemiology*, vol 3, ed Monath TP, CRC Press, Boca Raton FL, 117–36.

Renard A, Guiot C et al., 1985, Molecular cloning of bovine viral diarrhea viral sequences, *DNA*, **4:** 429–38.

Renard A, Schmetz DA et al., 1987, Molecular cloning of the bovine viral diarrhea virus genome RNA, *Ann Rech Vet*, **18:** 121–5.

Report, 1972, *Venezuelan Encephalitis*, Pan-American Health Organization, Washington DC.

Rey FA, Heinz FX et al., 1995, The envelope glycoprotein from tick-borne encephalitis virus at 2Å resolution, *Nature (London)*, **375:** 291–8.

Rice CM, Lenches EM et al., 1985, Nucleotide sequence of yellow fever virus: implications for flavivirus gene expression and evolution, *Science*, **229:** 726–33.

Rice CM, Lewis R et al., 1987, Production of infectious RNA transcripts from Sindbis virus cDNA clones: mapping of lethal mutations, rescue of temperature-sensitive marker, and *in vitro* mutagenesis to generate defined mutants, *J Virol*, **61:** 3809–19.

Roehrig JT, 1986, The use of monoclonal antibodies in studies of the structural proteins of togaviruses and flaviviruses, *The Togaviridae and* Flaviviridae, eds Schlesinger S, Schlesinger MJ, Plenum Press, New York, 251–78.

Roehrig JT, Hunt AR, 1988, *In vitro* mechanisms of monoclonal antibody neutralization of alphaviruses, *Virology*, **165:** 66–73.

Roehrig JT, Mathews JH, 1985, The neutralization site on the E2 glycoprotein of Venezuelan equine encephalomyelitis (TC-83) virus is composed of multiple conformationally stable epitopes, *Virology*, **142:** 347–56.

Roehrig JT, Hunt AR et al., 1990, Identification of monoclonal

antibodies capable of differentiating antigenic varieties of eastern equine encephalitis viruses, *Am J Trop Med Hyg*, **2:** 394–8.

Rosen L, 1986a, The natural history of Japanese encephalitis, *Annu Rev Microbiol*, **40:** 395–414.

Rosen L, 1986b, The pathogenesis of dengue hemorrhagic fever – a critical appraisal of current hypotheses, *S Afr Med J*, **suppl:** 40–2.

Rosen L, 1987, Overwintering mechanisms of mosquito-borne arboviruses in temperate climates, *Am J Trop Med Hyg*, **37:** 69–76S.

Rosen L, 1989, Disease exacerbation caused by sequential dengue infections: myth or reality?, *Rev Infect Dis*, **suppl:** 5840–2.

Rosen L, Gubler DJ, Bennett, PH, 1981, Epidemic polyarthritis (Ross River) virus infection in the Cook Islands, *Am J Trop Med Hyg*, **30:** 1294–302.

Rowson KEK, Mahy BWJ, 1985, Lactate dehydrogenase-elevating virus, *J Gen Virol*, **66:** 2297–312.

Rümanapf T, Unger G et al., 1993, Processing of the envelope glycoproteins of pestiviruses, *Virology*, **67:** 3288–94.

Russell PK, McCown J, 1972, Comparison of dengue-2 and dengue-3 virus strains by neutralization tests and identification of a subtype of dengue-3, *Am J Trop Med Hyg*, **21:** 97–9.

Sabin AB, 1952, Research on dengue during World War II, *Am J Trop Med Hyg*, **1:** 30–50.

St George TD, Standfast HA et al., 1977, The isolation of Saumarez Reef virus, a new flavivirus, from bird ticks *Ornithodoros capensis* and *Ixodes eudyptidis* in Australia, *Aust J Exp Biol Med Sci*, **55:** 493–9.

Schatzmayr HG, Nogueira RMR, Travassos da Rosa APA, 1986, An outbreak of dengue virus at Rio de Janeiro – 1986, *Mem Inst Oswaldo Cruz*, **81:** 245–6.

Siler JF, Hall MW, Hitchens AP, 1926, Dengue: its history, epidemiology, mechanisms of transmission, etiology, clinical manifestations, immunity and prevention, *Philippine J Sci*, **29:** 1–304.

Simmons JS, St John JH, Reynolds FHK, 1931, Experimental studies of dengue, *Philippine J Sci*, **44:** 1–251.

Smithburn KC, Haddow AJ, 1944, Semliki Forest virus, isolation and pathogenic properties, *J Immunol*, **49:** 141–57.

de Souza Lopes O, Sacchetta LA et al., 1981, Emergence of a new arbovirus disease in Brazil. 3. Isolation of Roccio virus from *Psorophora ferox* (Humboldt 1819), *Am J Epidemiol*, **113:** 122–5.

Sreenivasan MA, Bhat HR, Rajagopalan PK, 1979, Studies on the transmission of Kyasanur forest disease virus by partly fed ixodid ticks, *Indian J Med Sci*, **69:** 708–13.

Standfast HA, Dyce AL et al., 1984, Isolation of arboviruses from insects collected at Beatrice Hill, Northern Territory of Australia, 1974–1976, *Aust J Biol Sci*, **37:** 351–66.

Strauss EG, Rice CM, Strauss JH, 1984, Complete nucleotide sequence of the genomic RNA of Sindbis virus, *Virology*, **133:** 92–110.

Strauss EG, Stec DS et al., 1991, Identification of antigenically important domains in the glycoproteins of Sindbis virus by analysis of antibody escape variants, *J Virol*, **65:** 4654–64.

Strauss JH, Strauss EG, 1994, The alphaviruses: gene expression, replication, and evolution, *Microbiol Rev*, **58:** 491–562.

Strode GK, 1951, *Yellow Fever*, McGraw-Hill, New York.

Sumiyoshi H, Mori C et al., 1987, Complete nucleotide sequence of the Japanese encephalitis virus genome RNA, *Virology*, **161:** 497–510.

Taylor RM, Work TH et al., 1956, A study of the ecology of West Nile virus in Egypt, *Am J Trop Med Hyg*, **5:** 579–620.

Thiel H-J, Stark R et al., 1991, Hog cholera virus: molecular composition of virions from a pestivirus, *J Virol*, **65:** 4705–12.

Thomas LA, Patzer ER et al., 1980, Antibody development in garter snakes (*Thamnophis* spp.) experimentally infected with western equine encephalitis virus, *Am J Trop Med Hyg*, **29:** 112–17.

Tong L, Wengler G et al., 1993, Refined structure of Sindbis virus core protein and comparison with other chymotrypsin-like serine proteinase structures, *J Mol Biol*, **230:** 228–47.

Trent DW, Grant JA, 1980, A comparison of new world alphaviruses in the western equine encephalomyelitis virus complex by immunochemical and oligonucleotide fingerprint techniques, *J Gen Virol*, **47:** 261–82.

Trent DW, Grant JA et al., 1989, Genetic variation and microevolution of dengue 2 virus in southeast Asia, *Virology*, **172:** 523–35.

Umenai T, Krzysko R et al., 1985, Japanese encephalitis: current worldwide status, *Bull W H O*, **63:** 625–31.

Vogel RH, Provencher SW et al., 1986, Envelope structure of Semliki Forest virus reconstructed from cryoelectron micrographs, *Nature (London)*, **320:** 533–5.

Von Bonsdorff CH, Harrison SC, 1978, Hexagonal glycoprotein arrays from Sindbis virus membranes, *J Virol*, **28:** 578–83.

Wang KS, Kuhn RJ et al., 1992, High-affinity laminin receptor for Sindbis virus in mammalian cells, *J Virol*, **66:** 4992–5001.

Weiland E, Stark R et al., 1990, Pestivirus glycoprotein which induces neutralizing antibodies forms part of a disulfide-linked heterodimer, *J Virol*, **64:** 3563–9.

Weiland E, Ahl R et al., 1992, A second envelope glycoprotein mediates neutralization of a pestivirus, *J Virol*, **66:** 3677–82.

Wengler G, Castle E et al., 1985, Sequence analysis of the membrane protein V3 of the flavivirus West Nile virus and of its gene, *Virology*, **147:** 264–74.

Wengler G, Wengler G et al., 1987, Analysis of the influence of proteolytic cleavage on the structural organization of the surface of the West Nile flavivirus leads to the isolation of a protease-resistant E protein oligomer from the viral surface, *Virology*, **160:** 210–19.

Westaway EG, Brinton MA et al., 1985a, Togaviridae, *Intervirology*, **24:** 125–39.

Westaway EG, Brinton MA et al., 1985b, Flaviviridae, *Intervirology*, **24:** 183–92.

WHO, 1967, *Arboviruses and Human Disease*, World Health Organization Technical Report Series No 369, WHO, Geneva.

WHO, 1985, *Arthropod-borne and Rodent-borne Viral Diseases*, World Health Organization Technical Report Series No. 719, WHO, Geneva.

WHO, 1986, Dengue haemorrhagic fever: diagnosis, treatment and control, *World Health Organization Technical Report Series, No 721*, WHO, Geneva.

Wiebe ME, Scherer WF, 1980, Virion envelope glycoproteins as epidemiological markers of Venezuelan encephalitis virus isolates, *J Clin Microbiol*, **11:** 349–54.

Wildy P, 1971, *Monographs in Virology*, vol. 5, *Classification and Nomenclature of Viruses*, W Karger, Basel.

Willems WR, Kaluza G et al., 1979, Semliki Forest virus: cause of a fatal case of human encephalitis, *Science*, **203:** 1127–9.

Wiskerchen M, Collett MS, 1991, Pestivirus gene expression: protein p80 of bovine viral diarrhea virus is a proteinase involved in polyprotein processing, *Virology*, **184:** 341–50.

Wolfe MS, Calisher CH, McGuire K, 1982, Spondweni virus infection in a foreign resident of Upper Volta, *Lancet*, **2:** 1306–8.

Woodward TM, Miller BR et al., 1991, A single amino acid change in the E2 glycoprotein of Venezuelan equine encephalitis virus affects replication and dissemination in *Aedes aegypti* mosquitoes, *J Gen Virol*, **72:** 2431–5.

Yolken R, Dubovi E et al., 1989, Infantile gastroenteritis associated with excretion of pestivirus antigens, *Lancet*, **1:** 517–20.

Xin YY, Ming ZG et al., 1988, Safety of a live-attenuated Japanese encephalitis virus vaccine (SA14-14-2) for children, *Am J Trop Med Hyg*, **39:** 214–17.

Chapter 30

BUNYAVIRIDAE

Connie S Schmaljohn and James W LeDuc

1 Properties of the viruses	2 Clinical and pathological aspects

1 PROPERTIES OF THE VIRUSES

1.1 Introduction

Viruses of the family *Bunyaviridae* are enveloped, single-stranded RNA viruses with a tripartite genome. Approximately 300 distinct viruses are included in 5 genera of the family: *Bunyavirus, Hantavirus, Nairovirus, Phlebovirus* and *Tospovirus*. Viruses of the same genus share structural, genetic and antigenic characteristics, and often similar epidemiology. Many are arboviruses (**ar**thropod-**bo**rne viruses), transmitted between vertebrate hosts (or plants in the case of tospoviruses) by blood-feeding mosquitoes, ticks, gnats or thrips. A significant exception is the genus *Hantavirus*, whose known members are maintained in nature by chronically infected rodents, especially of the family *Muridae*, and are thought to be transmitted most commonly among rodents by bite and aerosol and to humans by aerosol. The most noteworthy human pathogens among the hantaviruses are Hantaan virus, the cause of haemorrhagic fever with renal syndrome (also known as epidemic haemorrhagic fever and Korean haemorrhagic fever) in Asia, and Sin Nombre virus (previously known as Four Corners virus), the recently discovered cause of hantavirus pulmonary syndrome. Other human diseases caused by viruses within the family include California encephalitis and La Crosse encephalitis (bunyavirus), sandfly fever and Rift Valley fever (phlebovirus), Crimean–Congo haemorrhagic fever (nairovirus) and others. Viruses of the genus *Tospovirus* are presently known only as plant pathogens. More than 360 plant species belonging to 50 families are known to be susceptible to infection with tomato spotted wilt virus.

The history of viruses of the family *Bunyaviridae* parallels that of arbovirology. Before 1950, many viruses were investigated because of their ability to cause human disease. Thus, during World War II, much was discovered about sandfly fever viruses, because these viruses were responsible for sig-

nificant morbidity among Allied troops stationed in the Middle East (Hertig and Sabin 1964). Sandfly (or phlebotomus) fever virus later became the prototype member of the genus *Phlebovirus*. A second complex of viruses destined to become a genus within the family also has links to military medicine. Viruses now known to be members of the genus *Hantavirus* played major roles in military campaigns in Asia, Yugoslavia and Scandinavia during World War II, and again during the Korean conflict. Indeed, today these viruses continue to infect soldiers in the Balkans and elsewhere. Likewise, university researchers in California isolated the prototype strain of California encephalitis in the mid-1940s, setting the stage for the discovery of many other closely related viruses, including significant human pathogens like La Crosse virus. Investigations of the California antigenic group of bunyaviruses led to the discovery of many of the fundamental characteristics of the family: the pathogenic potential of some viruses; transovarial transmission as a method of epidemiological maintenance; and the molecular basis for our current understanding of the group (LeDuc 1987).

The type species of the family, Bunyamwera virus, was first isolated in Uganda from a pool of *Aedes* mosquitoes collected during studies of yellow fever (Smithburn, Haddow and Mahaffy 1946). Bunyamwera virus was clearly unrelated either to yellow fever virus or to any other arbovirus then known, but subsequent studies showed that it shares structural and biochemical properties with many other viruses that now make up the family (Smithburn, Haddow and Mhaffy 1946, Murphy, Harrison and Whitfield 1973, Bishop et al. 1980, Elliott 1990). In the 1950s, the Rockefeller Foundation founded a series of international research stations dedicated to the study of viral diseases of humans, and during this time many of the viruses now recognized as members of the family were first discovered. For example, the laboratory in Belem, Brazil, was the source of many viruses then grouped antigenically as the 'group C' arboviruses through the classic work of Clarke and Casals (group A viruses evolved to the genus *Alphavirus*, in the family *Togaviridae*, while the group B viruses have become the genus *Flavivirus* in the family *Flaviviridae*). The group C arboviruses were known for a time as the 'Bunyamwera supergroup', then finally linked structurally and biochemically to form the family *Bunyaviridae*. Rockefeller-sponsored laboratories in Africa and India further contributed to the growing number of then known 'bunyaviruses'. Even today, 'new' viruses isolated from arthropods or vertebrates are often found to be members of the family.

1.2 Classification

Viruses of the family *Bunyaviridae* are classified according to structural similarities, antigenic characteristics, common biochemical properties and, more recently, genetic homology. Five genera are now recognized, the largest being the genus *Bunyavirus*, with c. 170 different viruses assigned to 18 groups (Table 30.1). The genus *Hantavirus* takes its name from Hantaan virus, the cause of haemorrhagic fever with renal syndrome. The hantaviruses are rapidly expanding in number, many 'new' viruses being identified by polymerase chain reaction (PCR) amplification of viral RNA obtained from field samples, but in several cases the actual viruses have yet to be isolated in a tractable form. At present, at least 16 serologically and/or genetically unique hantaviruses have been described, with many others almost certainly awaiting discovery (Table 30.2). The genus *Nairovirus* is named after the virus of Nairobi sheep disease (Montgomery 1917), and contains more than 30 viruses in 7 groups. The genus *Phlebovirus* has recently been expanded to include an earlier distinct genus, *Uukuvirus*, now merged with the phleboviruses on the basis of a common replication strategy and genetic similarities (Elliott et al. 1992). The most recent addition to the family is the genus *Tospovirus*, which takes its name from tomato spotted wilt virus. At present, this genus is limited to plant viruses and is transmitted by thrips. About 40 viruses are at present unassigned to any genus within the family.

Within each genus, viruses were historically divided on serological characteristics into group, complex, virus and subtype. 'Subtype' refers to viruses that can be serologically distinguished only with difficulty; named viruses can be easily distinguished; 'complex' refers to assemblies of viruses that are significantly cross-reactive; and 'group' or 'serogroup' encompasses complexes that are distantly related by serological activity (Peters and LeDuc 1991). More recent classification schemes have included the concept of a virus species, defined as a polythetic class of viruses. The interpretation of what constitutes a virus species is not consistent for each genus of the family, or among virus families in general.

1.3 Morphology and structure

Virions generally seem, by electron microscopy (EM), to be 80–120 nm spherical particles. Although pleomorphic particles are commonly observed by EM, such irregularity may be the result of desiccation, which occurs during specimen preparation, rather than inherent properties of viruses in the family (Hewlett and Chiu 1991). External features of the virions include a distinct bilaminar membrane, c. 5 nm thick, and a fringe of surface projections c. 5–10 nm long, comprised of the viral envelope glyco-

proteins, G1 and G2 (von Bonsdorff and Pettersson 1975, Hewlett and Chiu 1991) (Fig. 30.1). Because of differences in the G1 and G2 proteins of viruses in each genus, the characteristic appearance of virions varies. The surface area of the bunyavirus, La Crosse virus, was calculated to be able to accommodate from 4700 to 12 000 tightly packed G1 and G2 proteins; however, estimates from EM studies suggest that only 270–1400 proteins are present on a virion (Hewlett and Chiu 1991). The arrangement of the proteins, therefore, must include a wide spacing between each heterodimer of G1 and G2. The most comprehensive study of surface structure and chemical composition for a virus in the family was performed with the phlebovirus Uukuniemi virus. The virion surface units of Uukuniemi virus appeared as penton–hexon clusters with a T = 12, P = 3 icosahedral surface lattice and with hexon–hexon distances of c. 12.5–16 nm for stained viral particles and 17 nm for freeze-etched samples (von Bonsdorff and Pettersson 1975). The biochemical composition of Uukuniemi virus was estimated to be 2% RNA, 58% protein, 33% lipid and 7% carbohydrate (Obijeski and Murphy 1977).

All viruses in the family have tripartite, single-stranded RNA genomes, with segments designated large (L), medium (M) and small (S). Each RNA is complexed with many copies of the viral nucleocapsid protein (N) to form 3 distinct ribonucleocapsids, which seem to be helical (von Bonsdorff, Saikku and Oker-Blom 1970, von Bonsdorff and Pettersson 1975). Terminal, complementary, nucleotide sequences are conserved on the L, M and S segments for viruses within a particular genus and differ from those of viruses in other genera (Patterson et al. 1983, Collett et al. 1985, Schmaljohn et al. 1986, Rönnholm and Pettersson 1987, Schmaljohn, Schmaljohn and Dalrymple 1987, de Haan et al. 1990, 1991, Elliott, Schmaljohn and Collett 1991, Kormelink et al. 1992a) (Table 30.3). Base pairing of these RNAs to form panhandle structures (Fig. 30.2) can result in non-covalently closed circular RNAs and nucleocapsids (Pettersson and Bonsdorf 1975, Obijeski et al. 1976, Hewlett, Petterson and Baltimore 1977, Raju and Kolakofsky 1989) (see Fig. 30.1).

At least one each of the L, M and S ribonucleocapsids are required for viral infectivity; however, equal numbers of nucleocapsids may not always be packaged in mature virions (Bishop and Shope 1979). Differing complements of ribonucleocapsids were suggested to be related to virion size differences noted by EM (Talmon et al. 1987). Varying amounts of virus complementary-sense RNAs (cRNAs) were also identified in virions, but the significance, if any, of this finding is not known (Raju and Kolakofsky 1989, Simons, Hellman and Pettersson 1990, Kormelink et al. 1992a).

In addition to N, G1 and G2, virions also contain a polymerase protein (L) that is needed to copy the negative-sense viral genome into messenger-sense RNA(s) (Ranki and Pettersson 1975, Bouloy and Hannoun 1976, Schmaljohn and Dalrymple 1983, Patterson and Kolakofsky 1984, Gerbaud et al. 1987a, Adkins et al. 1995) (see Fig. 30.1). The exact place-

Table 30.1 Viruses of the *Bunyaviridae* known to cause disease in humans, domestic animals or plants and their geographic distribution and principal vectors (Numbers in parenthesis indicate the total viruses within that taxon)

	Geographic distribution	Associated illness	Principal vector
GENUS *BUNYAVIRUS*			
Anopheles A group (12)			
Tacaiuma	S America	Human	Mosquitoes
Bunyamwera group (32)			
Bunyamwera	Africa	Human	Mosquitoes
Cache valley	N America	Sheep, cattle	Mosquitoes
Fort Sherman	C America	Human	Mosquitoes
Germiston	Africa	Human	Mosquitoes
Ilesha	Africa	Human	Mosquitoes
Kairi	S America	Equine	Mosquitoes
Main Drain	N America	Equine	Mosquitoes, culicoid flies
Shokwe	Africa	Human	Mosquitoes
Wyeomyia	S America	Human	Mosquitoes
Xingu	S America	Human	Mosquitoes
Bwamba group (2)			
Bwamba	Africa	Human	Mosquitoes
Pongola	Africa	Human	Mosquitoes
Group C (14)			
Apeu	S America	Human	Mosquitoes
Caraparu	S & N America	Human	Mosquitoes
Itaqui	S America	Human	Mosquitoes
Madrid	N America	Human	Mosquitoes
Marituba	S America	Human	Mosquitoes
Murutucu	S America	Human	Mosquitoes
Nepuyo	S & N America	Human	Mosquitoes
Oriboca	S America	Human	Mosquitoes
Ossa	N America	Human	Mosquitoes
Restan	S America	Human	Mosquitoes
California group (14)			
California encephalitis	N America	Human	Mosquitoes
Guaroa	S & N America	Human	Mosquitoes
Inkoo	Europe	Human	Mosquitoes
Jamestown Canyon	N America	Human	Mosquitoes
La Crosse	N America	Human	Mosquitoes
Snowshoe hare	N America	Human	Mosquitoes
Tahyna	Europe	Human	Mosquitoes
Guama group (12)			
Catu	S America	Human	Mosquitoes
Guama	S & N America	Human	Mosquitoes
Nyando group (2)			
Nyando	Africa	Human	Mosquitoes
Simbu group (24)			
Akabane	Africa, Asia, Australia	Cattle	Mosquitoes, culicoid flies
Ingwavuma	Africa, Asia	Pigs	Mosquitoes
Oropouche	S America	Human	Culicoid flies, mosquitoes
GENUS *HANTAVIRUS* (14)			
Hantaan group			
Black Creek Canal	N America	Human	Rodent
Dobrava (Belgrade)	Europe	Human	Rodent
Hantaan	Asia, Europe	Human	Rodent
Puumala	Europe, Asia	Human	Rodent
Seoul	Asia, Europe, N & S America	Human	Rodent
Sin Nombre	N & S America	Human	Rodent

Table 30.1 Continued

	Geographic distribution	Associated illness	Principal vector
GENUS *NAIROVIRUS* (34)			
Crimean–Congo hemorrhagic fever (CCHF) group (3)			
CCHF	Africa, Asia, Europe	Human	Ticks
Hughes group (10)			
Hughes	N & S America	Sea birds	Ticks
Nairobi sheep disease group (2)			
Dugbe	Africa	Human, cattle	Ticks, culicoid flies, mosquitoes
Nairobi sheep disease	Africa, Asia	Human, cattle	Ticks, mosquitoes
GENUS *PHLEBOVIRUS* (51)			
Sandfly fever group (23)			
Candiru complex			
Alenquer	S America	Human	?
Candiru	S America	Human	?
Punta Toro complex			
Punta Toro	N & S & C America	Human	Phlebotomine flies
Rift Valley fever complex			
Rift Valley fever	Africa	Human, cattle	Mosquitoes
Sandfly fever Naples complex			
Sandfly fever Naples	Europe, Africa, Asia	Human	Phlebotomine flies
Toscana	Europe	Human	Phlebotomine flies
No complex assigned in sandfly fever group (16)			
Chagres	C America	Human	Phlebotomine flies
Sandfly fever Sicilian	Europe, Africa, Asia	Human	Phlebotomine flies
Uukuniemi group (12)			
St Abbs head	Europe	Sea birds	Ticks
GENUS *TOSPOVIRUS* (4)			
Tomato spotted wilt (3)	World-wide	Plants	Thrips
Impatiens necrotic spot (1)		Plants	
Grouped but unassigned viruses of *Bunyaviridae* (19)			
Bhanja group (3)			
Bhanja	Africa, Asia, Europe	Human	Ticks
Kasokero	Africa	Human	?
Yogue	Africa	Human	?
Ungrouped and unassigned viruses of *Bunyaviridae* (23)			
Bangui	Africa	Human	Mosquitoes
Issyk-Kul (Keterah)	Asia	Human	Mosquitoes, ticks
Tamdy	Asia	Human	Ticks
Tataguine	Africa	Human	Mosquitoes
Wanowrie	Africa, Asia	Human	Mosquitoes, ticks

Table 30.2 Serologically or genetically distinct viruses in the *Hantavirus*

Virus	Principal host	Distribution	Disease
Hantaan	*Apodemus agrarius*	China, Russia, Korea	HFRS
Dobrava	*Apodemus flavicolis*	Balkans	HFRS
Seoul	*Rattus norvegicus*	World-wide	HFRS
Puumala	*Clethrionomys glareolus*	Europe, Scandinavia, Russia	HFRS
Sin Nombre	*Peromyscus maniculatus*	USA, Canada, Mexico	HPS
New York 1[a]	*Peromyscus leucopus*	USA	HPS
Black Creek Canal	*Sigmodon hispidus*	USA	HPS
Bayou[a]	*Orizomys palustris*	USA	HPS
Thai-749	*Bandicota indica*	Thailand	?
Prospect Hill	*Microtus pennsylvanicus*	USA, Canada	?
Khabarovsk	*Microtus fortis*	Russia	?
Isla Vista[a]	*Microtus californicus*	USA	?
Bloodland Lake[a]	*Microtus ochrogaster*	USA	?
Thottapalayam	*Suncus murinus*	India	?
Tula[a]	*Microtus arvalis*	Europe	?
El Moro Canyon[a]	*Reithrodontomys* spp.	USA, Mexico, Central America	?

[a]A cell culture isolate has not been reported.
HFRS, haemorrhagic fever with renal syndrome; HPS, hantavirus pulmonary syndrome; ? it is not known if the virus causes human disease.
Data from: Lee, Lee and Johnson 1978, Avsic-Zupanc et al. 1992a, 1992b, Lee, Baek and Johnson 1982, Schmaljohn et al. 1985, Lee, Baek and Johnson 1982, Elliot et al. 1994, Schmaljohn et al. 1995, Song et al. 1994a, 1994b, Rollin et al. 1995, Torrez-Martinez and Hjelle 1995, Elwell et al. 1985, Torrez-Martinez, Song and Hjelle 1995, Plyusnin et al. 1994, Carey et al. 1971, Song et al. 1995.

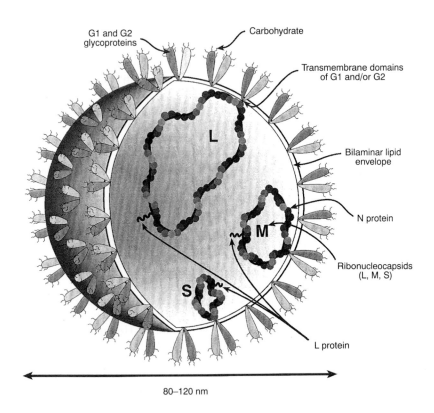

Fig. 30.1 Structure of a typical virus particle in the family *Bunyaviridae*. Individual components of the virus are described in the text.

ment of the L protein within virions is not known, but it is believed to be associated with each of the ribonucleocapsids.

1.4 Genome structure and function

The expression strategies of the L, M and S segments of viruses in the 5 genera of the family *Bunyaviridae* include both similarities and marked differences (Fig. 30.3). All viruses encode their structural proteins (N, G1/G2 and L) in the S, M and L cRNA, respectively. Viruses in each genus, except for those in the *Hantavirus* genus, also encode non-structural proteins in their M and/or S segment vRNA or cRNA. No functional significance has yet been clearly demonstrated for any of the non-structural proteins. The G1 and G2 proteins of all viruses are believed to be encoded as a polyprotein precursor that is cleaved co-translation-

Table 30.3 Consensus 3′ terminal nucleotide sequences of the L, M and S genome segments of representative members of the *Bunyaviridae*

Genus	Virus	Genome segment	Gene size (nucleotides)	Nucleotide[a] sequence	GenBank number
Bunyavirus	Bunyamwera	S	961	3′-UCAUCACAUGAGGUG	D00353
		M	4458	3′-UCAUCACAUGAUGGC	M11852
		L	6875	3′-UCAUCACAUGAGGAU	X14383
Hantavirus	Hantaan	S	1696	3′-AUCAUCAUCUGAGGG	M14626
		M	3616	3′-AUCAUCAUCUGAGGC	M14627
		L	6533	3′-AUCAUCAUCUGAGGG	X55901
Nairovirus	Dugbe	S	1712	3′-AGAGUUUCUGUUUGC	M25150
		M	4888	3′-AGAGUUUCUGUAUGG	M94133
		L	12255	3′-AGAGUUUCUGUAGUU	U15018
Phlebovirus	Rift Valley fever	S	1690	3′-UGUGUUUCGAGGGAUC	X53771
		M	3885	3′-UGUGUUUCUGCCACGU	M11157
		L	6404	3′-UGUGUUUCUGGCGGGU	X56464
Tospovirus	Tomato spotted wilt	S	2916	3′-UCUCGUUAGCACAGUU	D00645
		M	4821	3′-UCUCGUUAGUCACGUU	S48091
		L	8897	3′-UCUCGUUAGUCCAUUU	D10066

[a]Sequences identical on all 3 genome segments are underlined.

ally, although direct evidence for this has been obtained only for phleboviruses (Ulmanen, Seppala and Pettersson 1981, Rönnholm and Pettersson 1987, Suzich and Collett 1988). The L segments of all viruses described to date encode only the L protein and have <200 nucleotides of non-coding information (Elliott 1989, Schmaljohn 1990, de Haan, Kormelink et al. 1991, Muller et al. 1991). There is no evidence for additional coding regions in either the L segment cRNA or the vRNA.

BUNYAVIRUSES

Bunyaviruses produce both N and a non-structural protein, NS$_S$, from overlapping reading frames found in the S segment cRNA (Gentsch and Bishop 1978, Cash et al. 1979, Bishop et al. 1982, Fuller and Bishop 1982, Akashi and Bishop 1983, Cabradilla, Holloway and Obijeski 1983, Fuller, Bhown and Bishop 1983, Akashi et al. 1984, Bouloy et al. 1984, Elliott 1985, Gerbaud et al. 1987b). Only one S segment mRNA species was detected for the bunyaviruses; thus, a single mRNA must be used for translation of both N and NS$_S$ (Bouloy et al. 1984, Patterson and Kolakofsky 1984, Eshita et al. 1985). The bunyavirus M segment encodes an NS$_M$ protein between coding information for G2 and G1 (Eshita and Bishop 1984, Lees, Pringle and Elliott 1986, Grady, Sanders and Campbell 1987, Fazakerly et al. 1988, Nakitare and Elliott 1993).

HANTAVIRUSES

Hantaviruses seem to have the simplest genome expression strategy of viruses in the family *Bunyaviridae*, in that there is no clear evidence that nonstructural proteins are generated. The S segments of certain hantaviruses have an overlapping reading frame within N, which could encode a protein similar in size to that of the bunyavirus NS$_S$ protein; however, such a protein has not yet been found (Parrington and Kang 1990, Settergren et al. 1990, Stohwasser et

al. 1990, Spiropoulou et al. 1994, Li et al. 1995). Certain of the New World hantaviruses have very large S segment 3′ non-coding regions; i.e. >700 bases for Sin Nombre virus as compared to <400 bases for prototype Hantaan virus. Numerous repeated nucleotide sequences found in the Sin Nombre virus non-coding region are suggested to result from polymerase slippage, but a functional importance for their presence has not been discovered (Spiropoulou et al. 1994, Li et al. 1995, Morzunov et al. 1995, Ravkov et al. 1995). The M segments of hantaviruses have only a short potential intergenic region (e.g. ≤34 amino acids for Hantaan virus) between the sequences encoding G1 and G2, as well as little additional 5′ or 3′ non-coding information (Schmaljohn, Schmaljohn and Dalrymple 1987).

PHLEBOVIRUSES

Phleboviruses use ambisense coding to produce an NS$_S$ polypeptide. That is, NS$_S$ is encoded in vRNA in a reading frame that does not overlap the cRNA sequences encoding N (Ihara, Akashi and Bishop 1984, Overton, Ihara and Bishop 1987, Marriott, Ward and Nuttall 1989, Simons, Hellman and Pettersson 1990, Giorgi et al. 1991). The existence of NS$_S$ was verified in cells infected with numerous phleboviruses, including Uukuniemi virus, Rift Valley fever virus, Punta Toro virus and Karimabad virus (Parker and Hewlett 1981, Ulmanen, Seppala and Pettersson 1981, Smith and Pifat 1982, Struthers and Swanepoel 1982, Overton, Ihara and Pettersson 1987). In vitro translation studies and Northern blot analyses with viral RNAs demonstrated that N and NS$_S$ are generated from separate, subgenomic messages (Ulmanen, Seppala and Pettersson 1981, Parker, Smith and Dalrymple 1984, Ihara, Matsuura and Bishop 1985, Marriott et al. 1989, Simons, Hellman and Pettersson 1990). The M segment of some, but not all, phleboviruses encodes an NS$_M$ in cRNA in the same reading frame

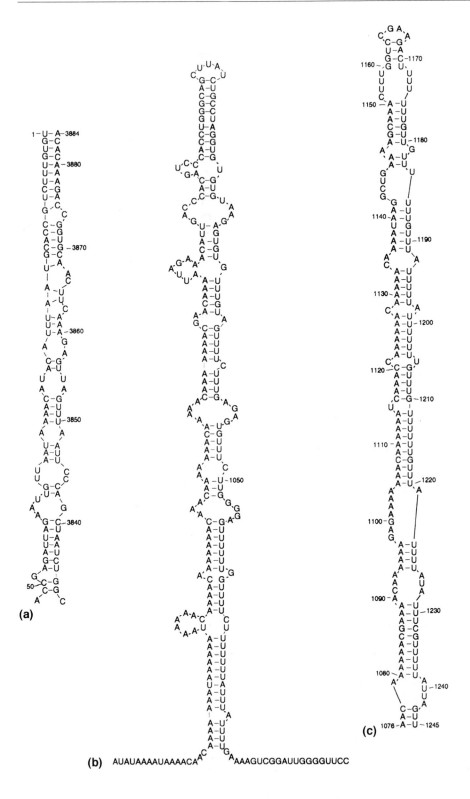

(b) AUAUAAAAUAAAACA ... AAAGUCGGAUUGGGGUUCC

Fig. 30.2 Predicted panhandle structures formed by base-pairing of complementary sequences. (a) Terminal sequences of the M genome segment of the phlebovirus Rift Valley fever virus (data from Collett et al. 1985). (b) Intergenic region of the ambisense S genome segment of the phlebovirus Punta Toro virus (data from Emery 1987). (c) Intergenic region of the M genome segment of the tospovirus tomato spotted wilt virus (data from Kormelink et al. 1992).

but preceding the coding information for G1 and G2 (Collett et al. 1985). For example, the cRNA open reading frame of Rift Valley fever virus has 5 in-frame translation initiation codons. Use of the first ATG resulted in production of uncleaved NS$_M$ G2 as well as G1, whereas use of the second ATG resulted in distinct NS$_M$ of c. 14 kDa, G2 and G1 proteins (Collett et al. 1985, Suzich and Collett 1988, Kakach, Suzich and Collett 1989, Schmaljohn et al. 1989, Suzich, Kakach and Collett 1990). Both the NS$_M$ G2 fusion protein and the NS$_M$ protein are readily observed in cell cultures infected with Rift Valley fever virus. An even larger potential NS$_M$ protein (c. 30 kDa) with 13 in-frame initiation codons is predicted from the M segment nucleotide sequence of Punta Toro virus; however, no polypeptide of this has been identified in cells

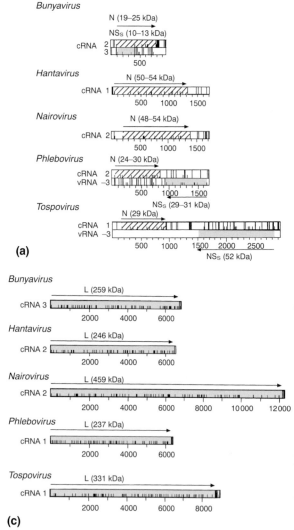

(a)

(b)

(c)

Fig. 30.3 Coding strategy and gene organization of the bunyaviruses. (a) S segment open reading frames encoding the N and NS_S proteins are indicated by striped and stippled boxes, respectively. (b) M segment open reading frames encoding G1, G2 and NS_M are indicated by stippled, cross-hatched and striped boxes, respectively. (c) L segment open reading frames encoding the L protein are indicated by stippled boxes. Translation initiation codons are represented by short hatch marks and stop codons are indicated by long hatch marks. The reading frame used, with respect to complementary sense RNA (cRNA, frames 1, 2, 3) or virus sense RNA (vRNA, frames –1, –2, –3) are listed to the left of the boxes. Nucleotide sequence numbers, with respect to the 5′ terminus of cRNA are shown below the boxes. Arrows indicate the direction of translation, 5′ to 3′, and predicted molecular weights of the gene products are shown above or below the arrows.

infected with Punta Toro virus (Ihara, Dalrymple and Bishop 1985). There is no apparent homology between the Rift Valley fever virus and Punta Toro virus NS_M proteins, and both Rift Valley fever virus and Punta Toro virus G1 and G2 proteins can be efficiently produced in vitro in the absence of the NS_M coding information (Matsuoka et al. 1988, Suzich and Collett 1988, Suzich, Kakach and Collett 1990).

In contrast to those of Punta Toro virus and Rift Valley fever virus, the M segment of the phlebovirus, Uukuniemi virus, has no preglycoprotein coding region, and the amino terminus of G1 is located 17 amino acids downstream of the first (and only) initiation codon (Rönnholm and Pettersson 1987). Thus, Uukuniemi virus G1 seems to be similar to the Rift Valley fever virus NS_M G2 fusion protein. Carboxyterminal sequence information has not been obtained for phlebovirus envelope proteins; consequently, the exact point of cleavage between G1 and G2 has not been identified. However, few or no extra coding sequences reside between G1 and G2 (e.g. <27 amino acids for Rift Valley fever virus and <81 amino acids for Uukuniemi virus) (Rönnholm and Pettersson 1987, Kakach, Suzich and Collett 1989).

NAIROVIRUSES

The S segment of nairoviruses, like that of hantaviruses, encodes only a large N protein and has no known non-structural protein coding information (Cash 1985, Ward et al. 1990, Marriott and Nuttall 1992). The M segment of the nairovirus, Dugbe virus, seems to encode only G2 and G1, although G1 was suggested to arise from post-translational cleavage of a slightly larger precursor (Marriott, el Ghorr and Nuttall 1992). The L segment of Dugbe virus is the largest gene of any member of the family *Bunyaviridae*. Why nairoviruses might need a polymerase protein almost twice the size of those of other viruses in the family is not known.

TOSPOVIRUSES

Both the S and the M segments of tospoviruses have ambisense coding strategies and separate subgenomic messages to generate structural and non-structural proteins (de Haan et al. 1990, Kormelink et al. 1992a, Law, Speck and Moyer 1992). Unlike the NS_S of phleboviruses, which is about the same size as N, that of tospoviruses is approximately twice the size of N (Fig. 30.3). Thus, the L segment of tospoviruses is the only one of the 3 gene segments that uses a strictly nega-tive-sense coding strategy (de Haan et al. 1991).

1.5 Replication

ATTACHMENT AND ENTRY

One or both of the integral viral envelope proteins, G1 and G2, are believed to mediate attachment of virions to host-cell receptors of unknown specificity. This was first demonstrated by proteolytic enzyme treatment of purified La Crosse virus, which resulted in 'spikeless' virus particles and a concomitant 5 $\log_{10}$ reduction in infectivity (Obijeski et al. 1976). For most viruses in the family, it is not known which of the envelope glycoproteins mediates attachment. To attempt to answer that question for bunyaviruses, La Crosse virus was treated with bromelain or Pronase, which degraded portions of G1 but left G2 uncleaved. Such treatment resulted in its complete loss of infec-tivity (Kingsford and Hill 1981). La Crosse virus G1 was also implicated as the attachment protein for mammalian cells because affinity-purified G1 protein could competitively inhibit attachment of radiolab-elled G1 to Vero cells (Ludwig et al. 1991). In contrast, G2 did not bind to Vero cells, but did bind to cultured mosquito cells and midguts. To competitively inhibit binding of G2, both G1 and G2 were required, which led to the speculation that the G1 protein might be the viral attachment protein for vertebrates, whereas G2 is used for arthropod infection (Ludwig et al. 1991). Confirmation of this as a general feature of the bunyaviruses is needed. Although no similar infor-mation exists for viruses in other genera, there is evi-dence that neutralizing and haemagglutination-inhibiting (HI) sites are present on both the G1 and G2 proteins of phleboviruses (Keegan and Collett 1986, Pifat, Osterling and Smith 1988) and hanta-viruses (Dantas et al. 1986, Arikawa et al. 1989), so it is possible that either or both of these proteins may be involved in attachment.

Fusion of infected cells at acidic pH has been reported for viruses in the *Bunyaviridae* (Gonzalez-Scarano, Pobjecky and Nathanson 1984, Arikawa, Takashima and Hashimoto 1985, Gonzalez-Scarano 1985, Gonzalez-Scarano et al. 1985). Such pH-dependent fusion is generally believed to relate to early events in internalization of viral particles. Electron microscopy of the infection process of Rift Valley fever virus revealed that virions seem to enter cells in phagocytic vacu-oles (Ellis et al. 1988). This observation is consistent with a mode of entry similar to that first described for alphaviruses in which the virus is endocytosed in coated vesicles which subsequently become acidified (Marsh and Helenius 1980, Tycko and Maxfield 1982). The acidification triggers a fusion of viral membranes and endosomal membranes, and results in the release of the viral nucleocapsid into the cell cyto-plasm. Whether one or both of the envelope proteins are necessary for fusion has not been determined for most mem-bers of the family. For the bunyavirus La Crosse virus, there is ample information to indicate that the G1 protein is involved in fusion. For example, it is known that monoclonal antibodies to G1 inhibit fusion, that G1 undergoes a confor-mational change at the pH of fusion and that a virus mutant with a defective G1 does not cause fusion (Gonzalez-Scarano

1985, Gonzalez-Scarano et al. 1985, Gonzalez-Scarano, Pob-jecky and Nathanson 1987). Consistent with this, expression of G1 in the absence of G2 with recombinant vaccinia viruses resulted in cell fusion in vitro (Jacoby et al. 1993). These functions defined for the G1 and G2 proteins of bunyaviruses do not imply like functions for viruses in other genera.

TRANSCRIPTION

After uncoating of viral genomes, primary transcrip-tion of negative-sense vRNA to complementary mRNA occurs through interaction of the virion-associated polymerase (L protein) and the 3 viral RNA templates (Ranki and Pettersson 1975, Bouloy and Hannoun 1976). Transcription occurs entirely in the cytoplasm and there is no requirement for ongoing cellular tran-scription, as indicated by the resistance of viruses in the family to actinomycin D, an inhibitor of DNA-dependent RNA polymerases, such as host-cell DNA-dependent RNA polymerase II (Obijeski and Murphy 1977). The L protein is believed to function first as an endonuclease to cleave capped oligonucleotides from host mRNAs to serve as transcription primers (Fig. 30.4). This priming results in the presence of 5′ ter-minal extensions of c. 10–18 heterogeneous nucleo-tides on the termini of viral mRNAs (Bishop, Gay and Matsuoko 1983, Bishop et al. 1984, Patterson and Kolakofsky 1984, Eshita et al. 1985, Ihara, Matsuura and Bishop 1985, Collett 1986, Bouloy et al. 1990, Simons and Pettersson 1991, Kormelink et al. 1992c, Dobbs and Kang 1993, Jin and Elliott 1993a, 1993b). For phleboviruses and tospoviruses, which have ambi-sense coding strategies, both the N and the NS$_S$ subgenomic mRNA have heterogeneous, non-viral, 5′ terminal extensions (Ihara, Matsuura and Bishop 1985, Simons and Pettersson 1991, Kormelink et al. 1992).

Direct evidence for the presence of capped struc-tures on the termini of the extensions was obtained by using anti-cap antibodies to immunoselect mRNAs (Hacker 1990, Vialat and Bouloy 1992). That the cleavage of capped oligonucleotides may not be an entirely random process is indicated by a preference for specific mono-, di- or trinucleotides at the −1 to −3 positions with respect to the 5′ terminus of mRNAs of particular viruses. For example, almost all cDNA clones of the S mRNA of the bunyavirus Germiston virus displayed U or G at the −1 position (Bouloy et al. 1990). Similarly, Bunyamwera virus preferred UG, but snowshoe hare virus was found to have A most commonly as the 3′ terminal nucleotide of the S mRNA extensions (Bishop et al. 1983, Eshita et al. 1985, Jin and Elliott 1993a). For phleboviruses, C was found most often at the −1 position of the M mRNA of Rift Valley fever virus and also at the −1 position of the N and NS$_S$ mRNAs of Uukuniemi virus (Collett 1986, Simons and Pettersson 1991). For Hantaan virus, the preferred −1 nucleotide was G (Dobbs and Kang 1993, Garcin et al. 1995) and for the nairovirus Dugbe virus, C (Jin and Elliott 1993b). The reason for such preferences could imply that a restricted or specific subset of host mRNAs is used for primers, per-

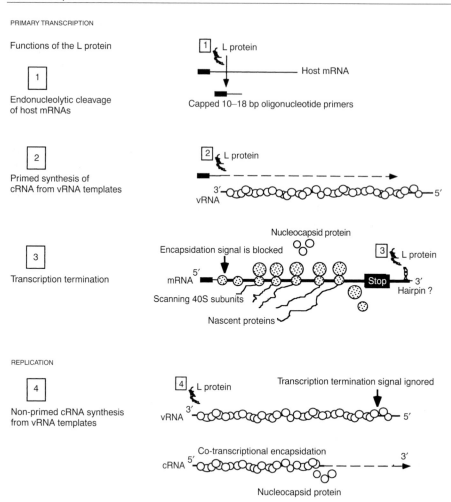

PRIMARY TRANSCRIPTION

Functions of the L protein

1

Endonucleolytic cleavage of host mRNAs

2

Primed synthesis of cRNA from vRNA templates

3

Transcription termination

REPLICATION

4

Non-primed cRNA synthesis from vRNA templates

Fig. 30.4 Transcription and replication of the bunyaviruses. 1. The L protein cleaves capped oligonucleotides from host cell mRNAs. 2. The capped oligonucleotides are used to prime transcription of cRNA from vRNA templates. 3. Transcription is terminated at signals that may involve secondary structure or primary sequence of the vRNA template. mRNAs are not encapsidated, perhaps owing to the presence of scanning 40S ribosomes or the caps. 4. For replication to proceed, the L protein must use non-primed synthesis and must ignore transcription termination signals to produce complete cRNA templates for further vRNA synthesis. The mechanism(s) of the switch from transcription to replication are not well defined.

haps because of a need for limited base pairing with the viral genome, but this has not been demonstrated.

Studies on the bunyaviruses Germiston virus and Bunyamwera virus revealed the insertion of U or GU between the primer and the 5′ terminal viral sequence. It was also noted that the 3′ most terminal nucleotides of the stolen host sequences were often similar to the 5′ terminal viral sequences, leading to the hypothesis that the insertions might arise from partial reiteration of the 5′ terminal sequences owing to a backward slippage of the viral polymerase after the first 2 or 3 nucleotides are transcribed (Vialat and Bouloy 1992, Jin and Elliott 1993a). In addition to such insertions, for bunyavirus and phlebovirus mRNAs, but not for the nairovirus mRNAs studied, the +1 nucleotide in the mRNA transcript is sometimes missing (Bishop et al. 1983, Bouloy et al. 1990, Simons and Pettersson 1991, Jin and Elliott 1993a, 1993b), and for hantavirus RNAs the first 3 nucleotides are often absent (Dobbs and Kang 1993). Whether this indicates primary transcription initiation at nucleotides other than the terminal one or perhaps artefacts of the cloning procedures remains to be determined.

At present, it is not clear what host functions are important for primary transcription of viruses in the family *Bunyaviridae*. Conflicting data concerning the

need for ongoing host protein synthesis for primary transcription (as defined by the inability to achieve full length transcripts in the presence of drugs such as cycloheximide and puromycin) were reported for viruses in the *Bunyavirus* genus (Abraham and Pattnaik 1983, Patterson and Kolakofsky 1984, Eshita et al. 1985, Raju and Kolakofsky 1986, 1989, Bellocq et al. 1987). Recent studies suggest that, if there is a need for ongoing protein synthesis, it may be at the level of ribosome scanning, rather than translation. This speculation was based on the finding that transcription was not inhibited by edeine, a drug that prevents 40S and 60S ribosomal subunits from complexing (Vialat and Bouloy 1992). These data are consistent with an earlier hypothesis that scanning ribosomes prevent premature termination by preventing base-pairing between the template RNA and the transcript, which would cause the polymerase to halt and terminate prematurely (Bellocq et al. 1987).

Termination of primary transcripts (i.e. mRNAs) occurs c. 100 nucleotides from the 5′ terminus of the vRNA template, resulting in mRNAs that are truncated at their 3′ termini, as compared to cRNA (Fig. 30.4) (Cash et al. 1979, Pattnaik and Abraham 1983, Bouloy et al. 1984, Patterson and Kolakofsky 1984, Eshita et al. 1985, Pettersson et al. 1985, Collett 1986, Raju and Kolakofsky 1987b, Bouloy et al. 1990). Potential transcription termination sites have been proposed for the S segments of La Crosse virus (Patterson and Kolakofsky 1984) and snowshoe hare virus (Eshita and Bishop 1984, Eshita et al. 1985) at or near the genomic sequence 3'-G/CUUUUU. Proposed U-rich transcription termination sites also are found on the M and S segments of Germiston virus (3'-AUGUUUUGUU and 3'-GGGGUUUGUU, respectively) (Bouloy et al. 1990). Although such transcription termination sites are similar to those resulting in polyadenylation of mRNAs of other viruses, mRNAs of viruses in the family *Bunyaviridae* are not known to be polyadenylated (Ulmanen, Seppala and Pettersson 1981, Pattnaik and Abraham 1983, Pettersson et al. 1985). Moreover, transcription termination sites without the homopolymeric U_5 or U_6 tract have been proposed for the S and M segment mRNAs of another bunyavirus, snowshoe hare virus (5'-GGUGGGGGGUGGGG and 5'-GGUGGGGGGUGGGG, respectively) (Eshita and Bishop 1984) and the M segments of the phleboviruses Rift Valley fever virus and Punta Toro virus (5'-UGGGGUGGUGGGGU and 5'-GGUGAGAGU-GUAGAAAG, respectively) (Collett 1986). Comparing the S segment sequences of a number of phleboviruses revealed that G-rich sequences and similar sequence motifs were found in the intergenic regions of some but not all phleboviruses (Giorgi et al. 1991).

Transcription termination of ambisense genes to yield structural and non-structural protein mRNAs may occur through recognition of RNA secondary structure rather than a specific gene sequence. For example, the transcription termination sites for both the N and the NS_S mRNAs of Punta Toro virus were mapped to within 40 nucleotides of one another, and predicted hairpin structures were found in this intergenic region as well as in the intergenic regions of the S segments of certain other phleboviruses and in both the S and the M segments of tospoviruses (de Haan et al. 1990, Kormelink et al. 1992, Law, Speck and Moyer 1992) (see Fig. 30.3). For the S segment of the phlebovirus Uukuniemi virus, although there is a non-coding region of 70 nucleotides between the N and the NS_S genes, hybridization studies demonstrated that the 3' ends of the subgenomic messages overlap one another by about 100 nucleotides. Thus the 3' end of the NS_S mRNA extends into the coding region of N and the 3' end of the N mRNA terminates just before the coding sequences for N. A short palindromic sequence in the intergenic region (including the 3' ends of each mRNA) is predicted to allow formation of an A/U-rich hairpin structure (Simons and Pettersson 1991). Such structures could affect transcription termination only if they can form while the genome is complexed with N; to date there is no direct evidence that this occurs.

Currently, there is no conclusive evidence that either of these mechanisms (i.e. secondary structure or gene sequence) is important for transcription termination with viruses in this family. Although the mechanism of transcription termination is not known, studies performed with the L protein of Bunyamwera virus expressed by vaccinia virus recombinants resulted infrequently in correct transcription termination, suggesting that an additional factor (or factors), of viral or cellular origin, may be required for consistent transcription termination (Jin and Elliott 1993a). One such factor might include interaction between the transcriptase and a newly synthesized viral protein, such as NS_S (Vialat and Bouloy 1992, Jin and Elliott 1993a). This could not be a familial characteristic, however, because hantaviruses and nairoviruses are not known to encode NS_S proteins. Also, for viruses using ambisense coding to produce NS_S, the kinetics of synthesis of N and NS_S, as well as the finding that only N mRNA can be detected in the presence of cycloheximide, suggest that replication of full-length, encapsidated cRNA

must occur before synthesis of the NS_S mRNA. Thus, because NS_S appears relatively late in infection, it is unlikely to have a role in primary transcription, unless it can be generated in small amounts directly by translation of the vRNA (Simons, Persson and Pettersson 1992).

GENOME REPLICATION

The switch from primary transcription to genome replication requires the L protein to switch from primed synthesis, by using capped host cell oligonucleotides, to a process of independently initiating transcription at the precise 3' end of the template and producing an encapsidated, full-length transcript. The factors dictating that vRNA and cRNA should complex with N to form nucleocapsid structures, while mRNAs should not, are not known, but it has been suggested that the added capped host cell sequences on the 5' ends of viral messages may somehow prevent encapsidation (Raju and Kolakofsky 1989).

Unlike primary transcription, secondary transcription is clearly sensitive to inhibitors of protein synthesis such as cycloheximide. The need for ongoing protein synthesis for replication to proceed is likely to be due to the need for continued viral protein synthesis rather than host cell protein synthesis. Although the factors that dictate that the L protein should begin genome replication are not known for viruses in the family *Bunyaviridae*, a mechanism similar to that proposed for rhabdoviruses and paramyxoviruses seems plausible: accumulating a sufficient quantity of N seems to trigger encapsidation and to serve as an antitermination signal, thus allowing full-length genome synthesis (Blumberg, Giorgi and Kolakofsky 1983, Wertz 1983, Patton, Davis and Wertz 1984a, 1984b, Arnheiter et al. 1985, Banerjee 1987, Vidal and Kolakofsky 1989). Non-structural proteins were suggested to control the availability of the N protein of rhabdoviruses, and, where available, they could possibly do the same for the *Bunyaviridae*. A model for transcription and replication based on information detailed above is presented in Fig. 30.4.

SYNTHESIS AND PROCESSING OF VIRAL PROTEINS

S segment gene products

As described above ('Bunyaviruses', p. 606; 'Phleboviruses', p. 606; 'Tospoviruses', p. 608), the N and NS_S proteins encoded by the vRNA and cRNA of the S segments of bunyaviruses, phleboviruses and tospoviruses do not originate from precursor polypeptides, and therefore processing of proteins is not required. Hantaviruses and nairoviruses encode only one product in their S segments. Post-translational modifications (e.g. phosphorylation or amidation) have not generally been defined for S segment products except for the NS_S of Rift Valley fever virus. For Rift Valley fever virus, the NS_S protein was reported to be phosphorylated (Parker, Smith and Dalrymple 1984) and to accumulate in the nuclei of infected cells where they seemed to aggregate as filamentous structures (Struthers and Swanepoel 1982). Although this is not known to be a general finding for phleboviruses, very few of them have been examined with immune sera specific for the NS$_S$ protein. The NS$_S$ of the tospovirus tomato spotted wilt virus was seen in association with fibrous structures in the cytoplasm of infected plants; however, it was not clear if the proteins actually formed the filaments or were just associated with them (Kormelink et al. 1991).

The function of the NS$_S$ protein has not been clearly defined for any virus in the family. For Rift Valley fever virus, a complete NS$_S$ was found to be nonessential for replication in that a mutant virus, isolated from mosquitoes, with an in-frame internal deletion of about 70% of NS$_S$, was still replication-competent in Vero and mosquito cells and in mosquitoes. However, it produced abortive infections in human lung cell cultures, and was attenuated when inoculated into mice (Muller et al. 1995).

M segment gene products

The designation of G1 and G2 comes from their relative migrations when analysed by sodium dodecyl sulphate polyacrylamide gel electrophoresis (SDS-PAGE). G1 is the more slowly migrating polypeptide. These designations, based on apparent polypeptide size, do not always correlate with the gene order, structure or function of G1 and G2. For example, for the 2 phleboviruses Rift Valley fever virus and Punta Toro virus it is known that G1 of Rift Valley fever virus is related to G2 of Punta Toro virus and vice versa (see Fig. 30.3).

Co-translational cleavage of G1 and G2 (and, in the *Bunyavirus* and *Phlebovirus* genera, NS$_M$) is believed to be mediated by a cellular signalase-like enzyme. Except for the nairovirus Dugbe virus, which may encode G1 as a precursor (see p. 608), all predicted polyprotein precursors have hydrophobic regions preceding both G1 and G2 that are consistent with signal sequences that allow transport of the nascent proteins through membranes. The precursors also have variable numbers of potential transmembrane regions, and a hydrophobic sequence at the carboxy terminus, indicative of a membrane anchor region (Eshita and Bishop 1984, Collett et al. 1985, Schmaljohn, Schmaljohn and Dalrymple 1987, Fazakerley and Ross 1989, Law, Speck and Moyer 1992, Marriott et al. 1992). Thus, these proteins are typical class 1 membrane proteins, i.e. with the amino terminus exposed on the surface of the virion and the C terminus anchored in the membrane.

A common property of all M segment gene products predicted from cDNA sequences studied so far is their high cysteine content (4–7%) and, in related viruses, the conservation of the position of the cysteine residues (Ihara, Dalrymple and Bishop 1985, Lees et al. 1986, Grady, Sanders and Campbell 1987, Rönnholm and Pettersson 1987, Antic et al. 1992, Kormelink et al. 1992, Law, Speck and Moyer 1992, Marriott et al. 1992). These findings suggest that extensive disulphide bridge formation may occur and that the positions may be crucial for determining correct polypeptide folding. The secondary structure of the proteins can also play a role in immunogenicity, in that neu-

tralizing or protective epitopes are often non-linear (Battles and Dalrymple 1988, Wang et al. 1993).

All of the envelope proteins examined to date possess *N*-linked oligosaccharides. The gene sequences that define a potential *N*-linked glycosylation site are those that encode Asn–X–Ser/Thr, where X is not Pro (Hubbard and Ivatt 1981). The number of potential glycosylation sites found in the predicted M segment gene product range from 4 sites for certain hantaviruses to 9 sites for some tospoviruses (Antic et al. 1992, Law, Speck and Moyer 1992). The number of sites actually used in mature virion proteins has not been defined for most viruses; however, G2 of the phlebovirus Rift Valley fever virus was demonstrated to be glycosylated at its single available site and at least 3 of 4 possible G1 sites (Kakach, Suzich and Collett 1989). Analysis of the predicted amino acid sequences of the envelope proteins of the bunyavirus snowshoe hare virus (Eshita and Bishop 1984, Fazakerly et al. 1988) and examination of glycosylated tryptic oligopeptides (Vorndam and Trent 1979) suggest that all 3 potential glycosylation sites on G2 are used and at least one of 2 sites on G1. The single glycosylation site available in the G2 protein of Hantaan virus is used, and this site is conserved among numerous other hantaviruses (Schmaljohn et al. 1986, Antic, Wright and Kang 1992). Where studied, the oligosaccharides attached to the G1 and G2 proteins were mostly high-mannose glycans, although complex and novel intermediate-type oligosaccharides were also identified on the G1 protein of Uukuniemi virus (Madoff and Lenard 1982, Pesonen, Kuismanen and Pettersson 1982, Schmaljohn et al. 1986, Antic, Wright and Kang 1992, Ruusala et al. 1992).

Although not studied extensively, the NS$_M$ proteins of the bunyavirus Bunyamwera virus and the phlebovirus Rift Valley fever virus were found not to be glycosylated (Lees et al. 1986, Collett et al. 1988, Kakach, Suzich and Collett 1989). For Rift Valley fever virus, however, another M segment gene product consisting of an uncleaved form of the NS$_M$ protein and G2 is also routinely generated, and the NS$_M$ portion of that fusion protein is glycosylated (Kakach, Suzich and Collett 1989).

L segment gene products

No post-translational modifications of L proteins for viruses in the *Bunyaviridae* have been described. As detailed above (p. 609), the L protein is a multifunctional enzyme. For Bunyamwera virus and Rift Valley fever virus, the L and N proteins are essential and sufficient for transcriptase activity (Dunn et al. 1995, Lopez et al. 1995). The Bunyamwera virus L protein transcribes a synthetic template in concert with the N proteins of closely related bunyaviruses, but only inefficiently with more dissimilar bunyavirus N proteins (Dunn et al. 1995). As described above (p. 607), the complementary terminal nucleotide sequences of viruses in the family *Bunyaviridae* that are predicted to form panhandle structures have been suggested as possible polymerase recognition structures. Although only limited information exists, in one study a point mutation resulting in disruption of the base-paired structure was found to drastically reduce Bunyamwera virus L transcriptase activity in vitro (Dunn et al. 1995).

Comparison of L protein sequences of viruses in the family *Bunyaviridae* with other RNA polymerases revealed the presence of 4 conserved 'polymerase motifs' (Poch et al. 1989, Jin and Elliott 1992). Mutational analysis of cDNA representing Bunyamwera virus L within these conserved regions was used to demonstrate that amino acid residues that are highly conserved among viruses in the family could not be changed, but that changes in non-conserved amino acids did not generally reduce the ability of the expressed L protein to transcribe authentic viral nucleocapsid templates in an in vitro assay (Jin and Elliott 1992, Dunn et al. 1995).

TRANSPORT

One of the earliest notable features found to distinguish bunyaviruses from all other negative-strand RNA viruses was that the viral particles are formed intracellularly by a budding process at smooth surface vesicles in the Golgi area (von Bonsdorff, Saikku and Oker-Blom 1970, Lyons and Heyduk 1973, Murphy, Harrison and Whitfield 1973, Bishop and Shope 1979). The reason(s) for virus maturation in the Golgi complex as opposed to the more usual mode of viral morphogenesis, i.e. budding at the plasma membrane, is not known. Because the ionophore monensin, which exchanges protons for sodium ions, inhibits budding of Uukuniemi virus, it was postulated that the pH or ionic conditions present in the Golgi complex might be critical for viral budding (Kuismanen, Saraste and Pettersson 1985, Pettersson 1991). It is also not known what signals are responsible for the accumulation of viral structural proteins in the Golgi complex; however, possibilities include a structural or molecular resemblance between G1 and/or G2 and Golgi-specific proteins, such as the glycosyltransferases that are normally retained in the Golgi (Gahmberg et al. 1986). Another possibility is that they may lack the signal required for transport from the Golgi to the plasma membrane (Kuismanen et al. 1982).

Dimerization of the G1 and G2 proteins in the endoplasmic reticulum (ER), shortly after their synthesis, is generally believed to be necessary for transport of the proteins to the Golgi complex. For Punta Toro virus, kinetic studies indicated that heterodimerization occurs between newly synthesized G1 and G2 within 3 min after protein synthesis and that the dimers are linked by disulphide bonds (Chen and Compans 1991). The NS_M proteins of the phleboviruses Rift Valley fever and Punta Toro viruses and the bunyavirus Bunyamwera virus were not needed for transport, because G1 and G2 were targeted to the Golgi when expressed from an M segment from which the NS_M coding region had been deleted (Matsuoka et al. 1988, Wasmoen, Kakach and Collett 1988, Lappin et al. 1994). However, when the entire M segment of Rift Valley fever virus was expressed, the NS_M proteins of Rift Valley fever virus did co-localize to the Golgi with the G1 and G2 proteins (Wasmoen, Kakach and Collett 1988). Similar findings with the NS_M proteins of La Crosse virus and Bunyamwera virus were reported, but in neither case was it determined whether the NS_M proteins served any role in morphogenesis (Nakitare and Elliott 1993, Lappin et al. 1994).

The Golgi transport and retention signals have not been defined for most viruses, although in some cases it is known that only one protein can move to the Golgi if dimerization does not occur (Matsuoka et al. 1988, Chen and Compans 1991, Matsuoka, Chen and Compans 1991, Rönnholm 1992, Ruusala et al. 1992). For example, in the absence of G1, G2 of Punta Toro virus was transported out of the ER and expressed on the cell surface. Removal of the carboxy-terminal anchor sequence of G1 resulted in secretion of this protein. When both proteins were expressed, however, both G1 and G2 were found in the Golgi. These studies suggest that the Golgi transport and retention signal is located on the G1 protein of Punta Toro virus (Chen, Matsuoka and Compans 1991). Similar results were obtained with the phlebovirus Uukuniemi virus, in that expression of G1 and G2 independently in COS cells resulted in translocation of only G1 to the Golgi, while G2 remained in the ER, suggesting that the signal for transport resides on G1 and that G2 is transported only by association with G1 (Rönnholm 1992). In contrast, independent expression of G1 and G2 of the hantavirus Hantaan virus resulted in the inability of either protein to leave the ER, but co-expression resulted in efficient transport of both proteins to the Golgi (Pensiero et al. 1988, Pensiero and Hay 1992, Ruusala et al. 1992).

The transport of tospovirus proteins within plant cells and insect cells has not been studied extensively. These viruses replicate in insects (Ullman et al. 1993, Wijkamp et al. 1993) as well as plants; therefore, in addition to possessing the transport mechanisms described for other arthropod-borne viruses in this family, tospoviruses must also be able to traverse the plant cell wall. For tomato spotted wilt virus, the NS_M protein was found to be associated with nucleocapsid aggregates and was postulated to be involved in cell-to-cell movement of non-enveloped ribonucleocapsids (Kormelink et al. 1994). It is likely that the G1 and G2 proteins (and envelope) of tospoviruses are required for replication in their insect vectors but not in plants (Verkleij and Peters 1983, Resende et al. 1991).

PROTEIN INTERACTIONS IN VIRUS ASSEMBLY AND RELEASE

Unlike viruses in families such as the *Rhabdoviridae*, *Orthomyxoviridae* and *Paramyxoviridae*, which utilize their matrix (M) protein to act as a nucleating step for assembly and to bridge the gap between the integral viral envelope proteins and their nucleocapsids, bunyaviruses that do not have an M protein must rely on direct interaction of the envelope proteins and ribonucleocapsids to trigger assembly (Smith and Pifat 1982). Because viral ribonucleocapsids and spike structures have been observed only on portions of

Golgi vesicle membranes directly involved in the budding process and not on adjacent areas of the same membranes, it is likely that some sort of transmembranal recognition between the viral glycoproteins and the N protein is required for budding. Candidate transmembrane regions have been predicted from hydropathic characteristics of derived amino acid sequences representing the envelope proteins of all members of the *Bunyaviridae* examined to date. For Uukuniemi virus, it has been suggested that the cytoplasmic tail of G1 (which is at least 70 residues long) is a logical candidate for interaction with the nucleocapsids (Rönnholm and Pettersson 1987, Pettersson 1991). Direct evidence for transmembrane regions of G1 and G2 was obtained by enzymatic digestion of exposed proteins of the phlebovirus Karimabad. In this study, it was determined that c. 12% of G1 or G2, or both, was exposed on the cytoplasmic face of membranes in infected cells and was accessible to digestion. A large protease-resistant fragment was identified, which was presumably sequestered in the membrane in a manner that rendered it safe from enzymatic digestion (Smith and Pifat 1982).

It is believed that, after the particles bud into the Golgi cisternae, they are released in individual small vesicles in a manner analogous to secretory granules of other cell types (Broadwell and Oliver 1981, Rothman 1981, Smith and Pifat 1982). The release of virus from infected cells presumably occurs when the cytoplasmic, virus-containing vesicles fuse with the cellular plasma membrane, i.e. by normal exocytosis.

The morphogenesis of tospoviruses in their insect vector, thrips, seems to be similar to that observed with other viruses in the family (Wijkamp et al. 1993). Differences, however, are seen in plants and plant cells. As indicated above, it is likely that the tospovirus envelope is needed only for replication in insects, and not in plants. Non-enveloped tospovirus particles are commonly seen in infected plants (Kitajima et al. 1992); defective tomato spotted wilt virus isolates, which are defective in glycoprotein synthesis and lack the lipid envelope, were found to retain the ability to spread through plant tissues at the same rate as non-defective viruses (Verkleij and Peters 1983, Resende et al. 1991). These findings, as well as the small pore size (c. 3 nm) of plants' plasmodesmata, suggest that infectious ribonucleocapsids, rather than complete tospovirus virions, are transported through the plant plasmodesmata (Kormelink et al. 1994).

1.6 Antigens and immune responses

The major viral antigens are the structural proteins, N, G1 and G2. Generally, the N protein is highly antigenic, and is usually the prominent antigen detected in serological assays such as complement fixation and ELISA of infected cell-culture lysates. The G1 and G2 proteins are the basis for serological assays such as haemagglutination inhibition and plaque-reduction neutralization.

For all animal-infecting bunyaviruses, the envelope glycoproteins, G1 and G2, are presumed to be the major antigens involved in induction of immunity. Three lines of evidence support this assumption: (1) monoclonal antibodies to G1 or G2 or both, but not to N, can neutralize viral infectivity in vitro; (2) passive transfer of neutralizing, but not non-neutralizing, monoclonal antibodies or monospecific polyclonal sera to G1 or G2 or both, protects animals from challenge with homologous viruses; and (3) immunization of animals with recombinant viruses expressing G1 or G2 (or both) results in protective immunity (Dantas et al. 1986, Collett et al. 1987, Pifat, Osterling and Smith 1988, Arikawa et al. 1989, Dalrymple et al. 1989, Schmaljohn et al. 1990, Arikawa et al. 1992, Pekosz et al. 1995) For some viruses, such as the phlebovirus Rift Valley fever virus, although monoclonal antibodies to both G1 and G2 will neutralize virus in cell culture, only those specific for G2 were able to passively protect animals. Passively transferred polyclonal, monospecific sera to G2 were also found to be protective, but sera to G1 were not (Dalrymple et al. 1981, 1989, Keegan and Collett 1986, Smith et al. 1987). This finding was substantiated in mice immunized with recombinant vaccinia or baculoviruses expressing either G1 or G2, in that only the G2 recombinants induced a protective immune response in the animals (Dalrymple et al. 1989, Schmaljohn et al. 1989). These findings suggest that a humoral response alone to one or both of the envelope glycoproteins may be sufficient for protection from infection with viruses in the family.

Little information is available concerning the importance of cell-mediated immune responses to members of the *Bunyaviridae*. For the hantavirus Hantaan virus-specific cytotoxic T lymphocytes (CTLs) were demonstrated after restimulation of immune mouse lymphocytes with Haantan virus antigen in vitro. The CTL response was also suggested to be involved in cross-reactive protection among hantaviruses. Evidence for this was obtained by restimulating, with Hantaan virus, spleen cells from mice immunized with heterologous hantaviruses. In one instance of cross-protection (i.e. immunization with Puumala virus and protection against Hantaan virus), evidence suggested that T cells may be particularly relevant (Asada et al. 1987, 1988, 1989). A non-neutralizing, presumably cell-mediated, protective immune response was also demonstrated in hamsters immunized with baculovirus-expressed Hantaan virus and challenged with virulent Hantaan virus (Schmaljohn et al. 1990)

For tospoviruses, resistance to infection was achieved by transforming plants with viral nucleoprotein (N) gene sequences (De Haan et al. 1992, Vaira et al. 1995). This protection was demonstrated to be RNA-mediated, i.e. owing to the presence of N transcripts rather than to the presence of N protein (De Haan et al. 1992).

2   CLINICAL AND PATHOLOGICAL ASPECTS

2.1   Clinical manifestations

Over 60 viruses of the family *Bunyaviridae* are known to cause disease in humans or animals. Most human infections are silent, and are detectable only by the appearance of specific antibodies. When clinical disease occurs, manifestation of infection ranges from self-limited febrile disease to potentially fatal fulminant haemorrhagic fever or encephalitis. Acute undifferentiated illness is often characterized by an abrupt onset of fever, usually accompanied by chills. Myalgia, arthralgia, headache with or without photophobia, malaise, anorexia and nausea are common; occasionally vomiting also occurs. Gastrointestinal symptoms rarely dominate the clinical picture, however, nor are respiratory symptoms often seen, although some patients may have sore throat, cough or even pulmonary infiltrates. A notable exception is hantavirus pulmonary syndrome, as described below (p. 617). Physical examination may reveal conjunctival injection, mild adenopathy and some abdominal tenderness. Clinical laboratory findings usually indicate a normal, decreased or moderately elevated white blood count. The typical duration of uncomplicated illness is 2–4 days, perhaps extending to a week. A second wave of fever may occur ('saddle-back fever'), but there is no residual illness seen, although convalescence may require several days.

More severe infections may include a maculopapular rash on the trunk appearing after the onset of illness and lasting a few days (Bwamba, Oropouche and others), bleeding (most severe in Crimean–Congo haemorrhagic fever and Rift Valley fever), encephalitis (Bhanja, California group and Rift Valley fever), hepatitis (hantaviruses and Rift Valley fever), acute kidney failure (hantaviruses), aseptic meningitis (Bwamba, Oropouche and others), respiratory distress due to acute pulmonary oedema (New World hantaviruses) and retinal vasculitis (unique to Rift Valley fever). Fatal infections have often been associated with California group viruses, especially La Crosse virus in children, Crimean–Congo haemorrhagic fever, hantaviral infections, especially hantavirus pulmonary syndrome in which case fatality rates exceed 50%, and Rift Valley fever virus.

The most important veterinary pathogens are Akabane virus, the cause of congenital malformations and abortions in cattle, sheep and goats in Japan, Australia, South Africa and Israel (Parsonson and McPhee 1985), Nairobi sheep disease and Rift Valley fever virus. Rift Valley fever, in addition to human infections, also causes abortion and death in domestic animals. Rift Valley fever virus is common throughout sub-Saharan Africa, with periodic epizootic/epidemic transmission in Egypt (Meegan 1979).

IMPORTANT INFECTIONS

California encephalitis and related viruses

California encephalitis is, in most years, the most important arboviral disease seen in the USA, the vast majority of cases being detected among children infected with La Crosse virus. For example, in 1994, of 100 laboratory-confirmed arboviral infections, 76 (76%) were due to California group viruses. In that year, the greatest number of cases occurred in West Virginia (32 cases) and Ohio (14), 11 other states having at least one case (Report 1995b). Other pathogenic California group viruses include prototype California encephalitis virus, Guaroa, Inkoo, Jamestown Canyon, snowshoe hare and Tahyna viruses. With the exception of Inkoo and Tahyna viruses, California group viruses are found predominantly in North America where they are transmitted by mosquitoes. Inkoo and Tahyna viruses are found in Europe, and there is serological evidence to suggest that viruses similar or identical to snowshoe hare virus are present in Asia. Tahyna-related viruses have been found in Africa. California group viruses are widely distributed, being found from the tropical zones to above the Arctic Circle (reviewed in LeDuc 1979).

The incubation period for California encephalitis patients is about 3–7 days after an infectious mosquito bite. Onset is abrupt with fever, headache and lethargy; nausea and vomiting are common. Rash, diarrhoea and arthralgia are uncommon. In milder cases, recovery occurs within a week, the only indication of neurological involvement being meningeal signs and perhaps disorientation. More severe cases develop seizures, convulsions and loss of consciousness, with coma in some instances. Mild neurological signs, which may still be present at discharge, manifest as irritability and other conditions, but usually resolve over the course of several weeks, with little in the way of permanent illness being reported. Of 166 cases reported, 2 died and 2 had lasting hemiparesis. Patients with seizures during acute disease are at greater risk for subsequent convulsions, usually seen within a year after recovery. Intellectual and social functions do not seem to be disturbed among recovered children (Matthews, Chun and Grabow 1968, Sabatino and Cramblett 1968, Grabow et al. 1969, Rie, Hilty and Cramblet 1973).

Tahyna virus is found primarily in Europe, with a related or identical virus being found in Africa ('Lumbo' virus). Antibodies in humans have been found in Sri Lanka, China and Russia. Human infection ranges from a mild febrile disease to aseptic meningitis. Pharyngitis, pulmonary involvement or gastrointestinal disturbances such as nausea and vomiting may be common. Although CNS involvement has been documented, serious illness or death has not been associated with Tahyna virus infections (Peters and LeDuc 1991).

Akabane virus

Akabane virus is an important veterinary pathogen causing congenital malformations, arthrogryposis, hydranencephaly and other deformities, as well as abortions in cattle, sheep and goats in Japan, Australia, South Africa and Israel (Parsonson and McPhee 1985). Antibodies to Akabane virus have been found in sera collected from 25 of 41 wildlife species in 11 sub-Saharan African countries (Al Busaidy, Hamblin and Taylor 1987). Both *Culex* mosquitoes and *Culicoides* are implicated in transmission.

Oropouche fever virus

Oropouche virus was first isolated in Trinidad from the blood of a forest worker with a mild febrile illness. Although now rare in Trinidad, the virus has become a major cause of rural and urban epidemics in the Amazon region of South America, a large percentage of the resident population being infected during outbreaks. More than 500 000 cases have been recorded, primarily from the Brazilian states of Para, Amazonas, Maranhao and Goias (Vasconcelos et al. 1989, Vasconcelos, Travassos da Rosa and Travassos da Rosa 1994). The disease is characterized by headache, fever, myalgia, arthralgia, photophobia, retrobulbar pain, nausea and dizziness. Rash occurs in less than 10% of the confirmed cases. Symptoms may recur in more than half those clinically ill, usually within 1–2 weeks of the initial onset. No deaths have been reported for Oropouche fever, but meningitis or meningismus has been reported. Patients are often debilitated and prostration is common (reviewed in LeDuc and Pinheiro 1988).

Hantavirus infections

Haemorrhagic fever with renal syndrome (HFRS) has long been recognized clinically in Asia, Russia and Scandinavia, but the aetiology of the syndrome has been known only since the late 1970s. Over 200 synonyms have been used to describe HFRS, including Korean haemorrhagic fever, epidemic haemorrhagic fever, nephropathia epidemica, epidemic nephrosonephritis, and many others, often referring to geographic locations. It was not until 1978, however, that the causative agent, Hantaan virus, was isolated from the lungs of the striped fieldmouse, *Apodemus agrarius* (Lee, Lee and Johnson 1978). Unlike other members of the family *Bunyaviridae*, the hantaviruses are maintained in nature by chronically infected rodents. No arthropod vector is involved in their transmission cycle. Hantaan virus was named after the Hantaan River, near the demilitarized zone dividing the Korean peninsula, where the infected field mice were first captured.

Subsequent studies have demonstrated that Hantaan virus represents an antigenically and genetically novel virus among the *Bunyaviridae* and was thus the prototype member for a new genus within the family (Schmaljohn and Dalrymple 1983, Schmaljohn et al. 1985). Subsequently, additional serologically related viruses have been isolated, many of which are known to cause human disease. Previously, human disease was thought to be limited to febrile illness followed by varying degrees of kidney failure. Recently, however, a new clinical presentation has been documented:

hantavirus pulmonary syndrome (Duchin et al. 1994). This syndrome is characterized by acute onset of febrile disease, followed by an often fatal respiratory distress syndrome. Recent studies have shown this new disease to be due also to hantaviral infections, but with a unique group of antigenically and genetically related viruses found only (to date) in the Americas. Thus, it appears that 2 basic lineages of hantaviruses have evolved, one occurring predominantly in the Old World, specifically evolving with rodent species found there, and leading to haemorrhagic fever with renal syndrome presentations, and one in the New World causing hantavirus pulmonary syndrome, maintained in nature by New World rodent species (Fig. 30.5; and see Table 30.2).

The most severe form of HFRS occurs in Asia and is caused by prototype Hantaan virus. It is associated with a mortality rate of c. 5%, although this may be much higher in certain rural areas. This disease is characterized by an abrupt onset of fever, chills, malaise, myalgia, headache, dizziness and anorexia after a variable incubation period of 2–42 days, but most often of 2–4 weeks. During this initial **febrile phase**, severe abdominal and back pain appear, accompanied by increasing nausea and vomiting, tenderness over the lower back, flushing of the face, neck and chest, and injection of the conjunctivae, palate and pharynx. Petechiae may appear on the axillae, face, neck, chest and soft palate, and haemorrhages into the conjuncti-

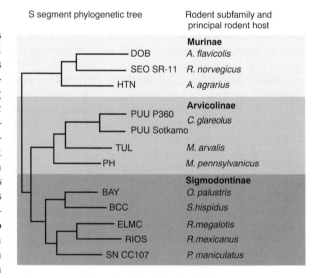

Fig. 30.5 Relationships of hantaviruses and their rodent hosts. Phylogenetic relationship of the complete S segments of hantaviruses is represented in a single most parsimonious tree derived by using PAUP 3.1.1 software. Horizontal lengths of branches are proportional to nucleotide sequence differences. Abbreviations for viruses and accession numbers for the S segment viral sequences are: Dobrava virus, DOB, L41916; Seoul virus, SEO, M34881; Hantaan virus, HTN, M14626; Puumala virus, PUU virus (strain P360), L11347; PUU (strain Sotkamo), X61035; Tula virus, TUL, Z30941; Prospect Hill virus, PH, X55128; Bayou virus, BAY, L36929; Black Creek Canal virus, BCC, L39949; El Moro Canyon virus, ELMC, U11427; Rio Segundo virus, RIOS, U18100; Sin Nombre virus (strain CC107) SN, L33683.

vae may occur. Clinical laboratory studies reveal normal or slightly elevated white blood cell counts, decreased platelets and rising haematocrit (packed cell volume) values. Proteinuria may appear towards the end of this phase of the disease (McKee et al. 1985).

Defervescence occurs after 3–7 days and marks the start of the **hypotensive phase**, which may last from several hours to a few days. This phase is characterized by tachycardia, falling arterial pressure and narrowing pulse pressure, mental changes and, in severe cases, classic shock. Bleeding tendencies continue with capillary haemorrhage and rising haematocrit values. Leucocytosis with a left shift, thrombocytopenia and prolonged bleeding times are seen; there are high levels of proteinuria and oliguria begins. About one-third of the fatalities occur during this phase. The **oliguric phase** follows and lasts for 3–7 days, during which blood pressure returns to normal or is slightly elevated due to relative hypervolaemia. The fall in urinary output is accompanied by elevated serum creatinine and blood urea nitrogen and other evidence of renal failure. Pulmonary oedema may occur and care must be taken in fluid management. Rash and facial flushing disappear during this phase, although nausea and vomiting may continue. Severe haemorrhagic manifestations may occur, gastrointestinal or CNS bleeding being especially serious. Almost half the deaths occur during this phase, often due to pulmonary oedema or infection, electrolyte imbalance, late shock or haemorrhage into the brain. Clinical recovery begins during the **diuretic phase**, with the normalization of clotting and return of renal function. For the next few hours or days there is diuresis, with outputs of 3–6 litres daily. Strength and appetite improve, but fluid management must be maintained to prevent negative fluid balances which may lead to shock. The **convalescent phase** may require several months, and hyposthenuria may persist for months to years (McKee et al. 1985). Although complete recovery has been assumed, recent studies with Seoul virus have called this assumption into question (Glass et al. 1993). Specific therapy is not available, and careful supportive care is essential to improving survival. Care must be consistent with the phase of the disease, careful attention being paid to fluid management. Recent studies have demonstrated that ribavirin is efficacious in treating HFRS if administered early in the course of illness (Huggins et al. 1991). Treated patients had significantly fewer deaths than those untreated, and they spent less time in each phase of the disease and were more likely to skip entire phases altogether.

Other Old World hantaviruses cause diseases similar to, though generally less severe than, classic Hantaan virus infections. These include Puumala virus, the cause of nephropathia epidemica of western Europe, Scandinavia and the western portions of Russia. Nephropathia epidemica may follow the same phases as classic HFRS, but is fatal in less than 1% of cases. In the Balkan region of Europe, Puumala virus overlaps in many areas with both classic Hantaan virus and local strains that are capable of causing very severe

disease with mortality rates at least as high as those seen in Asia. The severe HFRS of the Balkans has been associated with Dobrava virus, also reported as Belgrade virus (now known to be the same viruses) and is indistinguishable clinically from HFRS of Asia (Gligic et al. 1992, Avsic-Zupanc et al. 1992a, 1992b, 1995, Taller et al. 1993). Seoul virus, associated with *Rattus norvegicus* (brown rat), probably originated in Asia, but is now found throughout the world wherever large populations of rats exist (LeDuc et al. 1986). It causes a less severe form of HFRS that is characterized by greater liver involvement than classic Hantaan infections, and in general a lower mortality rate although deaths have been recorded. Seoul virus infections are especially common in China, but have been documented in many parts of the world, including Europe and the Americas. In the USA, careful studies have associated past Seoul virus infection with an increased risk of hypertensive renal disease (Glass et al. 1993), an observation that could have significant economic implications for many developed countries (LeDuc, Childs and Glass 1992).

Hantavirus pulmonary syndrome was first recognized in 1993, when an outbreak of an apparently new and highly fatal form of severe respiratory illness occurred in southwestern USA. As a result of subsequent field and laboratory investigations, the epidemiology and clinical characteristics of this new disease were described, and the name hantavirus pulmonary syndrome was proposed. It was caused by a previously unknown hantavirus, later named Sin Nombre virus (also reported as Four Corners or Muerto Canyon virus). By August 1995 there had been 115 confirmed cases of hantavirus pulmonary syndrome, with a case fatality rate of 51%. The mean age was 35 years, with a range of 11–69 years (Report 1995a).

Hantavirus pulmonary syndrome has a prodrome of fever and myalgia (all of 17 patients originally described), with cough or dyspnoea (76%), gastrointestinal symptoms (76%) and headache (71%) (Duchin et al. 1994). Physical characteristics seen among these original 17 cases include tachypnoea (100%), tachycardia (94%) and hypotension (50%). Laboratory findings reflect leucocytosis, increased haematocrit, thrombocytopenia, prolonged prothrombin and partial thromboplastin times, elevated serum lactate dehydrogenase, decreased serum protein concentrations and proteinuria. Fifteen (88%) cases rapidly progressed to acute pulmonary oedema, and 13 (76%) died. Predictors of death included increases in haematocrit and partial thromboplastin time, and all deaths occurred with profound hypotension (Duchin et al. 1994). Despite laboratory evidence strongly suggestive of disseminated intravascular coagulopathy, clinical signs of haemorrhage have rarely been reported (Zaki et al. 1995). Radiographic examination reveals bilateral pulmonary infiltrates in virtually all hospitalized patients, and pleural effusions in many. At postmortem examination, copious pleural effusions are often found (Zaki et al. 1995). Multi-organ involvement was found in all of 44 fatal cases examined, with generalized vascular congestion. The primary histo-pathological features were seen in the lung where microscopic examination revealed mild to moderate interstitial pneumonitis with variable degrees of congestion, oedema and mononuclear cell infiltrates (Zaki et al. 1995). Immunohistochemical examination of postmortem tissue from 44 fatal cases revealed viral antigen-positive cells widely distributed in various tissues, but seen predominantly within endothelial cells of capillaries and small vessels. The most intensive and extensive endothelial staining was in tissues of the lungs, where viral antigen was abundant and uniformly distributed; it involved most of the pulmonary microvasculature, although high densities of viral antigens were also observed in lymphoid follicles of the spleen and, to a lesser extent, in lymph node follicles (Zaki et al. 1995). The magnitude and extent, however, of pulmonary endothelial involvement reflect the difficulty experienced by clinicians in attempting to manage the often terminal shock syndrome.

Treatment has been prompt hospitalization, aggressive clinical management and early pulmonary support. Ribavirin, which can be efficacious in the treatment of HFRS patients, has been administered to hantavirus pulmonary syndrome patients, but at present there are insufficient data to indicate efficacy clearly.

Crimean–Congo haemorrhagic fever virus

Crimean–Congo haemorrhagic fever (CCHF) is a severe, tick-borne, acute haemorrhagic fever found throughout much of Africa, extending northward to Albania, the former Yugoslavia, Crimea and elsewhere in the former Soviet Union, Iraq and much of the Middle East, and eastward into Pakistan and western China. Clinical disease has been well described from cases seen in the former Soviet Union, and nosocomial outbreaks have been common among hospitalized patients, especially those undergoing surgery. The mortality rate originally described for cases occurring in Crimea was 15–30% (Chumakov 1946); other outbreaks have had mortality rates as high as 40% (Hoogstraal 1979). Cases usually occur singly among shepherds or others with rural exposure who have been fed on by ticks, or as small clusters among individuals involved in the slaughter of an infected animal (Swanepoel et al. 1985). Nosocomial outbreaks have occurred in the former Soviet Union, the former Yugoslavia, South Africa and the Middle East (Burney et al. 1976). They typically involve a severely ill patient with haemorrhage and a suspected acute abdomen, perforated ulcer or other diagnosis leading to surgical intervention. Inevitably the patient dies, and often the medical team, family members, or both, are infected, often with a fatal outcome.

The clinical picture of CCHF is an initial influenza-like illness followed by severe headache, joint and back pains, fever, nausea, vomiting and photophobia. The incubation period is typically 3–6 days in nosocomial infections, and 3–12 days following tick exposure. Initial symptoms may be followed by circu-latory collapse, shock and a variety of haemorrhagic manifestations such as epistaxis, haemoptysis, haematemesis, melaena and skin haemorrhage. Bleeding into the intestinal tract may cause the patient to present with acute abdominal pain, leading to surgical intervention and increased risk of nosocomial spread. Involvement of the central nervous system indicates a poor prognosis. Clinical laboratory data include leucopenia from the onset of illness, neutropenia, thrombocytopenia, and falling haemoglobin and erythrocyte counts in severely ill patients. The clinically apparent attack rate was estimated to be 5 infections per case of haemorrhagic fever in the former Soviet Union (Goldfarb et al. 1980).

Nairobi sheep disease virus

This acute, haemorrhagic gastroenteritis affecting sheep and goats in East Africa was described by Montgomery (1917), who correctly attributed transmission to the tick, *Rhipicephalus appendiculatus*. The mortality rate may be 70–90% in sheep, but goats are less seriously affected. Herdsmen tending infected animals may develop a mild, febrile illness, and laboratory infections with this virus have occurred (Swanepoel 1995). In India, Ganjam virus was isolated from ticks collected from sheep and goats in Orissa state (Karabatsos 1985). Ganjam virus is now considered to be synonymous with Nairobi sheep disease virus (Davies et al. 1978). Dugbe virus, another virus of the genus *Nairovirus*, has been isolated many times from cattle ticks in Nigeria (Kemp, Causey and Causey 1971), and there have been a few Dugbe virus isolations from humans.

Rift Valley fever virus

Epizootics of Rift Valley fever virus were first reported in the 1930s in the Rift Valley of Kenya, where sheep suffered fatal hepatic necrosis and abortion. Since then, there have been many epizootics throughout sub-Saharan Africa, and associated human disease has been described. In 1977, Rift Valley fever was first documented outside sub-Saharan Africa, when an outbreak occurred in Egypt (Hoogstraal 1979, Laughlin et al. 1979, Meegan 1979). Extensive human and animal disease occurred in Egypt, including the Nile delta region, between 1977 and 1979 but adjacent countries were spared; transmission appears to have ceased in 1979. In 1993, however, Rift Valley fever once again appeared in Egypt, initially in Upper Egypt near Aswan, and subsequently in the Nile delta (WHO 1994). This presumed importation has likewise not spread beyond Egypt's borders, and may have been contained or eliminated by an aggressive vaccination campaign.

Sheep, cattle and goats suffer 10–30% mortality from Rift Valley fever virus, and a large percentage of infected pregnant animals abort. Disease and death are most frequent in young animals. Native ungulates seem to be more resistant to lethal infection. Disease in humans is characterized by acute onset of fever, headache and myalgia with incapacitating prostration. The incubation period is typically 2–6 days; in most patients the illness resolves after 2–3 days' rest, although symptoms may persist for a week. A small portion, perhaps 1%, of cases develop haemorrhagic fever, encephalitis or retinal vasculitis. Haemorrhagic disease begins as typical Rift Valley fever, but patients develop gastrointestinal bleeding, become jaundiced and may die in shock. Disseminated vascular damage and hepatic failure may contribute to the cause of death. Fatal encephalitis may also follow Rift Valley fever, which typically develops a few days to 1–2 weeks after initial recovery from classic disease. Patients develop headache, confusion, return of fever and various neurological signs that may lead to residual illness or death. Similarly, ocular complications appear up to 3 weeks after acute disease, presenting with rapid onset of decreased visual acuity due to retinal haemorrhage, exudates and macular oedema. Vision returns as the oedema and exudates resolve, but about half the patients suffer some degree of permanent visual loss.

Sandfly fever and related viruses

Sandfly fever, also known as pappataci fever or phlebotomus fever, has been recognized as a militarily important disease since the Napoleonic Wars (Hertig and Sabin 1964). During both World Wars, foreign troops suffered significant incidence rates of sandfly fever in the Mediterranean theatres. These viruses are transmitted by the bite of infectious sandflies (genus *Phlebotomus*, thus 'phlebotomus fever'), and take their names from the sites of their original isolation. Sabin was the first to demonstrate that these 2 distinct viruses could cause virtually identical diseases in humans (Sabin 1951). The clinical syndrome after infections with either Naples virus or Sicilian virus is characterized by abrupt onset of fever lasting 2–4 days, headache, eye pain, photophobia, pain in the back and joints, anorexia and malaise. Nausea and vomiting, other abdominal symptoms, sore throat, drowsiness, dizziness and saddleback fever may also be seen, but rash or meningeal signs are uncommon (Sabin 1951, Hertig and Sabin 1964, Bartelloni and Tesh 1976). No deaths have been documented among several hundred cases studied, and no sequelae are recognized. Life-long homologous protection probably follows infection, but there is no cross-protection between Naples and Sicilian viruses.

Toscana virus was isolated in 1971 from sandflies (*Phlebotomus pernicious*) captured in the Tuscany region of central Italy (Verani et al. 1980). Subsequent investigations there have shown it to be the causative agent in many cases of summertime aseptic meningitis (Verani and Nicoletti 1995). Serological surveys have found antibodies to Toscana virus in other southern European countries as well, although its health impact in these areas is less well characterized (Balducci, Fausto and Verani 1985).

New World sandfly fever viruses
Alenquer, Candiru, Chagres and Punta Toro are all New World sandfly fever viruses originally isolated from febrile patients. The clinical disease following infection with any of these viruses is virtually indistinguishable from that seen in Naples or Sicilian infections. Human cases are not common owing to the secretive nature of their New World sandfly vectors (genus *Lutzomyia*), which inhabit tropical forests and are unlikely to come into contact with large numbers of humans. Even so, antibody prevalence rates ranging from 2% to 34% for Punta Toro virus were detected in serological surveys of residents of rural Panama, and about half those rates for Chagres virus (Le Duc, Cuevas and Garcia 1980).

Other infections

Bangui virus causes a febrile illness with rash in the Central African Republic. It has also been recovered from a bird in the same country (Digoutte et al. 1980).

Bhanja virus was first isolated in India from *Haemaphysalis intermedia* ticks collected from goats in Ganjam district, Orissa (Shah and Work 1969). Other isolations have been made from cattle and goat ticks in West Africa, and from blood samples collected there from cattle, sheep, ground squirrels and hedgehogs. Bhanja infection of goats is widespread in the former Czechoslovakia, Italy and the former Yugoslavia; and many animal sera collected in Sri Lanka have antibodies against this virus. Infection of humans caused severe neurological disease and death in at least 2 cases in the former Yugoslavia, and laboratory infections have occurred (Vesenjak-Hirjan et al. 1980).

Bwamba virus was first isolated from acutely ill febrile patients in Bwamba County, Uganda (Smithburn, Mahaffy and Paul 1941). Later serological studies have found high prevalence rates of antibodies to this and closely related viruses throughout East, Central, West and South Africa. Bwamba virus seems to be a common cause of febrile illness in humans in Africa, causing a self-limiting disease accompanied by rash and prostration, often with meningeal signs (Georges et al. 1980). Bwamba and a closely related virus, Pongola, have been isolated from various mosquito species, but little is known about their natural history. Kasokero virus has been isolated from bats in Uganda, where it may cause fever in humans (Kaluda et al. 1986). Laboratory infections have occurred.

Keterah virus, isolated in Malaysia from Argas ticks and from bats, is indistinguishable from Issyk-kul virus, which has been isolated from *Aedes caspius* mosquitoes and from bats (*Nyctalus noctula*, *Myotis blythii* and *Vespertilio serotinus*) and ticks (*Argas vespertilionsis*) in Kirghiz SSR, the former USSR. It has since been associated with epidemics of febrile disease in humans in that region (Lvov et al. 1984).

Nyando virus was isolated from mosquitoes in Kenya, and from humans in the Central African Republic, where it caused fever, myalgia and vomiting (Digoutte et al. 1980).

Tamdy virus is a tick-borne virus causing a febrile illness in humans in the Asiatic regions of the former USSR (Lvov et al. 1976).

Tataguine virus is a mosquito-borne virus that causes fever, joint pains and rash in humans in Africa (Digoutte et al. 1980).

Wanowrie virus was isolated from *Hyalomma marginatum isaaci* ticks collected from sheep in India, and from the brain of a 17 year old girl who died in Sri Lanka after a 2 day fever with abdominal pain and vomiting (Pavri et al. 1976). The virus is also present in Egypt and Iran (Sureau and Klein 1980).

2.2 Epidemiology

GENERAL CONSIDERATIONS

Viruses of the family *Bunyaviridae* are maintained in nature in a complex life cycle, usually involving an arthropod vector and a vertebrate host. The exceptions are viruses of the genus *Hantavirus*, which are maintained by chronic infection of rodents and other small mammals. In general, each virus is specifically associated with a particular arthropod species that serves to transmit the virus, and one or more species of vertebrate hosts that serve to amplify the virus following infection through a transient viraemia. Arthropod vectors, especially mosquitoes, are often seasonally abundant, which results in seasonal transmission of the viruses they transmit. During periods of adverse weather conditions, virus survival is often maintained by vertical or transovarial transmission whereby an infected female passes the viral infection on to the next generation of vectors. The virus survives in association with the dormant egg and, with hatching and subsequent development, virus transmission to vertebrate hosts takes place during blood feeding. Viruses may also be transmitted venereally from infected males to uninfected female vectors during mating. Vertebrate hosts serve to amplify the amount of virus in circulation by means of a viraemia of varying intensity and duration. Uninfected vector species become infected when ingesting a viraemic blood meal. Following an extrinsic incubation period of a few days' duration, during which the virus replicates and is disseminated throughout the vector, the newly infected vectors are then able to transmit the virus at subsequent blood feeding. Mosquitoes are the most important group of arthropod vectors, but ticks, sandflies and biting midges (*Culicoides* spp.) are also important vectors for certain viruses.

Most of the bunyaviruses are zoonotic in nature, and humans are usually only accidental hosts that generally do not facilitate amplification of the virus in nature. Exceptions are Oropouche virus and perhaps sandfly fever viruses, in which humans seem to be important sources of virus for uninfected vectors. Selected examples of the transmission cycles of representative viruses are presented below to demonstrate their complexity.

IMPORTANT INFECTIONS

California encephalitis due to La Crosse virus

Most viruses of the genus *Bunyavirus* are transmitted by mosquitoes, and California encephalitis due to La Crosse virus may serve as an example of one of the better understood transmission cycles (see Calisher and Thompson 1983 for overview). The mosquito *Aedes triseriatus* is the principal vector of La Crosse virus. This species is common in the hardwood forests of the upper midwestern United States, where it breeds primarily in tree holes. It survives the harsh winters in the egg stage; in late spring or early summer the first adults emerge, mate and begin to seek a blood meal. La Crosse virus is transmitted transovarially from infected adult female *Ae. triseriatus* to the next generation of eggs, so a proportion of those newly emerging adults are already infected with the virus (Watts et al. 1973, 1974). These infected females transmit the virus to susceptible vertebrate hosts at blood feeding, beginning the amplification cycle each year, whereas infected males may pass the virus to uninfected females during mating. (Male mosquitoes do not feed on blood, and thus cannot transmit the virus directly to an amplifying vertebrate host.) *Ae. triseriatus* females typically feed during the day, most frequently on squirrels, chipmunks, foxes and rabbits, and on humans if present. Susceptible squirrels and chipmunks circulate the virus in high enough titre to infect other *Ae. triseriatus*, thus serving to amplify the prevalence of virus in the vector population. Foxes, with their larger range, may both amplify the virus among local vector populations and also disseminate it to more distant vector populations (Yuill 1983). Humans are infected when they enter the woods for recreation or work, most clinical cases being seen among children less than 15 years old. As *Ae. triseriatus* breeds equally well in discarded tyres or other items that retain water, infected mosquito populations may flourish in close proximity to dwellings, increasing the risk of infection to residents. Prevention of California encephalitis due to La Crosse virus can be facilitated by clean-up campaigns to reduce the availability of mosquito breeding sites, but elimination of all breeding is probably impossible owing to the abundance of natural breeding sites (Francy 1983).

Oropouche virus

Although most viruses of the genus *Bunyavirus* are transmitted by mosquitoes, some, such as Oropouche and other members of the Simbu serogroup, are transmitted by biting midges (family *Ceratopogonidae*, genus *Culicoides*). Oropouche virus was first described from Trinidad, but in the past 2 decades has become a major public health problem in northern Brazil and adjacent Amazon Basin nations (for an overview, see LeDuc and Pinheiro 1988). This increase is almost certainly a result of the changing ecology of the Amazon Basin, deforestation leading to human settlements and large plantations of banana and cacao, with the organic waste from these and other crops serving as ideal breeding sites for the vector *Culicoides*. This has led to tremendous population densities of *C. paraensis* in many parts of the Amazon Basin. Oropouche virus is thought to be maintained in 2 distinct transmission cycles: silent sylvatic transmission involving non-human primates, sloths and perhaps other vertebrate hosts; and an urban cycle in which humans are the primary amplifying and disseminating host and *C. paraensis* serving as the primary vector (Pinheiro, Travassos da Rosa and Travassos da Rosa 1981). This species lives in close association with humans and readily feeds during daylight hours. Epidemics occur when midge populations are large, the majority of the human population is susceptible and Oropouche virus is introduced from the silent sylvatic cycle into the urban setting. Although only a small percentage of the midges are able to transmit the virus, it seems that the populations are often so abundant that transmission is sustained until the majority of those humans susceptible have been infected. Humans circulate virus in sufficiently high titres to infect feeding *C. paraensis*, and consequently may serve to introduce the virus to new areas through their travel. With the increasing deforestation of the Amazon Basin, epidemics of Oropouche and other previously uncommon viruses found there are likely to increase.

Hantaan and related hantaviruses

Unlike other viruses of the family *Bunyaviridae*, arthropod vectors do not seem to play a significant role in the transmission of the hantaviruses. It seems that the hantaviruses, perhaps like other members of the family, represent an excellent example of co-evolution of the virus with a specific vertebrate host. As information about each of the genetically unique hantaviruses accumulates, it is increasingly apparent that each virus is specifically linked to a particular species of rodent host. These associations are shown in Table 30.2. The virus lineages closely follow the origin of the rodent hosts. Within the rodent family *Muridae*, 3 subfamilies exist: *Murinae*, *Arvicolinae* and *Sigmodontinae*; the hantaviruses maintained by rodent species of each of these subfamilies are genetically most closely related to each other, and less so to those of viruses associated with rodents of the other subfamilies (see Fig. 30.5) (for an overview, see LeDuc 1995). Transmission of hantaviruses between rodent hosts is thought to occur by aerosol from infectious excreta, and perhaps by saliva (Glass et al. 1988, Nuzum et al. 1988). Biting may play an important role in transmission of hantaviruses among rodents as territories are set and mating occurs (Glass et al. 1988). Studies have failed to demonstrate direct transmission from infected parent rodents to their offspring. Humans are infected when they come into contact with infected rodent hosts. There is thus a strong occupational association with the risk of hantaviral infection, farmers, woodcutters, soldiers and others with significant rural exposure being most often infected. Hantaviral infections are also seasonal, infections due to Hantaan and Puumala virus being seen most often in late fall and early winter in Asia and Europe, respectively. Elsewhere, hantaviral infections may occur most frequently in warmer months when recreational activities and outdoor work bring people into close contact with infected rodents.

Crimean–Congo haemorrhagic fever virus

Crimean–Congo haemorrhagic fever (CCHF)virus serves as an excellent example of 2 aspects of the epidemiology of viruses in the family *Bunyaviridae*: the threat of nosocomial or other direct transmission from infected blood to susceptible humans, and transmission by ticks (for overviews, see Hoogstraal 1979, Watts et al. 1989, Swanepoel 1995). CCHF virus is widely distributed from eastern Europe to Asia and Africa. In general, its distribution follows closely that of the primary tick vectors of the genus *Hyalomma*.

Immature ticks acquire infection during feeding on viraemic hosts, often small mammals, or by vertical transmission from infected females to the progeny. As ticks develop, the virus may be transmitted transstadially to subsequent developmental stages, and infected ticks may pass the virus to uninfected females during mating. Adult females, including those infected venereally, may then pass the virus to subsequent generations transovarially (Gonzalez et al. 1992). Viraemia occurs after infection of small mammals as well as of domestic ruminants, which may serve to infect uninfected tick vectors. The proportion of uninfected ticks that becomes infected when feeding on a viraemic host generally increases with the intensity of viraemia. In addition, non-viraemic transmission, as described for Dugbe virus, is also thought to occur with CCHF (Jones et al. 1987, Jones, Hodgson and Nuttall 1989).

Humans become infected either through the bite of an infected tick or through direct contact with infectious blood from an infected animal. The original outbreak of CCHF described from the Crimean peninsula involved large numbers of people exposed to ticks during conditions of war. Today, however, most cases are seen among individuals in Bulgaria, Albania and adjacent parts of the former Yugoslavia, sporadically in the Middle East, and as isolated cases in Africa, especially in South Africa where the virus is well known and studied. Clusters of cases occur in hospitals, especially in remote or ill-equipped clinics and surgeries, where the disease may not be recognized initially, and staff are infected by direct contact with infectious bodily fluids. Transmission of CCHF virus to workers in the laboratory setting has also occurred, leading to severe disease and fatalities.

2.3 Pathogenesis, pathology and immune response

Human infection with a bunyavirus generally follows the bite of an infectious vector or, less frequently, inhalation of infectious virus. After an incubation period, a brief viraemia often occurs, which corresponds to the period of acute illness. Signs and symptoms probably result from direct effects of virus on target organs such as the liver or brain. Immunohistochemical analysis has found widespread hantaviral antigens in endothelial cells of the microvasculature of hantavirus pulmonary syndrome patients, which may reflect similar targets of infection with other hantaviruses (Zaki et al. 1995). Disseminated intravascular coagulopathy may occur in severe disease with haemorrhagic manifestations such as HFRS, CCHF or Rift Valley fever. A typical humoral immune response leads to cessation of viraemia and clinical recovery in most cases, with immunoglobulin M (IgM) predominating initially, followed by immunoglobulin G (IgG). The cellular immune response to bunyavirus infections is not well defined, nor is the role of cytokines. A brief discussion of the pathogenesis, pathology, and immune response of selected diseases is presented in section 2.1 (p. 615).

2.4 Diagnosis

Diagnosis is based on demonstration of the specific virus causing infection, by isolation, by detection of viral antigen or nucleic acids or by acquisition of antibody specific for the infecting virus. Classic virus isolation techniques such as inoculation of suckling mice or cell cultures of mammalian or insect origin have been often used with considerable success. Likewise, routine serological techniques such as haemagglutination inhibition, complement fixation, immunofluorescent antibody assays, neutralization tests in mice or cell culture have been used to demonstrate rising or falling titres of antibody in paired sera from patients. These techniques are generally time consuming and expensive, and do not offer a definitive diagnosis soon enough to influence clinical management. Recently, more rapid diagnostic procedures have been developed that can offer a presumptive diagnosis within a few hours of receipt of a single acute serum sample. With enzyme immunoassays, viral antigen may be detected directly, or virus-specific IgM antibody demonstrated, generally in time to influence clinical management. For example, patients with HFRS due to Hantaan virus are often positive for IgM antibodies at the time of hospital admission (LeDuc et al. 1990). Confirmation of the specific aetiology helps in forecasting the course of the illness and initiating antiviral therapy such as ribavirin, which is efficacious in the treatment of HFRS (Huggins et al. 1991). Direct detection of viral nucleic acid, most often through reverse transcriptase-polymerase chain reaction amplification, and subsequent sequencing or endonuclease digestion of amplified products, has recently been applied for diagnosis, especially of hantavirus infections (Nichol et al. 1993). Acute specimens and autopsy tissues have both been used successfully to establish the diagnosis; however, the value of the technique is limited by the need for specially designed primers and very careful laboratory techniques to minimize the risk of contamination (Grankvist et al. 1992, Feldmann et al. 1993, Nichol et al. 1993). At present, these techniques are limited to research or reference laboratories and not widely available.

2.5 Prevention and control

Diseases caused by bunyaviruses have, with few exceptions, a low incidence of human infection and thus do not justify development of vaccines. An exception is HFRS, especially that due to Hantaan virus in Asia, where several candidate vaccines are in development, under field trails or, in at least one case, commercially available (Lee et al. 1990, Schmaljohn et al. 1994). Most current candidates are inactivated whole virus vaccines that require multiple inoculations and boosters to ensure protection; however, recombinant candidates are also under development. Development of live attenuated vaccines for hantavirus infections has been hampered by the absence of a suitable animal model that would faithfully mimic human disease (WHO 1995). Vaccines for Rift Valley fever virus have also been developed, with both inactivated and live attenuated products available for veterinary use, and an inactivated vaccine available on a limited basis for humans (Smithburn 1949, Eddy et al. 1981, Kark et al. 1982, Morrill et al. 1987, 1991). A live attenuated candidate vaccine for humans is now in early clinical trails.

Most often, however, prevention and control of bunyaviruses are based on avoidance of human contact with infected arthropod or small mammal vectors. Infection usually occurs when people enter into the ecological setting where viruses are being transmitted silently among infected vectors and wild vertebrate hosts. In these situations, personal protective measures such as the liberal use of insect repellants and wearing appropriate clothing may reduce the risk of infection. Likewise, care should be taken to ensure that houses, vacation cabins or campsites do not attract or support breeding potential vectors. Thus, using screens on windows and doors and removing potential mosquito breeding sites such as used tyres or other water-holding containers will help prevent infections. In the case of rodent-borne hantaviruses, special precautions are needed to rodent-proof homes and to maintain clean campsites.

REFERENCES

Abraham G, Pattnaik A, 1983, Early RNA synthesis in Bunyamwera virus-infected cells, *J Gen Virol*, **64**: 1277–90.

Adkins S, Quadt R et al., 1995, An RNA-dependent RNA polymerase activity associated with virions of tomato spotted wilt virus, a plant- and insect-infecting bunyavirus, *Virology*, **207**: 308–11.

Akashi H, Bishop D, 1983, Comparison of the sequences and coding of La Crosse and snowshoe hare bunyavirus S RNA species, *J Virol*, **45**: 1155–8.

Akashi H, Gay M et al., 1984, Localized conserved regions of the S RNA gene products of bunyaviruses are revealed by sequence analysis of the Simbu serogroup Aino viruses, *Virus Res*, 1: 51–63.

Al Busaidy S, Hamblin C, Taylor W, 1987, Neutralising antibodies to Akabane virus in free-living wild animals in Africa, *Trop Anim Health Prod*, **19**: 197–202.

Antic D, Wright K, Kang C, 1992, Maturation of Hantaan virus glycoproteins G1 and G2, *Virology*, **189**: 324–8.

Antic D, Kang C et al., 1992, Comparison of the deduced gene products of the L, M and S genome segments of hantaviruses, *Virus Res*, **24**: 35–46.

Arikawa J, Takashima I, Hashimoto N, 1985, Cell fusion by haemorrhagic fever with renal syndrome (HFRS) viruses and its application for titration of virus infectivity and neutralizing antibody, *Arch Virol*, **86**: 303–13.

Arikawa J, Schmaljohn A et al., 1989, Characterization of Hantaan virus envelope glycoprotein antigenic determinants by monoclonal antibodies, *J Gen Virol*, **70**: 615–24.

Arikawa J, Yao J et al., 1992, Protective role of antigenic sites on the envelope protein of Hantaan virus defined by monoclonal antibodies, *Arch Virol*, **126**: 271–81.

Arnheiter H, Davis N et al., 1985, Role of the nucleocapsid proteins in regulating vesicular stomatitis virus RNA synthesis, *Cell*, **41**: 259–67.

Asada H, Tamura M et al., 1987, Role of T lymphocyte subsets in protection and recovery from Hantaan virus infection in mice, *J Gen Virol*, **68**: 1961–9.

Asada H, Tamura M et al., 1988, Cell-mediated immunity to virus causing haemorrhagic fever with renal syndrome: generation of cytotoxic T lymphocytes, *J Gen Virol*, **69**: 2179–88.

Asada H, Balachandra K et al., 1989, Cross-reactive immunity among different serotypes of virus causing haemorrhagic fever with renal syndrome, *J Gen Virol*, **70**: 819–25.

Avsic-Zupanc T, Poljak M et al., 1992a, Antigenic variation of hantavirus isolates from Slovenia [abstract], 2nd International Conference on Haemorrhagic Fever with Renal Syndrome, Beijing, China, October 26–28.

Avsic-Zupanc T, Xiao S et al., 1992b, Characterization of Dobrava virus: a hantavirus from Slovenia, Yugoslavia, *J Med Virol*, **38**: 132–7.

Avsic-Zupanc T, Toney AR et al., 1995, Genetic and antigenic properties of Dobrava virus: a unique member of the *Hantavirus* genus, family *Bunyaviridae*, *J Gen Virol*, **76**: 2801–8.

Balducci M, Fausto A, Verani P, 1985, Phlebotomus-transmitted viruses in Europe, *Proceedings of the International Congress for Infectious Diseases, Rome*, ed Pozzi EL.

Banerjee A, 1987, Transcription and replication of rhabdoviruses, *Microbiol Rev*, **51**: 66–87.

Bartelloni P, Tesh R, 1976, Clinical and serologic responses of volunteers infected with phlebotomus fever virus (Sicilian type), *Am J Trop Med Hyg*, **25**: 456–62.

Battles J, Dalrymple J, 1988, Genetic variation among geographic isolates of Rift Valley fever virus, *Am J Trop Med Hyg*, **39**: 617–31.

Bellocq C, Raju R et al., 1987, Translational requirement of La Crosse virus S-mRNA synthesis: in vitro studies, *J Virol*, **61**: 87–95.

Bishop D, Gay M, Matsuoko Y, 1983, Nonviral heterogeneous sequences are present at the 5′ ends of one species of snowshoe hare bunyavirus S complementary RNA, *Nucleic Acids Res*, **11**: 6409–19.

Bishop D, Shope R, 1979, *Bunyaviridae, Comprehensive Virology*, vol 14, eds Fraenkel-Conrat H, Wagner RR, Plenum Press, New York, 1–156.

Bishop D, Calisher C et al., 1980, *Bunyaviridae, Intervirology*, **14**: 125–43.

Bishop D, Gould K et al., 1982, The complete sequence and coding content of snowshoe hare bunyavirus small (S) viral RNA species, *Nucleic Acids Res*, **10**: 3703–13.

Bishop D, Rud E et al., 1984, Genome structure, transcription, and genetics, *Segmented Negative Strand Viruses, Arenavirus, Bunyaviruses and Orthomyxoviruses*, eds Compans RD, Bishop D, Academic Press, Orlando FL, 3–11.

Blumberg B, Giorgi C, Kolakofsky D, 1983, N protein of vesicular stomatitis virus selectively encapsidates leader RNA in vitro, *Cell*, **32**: 559–67.

von Bonsdorff C-H, Pettersson R, 1975, Surface structure of Uukuniemi virus, *J Virol*, **95**: 1–7.

von Bonsdorff C-H, Saikku P, Oker-Blom N, 1970, Electron microscopy study on development of Uukuniemi virus, *Acta Virol*, **14**: 109–14.

Bouloy M, Hannoun C, 1976, Studies on Lumbo virus replication. I. RNA-dependent RNA polymerase associated with virions, *Virology*, **69**: 258–64.

Bouloy M, Vialat M et al., 1984, A transcript from the S segment of the Germiston bunyavirus is uncapped and codes for the nucleoprotein and a nonstructural protein, *J Virol*, **49**: 717–23.

Bouloy M, Pardigon N et al., 1990, Characterization of the 5′ and 3′ ends of viral messenger RNAs isolated from BHK21 cells infected with Germiston virus (Bunyavirus), *Virology*, **175**: 50–8.

Broadwell R, Oliver C, 1981, Golgi apparatus, GERL, and secretory granule formation within neurons of the hypothalamo-neurohypophysial system of control and hyperosmotically stressed mice, *J Cell Biol*, **90**: 474–84.

Burney M, Ghafoor A et al., 1976, Nosocomial outbreak of viral hemorrhagic fever caused by Crimean hemorrhagic fever–Congo virus in Pakistan, *Am J Trop Med Hyg*, **29**: 941–7.

Cabradilla C, Holloway B, Obijeski J, 1983, Molecular cloning and sequencing of the La Crosse virus S RNA, *Virology*, **128**: 463–8.

Calisher C, Thompson W, eds, 1983, *California Serogroup Viruses*, Alan R Liss, New York.

Carey D, Reuben R et al., 1971, Thottapalayam virus: a presumptive arbovirus isolated from a shrew in India, *Indian J Med Res*, **59**: 1758–60.

Cash P, 1985, Polypeptide synthesis of Dugbe virus, a member of the *Nairovirus* genus of the *Bunyaviridae*, *J Gen Virol*, **66**: 141–8.

Cash P, Vezza A et al., 1979, Genome complexities of the three mRNA species of snowshoe hare bunyavirus and in vitro translation of S mRNA to viral N polypeptide, *J Virol*, **31**: 685–94.

Chen S, Compans R, 1991, Oligomerization, transport, and Golgi retention of Punta Toro virus glycoproteins, *J Virol*, **65**: 5902–9.

Chen S, Matsuoka Y, Compans R, 1991, Golgi complex localization of the Punta Toro virus G2 protein requires its association with the G1 protein, *Virology*, **183**: 351–65.

Chumakov M, 1946, *Vestnik Akademii Nauk SSSR*, **2**: 19.

Collett MS, 1986, Messenger RNA of the M segment RNA of Rift Valley fever virus, *Virology*, **151**: 151–6.

Collett MS, Purchio AF et al., 1985, Complete nucleotide sequence of the M RNA segment of Rift Valley fever virus, *Virology*, **144**: 228–45.

Collett M, Keegan K et al., 1987, Protective subunit immunogens to Rift Valley fever virus from bacteria and recombinant vaccina virus, *The Biology of Negative Strand Viruses*, eds Mahy BWJ, Kolakofsky D, Elsevier, Amsterdam, 321–9.

Collett MS, Kakach L et al., 1989, Protein structure and function, *Genetics and Pathogenicity of Negative Strand Viruses*, eds Mahy BWJ, Kolakofsky D, Elsevier, Amsterdam, 49–57.

Dalrymple J, Peters C et al., 1981, Bunyaviruses, *The Replication of Negative Strand Viruses*, eds Bishop DHL, Compans RW, Elsevier, New York, 167–72.

Dalrymple J, Hasty S et al., 1989, *Vaccines 89*, eds Brown F, Chanock RM et al., Cold Spring Harbor Laboratory, Cold Spring Harbor NY, 371–5.

Dantas JR, Okuno Y et al., 1986, Characterization of glycoproteins of virus causing hemorrhagic fever with renal syndrome (HFRS) using monoclonal antibodies, *Virology*, **151**: 379–84.

Davies F, Casals J et al., 1978, The serological relationships of Nairobi sheep disease virus, *J Comp Pathol*, **88**: 519–23.

Digoutte J-P, Salaum J-J et al., 1980, Les arboviroses mineures en Afrique Centrale et Occidentale, *Med Trop*, **40**: 523–33.

Dobbs M, Kang CY, 1993, Hantaan virus mRNAs contain non-viral 5′ end sequences and lack poly(A) at the 3′ end, *IXth International Congress of Virology*, Abstract P44-16: 280.

Duchin JS, Koster FT et al., 1994, Hantavirus pulmonary syndrome: a clinical description of 17 patients with a newly recognized disease, *N Engl J Med*, **330**: 949–55.

Dunn EF, Pritlove DC et al., 1995, Transcription of a recombinant bunyavirus RNA template by transiently expressed bunyavirus proteins, *Virology*, **211**: 133–43.

Eddy G, Peters C et al., 1981, Rift Valley fever vaccine for humans, *Contrib Epidemiol Biostat*, **3**: 124–41.

Elliot LH, Ksiazek TG et al., 1994, Isolation of the causative agent of hantavirus pulmonary syndrome, *Am J Trop Med Hyg*, **51**: 102–8.

Elliott RM, 1985, Identification of nonstructural proteins encoded by viruses of the bunyamwera serogroup (family *Bunyaviridae*), *Virology*, **143**: 119–26.

Elliott RM, 1989, Nucleotide sequence analysis of the large (L) genomic RNA segment of bunyamwera virus, the prototype of the family *Bunyaviridae*, *Virology*, **173**: 426–36.

Elliott RM, 1990, Molecular biology of the *Bunyaviridae, J Gen Virol*, **71**: 501–22.

Elliott RM, Schmaljohn CS, Collett MS, 1991, *Bunyaviridae* genome structure and gene expression, *Curr Top Microbiol Immunol*, **169**: 91–141.

Elliott RM, Dunn E et al., 1992, Nucleotide sequence and coding strategy of the Uukuniemi virus L RNA segment, *J Gen Virol*, **73**: 1745–52.

Ellis DS, Shirodaria PV et al., 1988, Morphology and development of Rift Valley fever virus in Vero cell cultures, *J Med Virol*, **24**: 161–74.

Elwell MR, Ward GS et al., 1985, Serologic evidence of Hantaan-like virus in rodents and man in Thailand, *Southeast Asian J Trop Med Public Health*, **16**: 349–54.

Emery VC, 1987, Characterization of Punta Toro S mRNA species and identification of an inverted complementary sequence in the intergenic region of Punta Toro phlebovirus ambisense S RNA that is involved in mRNA transcription termination, *Virology*, **156**: 1–11.

Eshita Y, Bishop DHL, 1984, The complete sequence of the M RNA of snowshoe hare bunyavirus reveals the presence of internal hydrophobic domains in the viral glycoprotein, *Virology*, **137**: 227–40.

Eshita Y, Ericson B et al., 1985, Analyses of the mRNA transcription processes of snowshoe hare bunyavirus S and M RNA species, *J Virol*, **55**: 681–9.

Fazakerley JK, Ross AM, 1989, Computer analysis suggests a role for signal sequences in processing polyproteins of enveloped RNA viruses and as a mechanism of viral fusion, *Virus Genes*, **2**: 223–39.

Fazakerly JK, Gonzalez-Scarano F et al., 1988, Organization of the middle RNA segment of snowshoe hare bunyavirus, *Virology*, **167**: 422–32.

Feldmann H, Sanchez A et al., 1993, Utilization of autopsy RNA for the synthesis of the nucleocapsid antigen of a newly recognized virus associated with hantavirus pulmonary syndrome, *Virus Res*, **30**: 351–67.

Francy D, 1983, *California Serogroup Viruses*, eds Calisher C, Thompson W, Alan R Liss, New York, 365–75.

Fuller F, Bhown AS, Bishop DHL, 1983, Bunyavirus nucleoprotein, N, and a non-structural protein, NS$_S$ are coded by overlapping reading frames in the S RNA, *J Gen Virol*, **64**: 1705–14.

Fuller F, Bishop DHL, 1982, Identification of virus-coded nonstructural polypeptides in bunyavirus-infected cells, *J Virol*, **41**: 643–8.

Gahmberg N, Kuismanen E et al., 1986, Uukuniemi virus glycoproteins accumulate in and cause morphological changes of the Golgi complex in the absence of virus maturation, *J Virol*, **57**: 899–906.

Garcin D, Lezzi M et al., 1995, The 5′ ends of Hantaan virus (*Bunyaviridae*) RNAs suggest a prime-and-realign mechanism for the initiation of RNA synthesis, *J Virol*, **69**: 5754–62.

Gentsch JR, Bishop DHL, 1978, Small viral RNA segment of bunyaviruses codes for viral nucleocapsid protein, *J Virol*, **28**: 417–19.

Georges A, Saluzzo J et al., 1980, Arboviruses from Central African Republic: incidence, diagnosis in human pathology, *Med Trop*, **40**: 561–8.

Gerbaud S, Pardigon N et al., 1987a, Gene expression, transcription and genome replication, *The Biology of Negative Strand Viruses*, eds Kolakofsky D, Mahy BWJ, Elsevier, Amsterdam, 191–8.

Gerbaud S, Vialat P et al., 1987b, The S segment of the Germiston virus RNA genome can code for three proteins, *Virus Res*, **8**: 1–13.

Giorgi C, Accardi L et al., 1991, Sequences and coding strategies of the S RNAs of Toscana and Rift Valley fever viruses compared to those of Punta Toro, Sicilian sandfly fever, and Uukuniemi viruses, *Virology*, **180**: 738–53.

Glass G, Childs J et al., 1988, Association of intraspecific wounding with hantaviral infection in wild rats (*Rattus norvegicus*), *Epidemiol Infect*, **101**: 459–72.

Glass GE, Watson AJ et al., 1993, Infection with a rat-borne hantavirus in United States residents is consistently associated with hypertensive renal disease, *J Infect Dis*, **167**: 614–20.

Gligic A, Dimkovic N et al., 1992, Belgrade virus: a new hantavirus causing severe hemorrhagic fever with renal syndrome in Yugoslavia, *J Infect Dis*, **166**: 113–20.

Goldfarb L, Chumakov M et al., 1980, An epidemiological model of Crimean hemorrhagic fever, *Am J Trop Med Hyg*, **29**: 260–4.

Gonzalez J, Le-Guenno B et al., 1992, Serological evidence in sheep suggesting phlebovirus circulation in a Rift Valley fever enzootic area in Burkina Faso, *Trans R Soc Trop Med Hyg*, **86**: 680–2.

Gonzalez-Scarano F, 1985, La Crosse virus G1 glycoprotein undergoes a conformational change at the pH of fusion, *Virology*, **140**: 209–16.

Gonzalez-Scarano F, Pobjecky N, Nathanson N, 1984, La Crosse bunyavirus can mediate pH-dependent fusion from without, *Virology*, **132**: 222–5.

Gonzalez-Scarano F, Pobjecky N, Nathanson N, 1987, Virus-membrane interactions, *The Biology of Negative Strand Viruses*, eds Kolakofsky D, Mahy BWJ, Elsevier, New York, 33–39.

Gonzalez-Scarano F, Janssen RS et al., 1985, An avirulent G1 glycoprotein variant of La Crosse bunyavirus with defective fusion function, *J Virol*, **54**: 757–63.

Grabow J, Matthews C et al., 1969, The electroencephalogram and clinical sequelae of California arbovirus encephalitis, *Neurology*, **19**: 394–404.

Grady LJ, Sanders ML, Campbell WP, 1987, The sequence of the M RNA of an isolate of La Crosse virus, *J Gen Virol*, **68**: 3057–71.

Grankvist O, Juto P et al., 1992, Detection of nephropathia epidemica virus RNA in patient samples using a nested primer-based polymerase chain reaction, *J Infect Dis*, **165**: 934–7.

de Haan P, Wagemakers L et al., 1990, The S RNA segment of tomato spotted wilt virus has an ambisense character, *J Gen Virol*, **71**: 1001–7.

de Haan P, Kormelink R et al., 1991, Tomato spotted wilt virus L RNA encodes a putative RNA polymerase, *J Gen Virol*, **72**: 2207–16.

de Haan P, Gielen J et al., 1992, Characterization of RNA-mediated resistance to tomato spotted wilt virus in transgenic tobacco plants, *BioTechnology*, **10**: 1133–7.

Hacker D, 1990, Anti-mRNAS in La Crosse bunyavirus-infected cells, *J Virol*, **64**: 5051–7.

Hertig M, Sabin A, 1964, *Preventive Medicine in World War II*, eds Coates J, Hoff E, Hoff P, Office of the Surgeon General, Washington DC, 109–74.

Hewlett MJ, Chiu W, 1991, Virion structure, *Curr Top Microbiol Immunol*, **169**: 79–90.

Hewlett MJ, Petterson RF, Baltimore D, 1977, Circular forms of Uukuniemi virion RNA: an electron microscopic study, *J Virol*, **21**: 1085–93.

Hoogstraal H, 1979, The epidemiology of tick-borne Crimean–Congo haemorrhagic fever in Asia, Europe and Africa, *J Med Entomol*, **15**: 307–417.

Hubbard S, Ivatt R, 1981, Synthesis and processing of asparagine-linked oligosaccharides, *Annu Rev Biochem*, **50**: 55–83.

Huggins JW, Hsiang CM et al., 1991, Prospective, double-blind, concurrent, placebo-controlled clinical trial of intravenous ribavirin therapy of hemorrhagic fever with renal syndrome, *J Infect Dis*, **164**: 1119–27.

Ihara T, Akashi H, Bishop D, 1984, Novel coding strategy (ambisense genomic RNA) revealed by sequence analysis of Punta Toro phlebovirus S RNA, *Virology*, **136**: 293–306.

Ihara T, Dalrymple JM, Bishop DHL, 1985, Complete sequences of the glycoprotein and M RNA of Punta Toro phlebovirus compared to those of Rift Valley fever virus, *Virology*, **144**: 246–59.

Ihara T, Matsuura Y, Bishop DHL, 1985, Analysis of the mRNA

transcription processes of Punta Toro phlebovirus (*Bunyaviridae*), *Virology*, **147**: 317–25.

Jacoby D, Cooke C et al., 1993, Expression of the La Crosse M segment proteins in a recombinant vaccinia expression system mediates pH-dependent cellular fusion, *Virology*, **193**: 993–6.

Jin H, Elliott R, 1992, Mutagenesis of the L protein encoded by bunyamwera virus and production of monospecific antibodies, *J Gen Virol*, **73**: 2235–44.

Jin H, Elliott RM, 1993a, Characterization of bunyamwera virus S RNA that is transcribed and replicated by the L protein expressed from recombinant vaccinia virus, *J Virol*, **67**: 1396–404.

Jin H, Elliott RM, 1993b, Non-viral sequences at the 5′ ends of Dugbe nairovirus S mRNAs, *J Gen Virol*, **74**: 2293–7.

Jones L, Hodgson E, Nuttall P, 1989, Enhancement of virus transmission by tick salivary glands, *J Gen Virol*, **70**: 1895–8.

Jones L, Davies C et al., 1987, A novel mode of arbovirus transmission involving a nonviremic host, *Science*, **237**: 775–7.

Kakach LT, Suzich JA, Collett MS, 1989, Rift Valley fever virus M segment: phlebovirus expression strategy and protein glycosylation, *Virology*, **170**: 505–10.

Kaluda M, Mukwaya L et al., 1986, Kasokero virus: a new human pathogen from bats (*Rousettus aegypticus*) in Uganda, *Am J Trop Med Hyg*, **35**: 387–92.

Karabatsos N, 1985, *International Catalog of Arboviruses including Certain Other Viruses of Vertebrates*, American Society of Tropical Medicine and Hygiene, San Antonio.

Kark JD, Aynor Y et al., 1982, A serological survey of Rift Valley fever antibodies in the northern Sinai, *Trans R Soc Med Hyg*, **76**: 427–30.

Keegan K, Collett MS, 1986, Use of bacterial expression cloning to define the amino acid sequences of antigenic determinants on the G2 glycoprotein of Rift Valley fever virus, *J Virol*, **58**: 263–70.

Kemp G, Causey O, Causey C, 1971, Virus isolations from trade cattle, sheep, goats and swine at Ibadan, Nigeria, 1964–68, *Bull Epizootic Dis Afr*, **19**: 131–5.

Kingsford L, Hill DW, 1981, *The Replication of Negative Strand Viruses*, eds Bishop D, Compans R, Elsevier, New York, 111–16.

Kitajima EW, De Avila AC et al., 1992, Comparative cytological and immunogold labelling studies on different isolates of tomato spotted wilt virus, *J Submicrosc Cytol Pathol*, **24**: 1–4.

Kormelink R, Kitajima EW et al., 1991, The nonstructural protein (NS_S) encoded by the ambisense S RNA segment of tomato spotted wilt virus is associated with fibrous structures in infected plant cells, *Virology*, **181**: 459–68.

Kormelink R, de Haan P et al., 1992a, The nucleotide sequence of the M RNA segment of tomato spotted wilt virus, a bunyavirus with two ambisense RNA segments, *J Gen Virol*, **73**: 2795–804.

Kormelink R, de Haan P et al., 1992b, Viral RNA synthesis in tomato spotted wilt virus-infected *Nicotiana rustica* plants, *J Gen Virol*, **73**: 687–93.

Kormelink R, Van Poelwijk F et al., 1992c, Non-viral heterogeneous sequences at the 5′ ends of tomato spotted wilt virus mRNAs, *J Gen Virol*, **73**: 2125–8.

Kormelink R, Storms M et al., 1994, Expression and subcellular location of the NS_M protein of tomato spotted wilt virus (TSWV), a putative viral movement protein, *Virology*, **200**: 56–65.

Kuismanen E, Saraste J, Pettersson RF, 1985, Effect of monensin on the assembly of Uukuniemi virus in the Golgi complex, *J Virol*, **55**: 813–22.

Kuismanen E, Hedman K et al., 1982, Uukuniemi virus maturation: accumulation of virus particles and viral antigens in the Golgi complex, *Mol Cell Biol*, **2**: 1444–58.

Lappin DF, Nakitare GW et al., 1994, Localization of Bunyamwera bunyavirus G1 glycoprotein to the Golgi requires association with G2 but not with NS_M, *J Gen Virol*, **75**: 3441–51.

Laughlin LW, Meegan JM et al., 1979, Epidemic Rift Valley fever in Egypt: observations of the spectrum of human illness, *Trans R Soc Trop Med Hyg*, **73**: 630–3.

Law MD, Speck J, Moyer JW, 1992, The M RNA of impatiens necrotic spot tospovirus (*Bunyaviridae*) has an ambisense genomic organization, *Virology*, **188**: 732–41.

LeDuc J, 1979, The ecology of California group viruses, *J Med Entomol*, **16**: 1–17.

LeDuc JW, Cuevas M, Garcia M, 1980, The incidence and prevalence of Phlebotomus fever group virus in Panama. In *Proceedings of International Symposium on Tropical Arboviruses and Hemorrhagic Fevers*. ed. Pinheiro FP, Academia Brasileira de Ciencias, 385–390.

LeDuc JW, 1987, Epidemiology and ecology of the California serogroup viruses, *Am J Trop Med Hyg*, **37**: 60S–8S.

LeDuc J, 1995, *Kass Handbook of Infectious Diseases: Exotic Viral Infections*, ed Porterfield J, Chapman & Hall Medical, Oxford, 261–84.

LeDuc JW, Childs JE, Glass GE, 1992, The hantaviruses, etiologic agents of hemorrhagic fever with renal syndrome: a possible cause of hypertension and chronic renal disease in the United States, *Annu Rev Public Health*, **13**: 79–98.

LeDuc J, Pinheiro F, 1988, *The Arboviruses: epidemiology and ecology*, CRC Press, Boca Raton FL.

LeDuc JW, Smith GA et al., 1986, Global survey of antibody to Hantaan-related viruses among peridomestic rodents, *Bull WHO*, **64**: 139–44.

LeDuc JW, Ksiazek TG et al., 1990, A retrospective analysis of sera collected by the Hemorrhagic Fever Commission during the Korean Conflict, *J Infect Dis*, **162**: 1182–4.

Lee H, Baek L, Johnson K, 1982, Isolation of Hantaan virus, the etiologic agent of Korean hemorrhagic fever, from wild urban rats, *J Infect Dis*, **146**: 638–44.

Lee HW, Lee PW, Johnson KM, 1978, Isolation of the etiologic agent of Korean hemorrhagic fever, *J Infect Dis*, **137**: 298–308.

Lee H, Ahn C et al., 1990, Field trial of an inactivated vaccine against hemorrhagic fever with renal syndrome in humans, *Arch Virol Suppl* **1**: 35–47.

Lees JF, Pringle CR, Elliott RM, 1986, Nucleotide sequence of the bunyamwera virus M RNA segment: conservation of structural features in the bunyavirus glycoprotein gene product, *Virology*, **148**: 1–14.

Li D, Schmaljohn AL et al., 1995, Complete nucleotide sequences of the M and S segments of two hantavirus isolates from California: evidence for reassortment in nature among viruses related to hantavirus pulmonary syndrome, *Virology*, **206**: 973–83.

Lopez N, Muller R et al., 1995, The L protein of Rift Valley fever virus can rescue viral ribonucleoproteins and transcribe synthetic genome-like RNA molecules, *J Virol*, **69**: 3972–9.

Ludwig GV, Israel BA et al., 1991, Role of La Crosse virus glycoproteins in attachment of virus to host cells, *Virology*, **181**: 564–71.

Lvov D, Sidorova G et al., 1976, Virus 'Tandy' – a new arbovirus, isolated in the Uzbec SSR and Turkmen SSR from ticks *Hyalamma asiaticum asiaticum* Schulce et Schlottke, 1929, and *Hyalomma plumbeum plumbeum* Panzer, 1796, *Arch Virol*, **51**: 15–21.

Lvov D, Kostyukov M et al., 1984, An outbreak of arbovirus infection in the Tajik SSR caused by Issyk-kyl virus (Issyk-kul fever), *Vopr Virusol*, **29**: 89–92.

Lyons MJ, Heyduk J, 1973, Aspects of the developmental morphology of California encephalitis virus in cultured vertebrate and arthropod cells and in mouse brain, *Virology*, **54**: 37–52.

McKee K Jr, MacDonald C et al., 1985, Hemorrhagic fever with renal syndrome, a clinical perspective, *Milit Med*, **150**: 640–7.

Madoff DH, Lenard J, 1982, A membrane glycoprotein that accumulates intracellularly: cellular processing of the large glycoprotein of La Crosse virus, *Cell*, **28**: 821–9.

Marriot A, El-Ghorr A, Nuttall P, 1992, Dugbe nairovirus M RNA: nucleotide sequence and coding strategy, *Virology*, **190**: 606–15.

Marriott AC, Nuttall PA, 1992, Comparison of the S RNA segments and nucleoprotein sequences of Crimean–Congo hemorrhagic fever, Hazara, and Dugbe viruses, *Virology*, **189**: 795–9.

Marriott A, Ward V, Nuttall P, 1989, The S RNA segment of sandfly fever Sicilian virus: evidence for an ambisense genome, *Virology*, **169**: 341–5.

Marsh M, Helenius A, 1980, Adsorptive endocytosis of Semliki Forest virus, *J Mol Biol*, **142**: 439–54.

Matsuoka Y, Chen SY, Compans RW, 1991, Bunyavirus protein transport and assembly, *Curr Top Microbiol Immunol*, **169**: 161–79.

Matsuoka Y, Ihara T et al., 1988, Intracellular accumulation of Punta Toro virus glycoproteins expressed from cloned cDNA, *Virology*, **167**: 251–60.

Matthews C, Chun R, Grabow J, 1968, Psychological sequelae in children following California arbovirus encephalitis, *Neurology*, **18**: 1023–30.

Meegan J, 1979, The Rift Valley fever epizootic in Egypt 1977–78. I. Description of the epizootic and virological studies, *Trans R Soc Trop Med Hyg*, **73**: 618–23.

Montgomery R, 1917, On a tick-borne gastro-enteritis of sheep and goats occurring in British East Africa, *J Comp Pathol*, **30**: 28–57.

Morrill JC, Jennings GB et al., 1987, Pathogenicity and immunogenicity of a mutagen-attenuated Rift Valley fever virus immunogen in pregnant ewes, *Am J Vet Res*, **48**: 1042–7.

Morrill JC, Carpenter L et al., 1991, Further evaluation of a mutagen-attenuated Rift Valley fever vaccine in sheep, *Vaccine*, **9**: 35–41.

Morzunov SP, Feldmann H et al., 1995, A newly recognized virus associated with a fatal case of hantavirus pulmonary syndrome in Louisiana, *J Virol*, **69**: 1980–3.

Muller R, Argentini C et al., 1991, Completion of the genome sequence of Rift Valley fever phlebovirus indicates that the L RNA is negative sense or ambisense and codes for a putative transcriptase-replicase, *Nucleic Acids Res*, **19**: 5433.

Muller R, Saluzzo J-F et al., 1995, Characterization of clone 13, a naturally attenuated avirulent isolate of Rift Valley fever virus, which is altered in the small segment, *Am J Trop Med Hyg*, **53**: 405–11.

Murphy FA, Harrison AK, Whitfield SG, 1973, Morphologic and morphogenetic similarities of bunyamwera serological supergroup viruses and several other arthropod-borne viruses, *Intervirology*, **1**: 297–316.

Nakitare GW, Elliott RM, 1993, Expression of the bunyamwera virus M genome segment and intracellular localization of NS$_M$, *Virology*, **195**: 511–20.

Nichol ST, Spiropoulou CF et al., 1993, Genetic identification of a novel hantavirus associated with an outbreak of acute respiratory illness in the southwestern United States, *Science*, **262**: 914–17.

Nuzum EO, Rossi CA et al., 1988, Aerosol transmission of Hantaan and related viruses to laboratory rats, *Am J Trop Med Hyg*, **38**: 636–40.

Obijeski JF, Murphy FA, 1977, *Bunyaviridae*: recent biochemical developments, *J Gen Virol*, **37**: 1–14.

Obijeski JF, Bishop DHL et al., 1976, Segmented genome and nucleocapsid of LaCrosse Virus, *J Virol*, **20**: 664–75.

Overton HA, Ihara T, Bishop DH, 1987, Identification of the N and NS$_S$ proteins coded by the ambisense S RNA of Punta Toro phlebovirus using monospecific antisera raised to baculovirus expressed N and NS$_S$ proteins, *Virology*, **157**: 338–50.

Parker MD, Hewlett MJ, 1981, Bunyaviruses, *Replication of Negative Strand Viruses*, eds Bishop D, Compans R, Elsevier, New York, 125–45.

Parker MD, Smith JF, Dalrymple JM, 1984, Genome structure, transcription and genetics, *Segmented Negative Strand Viruses*, eds Compans R, Bishop D, Academic Press, Orlando FL, 21–8.

Parrington MA, Kang CY, 1990, Nucleotide sequence analysis of the S genomic segment of Prospect Hill virus: comparison with the prototype hantavirus, *Virology*, **175**: 167–75.

Parsonson I, McPhee DA, 1985, Bunyavirus pathogenesis, *Adv Virus Res*, **30**: 279–316.

Patterson JL, Kolakofsky D, 1984, Characterization of La Crosse virus small-genome segment transcripts, *J Virol*, **49**: 680–5.

Patterson JL, Kolakofsky D et al., 1983, Isolation of the ends of La Crosse virus small RNA as a double-stranded structure, *J Virol*, **45**: 882–4.

Pattnaik AK, Abraham G, 1983, Identification of four complementary RNA species in Akabane virus-infected cells, *J Virol*, **47**: 452–62.

Patton JT, Davis NL, Wertz GW, 1984a, N protein alone satisfies the requirement for protein synthesis during RNA replication of vesicular stomatitis virus, *J Virol*, **49**: 303–9.

Patton JT, Davis NL, Wertz GW, 1984b, Transcription and replication, *Nonsegmented Negative Strand Viruses. Paramyxoviruses and Rhabdoviruses*, eds Bishop D, Compans R, Academic Press, Orlando FL, 147–52.

Pavri R, Anandarajah M et al., 1976, Isolation of Wanowrie virus from brain of a fatal human case from Sri Lanka, *Indian J Med Res*, **64**: 557–61.

Pekosz A, Griot C et al., 1995, Protection from La Crosse virus encephalitis with recombinant glycoproteins: role of neutralizing anti-G1 antibodies, *J Virol*, **69**: 3475–81.

Pensiero MN, Hay J, 1992, The Hantaan virus M-segment glycoproteins G1 and G2 can be expressed independently, *J Virol*, **66**: 1907–14.

Pensiero MN, Jennings GB et al., 1988, Expression of the Hantaan virus M genome segment by using a vaccinia virus recombinant, *J Virol*, **62**: 696–702.

Pesonen M, Kuismanen E, Pettersson RF, 1982, Monosaccharide sequence of protein-bound glycans of Uukuniemi virus, *J Virol*, **41**: 390–400.

Peters C, LeDuc J, 1991, Bunyaviruses, phleboviruses and related viruses, *Textbook of Human Virology*, ed Belshe R, Mosby Year-Book, St Louis MO, 571–614.

Pettersson RF, 1991, Protein localization and virus assembly at intracellular membranes, *Curr Top Microbiol Immunol*, **170**: 67–106.

Pettersson RF, Bonsdorf CH, 1975, Ribonucleoproteins of Uukuniemi virus are circular, *J Virol*, **15**: 386–92.

Pettersson RF, Kuismanen E et al., 1985, *Viral Messenger RNA Transcription, Processing, Splicing, and Molecular Structure*, ed Becker Y, Martinus Nijhoff, Boston MA, 283–300.

Pifat DY, Osterling MC, Smith JF, 1988, Antigenic analysis of Punta Toro virus and identification of protective determinants with monoclonal antibodies, *Virology*, **167**: 442–50.

Pinheiro FP, Travassos da Rosa APA, Travassos da Rosa JFS, 1981, Oropouche virus. I. A review of clinical, epidemiological and ecological findings, *Am J Trop Med Hyg*, **30**: 149–60.

Plyusnin A, Vapalahti O et al., 1994, Tula virus: a newly detected hantavirus carried by European common voles, *J Virol*, **68**: 7833–9.

Poch O, Sauvaget I et al., 1989, Identification of four conserved motifs among the RNA-dependent polymerase encoding elements, *EMBO J*, **8**: 3867–75.

Raju R, Kolakofsky D, 1986, Inhibitors of protein synthesis inhibit both La Crosse virus S-mRNA and S genome syntheses in vivo, *Virus Res*, **5**: 1–9.

Raju R, Kolakofsky D, 1987a, Translational requirement of La Crosse virus S-mRNA synthesis, *J Virol*, **63**: 122–8.

Raju R, Kolakofsky D, 1987b, Unusual transcripts in La Crosse virus-infected cells and the site for nucleocapsid assembly, *J Virol*, **61**: 667–72.

Raju R, Kolakofsky D, 1989, The ends of La Crosse virus genome and antigenome RNAs within nucleocapsids are base paired, *J Virol*, **63**: 122–8.

Ranki M, Pettersson RF, 1975, Uukuniemi virus contains an RNA polymerase, *J Virol*, **16**: 1420–5.

Ravkov EV, Rollin PE et al., 1995, Genetic and serologic analysis of Black Creek Canal virus and its association with human disease and *Sigmodon hispidus* infection, *Virology*, **210**: 482–9.

Report, 1995a, *115 Confirmed Cases of Hantavirus Pulmonary Syndrome*, Centers for Disease Control and Prevention, Atlanta GA.

Report, 1995b, *Arbovirus Surveillance Summary*, Centers for Disease Control and Prevention, Fort Collins CO.

Resende R deO, de Haan P et al., 1991, Generation of envelope and defective interfering RNA mutants of tomato spotted wilt virus by mechanical passage, *J Gen Virol*, **72**: 2375–83.

Rie H, Hilty M, Cramblet H, 1973, Intelligence and coordination following California encephalitis, *Am J Dis Child*, **125**: 824–7.

Rollin PE, Ksiazek TG et al., 1995, Isolation of Black Creek Canal virus, a new hantavirus from *Sigmodon hispidus* in Florida, *J Med Virol*, **46**: 35–9.

Rönnholm R, 1992, Localization to the Golgi complex of Uukuniemi virus glycoproteins G1 and G2 expressed from cloned cDNAs, *J Virol*, **66**: 4525–31.

Rönnholm R, Pettersson RF, 1987, Complete nucleotide sequence of the M RNA segment of Uukuniemi virus encoding the membrane glycoproteins G1 and G2, *Virology*, **160**: 191–202.

Rothman JE, 1981, The Golgi apparatus: two organelles in tandem, *Science*, **213**: 1212–18.

Ruusala A, Persson R et al., 1992, Coexpression of the membrane glycoproteins G1 and G2 of Hantaan virus is required for targeting to the Golgi complex, *Virology*, **186**: 53–64.

Sabatino D, Cramblett H, 1968, Behavioral sequelae of California encephalitis virus infection in children, *Dev Med Child Neurol*, **10**: 331–7.

Sabin A, 1951, Experimental studies on phlebotomus (pappataci, sandfly) fever during World War II, *Arch Virusforsch*, 367–410.

Schmaljohn C, 1990, Nucleotide sequence of the L genome segment of hantaan virus, *Nucleic Acids Res*, **18**: 6728.

Schmaljohn CS, Dalrymple JM, 1983, Analysis of Hantaan virus RNA: evidence for a new genus of *Bunyaviridae*, *Virology*, **131**: 482–91.

Schmaljohn CS, Schmaljohn AL, Dalrymple JM, 1987, Hantaan virus M RNA: coding strategy, nucleotide sequence, and gene order, *Virology*, **157**: 31–9.

Schmaljohn CS, Hasty SE et al., 1985, Antigenic and genetic properties of viruses linked to hemorrhagic fever with renal syndrome, *Science*, **227**: 1041–4.

Schmaljohn CS, Hasty SE et al., 1986a, Hantaan virus replication: effects of monensin, tunicamycin and endoglycosidases on the structural glycoproteins, *J Gen Virol*, **67**: 707–17.

Schmaljohn CS, Jennings GB et al., 1986b, Coding strategy of the S genome of Hantaan virus, *Virology*, **155**: 633–43.

Schmaljohn CS, Parker MD et al., 1989, Baculovirus expression of the M genome segment of Rift Valley fever virus and examination of antigenic and immunogenic properties of the expressed proteins, *Virology*, **170**: 184–92.

Schmaljohn CS, Chu YK et al., 1990, Antigenic subunits of Hantaan virus expressed by baculovirus and vaccinia virus recombinants, *J Virol*, **64**: 3162–70.

Schmaljohn C, Dalrymple J et al., 1994, *Recombinant and Synthetic Vaccines*, eds Talwar G, Rao K, Chauha V, Narosa Publishing, New Delhi, 332–9.

Schmaljohn AL, Li D et al., 1995, Isolation and initial characterization of a newfound hantavirus from California, *Virology*, **206**: 963–72.

Settergren B, Juto P et al., 1990, Molecular characterization of the RNA S segment of nephropathia epidemica virus strain Hallnas B1, *Virology*, **174**: 79–86.

Shah K, Work T, 1969, Bhanja virus: a new arbovirus from ticks *Haemaphysalis intermedia* Warburton and Nuttall, 1909, in Orissa, India, *Indian J Med Res*, **57**: 793–8.

Simons JF, Hellman U, Pettersson RF, 1990, Uukuniemi virus S RNA segment: ambisense coding strategy, packaging of

complementary strands into virions, and homology to members of the genus *Phlebovirus*, *J Virol*, **64**: 247–55.

Simons JF, Persson R, Pettersson RF, 1992, Association of the nonstructural protein NS$_S$ of Uukuniemi virus with the 40S ribosomal subunit, *J Virol*, **66**: 4233–41.

Simons JF, Pettersson RF, 1991, Host-derived 5′ ends and overlapping complementary 3′ ends of the two mRNAs transcribed from the ambisense S segment of Uukuniemi virus, *J Virol*, **65**: 4741–8.

Smith JF, Pifat DY, 1982, Morphogenesis of sandfly viruses (*Bunyaviridae* family), *Virology*, **121**: 61–81.

Smith JF, Hodson L et al., 1987, Induction of neutralizing antibodies to Rift Valley fever virus with synthetic peptides [abstract], *VIIth International Congress of Virology*, Edmonton, Alberta, Canada, 65.

Smithburn K, 1949, Rift Valley fever: the neurotropic adaptation of the virus and the experimental use of this modified virus as a vaccine, *Br J Exp Pathol*, **30**: 1–16.

Smithburn K, Haddow A, Mahaffy A, 1946, A neurotropic virus isolated from *Aedes* mosquitoes caught in the Semliki Forest, *Am J Trop Med Hyg*, **21**: 189–208.

Smithburn K, Mahaffy A, Paul J, 1941, Bwamba fever and its causative virus, *Am J Trop Med Hyg*, **21**: 75–90.

Song JW, Baek LJ et al., 1994, Isolation of pathogenic hantavirus from white-footed mouse (*Peromyscus leucopus*) [letter], *Lancet*, **344**: 1637.

Song W, Quintana M et al., 1995a, High genetic complexity of hantavirus radiation of New World microtine voles (*Rodentia microtus*) [abstract], *3rd International Conference on HFRS and Hantaviruses*, Helsinki, Finland.

Song W, Torrez-Martinez N et al., 1995b, Isla Vista virus: a genetically novel hantavirus of the California vole *Microtus californicus*, *J Gen Virol*, **76**: 3195–9.

Spiropoulou CF, Morzunov S et al., 1994, Genome structure and variability of a virus causing hantavirus pulmonary syndrome, *Virology*, **200**: 715–23.

Stohwasser, R, Giebel LB et al., 1990, Molecular characterization of the RNA S segment of nephropathia epidemica virus strain Hallnas B1, *Virology*, **174**: 79–86.

Struthers JK, Swanepoel R, 1982, Identification of a major nonstructural protein in the nuclei of Rift Valley fever virus-infected cells, *J Gen Virol*, **60**: 381–4.

Sureau P, Klein J-M, 1980, Arbovirus en Iran, *Med Trop*, **40**: 549–54.

Suzich JA, Collett MS, 1988, Rift Valley fever virus M segment: cell-free transcription and translation of virus-complementary RNA, *Virology*, **164**: 478–86.

Suzich JA, Kakach LT, Collett MS, 1990, Expression strategy of a phlebovirus: biogenesis of proteins from the Rift Valley fever virus M segment, *J Virol*, **64**: 1549–55.

Swanepoel R, 1995, *Kass Handbook of Infectious Diseases, Exotic Viral Infections*, ed Porterfield J, Chapman & Hall Medical, Oxford, 285–93.

Swanepoel R, Shepherd A et al., 1985, A common-source outbreak of Crimean–Congo haemorrhagic fever on a dairy farm, *S Afr Med J*, **68**: 635–7.

Taller AM, Xiao SY et al., 1993, Belgrade virus, a cause of hemorrhagic fever with renal syndrome in the Balkans, is closely related to Dobrava virus of field mice, *J Infect Dis*, **168**: 750–3.

Talmon Y, Prasad BV et al., 1987, Electron microscopy of vitrified-hydrated La Crosse virus, *J Virol*, **61**: 2319–21.

Torrez-Martinez N, Hjelle B, 1995, Enzootic of Bayou hantavirus in rice rats (*Oryzomys palustris*) in 1983 [letter], *Lancet*, **346**: 780–1.

Torrez-Martinez N, Song W, Hjelle B, 1995, Nucleotide sequence analysis of the M genomic segment of El Moro Canyon hantavirus: antigenic distinction from Four Corners hantavirus, *Virology*, **211**: 336–8.

Tycko B, Maxfield FR, 1982, Rapid acidification of endocytic vesicles containing alpha-2-macroglobulin, *Cell*, **28**: 643–51.

Ullman DE, German TL et al., 1993, Tospovirus replication in insect vector cells: immunocytochemical evidence that the nonstructural protein encoded by the S RNA of tomato spotted wilt tospovirus is present in thrips vector cells, *Phytopathology*, **83**: 456–63.

Ulmanen I, Seppala P, Pettersson RF, 1981, In vitro translation of Uukuniemi virus-specific RNAs: identification of a nonstructural protein and a precursor to the membrane glycoproteins, *J Virol*, **37**: 72–9.

Vaira AM, Semeria L et al., 1995, Resistance to tospoviruses in *Nicotiana benthamiana* transformed with the N gene of tomato spotted wilt virus: correlation between transgene expression and protection in primary transformants, *Mol Plant Microbe Interact*, **8**: 66–73.

Vasconcelos P, Travassos da Rosa J, Travassos da Rosa A, 1994, *Virologica 91: II Simposio Internacional Soubre Arbovirus dos Tropicos e Febres Hemorragicas*, eds Travassos da Rosa A, Ishak R, Instituto Evandro Chagas/Universidade Federal do Para/Sociedade Brasileira de Virologia, Belem, Brazil, 347–60.

Vasconcelos PF, Travassos da Rosa JF et al., 1989, 1st register of an epidemic caused by Oropouche virus in the states of Maranhao and Goias, Brazil, *Rev Inst Med Trop Sao Paulo*, **31**: 271–8.

Verani P, Nicoletti L, 1995, *Kass Handbook of Infectious Diseases, Exotic Viral Infections*, ed Porterfield J, Chapman & Hall Medical, Oxford, 295–317.

Verani P, Lopes M et al., 1980, Arboviruses in the Mediterranean countries, *Zentralbl Bakteriol Mikrobiol Hyg*, 195–201.

Verkleij FN, Peters D, 1983, Characterization of a defective form of tomato spotted wilt virus, *J Gen Virol*, **64**: 677–86.

Vesenjak-Hirjan J, Calisher C et al., 1980, Arboviruses in the Mediterranean Countries, *Zentralblatt Bakteriol, Parasit, Infect. Hyg.* **I Abt**, 297–301.

Vialat P, Bouloy M, 1992, Germiston virus transcriptase requires active 40S ribosomal subunits and utilizes capped cellular RNAs, *J Virol*, **66**: 685–93.

Vidal S, Kolakofsky D, 1989, Modified model for the switch from Sendai virus transcription to replication, *J Virol*, **63**: 1951–8.

Vorndam AV, Trent DW, 1979, Oligosaccharides of the California encephalitis viruses, *Virology*, **95**: 1–7.

Wang MW, Pennock DG et al., 1993, Epitope mapping studies with neutralizing and non-neutralizing monoclonal antibodies to the G1 and G2 envelope glycoproteins of Hantaan virus, *Virology*, **197**: 757–66.

Ward VK, Marriott AC et al., 1990, Coding strategy of the S RNA segment of Dugbe virus (*Nairovirus; Bunyaviridae*), *Virology*, **175**: 518–24.

Wasmoen TL, Kakach LT, Collett MS, 1988, Rift Valley fever virus M segment: cellular localization of M segment-encoded proteins, *Virology*, **166**: 275–80.

Watts D, Pantuwatana S et al., 1973, Transovarial transmission of La Crosse virus (California encephalitis group) in the mosquito, *Aedes triseriatus*, *Science*, **182**: 123–30.

Watts D, Thompson W et al., 1974, Overwintering of La Crosse virus in *Aedes triseriatus*, *Am J Trop Med Hyg*, **23**: 694–700.

Watts D, Ksiazek T et al., 1989, *The Arboviruses: epidemiology and ecology*, ed Monath T, CRC Press, Boca Raton FL, 177–222.

Wertz GW, 1983, Replication of vesicular stomatitis virus defective interfering particle RNA in vitro: transition from synthesis of defective interfering leader RNA to synthesis of full-length defective interfering RNA, *J Virol*, **46**: 513–22.

WHO, 1994, Weekly Epidemiological Record, *Wkly Epidemiol Rec*, 197–204.

WHO, 1995, *Report of a Meeting on Hantavirus Vaccine Development*, World Health Organization, Geneva.

Wijkamp I, van Lent J et al., 1993, Multiplication of tomato spotted wilt virus in its insect vector, *Frankliniella occidentalis*, *J Gen Virol*, **74**: 341–9.

Yuill T, 1983, *California Serogroup Viruses*, eds Calisher C, Thompson W, Alan R Liss, New York, 77–88.

Zaki SR, Greer PW et al., 1995, Hantavirus pulmonary syndrome. Pathogenesis of an emerging infectious disease, *Am J Pathol*, **146**: 552–79.

Chapter 31

ARENAVIRUSES

M S Salvato and S K Rai

1 Properties of the arenaviruses	2 Clinical and pathological aspects

1 PROPERTIES OF THE ARENAVIRUSES

1.1 Introduction

The arenaviruses are enveloped, single-stranded RNA viruses that are primarily carried by rodents and occasionally transmitted to humans. Old World and New World arenaviruses have been isolated on the African and American continents respectively (see Table 31.1). The arenaviruses are important clinically as human pathogens and experimentally as models for persistent infection and cellular immune responses. The prototype virus, lymphocytic choriomeningitis virus, was first isolated from a human diagnosed with St Louis encephalitis; tissue homogenates passaged through monkeys and mice caused fever and aseptic meningitis (Armstrong and Lillie 1934). A year later, a filterable agent was isolated from the cerebrospinal fluids of 2 patients; this agent elicited similar symptoms in mice (Rivers and Scott 1935). At the same time, Traub (1935) discovered a contaminant virus in the mouse colony of the Rockefeller Laboratories. Viruses were exchanged between the 3 laboratories and their identity was confirmed by neutralization in vitro and cross-protection in vivo (Rivers and Scott 1936). Lymphocytic choriomeningitis virus (LCMV) has frequently been found as a contaminant of laboratory mice, rats and hamsters in North America and Europe, and may have entered North America via mice from Europe. Studies of murine LCMV infection have contributed to a wealth of information on the mechanisms of viral persistence and the interactions of viruses with host immune systems (see section 2.4, p. 640).

In 1956, the non-pathogenic Tacaribe virus was isolated from Caribbean fruit bats (Downs et al. 1963). With the agricultural expansion in South America, 2 pathogenic arenaviruses emerged: Junin, isolated from humans with Argentine haemorrhagic fever (Parodi et al. 1958); and Machupo, isolated from humans with Bolivian haemorrhagic fever (Johnson et al. 1965). Collaboration between field workers, the Yale Arbovirus Laboratories and the Rockefeller Laboratories documented the morphology and antigenicity of the 'Tacaribe group' of viruses. A non-pathogenic member of this group, Pichinde virus, was isolated during a trapping programme in Colombia, and has since served in many biochemical studies.

It was not until the late 1960s that the morphological similarities between LCMV and the Tacaribe group of viruses were noted: both were enveloped viruses with a granular or sandy appearance. Serological tests later confirmed the relationship and they were named arenaviruses after the Latin *arena* for 'sandy' (Johnson et al. 1965, Dalton et al. 1968, Rowe et al. 1970). When Lassa fever virus emerged in Africa, it was quickly identified as an arenavirus on morphological and serological criteria (Murphy 1975). Arenaviruses are considered 'emerging pathogens' because new isolates are coming to our attention with great frequency (Coimbra et al. 1994). The following publications contain more details about the arenaviruses: Oldstone (1987a), Bishop (1990), McCormick (1990), Salvato (1993a), Southern (1996), Buchmeier (1996) and Peters (1996).

1.2 Classification

The *Arenaviridae* are one of 6 families of negative-strand RNA viruses, the others being *Filoviridae, Rhabdoviridae, Paramyxoviridae, Orthomyxoviridae* and *Bunyaviridae*. These viruses are characterized by single-stranded, non-infectious genomic RNA that requires a virus-encoded RNA transcriptase to initiate replication. Arenaviruses have been classified by a combination of morphological characteristics, biochemical analyses and immunological tests (Pfau 1974) and are the only family of negative-strand RNA viruses with a bisegmented genome (Pedersen 1979). Under the Old World and New World groupings are the 16 genera of arenaviruses (Table 31.1) with the probable

Table 31.1 *Arenaviridae*: carriers and geographical distribution

Virus	Virus carrier	Geographical distribution	Potential for human disease
New World			
Amapari	*Oryzomys goeldii*	Brazil	None reported
	Neacomys guinae	Brazil	
Flexal	*Neacomys* spp.	Brazil	None reported
Guanarito	*Oryzomys* spp.	Venezuela	Severe
Junin	*Calomys laucha*	Argentina	Severe
	Calomys musculinus	Argentina	
	Akodon azarae	Argentina	
Latino	*Calomys callosus*	Bolivia	None reported
Machupo	*Calomys callosus*	Bolivia	Severe
Parana	*Oryzomys buccinatus*	Paraguay	None reported
Pichinde	*Oryzomys albigularis*	Colombia	None
	Thomasomys fuscatus	Colombia	
Sabía	Not known	Brazil	Severe
Tacaribe	*Artibeus literatus*	Trinidad	None reported
	Artibeus jamaicensis	Trinidad	
Tamiami	*Sigmodon hispidus*	USA	None reported
Old World			
LCM	*Mus musculus*	World-wide	Mild to severe
Lassa	*Mastomys natalensis*	West Africa	Severe, often fatal
Mopeia	*Mastomys natalensis*	Mozambique Zimbabwe	None reported
Mobala	*Praomys jacksoni*	Central African Republic	None reported
Ippy	*Mastomys natalensis*	Central African Republic	None reported

addition of further viruses as the Asian continents are scrutinized and as human settlement of the globe expands. Within the genus LCMV, the Armstrong, Traub, UBC/WE and Pasteur strains and their isolates have been extensively characterized. Genetic relationships among the arenaviruses can be depicted by a phylogenetic tree based on the differences between the viral nucleocapsid protein sequences (Fig. 31.1).

1.3 Distribution

The worldwide distribution of arenaviruses follows the distribution of their natural reservoir hosts, primarily rodents (Fig. 31.2). Occasionally, infected humans

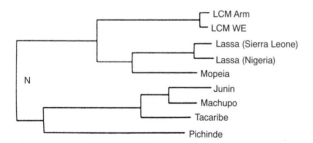

Fig. 31.1 Phylogenetic tree showing the genetic relatedness of arenaviruses based on the sequence of the nucleocapsid protein (N) genes. Old World arenaviruses LCM, Lassa and Mopeia are more closely related than New World arenaviruses Junin, Machupo, Tacaribe and Pichinde. (Reproduced from Clegg 1993.)

have travelled extensively, resulting in movement of the viruses (Holmes et al. 1990).

Although there are over 30 families of rodents, the arenaviruses are associated with only 2 major families: the *Muridae* (e.g. house mice and rats) and the *Cricetidae* (e.g. voles, deer mice and gerbils). The *Muridae* inhabit human dwellings and food stores, in contrast to the *Cricetidae* that live in the open grasslands. *Muridae* include *Mastomys*, that carries the Lassa-like viruses; *Praomys*, that carries Mobala; and *Mus*, that spread from the Old World to the rest of the globe, simultaneously dispersing LCMV. The cottonrat, *Sigmodon hispidus*, from which Tamiami was isolated in the USA, is related to the *Cricetidae* (*Calomys*, *Akodon*, *Oryzomys* and *Neocomys*) of South America. Tacaribe virus is an exception in that it was isolated from the fruit bat, *Artibeus*. It is notable that infections follow seasonal associations between humans and carriers; for example, the harvest season in Argentina, April to June, is also the peak time for the occurrence of Argentine haemorrhagic fever.

1.4 Morphology and structure

The envelope composition of an arenavirus derives from host cell membranes during maturation from the cell surface (Fig. 31.3a). The envelope is sensitive to organic solvents and detergents; treatment with these reagents can be used to separate viral cores from their envelopes. Virions are also sensitive to UV and γ-irradiation, to heating at 56°C, and to pH outside

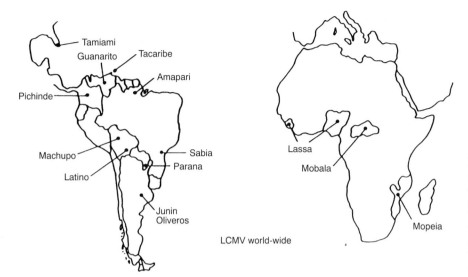

Fig. 31.2 Map of the distribution of Old World and New World arenaviruses. The Old World viruses originated on the European and African continents and the New World viruses originated in the Americas.

the range of 5.5–8.5. Acid or high salt treatment of LCMV causes one of the envelope glycoprotein chains, GP-1, to dissociate from the virion surface, whereas the other chain, GP-2, remains anchored in the envelope (Di Simone et al. 1994). Acid treatment of LCMV decreases its Vero cell infectivity, which is due to virus aggregation or the loss of GP-1. Virions are generally purified from the media surrounding infected cells by a combination of precipitation with 7% polyethylene glycol and centrifugation: buoyant densities are 1.9–1.2 g/cm^3 in caesium chloride, 1.17–1.18 g/cm^3 in sucrose and 1.14 g/cm^3 in amidotrizoate (Buchmeier, Elder and Oldstone 1978).

Originally, electron micrographs showed arenaviruses as highly pleiomorphic, probably because of their instability during fixation procedures. More recently, cryoelectron micrographs have revealed spherical particles with an average diameter of 90–110 nm (Burns and Buchmeier 1993) (Fig. 31.3b, c). Glycoproteins on the surface of the virion form T-shaped spikes extending 7–10 nm from the envelope. Electron-dense granules within arenaviruses, from which the name 'arena' derives, are ribonucleoprotein particles. These include ribosomal RNA, and perhaps whole ribosomes, and more of such particles are present in late viral harvests than in early harvests (Farber and Rawls 1975, Pedersen 1979, Dutko and Oldstone 1983, Southern et al. 1987). With Pichinde virus, virion-associated ribosomes are not essential for the infectious process; viruses produced in cells containing *ts* ribosomes are infectious even at the nonpermissive temperature (Leung and Rawls 1977). Electron microscopy of disrupted virions reveals circularized strings of ribonucleoproteins (Palmer et al. 1977) that may have resulted from the self-annealing of the RNA termini that encode approximately 20 bases of complementary nucleotides.

Arenaviruses produce defective interfering (DI) particles (reviewed by Buchmeier et al. 1980a). DI particles are generated rapidly during infection of tissue cultures with LCMV, and render the cells resistant to superinfection with LCMV, less resistant to Pichinde

and entirely susceptible to heterologous viruses (Lehmann-Grube, Slenczka and Tees 1969, Welsh and Buchmeier 1979). DI particles sediment to a lower density than infectious virus and have a smaller target size for UV inactivation, and their concentration can be measured by cytopathogenicity-reduction assays. DI particles of Pichinde lack conventional S RNA (Dutko, Wright and Pfau 1976).

1.5 Genome structure and function

The arenaviruses contain single-stranded RNA that consists of 2 RNA segments, L c. 7000 bases and S c. 3400 bases. Complete sequences are now available for LCMV, Tacaribe and Pichinde, and partial sequences for Lassa, Junin, Mopeia and other arenaviruses (Romanowski, Matsuura and Bishop 1985, Auperin, Sasso and McCormick 1986, Auperin and McCormick 1989, Iapalucci et al. 1989, Salvato and Shimomaye 1989, Salvato, Shimomaye and Oldstone 1989, Ghiringhelli et al. 1991, Harnish, Zheng and Polyak, unpublished; reviewed in Clegg 1993). Four open reading frames have been identified: a gene for the envelope glycoprotein is encoded at the 5′ end of the S RNA segment, and, in the negative sense, a gene for the nucleocapsid protein is encoded at the 3′ end of the S RNA. A gene for a small zinc-binding protein is encoded at the 5′ end of the L RNA, and, in the negative sense, a gene for the viral RNA polymerase is encoded at the 3′ end of the L RNA (Fig. 31.4).

A hallmark of the arenaviruses is their 'ambisense' coding strategy (Auperin et al. 1984). Each RNA segment encodes a gene in the positive (mRNA) sense and an additional non-overlapping gene in the negative sense, i.e. the latter gene must first be transcribed to obtain the mRNA sense. The viruses are classified as negative strand, because the mRNA sense genes cannot function in translation directly from the genomic RNA; subgenomic mRNA copies of these genes must first be produced by transcription (Fig. 31.5).

Strong secondary structures can be predicted for arenavirus genomic RNAs: stem–loops in the

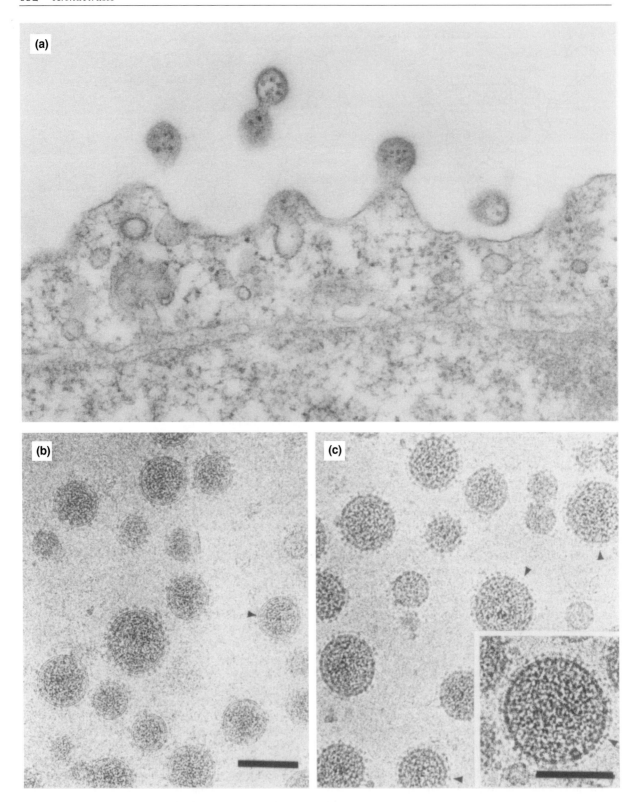

Fig. 31.3   Electron micrographs of LCM virions. (a) Thin section showing virions budding from infected BHK-21 cells. Typical 110 nm virions containing 20 nm electron-dense particles are evident. (b) Cryoelectron micrograph of unstained LCM virions at the 1.5 μm defocus level to emphasize lipid bilayer (see arrow) and in (c) cryoelectron micrograph of LCM at the 3 μm defocus level to emphasize surface topography. Bars = 100 nm. (Microscopy by R Milligan, Scripps Clinic and Research Foundation, San Diego. Reproduced from Burns and Buchmeier 1993.)

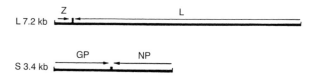

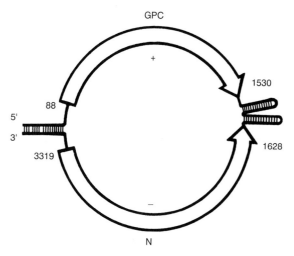

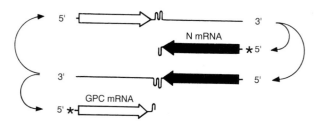

Fig. 31.4 The 2 arenavirus RNA segments, L and S, are depicted with the 4 encoded genes: Z (zinc-binding protein), L (polymerase), GP (envelope glycoprotein) and NP (nucleocapsid protein). (Reproduced from Salvato 1993.)

Fig. 31.5 The ambisense coding strategy of the arenaviruses is illustrated for the S RNA segment of Junin virus. First, the subgenomic nucleocapsid mRNA (N mRNA) is made and then the full-length antigenomic RNA is made (this is a 'replication intermediate'); finally, the subgenomic glycoprotein mRNA (GPC mRNA) is made. For the L RNA a similar sequence occurs with the L and Z subgenomic mRNAs. (Reproduced from Romanowski 1993.)

Fig. 31.6 The S RNA segment of Junin virus can be predicted to form strong secondary structures at the RNA terminus (a panhandle of the 3′ and 5′ ends) and at the intergenic region (a double stem–loop structure). The glycoprotein (GPC) and the nucleocapsid protein (N) open reading frames are in opposite coding sense on either side of the intergenic stem–loops. (Reproduced from Romanowski 1993.)

1.6 Replication

TROPISM AND VIRUS ENTRY

Arenaviruses replicate in a broad range of mammalian hosts and in almost every tissue of the host, reaching high titres in brain, kidney, liver and secondary lymphoid organs (see Fig. 31.9). Virus replication is restricted in lymphocytes, macrophages and terminally differentiated neurons, probably because of the absence of host cell factors (Borrow, Tishon and Oldstone 1991, de la Torre et al. 1993, Polyak, Zheng and Harnish 1995a). Arenaviruses are often propagated in adherent cell lines such as BHK-21 cells, mouse L cells or Vero cells. The broad range of mammalian cells that can be infected suggests that the receptor for virus entry is fairly well conserved. In attempts to find the receptor for LCMV, Borrow and Oldstone (1992) used a virus overlay blot assay to identify a 160 kDa glycoprotein from rodent fibroblasts. The normal function of this protein is not yet known, nor is it known whether this protein is broadly distributed across species and cell types.

Arenavirus entry into cultured cells is sensitive to lysosomotropic agents (Pichinde: Mifune, Carter and Rawls 1971; Lassa and Mopeia: Glushakova and Lukashevich 1989, Glushakova et al. 1992; LCMV: Borrow and Oldstone 1994, Di Simone, Zandonatti and Buchmeier 1994). In the case of LCMV, this uptake was not affected by cytochalasins, so does not require clathrin-coated pits and takes place in smooth-walled vesicles by 'viropexis'. Once the virus is in the cell, the life cycle of uncoating, mRNA transcription, translation, and genome replication takes place in the cytoplasm, with some contribution from host cell components for transcription and translation (Fig. 31.7).

intergenic regions and base-paired 'panhandles' at the termini of the RNA segments. The terminal 20 bases of the arenavirus genomic RNA are conserved between genera and almost identical within one arenavirus strain. It is possible to form intra- and extramolecular complexes, i.e. the 3′ and 5′ termini of the S RNA can anneal with each other or the 3′ of the S RNA can anneal with the 5′ of the L RNA, and so on. It has been suggested that this conserved terminal structure may represent a binding site for the viral RNA polymerase (Salvato 1993b) (Fig. 31.6).

Reassortment of the 2 genomic RNA segments has been used to map functions to one segment or the other. Production of reassortant viruses involves infection of cultured cells with 2 virus isolates at once and screening for progeny virus by nucleic acid hybridization, reverse transcription followed by polymerase chain reaction (RT-PCR), or by limited sequence analysis. Reassortant viruses that contain the S RNA of one parental virus and the L RNA of the other can usually be isolated. This approach was used to show that the virulence of LCMV WE for guinea-pigs mapped to the L RNA (Riviere 1986), that the S RNA of LCMV Armstrong is associated both with diminished growth in C3H mice (Oldstone et al. 1985) and with the emergence of insulin-dependent diabetes in non-obese diabetic mice (Oldstone, Ahmed and Salvato 1990), and that the persistence of an LCMV Armstrong isolate depends on the L RNA (Matloubian et al. 1993). The latter case illustrates one shortcoming of this approach in that the persistent phenotype is likely to be pleiotropic, with essential genetic components on both RNAs (Salvato et al. 1991).

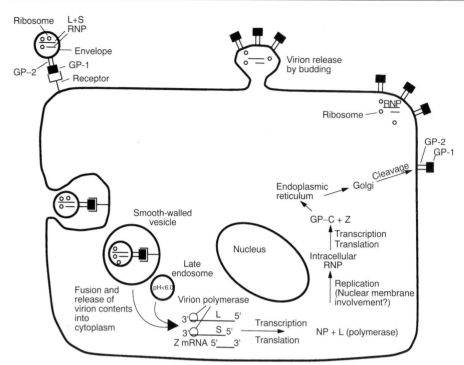

Fig. 31.7 Arenavirus life cycle. L, large RNA segment; RNP, ribonucleoprotein; S, small RNA segment. (Reproduced from Southern 1996.)

ARENAVIRUS GENE EXPRESSION

The ambisense coding arrangement of the arenavirus genome provides a mechanism for temporal regulation of gene expression: NP and L mRNAs can be transcribed from the incoming genomic RNA, whereas GP and Z mRNAs are transcribed only from RNA antigenomic templates that also function as replication intermediates. Kinetic analysis of LCMV replication shows simultaneous accumulation of NP and GP mRNA (Fuller-Pace and Southern 1988), but in Tacaribe, newly synthesized NP mRNA accumulates before the onset of RNA replication. Furthermore, inhibition of protein synthesis during early infection prevents RNA replication but allows the continued synthesis of NP mRNA (Lopez and Franze-Fernandez 1985, Franze-Fernandez et al. 1987). For LCMV, it has been shown that the Z mRNA is included in the virion, unlike mRNAs for the other viral genes, and may be essential at an early stage of the viral life cycle (Salvato and Shimomaye 1989). Further work with inhibitors of transcription and translation will be necessary to characterize the sequence of events in arenavirus replication.

Arenavirus mRNA transcription begins with 3–7 non-templated nucleotides: this has been demonstrated for the 5′ terminus of the NP mRNA in Tacaribe virus (Raju et al. 1990), the NP and GP mRNAs in LCMV (Meyer and Southern 1993) and the NP and GP mRNAs in Pichinde (Polyak, Zheng and Harnish 1995b). Genome and antigenomes generally have one non-templated base. These may arise either by *de novo* synthesis or by a cap stealing mechanism as has been described for the *Orthomyxoviridae* and the *Bunyaviridae* (Garcin and Kolakofsky 1990).

The non-coding regions of arenavirus genomic RNA have the potential to form several stem–loop structures that are well placed to regulate transcription and translation. LCMV, Lassa and Pichinde each have single intergenic stem–loops on the S RNA, whereas Mopeia, Tacaribe and Junin each predict double stem–looped structures (reviewed by Clegg 1993). Translation termination codons have been described on the proximal side of the intergenic stem–loops on the S RNA and L RNA. Transcription terminations for Tacaribe NP, GP, Z and L mRNAs have been described at the distal portion of each stem–loop, indicating that the secondary structure is not acting to stop transcription. Furthermore, since transcription termination has been described at multiple positions on the stem, it is likely that the polymerase is displaced from the RNA by an extragenomic factor rather than by a feature of the genome structure (Franze-Fernandez et al. 1993, Meyer and Southern 1993). Thus, since it appears that the intergenic stem–loops may help stop translation, in conjunction with the encoded stop codons, they are unlikely to serve as terminators or attenuators of transcription, and they may serve as recognition or nucleation points for virus assembly and encapsidation.

VIRUS–HOST INTERACTIONS DURING ARENAVIRUS REPLICATION

LCMV infections in carrier mice (covered more extensively in section 2, p. 637) can persist in a broad range of tissues, without detectable cellular damage or inflammation (see Fig. 31.9). However, some terminally differentiated cell functions or 'luxury functions' can be abolished by the presence of replicating virus. For example, a reduction of macrophage lymphokines, growth hormone, thyroid hormones and acetylcholinesterase have been observed in persistently infected murine systems (Jacobs and Cole 1976,

Oldstone, Holmstoen and Welsh 1977, Oldstone et al. 1982, Rodriguez et al. 1983, Oldstone et al. 1985, Klavinskis and Oldstone 1987). The ability of LCMV to affect differentiated functions of the immune, neural and endocrine systems depends on the genetic background of the host.

In tissue culture at low multiplicity of infection (i.e. moi <0.1) arenavirus replication is not detected for 6 hours, after which cell-associated virus increases exponentially. The titre of extracellular virus reaches a maximum 36–48 hours after infection. Infected cells undergo only limited cytopathic change during virus production with little or no change in the level of host protein synthesis. Long-term virus cultures are readily established.

Although arenavirus replication takes place in the host cell cytoplasm, enucleated cells fail to support virus production. Specifically, the host cell nucleus is required during the first 10 hours of Pichinde virus infection of BHK-21 cells (Banerjee, Buchmeier and Rawls 1976). Either enucleation removes a site of virus replication near the nuclear membrane or host nuclear products are required for viral replication. The latter is supported by the finding that α-amanitin, an inhibitor of host RNA polymerase II which is responsible for mRNA and hnRNA synthesis, prevents arenavirus replication. In contrast, actinomycin D, which primarily inhibits rRNA synthesis, has a lesser effect on Pichinde replication.

Host cell ribosomes that become incorporated into nascent virions retain their capacity to catalyse protein synthesis, but are not necessary for virus replication (Leung and Rawls 1977). In Pichinde, hybrid molecules between viral RNA and host cell ribosomal RNA have been observed (Shivraprakash et al. 1988) but their functional significance is unclear.

Host cell enzymes are essential for the maturation of arenavirus envelope glycoproteins. These are translated as a long precursor (GP-C) that undergoes glycosylation, transport and proteolysis involving host cell enzymes (Buchmeier and Oldstone 1979; reviewed in Burns and Buchmeier 1993). Initially, for LCMV, a 58-residue signal peptide is cleaved from the N terminus of GP-C. Further cleavage depends on glycosylation of the precursor in the Golgi or post-Golgi compartments with 5–6 N-linked glycosylations for the N-terminal portion of GP-C (to become GP-1) and 2 N-linked glycosylations for the C-terminal portion of GP-C (to become GP-2) (Wright, Salvato and Buchmeier 1989). Cleavage by a furin-like protease occurs at Arg_{262}–Arg_{263}. This cleavage is followed by trimming of the N-terminal portion of GP-2 (Burns and Buchmeier 1993). A protein kinase activity capable of phosphorylating the nucleocapsid protein has been identified in preparations of LCMV (Howard and Buchmeier 1983), but it is not known whether this is a cellular or viral enzyme or if it has any essential function.

1.7 Polypeptides: non-structural and structural

Arenavirus proteins include the 250 kDa RNA polymerase (L), the 11–14 kDa zinc-binding protein (Z) encoded on the L RNA, the 63 kDa nucleocapsid protein (N or NP) and the 75 kDa glycoprotein precursor (GP-C) encoded on the S RNA (see Fig. 31.4). These 4 proteins account for the coding capacity of the virus without overlap; however, overlapping open reading frames have been found and may yet be identified as gene products (Salvato and Shimomaye 1989). The stoichiometry of proteins in the LCM virion has been determined by metabolic labelling (Salvato et al. 1992). Per virion, there are about 30 copies of L protein, 1500 copies of NP, 650 copies of GP-1, 650 copies of GP-2 and 450 copies of Z protein (Fig. 31.8). According to cross-linking studies, NP and Z are associated (Salvato et al. 1992) and NP and GP-2 are associated (Burns and Buchmeier 1991).

NP is the most abundant virion protein as well as the most stable and abundant viral protein in infected cells. There are c. 1500–2000 copies of NP per virion, or one copy per 10–20 bases of viral genomic RNA (Bishop 1990). Among the negative-strand viruses, the nucleocapsid proteins usually function as the primary structural protein of viral cores and in mediating the interaction of the RNA polymerase with the viral RNA. A phosphorylated form of NP has been detected late in acute infection and in greater abundance in persist-

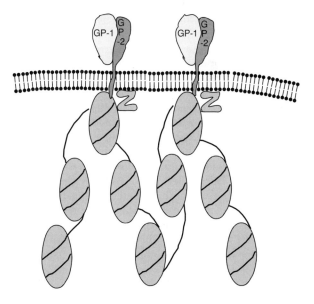

Fig. 31.8 Hypothetical scheme for the association of structural proteins in the LCM virion. The viral RNA is represented as a string winding around the beads that are the nucleocapsid protein molecules. The Z protein is depicted as a Z associated with the nucleocapsid proteins. GP-2 is anchored in the viral envelope and associated with NP. GP-1 is loosely associated with the surface of the virion. In each virion the proportions of Z, GP-1 and GP-2 in the virion are roughly equivalent, whereas NP is 3- to 5-fold more abundant. The polymerase or L protein accounts for only 30 molecules per virion. (Reproduced from Salvato 1993.)

ently infected cells (Bruns et al. 1986), leading to the suggestion that phosphorylation of NP is associated with attenuation of virus production and persistence. Breakdown products of NP have also been detected both in infected cells and in virions. It is conceivable, but not yet demonstrated, that fragments of NP serve as minor structural proteins (Coto et al. 1993). A 28 kDa degradation product of NP has been identified within the nuclei of Pichinde virus-infected cells, but no significance can yet be assigned to this (Howard 1993).

For LCMV, the envelope glycoprotein (GP) is synthesized as a 73 kDa precursor and cleaved into 43 kDa (GP-1) and 35 kDa (GP-2) polypeptides (Buchmeier and Oldstone 1979). Cleavage and maturation of the arenavirus glycoproteins, using host enzymes, has been described in the previous section (p. 635). All arenaviruses that have been examined so far have potential cleavage sites in the glycoprotein precursor and 2 cleavage products that can be identified in protein gels. Tamiami and Tacaribe viruses are an exception in which only one cleavage product is observed in gels; however, the situation was clarified for Tacaribe when it was shown that the 2 cleavage products co-migrate on gels but can be detected by analysis of the peptide termini (Burns and Buchmeier 1993).

The spikes of the virion are composed of GP-1 and GP-2: GP-2 is anchored in the membrane and associated with the nucleocapsid core through its C terminus and GP-1 is loosely attached to the virion surface through ionic interactions. Cross-linking studies indicate that GP-1 and GP-2 are present as homotetramers (Burns and Buchmeier 1991). Sequence analysis and antigenic cross-reactivity indicate that GP-2 contains a highly conserved sequence, whereas GP-1 contains the most variable sequence among the *Arenaviridae* (Weber and Buchmeier 1988, Clegg 1993). With Junin virus, rabbits and guinea-pigs inoculated with GP-2 produce neutralizing antibodies against the infectious virus (reviewed in Martinez Peralta et al. 1993). In contrast, for LCMV, neutralizing antibodies predominately recognize conformational epitopes within GP-1 (Parekh and Buchmeier 1986) and this recognition depends on glycosylation and retention of disulphide bonds (Wright, Salvato and Buchmeier 1989). It is likely that conformational changes of GP-1 expose domains on the spike glycoprotein that mediate virus entry into host cells (Di Simone, Zandonatti and Buchmeier 1994).

The zinc-binding protein of 11–14 kDa has a strongly conserved 'ring finger' motif in LCMV, Tacaribe and Pichinde (Iapalucci et al. 1989, Salvato and Shimomaye 1989, Harnish, Zheng and Polyak unpublished). This motif is characterized by the classic zinc-binding residues described in TFIIIA, and additional cysteine and histidine residues that help the molecule form a ring, i.e. C–X2–C–X(9–27)–C–X(1–3)–H–Y2–C–X2–C–X(4–48)–C–X2–C (Freemont 1993). Ring finger proteins generally have *trans*-regulatory functions and have been involved in protein–protein, protein–membrane and protein–nucleic acid

interactions. The LCMV Z protein is a significant structural component of the virion and is able to bind isotopic zinc (Salvato and Shimomaye 1989, Salvato et al. 1992). Garcin, Rochat and Kolakofsky (1993) have shown that the Tacaribe version of the Z protein is essential for mRNA and genome transcription. Thus, unlike some other negative-strand RNA viruses, where the transcription factor is usually a non-structural protein, the Z protein of the arenaviruses is both structural and functional in transcription.

1.8 Antigens

Highly accurate nucleic acid technologies (i.e. sequencing and RT-PCR) have recently superseded the use of viral antigens in identification and classification of arenaviruses. Nevertheless, complement fixation (CF), immunofluorescence (IF), enzyme-linked immunosorbent assay (ELISA) and neutralization/plaque-reduction assays have all been instrumental in the detection, diagnosis, characterization and classification of arenaviruses.

CF shows a strong relationship between Tacaribe, Junin and Machupo, and distant cross-reactivities between Pichinde and Tamiami: both are distant to each other and to other New World arenaviruses (Casals 1975, Casals et al. 1975). By the CF test, LCMV and Lassa viruses are related to each other, but very distantly related to the New World arenaviruses. The complement-fixing antigen is probably a portion of the nucleocapsid protein (Howard 1993).

IF with antisera raised against heterologous viral antigens afforded the first evidence that Tacaribe and LCMV are related. Serological cross-reactivities between the 'type-specific' envelope proteins have been determined by IF assays in which unfixed cells, displaying viral envelope antigens, are suspended with antisera. Cross-reactivities between 'group-specific' nucleocapsid proteins are determined from acetone-fixed cells, because the primary antigen within infected cells is NP. Serological cross-reactions in patients with Bolivian and Argentine haemorrhagic fevers are detected by IF tests with fixed cultures. Acute phase and early convalescent sera have been particularly valuable. A great deal of cross-reactivity can be seen between Machupo and Junin, closely followed by Tacaribe.

IF has played an important role in arenavirus diagnosis. In the case of Lassa fever virus, infected cells have been fixed to glass slides that are stable for months and can be used for field work in Africa (McCormick 1987). Infected cells on slides can be treated with UV and γ-irradiation and with acetone to ensure that they are not infectious. ELISA has also been useful for diagnosis in the field, but requires more viral antigen than the fixed-cell slides.

Cross-neutralization is the most specific test of antigen relatedness between arenaviruses. Neutralizing antibodies to Lassa appear late in convalescent sera, but are usually too specific or too weak to be detected in cross-neutralization (Peters 1984). High titre animal sera can effect cross-neutralization between Junin,

Tacaribe and Machupo viruses, but cross-neutraliz-ation has not been observed between Junin and Machupo with human convalescent sera, even though these are positive in CF assays. The sensitivity of the neutralization test can be increased for LCMV by adding complement or anti-γ-globulin to the test system. The incorporation of antibodies into the overlay for a plaque assay can also be used to detect neutralizing antibodies; for example, plaque size reduction was described for Pichinde virus (Chanas et al. 1980).

With the advent of monoclonal antibodies, many useful and specific reagents against arenavirus antigens became available. Initially they were used to demonstrate the relatedness or conservation of arenavirus antigens. Panels of monoclonal antibodies against LCMV and Pichinde showed distinct cross-reactivities with Lassa and Mopeia viruses (Buchmeier et al. 1981). Antibodies against GP-2 and NP are more broadly cross-reactive than antibodies against GP-1, which react only against a subset of the strains. For example, one LCMV GP-2 monoclonal cross-reacted with both Old World (LCMV, Lassa, Mopeia and Mobala) and New World (Pichinde, Junin, Tacaribe, Amapari, Parana and Machupo) viruses (Weber and Buchmeier 1988). In a similar comparison, mono-clonals raised to Lassa fever virus were tested against Mopeia and Mobala, and GP-2 cross-reactivity once again was notable (Gonzalez et al. 1984). Cross-reactivity of NP epitopes between Lassa and Mopeia has been confirmed, along with lesser reactivity to the envelope glycoprotein (Clegg and Lloyd 1984). Broad cross-reactivities observed between epitopes on Pichinde and Old World arenaviruses demonstrate that several surface antigens are conserved between the Old World and New World arenaviruses.

In recent studies, monoclonal and monospecific antibodies have been invaluable in determining the molecular structure and function of arenaviruses. For example, nucleic acid sequences have been confirmed to encode proteins by the use of peptide-specific antisera (Southern et al. 1987, Salvato, Shimomaye and Oldstone 1989), neutralizing antisera have been used to identify the viral structural proteins involved in neutralization (Burns and Buchmeier 1993, Martinez Peralta et al. 1993) and Z protein-specific antibodies have been used to demonstrate the need for Z protein during transcription in vitro (Garcin, Rochat and Kolakofsky 1993).

2 CLINICAL AND PATHOLOGICAL ASPECTS

2.1 Clinical manifestations

IN ANIMALS

All arenaviruses establish persistent infection in the natural rodent host after virus infection in utero or within a few days of birth. Adult mice inoculated intra-cerebrally with LCMV develop tremor with characteristic extensor spasm of the legs and they finally go into convulsions and die (Oldstone 1987b). When adult mice are inoculated peripherally, the outcome is variable with a marked loss of body weight. Lassa virus causes a silent persistent infection in its natural reservoir *Mastomys natalensis,* in the same way that LCMV infects mice. In hamsters, LCMV causes symptoms similar to those in mice. Guinea-pigs infected with Junin virus develop haemorrhagic disease with extensive necrosis of lymphatic tissue and a late development of neurological disease (Weissenbacher et al. 1975, Molinas et al. 1978). Guanarito virus causes mortality in suckling mice and adult guinea-pigs, but not in adult mice (Tesh et al. 1994). In rhesus and cynomolgus monkeys, LCMV and Lassa virus cause fever, anorexia, severe petechial rash on the face, progressive wasting and death within about 2 weeks, with a course similar to Lassa fever in humans (Jahrling et al. 1980, Peters et al. 1987). Junin and Machupo virus infections of non-human primates simulate the disease in humans, with fever, anorexia, weight loss and gastrointestinal symptoms. The animals die with cachexia and severe dehydration (Eddy et al. 1975, Kastello, Eddy and Kuehne 1976, Weissenbacher et al. 1979, Avila et al. 1987).

IN HUMANS

Arenavirus infections in humans range from a febrile disease with aseptic meningitis with LCMV (Armstrong and Sweet 1939) and Tacaribe (anecdotal laboratory-acquired infection in 1976; see Martinez Paralta, Coto and Weissenbacher 1993) to total collapse and death with circulatory and respiratory failure with the haemorrhagic fever viruses: Lassa fever (Rose 1956, Buckley, Casals and Downs 1970, Frame et al. 1970), Argentine haemorrhagic fever (Maiztegui 1975) and Bolivian haemorrhagic fever (MacKenzie et al. 1964, Johnson et al. 1965), Venezuelan haemorrhagic fever (Peters et al. 1974) and Sabía virus infection (Coimbra et al. 1994). The arenavirus haemorrhagic fevers are often severe, generalized febrile diseases with multi-organ involvement and fatality rates of about 16–30% in untreated hospitalized patients, characterized by tissue and pulmonary oedema with prominent hypovolaemic shock and adult respiratory distress syndrome (Fisher-Hoch 1993). Several of the South American arenaviruses have been found by screening rodent populations but are not associated with human disease; for example, Oliveros virus is carried by 20–30% of *Bolomys obscuras* in the Argentine haemorrhagic fever areas (Mills et al. 1996).

LCMV infection may be asymptomatic, mild or moderately severe with CNS manifestation. Lymphocytic choriomeningitis begins with fever, malaise, weakness, myalgia and headache associated with photophobia. Anorexia, nausea and dizziness are common (Farmer and Janeway 1942).

The onset of Lassa fever is characterized by generalized symptoms, including high fever, joint pain, back pain and severe headache, leading on to dry cough and exudative pharyngitis. In severe cases, patients have raised haematocrit (packed cell volume), vomiting and diarrhoea (Fisher-Hoch et al.

1985, Johnson et al. 1987, McCormick et al. 1987a). Oedema and bleeding may occur together or independently. Acute neurological manifestations ranging from unilateral or bilateral deafness to moderate or severe diffuse encephalopathy with or without seizures are common in Lassa fever. A febrile, systemic illness typically progresses in 4 days to subacute or chronic neuropsychiatric syndromes, including generalized seizures, dystonia and memory difficulties or seizures, agitation with personality and cognitive changes (McCormick et al. 1987a, Solbrig 1993). In pregnant women, Lassa fever is severe, especially during the third trimester, and fetal/neonatal loss is 87% (Price et al. 1988). In children, Lassa virus infection has been associated with a 'swollen baby syndrome' consisting of widespread oedema, abdominal distension and bleeding (Monson et al. 1987).

Argentine haemorrhagic fever, Bolivian haemorrhagic fever, Venezuelan haemorrhagic fever and the newly isolated Sabía virus infection are clinically very similar (Mackenzie et al. 1964, Johnson et al. 1965, Peters et al. 1974, Maiztegui 1975, Weissenbacher, Laguens and Coto 1987, Coimbra et al. 1994). Symptoms include malaise, high fever, severe myalgia, arthralgia, anorexia, relative bradycardia, lumbar pain, epigastric pain, abdominal tenderness, conjunctivitis and retro-orbital pain, with photophobia. In severe cases there is nausea, vomiting, diarrhoea, tremor and convulsions (Vainrub and Salas 1994). Proteinuria, microscopic haematuria with subsequent oliguria and uraemia are common. Fatal cases show haemorrhagic disorders due to vascular collapse with hypotensive shock, hypothermia and pulmonary oedema. In contrast to Lassa fever, bleeding with severe thrombocytopenia is more common in Argentine and Bolivian haemorrhagic fevers (Fisher-Hoch 1993).

2.2 **Epidemiology**

Arenaviruses are zoonotic agents maintained within rodent hosts in a chronic carrier state. The majority of the rodents associated with arenaviruses are commensals or semi-commensals, living within human dwellings or in cultivated fields. The habitat preferences of each species dictate the epidemiological patterns of the diseases they cause in humans with regard to occupational, sexual or seasonal bias (reviewed by Childs and Peters 1993).

In the case of LCMV, vertical transmission in utero is the major mechanism of viral maintenance in *Mus musculus* at the population level. Transmission through the gastrointestinal tract is the other possibility (Montali et al. 1993, Rai et al. 1996). Rodent-to-human infections probably occur through aerosols or contact with rodent blood, droplets and fomites. Infection through the gastrointestinal tract is the other possibility. Nosocomial spread of LCMV has not been reported. A longitudinal study in the USA from 1941 to 1958 implicated LCMV infections in about 8% of the patients diagnosed with suspected viral meningitis, and serological studies have suggested an incidence of LCMV infection in the general population of up to

10–15%. Most of these infections are probably mild or subclinical. Laboratory infections with LCMV are relatively common.

Human-to-human spread has been reported for Lassa fever in the community and in hospital settings (McCormick et al. 1987b), whereas only a few cases of nosocomial transmission have been reported for Bolivian haemorrhagic fever (Peters et al. 1974) and none for Argentine haemorrhagic fever virus. There have been reports suggestive of sexual transmission of Lassa and Machupo viruses from convalescing patients (Douglas, Wiebenga and Couch 1965). Aerosol spread and direct contact are the most likely routes of infection between humans. Neonates are at risk of infection through their mother's milk.

The aerosol stability of arenaviruses seems to be high. Studies with Lassa virus indicate a biological half-life of 55 minutes at 25°C and 30% relative humidity or 18 minutes at 25°C and 80% relative humidity (Stephenson, Larson and Dominik 1984). Arenaviruses are susceptible to heat and desiccation.

In natural primary hosts, arenaviruses can establish at least 2 types of chronic infections. LCM, Junin, Machupo and Lassa viruses can establish persistent infections resulting in long-term viraemia with few signs of disease in carriers. Other arenaviruses such as Latino virus and Tamiami virus cause chronic infections without persistent viraemia (Jennings et al. 1970, Webb et al. 1973). Strain and passage history of arenaviruses inoculated into experimental animals have a marked effect on lethality, tissue tropism and development of persistent infection (Traub 1938, Dutko and Oldstone 1983). The dose of arenavirus in conjunction with the route of exposure and age of the host can have a critical effect on the type of infection that results (Webb, Justines and Johnson 1975).

2.3 **Pathogenesis**

In animals

Adult mice infected intracerebrally with LCMV develop an acute inflammatory leptomeningitis, and choroiditis leading to death within 6–10 days (Oldstone 1987a). When adult mice are inoculated peripherally, viraemia peaks about 4–5 days after inoculation, usually causing widespread immune-mediated damage to the meninges, choroid plexus and ependyma (Cole and Johnson 1975). LCMV is known to infect and replicate in virtually every organ examined, particularly in the spleen, liver, kidney, brain, lung, uterus, thymus and lymph nodes (Fig. 31.9). Immunopathology characteristic of acute murine infection with LCMV is described in section 2.4 (see p. 640). In newborn mice, LCMV inoculation by any route leads to persistent infection. After replication in the brain, virus enters the circulation to reach tissues, serum and urine. The pathogenesis of Lassa virus in mice is minimal and similar to infection by LCMV, whereas Junin and Machupo viruses may cause either illness and death or may induce persistence in newborn mice (Webb, Justine and Johnson 1975, Sabatini et al. 1977). Junin and Machupo viruses in their natural rodent hosts, *Calomys*, cause up to 50% fatality of infected suckling animals. Machupo virus renders the animals sterile, causes fetal mortality and also induces haemolytic anaemia with significant splenomegaly.

Histological studies of LCMV infection in hamsters and guinea-pigs show that the virus is pantropic, with high titres of virus and little evidence of histological damage. In guinea-pigs, Lassa virus causes myocarditis, pulmonary oedema and hepatocellular damage (Walker et al. 1975, Jahrling et al. 1982). Junin virus is mainly viscerotropic in guinea-pigs without evidence of an immunopathological mechanism. The animals develop haemorrhagic disease with extensive necrosis of lymphatic tissue (Weissenbacher, de Guerrero and Boxaca 1975, Molinas et al. 1978). Monkeys infected with Lassa virus have mild hepatic focal necrosis, pulmonary interstitial pneumonitis with interstitial oedema and focal adrenal cortical necrosis (Walker et al. 1982). In rhesus and cynomolgus monkeys the infection causes death in 10–15 days due to vascular collapse and shock, with mild haemorrhage into mucosal surfaces (Fisher-Hoch et al. 1987).

In humans

The arenavirus haemorrhagic fevers in humans are often severe, generalized febrile diseases with multi-organ involvement. The haemostatic defect in these infections is characterized by platelet dysfunction and loss of integrity of the capillary bed. This presumably causes the leakage of fluids and macromolecules into the extravascular spaces and subsequent haemoconcentration, hypoalbuminaemia and hypovolaemic shock. There is no evidence for major hepatorenal failure or organ destruction by direct viral replication. Renal damage in Argentine and Bolivian haemorrhagic fevers is characterized by structural damage in the distal tubular cells and collecting ducts (Cossio et al. 1975). Lungs show large areas of intra-alveolar or bronchial haemorrhage. Microscopic examinations reveal a general alteration in endothelial cells and mild oedema of the vascular walls, with capillary swelling and perivascular haemorrhage (reviewed by Fisher-Hoch 1993). Necropsy findings from a single case of Sabía virus infection show diffuse pulmonary oedema and congestion with intraparenchymal haemorrhages, hepatic congestion with focal haemorrhage and necrosis, renal oedema and acute tubular necrosis, splenic enlargement and congestion, and massive gastrointestinal haemorrhage (Coimbra et al. 1994).

The pathogenesis of CNS disease in arenavirus infections is poorly understood. Seizures, delirium, memory difficulties and abnormal movements are the final common pathways of many metabolic changes. Failure of postmortem examinations to detect specific pathological changes in the brain of Lassa virus-infected individuals along with lower viral titres than other organs suggests that some of the neurological manifestations of these infections may not result from a direct viral effect but are due to some indirect cause (reviewed by Solbrig 1993).

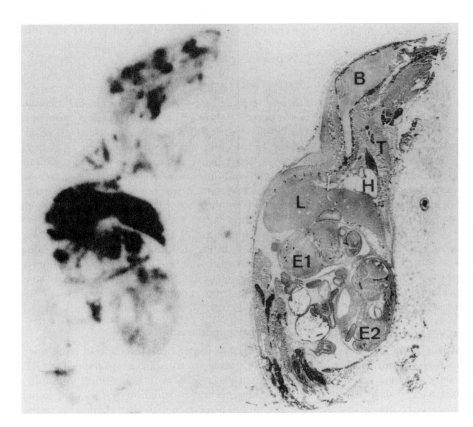

Fig. 31.9 Sagittal section of a pregnant mouse infected with LCMV. On the left is an autoradiograph of radioactive probes hybridizing to viral RNA within the section. On the right is the stained section: B, brain; E1, one embryo; E2, another embryo; H, heart; L, liver; T, thymus. (Reproduced from Southern, Blount and Oldstone 1984.)

2.4 Immune response

The LCMV murine model has proved to be invaluable for the study of acute and persistent infections in a natural host and also has brought to light several principles of viral immunobiology and viral immunopathology. As many of the studies on arenavirus immunology have been done in the LCMV murine model, the virus-specific immune responses in the LCMV context are summarized here.

Adult immunocompetent mice inoculated with LCMV either succumb to the disease or survive with permanent immunity. Neonatally infected mice or immunosuppressed mice inoculated with LCMV develop a lifelong persistent infection. Anti-LCMV antibodies are detectable by day 4 and LCMV-specific cytotoxic T lymphocytes (CTLs) peak around 7–9 days after infection (Hotchin 1971, Lehmann-Grube 1971, Bro-Jorgensen and Volkert 1974).

Protection against an acute LCMV infection is mediated almost exclusively by CD8+ CTLs (Zinkernagel and Doherty 1979, Buchmeier et al. 1980a, Lehmann-Grube, Moskophidis and Lohler 1988). The same CTLs may also cause immunopathology (Hotchin 1962, Cole, Nathanson and Pendergast 1972, Doherty and Zinkernagel 1974, Zinkernagel and Doherty 1979, Leist, Ruedi and Zinkernagel 1988). The kinetics of viral spread and the T cell response are important factors that affect the outcome of the disease (Hotchin 1962, Buchmeier et al. 1980a). After intracerebral infection, the T cell immune response is protective only when a large number of T cells are recruited early, while relatively few choriomeningeal cells are infected. When virus spreads rapidly and too many choriomeningeal cells are infected, immune T cells cause extensive lysis and therefore lethal immunopathological disease (Oehen, Hengartner and Zinkernagel 1991, Battegay et al. 1992).

During the acute LCMV infection, the H-2-restricted, LCMV-specific CD8+ CTL response peaks at 7–9 days after infection (Marker and Volkert 1973, Zinkernagel and Doherty 1974). These responses are accompanied by and depend on high levels of IL-2 gene transcription, IL-2 production and expression of the high affinity form of the IL-2 receptor (Kasaian and Biron 1990). A secondary stimulation of LCMV-immune mice with homologous virus results in a memory CTL response peaking earlier than in primary infections (Lehmann-Grube and Lohler 1981). The magnitude of secondary CTL response is often less than the acute response, probably because the virus is cleared so rapidly. CD8+ cells have a functional autonomy during the immune response to LCMV infection and do not depend on the presence of the majority of CD4+ cells to sustain either activation or proliferation in vivo (Kasaian, Leite-Morris and Biron 1991).

In contrast to the fatal meningitis mediated by CD8+ T cells, CD4+ T cells mediate a less severe form of choriomeningitis in response to intracerebral LCMV infection. Evaluation of the immune response against LCMV in CD8-defective mice reveals a CD4+ T cell-dependent immunopathology after intracerebral

infection with LCMV and the clearance of LCMV by mechanisms independent of CD8+ T cells (Fung-Leung et al. 1991).

Mice persistently infected with LCMV by congenital infection or neonatal inoculation do not develop a detectable CTL response and can be regarded as 'tolerant' at the level of CTLs. The characteristically subclinical persistent infections of these animals have given rise to the notion that persistence requires B cell tolerance (Hotchin 1971). However, these mice are not completely tolerant to LCMV, because they make antibody to all the LCMV structural proteins (Oldstone and Dixon 1967, Buchmeier, Elder and Oldstone 1978).

In Lassa fever there is a substantial macrophage response, with little if any lymphocytic infiltrate. The antibodies directed against the glycoprotein and nucleocapsid protein appear early in the illness in Lassa fever, with a classic primary IgG and IgM response. The antibodies are present simultaneously with viraemia in humans and primates (Fisher-Hoch et al. 1987, Johnson et al. 1987). Thus, though the antibodies are markers of acute illness, they are not involved in recovery. Neutralizing antibodies are found in only a minority of patients several months after the clearance of virus (Jahrling et al. 1980, Jahrling and Peters 1984). Thus clearance of virus presumably depends on cell-mediated immunity. In contrast, IgG antibodies to Junin and Machupo viruses appear 12–30 days after onset and are usually associated with clinical improvement and virus clearance, and the therapeutic efficacy of immune plasma in patients with Junin infection is directly associated with the titre of neutralizing antibodies in the plasma given (Peters. Webb and Johnson 1973, Enria et al. 1984). The role of cell-mediated immunity in viral clearance and subsequent protection from Junin and Machupo virus infections is not known.

IMMUNOPATHOLOGY

Efficient cell-mediated immunity is crucial for the recovery of a host from acute LCMV infection (Zinkernagel and Doherty 1979, Buchmeier et al. 1980a). In infections with a non-cytopathic virus such as LCMV, the balance between the virus spread and the T cell immune response determines whether either virus elimination (protection) or cell and tissue damage (immunopathology) predominates or whether a virus carrier state (no virus elimination, no cell and tissue damage) results. Acute LCM disease, chronic LCM-wasting disease and LCM carrier status in mice (Hotchin 1962, Zinkernagel and Doherty 1979, Buchmeier et al. 1980a) are examples of these varying equilibrium conditions between virus and immune response.

Effectors of immunopathology

Intraperitoneal or intravenous infection of adult mice with LCMV usually results in a virus-specific CTL response that clears virus with long-lasting immunity, whereas intracerebral inoculation results in a lethal leptomeningitis associated with virus replication in the brain and an intense mononuclear cell infiltrate. Death and the associated meningitis are blocked if the mice are treated with thymectomy, immunosuppressive irradiation or immunosuppressive drugs such as cyclophosphamide; this led to the suggestion that the disease is mediated by the immune response (Haas and Stewart 1956, Rowe, Black and Lercy 1963, Gilden et al. 1972). Subsequent investigations have supported the hypothesis that the pathology in acute LCMV disease is mediated by cellular immunity (Volkert and Lundstedt 1968, Cole, Nathanson and Pendergast 1972, Gilden et al. 1972).

Interferon (IFN) increases the susceptibility of LCMV-infected fibroblasts to lysis by H-2-restricted CTLs (Bukowski and Welsh 1985). This enhanced lysis correlates with increased cell surface expression of MHC antigens but not of LCMV antigen. IFN-γ is an especially potent inducer of MHC expression in most cell types (Wong et al. 1984). This indicates that the limiting component in the lytic interaction is the histocompatibility antigen and that physiological influences on the expression of antigen may affect the progress of host-mediated disease. Treatment of adult mice infected intracerebrally with LCMV with antibody to IFN prevents their death, whereas untreated control mice succumb to the same dose of lethal LCMV, thus showing the role of IFN in the pathogenesis of cell damage in murine LCM (Pfau, Gresser and Hunt 1983).

Murine LCMV infection is also considered the classic example of virus-induced immune complex disease. Persistent LCMV infection with circulating non-neutralizing antibodies in ratios and quantities that favour binding of complement and deposition in tissues results in immunopathology. This state is affected by host and viral genetic factors (Oldstone, Tishon and Buchmeier 1983). Large quantities of deposited immune complexes along with IFN-γ seem to cause development of glomerulonephritis (Walker and Murphy 1987). Strains of mice characterized as intermediate IFN responders, such as outbred Swiss mice, have higher levels of circulating immune complexes and develop much more severe immune complex-associated glomerulonephritis than strains of low IFN responder mice, such as BALB/c mice, after LCMV infection (Woodrow et al. 1982). Antibodies to IFN diminish glomerular damage without affecting levels of circulating immune complexes (Pfau, Gresser and Hunt 1983).

Progress of central nervous system pathology

CD8+ T cells along with macrophages are thought to be the main cells that contribute to meningeal inflammation after LCMV infection (Allan, Dixon and Doherty 1987). In addition, NK cells, CD4+ T cells, neutrophils and B cells are also present at the site of inflammation (Johnson, Monjan and Morse 1978). Large numbers of white blood cells, including CTLs, NK cells and macrophages, are found in the CSF, brain tissue and meningeal exudate. Although the integrity of the blood–brain barrier is destroyed, the relatively non-lytic LCMV itself is unlikely to disrupt

the barrier (Doherty 1973, Doherty and Zinkernagel 1974). It is more likely that the virus-induced IFN-γ initiates the infiltration of inflammatory cells across the blood–brain barrier.

The presence of CTLs in CSF has been shown by functional studies and by immunocytochemistry (Zinkernagel and Doherty 1973). CTL activity is also present in the CSF 3 days after immune-cell transfer to LCMV-infected, immunosuppressed animals. After CNS infection with LCMV, high levels of NK cell activity are detected in CSF and cervical lymph nodes. However, meningitis presumably does not occur before development of T cell response, as NK cells probably do not play an essential role in LCMV-induced immunopathology (Allan and Doherty 1986). NK cells do not influence LCMV synthesis in vivo, but do decrease the level of Pichinde virus (Welsh 1987, Brutkiewicz and Welsh 1995).

The CTLs present in cyclophosphamide-suppressed LCMV-infected mice after passive transfer of immune cells are of donor and not of recipient origin. So CD8+ T cells also seem to be essential for triggering infiltration into the CNS. Presumably, for a maximal inflammatory process to occur, class I MHC-restricted CD8+ T cells proliferate first in the peripheral lymphoid tissue and then enter the brain after recognition of class I MHC-compatible infected cells at the blood–CSF barrier (reviewed by Allan, Dixon and Doherty 1987).

Immunosuppressed mice that survive an ordinarily lethal dose of LCMV develop acute LCM disease and die when reconstituted with syngeneic LCMV-specific immune T cells (Gilden et al. 1972). Thus, it is possible to imitate the immunopathology observed in acute LCMV infection by inoculating LCMV-specific H-2-restricted CTLs into carrier mice, which in turn cause either viral clearance and recovery or CTL-mediated immunopathology and death (Allan and Doherty 1985). CD8+ T cells act directly rather than by the recruitment of circulating monocytes. Lethal LCM can be prevented in the uninfected mouse by intracerebral inoculation of cloned CD8+ T cells together with the virus (Baenziger et al. 1986). The co-injected CD8+ T cells gradually eliminate the virus-infected cells without causing the massive inflammation associated with the acute LCM disease. Severe meningitis ensues in the adoptive transfer of LCMV-specific CTLs only when there is matching of class I MHC antigens between donor and recipient mice. In comparison, compatibility of class II MHC antigens is less important (Doherty et al. 1976, Allan and Doherty 1985).

IMMUNOSUPPRESSION

Mechanism of immunosuppression

Acute infection of adult mice with LCMV leads to a general suppression of the immunological and mitogenic responses in vivo and in vitro, which persists for 2–3 months after infection (Mims and Wainwright 1968, Bro-Jorgensen and Volkert 1972, Jacobs and Cole 1976, Brenan and Zinkernagel 1983). Although different mechanisms have been postulated to explain this phenomenon, it is still poorly defined. LCMV infects different types of lymphocytes (Gartner et al. 1986, Rosenthal et al. 1986, Ahmed, King and Oldstone 1987b) and macrophages (Mims and Subrahmanyan 1966, Zinkernagel and Doherty 1979). The ability of LCMV to induce a virus carrier state conatally or neonatally and in adult mice may be due to these particular tropisms of LCMV (Ahmed, King and Oldstone 1987b). Depending on the virus isolate, the virus dose, the time after infection and the mouse strain infected, LCMV can cause a severe immune deficiency, rendering the mice more susceptible to secondary infections.

Mice persistently infected with LCMV are deficient in generating LCMV-specific CTLs and delayed type hypersensitivity responses and also make low levels of antibodies against LCMV (Buchmeier et al. 1980a). It is unlikely that LCMV-specific immune responses are inhibited by a lack of appropriate T-helper cells, because deletion of CD4+ T cells in a transgenic mouse model does not impair the CD8+ LCMV-specific CTL response (Rahemtulla et al. 1991). The different levels of cytokines in the brain and sera of acutely and persistently infected mice indicate that the 2 types of infections probably activate different types of cells.

A mechanism for generalized immunosuppression has been elucidated in the case of a particular LCMV isolate. For this isolate, LCMV Armstrong clone 13 (Ahmed et al. 1984), virus replicates to high titre in the spleen, causing immune-mediated destruction of dendritic cells; hence loss of the cells needed for immune responses to other pathogens (Tishon et al. 1993, Borrow, Evans and Oldstone 1995). Clonal deletion of LCMV-specific CTLs may occur subsequently (Moskophidis et al. 1993). The long-term effect of clone 13 infection is that reduced immune response capacity allows the virus to persist, in contrast to infection with other isolates of this strain that are cleared within weeks by a vigorous cellular immune response (Salvato et al. 1991). The persistent and rapidly cleared isolates of LCMV Armstrong are analogous to the Docile (viscerotropic) and Aggressive (neurotropic) isolates of LCMV UBC in which docility is associated with the tendency for high titre replication in the viscera that leads to suppression of the CTL response and persistent infection (Thomsen and Pfau 1993). It is important to note that viral tropism is crucial to the pathogenesis in these cases. The different tropisms of LCMV Armstrong and its variant isolate, clone 13, are shown in Fig. 31.10 (Plate 31.10).

Suppression of cell-mediated immunity

LCMV infection causes suppression of responses to T-dependent antigens in vivo (Mims and Wainwright 1968) and to allografts (Lehmann-Grube, Neimeyer and Lohler 1972, Guttler, Bro-Jorgensen and Jorgensen 1975). This may be due to a decreased number of mature T lymphocytes in lymphoid organs as a result of an alteration of T-progenitor cells in the bone marrow (Bro-Jorgensen and Volkert 1972, Thomsen, Bro-Jorgensen and Jensen 1982). Alterna-

tively, it is suggested that the immunosuppression may be related to the lysis of infected T lymphocytes and macrophages by virus-specific CTLs (Silberman, Jacobs and Cole 1978). In addition to unresponsiveness to antigens, the proliferative response to T and B cell mitogens is also depressed and a virus-induced macrophage defect is probably responsible for the abortive collaboration with T lymphocytes (Jacobs and Cole 1976).

Suppression of humoral immunity

The suppression of T-independent IgM and a strictly T help-dependent IgG immune response against a second infectious agent is observed in immunocompetent adult mice infected with LCMV but not in tolerant LCMV carrier mice or LCMV-infected mice that have been depleted of CD8+ T cells with monoclonal antibodies. Thus, the immune suppression is due not to LCMV itself nor to IFN induced by it but rather to the CD8+ T cell-dependent immune response against LCMV (Leist, Ruedi and Zinkernagel 1988).

Studies of the kinetics of T cell-mediated immunosuppressive effects of LCMV infection on primary and secondary antibody responses (to vesicular stomatitis virus, VSV) show that LCMV-WE induced immunosuppression is absolute for primary IgG responses induced during a limited time between days 2 and 11 after LCMV infection. The kinetics of induction of the T cell-independent IgM responses closely follow that of a normal CTL response to LCMV-WE (Roost et al. 1988). LCMV infection on the same day or before (but not after) VSV infection leads to suppression of IgG responses to VSV. However, primed IgG responses are not suppressed by a subsequent LCMV-WE infection and immunosuppression is not antigen specific but general (Ruedi, Hengartner and Zinkernagel 1990). LCMV-induced suppression is absolute to the extent that priming does not occur, since subsequent challenge with the identical VSV serotype triggers a strictly primary response.

The severity and duration of immunosuppressiveness depend on the virus dose, the virus isolate and the mouse strain used. LCMV-WE and LCMV Docile are the most and LCMV Armstrong the least immunosuppressive. Mouse strains differ considerably with respect to extent of suppression, depending on both the MHC and non-MHC genes. H-2q and H-2k seem to be more susceptible to immune suppression than H-2b or H-2d mice (Roost et al. 1988).

2.5 Diagnosis

Diagnosis of arenavirus infection relies mainly on isolation and subsequent identification of the virus. Serological tests can also be used to detect specific antibodies or antigens.

Virus can be isolated mainly from the blood or serum. In addition, throat swabs, CSF, urine, breast milk or other tissues taken by biopsy or at necropsy can also be used (Monath et al. 1974, Walker, McCormick and Johnson 1982, Johnson et al. 1987). The most successful system for isolating arenaviruses has

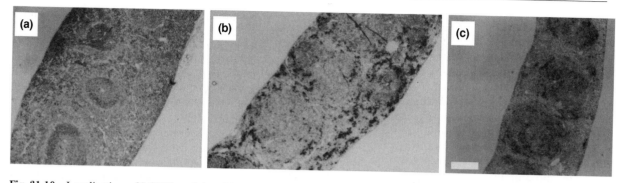

Fig. 31.10 Localization of LCMV nucleic acids in murine spleen by in situ hybridization with ^{35}S riboprobe specific for NP mRNA. (a) Spleen section from an uninfected control mouse (BALB/c ByJ). (b) Spleen section from a mouse infected i.v. with LCMV Armstrong for 3 days. (c) Spleen section from a mouse infected i.v. with the clone 13 variant of LCMV Armstrong for 3 days. For colour, see Plate 31.10. (Reproduced from Borrow et al. 1995.)

proved to be cell culture. In addition to cell culture, laboratory animals such as suckling mice, guinea-pigs and hamsters can also be used, although they are more expensive and increased safety precautions are necessary. The probability and timing of virus isolation vary with each arenavirus (Table 31.2).

Differential diagnosis for arenavirus infections, especially for Lassa fever, includes bacterial septi-caemia, typhoid, paratyphoid, typhus, trypanosomi-asis, streptococcal pharyngitis, leptospirosis, malignant malaria and other viral haemorrhagic fevers (Howard and Simpson 1990). Nucleic acid amplification by RT-PCR along with Southern blot hybridization with virus-specific DNA probe can be used as an early, rapid and sensitive method for detecting arenavirus nucleic acid in peripheral blood mononuclear cells (PBMCs) as well as from other tissues. Studies with Junin virus-infected PBMCs and tissues have shown that this assay allows detection of Junin virus RNA in RNA extracted from 100 μl of whole blood by guanidinium thiocyan-ate disruption and acid phenol extraction. As little as 0.01 pfu of Junin virus can be detected in a blood sample by this assay (Bockstahler et al. 1992, Lozano et al. 1993). In situ hybridization by viral sequence-specific radioactive probes can be done directly on biopsy or autopsy specimens to detect viral RNA and has proved to be highly sensitive in experimental LCMV infections of mice (see Fig. 31.9).

Antibodies to arenaviruses can be detected in serum by a variety of serological methods, including immunofluorescence assay, ELISA, immunoperoxid-ase labelling, radioimmunoassay, reverse phase haem-agglutination assay and haemagglutination inhibition tests. The complement fixation test is now rarely used because it is less sensitive than other methods (serological tests and antibody levels in arenavirus infections have been reviewed by McCormick 1990). The immunofluorescence assay is more often used in the serological diagnosis of arenaviruses in infected cell monolayers. At present, ELISA is increasingly used for the diagnosis of arenavirus infections. Alterna-tively, known antiserum or monoclonal antibodies can be used to detect viral antigens in biopsy or necropsy materials by immunohistochemical techniques.

Table 31.2 Arenavirus isolation from tissue specimens at different stages of illness

Virus	Tissue specimen	Stage of illness
LCMV	Blood	Initial febrile stage
	CSF	During acute illness
Junin	Blood	Up to 8 days in milder cases, up to 2 weeks in severely ill patients
	Throat swab	During acute illness
	Breast milk	During acute illness
Machupo	Blood	Up to 2 weeks (intermittent viraemia)
	Throat swabs	Sporadic detection
Lassa	Blood	3–5 days in milder cases, up to 4 weeks in severely ill patients
	Throat swabs	Days 5–12 of illness
	Breast milk	During acute illness
	CSF	During acute illness
	Pleural transudate	During acute illness
	Pericardial transudate	During acute illness
	Urine	Up to 1–2 months

Data adapted from McCormick (1990).

2.6 **Prophylaxis**

The development of a safe and effective vaccine for arenavirus infections of humans has proved difficult. Several killed and live attenuated vaccines have been tested for Lassa, Junin and Machupo viruses, none of which has proved suitable for widespread human use. Many of these vaccines are still in the stage of animal trials. A new live attenuated Junin virus vaccine, Candid:1, has been developed which has been shown to be safe and immunogenic in non-human primates (Barrera Oro and McKee 1991, Contigiani et al. 1991, McKee et al. 1993). Laboratory animals infected with various avirulent viruses serologically related to Lassa virus, including LCMV, Mopeia and Mobala viruses, survived a subsequent challenge with virulent Lassa virus (Walker et al. 1982, Jahrling and Peters 1986). Similar strategies for protection against Junin virus with heterologous live vaccines have repeatedly demonstrated protection against Junin virus in guinea-pigs and hamsters (reviewed by Barrera Oro and McKee 1991). Other vaccine trials with inactivated Lassa and Machupo viruses have given mixed results, although they are immunogenic. Immunization with inactivated Lassa virus protects *Papio hamadryas* monkeys from a subsequent challenge with Lassa virus (Krasnianski et al. 1993), but fails to protect rhesus monkeys even though there is a secondary, high titre antibody response to the major structural proteins of Lassa virus in these vaccinated monkeys (McCormick et al. 1992).

For Lassa virus, for which a killed antigen vaccine has proved ineffective and an attenuated virus vaccine is not available, a live recombinant virus vaccine provides a very attractive alternative. Recombinant vaccinia virus vaccines, which express either the Lassa virus nucleoprotein or the glycoprotein gene, successfully protect guinea-pigs from a lethal Lassa virus infection, but offer incomplete protection in primates (Auperin, Esposito and Lange 1988, Morrison et al. 1989, Auperin 1993). A weak but measurable cross-protection against LCMV intracranial challenge can be mediated by Lassa-specific CD4+ T cells (La Posta et al. 1993). Vaccine trials so far have suggested that cell-mediated immune response must be activated to protect against challenge with arenaviruses.

Immunization with recombinant vaccinia virus that expresses the LCMV glycoprotein (VV GP) or nucleoprotein (VV NP) protects mice from LCM disease by induction of a protective CTL response in an H-2 haplotype-dependent manner (Hany et al. 1989, Klavinskis et al. 1990, Oehen, Hengartner and Zinkernagel 1991). Mice can be specifically protected by subcutaneous inoculation of recombinant LCMV proteins (GP or NP) or just the T cell epitope of the LCMV nucleoprotein as an unmodified free synthetic peptide in incomplete Freund's adjuvant (Schulz et al. 1991, Bachmann et al. 1994). Vaccination with DNA encoding the LCMV nucleoprotein or the glycoprotein also confers protection against lethal LCMV challenge and against persistent LCMV infection in an MHC-dependent manner by priming CD8+ cytotoxic lymphocytes

(Martins et al. 1995, Yokoyama, Zhang and Whitton 1995).

In certain circumstances, however, immunization with VV GP or VV NP aggravates disease. For example, Balb/C mice infected with a high dose of the LCMV Docile isolate usually survive, unless they are preinjected with VV NP or VV GP (Oehen, Hengartner and Zinkernagel 1991). This suggests that low level immunization may accelerate development of disease. Vaccination may shift the balance from low (i.e. late) to high (i.e. early) responder status and may therefore prevent immunopathologically mediated disease or it may shift the balance only slightly from a non-responsive asymptomatic carrier to a low or intermediate responder status to cause immunopathology. Thus, as well as illustrating the potential value of CTL vaccines, these vaccine studies also highlight the limitations of subunit vaccines. To protect an outbred population in an MHC-restricted fashion, it will be necessary to make a vaccine that consists of a cocktail of relevant peptides and to ensure that none of its components aggravates the disease in a subsequent virus challenge.

2.7 **Treatment**

IMMUNOTHERAPY

LCMV-induced persistent infection in mice is a classic example of viral persistence and serves as a model to study basic principles of immune clearance in persistent and disseminated infections in general. This model system makes it possible to test the potential of specific immune therapy to clear virus from a chronically infected host and to study the effector mechanisms responsible for clearing such infections.

Volkert (1963) was the first to show that the adoptive transfer of spleen cells from LCMV-challenged immune adult mice results in reduction of infectious virus in carrier mice. This has been confirmed by a number of workers (Gilden et al. 1972, Allan and Doherty 1985, Baenziger et al. 1986). Distinct patterns of viral clearance and histopathology are observed in different organs after adaptive immunotherapy of persistently infected (carrier) mice. The clearance of viral materials from the CNS is distinct in pattern and timing with clearance from other organs. Clearance from the liver, lung, spleen, lymph nodes, pancreas etc. occurs within 30 days, whereas in the brain infectious virus is eliminated but viral antigen persists up to 90 days after immunotherapy (Ahmed, Jamieson and Porter 1987a). The urinary system is the most resistant to immunotherapy, and the viral antigen is localized within the renal tubules in the form of antigen–antibody complexes.

Clearance of viral materials (infectious virus, viral nucleic acid and proteins) from several organs of persistently infected mice probably occurs by reconstitution of LCMV-specific CTLs that have malfunctioned or have been deleted during viral infection. By using mice that are recombinant in the H-2 region and by selective depletion of lymphocyte subpopulations, it has been shown that viral clearance is mediated by co-operation between virus-specific CD8+

T cells and non-specific bone marrow-derived mononuclear cells from the carrier host (Ahmed, King and Oldstone 1987b). The effector mechanisms responsible for eliminating the persistent and disseminated LCMV infection of mice are dependent on the lytic ability of CTLs, because perforin-negative transgenic mice are unable to clear infection (Kagi et al. 1994).

Early success of Lassa virus immune plasma in the treatment of Lassa fever (Leifer, Goecke and Bourne 1970) and immunotherapy of Machupo virus infections in primates (Eddy et al. 1975) showed promise for the treatment of arenavirus infections in humans. Convalescent phase plasma from Junin virus patients reduced mortality from 16% to 1% in those who were treated in the first 8 days of illness (Maiztegui, Fernandez and de Damilano 1979), and the efficacy of the plasma seemed to be directly related to the concentration of neutralizing antibodies of the plasma. However, a better understanding of the limitations of this approach and reduced success in subsequent cases have restricted its use. A late neurological syndrome developed 4–6 weeks after the onset of acute illness in about 10% of the cases treated with Junin virus immune plasma. Passive antibody therapy depends on collection of plasma from people known to have had the disease, testing the plasma or screening the donor for antibodies to blood-borne agents such as hepatitis and proper storage of plasma until it is used. In addition, the existence of HIV and other retroviral diseases transmissible by blood products has made mandatory the further screening of plasma before use.

ANTIVIRAL AGENTS

The antiviral drug ribavirin has proved effective in the treatment of Lassa fever in laboratory animals (Jahrling et al. 1980, Jahrling, Peters and Stephens 1984) and in humans (McCormick, King and Webb 1986), especially when administered during the first 6 days after the onset of illness. Later the pathogenesis of the infection is less reversible. Patients presenting late in disease require more effective clinical management of physiological dysfunction and need other drugs which may be used to stabilize the state of shock sufficiently long to facilitate recovery and survival. Ribavirin is perhaps more effective if given intravenously than orally (McCormick, King and Webb 1986, McCormick 1990). It is the drug of choice for treatment and for prophylaxis in cases of possible exposure to Lassa virus, in laboratory or hospitals. Studies with Junin virus infections indicate that ribavirin may also have beneficial effect in Argentine haemorrhagic fever (Enria and Maiztegui 1994). A single case of laboratory-acquired Sabía virus infection was successfully treated with intravenous ribavirin (Barry et al. 1995) at a dosage recommended by the Centers for Disease Control and Prevention (CDC, USA) for other arenavirus infections (a loading dose of 30 mg/kg body weight, followed by a dose of 15 mg/kg every 6 hours for 4 days and then by a dose of 7.5 mg/kg 3 times daily for 6 days).

In addition, fluid, electrolyte and osmotic imbalances must be corrected, in anticipation of the development of clinical shock and broad spectrum antibiotics administered to prevent secondary bacterial infections. However, even vigorous support of this kind may be insufficient to prevent fatal progression of disease.

REFERENCES

Ahmed R, Jamieson BD, Porter DD, 1987a, Immune therapy of a persistent and disseminated viral infection, *J Virol*, **61:** 3920–9.

Ahmed R, King C-C, Oldstone MBA, 1987b, Virus–lymphocyte interaction: T cells of the helper subset are infected with lymphocytic choriomeningitis virus during persistent infection *in vivo*, *J Virol*, **61:** 1571–6.

Ahmed RA, Salmi A et al., 1984, Selection of genetic variants of lymphocytic choriomeningitis virus in spleens of persistently infected mice: role in suppression of cytotoxic T lymphocyte response and viral persistence, *J Exp Med*, **160:** 521–40.

Allan JE, Dixon JE, Doherty PC, 1987, Nature of the inflammatory process in the central nervous system of mice infected with LCMV, *Curr Top Microbiol Immunol*, **134:** 131–43.

Allan JE, Doherty PC, 1985, Consequences of cyclophosphamide treatment in murine lymphocytic choriomeningitis: evidence for cytotoxic T cell replication *in vivo*, *Scand J Immunol*, **22:** 367–74.

Allan JE, Doherty PC, 1986, Natural killer cells contribute to inflammation but do not appear to be essential for the induction of clinical lymphocytic choriomeningitis, *Scand J Immunol*, **24:** 153–62.

Armstrong C, Lillie RD, 1934, Experimental lymphocytic choriomeningitis of monkeys and mice produced by a virus encountered in studies of the 1933 St Louis encephalitis epidemic, *Pub Health Rep (Washington)*, **49:** 1019–27.

Armstrong C, Sweet LK, 1939, Lymphocytic choriomeningitis, *Pub Health Rep (Washington)*, **54:** 673–84.

Auperin DD, 1993, Construction and evaluation of recombinant virus vaccines for Lassa fever, *The Arenaviridae*, ed Salvato MS, Plenum Press, New York, 259–80.

Auperin DD, Esposito JJ, Lange JV, 1988, Construction of a recombinant vaccinia virus expressing the Lassa virus glycoprotein gene and protection of guinea pigs from a lethal Lassa virus infection, *Virus Res*, **9:** 233–43.

Auperin DD, McCormick JB, 1989, Nucleotide sequence of the Lassa virus (Josiah strain) S genome RNA and amino acid sequence comparison of the N and GPC proteins to other arenaviruses, *Virology*, **156:** 421–5.

Auperin DD, Sasso DR, McCormick JB, 1986, Nucleotide sequence of the glycoprotein gene and intergenic region of the Lassa virus S genome RNA, *Virology*, **154:** 155–67.

Auperin DD, Romanowski V et al., 1984, Sequence studies of Pichinde arenavirus S RNA indicate a novel coding strategy, ambisense viral S RNA, *J Virol*, **52:** 897–904.

Avila MM, Samailovich SR et al., 1987, Protection of Junin virus infected marmosets by passive administration of immune serum: association with late neurologic signs, *J Med Virol*, **21:** 67–74.

Bachmann MF, Kundig TM et al., 1994, Induction of protective cytotoxic T cells with viral proteins, *Eur J Immunol*, **24:** 2228–36.

Baenziger J, Hengartner H et al., 1986, Induction or prevention of immunopathological disease by cloned cytotoxic T cell lines specific for LCMV, *Eur J Immunol*, **16:** 387–93.

Banerjee SN, Buchmeier M, Rawls WE, 1976, Requirement of a cell nucleus for the replication of an arenavirus, *Intervirology*, **6:** 190–6.

Barrera Oro JG, McKee KT Jr, 1991, Toward a vaccine against Argentine hemorrhagic fever, *Bull Pan Am Hlth Org*, **25:** 118–26.

Barry M, Russi M et al., 1995, Brief report: treatment of a laboratory-acquired Sabía virus infection, *N Engl J Med*, **333:** 294–6.

Battegay M, Oehen S et al., 1992, Vaccination with a synthetic peptide modulates LCMV-mediated immunopathology, *J Virol*, **66:** 1199–201.

Bishop DHL, 1990, *Arenaviridae* and their replication, *Fields' Virology*, 2nd edn, eds Fields BN, Knipe DM, Raven Press, New York, 1231–43.

Bockstahler LE, Carney PG et al., 1992, Detection of Junin virus by the polymerase chain reaction, *J Virol Methods*, **39:** 231–5.

Borrow P, Evans CF, Oldstone MBA, 1995, Virus-induced immunosuppression: immune system-mediated destruction of virus-infected dendritic cells results in generalized immunosuppression, *J Virol*, **69:** 1059–70.

Borrow P, Oldstone MBA, 1992, Characterization of lymphocytic choriomeningitis virus-binding receptor protein(s): a candidate cellular receptor of the virus, *J Virol*, **66:** 7270–81.

Borrow P, Oldstone MBA, 1994, Mechanism of lymphocytic choriomeningitis virus entry into cells, *Virology*, **198:** 1–9.

Borrow P, Tishon A, Oldstone MBA, 1991, Infection of lymphocytes by a virus that aborts cytotoxic T lymphocyte activity and establishes persistent infection, *J Exp Med*, **174:** 203–12.

Brenan M, Zinkernagel RM, 1983, Influence of one virus infection on a second concurrent primary *in vivo* antiviral cytotoxic T cell response, *Infect Immun*, **41:** 470–5.

Bro-Jorgensen K, Volkert M, 1972, Haemopoietic defects in mice infected with lymphocytic choriomeningitis virus, *Acta Pathol Microbiol Scand*, **80:** 853–62.

Bro-Jorgensen K, Volkert M, 1974, Defects in the immune system of mice infected with LCMV, *Infect Immun*, **9:** 605–14.

Bruns M, Zeller W et al., 1986, Lymphocytic choriomeningitis virus. 9. Properties of the nucleocapsid, *Virology*, **151:** 77–85.

Brutkiewicz RR, Welsh RM, 1995, Major histocompatibility complex class I antigens and the control of viral infections by natural killer cells, *J Virol*, **69:** 3967–71.

Buchmeier MJ, Elder JH, Oldstone MBA, 1978, Protein structure of lymphocytic choriomeningitis virus: identification of the virus structural and cell-associated polypeptides, *Virology*, **89:** 133–45.

Buchmeier MJ, Oldstone MBA, 1979, Protein structure of lymphocytic choriomeningitis virus: evidence for a cell-associated precursor of the virion glycopeptides, *Virology*, **99:** 111–20.

Buchmeier MJ, Welsh RM et al., 1980a, The virology and immunobiology of lymphocytic choriomeningitis virus infection, *Adv Immunol*, **30:** 275–331.

Buchmeier MJ, Lewicki HA et al., 1980b, Monoclonal antibodies to lymphocytic choriomeningitis virus react with pathogenic arenaviruses, *Nature (London)*, **288:** 486–7.

Buchmeier MJ, Lewicki HA et al., 1981, Monoclonal antibodies to lymphocytic choriomeningitis and Pichinde virus: generation, characterization, and cross-reactivity with other arenaviruses, *Virology*, **113:** 73–85.

Buckley SM, Casals J, Downs WG, 1970, Isolation and antigenic characterization of Lassa virus, *Nature (London)*, **227:** 174–6.

Bukowski JF, Welsh RM, 1985, Inability of interferon to protect virus-infected cells against lysis by natural killer (NK) cells correlates with NK cell-mediated antiviral effects *in vivo*, *J Immunol*, **135:** 3537–41.

Burns JW, Buchmeier MJ, 1991, Protein–protein interactions in lymphocytic choriomeningitis virus, *Virology*, **183:** 620–9.

Burns JW, Buchmeier MJ, 1993, Glycoproteins of the arenaviruses, *The* Arenaviridae, ed Salvato MS, Plenum Press, New York, 17–35.

Casals J, 1975, Arenaviruses, *Yale J Biol Med*, **48:** 115–40.

Casals J, Buckley SM, Cedeno R, 1975, Antigenic properties of the arenaviruses, *Bull W H O*, **52:** 421–5.

Chanas AC, Young PR et al., 1980, Evaluation of plaque size reduction as a method for the detection of Pichinde virus antibody, *Arch Virol*, **65:** 157–67.

Childs JE, Peters CJ, 1993, Ecology and epidemiology of arena-viruses and their hosts, *The* Arenaviridae, ed Salvato MS, Plenum Press, New York, 331–84.

Clegg JCS, 1993, Molecular phylogeny of the arenaviruses and guide to published sequence data, *The* Arenaviridae, ed Salvato MS, Plenum Press, New York, 175–87.

Clegg JCS, Lloyd G, 1984, The African arenaviruses Lassa and Mopeia: biological and immunochemical comparisons, *Segmented Negative Strand RNA Viruses*, eds Compans RW, Bishop DHL, Academic Press, Orlando FL, 341–7.

Coimbra TLM, Nassar ES, 1994, New arenavirus isolated in Brazil, *Lancet*, **343:** 391–2.

Cole GA, Johnson ED, 1975, Immune responses to LCM virus infection *in vivo* and *in vitro*, *Bull W H O*, **52:** 465–70.

Cole GA, Nathanson N, Pendergast RA, 1972, Requirements for theta-bearing cells: lymphocytic choriomeningitis virus induced central nervous system disease, *Nature (London)*, **238:** 335–7.

Contigiani MS, Medeot SI et al., 1991, Rapid vascular clearance of two strains of Junin virus in *Calomys musculinus*: selective macrophage clearance, *Acta Virol*, **35:** 144–51.

Cossio PM, Laguens RP et al., 1975, Ultrastructural and immunohistochemical study of the human kidney in Argentine hemorrhagic fever, *Virchows Arch*, **368:** 1–9.

Coto CE, Damonte EB et al., 1993, Genetic variation in Junin virus, *The* Arenaviridae, ed Salvato MS, Plenum Press, New York, 85–101.

Dalton AJ, Rowe WP et al., 1968, Morphological and cytochemical studies on lymphocytic choriomeningitis virus, *J Virol*, **2:** 1465–78.

De la Torre JC, Rall G et al., 1993, Replication of LCMV is restricted in terminally differentiated neurons, *J Virol*, **67:** 7350–9.

Di Simone C, Zandonatti MA, Buchmeier MJ, 1994, Acidic pH triggers LCMV membrane fusion activity and conformational change in the glycoprotein spike, *Virology*, **198:** 455–65.

Doherty PC, 1973, Quantitative studies of the inflammatory process in fatal viral meningoencephalitis, *Am J Pathol*, **73:** 607–22.

Doherty PC, Zinkernagel RM, 1974, T-cell mediated immunopathology in viral infections, *Transplant Rev*, **19:** 89–120.

Doherty PC, Dunlop MBC et al., 1976, Inflammatory process in murine lymphocytic choriomeningitis is maximal in H-2K or H-2D compatible interactions, *J Immunol*, **117:** 187–90.

Douglas GR, Wiebenga NH, Couch RB, 1965, Bolivian hemorrhagic fever probably transmitted by personal contact, *Am J Epidemiol*, **82:** 85–91.

Downs WG, Anderson CR et al., 1963, Tacaribe virus: a new agent isolated from *Artibeus* bats and mosquitoes in Trinidad, West Indies, *Am J Trop Med Hyg*, **12:** 640–6.

Dutko F, Oldstone MBA, 1983, Genomic and biological variation among commonly used lymphocytic choriomeningitis virus strains, *J Gen Virol*, **64:** 1689–98.

Dutko FJ, Wright EA, Pfau CJ, 1976, The RNAs of the defective interfering Pichinde virus, *J Gen Virol*, **31:** 417–27.

Eddy GA, Scott SK et al., 1975, Pathogenesis of Machupo virus infection in primates, *Bull W H O*, **52:** 517–21.

Enria DA, Maiztegui JI, 1994, Antiviral treatment of Argentine hemorrhagic fever, *Antiviral Res*, **23:** 23–31.

Enria D, Brigiler AM et al., 1984, Importance of dose of neutralizing antibodies in treatment of Argentine hemorrhagic fever with immune plasma, *Lancet*, **2:** 255–6.

Farber RE, Rawls WE, 1975, Isolation of ribosome-like structures from Pichinde virus, *J Gen Virol*, **26:** 21–31.

Farmer TW, Janeway CA, 1942, Infections with the virus of lymphocytic choriomeningitis, *Medicine*, **21:** 1–64.

Fields BN, Knipe DM, eds, 1990, *Fields' Virology*, 2nd edn, Raven Press, New York.

Fields BN, Knipe DM et al., eds, 1996, *Fields' Virology*, 3rd edn, Raven Press, New York.

Fisher-Hoch SP, 1993, Arenavirus pathophysiology, *The* Arenaviridae, ed Salvato MS, Plenum Press, New York, 299–323.

Fisher-Hoch SP, Price MJ et al., 1985, Safe intensive care management of a severe case of Lassa fever using simple barrier nursing techniques, *Lancet*, **2**: 1227–9.

Fisher-Hoch SP, Mitchell SW et al., 1987, Physiologic and immunologic disturbances associated with shock in Lassa fever in a primate model, *J Infect Dis*, **155**: 465–74.

Frame JD, Baldwin MN et al., 1970, Lassa fever: a new virus disease of man from West Africa. 1. Clinical description and pathological findings, *Am J Trop Med Hyg*, **73**: 219–24.

Franze-Fernandez MT, Zetina C et al., 1987, Molecular structure and early events in the replication of Tacaribe arenavirus S RNA, *Virus Res*, **7**: 309–24.

Franze-Fernandez M-T, Iapalucci S et al., 1993, Subgenomic RNAs of Tacaribe virus, *The* Arenaviridae, ed Salvato MS, Plenum Press, New York.

Freemont PS, 1993, The ring finger: a novel protein sequence motif related to the zinc finger, *Ann N Y Acad Sci*, **47**: 174–84.

Fuller-Pace FV, Southern PJ, 1988, Temporal analysis of transcription and replication during acute infection with lymphocytic choriomeningitis virus, *Virology*, **162**: 260–3.

Fung-Leung WP, Kundig TM et al., 1991, Immune response against LCMV infection in mice without CD8 expression, *J Exp Med*, **174**: 1425–9.

Garcin D, Kolakofsky D, 1990, A novel mechanism for the initiation of Tacaribe arenavirus genome replication, *J Virol*, **64**: 6196–203.

Garcin D, Rochat S, Kolakofsky D, 1993, The Tacaribe *Arenavirus* small zinc finger protein is required for both mRNA synthesis and genome replication, *J Virol*, **67**: 807–12.

Gartner S, Markovits P et al., 1986, The role of mononuclear phagocytes in HTLV-III/LAV infection, *Science*, **233**: 215–19.

Ghiringhelli PE, Rivera-Pomar RV et al., 1991, Molecular organization of Junin virus S RNA: complete nucleotide sequence, relationship with other members of the *Arenaviridae* and unusual secondary structures, *J Gen Virol*, **72**: 2129–41.

Gilden DH, Cole GA et al., 1972, Immunopathogenesis of acute central nervous system disease produced by lymphocytic choriomeningitis virus. 1. Cyclophosphamide-mediated induction of virus-carrier state in adult mice, *J Exp Med*, **135**: 860–73.

Glushakova SE, Lukashevich IS, 1989, Early events in arenavirus replication are sensitive to lysosomotropic compounds, *Arch Virol*, **104**: 157–61.

Glushakova S, Omelyanenko V et al., 1992, The fusion of artificial lipid membranes induced by the synthetic arenavirus 'fusion peptide', *Biochim Biophys Acta*, **1110**: 202–8.

Gonzalez JP, Buchmeier MJ et al., 1984, Comparative analysis of Lassa and Lassa-like arenavirus isolates from Africa, *Segmented Negative Strand RNA Viruses*, eds Compans RW, Bishop DHL, Academic Press, Orlando FL, 210–18.

Guttler F, Bro-Jorgensen K, Jorgensen PN, 1975, Transient impaired cell-mediated tumor immunity after acute infection with lymphocytic choriomeningitis virus, *Scand J Immunol*, **4**: 327–36.

Haas VH, Stewart SE, 1956, Sparing effect of amethopterin and guanazolo in mice with the virus of lymphocytic choriomeningitis, *Virology*, **2**: 511–16.

Hany M, Oehen S, 1989, Anti-viral protection and prevention of lymphocytic choriomeningitis or of the local footpad swelling reaction in mice by immunization with vaccinia-recombinant virus expressing LCMV-WE nucleoprotein or glycoprotein, *Eur J Immunol*, **19**: 417–24.

Holmes GP, McCormick JB et al., 1990, Lassa fever in the United States, *N Engl J Med*, **323**: 1120–3.

Hotchin J, 1962, The foot pad reaction of mice to lymphocytic choriomeningitis virus, *Virology*, **17**: 214–16.

Hotchin J, 1971, Tolerance to lymphocytic choriomeningitis virus. 3. Persistent tolerant infection of LCM and other oncogenic viruses, *Ann N Y Acad Sci*, **181**: 159–82.

Howard CR, 1993, Antigenic diversity among the arenaviruses, *The* Arenaviridae, ed Salvato MS, Plenum Press, New York, 37–41.

Howard C, Buchmeier MJ, 1983, A protein kinase activity in lymphocytic choriomeningitis virus and identification of the phosphorylated product using monoclonal antibody, *Virology*, **126**: 538–47.

Howard CR, Simpson DIH, 1990, Arenaviruses, *Topley and Wilson's Principles of Bacteriology, Virology and Immunity*, 8th edn, vol 4, eds Collier LH, Timbury MC, Edward Arnold, London, 593–607.

Iapalucci S, Lopez N et al., 1989, The 5′ region of Tacaribe virus L RNA encodes a protein with a potential metal binding domain, *Virology*, **173**: 357–61.

Jacobs RP, Cole GA, 1976, Lymphocytic choriomeningitis virus-induced immunosuppression: a virus-induced macrophage defect, *J Immunol*, **117**: 1004–9.

Jahrling PB, Peters CJ, 1984, Passive antibody therapy of Lassa fever in cynomolgus monkeys: importance of neutralizing antibody and Lassa virus strain, *Infect Immun*, **44**: 528–33.

Jahrling PB, Peters CJ, 1986, Serology and virulence diversity among Old World arenaviruses, and the relevance to vaccine development, *Med Microbiol Immunol*, **175**: 165–7.

Jahrling PB, Peters CJ, Stephens EL, 1984, Enhanced treatment of Lassa fever by immune plasma combined with ribavirin in cynomolgus monkeys, *J Infect Dis*, **149**: 420–7.

Jahrling PB, Hesse RA et al., 1980, Lassa virus infection of rhesus monkeys: pathogenesis and treatment with ribavirin, *J Infect Dis*, **141**: 580–9.

Jahrling PB, Smith S et al., 1982, Pathogenesis of Lassa virus infection in guinea pigs, *Infect Immun*, **37**: 771–8.

Jennings WL, Lewis AL et al., 1970, Tamiami virus in the Tampa Bay area, *Am J Trop Med Hyg*, **19**: 527–36.

Johnson ED, Monjan AA, Morse HC, 1978, Lack of B cell participation in acute LCM disease of CNS, *Cell Immunol*, **36**: 143–50.

Johnson KM, Wiebenga NH et al., 1965, Virus isolation from human cases of hemorrhagic fever in Bolivia, *Proc Soc Exp Biol Med*, **118**: 113–18.

Johnson KM, McCormick JB et al., 1987, Lassa fever in Sierra Leone: clinical virology in hospitalized patients, *J Infect Dis*, **155**: 456–64.

Kagi D, Ledermann B et al., 1994, Cytotoxicity mediated by T cells and natural killer cells is greatly impaired in perforin-deficient mice, *Nature (London)*, **369**: 31–7.

Kasaian MT, Biron CA, 1990, Cyclosporin A inhibition of IL-2 gene expression, but not NK cell proliferation, after interferon induction *in vivo*, *J Exp Med*, **171**: 745–62.

Kasaian MT, Leite-Morris KA, Biron CA, 1991, The role of CD4+ cells in sustaining lymphocyte proliferation during LCMV infection, *J Immunol*, **146**: 1955–63.

Kastello MD, Eddy GA, Kuehne RW, 1976, A rhesus monkey model for the study of Bolivian hemorrhagic fever, *J Infect Dis*, **133**: 57–62.

Klavinskis LS, Oldstone MBA, 1987, Lymphocytic choriomeningitis virus can persistently infect thyroid epithelial cells and perturb thyroid hormone production, *J Gen Virol*, **68**: 1867–73.

Klavinskis LS, Whitton JL et al., 1990, Vaccination and protection from a lethal viral infection: identification, incorporation, and use of a cytotoxic T lymphocyte glycoprotein epitope, *Virology*, **178**: 393–8.

Krasnianski VP, Potryvaeva NV et al., 1993, A trial to produce an inactivated Lassa fever vaccine, *Vopr Virusol*, **38**: 276–9.

La Posta V, Auperin DD et al., 1993, Cross-protection against lymphocytic choriomeningitis virus mediated by a CD4+ T-cell clone specific for an envelope glycoprotein epitope of Lassa virus, *J Virol*, **67**: 3497–506.

Lehmann-Grube F, 1971, Lymphocytic choriomeningitis virus, *Virol Monogr*, **10**: 1–173.

Lehmann-Grube F, Lohler J, 1981, Immunopathologic alterations of lymphatic tissues of mice infected with lymphocytic choriomeningitis virus. 2. Pathogenetic mechanism, *Lab Invest*, **44**: 205–13.

Lehmann-Grube F, Moskophidis D, Lohler J, 1988, Recovery

from acute virus infection: role of cytotoxic T lymphocytes in the elimination of lymphocytic choriomeningitis virus from spleens of mice, *Ann N Y Acad Sci*, **532**: 238–56.

Lehmann-Grube F, Niemeyer IP, Lohler J, 1972, Lymphocytic choriomeningitis of the mouse. 4. Depression of the allograft reaction, *Med Microbiol Immunol*, **158**: 16–25.

Lehmann-Grube F, Slenczka W, Tees R, 1969, A persistent and inapparent infection of L cells with the virus of lymphocytic choriomeningitis, *J Gen Virol*, **5**: 63–81.

Leifer E, Goecke DJ, Bourne H, 1970, Lassa fever: a new virus disease of man from West Africa. 2. Report of a laboratory acquired infection treated with plasma from a person recently recovered from the disease, *Am J Trop Med Hyg*, **19**: 677–9.

Leist TP, Ruedi E, Zinkernagel RM, 1988, Virus-triggered immune suppression in mice caused by virus-specific cytotoxic T cells, *J Exp Med*, **167**: 1749–54.

Leung WC, Rawls WE, 1977, Virion associated ribosomes are not required for the replication of Pichinde virus, *Virology*, **81**: 174–6.

Lopez R, Franze-Fernandez M-T, 1985, Effect of Tacaribe virus infection on host cell protein and nucleic acid synthesis, *J Gen Virol*, **66**: 1753–61.

Lozano ME, Ghiringhelli PD et al., 1993, A simple nucleic acid amplification assay for the rapid detection of Junin virus in whole blood samples, *Virus Res*, **27**: 37–53.

McCormick JB, 1987, Epidemiology and control of Lassa fever, *Curr Top Microbiol Immunol*, **134**: 69–78.

McCormick JB, 1990, Arenaviruses, *Fields' Virology*, 2nd edn, eds Fields BN, Knipe DM, Raven Press, New York, 1245–67.

McCormick JB, King IJ, Webb PA, 1986, Lassa fever: effective therapy with ribavirin, *N Engl J Med*, **314**: 202–26.

McCormick JB, King IJ et al., 1987a, Lassa fever: a case control study of the clinical diagnosis and course, *J Infect Dis*, **155**: 445–55.

McCormick JB, Webb PA et al., 1987b, A prospective study of the epidemiology and ecology of Lassa fever, *J Infect Dis*, **155**: 437–44.

McCormick JB, Mitchell SW et al., 1992, Inactivated Lassa virus elicits a non protective immune response in rhesus monkeys, *J Med Virol*, **37**: 1–7.

McKee KTJ, Oro JG et al., 1993, Safety and immunogenicity of a live attenuated Junin (Argentine hemorrhagic fever) vaccine in rhesus macaques, *Am J Trop Med Hyg*, **48**: 403–11.

Mackenzie RB, Beye HK et al., 1964, Epidemic hemorrhagic fever in Bolivia. 1. A preliminary report of the epidemiologic and clinical findings in a new epidemic area South America, *Am J Trop Med Hyg*, **13**: 620–5.

Maiztegui JI, 1975, Clinical and epidemiological patterns of Argentine hemorrhagic fever, *Bull W H O*, **52**: 567–75.

Maiztegui JI, Fernandez NJ, de Damilano AJ, 1979, Efficacy of immune plasma in treatment of Argentine hemorrhagic fever and association between treatment and a late neurological syndrome, *Lancet*, **2**: 1216–17.

Marker O, Volkert M, 1973, Studies on cell mediated immunity to lymphocytic choriomeningitis virus in mice, *J Exp Med*, **137**: 1511–25.

Martinez Peralta LA, Coto CE, Weissenbacher MC, 1993, The Tacaribe complex: the close relationship between a pathogenic (Junin) and nonpathogenic (Tacaribe) arenavirus, *The Arenaviridae*, ed Salvato MS, Plenum Press, New York, 281–98.

Martins LP, Lau LL et al., 1995, DNA vaccination against persistent viral infection, *J Virol*, **69**: 2574–82.

Matloubian M, Kohlhekar SR et al., 1993, Molecular determinants of macrophage tropism and virus persistence: importance of single amino acid changes in the polymerase and glycoprotein of lymphocytic choriomeningitis virus, *J Virol*, **67**: 7340–9.

Meyer BJ, Southern PJ, 1993, Concurrent sequence analysis of 5′ and 3′ RNA termini by intramolecular circularization

reveals 5′ nontemplated bases and 3′ terminal heterogeneity for lymphocytic choriomeningitis mRNAs, *J Virol*, **67**: 2621–7.

Mifune K, Carter M, Rawls W, 1971, Characterization of the Pichinde virus – a member of the arenavirus group, *Proc Soc Exp Biol Med*, **136**: 637–44.

Mills JN, Barrera Oro JG et al, 1996, Characterization of Oliveros virus, a new member of the Tacaribe complex (*Arenaviridae*: arenavirus), *Am J Trop Med Hyg*, **54**: 399–404.

Mims CA, Subrahmanyan TP, 1966, Immunofluorescence study of the mechanism of resistance to superinfection in mice carrying the LCMV, *J Pathol Bacteriol*, **91**: 403–15.

Mims CA, Wainwright S, 1968, The immunodepressive action of lymphocytic choriomeningitis virus in mice, *J Immunol*, **101**: 717–24.

Molinas FC, Paz RA et al., 1978, Studies of blood coagulation and pathology in experimental infection of guinea pigs with Junin virus, *J Infect Dis*, **137**: 740–6.

Monath TP, Maher M et al., 1974, Lassa fever in the eastern province of Sierra Leone, 1970–1972. 2. Clinical observations and virological studies on selected hospital cases, *Am J Trop Med Hyg*, **23**: 1140–9.

Monson MH, Cole AD et al., 1987, Pediatric Lassa fever: a review of 33 Liberian cases, *Am J Trop Med Hyg*, **36**: 408–15.

Montali RJ, Scanga CA et al., 1993, A common source outbreak of callitrichid hepatitis in captive tamarins and marmosets, *J Infect Dis*, **167**: 946–50.

Morrison HG, Bauer SP et al., 1989, Protection of guinea pigs from Lassa fever by vaccinia virus recombinants expressing the nucleoprotein or the envelope glycoproteins of Lassa virus, *Virology*, **171**: 179–88.

Moskophidis D, Lechner F et al., 1993, Virus persistence in acutely infected immunocompetent mice by exhaustion of antiviral cytotoxic effector T cells, *Nature (London)*, **362**: 758–61.

Murphy FA, 1975, Arenavirus taxonomy: a review, *Bull W H O*, **52**: 389–91.

Oehen S, Hengartner H, Zinkernagel RM, 1991, Vaccination for disease, *Science*, **251**: 195–8.

Oldstone MBA, 1987a, Arenaviruses – an introduction, *Curr Top Microbiol Immunol*, **134**: 1–4.

Oldstone MBA, 1987b, Immunotherapy for virus infection, *Curr Top Microbiol Immunol*, **134**: 212–29.

Oldstone MBA, Ahmed R, Salvato M, 1990, Viruses as therapeutic agents. 2. Viral reassortants map prevention of insulin-dependent diabetes mellitus to the small RNA of lymphocytic choriomeningitis virus, *J Exp Med*, **171**: 2091–100.

Oldstone MBA, Dixon FJ, 1967, Lymphocytic choriomeningitis: production of antibody by 'tolerant' infected mice, *Science*, **158**: 1193–5.

Oldstone MBA, Holmstoen J, Welsh RM, 1977, Alterations of acetylcholine enzymes in neuroblastoma cells persistently infected with lymphocytic choriomeningitis virus, *J Cell Physiol*, **91**: 459–72.

Oldstone MBA, Tishon A, Buchmeier MJ, 1983, Virus induced immune complex disease: genetic control of C1q binding complexes in the circulations of mice persistently infected with LCMV, *J Immunol*, **130**: 912–18.

Oldstone MBA, Sinha YN et al., 1982, Virus induced alterations in homeostasis: alterations in differentiated functions of infected cells *in vivo*, *Science*, **218**: 1125–7.

Oldstone MBA, Ahmed R et al., 1985, Perturbation of differentiated functions during viral infection in vivo. 1. Relationship of lymphocytic choriomeningitis virus and host strains to growth hormone deficiency, *Virology*, **142**: 158–74.

Palmer EL, Obijeski JF et al., 1977, The circular segmented nucleocapsid of an arenavirus, Tacaribe virus, *J Gen Virol*, **36**: 541–5.

Parekh BS, Buchmeier MJ, 1986, Proteins of lymphocytic choriomeningitis virus: antigenic topography of the viral glycoproteins, *Virology*, **153**: 168–78.

Parodi AS, Greenway DJ et al., 1958, Sobre la etiologia del bute epidemico de Junin, *Diagn Med*, **30**: 2300–2.

Pedersen IR, 1979, Structural components and replication of arenaviruses, *Adv Virus Res*, **24**: 277–330.

Peters CJ, 1984, Arenaviruses, *Textbook of Human Virology*, ed Belshe RB, PSG, Littleton MA, 513–45.

Peters CJ, Webb PA, Johnson KM, 1973, Measurement of antibodies to Machupo virus by the indirect fluorescent technique, *Proc Soc Exp Biol Med*, **142**: 526–31.

Peters CJ, Kuehne RW et al., 1974, Hemorrhagic fever in Cochabamba, Bolivia, 1971, *Am J Epidemiol*, **99**: 425–32.

Peters CJ, Jahrling PB et al., 1987, Experimental studies of arenaviral hemorrhagic fevers, *Curr Top Microbiol Immunol*, **134**: 5–68.

Pfau CJ, 1974, Biochemical and biophysical properties of the arenaviruses, *Progr Med Virol*, **18**: 64–80.

Pfau CJ, Gresser I, Hunt KD, 1983, Lethal role of interferon in lymphocytic choriomeningitis virus induced encephalitis, *J Gen Virol*, **64**: 1827–32.

Polyak SJ, Zheng S, Harnish DG, 1995a, Analysis of Pichinde arenavirus transcription and replication in human THP-1 monocytic cells, *Virus Res*, **36**: 37–48.

Polyak SJ, Zheng S, Harnish DG, 1995b, 5′ termini of Pichinde arenavirus S RNAs and mRNAs contain nontemplated nucleotides, *J Virol*, **69**: 3211–15.

Price ME, Fisher-Hoch SP et al., 1988, Lassa fever in pregnancy, *Br Med J*, **297**: 584–8.

Rahemtulla A, Fung-Leung WP et al., 1991, Normal development and function of CD8+ cells but markedly decreased helper cell activity in mice lacking CD4+, *Nature (London)*, **353**: 180–4.

Rai SK, Cheung DS et al., 1996, Murine infection with LCMV following gastric inoculation, *J Virol*, **70**: 7213–8.

Raju R, Raju L et al., 1990, Nontemplated bases at the 5′ ends of Tacaribe virus mRNAs, *Virology*, **174**: 53–9.

Rivers TM, Scott TFM, 1935, Meningitis in man caused by a filterable virus, *Science*, **81**: 439–40.

Rivers TM, Scott TFM, 1936, Meningitis in man caused by a filterable virus. 2. Identification of the etiological agent, *J Exp Med*, **63**: 415–32.

Riviere Y, 1986, Mapping arenavirus genes causing virulence, *Curr Top Microbiol Immunol*, **133**: 59–66.

Rodriguez M, von Wedel RJ et al., 1983, Pituitary dwarfism in mice persistently infected with lymphocytic choriomeningitis virus, *Lab Invest*, **49**: 48–53.

Romanowski V, 1993, Genetic organization of Junin virus, the etiological agent of Argentine hemorrhagic fever, *The Arenaviridae*, ed Salvato MS, Plenum Press, New York, 51–83.

Romanowski V, Matsuura Y, Bishop DHL, 1985, Complete sequence of the S RNA of lymphocytic choriomeningitis virus (WE strain) compared to that of Pichinde arenavirus, *Virus Res*, **3**: 101–14.

Roost H, Charan S et al., 1988, An acquired immune suppression in mice caused by infection with lymphocytic choriomeningitis virus, *Eur J Immunol*, **18**: 511–18.

Rose JR, 1956, A new clinical entity?, *Lancet*, **2**: 197–9.

Rosenthal KL, Zinkernagel RM et al., 1986, Persistence of vesicular stomatitis virus in cloned interleukin-2 dependent NK cell lines, *J Virol*, **60**: 539–47.

Rowe WP, Black PH, Lercy RH, 1963, Protective effect of neonatal thymectomy on mouse LCM infection, *Proc Soc Exp Biol Med*, **114**: 248–51.

Rowe WP, Murphy FA et al., 1970, Arenaviruses: proposed name for a newly defined virus group, *J Virol*, **5**: 651–2.

Ruedi E, Hengartner H, Zinkernagel RM, 1990, Immunosuppression in mice by lymphocytic choriomeningitis virus infection: time dependence during primary and absence of effects on secondary antibody responses, *Cell Immunol*, **130**: 501–12.

Sabattini MS, de Rios LEG et al., 1977, Natural and experimental infection of rodents with Junin virus, *Medicina (Buenos Aires)*, **37**: 149–61.

Salvato MS, ed, 1993a, *The* Arenaviridae, Plenum Press, New York.

Salvato MS, 1993b, Molecular biology of the prototype arenavirus, lymphocytic choriomeningitis virus, *The* Arenaviridae, ed Salvato, MS, Plenum Press, New York, 133–56.

Salvato MS, Shimomaye EM, Oldstone MBA, 1989, The primary structure of the lymphocytic choriomeningitis virus L gene encodes a putative RNA polymerase, *Virology*, **169**: 377–84.

Salvato M, Borrow P et al., 1991, Molecular basis of viral persistence: a single amino acid change in the glycoprotein of lymphocytic choriomeningitis virus is associated with suppression of the antiviral cytotoxic T lymphocyte response and establishment of persistence, *J Virol*, **65**: 1863–9.

Salvato MS, Schweighofer KJ et al., 1992, Biochemical and immunological evidence that the 11 kDa zinc-binding protein of lymphocytic choriomeningitis virus is a structural component of the virus, *Virus Res*, **22**: 185–98.

Schulz M, Aichele P et al., 1991, Major histocompatibility complex binding and T cell recognition of a viral nonapeptide containing a minimal tetrapeptide, *Eur J Immunol*, **21**: 1181–6.

Shivraprakesh M, Harnish D, Rawls WE, 1988, Characterization of temperature-sensitive mutants of Pichinde virus, *J Virol*, **62**: 4037–43.

Silberman SL, Jacobs RP, Cole GA, 1978, Mechanisms of hemopoietic and immunological dysfunction induced by lymphocytic choriomeningitis virus, *Infect Immun*, **19**: 533–9.

Solbrig MV, 1993, Lassa virus and central nervous system diseases, *The* Arenaviridae, ed Salvato MS, Plenum Press, New York, 325–30.

Southern PJ, 1996, *Arenaviridae*: the viruses and their replication, *Fields' Virology*, 3rd edn, eds Fields BN, Knipe DM et al., Raven Press, New York, 1505–19.

Southern PJ, Blount P, Oldstone MBA, 1984, Analysis of persistent virus infections by in situ hybridization to whole-mouse sections, *Nature (London)*, **312**: 555–8.

Southern PJ, Singh MK et al., 1987, Molecular characterization of the genomic S RNA segment from lymphocytic choriomeningitis virus, *Virology*, **157**: 145–50.

Stephenson EH, Larson EW, Dominik JW, 1984, Effect of environmental factors on aerosol-induced Lassa virus infection, *J Med Virol*, **14**: 295–303.

Tesh RB, Jahrling PB et al., 1994, Description of Guanarito virus (*Arenaviridae*: *Arenavirus*), the etiologic agent of Venezuelan hemorrhagic fever, *Am J Trop Med Hyg*, **50**: 452–9.

Thomsen AR, Bro-Jorgensen K, Jensen BL, 1982, Lymphocytic choriomeningitis induced immunosuppression: evidence for viral interference with T cell maturation, *Infect Immun*, **37**: 981–6.

Thomsen AR, Pfau CJ, 1993, Influence of host genes on the outcome of murine lymphocytic choriomeningitis infection: a model for studying genetic control of virus-specific immune responses, *The* Arenaviridae, ed Salvato MS, Plenum Press, New York, 199–224.

Tishon A, Borrow P et al., 1993, Virus induced immunosuppression. 1. Age at infection relates to a selective or generalized defect, *Virology*, **195**: 397–405.

Traub E, 1935, A filterable virus recovered from white mice, *Science*, **81**: 298–9.

Traub E, 1938, Factors influencing the persistence of choriomeningitis virus in the blood of mice after clinical recovery, *J Exp Med*, **68**: 229–50.

Vainrub B, Salas R, 1994, Latin American hemorrhagic fever, *Infect Dis Clin North Am*, **8**: 47–59.

Volkert M, 1963, Studies on immunological tolerance to LCMV. 2. Treatment of virus carrier mice by adoptive immunization, *Acta Pathol Microbiol Scand*, **57**: 465–87.

Volkert M, Lundstedt C, 1968, The provocation of latent LCMV infections in mice by treatment with anti-lymphocytic serum, *J Exp Med*, **127**: 327–39.

Walker DH, McCormick JB, Johnson KM, 1982, Pathologic and virologic study of fatal Lassa fever in man, *Am J Pathol*, **107:** 349–56.

Walker DH, Murphy FA, 1987, Pathology and pathogenesis of arenavirus infections, *Curr Top Microbiol Immunol*, **133:** 89–113.

Walker DH, Wolff H et al., 1975, Comparative pathology of Lassa virus infection in monkeys, guinea pigs and *Mastomys natalensis*, *Bull W H O*, **52:** 523–34.

Walker DH, Johnson KM et al., 1982, Experimental infection of rhesus monkeys with Lassa virus and a closely related arenavirus, Mozambique virus, *J Infect Dis*, **146:** 360–80.

Webb PA, Justines G, Johnson KM, 1975, Infection of wild and laboratory animals with Machupo and Latino viruses, *Bull W H O*, **52:** 493–9.

Webb PA, Johnson KM et al., 1973, Behavior of Machupo and Latino viruses in *Calomys callosus* from two geographic areas of Bolivia, *Lymphocytic Choriomeningitis Virus and Other Arenaviruses*, ed Lehmann-Grube F, Springer Verlag, New York, 314–22.

Weber EB, Buchmeier MJ, 1988, Fine mapping of a peptide sequence containing an antigenic site conserved among arenaviruses, *Virology*, **164:** 30–8.

Weissenbacher MC, de Guerrero LB, Boxaca MC, 1975, Experimental biology and pathogenesis of Junin virus infection in animals and in man, *Bull W H O*, **52:** 507–15.

Weissenbacher MC, Laguens RP, Coto CE, 1987, Argentine hemorrhagic fever, *Curr Top Microbiol Immunol*, **133:** 79–116.

Weissenbacher MC, Calello MA et al., 1979, Argentine hemorrhagic fever: a primate model, *Intervirology*, **11:** 363–7.

Welsh RM, 1987, Regulation and role of large granular lymphocytes in arenavirus infections, *Curr Top Microb Immunol*, **134:** 185–209.

Welsh RM, Buchmeier MJ, 1979, Protein analysis of defective interfering lymphocytic choriomeningitis virus and persistently infected cells, *Virology*, **96:** 503–15.

Wong GHW, Bartlett PF et al., 1984, Inducible expression of H-2 and Ia antigens in brain cells, *Nature (London)*, **310:** 688–91.

Woodrow D, Ronco P et al., 1982, Severity of glomerulonephritis induced in different strains of suckling mice by infection with LCMV: correlation with amounts of endogenous interferon and circulating immune complexes, *J Pathol*, **138:** 325–36.

Wright KE, Salvato MS, Buchmeier MJ, 1989, Neutralizing epitopes of lymphocytic choriomeningitis virus are conformational and require both glycosylation and disulfide bonds for expression, *Virology*, **171:** 417–26.

Yokoyama M, Zhang J, Whitton JL, 1995, DNA immunization confers protection against lethal lymphocytic choriomeningitis virus infection, *J Virol*, **69:** 2684–8.

Zinkernagel RM, Doherty PC, 1973, Cytotoxic thymus derived lymphocytes in cerebrospinal fluid of mice with lymphocytic choriomeningitis, *J Exp Med*, **138:** 1266–9.

Zinkernagel RM, Doherty PC, 1974, Restriction of *in vitro* T cell-mediated cytotoxicity in LCMV with a syngeneic or semiallogeneic system, *Nature (London)*, **248:** 701–2.

Zinkernagel RM, Doherty PC, 1979, MHC-restricted cytotoxic T cells: studies on the biological role of polymorphic major transplantation antigens determining T-cell restriction-specificity, function and responsiveness, *Adv Immunol*, **27:** 51–177.

Chapter 32

FILOVIRUSES

Heinz Feldmann, Anthony Sanchez and Hans-Dieter Klenk

1 Properties of filoviruses	3 Clinical and pathological aspects
2 Filovirus replication	

1 PROPERTIES OF FILOVIRUSES

1.1 Introduction

In 1967, an outbreak of viral haemorrhagic fever occurred in Europe among laboratory workers exposed to tissues and blood from African green monkeys (*Cercopithecus aethiops*) imported from Uganda (Siegert et al. 1967, Martini and Siegert 1971). The virus, which had been isolated from a number of patients, has been called Marburg virus (MBGV), after the city with the first reported cases. This episode marked the first identified outbreak of disease caused by a member of a group of viruses classified in the family *Filoviridae*. It was nearly a decade later, in 1976, when 2 other major filovirus outbreaks occurred in southern Sudan and northern Zaire. These outbreaks occurred simultaneously, but involved 2 biologically distinct subtypes, Sudan and Zaire, of a new filovirus, Ebola virus (EBOV) (World Health Organization 1978a, 1978b, McCormick et al. 1983).

In 1989, a third subtype of EBOV (Reston) emerged as the causative agent of an epizootic among a group of cynomolgus monkeys (*Macaca fascicularis*) imported from the Philippines into the USA (Jahrling et al. 1990). A similar epizootic occurred in 1992 when cynomolgus monkeys were imported into Italy from the same supplier who had shipped the 1989 monkeys into the USA (World Health Organization 1992). By contrast with previous observations of filovirus infections of humans, EBOV Reston seemed to be less pathogenic, and no disease occurred in 4 humans who were infected with this subtype of EBOV (Peters et al. 1993). This is also reflected in a lower pathogenicity for non-human primates (Fisher-Hoch et al. 1992a).

In 1996, EBOV Reston was introduced into a private quarantine facility in Texas, USA. Two cynomolgus monkeys (*Macaca fascicularis*) imported from the Philippines were infected. Sequence analysis of the entire glycoprotein gene of the EBOV from one of the monkeys indicated a 98.9% nucleotide identity with the original 1989 EBOV Reston (Centers for Disease Control and Prevention 1996).

EBOV was first detected in western Africa (Ivory Coast) in the autumn of 1994, when a single human case was identified and a novel EBOV was isolated (LeGuenno et al. 1995). This person was presumed to have been infected with EBOV while she was performing a necropsy on a wild chimpanzee, whose troop had undergone increased mortality, presumably due to EBOV disease. In 1995, EBOV re-emerged in Zaire, causing a severe outbreak of haemorrhagic fever in the city of Kikwit and surrounding villages in Bandundu Province. A total of 315 cases of EBOV haemorrhagic fever were reported, of whom 244 died (77%) (World Health Organization 1995a). Molecular analysis identified the causative agent as EBOV subtype Zaire, the glycoprotein gene differing by only 1.6% from the virus that caused the 1976 outbreak in northern Zaire (Sanchez et al. 1996). In 1996 an outbreak of EBOV haemorrhagic fever was reported from Gabon. There were 37 cases, of whom 21 (56.8%) died. Infection was linked to the butchering, transport and preparation for consumption of a chimpanzee found dead in the forest (World Health Organization 1996a).

Recently (1994 to 1997) Gabon has suffered from three Ebola epidemics that occurred north and west of Makokou. Virus isolation and sequence analysis demonstrated that all epidemics were caused by subtype Zaire (World Health Oganization 1996b, 1997).

In addition to the major outbreaks described above, sporadic cases of filovirus haemorrhagic fever in humans have occurred in various parts of Africa. Incidences of filovirus disease in humans that have been confirmed by virus isolation are summarized in Table 32.1.

Table 32.1 Outbreaks of filoviral haemorrhagic fever

Location	Year	Virus/Subtype[a]	Cases (Mortality)	Epidemiology
Germany/ 'Yugoslavia'	1967	Marburg	32 (23%)[b]	Imported monkeys from Uganda the source of most human infections
Zimbabwe	1975	Marburg	3 (33%)[c]	Unknown origin; index case infected in Zimbabwe; secondary cases infected in South Africa
Southern Sudan	1976	Ebola/Sudan	284 (53%)[d]	Unknown origin; spread mainly by close contact; nosocomial transmission and infection of health care personnel
Northern Zaire	1976	Ebola/Zaire	318 (88%)[e]	Unknown origin; spread by close contact and by use of contaminated needles and syringes in hospitals
Tandala, Zaire	1977	Ebola/Zaire	1 (100%)[f]	Unknown origin; single case in missionary hospital; other cases might have occurred nearby
Southern Sudan	1979	Ebola/Sudan	34 (65%)[g]	Unknown origin; recurrent outbreak at the same site as the 1976 outbreak
Kenya	1980	Marburg	2 (50%)[h]	Unknown origin; index case infected in western Kenya died but physician secondarily infected survived
Kenya	1987	Marburg	1 (100%)[i]	Unknown origin; expatriate traveling in western Kenya
USA	1989	Ebola/Reston	4 (0%)[j]	Introduction of virus with imported monkeys from the Philippines, 4 humans asymptomatically infected
Italy	1992	Ebola/Reston	0 (0%)[k]	Introduction of virus with imported monkeys from the Philippines; no human infections associated
Ivory Coast	1994	Ebola/(Ivory Coast?)	1 (0%)[l]	Contact with chimpanzees; single case
Kikwit, Zaire	1995	Ebola/Zaire	315 (77%)[m]	Unknown origin; course of outbreak as in 1976
Gabon	1996	Ebola	37 (57%)[n]	Linked to a chimpanzee found dead in the forest

Besides the well documented episodes listed in this Table, 2 more suspected fatal and 2 non-fatal cases of Ebola haemorrhagic fever, including a laboratory infection have been reported.
[a]Subtypes of Marburg are not classified. [b]Martini and Siegert 1967; numbers include a primary case that was diagnosed some years after the epidemic (Slenzka W, personal communication). [c]Gear et al. 1975. [d]World Health Organization 1978a. [e]World Health Organization 1978b; [f]Heymann et al. 1980. [g]Baron et al. 1983. [h]Smith et al. 1982. [i]Johnson ED, personal communication. [j]Jahrling et al. 1990. [k]World Health Organization 1992. [l]LeGuenno et al. 1995. [m]World Health Organization 1995a. [n]World Health Organization 1996a.

1.2 Classification

Filoviruses are classified in the order Mononegavirales, a large group of viruses that have non-segmented negative-strand (NNS) RNA as their genomes. The family *Filoviridae* was created on the basis of unique morphological, morphogenetic, physicochemical and biological features of its members (Kiley et al. 1982). Filoviruses can be separated into 2 distinct types, Marburg and Ebola (Table 32.2). In general, the Marburg type seems to be more homogeneous and without known subtypes (Kiley et al. 1988), but at least 2 different genetic lineages coexist (Trappier et al. 1996). The Ebola type, however, can be divided into at least 3 subtypes: Zaire, Sudan and Reston (Feldmann, Klenk and Sanchez 1993, Feldmann et al. 1994). Molecular characterization of the Ivory Coast virus revealed a novel lineage suggesting a fourth subtype

of EBOV (Sanchez et al. 1996). Nucleotide sequence comparison between MGBV and EBOV shows only scattered similarities, in contrast to the strong similarities seen between amino acid sequences of the structural proteins. Despite this amino acid similarity, there is no indication that there is any significant serological (antigenic) cross-reactivity between EBOV and MBGV, although the subtypes of EBOV share common epitopes (Richman et al. 1983, Feldmann et al. 1994). It may be that the nucleotide sequences of these agents diverged at some point in the distant past but the structural proteins have maintained similar structures and functions. Significant differences within the EBOV type were first noted from peptide and oligonucleotide mapping (Buchmeier et al. 1983, Cox et al. 1983), and have been confirmed by sequence analysis of the glycoprotein genes (Sanchez et al. 1996). The study by Sanchez et al. showed that all 4 subtypes differ from each other to a comparable extent (37–41% nucleotide differences). This suggests that filoviruses have evolved into specific niches and may reflect a similar divergence in the natural hosts, assuming that they have co-evolved. The differences seen between the filovirus types are so extensive that a taxonomic re-evaluation of the genus *Filovirus* may be necessary.

Molecular analysis of the genomes of filoviruses has clearly demonstrated a close genetic relationship to other families of the order, especially the *Rhabdoviridae* and *Paramyxoviridae*. All NNS RNA viruses have a similar genome organization: the more conserved genes that encode core and L proteins are located at the 3' and the 5' ends, respectively, of the genomic RNA. In between these conserved areas is a more variable region that generally contains genes encoding envelope and certain membrane-associated proteins. The only exception occurs in the genomes of filoviruses, which contain a minor nucleoprotein (VP30) in this region (Fig. 32.1). Filovirus genomes are more complex than those of rhabdoviruses, and their organization is more like those of members of the genera *Paramyxovirus* and *Morbillivirus*. This relationship was confirmed by comparisons of the deduced amino acid sequences of the nucleoprotein and L protein (Feldmann, Klenk and Sanchez 1993, Sanchez et al. 1993). In conclusion, all data available today support the concept of an order Mononegavirales comprised of at least 3 distinct families (Murphy et al. 1995).

In terms of biohazard classification, filoviruses are classified as 'Biosafety Level 4' agents on the basis of their high mortality rate, person-to-person transmission, potential aerosol infectivity and absence of vaccines or chemotherapeutic agents. Maximum containment is required for all laboratory work with infectious material (Centers for Disease Control and Prevention 1993).

1.3 Morphology and structure

Filovirus virions are bacilliform in shape, but particles can also appear as branched, circular, U- or 6-shaped and long filamentous forms. This morphology is unusual for viruses and has been important in the classification and nomenclature (Latin *filo*: thread) (Fig. 32.2). Virions vary greatly in length but have a uniform diameter of c. 80 nm. Family members differ in length of virion particles but seem to be very similar in morphology. Peak infectivity has been associated with particles of 665 nm for MBGV and 805 nm for EBOV. Virions are composed of a central core formed by a nucleocapsid or ribonucleoprotein (RNP) complex, which is surrounded by a lipid envelope derived from the host cell plasma membrane. Electron micrographs reveal an axial channel (10–15 nm in diameter) surrounded by a central dark layer (20 nm in diameter) and an outer helical layer (50 nm in diameter) with cross-striations of 5 nm intervals. Spikes c. 7 nm in diameter and spaced at intervals of c. 10 nm are seen as globular structures on the surface of virions (Siegert et al. 1967, Peters, Müller and Slenczka 1971, Murphy et al. 1978, Kiley et al. 1982).

The RNP complex is composed of a genomic RNA molecule bound by 4 of the 7 virion structural proteins: the nucleoprotein (NP), virion structural protein (VP) 30, VP35 and the large (L) protein (see Fig. 32.1b). The genomic RNA has a molecular weight of 4200 kDa and constitutes 1.1% of the virion mass (Regnery, Johnson and Kiley 1980). The 3 remaining structural proteins are membrane-associated; the glycoprotein (GP) shows a type I transmembrane protein profile (Will et al. 1993), while VP24 and VP40 are probably located at the inner side of the membrane. Virus particles have a molecular weight of c. $3-6 \times 10^8$ and a density in potassium tartrate of 1.14 g/cm^3 (Kiley et al. 1988).

1.4 Genome structure and function

Genomes of filoviruses consist of a single negative-strand linear RNA molecule (Kiley et al. 1982, Regnery, Johnson and Kiley 1980). The RNA is not infectious, does not contain a poly(A) tail, and upon entry into the cytoplasm of host cells is transcribed to generate polyadenylated subgenomic mRNA species (Kiley et al. 1982, Feldmann et al. 1992, Sanchez et al. 1993). The complete nucleic acid sequences of 2

Table 32.2 Characteristics of 'Marburg' and 'Ebola' types of filoviruses

Features	Type 'Marburg'	Type 'Ebola'
Serological cross-reactivity to other type	No	No
Subtypes	1[b]	4[d]
Glycoprotein (SDS-PAGE)	c. 170 kDa	c. 140 kDa
Terminal sialylation of carbohydrates[a]	No	Yes
Nucleoprotein (SDS-PAGE)	c. 95 kDa	c. 105 kDa
Non-structural proteins	No	1[e]
Editing	No	Yes[f]
Gene overlaps	1[c]	>1[g]
Overlapping ORF in gene 2	Yes	No

[a]By propagation of viruses in Vero E6 and MA-104 cells (monkey kidney cell lines). [b]Type Marburg, subtype Marburg. [c]Between VP30 and VP24. [d]Type Ebola, subtypes Zaire, Sudan, Reston, Ivory Coast. [e]Small glycosylated protein encoded by gene 4. [f]Gene 4. [g]Between VP35 and VP40/GP and VP30/VP24 and L (Ebola, subtype Zaire).
SDS-PAGE, sodium dodecylsulfate-polyacrylamide gel electrophoresis; ORF, open reading frame

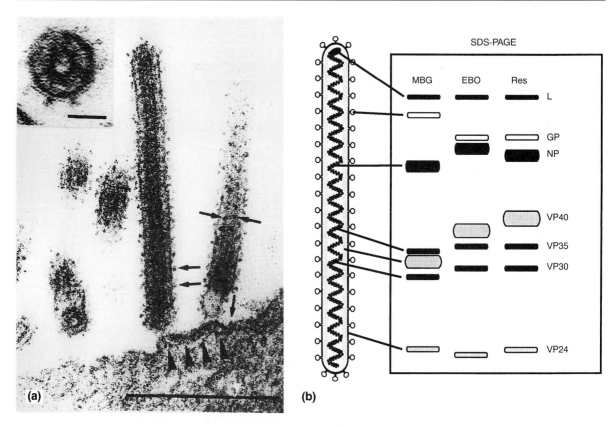

Fig. 32.1 Structure of filovirus particles. (a) Ultrathin sections obtained from primary cultures of human endothelial cells 3 days after infection with Marburg virus analysed by transmission electron microscopy. Particles consist of a nucleocapsid surrounded by a membrane in which spikes are inserted (arrows). The nucleocapsid contains a central channel (inset). The plasma membrane of infected cells is often thickened at locations were budding occurs (arrowheads) (bar = 0.5 μm; inset bar = 50 nm). (b) The non-segmented negative-strand RNA genome is associated with 4 viral proteins: the viral polymerase (L), the nucleoprotein (NP), and the virion structural proteins (VP) 35 and 30 (black). VP40 and VP24 are membrane-associated proteins (grey), and the spikes are formed by the glycoprotein (GP) (white). Differences in the electrophoretic mobility patterns (SDS-PAGE) of filovirus structural proteins are illustrated schematically. EBO, Ebola; MBG, Marburg; RES, Ebola subtype Reston.

different isolates of MBGV (Feldmann et al. 1992, Bukreyev et al. 1995), the Mayinga isolate of EBOV (subtype Zaire) (Sanchez et al. 1993), as well as partial sequences of EBOV Reston (subtype Reston) and EBOV Boniface isolates (subtype Sudan) (Sanchez et al. 1996) have been elucidated. Filovirus genomes are c. 19 kb (MBGV 19.1 kb; EBOV 18.9 kb) and are significantly longer than rhabdoviruses and paramyxoviruses. Genes have been delineated by transcriptional signals at their 3′ and 5′ ends that have been identified by their conservation and by analysis of mRNA sequences. The following order is characteristic for filoviruses: 3′ (leader)–N–VP35–VP40–GP–VP30–VP24–L–(trailer) 5′ (Fig. 32.2a).

Genes of filoviruses are usually separated from one another by intergenic regions that vary in length and nucleotide composition. However, some genes overlap, especially those of EBOV, and the positions and numbers of overlaps vary among filoviruses. Viruses belonging to the Zaire subtype of EBOV possess 3 overlaps, between the VP35 and VP40, GP and VP30, and VP24 and L genes, whereas MBGV isolates have only one overlap, involving the VP30 and VP24 genes (Fig. 32.2a). The length of the overlaps is centred on

5 highly conserved nucleotides within the transcriptional signals (3′–UAAUU–5′) that are found at the internal ends of the conserved sequences. Transcriptional start signals are conserved among filoviruses, and the sequence 3′–CUNCNUNUAAUU–5′ represents the consensus motif. Transcriptional stop signals are identical for all genes (3′–UAAUUCUUUUU–5′) except the VP40 gene of MBGV (Feldmann et al. 1992) and the L gene of EBOV, subtype Zaire (VE Volchkov 1996, personal communication) (Fig. 32.3). Most genes tend to possess long non-coding sequences at their 3′ and/or 5′ ends, which contribute to the increased length of the genome. Extragenic sequences are found at the 3′ (leader) and 5′ (trailer) ends of the genome. Those leader and trailer sequences are complementary to one another at the extreme ends (Kiley et al. 1986, Feldmann et al. 1992), a feature that is shared by all NNS RNA viruses.

1.5 Polypeptides

Nucleoprotein

The nucleoprotein (NP) is encoded close to the 3′ end of the linear RNA genome. The NPs from various

(a)

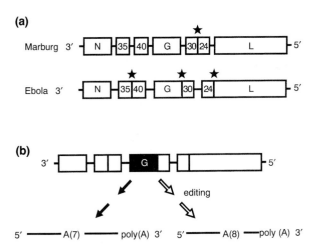

(b)

Fig. 32.2 (a) Filoviral genomes consist of a single, negative-strand, linear RNA molecule. Differences in organization between Marburg and Ebola type viruses are indicated. *, position of gene overlap. (b) Gene 4 of Ebola viruses is transcribed from 2 open reading frames. The primary gene product is a small glycoprotein (sGP). Full-length glycoprotein (GP) is expressed by RNA editing. A, adenosine residue; c, carboxy-terminal end of proteins; G, glycoprotein gene; L, polymerase (L) gene; n, amino-terminal end of proteins; N, nucleoprotein gene; ORF, open reading frame; 24 / 30 / 35 / 40, virion structural protein (VP) genes; 3′ and 5′, terminal ends of genomes and subgenomic RNAs.

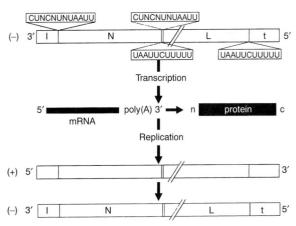

Fig. 32.3 The mode of transcription and replication of filoviruses, based on the data available to date. Each gene on the linear arranged non-segmented (–)-sense genome is flanked by conserved transcriptional start (3′–CUNCNUN-UAAUU–5′; indicated above) and termination signals (3′–UAAUUCUUUUU–5′; indicated underneath). Transcription starts at the 3′ end of the (–)-sense genome and leads to polyadenylated mRNA species. For replication a full-length (+)-sense antigenome is synthesized which serves as the template for the synthesis of progeny (–)-sense RNA anticomplementary to the parental RNA. c, carboxy-terminal end of proteins; l, 3′ untranslated region (leader); n, amino-terminal end of proteins; Poly(A), polyadenylation of mRNA species; t, 5′ untranslated region (trailer); NP, nucleoprotein; L, viral RNA-dependent RNA polymerase.

VP35: POLYMERASE COFACTOR?

The VP35 gene encodes a protein that ranges from 329 amino acids for MBGV to 340 for EBOV (Feldmann et al. 1992, Bukreyev et al. 1993, Sanchez et al. 1993). The association of this protein in the RNP complex is much weaker than that of the NP and VP30 (Elliott, Kiley and McCormick 1985, Kiley et al. 1988). With related viruses, the second gene usually encodes a phosphoprotein, but attempts to demonstrate phosphorylation of the VP35 in mammalian cell lines have failed (Elliott, Kiley and McCormick 1985, Elliott et al. 1993b). Hydropathy plots of MBGV VP35 and EBOV VP35 show similar profiles and a prominent common hydrophilic domain in close proximity to the N termini. This region may be involved in template binding. Despite the lack of phosphorylation and sequence homology, the genome position and its association in the RNP complex suggest that VP35 is functionally analogous to the P proteins of paramyxoviruses and rhabdoviruses (see Fig. 32.1b).

VP40: MATRIX PROTEIN

The VP40 of filoviruses is 303 and 326 amino acids long for MBGV and EBOV Zaire, respectively (Feldmann et al. 1992, Bukreyev et al. 1993, Sanchez et al. 1993). VP40 is not associated with the RNP complex and behaves like a membrane-associated protein when analysed after non-ionic detergent treatment of virion particles (Elliott, Kiley and McCormick 1985, Kiley et al. 1988). This finding together with a predominantly hydrophobic profile, the abundance in

filoviruses differ slightly in their electrophoretic mobility patterns, ranging from 95 kDa (MBGV) to 105 kDa (EBOV Zaire). The molecular weights calculated from the deduced amino acid sequences of the corresponding genes of MBGV (695 amino acids) and EBOV (739 amino acids) are 78 kDa and 83 kDa, respectively, and the differences in their lengths is related to the variable C termini of the protein (Sanchez et al. 1989, 1992). The NP proteins possess an unusually high molecular weight compared with other NNS virus nucleocapsid proteins, which range from 42 to 62 kDa. The NP protein is the major structural phosphoprotein, and only the phosphorylated form of the protein is incorporated into virions. This indicates that phosphorylation is needed to form stable virion RNP complexes (Elliott, Kiley and McCormick 1985, Elliott et al. 1993b, Becker et al. 1994). NP is the major component of the RNP complex and is tightly bound, but direct binding in vitro to vRNA has yet to be demonstrated. There is little doubt, however, that this protein is the functional analogue of the nucleocapsid proteins of paramyxoviruses and rhabdoviruses (see Fig. 32.1b).

virion particles and the genome position of the corresponding gene suggest that VP40 is the matrix protein analogue of filoviruses (see Fig. 32.1b).

GLYCOPROTEIN

The glycoprotein (GP) is encoded in the fourth gene, and is the only glycosylated structural protein of virions. GPs of MBGV and EBOV Zaire are 681 and 676 amino acids in length, respectively (Sanchez et al. 1993, Will et al. 1993, Volchkov et al. 1995). Filovirus GPs are type I transmembrane proteins that have a C terminal hydrophobic membrane anchor and an N terminal signal peptide that is cleaved by signal peptidases (Will et al. 1993). Filovirus GPs contain *N*- and *O*-glycans that account for up to 50% of the molecular weight of mature proteins (Feldmann et al. 1991, Geyer et al. 1992).

Comparison of amino acid sequences of filovirus GPs showed conservation at the N and C terminal ends of the proteins in which nearly all cysteine residues are located. The middle region is variable and extremely hydrophilic, and carries the bulk of the attachment sites for *N*- and *O*-glycans. The MBGV GP is acylated at 2 cysteine residues located at the border between the membrane anchor region and the cytoplasmic tail (Funke et al. 1995). The special arrangement of all cysteine residues in the molecule favours an intramolecular cysteine bridge formation between the 2 terminal regions of the molecule, resulting in a stem region with a crown-like domain on the top carrying the mass of the carbohydrate side chains. For MBGV the mature GP is inserted in the membrane as a homotrimer. Oligomerization may be mediated by intermolecular disulphide bridges, because complexes can be destroyed under reducing conditions (Feldmann et al. 1991). The fact that GP is the only surface protein of virions suggests a function in mediating binding to cellular receptors and fusion with cellular membranes. Furthermore, GP is discussed (see section 3.5, p. 660) as a major viral antigen and an important target for the host immune response (see Fig. 32.1b).

In general, filovirus GPs lack significant homologies with envelope proteins of other viruses. However, a region of 26 amino acids (and less conserved surrounding sequences) in the external domain close to the transmembrane region shows significant homology to an immunosuppressive domain in envelope proteins of several retroviruses (Volchkov, Blinov and Netesov 1992, Will et al. 1993). This is also the most conserved sequence between the GPs of MBGV and EBOV. It is not known whether this sequence in filovirus GPs has immunosuppressive properties.

VP30: MINOR NUCLEOPROTEIN?

The fifth gene encodes VP30, a protein intimately associated with the RNP complex (Elliott, Kiley and McCormick 1985, Kiley et al. 1988). The protein has a length of 260 and 281 amino acids with EBOV Zaire and MBGV, respectively (Feldmann et al. 1992, Sanchez et al. 1993). The VP30 of EBOV has been identified as a minor phosphoprotein of virions (Elliott,

Kiley and McCormick 1985, Elliott et al 1993b). VP30 may work as a functional unit in encapsidation of the RNA genome (Kiley et al. 1988). It could also have a role as an additional cofactor of the transcriptase/replicase complex (see Fig. 32.1b).

VP24: MEMBRANE-ASSOCIATED PROTEIN OF UNKNOWN FUNCTION

VP24 is expressed from the sixth gene, and is 253 amino acids long in MBGV and 251 in EBOV Zaire (Feldmann et al. 1992, Sanchez et al. 1993). Unlike VP40, VP24 is not completely removed from the RNP complex under isotonic conditions (Elliott, Kiley and McCormick 1985, Kiley et al. 1988). VP24 presumably serves as a second matrix protein and may bind to the cytoplasmic tail of GP or may link the membrane proteins (VP40 and/or GP) to the RNP (see Fig. 32.1b).

LARGE PROTEIN

The large (L) protein is encoded at the 5′ end of the linear genome and has a predicted molecular weight of 267 kDa (2331 amino acids) for MBGV (Mühlberger et al. 1992). Computer-assisted comparison revealed significant homologies to L proteins of other NNS RNA viruses. Homologies are mainly located in the N terminal half of the protein and concentrated within 3 common domains, named boxes A, B and C. Other common features are a high content of leucine and isoleucine residues, a large positive net charge, clusters of basic amino acids, putative ATP binding sites, 2 neighbouring cysteine residues located in the C terminal half of the protein, and the genome localization of the encoding gene. A highly conserved peptide motif, GDNQ, is located at the C terminal end of domain B (positions 744–747) and is flanked by hydrophobic amino acid residues, which for other viruses has been postulated to be a catalytic site of the protein. Similar motifs with alterations in the first amino acid have been described and discussed as catalytic sites for some RNA-dependent RNA polymerases of plant, animal and bacterial viruses. Even though transcriptase and replicase activities have not yet been demonstrated, the L protein is regarded as an RNA-dependent RNA polymerase (see Fig. 32.1b).

NON-STRUCTURAL GLYCOPROTEIN

A non-structural glycoprotein has recently been discovered for EBOV (Volchkov et al. 1995, Sanchez et al. 1996). This protein, designated sGP, is expressed from the glycoprotein gene by mechanisms discussed below (see section 2.3, p. 657) (Fig. 32.2b). The sGP shares about 300 N terminal amino acid residues with GP, but has a different C terminus (c. 70 amino acids) which contains many charged residues as well as conserved cysteines. The sGP contains N- and O-linked carbohydrate, although not as much as the GP, and is secreted into the culture medium in high quantities. The function of this non-structural protein is unknown, but may modulate the host immune response by binding antibodies or soluble factors. No expression of a similar protein has been detected in the MGB type viruses, nor is one predicted from analysis of the nucleotide sequence.

2 FILOVIRUS REPLICATION

2.1 Virus growth in cell cultures

The Vero cell line, especially the E6 clone, is most widely used for virus isolation and propagation. Primary virus isolation has also been successful in MA-104 and SW13 cells (McCormick et al. 1983, Jahrling et al. 1990). A variety of other cells have also been tested as substrates for filovirus replication (van der Groen et al. 1978, McCormick et al. 1983, Peters et al. 1992). These include a recently developed human microvascular endothelial cell line (HMEC-1), primary cultures of human umbilical cord vein endothelial cells (HUVEC) and human peripheral blood monocytes/macrophages (Schnittler et al. 1993, Feldmann et al. 1996a).

MBGV and EBOV (subtype Zaire) cause lytic infections in cell culture. The Sudan and Reston subtypes of EBOV replicate more slowly on primary isolation, and cytopathic effect (CPE) is not as prominent as with the Zaire subtype. The course of infection in tissue culture can be monitored by an indirect immunofluorescence assay (IFA) or by plaque assay. In cases of little or no CPE, reverse transcriptase-polymerase chain reaction (RT-PCR) on viral RNA isolated from infected cells and tissue culture supernatants can be helpful for quantification (Schnittler et al. 1993, Sanchez and Feldmann 1996).

Viral RNA synthesis in tissue culture is detectable at least 7 h after infection, reaches a maximum by 18 h, and declines thereafter; CPE is not seen before 48 h after infection. The first mRNA to be detected is NP-specific and reaches levels sufficient to produce protein 7 h after infection. All proteins are detectable by translation in vitro of polyadenylated RNA isolated 18 h after infection; thereafter the yield of translation products decreases (Sanchez and Kiley 1987). PCR assays of genomic RNA of MBGV particles in supernatants of infected cells have indicated that the replication cycle is c. 12 h (Schnittler et al. 1993).

2.2 Virus entry

Cell entry is presumably mediated by GP. The asialoglycoprotein receptor of hepatocytes might serve as a receptor for MBGV (Becker, Spiess and Klenk 1995). However, because the asialoglycoprotein receptor is not expressed on many cells that support the growth of filoviruses, other receptors may also be involved. The next step in virus entry presumably involves fusion, but it is not known whether this process occurs directly at the plasma membrane or in endocytic vesicles. The mechanism of uncoating is also unknown.

2.3 Transcription, translation and genome replication

Filovirus transcription and replication take place in the cytoplasm of infected cells, and the mechanisms resemble those of other NNS RNA viruses. As with other members of the order Mononegavirales, transcription is believed to start at the extreme 3′ end, leading to the synthesis of a short (+)-leader sequence that is terminated when the first transcription start site is encountered (Fig. 32.3). The 7 structural genes are subsequently transcribed to produce 7 monocistronic polyadenylated mRNA species. There is no evidence for larger amounts of bi- or multicistronic subgenomic RNA species (Sanchez and Kiley 1987, Feldmann et al. 1992, Sanchez et al. 1993). Analyses of MBGV mRNA species have shown that the 5′ ends of the transcripts are 2 bases shorter than previously published (Mühlberger et al. 1996). All start signals of filovirus genes contain the consensus sequence 3′–CUNCNUNUAAUU–5′. The 3′ ends of the transcripts carry a poly(A) tail generated by a stuttering mechanism of the viral polymerase at a run of 5 or 6 uridine residues located at the 5′ end of all transcription stop signals. Therefore, the sequence 3′–UAAUUCUUUUU(U)–5′ serves as a transcription stop and polyadenylation signal. Both signals carry the pentamer 3′–UAAUU–5′, a unique feature among NNS RNA viruses. The function of the pentamer is unknown, but it could serve as the recognition site for positioning the polymerase complex. The surrounding semiconserved sequences may then mediate the exact initiation of transcription and termination/polyadenylation events.

Filovirus transcripts contain unusually long untranslated regions, especially at the 3′ ends. The 5′ end untranslated regions show a potential for formation of stable hairpin structures, which might play a role in transcript stability and ribosome binding (Sanchez et al. 1993). The role of gene overlaps in regulation of transcription is unknown. Sanchez et al. (1993) proposed that, following mRNA synthesis, transcription is reinitiated by reposition of the polymerase at the downstream start site. This 'backup' mechanism is supported by the finding that attenuation of filovirus genes with start sites in overlaps does not occur to any higher degree, as has been noted for a much larger overlap found in the respiratory syncytial virus genome. Alternatively, the polymerase may occasionally terminate transcription without polyadenylation at the overlap and initiate transcription of the downstream gene, but there is no evidence for detectable levels of transcripts lacking poly(A) tails (see Fig. 32.3).

The switch mechanism between transcription and replication is unknown, but, as with other NNS viruses, synthesis of the NP protein could be a key factor. Encapsidation and polymerase complex entry sites are probably located on the leader sequence, and the fact that the ends of the genome are complementary suggests a single identical encapsidation site on genome and antigenome; this would function for transcription as well as for replication (Feldmann et al. 1992). Replication involves a full-length (+)-strand antigenome which serves as the template for synthesis of (−)-strand genome molecules. Encapsidated genomic RNA forms nucleocapsids that go into the formation of new infectious virions at the cell surface (see Fig. 32.3).

The organization and transcription of the GP genes of EBOV are unusual, and involve transcriptional editing. EBOV GP genes possess 2 open reading frames (see Fig. 32.2b). Full-length GP is expressed by the addition of a single non-templated adenosine residue at a run of 7 uridine residues on the vRNA template (Volchkov et al. 1995, Sanchez et al. 1996). The primary gene product is a small non-structural glycoprotein (sGP) that is secreted from infected cells. In addition, virus variants have been found after passaging in tissue culture and animals that express full-length GP from a single open reading frame. Those variants acquired a mutation that added a single uridine nucleotide at the editing site connecting the GP open reading frame (Sanchez et al. 1993, Volchkov et al. 1995). A smaller subgenomic RNA species was found in infected cells generated by polyadenylation at the mutation site. The MBGV GP is expressed in a single frame and the gene does not contain sequences favouring mechanisms such as editing or frameshifting. A second ORF has been described for MBGV (Musoke strain), but a corresponding gene product has not been identified (Will et al. 1993).

2.4 Virus assembly and exit

Virions usually bud at the plasma membrane, and the budding process is probably mediated at membrane locations where GP is incorporated. The cytoplasmic tail of GP is thought to interact with VP40 or VP24, or both. VP40 or VP24 may mediate the linkage between the RNP complexes and the membrane proteins. Particles mature preferentially in a vertical mode, but budding via the longitudinal axis has also been observed. In macrophages budding has also been observed at intracytoplasmic membranes surrounding vacuoles that form during infection (Feldmann et al. 1996a).

3 CLINICAL AND PATHOLOGICAL ASPECTS

3.1 Epidemiology

It is generally accepted that human filovirus outbreaks are of a zoonotic nature. Guinea-pigs, primates, bats and hard ticks have been suspected to be natural hosts, but the search for filoviruses in these and many other species has been so far unsuccessful.

MBGV and the Sudan and Zaire subtypes of EBOV seem to be indigenous to the African continent, and both EBOV subtypes have been isolated from human patients only in Africa. MBGV has been isolated from human patients in Africa and Europe, though the European cases were caused by a virus originating from Africa (Martini and Siegert 1971). The EBOV Reston outbreak provided the first evidence for the presence of a filovirus outside Africa (Hayes et al. 1992). Serological studies (IFA) among captive macaques in the Philippines indicated that the source of EBOV Reston might be wild non-human primates. However, IFA-detected antibodies seem to be spurious, and latent infection in non-human primates has never been observed (Fisher-Hoch et al. 1992b).

Serological studies suggest that filoviruses are endemic in many central African regions (summarized in Feldmann et al. 1996b). Recent sero-surveys in other countries, such as Germany, the USA and the Philippines, have identified antibodies to filoviruses in humans as well. Serological data based on IFA are of only limited reliability, as non-specific reactivity has been observed when filovirus antigens are used. Nevertheless, it is possible that subclinical infections caused by known or unknown filoviruses or a closely related virus (paramyxovirus?) may be responsible for a certain amount of the seropositivity detected in human populations.

3.2 Clinical manifestation

MODE OF TRANSMISSION

Person-to-person transmission by intimate contact is the main route of infection in human outbreaks. The EBOV outbreaks in 1976 and 1995 and the MBGV outbreak in 1967 all involved nosocomial transmission via contaminated syringes and needles. Therefore, extreme care should be taken with blood, secretions and excretions from infected patients. On the basis of experiences from these episodes, the isolation of patients, use of strict barrier nursing procedures (e.g. protective clothing, respirator) and measures to handle and disinfect contaminated material promptly are sufficient to prevent transmission to healthcare workers. Transmission by droplets and small-particle aerosols have been observed in outbreaks among experimentally infected and quarantined imported monkeys. This is confirmed by identification of filovirus particles in the alveoli of naturally and experimentally infected monkeys and humans (Peters, Johnson and McKee 1991, Pokhodyaeu, Gonchar and Psenichnov 1991, Geisbert et al. 1992, Zaki 1995). Epidemiological studies of human outbreaks, however, indicate that aerosols and droplets do not seem to be an important route of transmission.

CLINICAL SYNDROME

The onset of the disease is sudden with fever, chills, headache, myalgia and anorexia. These may be followed by symptoms such as abdominal pain, sore throat, nausea, vomiting, cough, arthralgia, diarrhoea, and pharyngeal and conjunctival injections. Patients are dehydrated, apathetic, disorientated, and may develop a characteristic, non-puritic, maculopapular centripetal rash associated with varying degrees of erythema that desquamates by day 5–7 of the illness. Haemorrhagic manifestations develop during the peak of the illness; they are of prognostic value. Bleeding into the gastrointestinal tract is most prominent, as well as petechiae and haemorrhages from puncture wounds and mucous membranes. Laboratory findings are less characteristic but the following are associated with the disease: leucopenia (as low as 1000/µl), left shift with atypical lymphocytes, thrombocytopenia (50 000–100 000/µl), markedly elevated serum transaminase levels (AST typically exceeding ALT), hyperproteinaemia and proteinuria. Prothrombin and partial thromboplastin times are prolonged and fibrin split products are detectable. In a later stage, secondary bacterial infection may lead to elevated white blood counts.

Non-fatal cases have fever for about 5–9 days; fatal cases develop clinical signs early during infection and death commonly occurs between days 6 and 16, due to haemorrhage and hypovolaemic shock. Mortality is high, varying between 22% and 88% depending on the virus. The highest rate has been reported for EBOV Zaire. MBGV infections are associated with the lowest mortality rates. However, one has to consider that most MBGV patients have been treated under European medical care standards, unlike most of the EBOV cases which occurred in Africa. EBOV Reston seems to possess a very low pathogenicity for humans or may even be apathogenic.

Convalescence is prolonged and sometimes associated with myelitis, recurrent hepatitis, psychosis or uveitis. There is an increased risk of abortion for pregnant women, and clinical observations indicate a high death rate for children of infected mothers (Martini and Siegert 1971, Pattyn 1978, Baron, McCormick and Zubeir 1983, Peters et al. 1996).

3.3 Pathology

PATHOLOGY IN EXPERIMENTAL ANIMALS

Monkeys, guinea-pigs, suckling mice and hamsters have been experimentally infected with filoviruses. MBGV and EBOV Zaire are highly virulent for most of these species. The Sudan and Reston subtypes of EBOV are less virulent, often causing a self-limited infection in guinea-pigs and monkeys.

The incubation period for rhesus and African green monkeys inoculated with MBGV and EBOV subtype Zaire is 4–16 days. High titres of virus can be detected in liver, spleen, lymph nodes and lungs by the onset of clinical symptoms. All these organs, especially liver, show severe necrosis due to virus replication in parenchymal cells. Little inflammatory response at those sites is typical and suggests that classic immunopathology may not be an important consideration. Interstitial haemorrhage occurs and is most prominent in the gastrointestinal tract. In infected non-human primates thrombocytopenia has been found accompanied by aggregation disorders of remaining platelets in response to agonists such as ADP and collagen (Murphy et al. 1971, Fisher-Hoch et al. 1985). Histopathological damage of the target organs is at odds with serum transferase levels showing increases in AST and ALT (AST/ALT = 7 : 1). This argues against hepatocellular dysfunction and raises the question for extrahepatic targets (Peters et al. 1996). Recent morphological studies on EBOV Reston-infected monkeys of the 1989 outbreak revealed extensive virus replication in tissue macrophages, interstitial fibroblasts of many organs, circulating monocytes/macrophages and less frequently in endothelial cells, hepatocytes, adrenal corticoid cells and renal tubular epithelium (Geisbert et al. 1992). Similar results have been reported from monkeys experimentally infected with MBGV and EBOV Zaire (Ryabchikova et al. 1994).

PATHOLOGY IN HUMANS

In fatal cases, generalized haemorrhage is found macroscopically in most organ systems. Microscopic changes include focal necrosis in liver, lymphatic organs, kidneys, testes and ovaries. The liver, although always involved with large eosinophilic intracytoplasmic inclusion bodies in hepatocytes and Councilman-like bodies within necrotic foci, is not the site of massive, potentially fatal necrosis. Generalized lymphoid necrosis is characteristic of the disease, and renal tubular necrosis is commonly found in the agonal stages. A diffuse encephalitis, as described for many viral infections, has been observed. In addition, focal haemorrhages have been observed in the brain. The clotting system is activated and intravascular fibrin thrombi have been observed. Viral antigen can be detected in many organs, predominantly in the liver, kidneys, spleen and adrenal glands. Viral persistence has been demonstrated for MBGV cases by isolation of virus from liver biopsy material, the anterior chamber of the eye (4–5 weeks) and semen (12 weeks), despite an apparently normal immune response (e.g. Martini and Siegert 1971, Pattyn 1978, Peters et al. 1996).

3.4 Pathophysiology

Pathophysiological changes that make filovirus infections so devastating are just beginning to be unravelled. Clinical and biochemical findings support the anatomical observations of extensive liver involvement, renal damage, changes in vascular permeability and activation of the clotting cascade. The necrosis of the visceral organs is a consequence of virus replication in parenchymal cells. However, no organ, not even the liver, shows sufficient damage to account for death. The role of disseminated intravascular coagulation (DIC) in pathogenesis is still controversial, because laboratory confirmation of DIC in human infections has never been demonstrated. In nonhuman primates the intrinsic clotting pathway is most affected, whereas the extrinsic pathway is spared.

Laboratory findings in the crucial early stage of filovirus haemorrhagic fever, such as a high AST/ALT ratio, normal bilirubin levels and marked lymphopenia followed by a dramatic neutrophilia with left shift, suggest extrahepatic targets in the infection. As with viral haemorrhagic fever with renal syndrome (HFRS), dengue haemorrhagic fever and Lassa fever, fluid distribution problems and platelet abnormalities are dominant clinical manifestations indicating dysfunction or damage of endothelial cells and platelets. Post mortem there is little monocyte/macrophage infiltration in sites of parenchymal necrosis, suggesting that a dysfunction of white blood cells, such as macrophages, occurs. Morphological studies on EBOV Reston-infected monkeys from the 1989 epizootic (Geisbert et al. 1992) and monkeys experimentally infected with EBOV Zaire (Ryabchikova et al. 1994) revealed that monocytes/macrophages and fibroblasts may be the preferred sites of virus replication in early stages, whereas other cell types may become involved as the disease progresses. Human monocytes/ macrophages in culture are also sensitive to infection, resulting in massive production of infectious virus and cell lysis (Feldmann et al. 1996a). Although the studies on infected non-human primates did not identify endothelial cells as sites of massive virus replication, in vitro studies and investigations on humans with EBOV haemorrhagic fever clearly demonstrated that endothelial cells of human origin are suitable targets for virus replication (Schnittler et al. 1993). Here, infection leads to complete cell lysis, indicating that damage to endothelial cells may occur during infection. Supernatants of MBGV-infected monocyte/macrophage cultures can increase paraendothelial permeability in an in vitro model (Feldmann et al. 1996a). Examination for mediators in those supernatants revealed increased levels of secreted TNF-α, the prototype cytokine of macrophages.

These data support a mechanism of a mediator-induced vascular instability that leads to increased permeability and a shock syndrome that is seen in severe/fatal cases. Haemorrhagic manifestations, however, are also likely to be caused in part by the damage inflicted on the reticuloendothelial system as a direct result of massive virus replication. Haemorrhages occur later in infection and could be due to extensive damage that cannot be repaired by wound-healing mechanisms. The bleeding tendency is reinforced by a decrease in blood pressure as a common consequence of shock. The combination of viral replication in endothelial cells and virus-induced cytokine release from macrophages may also promote a distinct proinflammatory endothelial phenotype that then triggers the coagulation cascade.

3.5 Immune responses

The mechanisms of recovery from filovirus infections in humans and in wild as well as laboratory animals are unknown. Neutralization in vitro has never been demonstrated by plaque reduction in cell culture systems, and protection by convalescence sera has not been evaluated in controlled clinical trials. Fatal filovirus infections usually end with high viraemia and no evidence of an immune response. In humans and monkeys there is extensive disruption of the parafollicular regions in the spleen and lymph nodes. EBOV Reston infection in monkeys is an exception, as there is a rise in non-productive antibodies shortly before death. Thus, cell-mediated immunity may mediate recovery from filovirus infections.

GP is assumed to be the major virion antigen. Its interaction with the host immune system may be modulated by the high content of carbohydrates. For EBOV, sGP production and secretion might interfere with the host immune response by neutralizing effective antibodies. As already mentioned (see p. 656), filovirus GP has a sequence close to the C terminus resembling an immunosuppressive domain in retrovirus glycoproteins. Peptides synthesized according to that 26 amino acid long region inhibited the blastogenesis of lymphocytes in response to mitogens, induced the production of cytokines and increased the proliferation of mononuclear cells in vitro. These findings are in line with the observation of immunosuppression in monkeys experimentally infected with MBGV and EBOV and of proliferation of filoviruses in macrophages and monocytes in vivo and in vitro (Murphy et al. 1971, Baskerville et al. 1985, Geisbert et al. 1992, Schnittler et al. 1993).

3.6 Diagnosis

In tropical settings identification of a filovirus haemorrhagic fever may be difficult, because the most common causes of severe, acute, febrile disease are malaria and typhoid fever. A wide range of infectious diseases must be considered next, such as shigellosis, meningococcal septicaemia, plague, leptospirosis, anthrax, relapsing fever, typhus, murine typhus, yellow fever, Chikungunya fever, Rift Valley fever, haemorrhagic fever with renal syndrome, Crimean–Congo haemorrhagic fever, Lassa fever and fulminant viral hepatitis. Travel, treatment in local hospitals, contact with sick people or wild and domestic monkeys are useful historical features in returning travellers, especially from Africa. Diagnosis of single cases is extremely difficult, but the occurrence of clusters of cases with prodromal fever followed by cases of haemorrhagic diatheses and person-to-person transmission are suggestive of viral haemorrhagic fever, and containment procedures have to be initiated. In filoviral haemorrhagic fever, prostration, lethargy, wasting and diarrhoea seem to be more severe than are observed in patients with other viral haemorrhagic fevers. The rash is characteristic and extremely useful in differential diagnosis.

Laboratory diagnosis can be achieved in 2 ways: measurement of the host-specific immune response to the infection; and detection of viral antigen and genomic RNA in the infected host (Table 32.3). The easiest and most commonly used assay to detect antibodies to filoviruses is the indirect immunofluorescence assay (IFA) on acetone-fixed infected cells inactivated by γ-irradiation. The use of this assay, however, has been quite misleading because a significant proportion of human and monkey sera will react with filovirus antigen without showing any symptoms of disease. A titre of at least 1 : 320 is required before an IFA test can be considered positive, and should be confirmed by another assay. Confirmatory tests include western blot (Becker et al. 1992, Elliott et al. 1993a), direct IgG and IgM enzyme-linked immunosorbent assays (ELISA) (Ksiazek 1991,

Table 32.3 Laboratory diagnosis

Test	Target	Source	Remarks
Indirect immunofluoresence assay (IFA)	Antiviral antibodies	Serum	Simple to perform, but prone to non-specific positives and subjective interpretation
Enzyme-linked immunosorbent assay (ELISA)	Antiviral antibodies	Serum	Specific and sensitive, but initial response slower than IFA
Immunoblot	Antiviral antibodies	Serum	Protein-specific, but interpretation sometimes difficult
Antigen ELISA	Viral antigen	Blood, serum, tissues	Rapid and sensitive, but requires special equipment
Immunohistochemistry	Viral antigen	Tissues (e.g. skin, liver)	Inactivated material, but requires time
Fluorescence assay (FA)	Viral antigen	Tissues (e.g. liver)	Rapid and easy, but interpretation is subjective
Polymerase chain reaction (PCR)	Viral nucleic acid	Blood, serum, tissues	Rapid and sensitive, but requires special equipment
Electron microscopy	Viral particle	Blood, tissues	Unique morphology (immunostaining possible), but insensitive and requires expensive equipment
Virus isolation	Viral particle	Blood, tissues	Virus available for studies, but requires time

Becker et al. 1992) and IgM capture assay (Ksiazek TG, personal communication).

Direct detection of virus antigen, virus particles and viral RNA can be achieved by several assays. Electron microscopy has been particularly useful in the diagnosis of filovirus infections (Siegert et al. 1967, Murphy et al. 1978, Jahrling et al. 1990). Viral structures can be visualized in culture fluid from initial passage cell cultures by negative staining, and in thin sections of any infected material. Immunohistochemistry on formalin-fixed material and paraffin-embedded tissues can be used for detection of filoviruses (Jahrling et al. 1990) as well as immunofluorescence on impression smears of tissues (Rollin et al. 1990). Antigen detection ELISA (Ksiazek et al. 1992) and RT-PCR (Sanchez and Feldmann 1996) have been used successfully to detect filoviruses in clinical material.

Attempts to isolate virus from serum or other clinical material should be performed using Vero or MA-104 cells (monkey kidney cells). However, most filoviruses do not cause an extensive cytopathic effect on primary isolation. Monkeys are the best animals for propagating filoviruses, but guinea-pigs are more cost-effective and convenient for primary isolation of filoviruses that initially do not grow well in tissue culture. Several passages in these animals is required to produce a uniformly fatal disease.

3.7 Patient management and control

There is no vaccination or chemotherapy against filovirus infections. Supportive therapy should be directed toward maintenance of effective blood volume and electrolyte balance. Shock, cerebral oedema, renal failure, coagulation disorders and secondary bacterial infection have to be managed and may be life-saving. Heparin treatment should be considered only in cases with clear evidence for DIC. Human interferon and human convalescence plasma have been used to treat patients, but there are no experimental data to support their use. On the contrary, filoviruses are resistant to the antiviral effects of interferon, and the administration of interferon to monkeys has failed to increase survival rate or achieve a reduction in virus titre. Ribavirin, a drug that is believed to interfere with capping of viral mRNAs, has no effect on filoviruses in vitro and is probably of no therapeutic value, which is in contrast to its effect with other viral haemorrhagic fevers.

Isolation of patients is recommended, and protection of medical and nursing staff is required. This can be achieved by strict barrier nursing techniques and the use of high-efficiency particulate air (HEPA) filter respirators for protection against aerosols when feasible. Detailed information has been published regarding the management of patients with suspected filoviral haemorrhagic fever and ways to minimize spread of virus outbreaks, especially in Africa (Centers for Disease Control and Prevention 1988, World Health Organization 1995b).

A protective vaccine would be extremely valuable for at-risk medical personnel in Africa and researchers working with infectious filoviruses. Cross-protection among different EBOV subtypes in experimental animal systems has been reported, suggesting a general value of vaccines (Bowen et al. 1980, Fisher-Hoch et al. 1992a). Inactivated vaccines have been developed with formalin or heat treatment of cell culture-propagated MBGV and EBOV (Sudan and Zaire subtypes) (Lupton et al. 1980, Agafonov et al. 1992). Because of the biohazard of filoviruses and the general lack of knowledge of the pathogenic processes involved in filovirus diseases, it is difficult to ensure the safety of attenuated strains of MBGV or EBOV. Immunizations of monkeys with purified NP and GP have induced humoral and cellular immune responses and protected animals against challenge with lethal doses. Those 2 proteins and perhaps the sGP (EBOV) may therefore be candidates for recombinant vaccines.

The importation of wild-caught monkeys is an important factor in the introduction of filoviruses into foreign human populations (Martini and Siegert 1971, Jahrling et al. 1990, World Health Organization 1992). Quarantine of imported non-human primates and professional handling and testing of these animals will help to minimize the risk of filovirus outbreaks in humans. Guidelines have been published for quarantine and proper handling of monkeys in medical research (Centers for Disease Control and Prevention 1990).

Filovirus infectivity is quite stable at room temperature (20°C), but is destroyed in 30 min at 60°C. Infectivity is also destroyed by UV and γ-irradiation, formalin (1%), lipid solvents (deoxycholate, ether), β-propiolactone, and hypochloric and phenolic disinfectants (Elliott et al. 1982, Centers for Disease Control and Prevention 1988, 1993).

REFERENCES

Agafonov AP, Ignatyev GM et al., 1992, The immunogenic properties of Marburg virus proteins, *Vopr Virusol*, **37**: 58–61.

Baron RC, McCormick JB, Zubeir OA, 1983, Ebola hemorrhagic fever in southern Sudan: hospital dissemination and intrafamilial spread, *Bull W H O*, **61**: 997–1003.

Baskerville A, Fisher-Hoch SP et al., 1985, Ultrastructural pathology of experimental Ebola haemorrhagic fever virus infection, *J Pathol*, **147**: 199–209.

Becker S, Spiess M, Klenk HD, 1995, The asialoglycoprotein receptor is a potential liver-specific receptor for Marburg virus, *J Gen Virol*, **76**: 393–9.

Becker S, Feldmann H et al., 1992, Evidence for occurrence of

filovirus antibodies in humans and imported monkeys: do subclinical filovirus infections occur worldwide? *Med Microbiol Immunol*, **181**: 43–55.

Becker S, Huppertz S et al., 1994, The nucleoprotein of Marburg virus is phosphorylated, *J Gen Virol*, **75**: 809–18.

Bowen ETW, Platt GS et al., 1980, A comparative study of strains of Ebola virus isolated from southern Sudan and northern Zaire in 1976, *J Med Virol*, **6**: 129–38.

Buchmeier MJ, DeFries R et al., 1983, Comparative analysis of the structural polypeptides of Ebola virus from Sudan and Zaire, *J Infect Dis*, **147**: 276–81.

Bukreyev AA, Volchkov VE et al., 1993, The VP35 and VP40 proteins of filoviruses: homology between Marburg and Ebola viruses, *FEBS Lett*, **322**: 41–6.

Bukreyev AA, Volchkov VE et al., 1995, The nucleotide sequence of the Popp (1967) strain of Marburg virus: a comparison with the Musoke (1980) strain, *Arch Virol*, **140**: 1589–600.

Centers for Disease Control and Prevention, 1988, Management of patients with suspected viral hemorrhagic fever, *Morbid Mortal Weekly Rep*, **37, suppl 3**: 1–16.

Centers for Disease Control and Prevention, 1990, Update: Ebola-related filovirus infection in nonhuman primates and interim guidelines for handling nonhuman primates during transit and quarantine, *Morbid Mortal Weekly Rep*, **39 (2)**: 22–24, 29–30.

Centers for Disease Control and Prevention, 1993, *Biosafety in Microbiology and Biomedical Laboratories*, US Department of Health and Human Services (HHS), publication (CDC) 93-8395, US Government Printing Office, Washington DC.

Centers for Disease Control and Prevention, 1996, Ebola-Reston virus infection among quarantined nonhuman primates – Texas, 1996, *Morb Mortal Weekly Rep*, **45**: 314–6.

Cox NJ, McCormick JB et al., 1983, Evidence for two subtypes of Ebola virus based on oligonucleotide mapping of RNA, *J Infect Dis*, **147**: 272–5.

Elliott LH, Kiley MP, McCormick JB, 1985, Descriptive analysis of Ebola virus proteins, *Virology*, **147**: 169–76.

Elliott LH, McCormick JB, Johnson KM, 1982, Inactivation of Lassa, Marburg, and Ebola viruses by gamma irradiation, *J Clin Microbiol*, **16**: 704–8.

Elliott LH, Bauer SP et al., 1993a, Improved specificity of testing methods for filovirus antibodies, *J Virol Methods*, **43**: 85–100.

Elliott LH, Sanchez A et al., 1993b, Ebola protein analysis for the determination of genetic organization, *Arch Virol*, **133**: 423–36.

Feldmann H, Klenk HD, Sanchez A, 1993, Molecular biology and evolution of filoviruses, *Arch Virol*, **suppl 7**: 81–100.

Feldmann H, Will C et al., 1991, Glycosylation and oligomerization of the spike protein of Marburg virus, *Virology*, **182**: 353–6.

Feldmann H, Mühlberger E et al., 1992, Marburg virus, a filovirus: messenger RNAs, gene order, and regulatory elements of the replication cycle, *Virus Res*, **24**: 1–19.

Feldmann H, Nichol ST et al., 1994, Characterization of filoviruses based on differences in structure and antigenicity of the virion glycoprotein, *Virology*, **199**: 469–73.

Feldmann H, Bugany H et al., 1996a, Filovirus-induced endothelial leakage triggered by infected monocytes/ macrophages, *J Virol*, **70**: 2208–14.

Feldmann H, Slenczka W, Klenk H-D, 1996b, Emerging and reemerging of filoviruses, *Arch Virol*, **suppl 11**: 77–100.

Fisher-Hoch SP, Platt GS et al., 1985, Pathophysiology of shock and hemorrhage in a fulminating viral infection (Ebola), *J Infect Dis*, **152**: 887–94.

Fisher-Hoch SP, Brammer L et al., 1992a, Pathogenic potential of filoviruses: role of geographic origin of primate host and virus strain, *J Infect Dis*, **166**: 753–63.

Fisher-Hoch SP, Perez-Oronoz GI et al., 1992b, Filovirus clearance in non-human primates, *Lancet*, **340**: 451–3.

Funke C, Becker S et al., 1995, Acylation of the Marburg virus glycoprotein, *Virology*, **208**: 289–97.

Gear JSS, Cassel GA et al., 1975, Outbreak of Marburg virus disease in Johannesburg, *Br Med J*, **4**: 489–93.

Geisbert TW, Jahrling PB et al., 1992, Association of Ebola-related Reston virus particles and antigen with tissue lesions of monkeys imported to the United States, *J Comp Pathol*, **106**: 137–52.

Geyer H, Will C et al., 1992, Carbohydrate structure of Marburg virus glycoprotein, *Glycobiology*, **2**: 299–312.

van der Groen G, Johnson KM et al., 1978, Results of Ebola antibody survey in various population groups, *Ebola Virus Hemorrhagic Fever*, ed Pattyn SR, Elsevier/North-Holland, Amsterdam, 203–8.

Hayes CG, Burans JP et al., 1992, Outbreak of fatal illness among captive macaques in the Philippines caused by an Ebola-related filovirus, *Am J Trop Med Hyg*, **46**: 664–71.

Heymann DL, Weisfeld JS et al., 1980, Ebola hemorrhagic fever: Tandala Zaire, 1977–78, *J Infect Dis*, **142**: 372–6.

Jahrling PB, Geisbert TW et al., 1990, Preliminary report: isolation of Ebola virus from monkeys imported to USA, *Lancet*, **335**: 502–5.

Kiley MP, Bowen ETW et al., 1982, Filoviridae: a taxonomic home for Marburg and Ebola viruses? *Intervirology*, **18**: 24–32.

Kiley MP, Wilusz J et al., 1986, Conservation of the 3′ terminal nucleotide sequence of Ebola and Marburg viruses, *Virology*, **149**: 251–4.

Kiley MP, Cox NJ et al., 1988, Physicochemical properties of Marburg virus: evidence for three distinct virus strains and their relationship to Ebola virus, *J Gen Virol*, **69**: 1957–67.

Ksiazek TG, 1991, Laboratory diagnosis of filovirus infections in non-human primates, *Lab Anim*, **20**: 34–46.

Ksiazek TG, Rollin PE et al., 1992, Enzyme immunosorbent assay for Ebola virus antigens in tissues of infected primates. *J Clin Microbiol*, **30**: 947–50.

LeGuenno B, Formentry P et al., 1995, Isolation and partial characterization of a new strain of Ebola virus, *Lancet*, **345**: 1271–4.

Lupton HW, Lambert RD et al., 1980, Inactivated vaccine for Ebola virus efficacious in guinea pig model, *Lancet*, **2**: 1294–5.

McCormick JB, Bauer SP et al., 1983, Biological differences between strains of Ebola virus from Zaire and Sudan, *J Infect Dis*, **147**: 264–7.

Martini GA, Siegert R, 1971, *Marburg Virus Disease*, Springer-Verlag, New York.

Mühlberger E, Sanchez A et al., 1992, The nucleotide sequence of the L gene of Marburg virus, a filovirus: homologies with paramyxoviruses and rhabdoviruses, *Virology*, **187**: 534–47.

Mühlberger E, Trommer S et al., 1996, Termini of all mRNA species of Marburg virus: sequence and secondary structure, *Virology* **223**: 376–80.

Murphy FA, Simpson DIH et al., 1971, Marburg virus infection in monkeys, *Lab Invest*, **24**: 279–91.

Murphy FA, van der Groen G et al., 1978, Ebola and Marburg virus morphology and taxonomy, *Ebola Virus Hemorrhagic Fever*, ed Pattyn SR, Elsevier/North-Holland, Amsterdam, 61–84.

Murphy FA, Fauquet CM et al., 1995, Virus taxonomy: classification and nomenclature of viruses, Sixth Report of the International Committee on Taxonomy of Viruses, *Arch Virol*, **suppl 10**: 265–92.

Pattyn SR, ed, 1978, *Ebola Virus Hemorrhagic Fever*, Elsevier/North-Holland, Amsterdam.

Peters CJ, Johnson ED, McKee KT, 1991, Filoviruses and management of viral hemorrhagic fevers, *Textbook of Human Virology*, ed Belshe RB, Mosby Year Book, St Louis MO, 699–712.

Peters CJ, Jahrling PB et al., 1992, Filovirus contamination of cell cultures, *Dev Biol Stand*, **76**: 267–74.

Peters CJ, Johnson ED et al., 1993, Filoviruses, *Emerging Viruses*, ed Morse SS, Oxford University Press, Oxford, 159–75.

Peters CJ, Sanchez A et al., 1996, *Filoviridae*: Marburg and Ebola viruses, *Fields' Virology*, 3rd edn, eds Fields BN, Knipe DM et al., Raven Press, New York, 1161–76.

Peters D, Müller G, Slenczka W, 1971, Morphology, development, and classification of Marburg virus, *Marburg Virus Disease*, eds Martini GA, Siegert R, Springer-Verlag, New York, 68–83.

Pokhodyaeu VA, Gonchar NI, Pshenichnov VA, 1991, Experimental study of Marburg virus contact transmission, *Vopr Virusol*, **36**: 506–8.

Regnery RL, Johnson KM, Kiley MP, 1980, Virion nucleic acid of Ebola virus, *J Virol*, **36**: 465–9.

Richman DD, Cleveland PH et al., 1983, Antigenic analysis of strains of Ebola viruses: identification of two Ebola virus subtypes, *J Infect Dis*, **147**: 268–71.

Rollin PE, Ksiazek TG et al., 1990, Detection of Ebola-like viruses by immunofluorescence, *Lancet*, **336**: 1591.

Ryabchikova EI, Kolesnikova LV et al., 1994, Ebola infection in four monkey species, *Ninth International Conference on Negative Strand RNA Viruses*, Estoril, Portugal, Abstract 246: 164.

Sanchez A, Feldmann H, 1996, Detection of Marburg and Ebola virus infections by polymerase chain reaction assays, *Frontiers of Virology – Diagnosis of human viruses by polymerase chain reaction technology*, 2nd edn, eds Becker Y, Darai G, Springer-Verlag, Berlin, Heidelberg, New York, 411–18.

Sanchez A, Kiley MP, 1987, Identification and analysis of Ebola virus messenger RNAs, *Virology*, **157**: 414–20.

Sanchez A, Kiley MP et al., 1989, The nucleoprotein gene of Ebola virus: cloning, sequencing, and in vitro expression, *Virology*, **170**: 81–91.

Sanchez A, Kiley MP et al., 1992, Sequence analysis of the Marburg virus nucleoprotein gene: comparison to Ebola virus and other non-segmented negative-strand RNA viruses, *J Gen Virol*, **73**, 347–57.

Sanchez A, Kiley MP et al., 1993, Sequence analysis of the Ebola virus genome: organization, genetic elements, and comparison with the genome of Marburg virus, *Virus Res*, **29**: 215–40.

Sanchez A, Trappier S et al., 1996, Glycoprotein genes of Ebola viruses: unusual organization and mechanisms of gene expression, *Proc Natl Acad Sci USA*, **93**: 3602–7.

Schnittler HJ, Mahner F et al., 1993, Replication of Marburg virus in human endothelial cells. A possible mechanism for the development of viral hemorrhagic disease, *J Clin Invest*, **91**: 1301–9.

Siegert R, Shu H-L et al., 1967, Zur äthiologie einer unbekannten von Affen ausgegangenen Infektionskrankheit, *Dtsch Med Wochenschr*, **92**: 2341–3.

Smith DH, Johnson BK et al., 1982, Marburg-virus disease in Kenya, *Lancet*, **1**: 816–20.

Trappier SG, Nichol ST et al., 1996, Genetic diversity in the glycoprotein genes of filoviruses, *15th Annual Meeting of the American Society for Virology*, ASV, London, Ontario, W34-1: 142.

Volchkov VE, Blinov VM, Netesov SV, 1992, The envelope glycoprotein of Ebola virus contains an immunosuppressive-like domain similar to oncogenic retroviruses, *FEBS Lett*, **305**: 181–4.

Volchkov VE, Becker S et al., 1995, GP mRNA of Ebola virus is edited by the Ebola virus polymerase and by T7 and vaccinia virus polymerases, *Virology*, **214**: 421–30.

Will C, Mühlberger E et al., 1993, Marburg virus gene four encodes for the virion membrane protein, a type I transmembrane glycoprotein, *J Virol*, **67**: 1203–10.

World Health Organization, 1978a, Ebola haemorrhagic fever in Sudan, 1976, *Bull WHO*, **56**: 247–70.

World Health Organization, 1978b, Ebola haemorrhagic fever in Zaire, 1976, *Bull WHO*, **56**: 271–93.

World Health Organization, 1992, Viral hemorrhagic fever in imported monkeys, *Wkly Epidemiol Rec*, **67**: 142–3.

World Health Organization, 1995a, Ebola haemorrhagic fever, *Wkly Epidemiol Rec*, **70**: 241–2.

World Health Organization, 1995b, Viral haemorrhagic fever – management of suspected cases, *Wkly Epidemiol Rec*, **70**: 249–56.

World Health Organization, 1996a, Outbreak of Ebola hemorrhagic fever in Gabon officially declared over. *Wkly Epidemiol Rec*, **71**: 125–6.

World Health Organization, 1996b, Ebola haemorrhagic fever, Gabon, *Wkly Epidemiol Rec*, **71**: 125–6.

World Health Organization, 1997, Ebola haemorrhagic fever – a summary of the outbreak in Gabon, *Wkly Epidemiol Rec*, **72**: 7–8.

Zaki S, 1995, Pathology of Ebola virus hemorrhagic fever, *European Conference on Tropical Medicine*, Hamburg, Germany, Abstract 22: 3.

Chapter 33

RHABDOVIRUSES: RABIES

N Tordo, K Charlton and A Wandeler

1 INTRODUCTION

The family *Rhabdoviridae* (from Greek *rhabdos*: rod) contains more than 200 viruses whose hosts vary widely among vertebrates, invertebrates and plants (Murphy et al. 1995) in which they give rise to various diseases (Fig. 33.1). This variability contrasts strongly with their striking similarity in morphology, structure and mechanisms of replication. Another common feature is that all members present a danger to humans, not only from direct disease but also from livestock and crop losses.

Arthropods are their most frequent vectors and probable original reservoirs, from which they adapted to plants and vertebrates. Traces of this evolution still exist: the sigma virus exclusively infects the fruitfly *Drosophila*; the plant rhabdoviruses have mixed arthropod–plant cycles; vesiculoviruses, ephemeroviruses and several lyssaviruses undergo mixed insect–mammal cycles; and some evidence even suggests that an aquatic arthropod could be involved in the transmission of fish rhabdovirus. Several insect species replicate both vertebrate and plant rhabdoviruses, but a triple insect–plant–vertebrate cycle has not so far been observed. Finally, rabies and rabies-related viruses became more narrowly adapted and now infect only mammals. The vast majority of rhabdoviruses are transmitted mechanically: in plants by injury or through arthropod or worm vectors and in vertebrates by aerosols, contact, bite or sexual transmission. A few viruses (e.g. the sigma virus of *Drosophila*) are vertically transmitted.

For historical reasons, studies on rabies virus contributed greatly to the development of vaccines, pathology and analysis of the immune response. Studies on vesicular stomatitis virus, which is comparatively safe to handle and replicates readily in most cell types, have provided much useful biochemical, biophysical and molecular data. The fish, plant and cattle rhabdoviruses, for long neglected, have recently attracted increased attention because of their economic importance.

2 PROPERTIES OF THE VIRUSES

2.1 The *Rhabdoviridae*

The family *Rhabdoviridae* belongs to the *Mononegavirales* order, which also embraces the families *Paramyxoviridae* and *Filoviridae*. These viruses share a linear non-segmented RNA genome of negative polarity embedded within a helical ribonucleoprotein complex (RNP). The criteria for rhabdovirus classification have been progressively sharpened, taking into account physical, chemical and structural properties, antigenicity and, finally, genetics. The viruses were first grouped into genera or other groups by serological cross-reactions between internal antigens and their antibodies. Subdivision into serotypes was performed by cross-reaction between envelope antigens (Schneider et al. 1973). The use of monoclonal antibodies further refined the classification (Rupprecht et al. 1991). Molecular biology techniques permitted phylogenetic studies and the definition of genotypes (Bourhy et al. 1993a, Morzunov et al. 1995, Tordo, Bourhy and Sacramento 1995, Wang, Cowley and Walker 1995). However, a considerable number of rhabdoviruses remain, classified only roughly on the basis of morphology, host or geographical distribution, or pathological features. Further analysis is needed to justify their inclusion in existing groups or the creation of new ones.

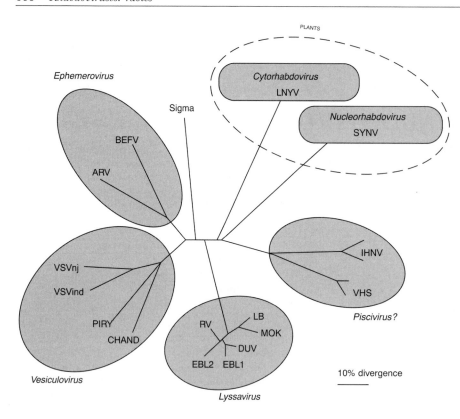

Fig. 33.1 Radial phylogenetic tree of the *Rhabdoviridae* family established from N protein sequence alignment using the Clustalw program (neighbour joining method). Grey circles outline the genera. ARV, Adelaide River virus; BEFV, bovine ephemeral fever virus; CHAND, Chandipura virus; DUV, Duvenhage virus; EBL1 and EBL2, European bat Lyssavirus, types 1 and 2; IHNV, infectious haematopoietic necrosis virus; LB, Lagos bat virus; LNYV, lettuce necrotic yellow virus; MOK, Mokola virus; PIRY, piry virus; RV, rabies virus; Sigma, sigma virus; SYNV, sonchus yellow net virus; VHS, viral haemorrhagic septicaemia; VSVind, vesicular stomatitis virus, Indiana; VSVnj, vesicular stomatitis virus, New Jersey.

Genus *Vesiculovirus*

The main member of the genus *Vesiculovirus* (Latin *vesicula*: blister) is vesicular stomatitis virus (VSV), which is frequently designated as the prototype of the entire family *Rhabdoviridae*. Five or 6 serotypes have been characterized, of which Indiana and New Jersey are the most recent (Murphy et al, 1995). VSV causes a febrile illness in cattle, horses and pigs, characterized by the appearance of blisters in the mouth which rapidly ulcerate (see section 3, p. 675). Similar lesions are caused by other 'vesicular viruses', which include members of other families: for example, *Picornaviridae* (foot-and-mouth disease and swine vesicular disease) and *Caliciviridae* (vesicular exanthema virus). These viruses, of great economic importance for farming, are readily distinguished by morphological or serological criteria.

Genus *Lyssavirus*

Until 1956 and the first isolations of rabies-related viruses in Africa (King, Meredith and Thomson 1994) and Europe (Schneider and Cox 1994), rabies virus (RV) was believed to be antigenically unique. This warranted the creation of the genus *Lyssavirus* (Greek *lyssa*: rabies) for viruses responsible for rabies-like encephalitis. The genus was at first divided into 4 serotypes by antigenic cross-reactivity with sera and monoclonal antibodies, but European bat lyssavirus (EBL) isolates remained unclassified (Dietzschold et al. 1988, Rupprecht et al. 1991, WHO 1992). Phylogenetic analysis of the nucleoprotein and glycoprotein genes further delineated 6 genotypes, the first 4 of which matched the serotypes (1) rabies, (2) Lagos bat, (3)

Mokola and (4) Duvenhage. The other 2 genotypes are EBL types 1 (5) and 2 (6) (Bourhy et al. 1993a).

Genotype 1 corresponds to classic RV. It encompasses laboratory strains used for vaccine seed or control (Challenge Virus Standard, CVS) and many viruses isolated from various rabid domestic or wild animals world-wide. Members of genotypes 2–6 are rabies-related viruses which so far have been isolated only in the Old World. They have a narrower geographic distribution than rabies and, although they occasionally infect humans and domestic animals, they seem to infect preferentially certain specific host species. Lagos bat, Mokola and Duvenhage viruses were isolated in sub-Saharan Africa, principally from frugivorous bats, small mammals (shrews and rodents) and insectivorous bats, respectively (King, Meredith and Thomson 1994). EBL1 and EBL2 are spreading widely in Europe, from the former USSR to Spain, and mainly infect insectivorous bats of the *Eptesicus* and *Myotis* species, respectively (Bourhy et al. 1992, 1993a, Schneider and Cox 1994).

In May 1996 a new lyssavirus was isolated from fruit-eating bats (flying foxes, *Pteropus alecto*) on the eastern coast of Australia, a country considered to be rabies-free since 1867. The same virus was also isolated from 2 other species of *Pteropus*, and from an insectivorous bat. In November 1996 a fatal case of human encephalitis caused by this new Australian bat lyssavirus was confirmed. Preliminary genetic and antigenic analysis of the virus as well as cross-seroneutralization suggested that this lyssavirus is closer to genotype 1, but distinct.

From the epizootiological point of view, rabies is

maintained and transmitted by mammalian species serving as reservoirs and vectors (Baer 1991a) (see section 4.3, p. 677). They are distinguished from other mammals which, although susceptible to infection, constitute epidemiological culs-de-sac. Rabies exists in 2 major epidemiological forms: (1) canine rabies, of which stray dogs are the vectors, is responsible for >95% of the human cases in developing countries (Plotkin 1992, Meslin, Fishbein and Matter 1994); and (2) sylvatic rabies, which involves wildlife world-wide. The wild vectors vary geographically and include terrestrial mammals and bats, the latter being possible vectors for most *Lyssavirus* genotypes. Polymerase chain reaction (PCR) technology has revolutionized the analysis of lyssavirus field isolates (Benmansour et al. 1992, Sacramento et al. 1992, Smith et al. 1992, Tordo, Bourhy and Sacramento 1992, 1995, Bourhy, Kissi and Tordo 1993, Bourhy et al. 1993, Nadin-Davies, Casey and Wandeler 1993, 1994, Kissi, Tordo and Bourhy 1995, Nel, Thomson and von Teicham 1993, Smith, Yager and Orciari 1993, Tordo et al. 1993a). In particular, phylogenetic analysis of genotype 1 strains (classic rabies) isolated world-wide indicated that they fall into various groups according to (1) geographical origin, (2) whether they are cosmopolitan or indigenous strains and (3) their vectors, suggesting that several variants are very well adapted to their hosts (e.g. vampire bat in Latin America, arctic fox in arctic regions).

GENUS *EPHEMEROVIRUS*

The genus *Ephemerovirus* was recently created to accommodate viruses in tropical and subtropical areas transmitted by haematophagous insects to cattle and water buffalo (Walker et al. 1992, 1994, Wunner et al. 1994). The name came from the prototype 'bovine ephemeral fever virus' (BEFV), which was initially reported to cause a brief, transient fever. However, ephemeroviruses have also been isolated from healthy insects and cattle, as well as from cattle with acute febrile illnesses of major economic importance. BEFV has been found in Australia, Japan, China and South Africa. Adelaide river (ARV), Kimberley and Berrimah viruses have been isolated in Australia, Makalal virus in Kenya and Puchong virus in Malaysia (Calisher et al. 1989).

Ephemeroviruses are genetically closer to vesiculoviruses (Wang, Cowley and Walker 1995) but are antigenically related to: (1) the unclassified rhabdoviruses Obodhiang, Kotonkan and Kolongo that were isolated from, respectively, mosquitoes in the Sudan, midges in Nigeria and birds in Central African Republic; and (2) the rabies-related Lagos bat virus (Calisher et al. 1989). Obodhiang and Kotonkan are in turn serologically linked to the rabies-related Mokola virus (Calisher et al. 1989), which is the only lyssavirus replicating in *Aedes albopictus* cell cultures (Buckley 1975). Taken together, these data suggest that Obodhiang and Kotonkan viruses may occupy an intermediate position between the genus *Lyssavirus*, adapted to mammals, and the genus *Ephemerovirus*, which has maintained a mixed arthropod–mammal cycle.

PLANT RHABDOVIRUSES

Although c. 100 plant viruses are listed as possible rhabdoviruses, their poor immunogenicity has hampered serological grouping. They are named according to the lesions they cause (e.g. necrosis, yellowing, mosaic). Most are still classified according to the type of arthropod vector (aphid, leafhopper, etc.) (Jackson, Francki and Zuidema 1987). Their transmission is mechanical, via arthropod or worm vectors, and most of those examined replicate efficiently in these vectors (Jackson et al. 1987). Two genera have so far been distinguished on replicative criteria. Members of the genus *Cytorhabdovirus* (prototype: lettuce necrotic yellows virus, LNYV) replicate in the cytoplasm in association with viroplasms, and their morphogenesis takes place in vesicles of the endoplasmic reticulum. Members of the genus *Nucleorhabdovirus* (prototype: sonchus yellow net virus, SYNV) replicate in the nucleus, morphogenesis takes place at the inner nuclear envelope and virions accumulate in the perinuclear spaces (Murphy et al. 1995).

FISH RHABDOVIRUSES

The rhabdoviruses of fish cause haematopoietic necrosis, haemorrhagic septicaemia, dropsy, swim bladder inflammation and hydrocephalus, diseases of major economic importance to the fish farming industry. They were initially classified as vesiculoviruses or lyssaviruses on the basis of structural similarities in protein composition and size. Recent phylogenetic analyses suggest placing them in a separate genus, *Piscivirus* (Benmansour et al. 1994, Morzunov, Winston and Nichol 1995, Schütze et al. 1995). Fish rhabdoviruses grow in cell cultures at the ambient temperature of fish. They may be transmitted by an aquatic arthropod.

SIGMA VIRUS

Sigma virus is unique among the rhabdoviruses. It is a hereditary factor endemic in 20% of natural populations of the fruitfly *Drosophila*, in which it is propagated via the gametes. Sigma virus is not cytopathic and only slightly pathogenic in the infected flies, except that it confers sensitivity to CO_2. Replication is partly under the control of an antiviral host gene, *ref(2)P*, which is also required for male fertility (Dezélée et al. 1989). It has been suggested that sigma was a rhabdovirus trapped by a non-biting fly and behaved as a hereditary factor to ensure its own survival (Brun 1984).

BIRD RHABDOVIRUSES

There have been rare isolations of rhabdoviruses from birds in Central Africa and India. Very little is known from them, except that they replicate quite efficiently in insect cells (Zeller and Mitchell 1989).

2.2 Morphology and chemical composition

MORPHOLOGY

Under the electron microscope (Fig. 33.2), animal rhabdoviruses are usually bullet-shaped with one round end and the other flat; plant rhabdoviruses are more frequently bacilliform (Figs 33.2 and 33.3); a few examples of conical forms have been observed in Obhodiang, Kotonkan and bovine ephemeral fever viruses and sometimes in RV. The virion diameter is almost constant (50–100 nm), but lengths vary (100–430 nm), depending on the species or on the presence of defective interfering (DI) particles, which appear when the multiplicity of infection is high. The DI particles possess a truncated genome, are therefore defective in various viral functions, and must depend on infectious virions to complement their deficiency (Lazzarini, Keene and Schubert 1981). Their smaller genomes compete efficiently with normal genomes for replication and packaging into virions. Although their role during natural infection remains unclear, these subgenomic deletion mutants have been mimicked extensively to generate non-infectious recombinant viruses for reverse genetic studies (reviewed by Conzelmann 1996).

The virion is composed of 2 structural units (Fig. 33.4). One is a **central cylinder** 50 nm in diameter with characteristic cross-striations composed of a tightly coiled ribonucleoprotein complex (RNP) with helical symmetry. This is contained within the second unit, a **lipoprotein membrane** 8 nm thick that is provided by the cell membrane during budding, and through which protrudes an array of knobbed glycoprotein spikes 10 nm in length.

CHEMICAL COMPOSITION

The chemical composition is c. 74% proteins, 20% lipids (composition dependent on the host cell), 3% carbohydrates and 3% RNA. The RNA is a single molecule of negative polarity (i.e. non-infectious). There are 5 major viral proteins with post-translational modifications that have been assigned either to the envelope or to the RNP structures by biochemical dissection of the virion with proteases and detergents (Delagneau, Perrin and Atanasin 1981, Tordo and Poch 1988b). From outside to inside:

1 The glycoprotein is glycosylated, and acylated with palmitic acid. It is membrane-anchored and constitutes the protruding spikes, each composed of 3 glycosylated ectodomains (Delagneau, Perrin and Atanasin 1981, Gaudin et al. 1992).

2 The central RNP is formed by an intimate association between the nucleoprotein (phosphorylated in RV) and the RNA genome, which is thereby rendered insensitive to nucleases. The heavily phosphorylated phosphoprotein and the large protein (polymerase) are also bound to the RNP, although less intimately.

3 The exact position of the palmytoylated and phosphorylated matrix protein remains controversial. It is unclear if it is embedded in the inner layer of the membrane, in the central axial channel of the RNP, or both (Barge et al. 1993, Gaudin et al. 1995a).

Recent data on RV and VSV suggest that matrix protein is both necessary and sufficient to impart the typical bullet shape (Justice et al. 1995, Lyles et al. 1996).

For historical reasons, the nomenclature of the 5 basic proteins differs between viruses; reports of their relative number per virion also vary owing to the different assay techniques used (reviewed by Coll 1995). Despite these discrepancies the proteins have similar functions and similar molecular weights. We shall use the conventional abbreviations N for nucleoprotein (50–55 kDa), P for phosphoprotein (35–40 kDa), M for matrix protein (25 kDa), G for glycoprotein (60–70 kDa) and L for the large polymerase (c. 200 kDa).

Besides these main viral proteins, several rhabdoviruses have developed additional polypeptides for

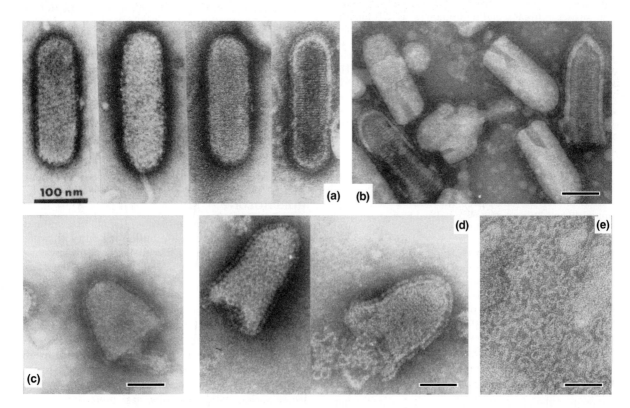

Fig. 33.2 Electron micrographs of rhabdoviruses. (a) Plant rhabdoviruses. (Courtesy of AO Jackson.) (b) Vesiculovirus. (c) Lyssavirus (rabies virus, PV strain). (d) Lyssavirus (Mokola); one damaged virion with ribonucleocapsid protruding from the basis). (e) Ribonucleocapsid RNP. All scale bars = 100 nm.

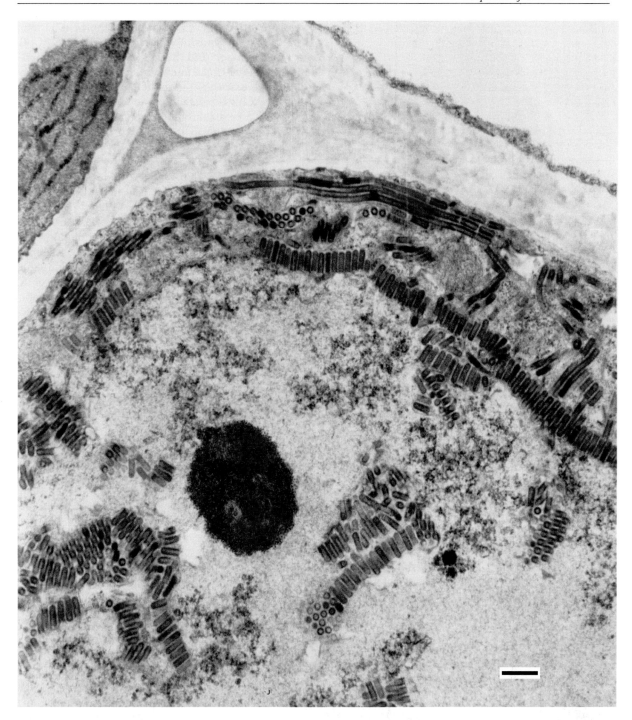

Fig. 33.3 Eggplant mottle dwarf virus within a cell nucleus. Note the long bacillary forms near the nuclear membrane. Bar = 4.5 μm. (Courtesy of R Hull.)

specific functions (see 'Implications for the structure of the genome', p. 673, and Fig. 33.7). These additional proteins are rarely found in the viral particle, suggesting their involvement in replicative functions or interaction with the host cell. Conversely, several cellular proteins are reported as being packaged in the RV and VSV virions, for example cellular kinases playing a major role in activation of the phosphoprotein for replicative functions (Gao and Lenard 1995b, Gupta, Das and Banerjee 1995) and heat shock proteins (Sagara and Kawai 1992). Cytoskeleton-associated proteins such as actin-binding proteins (from the ezrin–radizin–moesin family) are closely associated with the membrane glycoprotein and thereby promote incorporation of actin into the virion (Sagara et al. 1995). Their involvement in virion formation during the budding process is likely but the role of the cytoskeleton in the replication process remains unclear.

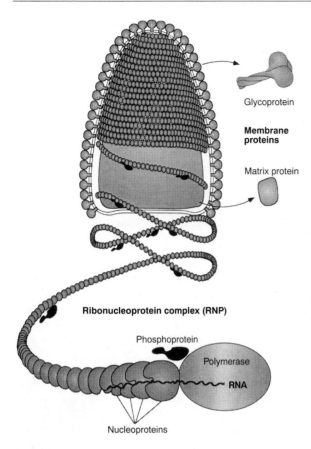

Fig. 33.4 Structure of the virion.

2.3 Infection cycle in the cell

Except for the sigma virus of *Drosophila*, which is passed vertically, the vast majority of rhabdoviruses are transmitted mechanically by injury, contacts, bite or aerosols. Tissue tropisms and pathogenicity vary with individual viruses. The main steps of cell infection, shared by all the rhabdoviruses, will now be described (Fig. 33.5). It should be noted that the data come mainly from studies on VSV and to some extent on RV; current researches on other rhabdoviruses may reveal variations.

Penetration into the cell

The attachment of the virus to the susceptible cell membrane is thought to be mediated by the trimers of glycoproteins, which recognize a specific receptor(s) (Coll 1995). There is, however, little evidence for variation in cell surface receptors as the only determinant of cellular specificity, even for very selective viruses such as the neurotropic RV. Indeed, cell susceptibility also depends on the intracellular environment required for replication. The accumulated data suggest complex receptor(s): phosphatidyl serine is important for VSV (Schlegel et al. 1983). Several studies indicate that the nicotinic acetylcholine receptor (AChR) is a receptor for RV (review: Baer and Lentz 1991). However, there is evidence that, in addition to the nicotinic AChR, other receptors (as yet undefined) bind RV and probably function in vivo.

Reagan and Wunner (1985) and Tsiang et al. (1986) found that RV binds to cells that do not have AChR (review: Wunner and Reagan 1986). From experiments with the Challenge Virus Standard (CVS) strain of RV and its avirulent mutant, AVO1, it was suggested that the AChR is not the unique receptor for RV, that CVS should be able to bind several receptors and that AVO1 is restricted in the types of neurons that can be penetrated (Lafay et al. 1991, review: Coulon et al. 1994).

Other studies to characterize cellular receptors for RV implicated carbohydrate moieties, phospholipids and gangliosides (review: Tsiang 1993). In a study using a solubilized preparation of normal rat brain, gangliosides were important but phospholipids were not always required; a role for proteins in virus binding could not be demonstrated (Conti et al. 1988). However, Broughan and Wunner (1995) recently demonstrated involvement of a cellular membrane protein or protein complex in virus binding to BHK-21 cells. The high molecular weight protein of an *n*-octylglucoside plasma membrane extract co-migrated with bovine fibronectin after reducing polyacrylamide gel electrophoresis.

Once bound, the virus is internalized into a cellular endosome. Then, as the pH decreases within the endosome, it fuses with the viral membrane and the RNP is freed into the cytoplasm. Fusion requires only the reduction in pH and no specific elements such as receptors or specific phospholipid (Perrin, Portnoi and Sureau 1982). The fusion ability depends on progressive conformational changes of the glycoprotein that have been measured by electron microscopy, sensitivity to proteases and monoclonal antibody assays (Gaudin et al. 1991b, 1993, Gaudin, Ruigrok and Brunner 1995). Two steps can be identified: (1) up to pH 6.7, hydrophobic regions of the glycoprotein start to interact with the membrane; and (2) under pH 6.2 fusion is complete. It is interesting that, in the absence of the target membrane, the conformational change occurs but the modified glycoprotein loses its fusion ability. However, this conformational change is reversible by raising the pH. Indeed, the fusion-active and fusion-inactive forms of the G protein are in dynamic equilibrium, 50% of each at pH 6.7, whereas at lower pH there is a shift toward the inactive form (Gaudin, Ruigrok and Brunner 1995). Once delivered into the cytoplasm the RNP is ready to serve as a template for gene expression. In the particular case of neuron infection by RV, the RNP is first transported by retrograde axonal flow and replicates only in the perikaryon. Expression takes place exclusively in the cytoplasm. Only a limited number of viral transcripts or proteins reach the nucleus, where they generally participate in the inhibition of host cell machinery, the degree of which depends on the virus concerned. VSV is deleterious to all types of cell, whereas such effects do not occur in most types infected with RV. This explains the preferential use of VSV for molecular studies.

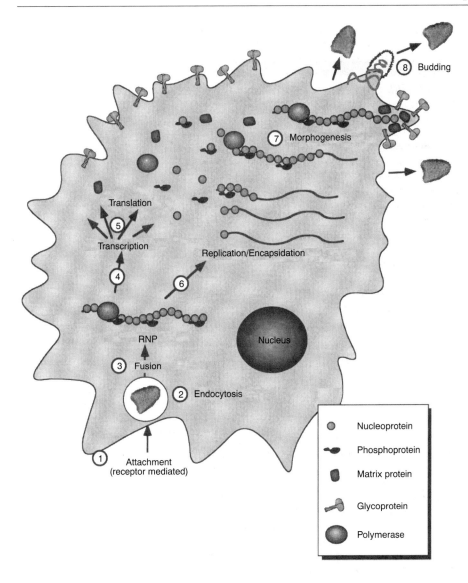

8 Budding

7 Morphogenesis

Translation

5

Transcription

Replication/Encapsidation

4

6

RNP

Nucleus

3 Fusion

2 Endocytosis

1 Attachment
(receptor mediated)

○ Nucleoprotein

Phosphoprotein

Matrix protein

Glycoprotein

● Polymerase

Fig. 33.5 Example of the rhabdoviral cell infection cycle (rabies virus).

Mechanism of genome expression

Because the rhabdovirus genome has negative polarity it must be transcribed to produce the complementary positive-strand mRNAs. The RNP serves as template for 2 successive RNA synthetic functions (Fig. 33.6): transcription then replication. For both, the viral polymerase seems to recognize the same promoter at the 3' end of the encapsidated genome, and to proceed toward the 5' end. The difference between transcription and replication is determined by the way in which the polymerase progresses either sequentially or continuously (reviews: Banerjee 1987, Tordo and Poch 1988b, Vidal and Kolakofsky 1989, Banerjee and Barik 1992, Tordo and Kouznetzoff 1993). Transcription gives rise to mostly monocistronic transcripts: first a short non-capped, non-polyadenylated leader RNA, then 5 (or more) mRNAs coding for the viral proteins (Fig. 33.6). This sequential progression depends on the recognition of short conserved signals, bordering the cistrons, which initiate start (and capping) and stop (and polyadenylation) of the mRNAs. It is thought that the transcriptase stops transcribing at each polyadenylation signal, scans through the

intergenic region, and recommences transcribing poorly at the next capping signal, resulting in a progressively decreased transcription rate. The length of the scanned intergenic region could itself influence the efficiency of reinitiation.

In contrast, the replicase acts continuously and generates a full-length positive-strand anti-genome that is in turn replicated into negative-strand genomes for the progeny virions. To become functional templates, the genomes and anti-genomes must be encapsidated into RNP, which protects them from the action of nuclease. This is why viral protein synthesis is a prerequisite for replication. There is an entry site for the nucleoprotein at its 5' end to promote the concomitant encapsidation of the growing RNA. During the transcription step, leader RNA carrying this entry site is released. During replication, the 5' end remains linked to the growing RNA, which is progressively encapsidated.

The main event influencing continuous synthesis by the polymerase and its switch from transcription to replication mode is the concomitant (anti)genome encapsidation. Here, the amount of nucleoprotein

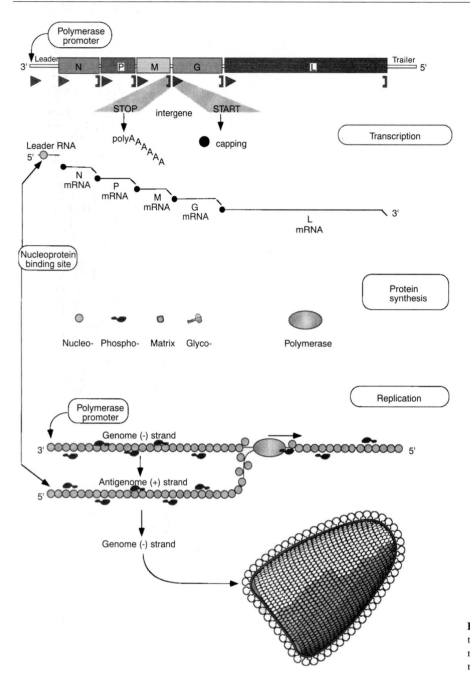

Fig. 33.6   Transcription, translation and replication mechanisms of rhabdoviruses.

available is decisive (Vidal and Kolakofsky 1989, Horikami et al. 1992). At low levels, the polymerase stops at the end of the leader RNA and immediately reinitiates at the start signal of the first mRNA. This reinitiation prevents encapsidation of the mRNAs and causes a shift to the sequential transcription mode, in which elongation is independent of encapsidation. This results in an increase in the amount of viral protein. At high levels of nucleoprotein, the concomitant encapsidation prevents the polymerase stopping at the end of the leader RNA, causing a switch into the continuous mode. For the same reason, the replicase becomes unable to recognize the following start and stop signals.

The translation step separating transcription from replication is ensured by cellular mechanisms. The

classic scanning model (Kozak 1989), predicting that ribosomes bind to the capped 5′ end of the mRNA and scan downstream, is generally accepted. Thus, most of the viral proteins start at the first AUG codon along the mRNA. Exceptions to this rule have, however, been noted during translation of the P mRNA. In addition to the normal P protein, VSV encodes 2 other polypeptides starting at distal AUGs, one in the same open reading frame (ORF) (Herman 1986) and one in another ORF (Spiropoulou and Nichol 1993). By contrast, RV uses at least 4 AUGs in the same ORF (Chenik, Chebli and Blondel 1995). All the viral proteins are expressed in the cytosol by free polyribosomes, except the glycoprotein which is synthesized as a transmembrane protein by polyribosomes associated with membranes of the rough endoplasmic reticulum (RER). It is then transported to the cytoplasmic membrane via the Golgi apparatus. Because of the acidity of the RER and Golgi compartments, the glycoprotein is synthesized in a conformation inactive for fusion, thus impairing its interaction with viral membranes during transport. Once at the cell surface, the pH increases and the conformation reverts to the native type (Gaudin, Ruigrok and Brunner 1995).

Several viruses have developed variations on this general model of expression. The ephemeroviruses use a polycistronic strategy to express both structural and regulatory genes (Wang and Walker 1993, Wang et al. 1994). In the case of vaccine strains of RV (PV, ERA, SAD) there are alternative terminations for the matrix and glycoprotein cistrons (Tordo and Poch 1988a, Morimoto, Ohkubo and Kawai 1989, Sacramento et al. 1992, Tordo et al. 1992, Tordo and Kouznetzoff 1993). Two consecutive stop (polyadenylation) signals are alternatively recognized by the transcriptase to produce either a small or a large mRNA. It has been proposed that alternative termination, by modifying the length of the scanned intergenic region, could influence the transcription level of the distal cistron, resulting in a regulation tool for genome expression (Tordo and Poch 1988a, Tordo et al. 1992, Tordo and Kouznetzoff 1993). This regulation could be partly under the control of specific cellular factors, reinforcing the importance of the intracellular environment for cell susceptibility noted above, and suggesting that it might be worth while to study rabies neurotropism at the transcriptional level.

Implications for the structure of the genome

The genome of rhabdoviruses varies in length between 11 kb (vesiculovirus) and 15 kb (ephemerovirus) (Fig. 33.7). Its structure subserves a typical expression mechanism. For both the minus-strand genome and the plus-strand anti-genome the promoter for the polymerase is located at the 3' end (Smallwood and Moyer 1993); the entry site of the nucleoprotein for encapsidation is at the 5' end (Moyer et al. 1991) (see Fig. 33.6). The consequence of the preservation of these important signals is that the extremities of both positive and negative strands are complementary although a hairpin structure was never evidenced in vivo. Indeed, a minigenome consisting of only 50 residues from each end is sufficient to ensure transcription, replication, encapsidation and envelopment (Pattnaik et al. 1995). In addition, when the complementarity between extremities is increased by mutagenesis, replication rather than transcription is favoured (Wertz et al. 1994). It is interesting that most of the DI particles effectively mimic such minigenomes; those with extensive complementary ends are the most efficient for interference.

Besides the conserved extremities, the genome possesses a modular structure with the juxtaposition of cistrons independently controlled by signal sequences. Indeed, the progressive decrease in the rate of transcription from the 3' to the 5' end implies that the position of a cistron directly influences its rate of expression. This explains why rhabdoviruses have conserved very similar genome organizations into 3 blocks (Fig. 33.7) (Tordo et al. 1992). Block 1 at the 3' end encodes proteins required in large quantities (N, P), particularly the nucleoprotein that balances the switch between transcription and replication. Block 2 encodes the membrane proteins (M, G). Block 3 at the 5' end encodes the viral polymerase (L), required in limited amounts. This modular structure accepts some flexibility, and in several viruses typical genes are inserted that are adapted to their particular biology. Between blocks 1 and 2, the plant rhabdo-

viruses encode a protease-like protein (sc4, 4b) that could correspond to the movement protein needed for passage of the virus through plasmodesmata, thus allowing cell-to-cell transmission despite the presence of the cell wall (Scholthof et al. 1994). At the same position the sigma virus encodes a protein related to the reverse transcriptase of retro-elements (ORF 3) (Landès-Devauchelle, Bras and Delézée 1995). Between blocks 2 and 3, the ephemeroviruses encode a second heavily glycosylated glycoprotein (Gns) which probably arose from a sequence duplication of the *G* gene (Wang and Walker 1993). Gns is non-structural and of unknown function, as are the additional small proteins (α, β, γ) encoded consecutively (Wang et al. 1994) and the NV protein of the fish rhabdovirus IHNV (Morzunov, Winton and Nichol 1995). It is interesting that, at the same position between blocks 2 and 3, lyssaviruses conserve a large non-coding area initially termed 'pseudogene' ψ because it could represent a vestige of the multiple changes occurring in this region during rhabdovirus evolution (Tordo et al. 1986, 1992b, Ravkov, Smith and Nichol 1995).

Exit from the cell

Before viral budding, transcription and replication are inhibited and, simultaneously, the RNP becomes intensively condensed and coiled. In parallel, glycoproteins are concentrated in particular regions of the plasma membrane. A considerable body of evidence suggests that this morphological role during virion assembly is played by the matrix protein (see section 2.4, below). After the cytoplasmic maturation step, the virion leaves the cell by budding, the lipid envelope being provided by the host cell membrane. Most rhabdoviruses bud from the plasma membrane and some from internal cell membranes. The plant rhabdoviruses bud either from the endoplasmic reticulum (cytorhabdoviruses) or from the inner nuclear envelope (nucleorhabdoviruses) and accumulate in perinuclear spaces (Jackson, Francki and Zuidema 1987).

2.4 Functional role of the viral polypeptides

The recent advances in genetic manipulation of negative-strand RNA viruses have greatly facilitated the functional dissection of viral genes and proteins by reverse genetics (see Conzelmann 1996 for a review, and also Lawson et al. 1995, Whelan et al. 1995, Kretzschmar et al. 1996, Schnell et al. 1996). The use of these viruses as stable vectors to express foreign genes now seems realistic (Schnell et al. 1996). In addition, studies of the interactions between the proteins and the backbone RNA genome are being pursued by various physical, biochemical and immunological methods.

THE RIBONUCLEOCAPSID COMPLEX (RNP)

The RNP is the minimum structure needed to mediate RNA synthesis. The N protein RNA is the template whereas the polymerase function is catalysed by the L and P proteins (Conzelmann and Schnell 1994). L is the RNA-dependent RNA polymerase that possesses most of the required enzymatic activities: RNA synthesis (De and Banerjee 1984); mRNA capping and methylation (Horikami and Moyer 1982); mRNA polyadenylation (Hunt, Smith and Buckley

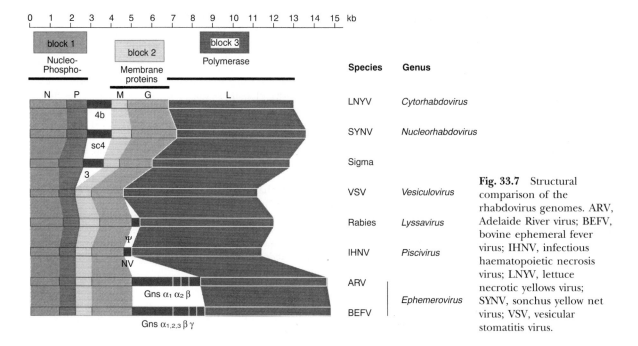

Fig. 33.7 Structural comparison of the rhabdovirus genomes. ARV, Adelaide River virus; BEFV, bovine ephemeral fever virus; IHNV, infectious haematopoietic necrosis virus; LNYV, lettuce necrotic yellows virus; SYNV, sonchus yellow net virus; VSV, vesicular stomatitis virus.

1984, Hunt and Hutchinson 1993); and possible kinase activity on the P protein (Barik and Banerjee 1992). P is a regulatory co-factor for which various functions have been proposed: helping the L protein to bind the promoter (Isaac and Keene 1982, De and Banerjee 1984); transiently displacing the N protein to gain access to the RNA (Hudson, Condra and Lazzarini 1986); complexing the free N protein in a convenient form (ratio 1N:1P) for encapsidation (La Ferla and Peluso 1989).

The N protein possesses a large NH_2 core strongly resistant to proteases and carrying the RNA binding site (Tordo 1996, personal observations). The COOH extremity is structurally independent and interacts with other proteins of the RNP, notably P, in order to gain specificity and prevent encapsidation of non-viral RNAs (Banerjee et al. 1989).

The P protein seems to be composed of 2 distal domains separated by a hinge region. Both domains are implicated in various interactions with the N and L proteins (Chenik et al. 1994, Fu et al. 1994, Gao and Lenard 1995a, Takacs and Banerjee 1995). The phosphorylation of P is essential for regulating its activity in transcription (Barik and Banerjee 1992, Beckes and Perrault 1992, Gao and Lenard 1995a) and replication (Chang, Reiss and Huang 1994). P subspecies varying in degree of phosphorylation and in physical state (soluble, multimeric or complexed with N or L) have different activities in relation to both functions (Gao and Lenard 1995a, Richardson and Peluso 1996). The primary phosphorylation step of P is ensured at precise sites by cellular kinases packaged in the virion: the casein kinase-II for VSV (Gao and Lenard 1995b, Gupta, Das and Banerjee 1995) and the protein kinase Cγ for RV (AK Banerjee 1995, personal communication). It is interesting that protein kinase Cγ is mostly found in nervous tissue, and could provide another tissue-specific element in the regulation of transcription. The primary phosphorylation is thought to promote conformational changes, initiating a secondary phosphorylation cascade in which the viral L polymerase is probably active (Barik and Banerjee 1992, Beckes and Perrault 1992, Gao and Lenard 1995a). In contrast to the primary phosphorylation, the L-associated kinase activity is without transcriptional effect on the P protein. Similarly, the small C and C′ basic proteins encoded in a second ORF on the *P* gene

(Spiropoulou and Nichol 1993, Kretzschmar et al. 1996) are unnecessary for VSV growth in tissue culture (Kretzschmar et al. 1996). It has been suggested that they play a role in viral pathogenesis or transmission by insect vectors (Kretzschmar et al. 1996).

The sequence alignment of L proteins from *Mononegavirales* has provided a structure consistent with its multifunctional nature: 6 conserved domains (probably carrying the catalytic activities) are concatenated by variable hinge regions (Poch et al. 1990). The domains seem to be autonomous as suggested by complementation between L mutants (Flamand 1980). Putative functions have been tentatively assigned to several domains (Poch et al. 1990). In particular, domain III possesses 4 or 5 hyperconserved motifs similar in structure and position to those found in all RNA-dependent polymerases (Poch et al. 1989, Müller et al. 1994) and also in DNA-dependent polymerases, although more distantly (Delarue et al. 1990). This predictive analysis has guided the first trials of site-directed mutagenesis which basically confirmed the functional importance of the predicted motifs (Sleat and Banerjee 1993, Schnell and Conzelmann 1995). A more systematic analysis by extensive sequence comparison between wild type and mutant strains of VSV suggests that residues in the interdomain V–VI are essential for polyadenylation and thermosensitivity (Hunt and Hutchinson 1993). Furthermore, it was recently suggested that host factor(s) may be required for the activity of the L protein (Mathur, Das and Banerjee 1996).

Membrane proteins

The M protein is involved in certain cytopathic effects of VSV: rounding of the cell by interaction with the tubulin of the microtubular network (Melki, Gaudin and Blondel 1994) and inhibition of host cell transcription (Black et al. 1993). In addition, the M protein is important during viral morphogenesis: it is responsible for condensation of the RNP (Newcomb et al. 1982) and inhibition of genome transcription (Clinton et al. 1978, De et al. 1982); it also interacts with the cell membrane (Chong and Rose 1994). The amino-terminal phosphorylated and basic domain of the M protein (Poch, Tordo and Keith 1988) seems to play an essential role in these activities (Ogden, Pal and Wagner 1986, Chong and

Rose 1994), although the phosphorylation *per se* does not (Kaptur et al. 1995).

The glycoprotein (reviewed by Coll 1995) has the typical structure of group I transmembrane proteins. An NH_2 terminal signal peptide 19 amino acids (aa) in length serves the translocation of nascent protein through the RER membrane and is cleaved in the mature protein. A hydrophobic transmembrane segment (c. 20 aa) remains embedded in the viral envelope. It separates the 'cytoplasmic' COOH domain (about 50 aa), interacting with internal viral proteins, from the glycosylated NH_2 ectodomain (c. 450 aa). The glycosylation and palmytoylation sites have been mapped (Gaudin et al. 1991a, Coll 1995), as have, tentatively, the important functions of the ectodomain. On the basis of sequence similarity with snake venom curare-mimetic neurotoxins (Lentz et al. 1984, Rustici et al. 1993, Tordo et al. 1993b), and further studies using anti-idiotypic antibodies (Hanham, Zhao and Tignor 1993), the 190–203 aa sequence of rabies glycoprotein ectodomain has been implicated in the recognition of the nicotinic AChR. However, as mentioned above, the rhabdovirus receptor is complex and probably consists of several molecules. Furthermore, the region involved in fusion has been searched by insertion and directed mutagenesis. Different sites modified the ectodomain structure in such a way that fusion activity was blocked or modified (Zhang and Ghosh 1994, Fredericksen and Whitt 1996). However, the exact locations of the fusion peptide were mapped by photolabelling or solid-phase binding assay to the following sequences: aa 102–179 for RV, 58–221 for VSV (Durrer et al. 1995, Gaudin, Ruigrok and Brunner 1995) and aa 82–109 for the fish rhabdovirus VHSV (Coll 1995, Espeta and Coll 1996). Finally, several residues of the ectodomain seem to play a crucial role in pathogenicity and virulence (Tordo et al. 1993b). For RV, neurovirulence is directly linked to the maintenance of a basic residue in position 333 (Tuffereau et al. 1989). Mutation at this residue reduced the categories of neurons sensitive to infection (Coulon et al. 1994).

2.5 Antigens

The immune response against lyssaviruses is complex; the response to RV has been extensively studied. Although all the viral proteins are antigenic, their roles in protection vary (Lafon 1994, Xiang et al. 1995). Their respective importance has been defined by recombinant DNA techniques (Tordo 1991). Two of them, G and N, are of primary importance, the phosphoprotein M1 being of less significance. Purified G protein protects against intracerebral challenge with RV, and is the only antigen that consistently induces virus-neutralizing antibody (Wiktor et al. 1973). This property mainly depends on the preservation of its 3-dimensional structure, although a linear neutralizing epitope has been identified (Bunschoten et al. 1989, Benmansour et al, 1991, Ni et al. 1995). On the other hand, the glycoprotein shares with the N and M1 proteins of RNP the capacity to induce a cellular immune response, involving respectively T helper cells (Th) and cytotoxic T cells (Tc) (Lafon 1994, Xiang et al. 1995). Purified RNP protects against challenge by peripheral routes, probably through a cross-help mechanism between N-specific Th lymphocytes and G-specific B lymphocytes producing neutralizing antibodies (Dietzschold et al. 1987, Lodmell

et al. 1991, Lodmell, Esposito and Ewalt 1993). An effective role of the Tc response in protection remains to be clearly demonstrated (Xiang et al. 1995). It is interesting that the G and N antigens conserve their immunogenic properties when administered orally (Hooper et al. 1994). This property is used extensively in large vaccination campaigns with vaccinia or adenoviruses expressing recombinant G protein (see section 4.7, p. 685).

Most of the current rabies vaccine strains derive from a wild strain isolated by Pasteur (Tordo 1991). This was initially passaged intracerebrally in rabbits until the incubation period shortened and became 'fixed' at 5–8 days. From this, multiple passages in animal brain and cell culture were performed. Vaccine strains belong to genotype 1 (causing classic rabies) and protect against homologous isolates (Lodmell et al. 1995), but do not protect efficiently against rabies-related viruses in genotypes 2–6 that also pose possible threats to humans. Work is in progress to improve the protection offered by the vaccine by increasing the number of genotypes against which it is effective. The conserved N protein, a strong inducer of Th cells, may be important in this respect. It behaves as a superantigen in humans and BALB/c mice, activating Vβ8 and Vβ6 T cells respectively (Lafon et al. 1992, Lafon 1994). The antigenic sites for B and T cell responses have been extensively mapped along the G, N and M1 viral antigens by sequencing mutants resistant to neutralizing antibodies or by measuring the reactivity of chemically cleaved or synthetic peptides (Bunschoten et al. 1989, Benmansour et al. 1991, Ertl, Dietzschold and Otvos 1991, Minamoto et al. 1994, Goto et al. 1995). The vast majority of the G protein antigenic sites seem to be conformational, sometimes involving regions that are distant from each other in the primary structure but which are brought in proximity by protein folding and disulphide bridges.

3 CLINICAL AND PATHOLOGICAL ASPECTS: VESICULOVIRUS INFECTION

3.1 Vesicular stomatitis

The interest in vesicular stomatitis viruses as models for basic studies in virology and molecular biology has tended to overshadow their natural history and their role as agents of disease. The disease was first reported in livestock in the USA in 1821 (Hanson 1981). It is largely confined to the western hemisphere and reports of its occurrence elsewhere are considered to be either of importations from the West or of doubtful authenticity (Brown and Crick 1979). The virus was first isolated by Cotton (1927) and its morphology established by Chow and co-workers (Chow, Chow and Hanson 1954).

3.2 Disease in animals

The clinical manifestations in horses and cattle are fever, development of vesicles on the tongue, gums and lips, and excessive salivation. Teats of milking cows may be infected and, less commonly, lesions may be seen on the feet. Animals have difficulty in eating and walking, and lose weight; milking cows stop lactating. The disease is rarely lethal except in pigs. Epizootics of vesicular stomatitis are sudden in onset (within c. 2 weeks) and quickly involve many animals in a herd but often do not spread to adjacent farms. In the USA it occurs in summer months in c. 10-year cycles. In Central America, outbreaks are more frequent and possibly associated with the change from wet to dry seasons.

3.3 Disease in humans

The virus can also infect humans, usually causing a mild influenza-like illness, although more severe forms are reported. The incubation period is 1–9 days after exposure and symptoms may last 3–4 days; occasionally there may be a relapse (Sellers 1984). Infections of humans have mostly been reported in laboratory workers after aerosol inhalation or accidental contamination of eyes or abrasions. However, in some areas of North and Central America 25–90 % of farmers have antibody to VSV (Hanson 1981)

3.4 Transmission

The virus is found in vesicle fluid and epithelium and does not persist after recovery. It is not excreted in urine, faeces or milk. Spread by direct contact with vesicle fluid is possible, and transfer from teat lesions by milkers and milking equipment is occasionally reported. However, experimental studies have failed to demonstrate direct animal-to-animal transmission, and Sellers (1984) noted many outbreaks in which the disease did not spread to neighbouring animals on the same farm. The bites of infected blood-sucking arthropods seem to be the most likely mode of transmission, demonstrated experimentally with several strains of the virus. Furthermore, many vesiculoviruses have been isolated in nature from mosquitoes, sandflies, midges, mites and ticks. There are no overt pathological signs in arthropods, and how they become infected is obscure. The disease in animals being brief, with minimal and transient viraemia, they are unlikely natural reservoirs of the virus. It has been suggested that some strains may be plant viruses and that animals are infected either directly, by eating infected plants, or by the bites of insects that have fed on such plants.

3.5 Vaccines

Vaccines ranging from live unmodified virus to vaccinia recombinants specific for the G protein have been used with poor success. Their development has not been pursued vigorously, both because of the self-limiting nature of the disease and because the durability of the immune response is uncertain.

4 CLINICAL AND PATHOLOGICAL ASPECTS: RABIES INFECTION

4.1 Introduction

Although the clinical signs of rabies have been recognized for many centuries, it is mainly since the late nineteenth century that significant progress has been made in laboratory diagnosis, human postexposure treatment, control of animal rabies, and studies of the epidemiology, pathogenesis and immune response. Currently, in most of the industrialized world, diagnostic systems are well organized, rapid and efficient; human postexposure treatment is very effective; host species are principally wildlife; and technologically, there are excellent prospects for control or eradication of the disease in large geographical areas. In spite of these remarkable advances, rabies is still a serious problem with significant economic losses and human deaths in large parts of Africa, Asia and South America.

4.2 Clinical aspects

FACTORS DETERMINING CLINICAL MANIFESTATIONS

Susceptibility, incubation and morbidity periods, clinical signs and viral excretion are all important when considering the clinical manifestations of rabies. Variation in these factors occurs with different strains of virus and the success of certain combinations of strain and host species in causing species-specific enzootics is due, at least partly, to favourable forms of clinical expression (see section 4.3, p. 677).

Although many species of mammals can be infected with RV, there are fairly wide variations in susceptibility. It has been customary to place species in groups of low, moderate, high and extremely high susceptibility (WHO 1973). Examples include: foxes, extremely high; cattle, high; non-human primates, moderate; opossums, low. The classification is based mainly on data collected before typing of street viruses with monoclonal antibodies was available. Although generally valid when testing was done with host-adapted viral strains, the classification may not reflect differences (largely untested) among several variants in a given host species.

CLINICAL MANIFESTATIONS IN ANIMALS

The incubation period in domestic animals usually ranges from 2 to 12 weeks and is probably similar in wild animals (Charlton, Casey and Campbell 1987); it is often shorter following bite wounds to the head region than after those at the extremities. Generally (but not always) there is an inverse correlation between the length of the incubation period and the dose of virus. However, even in animals experimentally inoculated with the same dose by the same route and site, the incubation period may vary widely. Periods much longer than 3 months have been observed in naturally exposed and experimentally infected animals. In humans, there are several recorded cases in which the circumstances strongly suggest incubation periods of several years (Fishbein 1991, Hemachuda 1994).

The range in length of illness in most species is 1–10 days. Rarely, longer periods have been recorded. In dogs inoculated with several strains of street virus from dogs, the clinical course was 1–14 days and was dose- but not strain-dependent (review: Fekadu 1991). In contrast, the average period of morbidity differed markedly in skunks inoculated with the mid-Atlantic raccoon strain (50 h) or the eastern Arctic strain (180 h) (Rupprecht and Charlton 1987, unpublished data). Most of the clinical signs of rabies are expressions of neurological dysfunction (impaired neurotransmission) (review: Charlton 1994). For complete descriptions of clinical signs in various species, see recent reviews (Baer 1991b, Blancou, Aubert and Artois 1991, Bunn 1991, Charlton, Webster and Casey 1991, Crandell 1991, Fekadu 1991, Fishbein 1991, Winkler and Jenkins 1991, Hemachuda 1994, Radostits, Blood and Gay 1994). Most clinicians are aware that the clinical signs are variable and may be non-specific in the early stages of the disease, thus contributing to the difficulty of diagnosis. The prodromal period (a few hours to a few days in humans) may include general malaise and symptoms suggestive of involvement of several organ systems; dogs and cats frequently undergo a change in temperament, becoming withdrawn and shy or more alert and restless. At some point, most animals become disorientated and wander aimlessly without regard for the social organization of the species.

Although there is variability in many clinical signs, paralysis is fairly consistent, and is seen in nearly all cases unless death occurs early. Paresis may be present initially, or develop later after an initial period of increased alertness, hyper-responsiveness to auditory, visual and tactile stimuli, and aggressive behaviour. Generally, paresis is evident as a wobbly, laboured gait, with or without paralysis of the muscles of mastication (dropped jaw syndrome), noted mainly in dogs. The paresis usually progresses to recumbency; terminally, the animal becomes comatose. On the criteria of the predominance of paralysis or of excitability and biting, the clinical syndrome has been classified either as **dumb (paralytic)** or **furious (encephalitic).** This is a useful distinction. However, it is appropriate to consider rabies primarily – perhaps universally – as paralytic, the encephalitic form being due to hyper-responsiveness and aggressive behaviour preceding and then superimposed on the paralytic stage. These variations in clinical presentation are induced or influenced by differences in immunopathology (see section 4.5, p. 683).

The above or closely similar clinical signs have been described in many mammalian species. Other signs include, for dogs, cats, or both: pupillary dilation, protrusion of the third eyelid, altered phonation (apparently due to paralysis of pharyngeal/laryngeal musculature), aimless wandering, drooling of saliva, convulsions, muscle twitching and tremors (reviews:

Tierkel 1975, Vaughn 1975, Bunn 1991, Fekadu 1991); skunks: mania and muscle tremors (review: Charlton, Webster and Casey 1991); cattle: altered phonation, sexual hyperactivity (Radostits, Blood and Gay 1994).

CLINICAL MANIFESTATIONS IN HUMANS

The early symptoms are frequently non-specific and may include general malaise, fever, chills, sore throat, cough, nausea, vomiting, diarrhoea, headache, anxiety, apprehension and irritability. Many patients have pain/paraesthesia at the site of the bite wound. If the disease develops as furious rabies, one or more forms of hyperactivity (agitation, hallucinations, threshing, running etc.) are common in the early stages. These signs may occur spontaneously or be precipitated by various visual, auditory, olfactory or tactile stimuli. Hydrophobia occurs in some patients. It can be precipitated by attempts to drink or even by the sight or mention of liquids. Periods of hyperactivity may be interspersed with periods of calm and lucidity. Unless the patient dies early, the 'encephalitic symptoms' progress to paralysis and coma. If the disease presents as dumb (paralytic) rabies, the prodrome may be similar but the main feature is paralysis. Hemachuda (1994) lists criteria that may be useful in diagnosing paralytic rabies. Unless intensive care is given, patients with encephalitic rabies usually die within 7 days; those with paralytic rabies may survive as long as 2–3 weeks. For detailed descriptions of human symptoms, see recent reviews (Fishbein 1991, Hemachuda 1994).

RELATION OF CLINICAL SIGNS TO SPECIFIC NEUROLOGICAL DYSFUNCTIONS

Only modest progress has been made in this area. Although there is little morphological evidence of neuronal injury, it is generally assumed that viral replication, possibly coupled with immunological mechanisms, results in specific neuronal dysfunctions, due at least in part to the sequence of infection of various groups of neurons, variations in susceptibility among different groups of neurons, or both. Rabies infection increases the inducible nitric oxide synthase in brain (Koprowski et al. 1993). Furthermore, altered expression of cellular mRNA has been detected in rabies-infected rat brain (Fu et al. 1993). These studies suggest basic mechanisms that may be involved in neuronal dysfunction.

4.3 Epizootiology and epidemiology

TRANSMISSION OF INFECTION

Transmission of the disease usually requires bite-inflicted deposition of virus-laden saliva into tissues of the recipient animal. Virus may be excreted several days before the onset of clinical signs. The maximum recorded times are: fox, 5 days; skunk, 6 days; dog, 7 days with a Mexican isolate and 13 days with an Ethiopian isolate; cat, 3 days; bat (*Tadarida brasiliensis mexicana*), 12 days (review: Charlton 1988). Excretion of virus before signs of illness is the justification for quarantine (usually 10–14 days) of clinically normal dogs and cats that have bitten humans. Occasionally, excretion of virus may be intermittent; some animals with virus-positive saliva on one or more days before or during overt illness may have negative saliva terminally. Furthermore, virus may not be isolated from glands of animals that had previously shed virus in saliva. Because of these features and the patchy nature of antigen-containing cells in salivary glands, examinations of saliva or salivary glands at the time of death may not be reliable indicators of virus transmitted in an earlier exposure to a rabid animal. There are very few data on the dose of virus received in natural infections. The carrier is defined as a clinically normal animal that secretes virus in saliva (not the immediately prodromal excretion of virus just described). There is no convincing evidence of the carrier state in field cases in North America. Most of the reports of rabies transmission by apparently healthy animals (usually dogs) and prolonged secretion in saliva are from Africa and Asia (review: Fekadu 1991).

FACTORS AFFECTING THE EPIZOOTIOLOGY OF RABIES

A particular species may serve as a principal host only in a limited part of its geographical distribution. The disease occurs regularly in a number of other mammalian species in addition to the species recognized as the principal host. The occurrence of rabies in these other species may have little or no influence on the course of an epizootic; however, their role is often not readily defined. Each principal host species has its specific pattern population biology and specific modes of social interaction. These host qualities determine which virus variants are capable of survival. It is essential that the virus be transmitted by an infected animal during a period of virus excretion to an adequate number of other susceptible individuals. For this to occur, lyssavirus strains must be adapted to the physiological traits and population biology of their hosts (Bacon 1985, Wandeler 1991a, Wandeler et al. 1994). They must have a host-specific pathogenicity and pathogenesis (length of incubation period, duration and magnitude of virus excretion, duration and extent of clinical illness). We assume that each principal host has its own virus variants adapted for persistence in its populations. Thus, within the area of a principal host, there is little virus variation among the isolates, even if they are performed in a species that is the principal host in another area. With the development of molecular and monoclonal antibody technologies it became possible to demonstrate that indeed antigenically distinct variants exhibiting phylogenetic relationships circulate in different host populations (Rupprecht et al. 1991, Benmansour et al. 1992, Sacramento et al. 1992, Smith et al. 1992, Bourhy, Kissi and Tordo 1993a, 1993b, Kissi, Tordo and Bourhy 1995, Nadin-Davies, Casey and Wandeler 1993, 1994, Nel, Thomson and von Teicham 1993, Smith, Yager and Orciari 1993, Tordo et al. 1993a).

RABIES IN DOGS

One can readily distinguish between areas of the world in which dogs are the predominant hosts and those where rabies is maintained in wild animals and in which only 0.1–5.0% of the rabies cases reported annually are in dogs. In large parts of Asia, Africa and Latin America, rabies in dogs is much more common, making up 95% or more of all diagnosed cases. Even though dog rabies is often termed 'urban rabies', it is clearly a rural problem in many developing countries (Fekadu 1991). Dogs are kept and tolerated at very high numbers in most human societies, sometimes reaching densities of several thousand/km²; this is considerably more than any wild carnivore population ever achieves. Such high densities could facilitate enzootic canine rabies, although it is also suspected that rabies in dogs could be linked with wildlife rabies. There is no doubt that rabid dogs are the major source of human infection (Beran 1991, Wandeler et al. 1993). In industrialized countries of North America and Europe, where the epizootic is maintained and spread by wild carnivores, 3 factors may account for the low incidence of rabies in dogs: most dogs are restricted in their movements; they are kept indoors or in enclosures and leashed when outside; dog vaccination is strongly recommended or even compulsory.

RABIES IN WILD *CARNIVORA*

The principal rabies hosts of the order *Carnivora* are all small to medium size (0.4–20 kg) omnivores, scavenging and foraging on small vertebrates, invertebrates, fruit and refuse produced by humans. They reach high population densities (often several individuals/km²) in and near human settlements. High intrinsic population growth rates allow rapid recovery of populations reduced by persecution or disease. They all are able to support initial epidemics of high case density and thereafter an oscillating prevalence over many years (Wandeler 1991a).

Areas for which an association of RV variants with populations of wild *Carnivora* are well documented are limited to North America, Europe, parts of southern Africa and some Caribbean islands. The red fox (*Vulpes vulpes*) is the principal rabies host in subarctic and northeastern North America, in all of central and eastern Europe, and in subarctic and temperate zones of Asia (Blancou et al. 1991). In arctic regions of North America and Asia, the arctic fox (*Alopex lagopus*) is the predominant rabies host (Crandell 1991). The viruses isolated from red and arctic foxes from fox rabies areas of North America are all closely related, but distinct from European fox isolates. Jackals (*Canis* sp.) are the principal hosts in southern Africa (Foggin 1985) and are probably involved in much larger areas in Africa and Asia. Other wildlife species that maintain independent cycles of distinct RV variants in southern Africa are various viverrids, especially the yellow mongoose (*Cynictis penicillata*), and possibly the bat-eared fox (*Otocyon megalotis*) (King, Meredith and Thomson 1994). The striped skunk (*Mephitis mephitis*) is the species most often diagnosed rabid in large areas of Canada and the USA (Charlton, Webster and Casey

1991). Raccoon (*Procyon lotor*) rabies is at present confined to the USA, but is spreading in the southeastern and in mid-Atlantic states (Winkler and Jenkins 1991). Mongooses (*Herpestes auropunctatus*) introduced to some Caribbean islands are now the principal reservoir there (Everard and Everard 1985). Grey foxes (*Urocyon cinereoargenteus*) in some North American areas (Carey, Giles and McLean 1978) and raccoon dogs (*Nyctereutes procyonides*) introduced to eastern and subarctic Europe (Cherkasskiy 1988) are sometimes suspected of supporting independent epizootics. Populations of a number of bat species in the Americas, Africa and Eurosiberia also support independent cycles of lyssavirus epizootics (Baer 1991b, Baer and Smith 1991).

RABIES IN BATS

The African bat *Lyssavirus* isolates are of genotypes (serotypes) 2 and 4, while those from bats in Europe were identified as genotypes 5 and 6. So far, American bat rabies viruses have been categorized as genotype 1, but a more detailed analysis of the large diversity of distinct isolates is still good for surprises. *Chiroptera* have life history traits that are quite different from those of carnivoran rabies hosts: they are small, long lived, have low intrinsic population growth rates and are ecological specialists. The properties of lyssaviruses adapted to bats must therefore be different from those of *Carnivora* rabies. This statement remains a hypothesis because the population biology and epidemiology of bat rabies is insufficiently explored. A notable exception is rabies in vampire bats as described by Lord et al. (1975). An interesting feature of bat rabies is the vast antigenic diversity of isolates. In Canada alone, 12 distinct variants are recognized with monoclonal antibodies. Several variants occur in a single species, and the geographical distribution of variants is overlapping. This is in sharp contrast to the pattern of rabies in *Carnivora*, where very little epitope variation is recognized over very large areas.

INCIDENCE OF RABIES IN HUMANS

In industrialized countries, rabies in humans is rare owing to low rates of exposure, high standards of health education and relatively easy access to postexposure treatment with potent vaccines. Even so, c. 35 000 people die from rabies every year world-wide. The number of people receiving postexposure treatment – mostly after dog bites – is about 3.5 million per year (Bögel and Motschwiller 1986, Bögel and Meslin 1990). Almost all deaths of humans from rabies and the vast majority of treated bite exposures occur in developing countries (Acha and Arambulo 1985). This may in part be due to a high rate of exposure to biting rabid dogs, but even if this assumption is correct, it does not fully explain the high number of rabies casualties. In view of the efficacy of modern postexposure treatment, nearly all cases of rabies in humans must be considered as failures of the medical system: for various reasons, including lack of availability or ignorance, the correct treatment was not applied or not applied in time (Wandeler et al. 1993).

4.4 Pathogenesis and pathology

The pathogenesis of rabies includes the following steps in movement of virus through the animal body: inoculation of virus (usually via a bite wound) into tissues of a susceptible animal, migration up peripheral nerves to the central nervous system (CNS), dissemination throughout the CNS and centrifugal migration in peripheral nerves to infect certain non-nervous tissues. Although there are many similarities in the pathogenesis in various hosts and under different experimental conditions, certain aspects may be modified by animal species, age, viral strain, dose, route of inoculation and the immune response.

THE CELLULAR INFECTION CYCLE

To a large extent the pathogenesis of rabies consists of the sequential infection of various types of neurons and some non-nervous cells. The cellular infection cycle of RV consists of: attachment of virus to the plasma membrane, entry of virus into the cell, replication, assembly of virions on intracytoplasmic membranes and plasma membrane; and release into the intercellular environment. For detailed descriptions, see section 2.3 (p. 670) and previous reviews (Tordo and Poch 1988b, Tsiang 1993, Kawai and Morimoto 1994).

Cellular receptors that bind RV to the plasma membrane are presumed to be important in the infection of cells throughout progression of the infection. Such receptor-mediated binding would have to occur on axon terminals, dendrites and perikarya of many different types of neurons and non-nervous cells. Although RV is widely considered to be highly neuronotropic, it will, in fact, infect many other types of cells (review: Charlton 1988). In various animals, they include cells of the myocardium, adrenal medulla, various exocrine glands and epithelia, including those of the skin, respiratory tract and urinary tract (reviews: Dierks 1975, Schneider 1975, Charlton 1988). In some salivary glands, replication is frequently more efficient than in brain (Charlton, Casey and Campbell 1987). Except for extrafusal muscle fibres at the inoculation site, nearly all the above cells are infected after viral replication in neurons and release of infectious virions from axon terminals.

INOCULATION SITE AND TRANSIT OF VIRUS TO THE CNS

Early studies of the initial events in rabies infection usually included inoculation of virus-containing preparations followed by a variety of procedures (neurectomy, leg amputation, virus isolation etc.) to determine the route(s) and tissues involved in migration of virus to the CNS (Dean, Evans and McClure 1963, Johnson 1965, Baer, Shanthaveerappa, Bourne 1965, 1968). These studies demonstrated that in many cases virus is en route to the CNS before there is time for replication to occur in non-nervous tissue at the inoculation site, thus indicating direct entrance of inoculated virus into peripheral nerves (reviews: Charlton 1988, 1994). Recent studies using immunohistochemical or molecular biological techniques have demonstrated antigen/viral RNA in the CNS, ganglia, or both, also at times inconsistent with prior replication at the inoculation site (Kucera et al. 1985, Coulon at al. 1989, Shankar, Dietzschold and Koprowski 1991). Thus, there is substantial evidence for direct uptake of inoculated virus by the peripheral nerves.

An alternative (indirect) mechanism would involve viral replication in non-nervous tissue and the transfer of progeny virions to peripheral nerves. Direct infection of myocytes by inoculation has been demonstrated in hamsters (Murphy et al. 1973) and in skunks (Charlton and Casey 1979). By electron microscopy, bodies of matrix, anomalous viral structures and a small number of virions are seen in the sarcoplasm of affected fibres (Fig. 33.8). However, neither of these studies nor any others have provided convincing evidence that myocyte infection is an essential link in the pathogenesis. Most of the above-mentioned studies used models with short incubation periods. Our own studies of the long incubation period in skunks (Charlton et al. 1997) strongly suggest that delay in the progression of infection in muscle at the incubation site plays a major role in the long incubation period. To account, at least partly, for the wide variation in incubation periods, the following mechanisms are proposed. With high doses of rabies virus, virions enter both axons of peripheral nerves and myocytes. In this scheme, myocyte infection is mainly incidental, the main course of infection proceeding up peripheral axons (directly to the CNS or to spinal ganglia en route to the CNS), resulting in short incubation periods within a narrow range. With lower doses of virus, there is an increasingly high probability that virions will enter either axons or muscle fibres (or occasionally neither). This could result in early transit directly via peripheral axons, or retention in muscle for varying periods before release and uptake by peripheral nerve axons resulting in a wide range of incubation periods from fairly short to long.

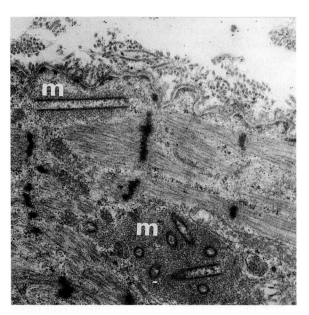

Fig. 33.8 Electron micrograph of 2 bodies of matrix (m) and anomalous tubular structures in a muscle cell of a skunk at the site of inoculation of street RV (×2000).

At the inoculation site, virus enters axons of peripheral nerve fibres and migrates via retrograde axoplasmic flow in sensory or motor nerve fibres to neuronal perikarya in relevant portions of the CNS, cerebrospinal ganglia or both. The rates of migration in various systems are: 3 mm/h or more in nerve trunks of a pelvic limb in mice (Dean, Evans and McClure 1963); 15–24 mm/day in neurites of cultured rat sensory neurons (Lyke and Tsiang 1987); and 50–100 mm/day in neurites of cultured human sensory neurons (Tsiang, Ceccaldi and Lyke 1991). Studies with the CVS strain and its avirulent derivative indicated that the slight changes in the glycoprotein of the derivative altered the neural uptake after intraocular inoculation (reviews: Coulon et al. 1994, Jackson 1994).

EVENTS IN THE CNS

The initial event in CNS infection is the arrival of virus into a region of the brain or spinal cord having direct neural connections to the inoculation site, as described above. The preponderance of evidence suggests that dissemination in the CNS occurs mainly through cycles of replication in neuronal perikarya and dendrites, transit of virions in axons via retrograde and anterograde axoplasmic flow, and transneuronal transfer of infection at and near synapses. Ultrastructural studies suggest that viral replication begins in Nissl granules (Yamamoto and Ohtani 1978, Charlton 1994). The morphological features in infected neurons include bodies of matrix (randomly orientated strands of viral nucleocapsid), mature virions, convoluted membranous profiles and bizarre tubular structures. All are in the cytoplasm. The Negri body is an inclusion body detectable by light microscopy. Its internal structure has been attributed to entrapment of cellular organelles and virions within a body of matrix (Fig. 33.9). Budding of RV occurs on intracytoplasmic membranes and on the plasma membrane. Some observations suggest an affinity of matrix for postsynaptic membrane (Charlton 1994). Budding on postsynaptic or adjacent plasma membrane with simultaneous endocytic uptake by the adjacent axon terminal is a mechanism of dendroaxonal transfer of virus (Fig. 33.10) (Iwasaki and Clark 1975, Charlton and Casey 1979). Subsequent retrograde axonal transport of virions to the perikaryon/dendrites of the recipient neuron and replication is a step in the continuing dissemination of infection. Anterograde viral migration can also occur in axons. This would require axodendritic or axosomatic transfer of infection, for which as yet there is no evidence for a specific mechanism. Movement in axons was demonstrated by stereotaxic inoculation of virus into rat striatum and subsequent infection of the substantia nigra (Gillet, Derer and Tsiang 1986). That axoplasmic flow was involved was demonstrated by the impedance of connecting brain structures by colchicine (Ceccaldi, Gillet and Tsiang 1989, Ceccaldi, Ermine and Tsiang 1990).

Although these details of the subcellular process are fairly well established, very little has been published on the transitways to and sequence of infection of

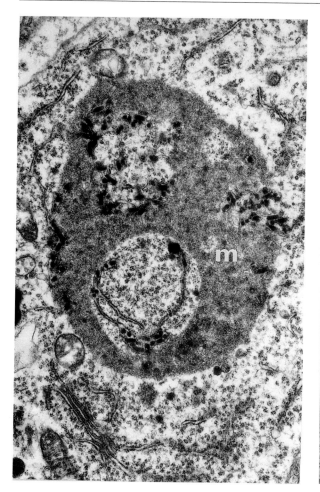

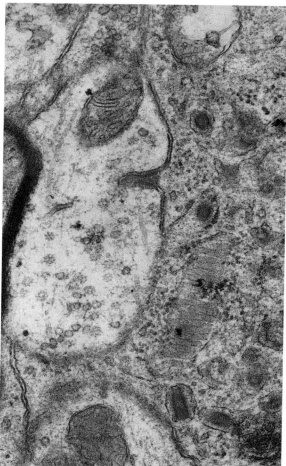

Fig. 33.9 Electron microscopic structure of Negri body in a neuron in skunk brain. Note the body of matrix (m) with entrapped rough endoplasmic reticulum, free ribosomes and virions (×15 000).

Fig. 33.10 Electron micrograph of skunk brain. Virion budding on neuronal plasma membrane and simultaneous endocytosis by an adjacent axon terminal (×25 000).

particular nuclei or other regions of the CNS. Recent studies in skunks experimentally inoculated in the right pelvic limb with street virus suggest the following events in early CNS infection (Charlton et al. 1996). After entering the caudal spinal cord, infection spreads locally (probably by propriospinal neurons) in the cord and also via long descending and ascending fibre tracts to the brain. Spread in the long tracts bypasses the grey matter of the rostral cord, and results in early infection of the following brain regions, as determined by the location of antigen-containing neurons: the reticular formation (bilateral), right nucleus interpositus, right lateral vestibular nucleus, left red nucleus, left motor cortex, left ventral posterolateral and reticular nucleus of the thalamus, and right nucleus gracilis. These mechanisms are consistent with early and rapid dissemination in the brain before an effective immune response develops, and could provide for induction of behavioural changes before the animal is incapacitated by spinal cord infection. The early distribution of antigen-containing neurons (ventral motor neurons, motor cortex, red nucleus, lateral vestibular nucleus) indicated early involvement of several neuronal groups (upper and lower motor neurons, pyramidal and extrapyramidal systems) concerned with control of voluntary muscle (important in the genesis of paralysis). There was relative sparing of pain pathways with concomitant infection of the medial reticular formation (involved in modulation of pain in the spinal cord), suggesting mechanisms in early hyper-responsiveness and, in humans, hyperaesthesia. Although there was early infection of the motor cortex, other parts of the cerebral cortex and hippocampus were devoid of antigen, features that are probably important in the increased alertness in early animal rabies and the retained lucidity in early human rabies. Several immunohistochemical studies indicate that, in terminal stages of the disease, antigen (as detected by antibodies to nucleoprotein) is very widespread in both the central and the peripheral nervous systems. Neurons are predominantly affected. Antigen occurs as fine to large granules and bodies in perikarya and dendrites and, to a lesser extent, in axons. A few oligodendroglia may contain antigen. In many cases, neurons contain truly massive amounts of antigen, suggesting the large extent to which RV has appropriated the protein-synthesizing machinery of the cell.

Inflammatory lesions

The polioencephalomyelitis of rabies is characterized by varying degrees of perivascular cuffing with mononuclear cells, focal and regional gliosis, slight neuronophagia and, usually, moderate accumulations of inflammatory cells in the meninges. These lesions have been described in several reviews (see Charlton 1988, Perl and Good 1991).

Spongiform lesions

Spongiform lesions in rabies were first described by Charlton (1984). This vacuolation of the neuropil of the grey matter was detected initially in experimental rabies in skunks and foxes, and later in spontaneous rabies in these and other animals. The lesion is considered to be a spongiform change as defined by Masters and Richardson (1978). The distribution of lesions is similar in all affected species, of which the skunk and fox have been studied most extensively. The thalamus (all nuclei) and cerebral cortex are the most frequently and severely affected regions (Fig. 33.11). Other less frequently affected areas include the reticular formation, brain stem nuclei caudal to the diencephalon, cerebellar cortex and nuclei, and olfactory bulbs. Rarely, other areas may be involved. The light and electron microscopic lesions are qualitatively similar to experimental scrapie in skunks. However, in scrapie the lesions are more extensive and a greater proportion of the vacuoles are small. The rabies spongiform lesions are considered to develop as follows. Early lesions consist of small membrane-bound vacuoles in dendrites (Fig. 33.12) and, less frequently, in axons and astrocytes. These intracytoplasmic vacuoles enlarge and both the vacuolar and surrounding plasma membranes rupture, resulting in small tissue spaces, most of which constitute the vacuoles detected by light microscopy. Vacuolation seems to develop rapidly, probably in <2–3 days, occurs after infection by several street virus variants, and is independent of the immune response, route of inoculation or viral preparation (Charlton et al. 1987). In affected regions of the brain, the degree of vacuolation was not correlated with the amount of antigen accumulation, suggesting that spongiform change in rabies is probably an indirect effect.

PERIPHERAL SPREAD OF VIRUS AND INFECTION OF NON-NERVOUS TISSUE

During viral dissemination in the CNS, beginning soon after arrival in the brain or spinal cord, infection is also spreading centrifugally in the axons of peripheral nerve fibres, which may be myelinated, unmyelinated, motor, sensory, sympathetic or parasympathetic, and of various calibres. The mechanism of transport is anterograde axoplasmic flow; the rate of transit (as determined in cultured rat dorsal root ganglia neurons) is 100–400 mm/day (Tsiang et al. 1989). Because of the lack of ribosomes, replication is not considered to occur in axons. Thus the mechanism of viral release from axon terminals must differ from that described for dendro-axonal transfer in the CNS in which virions bud on dendritic or perikaryal plasma

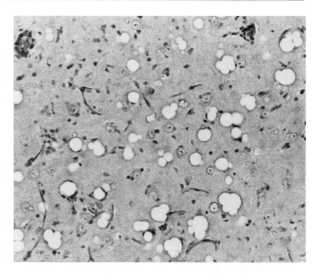

Fig. 33.11 Spongiform lesions in neuropil of thalamus of a skunk experimentally infected with street RV (H & E ×160). (Reproduced, with permission of the publisher, from Charlton 1984.)

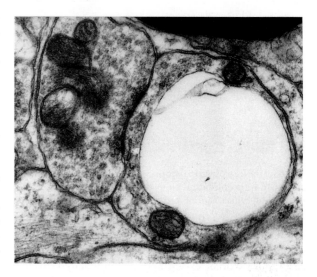

Fig. 33.12 Electron micrograph of a membrane-bound vacuole in the dendrite of a neuron in skunk brain (×30 000). (Reproduced, with permission of the publisher, from Charlton 1984).

membrane by incorporating nucleocapsid (synthesized in closely adjacent cytoplasm) into an everting portion of plasma membrane. Whether the mechanism in peripheral nerve fibres is via viral transport (probably in vesicles) and release of complete virions or via some other mechanism has not been reported. As described above, many non-nervous cells can be infected following centrifugal neural transport (reviews: Schneider 1975, Charlton 1988). Techniques for detecting antigen in the skin and cornea are useful for antemortem diagnosis. Obviously, infection of the salivary glands is essential for the usual mode of transmission of the disease. As with most other non-nervous tissues, infection occurs via peripheral nerves. There is evidence that extensive infection of salivary gland epithelial cells requires widespread release of infectious virus from axon terminals; thus, cell-to-cell spread among epithelial cells is not important even as an auxiliary mechanism in salivary gland infection. Most reports of salivary gland infection concern the submandibular glands. However, several other glands may contain antigen and virus. In naturally infected skunks they include the parotid, sublingual, zygomatic, molar and lingual glands. The nasal mucosa and nasal glands may also contain virus. Generally, titres are high in the submandibular, moderate in the parotid and low in the other salivary glands (review: Charlton 1988). Immunohistochemical studies indicate that staining of antigen-containing cells may be focal or regional, with variable numbers of cells affected in individual acini. The inflammatory response is variable, consisting mainly of focal accumulations of mononuclear cells in the interstitium and occasionally a few foci of necrosis of acinar cells. Electron microscopically, infection is chiefly in mucogenic cells. They contain much less viral matrix than neurons; viral budding is marked on the apical plasma membrane with release of virions into acinar lumens (Fig. 33.13) (Dierks 1975, Balachandran and Charlton 1994). In skunks, budding also occurred into secretory granules of epithelial cells of submandibular salivary glands and nasal glands (Fig. 33.14), suggesting a mechanism to augment the release of virions into the salivary ducts by exocytosis of virus-containing granules (Balachandran and Charlton 1994).

Negri bodies have been described in adrenal medul-

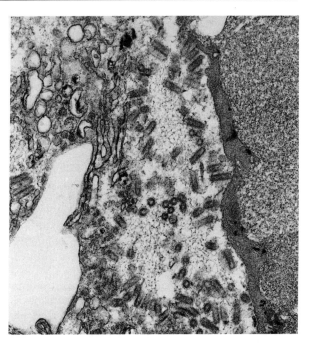

Fig. 33.14 Electron micrograph of mucous cell of submandibular salivary gland of skunk infected with street RV. Viral budding on the inner surface of secretory granules (×37 500).

lary cells (modified neurons). At least in skunks and foxes, many of these cells contain antigen, and foci of mononuclear cells are common in these species. Mononuclear cell accumulations have been described in the adrenal medulla of humans.

The above description is an overview of the usual type of rabies pathogenesis, i.e. undelayed progression of the disease characterized by spread of the agent through the above-mentioned sites, the development of clinical signs and death. In a minority of cases, there may be variations from this general pattern, consisting mainly in recovery from or delay in the progression of infection at one or more of the steps (review: Charlton 1988).

4.5 Immune responses

An important concern is the extent to which the expressions of the naturally occurring disease are the result of the immune response. Although conclusive evidence from natural infections is rather sparse, several reports of experimental studies suggest that the immune response can influence the susceptibility, incubation and morbidity periods, the type of clinical signs, excretion of virus and recovery from infection (before or, rarely, after clinical signs). Furthermore, these effects frequently depend on interactions of the immune response with other factors such as animal species and age, viral strain, route of inoculation and dose of virus.

NEUTRALIZING ANTIBODIES

Virus-neutralizing antibodies (VNA) are a critical component of immune resistance. They are produced

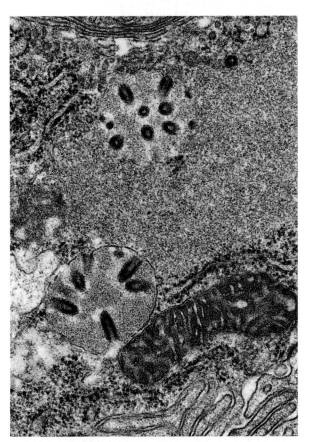

Fig. 33.13 Electron micrograph of rabies virions in acinar lumen of submandibular salivary gland (skunk) (×30 000).

in response to RV glycoprotein; production is T cell dependent, requiring CD4+ T cells as well as B cells. They are considered to be most effective in the early stages of infection, i.e. before viral entrance into peripheral nerves. However, some weakly pathogenic strains can be cleared from the CNS by VNA. Apparently, protection resides primarily with IgG rather than IgM (reviews: Turner 1990, Lafon 1994). Measurement of serum VNA has been and continues to be the predominant method for estimating immune resistance to rabies infection in humans, and in conjunction with challenge is frequently used in efficacy tests of vaccines in other animals.

Generally, VNA is not detected in infected humans until after the onset of clinical signs (reviews: Fishbein 1991, Hemachuda 1994). In animal experiments the relation of neutralizing antibody to outcome of infection is variable. There are several reports of VNA in a small proportion of apparently healthy foxes, skunks and raccoons in rabies enzootic areas, presumably as a result of previous exposure to the virus (reviews: McLean 1975, Winkler 1975, Blancou, Aubert and Artois 1991, Winkler and Jenkins 1991, Wandeler et al. 1994). The prevalence of VNA in mongooses in enzootic areas in Grenada may be high (up to 40%), and fluctuates with changes in the incidence of rabies. High titres of VNA may be indicative either of advanced CNS infection or of recovery. Evidence that the VNA response can influence susceptibility to rabies comes mainly from work with inbred strains of mice inoculated intraperitoneally with street RV (review: Lodmell 1988): resistant and susceptible strains were, respectively, good or poor responders in terms of VNA production.

N PROTEIN

Recent advances include the demonstration, originally by Dietzschold and co-workers (1987), that N protein can induce an immune response sufficient to protect animals against challenge in the absence of detectable VNA. Priming with N protein can augment the production of VNA on subsequent inoculation of live vaccines (review: Fu, Wunner and Dietzschold 1994). A recent study indicates that the nucleoprotein of RV is a superantigen (Lafon et al. 1992). The significance of this in immune resistance has not yet been determined (Lafon 1994).

IMMUNOSUPPRESSION AND CELL-MEDIATED IMMUNITY

Various features of rabies have been studied by immunosuppression or other manipulations of immune mechanisms in experimental animals. The findings include: an increase or a decrease in the incubation period due to immunosuppression (Tignor et al. 1974, Smith et al. 1982, Charlton, Casey and Campbell 1984); early death in mice due to antibody and not to immune T cells (Prabhakar and Nathanson 1981); optimum clearance of RV from the nervous system requires both B and T lymphocytes (Kaplan, Wiktor and Koprowski 1975, Miller et al. 1978, Prabhakar, Fischman and Nathanson 1981, Smith 1981);

immunosuppression-facilitated centrifugal neural migration of virus (Smith et al. 1982); and dissemination to the salivary glands (Charlton, Casey and Campbell 1987).

Cytotoxic T cells can be induced by rabies glycoprotein, nucleocapsid, N protein and NS protein (review: Lafon 1994). The precise role of cytotoxic T cells in immunoprotection has not been resolved. Under certain circumstances, they may be critical for host defence (Nathanson and Gonzalez-Scarano 1991). Lafon (1994) has indicated that, in the absence of neutralizing antibodies, cytotoxic T cells are not sufficient to protect the host; however, their participation in combination with other immune effector mechanisms cannot be excluded. Alternatively, they may contribute to immune injury in rabies.

INFLUENCE OF IMMUNE RESPONSE ON TYPE OF RABIES

The role of the immune response in the type of clinical signs, especially encephalitic vs paralytic rabies, is now being studied. As described above, in skunks inoculated with street virus, early spread in the CNS included ventral motor neurons in the lumbar cord, the motor cortex and other brain nuclei relevant to motor control of skeletal muscle. Assuming its deleterious effect on infected neurons, an early immune response might be more likely to induce paralytic rather than encephalitic signs. In fact, several studies do support a role for the immune response in paralytic rabies (Tignor et al. 1974, Iwasaki, Gerhard and Clark 1977, Smith et al. 1982, Sugamata et al. 1992, Weiland et al. 1992, Lafon et al. 1994); however, Hemachuda et al. (1988) suggested that in humans lymphocyte proliferative responses are associated with encephalitic rabies, and that paralysis in mice infected with the CVS strain of RV did not depend on the T cell system (Hovanessian et al. 1988). Still other studies suggest that the immune response has little effect on the type of clinical signs (Gourmelon et al. 1991, Charlton 1994).

4.6 Diagnosis

Because almost all human infections result from bites by rabid animals, the decision to initiate or continue postexposure treatment often depends on the results of laboratory diagnostic tests on the animal of concern. For maximum effectiveness, diagnostic programmes require efficient and well organized field inspection, specimen collection and reporting systems, adequately equipped laboratories and well trained laboratory personnel. Details of the following laboratory procedures are contained in several excellent reviews (Webster and Casey 1988, Sureau, Ravisse and Rollin 1991, Trimarchi and Debbie 1991, Bourhy et al. 1992).

NEGRI BODIES

Examination of brain tissue for Negri bodies was the principal laboratory test for most of the twentieth century, until immunofluorescent methods were introduced in the late 1950s and early 1960s. The Negri body methods were rapid, but there was a fairly high rate of false negatives (c. 12%) when compared to virus isolation by intracerebral inoculation of mice.

IMMUNOFLUORESCENCE

During the 1960s, immunofluorescence rapidly became the method of choice in most industrialized countries. The method can be performed on smears of brain tissue, is rapid (results in a few hours), is less labour-intensive than Negri body methods and, most important, is highly specific. With improvements in conjugates and microscopes, the rate of false negatives has gradually decreased to about 0.1%. Many laboratories use immunofluorescence as a primary test and either mouse inoculation or tissue culture as a confirmatory test on specimens from suspect animals.

OTHER METHODS

As mentioned elsewhere, monoclonal antibodies and molecular biological techniques (PCR) can be used to characterize street virus isolates for epizootiological studies and have potential for use in routine diagnosis (Sacramento, Bourhy and Tordo 1991, Tordo, Bourhy and Sacramento 1992, 1995, Kamolvarin et al. 1993). However, WHO (1992) does not at present recommend the use of PCR in routine diagnosis in view of the high degree of expertise required.

The recently developed rapid rabies enzyme immunodiagnosis (RREID) test has a high degree of accuracy, and has been advocated for laboratories (e.g. in developing countries) having difficulties in using the FA test, and for screening large numbers of specimens in epidemiological studies. It can be performed on heat-inactivated specimens but not on formalin-fixed specimens. Immunohistochemical (immunoperoxidase) methods are suitable when only formalin-fixed specimens are available.

Antemortem diagnosis is occasionally requested for humans with suspected rabies. Corneal impressions and skin biopsies (back of the neck above the hairline) are recommended for immunofluorescence and oral fluids for virus isolation. Here again, the use of PCR in the future seems promising (Tordo, Bourhy and Sacramento 1995).

4.7 Control

The ultimate purpose of rabies control is the protection of humans from both infection and economic loss. In humans, rabies can be controlled by prophylactic vaccination and postexposure treatment, by reducing the risk of human exposure or, conclusively, by eradication.

CONTROL OF RABIES IN DOMESTIC ANIMALS

Control measures include immunization, movement restrictions, reproduction control, habitat control and removal of stray dogs; they may be difficult or impossible to implement in some developing countries.

Immunization

An effective way of reducing the incidence of human infection is by prophylactic immunization of those domestic animals that are the most common source of human exposure. Rabies has a high incidence in dogs in enzootic areas where dog populations reach high densities. Well planned and executed vaccination campaigns may drastically reduce rabies incidence in dogs and may even eliminate the disease in areas where it is not maintained by wildlife. Vaccinations should be done by parenteral inoculation of a product approved by the national authorities, usually an inactivated vaccine conferring 2 years of immunity after one injection. Elimination of disease should be the goal rather than a temporary reduction in incidence. The most economical way to achieve it is by mass vaccination performed in accordance with a comprehensive national plan. When the appropriate technology and resources are available the immunization of individual domestic animals should be verifiable by certification, preferably in the form of an implanted microchip.

Whenever possible, modern inactivated tissue culture vaccines should be used for the immunization of dogs and other domestic animals. They combine safety with high immunogenicity. Cell lines and primary cell cultures are used as substrates for a number of virus strains. Several manufacturers include a variety of different antigens (distemper, adenovirus, leptospirosis, parainfluenza, parvovirus) in combined vaccines. No indication of competitive inhibition has been noted. The use of live attenuated vaccines is no longer recommended for dog immunization, except for special situations (e.g. national campaigns under economic constraints). Live recombinant vaccines and other products of genetic engineering will soon become available.

Quarantine

A number of rabies-free countries have prevented the importation of rabies by rigorous enforcement of quarantine measures; for example, a 6 month quarantine period for imported cats and dogs in the UK. This approach is often not feasible in countries with contiguous land borders and is now held by some to be unnecessary, given the availability of effective vaccines for pet animals and tests for an adequate antibody response.

IMMUNIZATION OF WILD ANIMALS

Control of wildlife rabies by reducing major host populations has been attempted. However, the resilience of these opportunistic *Carnivora* to persecution, their reproductive potential, and high densities in both rural and urban habitats often nullify such efforts. A more promising approach is mass vaccination of the main hosts, although immunization of free-living wild animals is not an easy task. The wild mammal has to be lured by some trick into vaccinating itself. This is possible by incorporating oral vaccines in baits targeted at the principal host species. The methods have to be simple and efficient, so that it becomes technically and economically possible to establish the level and distribution of herd immunity required to eliminate rabies.

The most important qualities of baits for proper vaccine delivery are that they should, as far as possible, be attractive for the target species and not for others. All baits tested so far have been picked up not only by various domestic and wild *Carnivora* but also by ruminants and rodents. The next requirement is a delivery system that ensures mass immunization of the target species and that takes into consideration technical resources, administrative structures and manpower needs, as well as constraints imposed by safety requirements, terrain, climate etc.

Wandeler (1991b) detailed the requirements for vaccines to be used for oral immunization of free-living wild animals, and the development of oral immunization of wildlife as an instrument for rabies control was described by Winkler (1992). More recently, Aubert et al. (1994) have reported the extent of wildlife rabies vaccination in Europe, and Campbell (1994) has given an account of the North American situation. Oral rabies immunization became attainable in the early 1970s when it was found that ingested attenuated rabies vaccine immunized foxes (Black and Lawson 1970, Baer, Abelseth and Debbie 1971). This discovery suggested the possibility of administering an oral rabies vaccine to wild carnivores by bait. The SAD and ERA strains and their derivatives mostly fulfilled the requirements for immunizing foxes. The first field trial with foxes was carried out in Switzerland in 1978, followed by additional campaigns (Steck et al. 1982). Most areas in Switzerland and, later, large areas of other European countries and Canada became free from rabies after oral immunization campaigns (Wandeler 1991b). More recently, genetically engineered recombinant vaccines have been prepared, with great potential for wildlife rabies control (Blancou et al. 1986, Rupprecht et al. 1986). A vaccinia–rabies glycoprotein recombinant (V–RG) has been used successfully in Belgium (Brochier et al. 1991) and Luxembourg and in parts of France (Aubert et al. 1994); the first limited field trials are being carried out in raccoon rabies areas of eastern USA.

The most important conclusion from the field applications of oral vaccination in Europe and Canada is that it seems to be possible to immunize enough foxes by bait to stop the spread of the disease into rabies-free areas and to eliminate it from enzootic areas. In areas freed of fox rabies the disease also disappeared from all other species except bats. It did not reappear spontaneously from an undetected reservoir after fox vaccination campaigns were discontinued, but was occasionally able to reinvade a fox population from infected contiguous areas.

RABIES PROPHYLAXIS IN HUMANS

The history of rabies vaccines and of postexposure treatment in humans from the time of Louis Pasteur to the modern era is well described (Vodopija and Clark 1992, Thraenhart, Marcus and Kreuzfelder 1994). Highly efficacious vaccines that usually provoke only minimal or no side effects are now available and can be used for pre- and postexposure immunization. All of them contain RV antigens in a concentrated and partially purified form. Preparations widely used are the human diploid cell strain (HDCS) or the Vero cell strain, which are inactivated with β-propiolactone. Unfortunately, because of economic considerations, the cheaper brain-tissue-derived vaccines are still predominant in large parts of the world. These vaccines are of inferior potency and may induce severe allergic reactions which can occasionally be difficult to distinguish from clinical rabies (Hemachudha 1989).

Pre-exposure prophylaxis

Pre-exposure immunization is generally encouraged only for people at potentially high risk of exposure; for example, laboratory personnel working with rabies, veterinarians, and animal control and wildlife officers. Pre-exposure immunization consists of a series of inoculations (usually 3) within 21–180 days with an approved and potent inactivated vaccine. Serum antibody titres should be monitored. For people at continuing high risk of exposure, it is recommended that booster injections are given when the serum antibody titre falls below 0.5 IU/ml (WHO 1992).

Postexposure prophylaxis

People bitten or licked by a mammal acting abnormally in a geographic area where rabies might occur must be considered as exposed and postexposure treatment should begin as soon as possible. Properly administered, it is highly effective. It consists of passive immunization with rabies immunoglobulin, and vaccination (WHO 1992). Instant thorough washing of bite and scratch wounds with water and soap or detergent is most important; the use of disinfectants is also recommended. Purified rabies immunoglobulin, of equine or, preferably, human origin (HRIG), and the first dose of a potent vaccine must be administered with as little delay as possible. Additional doses of vaccine at the officially specified intervals are necessary. Tetanus prophylaxis should also be given to people without definite evidence of recent immunization. Recommendations on what has to be considered an exposure, what vaccines to use, routes of vaccine administration and treatment schedules, and the application of immunoglobulins vary from country to country; the guidelines of the national health authority must be consulted.

REFERENCES

Acha PN, Arambulo PV, 1985, Rabies in the tropics: history and current status, *Rabies in the Tropics*, eds Kuwert E, Mérieux C et al., Springer-Verlag, Berlin, 343–59.

Aubert MFA, Masson E et al., 1994, Oral wildlife rabies vaccination field trials in Europe, with recent emphasis on France, *Lyssaviruses*, eds Rupprecht CE, Dietzschold B, Koprowski H, Springer-Verlag, Berlin, 219–43.

Bacon PJ, 1985, A systems analysis of wildlife rabies epizootics, *Population Dynamics of Rabies in Wildlife*, ed Bacon PJ, Academic Press, London, 109–30.

Baer GM (ed), 1991a, *The Natural History of Rabies*, CRC Press, Boca Raton FL.

Baer GM (ed), 1991b, Vampire bat and bovine paralytic rabies, *The Natural History of Rabies*, 2nd edn, CRC Press, Boca Raton FL, 389–403.

Baer GM, Abelseth MK, Debbie JG, 1971, Oral vaccination of foxes against rabies, *Am J Epidemiol*, **93:** 487–90.

Baer GM, Lentz TL, 1991, Rabies pathogenesis to the central nervous system, *The Natural History of Rabies*, 2nd edn, ed Baer GM, CRC Press, Boca Raton FL, 105–20.

Baer GM, Shanthaveerappa TR, Bourne GH, 1965, Studies on the pathogenesis of fixed rabies virus in rats, *Bull W H O*, **33:** 783–94.

Baer GM, Shanthaveerappa TR, Bourne GH, 1968, The pathogensis of street rabies virus in rats, *Bull W H O*, **38:** 119–25.

Baer GM, Smith JS, 1991, Rabies in nonhematophagous bats, *The Natural History of Rabies*, 2nd edn, ed Baer GM, CRC Press, Boca Raton FL, 341–66.

Balachandran A, Charlton KM, 1994, Experimental rabies infection of non-nervous tissues in skunks (*Mephitis mephitis*) and foxes (*Vulpes vulpes*), *Vet Pathol*, **31:** 93–102.

Banerjee AK, 1987, Transcription and replication of rhabdoviruses, *Microbiol Rev*, **51:** 66–87.

Banerjee AK, Barik S, 1992, Gene expression of vesicular stomatitis virus genome RNA, *Virology*, **188:** 417–28.

Banerjee AK, Masters PS et al., 1989, Specific interaction of vesicular stomatitis capsid protein (N) with the phosphoprotein (NS) prevents its binding with non-specific RNA, *Genetics and Pathogenicity of Negative Strand Viruses*, eds Kolakofsky D, Mahy BWJ, Elsevier, New York, 121–8.

Barge A, Gaudin Y et al., 1993, Vesicular stomatitis virus M protein may be inside the ribonucleocapsid coil, *Virology*, **67:** 7246–53.

Barik S, Banerjee AK, 1992, Sequential phosphorylation of the phosphoprotein of vesicular stomatitis virus by cellular and viral protein kinases is essential for transcription activation, *J Virol*, **66:** 1109–18.

Beckes JD, Perrault J, 1992, Stepwise phosphorylation of vesicular stomatitis virus P protein by virion-associated protein kinases and uncoupling of second step from in vitro transcription, *Virology*, **188:** 606–17.

Bell JF, 1975, Latency and abortive rabies, *The Natural History of Rabies*, vol 1, ed Baer GM, Academic Press, New York, 331–54.

Benmansour A, Leblois H et al., 1991, Antigenicity of rabies virus glycoprotein, *J Virol*, **65:** 4198–203.

Benmansour A, Brahimi M et al., 1992, Rapid sequence evolution of street rabies glycoprotein is related to the heterogeneous nature of the viral population, *Virology*, **187:** 33–45.

Benmansour A, Paubert G et al., 1994, The polymerase-associated protein (M1) and the matrix protein (M2) from a virulent and avirulent strain of viral hemorrhagic scepticemia virus (VHSV), a fish rhabdovirus, *Virology*, **198:** 602–12.

Beran GW, 1991, Urban rabies, *The Natural History of Rabies*, 2nd edn, ed Baer GM, CRC Press, Boca Raton FL, 427–43.

Black JG, Lawson KF, 1970, Sylvatic rabies studies in the silver fox (*Vulpes vulpes*): susceptibility and immune responses, *Can J Comp Med*, **34:** 309–11.

Black BL, Rhodes RB et al., 1993, The role of vesicular stomatitis virus matrix protein in inhibition of host-directed gene expression is genetically separable from its function in virus assembly, *J Virol*, **67:** 4814–21.

Blancou J, Aubert MFA, Artois M, 1991, Fox rabies, *The Natural History of Rabies*, 2nd edn, ed Baer GM, CRC Press, Boca Raton FL, 257–90.

Blancou J, Kieny MP et al., 1986, Oral vaccination of the fox against rabies using a live recombinant vaccinia virus, *Nature (London)*, **322:** 373–5.

Bögel K, Meslin F, 1990, Economics of human and canine rabies elimination: guidelines for programme orientation, *Bull W H O*, **68:** 281–91.

Bögel K, Motschwiller E, 1986, Incidence of rabies and post-exposure treatment in developing countries, *Bull W H O*, **64:** 883–7.

Bourhy H, Kissi B, Tordo N, 1993a, Molecular diversity of the *Lyssavirus* genus, *Virology*, **194:** 70–81.

Bourhy H, Kissi B, Tordo N, 1993b, Taxonomy and evolutionary studies on lyssaviruses with special reference to Africa, *Onderstepoort J Vet Res*, **60:** 277–82.

Bourhy H, Kissi B et al., 1992, Antigenic and molecular characterization of bat rabies virus in Europe, *J Clin Microbiol*, **30:** 2419–26.

Brochier B, Kieny MP et al., 1991, Large scale eradication of rabies using recombinant vaccinia–rabies vaccine, *Nature (London)*, **354:** 520–2.

Broughan JH, Wunner WH, 1995, Characterization of protein involvement in rabies virus binding to BHK-21 cells, *Arch Virol*, **140:** 75–93.

Brown F, Crick J, 1979, Natural history of rhabdoviruses of vertebrates and invertebrates, *The Rhabdoviruses*, vol 1, ed Bishop DHL, CRC Press, Boca Raton FL, 1–22.

Brun G, 1984, Host-range mutants of Pincy virus, a new type of mutant in drosophila, *Non-segmented negative strand viruses*, eds Bishop DHL, Compans RW, Academic Press, Orlando FL, 921–6.

Buckley SM, 1975, Arbovirus infection of vertebrate and insect cell cultures, with special emphasis on Mokola, Obodhiang and Kotonkan viruses of the rabies serogroup, *Ann NY Acad Sci*, **266:** 241–50.

Bunn TO, 1991, Cat rabies, *The Natural History of Rabies*, 2nd edn, ed Baer GM, CRC Press, Boca Raton FL, 379–87.

Bunschoten H, Gore M et al., 1989, Characterization of a new virus-neutralization epitope that denotes a sequential determinant on rabies virus glycoprotein, *J Gen Virol*, **70:** 291–8.

Calisher CH, Karabatsos N et al., 1989, Antigenic relationships among rhabdoviruses from vertebrates and hematophagous arthropods, *Intervirology*, **49:** 241–57.

Campbell JB, 1994, Oral rabies immunization of wildlife and dogs: challenges to the Americas, *Lyssaviruses*, eds Rupprecht CE, Dietzschold B, Koprowski H, Springer-Verlag, Berlin, 245–66.

Carey AB, Giles RH, McLean RG, 1978, The landscape epidemiology of rabies in Virginia, *Am J Trop Med Hyg*, **27:** 573–80.

Ceccaldi P-E, Ermine A, Tsiang H, 1990, Continuous delivery of colchicine in the rat brain with osmotic pumps for inhibition of rabies virus transport, *J Virol Methods*, **28:** 79–84.

Ceccaldi P-E, Gillet JP, Tsiang H, 1989, Inhibition of the transport of rabies virus in the central nervous system, *J Neuropathol Exp Neurol*, **48:** 620–30.

Chang TL, Reiss CS, Huang AS, 1994, Inhibition of vesicular stomatitis virus RNA synthesis by protein hyperphosphorylation, *J Virol*, **68:** 4980–7.

Charlton KM, 1984, Rabies: spongiform lesions in the brain, *Acta Neuropathol (Berl)*, **63:** 198–202.

Charlton KM, 1988, The pathogenesis of rabies, *Rabies*, eds Campbell JB, Charlton KM, Kluwer Academic, Boston MA, 101–50.

Charlton KM, 1994, The pathogenesis of rabies and other lyssaviral infections, *Lyssaviruses*, eds Rupprecht CE, Dietzschold B, Koprowski H, Springer-Verlag, Berlin, 95–119.

Charlton KM, Casey GA, 1979, Experimental rabies in skunks: immunofluorescent, light and electron microscopic studies, *Lab Invest*, **41**: 36–44.

Charlton KM, Casey GA, Campbell JB, 1984, Experimental rabies in skunks: effects of immunosuppression induced by cyclophosphamide, *Can J Comp Med*, **48**: 72–7.

Charlton KM, Casey GA, Campbell JB, 1987, Experimental rabies in skunks: immune response and salivary gland infection, *Comp Immunol Microbiol Infect Dis*, **10**: 227–35.

Charlton KM, Webster WA, Casey GA, 1991, Skunk rabies, *The Natural History of Rabies*, 2nd edn, ed Baer GM, CRC Press, Boca Raton FL, 307–24.

Charlton KM, Casey GA et al., 1987, Experimental rabies in skunks and foxes: pathogenesis of the spongiform lesions, *Lab Invest*, **57**: 634–45.

Charlton KM, Casey GA et al., 1994, Early events in rabies infection of the CNS in skunks, *Vet Pathol*, **31**: 601.

Charlton KM, Casey GA et al., 1996, Early events in rabies virus infection of the central nervous system in skunks (*Mephitis mephitis*), *Acta Neuropathol*, **91**: 89–98.

Charlton KM, Nadin-Davis S et al., 1997, The long incubation period in rabies. Delayed progression of infection in muscle at the inoculation site, *Acta Neuropathol*, in press.

Chenik M, Chebli K, Blondel D, 1995, Translation initiation at alternate in-frame AUG codons in the rabies virus phosphoprotein mRNA is mediated by a ribosomal leaky scanning mechanism, *J Virol*, **69**: 707–12.

Chenik M, Chebli K et al., 1994, In vivo interaction of rabies virus phosphoprotein (P) and nucleoprotein (N): existence of two N-binding sites on P protein, *J Gen Virol*, **75**: 2889–96.

Cherkasskiy BL, 1988, Roles of the wolf and the raccoon dog in the ecology and epidemiology of rabies in the USSR, *Rev Infect Dis*, **10**: S634–6.

Chong LD, Rose JK, 1994, Interactions of normal and mutant vesicular stomatitis matrix proteins with the plasma membrane and nucleocapsids, *J Virol*, **68**: 441–7.

Chow TL, Chow FH, Hanson RP, 1954, Morphology of vesicular stomatitis virus, *J Bacteriol*, **68**: 724–6.

Clinton GM, Little SP et al., 1978, The matrix (M) protein of vesicular stomatitis virus regulates transcription, *Cell*, **15**: 1455–62.

Coll JM, 1995, The glycoprotein G of rhabdoviruses, *Arch Virol*, **140**: 827–51.

Conti C, Hauttecoeur B et al., 1988, Inhibition of rabies virus infection by a soluble membrane fraction from the rat central nervous system, *Arch Virol*, **98**: 73–86.

Conzelmann KK, 1996, Genetic manipulation of non-segmented negative-strand RNA viruses, *J Gen Virol*, **77**: 381–9.

Conzelmann K, Schnell M, 1994, Rescue of synthetic genomic RNA analogs of rabies virus by plasmid-encoded proteins, *J Virol*, **68**: 713–19.

Coulon P, Derbin C et al., 1989, Invasion of the peripheral nervous systems of adult mice by the CVS strain of rabies virus and its avirulent derivative Av01, *J Virol*, **63**: 3550–4.

Coulon P, Lafay F et al., 1994, The molecular basis for altered pathogenicity of lyssavirus variants, *Lyssaviruses*, eds Rupprecht CE, Dietzschold B, Koprowski H, Springer-Verlag, Berlin, 69–84.

Crandall RA, 1991, Arctic fox rabies, *The Natural History of Rabies*, 2nd edn, ed Baer GM, CRC Press, Boca Raton FL, 291–306.

De BP, Banerjee AK, 1984, Specific interactions of vesicular stomatitis virus L and NS proteins with heterologous genome ribonucleoprotein template lead to mRNA synthesis in vitro, *J Virol*, **51**: 628–34.

De BP, Thornton GB et al., 1982, Purified matrix protein of vesicular stomatitis virus blocks viral transcription in vitro, *Proc Natl Acad Sci USA*, **79**: 7137–41.

Dean DJ, Evans WM, McClure RC, 1963, Pathogenesis of rabies, *Bull W H O*, **29**: 803–11.

Delagneau JF, Perrin P and Atanasin A, 1981, Structure of the rabies virus: spatial relationships of the proteins 6, M_1, M_2 and N, *Ann Virol (Inst Pasteur)*, **132E**: 473–93.

Delarue M, Poch O et al., 1990, An attempt to unify the structure of polymerases, *Protein Eng*, **3**: 461–7.

Dezélée S, Bras F et al., 1989, Molecular analysis of *ref(2)p*, a *Drosophila* gene implicated in sigma rhabdovirus multiplication and necessary for male fertility, *EMBO J*, **8**: 3437–46.

Dierks RE, 1975, Electron microscopy of extraneural rabies infection, *The Natural History of Rabies*, vol 1, ed Baer GM, Academic Press, New York, 303–18.

Dietzschold B, Wang H et al., 1987, Induction of protective immunity against rabies by immunization with rabies virus ribonucleoprotein, *Proc Natl Acad Sci USA*, **84**: 9165–9.

Dietzschold B, Rupprecht CE et al., 1988, Antigenic diversity of the glycoprotein and nucleocapsid proteins of rabies and rabies-related viruses: implications for epidemiology and control of rabies, *Rev Infect Dis*, **10**: S785–98.

Durrer P, Gaudin Y, 1995, Photolabeling identifies a putative fusion domain in the envelope glycoprotein of rabies and vesicular stomatitis virus, *J Biol Chem*, **270**: 17575–81.

Ertl HCJ, Dietzschold B, Otvos J, 1991, T-helper cell epitopes of rabies virus nucleoprotein defined by tri- and tetrapeptides, *Eur J Immunol*, **21**: 1–10.

Espeta A, Coll JM, 1996, Pepscan mapping and fusion-related properties of the major phosphatidylserine-binding domain of the glycoprotein of viral hemorrhagic scepticemia virus, a salmonid rhabdovirus, *Virology*, **216**: 60–70.

Everard COR, Everard JD, 1985, Mongoose rabies in Grenada, *Population Dynamics of Rabies in Wildlife*, ed Bacon PJ, Academic Press, London, 43–69.

Fedaku M, 1991, Canine rabies, *The Natural History of Rabies*, 2nd edn, ed Baer GM, CRC Press, Boca Raton FL, 367–87.

Fishbein DB, 1991, Rabies in humans, *The Natural History of Rabies*, 2nd edn, ed Baer GM, CRC Press, Boca Raton FL, 519–49.

Flamand A, 1980, Rhabdovirus genetics, *Rhabdoviruses*, ed Bishop DHL, CRC Press, Boca Raton FL, 115–39.

Foggin CM, 1985, The epidemiological significance of jackal rabies in Zimbabwe, *Rabies in the Tropics*, eds Kuwert E, Mérieux C et al., Springer-Verlag, Berlin, 399–405.

Fredericksen BL, Whitt MA, 1996, Mutations at two conserved acidic amino acids in the glycoprotein of vesicular stomatitis virus affect pH-dependent conformational changes and reduce the pH threshold for membrane fusion, *Virology*, **217**: 49–57.

Fu ZF, Wunner WH, Dietzschold B, 1994, Immunoprotection by rabies virus nucleoprotein, *Lyssaviruses*, eds Rupprecht CE, Dietzschold B, Koprowski H, Springer-Verlag, Berlin, 161–72.

Fu ZF, Weihe E et al., 1993, Differential effects of rabies and Borna disease viruses on immediate-early response and late-response gene expression in brain tissues, *J Virol*, **67**: 6674–81.

Fu ZF, Zengh Y et al., 1994, Both the N- and the C-terminal domains of the nominal phosphoprotein of rabies virus are involved in the binding to the N protein, *Virology*, **200**: 590–7.

Gao Y, Lenard J, 1995a, Cooperative binding of multimeric phosphoprotein (P) of vesicular stomatitis virus to polymerase (L) and template: pathway and assembly, *J Virol*, **69**: 7718–23.

Gao Y, Lenard J, 1995b, Multimerization and transcriptional activation of the phosphoprotein (P) of vesicular stomatitis virus by casein kinase-II, *EMBO J*, **14**: 1240–7.

Gaudin Y, Ruigrok RWH, Brunner J, 1995, Low-pH induced conformational changes in viral fusion proteins: implications for the fusion mechanism, *J Gen Virol*, **76**: 1541–56.

Gaudin Y, Tuffereau C et al., 1991a, Fatty acylation of rabies virus proteins, *Virology*, **184**: 441–4.

Gaudin Y, Tuffereau C et al., 1991b, Reversible changes and fusion activity of the rabies virus glycoprotein, *J Virol*, **65**: 4853–9.

Gaudin Y, Ruigrok RWH et al., 1992, Rabies virus glycoprotein is a trimer, *Virology*, **187**: 627–32.

Gaudin Y, Ruigrok RWH et al., 1993, Low-pH conformational changes of rabies virus glycoprotein and their role in membrane fusion, *J Virol*, **67**: 1365–72.

Gaudin Y, Barge A et al., 1995, Aggregation of VSV M protein is reversible and mediated by nucleation sites: implications for viral assembly, *Virology*, **206**: 28–37.

Gillet JP, Derer P, Tsiang H, 1986, Axonal transport of rabies virus in the central nervous system of the rat, *J Neuropathol Exp Neurol*, **45**: 619–34.

Goto H, Nimamoto N et al., 1995, Expression of the nucleoprotein of rabies virus in *Escherichia coli* and mapping of antigenic sites, *Arch Virol*, **140**: 1061–74.

Gourmelon P, Briet D et al., 1991, Sleep alterations in experimental street rabies virus infection occur in the absence of major EEG abnormalities, *Brain Res*, **554**: 159–65.

Gupta AK, Das T, Banerjee AK, 1995, Casein kinase II is the protein phosphorylating cellular kinase associated with the ribonucleoprotein complex of purified vesicular stomatitis virus, *J Gen Virol*, **76**: 365–72.

Hanham CA, Zhao F, Tignor GH, 1993, Evidence from the anti-idiotypic network that the acetylcholine receptor is a rabies virus receptor, *J Virol*, **67**: 530–42.

Hanson RP, 1981, *Virus diseases of food animals*, vol 2, ed Gibbs EPJ, Academic Press, London.

Hemachudha T, 1989, Rabies, *Handbook of Clinical Neurology*, eds Vinken PJ, Bruyn GW, Klawans HL, Elsevier Science, Amsterdam, 383–404.

Hemachudha T, 1994, Human rabies: clinical aspects, pathogenesis and potential therapy, *Lyssaviruses*, eds Rupprecht CE, Dietzschold B, Koprowski H, Springer-Verlag, Berlin, 121–43.

Hemachudha T, Phanuphak P et al., 1988, Immunologic study of human encephalitic and paralytic rabies, *Am J Med*, **84**: 673–7.

Herman RC, 1986, Internal initiation of translation on the vesicular stomatitis virus phosphoprotein mRNA yields a second protein, *J Virol*, **58**: 797–804.

Hooper DC, Pierard I et al., 1994, Rabies ribonucleocapsid as an oral immunogen and immunological enhancer, *Proc Natl Acad Sci USA*, **91**: 10908–12.

Horikami SM, Moyer SA, 1982, Host range mutants of vesicular stomatitis virus defective in in vitro RNA methylation, *Proc Natl Acad Sci USA*, **79**: 7694–8.

Horikami SM, Curran J et al., 1992, Complexes of Sendai virus NP-P and P-L proteins are required for defective interfering particle genome replication in vitro, *J Virol*, **66**: 4901–8.

Hovanessian AR, Marcovistz R et al., 1988, Production and action of interferon in rabies virus infection, *Interferon Treatment of Neurologic Disorders*, ed Smith RA, Dekker, New York, 157–86.

Hudson LD, Condra C, Lazzarini RA, 1986, Cloning and expression of viral phosphoprotein: structure suggests vesicular stomatitis virus NS may function by mimicking an RNA template, *J Virol*, **67**: 1571–9.

Hunt DM, Hutchinson K , 1993, Amino acid changes in the L polymerase protein of vesicular stomatitis virus which confer aberrant polyadenylation and temperature-sensitive phenotypes, *Virology*, **193**: 786–93.

Hunt DM, Smith EF, Buckley DW, 1984, Aberrant polyadenylation by a vesicular stomatitis virus mutant is due to an altered L protein, *J Virol*, **52**: 515–21.

Isaac CL, Keene JD, 1982, RNA polymerase-associated interactions near template promoter sequences of defective interfering particles of vesicular stomatitis virus, *J Virol*, **43**: 241–9.

Iwasaki Y, Clark HF, 1975, Cell to cell transmission of virus in the central nervous system. II. Experimental rabies in mouse, *Lab Invest*, **33**: 391–9.

Iwasaki Y, Gerhard W, Clark HF, 1977, Role of the host immune response in the development of either encephalitic or paralytic disease after experimental rabies infection in mice, *Infect Immun*, **18**: 220–5.

Jackson AC, 1994, Animal models of rabies virus neurovirulence, *Lyssaviruses*, eds Rupprecht CE, Dietzschold B, Koprowski H, Springer-Verlag, Berlin, 85–93.

Jackson AO, Francki RIB, Zuidema D, 1987, Biology, structure, and replication of plant rhabdoviruses, *The Rhabdoviruses*, ed Wagner RR, Plenum Press, New York, 427–508.

Johnson RT, 1965, Studies of cellular vulnerability and pathogenesis using fluorescent antibody staining, *J Neuropathol Exp Neurol*, **24**: 662–74.

Justice PA, Sun W et al., 1995, Membrane vesiculation function of wild-type and mutant matrix proteins of vesicular stomatitis virus, *J Virol*, **69**: 3156–60.

Kamolvarin N, Tirawatnpong T et al., 1993, Diagnosis of rabies by polymerase chain reaction with nested primers, *J Infect Dis*, **167**: 207–10.

Kaplan MM, Wiktor TJ, Koprowski H, 1975, Pathogenesis of rabies in immunodeficient mice, *J Immumol*, **114**: 1761–5.

Kaptur PE, McKenzie MO et al., 1995, Assembly functions of vesicular stomatits virus matrix protein are not disrupted by mutations at major sites of phosphorylation, *Virology*, **206**: 894–903.

Kawai A, Morimoto K, 1994, Functional aspects of lyssavirus proteins, *Lyssaviruses*, eds Rupprecht CE, Dietzschold B, Koprowski H, Springer-Verlag, Berlin, 27–42.

King AA, Meredith CD, Thomson GR, 1994, The biology of southern African Lyssavirus variants, *Lyssaviruses*, eds Rupprecht CE, Dietzschold B, Koprowski H, Springer-Verlag, Berlin, 267–95.

King AA, Turner GS, 1993, Rabies: a review, *J Comp Pathol*, **108**: 1–39.

Kissi B, Tordo N, Bourhy H, 1995, Genetic polymorphism in the rabies virus nucleoprotein gene, *Virology*, **209**: 526–37.

Koprowski H, Zheng YM et al., 1993, In vivo expression of inducible nitric oxide synthase in experimentally induced neurologic diseases, *Proc Natl Acad Sci USA*, **90**: 3024–7.

Kozak M, 1989, The scanning model of translation: an update, *J Cell Biol*, **108**: 229–41.

Kretzschmar E, Peluso R et al., 1996, Normal replication of vesicular stomatitis virus without C proteins, *Virology*, **216**: 309–16.

Kucera P, Dolivo M et al., 1985, Pathways of the early propagation of virulent and avirulent rabies strains from the eye to the brain, *J Virol*, **55**: 158–62.

Lafay F, Coulon P et al., 1991, Spread of CVS strain of rabies virus and of the avirulent mutant AV01 along the olfactory pathways of the mouse after intranasal inoculation, *Virology*, **183**: 320–30.

La Ferla F, Peluso R, 1989, The 1:1 N–NS protein complex of vesicular stomatitis virus is essential for efficent genome replication, *J Virol*, **63**: 3852–7.

Lafon M, 1994, Immunobiology of lyssaviruses: the basis for immunoprotection, *Lyssaviruses*, eds Rupprecht CE, Dietzschold B, Koprowski H, Springer-Verlag, Berlin, 145–60.

Lafon M, Lafage M et al., 1992, Evidence in humans of a viral superantigen, *Nature (London)*, **358**: 507–9.

Lafon M, Scott-Algara D et al., 1994, Neonatal deletion and selective expansion of mouse T-cells by exposure to rabies virus nucleocapsid superantigen, *J Exp Med*, **180**: 1207–15.

Landès-Devauchelle C, Bras F et al., 1995, Gene 2 of the sigma rhabdovirus genome encodes the PO protein, and gene 3 encodes a protein related to the reverse transcriptase of retroelements, *Virology*, **213**: 300–12.

Lawson DL, Stillman EA et al., 1995, Recombinant vesicular stomatitis viruses from DNA, *Proc Natl Acad Sci USA*, **92**: 4477–81.

Lazzarini RA, Keene JD, Schubert M, 1981, The origins of defective interfering particles of the negative strand RNA viruses, *Cell*, **26**: 145–54.

Lentz TL, Wilson PT et al., 1984, Amino acid sequence similarity between rabies virus glycoprotein and snake venom curaremimetic neurotoxins, *Science*, **226**: 847–8.

Lodmell DL, 1988, Genetic control of resistance to rabies, *Rabies*, eds Campbell JB, Charlton KM, Kluwer Academic, Boston MA, 151–61.

Lodmell DL, Esposito JJ, Ewalt LC, 1993, Rabies virus antinucleoprotein antibody protects against rabies challenge in vivo and inhibits rabies virus replication in vitro, *J Virol*, **67:** 6080–6.

Lodmell DL, Sumner JW et al., 1991, Raccoon poxvirus recombinants expressing the rabies virus nucleoprotein protect mice against lethal rabies virus infection, *J Virol*, **65:** 3400–5.

Lodmell DL, Smith JS et al., 1995, Cross-protection of mice against a global spectrum of rabies virus variants, *J Virol*, **69:** 4957–62.

Lord RD, Fuenzalida E et al., 1975, Observations on the epizootiology of vampire bat rabies, *Bull Pan Am Health Org*, **9:** 189–95.

Lycke E, Tsiang H, 1987, Rabies virus infection of cultured rat sensory neurons, *J Virol*, **61:** 2733–41.

Lyles DS, McKenzie MO et al., 1996, Complementation of M gene mutants of vesicular stomatitis virus by plasmid-derived M proteins converts spherical extracellular particles into native bullet shapes, *Virology*, **217:** 76–87.

McLean RG, 1975, Raccoon rabies, *The Natural History of Rabies*, vol 2, ed Baer GM, Academic Press, New York, 53–77.

Masters CL, Richardson EP Jr, 1978, Subacute spongiform encephalopathy (Creutzfeld–Jakob disease). The nature and progression of spongiform change, *Brain*, **101:** 333–44.

Mathur M, Das T, Banerjee AK, 1996, Expression of the L protein of vesicular stomatitis virus Indiana serotype from recombinant baculovirus in insect cells: requirement of host factor(s) for its biological activity in vitro, *J Virol*, **70:** 2252–9.

Melki R, Gaudin Y, Blondel D, 1994, Interaction between tubulin and the matrix protein of vesicular stomatitis virus: possible implications in the viral cytopathic effect, *Virology*, **202:** 339–47.

Meslin F-X, Fishbein DB, Matter HC, 1994, Rationale and prospects for rabies elimination in developing countries, *Lyssaviruses*, eds Rupprecht CE, Dietzschold B, Koprowski H, Springer-Verlag, Berlin, 1–26.

Meslin FX, Kaplan MM, Koprowski H (eds), 1995, *Laboratory Techniques in Rabies*, 4th edn, WHO, Geneva.

Miller A, Morse HC et al., 1978, The role of antibody in recovery from experimental rabies. I. Effect of depletion of B and T cells, *J Immunol*, **121:** 321–6.

Minamoto N, Tanaka H et al., 1994, Linear and conformational-dependent antigenic sites on the nucleoprotein of rabies virus, *Microbiol Immunol*, **38:** 449–55.

Morimoto K, Ohkubo A, Kawai A, 1989, Structure and transcription of the glycoprotein gene of attenuated HEP-Flury strain of rabies virus, *Virology*, **173:** 465–77.

Morzunov SP, Winton JR, Nichol ST, 1995, The complete genome structure and phylogenetic relationships of infectious hematopoietic necrosis virus, *Virus Res*, **38:** 175–92.

Moyer SA, Smallwood-Kentro S et al., 1991, Assembly and transcription of synthetic vesicular stomatitis virus nucleocapsids, *J Virol*, **65:** 2170–8.

Müller R, Poch O et al., 1994, Rift valley fever virus L segment: correction of the sequence and possible functional role of newly identified regions conserved in RNA-dependent polymerases, *J Gen Virol*, **75:** 1345–52.

Murphy FA, Bauer SP et al., 1973, Comparative pathogenesis of rabies and rabies-like virus. Viral infection and transit from inoculation site to the central nervous system, *Lab Invest*, **28:** 361–76.

Murphy FA, Fauquet CM et al., 1995, *Virus Taxonomy*, Springer-Verlag, Vienna.

Nadin-Davies SA, Casey GA, Wandeler A, 1993, Identification of regional variants of the rabies virus within the Canadian province of Ontario, *J Gen Virol*, **74:** 829–37.

Nadin-Davies SA, Casey GA, Wandeler AI, 1994, A molecular epidemiological study of rabies virus in central Ontario and western Quebec, *J Gen Virol*, **75:** 2575–83.

Nathanson N, Gonzalez-Scarano F, 1991, Immune response to

rabies virus, *The Natural History of Rabies*, 2nd edn, ed Baer GM, CRC Press, Boca Raton FL, 145–61.

Nel LH, Thomson GR, Von Teicham BF, 1993, Molecular epidemiology of rabies virus in South Africa, *Onderstepoort J Vet Res*, **60:** 301–6.

Newcomb WW, Tobin TJ et al., 1982, In vitro reassembly of vesicular stomatitis virus skeletons, *J Virol*, **41:** 1055–62.

Ni Y, Tominaga Y et al., 1995, Mapping and characterization of a sequential epitope on the rabies virus glycoprotein which is recognized by a neutralizing monoclonal antibody RG719, *Microbiol Immunol*, **39:** 693–702.

Ogden JR, Pal R, Wagner RR, 1986, Mapping regions of the matrix protein of vesicular stomatitis virus which bind to the ribonucleocapsids, liposomes, and monoclonal antibodies, *J Virol*, **58:** 860–8.

Pattnaik AK, Ball AL et al., 1995, The termini of VSV DI particle RNAs are sufficient to signal encapsidation, replication, and budding to generate infectious particles, *Virology*, **206:** 760–4.

Perl DP, Good PF, 1991, The pathology of rabies in the CNS, *The Natural History of Rabies*, 2nd edn, ed Baer GM, CRC Press, Boca Raton FL, 163–90.

Perrin P, Portmoi D and Sureau P, 1982, Étude de l'adsorption et de la pénétration du virus rabique: interactions avec les cellules BHK21 et des membranes artificielles, *Ann Virol (Inst Pasteur)*, **133E:** 403–22.

Plotkin SA, 1993, Vaccination in the 21st century, *J Infect Dis*, **168:** 29–57.

Poch O, Tordo N, Keith G, 1988, Sequence of the 3386 3′ nucleotides of the genome of the Av01 strain rabies virus: structural similarities of the protein regions involved in transcription, *Biochimie*, **70:** 1019–29.

Poch O, Sauvaget I et al., 1989, Identification of four conserved motifs among the RNA-dependent polymerase encoding elements, *EMBO J*, **8:** 3867–74.

Poch O, Blumberg BM et al., 1990, Sequence comparison of five polymerases (L proteins) of unsegmented negative-strand RNA viruses: theoretical assignments of functional domains, *J Gen Virol*, **71:** 1153–62.

Prabhakar BS, Fischman HR, Nathanson N, 1981, Recovery from experimental rabies by adoptive transfer of immune cells, *J Gen Virol*, **56:** 25–31.

Prabhakar BS, Nathanson N, 1981, Acute rabies death mediated by antibody, *Nature (London)*, **290:** 590–1.

Radostits OM, Blood DC, Gay CC, 1994, *Veterinary Medicine*, 8th edn, Baillière Tindall, London, 1087–94.

Rando RF, Hotkins AL, 1994, Production of human monoclonal antibodies against rabies virus, *Lyssaviruses*, eds Rupprecht CE, Dietzschold B, Koprowski H, Springer-Verlag, Berlin, 195–205.

Ravkov EV, Smith JS, Nichol ST, 1995, Rabies virus glycoprotein gene contains a long 3′ noncoding region which lacks pseudogene properties, *Virology*, **206:** 718–23.

Reagan KJ, Wunner WH, 1985, Rabies virus interaction with various cell lines is independent of the acetylcholine receptor, *Arch Virol*, **84:** 277–82.

Richardson JC, Peluso RW, 1996, Inhibition of VSV genome RNA replication but not transcription by monoclonal antibodies specific for the viral P protein, *Virology*, **216:** 26–34.

Rupprecht CE, Wiktor TJ et al., 1986, Oral immunization and protection of raccoons (*Procyon lotor*) with a vaccinia–rabies glycoprotein recombinant virus vaccine, *Proc Natl Acad Sci USA*, **83:** 7947–50.

Rupprecht CE, Dietzschold B et al., 1991, Antigenic relationships of lyssaviruses, *The Natural History of Rabies*, 2nd edn, ed Baer GM, CRC Press, Boca Raton FL, 69–100.

Rustici M, Bracci L et al., 1993, A model of the rabies glycoprotein active site, *Biopolymers*, **3:** 961–9.

Sacramento D, Bourhy H, Tordo N, 1991, PCR technique as an alternative method for diagnosis and molecular epidemiology of rabies virus, *Mol Cell Probes*, **6:** 229–40.

Sacramento D, Badrane H et al., 1992, Molecular epidemiology of rabies in France: comparison with vaccinal strains, *J Gen Virol*, **73**: 1149–58.

Sagara J, Kawai A, 1992, Identification of heat shock protein 70 in the rabies virion, *Virology*, **190**: 845–8.

Sagara J, Tsukita S et al., 1995, Cellular actin-binding ezrin–radixin–moesin (ERM) family proteins are incorporated into the rabies virion and closely associated with viral envelope proteins in the cell, *Virology*, **206**: 485–94.

Schlegel R, Tralka M et al., 1983, Inhibition of VSV binding and infectivity by phosphatidylserine: is phosphatidylserine a VSV-binding site?, *Cell*, **32**: 639–46.

Schneider LG, 1975, Spread of virus from the central nervous system, *The Natural History of Rabies*, vol 1, ed Baer GM, Academic Press, Boca Raton FL, 273–301.

Schneider LG, Cox JH, 1994, Bat lyssaviruses in Europe, *Lyssaviruses*, eds Rupprecht CE, Dietzschold B, Koprowski H, Springer-Verlag, Berlin, 207–18.

Schneider LG, Dietzschold B et al., 1973, Rabies group-specific ribonucleoprotein antigen and a test system for grouping and typing of rhabdoviruses, *J Virol*, **11**: 748–55.

Schnell M, Conzelmann KK, 1995, Polymerase activity of in vitro mutated rabies virus L protein, *Virology*, **214**: 522–30.

Schnell MJ, Buonocore L et al., 1996, The minimal conserved transcription stop–start signal promotes stable expression of a foreign gene in vesicular stomatitis virus, *J Virol*, **70**: 2318–23.

Scholthof KBG, Hillman B et al., 1994, Characterization and detection of sc4: a sixth gene encoded by sonchus yellow net virus, *Virology*, **204**: 279–88.

Schütze H, Enzmann P-J et al., 1995, Complete genomic sequence of the fish rhabdovirus infectious haematopoietic necrosis virus, *J Gen Virol*, **76**: 2519–27.

Sellers RF, 1984, Vesicular viruses, *Topley and Wilson's Principles of Bacteriology, Virology and Immunity*, 7th edn, vol 4, eds Brown F, Wilson GS, Edward Arnold, London, 213–32.

Shankar V, Dietzschold B, Koprowski H, 1991, Direct entry of rabies virus into the central nervous system without prior local replication, *J Virol*, **65**: 2736–8.

Sikes RK, 1962, Pathogenesis of rabies in wildlife. I. Comparative effect of varying doses of rabies virus inoculated into foxes and skunks, *Am J Vet Res*, **23**: 1041–7.

Sleat DE, Banerjee AK, 1993, Transcriptional activity and mutational analysis of recombinant vesicular stomatitis virus RNA polymerase, *J Virol*, **67**: 1334–9.

Smallwood S, Moyer SA, 1993, Promoter analysis of vesicular stomatitis virus RNA polymerase, *Virology*, **192**: 254–63.

Smith JS, 1981, Mouse model for abortive rabies infection of the central nervous system, *Infect Immun*, **31**: 297–308.

Smith JS, Yager PA, Orciari LA, 1993, Rabies in wild and domestic carnivores of Africa: epidemiological and historical associations determined by limited sequence analysis, *Onderstepoort J Vet Res*, **60**: 307–14.

Smith JS, McClelland CL et al., 1982, Dual role of the immune response in street rabies virus infection of mice, *Infect Immun*, **35**: 213–21.

Smith JS, Orciari LA et al., 1992, Epidemiologic and historical relationships among 97 rabies virus isolates as determined by limited sequence analysis, *J Infect Dis*, **166**: 296–307.

Spiropoulou CF, Nichol ST, 1993, A small highly basic protein is encoded in overlapping frame within the P gene of vesicular stomatitis virus, *J Virol*, **67**: 3103–10.

Steck F, Wandeler A et al., 1982, Oral immunization of foxes against rabies: a field study, *Zentralbl Veterinär-Med, B*, **29**: 372–96.

Sugamata M, Miyazawa M et al., 1992, Paralysis of street rabies virus-infected mice is dependent on T lymphocytes, *J Virol*, **66**: 1252–60.

Sureau P, Ravisse P, Rollin PE, 1991, Rabies diagnosis by animal inoculation, identification of Negri bodies, or ELISA, *The Natural History of Rabies*, 2nd edn, ed Baer GM, CRC Press, Boca Raton FL, 203–17.

Takacs AM, Banerjee AK, 1995, Efficient interaction of the ves-

icular stomatitis virus P protein or the N protein in cell expressing the recombinant proteins, *Virology*, **208**: 821–6.

Thraenhart O, Marcus I, Kreuzfelder E, 1994, Current and future immunoprophylaxis against rabies: reduction of treatment failure and errors, *Lyssaviruses*, eds Rupprecht CE, Dietzschold B, Koprowski H, Springer-Verlag, Berlin, 173–94.

Tierkel ES, 1975, Canine rabies, *The Natural History of Rabies*, vol 2, ed Baer GM, Academic Press, New York, 123–37.

Tignor GH, Shope RE et al., 1974, Immunopathologic aspects of infection with Lagos bat virus of the rabies serogroup, *J Immunol*, **112**: 260–5.

Tordo N, 1991, Contribution of molecular biology to vaccine development and molecular epidemiology of rabies disease, *Mem Inst Butantan*, **53**: 31–51.

Tordo N, Bourhy H, Sacramento D, 1992, Polymerase chain reaction technology for rabies virus, *Frontiers in Virology*, eds Becker Y, Darai G, Springer-Verlag, Berlin, 389–405.

Tordo N, Bourhy H, Sacramento D, 1995, PCR technology for lyssavirus diagnosis, *The Polymerase Chain Reaction for Human Diagnosis*, ed Clewley JP, CRC Press, Boca Raton FL, 125–45.

Tordo N, Kouznetzoff A, 1993, The rabies virus genome: an overview, *Onderstepoort J Vet Res*, **60**: 263–9.

Tordo N, Poch O, 1988a, Strong and weak transcription signals within the rabies genome, *Virus Res Suppl*, **2**: 30.

Tordo N, Poch O, 1988b, The structure of rabies virus, *Rabies*, eds Campbell JB, Charlton KM, Kluwer Academic, Boston MA, 25–45.

Tordo N, Poch O et al., 1986, Walking along the rabies genome: is the large G–L intergenic region a remnant gene?, *Proc Natl Acad Sci USA*, **83**: 3914–18.

Tordo N, De Haan P et al., 1992, Evolution of negative-stranded RNA genomes, *Semin Virol*, **3**: 311–417.

Tordo N, Badrane H et al., 1993a, Molecular epidemiology of lyssaviruses: focus on the glycoprotein and pseudogenes, *Onderstepoort J Vet Res*, **60**: 315–23.

Tordo N, Bourhy H et al., 1993b, Structure and expression in the baculovirus of the Mokola virus glycoprotein: an efficient recombinant vaccine, *Virology*, **194**: 59–69.

Trimarchi CV, Debbie JG, 1991, The fluorescent antibody in rabies, *The Natural History of Rabies*, 2nd edn, ed Baer GM, CRC Press, Boca Raton FL, 219–33.

Tsiang H, 1993, Pathophysiology of rabies virus infection of the central nervous system, *Adv Virus Res*, **42**: 375–412.

Tsiang H, Ceccaldi PE, Lycke E, 1991, Rabies virus infection and transport in human sensory dorsal root ganglia neurons, *J Gen Virol*, **72**: 1191–4.

Tsiang H, de la Port S et al., 1986, Infection of rat myotubes and neurons from the spinal cord by rabies virus, *J Neuropathol Exp Neurol*, **45**: 28–42.

Tsiang H, Lycke E et al., 1989, The anterograde transport of rabies virus in rat sensory dorsal root ganglia neurons, *J Gen Virol*, **70**: 2075–85.

Tuffereau C, Leblois H et al., 1989, Arginine or lysine in position 333 of ERA and CVS glycoprotein is necessary for rabies virulence in adult mice, *Virology*, **172**: 206–12.

Turner GS, 1990, Rhabdoviridae and rabies, *Topley & Wilson's Principles of Bacteriology, Virology and Immunity*, 8th edn, vol 4, eds Collier LH, Timbury MC, Edward Arnold, London, 479–98.

Vaughn JB, 1975, Cat rabies, *The Natural History of Rabies*, vol 2, ed Baer GM, Academic Press, New York, 139–54.

Vidal S, Kolakofsky D, 1989, Modified model for the switch from Sendai virus transcription to replication, *J Virol*, **63**: 1951–8.

Vodopija I, Clark HF, 1991, Human vaccination against rabies, *The Natural History of Rabies*, 2nd edn, ed Baer GM, CRC Press, Boca Raton FL, 571–95.

Walker PJ, Byrne KE et al., 1992, The genome of bovine ephemeral fever rhabdovirus contains two related glycoproteins, *Virology*, **191**: 49–61.

Walker PJ, Wang Y et al., 1994, Structural and antigenic analysis of the nucleoprotein of bovine ephemeral fever rhabdovirus, *J Gen Virol*, **75:** 1889–99.

Wandeler AI, 1988, Control of wildlife rabies: Europe, *Rabies*, eds Campbell JB, Charlton KM, Kluwer Academic, Boston MA, 365–80.

Wandeler AI, 1991a, Carnivore rabies: ecological and evolutionary aspects, *Hystrix*, **3:** 121–35.

Wandeler AI, 1991b, Oral immunization of wildlife, *The Natural History of Rabies*, 2nd edn, ed Baer GM, CRC Press, Boca Raton FL, 485–503.

Wandeler AI, Matter HC et al., 1993, The ecology of dogs and canine rabies: a selective review, *Rev Sci Tech*, **12:** 51–71.

Wandeler AI, Nadin-Davis SA et al., 1994, Rabies epidemiology: some ecological and evolutionary perspectives, *Lyssaviruses*, eds Rupprecht CE, Dietzschold B, Koprowski H, Springer-Verlag, Berlin, 297–324.

Wang Y, Cowley JA, Walker PJ, 1995, Adelaide river virus nucleoprotein gene: analysis of phylogenetic relationships of ephemeroviruses and other rhabdoviruses, *J Gen Virol*, **76:** 995–9.

Wang Y, Walker PJ, 1993, Adelaide river rhabdovirus expresses consecutive glycoprotein genes as polycistronic mRNAs: new evidence of gene duplication as an evolutionary process, *Virology*, **195:** 719–31.

Wang Y, McWilliam SM et al., 1994, Complex genome organization in the Gns–L intergenic region of Adelaide river rhabdovirus, *Virology*, **203:** 63–72.

Webster WA, Casey GA, 1988, Diagnosis of rabies infection, *Rabies*, eds Campbell JB, Charlton KM, Kluwer Academic, Boston MA, 201–22.

Weiland F, Cox JH et al., 1992, Rabies virus neuritic paralysis: immunopathogenesis of non fatal paralytic rabies, *J Virol*, **66:** 5096–9.

Wertz GW, Whelan S et al., 1994, Extent of terminal complementarity modulates the balance between transcription and replication of vesicular stomatitis virus RNA, *Proc Natl Acad Sci USA*, **91:** 8587–91.

Whelan SPJ, Ball LA et al., 1995, Efficient recovery of infectious vesicular stomatitis virus entirely from cDNA clones, *Proc Natl Acad Sci USA*, **92:** 8388–92.

WHO, 1973, *WHO Expert Committee on Rabies – Sixth Report*, WHO, Geneva.

WHO, 1983, *Guidelines for Dog Rabies Control*, Seventh Report of the WHO Expert Committee on Rabies, WHO, Geneva.

WHO, 1992, *WHO Expert Committee on Rabies – Eighth Report*, WHO, Geneva.

Wiktor TJ, Gyorgy E et al., 1973, Antigenic properties of rabies virus components, *J Immunol*, **110:** 269–76.

Winkler WG, 1975, Fox rabies, *The Natural History of Rabies*, vol 2, ed Baer GM, Academic Press, New York, 3–22.

Winkler WG, 1992, A review of the development of the oral vaccination technique for immunizing wildlife against rabies, *Wildlife Rabies Control*, eds Bögel K, Meslin F-X, Kaplan M, Wells Medical, Chapel Place, 82–96.

Winkler WG, Jenkins SR, 1991, Raccoon rabies, *The Natural History of Rabies*, 2nd edn, ed Baer GM, CRC Press, Boca Raton FL, 325–40.

Wunner WH, Reagan KJ, 1986, Nature of the rabies virus cellular receptor, *Virus Attachment and Entry into Cells*, eds Crowell RL, Lonberg-Holm K, American Society for Microbiology, Washington DC, 152–9.

Xiang ZQ, Spitalnik SL et al., 1995, Immune responses to nucleic acids vaccines to rabies virus, *Virology*, **209:** 569–79.

Yamamoto T, Ohtani S, 1978, Ultrastructural localization of rabies virus antigens in infected trigeminal ganglion of hamsters, *Acta Neuropathol (Berl)*, **43:** 229–33.

Zeller HG, Mitchell CJ, 1989, Replication of certain recently classified viruses in toxorhynchites amboinensis mosquitoes and in mosquito and mammalian cell lines, with implications for their arthropod-borne status, *Res Virol*, **140:** 563–70.

Zhang L, Ghosh HP, 1994, Characterization of the putative fusogenic domain in vesicular stomatitis virus glycoprotein G, *J Virol*, **68:** 2186–93.

Chapter 34

HEPATITIS A AND E

Betty H Robertson and Stanley M Lemon

1 INTRODUCTION

1.1 Enterically transmitted viral hepatitis

Although descriptions of epidemic jaundice go back to earliest recorded human history, the infectious nature of hepatitis was not widely appreciated until this century. Investigations during the Second World War led to the first clear recognition that there were distinct forms of transmissible hepatitis: one that was acquired through ingestion of contaminated food or water ('infectious jaundice') and another that was associated with the administration of blood or blood products ('homologous serum jaundice') (Havens 1944, Barker, Capps and Allen 1945). MacCallum classified these as type A and type B hepatitis, setting in place a classification scheme that still exists. The distinguishing epidemiological features of these infectious diseases and the lack of cross-protection engendered by their respective agents were confirmed by Krugman and his associates in a classic series of studies carried out among institutionalized children (Krugman and Ward 1958, Ward et al. 1958, Krugman et al. 1960). However, the modern era of hepatitis A virology began with the identification of virus particles in human faecal samples (Feinstone, Kapikian and Purcell 1973).

The subsequent development of an immune electron microscopy assay for virus-aggregating antibodies resulted in a variety of increasingly sophisticated diagnostic tests for hepatitis A virus (HAV) infection. Widespread application of these new serologies, coupled with recently developed assays for hepatitis B virus (HBV) and its related antibody responses, led to the recognition that there were at least 2 additional human viruses responsible for reported cases of 'non-A, non-B' (NANB) hepatitis. One type of NANB hepatitis, now recognized to be due to infection with hepatitis C virus (HCV), resembled hepatitis B in that it was frequently associated with chronic liver disease and often transmitted by transfusion or other parenteral blood exposures (Choo et al. 1989). However, a distinctive agent responsible for water-borne or enterically transmitted NANB hepatitis was recognized to be the cause of large outbreaks of acute hepatitis in the Indian subcontinent and subsequently elsewhere (Khuroo 1980). These outbreaks included an epidemic in Delhi in 1955 that involved over 30 000 people and was associated with a breach in the city's sanitary water supply system. Although for many years this epidemic was considered to be due to type A 'infectious' hepatitis, serological tests carried out in the late 1970s indicated otherwise (Wong et al. 1980). The responsible agent, hepatitis E virus (HEV), was identified by Balayan et al. (1983) in human faecal samples.

1.2 Similar and contrasting properties of HAV and HEV

HAV and HEV share a number of physical and biological characteristics (Table 34.1). Both are non-enveloped, RNA viruses with single-stranded genomes of positive polarity. Both display strong tropism for the liver (hepatocytes) and typically cause self-limited infections associated with acute hepatic inflammation. Above all, however, it is the faecal–oral transmission of HAV and HEV that distinguishes these viruses from other human hepatitis viruses, including HBV, hepatitis delta virus (HDV) and HCV. Both HAV and HEV are shed at high titres in the faeces of infected individuals. In each case, the virus present in faeces is replicated primarily in the liver and reaches the intestinal tract following secretion from the hepatocytes into biliary canaliculi and passage through the bile ducts. The absence of a lipid envelope is an important factor in this process, as it renders both HAV and HEV stable when suspended in bile. In contrast, the other human hepatitis viruses possess an outer lipid envelope and are likely to be rapidly inactivated in bile. Therefore, newly replicated HAV and HEV particles have a direct route to the outside environment that is denied the other hepatitis viruses. This allows HAV and HEV to cause explosive outbreaks of disease that are not seen with other types of hepatitis. However, neither HAV nor HEV causes persistent infections in humans and thus, unlike HBV and HCV, they have no association with chronic viral hepatitis or hepatocellular carcinoma.

Despite these similarities, HAV and HEV are very different viruses with a number of distinguishing features that result in their classification within different virus families (Table 34.1). These differences include fundamental aspects of virion structure and genome organization, as well as molecular mechanisms of translation and RNA replication.

2 HEPATITIS A VIRUS

2.1 Classification

On the basis of several features that distinguish HAV from other picornaviruses (Table 34.2), it is classified as the only member of the *Hepatovirus* genus of the *Picornaviridae* family (Minor 1991). Unique attributes of HAV include its tropism for the liver, its unusually slow and usually non-cytolytic replication cycle, and its lack of close genetic relatedness to any other picornavirus.

2.2 Morphology of the HAV particle

The HAV virion appears as a relatively smooth, 27–30 nm rounded particle when viewed by electron microscopy in negatively stained preparations (Fig. 34.1). Icosahedral symmetry is evident in many particles, but information concerning finer aspects of the capsid structure is limited (see p. 697). Infectious virions have a sedimentation constant of c. 150S and band in CsCl at c. 1.325 g/cm³ (Lemon, Jansen and Newbold 1985). Most virus preparations contain a large proportion of empty 70S capsids that are antigenically identical to virions.

2.3 Genome organization

The genomic RNA is single-stranded, c. 7.5 kb in length and of positive polarity. The extreme 5′ end of the virion RNA is covalently coupled to a small viral protein, 3B (VPg, see p. 700), which is presumed to be removed from the RNA after its release from the capsid. The organization of the genome is similar to that of all picornaviruses (Fig. 34.2) (Najarian et al. 1985, Cohen et al. 1987c), but there are several unique features. There are at least 3 functionally separate domains: the 5′ and 3′ non-translated RNA (5′NTR) and a single, intervening, long open reading frame (ORF) which encodes the viral polyprotein.

5′ NON-TRANSLATED RNA

The 5′NTR is approximately 735 nt long and contains an extensive secondary and tertiary RNA structure (Fig. 34.3). The segment from nucleotides 1–94 contains a 5′ terminal hairpin followed by 2 RNA pseudoknots (Brown et al. 1991, Shaffer, Brown and Lemon 1994) that, on the basis of studies of the corresponding cloverleaf-like RNA structure in poliovirus, probably play a controlling role in the initiation of positive-strand RNA synthesis (Andino et al. 1993). At nucleotides 95–154 there is a unique pyrimidine-rich tract (pY1) that contains a series of repetitive (U)UUCC(C) sequence motifs assuming a poorly defined higher ordered structure, followed by a short, single-stranded domain (Shaffer, Brown and Lemon 1994). Both in location and in base composition, the pY1 domain resembles the much longer, nearly pure poly(C) tracts of the cardioviruses and aphthoviruses, other genera within the *Picornaviridae*. It seems that the pY1 tract is dispensable for viral replication, both in primates in vivo and in cultured cells (Shaffer, Brown and Lemon 1994, Shaffer et al. 1995). The single-stranded domain located at nucleotides 135–155 seems to play a functional role in viral RNA replication, as deletion

Table 34.1 Similar and contrasting properties of HAV and HEV

Common properties		
Particle shape	Icosahedral	
Particle size	27–32 nm	
Chloroform sensitivity	Resistant	
Genome	ss (+)* 7.5 kb RNA	
Predominant transmission	Faecal–oral	
Liver disease	Acute, self-limited	
Unique properties	**HAV**	**HEV**
$S_{20,w}$	157S	183S
Density (g/ml)	1.33	1.29
Polypeptides	3–4 structural, 7 non-structural	1–2 structural, 4–5 non-structural
Stability	60°C, 1 hour	Unknown
ORF	Single ORF	3 overlapping ORFs
5′ End structure	VPg	5′ Methylated cap (?)

*ss (+), single-stranded, positive-sense.

Table 34.2 Properties of hepatoviruses and other picornaviral genera

	Hepatoviruses	Aphthoviruses	Cardioviruses	Enteroviruses	Rhinoviruses
Primary host	Humans and higher primates	Cloven-hoofed mammals	Mammals	Higher primates	Mammals
Host species restriction	Strict	Relatively strict	Relatively broad	Strict	Strict
Primary target organ	Liver (gut)	Systemic	CNS, liver	CNS, muscle (gut)	Respiratory mucosa
Dominant mode of transmission	Faecal–oral	Respiratory	??	Faecal–oral and respiratory	Respiratory
Serotypes	1	7	2	>70	>100
Particle size	27–30 nm	23–25 nm	24–30 nm	22–28 nm	24–30 nm
Buoyant density	1.33 g/cm^3	1.44 g/cm^3	1.34 g/cm^3	1.34 g/cm^3	1.41 g/cm^3
Stability <pH 7.0	pH 1.0	Nil	pH 3.0	pH 3.0	Nil
Stability >60°C	+	–	–	–	–
Genome RNA	7.5 kb	8.4 kb	7.8 kb	7.4 kb	7.2 kb
Sequence relatedness*	None	Cardioviruses	Aphthoviruses	Rhinoviruses	Enteroviruses
% G + C content	38	43	50	47	40
5′ poly(Y) tract	Poly(UUCC)	Poly(C)	Poly(C)	No	No
IRES structure	Type II	Type II	Type II	Type I	Type I
Leader (L) protein	Probably not	Yes	Yes	No	No
2A protease	No	Yes	Yes	Yes	Yes
Replication cycle	Very slow	Very fast	Very fast	Fast	Fast

*to other *Picornaviridae*; Palmenberg, 1989.

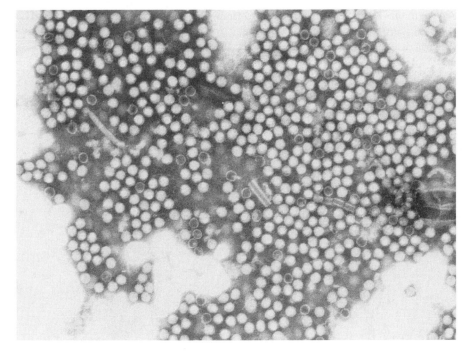

Fig. 34.1 Hepatitis A particle morphology demonstrated by electron microscopy. Negative-stained preparation.

mutations in this region confer a temperature-sensitive viral replication phenotype due to a defect in RNA synthesis (Shaffer and Lemon 1995). Further downstream, the segment of 155–735 nt contains several complex stem–loops that comprise an internal ribosomal entry site (IRES) and direct the cap-independent translation of the long ORF (pp 696 and 699) (Brown et al. 1991, Glass and Summers 1992, Brown, Zajac and Lemon 1994).

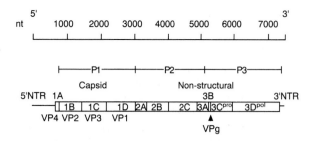

Fig. 34.2 Organization of the single-stranded positive-sense RNA genome of HAV. See pp 694 to 696 for details.

LONG OPEN READING FRAME

The long ORF encodes a large polyprotein of c. 2200 amino acid residues that is proteolytically cleaved cotranslationally and post-translationally to generate mature viral proteins. As illustrated in Fig. 34.2, the polyprotein can be functionally divided into 3 segments, P1, P2 and P3, as defined for other picornaviruses (Rueckert and Wimmer 1984). The P1 segment contains the structural proteins that form the viral capsid: 1A (also known as VP4), which is very small and not yet demonstrated to be a component of the HAV virion; 1B (VP2); 1C (VP3); and 1D (VP4). The P2 segment contains 3 non-structural polypeptides, 2A, 2B and 2C, the functions of which are not well understood. 2A may play a role in viral assembly and is present in some immature virions as uncleaved 1D2A (Borovec and Anderson 1993), whereas 2B and 2C have functions related to RNA replication (see section 2.5, p. 699). The P3 segment contains 4

additional non-structural proteins, including 3A (which probably helps anchor replication complexes to cellular membranes), 3B (VPg, the genome-linked protein), 3C^{pro} (a cysteine protease) and 3D^{pol} (an RNA-dependent RNA polymerase). Some precursor proteins (e.g. 3AB or 3CD) may have functions distinct from their processing products, but little is known of these activities in the HAV system. The primary cleavage of the polyprotein occurs at the 2A/2B junction (see p. 697).

3′ NON-TRANSLATED RNA

The 3′NTR is c. 60 nt in length and is polyadenylated at its 3′ terminus. Little is known about the functions of the 3′NTR sequence in virus replication. As with the 5′NTR, the 3′NTR is suspected to have substantial secondary structure and to interact with specific viral or host cell proteins (Nuesch, Weitz and Siegl 1993).

GENETIC VARIATION AMONG HAV STRAINS

Although the nucleotide sequences of different HAV strains have a relatively high degree of conservation, there is sufficient sequence heterogeneity to distinguish distinct phylogenetic lineages (Jansen, Siegl and Lemon 1990, Robertson et al. 1991, 1992). A comparison of the sequences of a 168 nt segment near the 1D/2A junction of 152 different strains of HAV revealed 7 distinct 'genotypes' that differed from each other at >15% of base positions (Fig. 34.4) (Robertson et al. 1992). Representatives of 3 of these genotypes (I, II, VII) have been recovered only from human sources, whereas another genotype (III)

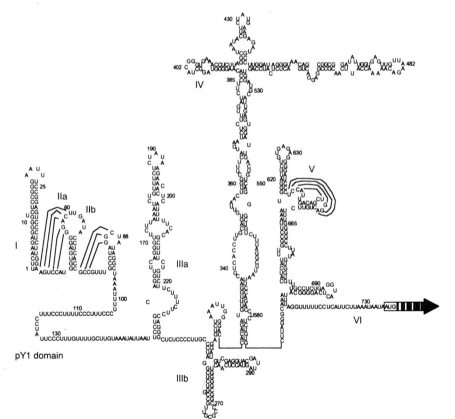

Fig. 34.3 Secondary and tertiary structure within the 5′ non-translated RNA of HAV (Brown et al. 1991).

contains viruses isolated both from humans and from captive Panamanian owl monkeys. The remaining 3 genotypes (IV, V, VI) are represented by single strains of simian HAV recovered from non-human primates (African green and cynomolgus monkeys). Genotypes I and III include the vast majority of identified human strains and each contains 2 subgroups that differ at >7.5% of base positions. These have been designated subgenotypes IA and IB, and so on.

Studies examining the genetic relatedness of HAV strains have revealed clues regarding patterns of virus spread in different regions of the world (Jansen, Siegl and Lemon 1990, Robertson et al. 1991, 1992). For example, many virus strains recovered in China and North America comprise separate, phylogenetically and geographically related clusters within genotype IA. The generally close genetic relatedness of HAV strains within these regions seems likely to reflect the endemic spread of dominant viruses. In contrast, most HAV strains recovered in Europe show extensive genetic divergence, suggesting the absence of a dominant circulating virus and consistent with a large proportion of cases being caused by virus strains imported from regions outside Europe (Jansen, Siegl and Lemon 1990, Robertson et al. 1992). Virus strains recovered from drug abusers in Sweden represent an interesting exception, however; the close genetic relatedness of HAV strains obtained from these people over a number of years suggests the continued circulation of a single virus within this apparently closed population (Robertson et al. 1992).

2.4 Structure of HAV

STRUCTURAL POLYPEPTIDES

The structural (capsid) proteins of HAV are encoded by the most 5′ (P1) region of the long ORF (see pp 695 and 696). The primary proteolytic cleavage of the nascent viral polyprotein seems to occur between the 2A and 2B polypeptides (Almela, Gonzalez and Carrasco 1991, Cho and Ehrenfeld 1991, Winokur, McLinden and Stapleton 1991, Borovec and Anderson 1993). The site of this cleavage, which is mediated by the viral protease 3C^{pro}, was recently shown to occur at residue 867 of the polyprotein, making 2B considerably larger than in other picornaviruses (Martin et al. 1996). Subsequent cleavage of the P12A precursor at the 1B/1C and 1C/1D junctions by 3C^{pro} results in 1AB (also known as VP0), 1C and 1D2A (otherwise known as PX). 1D2A seems to be an intermediate in virus assembly, as it can be detected within infected cells in pentameric subunits and possibly in some early virions (Borovec and Anderson 1993). It is possible that the subsequent cleavage of 1D2A to yield 1D and 2A is also mediated by the viral protease 3C^{pro}, but there are few data directly supporting this hypothesis and some evidence that this cleavage may take place at multiple sites. The 2A protein of HAV does not seem to have protease activity as it does in other picornaviruses, and a functional role other than in assembly has not been defined for this protein.

The 1A (VP4) sequence, located at the extreme amino terminus of the polyprotein, includes 2

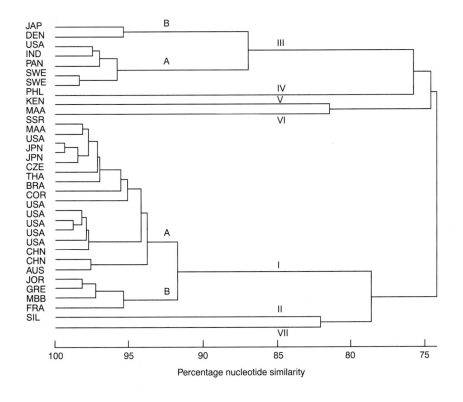

Fig. 34.4 Phylogenetic analysis of RNA sequences near the 1D/2A junctions of hepatovirus strains recovered from human sources in different geographic regions (genotypes I, II, III and VII) or simian sources (genotypes IV, V and VI) (Robertson et al. 1992).

potential methionine initiation codons (codons 1 and 3) which precede a consensus myristylation signal (GxxxT/S) (Chow et al. 1987). This has led to speculation that '1A' might be cleaved during replication to place the myristylation signal at the N terminus of the polyprotein, as such a signal is present at the amino terminus of the 1A proteins of enteroviruses and rhinoviruses. Moreover, in the aphthovirus and cardiovirus genera of the *Picornaviridae*, a 'leader' (L) protein, located at the amino terminus of the polyprotein, is proteolytically removed to yield the free amino end of 1A, which is then myristylated (Chow et al. 1987). Thus, the 1A proteins of all other picornaviruses are N terminally myristylated. However, despite numerous attempts, no one has yet been able to demonstrate the presence of 1A within the HAV particle, or to determine by labelling experiments whether any of the viral capsid proteins are myristylated. In addition, site-directed mutagenesis of the 2 potential initiator methionines resulted in a change in the size of 1AB (VP0), proving that there is no early cleavage within the sequence of 1A and strongly suggesting that HAV 1A is not myristylated (Tesar et al. 1992, 1993). Thus, although myristylation of VP4 seems to be important for the assembly of other picornaviruses, it does not seem to be necessary for HAV morphogenesis.

As in other picornaviruses, cleavage of 1AB (VP0) to 1A and 1B occurs after the encapsidation of viral RNA (Bishop and Anderson 1993), resulting in a difference in the protein profile of empty capsids and complete virions. However, this cleavage occurs slowly with HAV, a feature that might be important to pathogenesis as it may prevent the infection of intestinal epithelial cells by virus secreted in the bile into the upper intestinal tract. The arrangement of the polypeptides within the assembled capsid is not known, as the hepatoviruses represent the only genus of the *Picornaviridae* for which the capsid structure has not been solved by x-ray crystallography. A hypothetical structure has been proposed, modelled after the structures of mengovirus and rhinovirus (Luo, Rossman and Palmenburg 1988). However, this model does not correlate particularly well with experimental data obtained from biochemical and enzymatic studies, or with analysis of neutralization-resistant escape mutants (see below). Extended incubation of virus (up to 24 h) in the presence of large amounts of protease (1–10 mg/ml) results in the cleavage of VP2 by chymotrypsin and of 1D and 1B by trypsin. However, protease digestion has no effect on infectivity or antigenicity of the virus (Lemon, Amphlett and Sangar 1991). Chemical iodination of exposed tyrosine residues occurs at 2 surface sites, one involving 1D and the other, 1B. The 1D residue is located between amino acids 233 and 273, whereas the 1B site was at Tyr[100] (Robertson et al. 1989).

ANTIGENIC STRUCTURE

Available evidence indicates that HAV strains comprise a single serotype, and that infection or immunization with any one strain confers protection against all others (LeDuc et al. 1983, Lemon and Binn 1983a, Lemon, Jansen and Brown 1992). Although significant antigenic differences between human and simian viruses can be detected with selected monoclonal antibodies (mAbs) (Nainan et al. 1991, Tsarev et al. 1991), the simian viruses react with other mAbs as well as polyclonal antibodies raised to human strains. The dominant antigenic determinants of HAV are highly conformational, as mAbs to the virus fail to recognize any capsid polypeptide in immunoblot assays. In addition, the antigenicity of the virus is curiously monotonic. Many mAbs are able to inhibit competitively by >50% the binding of polyclonal antibodies to the virus, and mAbs can be classified into several different groups on the basis of their ability to block the binding of 2 reference monoclonals (Stapleton and Lemon 1987, Ping and Lemon 1992). Some mAbs recognize antigenic determinants common to 70S empty particles and 14S pentamer subunits (which are formed by 5 copies of the 1B–1C–1D protomer subunit), whereas others recognize an antigenic determinant that is present only on 70S particles and is thus likely to span pentamer–pentamer interfaces (Stapleton et al. 1993). With few exceptions, mAbs to the virus are able to neutralize infectivity (Ping and Lemon 1992).

Neutralization-resistant HAV mutants have been produced by successive rounds of neutralization and passage of virus in the presence of mAbs (Stapleton and Lemon 1987). These mutants have only a limited number of amino substitutions, all in 1C or 1D (Ping et al. 1988, Ping and Lemon 1992, Nainan, Brinton and Margolis 1992). Most, if not all, of these amino acid substitutions are likely to be at residues that interact directly with the complementarity-determining regions of the cognate mAbs. They thus serve to map the neutralizing epitopes of the virus. The most frequently identified mutations are at Asp[70] of 1C, but escape mutations also have been found at Pro[65], Ser[71] and Glu[74] of this protein. Mutation at Asp[70] profoundly alters the antigenicity of the virus, significantly reducing the reactivity of the virus with most polyclonal antibodies (Lemon et al. 1991a, Ping and Lemon 1992). Several different amino acid substitutions have been identified at this residue. Other neutralization escape mutants have substitutions within the 1D sequence, at Ser[102], Asp[104], Lys[105], Val[171], Ala[176] or Lys[221]. Substitutions at Glu[174] and Ser[178] of 1D may contribute to antigenic differences present in some simian strains of HAV. Except for several mutants with different amino acid substitutions at Lys[221] of 1D (all of which determine resistance to a single mAb), most escape mutants demonstrate extensive cross-resistance to multiple mAbs (Ping and Lemon 1992). These data suggest that residues 65–74 of 1C (centring on Asp[70]) and 102–105 and 171–176 of 1D contribute to a single immunodominant antigenic site that contains a limited number of closely related and overlapping epitopes. This interpretation is consistent with the monotonicity of the polyclonal antibody response to the virus noted above.

There is also limited evidence for a neutralization

epitope located near the amino terminus of 1D. Antibodies raised against a synthetic peptide representing residues 13–24 of 1D generated neutralizing antibodies (Emini et al. 1985), and low levels of neutralizing antibodies were found in some animals immunized with a chimaeric poliovirus containing this segment of the HAV 1D molecule placed within an antigenic surface loop of poliovirus 1D (Lemon et al. 1992). Because the amino terminal domain of 1D is located internally within the crystallographically determined structures of other picornaviruses, it is likely that this epitope becomes exposed only after interaction of the virus with its putative cellular receptor.

Consistent with the conformational nature of HAV epitopes, individual recombinant HAV capsid proteins generally fail to elicit antibody responses that are reactive with the viral capsid. However, such proteins may prime for B cell responses in small animals (Johnston et al. 1988). Epitope(s) responsible for such priming reside within the carboxy terminal 156 residues of 1D (Harmon et al. 1993). Also consistent with the conformational nature of HAV epitopes, a large number of synthetic peptides representing different segments of the HAV capsid proteins have been shown not to express any relevant HAV antigenic activity (Lemon et al. 1991b). However, a recent (though unconfirmed) report suggests that a synthetic peptide 'mimotope' selected using a combinatorial approach may be able to stimulate production of antibodies that are reactive with the virus capsid.

The epitopes of HAV are highly conserved among human strains of HAV, indicating that residues that contribute to these structures may play an important role in maintaining the viability of the virus. A neutralization escape mutant containing a mutation at Asp^{70} of 1D was markedly impaired in its ability to replicate in otherwise susceptible New World owl monkeys, suggesting a possible role in recognition of the cellular receptor for HAV (Lemon et al. 1990). Although this mutation is relatively stable during passage of virus in cultured cells, there was rapid reversion to the wild type sequence in infected primates.

2.5 Replication of HAV

PROPAGATION OF VIRUS IN CULTURED CELLS

Replication of wild type HAV is very slow and inefficient in cell culture, typically taking days to weeks to reach maximum virus yields (Provost and Hilleman 1979, Daemer et al. 1981, Binn et al. 1984). However, with patience and continued passage, virus yields are increased and the otherwise lengthy replication period is shortened. HAV variants that have been adapted to cell culture will replicate in many primate cell lines, but certain cell lines derived from African green monkey (BS-C-1 or CV-1) or fetal rhesus monkey kidney (FRhK-4) seem to be most permissive for virus growth (Provost and Hilleman 1979, Daemer et al. 1981, Binn et al. 1984). Other mammalian cell types are also permissive for limited replication of the virus (Dotzauer, Feinstone and Kaplan 1994). Thus there does not

seem to be a strict host species requirement in cell culture. Viruses that are well adapted to growth in monkey kidney cell cultures are often highly attenuated when inoculated into susceptible primates or humans (Provost et al. 1982, Karron et al. 1986) (see below).

The specific cell culture infectivity (cell culture infectious units per genome copy) of one virus variant (HM175/P16) that had been adapted to growth in cultured cells during 16 sequential passages in African green monkey kidney cells was >3000 times that of the related wild type virus (Jansen, Newbold and Lemon 1988). However, even virus isolates that are well adapted to growth in cultured cells replicate much more slowly than picornaviruses such as encephalomyocarditis virus (EMCV) or poliovirus (Lemon et al. 1991a). Most HAV strains fail to induce a cytopathic effect in cultured cells, although this is seen with some cytopathic variants that are highly adapted to growth in cultured cells (Anderson 1987, Cromeans, Sobsey and Fields 1987, Lemon et al. 1991a). Such cytopathic variants may reach maximum yields in <24 h under one-step growth conditions, and have been described as having a 'rapidly replicating, cytopathic', or rr/cpe^+, phenotype (Lemon et al. 1991a). However, even these strains of HAV do not induce a specific shutdown in host cell macromolecular synthesis. To a considerable extent, the poor growth of HAV in cultured cells has limited investigations of the replication cycle.

In most cases, the replication of HAV in cell cultures can be detected only by immunological techniques or demonstration of the viral RNA by nucleic acid hybridization. The quantal, radioimmunofocus assay allows accurate titration of viral infectivity by immunostaining of viral replication foci developing beneath an agarose overlay over a period of 6–14 days (Lemon, Binn and Marchwicki 1983).

EARLY EVENTS IN VIRAL REPLICATION

Viral attachment is mediated through interactions with a putative specific cellular receptor, which is yet to be formally identified (Stapleton, Jansen and Lemon 1991, Zajac et al. 1991). Penetration is likely to be accomplished by receptor-mediated endocytosis, but nothing is known of this or subsequent steps in the uncoating of the viral genome.

CAP-INDEPENDENT TRANSLATION OF THE VIRAL POLYPROTEIN

The first step in replication following the uncoating of the viral RNA is the cap-independent translation of the viral polyprotein. The initiation of translation is carried out under direction of the IRES located between nucleotides 155 and 735 of the 5'NTR (Brown et al. 1991, Brown, Zajac and Lemon 1994). Although the IRES shares several structural features with that of EMCV, it is c. 50–100-fold less active in directing translation than the EMCV IRES, even in HAV permissive cells (Brown, Zajac and Lemon 1994, Whetter et al. 1994, Schultz et al. 1996). It is likely that weak IRES activity contributes to the slow and noncytopathic growth of HAV (see p. 700), because studies indicate that translation is rate limiting in infection of cultured African green monkey kidney cells with wild type virus (Schultz et al. 1996).

The IRES of HAV binds specifically to several cellular proteins, including polypyrimidine tract-binding protein (PTB) and glyceraldehyde-3-phosphate dehydrogenase (GAPDH, p39) (Chang, Brown and Lemon 1993, Schultz, Hardin and Lemon 1996). PTB enhances HAV IRES activity in transfected cell cultures (Gossert, Chang and Lemon, unpublished data 1997), whereas experimental data indicate that the binding of GAPDH destabilizes RNA secondary structure and is thus likely to be detrimental to IRES-directed translation (Schultz, Hardin and Lemon 1996). PTB and GAPDH compete with each other for binding to certain stem–loop structures within the 5′NTR, and the relative levels of these cellular proteins may be important in determining the translational activity of the HAV IRES. Specific hepatocyte factors may enhance translation directed by the HAV IRES (Glass and Summers 1993).

REPLICATION FUNCTIONS ASSOCIATED WITH NON-STRUCTURAL PROTEINS

The non-structural proteins of HAV are responsible for proteolytic processing of the polyprotein and replication of the viral RNA. There are at least 7 distinct non-structural proteins: 2A, 2B, 2C, 3A, 3B (the genome-linked protein, VPg, which is covalently attached to the 5′ end of virion RNA), 3C^{pro} (the viral protease) and 3D^{pol} (putatively an RNA-dependent RNA polymerase). Many of the specific functions of these proteins are not well understood.

Although the 2A proteins of other picornaviruses have protease activities and are responsible for the primary *cis*-active cleavage of the polyprotein (at either 1D/2A or 2A/2B), this is not the case for HAV. The HAV 2A protein shares no sequence identity with these other picornaviral 2A proteins and does not seem to have proteolytic activity. It may have a structural role in viral assembly (see p. 697). Recent evidence indicates that large (15 amino acid) deletions within 2A do not impair virus growth in cultured cells (Harmon et al. 1995). Whereas the 2A/2B cleavage site has been identified and shown to be mediated by 3C^{pro} (Martin et al. 1996), the 1D/2A cleavage remains poorly defined and may occur at multiple sites. Although this cleavage may be mediated by 3C^{pro} (Schultheiss, Kusov and Gauss-Müller 1994, Schultheiss et al. 1995), it has not been linked definitively to any specific protease.

The 2B and 2C proteins of HAV have functions related to replication of the viral RNA and, on the basis of studies with poliovirus, presumably play essential roles in directing the assembly of a membrane-based replicase complex (Bienz et al. 1992, Cho et al. 1994). Since mutations in 2B and 2C are important for adaptation of wild type HAV to replication in cultured cells (see p. 701) (Emerson et al. 1992a, Emerson, Huang and Purcell 1993), it is very likely that these proteins interact in an as yet undefined but highly specific fashion with cellular proteins or other components of the intracellular membrane. 2C contains a 'DEAD' motif, suggesting that it may have RNA helicase activity, and has been shown to be an NTPase. The HAV 2B and 2C proteins most probably function as a complex, as mutations in these proteins which play an important role in defining the replication properties of *rr/cpe*$^+$ viruses act in a highly co-operative fashion (Zhang et al. 1995). The 2C proteins of HAV and poliovirus are clearly related phylogenetically, and mutations that confer resistance of poliovirus to guanidine (an inhibitor of poliovirus RNA replication) map to the 2C protein. HAV replication has been suggested to be sensitive to guanidine (Cho and Ehrenfeld 1991), but this has not been found to be the case by other investigators (Siegl and Eggers 1982, SM Lemon 1992, unpublished data).

The function of the 3A protein in viral replication is also poorly defined, but it is likely to serve as an anchor for 3AB or 3ABCD within the membranous replication complexes. Mutations in 3A may play a role in determining the *rr/cpe*$^+$ phenotype, as multiple cytopathic strains that have been sequenced in this region contain deletions of one or more amino acids near the amino terminus of 3A (Lemon et al. 1991a, Beneduce et al. 1995). However, any role that mutations in 3A may play in determining this phenotype is of secondary importance to the role played by mutations in 2BC (Zhang et al. 1995). The 3B (VPg) protein is covalently attached to the 5′ nucleotide of the virion RNA (Weitz et al. 1986). Studies with other picornaviruses suggest that it is removed shortly after uncoating of the viral RNA, and that it is also likely to be present at the 5′ end of newly synthesized minus-strand RNAs. Its precise functions may include a role in priming for RNA synthesis, or possibly in cleavage of the RNA if negative-strand synthesis originates from a snap-back, self-priming mechanism.

3C^{pro} is clearly the best studied of the non-structural proteins of HAV because its 3-dimensional structure has been determined by x-ray crystallography (Allaire et al. 1994). It is a cysteine protease with both structural and functional relatedness to chymotrypsin and the serine proteases. 3C^{pro} seems to be responsible for each of the proteolytic cleavages of the viral polyprotein (Harmon et al. 1992, Kusov et al. 1992, Schultheiss, Kusov and Gauss-Müller 1994, Tesar et al. 1994), with the exception of the 1A/1B (VP4/VP2) cleavage (Bishop and Anderson 1993) and possibly also 1D/2A (VP1/2A) as indicated above. The substrate specificity of the 3C^{pro} enzyme has been studied extensively using synthetic peptide substrates (Jewell et al. 1992, Malcolm et al. 1992). The dipeptide sequences present at the various HAV cleavage sites are considerably more variable than in other picornaviruses. Studies with poliovirus suggest that 3C^{pro} has specific RNA-binding activity and interacts with the 5′NTR during initiation of plus-strand RNA synthesis; structural studies indicate that the RNA-binding site is located on the opposite side of the molecule from the protease active site. Poliovirus 3C^{pro} has also been considered to contribute to host cell shutdown at the transcriptional level by directing cleavage of the human

TATA-binding protein (Clark et al. 1993, Das and Dasgupta 1993). However, either the HAV 3C^{pro} protein lacks this activity or it is expressed at much lower levels during viral replication, because HAV infection has never been shown specifically to impair host cell metabolic processes. The putative RNA-dependent RNA polymerase activity of 3D^{pol} is suggested by the presence of a conserved 'GDD' amino acid motif. Thus far, however, attempts to express an active polymerase have resulted in an insoluble product with no detectable activity.

GENETIC CHANGES ASSOCIATED WITH ADAPTATION TO GROWTH IN CULTURED CELLS

The genetic changes associated with adaptation of the HM175 and GBM strains of HAV to growth in cell culture have been identified by comparisons of the nucleotide sequences of wild type and cell culture-adapted variants (Cohen et al. 1987a, Jansen, Newbold and Lemon 1988, Ross et al. 1989, Graff et al. 1994). These studies are important because cell culture-adapted viruses often are highly attenuated and have been used as candidate vaccines in humans (see p. 705). The HM175 strain has been studied intensively, with complete genomic sequences determined for 3 independently isolated, cell culture-adapted viruses (Cohen et al. 1987a, Jansen, Newbold and Lemon 1988, Ross et al. 1989). The mutations associated with cell culture adaptation are scattered throughout the genome, but tend to concentrate in the 5'NTR and P2 domains. Several individual mutations are present in multiple, independent cell culture-adapted isolates, signifying their importance to efficient replication in cell culture. The construction of an infectious cDNA clone of the HM175 virus (Cohen et al. 1987b) has allowed a detailed molecular genetics analysis of mutations that are associated with the adaptation of HAV to growth in cultured cells. Emerson and colleagues (Emerson et al. 1991, 1992a, 1992b) found that mutations within the P2 region (2B and 2C proteins) are necessary for efficient growth in cultured cells. A relatively conservative Val to Ala substitution in 2B seems to be the most important single mutation with respect to growth in cultured cells. It is present in all cell culture-adapted isolates of HAV. These P2 mutations probably facilitate interactions between these viral proteins and a host cell-specific factor(s) required for replication, but further details are lacking.

Mutations within the 5'NTR of cell culture-adapted virus significantly enhance replication in CV-1 or BS-C-1 cells derived from African green monkey kidney, but not in permissive FRhK-4 cells derived from fetal rhesus kidney (Day and Lemon 1990, Day et al. 1992, Emerson et al. 1992a). The mutations responsible for this effect (Day et al. 1992) are located in or near the viral IRES, and enhance cap-independent translation in BS-C-1 cells (Schultz et al. 1996). These results indicate that there are cell type-specific factors that influence the efficiency of translation directed by the HAV IRES. Differing cytoplasmic levels of GAPDH and PTB

may play an important role in determining the activity of these 5'NTR mutations, as these 2 cellular proteins compete for binding to the 5'NTR with opposing effects on viral translation (see p. 700) (Chang, Brown and Lemon 1993, Schultz, Hardin and Lemon 1996). Additional nucleotide substitutions within the 3' distal portion of the 5'NTR are important for efficient growth of the HM175/P35 virus in MRC-5 cells (Funkhouser et al. 1994). These mutations probably also enhance IRES-directed translation in these cells.

The nearly complete nucleotide sequences have been determined for 3 rr/cpe$^+$ variants recovered from cells that were persistently infected with the HM175 virus (Lemon et al. 1991a). These clonally isolated variants contained identical mutations within the 5' and 3' NTRs as well as within the RNA encoding the P2 and P3 proteins (2B, 2C, 3A and 3D), while the intervening genomic sequences contained unique silent and non-silent mutations. This suggested that the mutations that were common to the 3 cytopathic variants were likely to be responsible for the rr/cpe$^+$ phenotype. The presence of identical non-silent as well as silent mutations in these specific genomic regions was probably due to recombination between viral RNAs during persistent infection. It is interesting that one of the cytopathic variants (HM175/43c) had a mutation at Asp^{70} of 1C which eliminates an immunodominant epitope on the viral surface (see p. 698). Although this variant predominated during mixed infections of persistently infected cells, it was strongly selected against during serial passage of cell-free virus harvests (Lemon et al. 1991a). To determine which mutations are responsible for the rr/cpe$^+$ phenotype, infectious cDNA chimaeras were constructed that contained various segments of one of these cytopathic variants (HM175/18f) in the genetic background of a noncytopathic virus (Zhang et al. 1995). Analysis of the chimaeric viruses recovered from these clones demonstrated that complete expression of the rr/cpe$^+$ phenotype required the co-operative effects of multiple mutations in 2B, 2C, the 5'NTR and the P3 regions of the genome. Thus, the rr/cpe$^+$ phenotype represents a super-adaptation of HAV to growth in cell culture, and reflects changes in multiple virus functions. Virus rescued from a genomic-length cDNA clone containing all but the P1 and 3'NTR mutations of the cytopathic HM175/18f virus replicated rapidly, causing large radioimmunofoci as well as visible plaques that could be demonstrated by neutral red staining within 6 days of inoculation of BS-C-1 or FRhK-4 cells.

2.6 Clinical and pathological aspects of HAV infection

PATHOGENESIS OF HEPATITIS A

To a considerable extent, present understanding of the pathogenesis of hepatitis A derives from studies of HAV infections in several species of susceptible non-human primates: chimpanzees, certain species of tamarins and New World owl monkeys (Dienstag, Popper and Purcell 1975, Dienstag et al. 1976, Bradley et al. 1977, Cohen, Feinstone and Purcell 1989). Although these primate species can be infected either by oral or by intravenous challenge with virus, HAV infection typically follows oral exposure to the virus in humans, due either to close personal contact with an infected individual or to the ingestion of faecally contaminated water or food. Viral replication occurs primarily within hepatocytes, and the secretion of virus into bile results in large quantities of virus being shed in the faeces. The titre of virus excreted in stool may be at least as high as 10^8 particles or 10^6 infectious virions/g (Purcell et al. 1984, Lemon et al. 1990). A sustained viraemia throughout the incubation period and the early stages of acute liver disease parallels the faecal shedding of virus, but at titres that are 100–1000-fold lower (Cohen, Feinstone and Purcell 1989, Lemon et al. 1990) (Fig. 34.5). Early studies demonstrated viral antigen within the liver, in hepatocytes and Kupffer cells, as well as in splenic macrophages and along the glomerular basement membrane in the kidney (Dienstag et al. 1976, Mathiesen et al. 1978a, 1980, Shimizu et al. 1982). However, it is not clear whether the presence of viral antigen in phagocytic cells reflects non-specific trapping of viral antigen or replication of virus.

Although most if not all of the virus found in faeces and blood is likely to be replicated within hepatocytes, there are limited data that indicate that HAV also infects intestinal epithelial cells in vivo. The early events in hepatitis A infection and the mechanism by which the virus reaches the liver remained poorly defined. HAV antigen has been identified within intestinal epithelial cells of experimentally infected tamarins (Karayiannis et al. 1986) as well as orally inoculated owl monkeys (Asher et al. 1995). In owl monkeys, viral antigen was observed in epithelial cells lining crypts in the small intestine within 3 days of inoculation. These findings in vivo are supported by studies demonstrating the growth of cell culture-adapted HAV in polarized cultures of colonic carcinoma cells (CaCo-2) grown on semipermeable membranes (Blank and Lemon, unpublished data 1997). Such cells could be infected only from their apical surface, and released progeny virus in a vectorial fashion only from the apical surface. Infectious virus has also been detected at low levels within pharyngeal secretions, but later in infection when viraemia was also present (Cohen, Feinstone and Purcell 1989, Asher et al. 1995). It is difficult to be certain whether this reflects virus produced locally or simply secretion of virus into saliva from the blood.

The light microscopic findings in acute hepatitis A

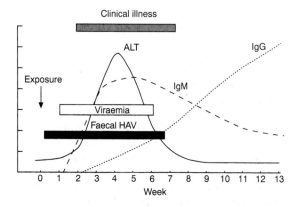

Fig. 34.5 Virological and pathological events during a typical infection with HAV.

include features common to all forms of acute viral hepatitis, including inflammatory cell infiltration, hepatocellular necrosis and liver cell regeneration. Studies in chimpanzees demonstrated that the early histological lesions of hepatitis A infection involve periportal liver cell necrosis with relative sparing of the perivenular area of the lobule (Dienstag, Popper and Purcell 1976). These histological observations have been confirmed in humans undergoing biopsies at different stages of the acute disease. Portal infiltration by lymphocytes, plasma cells and periodic acid–Schiff (PAS)-positive macrophages are prominent features in early biopsies. These features are more pronounced in later biopsies (Abe et al. 1982, Teixera et al. 1982). Some biopsies taken during acute hepatitis A infection demonstrate extension of the inflammatory infiltrate from the periportal region into the hepatic parenchyma, with significant erosion of the limiting plate. Although this histological picture is more suggestive of chronic hepatitis, the histopathological features of hepatitis A are reversible and generally resolve completely given sufficient time.

CELLULAR IMMUNE RESPONSE TO HAV INFECTION

Because infection of cultured cells with wild type HAV does not result in the cytopathic effects observed with many other well characterized picornaviruses, it is generally assumed that HAV infection is also non-cytopathic in vivo and that hepatitis A is an immunopathologically mediated disease. This is probably correct, as virus replication and faecal virus shedding are maximal in the late incubation period, before the onset of symptoms or biochemical evidence of liver injury. Thus, liver injury and viral clearance are closely related. CD8+, class I-dependent, cytotoxic T cells that are capable of lysing autologous HAV infected cells, but not of controlling uninfected cells, are present both in the circulation and in the liver at the site of disease (Vallbracht et al. 1986, Vallbracht et al. 1989, Fleischer et al. 1990). These virus-specific T cells also produce interferon-γ (Maier et al. 1988). It is likely that interferon-γ and other cytokines secreted by virus-specific CD8+ cells serve to recruit additional, less specific, inflammatory cells to the site of the infection that may be responsible for much of the liver injury. The exact mechanism by which the infection is cleared is inadequately defined, but this process probably involves a combination of antibody-mediated neutralization of infection, interferon-mediated inhibition of viral replication and cytotoxic T cell-induction of cellular apoptosis. A prominent feature of this response may be the up-regulation of the normally low levels of class I markers displayed by hepatocytes in response to interferon-γ and other cytokines. Specific T cell epitopes of HAV have not been identified.

HUMORAL IMMUNE RESPONSE TO HAV

In addition to the cellular immune responses described above, there is a vigorous antibody response to the virus during the later stages of infection. These antibodies are directed against conformational epitopes that are displayed by intact virions as well as empty viral capsids (see p. 698). Serum-neutralizing antibodies provide protection against reinfection with HAV, whereas cell-mediated immunity seems to be involved in viral clearance once infection has been established. Serum antibody responses are first noted at the onset of symptoms and include virus-specific IgM as well as IgG and IgA. IgM anti-HAV is detected concurrently with the onset of clinical symptoms, but IgG is also present during the acute symptomatic phase of the infection (Locarnini et al. 1979, Lemon et al. 1980). Both IgM and IgG antibodies have virus-neutralizing activities (Lemon and Binn 1983b, Lemon 1985b). The IgG response is durable and provides longstanding protection against reinfection. However, there are suggestions that it may decline to low and potentially non-detectable levels after many decades, particularly in people infected early in life. Upon re-exposure, such individuals may experience asymptomatic reinfections associated with anamnestic IgG antibody responses in the absence of detectable IgM (Villarejos et al. 1982). Although coproantibodies have been detected by immunoassay, saliva and stool do not contain virus-specific neutralizing antibodies (Locarnini et al. 1980, Stapleton et al. 1991). These data suggest that secretory antibody plays little if any role in protection against hepatitis A.

Sensitive and specific immunoassays are widely available for the detection of total and IgM-specific antibody to HAV (see p. 704). However, measurements of virus-neutralizing antibody are tedious and labour intensive. The radioimmunofocus reduction assay (Lemon and Binn 1983b) or HAV antigen reduction assay (Krah et al. 1991) are the most accurate methods available for determination of virus-neutralizing antibody. In addition to antibodies directed against the virus capsid, antibodies reactive with non-structural proteins (especially 3C^{pro}) have also been detected. The presence of such antibodies may differentiate immunity due to natural infection from that gained by immunization with inactivated HAV vaccine (Robertson et al. 1993).

CLINICAL MANIFESTATIONS

HAV causes an acute, self-limiting infection that does not progress to a chronic phase. Manifestations of the disease are generally restricted to the liver. However, although extrahepatic manifestations suggesting involvement of the central nervous system or kidneys are rare, their occurrence is well documented (Bromberg, Newhall and Peter 1982, Hammond et al. 1982, Malbrain et al. 1994, Ogawa et al. 1994, Zikos et al. 1995). The typical clinical course of type A hepatitis is shown in Fig. 34.5. Following exposure, an incubation period of 15–45 days precedes the development of clinical symptoms. However, virus is present in the blood and shed in the stools within a few days of exposure (Asher et al. 1995, Ward et al. 1958, Krugman, Ward and Giles 1962, Lemon et al. 1990). The magnitude of the viraemia and the amount of virus shed in the faeces continues to increase until just before the onset of symptoms. Symptoms typically occur abruptly, with liver injury heralded by fever, myalgia, malaise, nausea, anorexia and vomiting, accompanied occasionally by abdominal pain in the right upper quadrant. More distinctive signs of hepatitis and the disruption of normal hepatobiliary metabolism appear rapidly thereafter, including the passage of dark, 'Coca-Cola'-like urine, light, clay-coloured stools and frank icterus. These clinical findings coincide with the appearance of characteristic biochemical abnormalities, including abnormal elevations of serum levels of the liver-derived enzymes alanine aminotransferase (ALT), alkaline phosphatase (AST), and γ-glutamyl transpeptidase (GGTP), as well as increased levels of serum bilirubin. All these events signal the host immune response to the infection, including the appearance of virus-specific neutralizing antibodies (Lemon and Binn 1983b). Resolution is marked by slow recovery and often a prolonged period of convalescence. Nevertheless, serum enzyme levels are almost always normal by 6–12 months after onset of the disease, often much sooner. Rarely, however, HAV infection may trigger the onset of a chronic, autoimmune hepatitis (Vento et al. 1991).

The severity of symptoms associated with HAV infection is closely correlated with age. Acute, symptomatic, icteric infections seem to be the rule in older adolescents and adults (Lednar et al. 1985). On the other hand, infection in children under 2 years of age is almost never recognized clinically as hepatitis (Hadler et al. 1980). Most people with antibodies to HAV have no history of acute hepatitis, probably reflecting infection at an early age many years previously. Individuals over 50 years of age at the time of infection are at substantially increased risk of developing fulminant hepatitis, and clinical evidence of hepatic failure such as ascites, bleeding diathesis or hepatic coma (Forbes and Williams 1990, Hadler 1991, Lemon and Shapiro 1994). A systematic study has not been done, but patients with pre-existing chronic liver disease due to any cause may be at increased risk of fulminant disease when infected with HAV. Fortunately, fulminant hepatitis A is relatively rare, and accounts for fewer than 100 deaths annually in the USA (Lemon and Shapiro 1994).

Cholestatic hepatitis A and relapsing hepatitis A represent 2 less severe complications of type A hepatitis. Cholestatic hepatitis is characterized by persistent jaundice associated with pruritus, anorexia and weight loss. Patients eventually recover after several weeks to months, but may recover more rapidly following a brief course of corticosteroids (Gordon et al. 1984). Such therapy should be attempted with caution, and only when there is no doubt about the diagnosis. There are many reports of clinical relapses 1–3 months after apparent recovery from acute hepatitis A. Relapsing hepatitis A is characterized by secondary rises in levels of serum enzyme, persistence of IgM anti-HAV, and possibly recurrent viraemia and faecal virus shedding (Sjogren et al. 1987, Glikson et al. 1992). The pathogenesis of relapsing hepatitis A is unknown, but may involve viral escape from immune surveillance.

DIAGNOSIS

The diagnosis of acute viral hepatitis is usually suggested by the presence of the typical constellation of signs and symptoms associated with elevation of serum ALT activities. However, in the absence of a specific epidemiological setting suggestive of hepatitis A, the clinical manifestations of HAV infection are not sufficiently different from those of other types of acute viral hepatitis to allow a virus-specific diagnosis to be made without serological testing. Generally, the diagnosis is confirmed by the demonstration of IgM antibodies to the virus, which are almost always present at the onset of symptoms and which persist for up to 6 months following infection. These antibodies are usually measured by solid phase, IgM-capture immunoassays (Lemon et al. 1980, Decker et al. 1981). Competitive-inhibition immunoassays allow non-isotype-specific detection of viral antibodies (Mathiesen et al. 1978b, Decker et al. 1979). When such tests are positive in the absence of IgM antibodies, they are considered indicative of the presence of IgG antibodies to the virus. This result is consistent with immunity due to prior infection or immunization against HAV.

2.7 Epidemiology of hepatitis A

TRANSMISSION OF HEPATITIS A

Almost all transmission occurs by the faecal–oral route. Within the USA the most common risk factor for infection is close contact with a person with hepatitis A (Centers for Disease Control 1994). Person-to-person transmission accounts for most infections among household contacts as well as institutionalized individuals and children and staff in preschool daycare centres (Hadler et al. 1980). Handlers of non-human primates may be at risk for similar reasons. Not surprisingly, sexual behaviour can influence the spread of infection, particularly among male homosexuals (Corey and Holmes 1980). Food- and waterborne transmission of HAV is also common, facilitated by the stability of the HAV virion and its relative resistance to drying (Siegl, Weitz and Kronauer 1984, Lemon et al. 1991a). Food-borne transmission of HAV may follow contamination of uncooked foods by infected food handlers, and is not infrequently implicated in common source outbreaks of disease. However, fresh produce may also be contaminated at its source, before distribution (Rosenblum et al. 1990). Finally, infection may occur following ingestion of raw or partially cooked filter-feeding shellfish collected from polluted waters, as these organisms have the ability to concentrate the virus. All these modes of transmission pose risks for travellers to HAV-endemic regions.

Although uncommon, parenteral transmission of the virus is also possible. Injecting drug users have represented a substantial proportion of cases of hepatitis A in some studies, and there is little doubt that they are at increased risk of HAV infection (Widell et al. 1983, Centers for Disease Control 1988). These infec-

tions are probably related to sharing of contaminated needles and thus to parenteral transmission of the virus, given that a relatively high level viraemia is present for several weeks throughout the asymptomatic incubation period of the hepatitis A (Lemon et al. 1990). This conclusion is strongly supported by remarkable concurrent declines in the incidence of drug use-associated cases of hepatitis A, hepatitis B and hepatitis C in the USA since 1988. This would be unexpected if cases of hepatitis A among drug users related primarily to poor sanitation. Transmission of virus by blood and blood products is also well documented, although it is much less common than with other hepatitis agents. Many such infections have been recognized in neonates who may receive split units of blood (Rosenblum et al. 1991), but transfusion-related infections have also been observed rarely in adults (Hollinger et al. 1983, Sherertz, Russell and Reuman 1984). Parenterally transmitted infections have been described in haemophiliacs receiving high-purity, solvent-detergent inactivated factor VIII (Mannucci et al. 1994, Robertson et al. 1994b), and cancer patients who received IL-2 produced in LAK cells maintained in 'normal human serum' (Weisfuse et al. 1990). With the possible exception of infections among drug users, however, parenteral transmission of HAV does not contribute significantly to the overall spread of the infection.

PREVALENCE OF HEPATITIS A

The prevalence of HAV infection varies widely by geographical region and depends on factors such as population density and the quality of public health sanitation and sewage disposal (Lemon and Shapiro 1994). It may be greatly increased during periods of social upheaval and war. The poorest of developing countries are characterized by the type I seroprevalence curve shown in Fig. 34.6. In these countries, including many in Africa, Asia and Central America, infections occur predominantly in very young children and are thus generally clinically inapparent. As a result, most children have antibodies against HAV by the age of 5–10 years, and disease is very infrequent in older people. With improved sanitary conditions, as found in the emerging economies of eastern Europe, the republics of the former Soviet Union and China, HAV infections tend to occur at a somewhat older age, resulting in the type II seroprevalence curve in Fig. 34.6. In these regions, the probability of exposure and infection remains relatively high, but an increase in the mean age at infection results in a greater disease burden as adolescents and young adults are more likely to experience clinical symptoms when infected (Szmuness et al. 1977, Frosner et al. 1979, Lemon 1985a). In recent decades, improving economic conditions have resulted in changing epidemiological patterns in many developing nations (Innis et al. 1991), with the result that epidemics of hepatitis A among older children, adolescents and young adults, previously unheard of, are now becoming apparent. Older adults and the elderly are protected from infection by virtue of the antibody they carry from infections acquired in earlier, more endemic periods.

This trend continues in relatively well developed countries such as the USA and much of western Europe, where young children are no longer commonly infected (except in the setting of daycare centres), and the burden of disease is found among adolescents and young adults (Szmuness et al. 1977, Frosner et al. 1979, Lemon and Shapiro 1994). In these countries, symptomatic HAV infections in older individuals result in substantial absence from work and associated medical expenses. The major sources of infection in these populations are community-wide outbreaks, daycare centres and common source outbreaks. Relatively high seroprevalence in the older age groups (Fig. 34.6) signifies not continued risk of infection over time, but rather a cohort effect from infection in previous decades when HAV infections were more prevalent (Frosner et al. 1978). Finally, in highly developed regions such as the Scandinavian countries, seroprevalence tends to follow the type IV curve shown in Fig. 34.6. There is little endemic transmission of the virus, and disease occurs primarily in travellers to other regions and in certain high risk groups such as intravenous drug users (Frosner et al. 1979, Siebke et al. 1982, Widell et al. 1983). Despite this convenient classification, it is important to note that prevalence patterns do not follow political as much as socioeconomic borders. For example, within the USA there are communities that would fit each of the type II, III and IV patterns.

2.8 Prevention of hepatitis A

To a considerable extent, hepatitis A can be prevented by good personal hygiene, adequate disposal and treatment of human waste, and provision of safe drinking water. As indicated above, HAV is rarely transmitted endemically in countries where these standards are met. However, specific measures are also available for the prevention of hepatitis A. These include pass-

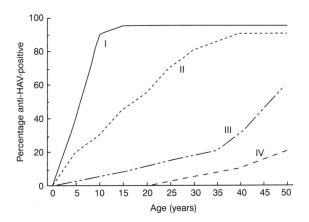

Fig. 34.6 Typical age-related seroprevalence curves found in populations residing in regions with high (I), intermediate (II) or low (III) endemicity for HAV infections, and in regions such as Scandinavia where endogenous transmission of HAV is now very uncommon (IV).

ive immunoprophylaxis with pooled human immunoglobulin (IG) and active immunization with hepatitis A vaccines.

POOLED HUMAN IMMUNOGLOBULIN

Postexposure prophylaxis is generally accomplished with human immunoglobulin (IG) (0.2 ml/kg), which should be given to people who are household members or sexual contacts of an infected individual (Gellis et al. 1945, Winokur and Stapleton 1992, Immunization Practices Advisory Committee 1990). Postexposure prophylaxis with IG may not prevent infection but it is remarkably effective in reducing or eliminating symptoms. It probably exerts this effect by reducing the level of viraemia, thereby reducing spread of virus within the liver (Lemon 1985a). To be optimally effective, it must be given within 2 weeks of exposure to the virus. IG is also useful for pre-exposure prophylaxis (0.2–0.5 ml/kg) and has been administered routinely to individuals travelling to HAV-endemic regions. If given before exposure, IG prevents disease for up to 4–6 months (Conrad and Lemon 1987). In this setting it is more likely to prevent infection as well as symptoms of hepatitis A, but this depends on the dose administered, the time elapsed between administration of IG and exposure to the virus, as well as the magnitude of the viral inoculum. Except for very limited travel, the use of inactivated hepatitis A vaccine is preferable and is largely replacing pre-exposure prophylaxis with IG.

HEPATITIS A VACCINES

Inactivated whole virus vaccines contain purified HAV particles (both complete virions and empty capsids) produced in cell culture and inactivated with formalin (Binn et al. 1986, Andre, Hepburn and D'Hondt 1990, Lewis et al. 1991). Several inactivated vaccines are licensed in their countries of origin and elsewhere, making inactivated HAV vaccine available world-wide. Most of these vaccines are adsorbed with alum (aluminium hydroxide) and all seem to be very immunogenic when administered by intramuscular injection. They are generally safe, and 2 have been shown in well designed clinical trials to provide a high level of protection against symptomatic hepatitis A in children (Werzberger et al. 1992, Innis et al. 1994, Lemon 1994). Antibody levels exceeding that produced by a single injection of IG are often present within 2–4 weeks of the first vaccine dose. Booster doses, given as early as one month following primary immunization, enhance the titre of neutralizing antibody and thus are likely to extend the duration of protection. Although the minimal protective level of antibody is not well defined, it is very low (<45 mIU/ml) (Stapleton, Jansen and Lemon 1985, Werzberger et al. 1992). Although inactivated vaccines do not produce detectable secretory antibody, the prevention of intrahepatic virus replication is likely to prevent or substantially reduce the faecal shedding of virus. Thus, in contrast to inactivated poliovirus vaccines, immunization with inactivated hepatitis A vaccines should render an individual unable to transmit the infection if exposed to the virus.

The major shortcoming of inactivated HAV vaccines is that they are quite expensive and thus not available for the control of hepatitis A on a population-wide basis in countries where immunization is most needed. Although inactivated vaccines are likely to be more effective than IG in controlling community-wide outbreaks of disease (Werzberger et al. 1992, Lemon and Shapiro 1994, Prikazsky et al. 1994), the use of the vaccine in this setting is also likely to be limited by cost. Although data are limited, immunization may provide some level of protection against hepatitis A if it is administered immediately after exposure to the virus (Werzberger et al. 1992, Robertson et al. 1994a).

Several candidate attenuated HAV vaccines have been evaluated in clinical trials (Provost et al. 1986, Midthun et al. 1991, Sjogren et al. 1992). The virus strains included in these vaccines have been attenuated by passage in cell culture and require parenteral injection to initiate infection uniformly in human recipients. In general, the immune response to these candidate vaccines has been disappointing with slow, low magnitude antibody responses. This probably reflects the fact that these virus strains are highly restricted in their ability to replicate in human hosts. Although they seem quite safe in clinical trials involving limited numbers of people and are likely to be effective clinically, these candidate attenuated vaccines have generally been abandoned by commercial manufacturers in favour of the development of more profitable inactivated vaccines. However, one such vaccine has been used extensively in China (Mao et al. 1989, 1991).

A fresh approach to the selection of candidate attenuated HAV vaccine strains is likely to be required for the development of highly immunogenic attenuated vaccines. One such approach has been the creation of large deletion mutations within the 5′NTR of a virulent, but minimally cell culture-adapted, variant of HAV (Shaffer, Brown and Lemon 1994). Some of these mutants have a strongly temperature-sensitive replication phenotype. However, there is no evidence thus far that these large 5′NTR deletions result in significant attenuation of the virus in primates (Shaffer et al. 1996). An alternative approach is to consider the use of simian strains of HAV, some of which seem to be naturally restricted in their ability to cause disease in chimpanzees (Purcell 1991), or chimaeric viruses containing selected sequences of human and simian HAVs.

Similarly, there has been little success in developing recombinant hepatitis A vaccines. This reflects the fact that the protective epitopes present on the surface of this picornavirus are conformationally defined by interactions between the individual capsid proteins in the assembled virus particle (see p. 698). However, Winokur and colleagues (Winokur, McLinden and Stapleton 1991) have demonstrated that it is possible to produce immunogenic, assembled virus-like capsids following expression of the P1 protein precursor and 3C^pro by recombinant vaccinia virus. Moreover, pre-liminary studies with synthetic peptide mimotopes (Mattioli et al. 1995) indicate that certain peptide motifs may successfully mimic the conformational, immunodominant antigenic site of HAV, suggesting the ultimate feasibility of a synthetic peptide-based vaccine.

3 HEPATITIS E VIRUS (HEV)

3.1 Classification of HEV

On the basis of the morphology of the HEV particle, the absence of a lipid envelope, the type and length of its nucleic acid and the general organization of its genome, HEV has been classified within the *Caliciviridae* (Cubitt 1995) (Table 34.3). However, a phylogenetic analysis of the nucleotide sequence of HEV shows that it is related more closely to the alphavirus superfamily of positive-strand RNA viruses, in particular the rubiviruses (Koonin et al. 1992).

3.2 Morphology and structure

As with many other features of HEV, details of the structure of the virion remain elusive owing to the absence of a cell culture system that is permissive for its replication and to difficulties in obtaining large quantities of stable particles from human and non-human primate samples. The HEV particle is chloroform-resistant and has a morphology resembling that of human caliciviruses and Norwalk virus (Fig. 34.7; and see Table 34.1). Although early reports suggested the diameter of HEV particles to be c. 27 nm (Balayan et al. 1983), subsequent studies have shown the average diameter to be closer to 32 nm (Bradley et al. 1988). Smaller particles may result from proteolytic degradation as the virus passes through the intestine, as both particle sizes have been observed in single stool suspensions (Bradley et al. 1987). HEV-specific antibodies recognize both forms. The characteristic cup-like surface of caliciviruses is less prominent in HEV, but Markham rotational enhancement clearly indicates surface projections and valleys (Ticehurst 1991).

3.3 Genome structure and function

GENOME ORGANIZATION

The genome of HEV is a single-stranded, 7.5 kb, positive-sense RNA that is polyadenylated at its 3′ terminus (Reyes et al. 1990, Tam et al. 1991). It contains 3 separate ORFs flanked by short 5′ and 3′ NTRs of 27 and 68 nt, respectively (Fig. 34.8). The presence of a methyltransferase motif within the non-structural proteins encoded by the most 5′ ORF (ORF1) closest to the 5′ terminus suggests that this region of the genomic RNA may contain a methylated cap structure (Koonin et al. 1992). The ORF closest to the 3′ terminus (ORF2) is thought to encode the major structural protein. There is an additional short ORF (ORF3), which overlaps ORF1 by a single nucleotide

Table 34.3 Properties of hepatitis E virus, calicivirus and rubivirus

	Calicivirus	**Hepatitis E virus**	**Rubivirus**
Morphology	Icosahedral	Icosahedral	Spherical
Envelope	No	No	Yes
Size	35–39 nm	27–32 nm	60 nm
Density	1.33–1.39 g/cm^3	1.29 g/cm^3	1.2 g/cm^3 (?)
$S_{20,w}$	170–183S	183S	280S (?)
RNA genome:	ss (+) RNA	ss (+) RNA	ss (+) RNA
5′ structure	VPg	5′ methylated cap (?)	5′ methylated cap
3′ structure	Poly(A)	Poly(A)	Poly(A)
length	8.2 kb	7.5 kb	9.8 kb
Subgenomic RNAs	2	2	1
Structural proteins	1 capsid protein	2 (?)	1 capsid protein
		(1 glycosylated)	2 glycoproteins
Non-structural proteins	Picorna-like protease	Papain-like protease	Papain-like protease
	RDRP	RDRP	RDRP
		Methyltransferase	Methyltransferase

RDRP, RNA-dependent RNA polymerase; ss(+), single-stranded, positive-sense.

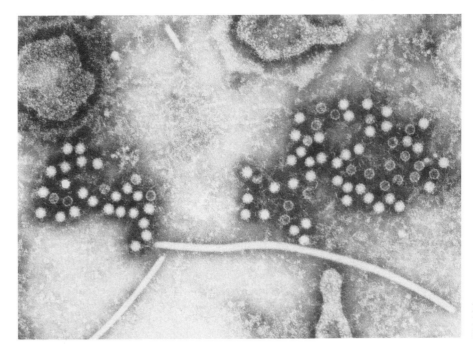

Fig. 34.7 Morphology of HEV particles demonstrated by electron microscopy.

and ORF2 by most of its length. ORF3 encodes a small protein of unknown function. The 5′ end of HEV RNA may contain a secondary structure analogous to that predicted to be present in alphaviruses. In addition, the sequence between 150 and 208 nt of HEV resembles a conserved 51 nt alphavirus sequence, whilst homology at 3602–3632 nt of HEV and junction sequences of alphaviruses suggests that this region may contain a promoter for transcription of a subgenomic RNA.

HEV PROTEINS

Most information about the proteins of HEV has been obtained from analysis of the nucleotide sequence of the virus. ORF1 encodes a relatively large polyprotein that contains consensus motifs for a methyltransferase,

a papain-like cysteine protease, a helicase (NTP binding site), and an RNA-dependent RNA polymerase similar to those found in the alphaviruses (Koonin et al. 1992). Also present in the ORF1 polyprotein is a polyproline 'hinge', which is also found in rubiviruses, and a conserved 'X' domain, which is of unknown function but is found flanking the papain-like protease domain in other positive-strand RNA viruses. Although this polyprotein is almost certainly proteolytically cleaved into 4–5 individual polypeptides with distinct functions in replication, the details of this process are not understood. Several unusual features of this polyprotein distinguish HEV from members of the alphavirus family (Koonin et al. 1992). For example, a peculiar domain ('Y' domain) located downstream of the methyltransferase motif has no equivalent in

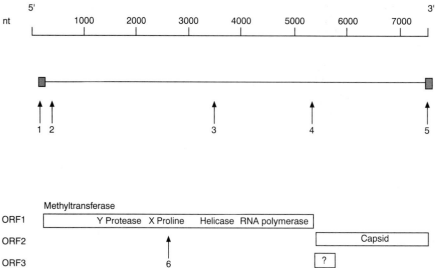

Fig. 34.8 Organization of the 7.5 kb single-stranded RNA genome of HEV.

the alphaviruses, although a similar domain is found in the plant virus beet necrotic yellow vein virus. The function of this domain is unknown.

ORF2 is thought to encode a 72 kDa capsid polypeptide, although direct evidence supporting this assumption is still lacking. This protein contains a signal peptide sequence and 3 potential glycosylation sites (Tam et al. 1991, Yarbough et al. 1991), and recent studies indicate that it is translocated into the endoplasmic reticulum, cleaved by signal peptidase and glycosylated (Jameel et al. 1996). Although the ORF2 protein is found on the cell surface (Asher et al. 1995), it is important to note that any surface lipid components of the virus would be unstable and almost certainly removed during passage of the virus through the bile. Thus it is not clear how these findings relate to the structure of HEV. The amino half of the ORF2 protein is rich in arginine residues, suggesting that it may associate with viral RNA. Overlapping ORF1 and ORF2 is a small open reading frame (ORF3) that encodes a 13 kDa, cysteine-rich polypeptide that is immunoreactive with many patient sera. Because antibodies raised to synthetic peptides representing segments of this protein are able to capture virus in antigen capture/PCR assays (McCaustland et al., in preparation), it may represent a structural protein present on the surface of the virus. Surprisingly, large deletions have been described within this ORF in viruses recovered from 2 separate epidemics in India (Ray, Jameel and Manivel 1992).

REPLICATION OF HEV

Although there are reports of HEV replication in conventional cell cultures (RT Huang et al. 1992, Kazachkov et al. 1992), they have not been confirmed. However, replication has been documented recently in primary cultures of hepatocytes taken from cynomolgus monkeys infected in vivo (Tam et al. 1996). The absence of a well characterized and readily available permissive cell culture system has severely limited studies of the molecular mechanisms of replication. The non-structural proteins are presumably translated

from newly uncoated RNA by a 5′ cap-dependent mechanism, providing the enzymes required for subsequent synthesis of both negative- and positive-strand RNAs. Two 3′ co-terminal, subgenomic messenger RNAs of 3.7 and 2.0 kb seem to be transcribed from the full-length negative-strand RNA, with the 2.0 kb message present in greater abundance than the 3.7 kb product (Tam et al. 1991). However, the role of these subgenomic RNAs in directing translation of the ORF2 and ORF3 proteins remains unclear. There is no understanding of how these processes are regulated.

GENETIC AND ANTIGENIC VARIANTS OF HEV

HEV strains seem to comprise a single serotype of antigenically related viruses, as all well characterized strains share cross-reacting epitopes. Despite this, there are distinct genetic clusters of HEV strains, as those recovered in the eastern hemisphere (Myanmar, Pakistan, Afghanistan, China and India) are much more closely related genetically to each other than to a strain recovered in Mexico. Nucleotide sequence identity among strains from the eastern hemisphere approximates 90%, whereas these strains differ from the Mexico strain at about 24% of base positions. At the amino acid level, there is about 87% similarity between the protein sequences of these viruses. Sequence diversity is not evenly distributed throughout the genome, as there is a hypervariable region located near the 'proline hinge' (Fry et al. 1992, C-C Huang et al. 1992, Tsarev et al. 1992, Yin et al. 1993). Recently, a genetically distinct HEV strain has been recovered in the USA.

Several studies have examined the reactivity of acute or convalescent sera with synthetic peptides or recombinant proteins expressed from ORF2 and ORF3 of different HEV strains (Yarbough et al. 1991, Kaur et al. 1992, Khudyakov et al. 1993, Li et al. 1994). Antigenic epitopes have been identified at the carboxy termini of both ORF2 and ORF3 protein products. The ORF3 epitope seems to differ between eastern and western hemisphere strains (Yarbough et al. 1991). However, the biological relevance of this finding is unclear, as the absence of a virus neutralization assay significantly hinders formal serological comparisons. Although it is not known how well recombinant or synthetic polypeptides reflect the immunodominant, presumably conformational, epitopes of the native virus capsid, such materials have been used as antigens in diagnostic assays (see below).

3.4 Clinical and pathological aspects of HEV infection

Pathogenesis of hepatitis E

Chimpanzees and several species of monkeys are susceptible to HEV infection and have served as experimental models of hepatitis E in humans (Bradley et al. 1987, Ticehurst et al. 1992, Tsarev et al. 1993a). In addition, swine, rats and possibly other mammalian species may support replication of the virus (Balayan et al. 1990). The most reliable animal models have been the rhesus and cynomolgus macaques, and much of our understanding of the pathogenesis of this disease is derived from experimental infections of these animals. Following intravenous inoculation of cynomolgus macaques, there is an incubation period of 2–6 weeks, which precedes the development of raised liver enzymes (Fig. 34.9). During this period there are viraemia and faecal excretion of virus, reflecting replication of virus within hepatocytes. Antibodies to HEV develop just before elevations of liver enzymes, coincident with resolution of the viraemia and faecal virus shedding and reductions in the quantity of viral antigen present in the liver. A biphasic pattern of liver disease has been observed in some animals, the initial period of enzyme elevation occurring within the first 2 weeks after inoculation. Pathological changes in the liver are consistent with acute viral hepatitis (Longer et al. 1993), but not specific for any aetiological agent, and include hepatocyte necrosis and inflammatory cell infiltration. In general, the overall pattern and severity of disease do not seem to be as dramatic as in humans. Although limited evidence supports the theory of replication of the virus within the gastrointestinal tract of swine, an inoculum containing $10^{6.8}$ infectious units by intravenous inoculation failed to initiate infection when administered orally to macaques (Tsarev et al. 1994b).

There are few data about virological events in infected humans. In one of two reported human volunteer infections, raised liver enzymes and jaundice persisted for 3 months (Chauhan et al. 1993). Viraemia was first detected at day 22, and terminated at day 46 when liver enzymes reached their peak value. Antibodies against HEV were first detected at day 41; their appearance was followed by declining levels of liver enzyme. Excretion of virus in stool samples was detected by RT-PCR between 30 and 50 days after ingestion. Disease was limited to a one month period in the other reported experimental human infection (Balayan et al. 1983). Examination of liver specimens from patients involved in outbreaks of disease attri-

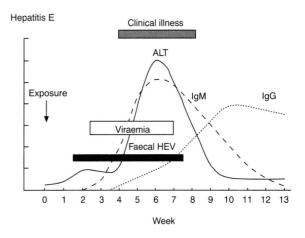

Fig. 34.9 Typical course of virological and pathological events during infection with HEV.

buted to HEV in Delhi, the Kashmir and (putatively) Ghana have revealed 2 general types of histopathological change (Gupta and Smetana 1955, Morrow et al. 1968, Khuroo 1980). A cholestatic pattern is characterized by prominent bile stasis within canaliculi and a unique gland-like transformation of parenchymal cells. There is portal and, to a lesser extent, parenchymal infiltration of lymphocytes and polymorphonuclear leucocytes. A second histopathological pattern is similar to that found in other types of acute hepatitis, and includes ballooning degeneration of hepatocytes and formation of acidophilic bodies.

Immune response to HEV infection

Antibodies to HEV develop during convalescence from the disease and are reactive with both linear and conformational epitopes of the virus. A wide variety of assays have been developed for detection of these antibodies, including various ELISAs using as antigen synthetic peptides (Coursaget et al. 1994, Favorov et al. 1994), recombinant proteins (Goldsmith et al. 1992, He et al. 1993, Tsarev et al. 1993b) or combinations of peptides and recombinant antigens (Sallie et al. 1992, Paul et al. 1994). In addition, immunoblot assays have been developed using recombinant antigens (Favorov et al. 1992, Li et al. 1994). These assays seem to vary considerably in their sensitivity and specificity, with relatively low overall concordance between results in a recent collaborative study. Synthetic peptides representing linear epitopes within the protein products of all 3 ORFs seem to react with sera from infected individuals (Kaur et al. 1992, Favorov et al. 1994), but peptide-based assays performed poorly over all against a reference panel of anti-HEV sera. A baculovirus-expressed, nearly complete ORF2 product was suggested to form virus-like particles and is likely to be a superior antigen because it may display conformation-dependent epitopes (Tsarev et al. 1993b). The early antibody response to this antigen includes both IgM and IgG antibodies to the virus (Tsarev et al. 1993b, 1994a). Antibody to the ORF2 protein was detectable in immunoblots for more than 12 months after infection, whereas antibody to ORF3 disappeared following resolution of the disease (Li et al. 1994). Nothing is known of the cellular immune responses, and there is controversy regarding the longevity of natural immunity after infection with HEV (Bryan et al. 1994, Arankalle et al. 1995).

CLINICAL MANIFESTATIONS OF HEPATITIS E

HEV, like HAV, causes an acute, self-limited disease that does not progress to a chronic phase. As shown in Fig. 34.9, the incubation period is somewhat longer than that for HAV, averaging c. 40 days. The prodromal symptoms of infection are similar to hepatitis A, including malaise, anorexia and abdominal discomfort. A 15–20% case-fatality rate has been observed among women who become infected during the third trimester of pregnancy (Khuroo et al. 1981), although the clinical features of fatal disease are not well described. Fulminant disease also occurs in other settings. About 60% of sporadic cases of fulminant hepatitis in India are due to HEV infection (Nanda et al. 1994). The much less frequent involvement of HEV in fulminant hepatitis in developed countries (Liang et al. 1993, Sallie et al. 1994) reflects the rarity of the infection in these regions.

DIAGNOSIS

Serological diagnosis of acute infection is relatively straightforward with the assays currently available. Detection of IgG anti-HEV in the absence of markers of other types of acute viral hepatitis is generally indicative of HEV infection. Tests for IgM antibodies have marginal sensitivity and are therefore of limited usefulness. In addition, lack of standardization and poor concordance between many available assays for IgG anti-HEV severely limit their usefulness in population-based studies and epidemiological investigations.

3.5 Epidemiology of HEV

The earliest documented outbreak of hepatitis E occurred in Delhi, India, in 1955, after heavy flooding of the Yamuna River (Viswanathan 1957). Subsequent outbreaks of disease and sporadic cases of hepatitis E have been confirmed in a wide variety of tropical and developing regions, including India, China, Nepal, Pakistan, Myanmar, Indonesia, the Central Asian region of the former Soviet Union, Egypt, Ethiopia, Jordan, Algeria, the Ivory Coast, Chad, Sudan, Somalia, Ethiopia and Mexico. In most outbreaks, contaminated drinking water has been incriminated as the source of infection. However, sporadic cases of hepatitis E cases also occur in these regions (Hyams et al. 1992a, 1992b, Bile et al. 1994), suggesting that the virus is endemic. Clinically apparent hepatitis E generally occurs in individuals 25–40 years of age (Bradley 1992, Jameel et al. 1992), and the mean age at infection with HEV seems to differ markedly from the mean age of infection with HAV in regions that are endemic for both viruses. Surveys of sera collected over an interval of 10 years from an HEV-endemic region of India demonstrated that most HAV infec-

tions occurred before the age of 5 years, whereas HEV infections generally occurred after the age of 16 years (Arankalle et al. 1995). The reason for this difference is not known; serologically determined rates of infection are similar in children and adults during disease outbreaks, although adults are more likely to develop clinical evidence of hepatitis (Mast et al. 1993). Hepatitis E is an extraordinarily rare disease in the USA and Europe, although seroprevalence studies with currently available assays indicate that limited exposure to HEV or a closely related virus may indeed occur. In these regions of the world, almost all reported cases have been in travellers who have recently returned from endemic regions.

The apparent low level, endemic circulation of the virus in some regions contrasts with the fact that person-to-person transmission of HEV is unusual during epidemics (Mast et al. 1993, Aggarwal and Naik 1994). This has led to speculation that HEV may represent a zoonotic pathogen, confined to its ecological niche until adverse circumstances, such as flooding, result in faecal contamination of the water supply (Bile et al. 1994). Another possibility is that certain individuals may shed virus for extended periods and thereby serve as reservoirs of infection (Nanda et al. 1995).

3.6 Control of hepatitis E

As with HAV, primary prevention of HEV infection rests with the provision of safe drinking water and the sanitary disposal of human waste (Bile et al. 1994), but most cases of hepatitis E occur in regions of the world where these conditions are difficult to achieve. Data concerning the protective efficacy of IG are limited and difficult to interpret (Joshi et al. 1985, Khuroo and Dar 1992). However, it is likely that anti-HEV is not present in significant titres in IG prepared from plasma collected in well developed, industrialized countries. Passive immunoprophylaxis of non-human primates with hyperimmune globulin has prevented biochemical and histological evidence of hepatitis although it did not prevent infection (Tsarev et al. 1994a). Both viraemia and faecal virus excretion were documented in animals receiving hyperimmune globulin.

Because HEV cannot be propagated efficiently in cell culture, vaccine development has focused on recombinant immunogens. Preliminary studies suggested that immunization of cynomolgus monkeys with a recombinant, partial ORF2 protein product may have provided protection against disease, but not virus replication following challenge with a heterologous inoculum (Purdy et al. 1993). More recently, immunization of cynomolgus macaques with 2 doses of a baculovirus-expressed recombinant ORF2 immunogen resulted in high titres of antibody and protection against both infection and disease (Tsarev et al. 1994a). These data are encouraging for the development of a vaccine.

ACKNOWLEDGEMENT

This work was supported in part by a grant from the US Public Health Service (RO1-AI32599).

REFERENCES

Abe H, Beninger PR et al., 1982, Light microscopic findings of liver biopsy specimens from patients with hepatitis type A and comparison with type B, *Gastroenterology*, **82**: 938–47.

Aggarwal R, Naik SR, 1994, Hepatitis E: intrafamilial transmission *versus* waterborne spread, *J Hepatol*, **21**: 718–23.

Allaire M, Chernala MM et al., 1994, Picornaviral 3C cysteine proteinases have a fold similar to chymotrypsin-like serine proteinases, *Nature (London)*, **369**: 72–6.

Almela MJ, González ME, Carrasco L, 1991, Inhibitors of poliovirus uncoating efficiently block the early membrane permeabilization induced by virus particles, *J Virol*, **65**: 2572–7.

Anderson DA, 1987, Cytopathology, plaque assay, and heat inactivation of hepatitis A virus strain HM175, *J Med Virol*, **22**: 35–44.

Andino R, Rieckhof GE et al., 1993, Poliovirus RNA synthesis utilizes an RNP complex formed around the 5′ end of viral RNA, *EMBO J*, **12**: 3587–98.

Andre FE, Hepburn A, D'Hondt E, 1990, Inactivated candidate vaccines for hepatitis A, *Prog Med Virol*, **37**: 72–95.

Arankalle VA, Tsarev SA et al., 1995, Age-specific prevalence of antibodies to hepatitis A and E viruses in Pune, India, 1982 and 1992, *J Infect Dis*, **171**: 447–50.

Asher LVS, Binn LN et al., 1995, Pathogenesis of hepatitis A in orally inoculated owl monkeys (*Aotus trivergatus*), *J Med Virol*, **47**: 260–8.

Balayan MS, Andzhaparidze AG et al., 1983, Evidence for a virus in non-A, non-B hepatitis transmitted via the fecal–oral route, *Intervirology*, **20**: 23–31.

Balayan MS, Usmanov RK et al., 1990, Brief report: experimental hepatitis E infection in domestic pigs, *J Med Virol*, **32**: 58–9.

Barker MH, Capps RB, Allen F, 1945, Acute infectious hepatitis in the Mediterranean theater: including acute hepatitis without jaundice, *JAMA*, **128**: 997–1003.

Beneduce F, Pisani G et al., 1995, Complete nucleotide sequence of a cytopathic hepatitis A virus strain isolated in Italy, *Virus Res*, **36**: 299–309.

Bienz K, Egger D et al., 1992, Structural and functional characterization of the poliovirus replication complex, *J Virol*, **66**: 2740–7.

Bile K, Isse A et al., 1994, Contrasting roles of rivers and wells as sources of drinking water on attack and fatality rates in a hepatitis E epidemic in Somalia, *Am J Trop Med Hyg*, **51**: 466–74.

Binn LN, Lemon SM et al., 1984, Primary isolation and serial passage of hepatitis A virus strains in primate cell cultures, *J Clin Microbiol*, **20**: 28–33.

Binn LN, Bancroft WH et al., 1986, Preparation of a prototype inactivated hepatitis A virus vaccine from infected cell cultures, *J Infect Dis*, **153**: 749–56.

Bishop NE, Anderson DA, 1993, RNA-dependent cleavage of VP0 capsid protein in provirions of hepatitis A virus, *Virology*, **197**: 616–23.

Borovec SV, Anderson DA, 1993, Synthesis and assembly of hepatitis A virus-specific proteins in BS-C-1 cells, *J Virol*, **67**: 3095–102.

Bradley DW, 1992, Hepatitis E: epidemiology, aetiology and molecular biology, *Rev Med Virol*, **2**: 19–28.

Bradley DW, Gravelle CR et al., 1977, Cyclic excretion of hepatitis A virus in experimentally infected chimpanzees: biophys-

ical characterization of the associated HAV particles, *J Med Virol*, **1**: 133–8.

Bradley DW, Krawczynski K et al., 1987, Enterically transmitted non-A, non-B hepatitis: serial passage of disease in cynomolgus macaques and tamarins and recovery of disease-associated 27- to 34-nm viruslike particles, *Proc Natl Acad Sci USA*, **84**: 6277–81.

Bradley D, Andjaparidze A et al., 1988, Aetiological agent of enterically transmitted non-A, non-B hepatitis, *J Gen Virol*, **69**: 731–8.

Bromberg K, Newhall DN, Peter G, 1982, Hepatitis A and meningoencephalitis, *JAMA*, **247**: 815.

Brown EA, Zajac AJ, Lemon SM, 1994, In vitro characterization of an internal ribosomal entry site (IRES) present within the 5′ nontranslated region of hepatitis A virus RNA: comparison with the IRES of encephalomyocarditis virus, *J Virol*, **68**: 1066–74.

Brown EA, Day SP et al., 1991, The 5′ nontranslated region of hepatitis A virus: secondary structure and elements required for translation in vitro, *J Virol*, **65**: 5828–38.

Bryan JP, Tsarev SA et al., 1994, Epidemic hepatitis E in Pakistan: patterns of serologic response and evidence that antibody to hepatitis E virus protects against disease, *J Infect Dis*, **170**: 517–21.

Centers for Disease Control, 1988, Hepatitis A among drug abusers, *Morbid Mortal Weekly Rep*, **37**: 297–305.

Centers for Disease Control, 1994, *Hepatitis Surveillance Report No 55*, Centers for Disease Control and Prevention, Atlanta GA.

Chang KH, Brown EA, Lemon SM, 1993, Cell type-specific proteins which interact with the 5′ nontranslated region of hepatitis A virus RNA, *J Virol*, **67**: 6716–25.

Chauhan A, Jameel S et al., 1993, Hepatitis E virus transmission to a volunteer, *Lancet*, **341**: 149–50.

Cho MW, Ehrenfeld E, 1991, Rapid completion of the replication cycle of hepatitis A virus subsequent to reversal of guanidine inhibition, *Virology*, **180**: 770–80.

Cho MW, Teterina N et al., 1994, Membrane rearrangement and vesicle induction by recombinant poliovirus 2C and 2BC in human cells, *Virology*, **202**: 129–45.

Choo Q-L, Kuo G et al., 1989, Isolation of a cDNA clone derived from a blood-borne non-A, non-B viral hepatitis genome, *Science*, **244**: 359–62.

Chow M, Newman JFE et al., 1987, Myristylation of picornavirus capsid protein VP4 and its structural significance, *Nature (London)*, **327**: 482–6.

Clark ME, Lieberman PM et al., 1993, Direct cleavage of human TATA-binding protein by poliovirus protease 3C in vivo and in vitro, *Mol Cell Biol*, **13**: 1232–7.

Cohen JI, Feinstone S, Purcell RH, 1989, Hepatitis A virus infection in a chimpanzee: duration of viremia and detection of virus in saliva and throat swabs, *J Infect Dis*, **160**: 887–90.

Cohen JI, Rosenblum B et al., 1987a, Complete nucleotide sequence of an attenuated hepatitis A virus: comparison with wild-type virus, *Proc Natl Acad Sci USA*, **84**: 2497–501.

Cohen JI, Ticehurst JR et al., 1987b, Hepatitis A virus cDNA and its RNA transcripts are infectious in cell culture, *J Virol*, **61**: 3035–9.

Cohen JI, Ticehurst JR et al., 1987c, Complete nucleotide sequence of wild-type hepatitis A virus: comparison with different strains of hepatitis A virus and other picornaviruses, *J Virol*, **61**: 50–9.

Conrad ME, Lemon SM, 1987, Prevention of endemic icteric viral hepatitis by administration of immune serum globulin, *J Infect Dis*, **156**: 56–63.

Corey L, Holmes KK, 1980, Sexual transmission of hepatitis A in homosexual men: incidence and mechanism, *N Engl J Med*, **302**: 435–8.

Coursaget P, Depril N et al., 1994, Hepatitis type E in a French population: detection of anti-HEV by a synthetic peptide-based enzyme-linked immunosorbent assay, *Res Virol*, **145**: 51–7.

Cromeans T, Sobsey MD, Fields HA, 1987, Development of a plaque assay for a cytopathic, rapidly replicating isolate of hepatitis A virus, *J Med Virol*, **22**: 45–56.

Cubitt D, Bradley DW et al., 1995, *Caliciviridae*. Virus Taxonomy: Classification and Nomenclature of Viruses, eds Murphy FA, Fauquet CM et al., *Arch Virol Suppl*, **10**: 359–63.

Daemer RJ, Feinstone SM et al., 1981, Propagation of human hepatitis A virus in African green monkey kidney cell culture: primary isolation and serial passage, *Infect Immun*, **32**: 388–93.

Das S, Dasgupta A, 1993, Identification of the cleavage site and determinants required for poliovirus 3C^{Pro}-catalyzed cleavage of human TATA-binding transcription factor TBP, *J Virol*, **67**: 3326–31.

Day SP, Lemon SM, 1990, A single base mutation in the 5′ non-coding region of HAV enhances replication of virus in vitro, *Vaccines 90: modern approaches to new vaccines, including prevention of AIDS*, eds Brown F, Chanock RM et al., Cold Spring Harbor Laboratory Press, Cold Spring Harbor NY, 175–8.

Day SP, Murphy P et al., 1992, Mutations within the 5′ nontranslated region of hepatitis A virus RNA which enhance replication in BS-C-1 cells, *J Virol*, **66**: 6533–40.

Decker RH, Overby LR et al., 1979, Serologic studies of transmission of hepatitis A in humans, *J Infect Dis*, **139**: 74–82.

Decker RH, Kosakowski SM et al., 1981, Diagnosis of acute hepatitis A by HAVAB$^{(R)}$-M, a direct radioimmunoassay for IgM anti-HAV, *Am J Clin Path*, **76**: 140–7.

Dienstag JL, Popper H, Purcell RH, 1976, The pathology of viral hepatitis types A and B in chimpanzees, *Am J Pathol*, **85**: 131–44.

Dienstag JL, Feinstone SM et al., 1975, Experimental infection of chimpanzees with hepatitis A virus, *J Infect Dis*, **132**: 532–45.

Dienstag JL, Schulman AN et al., 1976, Hepatitis A antigen isolated from liver and stool: immunologic comparison of antisera prepared in guinea pigs, *J Immunol*, **117**: 876–81.

Dotzauer A, Feinstone SM, Kaplan G, 1994, Susceptibility of nonprimate cell lines to hepatitis A virus infection, *J Virol*, **68**: 6064–8.

Emerson SU, Huang YK, Purcell RH, 1993, 2B and 2C mutations are essential but mutations throughout the genome of HAV contribute to adaptation to cell culture, *Virology*, **194**: 475–80.

Emerson SU, McRill C et al., 1991, Mutations responsible for adaptation of hepatitis A virus to efficient growth in cell culture, *J Virol*, **65**: 4882–6.

Emerson SU, Huang YK et al., 1992a, Mutations in both the 2B and 2C genes of hepatitis A virus are involved in adaptation to growth in cell culture, *J Virol*, **66**: 650–4.

Emerson SU, Huang YK et al., 1992b, Molecular basis of virulence and growth of hepatitis A virus in cell culture, *Vaccine*, **10, suppl 1**: S36–9.

Emini EA, Hughes JV et al., 1985, Induction of hepatitis A virus-neutralizing antibody by a virus-specific synthetic peptide, *J Virol*, **55**: 836–9.

Favorov MO, Fields HA et al., 1992, Serologic identification of hepatitis E virus infections in epidemic and endemic settings, *J Med Virol*, **36**: 246–50.

Favorov MO, Khudyakov YE et al., 1994, Enzyme immunoassay for the detection of antibody to hepatitis E virus based on synthetic peptides, *J Virol Methods*, **46**: 237–50.

Feinstone SM, Kapikian AZ, Purcell RH, 1973, Hepatitis A: detection by immune electron microscopy of a viruslike antigen associated with acute illness, *Science*, **182**: 1026–8.

Fleischer B, Fleischer S et al., 1990, Clonal analysis of infiltrating T lymphocytes in liver tissue in viral hepatitis A, *Immunology*, **69**: 14–19.

Forbes A, Williams R, 1990, Changing epidemiology and clinical aspects of hepatitis A, *Br Med Bull*, **46**: 303–18.

Frosner GG, Willers H et al., 1978, Decrease in incidence of hepatitis A infections in Germany, *Infection*, **6**: 259–60.

Frosner GG, Papaevangelou G et al., 1979, Antibody against hepatitis A in seven European countries. I. Comparison of prevalence data in different age groups, *Am J Epidemiol*, **110**: 63–9.

Fry KE, Tam AW et al., 1992, Hepatitis E virus (HEV): strain variation in the nonstructural gene region encoding a consensus RNA-dependent RNA polymerase and a helicase domain, *Virus Genes*, **6**: 173–85.

Funkhouser AW, Purcell RH et al., 1994, Attenuated hepatitis A virus: genetic determinants of adaptation to growth in MRC-5 cells, *J Virol*, **68**: 148–57.

Gellis SS, Stokes J Jr et al., 1945, The use of human immune serum globulin (gamma globulin) in infectious (epidemic) hepatitis in the Mediterranean theater of operations. I. Studies on prophylaxis in two epidemics of infectious hepatitis, *JAMA*, **128**: 1062–3.

Glass MJ, Summers DF, 1992, A *cis*-acting element within the hepatitis A virus 5′-non-coding region required for in vitro translation, *Virus Res*, **26**: 15–31.

Glass MJ, Summers DF, 1993, Identification of a *trans*-acting activity from liver that stimulates hepatitis A virus translation *in vitro*, *Virology*, **193**: 1047–50.

Glikson M, Galun E et al., 1992, Relapsing hepatitis A. Review of 14 cases and literature survey, *Medicine (Baltimore)*, **71**: 14–23.

Goldsmith R, Yarbough PO et al., 1992, Enzyme-linked immunosorbent assay for diagnosis of acute sporadic hepatitis E in Egyptian children, *Lancet*, **339**: 328–31.

Gordon SC, Reddy KR et al., 1984, Prolonged intrahepatic cholestasis secondary to acute hepatitis A, *Ann Intern Med*, **101**: 635–7.

Graff J, Normann A et al., 1994, Nucleotide sequence of wild-type hepatitis A virus GBM in comparison with two cell culture-adapted variants, *J Virol*, **68**: 548–54.

Gupta DN, Smetana HF, 1955, The histopathology of viral hepatitis as seen in Delhi epidemic, *Indian J Med Res*, **45, suppl**: 101–13.

Hadler SC, 1991, Global impact of hepatitis A virus infection: changing patterns, *Viral Hepatitis and Liver Disease*, eds Hollinger FB, Lemon SM, Margolis HS, Williams & Wilkins, Baltimore MD, 14–20.

Hadler SC, Webster HM et al., 1980, Hepatitis A in day-care centers: a community-wide assessment, *N Engl J Med*, **302**: 1222–7.

Hammond GW, MacDougall BK et al., 1982, Encephalitis during the prodromal stage of acute hepatitis A, *Can Med Assoc J*, **126**: 269–70.

Harmon SA, Updike W et al., 1992, Polyprotein processing in *cis* and in *trans* by hepatitis A virus 3C protease cloned and expressed in *Escherichia coli*, *J Virol*, **66**: 5242–7.

Harmon SA, Broman B et al., 1993, Localization of priming epitope to the C-terminal portion of hepatitis A virus VP1, *J Infect Dis*, **167**: 990–2.

Harmon SA, Emerson SU et al., 1995, Hepatitis A viruses with deletions in the 2A gene are infectious in cultured cells and marmosets., *J Virol*, **69**: 5576–81.

Havens WP Jr, 1944, Infectious hepatitis in the Middle East: a clinical review of 200 cases seen in a military hospital, *JAMA*, **126**: 17–23.

He J, Tam AW et al., 1993, Expression and diagnostic utility of hepatitis E virus putative structural proteins expressed in insect cells, *J Clin Microbiol*, **31**: 2167–73.

Hollinger FB, Khan NC et al., 1983, Posttransfusion hepatitis type A, *JAMA*, **250**: 2313–17.

Huang C-C, Nguyen D et al., 1992, Molecular cloning and

sequencing of the Mexico isolate of hepatitis E virus (HEV), *Virology*, **191**: 550–8.

Huang RT, Li DR et al., 1992, Isolation and identification of hepatitis E virus in Xinjiang, China, *J Gen Virol*, **73**: 1143–8.

Hyams KC, McCarthy MC et al., 1992a, Acute sporadic hepatitis E in children living in Cairo, Egypt, *J Med Virol*, **37**: 274–7.

Hyams KC, Purdy MA et al., 1992b, Acute sporadic hepatitis E in Sudanese children: analysis based on a new Western blot assay, *J Infect Dis*, **165**: 1001–5.

Immunization Practices Advisory Committee, 1990, Protection against viral hepatitis, *Morbid Mortal Weekly Rep*, **39**: 1–26.

Innis BL, Snitbhan R et al., 1991, The declining transmission of hepatitis A in Thailand, *J Infect Dis*, **163**: 989–95.

Innis BL, Snitbhan R et al., 1994, Protection against hepatitis A by an inactivated vaccine, *JAMA*, **271**: 1328–34.

Jameel S, Durgapal H et al., 1992, Enteric non-A, non-B hepatitis: epidemics, animal transmission, and hepatitis E virus detection by the polymerase chain reaction, *J Med Virol*, **37**: 263–70.

Jameel S, Zafrullah M et al., 1996, Expression in animal cells and characterization of the hepatitis E virus structural proteins, *J Virol*, **70**: 207–16.

Jansen RW, Newbold JE, Lemon SM, 1988, Complete nucleotide sequence of a cell culture-adapted variant of hepatitis A virus: comparison with wild-type virus with restricted capacity for *in vitro* replication, *Virology*, **163**: 299–307.

Jansen RW, Siegl G, Lemon SM, 1990, Molecular epidemiology of human hepatitis A virus defined by an antigen-capture polymerase chain reaction method, *Proc Natl Acad Sci USA*, **87**: 2867–71.

Jewell DA, Swietnicki W et al., 1992, Hepatitis A virus 3C proteinase substrate specificity, *Biochemistry*, **31**: 7862–9.

Johnston JM, Harmon SA et al., 1988, Antigenic and immunogenic properties of a hepatitis A virus capsid protein expressed in *Escherichia coli*, *J Infect Dis*, **157**: 1203–11.

Joshi YK, Babu S et al., 1985, Immunoprophylaxis of epidemic non-A non-B hepatitis, *Indian J Med Res*, **81**: 18–19.

Karayiannis P, Jowett T et al., 1986, Hepatitis A virus replication in tamarins and host immune response in relation to pathogenesis of liver cell damage, *J Med Virol*, **18**: 261–76.

Karron RA, Ticehurst JR et al., 1986, Evaluation of attenuation of hepatitis A virus in primates, *Abstracts of the 1986 Interscience Conference on Antimicrobial Agents and Chemotherapy*, American Society for Microbiology, Washington, 278.

Kaur M, Hyams KC et al., 1992, Human linear B-cell epitopes encoded by the hepatitis E virus include determinants in the RNA-dependent RNA polymerase, *Proc Natl Acad Sci USA*, **89**: 3855–8.

Kazachkov Y, Balayan MS et al., 1992, Hepatitis E virus in cultivated cells, *Arch Virol*, **127**: 399–402.

Khudyakov YE, Khudyakova NS et al., 1993, Epitope mapping in proteins of hepatitis E virus, *Virology*, **194**: 89–96.

Khuroo MS, 1980, Study of an epidemic of non-A, non-B hepatitis: possibility of another human hepatitis virus distinct from post-transfusion non-A, non-B type, *Am J Med*, **68**: 818–24.

Khuroo MS, Dar MV, 1992, Hepatitis E: evidence for person-to-person transmission and inability of low dose immune serum globulin from an Indian source to prevent it, *Indian J Gastroenterol*, **11**: 109–12.

Khuroo MS, Teli MR et al., 1981, Incidence and severity of viral hepatitis in pregnancy, *Am J Med*, **70**: 252–5.

Koonin EV, Gorbalenya AE et al., 1992, Computer-assisted assignment of functional domains in the nonstructural polyprotein of hepatitis E virus: delineation of an additional group of positive-strand RNA plant and animal viruses, *Proc Natl Acad Sci USA*, **89**: 8259–63.

Krah DL, Amin RD et al., 1991, A simple antigen-reduction assay for the measurement of neutralizing antibodies to hepatitis A virus, *J Infect Dis*, **163**: 634–7.

Krugman S, Ward R, 1958, Clinical and experimental studies of infectious hepatitis, *Pediatrics*, **22**: 1016–22.

Krugman S, Ward R, Giles JP, 1962, The natural history of infectious hepatitis, *Am J Med*, **32**: 717–28.

Krugman S, Ward R et al., 1960, Infectious hepatitis: studies on the effect of gammaglobulin and on the incidence of inapparent infection, *JAMA*, **174**: 323–30.

Kusov YY, Sommergruber W et al., 1992, Intermolecular cleavage of hepatitis A virus (HAV) precursor protein P1-P2 by recombinant HAV proteinase 3C, *J Virol*, **66**: 6794–6.

Lednar WM, Lemon SM et al., 1985, Frequency of illness associated with epidemic hepatitis A virus infections in adults, *Am J Epidemiol*, **122**: 226–33.

LeDuc JW, Lemon SM et al., 1983, Experimental infection of the New World owl monkey (*Aotus trivirgatus*) with hepatitis A virus, *Infect Immun*, **40**: 766–72.

Lemon SM, 1985a, IgM neutralizing antibody to hepatitis A virus, *J Infect Dis*, **152**: 1353–4.

Lemon SM, 1985b, Type A viral hepatitis: new developments in an old disease, *N Engl J Med*, **313**: 1059–67.

Lemon SM, 1994, Inactivated hepatitis A vaccines, *JAMA*, **271**: 1363–4.

Lemon SM, Amphlett E, Sangar D, 1991, Protease digestion of hepatitis A virus: disparate effects on capsid proteins, antigenicity, and infectivity, *J Virol*, **65**: 5636–40.

Lemon SM, Binn LN, 1983a, Antigenic relatedness of two strains of hepatitis A virus determined by cross-neutralization, *Infect Immun*, **42**: 418–20.

Lemon SM, Binn LN, 1983b, Serum neutralizing antibody response to hepatitis A virus, *J Infect Dis*, **148**: 1033–9.

Lemon SM, Binn LN, Marchwicki RH, 1983, Radioimmunofocus assay for quantitation of hepatitis A virus in cell cultures, *J Clin Microbiol*, **17**: 834–9.

Lemon SM, Jansen RW, Brown EA, 1992, Genetic, antigenic, and biologic differences between strains of hepatitis A virus, *Vaccine*, **10**: S40–4.

Lemon SM, Jansen RW, Newbold JE, 1985, Infectious hepatitis A virus particles produced in cell culture consist of three distinct types with different buoyant densities in CsCl, *J Virol*, **54**: 78–85.

Lemon SM, Shapiro CN, 1994, The value of immunization against hepatitis A, *Infect Agents Dis*, **3**: 38–49.

Lemon SM, Brown CD et al., 1980, Specific immunoglobulin M response to hepatitis A virus determined by solid-phase radioimmunoassay, *Infect Immun*, **28**: 927–36.

Lemon SM, Binn LN et al., 1990, *In vivo* replication and reversion to wild-type of a neutralization-resistant variant of hepatitis A virus., *J Infect Dis*, **161**: 7–13.

Lemon SM, Murphy PC et al., 1991a, Antigenic and genetic variation in cytopathic hepatitis A virus variants arising during persistent infection: evidence for genetic recombination, *J Virol*, **65**: 2056–65.

Lemon SM, Ping L-H et al., 1991b, Immunobiology of hepatitis A virus, *Viral Hepatitis and Liver Disease*, eds Hollinger FB, Lemon SM, Margolis HS, Williams & Wilkins, Baltimore MD, 20–4.

Lemon SM, Barclay W et al., 1992, Immunogenicity and antigenicity of chimeric picornaviruses which express hepatitis A virus (HAV) peptide sequences: evidence for a neutralization domain near the amino terminus of VP1 of HAV, *Virology*, **188**: 285–95.

Lewis JA, Armstrong ME et al., 1991, Use of a live attenuated hepatitis A vaccine to prepare a highly purified, formalin-inactivated hepatitis A vaccine, *Viral Hepatitis and Liver Disease*, eds Hollinger FB, Lemon SM, Margolis HS, Williams & Wilkins, Baltimore MD, 94–7.

Li F, Zhuang H et al., 1994, Persistent and transient antibody responses to hepatitis E virus detected by Western immunoblot using open reading frame 2 and 3 and glutathione S-transferase fusion proteins, *J Clin Microbiol*, **32**: 2060–6.

Liang TJ, Jeffers L et al., 1993, Fulminant or subfulminant non-A, non-B viral hepatitis: the role of hepatitis C and E viruses, *Gastroenterology*, **104**: 556–62.

Locarnini SA, Coulepis AG et al., 1979, Solid-phase enzyme-linked immunosorbent assay for detection of hepatitis A-specific immunoglobulin M, *J Clin Microbiol*, **9:** 459–65.

Locarnini SA, Coulepis AG et al., 1980, Coproantibodies in hepatitis A: detection of enzyme-linked immunosorbent assay and immune electron microscopy, *J Clin Microbiol*, **11:** 710–16.

Longer CF, Denny SL et al., 1993, Experimental hepatitis E: pathogenesis in cynomolgus macaques (*Macaca fascicularis*), *J Infect Dis*, **168:** 602–9.

Luo M, Rossmann MG, Palmenberg AC, 1988, Prediction of three-dimensional models for foot-and-mouth disease virus and hepatitis A virus, *Virology*, **166:** 503–14.

MacCallum FO, Bradley WH, 1944, Transmission of infective hepatitis to human volunteers, *Lancet*, **2:** 228.

Maier K, Gabriel P et al., 1988, Human gamma interferon production by cytotoxic T lymphocytes sensitized during hepatitis A virus infection, *J Virol*, **62:** 3756–63.

Malbrain MLNG, Lambrecht GLY et al., 1994, Acute renal failure in non-fulminant hepatitis A, *Clin Nephrol*, **41:** 180–1.

Malcolm BA, Chin SM et al., 1992, Expression and characterization of recombinant hepatitis A virus 3C proteinase, *Biochemistry*, **31:** 3358–63.

Mannucci PM, Gdovin S et al., 1994, Transmission of hepatitis A to patients with hemophilia by factor VIII concentrates treated with organic solvent and detergent to inactivate viruses, *Ann Intern Med*, **120:** 1–7.

Mao JS, Dong DX et al., 1989, Primary study of attenuated live hepatitis A vaccine (H2 strain) in humans, *J Infect Dis*, **159:** 621–4.

Mao JS, Dong DX et al., 1991, Further studies of attenuated live hepatitis A vaccine (H2 strain) in humans, *Viral Hepatitis and Liver Disease*, eds Hollinger FB, Lemon SM, Margolis HS, Williams & Wilkins, Baltimore MD, 110–11.

Martin A, Escriou N et al., 1996, Identification and site-direct mutagenesis of the primary (2A/2B) cleavage site of the hepatitis A virus polyprotein: functional impact on the infectivity of HAV transcripts, *Virology*, **213:** 213–22.

Mast EE, Polish LB et al., 1993, Hepatitis E among refugees in Kenya: minimal apparent person-to-person transmission, evidence for age-dependent disease expression and new serologic assays, *Viral Hepatitis and Liver Disease*, eds Nishioka K, Suzuki H et al., Springer-Verlag, Tokyo, 375–8.

Mathiesen LR, Drucker J et al., 1978a, Localization of hepatitis A antigen in marmoset organs during acute infection with hepatitis A virus, *J Infect Dis*, **138:** 369–77.

Mathiesen LR, Feinstone SM et al., 1978b, Enzyme-linked immunosorbent assay for detection of hepatitis A antigen in stool and antibody to hepatitis A antigen in sera: comparison with solid-phase radioimmunoassay, immune electron microscopy, and immune adherence hemagglutination assay, *J Clin Microbiol*, **7:** 184–93.

Mathiesen LR, Moller AM et al., 1980, Hepatitis A virus in the liver and intestine of marmosets after oral inoculation, *Infect Immun*, **28:** 45–8.

Mattioli S, Imberti L et al., 1995, Mimicry of the immunodominant conformation-dependent antigenic site of hepatitis A virus by motifs selected from synthetic peptide libraries, *J Virol*, **69:** 5294–9.

Midthun K, Ellerbeck E et al., 1991, Safety and immunogenicity of a live attenuated hepatitis A virus vaccine in seronegative volunteers, *J Infect Dis*, **163:** 735–9.

Minor PD, 1991, *Picornaviridae*. Classification and Nomenclature of Viruses: the Fifth Report of the International Committee on Taxonomy of Viruses, eds Francki RIB, Fauquet CM et al., *Arch Virol Suppl*, **2:** 320–6.

Morrow RH Jr, Smetana HF et al., 1968, Unusual features of viral hepatitis in Accra, Ghana, *Ann Intern Med*, **68:** 1250–64.

Nainan OV, Brinton MA, Margolis HS, 1992, Identification of amino acids located in the antibody binding sites of human hepatitis A virus, *Virology*, **191:** 984–7.

Nainan OV, Margolis HS et al., 1991, Sequence analysis of a new

hepatitis A virus naturally infecting cynomolgus macaques (*Macaca fascicularis*), *J Gen Virol*, **72:** 1685–9.

Najarian R, Caput D et al., 1985, Primary structure and gene organization of human hepatitis A virus, *Proc Natl Acad Sci USA*, **82:** 2627–31.

Nanda SK, Yalcinkaya K et al., 1994, Etiological role of hepatitis E virus in sporadic fulminant hepatitis, *J Med Virol*, **42:** 133–7.

Nanda SK, Ansari IH et al., 1995, Protracted viremia during acute sporadic hepatitis E virus infection, *Gastroenterology*, **108:** 225–30.

Nuesch JP, Weitz M, Siegl G, 1993, Proteins specifically binding to the 3' untranslated region of hepatitis A virus RNA in persistently infected cells, *Arch Virol*, **128:** 65–79.

Ogawa M, Hori J et al., 1994, A fatal case of acute renal failure associated with non-fulminant hepatitis A, *Clin Nephrol*, **42:** 205–6.

Palmenberg AC, 1989, Sequence alignments of picornavirus capsid proteins, *Molecular Aspects of Picornavirus Infections and Detections*, eds Semler BL, Ehrenfeld E, American Society for Microbiology, Washington, 211–41.

Paul DA, Knigge MF et al., 1994, Determination of hepatitis E virus seroprevalence by using recombinant fusion proteins and synthetic peptides, *J Infect Dis*, **169:** 801–6.

Ping L-H, Lemon SM, 1992, Antigenic structure of human hepatitis A virus defined by analysis of escape mutants selected against murine monoclonal antibodies, *J Virol*, **66:** 2208–16.

Ping L-H, Jansen RW et al., 1988, Identification of an immunodominant antigenic site involving the capsid protein VP3 of hepatitis A virus, *Proc Natl Acad Sci USA*, **85:** 8281–5.

Prikazsky V, Olear V et al., 1994, Interruption of an outbreak of hepatitis A in two villages by vaccination, *J Med Virol*, **44:** 457–9.

Provost PJ, Hilleman MR, 1979, Propagation of human hepatitis A virus in cell culture *in vitro*, *Proc Soc Exp Biol Med*, **160:** 213–21.

Provost PJ, Banker FS et al., 1982, Progress toward a live, attenuated human hepatitis A vaccine, *Proc Soc Exp Biol Med*, **170:** 8–14.

Provost PJ, Bishop RP et al., 1986, New findings in live, attenuated hepatitis A vaccine development, *J Med Virol*, **20:** 165–75.

Purcell RH, 1991, Approaches to immunization against hepatitis A virus, *Viral Hepatitis and Liver Disease*, eds Hollinger FB, Lemon SM, Margolis HS, Williams & Wilkins, Baltimore MD, 41–6.

Purcell RH, Feinstone SM et al., 1984, Hepatitis A virus, *Viral Hepatitis and Liver Disease*, eds Vyas GN, Dienstag JL, Hoofnagle JH, Grune & Stratton, Orlando FL, 9–22.

Purdy MA, McCaustland KA et al., 1993, Preliminary evidence that a *trpE*-HEV fusion protein protects cynomolgus macaques against challenge with wild-type hepatitis E virus (HEV), *J Med Virol*, **41:** 90–4.

Ray R, Jameel S, Manivel V, 1992, Indian hepatitis E virus shows a major deletion in the small open reading frame, *Virology*, **189:** 359–62.

Reyes GR, Purdy MA et al., 1990, Isolation of a cDNA from the virus responsible for enterically transmitted non-A, non-B hepatitis, *Science*, **247:** 1335–9.

Robertson BH, Brown VK et al., 1989, Structure of the hepatitis A virion: identification of potential surface-exposed regions, *Arch Virol*, **104:** 117–28.

Robertson BH, Khanna B et al., 1991, Epidemiologic patterns of wild-type hepatitis A virus determined by genetic variation, *J Infect Dis*, **163:** 286–92.

Robertson BH, Jansen RW et al., 1992, Genetic relatedness of hepatitis A virus strains recovered from different geographic regions, *J Gen Virol*, **73:** 1365–77.

Robertson BH, Jia X-Y et al., 1993, Antibody response to nonstructural proteins of hepatitis A virus following infection, *J Med Virol*, **40:** 76–82.

Robertson BH, D'Hondt EH et al., 1994a, Effect of postexposure vaccination in a chimpanzee model of hepatitis A virus infection, *J Med Virol*, **43**: 249–51.

Robertson BH, Friedberg D et al., 1994b, Sequence variability of hepatitis A virus and factor VIII associated hepatitis A infections in hemophilia patients in Europe. An update, *Vox Sang*, **67, suppl 1**: 39–46.

Rosenblum LS, Mirkin IR et al., 1990, A multifocal outbreak of hepatitis A traced to commercially distributed lettuce, *Am J Public Hlth*, **80**: 1075–9.

Rosenblum LS, Villarino ME et al., 1991, Hepatitis A outbreak in a neonatal intensive care unit: risk factors for transmission and evidence of prolonged viral excretion among preterm infants, *J Infect Dis*, **164**: 476–82.

Ross BC, Anderson RN et al., 1989, Nucleotide sequence of high-passage hepatitis A virus strain HM175: comparison with wild-type and cell culture-adapted strains, *J Gen Virol*, **70**: 2805–10.

Rueckert RR, Wimmer E, 1984, Systematic nomenclature of picornavirus proteins, *J Virol*, **50**: 957–9.

Sallie R, Rayner A et al., 1992, Detection of hepatitis 'C' virus in formalin-fixed liver tissue by nested polymerase chain reaction, *J Med Virol*, **37**: 310–14.

Sallie R, Silva AE et al., 1994, Hepatitis C and E in non-A non-B fulminant hepatic failure: a polymerase chain reaction and serological study, *J Hepatol*, **20**: 580–8.

Schultheiss T, Kusov YY, Gauss-Müller V, 1994, Proteinase 3C of hepatitis A virus (HAV) cleaves the HAV polyprotein P2-P3 at all sites including VP1/2A and 2A/2B, *Virology*, **198**: 275–81.

Schultheiss T, Sommergruber W et al., 1995, Cleavage specificity of purified recombinant hepatitis A virus 3C proteinase on natural substrates, *J Virol*, **9**: 1727–33.

Schultz DE, Hardin CC, Lemon SM, 1996, Specific interaction of glyceraldehyde 3-phosphate dehydrogenase with the 5' nontranslated RNA of hepatitis A virus, *J Biol Chem*, **271**: 14134–42.

Schultz DE, Honda M et al., 1996, Mutations within the 5' nontranslated RNA of cell culture-adapted hepatitis A virus which enhance cap-independent translation in cultured African green monkey kidney cells, *J Virol*, **70**: 1041–9.

Shaffer DR, Brown EA, Lemon SM, 1994, Large deletion mutations involving the first pyrimidine-rich tract of the 5' nontranslated RNA of hepatitis A virus define two adjacent domains associated with distinct replication phenotypes, *J Virol*, **68**: 5568–78.

Shaffer DR, Lemon SM, 1995, Temperature-sensitive hepatitis A virus mutants with deletions downstream of the first pyrimidine-rich tract of the 5' nontranslated RNA are impaired in RNA synthesis, *J Virol*, **69**: 6498–506.

Shaffer DR, Emerson SU et al., 1995, A hepatitis A virus deletion mutant which lacks the first pyrimidine-rich tract of the 5' nontranslated RNA remains virulent in primates following direct intrahepatic nucleic acid transfection, *J Virol*, **69**: 6600–4.

Sherertz RJ, Russell BA, Reuman PD, 1984, Transmission of hepatitis A by tranfusion of blood products, *Arch Intern Med*, **144**: 1579–80.

Shimizu YK, Shikata T et al., 1982, Detection of hepatitis A antigen in human liver, *Infect Immun*, **36**: 320–4.

Siebke JC, Degre M et al., 1982, Prevalence of hepatitis A antibodies in a normal population and some selected groups of patients in Norway, *Am J Epidemiol*, **115**: 185–91.

Siegl G, Eggers HJ, 1982, Failure of guanidine and 2-(α-hydroxybenzyl)benzimidazole to inhibit replication of hepatitis A virus *in vitro*, *J Gen Virol*, **61**: 111–14.

Siegl G, Weitz M, Kronauer G, 1984, Stability of hepatitis A virus, *Intervirology*, **22**: 218–26.

Sjogren MH, Tanno H et al., 1987, Hepatitis A virus in stool during clinical relapse, *Ann Intern Med*, **106**: 221–6.

Sjogren MH, Purcell RH et al., 1992, Clinical and laboratory observations following oral or intramuscular administration of a live, attenuated hepatitis A vaccine candidate, *Vaccine*, **10, suppl 1**: S135–7.

Stapleton JT, Frederick J, Meyer B, 1991, Hepatitis A virus attachment to cultured cell lines, *J Infect Dis*, **164**: 1098–103.

Stapleton JT, Jansen RW, Lemon SM, 1985, Neutralizing antibody to hepatitis A virus in immune serum globulin and in the sera of human recipients of immune serum globulin, *Gastroenterology*, **89**: 637–42.

Stapleton JT, Lemon SM, 1987, Neutralization escape mutants define a dominant immunogenic neutralization site on hepatitis A virus, *J Virol*, **61**: 491–8.

Stapleton JT, Lange DK et al., 1991, The role of secretory immunity in hepatitis A virus infection, *J Infect Dis*, **163**: 7–11.

Stapleton JT, Raina V et al., 1993, Antigenic and immunogenic properties of recombinant hepatitis A virus 14S and 70S subviral particles, *J Virol*, **67**: 1080–5.

Szmuness W, Dienstag JL et al., 1977, The prevalence of antibody to hepatitis A antigen in various parts of the world: a pilot study, *Am J Epidemiol*, **106**: 392–8.

Tam AW, Smith MM et al., 1991, Hepatitis E virus (HEV): molecular cloning and sequencing of the full-length viral genome, *Virology*, **185**: 120–31.

Tam AW, White R et al., 1996, In vitro propagation and production of hepatitis E virus from in vivo infected primary macaque hepatocytes, *Virology*, **215**: 1–9.

Teixera MR Jr, Weller IVD et al., 1982, The pathology of hepatitis A in man, *Liver*, **2**: 53–60.

Tesar M, Harmon SA et al., 1992, Hepatitis A virus polyprotein synthesis initiates from two alternative AUG codons, *Virology*, **186**: 609–18.

Tesar M, Jia X-Y et al., 1993, Analysis of a potential myristoylation site in hepatitis A virus capsid protein VP4, *Virology*, **194**: 616–26.

Tesar M, Pak I et al., 1994, Expression of hepatitis A virus precursor protein P3 *in vivo* and *in vitro*: polyprotein processing of the 3CD cleavage site, *Virology*, **198**: 524–33.

Ticehurst J, 1991, Identification and characterization of hepatitis E virus, *Viral Hepatitis and Liver Disease*, eds Hollinger FB, Lemon SM, Margolis HS, Williams & Wilkins, Baltimore MD, 501–13.

Ticehurst J, Rhodes LL Jr et al., 1992, Infection of owl monkeys (*Aotus trivirgatus*) and cynomolgus monkeys (*Macaca fascicularis*) with hepatitis E virus from Mexico, *J Infect Dis*, **165**: 835–45.

Tsarev SA, Emerson SU et al., 1991, Simian hepatitis A virus (HAV) strain AGM-27: comparison of genome structure and growth in cell culture with other HAV strains, *J Gen Virol*, **72**: 1677–83.

Tsarev SA, Emerson SU et al., 1992, Characterization of a prototype strain of hepatitis E virus, *Proc Natl Acad Sci USA*, **89**: 559–63.

Tsarev SA, Emerson SU et al., 1993a, Variation in course of hepatitis E in experimentally infected cynomolgus monkeys, *J Infect Dis*, **167**: 1302–6.

Tsarev SA, Tsareva TS et al., 1993b, ELISA for antibody to hepatitis E virus (HEV) based on complete open-reading frame-2 protein expressed in insect cells: identification of HEV infection in primates, *J Infect Dis*, **168**: 369–78.

Tsarev SA, Tsareva TS et al., 1994a, Successful passive and active immunization of cynomolgus monkeys against hepatitis E, *Proc Natl Acad Sci USA*, **91**: 10198–202.

Tsarev SA, Tsareva TS et al., 1994b, Infectivity titration of a prototype strain of hepatitis E virus in cynomolgus monkeys, *J Med Virol*, **43**: 135–42.

Vallbracht A, Gabriel P et al., 1986, Cell-mediated cytotoxicity in hepatitis A virus infection, *Hepatology*, **6**: 1308–14.

Vallbracht A, Maier K et al., 1989, Liver-derived cytotoxic T cells in hepatitis A virus infection, *J Infect Dis*, **160**: 209–17.

Vento S, Garofano T et al., 1991, Identification of hepatitis A virus as a trigger for autoimmune chronic hepatitis type 1 in susceptible individuals, *Lancet*, **337**: 1183–7.

Villarejos VM, Serra C J et al., 1982, Hepatitis A virus infection in households, *Am J Epidemiol*, **115**: 577–86.

Viswanathan R, 1957, Epidemiology [of an 'explosive' epidemic of infectious hepatitis in Delhi during Dec–Jan, 1955–56], *Indian J Med Res*, **45, suppl:** 1–29.

Ward R, Krugman S et al., 1958, Infectious hepatitis: studies of its natural history and prevention, *N Engl J Med*, **258:** 407–16.

Weisfuse IB, Graham DJ et al., 1990, An outbreak of hepatitis A among cancer patients treated with interleukin-2 and lymphokine activated killer cells, *J Infect Dis*, **161:** 647–52.

Weitz M, Baroudy BM et al., 1986, Detection of a genome-linked protein (VPg) of hepatitis A virus and its comparison with other picornaviral VPgs, *J Virol*, **60:** 124–30.

Werzberger A, Mensch B et al., 1992, A controlled trial of a formalin-inactivated hepatitis A vaccine in healthy children, *N Engl J Med*, **327:** 453–7.

Whetter LE, Day SP et al., 1994, Low efficiency of the 5' non-translated region of hepatitis A virus RNA in directing cap-independent translation in permissive monkey kidney cells, *J Virol*, **68:** 5253–63.

Widell A, Hansson BG et al., 1983, Increased occurrence of hepatitis A with cyclic outbreaks among drug addicts in a Swedish community, *Infection*, **11:** 198–200.

Winokur PL, McLinden JH, Stapleton JT, 1991, The hepatitis A virus polyprotein expressed by a recombinant vaccinia virus undergoes proteolytic processing and assembly into viruslike particles, *J Virol*, **65:** 5029–36.

Winokur PL, Stapleton JT, 1992, Immunoglobulin prophylaxis for hepatitis A, *Clin Infect Dis*, **14:** 580–6.

Wong DC, Purcell RH et al., 1980, Epidemic and endemic hepatitis A in India: evidence for a non-A, non-B hepatitis virus etiology, *Lancet*, **2:** 876–9.

Yarbough PO, Tam AW et al., 1991, Hepatitis E virus: identification of type-common epitopes, *J Virol*, **65:** 5790–7.

Yin S, Tsarev SA et al., 1993, Partial sequence comparison of eight new Chinese strains of hepatitis E virus suggests the genome sequence is relatively stable, *J Med Virol*, **41:** 230–41.

Zajac AJ, Amphlett EM et al., 1991, Parameters influencing the attachment of hepatitis A virus to a variety of continuous cell lines, *J Gen Virol*, **72:** 1667–75.

Zhang H, Chao S-F et al., 1995, An infectious cDNA clone of a cytopathic hepatitis A virus: genomic regions associated with rapid replication and cytopathic effect, *Virology*, **212:** 686–97.

Zikos D, Grewal KS et al., 1995, Nephrotic syndrome and acute renal failure associated with hepatitis A virus infection, *Am J Gastroenterol*, **90:** 295–8.

Chapter 35

HEPATITIS C

Peter Simmonds, David Mutimer and Edward A C Follett

| 1 Properties of the virus | 2 Clinical and pathological aspects |

1 PROPERTIES OF THE VIRUS

1.1 Introduction

The discovery of hepatitis C virus (HCV) in 1989 was the culmination of a large research endeavour to find the causes of post-transfusion hepatitis. In the 1970s, several groups produced evidence for an infectious agent, distinct from the hepatitis A and hepatitis B viruses (HAV, HBV), that caused chronic hepatitis and was frequently transmitted by blood and blood products (Prince et al. 1974, Alter et al. 1975, Feinstone, Kapikian and Purcell 1975). The diagnosis of non-A, non-B hepatitis (NANBH) was made by exclusion of HAV, HBV, herpesviruses such as cytomegalovirus and Epstein–Barr virus and other infectious causes of hepatitis.

Typically, NANBH is a mild disease that causes jaundice in less than half of cases, and is frequently asymptomatic. Its clinical features differ in several respects from acute HAV and HBV infection, with a longer incubation period from exposure to liver function abnormalities (c. 8 weeks) than is usually observed for HAV (4 weeks) but shorter than that for HBV (12 weeks). There is a high rate of chronicity following acute infection (at least 50% of cases, compared with c. 5% for adult HBV infection). Chronic infection is generally asymptomatic at first, although a large proportion of cases eventually progress to cirrhosis.

Progress towards identifying the cause of NANBH was hampered by the difficulty in culturing the agent in cell or organ culture; the eventual characterization of the infectious agent of NANBH followed the successful transmission of the agent into chimpanzees. Experimental data were then obtained that the agent passed through an 80 nm filter and was inactivated by lipid solvents such as chloroform, suggesting a small enveloped virus. Examination of liver biopsies from patients with NANBH and of experimentally infected

chimpanzees helped to define the histological features of acute and chronic disease and to differentiate it from other causes of hepatitis. Passaging and titration of the NANBH agent in chimpanzees eventually provided high titre stocks of virus that were necessary for cloning and sequence analysis of the infectious agent (Bradley et al. 1979, Bradley and Maynard 1986).

Nucleic acid (both DNA and RNA) was extracted following ultracentrifugation from a large volume of a plasma sample with a high infectivity titre in chimpanzees (c. 10^6 infectious units/ml). The nucleic acid was reverse transcribed and the resulting DNA fragments cloned into the λgt11 bacteriophage. The DNA sequences in the resulting library were expressed as fusion proteins during replication of the bacteriophage in *Escherichia coli*. Immunoscreening of large numbers of bacteriophage plaques with antisera from patients with NANBH led to the eventual identification of an immunoreactive clone (designated 5-1-1) that seemed to be specific for the NANBH agent, HCV (Choo et al. 1989). This clone showed no similarity with any human or *E. coli* genomic sequences and produced a protein that was consistently recognized by sera from patients with NANBH, but not by sera from control individuals or those with hepatitis of other aetiologies (Kuo et al. 1989).

The 5-1-1 clone was then used as a probe to identify overlapping sequences in the λgt11 library and this led to the assembly of a nearly complete nucleotide sequence of the NANBH agent (Choo et al. 1991). Knowledge of the length, nucleic acid composition and genome organization of HCV has since provided the basis for its proposed classification in the *Flaviviridae* family (see section 1.2, p. 718) and its likely method of replication (see section 1.4, p. 722). From the sequence of HCV it was possible to design hybridization probes and primers for amplification of the HCV genome by polymerase chain reaction (PCR) that can be used to detect HCV RNA in sera and liver biopsies from hepatitis patients (see 'Genome detection', p. 736). The original 5-1-1 clone, together with an overlapping clone, c100-3, and more recently with clones from other parts of the genome, has been used to manufacture recombinant proteins for assays for antibody to HCV. This has enabled effective screening of blood donors for HCV infection to be adopted world-wide (see section 2.3, p. 734, and 'Prevention of infection', p. 738).

1.2 Classification

COMPARISON WITH POSITIVE-STRAND RNA VIRUSES

The sequence of the HCV genome shares several features with other positive-strand RNA viruses. Most striking is the existence of a single continuous open reading frame that occupies almost the entire genome. By analogy with other positive-strand RNA viruses, this would be cleaved into individual proteins that are enzymes necessary for virus replication or are structural components of the virion (Fig. 35.1). In overall genome organization and presumed method of replication, HCV is most like members of the *Flaviviridae*. The roles of the different proteins encoded by HCV have been inferred by comparison with homologues in other flaviviruses and, more directly, by expression in vitro of cloned HCV sequences in prokaryotic and eukaryotic systems. For example, expression in vitro has allowed the investigation of protease activity of the NS3 protein and, more recently, the RNA polymerase activity of NS5b (see 'Non-structural proteins', p. 723).

Comparison with other positive-strand RNA virus groups whose coding capacity is contained within a single open reading frame provides several clues about the replication of HCV (Table 35.1). The genomes of *Picornaviridae* (e.g. poliovirus, Coxsackie A, B, hepatitis A virus) and *Flaviviridae* (e.g. dengue fever, yellow fever virus) all have a similar organization with structural proteins at the 5′ end and non-structural proteins at the 3′ end. However, these virus families differ in their genome size, the number of proteins produced, the mechanism by which the polyprotein is cleaved and the detailed mechanism of genome replication.

Members of the *Flaviviridae* have many features in common with HCV. They have a similar genome size to HCV (yellow fever virus: 10 862 bases (Rice et al. 1985), compared with 9379 of HCV (Choo et al. 1991)), and the virus envelope contains a viral encoded glycoprotein (E1). However, the homologue of HCV E2 in flaviviruses (also a membrane-bound glycoprotein: NS1) is expressed only on the infected cell surface. Like HCV, the polyprotein of flaviviruses is cleaved by a combination of viral and host cell proteases. Although there is no close sequence similarity between HCV and other viruses, there are at least 2 regions with conserved amino acid residues that provide information about potential protein functions. The NS5b protein of HCV contains the GDD (glycine–aspartate–aspartate) motif associated with the active site in virus RNA-dependent RNA polymerases (RdRp)

of positive-strand RNA viruses (Miller and Purcell 1990, Koonin 1991). There is also amino acid sequence similarity in part of NS3 to virus helicase polypeptides (Miller and Purcell 1990) (see 'Non-structural proteins', p. 723).

FEATURES OF HCV SHARED WITH PESTIVIRUSES

A fundamental aspect of genome organization that differs among members of the *Flaviviridae* is the structure of the 5′ and 3′ untranslated regions (UTRs). These parts of the genome are involved in replication (see section 1.4, p. 722) and in the initiation of translation of the virus genome by cellular ribosomes. There is evidence that both pestiviruses and HCV have a highly structured 5′UTR, in which internal base-pairing produces a complex set of stem–loop structures that are thought to interact with various host cell and virus proteins during replication and translation (Brown et al. 1992, Tsukiyama Kohara et al. 1992, Wang, Sarnow and Siddiqui 1994, Poole et al. 1995). In both viruses there is evidence for internal initiation of translation, in which binding to the host cell ribosome directs translation to an internal methionine (AUG) codon (see 'HCV translation', p. 722). This contrasts strongly with translation of flavivirus genomes which act much like cellular mRNAs, in which ribosomal binding occurs at the capped 5′ end of the RNA, followed by scanning of the sequence in the 5′ to 3′ direction with translation commencing at the first AUG codon.

Structurally, HCV is more like the pestiviruses than the flaviviruses, with a low buoyant density in sucrose (see 'Physicochemical properties', p. 721) similar to that reported for pestiviruses and attributable in both cases to extensively glycosylated proteins in the virus envelope. By contrast, flavivirus envelope glycoproteins contain few sites for N-linked glycosylation, and the virion itself is relatively dense (1.2 g/cm^3). Finally, the arrangement and number of cleavage sites of the HCV polyprotein are more like those of the pestiviruses, particularly in the cleavage of NS5 into 2 subunits, NS5b corresponding to the RNA polymerase.

RELATIONSHIP OF HCV TO NEWLY DISCOVERED HEPATITIS VIRUSES

Recently, 2 distinct RNA viruses have been discovered in the tamarin (*Sanguinis* spp.), a New World primate. This species had previously been shown to harbour an infectious agent causing chronic hepatitis after inoculation with plasma from a surgeon (initials GB) who had developed a chronic hepatitis of unknown aetiology (Simons et al. 1995b). Parts of the genome of 2 viruses isolated from infected tamarins (provisionally termed GBV-A and GBV-B) have measurable sequence similarity to certain regions of HCV. For example, a 200 amino acid sequence within NS3 of GBV-A and GBV-B shows 47% and 55% sequence identity similarity with the homologous region in HCV (positions 1298–1497 in the HCV polyprotein; Choo et al. 1991) and 43.5% identity to each other. Similarly in NS5,

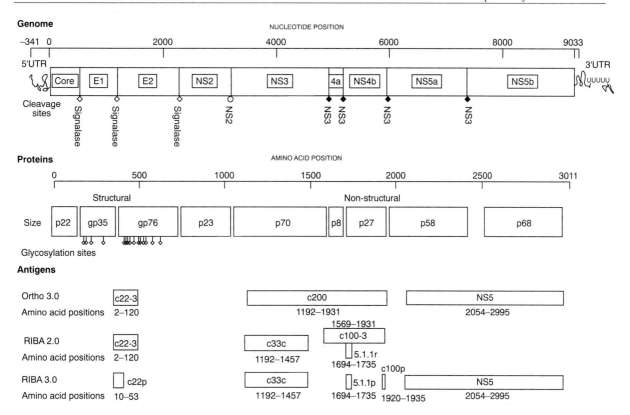

Fig. 35.1 Organization of HCV genome, showing polyprotein cleavage sites, the relative sizes of the encoded proteins and regions of the genome expressed as recombinant antigens for serological assays. Nucleotide and amino acid positions are numbered as in Choo et al. (1991). The properties and functions of the HCV proteins are summarized in Table 35.2.

the region around the active site of the RdRp (including the canonical GDD motif; positions 2662–2761 in HCV) shows 36% and 41% sequence identity, and 43% between GBV-A and B (Simons et al. 1995b). More recently there have been descriptions of additional viruses infecting humans that are closely related to GBV-A and which may be associated with chronic hepatitis: GBV-C (Simons et al. 1995a, Leary et al. 1996) and hepatitis G virus (Linnen et al. 1996).

The degree of relatedness between HCV and the GB agent and with other flaviviruses can be investigated using phylogenetic analysis of the RdRp. Analysis of a 100 amino acid sequence surrounding the GDD motif reveals a close relationship between HCV and GBV-A and GBV-B, whereas pestiviruses such as bovine viral diarrhoea virus (BVDV) and flaviviruses are more distinct (Fig. 35.2). Using such information and differences in genome organization, the International Committee on the Taxonomy of Viruses currently proposes to divide the *Flaviviridae* into three genera, the flaviviruses, the pestiviruses and the hepaciviruses, the last group consisting of HCV, with perhaps GBV-A and related viruses forming several subgenera within it.

1.3 Morphology and structure

PROPERTIES OF THE GENOME

The genome of HCV is single-stranded RNA of positive (protein coding) polarity. Although the genomic

RNA of most positive-strand RNA viruses is infectious, this has not yet been unequivocally demonstrated for HCV. Around 96% of the HCV genome codes for virus proteins (9033 of 9397 bases of the HCV-PT genome; Choo et al. 1991), with non-coding regions at both the 5′ and the 3′ end. The 5′UTR is 341–344 bases long, but it is not known whether the bases at this end of the RNA molecule are modified, for example by capping with a methyl[7]guanosine residue as in flaviviruses and in eukaryotic mRNAs. There is no evidence that the HCV genome encodes a homologue of the Vpg protein of picornaviruses that initiates transcription from a poly(U) primer.

Most published HCV sequences contain a relatively short 3′ untranslated region, typically containing 25–30 nucleotides and followed by a variable number of uridine residues. This homopolymeric tail was originally considered to represent the end of the genome, but recent evidence suggests that a 90 base sequence occurs beyond these residues (T Tanaka et al. 1995) and may form a stable, internally base-paired stem–loop structure, which may be involved in initiation of RNA transcription. Similarly, for GBV-B, the 3′ terminal poly(U) stretch is followed by a sequence of 49 nucleotides. Both the pestiviruses and the flaviviruses lack a poly(U) tract and have 3′UTR sequences that are longer than that of HCV (261 and 511 bases for BVDV and YFV, respectively; Rice et al. 1985, Collett et al. 1988).

Table 35.1 Comparison of the genome organization of HCV with other positive-stranded RNA viruses

Family	Genus	Example	Genome size	RNA modifications	Structural proteins	Non-structural proteins	Enveloped	Protease	Translation initiation
Picornaviridae	Enterovirus	Polio	7433	5': VpG, 3': poly(A)	VP1–VP4 (nucleocapsid)	2A–2C, 3A–3D	No	Viral: 2A, 3C	IRES element
	Hepadnavirus	Hepatitis A	7478	5': VpG 3': poly(A)	VP1–VP4	2A–2C, 3A–3D	No	Viral: 2A, 3C	IRES element
Flaviviridae	*Flavivirus*	Yellow fever	10862	5': capped 3': no poly(A)	Core, matrix, E1	NS1–NS5	Yes, E1	Host: signalase Viral: NS3	Ribosomal scanning
	Pestivirus	Bovine viral diarrhoea	12480	5': uncapped 3': no poly(A)	Core, gp48 gp25, gp53	p54, p80, p10 (38K), p54, p75	Yes, gp48 gp25, gp53	Host: signalase Viral: p54, p80	IRES element
	Hepacivirus	Hepatitis C	9379	5': uncapped 3': poly (U)/(A)	Core, E1, E2	NS2, 3, 4a, 4b NS5a, 5b	Yes, E1, E2	Host: signalase Viral: NS2, NS3	IRES element
		GB virus-B	9143	(5': uncapped) 3': poly(U)	(Core, E1 E2)	(NS2, 3, 4a, 4b NS5a, 5b)	(Yes, E1, E2)	(NS3)	(IRES element)

Information for GBV-B in parentheses inferred from sequence comparison with HCV (Muerhoff et al. 1995).

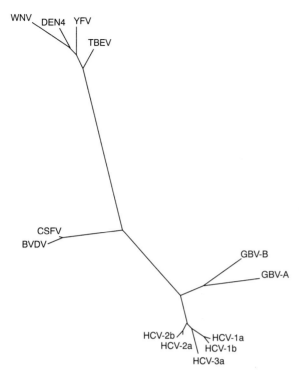

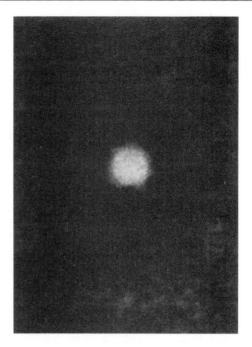

Fig. 35.3 Visualization of an isolated virus particle of HCV by surface staining using 2% phosphotungstic acid, pH 6.5 (Kaito et al. 1994). Fine spike-like projections can be seen around the edge of the virus particle of measured diameter of c. 60 nm. × 200 000 (Courtesy of M Kaito and S Watanabe.)

Fig. 35.2 Phylogenetic analysis of amino acid sequences of the region of NS5b encoding the RdRp (positions 2662-2761 in HCV-1) (Choo et al. 1991). HCV was compared with homologous sequences from flaviviruses (DEN4, dengue virus, serotype 4; TBEV, tick-borne encephalitis virus; WNV, West Nile virus; YFV, yellow fever virus), pestiviruses (BVDV, bovine viral diarrhoea virus (Collett et al. 1988); CSFV, classic swine fever virus [GenBank accession number X87939]) and GB viruses (GBV-A, GBV-B [GenBank accession numbers U22303 and U22304]) using optimized alignment described previously (Koonin 1991). Phylogenetic analysis was carried out using the programs PROTDIST, NEIGHBOR and DRAWTREE in the PHYLIP package (Felsenstein 1993).

MORPHOLOGY

HCV is difficult to visualize by electron microscopy. Recently, negative staining of HCV purified from a high titre plasma revealed virus-like particles of 55–65 nm in diameter (Fig. 35.3). Although this and other studies do not provide a detailed image of internal structures, by analogy with other viruses it is likely that HCV has an internal nucleocapsid containing the RNA genome, closely surrounded by a lipid envelope containing the E1 and E2 glycoproteins.

In appearance and size they closely resemble pestiviruses (Stott, Almeida and O'Reilly 1974), particularly in the 6 nm spike-like projections from the virion surface that may correspond to the envelope glycoproteins. The envelope glycoproteins of HCV show several potential sites for N-linked glycosylation (4 sites in E1, 11 sites in E2) (see Fig. 35.1) and it is likely that the addition of relatively large carbohydrate groups is a major structural feature of the virus surface that may influence the ability of antibody to neutralize infectivity.

PHYSICOCHEMICAL PROPERTIES

At present, the density of HCV cannot be measured accurately because in plasma (currently the only source of HCV) it associates to a variable extent with β-lipoprotein that reduces its density (Bradley et al. 1991, Thomssen et al. 1992), and also with antibody that increases its density (Hijikata et al. 1993b). Measurements of the density of HCV in anti-HCV-positive samples range from 1.03 to 1.14 g/cm³, although a second peak can be detected with a density of around 1.20–1.25 g/cm³, representing immune complexed virus (Bradley et al. 1991, Carrick et al. 1992, Miyamoto et al. 1992, Hijikata et al. 1993b). For comparison, pestivirus virions derived from cell culture show a density of 1.11 g/cm³ (Stott, Almeida and O'Reilly 1974) whereas that of flaviviruses is greater (c. 1.20 g/cm³).

HCV is inactivated by exposure to chloroform, ether and other organic solvents and by detergents. The effects of heat and other inactivating procedures have been discovered by studies of the infectivity of products manufactured from plasma such as the factor VIII and IX concentrates used to treat clotting disorders. For example, dry heat treatment at 80°C or wet-heat treatment at 60°C, organic solvents (*n*-heptane) and detergents efficiently remove infectivity for HCV in recipients (Mannucci 1993).

1.4 Replication of HCV

CULTURE OF HCV IN VITRO

Despite considerable efforts, very little progress has yet been made toward the development of a system for the culture of HCV in vitro. HCV does not produce obvious cytopathology, and the amounts of HCV released from cells infected in vitro are often low (Shimizu et al. 1992, Shimizu, Purcell and Yoshikura 1993, Carloni et al. 1993, Shimizu and Yoshikura 1994, Kato et al. 1995). This might be because the cells used for culture are not representative of those infected in vivo, or because productive infection requires a combination of cytokines and growth factors found in the liver that is not reproduced in cell culture. Low levels of HCV replication have been detected in lymphocytes in vitro (Shimizu et al. 1992, Kato et al. 1995).

Transfection of full length DNA sequences of the HCV genome might be expected to initiate the full replicative cycle of HCV, as it does when similar experiments are carried out with picornavirus sequences. However, only a very low level of expression of virus proteins was observed when a complete HCV sequence was transfected into a transformed hepatocyte (hepatoma) cell line (Huh7). These experiments used a clone of HCV that lacked the 90 bases 3′ to the poly(U) sequence (T Tanaka et al. 1995) that are probably essential for transcription initiation on the positive strand. Despite this, there was evidence for replication of the HCV genome and for the production of low numbers of progeny virus particles (Yoo et al. 1995). Such models will provide an important experimental system for the investigation of HCV replication in the future.

TRANSCRIPTION OF THE HCV GENOME

In common with other positive-strand RNA viruses, HCV is presumed to replicate its RNA genome through the production of a minus-strand replication intermediate, i.e. an RNA copy of the complete genome that is synthesized by the activity of a virus-encoded RdRp (NS5b; Table 35.2). The minus-strand copy would then become the template for the generation of positive-strand copies. Because the RNA template can be transcribed several times, many minus-strand copies could be copied from the infecting positive strand, and each of these transcripts used several times to produce positive-strand progeny sequences. In this way, a single input sequence could be amplified several thousand-fold during the course of replication within a cell.

Using a highly strand-specific PCR method, antisense HCV RNA sequences have been detected in the liver of HCV-infected individuals, confirming the presumed method of replication of HCV via a replication intermediate (Lanford et al. 1994). Although initiation of transcription is well understood for some positive-strand RNA viruses (such as the *Picornaviridae*), there is currently no information on how RNA synthesis of HCV or other flaviviruses may be primed.

HCV TRANSLATION

The 5′UTR is thought to play a major role in the initiation and regulation of translation of the large open reading frame of HCV. The region is 341–344 bases in length, and a combination of computer analysis, nuclease mapping experiments and studies of covariance allows the secondary structure to be predicted (Tsukiyama Kohara et al. 1992, Smith et al. 1995, Wang et al. 1995). A remarkably similar structure has been predicted for pestiviruses (Brown et al. 1992, Wang et al. 1995) despite the virtual absence of nucleotide sequence similarities with HCV, indicating the importance of the higher order structure of this region in interactions with viral and cellular proteins or other RNA sequences.

Evidence that the 5′UTR can direct the internal initiation of translation has been obtained by translation in vitro of reporter genes downstream from the 5′UTR sequence placed in mono- or dicistronic vectors (Wang, Sarnow and Siddiqui 1993, 1994, Fukushi et al. 1994). The internal ribosomal entry site (IRES) activity of the 5′UTR is consistent with the hypothesis that translation is initiated from the AUG methionine codon at position 341. There is no evidence for translation from any of the variable number of AUG triplets upstream from this site, although it was originally proposed that the production of the very small proteins from these upstream potential open reading frames (ORFs) played some role in regulating expression of the large ORFs (Yoo et al. 1992).

VIRUS ENTRY, UNCOATING, ASSEMBLY AND RELEASE

There is currently little or no information available on the nature of the cellular receptor for HCV, nor about the process by which HCV enters the cell. Once within the cell, replication has been observed to occur in the cytoplasm while assembly occurs in association with internal membranes of the rough endoplasmic reticulum and Golgi compartment. Steps in the assembly and release of HCV from the cell are unknown, although it is likely that the mature virus particle is formed by budding of the assembled nucleocapsid through the lipid membrane of the cell into which the E1 and E2 glycoproteins have inserted. Whether budding occurs through internal membranes or on the cell surface is not known.

1.5 Proteins of HCV

The genome of HCV is thought to encode at least 9 proteins, of which 3 are structural (core, E1 and E2) and 6 non-structural (NS2, NS3, NS4a, NS4b, NS5a and NS5b) (see Fig. 35.1 and Table 35.2). Most information about the function and enzymatic activities of the non-structural proteins has been obtained by expression of DNA sequences corresponding to the different proteins, and by direct observations of the cellular distributions and properties of HCV proteins detected in liver or plasma in vivo.

Table 35.2 Properties of HCV proteins

Protein	Nucleotide position[a]	Size[b]	Virion	Antigen[c]	Function
Core	1–573	191	Yes	c22–3	Thought to form the virus nucleocapsid, and shows RNA-binding activity. Highly conserved between HCV genotypes
E1	574–1149	192	Yes	...	Sequence predicts a membrane anchored glycoprotein, with several potential N-linked glycosylation sites. Highly variable between genotypes
E2/NS1	1150–2187	327 (?)	Yes (?)	...	Another membrane-bound glycoprotein, with prominent 'hypervariable' region. The homologue in pestiviruses is a virion component, but is non-structural in flaviviruses
NS2	2431–3078	316	No	...	Proteinase (Zn^{2+}-dependent)
NS3	3079–4971	631	No	c33c	Multi-functional protein with protease activity, and with sequence motifs suggesting a helicase activity
NS4a	4972–5133	54	No	c100–3	Co-factor for NS3 protease
NS4b	5134–5916	261	No	...	Unknown
NS5a	5917–7260	448	No	NS5	Unknown
NS5b	7261–9033	591	No	...	RNA-dependent RNA polymerase necessary for genome replication

[a] Amino acid positions numbered as in Choo et al. (1991).
[b] Size expressed in number of amino acid residues.
[c] Origin of HCV antigens used in current 2nd and 3rd generation assays for antibody to HCV (see Fig. 35.1).

STRUCTURAL PROTEINS

The structural proteins of HCV are encoded by sequences at the 5′ end of the genome and so are translated first (see Fig. 35.1; Table 35.2). Expression of this part of the genome in cells (Grakoui et al. 1993c, Ralston et al. 1993, Selby et al. 1993) or in reticulocyte lysate containing microsomal membranes (Hijikata et al. 1991b, Santolini et al. 1994) leads to the synthesis of a polyprotein followed by proteolytic cleavage into the core, E1 and E2 proteins. Cleavage between the capsid protein and E1, E1 and E2, and E2 and NS2 depends on the addition of microsomal membranes, implying the role of the host cell signalase in these processing steps. The capsid protein has a size of 21–22 kDa and contains several basic (positively charged) amino acids at its amino terminus that may confer RNA-binding properties required for encapsidation of HCV RNA during virus assembly. It is not known how core proteins bind together to form the HCV nucleocapsid.

The envelope proteins of HCV (E1, E2) are synthesized in mammalian cells as proteins with sizes ranging from 31 to 35 kDa and 68 to 72 kDa respectively (Hijikata et al. 1991b, Grakoui et al. 1993c, Ralston et al. 1993, Selby et al. 1993, Santolini et al. 1994). The sizes of E1 and E2 are greater than could be accounted for by their amino acid sequences alone, which supports biochemical evidence for extensive glycosylation of both proteins after translation. Both E1 and E2 have a large number of potential N-linked glycosylation sites, although the details of which sites are used, the extent to which the glycoprotein moieties are modified, and whether there is also O-linked glycosylation awaits further biochemical analysis. Two microsome-dependent cleavage sites between E2 and NS2 have been identified (Mizushima et al. 1994), by which E2 may be produced in 2 forms differing in size by 80 amino acid residues and possibly a cleavage product, p9 (Selby et al. 1994).

Evidence for interactions between E1 and E2 has been obtained by immunoprecipitation experiments, in which antibody to E1 or E2 could precipitate both proteins under non-denaturing conditions (Grakoui et al. 1993c, Ralston et al. 1993, Dubuisson et al. 1994). The nature or the significance of this association is unclear, although it is possible that this association leads to heterodimeric structures in the virus envelope. Current evidence suggests that the association is predominantly non-covalent (Dubuisson et al. 1994) and does not occur simply though hydrophobic interactions between the membrane anchors of the 2 proteins (Matsuura et al. 1994, Selby et al. 1994). The envelope proteins probably form the principal target of antibody-mediated neutralization of virus infectivity, although this cannot be demonstrated experimentally at present. Rapid sequence change at the amino terminus of E2 has been proposed to contribute to the ability of HCV to establish persistent infection in humans (see 'Mechanism of persistence', p. 729).

NON-STRUCTURAL PROTEINS

Translation in vitro of the rest of the genome leads to the production of proteins of sizes 23, 70–72, 4, 27, 56–58 and 66 kDa, corresponding to NS2, NS3, NS4a, NS4b, NS5a and NS5b respectively (see Fig. 35.1 and

Table 35.2). Proteolytic cleavage pathways that generate the non-structural proteins are mediated by NS2 and NS3 (Hijikata et al. 1993a), and have been studied extensively by several groups as possible targets of antiviral treatment. NS3 is a serine protease that catalyses cleavage reactions between NS3/NS4a, NS4a/NS4b, NS4b/NS5a and NS5a/NS5b (Bartenschlager et al. 1993, Eckart et al. 1993, Grakoui et al. 1993a, Hijikata et al. 1993a, Tomei et al. 1993). NS2 is a metalloproteinase that cleaves the NS2/NS3 junction (Grakoui et al. 1993b, Hijikata et al. 1993a). Both the NS3/NS4a cleavage reaction mediated by NS3 and the NS2/NS3 cleavage by NS2 occur in *cis*, while other reactions can occur through intermolecular associations between NS3 and the rest of the polyprotein.

Accounts of the complex sequence of events and the interactions between non-structural proteins involved in cleavage reactions differ in detail depending on the experimental methods used. However, there is evidence that cleavage may be a sequential process, and that it is modulated by the activities of other proteins such as NS4a. The NS2 protease activity is zinc-dependent and contains an active site that is dependent on residues in NS3. Therefore following the *cis* cleavage of the NS2/NS3 junction, the protease is inactivated, and will not act in *trans* on other substrates. It has recently been shown that cleavage at NS2/NS3 is essential for activation of the NS3 protease. It is possible that natural variation in the efficiency of reaction may serve to modulate the pathogenicity of HCV in vivo (Lin et al. 1994).

NS3 when released cleaves other sites with varying efficiency. The active site of NS3 has been mapped by deletion experiments to lie at the amino terminus of the protein (residues 1409–1215) (Tanji et al. 1994). The substrate specificity of the serine protease activity has been defined by sequence comparisons and by mutagenesis experiments (Kolykhalov, Agapov and Rice 1994, Komoda et al. 1994, Leinbach et al. 1994, Bartenschlager et al. 1995), and generally conforms to the consensus sequence $D/E(X_4)C/T{\downarrow}S/A$ in the target protein. There is some evidence for a less stringent requirement for specific amino acids around the *cis* cleavage site (NS3/NS4a) than those cleaved in *trans* (Bartenschlager et al. 1995). Several investigators have described the requirement for other protein cofactors for the activity of NS3. In particular, it appears that binding of NS4a to NS3 (Failla, Tomei and Defrancesco 1995, Tanji et al. 1995) is necessary at least for the cleavage of NS4b/NS5a, and may modulate activity of NS3 in other ways.

As well as acting as a protease, NS3 contains sequence motifs that are found in helicase enzymes. Helicases displace base-paired RNA or DNA sequences from a template strand, usually in a 3′ to 5′ direction. This process requires the presence of Mg^{2+} ions and energy provided by hydrolysis of ATP by an NTPase activity of the enzyme. An assay in vitro has demonstrated a combined helicase/NTPase activity in the NS3 homologue of pestiviruses (p80) (Warrener and Collett 1995). NS3 is probably essential for the replication of HCV RNA, because repeated copying of RNA templates requires that the previously synthesized strand is displaced by an unwinding activity acting immediately downstream of the RNA polymerase.

The NS5b protein has sequence similarities to RdRp of other positive-strand viruses (see section 1.2, p. 718). Recently, RNA polymerase activity was detected by expression of this protein in vitro and using a variety of artificial RNA templates (Bartholomeusz et al. 1995, Chung,

Kawashima and Kaplan 1995). Such methods will provide the means to investigate the mechanism of initiation of replication at the termini of the HCV genome and its dependence on the complex secondary structures found in the 5′ and 3′UTRs, and will allow the testing of polymerase inhibitors that might be developed as antiviral agents.

The functions of NS4b and NS5a are unknown, both for HCV and for their homologues in pestiviruses. It has been suggested that NS5a contains an interferon response element, on the basis that the presence of certain amino acid residues between positions 2209 and 2248 has been reported to correlate with the likelihood of responding to interferon treatment (Enomoto et al. 1995). The mechanism for this is currently unknown.

1.6 Classification of HCV into genotypes

Nucleotide sequence variation

The first indication of the genetic heterogeneity of HCV came from comparisons of nucleotide sequences of HCV variants from Japan with that of the prototype HCV variant obtained from the USA, HCV-PT (Choo et al. 1991). For example, the complete genome sequences of HCV-J (Kato et al. 1990) and HCV-BK (Takamizawa et al. 1991) from Japan showed 92% similarity to each other but only 79% with HCV-PT. At that time, the former were referred to as the 'Japanese' type (or type II), and those from the USA (HCV-PT and HCV-H) were classified as type I. However, far more divergent variants of HCV have since been found in Japan (Okamoto et al. 1991, 1992b) and elsewhere (Chan et al. 1992, Mori et al. 1992), leading to the adoption of an extended classification of HCV into types and subtypes.

Phylogenetic analysis of a 222 base fragment of NS5b from a series of HCV-infected individuals in Europe, North and South America and the Far East showed HCV to be structured into 6 approximately equally divergent groups of sequences, many of which were comprised of more closely related groups (Fig. 35.4). Similar relationships exist between variants if analysis is carried out in E1 (Bukh, Purcell and Miller 1993), NS4 (Bhattacherjee et al. 1995) or core regions (Bukh, Purcell and Miller 1994), and it currently seems that the sequences of any of these genes could be used for classification into genotypes.

Nomenclature of HCV genotypes

A current proposal for the nomenclature of HCV genotypes is to divide HCV into types, corresponding to the main branches in the phylogenetic tree, and subtypes corresponding to the more closely related sequences within some of the major groups (Enomoto et al. 1990, Simmonds et al. 1993a, 1994). The types have been numbered 1 to 6, and the subtypes a, b and c, in both cases in order of discovery. Therefore, the sequence cloned by Choo (1989) is assigned type 1a, HCV-J and BK are 1b, HC-J6 is type 2a and HC-J8 is 2b.

The distinction between type and subtype was originally made on the basis of phylogenetic analysis, where 2 levels of branching were found on analysis of NS5b, NS3 and core sequences (Enomoto et al. 1990, Chan et al. 1992). For genotypes 1–6 the sets of

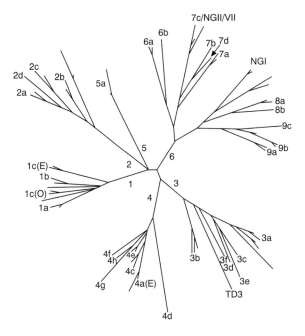

Fig. 35.4 Phylogenetic analysis of nucleotide sequences from part of the HCV NS5b region amplified from samples of HCV-infected blood donors and hepatitis patients from several countries. Six main groups of sequence variants are found corresponding to types 1–6; each group contains a number of more closely related subtypes (a, b, c...). Nomenclature of types 1–5 and 6a follows the consensus proposal for classification of HCV (Simmonds et al. 1994). Recently discovered variants from southeast Asia cluster with type 6a but are labelled according to the original publications (Tokita et al. 1994, Mellor et al. 1995, Sugiyama et al. 1995, Tokita et al. 1995) (see text, p. 725 and p. 733). TD3 is currently unclassified. See Mellor et al. (1995) for a more detailed discussion of current issues in HCV classification.

sequence distances between sequences of the same subtype, between different subtypes and finally between different major genotypes form three non-overlapping ranges. For example, sequence divergences of the 222 base fragment in NS5b between members of the same subtype range from 0 to 12%, between subtypes from 12% to 22% and between types from 28% to 44% (Simmonds et al. 1993a). Similar non-overlapping ranges can be computed for other regions of the genome, although their degree of variability affects the values observed. For example, the ranges for the 3 categories are slightly larger for E1 (Bukh et al. 1993, Stuyver et al. 1994) and smaller (and partially overlapping between type and subtype) for the core region (Bukh, Purcell and Miller 1994, Mellor et al. 1995). Since the original classification of HCV into 6 major genotypes, sequence comparisons of HCV obtained from a much wider range of geographic locations has provided evidence for the existence of an extremely large number of variants (Fig. 35.4). The majority of new variants can be classified as further subtypes of the 6 major HCV genotypes by the criteria described above. However, there is currently considerable discussion about how to classify

variants from southeast Asia (Thailand, Vietnam and Burma) that group with type 6a by phylogenetic analysis but which are more divergent from each other than subtypes of other genotypes.

VIROLOGICAL DIFFERENCES BETWEEN GENOTYPES

Despite the sequence diversity found among variants of HCV, there are few differences in overall genome organization between genotypes. For example, the genomes of HCV types 1, 2 and 3 are very similar in size and all genes are co-linear with few insertions or deletions. On current evidence there is no reason why there could not be extensive complementation of replicative functions and packaging if a cell were multiply infected by different genotypes of HCV. Similarly, a recombinant virus formed between 2 genotypes may be functionally equivalent to the parental genotypes, as seems to be the case for variants of other RNA viruses that show similar levels of heterogeneity as HCV (e.g. poliovirus serotypes 1, 2 and 3). However, to date there is no evidence for recombination between different HCV types.

Although the proteins of HCV may be functionally equivalent, the extensive amino acid sequence variability found in both structural and non-structural proteins would be expected to modify profoundly immunological recognition by both antibody and T cell receptors. For example, the envelope proteins of genotypes differ from each other in amino acid sequence by 34–40% and 26–29% for E1 and E2, similar to that between different serotypes of dengue fever virus (26–40%). For dengue, this degree of sequence variability is sufficient to prevent neutralization of one subtype by antibody elicited by a heterologous serotype. The absence of a suitable culture system in vitro for HCV prevents such genotype-specific differences in neutralization being investigated experimentally. However, there is clear evidence for antigenic differences between recombinant proteins or peptides from different genotypes in enzyme-linked immunosorbent assays (McOmish et al. 1993, Simmonds et al. 1993c, Tsukiyama Kohara et al. 1993, Mondelli et al. 1994). Antigenic differences between genotypes have implications for the development of vaccines for HCV and for the optimal design of serological screening and confirmatory assays for HCV (see section 2.3, p. 734).

HCV GENOTYPING ASSAYS

Although nucleotide sequence analysis is the most reliable method for identifying different genotypes of HCV, it is not practical for large clinical studies. Many of the published methods for 'genotyping' are based upon PCR amplification of virus sequences in clinical specimens, using type-specific primers that selectively amplify different genotypes (Okamoto et al. 1992c, Okamoto et al. 1993) or by analysis of the PCR product by hybridization with genotype-specific probes (Stuyver et al. 1993, Tisminetzky et al. 1994) or through restriction fragment length polymorphisms (McOmish et al. 1993, Davidson et al. 1995).

Serological typing methods are based on the detection of type-specific antibody to epitopes of HCV that differ between genotypes (see 'Virological differences between genotypes', p. 725, and 'Antigens', p. 734). They have advantages over PCR-based methods in terms of speed and simplicity of sample preparation and in the use of simple equipment that is found in any diagnostic virology laboratory. By careful optimization of reagents, such assays may show high sensitivity and reproducibility. For example, type-specific antibody to NS4 peptides of genotypes 1–6 can be detected in c. 85–90% of NANB patients (Bhattacherjee et al. 1995). However, antigenic similarity currently precludes the separate identification of subtypes such as 1a and 1b or 2a and 2b using the NS4 peptides alone.

A crucial assumption of all genotyping assays is that the region analysed (5'UTR, core, NS4, NS5b) is representative of the genome as a whole. This assumption would break down if recombination between HCV genotypes occurred during virus replication, so producing hybrid viruses containing contributions from different genotypes in different parts of the genome. So far, remarkably consistent results have been obtained by comparing results of genotyping assays based on sequence analysis of different regions of the genome, and between PCR-based and serological typing assays (Simmonds et al. 1993c, Tanaka et al. 1994, Bhattacherjee et al. 1995, Lau et al. 1995). These findings suggest that genotyping is a valid procedure despite the theoretical possibility of recombination. Many assays can reliably identify infection with those HCV genotypes likely to be encountered in clinical practice in the western world (1a, 1b, 2a, 2b and 3a).

2 CLINICAL AND PATHOLOGICAL ASPECTS

2.1 Clinical and pathological features of HCV infection

Hepatitis C infection causes an indolent and slowly progressive liver disease that is asymptomatic until the development of decompensated liver disease and, often, liver cancer. The following sections review the clinical and pathological features associated with acute and chronic hepatitis, the replication of HCV in liver and possibly at extrahepatic sites, and describes proposed mechanisms of liver damage and of persistence.

ACUTE HEPATITIS

Percutaneous exposure to HCV usually results in an asymptomatic infection (not associated with jaundice), and most people become chronic carriers of the virus (Fig. 35.5). This contrasts strongly with the observation that few adults infected with hepatitis B virus (HBV) become chronically infected. The period from exposure to the development of hepatitis has been measured in a number of investigations of post-transfusional hepatitis. Most studies have reported an interval of about 8 weeks to the development of abnormal liver function tests (such as alanine aminotransferase

(ALT) levels), although viraemia can be detected earlier (Fig. 35.5).

Only 5% of individuals with acute HCV infection have symptomatic disease, although in some cases it may be severe. HCV is very rarely associated with acute fulminant hepatic failure (TL Wright et al. 1991, Mutimer et al. 1995a). Clinically, hepatitis caused by HCV is indistinguishable from that caused by other hepatitis viruses; jaundice may develop, but more usually symptoms are non-specific such as fatigue, anorexia and nausea. Most HCV-infected individuals cannot recall a history of jaundice, and HCV accounts for a small proportion of clinically apparent hepatitis cases in the community.

Viraemia can be detected by PCR in the early stages of acute hepatitis, appearing at the same time or slightly earlier than abnormal levels of ALT (Fig. 35.6). In contrast, seroconversion for antibody may be delayed for several weeks or months after the onset of hepatitis (Lelie et al. 1992), although second and third generation assays have closed this 'window' period to some extent (see p. 734 and p. 735). Nevertheless, reliable identification of HCV as a cause of acute hepatitis depends on the use of PCR, in contrast to acute HAV infection where IgM is generally detectable at the onset of clinical hepatitis. Histological features of acute HCV are similar to those associated with acute HAV and HBV infection; liver biopsy is rarely indicated to make a diagnosis of acute HCV infection.

CHRONIC HEPATITIS

The frequency of chronic infection following exposure to HCV is high, although there are difficulties in estimating a precise figure. For example, HCV may be identified more frequently in those with symp-

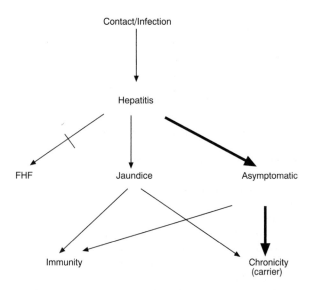

Fig. 35.5 Outcome of infection with HCV. Hepatitis can be detected by blood tests c. 2 months after exposure to HCV. Most infections are asymptomatic, and a few patients develop jaundice. At least 80% of infected patients have persistent infection, i.e. they become HCV carriers. Fulminant hepatic failure (FHF) is an extremely rare consequence of HCV infection.

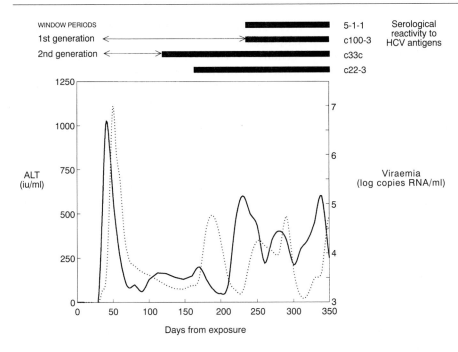

Fig. 35.6 Virological and biochemical markers of acute HCV infection. HCV RNA (solid line) and abnormal ALT levels (dotted line) appear c. 50 days after exposure to HCV in a typical individual. The subsequent development of chronic hepatitis is indicated by persistent viraemia and by fluctuating abnormal ALT levels. Antibody to HCV first appears after the onset of acute hepatitis, in this example leading to 'window periods' of c. 200 days for the first generation serological assay (containing only c100-3 as antigen) and c. 65 days for a second generation assay. The antibody profile elicited by infection is highly variable between individuals, although antibody to c33c is normally the first to appear.

tomatic primary infection or those with post-transfusion hepatitis (Kiyosawa et al. 1990, Gilletterver et al. 1995), both of which may be associated with an increased likelihood of chronic infection (Gordon et al. 1993, Mutimer et al. 1995b).

Individuals infected through blood transfusion and haemophiliacs, many of whom have been repeatedly exposed to HCV through the use of non-virally inactivated clotting factor concentrates, have a high rate of persistent infection associated with active liver disease (60–80%). In contrast, lower rates of chronic infection and more slowly progressive disease are observed in individuals with lesser exposure to HCV. For example, only 50% of women exposed to a particular batch of anti-D immunoglobulin had persistent infection (Meisel et al. 1995), whereas in a similar outbreak in Ireland, also associated with the use of anti-D (Power et al. 1994), viraemia was detected by PCR in only 50% of people remaining seropositive 17 years after exposure. Given the tendency for antibody to become undetectable following clearance of viraemia, the true frequency of persistent infection in these 2 cohorts may be even lower.

Persistent infection with HCV is generally associated with persistent and progressive hepatitis. Chronically infected individuals generally have fluctuating or continuously abnormal levels of ALT and are viraemic. However, it has been difficult to establish a correlation between the level of viraemia and the severity of liver disease. For example, HCV RNA levels in asymptomatic blood donors are similar to those found in patients treated for liver disease (Lau et al. 1995, Smith et al. 1996). Moreover, several studies have failed to document any association between the degree of viraemia and level of ALT or other biochemical abnormalities associated with hepatitis.

HISTOLOGICAL FEATURES

HCV infection causes a range of characteristic histological changes in the liver, although none allows a specific diagnosis of HCV infection to be made. The most striking feature of HCV infection of the liver is the presence of lymphoid follicles within the portal tracts (Fig. 35.7); these are rarely observed in hepatitis from other viral causes. Biopsies also typically reveal a dense periportal inflammatory process, associated with the infiltration of lymphocytes and plasma cells. Bile duct damage is often found in association with the infiltration, with vacuolization and ballooning of epithelial cells lining small bile ducts. Another common observation is the appearance of lobular hepatitis, with lymphocyte infiltration within sinusoids surrounding the hepatocytes.

The extent of histological abnormalities within biopsies is normally summarized by descriptions such as lobular, chronic persistent hepatitis (CPH) and chronic active hepatitis (CAH), with or without cirrhosis, although more informative scoring systems such as the Knodell score have also been devised (Knodell et al. 1981). Cross-sectional studies of patients with chronic hepatitis C typically show c. 40% with CPH or lobular hepatitis, 40% with CAH while the remainder have CAH and cirrhosis. A spectrum of milder disease is generally observed in studies of asymptomatic individuals, such as those identified by blood donor screening, possibly reflecting a shorter duration of infection.

Virus-induced cytopathic changes in cells of the

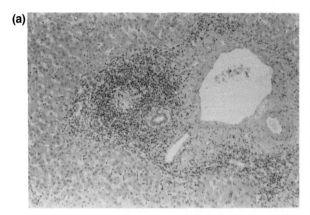

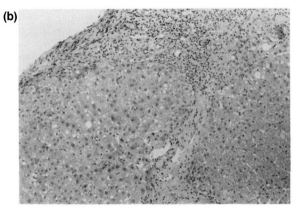

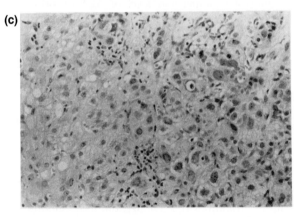

Fig. 35.7 Typical histopathological feature of HCV infection of the liver. (a) Typical HCV hepatitis with a large lymphoid aggregate within a portal tract showing reactive germinal centre formation. Although the aggregate is close to a bile duct and adjacent to the limiting plate of the tract, there is little evidence of bile duct damage and none of interface hepatitis (piecemeal necrosis). Plasma cells and macrophages are also commonly present. (b) Cirrhosis. This is characterized by coarse fibrous septa separating nodules of regenerating hepatocytes. (c) Hepatocellular carcinoma. Tumour cells (right) are pleomorphic and hyperchromatic adjacent to regenerating hepatocytes in a cirrhotic nodule. There is a patchy chronic inflammatory infiltrate at the interface between them. (Sections kindly provided by Dr D J Harrison, Department of Pathology, University of Edinburgh.)

liver cannot be directly observed. Recently, methods have been developed for the in situ detection in liver sections of HCV antigens by antisera and RNA sequences by hybridization. HCV proteins and RNA have a cytoplasmic distribution within infected hepatocytes, consistent with their presumed method of replication. Although results from different studies have occasionally produced conflicting results, it has been consistently observed that only a small number of hepatocytes (1%) are productively infected with HCV, while there is little evidence of infection of cells in the biliary epithelium (reviewed in Lau et al. 1996). There is generally no correlation between HCV infection and areas of observable liver damage. Conversely, inflammatory infiltration may occur in areas of the liver without evidence of HCV infection.

PROGRESSION OF DISEASE

The percentage of chronically infected individuals who progress to cirrhosis and liver failure is not known. Progression to clinically significant liver damage is almost invariably very slow, although it may be faster in the context of immunosuppression. Particularly aggressive liver disease associated with HCV has been observed in immunosuppressed recipients of organ transplants and in patients with inherited immunodeficiency states (Healey et al. 1994). Studies of post-transfusion HCV highlight the following important clinical features. Many transfusion recipients are elderly (often suffering significant non-hepatic diseases) and die within 2 decades of infection but not as a consequence of HCV infection. HCV-related mortality is rare within 20 years of infection; in one study, no excess mortality of HCV-infected individuals was observed over a period of 17 years (Fig. 35.8) (Seef, Buskell-Bales and Wright 1992). Cirrhosis is rarely observed within 10 years of infection, and as few as 20% of infected patients have cirrhosis after 20 years' follow-up. Cirrhosis may be complicated by hepatocellular carcinoma, but this rarely develops within 15 years of HCV infection (see 'Hepatocellular carcinoma', p. 729). Some patients have asymptomatic infection, with normal liver function tests and mild hepatitis, despite 30 years of infection.

HCV may be associated with more aggressive liver disease in older than in younger people. Prognosis may also depend on viral genotype, although this is interrelated with other factors such as age at acquisition. For example, most transfusion recipients are elderly, and HCV genotype 1b is most commonly isolated from the serum of patients with transfusion-associated infection (Mahaney et al. 1994). Although it is not possible to estimate long-term prognosis at the time of infection, it is more feasible for patients with a known long duration of infection. For instance, when a 30 year old patient has cirrhosis within 10 years of infection, there is a high likelihood that liver failure will eventually develop. However, for a 70 year old patient with mild hepatitis despite 30 years' duration of infection, HCV is unlikely to cause death. Assessment of prognosis is an important aspect of selecting patients for treatment.

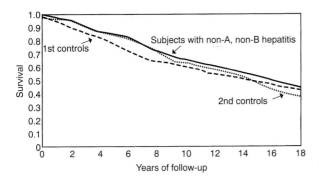

Fig. 35.8 Mortality associated with chronic post-transfusion hepatitis. The authors studied patients with transfusion-related non-A, non-B hepatitis (principally hepatitis C) who had been identified in 5 major prospective studies conducted in the USA between 1967 and 1980. Each index case was matched with 2 groups of non-infected transfusion recipients (1st and 2nd), and mortality rates from all causes were determined during an average follow-up of 18 years. Mortality from all causes was high (about 50% in all groups), and the survival curves for the 3 groups were the same (reproduced from Seef et al. 1992). Death from liver disease was low in all 3 groups, but was significantly higher in those originally given a diagnosis of non-A, non-B hepatitis (data not shown).

After many years, liver failure may develop in patients with cirrhosis (also known as decompensated cirrhosis). Decompensation may be manifest as hepatic encephalopathy, variceal haemorrhage or ascites. Clinical manifestations of liver failure are not specific for HCV-induced liver disease but are common to all forms of cirrhosis. Hepatocellular carcinoma may develop in an HCV-infected liver, but is very rarely observed in the absence of cirrhosis (see below).

In summary, most HCV infection is asymptomatic; when symptoms do develop, they are the non-specific symptoms of liver failure.

HEPATOCELLULAR CARCINOMA

Hepatocellular carcinoma (HCC) is a frequent complication of long-standing HCV infection. In many Western countries such as Spain and Italy, and in Japan, HCV infection is found in 60–90% of cases of HCC. HCC develops slowly, typically appearing 30 years after infection, and being rare within 15 years (Kiyosawa et al. 1990). In most studies, HCC usually, although not invariably (Demitri et al. 1995), occurs in patients with pre-existing cirrhosis.

For these reasons, the mechanism by which HCV causes HCC is generally considered to be indirect, arising as a consequence of chronic damage and inflammation of liver cells. Unlike HBV, replication of HCV does not produce DNA sequences that could be integrated into the host genome, nor is there any evidence for transforming activity of any of the HCV gene products. Treatment of hepatitis C patients with interferon-α has been reported to greatly reduce the subsequent risk of developing HCC, even in those conventionally regarded as 'non-responders', in whom long-term normalization of ALT was not achieved (Nishiguchi et al. 1995).

IMMUNE RESPONSE TO HCV INFECTION

Infection with HCV elicits humoral and T cell-mediated immune responses. Antibody reactivity to several HCV proteins can be detected in most infected individuals, although the response is highly variable and generally weak. There seems to be no specific pattern of antibody response that is predictive of the long-term outcome of infection. Greater serological reactivity to antigens used in second and third generation screening assays was observed in viraemic individuals compared with those who had cleared infection (Dhaliwal et al. 1996), suggesting that the major component of the antibody response is not directly protective. Neutralization assays remain insufficiently developed to explore their association with virus clearance and protection from reinfection.

A vigorous cellular immune response to HCV can be detected in infected individuals. T-helper cells obtained from peripheral blood of most HCV-infected people proliferate when exposed to recombinant HCV proteins such as core, E1, E2, NS3, NS4 and NS5 (Botarelli et al. 1993, Schupper et al. 1993, Ferrari et al. 1994). Proliferative responses were detected more frequently in individuals who had cleared infection, suggesting that the cellular immune response is important in the control of virus replication in vivo. Proliferative responses of T-helper cells obtained from the liver showed a highly restricted reactivity to NS4, compared with the responses found in mononuclear cells of peripheral blood (Minutello et al. 1993). Cytotoxic T lymphocytes (CTLs) from the liver and peripheral blood of HCV-infected individuals react with a wide range of epitopes from both structural and non-structural proteins (Koziel et al. 1992, 1993, Battegay et al. 1995, Cerny et al. 1995b). CTLs are likely to be important in both the control of and recovery from HCV infection and in the pathogenesis of liver disease (see below).

MECHANISM OF PERSISTENCE

Although humoral and cellular immune responses to HCV occur upon infection, these seem to be unable to clear the infection (see 'Chronic hepatitis', p. 726) or to protect an individual from reinfection. For example, it is possible to reinfect chimpanzees repeatedly with the same strain of HCV (Farci et al. 1992, Prince et al. 1992), producing hepatitis *de novo* similar to that observed on primary infection. Repeated exposure of humans to HCV may also produce recurrent episodes of infection, observed for example in thalassaemic patients transfused with HCV-contaminated blood (Lai et al. 1994). Infection with more than one HCV genotype is frequently observed in other multiply exposed individuals such as haemophiliacs (Jarvis et al. 1994).

Persistence of HCV and the observed susceptibility of individuals to reinfection may result from a weak or ineffective humoral response to envelope proteins that fails to neutralize virus infectivity. The 2 envelope genes are highly divergent between variants of HCV and have a higher rate of sequence change than other parts of the genome in a persistently infected chimpanzee (Okamoto et al. 1992a). The envelope proteins are the principal targets of humoral immune responses, and it has been hypothesized that changes in E1 and E2 alter the antigenic properties of the proteins, thereby allowing the virus to 'escape' from neutralizing antibodies (Weiner et al. 1992). In this model, persistent virus replication is achieved by continuous diversification of HCV in regions particularly sensitive to neutralizing antibody; this hypothesis is supported by the observation that much of the variability in the *E2* gene is concentrated in discrete 'hypervariable' regions (Hijikata et al. 1991a, Kato et al. 1992, Weiner et al. 1992) that may be in close proximity to parts of the protein involved in virus/cellular receptor interactions, as in influenza A virus. It has also been proposed that HCV may escape from CTL responses by changes in T cell epitopes. For example, an amino acid substitution in NS3 occurred shortly after experimental infection of a chimpanzee, which led to a loss of recognition of the epitope by CTLs (Weiner et al. 1995).

Experimental confirmation that immune pressure drives sequence change is difficult to obtain without a neutralization assay in vitro. However, it has been shown that novel E1 and E2 variants appearing over the course of infection in an individual are antigenically distinct from previous variants, and that their appearance is followed by the development of antibodies that specifically recognize the new variants (Weiner et al. 1992, Kato et al. 1993, Lesniewski et al. 1993, Taniguchi et al. 1993).

Another explanation for persistence is that it is difficult to neutralize the infectivity of HCV due to the structure of the virus. The extensive N-linked glycosylation of both E1 and E2 may shield amino acid epitopes from antibody, and prevent neutralization. It may be significant that HIV, another RNA virus that causes a persistent infection in humans, also has an extensively glycosylated outer membrane protein (c. 24 sites in a protein of 481 amino acids). A further contributing factor may be the binding of HCV to plasma lipoproteins (Miyamoto et al. 1992, Thomssen, Bonk and Thiele 1993), an association that may prevent effective neutralization. Binding of HCV to lipid need not eliminate its infectivity; indeed the process by which lipid micelles are specifically taken up by hepatocytes as part of normal cellular metabolism could provide a route by which HCV might gain entry into the liver. This would explain why HCV is so difficult to culture in vitro.

In the future, a full explanation of HCV persistence will have to account for the difference between HCV (and possibly hepatitis G virus and GB agents) and other flaviviruses, where infection is transient. For example, pestiviruses are incapable of persistence in immunocompetent animals, despite the fact that the virus is structurally similar to HCV with heavily glycosylated envelope proteins. Similarly, there is no reason to suppose that pestiviruses are any less genetically plastic than HCV, and therefore should be equally capable of immune escape.

MECHANISM OF LIVER DAMAGE

It is likely that direct cytopathic infection of cells in the liver as well as damage secondary to the inflammatory process contributes to HCV-associated liver disease. Evidence that HCV replication itself is directly cytopathic includes the clinical observation of more severe and rapidly progressive liver disease in individuals who are immunosuppressed and who have high levels of viraemia. Secondly, there is generally a direct correlation between clearance of viraemia and normalization of ALT levels in people who respond to interferon treatment (see 'Disease progression', p. 728), implying that it is virus replication itself that is responsible for the hepatitis. These observations contrast with HBV, in which successful treatment with interferon is thought to result from augmenting CTL activity in the liver and is associated with elevated ALT levels and a transient exacerbation of hepatitis.

On the other hand, there is also evidence that many aspects of the pathology of HCV infection result from the host immune response. For example, the frequency of infected hepatocytes in the liver is low, and there is often a complete absence of HCV infection in areas of the liver with lymphocyte infiltration. In a recent study, severe liver disease and failure to respond to antiviral treatment with interferon were associated with increased expression of MHC class I on the surface of hepatocytes, but were not associated with the numbers of HCV-infected cells as determined by immunocytochemistry (Ballardini et al. 1995).

Immunopathology may result from cytotoxic T cell reactivity against HCV-infected cells, or the process of HCV infection might trigger an autoimmune disease in which uninfected cells become the targets. The development of an immune response to the cellular protein, GOR, in association with HCV infection could be an example of this process (Mishiro et al. 1991). Understanding the mechanism of liver disease would assist the rational development of HCV treatment (see 'Antiviral treatment', p. 736). Standard treatment schedules with interferon-α have been shown empirically to clear hepatitis in some individuals (Davis et al. 1989, Di Bisceglie et al. 1989), although it is not known whether it acts as a virucidal agent or if its action depends on its immunomodulatory properties such as up-regulating expression of MHC class I on hepatocytes. At present it is not clear whether the further research into HCV treatment should concentrate on specific antivirals or if there is a therapeutic role of other immunomodulatory agents such as interleukins.

EXTRAHEPATIC MANIFESTATIONS

In a few infected patients, HCV may be responsible for extrahepatic clinical manifestations and disease (Martin 1993). The underlying pathogenic mechanisms for these extrahepatic manifestations are varied and often poorly understood. There are at least 3 mechanisms by which HCV could cause such disease. First, it is possible that HCV is capable of cytopathic replication in cell types outside of the liver. Secondly, HCV may trigger an autoimmune process that is directed against antigens expressed on non-hepatic cells. Thirdly, persistent HCV infection could lead to immune-complex formation with antibodies followed by deposition in small vessels.

Methods to detect extrahepatic replication of HCV include the detection of HCV protein expression by immunocytochemistry and the detection of replication intermediates by strand-specific PCR. Simple detection of HCV RNA sequences is generally insufficient evidence, as HCV may non-specifically associate or bind to cells such as macrophages or B lymphocytes in the peripheral circulation. The detection of HCV in tissues may reflect a process of immune-complex deposition rather than replication.

Many published studies reporting the detection of replication intermediates (complementary RNA sequences) in a range of cell types used methods that were insufficiently specific. However, using a PCR-based method for detection of sequences from the core region, Lerat and co-workers recently reported that replication may occur in certain lymphoid cells (Lerat et al. 1996). In contrast, no evidence for extrahepatic replication was observed in chimpanzees, using a similar assay (Lanford et al. 1995). In other studies, HCV was detected in lymphocytes infiltrating the liver by immunocytochemical and hybridization methods (Blight et al. 1994).

HCV infection is clearly associated with certain types of vasculitis and glomerulonephritis, which are caused by immune complex deposition. In southern Europe, HCV infection seems to be associated with porphyria cutanea tarda, a potentially disfiguring skin condition associated with an acquired deficiency of the liver enzyme uroporphyrinogen decarboxylase (Herrero et al. 1993). There is a putative association of HCV with other non-hepatic conditions, including Sjögren's syndrome, rheumatoid arthritis, pulmonary fibrosis, corneal ulceration, aplastic anaemia and non-Hodgkin's lymphoma. Vasculitis and glomerulonephritis are more frequent in patients with established cirrhosis.

HCV is classically associated with the small vessel vasculitis known as 'essential mixed cryoglobulinaemia' (Agnello, Chung and Kaplan 1992) (also observed in patients with chronic HBV infection). Laboratory features include the presence of rheumatoid factor activity in serum, the presence of a cryoprecipitate, complement activation and proteinuria/haematuria. The most important clinical manifestation is purpura, which is nearly always present, and 25–50% of patients have renal disease. Most patients have constitutional symptoms, especially weakness and arthralgia; Raynaud's phenomenon, Sjögren's syndrome and neuritis may also be present. Purpura may resolve with interferon-α therapy (Misiani et al. 1994).

HCV infection is also associated with membranoproliferative glomerulonephritis (MPGN) type 1 (Johnson et al. 1993), which is a consequence of immune complex deposition in the glomerular capillaries. It is associated with serum rheumatoid factor positivity, with complement activation, and with cryoglobulinaemia. MPGN is classically associated with heavy proteinuria, often in the nephrotic range (more than 3.5 g per 24

h), whilst creatinine clearance is modestly impaired. Treatment with interferon-α reduces urinary protein loss, but the impact of treatment on renal outcome is uncertain (Johnson et al. 1993). It should be emphasized that HCV infection is a relatively common cause of mixed essential cryoglobulinaemia and MPGN, but that HCV infection is rarely complicated by these conditions.

2.2 Epidemiology

PARENTERAL ROUTES OF TRANSMISSION

In western Europe, Australia and North America, most HCV-infected patients have a history of percutaneous exposure to the virus, and most are (or have been) intravenous drug users (IVDUs). The seroconversion rate of IVDUs has been estimated at 20% per year, so long-term drug users are almost invariably HCV-infected. Drug use was uncommon before the 1960s, so drug users tend to be younger than patients infected through transfusion and are also more likely to be infected with genotypes other than type 1b. Most drug users have asymptomatic infection with no history of jaundice but have chronic hepatitis whereas some have developed cirrhosis and a few have progressed to liver failure. If drug use is associated with a less aggressive form of hepatitis than that with transfusion-acquired infection, few IVDUs would progress to liver failure within 2 (or even 3) decades of infection. However, because of the lower average age of IVDUs, their life expectancy from the time of infection is 5 or 6 decades; despite less aggressive infection, many will survive long enough to develop significant liver disease.

In the 1960s, clotting factor concentrates became more widely used and most patients with coagulation disorders became infected with HCV. Thousands of donors contribute to each factor concentrate, so contamination with HCV and HIV was very likely. Many recipients were young, and most developed liver disease. Some have progressed to liver failure, and died or undergone liver transplantation (Telfer et al. 1994), although for many the prognosis may have been affected by HIV co-infection. Since the introduction of effective virus inactivation for blood products in the 1980s, factor concentrates have not transmitted HCV infection.

Repeated exposure to blood and blood products (in the absence of serological screening and/or heat treatment) is clearly associated with a high risk of HCV exposure and infection. The risk associated with exposure to a single donor product (e.g. one unit of blood) was already diminishing before the availability of specific serological tests for HCV, but varied significantly from country to country. Mercenary donors are more likely to be HCV-infected, and the prevalence of donor seropositivity was significantly reduced when 'self-exclusion' policies were introduced to combat the risk of HIV transmission. For example, by the mid-1980s fewer than 1% of UK donors were HCV-positive (Contreras et al. 1991).

Screening of blood donors for antibodies to HCV was introduced by most blood transfusion services in 1990 and 1991. Blood donors are clearly not representative of the entire population, but scrutiny of HCV-positive donors provides some insights into the epidemiology of this infection (Alter 1995, Mansell and Locarnini 1995). The lowest seroprevalence is observed in Scandinavia and in the UK with slightly higher prevalence in North America, western Europe and Australia. Prevalence is intermediate in eastern and southern European countries, even higher in Japan, and most prevalent in Middle Eastern (especially Egyptian) blood donors. When donor seroprevalence is low, the seropositive donor is more likely to have an identifiable risk factor for parenteral exposure (Mutimer et al. 1995b) but, as donor seroprevalence increases, prior parenteral exposure becomes more difficult to identify (Esteban et al. 1991).

In countries of low and intermediate seroprevalence, seropositive donors frequently admit to prior intravenous drug use; sometimes a single exposure, 20–30 years previously. Investigation of seropositive donors confirms that the majority are viraemic, and that many have chronic hepatitis and cirrhosis (Esteban et al. 1991, Irving et al. 1994, Mutimer et al. 1995b). As seropositive donors are excluded from the blood donor panels, the frequency of seropositivity falls; in the UK, for instance, true seropositivity fell from an initial rate of 0.60% to 0.15%.

In some countries, blood transfusion service and hospital records permit identification of the recipients of blood products that were donated before the introduction of HCV screening by a donor who was subsequently found to be HCV-positive (a policy sometimes referred to as 'HCV lookback'). Preliminary studies suggest that most living recipients will be HCV-infected (Jones et al. 1992, Ayob et al. 1994). When donor HCV infection is uncommon, living recipients with transfusion-associated HCV infection will also be uncommon. In the UK, for instance, as few as 3000 infected people will be traced by 'lookback', and this represents a very small fraction of all HCV-infected individuals in the community.

Transplanted organs may also transmit HCV infection, and studies in the USA and UK suggest that organ donors have a higher seropositivity rate than blood donors (Pereira et al. 1992, Wreghitt et al. 1994). The majority of high-risk blood donors are subject to self-exclusion, an option that is not available to the brain-dead organ donor. In one study, 6 of 554 (1.08%) British organ donors were HCV-seropositive in the screening assay, and 4 of these 6 infected an organ recipient.

OTHER ROUTES OF TRANSMISSION

Most studies (and this discussion) have focused on groups at risk for HCV infection as a result of percutaneous exposure. These groups include IVDUs, transfusion recipients (especially recipients of pooled plasma products such as factor VIII, anti-D) (Power et al. 1995), immunoglobulin (Healey et al. 1994), transplant recipients, haemodialysis patients and healthcare workers (Klein et al. 1991, Zuckerman et al. 1994). Tattooing and acupuncture may also be responsible for some percutaneous exposure, and in countries of high prevalence the use of unsterilized needles for cultural rituals, medical treatment or vaccination programmes may result in HCV infection. For example, bilharzia treatment using reusable and unsterile needles in the past has frequently been suggested as a cause for the very high population prevalence of HCV infection in Egypt.

However, for many people, overt percutaneous exposure cannot be identified. For example, detailed questioning failed to identify such a cause of infection in approximately one-third of HCV-infected Scottish blood donors (Crawford et al. 1994), and this has prompted the search for other routes of transmission. There seems to be a low risk of infection associated with sexual contact with an HCV carrier. Evidence suggesting that sexual transmission may occur includes the observation that HCV seems to be more common in people who have multiple sexual partners, such as prostitutes and male homosexuals (Tedder et al. 1991, Buchbinder et al. 1994). Large-scale studies of sexual partners of HCV-positive people generally show a slightly increased likelihood of HCV infection compared with the background population (Daikos, Lai and Fischl 1994, Soto et al. 1994, Cerny et al. 1995a, Utsumi et al. 1995), although in 2 studies (both of wives of haemophiliacs) no transmissions were documented (Bresters et al. 1993a, Hallam et al. 1993). Other sexually transmitted diseases may facilitate sexual transmission of HCV, as is the case for HIV.

Barrier methods of contraception/protection are likely to prevent transmission of HCV. For casual sexual contact, such precautions are mandatory (for mutual protection from all sexually transmitted infection). When one member of a long-term sexual partnership is identified as a carrier of HCV, both members should be counselled appropriately. The other partner might request serological testing. It seems likely that most couples will not elect to change their sexual practices. HIV/HCV co-infection may increase the risk for sexual transmission of HCV, and this may be a function of the higher HCV titre which is measured in the blood of HIV co-infected patients. In this setting, barrier methods of protection are clearly appropriate.

Early studies documented a low but detectable rate (5–15%) of mother-to-child transmission of HCV (Novati et al. 1992, Wejstal et al. 1992, Lam et al. 1993). However, it remains unclear whether this is true vertical transmission (in utero or during birth) or if it occurs through close contact (and possibly inapparent parenteral exposure) during the postnatal period. The risk of infant infection seems to be increased when the mother is HIV/HCV co-infected, and again this may be secondary to higher virus loads associated with immunosuppression (Ohto et al. 1994). HCV transmission may also occur as a result of 'household' contact. In this setting, it is almost impossible to distinguish vertical and sexual transmission from other 'household' contact. The parents of an index case are most likely to be infected. Relative risk is lower for spouses and siblings, and lowest for children of the index case.

In western Europe, most patients with liver failure will be referred for liver transplantation. Examination of the liver transplant experience during the 1980s and 1990s suggests that HCV has been an uncommon cause of liver failure in the UK. This observation suggests the relatively recent introduction of this virus into the western European population. It is evident that HCV infection was rare in western Europe and in North America before the emergence of intravenous drug use in the 1960s. However, it is calculated that the USA experienced an annual incidence of 15 cases per 100 000 population during the 1980s (Alter 1995), predicting a national reservoir of HCV carriers of as many as 3.5 million people. That HCV currently poses less of a clinical problem in the USA and northern Europe than in southern Europe, Japan and the Middle East is probably due to its later introduction in these populations. In the future, all countries can expect higher rates of significant liver disease from HCV, including liver cancer.

GEOGRAPHICAL DISTRIBUTION OF HCV GENOTYPES

Some genotypes of HCV (types 1a, 2a, 2b) show a broad worldwide distribution, whereas others (such as type 5a and 6a) are found only in specific geographical regions. HCV-infected blood donors and patients with chronic hepatitis from countries in western Europe and the USA often have genotypes 1a, 1b, 2a, 2b and 3a, although the relative frequencies of each may vary (e.g. infection with type 1b is more common in southern and eastern Europe). In many European countries genotype distributions vary with the age of the patients, reflecting rapid changes in genotype distribution with time within a single geographic area.

A striking geographical change in genotype distribution is apparent between southeast Europe and Turkey (both mainly type 1b) and several countries in the Middle East and parts of North and Central Africa where type 4 predominates. For example, a high frequency of HCV infection is found in Egypt (20–30%) (Saeed et al. 1991, Kamel et al. 1992, Darwish et al. 1993), of which almost all correspond to type 4a (Simmonds et al. 1993b, McOmish et al. 1994). HCV genotype 5a is frequently found among NANB patients and blood donors in South Africa but is found only rarely in other parts of Africa or elsewhere.

In Japan, Taiwan and probably parts of China, genotypes 1b, 2a and 2b are the most common. Infection with type 1a in Japan seems to be confined to haemophiliacs who have received commercial blood products such as factor VIII and IX clotting concentrates provided in the USA. A genotype with a highly restricted geographical range is type 6a: it was originally found in Hong Kong, where approximately one-third of anti-HCV-positive blood donors are infected with this genotype, as are an equivalent proportion in neighbouring Macau and Vietnam. A series of novel genotypes have recently been found in Vietnam

(Tokita et al. 1994) and Thailand (Mellor et al. 1995), distinct from types 1–6 but related more closely to type 6 than to other genotypes (Tokita et al. 1994). These variants currently pose a problem for HCV classification, as they seem to be intermediate in variability between the type and subtype categories described above (see 'Nomenclature of HCV genotypes', p. 724).

MOLECULAR EPIDEMIOLOGY OF HCV INFECTION

Persistent infection with HCV entails continuous replication of HCV over years or decades; the large number of replication cycles, combined with the relatively error prone RdRp leads to measurable sequence drift of HCV over time. For example, over an 8 year period of persistent infection in a chimpanzee, the rate of sequence change for the genome as a whole was 0.144% per site per year (Okamoto et al. 1992a), similar to the rate observed in the 5′ half of the genome over 3 years in a human carrier (0.192%) (Ogata et al. 1991). Using this 'molecular clock', it is in principle possible to calculate times of divergence between HCV variants, and therefore to establish their degree of epidemiological relatedness. Similarly, phylogenetic analysis of sequences from individuals exposed to HCV can be used as evidence for a common source of infection. Sequence comparisons in variable regions of the HCV genome such as E2 and NS5 have been used to document transmission between individuals, and to explore the possibility of non-parenteral routes of transmission such as mother to child (Weiner et al. 1993) and within families (Honda et al. 1993) and by sexual contact (Rice et al. 1993, Setoguchi et al. 1994, Healey et al. 1995). For example, clustering of HCV sequences into a single phylogenetic group among recipients of an HCV-contaminated blood product (anti-D immunoglobulin) was still apparent 17 years after exposure (Power et al. 1995).

ORIGINS OF HCV GENOTYPES

As with other RNA viruses, it is difficult to place a specific geographical or temporal origin for the common ancestor of the existing HCV genotypes. However, the preponderance of types 3 and 6 in India and southeast Asia and of types 1, 2 and 4 in Central and West Africa provides some clues, particularly as their presence is associated with a diversity of subtypes not observed in Europe, the USA or the Far East, and which may be associated with their long-term presence within these human populations. The sequence differences between subtypes (e.g. type 1a and 1b) imply a common ancestor for these variants at least 200 years ago, whereas the much greater differences between genotypes (such as between types 1 and 2) probably represent an interval of at least several thousand years. The existence of ancient lineages heightens the difficulties in understanding the persistence of a virus infection within human societies in which parenteral exposure has been documented to be the only efficient route of transmission.

2.3 Diagnosis of HCV infection

ANTIGENS

Antibody reactivity can be detected to a wide range of linear and conformational epitopes present on both structural and non-structural proteins of HCV. Recombinant proteins or peptides containing these antigenic regions are used for serological tests for antibody to HCV (see Fig. 35.1), and much of our current knowledge of antibody responses to HCV has arisen from research aimed at improving antibody tests to enable effective screening of blood donors and diagnosis in patients. Cytotoxic T cell and proliferative responses have also been detected to several peptides or recombinant proteins.

NS4

The original HCV-specific clone isolated from chimpanzee plasma was expressed in *E. coli*, the derived protein of 42 amino acids (1694–1735) being encoded by the NS4 region of the genome (see Fig. 35.1). A larger clone (c100-3) assembled from several overlapping clones was expressed in yeast and formed the basis of the first commercial tests for HCV antibody. The antigen was derived from amino acids 1569–1931, thus spanning a small section of the NS3 region as well as almost all of 4a and 4b. Despite its being a somewhat unnatural hybrid, use of the antigen in screening assays provided the first evidence of the importance and widespread occurrence of HCV infection. Antigen from NS4 is present in all current screening ELISAs, whether singly, in combination with NS3 or in synthetic peptide form. Likewise, all commercial supplementary immunoblot assays contain NS4 components either as recombinant antigens (Chiron RIBA-2, Murex Western blot, Abbott Matrix) or as synthetic peptides (Chiron RIBA-3, Organon Liatek III), which show improved specificity.

Many of the antigenic determinants in the NS4 region show considerable amino acid sequence variability between genotypes of HCV; serological reactivity to the 5-1-1 protein is absent or weak in samples from individuals infected with types 2 or 3 (Chan et al. 1991, McOmish et al. 1993). Indeed, type-specific reactivity to NS4 forms the basis for serological typing assays that can differentiate between the antibody responses elicited by different genotypes (Simmonds et al. 1993c, Tanaka et al. 1994, Bhattacherjee et al. 1995)

Core

Infection with HCV elicits a strong humoral antibody response to the core protein, predominantly to a series of linear epitopes at the N terminus of the protein (Nasoff et al. 1991, Sallberg et al. 1992). The incorporation of either recombinant proteins or synthetic peptides from the core region led to a great improvement in the sensitivity of screening assays for HCV antibody (Chiba et al. 1991, Hosein et al. 1991, Ishida et al. 1993). Commercial screening assays have mainly used recombinant antigen (c22) comprising a major portion of the core region (Ortho 3.0, amino acids 2–120;

Abbott 3.0 amino acids 1–150, Murex VK47/48) but the Sanofi Pasteur New Antigen ELISA use instead 2 synthetic peptides. The most recent version of the Chiron RIBA supplementary test, RIBA-3, replaces the recombinant antigen of RIBA-2 with one synthetic peptide using amino acids 10–53, resulting in much improved specificity. Liatek III incorporates 2 peptides from the core region, whilst the Murex and Matrix blots retain recombinant antigen. The amino acid sequence of the core region is highly conserved between different genotypes of HCV; consequently, most epitopes are cross-reactive, similar reactivity being observed for individuals infected with different genotypes. The differences that do exist have been exploited in a typing assay to distinguish antibody to type 1 and type 2 (Tsukiyama Kohara et al. 1993), although the core proteins of types 1, 3, 4, 5 and 6 are probably too similar to allow this assay to be extended further.

NS3

Antibody to epitopes in the NS3 region of HCV is produced early in infection and is the first detectable in many seroconversions; in established infections, it is as common as core antibody and seen more frequently than antibody to c100 or NS5. Several manufacturers were slow to realize the benefits of incorporating antigen from this region in their screening tests and some early tests had either none or too little to be effective, thus missing viraemic samples (Dow et al. 1993, Courouce et al. 1995). All current screening assays contain recombinant antigen either singly or in combination with NS4 sequences (Ortho 3.0) or c22 sequences (Abbott 3.0). In Ortho 3.0 the NS3 antigen has been modified biochemically to give increased sensitivity for NS3 antibody, enabling earlier detection of seroconversions (Courouce et al. 1994) and the detection of chronically infected patients with low levels of NS3 antibody (Dow et al. 1996b). All supplementary immunoblots use recombinant antigen from the NS3 region. Changes in the concentration of the coating antigen, c33c, in RIBA-3 have made this test particularly sensitive to NS3 antibody (Courouce et al. 1994).

NS5

Recombinant antigen from the NS5 region was incorporated in the first Wellcozyme/Murex ELISA but appeared in the Abbott and Ortho tests only with the third generation. Both Abbott and Ortho tests use recombinant antigen from almost the whole NS5 region (amino acids 2054–2995), whereas in the Murex assay the size of the recombinant protein has been reduced with each succeeding test and the present Murex test contains protein from only a small segment of the NS5a region. Of the current supplementary tests, RIBA-3 and Murex blot incorporate recombinant antigen whilst in Liatek III it is a peptide. The contribution of NS5 antigens to improved specificity and sensitivity in screening tests has been difficult to quantify. Seroconversions in which antibody to NS5 occurs first are rare, and no chronically infected patient has been found with NS5 antibody as the only marker. Specificity is not enhanced, as these tests produce significant numbers of a new population of RIBA-3, NS5 indeterminates, that are all PCR-negative; it is generally agreed that improvements in sensitivity with third generation ELISAs are associated with improved NS3 antibody detection. Inclusion in supplementary tests may have value in providing extra evidence of positivity but the poorer specificity of NS5 antigens in these tests may compromise interpretation.

Other proteins

The ultimate serological test for HCV will have all antigenic domains of HCV represented. The current Liatek III assay contains a peptide derived from the E2/NS1 region. This antigen did not contribute to earlier detection of antibody in seroconversion, nor was it essential for obtaining positive results on formerly indeterminate (RIBA-2) samples (Zaaijer et al. 1994a). However, a preliminary study of a recombinant E2 antigen in ELISA format has been encouraging (Zaaijer et al. 1994b).

Summary

The battery of antigens used in current screening and supplementary tests will detect the vast majority of chronic, established infections. Where improvement is required is in earlier detection of seroconversion. In addition, manufacturers need to address the problems associated with antigenic variation between different genotypes. All current screening tests are based on genotype 1 antigens, and, although this genotype is widely distributed throughout the world, it is not the only nor the predominant genotype in many countries. Diminished sensitivity to genotype 3 is seen in RIBA-2 (Damen et al. 1995) and, to a lesser extent, RIBA-3 (Dow et al. 1996a), and this may also be reflected in the sensitivity of screening ELISAs (Dhaliwal et al. 1996). Future tests will need to incorporate antigens from various genotypes to ensure an optimal sensitivity for all.

FIRST GENERATION TESTS

The first test to specifically detect antibody to HCV was based on the c100-3 antigen (Kuo et al. 1989). Use of this simple, single antigen test in ELISA format confirmed that HCV was the major cause of post-transfusion non-A, non-B hepatitis in the USA and elsewhere (Alter et al. 1989, Esteban et al. 1990, Hopf et al. 1990, van der Poel et al. 1990), and that prevalence of antibody to the c100-3 antigen was high in haemophiliacs (Brettler et al. 1990), in drug abusers (Esteban et al. 1990) and in patients with hepatocellular carcinoma (Bruix et al. 1989, Colombo et al. 1989, Nishioka et al. 1991). The simple first generation tests for anti-HCV were valuable in establishing the importance of HCV infection world-wide, its identity with non-A, non-B hepatitis and its wider spread in the community usually via drug abuse.

A difficulty with the first generation tests was that they were prone to non-specificity, especially when used to screen low risk populations or stored serum samples. A true confirmatory test for HCV antibody (demonstration of neutralization of virus or reactivity to viral antigens different from those used for screening) was not possible. Most investigators

used a supplementary recombinant immunoblot test nitrocellulose strip containing bands of 2 HCV recombinant antigens (5-1-1 and c100-3). Reactivity with one band was taken as 'confirmation' of HCV antibody positivity (Chiron Corp., RIBA-1). However, in many early studies of HCV antibody prevalence, this supplementary test was not used or not yet available, so data from such studies should be interpreted with care.

SECOND GENERATION TESTS

Once the HCV genome had been fully sequenced and the structural and non-structural regions identified (Choo et al. 1991), several manufacturers developed second generation tests, which included antigen to the core region (c22c) and one or more further non-structural regions NS3 (c33), NS4 (c100-3) or NS5. The most widely used tests, those manufactured by Ortho Diagnostics and Abbott Laboratories, contained 4 antigens (5-1-1, c100-3, c22 and c33c). These tests were significantly more sensitive and specific than their first generation equivalents, and their use for screening blood donations virtually eliminated post-transfusion HCV infection as a complication of transfusion (Aach et al. 1991). The improved sensitivity allowed earlier detection of seroconverting patients by some weeks (van der Poel et al. 1992) (see Fig. 35.6) and the detection of HCV antibody positivity in donors and patients previously reported as negative in the first generation assays (Yuki et al. 1992, Aoki et al. 1994).

The same series of antigens present in the second generation Ortho and Abbott tests were incorporated in an improved RIBA test by Chiron: RIBA-2, often referred to as 4-RIBA in early reports. In this test, 2 bands were required for positivity; 1 band was termed an indeterminate result. This test was very effective in identifying ELISA false positives in first generation tests where it represented a truer confirmatory test in that it incorporated new antigens (c33c and c22) not present in the ELISA screening test (Courouce, Janot and Hepatitis Study Group FSBT 1991, van der Poel et al. 1991). There was a strong correlation between RIBA-2 positivity and viraemia as detected by PCR tests (Garson et al. 1992, Larsen, Skaug and Maeland 1992, Bresters et al. 1993b, Yun et al. 1993). The interpretation of the RIBA-2 indeterminate result (of which there were significant numbers in low risk populations such as blood donors) and the advice to give the patient/donor has proved controversial. Only PCR testing could clearly define the association with HCV infection, but few PCR-positive indeterminate individuals were found in low risk groups (Follett et al. 1991) and these were almost always associated with the c22 or c33 band (Bresters et al. 1993b). Most of the indeterminate reactivity to c22 was due to non-specific cross-reactivity to restricted, N-terminal, regions of the core antigen (Tobler et al. 1994). RIBA-2 is less likely to 'confirm' samples from individuals infected with type 1 genotypes (Pawlotsky et al. 1995, Dow et al. 1996a) owing to the predominantly type-specific reactivity to the NS3 and particularly NS4 proteins.

THIRD GENERATION TESTS

Current tests for HCV antibody omit the original 5-1-1 antigen and include the NS5 antigen, although the value of this addition is questionable. Third generation ELISAs are more sensitive and detect seroconversions significantly earlier (Courouce et al. 1994, Uyttendaele et al. 1994, Vrielink et al. 1995c) but this improvement is associated with an improved reactivity of the c33 antigen component and not with the presence of the NS5 antigen (Barrera et al. 1995, Courouce et al. 1995, Lee et al. 1995). Counterbalancing this improvement in sensitivity is some loss in specificity related to a new population of indeterminate samples associated with the NS5 antigen. At the time of writing, no NS5 indeterminate sample has been found to be PCR-positive in a chronically infected patient.

Significant changes were made in the updated RIBA test, RIBA-3, introduced in Europe in 1994. As well as NS5 recombinant antigen, RIBA-3 incorporates synthetic peptides for c22 and c100, replacing the recombinant antigens of RIBA-2. Improved sensitivity is again apparent and associated with the NS3 component (Courouce et al. 1994, Zaaijer et al. 1994b). Specificity is greatly enhanced, and use of RIBA-3 resolves many of the non-specific problems associated with RIBA-2 (Dow et al. 1993, Zaaijer et al. 1994b). Viraemia and RIBA-3 positivity are strongly associated when 3 and 4 bands are present but much less so for 2 band positives (Dow et al. 1996a). Care is required with all PCR-negative, 2 band positives, and further ELISA and supplementary tests are necessary before equating such reactivity with HCV infection, because false positives are known (Damen et al. 1995, Dow et al. 1996a). Although RIBA-3 has improved sensitivity for genotypes 2 and 3 compared with RIBA-2, some lack of sensitivity to type 3 is still apparent (Dow et al. 1996b).

There remains a considerable window period in HCV infection between exposure and development of antibody detectable by the best current ELISAs. Viraemia can be detected in this period (Dow et al. 1994) and transmission by blood donated in this period is known (Vrielink et al. 1995a).

Alternative antigen tests

Manufacturers of HCV serological assays use recombinant proteins and peptides from type 1a, although some in the USA and Europe have cloned HCV independently and produced commercial products based on differently sourced HCV antigens. These produce tests that show non-specific reactivity on screening different from that produced by the Chiron-based tests. Consequently, using one such test to screen ELISA reactives from an alternatively sourced antigen test could help to resolve many of the specificity problems associated with HCV ELISAs (Craske, Paver and Farmer 1993). However, patent regulations have forced the removal of these tests from the market place and only 2 commercially available ELISAs with independently sourced antigen are widely available (Murex, Sanofi-Pasteur).

Alternative supplementary tests to the Chiron RIBA products are produced by several manufacturers, based either on the Chiron isolate (Abbott Matrix) or independently sourced antigen (Murex Western Blot, Organon Liatek line immunoassay, Diagnostic Biotechnology blot assay). The Liatek assay most closely approaches RIBA-3 for sensitivity and specificity (Zaaijer et al. 1994b). A new antigen from the *E2/NS1* region of the genome incorporated into this test did not contribute to earlier detection of HCV antibody in seroconversion. Whether use of recombinant envelope antigens is helpful must await further studies. All these supplementary tests can be valuable when investigating a doubtful ELISA or RIBA result.

Genome detection

Detection of the HCV genome is indispensable for the accurate diagnosis and the complete characterization of HCV infection in a patient. Our knowledge of HCV infection has benefited immensely from use of the PCR for HCV RNA. The PCR test or equivalent is the only method of confirming HCV infection in equivocal ELISA reactives such as RIBA indeterminates, and is the only method for distinguishing between chronic and resolved infections. 'Lookback' studies on recipients of blood donations known to be RIBA positive or

indeterminate indicate that transmission is associated only with PCR positivity (Vrielink et al. 1995b). Detection of the virus genome is the only reliable method of following the effect of treatment with antiviral drugs on patients with chronic infection, because normalization of biochemical liver function tests is not always associated with virus clearance. Similarly, chronic HCV infection with associated disease is known in patients with normal liver function tests (Nalpas et al. 1995). Patients in early seroconversion or with an impaired immune response can appear falsely negative in current HCV ELISA tests, and PCR is necessary for complete diagnosis in such cases (Bukh et al. 1993). In chimpanzees, viraemia can be detected by PCR within the first week after infection (Shimizu et al. 1990, Beach et al. 1992), providing a long window period when the blood is infectious but no antibody can be detected. In blood donor populations at high risk of HCV infection PCR testing may be the only method of ensuring the safety of donated blood.

Most PCR data on HCV infection has been derived from the use of 'in-house' tests. PCR technology is complex and prone to errors producing false positivity and lack of sensitivity, particularly from laboratories where PCR testing is infrequent. A study of laboratory proficiency for HCV PCR in laboratories throughout Europe has shown only 16% to be performing optimally for specificity and sensitivity (Zaaijer et al. 1994a). Availability of simpler or automated commercial genome amplification or detection tests will help to raise the figure to a more acceptable level, but genome detection by whatever method is not yet comparable to ELISA testing for reliability and a second opinion from another laboratory on unusual or unexpected results is often helpful. Despite the enormous amplification achieved by PCR technology the tests do have a limit to their sensitivity, and this value should be measured and quoted when data are published.

Quantification of the virus genome titre is now increasingly possible with commercial tests and has a place in following patients receiving antiviral therapy. An alternative technology to PCR, the use of branched chain DNA (bDNA, Quantiplex, Chiron) to amplify the signal rather than the viral genome, is particularly suited to quantitative work. This assay is based on HCV genome material from a type 1 American isolate; the test is less sensitive for types 2 and 3, and a correction factor is required for accurate comparison of quantitative data from patients infected with different genotypes (Lau, Simmonds and Urdea 1995). It is not yet known whether the commercially available semi-quantitative PCR assay (Roche Monitor) is similarly less sensitive for type 2 and type 3 sequences.

2.4 Control of HCV infection

Antiviral treatment

Since the introduction of serological screening of blood products, acute HCV infection is seldom encountered in clinical practice. Small studies suggest that treatment with interferon (interferon-α and β have been used) during the acute phase may be beneficial, and may reduce the risk of chronic infection (Omata et al. 1991, Lampertico et al. 1994).

Interferon-α is now widely prescribed for the treatment of chronic hepatitis associated with HCV infection. An enormous number of studies have been conducted, and both lymphoblastoid and recombinant interferons have been used (Fried and Hoofnagle 1993). Most physicians use 3–6 MU thrice weekly for 6–12 months, and it seems likely that treatment response may be enhanced by the use of higher doses for longer durations. Before the availability of PCR tests for HCV RNA, serum transaminases served as surrogate markers of response to treatment. Most physicians still rely on serum alanine transaminase (ALT) to monitor interferon treatment, and the principal aim of treatment is the normalization of ALT levels. The application of qualitative and quantitative PCR assays now permits virological assessment of response. These have shown that (1) persistently elevated ALT is associated with persistent HCV RNA positivity, (2) normalization of ALT is frequently associated with RNA clearance, (3) biochemical relapse is associated with reappearance of RNA, and (4) viral RNA may be detected in the follow-up serum of patients with apparent biochemical remission.

Three patterns of response are observed (Fig. 35.9). In a typical study, c. 50% of treated patients have persistently elevated ALT and remain RNA-positive despite treatment, whereas the remaining 50% respond with normalization of ALT and RNA becoming undetectable. At least half of this latter group relapse during therapy or when therapy is withdrawn. The treatment objective is a sustained response, which implies persistently normal ALT with RNA clearance after treatment is concluded, but fewer than 20% of 'all-comers' achieve this objective. In an attempt to improve response rates, and to prevent the unnecessary treatment of potential non-responders, clinical and virological features associated with sustained response have been defined (see 'Predictive factors for response to treatment'). Improved response rates may be observed for young patients with a short duration of infection whereas a sustained response is seldom observed for patients with cirrhosis and portal hypertension.

Interferon-α may also be indicated for the treatment of extrahepatic manifestations of HCV infection such as essential cryoglobulinaemia and glomerulonephritis. The nucleoside analogue ribavirin has also been used for the treatment of chronic HCV infection (Reichard et al. 1991, Di Bisceglie, Shindo and Fong 1992, Camps et al. 1993). The biochemical response may be observed for the duration of therapy, but relapse occurs when therapy is withdrawn. Because viral RNA persists despite the biochemical response, treatment with ribavirin as single-agent therapy cannot be recommended. However, combination therapy using interferon-α and ribavirin may achieve a better response rate than treatment with interferon alone (Brillianti, Garson and Foli 1994).

PREDICTIVE FACTORS FOR RESPONSE TO TREATMENT

Several clinical studies have catalogued a variety of factors (including virus genotype) that correlate with severity of liver disease and which show predictive value for the response to antiviral treatment. Factors that have frequently been shown to influence response to interferon treatment include patient age and duration of infection, presence of cirrhosis before treatment, virus genotype and pretreatment level of circulating viral RNA in plasma. A consistent finding is the greatly increased rate of long-term response found on treating patients infected with genotypes 2a, 2b and 3a, compared with type 1. Normalization of ALT levels (>12 months) is typically observed in 20–30% of patients infected with type 1 variants, compared with 50–70% of those with type 2 and 3 infections (reviewed in Simmonds 1995, Bukh 1995). Using multivariate analysis, infection with type 1b, the presence of cirrhosis and a high pretreatment virus load were each independently associated with a reduced chance of response. In a Japanese study, the relative risks for these 3 factors were 16, 5 and 4 respectively (Tsubota et al. 1994).

The mechanism by which different genotypes might differ in responsiveness to treatment remains obscure, particularly as it is still unclear whether interferon acts as an antiviral or as an immunomodulatory agent (see 'Antiviral treatment', p. 736). Infection with genotypes 1, 2 and 3 all cause progressive liver disease with no evidence that type 1 is significantly more pathogenic than other variants. Similarly, studies of both blood donors and patients have indicated that virus loads are similar among individuals infected with different genotypes (Lau, Simmonds and Urdea 1995, Smith et al. 1996). It is therefore unlikely that the greater response rates achieved with types 2 and 3 are simply secondary to differences in disease severity. Recently, sequence comparisons demonstrated a cluster of amino acids in the NS5a region that consistently differed between responders and non-responders to interferon treatment (Enomoto et al. 1995). This observation may provide a basis for future investigations of genotype-specific differences in response and the nature of the resistance mechanism that currently limits the effectiveness of treatment.

LIVER TRANSPLANTATION

Liver transplantation is indicated for patients with decompensated HCV cirrhosis and for some patients with hepatocellular carcinoma complicating HCV infection. Liver transplantation does not cure HCV infection, and reinfection of the graft is probably inevitable (TL Wright, Gavaler and van Theil 1992). Recurrence may be associated with hepatitis of the graft, which typically occurs within 6 months of transplantation. Short-term and intermediate-term outcomes of graft infection are excellent, and reinfection has no discernible effect on patient morbidity or mortality during the first 3 years or so after transplantation. Liver disease may be more aggressive in the

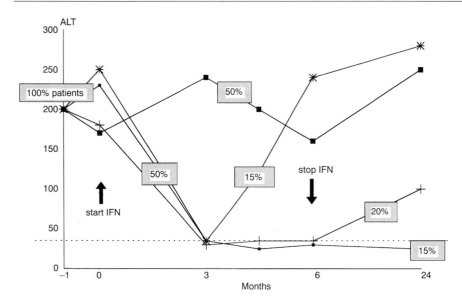

Fig. 35.9 Response rate of chronic HCV infection to interferon-α therapy. For 50% of treated patients, biochemical improvement is not observed after institution of a standard dose of interferon (3 megaunits thrice weekly); 50% respond during therapy with normalization of serum transaminases. About 15% relapse during therapy, and a further 20% relapse at conclusion of therapy; 18 months after a standard 6 month course of interferon-α, only 15% of treated patients have sustained biochemical and virological remission. This fraction might be cured.

setting of immunosuppression, especially when HCV genotype 1b is involved. There is a need to develop strategies for the treatment of HCV reinfection of the transplanted liver, which might also be applied to the treatment of other immunosuppressed patients (e.g. renal transplant patients) with hepatitis due to HCV infection.

Both interferon-α (HI Wright, Gavaler and van Theil 1992) and ribavirin (Gane et al. 1995) have been used to treat graft reinfection, but neither has been assessed in a controlled study and it seems unlikely that these agents can eradicate HCV in the setting of immunosuppression.

PREVENTION

Screening of blood donors has proved to be effective in preventing transmission of HCV infection through blood transfusion. For example, the incidence of post-transfusion hepatitis fell from 10.7% to 1.9% in Spain (Gonzalez et al. 1995) and from 7.7% to 2.1% in Japan (Japanese Red Cross Non-A Non-B Hepatitis Research Group 1991) following the introduction of first generation screening assays. Most of the donations that were missed using this initial test would have been identified as positive by second or third generation assays (Aach et al. 1991, Yuki et al. 1992, Aoki et al. 1994, Gonzalez et al. 1995). A combination of blood donor screening and virus inactivation has virtually eliminated HCV transmission by blood products such as clotting factor concentrates and immunoglobulins.

The main continuing risks for HCV transmission are intravenous drug abuse and the use of unsterile needles for medical and dental procedures, tattooing and other percutaneous exposures. Much of this could be prevented by education, greater availability of disposable needles and, for drug abusers, needle exchange programmes. Many of the public health measures adopted to prevent transmission of HIV by parenteral routes will assist efforts at controlling HCV.

IMMUNIZATION

The development of a vaccine for HCV faces a series of formidable obstacles. HCV is highly heterogeneous, and effective vaccines may need to be multivalent in a way analogous to poliovirus vaccine in order to be protective against multiple serotypes. There is no in vitro neutralization assay currently available to determine the most effective antigen(s) to use to induce protective antibody. Furthermore, the high rate of chronicity and the continued susceptibility of HCV-infected individuals to reinfection (see 'Chronic hepatitis', p. 726) suggests that a protective immune response may be difficult to achieve by immunization. At a practical level, the absence of a widely available and inexpensive animal model for HCV infection, and the resulting requirement to use chimpanzees, has greatly curtailed the number of experiments that can be done.

Despite these difficulties, encouraging results have been obtained using recombinant envelope proteins (E1 and E2) expressed in mammalian cells as immunogens. These induce a short-lived specific anti-E1 and E2 response in immunized chimpanzees, and a protective effect from challenge with low titres of the homologous virus (Choo et al. 1994). Further research is currently concentrated on investigations of the duration and immunological basis of the observed protection, and the extent to which the chimpanzees are protected from challenge by different HCV variants.

Infection with HCV is a growing medical problem world-wide. A combination of public health preventative measures, improved diagnosis, screening, antiviral treatment and immunization will undoubtedly all be required to combat its spread in the future.

REFERENCES

Aach RD, Stevens CE et al., 1991, Hepatitis C virus infection in post-transfusion hepatitis. An analysis with first- and second-generation assays, *N Engl J Med*, **325**: 1325–9.

Agnello V, Chung RT, Kaplan LM, 1992, A role for hepatitis C virus infection in type-II cryoglobulinemia, *N Engl J Med*, **327**: 1490–5.

Alter MJ, 1995, Epidemiology of hepatitis C in the west, *Semin Liver Dis*, **15**: 5–14.

Alter HJ, Holland PV et al., 1975, Clinical and serological analysis of transfusion-associated hepatitis, *Lancet*, **2**: 838–41.

Alter HJ, Purcell RH et al., 1989, Detection of antibody to hepatitis C virus in prospectively followed transfusion recipients with acute and chronic non-A, non-B hepatitis, *N Engl J Med*, **321**: 1494–500.

Aoki SK, Kuramoto IK et al., 1994, Evidence that use of a second-generation hepatitis C antibody assay prevents additional cases of transfusion-transmitted hepatitis, *J Viral Hepatitis*, **1**: 73–7.

Ayob Y, Davidson JI et al., 1994, Risk of hepatitis C in patients who received blood from donors subsequently shown to be carriers of hepatitis C virus, *Transfusion Med*, **4**: 269–72.

Ballardini G, Groff P et al., 1995, Hepatitis C virus (HCV) genotype, tissue HCV antigens, hepatocellular expression of HLA-a,b,c, and intercellular adhesion-1 molecules – clues to pathogenesis of hepatocellular damage and response to interferon treatment in patients with chronic hepatitis C, *J Clin Invest*, **95**: 2067–75.

Barrera JM, Francis B et al., 1995, Improved detection of anti-HCV in post-transfusion hepatitis by a third-generation ELISA, *Vox Sang*, **68**: 15–18.

Bartenschlager R, Ahlbornlaake L et al., 1993, Nonstructural protein-3 of the hepatitis C virus encodes a serine-type proteinase required for cleavage at the NS3/4 and NS4/5 junctions, *J Virol*, **67**: 3835–44.

Bartenschlager R, Ahlbornlaake L et al., 1995, Substrate determinants for cleavage in *cis* and in *trans* by the hepatitis C virus NS3 proteinase, *J Virol*, **69**: 198–205.

Bartholomeusz AI, Guo K-J et al., 1995, An HCV polymerase assay used cloned HCV non-structural proteins, *3rd International Meeting on Hepatitis C and Related Viruses*, Brisbane, Australia, September 1995, Abstract C8.

Battegay M, Fikes J et al., 1995, Patients with chronic hepatitis C have circulating cytotoxic T cells which recognize hepatitis C virus-encoded peptides binding to HLA-a2.1 molecules, *J Virol*, **69**: 2462–70.

Beach MJ, Meeks EL et al., 1992, Temporal relationships of hepatitis C virus RNA and antibody responses following experimental infection of chimpanzees, *J Med Virol*, **36**: 226–37.

Bhattacherjee V, Prescott LE et al., 1995, Use of NS4 peptides to identify type-specific antibody to hepatitis C virus genotypes 1, 2, 3, 4, 5 and 6, *J Gen Virol*, **76**: 1737–48.

Blight K, Lesniewski RR et al., 1994, Detection and distribution of hepatitis C-specific antigens in naturally infected liver, *Hepatology*, **20**: 553–7.

Botarelli P, Brunetto MR et al., 1993, Lymphocyte-T response to hepatitis C virus in different clinical courses of infection, *Gastroenterology*, **104**: 580–7.

Bradley DW, Maynard JE, 1986, Etiology and natural history of post-transfusion and enterically transmitted non-A, non-B hepatitis, *Semin Liver Dis*, **6**: 56–66.

Bradley DW, Cook EH et al., 1979, Experimental infection of chimpanzees with antihemophilic (factor VIII) materials: recovery of virus-like particles associated with non-A, non-B hepatitis, *J Med Virol*, **3**: 253–69.

Bradley D, McCaustland K et al., 1991, Hepatitis C virus: buoyant density of the factor VIII-derived isolate in sucrose, *J Med Virol*, **34**: 206–8.

Bresters D, Mauserbunschoten EP et al., 1993a, Sexual transmission of hepatitis C virus, *Lancet*, **342**: 210–11.

Bresters D, Zaaijer HL et al., 1993b, Recombinant immunoblot assay reaction patterns and hepatitis C virus RNA in blood donors and non-A, non-B hepatitis patients, *Transfusion*, **33**: 634–8.

Brettler DB, Alter HJ et al., 1990, Prevalence of hepatitis C virus antibody in a cohort of hemophilia patients, *Blood*, **76**: 254–6.

Brillianti S, Garson J, Foli M, 1994, A pilot study of combination therapy with ribavirin plus interferon-alpha for interferon-alpha resistant chronic hepatitis C, *Gastroenterology*, **107**: 812–17.

Brown EA, Zhang H et al., 1992, Secondary structure of the 5′ nontranslated region of hepatitis C virus and pestivirus genomic RNAs, *Nucleic Acids Res*, **20**: 5041–5.

Bruix J, Barrera JM et al., 1989, Prevalence of antibodies to hepatitis C virus in Spanish patients with hepatocellular carcinoma and hepatic cirrhosis, *Lancet*, **2**: 1004–6.

Buchbinder SP, Katz MH et al., 1994, Hepatitis C virus infection in sexually active homosexual men, *J Infect*, **29**: 263–9.

Bukh J, 1995, Genetic heterogeneity of hepatitis C virus: quasi-species and genotypes, *Semin Liver Dis*, **15**: 41–63.

Bukh J, Purcell RH, Miller RH, 1993, At least 12 genotypes of hepatitis C virus predicted by sequence analysis of the putative E1 gene of isolates collected worldwide, *Proc Natl Acad Sci USA*, **90**: 8234–8.

Bukh J, Wantzin P et al., 1993, High prevalence of hepatitis C virus (HCV) RNA in dialysis patients – failure of commercially available antibody tests to identify a significant number of patients with HCV infection, *J Infect Dis*, **168**: 1343–8.

Bukh J, Purcell RH, Miller RH, 1994, Sequence analysis of the core gene of 14 hepatitis C virus genotypes, *Proc Natl Acad Sci USA*, **91**: 8239–43.

Camps J, Garcia N et al., 1993, Ribavirin in the treatment of chronic hepatitis C unresponsive to α interferon, *J Hepatol*, **19**: 408–12.

Carloni G, Iacovacci S et al., 1993, Susceptibility of human liver cell cultures to hepatitis C virus infection, *Arch Virol Suppl*, **8**: 31–9.

Carrick RJ, Schlauder GG et al., 1992, Examination of the buoyant density of hepatitis-C virus by the polymerase chain reaction, *J Virol Methods*, **39**: 279–90.

Cerny A, Fowler P et al., 1995a, Induction in vitro of a primary human antiviral cytotoxic T cell response, *Eur J Immunol*, **25**: 627–30.

Cerny A, McHutchison JG et al., 1995b, Cytotoxic T lymphocyte response to hepatitis C virus-derived peptides containing the HLA a2.1 binding motif, *J Clin Invest*, **95**: 521–30.

Chan S-W, Simmonds P et al., 1991, Serological reactivity of blood donors infected with three different types of hepatitis C virus, *Lancet*, **338**: 1391.

Chan S-W, McOmish F et al., 1992, Analysis of a new hepatitis C virus type and its phylogenetic relationship to existing variants, *J Gen Virol*, **73**: 1131–41.

Chiba J, Ohba H et al., 1991, Serodiagnosis of hepatitis C virus (HCV) infection with an HCV core protein molecularly expressed by a recombinant baculovirus, *Proc Natl Acad Sci USA*, **88**: 4641–5.

Choo QL, Kuo G et al., 1989, Isolation of a cDNA derived from a blood-borne non-A, non-B hepatitis genome, *Science*, **244**: 359–62.

Choo QL, Richman KH et al., 1991, Genetic organization and diversity of the hepatitis C virus, *Proc Natl Acad Sci USA*, **88**: 2451–5.

Choo QL, Kuo G et al., 1994, Vaccination of chimpanzees against infection by the hepatitis C virus, *Proc Natl Acad Sci USA*, **91**: 1294–8.

Chung RT, Kawashima T, Kaplan LM, 1995, Expressed hepatitis C virus NS5b exhibits RNA-dependent RNA polymerase activity, *3rd International Meeting on Hepatitis C and Related Viruses*, Brisbane, Australia, September, Abstract C7.

Collett MS, Larson R et al., 1988, Molecular cloning and nucleotide sequence of the pestivirus bovine viral diarrhoea virus, *Virology*, **165**: 191–9.

Colombo M, Kuo G et al., 1989, Prevalence of antibodies to hepatitis C virus in Italian patients with hepatocellular carcinoma, *Lancet*, **2**: 1006–8.

Contreras M, Barbara JA et al., 1991, Low incidence of non-A, non-B post-transfusion hepatitis in London confirmed by hepatitis C virus serology, *Lancet*, **337**: 753–7.

Courouce A, Janot C, Hepatitis Study Group FSBT, 1991, Recombinant immunoblot assay first and second generations on 732 blood donors reactive for antibodies to hepatitis C virus by ELISA, *Vox Sang*, **61**: 177–80.

Courouce AM, Le Marrec N et al., 1994, Anti-hepatitis C virus (anti-HCV) seroconversion in patients undergoing hemodialysis: comparison of second- and third-generation anti-HCV assays, *Transfusion*, **34**: 790–5.

Courouce AM, Barin F et al., 1995, A comparative evaluation of the sensitivity of seven anti-hepatitis C virus screening tests, *Vox Sang*, **69**: 213–16.

Craske J, Paver WK, Farmer D, 1993, An algorithm for confirming screen reactivity in blood donors in enzyme immunoassays for antibodies to hepatitis C virus, *J Immunol Methods*, **160**: 227–35.

Crawford RJ, Gillon J et al., 1994, Prevalence and epidemiological characteristics of hepatitis C in Scottish blood donors, *Transfusion Med*, **4**: 121–4.

Daikos GL, Lai S, Fischl MS, 1994, Hepatitis C virus infection in a sexually active inner city population – the potential for heterosexual transmission, *Infection*, **22**: 72–6.

Damen M, Zaaijer HL et al., 1995, Reliability of the third-generation recombinant immunoblot assay for hepatitis C virus, *Transfusion*, **35**: 745–9.

Darwish MA, Raouf TA et al., 1993, Risk factors associated with a high seroprevalence of hepatitis C virus infection in Egyptian blood donors, *Am J Trop Med Hyg*, **49**: 440–7.

Davidson F, Simmonds P et al., 1995, Survey of major genotypes and subtypes of hepatitis C virus using RFLP of sequences amplified from the 5′ non-coding region, *J Gen Virol*, **76**: 1197–204.

Davis GL, Balart LA et al., 1989, Treatment of chronic hepatitis C with recombinant interferon α. A multicenter randomized, controlled trial. Hepatitis Interventional Therapy Group, *N Engl J Med*, **321**: 1501–6.

Demitri MS, Poussin K et al., 1995, HCV-associated liver cancer without cirrhosis, *Lancet*, **345**: 413–15.

Dhaliwal SK, Prescott LE et al., 1996, Influence of viraemia and genotype upon serological reactivity in screening assays for antibody to hepatitis C virus, *J Med Virol*, **48**: 184–90.

Di Bisceglie AM, Martin P et al., 1989, Recombinant interferon α therapy for chronic hepatitis C. A randomized, double-blind, placebo-controlled trial, *N Engl J Med*, **321**: 1506–10.

Di Bisceglie AM, Shindo M, Fong TL, 1992, A pilot study of ribavirin therapy for chronic hepatitis C, *Hepatology*, **16**: 649–54.

Dow BC, Coote I et al., 1993, Confirmation of hepatitis C virus antibody in blood donors, *J Med Virol*, **41**: 215–20.

Dow BC, Follett EAC et al., 1994, Failure of 2nd- and 3rd-generation HCV ELISA and RIBA to detect HCV polymerase chain reaction-positive donations, *Vox Sang*, **67**: 236–7.

Dow BC, Buchanan I et al., 1996a, Relevance of RIBA-3 supplementary test to HCV PCR positivity and genotypes in HCV confirmation of blood donors, *J Med Virol*, **49**: 132–6.

Dow BC, Munro H et al., 1996b, Third-generation recombinant immunoblot assay: comparison of reactives according to hepatitis B virus genotype, *Transfusion*, **36**: 547–51.

Dubuisson J, Hsu HH et al., 1994, Formation and intracellular localization of hepatitis C virus envelope glycoprotein complexes expressed by recombinant vaccinia and Sindbis viruses, *J Virol*, **68**: 6147–60.

Eckart MR, Selby M et al., 1993, The hepatitis C virus encodes a serine protease involved in processing of the putative non-structural proteins from the viral polyprotein precursor, *Biochem Biophys Res Commun*, **192**: 399–406.

Enomoto N, Takada A et al., 1990, There are two major types of hepatitis C virus in Japan, *Biochem Biophys Res Commun*, **170**: 1021–5.

Enomoto N, Sakuma I et al., 1995, Comparison of full-length sequences of interferon-sensitive and resistant hepatitis C virus 1b – sensitivity to interferon is conferred by amino acid substitutions in the NS5a region, *J Clin Invest*, **96**: 224–30.

Esteban JI, Gonzalez A et al., 1990, Evaluation of antibodies to hepatitis C virus in a study of transfusion-associated hepatitis, *N Engl J Med*, **323**: 1107–12.

Esteban JI, Lopez Talavera JC et al., 1991, High rate of infectivity and liver disease in blood donors with antibodies to hepatitis C virus, *Ann Intern Med*, **115**: 443–9.

Failla C, Tomei L, Defrancesco R, 1995, An amino-terminal domain of the hepatitis C virus NS3 protease is essential for interaction with NS4A, *J Virol*, **69**: 1769–77.

Farci P, Alter HJ et al., 1992, Lack of protective immunity against reinfection with hepatitis C virus, *Science*, **258**: 135–40.

Feinstone SM, Kapikian AZ, Purcell RH, 1975, Transfusion-associated hepatitis not due to viral hepatitis A or B, *N Engl J Med*, **292**: 767–70.

Felsenstein J, 1993, *PHYLIP Inference Package version 3.5*, Department of Genetics, University of Washington, Seattle.

Ferrari C, Valli A et al., 1994, T-cell response to structural and nonstructural hepatitis C virus antigens in persistent and self-limited hepatitis C virus infections, *Hepatology*, **19**: 286–95.

Follett EAC, Dow BC et al., 1991, HCV confirmatory testing of blood donors, *Lancet*, **338**: 1024.

Fried MW, Hoofnagle JH, 1993, Therapy of hepatitis C, *Semin Liver Dis*, **341**: 1501–4.

Fukushi S, Katayama K et al., 1994, Complete 5′ noncoding region is necessary for the efficient internal initiation of hepatitis C virus RNA, *Biochem Biophys Res Commun*, **199**: 425–32.

Gane E, Tibbs CJ et al., 1995, Ribavirin therapy for hepatitis C infection following liver transplantation, *Transplant Intern*, **8**: 61–4.

Garson JA, Clewley JP et al., 1992, Hepatitis C viraemia in United Kingdom blood donors – a multicentre study, *Vox Sang*, **62**: 218–23.

Gilletterver MN, Modiano P et al., 1995, Periarthrite nodosa revealing chronic active hepatitis, *Presse Med*, **24**: 1221.

Gonzalez A, Esteban JI et al., 1995, Efficacy of screening donors for antibodies to the hepatitis C virus to prevent transfusion-associated hepatitis: final report of a prospective trial, *Hepatology*, **22**: 439–45.

Gordon SC, Elloway RS et al., 1993, The pathology of hepatitis C as a function of mode of transmission – blood transfusion vs intravenous drug use, *Hepatology*, **18**: 1338–43.

Grakoui A, Mccourt DW et al., 1993a, Characterization of the hepatitis C virus-encoded serine proteinase – determination of proteinase-dependent polyprotein cleavage sites, *J Virol*, **67**: 2832–43.

Grakoui A, Mccourt DW et al., 1993b, A second hepatitis C virus-encoded proteinase, *Proc Natl Acad Sci USA*, **90**: 10583–7.

Grakoui A, Wychowski C et al., 1993c, Expression and identification of hepatitis C virus polyprotein cleavage products, *J Virol*, **67**: 1385–95.

Hallam NF, Fletcher ML et al., 1993, Low risk of sexual transmission of hepatitis C virus, *J Med Virol*, **40**: 251–3.

Healey CJ, Sabharwal NK et al., 1994, Outbreak of acute hepatitis C following intravenous immunoglobulin therapy, *Hepatology*, **20**: 249A.

Healey CJ, Smith DB et al., 1995, Acute hepatitis C infection after sexual exposure, *Gut*, **36**: 148–50.

Herrero C, Vicente A et al., 1993, Is hepatitis C virus infection a trigger of porphyria cutanea tarda?, *Lancet*, **341**: 788–9.

Hijikata M, Kato N et al., 1991a, Hypervariable regions in the putative glycoprotein of hepatitis C virus, *Biochem Biophys Res Commun*, **175**: 220–8.

Hijikata M, Kato N et al., 1991b, Gene mapping of the putative structural region of the hepatitis C virus genome by in vitro processing analysis, *Proc Natl Acad Sci USA*, **88**: 5547–51.

Hijikata M, Mizushima H et al., 1993a, Two distinct proteinase activities required for the processing of a putative nonstructural precursor protein of hepatitis C virus, *J Virol*, **67**: 4665–75.

Hijikata M, Shimizu YK et al., 1993b, Equilibrium centrifugation studies of hepatitis C virus – evidence for circulating immune complexes, *J Virol*, **67**: 1953–8.

Honda M, Kaneko S et al., 1993, Risk of hepatitis C virus infections through household contact with chronic carriers – analysis of nucleotide sequences, *Hepatology*, **17**: 971–6.

Hopf U, Moller B et al., 1990, Long-term follow-up of posttransfusion and sporadic chronic hepatitis non-A, non-B and frequency of circulating antibodies to hepatitis C virus (HCV), *J Hepatol*, **10**: 69–76.

Hosein B, Fang CT et al., 1991, Improved serodiagnosis of hepatitis C virus infection with synthetic peptide antigen from capsid protein, *Proc Natl Acad Sci USA*, **88**: 3647–51.

Irving WL, Neal KR et al., 1994, Chronic hepatitis in United Kingdom blood donors infected with hepatitis C virus, *Br Med J*, **308**: 695–6.

Ishida C, Matsumoto K et al., 1993, Detection of antibodies to hepatitis C virus (HCV) structural proteins in anti-HCV-positive sera by an enzyme-linked immunosorbent assay using synthetic peptides as antigens, *J Clin Microbiol*, **31**: 936–40.

Japanese Red Cross Non-A Non-B Hepatitis Research Group, 1991, Effect of screening for hepatitis C virus antibody and hepatitis B virus core antibody on the incidence of post-transfusion hepatitis, *Lancet*, **338**: 1040–1.

Jarvis LM, Watson HG et al., 1994, Frequent reinfection and reactivation of hepatitis C virus genotypes in multitransfused hemophiliacs, *J Infect Dis*, **170**: 1018–22.

Johnson RJ, Gretch DR et al., 1993, Membranoproliferative glomerulonephritis associated with hepatitis C virus infection, *N Engl J Med*, **328**: 465–70.

Jones AP, Meech RJ et al., 1992, Hepatitis C: the tracing dilemma, *Transfusion Med*, **327**: 910–15.

Kaito M, Watanabe S et al., 1994, Hepatitis C virus particle detected by immunoelectron microscopic study, *J Gen Virol*, **75**: 1755–60.

Kamel MA, Ghaffar YA et al., 1992, High HCV prevalence in Egyptian blood donors, *Lancet*, **340**: 427.

Kato N, Hijikata M et al., 1990, Molecular cloning of the human hepatitis C virus genome from Japanese patients with non-A, non-B hepatitis, *Proc Natl Acad Sci USA*, **87**: 9524–8.

Kato N, Ootsuyama Y et al., 1992, Marked sequence diversity in the putative envelope proteins of hepatitis C viruses, *Virus Res*, **22**: 107–23.

Kato N, Sekiya H et al., 1993, Humoral immune response to hypervariable region-1 of the putative envelope glycoprotein (gp70) of hepatitis C virus, *J Virol*, **67**: 3923–30.

Kato N, Nakazawa T et al., 1995, Susceptibility of human T-lymphotropic virus type I infected cell line MT-2 to hepatitis C virus infection, *Biochem Biophys Res Commun*, **206**: 863–9.

Kiyosawa K, Sodeyama T et al., 1990, Interrelationship of blood transfusion, non-A, non-B hepatitis and hepatocellular carcinoma: analysis by detection of antibody to hepatitis C virus, *Hepatology*, **12**: 671–5.

Klein RS, Freeman K et al., 1991, Occupational risk for hepatitis C virus infection among New York City dentists, *Lancet*, **338**: 1539–42.

Knodell RG, Ishak KG et al., 1981, Formulation and application of a numerical scoring system for assessing histological activity in asymptomatic chronic active hepatitis, *Hepatology*, **1**: 431–5.

Kolykhalov AA, Agapov EV, Rice CM, 1994, Specificity of the hepatitis C virus NS3 serine protease: effects of substitutions

at the 3/4a, 4a/4b, 4b/5a, and 5a/5b cleavage sites on polyprotein processing, *J Virol*, **68**: 7525–33.

Komoda Y, Hijikata M et al., 1994, Substrate requirements of hepatitis C virus serine proteinase for intermolecular polypeptide cleavage in *Escherichia coli*, *J Virol*, **68**: 7351–7.

Koonin EV, 1991, The phylogeny of RNA-dependent RNA polymerases of positive-strand RNA viruses, *J Gen Virol*, **72**: 2197–206.

Koziel MJ, Dudley D et al., 1992, Intrahepatic cytotoxic T lymphocytes specific for hepatitis-C virus in persons with chronic hepatitis, *J Immunol*, **149**: 3339–44.

Koziel MJ, Dudley D et al., 1993, Hepatitis C virus (HCV)-specific cytotoxic T lymphocytes recognize epitopes in the core and envelope proteins of HCV, *J Virol*, **67**: 7522–32.

Kuo G, Choo QL et al., 1989, An assay for circulating antibodies to a major etiologic virus of human non-A, non-B hepatitis, *Science*, **244**: 362–4.

Lai ME, Mazzoleni AP et al., 1994, Hepatitis C virus in multiple episodes of acute hepatitis in polytransfused thalassaemic children, *Lancet*, **343**: 388–90.

Lam JPH, McOmish F et al., 1993, Infrequent vertical transmission of hepatitis C virus, *J Infect Dis*, **167**: 572–6.

Lampertico P, Rumi M et al., 1994, A multicenter randomized controlled trial of recombinant interferon-α2b in patients with acute transfusion-associated hepatitis C, *Hepatology*, **19**: 19–22.

Lanford RE, Sureau C et al., 1994, Demonstration of in vitro infection of chimpanzee hepatocytes with hepatitis C virus using strand-specific RT/PCR, *Virology*, **202**: 606–14.

Lanford RE, Chavez D et al., 1995, Lack of detection of negative-strand hepatitis C virus RNA in peripheral blood mononuclear cells and other extrahepatic tissues by the highly strand-specific rTth reverse transcriptase PCR, *J Virol*, **69**: 8079–83.

Larsen J, Skaug K, Maeland A, 1992, Second generation anti-HCV tests predict infectivity, *Vox Sang*, **63**: 39–42.

Lau JYN, Mizokami M et al., 1995, Application of six hepatitis C virus genotyping systems to sera from chronic hepatitis C patients in the United States, *J Infect Dis*, **171**: 281–9.

Lau JYN, Simmonds P, Urdea MS, 1995, Implications of variations of 'conserved' regions of hepatitis C virus genome, *Lancet*, **346**: 425–6.

Lau JYN, Krawczynski K et al., 1996, In situ detection of hepatitis C virus: a critical appraisal, *J Hepatol*, **24, Suppl. 2**: 43–51.

Leary TP, Muerhoff AS et al., 1996, Sequence and genomic organisation of GBV-C: a novel member of the *Flaviviridae* associated with non-A–E hepatitis, *J Med Virol*, **48**: 60–7.

Lee SR, Wood CL et al., 1995, Increased detection of hepatitis C virus infection in commercial plasma donors by a third-generation screening assay, *Transfusion*, **35**: 845–9.

Leinbach SS, Bhat RA et al., 1994, Substrate specificity of the NS3 serine proteinase of hepatitis C virus as determined by mutagenesis at the NS3/NS4a junction, *Virology*, **204**: 163–9.

Lelie PN, Cuypers HTM et al., 1992, Patterns of serological markers in transfusion-transmitted hepatitis C virus infection using 2nd-generation HCV assays, *J Med Virol*, **37**: 203–9.

Lerat H, Berby F et al., 1996, Specific detection of hepatitis C virus minus-strand RNA in haematopoietic cells, *J Clin Invest*, **97**: 845–51.

Lesniewski RR, Boardway KM et al., 1993, Hypervariable 5'-terminus of hepatitis C virus E2/NS1 encodes antigenically distinct variants, *J Med Virol*, **40**: 150–6.

Lin C, Pragai BM et al., 1994, Hepatitis C virus NS3 serine proteinase: *trans*-cleavage requirements and processing kinetics, *J Virol*, **68**: 8147–57.

Linnen J, Wages J et al., 1996, Molecular cloning and disease association of hepatitis G virus: a transfusion-transmissible virus, *Science*, **271**: 505–8.

McOmish F, Chan S-W et al., 1993, Detection of three types of hepatitis C virus in blood donors: investigation of type-

specific differences in serological reactivity and rate of alanine aminotransferase abnormalities, *Transfusion*, **33**: 7–13.

McOmish F, Yap PL et al., 1994, Geographical distribution of
hepatitis C virus genotypes in blood donors – an international
collaborative survey, *J Clin Microbiol*, **32**: 884–92.

Mahaney K, Tedeschi V et al., 1994, Genotypic analysis of hepatitis C virus in American patients, *Hepatology*, **20**: 1405–11.

Mannucci PM, 1993, Clinical evaluation of viral safety of coagulation factor VIII and IX concentrates, *Transfusion*, **64**: 197–
203.

Mansell CJ, Locarnini SA, 1995, Epidemiology of hepatitis C in
the east, *Semin Liver Dis*, **15**: 15–32.

Martin P, 1993, Hepatitis C – more than just a liver disease, *Gastroenterology*, **104**: 320–3.

Matsuura Y, Suzuki T et al., 1994, Processing of E1 and E2 glycoproteins of hepatitis C virus expressed in mammalian and
insect cells, *Virology*, **205**: 141–50.

Meisel H, Reip A et al., 1995, Transmission of hepatitis C virus to
children and husbands by women infected with contaminated
anti-D immunoglobulin, *Lancet*, **345**: 1209–11.

Mellor J, Holmes EC et al., 1995, Investigation of the pattern of
hepatitis C virus sequence diversity in different geographical
regions: implications for virus classification, *J Gen Virol*, **76**:
2493–507.

Miller RH, Purcell RH, 1990, Hepatitis C virus shares amino acid
sequence similarity with pestiviruses and flaviviruses as well
as members of two plant virus supergroups, *Proc Natl Acad Sci
USA*, **87**: 2057–61.

Minutello MA, Pileri P et al., 1993, Compartmentalization of T
lymphocytes to the site of disease – intrahepatic CD4+ T-cells
specific for the protein NS4 of hepatitis C virus in patients
with chronic hepatitis C, *J Exp Med*, **178**: 17–25.

Mishiro S, Takeda K et al., 1991, An autoantibody cross-reactive
to hepatitis C virus core and a host nuclear antigen, *Autoimmunity*, **10**: 269–73.

Misiani R, Bellavita P et al., 1994, Interferon-α2a therapy in cryoglobulinemia associated with hepatitis C virus, *N Engl J Med*,
330: 751–6.

Miyamoto H, Okamoto H et al., 1992, Extraordinarily low density
of hepatitis C virus estimated by sucrose density gradient centrifugation and the polymerase chain reaction, *J Gen Virol*, **73**:
715–18.

Mizushima H, Hijikata M et al., 1994, Analysis of N-terminal processing of hepatitis C virus nonstructural protein 2, *J Virol*,
68: 2731–4.

Mondelli MU, Cerino A et al., 1994, Hepatitis C virus (HCV)
core serotypes in chronic HCV infection, *J Clin Microbiol*, **32**:
2523–7.

Mori S, Kato N et al., 1992, A new type of hepatitis C virus in
patients in Thailand, *Biochem Biophys Res Commun*, **183**: 334–
42.

Muerhoff AS, Leary TP et al., 1995, Genomic organization of
GB viruses A and B: two new members of the *Flaviviridae* associated with GB agent hepatitis, *J Virol*, **69**: 5621–30.

Mutimer D, Shaw J et al., 1995a, Failure to incriminate hepatitis
B, hepatitis C, and hepatitis E viruses in the aetiology of fulminant non-A non-B hepatitis, *Gut*, **36**: 433–6.

Mutimer DJ, Harrison RF et al., 1995b, Hepatitis C virus infection in the asymptomatic British blood donor, *J Viral Hepatitis*,
2: 47–53.

Nalpas B, Romeo R et al., 1995, Serum hepatitis C virus (HCV)
RNA: a reliable tool for evaluating HCV-related liver disease
in anti-HCV positive blood donors with persistently normal
alanine aminotransferase values, *Transfusion*, **35**: 750–3.

Nasoff MS, Zebedee SL et al., 1991, Identification of an immunodominant epitope within the capsid protein of hepatitis C
virus, *Proc Natl Acad Sci USA*, **88**: 5462–6.

Nishiguchi S, Kuroki T et al., 1995, Randomised trial of effects
of interferon-α on incidence of hepatocellular carcinoma in
chronic active hepatitis C with cirrhosis, *Lancet*, **346**: 1051–5.

Nishioka K, Watanabe J et al., 1991, A high prevalence of anti-

body to the hepatitis C virus in patients with hepatocellular
carcinoma in Japan, *Cancer*, **67**: 429–33.

Novati R, Thiers V et al., 1992, Mother-to-child transmission of
hepatitis C virus detected by nested polymerase chain reaction, *J Infect Dis*, **165**: 720–3.

Ogata N, Alter HJ et al., 1991, Nucleotide sequence and
mutation rate of the H strain of hepatitis C virus, *Proc Natl
Acad Sci USA*, **88**: 3392–6.

Ohto H, Terazawa S et al., 1994, Transmission of hepatitis C
virus from mothers to infants, *N Engl J Med*, **330**: 744–50.

Okamoto H, Okada S et al., 1991, Nucleotide sequence of the
genomic RNA of hepatitis C virus isolated from a human carrier: comparison with reported isolates for conserved and
divergent regions, *J Gen Virol*, **72**: 2697–704.

Okamoto H, Kojima M et al., 1992a, Genetic drift of hepatitis C
virus during an 8.2 year infection in a chimpanzee: variability
and stability, *Virology*, **190**: 894–9.

Okamoto H, Kurai K et al., 1992b, Full-length sequence of a
hepatitis C virus genome having poor homology to reported
isolates: comparative study of four distinct genotypes, *Virology*,
188: 331–41.

Okamoto H, Sugiyama Y et al., 1992c, Typing hepatitis C virus
by polymerase chain reaction with type-specific primers:
application to clinical surveys and tracing infectious sources,
J Gen Virol, **73**: 673–9.

Okamoto H, Tokita H et al., 1993, Characterization of the genomic sequence of type V (or 3a) hepatitis C virus isolates and
PCR primers for specific detection, *J Gen Virol*, **74**: 2385–90.

Omata M, Yokosuka O et al., 1991, Resolution of acute hepatitis
C after therapy with natural beta interferon, *Lancet*, **338**:
914–15.

Pawlotsky JM, Roudot-Thoraval F et al., 1995, Influence of hepatitis C virus (HCV) genotypes on HCV recombinant immunoblot assay patterns, *J Clin Microbiol*, **33**: 1357–9.

Pereira BJG, Milford EL et al., 1992, Prevalence of hepatitis-C
virus RNA in organ donors positive for hepatitis-C antibody
and in the recipients of their organs, *N Engl J Med*, **327**:
910–15.

van der Poel CL, Reesink HW et al., 1990, Infectivity of blood
seropositive for hepatitis C virus antibodies, *Lancet*, **335**:
558–60.

van der Poel CL, Cuypers HT et al., 1991, Confirmation of hepatitis C virus infection by new four-antigen recombinant immunoblot assay, *Lancet*, **337**: 317–19.

van der Poel CL, Bresters D et al., 1992, Early anti-hepatitis C
virus response with 2nd generation C200/C22 ELISA, *Vox
Sang*, **62**: 208–12.

Poole TL, Wang CY et al., 1995, Pestivirus translation initiation
occurs by internal ribosome entry, *Virology*, **206**: 750–4.

Power JP, Lawlor E et al., 1994, Hepatitis C viraemia in recipients
of Irish intravenous anti-D immunoglobulin, *Lancet*, **344**:
1166–7.

Power JP, Lawlor E et al., 1995, Molecular epidemiology of an
outbreak of infection with hepatitis C virus in recipients of
anti-D immunoglobulin, *Lancet*, **345**: 1211–13.

Prince AM, Brotman B et al., 1974, Long incubation post-transfusion hepatitis with evidence of exposure to hepatitis B virus,
Lancet, **2**: 241–6.

Prince AM, Brotman B et al., 1992, Immunity in hepatitis C
infection, *J Infect Dis*, **165**: 438–43.

Ralston R, Thudium K et al., 1993, Characterization of hepatitis
C virus envelope glycoprotein complexes expressed by recombinant vaccinia viruses, *J Virol*, **67**: 6753–61.

Reichard O, Andersson J et al., 1991, Ribavirin treatment for
chronic hepatitis C, *Lancet*, **337**: 1058–61.

Rice CM, Lenches EM et al., 1985, Nucleotide sequence of yellow
fever virus: implications for flavivirus gene expression and
evolution, *Science*, **229**: 726–33.

Rice PS, Smith DB et al., 1993, Heterosexual transmission of
hepatitis C virus, *Lancet*, **342**: 1052–3.

Saeed AA, al Admawi AM et al., 1991, Hepatitis C virus infection in Egyptian volunteer blood donors in Riyadh, *Lancet*, **338**: 459–60.

Sallberg M, Ruden U et al., 1992, Immunodominant regions within the hepatitis C virus core and putative matrix proteins, *J Clin Microbiol*, **30**: 1989–94.

Santolini E, Migliaccio G et al., 1994, Biosynthesis and biochemical properties of the hepatitis C virus core protein, *J Virol*, **68**: 3631–41.

Schupper H, Hayashi P et al., 1993, Peripheral-blood mononuclear cell responses to recombinant hepatitis C virus antigens in patients with chronic hepatitis C, *Hepatology*, **18**: 1055–60.

Seef LB, Buskell-Bales Z et al., 1992, Long term mortality after transfusion-associated non-A, non-B hepatitis, *N Engl J Med*, **327**: 1906–11.

Selby MJ, Choo QL et al., 1993, Expression, identification and subcellular localization of the proteins encoded by the hepatitis C viral genome, *J Gen Virol*, **74**: 1103–13.

Selby MJ, Glazer E et al., 1994, Complex processing and protein:protein interactions in the E2:NS2 region of HCV, *Virology*, **204**: 114–22.

Setoguchi Y, Kajihara S et al., 1994, Analysis of nucleotide sequences of hepatitis C virus isolates from husband–wife pairs, *J Gastroenterol Hepatol*, **9**: 468–71.

Shimizu YK, Yoshikura H, 1994, Multicycle infection of hepatitis C virus in cell culture and inhibition by alpha and beta interferons, *J Virol*, **68**: 8406–8.

Shimizu YK, Weiner AJ et al., 1990, Early events in hepatitis C virus infection of chimpanzees, *Proc Natl Acad Sci USA*, **87**: 6441–4.

Shimizu YK, Iwamoto A et al., 1992, Evidence for in vitro replication of hepatitis C virus genome in a human T-cell line, *Proc Natl Acad Sci USA*, **89**: 5477–81.

Shimizu YK, Purcell RH, Yoshikura H, 1993, Correlation between the infectivity of hepatitis C virus in vivo and its infectivity in vitro, *Proc Natl Acad Sci USA*, **90**: 6037–41.

Simmonds P, 1995, Variability of hepatitis C virus, *Hepatology*, **21**: 570–83.

Simmonds P, Holmes EC et al., 1993a, Classification of hepatitis C virus into six major genotypes and a series of subtypes by phylogenetic analysis of the NS-5 region, *J Gen Virol*, **74**: 2391–9.

Simmonds P, McOmish F et al., 1993b, Sequence variability in the 5′ non coding region of hepatitis C virus: identification of a new virus type and restrictions on sequence diversity, *J Gen Virol*, **74**: 661–8.

Simmonds P, Rose KA et al., 1993c, Mapping of serotype-specific, immunodominant epitopes in the NS-4 region of hepatitis C virus (HCV) – use of type-specific peptides to serologically differentiate infections with HCV type 1, type 2, and type 3, *J Clin Microbiol*, **31**: 1493–503.

Simmonds P, Alberti A et al., 1994, A proposed system for the nomenclature of hepatitis C viral genotypes, *Hepatology*, **19**: 1321–4.

Simons JN, Leary TP et al., 1995a, Isolation of novel virus-like sequences associated with human hepatitis, *Nature Med*, **1**: 564–9.

Simons JN, Pilot-Matias TJ et al., 1995b, Identification of two flavivirus-like genomes in the GB hepatitis agent, *Proc Natl Acad Sci USA*, **92**: 3401–5.

Smith DB, Mellor J et al., 1995, Variation of the hepatitis C virus 5′ non-coding region: implications for secondary structure, virus detection and typing, *J Gen Virol*, **76**: 1749–61.

Smith DB, Davidson F et al., 1996, Levels of hepatitis C virus in blood donors infected with different viral genotypes, *J Infect Dis*, **173**: 727–30.

Soto B, Rodrigo L et al., 1994, Heterosexual transmission of hepatitis C virus and the possible role of coexistent human immunodeficiency virus infection in the index case – a multicentre study of 423 pairings, *J Intern Med*, **236**: 515–19.

Stott EJ, Almeida JD, O'Reilly KJ, 1974, Characterisation of mucosal disease virus as a togavirus by electronmicroscopy, *Microbios*, **11A**: 79–83.

Stuyver L, Rossau R et al., 1993, Typing of hepatitis C virus isolates and characterization of new subtypes using a line probe assay, *J Gen Virol*, **74**: 1093–102.

Stuyver L, Vanarnhem W et al., 1994, Classification of hepatitis C viruses based on phylogenetic analysis of the envelope 1 and nonstructural 5b regions and identification of five additional subtypes, *Proc Natl Acad Sci USA*, **91**: 10134–8.

Sugiyama K, Kato N et al., 1995, Novel genotypes of hepatitis C virus in Thailand, *J Gen Virol*, **76**: 2323–7.

Takamizawa A, Mori C et al., 1991, Structure and organization of the hepatitis C virus genome isolated from human carriers, *J Virol*, **65**: 1105–13.

Tanaka M, Sato S et al., 1995, Clinical study of IgA antibody against hepatitis C virus core antigen in patients with type C chronic liver disease, *Dig Dis Sci*, **40**: 457–64.

Tanaka T, Tsukiyamakohara K et al., 1994, Significance of specific antibody assay for genotyping of hepatitis C virus, *Hepatology*, **19**: 1347–53.

Tanaka T, Kato N et al., 1995, A novel sequence found at the end of the 3′ terminus of hepatitis C virus genome, *Biochem Biophys Res Commun*, **215**: 744–9.

Taniguchi S, Okamoto H et al., 1993, A structurally flexible and antigenically variable N terminal domain of the hepatitis C virus e2/NS1 protein – implication for an escape from antibody, *Virology*, **195**: 297–301.

Tanji Y, Hijikata M et al., 1994, Identification of the domain required for *trans*-cleavage activity of hepatitis C viral serine proteinase, *Gene*, **145**: 215–19.

Tanji Y, Hijikata M et al., 1995, Hepatitis C virus-encoded nonstructural protein NS4a has versatile functions in viral protein processing, *J Virol*, **69**: 1575–81.

Tedder RS, Gilson RJC et al., 1991, Hepatitis C virus: evidence for sexual transmission, *Br Med J*, **302**: 1299–302.

Telfer P, Sabin C et al., 1994, The progression of HCV-associated liver disease in a cohort of haemophilic patients, *Br J Haematol*, **87**: 555–61.

Thomssen R, Bonk S et al., 1992, Association of hepatitis C virus in human sera with beta-lipoprotein, *Med Microbiol Immunol*, **181**: 293–300.

Thomssen R, Bonk S, Thiele A, 1993, Density heterogeneities of hepatitis C virus in human sera due to the binding of beta-lipoproteins and immunoglobulins, *Med Microbiol Immunol*, **182**: 329–34.

Tisminetzky SG, Gerotto M et al., 1994, Genotypes of hepatitis C virus in Italian patients with chronic hepatitis C, *Int Hepatol Commun*, **2**: 105–12.

Tobler LH, Busch MP et al., 1994, Evaluation of indeterminate c22-3 reactivity in volunteer blood donors, *Transfusion*, **34**: 130–4.

Tokita H, Okamoto H et al., 1994, Hepatitis C virus variants from Vietnam are classifiable into the seventh, eighth, and ninth major genetic groups, *Proc Natl Acad Sci USA*, **91**: 11022–6.

Tokita H, Okamoto H et al., 1995, Hepatitis C virus variants from Thailand classifiable into five novel genotypes in the sixth (6b), seventh (7c, 7d) and ninth (9b, 9c) major genetic groups, *J Gen Virol*, **76**: 2329–35.

Tomei L, Failla C et al., 1993, NS3 is a serine protease required for processing of hepatitis C virus polyprotein, *J Virol*, **67**: 4017–26.

Tsubota A, Chayama K et al., 1994, Factors predictive of response to interferon-alpha therapy in hepatitis C virus infection, *Hepatology*, **19**: 1088–94.

Tsukiyama Kohara K, Iizuka N et al., 1992, Internal ribosome entry site within hepatitis C virus RNA, *J Virol*, **66**: 1476–83.

Tsukiyama Kohara K, Yamaguchi K et al., 1993, Antigenicities of group I and group II hepatitis C virus polypeptides – molecular basis of diagnosis, *Virology*, **192**: 430–7.

Utsumi T, Hashimoto E et al., 1995, Heterosexual activity as a risk factor for the transmission of hepatitis C virus, *J Med Virol*, **46**: 122–5.

Uyttendaele S, Claeys H et al., 1994, Evaluation of third-generation screening and confirmatory assays for HCV antibodies, *Vox Sang*, **66**: 122–9.

Vrielink H, van der Poel CL et al., 1995a, Transmission of hepatitis C virus by anti-HCV-negative blood transfusion – case report, *Vox Sang*, **68**: 55–6.

Vrielink H, van der Poel CL et al., 1995b, Look-back study of infectivity of anti-HCV ELISA-positive blood components, *Lancet*, **345**: 95–6.

Vrielink H, Zaaijer HL et al., 1995c, Comparison of two anti-hepatitis C virus enzyme-linked immunosorbent assays, *Transfusion*, **35**: 601–4.

Wang CY, Sarnow P, Siddiqui A, 1993, Translation of human hepatitis C virus RNA in cultured cells is mediated by an internal ribosome-binding mechanism, *J Virol*, **67**: 3338–44.

Wang CY, Sarnow P, Siddiqui A, 1994, A conserved helical element is essential for internal initiation of translation of hepatitis C virus RNA, *J Virol*, **68**: 7301–7.

Wang CY, Le SY et al., 1995, An RNA pseudoknot is an essential structural element of the internal ribosome entry site located within the hepatitis C virus 5′ noncoding region, *RNA*, **1**: 526–37.

Warrener P, Collett MS, 1995, Pestivirus NS3 (p80) protein possesses RNA helicase activity, *J Virol*, **69**: 1720–6.

Weiner AJ, Geysen HM et al., 1992, Evidence for immune selection of hepatitis C virus (HCV) putative envelope glycoprotein variants: potential role in chronic HCV infections, *Proc Natl Acad Sci USA*, **89**: 3468–72.

Weiner AJ, Thaler MM et al., 1993, A unique, predominant hepatitis C virus variant found in an infant born to a mother with multiple variants, *J Virol*, **67**: 4365–8.

Weiner A, Erickson AL et al., 1995, Persistent hepatitis C virus infection in a chimpanzee is associated with emergence of a cytotoxic T lymphocyte escape variant, *Proc Natl Acad Sci USA*, **92**: 2755–9.

Wejstal R, Widell A et al., 1992, Mother-to-infant transmission of hepatitis C virus, *Ann Intern Med*, **117**: 887–90.

Wreghitt TG, Gray JJ et al., 1994, Transmission of hepatitis C virus by organ transplantation in the United Kingdom, *J Hepatol*, **20**: 768–72.

Wright HI, Gavaler JS, van Theil DH, 1992, Preliminary experience with alpha-2b-interferon therapy of viral hepatitis in liver allograft recipients, *Transplantation*, **53**: 121–4.

Wright TL, Hsu H et al., 1991, Hepatitis C virus not found in fulminant non-A, non-B hepatitis, *Ann Intern Med*, **115**: 111–2.

Wright TL, Donegan E et al., 1992, Recurrent and acquired hepatitis C viral infection in liver transplant recipients, *Gastroenterology*, **103**: 317–22.

Yoo BJ, Spaete RR et al., 1992, 5′ end-dependent translation initiation of hepatitis C viral RNA and the presence of putative positive and negative translational control elements within the 5′ untranslated region, *Virology*, **191**: 889–99.

Yoo BJ, Selby MJ et al., 1995, Transfection of a differentiated human hepatoma cell line (huh7) with in vitro-transcribed hepatitis C virus (HCV) RNA and establishment of a long-term culture persistently infected with HCV, *J Virol*, **69**: 32–8.

Yuki N, Hayashi N et al., 1992, Improved serodiagnosis of chronic hepatitis C in Japan by a 2nd-generation enzyme-linked immunosorbent assay, *J Med Virol*, **37**: 237–40.

Yun ZB, Lindh G et al., 1993, Detection of hepatitis C virus (HCV) RNA by PCR related to HCV antibodies in serum and liver histology in Swedish blood donors, *J Med Virol*, **39**: 57–61.

Zaaijer HL, Cuypers HTM et al., 1994a, New immunoblot resolves indeterminate results for antibody to hepatitis C virus, *Transfusion*, **34**: 184.

Zaaijer HL, Vrielink H et al., 1994b, Confirmation of hepatitis C infection: a comparison of five immunoblot assays, *Transfusion*, **34**: 603–7.

Zuckerman J, Clewley G et al., 1994, Prevalence of hepatitis C antibodies in clinical health-care workers, *Lancet*, **343**: 1618–20.

Chapter 36

HEPATITIS B

M Kann and W H Gerlich

1 Introduction	3 Clinical and pathological aspects
2 Properties of the virus	

1 INTRODUCTION

Epidemic jaundice was described by the Babylonians, but the infectious nature of the disease and the involvement of the liver were not recognized until the late nineteenth century. In general it was believed that bad living conditions, particularly during wars, generated the catarrhal jaundice. In 1885, Lürmann observed an outbreak of jaundice 2–8 months after people had been given smallpox vaccine. This outbreak was probably caused by hepatitis B virus, the vaccine having been prepared from human lymph. A larger outbreak of hepatitis caused by vaccination occurred in 1937 when soldiers developed severe jaundice after receiving a yellow fever vaccine containing human serum (Findlay and MacCallum 1937). On the basis of epidemiological studies, 2 types of agents were suggested: type A, causing large outbreaks via the faecal–oral route, and type B, transmitted mainly by human serum. Hepatitis B was therefore also called serum hepatitis. During the 1970s it became apparent that more than one virus species may transmit hepatitis parenterally (hepatitis C virus (HCV), HDV and possibly HGV or GB-C virus), but the first identified virus of parenterally transmissible hepatitis was called hepatitis B virus (HBV).

Early efforts to identify HBV failed because it did not grow in tissue cultures or the usual experimental animals. Only humans and chimpanzees are reliably susceptible to HBV. Thus, HBV was not discovered by these methods. The surface protein of HBV was discovered accidentally in 1965 during the search by an anthropologist for polymorphic serum proteins as genetic markers in the blood of an Australian aborigine (Blumberg, Alter and Visnich 1965), and was called Australia antigen. Two years later the association between the occurrence of the Australia antigen and serum hepatitis infection was detected (Blumberg et al. 1967). Australia antigen was exposed at the surface of pleomorphic, spherical or filamentous 20 nm

particles, which did not contain nucleic acid and were therefore probably not infectious agents. Among the more numerous particles, Dane and colleagues (Dane, Cameron and Briggs 1970) detected some larger double-shelled virus-like particles 42 nm in diameter (Fig. 36.1). The surface of these so-called Dane particles cross-reacted with antibodies against Australia antigen. Their significance as the potential viral agent of hepatitis B was confirmed by the detection of antibodies against the inner shell, termed core or nucleocapsid, of the Dane particle in patients with acute hepatitis B. The core antigen was called HBcAg; the Australia antigen was called hepatitis B surface antigen or HBsAg, inducing the corresponding antibodies anti-HBc and anti-HBs. Anti-HBc is a serological marker for previous and current HBV infections, whereas HBsAg is a marker for a current HBV infection. Using these epidemiological markers it became apparent that HBV is a common human pathogen that causes acute and chronic liver disease throughout the world, particularly in southeast Asia and Central Africa. Chronic illness develops in 5–10% of infected adolescents or adults, but in up to 90% of infected neonates. Chronic HBV infection is a major cause of liver cirrhosis and primary liver cell carcinoma (Beasley et al. 1981, Robinson, Miller and Marion 1987). About half of the world's population has had contact with HBV.

2 PROPERTIES OF THE VIRUS

2.1 Classification

In 1973, an endogenous DNA polymerase activity (i.e. an enzyme that incorporates nucleotides into DNA without addition of an exogenous template) was discovered within Dane particles. The endogenous template was a circular partially double-stranded DNA of c. 3200 nucleotides (nt). It was found that the DNA

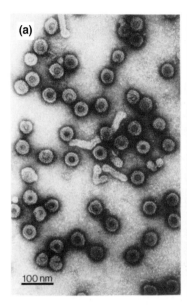
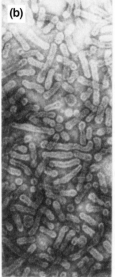
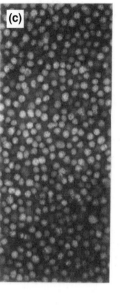

Fig. 36.1 Electron microscopy of (**a**) hepatitis B viruses (Dane particles), (**b**) HBs filaments and (**c**) 20 nm particles purified from HBV carrier plasma. Note the double-shelled structure of the HBV particles. Bar = 100 nm.

strand of negative polarity was transcribed inside the core particle from an encapsidated RNA-template, suggesting a similarity to retroviruses (Summers and Mason 1982).

The observation that liver carcinoma occurred in the Eastern woodchuck (a marmot of the North American east coast) led to the discovery of the HBV-like woodchuck hepatitis virus (WHV) and the closely related ground squirrel hepatitis virus (GSHV). HBV-like viruses were also found in Pekin ducks (DHBV), grey herons (HHBV) and have been reported in Arctic squirrels. All these viruses are highly species specific; for example, the heron HBV does not infect ducks, and the woodchuck virus does not infect ground squirrels. Some of these animal models are very useful for elucidating the replication and pathogenesis of HBV. The great molecular and biological similarity of these viruses led to the definition of a common virus family, *Hepadnaviridae* (from *hepa*, liver, and DNA, for the type of the genome) (Howard et al. 1995). The mammalian viruses form the genus *Orthohepadnavirus* (HBV, WHV, GSHV). Because of significant structural differences the avian viruses form a separate genus, *Avihepadnavirus* (DHBV, HHBV).

Although the genome organization, biology and replication of hepadnaviruses are quite different from those of the *Retroviridae*, the common strategy of reverse transcription places them and the *Caulimoviridae* of plants (Toh, Hayashida and Miyata 1983) into one group (which could possibly be defined as virus order 'retrovirales'). *Hepadnaviridae* and *Caulimoviridae* with their DNA genomes have also been called pararetroviruses, in contrast to the orthoretroviruses with an RNA genome.

2.2 Morphology and structure

All 5 well characterized hepadnavirus species are double-shelled particles of c. 42 nm diameter (Fig. 36.1). In mammalian hepadnaviruses the surface of the virions consists of c. 240 subunits comprising 5

different membrane-spanning proteins, termed L(arge), M(iddle) and S(mall) surface (HBs) proteins (Fig. 36.2; and see Fig. 36.7). These proteins are carboxy-terminally co-terminal and differ in additional amino-terminal domains. Thus, LHBs consists of an S domain and a preS domain (i.e. preS1 plus preS2 domain) (Heermann et al. 1984). The preS domain of LHBs can be localized externally or internally (Bruss et al. 1994). MHBs contains only the preS2 and the S domain and SHBs consists only of the S domain (Fig. 36.2). Because all proteins can be glycosylated at one or 2 positions, 6 different proteins, GP42, P39, GP36, GP33, GP27 and P24 kDa, can be distinguished whereby G indicates glycosylation and the number the molecular weight. Compared with the amount of core particles, these HBs proteins are overexpressed and assemble either to subviral spheres of 20 nm diameter or to filamentous structures, depending on the composition of the different surface proteins (Fig. 36.2). In serum samples of highly viraemic individuals, these particles can be found in up to a 1000-fold excess.

In contrast to the mammalian hepadnaviruses, the avian hepadnaviruses have only a large 36 kDa and a small 18 kDa surface protein and thus do not have division of the preS domain into preS1 and preS2 subdomains. Like the mammalian hepatitis B viruses, these proteins are overexpressed, resulting in the secretion of spherical particles of c. 60 nm diameter.

Both the virion and the surface antigen particle are assembled at the endoplasmic reticulum (ER) and bud to the lumen of a post-ER intermediate compartment. Thus the lipid in the outer protein shell or the HBs particles is derived from an intracellular compartment and not from the plasma membrane. In contrast to other enveloped viruses the lipid content seems to be lower, resulting in a relatively high density of 1.16 g/ml in sucrose. Furthermore, the HBs subunits of blood plasma-derived HBs particles are cross-linked by disulphide bonds and do not disassemble after the addition of detergent.

Within virions the surface proteins enclose the core

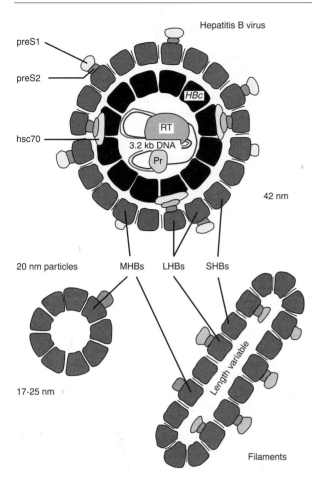

preS1

preS2

Hepatitis B virus

HBc

hsc70

RT

3.2 kb DNA

Pr

42 nm

20 nm particles

MHBs LHBs SHBs

17-25 nm

Length variable

Filaments

Fig. 36.2 Schematic presentation of hepatitis B virus. DNA. DNA is drawn as a single or double line. Structural proteins: the viral polymerase is depicted in grey with a priming domain (Pr) and the catalytic domain (RT). The nucleocapsid (core or HBc) is shown in black. Each block represents a dimer; 90 or 120 dimers comprise a particle. The surface proteins are shown in grey, with a dark grey S domain, a middle grey preS2 domain and a light grey preS1 domain. For the topology of the surface proteins, see Fig. 36.7. The virus particles also contain the cellular chaperone hsc70.

which encapsidates the viral genome. The core particles probably interact with the internally localized preS domain of LHBs (Figs. 36.2 and 36.7d), eventually mediated by the heat shock protein hsc70, which has been found at the internally localized preS domain of DHBV. The core protein consists of c. 185 amino acids (HBV) with a basic carboxy-terminus of 4 arginine-rich clusters, localized inside the lumen of the particles. The core molecules form dimers in the cytosol, which are linked by disulphide bridges after release from the reducing environment in the cytosol (Jeng, Hu and Chang 1991). Ninety or 120 dimers assemble spontaneously, so that 2 populations of core particles appear, having an icosahedral structure with a T = 3 and a T = 4 symmetry (Crowther et al. 1994, Kenney et al. 1995). In a patient's liver or in other eukaryotic cells, but not in bacteria, the assembly of the core particles is combined with the encapsidation of a cellular protein kinase C (PKC) (Kann and Gerlich 1994).

In human liver, or artificial genome-expressing cell cultures, most core particles encapsidate a complex of the pregenomic RNA and the viral polymerase. The polymerase transcribes the pregenomic RNA into a negative DNA strand, which is used as the template for second strand DNA synthesis. The viral polymerase consists of 4 domains: (1) the priming domain; (2) a so-called spacer or tether; (3) the reverse transcriptase domain, which catalyses RNA-dependent DNA synthesis; and (4) the RNase H domain, which degrades the RNA from the resulting DNA–RNA hybrid (for review, see Nassal and Schaller 1996). Because HBV DNA in infected hepatocytes remains unintegrated as an episomal minichromosome (Newbold et al. 1995) the HBV polymerase is, in contrast to retroviral polymerases, devoid of an integrase domain. Furthermore, no protease domain has been identified such as is found in retroviruses.

2.3 Genome structure and function

The HBV genome consists of a circular, partially double-stranded DNA in which the longer strand of negative polarity is c. 3200 nt long (Fig. 36.3). The 5′ end of this strand has a terminal redundancy of 8–10 nt. It is covalently bound to the primer domain of the viral polymerase. The polymerase presents the hydroxyl residue of tyrosine 96 (DHBV) or tyrosine 63 (HBV) as the acceptor for phosphodiester linkage to the first nucleotide of the negative DNA strand. The 5′ and 3′ end of this DNA strand are not covalently linked. The circular structure is caused by base pairing of the negative with the positive DNA strand at the discontinuity around the 2 ends of the negative DNA strand. The positive DNA strand has a defined 5′ end c. 230 nt (HBV) upstream of the 3′ end of the negative DNA strand. The 5′ end is linked to a capped RNA oligonucleotide, 18 nt long, which acts as a primer for second strand DNA synthesis and represents the undegraded 5′ end of the pregenomic RNA (see section 2.4, p. 748, and Fig. 36.3). The length of the positive DNA strand varies between 1100 and 2600 nt, depending on how far the viral polymerase has proceeded. Therefore a single-stranded region of 600–2100 nt is left and this gap can be partially filled in vitro by the viral polymerase after the addition of deoxynucleotides.

Cloning and sequencing of HBV DNA by many groups of workers confirmed the physical structure of the DNA. The genome of wild type orthohepadnaviruses contains 4 conserved, partially overlapping, open reading frames (ORFs) (Fig. 36.3), all on the negative DNA strand (Schlicht and Schaller 1989). Thus, the coding capacity of the 3200 nt corresponds to 5500 nt (had the ORFs been arranged in a linear manner). The ORFs encode:

1. The core protein and an additional precore region which includes a signal peptide sequence; this additional precore peptide results in a secreted, proteolytically modified form of the core protein, called HBe (see section 2.5, p. 755).

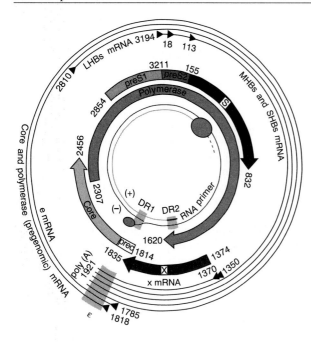

Fig. 36.3 Genome organization of the genus *Orthohepadnavirus* (HBV, WHV, GSHV). The HBV genome (isolate 991) is represented in the centre with a negative DNA strand and an incomplete positive DNA strand, as is found in mature viruses. The structural elements direct repeat 1 and 2 are designated DR1 and DR2. The primer domain of the viral polymerase is drawn as a separate protein although it is covalently linked to the polymerase. The ORFs are drawn with corresponding start and termination sites according to the notation of Galibert et al. (1979). In the outer region the transcribed HBV RNAs are shown. The black triangles represent the different 5′ ends of the RNAs; the common 3′ end is located at position 1921, followed by a ≈300 b poly(A) sequence. The primary sequence of the encapsidation signal ε is drawn as a dotted box.

2   The DNA polymerase.
3   The nested set of surface proteins.
4   A protein of unknown function, X protein (HBx), which is absent in the avian hepadnaviruses.

The expression of the ORFs is controlled by at least 4 promoters, enhancers I and II (for review, see McLachlan 1991), glucocorticoid-responsive elements, a partially leaky polyadenylation signal, and a genome region that suppresses splicing of the transcribed RNAs (Huang and Liang 1993). Due to the viral replication strategy, 2 direct repeats (DR) of 11 nt (mammalian hepadnaviruses) or 12 nt (avian hepadnaviruses) exist, termed DR1 and DR2 (Fig. 36.3) (see section 2.4, below).

2.4   Replication

OVERVIEW OF THE VIRAL LIFE CYCLE

Figure 36.4 outlines the essential steps in the viral life cycle. The mode of attachment and entry is not known. In Fig. 36.4 endocytosis and the release of capsids from endosomes are shown as a possible mechanism. Because hepadnaviruses multiply via RNA generated by the cellular RNA polymerase II, the DNA

genome must be uncoated and transported into the nucleus. From this DNA at least 5 or 4 different sets of mRNAs are synthesized in mammalian or avian hepadnaviruses respectively. For genome replication, one mRNA species of supergenomic length is used. This mRNA is first translated into core protein and, in an overlapping reading frame, into the viral polymerase. This RNA can then specifically interact with the viral polymerase and this RNA–polymerase complex is specifically encapsidated by the core protein into particles. Within the core particle the encapsidated RNA serves thereafter as the template for reverse transcription and is therefore also called pregenomic RNA. The core particle containing the mature DNA genome can be either enveloped into the surface proteins and secreted as mature virus into the blood stream or released into the nucleus of the infected cell, leading to an amplification of the episomal viral DNA.

ATTACHMENT

Because HBV can be produced by non-primate liver cells after transfection of the naked HBV genome, the high species specificity of the virus must be determined by the attachment and uptake of the virus into the hepatocytes. These studies have been hampered by the lack of susceptible established hepatocyte cell lines for all the *Hepadnaviridae*. Therefore, a variety of different techniques, such as the infection of primary hepatocyte cultures and binding to liver plasma membranes, have been used to search for the receptor. Subviral HBsAg filaments rich in LHBs bind strongly to liver plasma membranes, while 20 nm particles, consisting mainly of SHBs, bind to a much lesser degree (Pontisso et al. 1989). Inhibition of the binding with monoclonal antibodies against amino acids 31–34 of the preS1 domain (Pontisso et al. 1989) or inhibition of in vitro uptake with antibodies against amino acids 21–47 (Neurath, Strick and Sproul 1992) confirmed the importance of LHBs. Persistently infected patients may contain natural viable HBV variants, which are devoid of MHBs (Fernholz et al. 1993), whereas infectious variants devoid of L- or SHBs have never been observed. Thus, attachment mediated by LHBs or SHBs, or both, seems to be essential. Infection experiments with HDV in vitro (hepatitis D virus uses the surface proteins of HBV as envelope) confirmed that MHBs was, in contrast to LHBs, dispensable for infection (Sureau and Lanford 1993). Because the preS1 domain represents the additional sequence, differentiating LHBs from MHBs, attachment is probably mediated by preS1.

These data on HBV are in accord with investigations on DHBV, which does not possess an MHBs. Here, LHBs also mediates the attachment to the cell surface (Ishikawa et al. 1994). Furthermore, LHBs, at least in DHBV, determines host and tissue specificity. Heron HBV became infectious for ducks when its preS region was replaced by the DHBV preS region (Kuroki et al. 1994). However, several studies suggest SHBs as the essential ligand for hepadnaviral attachment (de Bruin et al. 1994, Hertogs et al. 1994, Mehdi et al.

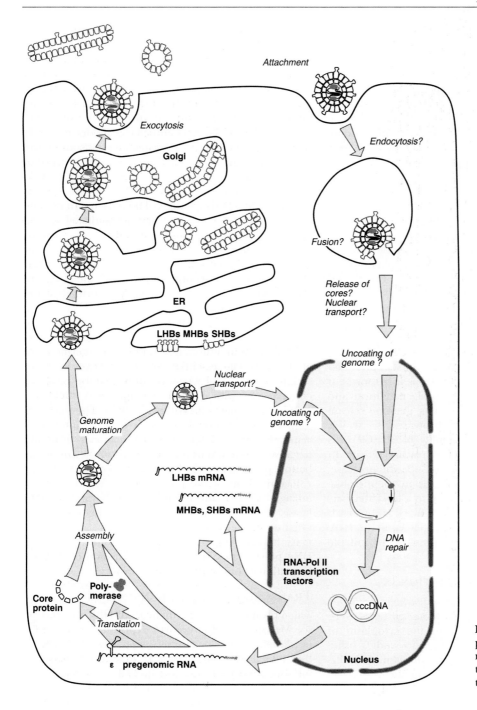

Fig. 36.4 Schematic presentation of the HBV replication cycle. Details of the Figure are given in the text (p. 748).

1994), using the same types of experiments used to obtain the results described above.

The non-essential preS2 domain of MHBs may have a supportive function in viral attachment. An enhancement of viral attachment to human liver membranes, mediated by the binding of preS2 to monomeric or polymerized human serum albumin (pHSA), was observed. Hepatocytes have receptors for polymerized serum albumin (Trevisan et al. 1988) and the preS2 domain binds in a species-specific manner to human or chimpanzee albumin (Machida et al. 1984). Fibronectin of human liver sinusoids is also a ligand for preS2 (Budkowska et al. 1995). It is noteworthy that mammalian hepadnaviruses have conserved MHBs with a glycosylated surface-exposed preS2 domain.

At the time of writing the published data on the viral receptors for HBV are inconclusive and are, therefore, not discussed here. For DHBV a membrane-bound carboxypeptidase was identified as part of a receptor (Kuroki et al. 1995).

VIRUS UPTAKE

Most research on virus uptake has used primary hepatocyte cultures. In contrast to the established hepatic cell lines, these hepatocytes are susceptible for the first days after being taken into culture. In primary duck hepatocytes, *de novo* synthesized DHBV is secreted 2 days after infection. These data were confirmed for primary woodchuck hepatocytes by infection with WHV and GSHV and for HBV, using primary human hepatocytes of fetal or adult origin. In all experiments only c. 10% of the cells were susceptible. This rate can be extended artificially to nearly 100% by adding dimethyl sulphoxide or polyethylene glycol to the culture medium. These treatments also extend susceptibility of the primary duck hepatocytes for at least 2 weeks.

Treatment of primary duck hepatocytes with lysosomatropic agents and actin-depolymerizing and energy-depleting substances showed that both energy depletion, and actin depolymerization completely prevented uptake of DHBV, whereas lysosomatropic agents had no effect. Thus, an endocytotic pathway without the necessity of an acidic intracellular pH is postulated for DHBV uptake (Köck, Borst and Schlicht 1996).

Besides the limited availability of human, primate or marmot liver, the cultivation of primary hepatocytes remains difficult. Therefore, infection of well established human hepatoma cell lines, such as HEp-G2 cells, has been attempted. These cells bound and internalized the virions in a preS1-dependent way, but replication did not occur (Qiao, Macnaughton and Gowans 1994). As with adenoviruses, genome release may involve viral or cellular proteases, so it was assumed that the non-susceptibility of HepG2 cells might be caused by the lack of a protease activity. In fact, treatment of HBV with a Glu–C-specific protease, which cleaves adjacent to a fusion peptide-like sequence within the S domain, led to a low infectivity of the viruses for HepG2 cells (Lu, Block and Gerlich 1996). Thus, the susceptibility of cell lines for HBV may also be determined by the presence of suitable proteases.

NUCLEAR ENTRY AND FORMATION OF EPISOMAL VIRAL DNA

Using immune histology, HBV core particles were found in both the nucleus and the cytoplasm of infected patients' hepatocytes. In vitro studies using HepG2 cells showed nuclear and cytoplasmic localization of the particles, dependent on the cell cycle. Core protein contains a nuclear localization signal on its carboxy-terminal portion. However, several observations make it unlikely that the entire core particle enters the nucleus:

1 Core particles consist of 2 populations, of 30 nm and 34 nm diameter. Because nuclear pores have an upper limit of c. 25 nm, nuclear transport of core particles seems to be impossible.
2 Core particles from human liver nuclei have a low density and are devoid of nucleic acids.
3 Core particles of rodent and avian hepadnaviruses do not accumulate in the nucleus.
4 In mice transgenic for HBV core, core particles are almost exclusively localized in the nucleus (Guidotti et al. 1994).

In transgenic mice the appearance of cytosolic cores is strictly correlated with cell division, indicating that the assembled core particles are not able to cross the nuclear membrane. These data indicate that (1) the nuclear core particles have been assembled from dimers of core protein **within** the nucleus and (2) genome release from the infecting core particle occurs before nuclear transport. In vitro assays using digitonin-permeabilized cells indicate a model in which phosphorylated core particles mediate transport of the encapsidated genome to the nuclear pore. Because of the size of HBV core particles a disassembly of particle structure must be proposed, resulting in the release of polymerase–DNA complex. The subsequent passage through the nuclear pore may be mediated by the viral polymerase (Kann, Bischof and Gerlich 1997).

In order to initiate expression of viral proteins and genome replication the partially double-stranded DNA genome with its protein primer at the 5′ end of the negative DNA strand and its RNA primer at the 5′ end of viral positive strand must be converted to a covalently closed circular (ccc) DNA. After infection, formation of cccDNA occurs as a first marker of successful infection, followed by replication intermediates after 24 h. The essential role of cccDNA for transcription of viral RNAs was confirmed by infecting chimpanzees with cloned, circular HBV DNA via intrahepatic injection (Will et al. 1985). The following steps for the generation of cccDNA are implied: (1) removal of the 5′ terminal redundancies from the negative strand and deproteinization of the covalently bound polymerase; (2) removal of the RNA primer; (3) completion of the positive DNA strand; and (4) linkage of the 5′ and 3′ ends of each strand by DNA ligase. The positive DNA strand could theoretically be filled up by the viral polymerase, but treatment of primary hepatocytes with ddG, an inhibitor of cellular DNA polymerases, resulted in suppression of cccDNA formation (Köck and Schlicht 1993).

TRANSCRIPTION AND TRANSLATION

The 4 promoters and 2 enhancers of HBV (for review, see McLachlan 1991) control expression of at least 5 overlapping RNAs of different sizes (see Fig. 36.3) by the cellular RNA polymerase II. Like most eukaryotic mRNAs, the viral transcripts include a CAP structure at their 5′ terminus and are polyadenylated at their 3′ end. Because of the unique polyadenylation signal TATAAA, which is conserved in all mammalian hepadnaviruses, all viral transcripts share a common 3′ end. The transcripts contain many potential splice donor and acceptor sites, but they also contain a splice-suppressing sequence, homologous to the rev-responsive element of HIV. As in most eukaryotic mRNAs, only the first reading frame is efficiently translated. Thus, the different mRNAs are named after the first encoded ORF HBe-: HBc/pol-, preS1-, preS2/S- and X-RNA. Among these RNAs, 2 sets can be discriminated: RNAs of subgenomic length, encoding X and the surface proteins; and RNAs longer than the genome (supergenomic RNAs), encoding HBe, core and polymerase. Regulation of transcription from the HBV genome has been studied in great detail. A summary of the sites identified for various transcription factors is given in Fig. 36.5.

The HBx RNA, present only in mammalian hepadnaviruses, is c. 700 nt long, and starts at 2 closely situated initiation sites (Schaller and Fischer 1991). The presence of multiple binding sites for liver-specific transcription factors (hepatonuclear factors 3 and 4 = HNF3 and HNF4; C/EBP) (Fig. 36.5) in its promoter, which overlaps the enhancer I, make it likely that the transcription of this RNA is regulated in a tissue-specific manner, but it can also be expressed in a large variety of non-hepatic cell lines.

The major transcript of the HBV genome of c. 2.1 kb does not contain a clearly defined 5′ end, and is well transcribed in a large variety of hepatic and non-hepatic cell lines. This subspecies of mRNA contains the preS2 and S regions with their start codons, resulting in the expression of MHBs when the first AUG is used. In most translation events, the second AUG is used, leading to the expression of the major surface protein, SHBs. Its promoter is called preS2/S promoter and consists mainly of ubiquitous SP1 binding sites, which explains the wide variety of cell lines and tissues in which the SHBs can be expressed.

Enh1/X promoter

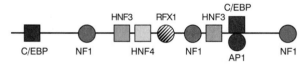

Enh2/c promoter

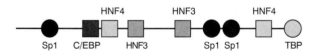

preS1 promoter

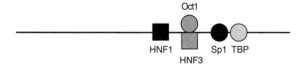

preS2/S promoter

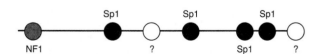

Fig. 36.5 Binding sites for transcription factors in the enhancers and promoters of hepatitis B virus. AP1: activator protein 1; C/EBP: CCAAT/enhancer binding protein; HNF4: hepatocyte nuclear factor 4; NF1: nuclear factor 1; Sp1: SV40 promotor protein 1; TBP: TATA-box binding protein. Squares represent liver specific/liver enriched transcription factors; circles represent ubiquitous transcription factors. (After McLachlan personal communication.)

In contrast to the above-mentioned transcripts, the LHBs-encoding mRNA of c. 2.4 kb is transcribed in a liver-specific manner (Antonucci and Rutter 1989), requiring the presence of the liver-specific transcription factors HNF1 and 3. Because the expression of the encoded LHBs protein is essential for virus secretion (Bruss and Ganem 1991), activation of the LHBs promoter seems to be an essential element in HBV-host cell restriction. In DHBV-transfected cells and DHBV-infected ducks a common additional spliced mRNA is found, with the start site of the pregenomic transcript, which seems to be essential for virus production (Obert et al. 1996). Because the resulting mRNA is the same length as the major LHBs mRNA, splicing of a 1.1 kb intron seems to be most probable.

Two sets of supergenomic mRNAs exist, both of c. 3.3 kb in length, being terminally redundant in c. 150 nt. Owing to the redundancy of the RNAs, the polyadenylation signal, localized downstream of the AUG of the core ORF, must be ignored on the first passage of the transcription machinery. Apparently, this phenomenon is caused by the surrounding nucleotide sequences and by the length of the upstream region (Cherrington, Russnak and Ganem 1992).

The transcription of these supergenomic RNAs is controlled by the core promoter, which is liver specific owing to the presence of C/EBP and HNF3 and HNF4 binding sites. This promoter initiates the transcription of a subset of 2 classes of RNAs, which differ by c. 30 nt at their 5′ end but have completely different biological functions. Only the longer mRNAs contain the AUG start codon of the preC region at their 5′ end, which is in frame with the AUG of the core reading frame. Therefore, these RNAs encode a primary translation product that differs from the core protein by 29 additional amino acids at the amino-terminal end. This additional domain, called preC, contains a hydrophobic sequence that serves as a signal sequence for secretion into the ER (see section 2.5, p. 755).

For genome replication, only the other supergenomic transcript is essential which does not contain the preC AUG, but includes the initiation AUG at nt 1900 for core protein (Ou et al. 1990). From this RNA, the overlapping pol ORF, beginning 407 nt downstream of the core AUG, is also translated, probably with less efficiency. In contrast to retroviruses which also have overlapping polymerase and nucleocapsid ORFs, expression of hepadnaviral polymerase occurs by *de novo* translational initiation and not by ribosomal frameshifting (Chang, Ganem and Varmus 1990). The exact mechanism of pol translation remains unsolved because conflicting evidence has been reported for both an internal entry of the ribosomes at or near the pol AUG and for leaky scanning from the 5′ end of core/pol mRNA.

ASSEMBLY OF THE VIRAL NUCLEOCAPSID AND GENOME MATURATION

Expression of the viral nucleocapsid in *Escherichia coli* leads to core particles that, by electron microscopy, are indistinguishable from natural nucleocapsids found in infected liver (Kenney et al. 1995). In these expression systems, devoid of any other viral protein, assembly is combined with non-specific encapsidation of RNA. Specific encapsidation of the pregenomic RNA, as it occurs in vivo, is mediated by the viral polymerase (Bartenschlager, Junker-Niepmann and Schaller 1990, Hirsch et al. 1990). Mutations throughout the whole polymerase gene affect the ability for specific RNA encapsidation, suggesting a complex interaction between viral polymerase with pregenomic RNA and the core particle in which other proteins such as the cellular chaperone Hsp90 may be involved (Hu and Seeger 1996).

An encapsidation signal ε of the pregenomic RNA was mapped within the preC region of DHBV and HBV (Nassal and Schaller 1996). Although ε is present in all HBV RNAs at the 3′ end and redundant at the 5′ and 3′ ends of the supergenomic transcripts, only the 5′ terminal ε supports encapsidation (Junker-Niepmann, Bartenschlager and Schaller 1990). ε forms a base-paired stem–loop (see Fig. 36.6a), conserved in its structure throughout all hepadnaviruses. Although ε seems to be sufficient for pregenome encapsidation by viral polymerase, additional sequence elements downstream increase the encapsidation efficiency (Hirsch et al. 1991, Calvert and Summers 1994). These elements may explain how the viral polymerase discriminates between the 5′ terminal ε from the 3′ terminal ε in the super- and subgenomic RNAs. The non-reactivity of the HBe mRNA despite the 5′ terminal ε in encapsidation is caused by the translating ribosomes on the HBe RNA which prevent the folding of ε or its interaction with the polymerase (Nassal, Junker-Niepman and Schaller 1990). This indicates that only complete, translating 80S ribosomes are able to displace the ε-bound polymerase, because the pregenomic RNA must be scanned by the 40S ribosomal initiation complex for the initiation of core protein synthesis.

In addition to the polymerase and the pregenomic RNA, a protein kinase is encapsidated within core particles (Gerlich et al. 1982). This activity is associated with nucleocapsids, even when expressing the core gene alone in insect cells (Lanford and Notvall 1990), and has been identified as protein kinase C (Kann and Gerlich 1994) phosphorylating the carboxy-terminal domain of the core protein inside the lumen of the core particle. Both in vitro and in vivo, phosphorylation inhibits interaction of nucleic acids and the core protein. Therefore phosphorylation probably occurs after encapsidation of pregenomic RNA (Kann and Gerlich 1994). Because phosphorylation is inhibited by RNA binding to the carboxy-terminus of the core proteins, RNA must be removed from the core, probably during reverse transcription. Thus, phosphorylation is presumably linked to genome maturation, and its function may be deduced by the significance of the carboxy-terminal region. Deletions in this region inhibit DNA maturation, probably caused by conformational changes of the core molecules (Yu and Summers 1994).

The complex events that convert the linear RNA pregenome to the circular double-stranded DNA in the virion are outlined in Fig. 36.6 (for review, see Ganem, Pollack and Tavis 1994). Previous observations on the endogenous polymerase activity suggested that this enzyme is active only within nucleocapsids. However, DHBV RNA, which contains the ε signal, and the polymerase ORF can be used in a cell-free translation system to express an active DHBV polymerase that can prime and elongate the first nucleotides of the negative-strand DNA (Wang and Seeger 1993). The polymerase starts at the bulge of the ε signal (Fig. 36.6a) and not, as originally concluded from primer extension experiments, within the 3′ terminal DR1. For the priming of the negative-strand DNA, the hydroxyl group of tyrosine 96 of the DHBV polymerase serves as the acceptor for the synthesis of a phosphodiester bridge with the first nucleotide. After the addition of the first 4 nt (DHBV) encoded by the bulge, the oligonucleotide polymerase complex dissociates from the bulge, and reanneals with a sequence complementary to the 3′ terminal DR1 (Fig. 36.6b). These findings were confirmed for the HBV polymerase by expression in yeast. However, because there are many complementary sequences to the 3 or 4 initial bases of the negative DNA strand within the hepadnavirus genomes, additional factors such as the primary and secondary structure of the surrounding RNA sequences of the DR1 as well as the distance between initiation site and DR1 regulate the transfer of the polymerase nucleotide complex from ε to the 3′ terminal DR1.

The process of genome maturation includes the steps of negative-strand DNA elongation by reverse transcription proceeding from DR1, followed by positive-strand DNA synthesis. These steps seem to occur only inside the lumen of the nucleocapsid. As with retroviruses, the elongation of the negative DNA strand is combined with degradation of the RNA strand in the resulting DNA–RNA hybrid.

Mapping of the 3′ end of the negative DNA strand showed that it nearly coincides with the 5′ end of the pregenomic RNA. Thus, the 3′ end of the negative DNA strand is obviously specified by 'run off', when the polymerase reaches the end of its RNA template, resulting in the terminal redundancy of the negative DNA strand of 8–10 nt (Fig. 36.6c).

The positive strand contains a 17–18 nt long 5′ capped RNA, covalently attached to its 5′ end. This RNA oligonucleotide is derived from the 5′ end of the pregenomic RNA and functions as a primer for synthesis at DR2 (Fig. 36.6d, e). Because the negative DNA strand which serves as a template for positive DNA strand synthesis is linear, second-strand synthesis could run off at the 5′ end of the template, but mature HBV genome in core particles is predominantly circular. Thus, the polymerase is able to bridge the gap between the 3′ and the 5′ end of the negative DNA strand. On the basis of its mutational analysis, a melting of the 3′ end of the positive DNA strand and the 5′ end of the negative DNA strand (Fig. 36.6f) was suggested, followed by an annealing of the 3′ end of the positive DNA strand with the complementary 3′

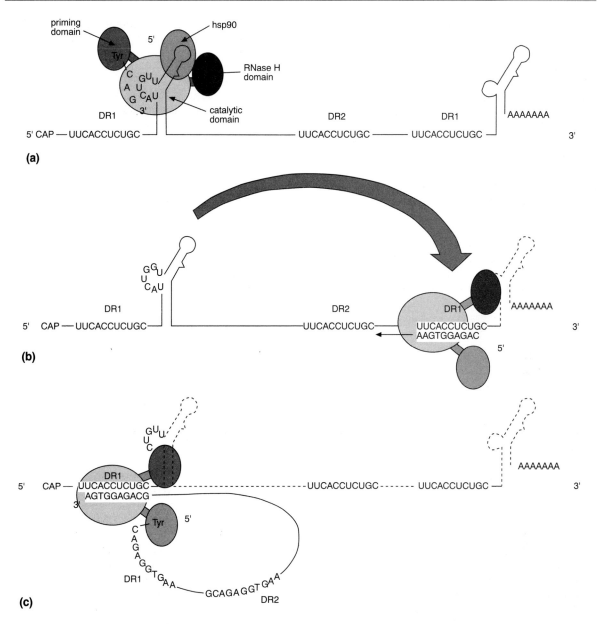

Fig. 36.6 Generation of the viral genome from the pregenomic RNA. (**a**) Binding of the viral polymerase and the cellular factor hsp90 to the encapsidation signal ε on the pregenomic RNA. Reverse transcription for the first 3 DNA nucleotides starts at the bulge of the stem–loop structure. The first nucleotide (C) is covalently linked to a hydroxyl group of a tyrosine within the priming domain of the polymerase. (**b**) Translocation (large arrow) of the polymerase–nucleotide complex to a complementary sequence on the DR1. Further negative DNA strand synthesis. (**c**) Completion of negative DNA strand synthesis. The degraded RNA template is depicted as a dotted line. The remaining undegraded RNA oligomer is shown in black.

end of the negative DNA strand (Fig. 36.6g) which allowed positive DNA strand synthesis to proceed (Fig. 36.6h).

ENVELOPMENT AND SECRETION OF HBV

Mature core particles may enter 2 different pathways which are important for the viral life cycle. Because the HBV cccDNA in the nucleus is subject to degradation, the pool of intranuclear HBV genomes must be restored permanently to ensure viral persistence. The restoration of the pool is usually possible either by new infection of the hepatocyte with HBV or by re-

entry of viral DNA after release from the viral nucleocapsid. Amplification of cccDNA between 10 and 50 copies per cell occurs even in cultured hepatocytes that are not susceptible to DHBV and HBV infection, so it obviously does not require re-infection but nuclear entry of viral genomes from newly synthesized core particles in the cytoplasm.

The second pathway for core particles is the envelopment into the surface proteins, followed by virus secretion. Mutants defective for envelope proteins but competent for replication lead to intranuclear cccDNA accumulation up to 50 times the natural copy

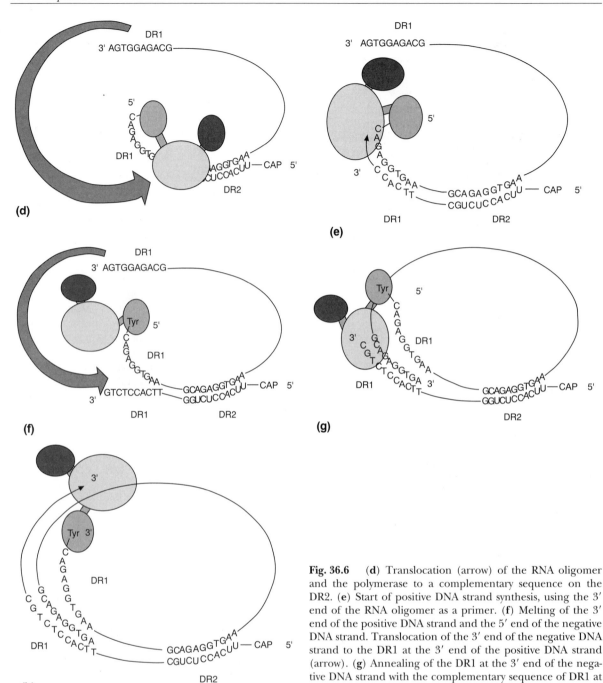

Fig. 36.6 (**d**) Translocation (arrow) of the RNA oligomer and the polymerase to a complementary sequence on the DR2. (**e**) Start of positive DNA strand synthesis, using the 3′ end of the RNA oligomer as a primer. (**f**) Melting of the 3′ end of the positive DNA strand and the 5′ end of the negative DNA strand. Translocation of the 3′ end of the negative DNA strand to the DR1 at the 3′ end of the positive DNA strand (arrow). (**g**) Annealing of the DR1 at the 3′ end of the negative DNA strand with the complementary sequence of DR1 at the 3′ end of the positive DNA strand (arrow). (**h**) Further positive DNA strand synthesis.

number. The expression of surface proteins results in enhanced encapsidation of core particles and secretion of virus, and regulates amplification of cccDNA (Summers, Smith and Horwich 1990). After *de novo* infection of hepatocytes, transcription of HBs mRNA is a late event (Tuttleman, Pourcel and Summers 1986). Thus, the regulation of cccDNA amplification via surface protein synthesis guarantees that a large pool of cccDNA has been generated in the infected cell, resulting in persistent infection.

In contrast to HDV, where only SHBs is required for assembly and secretion, assembly of HBV requires LHBs and SHBs (Bruss and Ganem 1991). Stepwise

truncation of LHBs showed that only sequences proximal to amino acid 108 of preS are required for HBV assembly. In the current model of HBV (Fig. 36.7c, d; and see Fig. 36.2), the preS domains in LHBs have a dual topology. The preS domain in part of the LHBs molecule is cytosolic; the other part is exposed at the surface of HBV, allowing multiple functions of LHBs:

1 Like matrix proteins of many other enveloped proteins, it mediates the budding of core particles together with their envelope proteins. For this task, a matrix protein must be fixed at the membrane, but its binding site for the viral capsid should be located on the cytosolic side.

2 The preS1 domain seems also to be the attachment site to the cell surface during infection. For this purpose the preS domain has to be accessible on the surface of the particle.

The mechanism by which the preS domain post-translationally passes through the ER or post-ER membrane is unclear. Direct passage through the lipid bilayer without the involvement of signal recognition particles (SRP) and secretion factors (sec) has been described for small amphipathic proteins, but the preS domain does not have this type of structure (Bruss et al. 1994). Another possibility for passing through the ER membrane may be the transport of the polypeptide chain through hydrophilic channels formed by the S domain. The S domain contains 4 or 5 putative transmembrane α-helices, 3 of which are amphipathic (Fig. 36.7). According to computer models, dimers of the S domain or the SHBs could assemble in a manner by which 6 amphipathic helices form a channel large enough for peptides to pass (Berting et al. 1995). Incubation at low pH favours translocation of interior preS domains to the surface of virions.

The forces that drive the budding and assembly of HBV and HBs particles are not yet well understood. The carboxy-terminal part and parts of the 2 hydrophilic loops in the S domain can be deleted or substituted, but most of the cysteine residues in the internal loop are essential. The high sequence conservation in the 4 α-helices suggest a coil-to-coil interaction which may contribute to the morphogenesis of virions and HBs particles (Berting et al. 1995).

The HBs particles mature in a pre-Golgi compartment. The *N*-linked glycoside of SHBs protein or the S domain is trimmed and modified to a complex biantennary oligosaccharide, whereas the preS2-linked glycan is of the hybrid type with one mannose chain and 2 modified chains (Lu and Gerlich 1995, unpublished). Cultivation of HBV-expressing cells with inhibitors of glucosidase I (e.g. *N*-butyldeoxynojirimycin) blocks the trimming and prevents the secretion of HBV (Block et al. 1994). MHBs is a specific target for this block of secretion (Lu et al. 1995). HBsAg 20 nm spheres are constitutively secreted. However, HBs-filaments may be retained in the ER if they contain more LHBs than SHBs. The retention signal resides in the preS1 region (Gallina, Gazina and Milanese 1995). MHBs does not significantly alter the secretion behaviour if properly glycosylated.

Certain hepatocytes in HBsAg carriers seem to overexpress LHBs, relative to SHBs, and contain a dilated ER which gives them a ground glass appearance under the light microscope. Such cells probably do not contribute to HBV production and are often found in so-called healthy HBsAg carriers with low viraemia (Dienes et al. 1990). Only cells that express core protein, polymerase, SHBs and LHBs protein in a well balanced mixture are able to assemble and secrete HBV.

2.5 Non-structural proteins

In contrast to the positive-strand RNA viruses that do not use reverse transcription, retroviruses and retrovirus-like viruses such as the hepadnaviruses do not use a major part of their coding capacity for non-structural proteins. However, LHBs and SHBs are not only essential structural components of the virion; they occur also as secreted antigens. Furthermore, MHBs is a non-essential structural protein of mammalian hepadnaviruses, which encode 2 further proteins that are not essential for replication in cell cultures, HBe protein and HBx protein. Avian HBVs do not have HBx protein. Neither HBe protein nor HBx protein has yet been identified as a structural component of the virions. They are therefore considered here as non-structural proteins, although their presence in low amounts in virions cannot be excluded.

HBs PROTEINS

A peculiarity of all wild type hepadnaviruses is expression of the HBs proteins in a large excess. Even in HBV carriers producing many virions, empty HBs particles are present in c. 1000-fold greater number than virions and may reach concentrations of 1 g/l, like major serum proteins such as IgM. In low viraemic HBsAg carriers, HBsAg may be present in particle numbers up to 10^{12}/ml even when HBV DNA is undetectable by PCR. Thus, in a way, HBs proteins are non-structural as well as structural proteins of the virions. HBsAg particles have a much longer half-life than virions, which disappear within 1 to 3 days from the serum if replication is blocked. However, HBV-transfected hepatoma cells also produce an excess of HBs proteins. Thus, the excess of non-structural HBs protein over virion-bound HBs protein is not only due to more rapid removal of virions from the circulation. The significance of this overexpression is not clear. It may contribute to an immune tolerance that is a precondition for highly productive persistent infection in an immunocompetent host. The excess HBs proteins may block the HBV receptors of the host during late or persistent stages of infection and thereby allow the circulation of virions, which is another precondition for efficient transmissibility. The long delay of several weeks or even months between infection and the first appearance of virions and HBs protein is probably due to the slow replication of HBV, but may also be due in part to immediate readsorption to receptors not yet blocked.

The proportion of HBs proteins is different in the 3 morphological forms of HBs particles. Virions contain a high proportion of LHBs, HBs filaments in intermediate amounts, but few 20 nm particles. The proportion of MHBs may be variable and is usually higher in HBs particles from high viraemic carriers.

HBe PROTEIN

HBe protein was discovered by the analysis of HBsAg-positive sera from different donors by double diffusion in agar gels (Magnius and Espmark 1972). Some HBsAg carriers contained a precipitating antibody

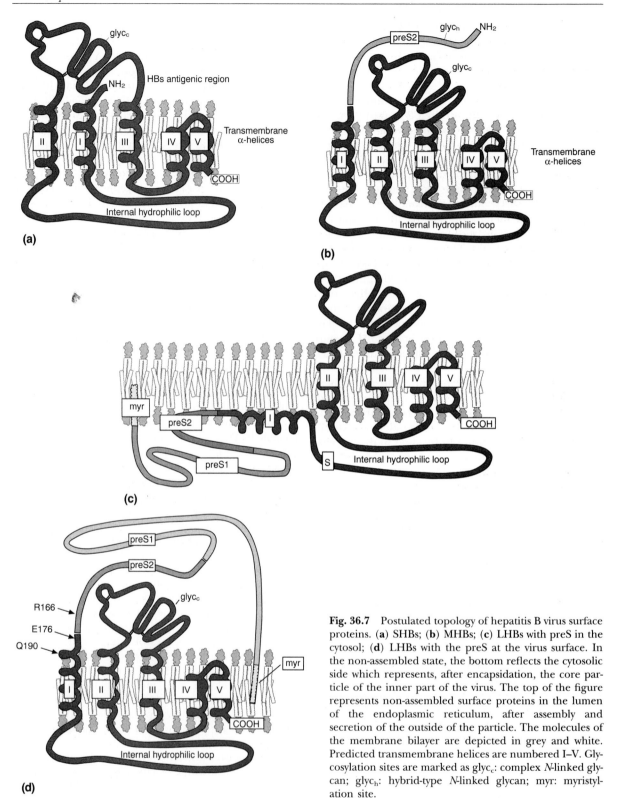

Fig. 36.7 Postulated topology of hepatitis B virus surface proteins. (**a**) SHBs; (**b**) MHBs; (**c**) LHBs with preS in the cytosol; (**d**) LHBs with the preS at the virus surface. In the non-assembled state, the bottom reflects the cytosolic side which represents, after encapsidation, the core particle of the inner part of the virus. The top of the figure represents non-assembled surface proteins in the lumen of the endoplasmic reticulum, after assembly and secretion of the outside of the particle. The molecules of the membrane bilayer are depicted in grey and white. Predicted transmembrane helices are numbered I–V. Glycosylation sites are marked as glyc$_c$: complex *N*-linked glycan; glyc$_h$: hybrid-type *N*-linked glycan; myr: myristylation site.

against a novel antigen called e antigen (HBeAg). HBeAg was found predominantly in highly productive HBV carriers with a detectable endogenous HBV DNA polymerase, whereas anti-HBe was usually found in 'healthy' low viraemic carriers. Sera from HBeAg-positive carriers typically have infectivity titres for chimpanzees of 10^8/ml or more and genome titres of 10^9–10^{10}/ml, whereas anti-HBe- and HBsAg-positive sera have only 10 infectious doses/ml (Shikata et al. 1977). The biochemical nature of HBe protein remained unclear until 1982, when recombinant HBc particles, devoid of any other viral component, were converted into HBeAg by treatment with protease and ionic detergents. Characterization of isolated HBe protein from the serum of HBV carriers revealed that it had an amino acid composition similar to that of HBc protein, but it was only c. 15 kDa owing to a carboxy-terminal truncation at val 149 of HBc.

It cannot be ruled out that a minor part of HBe protein in serum may be derived from degraded nucleocapsids or non-assembled HBc protein, but at least the major part of HBeAg, if not all, is generated by a biosynthetic pathway different from that of HBc protein. As mentioned in section 2.3 (p. 747), HBV-containing cells express, besides the pregenomic RNA, a slightly longer RNA which contains not only the AUG for the HBc protein but also the AUG for the preC region 29 codon upstream. The preC sequence has the property of a signal peptide which directs the nascent polypeptide to the membrane of the ER and causes its translocation to the ER lumen. The translocation is, however, incomplete, thus allowing the re-entry of part of the full-length HBe protein molecules with 25 kDa to the cytosol. This HBe protein may be transported to the nucleus because of its carboxy-terminal nuclear localization signals.

The major part of ER-associated HBe protein is cleaved at ala 19, thus generating a 22 kDa protein. During passage through the Golgi apparatus a protease cleaves HBe at val 149 or sites downstream, generating proteins of 16–18 kDa. This cleavage is a precondition for release from the cell. HBe protein may oligomerize but, in contrast to HBc, does not assemble to a closed particle. The tryptophane and cysteine residues in the remaining preC peptide prevent assembly to core-like particles (Schlicht and Wasenauer 1991). The amount of HBeAg in the serum of HBV carriers by far exceeds the amount of HBc protein within circulating virions. Titres in enzyme immune assay (EIA) often reach 1 : 8000, and detection by agar gel immune precipitation suggests amounts of several milligrams per millilitre. Thus, both major structural proteins HBs and HBc of the virion are accompanied by a large excess of slightly altered non-viral forms.

It is doubtful whether HBe protein has a direct function in the viral life cycle. The HBe mRNA does not support genome replication. HBe-negative mutated genomes of DHBV and WHV replicate in the natural hosts. Naturally occurring HBe-negative variants of HBV are present in many patients (see section 3, p. 759). It has even been found that preC-containing wild type genomes replicate less efficiently in transfected hepatoma cells than preC-negative genomes.

The conservation of HBe protein in all known hepadnaviruses in spite of its being non-essential suggests that it provides an important advantage for the survival and spread of hepadnaviruses in their host population. A clue to the function of HBe protein may be the observation that newborn woodchucks infected with an HBe-negative mutant develop acute but not chronic infection as occurs with wild type virus. It may be that HBe protein suppresses immune elimination of HBV, thus contributing to the development of a carrier state.

HBx PROTEIN

Mammalian hepadnaviruses encode a protein of 154 amino acids (141 in woodchuck and 138 in ground squirrel hepadnavirus), the function of which is essentially unknown. The absence of HBx in avian hepadnaviruses suggests that it is not essential for the molecular events during hepadnaviral replication but that it somehow alters the host organism in a way that it is more permissive for viral replication. HBx is not essential for efficient HBV production in transfected permanent cell lines (Yaginuma et al 1987) or primary rat hepatocyte cultures (Blum et al. 1992). However, WHV genomes without a functional *HBx* gene do not replicate efficiently in woodchucks (Chen et al. 1993, Zoulim, Saputelli and Seeger 1994). In some instances WHV was found late after infection with the HBx-negative mutants, but these were revertants in which the *HBx* gene had been restored (Chen et al. 1993). This observation suggests that HBx protein is not essential for low-level replication in vivo, but is necessary to establish overt infection. It may be that gene expression of hepatocytes in vivo is partially controlled by mechanisms in the liver that are absent in primary hepatocyte culture. HBx may counteract such negative control mechanisms. There may, however, also exist an effect of HBx on the immune system favouring tolerance against HBV, because HBV genomes with a truncated HBx have been observed in immunodeficient patients. Evolution of such HBV genomes without a complete *HBx* gene in immunocompromised patients may indicate that HBx protein is not so necessary in patients without an efficient immune defence as in normal hosts. HBx has been found to enhance expression of class I and II MHC molecules. In the absence of a second signal for T cell stimulation this may favour development of immune tolerance.

The position of the *HBx* gene and promoter next to HBV enhancer I is reminiscent of the genome position of the early 1A (*E1A*) gene of adenoviruses and of other immediate early genes of DNA viruses. *E1A* is essential for adenovirus replication in most but not all cell types by *trans*-activating the early promoters of E2 and E4 in the adenovirus genomes.

The *trans*-activating activity of HBx on HBV enhancer I and on various viral or cellular enhancers was first described in 1988 by Spandau and Lee and by Zahm and colleagues. Numerous further studies (reviewed by Henkler and Koshy 1996) confirmed the non-specific promiscuous *trans*-activating activity of HBx, but usually the activation factor is low. HBx does not bind directly to DNA. If artificially expressed in the absence of other HBV genes, it is found most abundantly in the cytoplasm, but it is also present in the nucleus. Current evidence suggests that cytoplasmic HBx may act either via *ras* or protein kinase C on the MAP kinase signalling cascade, but other pathways also seem to exist. However, the *trans*-activating activity seems to be maintained in some systems if a nuclear localization signal is added. Many potential nuclear binding partners of HBx protein have been identified in vitro: transcription factors (TF), ATF II and CREB, the TATA binding protein TFIID, TFIIB, RNA polymerase subunit RPB5, a novel X-associated protein XAP-1 which may be involved in DNA repair, the ubiquitous transcription factor Oct 1, tumour suppressor protein p53, DNA repair-associated transcription factor ERCC3, and single-stranded RNA. Furthermore, binding of HBx to XAP-C7, an α-subunit of the proteasome, or to XAP-P13 a subunit of the regulatory 26S complex of the proteasome, or to a liver-specific HBx-interacting protein XIP were reported. The highly divergent results of the in vitro binding studies allow, for the moment, only one conclusion: that HBx is very sticky. The association with the proteasome may be significant, but it might only be a result of the rapid turnover of HBx. A problem with all the *trans*-activation studies is that they depend on heavy overexpression of both HBx proteins and the target sequence. Moreover, they were carried out in cultures that produce HBV without the need for HBx and may thus be irrelevant to the viral life cycle.

Many viral immediate early transcription-activating factors, such as E1A of certain adenoviruses or P6 and P7 of certain papillomavirus types, are also tumour proteins. They bind and inactivate tumour suppressor proteins such as Rb or p53. HBx was reported to bind and inactivate essential functions of p53. An Rb-inactivating factor of HBV has not yet been reported. HBx transforms an SV40 TAg-immortalized fetal mouse hepatocyte line FMH 202 to overt malignancy if expressed in large amounts. Of several strains of mice transgenic for HBx protein, only one strain developed liver tumours; high expression of HBx in these mice was necessary. In one transgenic mouse line an enhanced susceptibility against chemical carcinogens was noted (reviewed by Schaefer and Gerlich 1995). In natural infection, HBx mRNA is usually expressed in low levels. Furthermore, the half-life of HBx seems to be very low – at least in systems where it is overexpressed. Acutely infected patients and chronically infected HBV patients with high replication do not develop hepatocellular carcinoma. It is open to question whether HBx is not oncogenic at all in natural settings, or its expression is too low, or viral factors suppress the activity of HBx. With regard to the last possibility, it is observed that the core gene of HBV, if co-expressed, suppresses the *trans*-activating activities of the *HBx* gene on a variety of promoters. As with oncogenes from other viruses, *HBx* may be negatively controlled by viral genes the expression of which is stimulated by *HBx*. *HBx* may be expressed in *trans*-acting form from HBV DNA integrates, which often do not encode other complete HBV ORFs. Furthermore, defective episomal HBV genomes with a complete HBx ORF may be generated by reverse transcription of spliced pregenomes. Expression of HBx may be negatively controlled by cell-specific factors as well, p53 being one of them.

In summary, HBx probably has a role in liver-specific expression of HBV and a weak oncogenic potential which, however, can be effective only in combination with other oncogenesis-favouring events.

2.6 Integration of HBV DNA and liver cancer

Integration of the viral genome into the host genome is not part of the hepadnaviral life cycle, in contrast to the retroviruses. Nevertheless, integration of HBV DNA fragments into the hepatocyte genome is a frequent event during HBV infection. The circular HBV genome is thereby disrupted and no longer able to express a viable pregenomic RNA even if a full-length genome would be integrated. (Viable HBV DNA can be integrated for experimental purposes in the form of artificial linear constructs covering the sequence of the pregenome plus homologous or heterologous upstream transcription signals.) However, subgenomic mRNAs and viral proteins may be expressed from integrated HBV DNA fragments. Integration sites in the viral genome are very often around DR1 at one end and at variable sites at the other end. These integrates may express a carboxy-terminally truncated HBx fused to cellular sequences protein which still has *trans*-activating activity in experimental systems (Wollersheim, Debelka and Hofschneider 1988). Furthermore, a cryptic polyadenylation site may be used that generates a polylysine tail at the carboxy-terminal end of a truncated HBx protein (Rakotomahanina et al. 1994).

The integrated HBV DNA is quite often composed of 2 or even more fragments that are linked together in a head to tail arrangement or in other complex rearrangements. Occasionally such a rearranged HBV DNA fragment may express truncated forms of preS/S proteins in particular truncated MHBs. Such truncated LHBs or MHBs proteins have been found to *trans*-activate transcription factor AP1 and others, suggesting an additional growth-stimulating effect of these defective HBV proteins (Hildt, Hofschneider and Urban 1997).

With human HBV DNA no clear preference for a defined integration site has been identified and it was noted that the integration site may be rearranged. It seems that integration of HBV DNA destabilizes the host genome (Hino, Tabata and Hotta 1991) but it is not yet clear whether this is due to a property of HBV DNA or an effect of the HBx protein on p53. A model has been proposed that topoisomerase I mediates the integration of HBV DNA around the DR1 site. A role of the integrated HBV DNA in the development of hepatocellular carcinoma (HCC) is suggested by the fact that virtually all HCC-derived cell lines from HBV carriers contain one or usually more HBV DNA fragments and that the HCCs are usually of monoclonal origin (Bréchot et al. 1980). The model of insertional mutagenesis leading to deregulation of growth control genes has, however, been verified for very few human HCCs. One example is the fusion of a retinoic acid receptor β chain with 29 amino-terminal residues from preS1, which may lead to uncontrolled expression of this differentiation factor (Dejean et al. 1986). Another example is the insertion of preS2/S sequences of HBV into an intron of cyclin A, generating a preS2/2 fusion with cyclin A devoid of its amino-terminal degradation signals (Wang et al. 1990). This altered cyclin A has transforming properties in cell cultures. A third example is the activation of mevalonate kinase (Graef et al. 1994). More typical are integrations into Alu-type repeats, minisatellite-like, satellite III or a variable number of tandem repeat sequences, suggesting a preference of HBV DNA integration into sites where other multiple insertions have already occurred during evolution (Rogler and Chisari 1992).

Development of HCC is a regular event in woodchucks chronically infected with WHV. In HCCs of this animal, insertion of WHV DNA very often occurs upstream of a functional retrotransposon encoding cellular N-*myc*2. Insertion of hepadnaviral DNA into c-*myc* sequences was observed both in woodchucks and in ground squirrels. However, in human HCC c-*myc* or N-*myc* activation was found only occasionally (Buendia et al. 1993).

Hepadnaviral DNA integration has also been found in HCC from ducks, but development of HCC seems to be correlated to exposure to aflatoxin B. In humans, HBV raises the risk of HCC development by a factor of c. 100 compared to non-infected individuals. Without additional specific risk HCC is still rare in chronic HBV carriers and usually has a latency period of several decades, but additional risks such as aflatoxin B exposure or HCV co-infection raise the risk to 40% or more during a lifetime.

2.7 HBV genotypes, HBsAg subtypes and HBV variants

The sequencing of numerous HBV isolates in the late 1970s and early 1980s has revealed a surprisingly high degree of conservation; even rodent hepadnaviruses are c. 60% homologous to human HBV. Human HBV splits into 6 identified genotypes, A to F, which diverge by 8–15% by DNA sequence (Magnius and Norder 1995). Avian hepadnaviruses are only distantly related to mammalian hepadnaviruses, despite their similar genomic organization and replication strategy. The multiple functions of the viral DNA sequence for the coding of overlapping genes, regulation of transcription and assembly of the virions prevents excessive variability. A hot spot of variability between virus species is the preS1 region, probably because of its role in host specificity and because the overlapping polymerase sequence functions in this region only as spacer.

Variability in the hydrophilic loop of the SHBs protein on the virion surface or on HBs particles, respectively, determines the serological HBsAg subtype. Besides the common antigenic determinant *a*, subtype-specific alleles *d* or *y*, and *w1*, *w2*, *w3*, *w4* or *r* are described. Combinations of these alleles define 9 HBsAg subtypes according to a workshop held in 1975 in Paris. Position 122 of SHBs is lysine for determinant *d* and arginine for determinant *y*. Position 160 is lysine for the 4 *w* alleles and arginine for *r*. Differentiation into *w1* to *w4* is mainly based on exchanges at position 127 (Norder, Courouce and Magnius 1994). As a consequence of this lack of correlation between genotype and HBsAg reactivity, HBV genomes should preferably be characterized by their genotype. Antigenic differences, defined by reactivity with monoclonal antibodies, exist also in the preS2 and preS1 regions. The predominant sequences of an HBV isolate are usually conserved within an infection chain from person to person, suggesting low variability. Obviously the existing genotypes of HBV are optimally adapted to replication in their host population. However, HBV turns out to be a quasispecies at all stages of infection if a large number of cloned genomes is analysed.

Despite the splice-suppressing element of the HBV genome, spliced variants with large deletions between the *C* and the *S* or *X* gene have been detected (Rosmorduc et al. 1995). Such encapsidation-competent variants obviously capture the polymerase from wild type virus and are, thus, defective interfering particles. In chronically infected patients with immunosuppression, deletions in the *HBx* gene or HBc/e promoter region have been found that generate a truncated HBx protein. Deletions of T or B cell epitopes, or both, in the central part of the core gene are also typical in these patients (Carman 1995).

3 CLINICAL AND PATHOLOGICAL ASPECTS

3.1 Introduction

Normal ('wild') types of *Hepadnavirus* species are not overtly cytopathogenic. Inflammatory liver disease is caused by the host immune response against viral antigens whereby cellular cytotoxic lymphocytes exert the strongest effect (Chisari and Ferrari 1995). Consequently, symptomatic liver disease is absent in persistently infected individuals whose immune system is either immature at birth or severely impaired. Some healthy adults may also develop persistent oligosymptomatic infection without an efficient immune response, and possibly immunogenetic factors predispose for persistent infection.

Another type of oligosymptomatic infection occurs when the infectious dose is very low or the immune response is rapid and efficient, or both. In such cases, silent immunization results. Acute hepatitis occurs in most immunocompetent adults who are infected by the percutaneous route with highly infectious serum or blood. A variable, but usually small, proportion of such patients develop chronic disease after acute hepatitis B. Depending on the balance between viral replication and host defence, chronic disease may cease spontaneously or proceed over years or decades to liver cirrhosis or HCC, or both. HCC usually develops in cirrhotic liver but may also appear independently of cirrhosis. In infections with high virus replication, extrahepatic manifestation (e.g. glomerulonephritis and periarteritis nodosa) due to circulating immune complexes may occur. Figure 36.8 illustrates the possible courses of HBV infection.

3.2 Clinical course of HBV infection

For more detailed descriptions and original literature, see textbooks on hepatology (e.g. McIntyre et al. 1991) or on hepatitis viruses (Zuckerman and Thomas 1993).

ACUTE HEPATITIS B

Diagnosis of acute hepatitis based merely on clinical symptoms is unreliable. Early non-specific symptoms are malaise, poor appetite, nausea and right upper quadrant pain which lasts for several days. In c. 10% of patients with acute hepatitis B a prolonged prodromal phase of up to 4 weeks occurs with serum-like sickness,

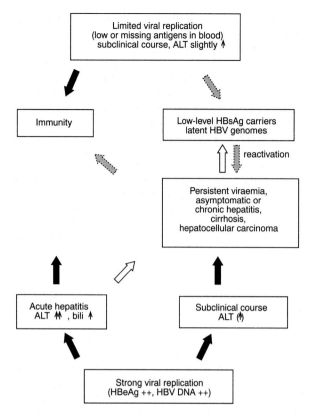

Fig. 36.8 Possible courses of hepatitis B virus infection. Black arrows show frequent courses, white arrows possible courses and shaded arrows rare or hypothetical events.

including arthralgia or even frank arthritis, fever and skin rash. After 3–6 days, fatigue and anorexia worsen and jaundice develops in the more severe cases. Essential for the diagnosis is the determination of the alanine amino transferase (ALT) in the serum. The upper limit of the normal range is 22 IU/l for men and 18 IU/l for women if measured at 25°C. Clinical hepatitis is associated with values higher than 300 IU/l, reaching several thousand IU/l in severe cases. The level of ALT indicates the degree of hepatocyte damage. It increases sharply at the end of the prodromal phase and usually reaches peak values shortly before the appearance of jaundice caused by levels of high bilirubin in the serum. In less severe cases bilirubin concentrations are below 50 μmol/l; in severe cases >340 μmol/l. In contrast to cholestatic jaundice, alkaline phosphatase is only moderately increased in the serum.

The **time course** of a typical acute hepatitis B is shown in Fig. 36.9a. Clinical and biochemical data do not allow distinction between infections by the various hepatitis viruses. The most reliable serological marker for acute hepatitis B is IgM antibody against HBcAg (IgM anti-HBc). With the onset of symptoms, IgM anti-HBc appears and reaches peak values within a few days.

Many clinicians rely more on the detection of HBsAg in the serum. HBsAg appears during the incubation phase (Fig. 36.9), depending on the infective dose and the mode of exposure, several weeks or

months after the infective event. It increases over several weeks, typically to peak levels of 10 000–100 000 PEI units/ml of HBsAg (PEI = Paul Ehrlich Institute, Germany). Decrease of HBsAg concentration starts with the onset of the prodromal phase and continues until complete recovery. Most patients remain HBsAg positive for several months.

In 2–10% of acute cases, HBsAg may have been eliminated so rapidly that it is already negative in the first available serum sample. To identify HBV as the aetiological agent in these cases, it is essential to

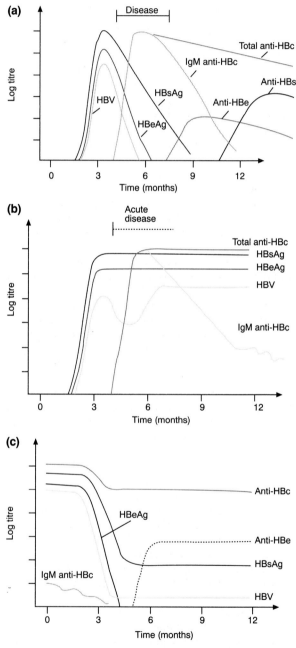

Fig. 36.9 Serological markers during the different courses of hepatitis B in arbitrary units: (**a**) acute hepatitis B, resolving; (**b**) acute hepatitis B, chronic evolution; (**c**) HBe seroconversion in chronic hepatitis B; (**d**) subclinical course of transient HBV infection.

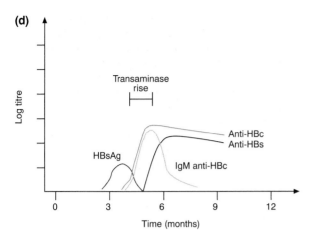

(d)

Log titre

Transaminase rise

HBsAg

Anti-HBc
Anti-HBs

IgM anti-HBc

0   3   6   9   12

Time (months)

Fig. 36.9 Continued.

obtain a quantitative IgM anti-HBc result if no other cause for the hepatitis has been identified. Some EIAs for HBsAg may detect less well with variants of HBsAg with altered determinant, but these variants are rare in acute hepatitis B.

Persistence of HBsAg for more than 6 months after onset in high concentrations (>100 PEI units/ml) means that (1) the acute hepatitis B evolved to chronicity (Fig. 36.9b); (2) a pre-existing chronic HBV infection was superimposed by an acute hepatitis of another aetiology; or (3) the acute disease may actually be an exacerbation of chronic hepatitis B. Again, a high IgM anti-HBc during the early acute phase confirms recent acute HBV infection whereas moderate or absent amounts indicate previous HBV infection.

Full recovery is assumed if the ALT reaches normal or close to normal levels and if HBsAg becomes negative in EIA. This takes more than 6 months in some cases of protracted disease. Anti-HBs appears several weeks or even months after the disappearance of HBsAg. IgM anti-HBc falls to levels <100 PEI units, but may occasionally remain positive at low levels for several years. Anti-HBc of the IgG class may either persist life-long or disappear after several years or decades.

HBV itself appears in the serum during the incubation period several weeks before HBsAg in numbers that allow its DNA to be detected by sensitive PCR techniques. Hybridization assays are not usually sensitive enough to detect HBV before HBsAg. Maximum concentration of 10^6–10^9 genomes/ml is reached before the onset of symptoms. About 40% of the patients are already negative in hybridization assays (<10^6 genomes/ml) when the first serum sample is available.

Subclinical course. The mild courses of transient HBV infection (Fig. 36.9d) will usually go unnoticed unless sought after known exposure. Serology will show for a few days low amounts of HBV DNA, HBsAg, IgM anti-HBc and a moderate transient rise of ALT to levels <300 IU/l for less than 4 weeks. Anti-HBc appears at the peak of ALT, anti-HBs somewhat later. This inapparent course will often develop in healthy people who were exposed to low doses or mucocutaneously.

Fulminant course. About 0.2% of clinically apparent cases of acute hepatitis B are so severe that the patients develop symptoms of hepatic failure within a few days, with hepatic coma. This course is often fatal. Survivors recover completely and develop immunity to HBV characterized by anti-HBs and anti-HBc. Fulminant cases are often associated with co-infection by hepatitis delta virus (see Chapter 37) or possibly other hepatitis viruses. The significance of HBe-negative HBV variants for the development of fulminant hepatitis B is controversial. Although these variants are often found in fulminant hepatitis, it is possible that they are not the cause of the severe disease but a result of immune selection. The cytotoxic immune response seems to be too vigorous in these patients.

CHRONIC HEPATITIS B

Clinical signs of chronic hepatitis are usually mild and non-specific. They include lack of energy, easy fatiguability and malaise. Myalgias, arthralgias and skin rash may be present in cases with high virus replication due to circulating immune complexes. HBV-associated immune complex disease is an important cause of glomerulonephritis in tropical countries. The course of the disease is usually intermittent with acute exacerbations during which abdominal discomfort, nausea, weight loss, dark urine, jaundice and mild fever may occur.

However, chronic HBV infection may go unnoticed until compensated or even decompensated cirrhosis is present. In this late disease phase the above-mentioned symptoms are enhanced and signs of hepatic encephalopathy may be present. Blood coagulation is decreased due to reduced synthesis of coagulation factors in the liver. Serum albumin is also decreased whereas IgG is increased, probably due to impaired degradation in the liver. The ALT levels are usually only moderately enhanced to, at the most, several hundred IU/l and often fluctuate. A major complication is the collateral blood circulation due to impaired blood flow through the cirrhotic liver. Breakages of the oesophageal varices are a life-threatening event and are a result of portal hypertension. A further consequence of portal hypertension is the development of ascites in some cases.

It is important to distinguish between disease activity reflected by markers of viral replication, antiviral immune response and hepatocyte damage, on the one hand, and symptoms caused by the lack of functional hepatocytes and the replacement of normal liver tissue by connective tissue on the other. Whereas the disease activity may come to an end either spontaneously or as a result of treatment, the conversion of normal liver tissue to cirrhotic tissue is irreversible. The liver status can be assessed only by histology, liver function tests and determination of serum proteins synthesized or metabolized by the liver. Sonography describes the shape and density of the liver and may detect an increased diameter of the portal vein due to portal hypertension.

Most patients are not aware of an acute hepatitis B before the development of persistent HBV infection. As pointed out above, HBV persistence very often develops in individuals who are immunologically immature or somehow impaired. Perinatal HBV infection is virtually always persistent, unless HBe-negative variants are predominant. In the early years of life, symptoms are usually absent in HBV carriers despite high virus replication. The same is true for patients who were infected when in a state of significant immune deficiency. However, in otherwise healthy HBV carriers a cytotoxic immune response will eventually develop and cause chronic disease. This cytotoxic immune response is directed primarily against the HBc protein or the polymerase of HBV, whereas the HBs protein seems to be a minor target in chronic hepatitis B. The HBc-specific T cell response suppresses HBV replication and may even eliminate HBV-expressing cells. As a result, an exacerbation of chronic hepatitis B may lead to a new state of persistent HBV infection, in which HBsAg is still present in the serum but the number of virions is much lower than in the high viraemic phase combined with the disappearance of HBeAg. Anti-HBe is often present in this phase. If HBV replication is constantly controlled by the immune system at low levels, the so-called healthy HBsAg carrier status is reached. Eventually HBsAg may also disappear from the serum. In these cases anti-HBc is often the only marker of HBV infection. This phase of low viral activity may be reached at all degrees of irreversible liver disease. Thus, a seemingly favourable serological constellation suggesting low viral replication does not necessarily mean insignificant liver disease.

During the high viraemic HBeAg-positive phase, variability of the HBV epitope regions is low. In HBeAg-negative cases, however, considerable variability, particularly in the HBc/e sequence and the HBs and preS epitope regions, is observed. This variability may be generated by the immune elimination of the original strains (Carman 1995).

A dangerous clinical situation occurs if a low viraemic HBV carrier (with or without symptoms) is therapeutically immunosuppressed because of autoimmune disease, organ transplantation or in anti-cancer therapy. In such cases high HBV replication reappears, but, as soon as the immune suppression is terminated, the existing memory cells induce a vigorous cytotoxic immune response that often results in fatal fulminant hepatitis B.

HEPATOCELLULAR CARCINOMA (HCC)

HBV is the major cause of hepatocellular carcinoma (HCC) in regions with high HBV prevalence. HCC is usually the consequence of cirrhosis, but may also develop without cirrhosis. The involvement of HBV may not be recognized by the assay of HBsAg in the serum, requiring detection of anti-HBc or anti-HBs, or both. In some cases in which the HCC contains integrated HBV DNA fragments no classic serological HBV marker may be present. However, in highly endemic areas of the world, people positive for HBsAg are 100 times more likely to develop HCC compared to those who have anti-HBc/s but not HBsAg (Beasley et al. 1981). In low endemic areas the relative risk of HBsAg carriers to develop HCC is also increased c. 100-fold in comparison with HBsAg-negative blood donors but at a lower level.

The development of HCC may be diagnosed early by quantitative measurement of α-fetoprotein (AFP) in the serum, but levels may be normal (<20 ng) before the HCC reaches a size of 3 cm. Levels above 1000 ng/ml or a sharp rise of AFP indicates HCC. Abdominal imaging by ultrasound of HBsAg-positive patients, particularly those with liver cirrhosis, is advisable at intervals of 3–4 months.

In countries with intermediate HBV prevalence, HCV may be the major cause of HCC more often than HBV, but co-infection with HBV, HCV and even HDV is quite common in HCC patients. An important co-factor is exposure to aflatoxin B.

3.3 Pathogenesis and immune response

Pathogenesis of HBV is caused mainly by the immune reaction. Virus replication itself is not overly pathogenic but subtle effects on hepatocyte function cannot be excluded. Transgenic mice expressing HBV or single HBV proteins are normal or almost normal. However, selective expression of LHBs in transgenic mice leads to storage of LHBs containing filaments in the ER and pre-Golgi compartments. The LHBs-storing hepatocyte acquires a ground glass-like appearance. In mouse strains with very high expression of LHBs, hepatocytes become very sensitive to interferon-γ. Inflammatory liver disease and eventually HCC develop whereby the tumours no longer express LHBs (Rogler and Chisari 1992). LHBs containing ground glass hepatocytes are often found in healthy HBsAg carriers but their diagnostic or pathogenetic significance in humans is not clear.

Selective overexpression of HBx protein in a certain mouse strain has generated HCC late in life, but other mouse strains did not develop HCC. However, one HBx-expressing mouse lineage was more susceptible to chemical carcinogens.

SHBs, HBc and HBe proteins are not pathogenic when expressed in transgenic mice. SHBs and HBe protein are secreted whereas HBc protein is stored as HBc particles in the nucleus. Cytoplasmic HBc particles are rapidly degraded whereas nuclear HBc protein has a longer half-life. All these findings are in accordance with observations on human HBV. HBsAg, secreted HBeAg and nuclear HBcAg are not associated with disease *per se*.

No clear differences exist in the pathogenicity of various genotypes, but *de novo* infection with HBe-negative variants may result in a more serious course of acute hepatitis B.

Virtually all infected people develop anti-HBc antibodies. Development of IgM anti-HBc indicates significant ongoing HBV replication and is a serological marker of inflammatory disease. The appearance of anti-HBs shows that HBsAg production is low or absent, unless HBs escape mutants are present. Anti-preS1 and anti-preS2 appear during recovery from acute hepatitis B, earlier than anti-SHBs. These antibodies may also contribute to the formation of circulating HBs immune complexes in chronic HBV carriers. Anti-HBx and anti-HBpol antibodies are detected in many but not all patients with acute or chronic hepatitis B, and are neither diagnostically nor pathogenetically important. HBs and HBe immune complexes may contribute to extrahepatic manifestations of HBV, but are probably not a major pathogenic factor in viral hepatitis.

Administration of anti-SHBs in high doses protects against *de novo* infection with HBV. The administration of anti-SHBs to individuals already infected (e.g. liver transplant recipients or some HBV-infected patients) favours outgrowth of HBs escape mutants. In vitro experiments with infection of cell cultures suggest that anti-preS2 and anti-preS1 are also neutralizing antibodies, but their protective function in vivo is not well established.

Pathogenesis and immune elimination of HBV-producing cells during acute hepatitis B are mediated mainly by a strong CD8 T cell response to HBc/e and HBs proteins (Chisari and Ferrari 1995). Passive transfer of HBs-specific T cell clones from immunized mice to HBs-transgenic mice induces acute hepatitis. The severity of the disease correlates directly with the dose of cytotoxic CD8 cells against HBs and the amount of HBs protein in the liver. It may result in fulminant hepatitis, as shown in animals with LHBs storage. The cytotoxic CD8 cells stimulate non-specific inflammatory cells which form necroinflammatory foci, inducing necrosis of hepatocytes. The histological picture of this CD8 cell-induced disease in transgenic mice is similar to that in acute or fulminant hepatitis B of humans. HBc/e- and HBs-specific CD8 cells have been isolated readily from the blood of patients with acute hepatitis B. In contrast, chronic hepatitis B patients have only low numbers of circulating or intrahepatic CD8+ cells specific for HBs or HBc. This low number may explain the persistence of HBV and the continuous inflammation at moderate levels. Control of HBV replication in liver cells does not necessarily require the elimination of all HBV-expressing cells. Activated CD8 cells secrete interferon-γ and interleukin 2 which induces secretion of tumour necrosis factor α (TNF-α). TNF-α reduces the stability of HBV mRNAs and suppresses expression of HBV or its proteins, or both, without necessarily inducing cytolysis or apoptosis. CD4+ lymphocytes against HBc/e are present in many patients with acute resolving hepatitis, but in few during chronic hepatitis B. CD4 cells against HBs proteins are less abundant than those against HBc/e.

Both CD4+ and CD8+ lymphocytes against HBV proteins have been cloned and their epitopes mapped. The lack of HBV-specific CD4+ cells may be responsible for insufficient cytotoxic and humoral immune responses.

HBV persistence seems to be caused by immune evasion and non-pathogenicity of the wild type virus. It has been suggested that intrauterine transfer of maternal HBV antigens, particularly HBeAg, generates immune tolerance to HBV in the newborn, but such a transfer has not been shown experimentally and most newborns of HBeAg-positive mothers respond very well to an HBsAg vaccine. HBeAg may be involved in

the suppression of a vigorous cytotoxic immune response, because newborns (both human and woodchuck) develop persistent infection only if the infecting HBV-positive serum is also HBeAg positive.

3.4 Diagnosis

A survey of the significance of HBV parameters for different diagnostic problems is given in Table 36.1.

ACUTE HEPATITIS

According to the description in 'Acute hepatitis B' (p. 760), every case of acute hepatitis B starts at the onset of symptoms with easily detectable levels of anti-HBc. Thus, a test for anti-HBc clarifies whether a patient with hepatitis is infected with HBV. Lack of anti-HBc excludes HBV as the causative agent of an existing acute hepatitis or of a subclinical transaminase rise (Table 36.1).

If anti-HBc is positive, a test for HBsAg and IgM anti-HBc should follow (Table 36.1). A negative or low IgM anti-HBc (<600 PEI units) excludes HBV as the cause of a clinically apparent acute hepatitis, but points to previous HBV infection, which may be resolved or persistent. (Persistent infection is recognized by a positive HBsAg test, immunity by a positive anti-HBs.) During early or very late phases of the acute disease, IgM anti-HBc may have lower concentrations. In mild HBV infections, IgM anti-HBc may also be lower (Gerlich et al. 1986).

HBsAg is positive in most hepatitis B-infected individuals and may be eliminated very rapidly in fulminant hepatitis or in very mild infections. Alternatively, HBsAg may be present but undetectable by the usual EIAs because of mutations in the major epitopes. Such cases can be diagnosed by the quantitative assay of IgM anti-HBc and by the assay of HBV DNA using PCR. HBV in a patient suggests, in addition, a risk of HDV, HCV and HIV, and appropriate tests for these infections may be advisable.

The patient's disease status should be followed by determination of the ALT level until it is close to normal. An early favourable prognosis is possible if the patient is already HBeAg negative, or HBV DNA negative in hybridization assays. These 2 parameters become negative in resolving cases within 4–6 weeks. Thus, a second assay of HBeAg or HBV DNA after 6 weeks is advisable. Alternatively, the HBsAg quantity may be measured accurately by electroimmunodiffu-

Table 36.1 Serological parameters of HBV infection

Prevalence	Anti-HBc
Infection	HBsAg
Time of infection	IgM anti-HBc (quantitative)
Infectivity	HBV DNA
Natural immunity	Anti-HBc and anti-HBs
Immunity after vaccination	Anti-HBs (quantitative)

sion or a quantitative EIA. In resolving cases HBsAg drops within 6 weeks by more than 60%. A definitive resolution may be assumed if HBsAg is negative in EIA and anti-HBs is positive but this may take up to one year.

CHRONIC HEPATITIS

Patients with symptoms of chronic hepatitis need a thorough examination of the liver, including liver function tests and, possibly, liver biopsy. The viral activity is not clearly correlated to disease activity or the histological appearance of the liver, but HBsAg is virtually always detectable. In early phases of chronic infection HBeAg is often present and HBV DNA detectable even by insensitive hybridization assays. Quantities of ALT, HBV DNA, HBeAg and IgM anti-HBc are often unstable, fluctuate or are occasionally even negative. HBeAg may be absent, but HBV DNA is usually still detectable. Sometimes PCR may be required as a more sensitive technique for the detection of HBV DNA.

VARIANTS

A typical feature of late phase chronic hepatitis B is the selection of variants with deletions or mutations leading to an altered expression of HBV or to altered gene products. Most frequent are mutations (stop codons, promoter inactivation, frameshifts) that abolish expression of HBeAg. Deletions also occur quite often in the B cell epitope region of HBcAg and preS. *HBx* gene deletions are common in patients with impaired immune reactions and are often the only mutation in these people.

Escape mutants arise if HBV replicates in the presence of anti-HBs. This setting occurs in babies of HBsAg-positive mothers who are vaccinated at birth. Passive immunization of liver transplant patients, who have chronic HBV infection, with hepatitis B immunoglobulin often also leads to escape mutants with altered SHBs epitopes. Replacement of glycine 145 of the S domain with arginine is a frequent escape mutation, but other point mutations or small insertions occur between amino acids 120 and 145 (Wallace and Carman 1996). Variant HBV genomes may also be detected in patients without HBsAg or even without any serological marker of HBV infection (i.e. anti-HBc or anti-HBs). In this case point mutations lead to low level replication; the clinical significance of these variants is unknown. They may occasionally be transmitted by blood transfusion or organ transplantation. Deletions in the HBV genome may be detected by a smaller than expected size of PCR products. Other mutations usually require direct sequencing after amplification or sequencing after cloning if less abundant mutants are sought.

INAPPARENT HBV INFECTION

HBV infection is often not recognized subjectively. Thus, HBV carriers are often detected accidentally – during blood donation, because of an occupational risk, before operations or during search for a possible source of HBV infection. The most universal test to detect an ongoing or previous HBV infection is anti-HBc. However, anti-HBc may remain negative for up to 6 months, whereas HBsAg is positive much earlier. The earliest marker of HBV infection is HBV DNA in the serum if detected by a highly sensitive nucleic acid amplification technique (NAAT) such as nested PCR.

If an HBsAg-positive person is identified he or she should be tested for anti-HBc. Negative anti-HBc suggests an early phase of infection with a possible acute hepatitis B still to come, or a severe state of immune deficiency which, however, would usually be known for other reasons. Absent IgM anti-HBc in the presence of IgG anti-HBc suggests low disease activity and a stable carrier state (Table 36.2). HBsAg carriers stay, by definition, HBsAg positive for more than 6 months. Positive HBeAg suggests high viraemia and high infectivity, but some HBeAg-positive carriers have only moderate viraemia ($<10^8$ genomes/ml) and are less infectious. A quantitative HBV DNA assay is therefore recommended. DNA hybridization allows more accurate quantification and is sufficiently sensitive for estimation of infectivity. Most HBeAg-positive carriers and some HBeAg-negative carriers reach viraemia levels of 10^9–10^{10} genome-containing HBV particles.

HBV carriers may be divided into 3 groups, as shown in Table 36.2. The immunotolerant type is highly infectious but oligosymptomatic. The HBsAg carrier is also healthy and non-infectious (except for blood donation). A status between these 2 extremes is usually associated with liver disease which, however, may be unrecognized. In this phase, disease activity is often fluctuating. Silent HBsAg carrier-like phases may change with flare-ups. Viraemic HBV carriers often spontaneously reach the HBsAg carrier state by one or more episodes of recurrent liver disease. Unfortunately, this disease phase may be long-lasting and result in liver cirrhosis or HCC. Thus, regular monitoring of ALT levels in persistently HBsAg-positive people is advisable until it is known whether a stable state is present. HBeAg and HBV DNA should also be regularly checked if positive.

NATURAL IMMUNITY

People who have been at risk from HBV may have acquired immunity by silent HBV infection. In order to detect natural immunity the person's blood should be tested for anti-HBc, and then, if positive, for anti-HBs. Naturally immune people should be anti-HBc and anti-HBs positive (see Table 36.1). It has, however, been noted that anti-HBs may occasionally disappear several years after an acute hepatitis B infection. It is not known whether immunity is still solid in this case. Isolated anti-HBs without previous vaccination may be non-specific and non-protective. Isolated anti-HBc may have different meanings:

1 The person may be in the phase after disappearance of HBsAg but before the appearance of anti-HBs (so-called window period). In this case the titre should be high.
2 It may be present long after previous HBV infection in which anti-HBs has already disappeared. In this case, the titre should be low.

Table 36.2 Three states of HBsAg carriership – typical parameters

Parameters	Immune tolerance	Chronic disease	'Healthy' HBsAg carrier
Serum			
HBsAg µg/ml[a]	30–150	<30	<30
HBeAg PEI[b] U/ml	2000–10 000	<2000	Negative, anti HBe+
HBV- DNA g.e./ml[c]	10^9–10^{10}	10^6–10^9	<10^6
pg/ml[d]	3000–30 000	<3000	<3
Anti-HBc	+ to ++	+++	+ to ++
IgM-antiHBc			
PEI units	<50	10–500	<10
ALT IU/ml 25°C	<60	>60, variable	<25
Liver			
HBcAg+ cells	90–100%	Variable, low	Negative
HBsAg+ cells	90–100%	Variable, low	Variable, frequent ground glass cells, LHBs+
Dynamics	Stable	Unstable	Stable
Interferon response	Transient or none	Often sustained	No treatment required

[a] 1 µg HBsAg = 1000 PEI units or 2000 WHO units. So-called ng units are often inaccurate.
[b] PEI: Paul Ehrlich Institute for Sera and Vaccines, Langen, Germany.
[c] g.e.: genome equivalents.
[d] Abbott's pg unit is too low by a factor of 50 and should not be used.

3   It may be a response to an HBV infection, in which HBsAg is mutated, bound in immune complexes or below the detection limit. In this case, the titre should be intermediate. Anti-HBe may be present.
4   The anti-HBc test may react non-specifically.

If distinction between the 4 situations seems to be required because of liver disease, an HBV DNA assay by NAAT may be helpful. If it is necessary to decide whether a person is immune, vaccination against HBV with one dose of vaccine is recommended and a test for acute HBs should be done 1–2 weeks later. Situation (2) will lead to a rapid anamnestic response with a reappearance of anti-HBs at high titres. If this does not occur, vaccination should be continued by the regular schedule with 2 or 3 further doses. In situation (3) no anti-HBs may develop. For the discussion of vaccine-induced immunity see 'Active immunization' (p. 769).

DETECTION OF HBV IN TISSUE SPECIMENS

Because of its ability to generate high viraemia and antigenaemia, HBV infection is usually easy to diagnose with the aid of serum samples. Liver biopsies are necessary to examine the degree of inflammation, necrosis and fibrosis, and repeated biopsies are required to follow the progression of the disease or the success of an antiviral therapy. Because of the risk associated with biopsy, it should be done only if the clinical, biochemical and virological data suggest severe, progressive disease. Once the biopsy is available, it may be stained for HBsAg, preS1 antigen, HBcAg or HBV DNA. In HBsAg-positive patients, usually no more information can be derived from these stainings than from a complete quantitative HBV serology. The situation is different in HBsAg-negative patients with liver cirrhosis or HCC. Here, a liver biopsy or tumour tissue may allow detection of extracted HBV DNA by

NAAT and, if positive, by Southern blot. Distinct bands in a Southern blot prove mono- or oligoclonal outgrowth of hepatocytes with integrated HBV DNA and, thus, HBV-associated liver disease. In this phase replication HBV may be absent from the liver.

DIAGNOSTIC TESTS FOR HBV

HBsAg is detected qualitatively by solid phase EIA with unlabelled anti-HBs at the surface and labelled anti-HBs for detection. Commercially available test kits are highly specific. The detection limit is between 0.05 and 1 PEI units/ml. Non-specific reactions are rare (<0.1%) and may be detected by inhibition with polyvalent anti-HBs. Quantification may be achieved by using reference samples and appropriate dilutions of the sample which give a result in the proportionality range (<100 PEI units/ml) of the EIA. Results may be expressed either in PEI or in WHO units/ml. One WHO unit is 0.55 PEI unit. One PEI unit corresponds to 1 ng of fully native HBsAg. Unfortunately, many test kit producers use 'ng' units, which are calibrated with partially denatured HBsAg. Test kits may react differently with various subtypes of HBsAg or with variants of HBsAg. A useful technique for quantifying HBsAg in the range of 1000–100 000 PEI units/ml is Laurell electrophoresis. This is the relevant range for quantitative assessment of acute and chronic hepatitis B.

Anti-HBc is usually determined by inhibition EIAs with recombinant HBcAg (expressed in *E. coli*) at the solid phase and labelled anti-HBc, the binding of which is inhibited by the samples anti-HBc. There are non-specific inhibitors of HBcAg in human sera; non-specific reactions may therefore be as frequent as 1% in the normal population. Repetition of the test using a test kit from a second producer usually yields a positive result if the reaction is specific, but a false-negative result in this second assay cannot completely be excluded. Western blotting is not helpful and quantification of anti-HBc is not usually done. Chronic HBV carriers and acute hepatitis B patients may have end point titres up to 1 : 1 000 000 whereas immune people usually have titres below 1 : 1000.

IgM anti-HBc is usually detected by the anti-μ capture EIA. This type of EIA binds via anti-μ antibodies IgM from the sample to the solid phase; thereafter labelled HBcAg is added. If the sample contains IgM anti-HBc, labelled HBcAg will be bound and quantification is necessary. Results may be expressed in PEI units/ml or as an EIA index. Some commercial test kits were made artificially insensitive to give a positive result only with sera from acute hepatitis B, but all test kits react significantly with sera from patients with active chronic hepatitis giving values up to 600 PEI units/ml. Testing for IgM anti-HBc is advisable only if the screening for total anti-HBc was positive.

Anti-HBs is usually detected by a sandwich EIA with HBsAg at the solid phase and labelled HBsAg. Some producers use naturally purified HBsAg from HBV carrier plasma; others use recombinant HBsAg particles from yeast or from mammalian cells devoid of preS antigen. Thus, quantitative results obtained for one serum using various test kits may differ by a factor of 2–4. The detection limit is usually between 1 and 10 mIU/ml and saturation of the assay is reached at 100–1000 mIU/ml. Sera may contain more than 100 000 mIU/ml after vaccination with HBsAg and although non-specific results are possible they are rare. Coincident positivity of HBsAg and anti-HBs may occur in patients with chronic hepatitis B and is not non-specific. The anti-HBs in these patients usually reacts with the HBsAg subtype not present in the HBV carrier. Anti-HBs should be assayed in anti-HBc-positive people or after vaccination.

HBeAg should be determined only in people with HBsAg. It is tested by EIA and may be quantified using PEI units. Detection limits of commercial assays are between 1 and 10 PEI units/ml and high viraemia is usually associated with high HBeAg titres (>2000 PEI units/ml). Anti-HBe is a less important marker of HBV infection, and only monitoring of chronic hepatitis B patients for seroconversion (Fig. 36.9c) from HBeAg to anti-HBe is clinically relevant.

HBV DNA has become more and more important in the diagnosis of HBV infections. For the detection of clinically relevant infection and infectivity (except blood donation) quantitative hybridization assays are advisable. The detection limit of these assays is 10^5–10^6 genomes/ml. For therapeutic decisions and monitoring of therapy it is important to follow the range between 10^6 and 10^{10}/ml. More sensitive NAAT is useful for very early or very late samples from an infection. NAAT allows early detection of HBV during incubation and in cases with atypical serology. Performance of NAAT was often plagued by false-positive and false-negative results (Quint et al. 1995) and calibration of some test kits has been faulty in the past;

for example, one often-used test kit underestimated the pg HBV DNA/ml by a factor of 50 (Gerlich et al. 1995). Thus, data from the literature have to be compared with reservation. Reference preparations for HBV genotypes A and D are available and are now used for calibrating test kits.

3.5 Epidemiology

PREVALENCE

It is estimated that 50% of the world's population have had contact with HBV and about 10% (i.e. c. 350 million of these) have developed persistent infection. These HBV carriers have a high risk of developing liver cirrhosis and a 100-fold greater risk of developing HCC. Mortality from acute hepatitis B is <1%, but much higher from chronic hepatitis. It is estimated that 1 million people per year die of chronic hepatitis B and its sequelae. Prevalence is highly variable in different geographic regions, ethnic or behavioural groups. Areas of low prevalence (<1%) are Northern Europe, North America and parts of South America; areas with a particularly high prevalence (>50%) are sub-Saharan Africa, southeast Asia and Oceania, where more than 10% of the adult population are HBsAg carriers. In Australia, New Zealand and Alaska the native population is much more affected than the Caucasian immigrants. There may also be very large differences within a country; for example, southern Italy has a much higher prevalence than most northern areas. There are no hints that certain races are more susceptible to persistent infection. Lower socioeconomic status is often (but not always) connected with higher prevalence. In areas of low or moderate endemicity, prevalence increases gradually with age, being very low during childhood. In areas of high prevalence most individuals have acquired the infection before school age (Nishioka et al. 1993).

INCIDENCE

In many countries cases of acute hepatitis B are registered, and in the USA and Germany 30–50% of all registered hepatitis cases are classified as hepatitis B (6/100 000 in Germany in 1995). The incidence of acute hepatitis B was higher in the early 1980s, decreased in the late 1980s as a result of altered sexual behaviours and fewer nosocomial infections, but has now reached a stable level in these countries. It is almost certain that acute hepatitis is under-reported, so the true number is probably 2 or 3 times higher. The number of new HBV infections is difficult to determine, because most infections are subclinical, even those that finally lead to chronic hepatitis. On the basis of 3–5% prevalence of anti-HBc in blood donors in Germany, even this low-risk population must have had an incidence of 100–500 inapparent HBV infections per 10^5 individuals per year. However, it seems that today's incidence is lower, because seroconversions of HBsAg are very rarely observed in blood donors.

Genotypes and HBsAg subtypes

HBV has a relatively low variability compared to other persistent viruses. Within infection chains usually no, or very few, base changes are observed in the predominant genome species. There exist, however, at least 6 defined genotypes, A to F. Genotypes seem to be stable within ethnic groups, but in recent decades genotypes have spread to some extent all over the world. Genotype A is most prevalent in the older population of northern Europe, and in North America and Central Africa; genotypes B and C are in eastern Asia and Oceania; genotype D is in southern Europe, the Mediterranean area, the Middle East and India; genotype E is in West Africa and genotype F in native Americans (particularly of South America) (Magnius and Norder, 1995).

In Germany young HBsAg carriers usually have the genotype D, indicating a different source of infection for genotypes A and D. The genotypes do not clearly differ in pathogenicity, but some differences should be noted: in southern Asia and Oceania transmission is mostly vertical from mother to child, which means that many women remain infectious until childbearing age. In Africa, transmission is mostly horizontal from child to child at an early age, because most HBsAg carrier mothers are already HBeAg negative and non-infectious for their newborn. Because of structural restraints genotype A cannot evolve as easily as HBe negative or HBs escape variants as the other genotypes. The genotypes express different HBsAg sero-subtypes, but there is no clear correlation with single HBsAg determinants. The determinant d (specified by lysine 122 in SHBs) occurs in all genotypes except D. Genotype A typically has the HBsAg subtype composition *adw2* or *ayw1*; B, *adw2* or *ayw1*; G, *adw2*, *adr* or *ayr*; D, *ayw2* or *ayw3*; E, *ayw4*; and F, *adw4*. Variability within genotypes is usually below 5%, and even less within one defined region; therefore, sequence identity does not exclude different sources of infections, but even minor differences suggest strongly different sources of infection.

Double infections with 2 genotypes are rare. Coexistence of HBsAg and a heterologous anti-HBs is probably caused by low affinity of the anti-HBs, and not by superinfection with another subtype. Persistent infections with one genotype obviously protect against infection by another genotype, possibly by competing for receptors.

Modes of transmission

Current knowledge indicates that transmission occurs exclusively by infectious blood serum or plasma. Because of the extremely high infectivity titre of $>10^8$/ml serum, even the slightest trace of serum or other bodily secretions such as saliva, ejaculate, vaginal secretion or menstrual blood may also cause transmission, and titres of 10^6/ml may be present in these secretions. Transmission is most efficient by intravenous injection, 100 times less efficient by the intramuscular or percutaneous route and least efficient by mucosal contact. Intact skin is impermeable to HBV but open wounds allow efficient entrance. Assuming an infectivity titre of 10^8/ml in an unrecognized HBV carrier, 1 nl of this serum (an invisible amount) would still contain 100 infectious doses, which would almost certainly cause infection if administered by a contaminated syringe or other medical device. Even dilution of this serum by $1:10^5$ (e.g. a blood spill of 0.1 ml has been removed with 10 litres of water) would leave 1 ml of this liquid still infectious when administered percutaneously. Swallowing highly infectious blood or serum, blood splashes into the eyes and contact with open wounds lead almost invariably to infection of susceptible individuals. Heterosexual contacts are a less reliable but still relatively efficient way of transmission. Transmission has been very frequent between male homosexuals, depending on their sexual practices. The danger of transmission by kissing is unknown whereas bites transmit very efficiently. Experience suggests that the rate of transmission from HBV carriers to contacts is proportional to the genome titre, frequency and intensity of exposure. Genome titres $<10^6$/ml obviously pose no risk to even the closest contact person unless contaminated syringes or similar devices are involved. HBsAg-positive mothers with a negative HBV DNA hybridization test ($<10^6$/ml) do not transmit HBV to their newborn babies (Ip et al. 1989). Thus, sources of infection are almost invariably (except for iatrogenic infections) highly viraemic HBV carriers. Even with very high titres, transmission to household contacts usually requires time and special situations; normal school contact or professional contact is not a risk. Transmissions occur more easily in nursery school or in injury-associated sports or jobs; for example, a young HBV carrier infected his co-pathfinders by hiking along the same thorny trail, and an HBV-positive butcher infected all his colleagues within a short time because of the many skin injuries received during the course of their work. Transmission of HBV from patients to medical staff is a well known risk, but the reverse is also well documented. In recreational activities, devices for ear or nose piercing or tattooing have been a source of transmission, but the most significant are shared syringe and needles for intravenous drug use.

3.6 Control

Control of HBV includes counselling HBV carriers, general hygiene, disinfection, blood screening, active and passive vaccination, and treatment of persistent infection.

Counselling of HBV carriers

As pointed out in 'Modes of transmission', even the slightest trace of highly infectious blood on a sharp item will transmit HBV if it penetrates the skin of a susceptible person. The job and the life style of a highly viraemic HBV carrier must be analysed as to whether their blood might contaminate sharp items that may percutaneously infect other people. The carrier should be informed that simple cleaning by wiping the blood away or washing with water will be insufficient to remove infectivity reliably. All highly viraemic HBV carriers should be instructed to avoid injuries, to keep lost blood under control and to disinfect items that are contaminated by their blood if they cannot be cleaned by regular washing.

Surgeons who have their hands and sharp instruments within the body cannot completely avoid small, often unnoticed, injuries. Thus, highly viraemic carriers (HBeAg positive or HBV DNA hybridization positive ($>10^6$/ml)) should not operate or work as dentists. HBV transmission by HBeAg and HBV DNA hybridization-negative ($<10^6$/ml) carriers has not yet been reported and should be safe if combined with wearing two pairs of gloves and an injury-avoiding technique. No restrictions are necessary for non-invasive medical procedures.

Household contacts, close friends and sexual partners should be vaccinated or (if appropriate) tested for anti-HBc and HBsAg, or both. Physicians should be informed before they do invasive procedures with the HBV carrier. To enable them to take appropriate precautions, it would be desirable that sexual partners and close social contacts should know that a person is a carrier of HBV; they may, however, fail to understand the nature of the risk and discriminate against the carrier. The HBeAg and HBV DNA status should be checked at least twice a year. The usefulness of antiviral therapy should be considered carefully, because an unsuccessful treatment might cause more harm than good.

HYGIENE

Human blood is almost ubiquitous in medical practice and laboratories, and HBV infections were once very frequent in the medical profession. Protection against the ingestion of blood is now observed more strictly since the occurrence of HIV; this includes wearing gloves and face-masks and using safer equipment (e.g. for blood taking) that causes fewer injuries.

Patients are now better protected by the use of disposable items, in particular syringes and needles, and by a generally higher awareness of hygiene. Non-disposable devices that cannot be autoclaved (e.g. endoscopes) still pose a problem.

In dialysis centres HBV carriers must have their own room with their own dialysis machine. Furthermore, dialysis patients should be vaccinated or – if non-responders – monitored for HBsAg. Outbreaks of HBV despite good hygiene have been observed in paediatric oncology wards. Here patient-to-patient contact is common but usually goes unnoticed if the patients are not screened for HBsAg. General screening of all patients, or at least of all those who undergo surgery, is considered to be cost-inefficient.

Isolation of patients with acute or chronic HBV infection is not essential if they are instructed as described above, behave responsibly and do not lose blood in an uncontrolled fashion. However, HBV carrier children should be supervised carefully.

DISINFECTION

Modern disinfectants should be validated with test organisms. In the European Community a standard test is required in which a disinfectant must reduce at a working dilution the infectivity titre of poliovirus by a factor of $>10^4$ within one hour at room temperature. Because there is no feasible infectivity test for HBV, no disinfectant is formally validated for HBV even though it is one of the largest disinfection problems in medicine. The use of duck HBV as a model that can be titrated has been suggested, but its structural proteins (which are the targets) and its mode of transmission (almost exclusively vertical) are very different. A better model would be woodchuck HBV but it is more difficult to test. Inactivation of HBsAg or of the viral endogenous DNA polymerase is an inadequate substitute because their connection with infectivity is not established and a reduction by a factor of $>10^4$ has not been measured. The morphological alteration and disintegration test (MADT) using purified HBV particles and electron microscopy has been of some value. Disinfectants that inactivate simian virus 40 would also be expected to inactivate HBV, whereas adenovirus may be a more sensitive model than HBV.

Good results have been obtained with glutaraldehyde-containing disinfectants in the MADT and in chimpanzee infection experiments. Ionic detergents and oxidants are probably also active in high concentrations, at elevated temperatures and with prolonged reaction time (Prince et al. 1993). Heating for 2 min at 98°C reliably inactivates HBV at even the highest possible concentrations; heating at 60°C for 10 h is insufficient.

Effective cleaning of the surface thought to be infected is essential. In particular, the lumina of hollow devices such as biopsy needles, endoscopes, electrodes and certain surgical instruments require the meticulous removal of tissue or blood clots. Disinfection by heat requires control of the temperature within the material to be disinfected.

SAFETY OF BLOOD PRODUCTS

All blood or plasma donations must be tested by licensed highly sensitive tests for HBsAg; HBsAg-positive blood or plasma must not be used. However, in developing countries with very high HBV prevalence and very limited financial resources, HBsAg testing is often not done because it is assumed that almost every recipient will be either infected or immune.

Donor blood may (very rarely) contain HBV despite HBsAg screening, because of (1) a mix-up in the blood bank, (2) a very early phase of HBV infection, (3) a late phase of HBV infection, (4) an escape mutant of HBV or (5) immune complexing of HBsAg. In cases (2) to (5) NAAT may detect HBV DNA; in cases (3) to (5) anti-HBc should be also positive. Screening of every blood donation for HBV DNA by NAAT is, at the time of writing, not yet feasible. Screening for anti-HBc by EIA is technically feasible but large-scale screening in low prevalence areas has prevented only a few additional cases of HBV infection in the recipients, and caused a large loss of donors. In high prevalence areas it is not feasible because most donors would be positive. Anti-HBc-positive donors should be tested for anti-HBs and only anti-HBs-negative donors excluded. Anti-HBs-positive blood is also thought to transfer protective antibody.

Anti-HBs in large plasma pools cannot exclude infectious HBV. In 1994, a clotting factor IX preparation transmitted HBV to at least 30 people although the donors were screened for HBsAg, the pool was anti-HBs positive and the transmitted HBV was not an escape mutant. The pool was, however, HBV DNA positive when tested by a highly sensitive NAAT (detection limit 10 genomes/ml). Several producers of plasma protein preparations now test pooled samples of the plasma donation by NAAT in order to identify HBV DNA-positive donations and exclude them from the main pool.

Since 1995 virtually all plasma protein products have been required to be treated with one or more virus inactivation steps, i.e. by heat at 60–70°C for 10–30 h in the presence of protective factors. Experience suggests that low contamination by HBV ($<10^4$ infectious doses/ml) can be completely inactivated by heat treatment, but inactivation has not always been complete. High contamination can be prevented by donor screening for HBsAg and NAAT testing of plasma pools. Treatment of plasma with solvent/detergent is probably effective against HBV as against other enveloped viruses. Chemical inactivation is not well validated. HBV transmission by blood or blood products should be rare exceptions today. However, if a **new** HBV infection occurs in a recipient, the producer of the product and the responsible public health institution should be notified and the source of infection identified.

ACTIVE IMMUNIZATION

All aspects of active and passive immunization have been described in detail by Ellis (1993). The first attempt to vaccinate against HBV used boiled HBsAg-containing serum as inactivated vaccine. More convincing success was obtained with HBsAg 20 nm particles purified from the plasma of HBV carriers. Residual infectivity of HBV and of other viruses potentially present was minimized by various procedures. The most frequently applied plasma-derived vaccine was treated with pepsin at pH 2, urea and formalin. Other products were inactivated with higher doses of formalin or heating to 100°C. Plasma-derived HBsAg has been used in millions of recipients without any known transmission of viruses. Meanwhile most countries use 'recombinant' HBsAg that has been expressed in transformed yeast cells. HBsAg expressed in mammalian cells is also used as a vaccine, but is more expensive and not generally available. Today all vaccines contain 10–20 µg purified 20 nm HBsAg particles as a standard dose, adsorbed to aluminium hydroxide as an adjuvant, and an antibacterial substance; some products are treated with formalin. Usually 3 doses, the second 1 month after the first and the third at 6 months, are recommended for adults. For infants of HBsAg-negative mothers combination with other vaccinations is recommended. The exact duration of the intervals is not essential, but long intervals between the second and the third dose favour development of high titres of anti-HBs. When rapid protection is required, or after exposure, a shortened schedule of 0, 1 and 2 months and a fourth dose after 6 or 12 months should be used. For infants smaller doses (2.5–10 µg) are advisable, and for immunodeficient recipients larger doses of 40 µg HBsAg.

Indications

WHO has recommended the vaccination of all children world-wide during the first year of life. In areas where perinatal transmission is frequent, vaccination should start soon after birth. The same is true for children whose mothers are known to be HBsAg positive. Post-exposure vaccination with 4 doses of 10 µg recombinant yeast-derived HBsAg (at 0, 1, 2 and 12 months) was reported to protect 95% of the babies born to HBsAg- and HBeAg-positive mothers. Most other studies on the prevention of perinatal HBV infection combined HBsAg vaccine with passive immunization (see 'Passive vaccination', p. 770), but it is not clear whether immunoglobulins against HBV (HBIG) really improve the protection rate if highly efficacious active vaccines are used (for review, see West 1993). In 1996, 80 countries are following the WHO programme, but many countries with high prevalence have financial limitations and are not able to take part. Some countries with low prevalence do not consider early childhood vaccination to be necessary.

Among adults, vaccination is strongly recommended for people at risk. Everyone who is or will be in professional contact with blood from other persons, whether directly or indirectly, should be offered free vaccination against HBV by their employer or teaching institution. This includes not only medical and paramedical professions but also people in the armed forces, the police, staff and inmates of prisons or other closed institutions and social workers. Patients who need continuous invasive or infusion therapy should be vaccinated, as should relatives and close contacts of HBV carriers. Intravenous drug abusers should be offered free vaccination and also free access to syringes and needles.

Travel to high prevalence countries does not require hepatitis B vaccination unless close contacts or a long stay is expected. Male homosexuals have a high risk of HBV infection and heterosexual promiscuity poses a greater risk than non-promiscuous heterosexual activity.

Side effects

The vaccine causes no local side effects except moderate pain at the injection site. Generalized non-specific side effects are rare or mild. Recipients should be questioned about hypersensitivity to yeast components, formalin or the antibacterial substance, but such reactions are very rare. Induction of neurological autoimmune disorder has been suspected in some cases of being associated with hepatitis B vaccine, but there is no statistical or theoretical evidence for this.

It should be noted that HBsAg may be detected in the serum for a few days after vaccination.

Pre- and post-testing

People to be vaccinated because of high risk should be tested for anti-HBc before vaccination, if the risk is substantial. Having come from a high prevalence area is also a risk. If anti-HBc is positive the serum sample should be tested further and the person vaccinated as described in 'Natural immunity' (p. 765). If anti-HBc is negative, vaccination should be started, following the schedule of the vaccine producers. If there is a high probability that HBV infection is already present, the person should be tested for HBsAg, even if negative for anti-HBc. An HBsAg-positive person should not be vaccinated, although accidental vaccination is not known to be harmful.

The immune response should be controlled by a semiquantitative anti-HBs test 4 weeks after the third dose in anyone who is at greater than average risk. Although T cell responses and immunological memory may be more important than the anti-HBs itself, an easily detectable anti-HBs level is a marker of protection. The detection limit is 1–5 IU/l; 10 IU/l is considered to be a marker of protection. People with less or no anti-HBs should be re-vaccinated immediately with another dose. Low responders with <100 IU/l should be re-vaccinated after one year, all others after 5–7 years if the special risk is still present.

Children who have been vaccinated during the first year of life should be re-vaccinated at the onset of adolescence because they are then again at increased risk. Non-responders after 4 doses may receive further doses if protection is urgently requested. Vaccines with preS antigen or other adjuvants may induce a better response but are not yet generally available at the time of writing.

Escape mutants

Post-exposure prophylaxis by active and passive vaccination is usually successful if given soon after injury (e.g. needle-sticks) with HBV-contaminated items. Active vaccination of newborns from HBsAg-positive mothers is also successful in 95% of cases. In c. 5% of the children HBsAg may appear in spite of vaccination or never be positive from the first day. Such infants may have already been infected in utero. In some children HBsAg appears despite protective levels of anti-HBs. These children have escape variants, detectable by sequencing of the SHBs gene, with mutations in the major HBs epitopes between amino acid 120 and 150. Escape variants have been described with various genotypes except for genotype A. A frequent escape mutation is glycine 145 of S to arginine (Wallace and Carman 1996).

Although early experiments in chimpanzees suggested that immunization with one HBsAg subtype protected against all HBV genotypes, it should be noted that most recombinant vaccines had genotype A or HBsAg *adw2* respectively. It is possible that genotype-specific antibodies may contribute to protection.

Experiments in chimpanzees and in cell culture suggest that anti-preS1 and anti-preS2 contribute to protection. Experiments with transgenic mice suggest that helper cell epitopes of the preS region may induce a better B cell response against SHBs. The potentially better protection of humans by preS-containing vaccines has not been confirmed by field studies. Induction of anti-HBs in many non-responders to the normal recombinant SHBs vaccine has been found with a vaccine containing preS1 and preS2.

PASSIVE VACCINATION

Normal immunoglobulin does not contain enough anti-HBs to be used for passive vaccination. A special immunoglobulin is produced from donors who are naturally immune and boosted with plasma-derived vaccine: 15% HBIG for intramuscular administration must contain 200 IU/ml; 5% HBIG for intravenous application must contain at least 50 IU/ml. Studies in the 1970s and 1980s showed that HBV infection was prevented in newborns from HBsAg- and HBeAg-positive mothers if HBIG was given within 24 h after birth. Active vaccination seems to be more effective and does not require complementation by passive immunization, but in many countries both active and passive vaccination are still used. Passive immunization of HBeAg-positive liver transplant recipients usually fails, but in HBeAg-negative patients continuous levels of 100 IU/l passively administered anti-HBs prevent recurrence of liver disease. Passive immunization is recommended together with active immunization after proven accidental exposure of a non-immune person. In these situations the blood of the 'donor' should be rapidly tested for HBsAg and, if positive, the 'recipient' should be vaccinated passively and actively, after a blood sample has been taken for anti-HBc and anti-HBs testing.

TREATMENT

The treatment of acute hepatitis B can only be symptomatic, but is usually not necessary. Antiviral therapy of fulminant cases has not been successful. The aim of antiviral or immunotherapy is to stop persistent viral replication at high levels. Interferon-α and interferon-β have been used for the treatment of chronic hepatitis B (Jacyna and Thomas 1993).

Success depends very much on the status of the patient: patients with the so-called immunotolerant state (see Table 36.2) cannot usually be cured and should be monitored until they reach the state of chronic active disease, when the success rate of interferon therapy is much higher. Patients with a high probability of sustained response have <10^9 genomes/ml, low or absent HBeAg (<2000 PEI units), low HBsAg (<30 000 PEI units/ml) and relatively high ALT levels (<60 IU/l, 25°C) (Burczynska et al. 1994). Treatment is undertaken with quite high doses (2.5–10 MU/m^2 3 times a week) if the patient tolerates the severe side effects such as flu-like symptoms, depression, hair loss and leucopenia and thrombopenia. Autoimmune antibodies should be monitored. Usually the HBV DNA concentration will fall within few days to levels $<10^6$ genomes/ml. Some patients do not respond at all, some may develop high levels of viraemia even during therapy and others may become positive soon after withdrawal of interferon. Six months of therapy are considered the minimum in responders before withdrawal is attempted. A relapse is not rare and a second course of interferon may be tried.

Interferon may be harmful to patients with cirrhosis and so is not useful in the terminal phases of chronic liver disease. In this situation liver transplantation may be the only cure. In order to prevent reinfection of the graft, patients should be infused with large amounts of HBIG (Samuel et al. 1993) and the level should be maintained at 100 IU/l. Reinfection of the graft is often associated with fibrosing cholestatic hepatitis.

Recently, effective non-toxic inhibitors of the HBV DNA polymerase have been developed. These nucleoside analogues (at the time of writing lamivudine and famciclovir) suppress HBV DNA synthesis and viraemia, and are particularly useful in liver transplant recipients (Grellier et al. 1996). After withdrawal the viraemia usually returns very rapidly (Dienstag et al. 1995), because the HBV cccDNA in the hepatocytes has a long half-life. Furthermore, the expression of the HBV RNA pregenome and the formation of the HBV DNA polymerase or of other proteins is not inhibited (Averett and Mason 1995). Therefore resistant variants can easily develop and have already been observed in clinical trials. Combination therapy as with HIV may be more promising.

An interesting possibility is treatment with antisense oligonucleotides or ribozymes, but this has not yet reached the phase of clinical testing. Immune stimulation using HBsAg vaccines with anti-preS antigen, with HBcAg or with core peptides is still in the experimental phase.

REFERENCES

Antonucci TK, Rutter WJ, 1989, Hepatitis B virus (HBV) promoters are regulated by the HBV enhancer in a tissue specific manner, *J Virol*, **63:** 579–83.

Averett DR, Mason WS, 1995, Evaluation of drugs for antiviral activity against hepatitis B virus, *Viral Hepatitis Rev*, **2:** 129–43.

Ayoola AE, 1993, Viral hepatitis in Africa in the 90s: facing realities, *Viral Hepatitis and Liver Disease*, eds Nishioka K, Suzuki H et al., Springer-Verlag, Tokyo, 381–495.

Bartenschlager R, Junker-Niepmann M, Schaller H, 1990, The P gene product of hepatitis B virus is required as a structural component for genomic RNA encapsidation, *J Virol*, **64:** 5324–32.

Beasley RP, Hwang LY et al., 1981, Hepatocellular carcinoma and hepatitis B virus. A prospective study of 22 707 men in Taiwan, *Lancet*, **2:** 1129–33.

Berting A, Hahnen J et al., 1995, Computer-aided studies on the spatial structure of the small hepatitis B surface protein, *Intervirology*, **38:** 8–15.

Block TM, Lu X et al., 1994, Secretion of human hepatitis B virus is inhibited by the imino sugar *N*-butyldeoxynojirimycin, *Proc Natl Acad Sci USA*, **91:** 2235–9.

Blum HE, Zhang ZS et al., 1992, Hepatitis B virus X protein is not central to the viral life cycle in vitro, *J Virol*, **66:** 1223–7.

Blumberg BS, Alter HJ, Visnich SA, 1965, A 'new' antigen in leukemia sera, *JAMA*, **191:** 541–6.

Blumberg BS, Gerstley BJ et al., 1967, A serum antigen (Australia antigen) in Down's syndrome, leukemia, and hepatitis, *Ann Intern Med*, **66:** 924–31.

Bréchot C, Pourcel C et al., 1980, Presence of integrated hepatitis B virus DNA sequences in cellular DNA in human hepatocellular carcinoma, *Nature (London)*, **286:** 533–5.

de Bruin W, Leenders TK et al., 1994, Hepatitis δ virus attaches to human hepatocytes via human liver endonexin II, a specific HBsAg binding protein, *J Viral Hepatitis*, **1:** 33–8.

Bruss V, Ganem D, 1991, The role of envelope proteins in hepatitis B virus assembly, *Proc Natl Acad Sci USA*, **88:** 1059–63.

Bruss V, Lu X et al., 1994, Post-translational alterations in transmembrane topology of the hepatitis B virus large envelope protein, *EMBO J*, **13:** 2273–9.

Budkowska A, Bedossa P et al., 1995, Fibronectin of human liver sinusoids binds hepatitis B virus: identification by an anti-idiotypic antibody bearing the internal image of the pre-S2 domain, *J Virol*, **69:** 840–8.

Buendia MA, Paterlini P et al., 1993, Liver cancer, *Viral Hepatitis – Scientific basis and management*, eds Zuckerman AJ, Thomas HC, Churchill Livingstone, Edinburgh, 137–64.

Burczynska B, Madalinski K et al., 1994, The value of quantitative measurement of HBeAg and HBsAg before interferon-α treatment of chronic hepatitis B in children, *J Hepatol*, **21:** 1097–102.

Calvert J, Summers J, 1994, Two regions of the avian hepadnavirus RNA pregenome are required in *cis* for encapsidation, *J Virol*, **68:** 2084–90.

Carman WF, 1995, Variations in the core and X genes of hepatitis B virus, *Intervirology*, **38:** 75–88.

Chang LJ, Ganem D, Varmus HE, 1990, Mechanism of translation of the hepadnaviral polymerase (P) gene, *Proc Natl Acad Sci USA*, **87:** 5158–62.

Chen HS, Kaneko S et al, 1993, The woodchuck hepatitis virus X gene is important for establishment of virus infection in woodchucks, *J Virol*, **66:** 1218–26.

Cherrington J, Russnak R, Ganem D, 1992, Upstream sequences and cap proximity in the regulation of polyadenylation in ground squirrel hepatitis virus, *J Virol*, **66:** 7589–96.

Chisari FV, Ferrari C, 1995, Hepatitis B virus immunopathogenesis, *Annu Rev Immunol*, **13:** 29–60.

Crowther RA, Kiselev NA et al., 1994, Three-dimensional structure of hepatitis B virus core particles determined by electron cryomicroscopy, *Cell*, **77:** 943–50.

Dane DS, Cameron CH, Briggs M, 1970, Virus-like particles in serum of patients with Australia-antigen-associated hepatitis, *Lancet*, **1:** 695–8.

Dejean A, Bougueleret L et al., 1986, Hepatitis B virus DNA integration in a sequence homologous to v-erb-A and steroid receptor genes in a hepatocellular carcinoma, *Nature (London)*, **322:** 70–2.

Dienes HP, Gerlich WH et al., 1990, Hepatic pre-S1 and pre-S2 expression pattern in viremic and non-viremic chronic hepatitis B, *Gastroenterology*, **98:** 1017–23.

Dienstag JL, Perillo RP et al., 1995, A preliminary trial of lamivudine for chronic hepatitis B infection, *N Engl J Med*, **333:** 1657–61.

Ellis RW (ed), 1993, *Hepatitis B Vaccines in Clinical Practice*, Marcel Dekker, New York.

Fernholz D, Galle PR et al., 1993, Infectious hepatitis B virus variant defective in pre-S2 protein expression in a chronic carrier, *Virology*, **194:** 137–48.

Findlay GM, MacCallum FO, 1937, Note on acute hepatitis and yellow fever immunization, *Trans R Soc Trop Med Hyg*, **31:** 297–308.

Galibert F, Mandart E et al., 1979, Nucleotide sequence of the hepatitis B virus genome (subtype *ayw*) cloned in *E. coli*, *Nature (London)*, **281**: 646–50.

Gallina A, Gazina E, Milanese G, 1995, A C-terminal preS1 sequence is sufficient to retain hepatitis B virus L protein in 293 cells, *Virology*, **213**: 57–69.

Ganem D, Pollack JR, Tavis J, 1994, Hepatitis B virus reverse transcriptase and its many roles in hepadnaviral genomic replication, *Infect Agents Dis*, **3**: 85–93.

Gerlich WH, Goldmann U et al., 1982, Specificity and localization of the hepatitis B virus-associated protein kinase, *J Virol*, **42**: 761–6.

Gerlich WH, Uy A et al., 1986, Cutoff levels of immunoglobulin M antibody against viral core antigen for differentiation of acute, chronic and past hepatitis B virus infections, *J Clin Microbiol*, **24**: 288–93.

Gerlich WH, Heermann KH et al., 1995, Quantitative assays for hepatitis B virus DNA: standardization and quality control, *Viral Hepatitis Rev*, **1**: 53–7.

Graef E, Caselmann WH et al., 1994, Insertional activation of mevalonate kinase by hepatitis B virus DNA in a human hepatoma cell line, *Oncogene*, **9**: 81–7.

Grellier L, Mutimer D et al., 1996, Lamivudine prophylaxis against reinfection in liver transplantation for hepatitis B cirrhosis, *Lancet*, **348**: 1212–15.

Guidotti LG, Martinez V et al., 1994, Hepatitis B virus nucleocapsid particles do not cross the hepatocyte nuclear membrane in transgenic mice, *J Virol*, **68**: 5469–75.

Heermann KH, Goldmann U et al., 1984, Large surface proteins of hepatitis B virus containing the pre-S sequence, *J Virol*, **52**: 396–402.

Henkler F, Koshy R, 1996, Multiple functions of the hepatitis B virus X protein, *Viral Hepatitis Rev*, **2**: 143–59.

Hertogs K, Depla E et al., 1994, Spontaneous development of anti-hepatitis B virus envelope (anti-idiotypic) antibodies in animals immunized with human liver endonexin II or with the F(ab′)2 fragment of anti-human liver endonexin II immunoglobulin G: evidence for a receptor-ligand-like relationship between small hepatitis B surface antigen and endonexin II, *J Virol*, **68**: 1516–21.

Hildt E, Hofschneider PH, Urban S, 1997, The role of hepatitis B virus (HBV) in the development of hepatocellular carcinoma, *Semin Virology*, **7**: 333–47.

Hino O, Tabata S, Hotta Y, 1991, Evidence for increased in vitro recombination with insertion of human hepatitis B virus DNA, *Proc Natl Acad Sci USA*, **88**: 9248–52.

Hirsch RC, Lavine JE et al., 1990, Polymerase gene products of hepatitis B viruses are required for genomic RNA packaging as well as for reverse transcription, *Nature (London)*, **344**: 552–5.

Hirsch RC, Loeb DD et al., 1991, *cis*-acting sequences required for encapsidation of duck hepatitis B virus pregenomic RNA, *J Virol*, **65**: 3309–16.

Howard C, Burell CJ et al., 1995, International Committee on Taxonomy of Viruses, *Arch Virol*, **suppl 10**: 179–84.

Hu J, Seeger C, 1996, Hsp90 is required for the activity of a hepatitis B virus reverse transcriptase, *Proc Natl Acad Sci USA*, **93**: 1060–4.

Huang J, Liang TJ, 1993, A novel hepatitis B virus (HBV) genetic element with Rev response element-like properties that is essential for expression of HBV gene products, *Mol Cell Biol*, **13**: 7476–86.

Ip HM, Lelie PN et al., 1989, Prevention of hepatitis B virus carrier state in infants according to maternal serum levels of HBV DNA, *Lancet*, **1**: 406–10.

Ishikawa T, Kuroki K et al., 1994, Analysis of the binding of a host cell surface glycoprotein to the preS protein of duck hepatitis B virus, *Virology*, **202**: 1061–4.

Jacyna MR, Thomas HC, 1993, Pathogenesis and treatment of chronic infection, *Viral Hepatitis – Scientific basis and management*, eds Zuckerman AJ, Thomas HC, Churchill Livingstone, Edinburgh, 185–205.

Jeng KS, Hu CP, Chang C, 1991, Different formation of disulfide linkages in the core antigen of extracellular and intracellular hepatitis B virus core particles, *J Virol*, **65**: 3924–7.

Junker-Niepmann M, Bartenschlager R, Schaller H, 1990, A short *cis*-acting sequence is required for hepatitis B virus pregenome encapsidation and sufficient for packaging of foreign RNA, *EMBO J*, **9**: 3389–96.

Kann M, Bischof A, Gerlich WH, 1997, In vitro model for the nuclear transport of the hepadnavirus genome, *J Virol*, **71**: 1310–16.

Kann M, Gerlich WH, 1994, Effect of core protein phosphorylation by protein kinase C on encapsidation of RNA within core particles of hepatitis B virus, *J Virol*, **68**: 7993–8000.

Kenney JM, von Bonsdorff CH et al., 1995, Evolutionary conservation in the hepatitis B virus core structure: comparison of human and duck cores, *Structure*, **3**: 1009–19.

Köck J, Borst EM, Schlicht HJ, 1996, Uptake of duck hepatitis B virus into hepatocytes occurs by endocytosis but does not require passage of the virus through an acidic intracellular compartment, *J Virol*, **70**: 5827–31.

Köck J, Schlicht HJ, 1993, Analysis of the earliest steps of hepadnavirus replication: genome repair after infectious entry into hepatocytes does not depend on viral polymerase activity, *J Virol*, **67**: 4867–74.

Kuroki K, Cheung R et al., 1994, A cell surface protein that binds avian hepatitis B virus particles, *J Virol*, **68**: 2091–6.

Kuroki K, Eng F et al., 1995, gp180, a host cell glycoprotein that binds duck hepatitis B virus particles, is encoded by a member of the carboxypeptidase gene family, *J Biol Chem*, **270**: 15022–8.

Lanford RE, Notvall L, 1990, Expression of hepatitis B virus core and precore antigens in insect cells and characterization of a core-associated kinase activity, *Virology*, **176**: 222–33.

Lu X, Block TM, Gerlich WH, 1996, Protease-induced infectivity of hepatitis B virus for a human hepatoblastoma cell line, *J Virol*, **70**: 2277–85.

Lu X, Mehta A et al., 1995, Evidence that N-linked glycosylation is necessary for hepatitis B virus secretion, *Virology*, **213**: 660–5.

Lürmann A, 1885, Eine Icterusepidemie, *Berl Klin Wochenschr*, **22**: 20–3.

McIntyre N, Benhamou JP et al. (eds), 1991, *Oxford Textbook of Clinical Hepatology*, Oxford University Press, Oxford.

McLachlan A, 1991, *Molecular Biology of the Hepatitis B Virus*, CRC Press, Boca Raton FL.

Machida A, Kishimoto S et al., 1984, A polypeptide containing 55 amino acid residues coded by the pre-S region of hepatitis B virus deoxyribonucleic acid bears the receptor for polymerized human as well as chimpanzee albumins, *Gastroenterology*, **86**: 9101–8.

Magnius LO, Espmark JA, 1972, A new antigen complex cooccurring with Australian antigen, *Acta Pathol Microbiol Scand*, **B80**: 335–7.

Magnius LO, Norder H, 1995, Subtypes, genotypes and molecular epidemiology of the hepatitis B virus as reflected by sequence variability of the S-gene, *Intervirology*, **38**: 24–34.

Mehdi H, Kaplan MJ et al., 1994, Hepatitis B virus surface antigen binds to apolipoprotein H, *J Virol*, **68**: 2415–24.

Nassal M, Junker-Niepmann M, Schaller H, 1990, Translational inactivation of RNA function: discrimination against a subset of genomic transcripts during HBV nucleocapsid assembly, *Cell*, **63**: 1357–63.

Nassal M, Schaller H, 1996, Hepatitis B virus replication – an update, *J Viral Hepatitis*, **3**: 217–26.

Neurath AR, Strick N, Sproul P, 1992, Search for hepatitis B virus cell receptors reveals binding sites for interleukin 6 on the virus envelope protein, *J Exp Med*, **175**: 461–9.

Newbold JE, Xin H et al., 1995, The covalently closed duplex form of the hepadnavirus genome exists in situ as a heterogeneous population of viral minichromosomes, *J Virol*, **69**: 3350–7.

Norder H, Courouce AM, Magnius LO, 1994, Complete genomes, phylogenetic relatedness, and structural proteins of six strains of the hepatitis B virus, four of which represent two new genotypes, *Virology*, **198:** 489–503.

Obert S, Zachmann Brand B et al., 1996, A splice hepadnavirus RNA that is essential for virus replication, *EMBO J*, **15:** 2565–74.

Ou JH, Bao H et al., 1990, Preferred translation of human hepatitis B virus polymerase from core protein – but not from precore protein-specific transcript, *J Virol*, **64:** 4578–81.

Pontisso P, Ruvoletto MG et al., 1989, Identification of an attachment site for human liver plasma membranes on hepatitis B virus particles, *Virology*, **173:** 522–30.

Prince DL, Prince HN et al., 1993, Methodological approaches to disinfection of human hepatitis B virus, *J Clin Microbiol*, **31:** 3296–304.

Qiao M, Macnaughton TB, Gowans EJ, 1994, Adsorption and penetration of hepatitis B virus in a nonpermissive cell line, *Virology*, **201:** 356–63.

Quint WG, Heijtink RA et al., 1995, Reliability of methods for hepatitis B virus DNA detection, *J Clin Microbiol*, **33:** 225–8.

Rakotomahanina CK, Hilger C et al., 1994, Biological activities of a putative truncated hepatitis B virus X gene product fused to a polylysin stretch, *Oncogene*, **9:** 2613–21.

Robinson WS, Miller RH, Marion PL, 1987, The role of hepadnaviruses in hepatocellular carcinoma, *Pharmacol Ther*, **35:** 1–26.

Rogler CE, Chisari FV, 1992, Cellular and molecular mechanisms of hepatocarcinogenesis, *Semin Liver Dis*, **12:** 265–78.

Rosmorduc O, Petit MA et al., 1995, In vivo and in vitro expression of defective hepatitis B virus particles generated by spliced hepatitis B virus RNA, *Hepatology*, **22:** 10–19.

Samuel D, Müller R et al., 1993, Liver transplantation in European patients with the hepatitis B surface antigen, *N Engl J Med*, **329:** 1824–47.

Schaefer S, Gerlich WH, 1995, In vitro transformation by hepatitis B virus DNA, *Intervirology*, **38:** 143–54.

Schaller H, Fischer M, 1991, Hepatitis B virus, *Curr Top Microbiol Immunol*, **168:** 21–39.

Schlicht HJ, Schaller H, 1989, Analysis of hepatitis B virus gene functions in tissue culture and in vivo, *Curr Top Microbiol Immunol*, **144:** 253–63.

Schlicht HJ, Wasenauer G, 1991, The quaternary structure, antigenicity, and aggregational behavior of the secretory core protein of human hepatitis B virus are determined by its signal sequence, *J Virol*, **65:** 6817–25.

Shikata T, Karasawa T et al., 1977, Hepatitis B e antigen and infectivity of hepatitis B virus, *J Infect Dis*, **136:** 571–6.

Summers J, Mason WS, 1982, Replication of the genome of a hepatitis B-like virus by reverse transcription of an RNA intermediate, *Cell*, **29:** 403–15.

Summers J, Smith PM, Horwich AL, 1990, Hepadnavirus envelope proteins regulate covalently closed circular DNA amplification, *J Virol*, **64:** 2819–24.

Sureau C, Lanford R, 1993, Analysis of hepatitis B virus envelope proteins in assembly and infectivity of human hepatitis delta virus, *Prog Clin Biol Res*, **382:** 45–51.

Toh H, Hayashida H, Miyata T, 1983, Sequence homology between retroviral reverse transcriptase and putative polymerases of hepatitis B virus and cauliflower mosaic virus, *Nature (London)*, **305:** 827–9.

Trevisan A, Cavigli R et al., 1988, Hepatocyte receptors for polymerized albumin. Experimental study on isolated hepatocytes and in vivo animals, *Minerva Med*, **79:** 81–90.

Tuttleman JS, Pourcel C, Summers J, 1986, Formation of the pool of covalently closed circular viral DNA in hepadnavirus-infected cells, *Cell*, **47:** 451–60.

Wallace L, Carman WF, 1997, Clinical implications of surface gene variation of HBV, *Viral Hepatitis Rev*, **3(1):** in press.

Wang GH, Seeger C, 1993, Novel mechanism for reverse transcription in hepatitis B viruses, *J Virol*, **67:** 6507–12.

Wang J, Chenivesse X et al., 1990, Hepatitis B virus integration in a cyclin A gene in a hepatocellular carcinoma, *Nature (London)*, **343:** 555–7.

West DJ, 1993, Scope and design of hepatitis B vaccine clinical trials, *Hepatitis B Virus in Clinical Practice*, ed Ellis EW, Marcel Dekker, New York, Basel, Hong Kong, 159–78.

Will H, Cattaneo R et al., 1985, Infectious hepatitis B virus from cloned DNA of known nucleotide sequence, *Proc Natl Acad Sci USA*, **82:** 891–5.

Wollersheim M, Debelka U, Hofschneider PH, 1988, A transactivating function encoded in the hepatitis B virus X gene is conserved in the integrated state, *Oncogene*, **3:** 545–52.

Yaginuma K, Shirakata Y et al., 1987, Hepatitis B virus (HBV) particles are produced in a cell culture system by transient expression of transfected HBV DNA, *Proc Natl Acad Sci USA*, **84:** 2678–82.

Yu M, Summers J, 1994, Multiple functions of capsid protein phosphorylation in duck hepatitis B virus replication, *J Virol*, **68:** 4341–8.

Zoulim F, Saputelli J, Seeger C, 1994, Woodchuck hepatitis virus X protein is required for viral infection in vivo, *J Virol*, **68:** 2026–30.

Zuckerman AJ, Thomas HC (eds), 1993, *Viral Hepatitis – Scientific basis and clinical management*, Churchill Livingstone, Edinburgh.

Chapter 37

HEPATITIS DELTA

J M Taylor

1 INTRODUCTION

The first clue to the existence of the virus came in 1977. Acute exacerbations of liver disease were being observed in patients chronically infected with hepatitis B virus (HBV), and it was speculated that these were due to infection by another virus. To test this hypothesis, convalescent sera were tested for antibodies that would react with liver biopsies taken at the peak of the disease. A novel nuclear antigen, called delta antigen, was found (Rizzetto et al. 1977). An initial interpretation was that the delta antigen might be a new variant of HBV. However, a more surprising explanation was subsequently obtained. By 1980, it was shown that this antigen was not only in the nucleus of infected hepatocytes but also within serum particles, and that it was part of an infectious agent that could be transmitted to chimpanzees (Rizzetto et al. 1980). Sometimes called the hepatitis delta agent, it is more commonly known as the hepatitis delta virus or hepatitis D virus (HDV). However, this nomenclature can be confusing, because we now know that HDV is a subviral agent that depends on HBV to provide the envelope proteins needed for the assembly of new virions. On the one hand, this dependence of HDV replication on HBV means that many aspects of HDV and HBV biology overlap. On the other hand, the RNA genome of HDV and its strategy of replication have proven to have features unlike those of the helper HBV or any other infectious agent of animals.

2 PROPERTIES OF THE VIRUS

2.1 Classification

HDV is classified as a **satellite** rather than a virus, because HBV acts as an essential helper. The RNA genome of HDV and its mechanism of replication are unique relative to RNA viruses but, as discussed in section 2.5 (p. 777), they have important similarities to certain infectious agents of plants. Nevertheless, there are also significant differences between these plant agents and HDV, leading to its classification in the new floating genus *Deltavirus*.

2.2 Virion structure

In the serum of an HDV-infected individual there are not only HDV particles but also the non-infectious empty surface antigen particles characteristic of HBV infection. The 42 nm diameter HBV may also be found, though surface antigen particles are always in at least 100-fold excess. The hepatitis B surface antigen particles (HBsAg) include both roughly spherical particles of 22 nm diameter and elongated filaments. Several groups of workers have tried to purify the HDV particles away from HBV and HBsAg particles. HDV was thus estimated to be c. 38–43 nm in diameter (Bonino et al. 1984, He et al. 1989, Ryu, Bayer and Taylor 1992). The envelope proteins of these particles include the same 3 found in HBV. Inside the HDV particle is the RNA genome, and c. 70 copies of the delta antigen (Ryu et al. 1993). The size and shape of this HDV ribonucleoprotein structure may be more heterogeneous than initially claimed; it is certainly not like the more defined icosahedral core structures of HBV.

The single-stranded RNA genome of HDV is, in several ways, fundamentally different from those of other RNA viruses of animals (Lai 1995):

1 At c. 1700 nt it is the smallest.
2 The genome has a circular conformation whereas the other viral genomes are linear.
3 The circle is able to fold on itself, with Watson and Crick base pairing of c. 70% of the nucleotides, forming an unbranched rod-like structure.
4 On the genome is a domain of c. 85 nt, which acts as a self-cleaving ribozyme. When heated in vitro,

in the presence of magnesium ions, this domain undergoes a specific transesterification reaction. The reaction can also be reversed in vitro, achieving self-ligation.

2.3 Replication

HBV is a hepatotropic virus but we do not yet know the receptor(s) by which it enters hepatocytes. We do know, however, that antibodies against epitopes within the preS1 and preS2 domains of the HBV envelope proteins neutralize the virus. The same is true for HDV (Sureau et al. 1992). The replication of HDV in an infected animal is limited to the liver (Netter et al. 1994).

Replication of the HDV genome is basically different from that of HBV; there is no involvement of reverse transcription. HDV replication occurs via RNA-directed RNA synthesis. There is evidence to suggest that the enzyme involved is the host RNA polymerase II, which by some mechanism has somehow been redirected or captured by the HDV RNA to carry out RNA- rather than DNA-directed transcription (Macnaughton et al. 1991, Fu and Taylor 1993).

Inside infected cells there are not only HDV genomes but also complementary copies, called antigenomes. These have the same 4 properties mentioned for the genomes in section 2.2 (p. 775). In addition, the antigenomic RNA encodes, down one side of the rod-like structure, the 195 amino acid (aa) delta antigen. However, the antigenomic RNA, like the genomic RNA, is located in the nucleus and is not translated; the circular confirmation of this molecule is likewise inconsistent with translation. Translation of the delta antigen is considered to depend on a third HDV RNA. This RNA is polyadenylated and cytoplasmic. Its size and sequence include the appropriate side of the antigenome; it is thus considered to be the mRNA for the delta antigen (Hsieh and Chao 1990). It has been estimated that an infected liver cell contains 300 000, 50 000 and 600 copies of the genome, antigenome and mRNA, respectively (Chen et al. 1986).

During genome replication an ever-increasing fraction of the antigenomes undergoes one or more post-transcriptional RNA-editing events. One such event is specific and essential for the life cycle. The adenosine located in the middle of the amber termination codon for the 195 aa delta antigen is deaminated by a host enzyme (Polson, Bass and Casey 1996). Ultimately this gives rise to molecules of mRNA in which the amber termination codon is replaced by one for tryptophan. This altered mRNA encodes a somewhat longer protein, the 214 aa delta antigen. Both the small and the large forms of the delta antigen are essential for HDV replication.

The small form of the delta antigen is required for genome replication (Kuo, Chao and Taylor 1989). The large delta antigen, which appears later in infection, does not support genome replication and, instead, is a dominant negative inhibitor of such replication (Chao, Hsieh and Taylor 1990). This inhibition may be associated with the fact that the large delta antigen is essential for the assembly of HDV ribonucleoprotein particles into new virions containing envelope proteins of the helper HBV (Chang et al. 1991). Another important property of the large form is that it becomes farnesylated at a site 4 aa from the new C terminus (Otto and Casey 1996). This modification is essential for virion formation (Glenn 1995), presumably because it facilitates interaction with membranes or HBV envelope proteins, or both. A monophosphorylated form of the large delta antigen has been detected, but only inside infected cells and not in serum particles (Bichko, Barik and Taylor 1997).

The two forms of the delta antigen thus have distinct biological functions. At the same time, because they share the same 195 aa antigen, they have some properties in common (Hwang, Jeng and Lai 1995). These include (1) a domain involved in protein–protein dimerization and multimerization; (2) a bipartite signal that acts as a signal for localization to the nucleus; and (3) a bipartite signal for protein–RNA interactions; the delta antigens have some specificity for recognizing HDV rod-like RNAs relative to other RNAs. Both proteins are highly basic.

2.4 Experimental systems

The HBV envelope proteins are essential for virion formation, but replication of the HDV genome can be achieved in cells independent of the helper virus. Genome replication can be studied in simple cell culture and even in vitro.

Other than humans, the only hosts that are known to allow complete replication of HDV are the chimpanzee and the woodchuck. The woodchuck hepatitis virus (WHV) is a near relative of HBV, and HDV can replicate in woodchucks with WHV replacing HBV as helper (Ponzetto et al. 1984). Other hepadnaviruses, such as duck HBV, are not able to support HDV replication.

The only cultured animal cells that can be infected with HDV are primary hepatocytes. This is considered to reflect the need for the same receptors as used by the helper HBV. Thus, natural HDV will infect human or chimpanzee hepatocytes, and HDV that has been passaged in woodchucks will infect woodchuck hepatocytes.

If one avoids the need for a receptor interaction by using techniques that directly fuse viral and cell membranes, HDV can be introduced into established cell lines that are not necessarily of liver origin (Bichko, Netter and Taylor 1994). Under such conditions, HDV genome replication occurs. This can also be achieved by transfection of cells with HDV RNA or cDNA constructs. For RNA transfections the small form of the delta antigen must either be present in the transfected cells or enter with the RNA. One interpretation is that HDV RNA will only migrate to the nucleus as a ribonucleoprotein complex with the delta antigen. If the transfected cells are also expressing the envelope proteins of the helper virus, HDV virus-like particles can be released. These will be infectious if not only the small but also the large envelope proteins of HBV are present; the large envelope protein contains the preS1 domain, which is essential for HBV receptor interactions (Sureau et al. 1992).

2.5 Plant viroid analogy

Even though HDV is in many respects unique among RNA viruses of animals, it does seem to have some relatives in the plant world. Viroids, of which more than 25 have been described, are subviral agents of plants. Like HDV, they have small single-stranded RNA genomes that are circular in conformation and able to replicate via redirection of the host RNA polymerase II. In some cases they contain both self-cleavage domains and the ability to self-ligate. However, unlike HDV, they are much smaller (only 240–375 nt), encode no proteins and are not dependent in any way on a helper virus (Taylor et al. 1990).

3 CLINICAL AND PATHOLOGICAL ASPECTS

3.1 Transmission

Like HBV, HDV is a blood-borne pathogen. Cycles of HDV replication depend on the envelope proteins produced by HBV; nevertheless, the modes of successful HDV transmission can be somewhat different from those of HBV. (Theoretically, expression of envelope proteins via integrated copies of HBV DNA might be able to support HDV replication cycles.) HDV is transmitted among drug abusers via contaminated needles and by blood products and transfusions. Sexual and perinatal transmission are rare.

In natural situations, cycles of HDV replication fall into two classes: **superinfections**, in which the person is already infected with HBV; or **co-infections**, in which the person receives both HDV and the helper HBV at the same time. For some time it was considered that superinfections were more likely than co-infections to lead to fulminant hepatitis. More recently, it has been hypothesized that, as HDV replication may be aided by a more aggressive HBV replication, it could be the response of the host to the HBV replication that is the principal element in pathogenesis (Casey et al. 1996). Some HDV infections pass through the acute phase and survive as a chronic infection. Such chronicity also depends on a chronic HBV infection; thus it is not surprising that HDV superinfections of patients already chronically infected with HBV are more likely, after the acute phase, to proceed to chronicity.

A third mechanism of HDV infection is believed to arise in some patients with terminal HDV-associated cirrhosis who are given a liver transplant from a virus-free donor. The interpretation is that hepatocytes of the new liver can first become infected by HDV alone; these would be non-productive or **latent** infections, in which genome replication occurs but no particles are

produced. Later, superinfection of such hepatocytes with HBV leads to rescue and spread of the HDV (Rizzetto and Ponzetto 1995). Analogous latent infections have also been produced in experimental animals (Netter et al. 1994).

3.2 Detection and clinical manifestations

There are several serum-based, commercially available assays for HDV infection. The most widely used test is for antibodies (IgM, IgG or both) directed against the delta antigen. More expensive tests are available for detection in serum of the delta antigen or the genomic RNA. Hybridization assays typically need more than 10^5 viral genomes per sample. By using reverse transcriptase to produce cDNA copies and the subsequent amplification of this cDNA with the polymerase chain reaction, as few as 10 molecules of the genome can be detected; however, sequence heterogeneity between isolates can render difficult the choice of appropriate oligonucleotide primers.

At one time, liver biopsy, with direct detection of delta antigen by immunohistochemistry, was considered the gold standard for the detection of HDV infections (Rizzetto and Ponzetto 1994). However, in chronic infections the number of infected hepatocytes and the level of replication per infected hepatocyte can be too low for easy detection. Not surprisingly, with more sophisticated in situ hybridization procedures, the sensitivity of detection can be increased. The possibility of adverse consequences of liver biopsy weighs against the use of the approach for routine purposes.

HDV infections may or may not have any pathogenic effect. For example, on one Greek island there was an endemic chronic infection with both HBV and HDV, yet infected individuals had no detectable signs of liver damage (Hadziyannis et al. 1993). In contrast, there have been local epidemics of HDV in the Amazon basin of South America associated with a high incidence of fulminant hepatitis and death. It is possible that in such individuals there is an excessive HBV replication with associated immune response and liver damage, and that the HDV – which after all depends on HBV – replicates more efficiently (Casey et al. 1996). Early studies ascribed for such patients specific histological lesions, such as cytoplasmic eosinophilia, and microvesicular steatosis without an inflammatory infiltrate. More recent studies argue against any direct involvement of HDV markers in such lesions. The lesions may reflect derangement in the secretory pathway of certain hepatocytes (Rizzetto and Ponzetto 1995) or the consequences of exposure to interferon presumably induced in response to the viral infection (Shimizu and Purcell 1989).

The incubation period before an acute HDV infection is c. 3–7 weeks (Purcell and Gerin 1996). This is followed by a preicteric phase of c. 1 week, during which there can be various non-specific symptoms such as fatigue, lethargy, anorexia and nausea. During this time the levels of virus in serum rise to a peak, and then fall, usually within a few days. Peak titres of

10^{10}–10^{12} HDV particles/ml can be detected in the serum. Such titres are much higher than for HBV, which usually do not exceed 10^9–10^{10} particles/ml, but are similar to the titre of HBsAg 22 nm particles. Also detected in serum is an increase in biochemical markers of liver damage, such as alanine and aspartate aminotransferases. The appearance of jaundice defines the next phase, the icteric phase. Fatigue and nausea may persist. Serum bilirubin levels may become abnormal. Even though the markers of HDV replication are decreasing, this phase may be the most severe clinical stage. At this point a fulminant hepatitis may occur, but this is rare, though c. 10 times more frequent than for hepatitis induced by HBV alone or by other hepatitis viruses. For most co-infections the patient recovers over a period of weeks to months, and HDV infection is cleared. In superinfections, however, the acute phase is usually followed by a chronic HDV infection. Such chronicity has a high chance of proceeding to cirrhosis and even hepatic failure. It has been thought that chronic HDV infections can progress not only to cirrhosis but also to hepatocellular carcinoma (Fattovich et al. 1987). A more recent evaluation suggests that, although chronic HDV infections frequently increase the risk of cirrhosis, they may only indirectly, via the HBV, increase the risk of hepatocellular carcinoma (Kew 1996).

3.3 Epidemiology and phylogenetics

As mentioned in Chapter 36 (section 3.5), chronic HBV infections number c. 350 million world-wide. Of these, it has been estimated that c. 25 million also involve HDV (Alter and Hadler 1993). HDV has been detected in many parts of the world, including Europe (Italy, Spain), Asia (China, Taiwan, Japan), the former USSR and South America (Amazon basin, Peru). The incidence in the USA is relatively low. World-wide the levels are decreasing with the impact of HBV vaccination (which also protects against HDV), testing of blood before transfusion and, in some cases, altered patterns of intravenous drug use.

Primary sequence differences between isolates can be as much as 35%. Such sequence differences have been used to group isolates into 3 genotypes. Genotype I contains the majority of isolates and has been divided further into subgroups (Niro et al. 1997). Genotype II consists of several isolates from east Asia. Genotype III includes only a small number of isolates from life-threatening infections in the Amazon basin. It was first thought that this was a more virulent HDV. Now it is believed that the replication of the associated HBV, of genotype F (Chapter 36, section 2.7), might be largely responsible for the high degree of pathogenicity.

3.4 Pathogenicity and interactions with the helper virus

It has been reported that when the small form of the delta antigen is expressed in cultured cells there can be an associated cytopathic effect (Cole et al. 1991). In contrast, mice made transgenic for the expression of either the small or the large forms of the delta antigen fail to show any associated pathology (Guilhot et al. 1994). It is generally agreed that there are no striking direct cytopathic effects of replication for HDV (or HBV) (Gowans and Bonino 1993).

Nevertheless, HDV replication is not without consequences for the infected cell. For example, in mice experimentally infected with HDV a small fraction of hepatocytes became infected and were somehow replaced within several days, even in mice with a severe combined immunodeficiency (Netter, Kajino and Taylor 1993). Also, some studies in tissue culture support the interpretation that in cells replicating the HDV genome the rate of cell division is decreased (Bichko and Taylor 1996).

It has been noted that, at the peak of an acute HDV infection, replication of the helper virus can be suppressed transiently (Purcell and Gerin 1996). However, in some cases this suppression can be as little as several-fold (Netter et al. 1994).

3.5 Treatment

Treatment with interferon-α is known to suppress particle production. However, the doses have to be very high and the side effects are substantial. Moreover, when therapy is withdrawn, the patient's HDV production usually resumes promptly. The cure rate that can be ascribed to such treatment, after subtracting spontaneous cures, is probably <20% (Rizzetto and Ponzetto 1995).

It is reasonable to expect that suppression of HBV replication and assembly would indirectly suppress HDV replication. Some of the inhibitors, such as lamivudine, have potent action on HBV replication and should therefore inhibit HDV (Luscombe and Locarnini 1996). Even the effects of interferon-α on HDV might in large part be indirect, via suppression of the HBV.

3.6 Vaccination

In most cases, an HDV-specific vaccine is not needed because that for HBV is effective, indirectly. However, for those already chronically infected with HBV, an HDV vaccine might be of use. In several preliminary studies the delta antigen was used for vaccination, with variable success (Rizzetto and Ponzetto 1995).

REFERENCES

Alter M, Hadler SC, 1993, Delta hepatitis and infection in North America, *Prog Clin Biol Res*, **382:** 243–50.

Bichko V, Barik S, Taylor J, 1997, Phosphorylation of the hepatitis delta virus antigens, *J Virol*, **71:** 512–18.

Bichko V, Netter HJ, Taylor J, 1994, Introduction of hepatitis delta virus into animal cell lines via cationic liposomes, *J Virol*, **68:** 5247–52.

Bichko V, Taylor JM, 1996, Redistribution of the delta antigens in cells replicating the genome of hepatitis delta virus, *J Virol*, **70:** 8064–70.

Bonino F, Hoyer W et al., 1984, Delta hepatitis agent: structural and antigenic properties of the delta-associated particles, *Infect Immun*, **43:** 1000–5.

Casey JL, Niro GA et al., 1996, Hepatitis B virus/hepatitis D virus (HDV) coinfection in outbreaks of acute hepatitis in the Peruvian Amazon basin: the roles of HDV genotype III and HBV genotype F, *J Infect Dis*, **174:** 920–6.

Chang FL, Chen PJ et al., 1991, The large form of hepatitis δ antigen is crucial for the assembly of hepatitis δ virus, *Proc Natl Acad Sci USA*, **88:** 8490–4.

Chao M, Hsieh S-Y, Taylor J, 1990, Role of two forms of the hepatitis delta virus antigen; evidence for a mechanism of self-limiting genome replication, *J Virol*, **64:** 5066–9.

Chen P-J, Kalpana G et al., 19886, Structure and replication of the genome of hepatitis δ virus, *Proc Natl Acad Sci USA*, **83:** 8774–8.

Cole S, Gowans EJ et al., 1991, Direct evidence for cytotoxicity associated with expression of hepatitis delta virus antigen, *Hepatology*, **13:** 845–51.

Fattovich G, Boscaro S et al., 1987, Influence of hepatitis delta virus infection on progression to cirrhosis in chronic hepatitis B type, *J Infect Dis*, **155:** 931–5.

Fu TB, Taylor J, 1993, The RNAs of hepatitis delta virus are copied by RNA polymerase II in nuclear homogenates, *J Virol*, **67:** 6965–72.

Glenn JS, 1995, Prenylation and virion morphogenesis, *The Unique Hepatitis Delta Virus*, ed Dinter-Gottlieb G, Landes, Austin TX, 83–94.

Gowans EJ, Bonino F, 1993, Hepatitis delta virus pathogenicity, *Prog Clin Biol Res*, **382:** 125–30.

Guilhot S, Huang S-N et al., 1994, Expression of hepatitis delta virus large and small antigens in transgenic mice, *J Virol*, **68:** 1052–8.

Hadziyannis SJ, Dourakis SP et al., 1993, Changing epidemiology and spreading modalities of hepatitis delta infection in Greece, *Prog Clin Biol Res*, **382:** 259–66.

He L-F, Ford E et al., 1989, The size of the hepatitis delta agent, *J Med Virol*, **27:** 31–3.

Hsieh S-Y, Chao M, 1990, Hepatitis delta virus genome replication: a polyadenylated mRNA for delta antigen, *J Virol*, **64:** 3192–8.

Hwang SB, Jeng K-S, Lai MMC, 1995, Studies of functional roles of hepatitis delta antigen in delta virus RNA replication, *The Unique Hepatitis Delta Virus*, ed Dinter-Gottlieb G, Landes, Austin TX, 95–110.

Kew MC, 1996, Hepatitis delta virus and hepatocellular carcinoma, *Viral Hepatitis Rev*, **2:** 285–90.

Kuo MY-P, Chao M, Taylor J, 1989, Initiation of replication of the human hepatitis delta virus genome from cloned DNA: role of delta antigen, *J Virol*, **63:** 1945–50.

Lai MMC, 1995, The molecular biology of hepatitis delta virus, *Annu Rev Biochem*, **64:** 259–86.

Luscombe CA, Locarnini SA, 1996, The mechanism of action of antiviral agents in chronic hepatitis B, *Viral Hepatitis Rev*, **2:** 1–3.

Macnaughton TB, Gowans EJ et al., 1991, Hepatitis delta antigen is necessary for access of hepatitis delta virus RNA to the cell transcriptional machinery but is not part of the transcriptional complex, *Virology*, **184:** 387–90.

Netter HJ, Kajino K, Taylor J, 1993, Experimental transmission of human hepatitis delta virus to the laboratory mouse, *J Virol*, **67:** 3357–62.

Netter HJ, Gerin JL et al., 1994, Apparent helper-independent infection of woodchucks by hepatitis delta virus and subsequent rescue with woodchuck hepatitis virus, *J Virol*, **68:** 5344–50.

Niro GA, Smedile A et al., 1997, The predominance of hepatitis delta virus genotype I among chronically infected Italian parents, *Hepatology*, **25:** 728–34.

Otto JC, Casey PJ, 1996, The hepatitis delta virus large antigen is farnesylated both in vitro and in animal cells, *J Biol Chem*, **271:** 4659–72.

Polson AG, Bass BL, Casey JL, 1996, RNA editing of hepatitis delta virus antigenome by dsRNA-adenosine deaminase, *Nature (London)*, **380:** 454–5.

Ponzetto A, Cote PJ et al., 1984, Transmission of the hepatitis B virus-associated δ agent to the eastern woodchuck, *Proc Natl Acad Sci USA*, **81:** 2208–12.

Purcell RH, Gerin JL, 1996, Hepatitis delta virus, *Fields' Virology*, 3rd edn, eds Fields BN, Knipe DM et al., Raven Press, New York, 2819–29.

Rizzetto M, Ponzetto A, 1995, Hepatitis delta virus infection: medical aspects, *The Unique Hepatitis Delta Virus*, ed Dinter-Gottlieb G, Landes, Austin TX, 125–39.

Rizzetto M, Hoyer B et al., 1980, δ agent: association of δ antigen with hepatitis B surface antigen and RNA in serum of δ-infected chimpanzees, *Proc Natl Acad Sci USA*, **77:** 6124–8.

Rizzetto M, Canese MG et al., 1997, Immunofluorescence detection of a new antigen–antibody system associated to the hepatitis B virus in the liver and in the serum of HBsAg carriers, *Gut*, **18:** 994–1003.

Ryu WS, Netter HJ et al., 1992, Assembly of hepatitis delta virus particles, *J Virol*, **66:** 2310–15.

Ryu WS, Netter HJ et al., 1993, Ribonucleoprotein complexes of hepatitis delta virus, *J Virol*, **67:** 3281–7.

Shimizu YK, Purcell RH, 1989, Cytoplasmic antigen of hepatocytes infected with non-A, non-B hepatitis or hepatitis delta virus: relationship to interferon, *Hepatology*, **10:** 764–8.

Sureau C, Moriarty AM et al., 1992, Production of infectious hepatitis delta virus in vitro and neutralization with antibodies directed against hepatitis B virus pre-S antigens, *J Virol*, **66:** 1241–5.

Taylor J, Chao M et al., 1990, Human hepatitis delta: unique or not unique, *New Aspects of Positive-strand Viruses*, eds Brinton M, Heinz FX, ASM Publications, Washington DC, 20–4.

RETROVIRUSES AND ASSOCIATED DISEASES IN HUMANS

Thomas M Folks and Rima F Khabbaz

1 Introduction	4 Clinical and pathological aspects
2 General properties of the *Retroviridae*	5 Epidemiology
3 Human T lymphotropic and	6 Laboratory diagnosis
immunodeficiency viruses	7 Treatment and control

1 INTRODUCTION

Retroviruses seem to have played a role in the evolution of human genetics, considering the large number of retroviral remnants lacing the human genome. Why, where and how these viral residues came about are a curious enigma of our genetic structure. Did they arise from multiple infections which over time devastated new evolving species of hominoids? Did such an occurrence result in survivors who either were infected with defective retroviruses or had modified their receptors to be resistant to primary infection? The answers may become apparent if, in several thousand years, remnants of human immunodeficiency virus (HIV) are determined to be 'fixed' in the human genome.

Within the large family of retroviruses, lentiviruses, which include the HIVs, are unusual in that they possess complexities and degeneracies that differ from the biological properties of other, more stable, primate retroviruses, such as the human T lymphotropic viruses (HTLVs) and the spumaviruses. Nevertheless, these agents share common features that place them in the taxonomic category of *Retroviridae*.

Retroviruses replicate in a unique manner. An enzyme carried by the viruses reverses the usual flow of genetic information (normally from DNA to RNA (messenger RNA) and then to protein) by causing the RNA genetic information of the virus to be transcribed into DNA. This enzyme, the reverse transcriptase, is a characteristic feature of all retroviruses. Viral genetic information in the DNA form is contained in the provirus, which can be integrated into the genome of the host cell, where it may remain latent or non-expressing for variable periods. Only when the pro-

virus is activated, often by first messenger signals such as cytokines or antigens, are viral proteins and new viruses made.

Among the viruses, retroviruses and the diseases they cause were some of the earliest to be described in detail (Weiss et al. 1985). At the turn of the century, equine infectious anaemia was one of the first animal infections recognized as having a viral aetiology. Shortly afterwards, there were descriptions of filterable, transmissible agents associated with cancers among chickens that related both leukaemias (avian leukosis, 1908) and solid tumours (Rous sarcoma, 1911) to infections with viruses. In 1936, breast cancer in mice was found to be transmitted by a virus in the animal's breast milk, and from the 1950s onwards leukaemias in mice, cats, fish, apes and other vertebrate hosts were found to be caused by retroviruses. Knowledge of these cancer-causing viruses has yielded important insights into the nature of neoplasia and catalysed the search for similar agents as a cause of malignancy in humans. Despite the attraction of this idea, which implied the possibility of vaccines to prevent cancer, it was not until 1980 that the relationship between a retrovirus infection and human neoplasia was documented, leading to the eventual characterization of the HTLV.

In southwestern Japan there is a relatively high incidence of an aggressive T cell leukaemia among adults. This leukaemia, adult T cell leukaemia/lymphoma (ATL), became the first human neoplasm identified as being caused by a retrovirus. Previously, human cancers had been linked to infections with DNA viruses only; for example, hepatoma with hepatitis B virus (HBV) and Burkitt's lymphoma with Epstein–Barr virus (EBV). Cells from patients with ATL were shown by Japanese workers to produce, albeit in small quantities, a virus in tissue culture with retroviral characteristics (Miyoshi et al. 1981). A year earlier, US workers culturing cells from a patient with an aggressive cutaneous T cell tumour had identified a similar retrovirus in tissue culture (Poiesz et al. 1980). These 2 isolates were shown to be HTLV-I, and it became evident that the US patients had a type of leukaemia indistinguishable from that in Japan. After West Indian immigrants with ATL in London were found to be seropositive for antibodies to HTLV-I (anti-HTLV-I), it was recognized that the infection was also prevalent in the Caribbean basin. A second disease, HTLV-I-associated myelopathy/tropical spastic paraparesis (HAM/TSP), has more recently been associated with HTLV-I. No genetic variation of HTLV-I has been documented that would explain these different disease presentations. Since the identification of HTLV-I, a second virus of the same group, HTLV type II (HTLV-II), has been described. No disease has been clearly associated with HTLV-II.

Retroviruses have also been known for some time to cause chronic progressive degenerative diseases with long incubation periods in animals. The recognition of these features led to the concept of 'slow virus diseases' and the term 'slow viruses'. Although the disease may in fact be slow in its progression, viral replication starts early and persists after infection. Thus, the term 'slow virus' is perhaps inappropriate.

The recent transmission of a lentivirus into humans has caused the pandemic of the novel human virus disease now known as the acquired immunodeficiency syndrome, or AIDS. Although retrospective searching of the medical literature indicates the possibility of earlier cases, the first accepted indications of this new disease were reports in June 1981 to the Centers for Disease Control (CDC), Atlanta, of an abrupt increase in requests for an experimental drug, pentamidine hydrochloride, needed to treat 5 cases of a hitherto rare protozoal lung infection, *Pneumocystis carinii* pneumonia, previously seen only in immunosuppressed patients. The patients were homosexual men living in Los Angeles.

In the same year, there was also increased reporting of a rare skin tumour, Kaposi's sarcoma, among young homosexual men in California and New York. A new underlying clinical entity, characterized by profound loss of immune function associated with a depletion of CD4 helper T lymphocytes, was soon recognized. As early as 1982, the associations between this syndrome and sexual contact between homosexual/bisexual men, drug addiction and blood transfusion (including the use of pooled blood products) reinforced the concept that AIDS had an infectious aetiology.

Initially, one candidate as a causative agent of AIDS was HTLV or a related virus. In 1983, searching for this or a similar virus, French scientists identified a lymphadenopathy-associated virus (LAV) from cells taken from a homosexual patient whose lymph nodes were persistently enlarged (Barré-Sinoussi et al. 1983). LAV was at first difficult to propagate productively in

culture, a problem that greatly hampered serological investigations and to some extent obscured its significance. In 1984, US scientists developed a continuous cell line that permitted large-scale production of LAV and the development of the first serological test for mass screening. Seroprevalence studies demonstrated unequivocally the association between AIDS and infection with LAV-1. These viruses and their variants represent the group now called human immunodeficiency virus type 1 (HIV-1). In the USA and Europe in the same year, serological findings revealed an alarming level of infection among patients who reported engaging in high-risk behaviours, indicating just how effectively the virus had been spreading at a time when, in view of the small number of AIDS cases, the need for a heightened awareness was not yet evident. Since then, another AIDS-related virus (HIV-2), serologically distinct from HIV-1 but in the same family (Clavel et al. 1986), has been identified in patients with AIDS. Sera from these patients contained antibody to HIV-2 but not to HIV-1. HIV-2, closely related to simian immunodeficiency virus (SIV), is currently limited geographically mainly to certain countries in West Africa, although infections are now beginning to be found occasionally in people in Europe and the USA.

In addition to HIV-2, clades of HIV-1 have been identified that can be distinguished genetically. Recently, a type 'O' clade has emerged in Africa that cannot be identified by standard serological assays. A chimpanzee SIV has also been identified that bears a greater genetic resemblance to HIV-1 than to HIV-2. The emergence and discovery of primate lentiviruses provide the fuel for studies of the natural history of HIV and of the origin of AIDS.

2 GENERAL PROPERTIES OF THE RETROVIRIDAE

Retroviruses all have similar morphological and biochemical properties, justifying their inclusion into a single family (Martin 1993). By definition, a retrovirus depends on reverse transcription of its genetic information (carried in the mature virion as RNA) into DNA in order for replication to proceed. The reverse transcriptase (RT) serves the function of an RNA-directed DNA polymerase and is responsible for making a DNA copy of the virus. RT is carried as a functional enzyme within the mature virion, and the presence of detectable RT activity in the supernatant fluid of tissue culture is considered to be a reliable indicator of the presence of retrovirus. RT analysis coupled with the powerful polymerase chain reaction (PCR) technology (Heneine et al. 1995) now permits the detection of retroviruses with a 10 000-fold increase in sensitivity over standard RT assays.

In the mature virion the genome is diploid, carried as a 60–70S dimer complex of 2 identical, positive-sense, single-stranded RNA copies, whereas RT is a meiotic event, resulting in a double-stranded haploid DNA provirus. The proviral genome structure of retroviruses is characterized by repeated sequences at either end of the genome, the long terminal repeats (LTRs). These structures play an important role in viral expression because they contain promoter and enhancer elements. The genomes of all retroviruses that are able to replicate fully always include 3 genes coding for the 3 sets of structural proteins: those of the core proteins (*gag*), the envelope proteins (*env*) and the polymerase enzyme (*pol*). The genome arrangement LTR–*gag–pol–env*–LTR is common to all known retroviruses. A simplified retroviral life cycle is depicted in Fig. 38.1.

2.1   Classification

The family *Retroviridae* is divided into 3 subfamilies: the *Oncovirinae, Lentivirinae* and *Spumavirinae.* Oncoviruses can also be divided epidemiologically into those capable of transmission between members of the host species and those that can be passed only between parent and offspring as an integrated provirus in the germ line, termed **exogenous** and **endogenous**, respectively (Weiss et al. 1985).

2.2   Retroviruses infecting humans

Retroviruses currently recognized as important in terms of human disease include exogenous virus representatives of 2 of the subfamilies, *Oncovirinae* and *Lentivirinae.* In addition, humans have been found to be seropositive for *Spumavirinae.* Endogenous *Oncoviri-*

nae fragments can be found only as remnants of retroviruses in the human genome.

EXOGENOUS *ONCOVIRINAE*: HUMAN T LYMPHOTROPIC VIRUSES

Like animal *Oncovirinae,* the human viruses HTLV-I and II have the classic genome arrangement of retroviruses but have an extra (X) region of the genome between *env* and the 3′ LTR coding for at least 2 control proteins (tax and rex). Both viruses infect humans, but only HTLV-I is definitely known to be associated with disease.

LENTIVIRINAE: HUMAN LENTIVIRUSES

Like the HTLVs, HIV-1 and 2 have genes coding for a series of control proteins as well as containing the normal *gag, pol* and *env* genes of the conventional retrovirus. Both HIVs cause disease in humans. HIV-1 is the virus responsible for the global pandemic of AIDS; HIV-2 also causes AIDS but with much slower progression and is essentially limited to various countries in West Africa and to Portugal.

SPUMAVIRINAE: HUMAN FOAMY VIRUSES

Foamy viruses, so called because of their characteristic foamy degeneration in cell culture, infect a number of mammalian species. Retroviruses causing this 'foamy' cytopathic effect (CPE) have been reported in several human cell lines; antibodies to human foamy viruses (HFV) can be detected in human sera. Foamy viruses are frequently found in monkey tissues, especially

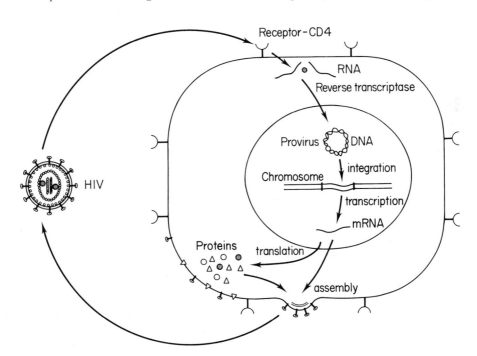

Fig. 38.1 Schematic representation of the life cycle of HIV. Virions attach to specific cell surface receptors. Following internalization and uncoating either via receptor-mediated endocytosis or by fusion at the plasma membrane, the reverse transcriptase in the core of the virion becomes activated and synthesizes a double-stranded DNA provirus. Circularized and linear forms of the provirus migrate to the nucleus and integrate in host chromosomal DNA. The integrated proviral genome may remain latent, but, if active, particularly in proliferating cells, it expresses positive-strand RNA. Full-length transcripts become packaged into progeny virions budding from the plasma membrane. Messenger RNA (mRNA) transcripts encode the structural and regulatory viral proteins, which can be recognized as antigens within infected cells.

brain and kidney cultures, and there is still some controversy as to whether the human isolates are similar culture contaminants. Although one HFV has been characterized (Mauser and Flugel 1988), little is known about their association with disease or their epidemiology and we shall not discuss them further.

ENDOGENOUS *ONCOVIRINAE*

Endogenous human retrovirus particles resembling animal oncogenic viruses have been detected in normal human placenta and some human teratocarcinoma cell lines. Although RT activity was detectable, these viruses have not been isolated as infectious particles. Cloning and sequence studies of human DNA have led to the identification of a number of distinct genetic elements that seem to be similar to certain sequences in retroviruses, ranging from full-length copies to highly defective sequences represented solely by LTRs or what seem to be single retroviral genes (most similar to *pol*). It is likely that at least some of these elements may be expressed during cell growth and differentiation of tissues, although no significance can be attributed to this expression. Little is known about their biology, other than that their proviral DNA is common to all Old World primates, and that at least one env protein is expressed in the syncytial trophoblast of the placenta.

We shall not discuss these viruses further, but it is noteworthy that a human AIDS patient has been selected for xenotransplantation treatment with bone marrow from a baboon. Baboons are known to be infected with foamy viruses, and an endogenous retrovirus is known to infect human cells in culture. Ongoing research in this area may soon improve our understanding of how these viruses behave in vivo in humans.

3 HUMAN T LYMPHOTROPIC AND IMMUNODEFICIENCY VIRUSES

3.1 Morphology

The mature virions of human retroviruses HTLV and HIV comprise icosahedral cores, containing the RNA genome, the RT enzyme and gag proteins, surrounded by an envelope acquired as the virion buds through the host cell membrane. Immature forms of both viruses can be identified budding from the periphery of infected cells; gag proteins alone can produce budding structures. The first recognizable stage of virus formation to appear is the condensation of core proteins in a semi-lunar structure beneath the cell membrane (Fig. 38.2, inset), probably as a function of the gag matrix protein. Envelope glycoproteins are inserted into the overlying cell membrane. As the core continues to condense around the genomic RNA, the immature virus particle rounds up until it is finally released into the extracellular spaces (Fig. 38.2). It is at this stage that the fine structure of the core component completes its final processing and becomes reco-

gnizable as either HTLV- or HIV-like. In the former, the nucleoid or dense inner part of the core condenses centrally within the core, whereas in the latter the core attains a cone or bar shape, often eccentrically placed. The overall diameter of the mature particles in both instances is 100–120 nm.

Host molecules, such as the class II major histocompatibility complex (MHC) (HLA-Dr), are inserted within the membrane that surrounds the virus. Host-derived glycoproteins are incorporated during morphogenesis. Membrane-bound glycoprotein spikes can be visualized for HIV, but it seems that for HTLV the binding of the spikes to the envelope is too unstable or in too low a density to allow this feature to be observed. Both viruses have been examined by negative staining for envelope spikes, but it has been difficult to resolve them owing to their fragility. Recently, cores of HIV have been visualized after mild treatment with detergents and have shown the predicted conical structure. In practice, however, most of our understanding of the structure of these viruses comes from the study of thin sections.

3.2 Genome organization

HTLV

Analysis of the complete sequence of this virus reveals an 8.3 kb genome. LTRs flank the open reading frames (ORFs), of which *gag*, *pol* and *env* are in the usual order for retroviruses and code for 48 kDa, 99 kDa and 68 kDa proteins, respectively (Fig. 38.3). In addition, there are coding frames that flank the *env* gene, the larger of which is a long reading frame between the *env* gene and the 3' LTR, called pX. This pX region contains 4 ORFs, of which at least the 2 largest, *rex* and *tax*, encode regulatory proteins, with functions similar to those of HIV rev and tat, described below. Two additional proteins have recently been described that are encoded by double spliced mRNA. One, Tof, uses the *Tax* initiation codon while the other, Rof, uses the *Rex* initiation codon. In leukaemia cells transformed by HTLV, proviral DNA can be detected within the proliferating cells, which themselves are clonal. There is, however, no integration site common to HTLV-related leukaemias. It has been speculated that one or the other of the pX proteins that transactivate the HTLV genome by interacting with the LTR may also activate specific T cell genes, leading to neoplastic transformation. HTLV-I *tax* can transactivate heterologous promoters, such as adenovirus and equine infectious anaemia and E3 promoters. As an explanation of leukaemogenesis, ATL cells have a vast overexpression of the receptor for interleukin 2 (IL-2R) as well as of IL-2 and GM-CSF. It seems that the p40 tax gene product activates IL-2R expression and possibly other cellular genes (Table 38.1), thus allowing autocrine and other factors to drive ATL cell proliferation (Gitlin et al. 1993).

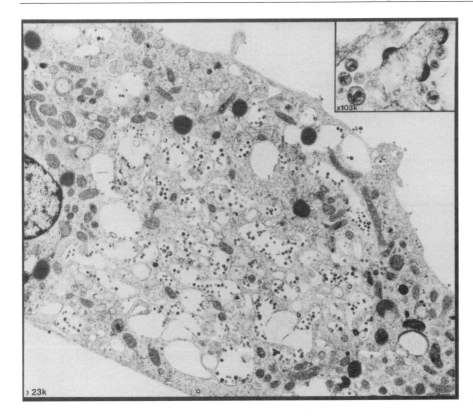

Fig. 38.2 Electron micrographs of an HIV-1-infected cell. Note budding structures (inset) at the intracellular and plasma membranes. (Courtesy of Jan Orenstein.)

HIV

The complete sequence of HIV-1 contains a 9.2 kb genome. LTRs flank the genes for *gag*, *pol* and *env* which lie in the standard order for retroviruses and code for 55 kDa, 66 kDa and 160 kDa proteins, respectively (Fig. 38.3). However, there are additional frames on either side of the *env* gene coding for at least 6 proteins, of which 5 are involved in the regulation or accessory function (Subbramanian and Cohen 1994) of HIV expression. Although much remains to be resolved about the pathways for controlling HIV expression in infected cells, some of these

Table 38.1 Cellular genes transactivated by Tax

HTLV-I Tax$_1$	HTLV-II Tax$_2$
IL-2	IL-2
IL-2Rα	IL-2Rα
GM-CSF	GM-CSF
IL-3	
Vimentin	
c-*fos*	
c-*sis*	
TGF-β1	
β-globin	
Act-2 cytokine	
egr-1	
egr-2	
Class I MHC	
NF-κB	
Nerve growth factor	

proteins are becoming quite well characterized and certain of their functions understood (Martin 1993, Antoni et al. 1994). These include the products of the following genes: *tat, rev, nef, vif, vpu, vpx* and VPR.

***tat* (transactivation gene)** The *tat* gene encodes a peptide of 14 kDa, which acts in a positive feedback loop by binding to the stem–loop region of LTR–RNA in association with cellular proteins at a defined target sequence (tar). Binding of tat results in as much as a 1000-fold increase in expression of all viral genes.

***rev* (regulator of virus gene)** The protein encoded by this spliced gene is a peptide of 19 kDa. Rev has an important function in regulating virus expression by allowing the transport of full-length, spliced mRNA from the nucleus to the cytoplasm. These mRNA transcripts (*gag, pol* and *env*) have specific rev-responsive element (RRE) sequences which require the presence of rev for transport, and in its absence become rapidly degraded in the nucleus. In contrast, the RNA sequences for non-structural proteins do not require these sequences. Thus, in the absence of rev, viral mRNA is either degraded or rapidly spliced into RNAs that can be fully transcribed. These resultant products are non-structural regulatory proteins.

***nef* (negative factor gene)** The protein encoded by this gene is a peptide of 27 kDa. The actual function of the nef protein remains unclear. It seems to be non-essential in vitro. Recently, it has been shown to down-modulate surface CD4 expression by lysosomal degradation. Additionally, nef has been identified as having considerable kinase activity and contributing to viral expression in the absence of cellular activation. Most

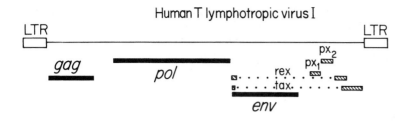

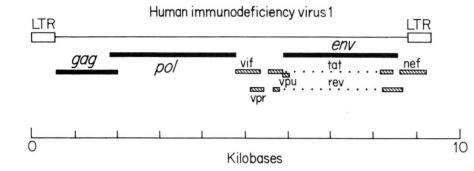

Fig. 38.3 Genome arrangement of HTLV-I and HIV-1. Genes coding for structural proteins are in solid bars, genes coding for non-structural and control proteins are cross-hatched. Dotted lines mark spliced genes.

importantly, mutations in SIV *nef* have resulted in survival of infected rhesus macaques, implying that this gene plays a larger role as a contributor to pathogenesis in vivo.

***vif* (viral infectivity factor gene)** The gene product is incorporated into virus particles in a way that confers infectivity on the virion, possibly influencing uncoating early in infection. HTLV-I and other oncoviruses lack *vif* genes. Cell-to-cell transmission is not impaired in HIV defective for *vif*, but transmission of free virus to cells is impaired. It seems likely that vif acts late in the viral life cycle, during virion assembly.

vpu* and *vpx The *vpu* (in HIV-1; 16 kDa) and *vpx* (in HIV-2; 12–16 kDa) are genes that code for viral proteins of less well defined function. Because the 2 proteins differ from each other but are both antigenic, they can be exploited in serological tests to distinguish between infection by either virus. By contrast, the detection of unique type-specific sequences *vpu* for HIV-1 and *vpx* for HIV-2 has proved most useful in distinguishing between infections by these viruses. Vpu is an accessory protein that shares a function with nef by degrading CD4. In addition, vpu shares functions with a non-retrovirus protein, M2, from influenza virus. Both proteins have ion channel functions and may affect Golgi compartment pH.

VPR (viral protein R) VPR is a 14 kDa protein that imparts a rapid growth advantage to HIV-1. It is assembled in the virion and may be associated with *gag* during transport. VPR seems to play a role with respect to nuclear import of the preintegration complex in unactivated cells. Another function attributed to VPR has been its ability to block cells in the replication cycle. The purpose of this function is not understood.

3.3 Replication strategy

Although the genomes of HTLV and HIV are both single-stranded, positive-sense mRNA and are capable of coding for protein synthesis in translation assays in vitro, linear translation of the sequence is unlikely to lead to comprehensive expression of viral proteins. The functionality of the proteins produced relies on splicing of their mRNAs. RT enzymatic action and reverse transcription seem to be required to produce a DNA intermediate. Once reverse transcription occurs, retrovirus DNA can be found in the nucleus, either as closed circular, supercoiled copies or as linear provirus copies, both unintegrated and integrated. Because both HTLV and HIV use the normal mechanisms of cellular protein synthesis for expression, it seems likely that, in addition to the regulatory proteins already described, the internal and external environment of the cell influence virus expression, possibly through interaction of certain normal intracellular proteins with the virus LTR. Such mechanisms may explain the cellular activation requirements for virus replication in HIV-infected T cells stimulated externally by antigens, superantigens or cytokines. As another example, the HIV LTR is known to have a sequence to which the lymphoid-specific cellular enhancer, NF-κB, binds. These interactions also leave open the possibility for co-factors, such as infections and non-specific cellular activators, in the progression of disease in infected individuals.

HIV expression and replication are not continuous but are likely to be stepwise. In a resting cell, there is little transcription of virus. Cell activation leads to the transcription of HIV mRNA in general, but the expression of structural viral proteins is repressed by the inhibitory sequences, RRE, in the mRNA, so that only low levels of prematurely truncated short transcripts are synthesized. However, the mRNA species that code for the regulatory proteins, including tat and rev, are transcribed. As the expression of tat and rev increases, a threshold is achieved when the positive feedback loop becomes active and transactivation is mediated by tat. At the same time, the action of rev allows the transport of functional mRNA transcripts into the cytoplasm where they are translated into proteins. As these are expressed, viral structural proteins are abundantly synthesized. Intense expression of virions leads to programmed cell death, usually with the accumulation of episomal proviruses. Cell cycle blockade in the G2/M phase macrophages seems to be more likely to sustain low levels of persistent virus release without cell death, as do lymphocytes infected with the HTLVs.

3.4 Antigens

In the course of replication, many viral proteins are expressed in the infected cell, only some of which are incorporated into the intact virion. As a result, sera from infected patients usually have antibody to more antigens than are carried on the structural proteins of the mature virions. In this section we discuss the antigenic make-up of the intact virus particle and refer to some of the precursor proteins and non-structural antigens as well as the structural proteins. In both HTLV and HIV the structural proteins arise from enzymatic cleavage of large polyprotein precursors, which can be detected in infected cells. The antigenic structure of the virus itself can be determined by disruption of purified virions. The individual proteins of the virus are separated by size, and their antigenicity is determined with specific antibodies.

HTLV STRUCTURAL ANTIGENS

Core antigens are synthesized as a 48 kDa polyprotein precursor. The nucleocapsid of the virus includes a shell of the smaller cleavage product, pl9. In addition, p24 and small amounts of pl5 are present in the inner core of the virus. Sera from infected patients usually contain antibodies to p24 and pl9, and occasionally to pl5 antigens. The cleavage of the 48 kDa precursor depends on the activity of a viral proteinase encoded in the *pol* gene.

Envelope antigens are synthesized and glycosylated to form a 68 kDa glycoprotein precursor that can be found in membranes of infected cells. Cleavage by cellular proteinases results in a 46 kDa outer glycoprotein (gp46) and a 21 kDa transmembrane protein (p21), which are the major antigens carried in the envelope of the mature virion. Sera from infected asymptomatic subjects, ATL patients and HAM/TSP patients usually contain antibodies to gp46. Some of these antibodies are also able to neutralize in vitro the infectivity of the virus. In addition to virus-specific antigens, some cell-specific surface proteins are incorporated into the envelope, including MHC antigens.

RT antigen is synthesized as a polyprotein precursor, which is cleaved autocatalytically to form the protease, RT and endonuclease ('integrase') required for viral integration. The RT is a protein of 62 kDa carried within the core and bound to the genomic RNA. Although only a few copies of this enzyme are carried in the intact virion, it is quite immunogenic and sera from infected patients frequently contain antibody to it.

HIV STRUCTURAL ANTIGENS

Although some of the HIV proteins differ in size from those of HTLV, the strategy of HIV structural antigen synthesis is essentially the same as for HTLV (Fig. 38.4).

Core antigens are synthesized as a 55 kDa polyprotein. The inner cone-shaped component of the nucleocapsid consists of a shell of the gag cleavage product p24. Besides being found in the intact virion, this protein is shed in vivo into the serum, where it can be detected as free p24 antigen in patients during early infection or as free antigen and immune complement during late stages of the infection. Its presence is a marker for viral replication, and absence of p24 antigen is often associated with patients treated successfully with antiviral agents. In addition to p24, another cleavage product, p18, makes up the icosahedral shell of the virus core. Smaller amounts of p15, further cleaved to p7 and p9, are also present in the virus. Sera from most, but not all, virus-infected patients contain antibody to a range of the gag proteins, so there is a characteristic pattern of antibody to p55, p24 and pl8. In addition, virions seem to contain variable amounts of intermediate gag cleavage products (43, 41, 39 and 35 kDa), the significance of which remains unknown.

Envelope antigens are synthesized as a heavily glycosylated polyprotein precursor of 160 kDa, detectable in infected cells. In the envelope of the virion this protein is present as 2 cleavage products: a transmembrane glycoprotein, gp4l, and an external glycoprotein, gpl20. These 2 proteins are the major envelope antigens of HIV and have the functions of attachment of virus to the target cell (gpl20) and fusion of virus envelope and cell membrane (gp4l).

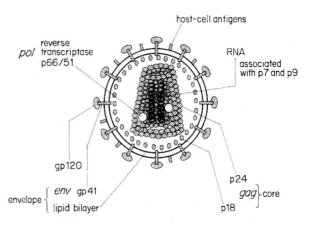

Fig. 38.4 Representation of the structure of the human immunodeficiency virus.

Besides these virus-specific proteins, host antigens of the MHC are also carried into the virus envelope during morphogenesis. Antibodies to gp41 and gp120 are almost always present in sera from infected patients.

RT antigen The biosynthesis of RT and associated enzymes of the *pol* gene is complex. The precursor is a fusion protein comprising a small C terminal portion of the gag protein and the entire pol sequence; it arises through a ribosomal frameshift as reading proceeds from the 5′ end of the *gag* gene. Autocatalytic post-translational cleavage by the protease at the N terminal end of the pol precursor protein first removes the gag sequences and then splits the precursor protein into an N terminal 10 kDa proteinase, a C terminal 32 kDa endonuclease (necessary for proviral integration) and the central 65 kDa RT protein (necessary for reverse transcription). The RT enzyme comprises a dimer of p65 protein subunits, one of which is autocatalytically cleaved to p51, and so, in the intact virus, RT is represented by a p65/51 complex. Antibodies to all these proteins are usually found in sera from infected patients.

3.5 Virus–cell interactions

For a cell to be susceptible to infection, 2 conditions have to be fulfilled. First, the envelope of the virus has to react with the cell surface and the cell must be capable of supporting viral replication. Receptors for both HTLV-I and HTLV-II are present in a wide variety of lymphoid and non-lymphoid cells of both human and non-human origin. This feature suggests that the tropism displayed by HTLV for CD4 cells is not determined at the receptor level but by the requirement for cell promoters able to recognize the LTRs of the HTLV provirus. Attachment to cells and the formation of HTLV-induced syncytia are the functions of the gp46 and gp21 envelope proteins. Inhibition of this effect by antibody to gp46 is the basis of neutralization assays for HTLV. These assays have an additional advantage of being able to distinguish between HTLV-I and HTLV-II.

The HIV receptor

Concomitant observations in 1984 of in vitro tropism of HIV for CD4 helper cells and the finding of CD4-positive lymphocyte depletion in infected patients stimulated investigations into the relationship between CD4-positive cells and HIV. Studies with monoclonal antibodies to CD4 showed conclusively that this antigen was responsible for the attachment of HIV to the target cell (Dalgleish et al. 1984). The precise binding site for the virus on CD4 has been mapped with anti-CD4 monoclonal antibodies and site-specific mutagenesis of the cloned CD4 gene. The initial function of the virus envelope is to bind to the CD4 as receptor; by use of recombinant HIV envelope gp120, mutated at known points, the site of its interaction with CD4 has also been localized to a specific region in the envelope sequence. Attachment to CD4 is not, however, sufficient for viral infection, because mouse cells

genetically engineered to express human CD4 allow attachment of virions but not internalization or HIV-induced cell fusion. A second human receptor component may thus be required for further steps in viral entry, possibly mediated by gp41. This second function of the viral envelope produces fusion between adjacent membranes brought into juxtaposition by binding of gp120, and in culture is seen as the typical CPE of syncytium formation, which is now thought to result from the function of the gp41 transmembrane protein (Fig. 38.5; see also Plate 38.5). This is the smaller of the 2 cleavage products of gp160 and is anchored in the envelope by a hydrophobic sequence towards its C terminal region. Following interaction with CD4, a steric change in the envelope gp41/120 complex brings about approximation of a hydrophobic domain of gp41 to the cell membrane and elicits membrane fusion.

The observation that HIV uses the CD4 antigen as a cell surface receptor explains much about the cell tropisms of HIV infection. T-helper lymphocytes are characterized by expression of CD4; c. 40% of blood monocytes and tissue macrophages, another major reservoir of HIV infection in vivo, are CD4+. Dendritic cells in the lymph nodes (follicular dendritic cells) adsorb large quantities of virus, and cells in the skin (Langerhans cells) become infected with HIV, both probably via the CD4 receptor. In the brain, microglia (which may represent macrophages of blood origin) are the cells chiefly infected. However, CD4– astroglial cell lines of genuine neuroectodermal origin can be infected with HIV. These cells are CD4– by immunofluorescence, although they express low levels of CD4 RNA. As soluble CD4 protein does not inhibit HIV infection of these cell types, it seems that alternative mechanisms of HIV entry are possible. A number of other cell-surface molecules have been implicated as at least having an accessory HIV-1 binding function. Such examples are the MHC antigens and the adhesion molecules CD44 and LFA-1.

The nature of infection

The hallmark of infection by both HTLV and HIV is persistence. As these retroviruses are able to integrate into host DNA it is not surprising that, once a person is infected with either of them, the virus is usually expressed continuously. In the case of HIV, the degree of virus expression can be measured indirectly by the amounts of circulating viral antigen, p24 antigen, and viral genomic RNA, which vary during the course of infection. As a consequence of the persistence of both these viruses, a person once infected will thereafter remain at risk of virus-related disease and will remain infectious. These attributes govern the epidemiology both of virus-related disease and of the rates of transmission of virus infection within the population.

3.6 Expression of genes

Little is known about the degree of expression of gene products in HTLV infections, and our knowledge of gene expression in HIV infections is based on longi-

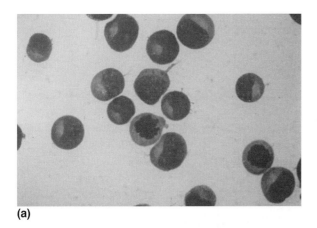

(a)

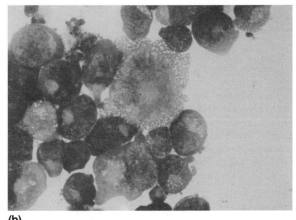

(b)

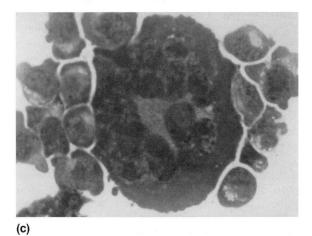

(c)

Fig. 38.5 Sequential cytopathic effects of human lympho-cytes infected in vitro by HIV-1: (a) uninfected cells; (b) day 5 after infection; (c) day 9 after infection (note multinucleated giant cell). For colour, see Plate 38.5. (Courtesy of Douglas Powell.)

tudinal studies of patients infected with HIV. It seems that, for HIV, the levels of virus expression, and perhaps of infectivity, change with time. This notion is based in the first instance on observation of virus in the blood of infected patients (Fig. 38.6). Shortly after infection, and before any immune response to the virus is detectable, free virus and viral antigens circulate in the blood. As antibody titres increase, the

amounts of free virus decrease (often to undetectable levels), indicating a degree of immunological suppression of virus replication and possibly retrafficking of virus load. Recent studies have shown virus to be sequestered in the lymph nodes after the early viraemic burst (Pantaleo et al. 1993). At no point in the progression of HIV disease is there non-expression of virus, implying that over time viral replication is continual and persistent (Embretson et al. 1993). HTLV is thought to have a similar property, although the tropism range, type of virus (oncogene vs lentivirus) and magnitude of replication result in a mechanism of pathogenesis different from that for HIV. Studies of the kinetics of viral turnover and viral body burden in healthy HIV seropositive individuals, as examined by recent advances in quantitative viral RNA analysis, estimate that 10^7–10^9 virions are produced each day. This translates roughly into 10^4–10^7 virion RNA copies/ml of blood. Furthermore, calculations based on CD4 T cell loss predict that c. 2×10^9 CD4 cells are destroyed per day (Ho et al. 1995, Wei et al. 1995). Most, but not all, patients maintain a reduced level of viral replication in the first few years of infection, but, as the damage to the immune system becomes more marked, viral replication increases.

Moreover, it seems that isolates from infected but asymptomatic patients grow slowly and infect only peripheral blood leucocytes. These isolates have been referred to as 'slow-low' strains. In contrast, isolates from symptomatic patients can infect established CD4+ cell lines of multiple origins possessing rapid growth characteristics and attain high viral titres in culture. These isolates have been termed 'rapid-high'. It is tempting to speculate that this change in growth characteristics may be a primary event that leads to disease in the host and is thus also a marker for virulence.

3.7 Diversity of HIV in vivo

There may be differences between HIV isolates from individuals in an infected population, between sequential isolates from an infected individual, and even between those from different sites in the same person. These differences can be measured in terms of variations in nucleotide sequences, antigens, cell tropism, growth characteristics and cytopathology.

As the virus is disseminated throughout the body shortly after infection, it is not surprising that isolates from lymphocytes in peripheral blood may exhibit lymphotropism, whereas those from macrophages may grow better in cells of a monocyte–macrophage lineage. By contrast, and perhaps as a result of such selection in vivo, the rate and degree of replication of some isolates in cells may be constant; virus isolated in the later stages of the disease tends to grow faster and more efficiently in lymphocytes and is able to infect a wider range of cells, characteristics that suggest an increase in virulence. It is likely that, in vivo, selection of variants occurs in any given tissue and that selective tropism is a feature of HIV infection. Recent evidence supporting this concept indicates that in some cases

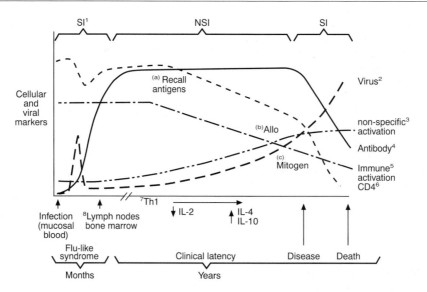

Fig. 38.6 Stages of HIV disease. During the course of HIV infection many cellular and viral markers reflect the states of disease progression. 1. SI (syncytium inducing), NSI (non-syncytium inducing): indicate the phenotype of HIV isolated at various times after infection. 2. Virus: indicates viral burden as detected by viral RNA, infectious virus titre, p24 antigen or reverse transcriptase (RT). 3. Non-specific activation: implies the level of activation markers, such as β2-microglobulin, neopterin, soluble TNF receptor, CD4 cell surface HLA-Dr, and IL-2 receptor expression. 4. Antibody: anti-p24 and anti-gp120 antibodies. 5. Immune activation: reflects the loss over time of host's immunological response to specific antigens (a), allogeneic (Allo) antigens such as MHC (b) and non-specific stimuli (mitogens) (c). 6. CD4: indicates loss of CD4 cells during disease progression. 7. Th1: shows the predominant CD4 Th1, IL-2 producing cells lost while the CD4 Th2, IL-4 and IL-10 producing cells increase over the course of disease. 8. Lymph nodes/bone marrow: indicates where virus can be found replicating after infection and primary antibody response.

the virus infecting the central nervous system (CNS) contains variants defective in the envelope gene. The generation of large numbers of defective virions during virus replication is a characteristic of retroviruses.

Diversity of HIV can be generated by the error-prone nature of reverse transcription, which allows mutations to accumulate, and by recombination between the diploid RNA genomes, if they are heterozygous, during their reverse transcription to form a provirus. Variants may then be selected in vivo by the ecology of the immune system of the infected individual. In vitro, neutralization-resistant mutants can be selected by culture in the presence of neutralizing antibody, and a similar process probably occurs in vivo. It is tempting to speculate that the occasional severe fluctuations in viral body burden may reflect increased replication of variants temporarily able to escape the immune system. HTLV-I is much less variable, possibly because it undergoes fewer rounds of replication in vivo.

3.8 Pathogenesis of HIV

As the AIDS pandemic moves into its second decade, concepts regarding the mechanisms of HIV pathogenesis have made important contributions to our understanding of the disease (Levy 1993). Many of these advances have revolved around correlations of disease progression and viral body burden, as mentioned above (Coffin 1995). However, several other areas related to disease progression have emerged as important (Fig. 38.6). For instance, changes in CD4 T

cell subtypes have been observed that may provide an understanding of the mechanisms of cell biology of AIDS. These findings, which show a steady decline in Th1 cells (those that mediate delayed type hypersensitivity cells) whereas Th2 cells (those that provide help for antibody-producing B cells) seem to remain at steady levels, provide insight into lymphoid subset profiles. Likewise, the finding that naive CD4 T cells (CD45 Ra) are lost during disease progression at a higher rate than CD45 Ro memory cells may imply a more central immunological defect. This effect may be further exemplified by an infected individual's loss of immune responsiveness first to specific recall antigens, then to allogeneic antigens and finally to mitogen stimulation.

The mechanism explaining the actual loss of CD4 T cells is still unresolved. Specifically, it remains to be determined whether the virus can directly account for CD4 cell loss via infection followed by programmed cell death (apoptosis) or whether indirect mechanisms, such as gp120–CD4 antibody cross-linking, viral protein-induced cellular dysregulation or antiviral bystander effects are involved.

Finally, it should be mentioned that, as a prerequisite for HIV or HTLV replication, cellular activation and proliferation are important factors. The role of cellular activation, whether induced by antigens via the specific T cell receptor or cytokines, remains a new and unexplained phenomenon of the cell's control over virus expression. Cellular models have been developed that permit synchronization of replicating virus for studies of potential therapeutic targets that may be sought to interrupt the viral life cycle (Butera and Folks 1992). Concepts regarding intervening illnesses and infections as non-specific activators of T cells from HIV-infected individuals are currently being investigated to explain differences observed between those who progress to disease rapidly compared with those who progress more slowly.

Sera from infected patients are able to inhibit both functions of the envelope proteins, i.e. fusion and virus attachment or internalization. As a result, some sera from infected patients neutralize virus infection in vitro. Variability in antigenic expression by the virus could influence the degree of neutralization, although some neutralizing activity for all HIV-1 strains is present albeit at low levels, in sera from infected humans. Furthermore, recent studies demonstrate that many HIV isolates in culture show passive shedding of free gp120 into the tissue culture fluid from infected cells. This in turn leads to blocking of antibody neutralization.

4 CLINICAL AND PATHOLOGICAL ASPECTS

The clinical and pathological correlates of HIV infection are markedly different from those of the HTLVs. Although most HIV-infected people eventually become ill, no more than 5% of those infected with HTLV-I develop clinical disease during a life-long infection. For HTLV-II, no firm disease association is currently recognized.

Similarly, although HIVs and the HTLVs share common modes of transmission, they have different epidemiological features, in part because of some biological differences but also because of a different distribution in human populations. Diagnosis relies on similar but different laboratory tests and reagents, and approaches to management of infection are different.

4.1 HTLV-I-associated diseases

HTLV-I has been definitively associated with 2 diseases: a leukaemia referred to as adult T cell leukaemia/lymphoma (ATL) and a neurological illness known as HTLV-I-associated myelopathy/tropical spastic paraparesis (HAM/TSP).

Adult T cell leukaemia/lymphoma ATL is a malignancy of HTLV-I-infected, CD4+ T lymphocytes. The HTLV-I provirus is monoclonally integrated into the DNA of the malignant cells. Patients with HTLV-I-related ATL can be identified reliably via the detection of virus-specific antibody (anti-HTLV-I) in their sera. Acute and chronic lymphoma and smouldering forms of ATL have been described. Acute ATL, the most aggressive form of the disease, is characterized by infiltration of lymph nodes, viscera and skin with malignant T lymphocytes, resulting in a constellation of clinical features, including lymphadenopathy, hepatosplenomegaly, skin lesions, lytic bone lesions, hypercalcaemia and abnormal liver function tests. Characteristic lymphocytes with lobulated nuclei, called

flower cells, are generally seen on the peripheral blood smear (Fig. 38.7a). The amount of calcium in the serum is often sufficiently elevated to cause symptoms of hypercalcaemia. Median survival in acute ATL is 11 months from diagnosis. Conventional chemotherapy is not curative, and relapses often occur quickly, although prolonged survival has been reported. ATL has been estimated to occur in 2–4% of individuals infected with HTLV-I in regions where it is endemic and where early childhood infection is common. The disease occurs most frequently in people aged 40–60 years, suggesting that a latent period as long as a few decades is required for it to develop. Males and females are affected equally. One case of ATL in an immunocompromised patient has been reported in which infection seems to have been acquired by blood transfusion.

Before the onset of frank leukaemia, early oligoclonal expansion can be recognized, and has been described by the Japanese as 'smouldering lymphocy-

(a)

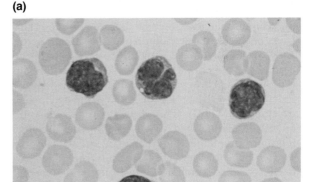

(b)

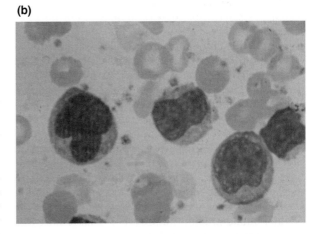

Fig. 38.7 Peripheral blood film of retrovirus infected patients. (a) Peripheral film of a patient with HTLV-I-associated adult T cell leukaemia/lymphoma (ATLL) showing lymphocytes with cleaved nuclei. ×1000. (Courtesy of Professor D Gatovsky.) (b) Film of patient presenting with acute glandular fever illness during HIV seroconversion. Marked lymphocytosis with many abnormal immature-looking lymphocytes. ×1500. (Courtesy of Dr C Ludlam.)

tosis'. In this condition there is a persisting lympho-cytosis in which most cells have normal morphological features, with 0.5–3% circulating flower cells. Some of the lymphocytes express HTLV-I antigens. It is assumed that this condition is a precursor to ATL, although early treatment is not indicated. Chronic ATL is characterized by >10% flower cells circulating in the peripheral blood and has a more slowly pro-gressive clinical course than acute ATL. Lymphoma ATL is a diffuse T cell lymphoma without the other clinical manifestations of ATL.

HTLV-I-associated myelopathy/tropical spastic para-paresis   HAM/TSP is a chronic, degenerative, neuro-logical disease associated predominantly with upper motor neuron lesions, characterized by progressive and permanent lower extremity weakness, spasticity, hyper-reflexia, sensory disturbances and urinary incontinence. Unlike the clinical manifestations in patients with multiple sclerosis, the signs and symp-toms in HAM/TSP do not wax and wane, cranial nerves are not involved and cognitive function is not affected. Disability increases with time, and patients may become wheelchair-bound. HAM/TSP is believed to be immunologically mediated. Antibodies to HTLV-I are characteristically found in high titre in serum and CSF, and treatment with corticosteroids has bene-fited some patients. Danazol, a synthetic androgen, reportedly improves symptoms, including bladder dys-function. Fewer than 1% of HTLV-I-infected people develop HAM/TSP. The disease occurs most fre-quently in people aged 40–60 years; women are affec-ted more frequently than men. The latency period is shorter than that for ATL; cases of HAM/TSP have been associated with blood transfusion, with a median interval of 3.3 years between transfusion and the devel-opment of neurological illness.

Other HTLV-I-associated diseases   The full spectrum of HTLV-I-associated diseases seems to include dis-orders related to hyperimmunity. Polymyositis, arthritis, pulmonary alveolitis and uveitis have been reported in HTLV-I-infected individuals, frequently in association with HAM/TSP. In addition, a mild immune deficiency may be associated with HTLV-I infection. There is a documented association between HTLV-I infection and unresolving systemic infections with the nematode *Strongyloides*, suggesting that HTLV-I-related damage to the immune system prevents the patient from clearing the strongyloides infection. Recently, case–control studies in Japan, corrected for age and gender, have shown a clear association between HTLV-I infection and loss of delayed skin reactivity to tuberculin, lending further support to the idea of a mild immunosuppressive sequel to long per-iods of infection with HTLV-I.

4.2   HTLV-II

HTLV-II infection has not been clearly associated with any disease. The virus was first isolated from 2 patients with atypical T cell hairy cell leukaemia, but no evi-dence of HTLV-II infection was found in 21 patients

with the more common B cell form of the disease. Cases of HAM/TSP-like neurological illnesses and of mycosis fungoides and large granular lymphocyte leukaemia have been reported in people infected with HTLV-II, but no definitive association with infection has been established. Similarly, cases of erythroderma-titis and bacterial skin infections have been reported in HIV-1- and HTLV-II-co-infected individuals.

4.3   HIV-associated disease

The primary clinical problems associated with HIV infection are the opportunistic infections and neo-plasms that occur as a result of the progressively severe immunodeficiency that develops in the course of the disease. The immunodeficiency is generally measured by the CD4 lymphocyte count, but in reality decreases in both the quantity and the function of CD4+ lym-phocytes occur over time.

ACUTE RETROVIRAL SYNDROME

One-half to two-thirds of people recently infected with HIV develop an acute mononucleosis-like illness. The illness occurs 2–4 weeks after infection and lasts 1–2 weeks. Its clinical features are variable and non-specific, and include fever, generalized lymphadeno-pathy, malaise, myalgias, anorexia, nausea, diarrhoea and a non-exudative pharyngitis. A rash on the trunk develops in two-thirds of patients, which may be macu-lopapular, roseola-like or urticarial. Aseptic meningitis and other neurological symptoms, such as encepha-litis, peripheral neuropathy and the Guillain–Barré syndrome, occur in a smaller proportion of patients. High-level viraemia is seen during this symptomatic stage of acute infection. Viral proteins and infectious virus can be detected in both CSF and serum at this time, and seroconversion for antibody coincides with or follows shortly after resolution. Recovery is the rule, with no apparent long-term sequelae.

CHRONIC ILLNESSES

The chronic clinical sequelae of HIV infection are many and varied. Most are secondary to the progress-ively severe immunodeficiency that results from HIV infection, and only a few, most prominent ones involv-ing the nervous systems are primarily due to the direct, immunological effect of HIV.

Staging of HIV disease   HIV infection represents an underlying progressive immunodeficiency disease pro-cess. The most severe sequelae of this immuno-suppression are gathered under the umbrella term acquired immunodeficiency syndrome. Although his-torically AIDS has been defined clinically, such defi-nition is limited and clearly represents only a small proportion of the illness caused at any time by HIV. Furthermore, it does not capture the broader group of HIV-infected patients who may benefit from anti-retroviral and other prophylactic treatment.

A number of systems have been proposed to classify HIV infection and disease. The 1986 CDC classi-fication system offered 4 broad, mutually exclusive groups or stages that are hierarchical in the sense that a person in one group is not intended to be reclassified to a preceding group if their symptoms subside. The 4 stages of this system are: group I, acute infection; group II, asymptomatic seropositive; group III, persistent generalized lymphadenopathy; and group IV, symptomatic HIV disease. This classification scheme has had limited use in prognosis. In 1993, CDC revised the AIDS surveillance case definition and added pulmonary tuberculosis, recurrent bacterial pneumonia and invasive cervical cancer to the list of AIDS-indicator conditions (Table 38.2). In conjunction with the revised definition, CDC also developed a revised classification system for HIV-infected adolescents and adults that incorporates both evolving knowledge about the spectrum and progression of HIV infection and current standards of medical care for infected people (Table 38.3). HIV-infected individuals are classified on the basis of CD4 lymphocyte counts and clinical categories. The continuum of HIV infection is accordingly divided into mutually exclusive categories. Additional classification schemes are also in use (Redfield, Wright and Tramont 1986, Yarchoan et al. 1991).

Acquired immunodeficiency syndrome The term AIDS is used to refer to the constellation of diseases that reflect the severe late manifestations of HIV infection (Table 38.2). The 1993 revised surveillance case definition for AIDS includes adolescents and adults with severe immunosuppression (<200 CD4/μl or <14 CD4 as a percentage of total lymphocyte count), recurrent bacterial infections, pulmonary tuberculosis and invasive cervical cancer (Table 38.3). These added clinical conditions have potential importance for the health of HIV-infected people. Moreover, measures of CD4 lymphocytes are an important guide for their clinical and therapeutic management.

HIV/AIDS in children The spectrum of AIDS-defining opportunistic infections and malignancies in children <13 years of age overlaps that of adults and adolescents; however, important differences exist. For instance, pulmonary disease accounts for a great proportion of the mortality and morbidity in children. Most AIDS-associated pulmonary disease diagnosed in infants ≤12 months of age is due to *Pneumocystis carinii* pneumonia (PCP), whereas most pulmonary disease in older children (1–4 years of age) is due to lymphoid interstitial pneumonitis (LIP). CD4 lymphocyte counts are higher in infants and younger children, and decline over the first few years of life. Moreover, opportunistic infections seem to develop at higher CD4 counts in children than in adults. In addition, HIV infection is difficult to diagnose before 18 months of age, owing to the presence of maternal anti-HIV IgG antibodies that cross the placenta. Because of these differences, a classification system for staging paediatric HIV disease was developed by CDC in 1987 and revised in 1994 to reflect the current understanding of clinical and prognostic aspects of HIV/AIDS. Like the system for adolescents and adults, the newer scheme classifies HIV-infected children into 4 hier-

Table 38.2 Clinical conditions included in the 1993 AIDS surveillance case definition

Bacterial infections, multiple or recurrent[a]
Candidiasis
of bronchi, trachea or lungs
oesophageal
Cervical cancer, invasive[a]
Coccidioidomycosis, disseminated or extrapulmonary
Cryptococcosis, extrapulmonary
Cryptosporidiosis, chronic intestinal (<1 month duration)
Cytomegalovirus disease (other than liver, spleen or nodes)
Cytomegalovirus retinitis (with loss of vision)
Encephalopathy, HIV-related
Herpes simplex, chronic ulcer(s) (>1 month duration); or bronchitis, pneumonitis or oesophagitis
Histoplasmosis, disseminated or extrapulmonary
Isosporiasis, chronic intestinal (>1 month duration)
Kaposi's sarcoma
Lymphoid interstitial pneumonia and/or pulmonary lymphoid hyperplasia[b]
Lymphoma
Burkitt's (or equivalent term)
immunoblastic (or equivalent term)
primary, of brain
Mycobacterium avium–intracellulare complex or *M. kansasii*, disseminated or extrapulmonary
Pneumocystis carinii pneumonia
Pneumonia, recurrent[a]
Progressive multifocal leucoencephalopathy
Salmonella septicaemia, recurrent
Toxoplasmosis of brain
Wasting syndrome due to HIV

[a]Added in the 1993 expansion of the AIDS surveillance case definition for adolescents and adults.
[b]Children less than 13 years old.
(From CDC 1992).

archical, mutually exclusive categories according to infection status, clinical status and immune status (Table 38.4). Classification by CD4 count for HIV-infected children takes into account the age of the child (Table 38.5).

Natural history of HIV infection The incubation time from infection to development of AIDS has been estimated in a number of studies and seems to range from 6 to 13 years (median 10 years). Progression rates vary with age, route of HIV infection and the underlying immune status of the host. The rate of progression of disease is faster for newborns and older people than for other groups. Transfusion recipients, whose initial inoculum of HIV is probably larger than that of people infected sexually or by needles, have a median incubation interval of only 6 years. In addition, the rate of disease progression in the recipient is associated with the stage of disease in the HIV-

Table 38.3 1993 revised classification system for HIV infection and expanded AIDS surveillance case definition for adolescents and adults[a]

| CD4+ T cell categories | Clinical categories | | |
	A Asymptomatic Acute (primary) HIV or PGL	B Symptomatic Not A or C conditions	C[b] AIDS-indicator conditions
1 ≥500/μl	A1	B1	C1
2 200–499/μl	A2	B2	C2
3 <200/μl	A3	B3	C3
(AIDS-indicator T cell count)[a]			

PGL, persistent generalized lymphadenopathy.
[a]C1, C2, C3, A3 and B3 indicate conditions included in the 1993 AIDS surveillance case definition for adolescents and adults.
[b]Clinical conditions in category C are listed in Table 38.2.
(From CDC 1992).

Table 38.4 Classification of human immunodeficiency virus (HIV) in children[a]

| Immunological categories | Clinical categories | | | |
	N: No signs/symptoms	A: Mild signs/symptoms	B: Moderate[b] signs/symptoms	C: Severe[b] signs/symptoms
1 No evidence of suppression	N1	A1	B1	C1
2 Evidence of moderate suppression	N2	A2	B2	C2
3 Severe suppression	N3	A3	B3	C3

[a]Children whose HIV infection status is not confirmed are classified by using the above grid with a letter E (for perinatally exposed) placed before the appropriate classification code (e.g. EN2).
[b]Both category C and lymphoid interstitial pneumonitis in category B are reportable to state and local health departments as acquired immunodeficiency syndrome.
(From CDC 1994a).

Table 38.5 Immunological categorization of HIV-infected children

| Immunological category | CD4+ count/μl (%) in indicated age group | | |
	<12 mo	1–5 y	6–12 y
No evidence of suppression	≥1500 (≥25)	≥1000 (≥25)	≥500 (≥25)
Moderate suppression	750–1499 (15–24)	500–999 (15–24)	200–499 (15–24)
Severe suppression	<750 (<15)	<500 (<15)	<200 (<15)

Categorized on the basis of age-specific CD4+ lymphocyte count and percentage of total lymphocytes bearing the CD4 marker.
(From CDC 1994a).

infected donor. The role of exogenous biological and behavioural co-factors in the progression to AIDS remains unclear. Limited evidence suggests a possible role for various antigenic stimulants, including sexually transmitted diseases, injecting drug use, intervening illnesses or non-specific immune stimulation. Because the natural history of HIV infection can vary considerably, clinical and laboratory indicators are useful predictors of progression. Oral candidiasis (thrush), oral hairy leucoplakia and severe recurrent herpes zoster infection have been associated with an increased likelihood of developing AIDS.

Among the laboratory tests that are used to measure HIV-related immunosuppression, CD4 cell counts are the most specific laboratory marker that predicts progression (Stein, Korvick and Vermund 1992). However, plasma viral burden, which identifies the number of viral genomic copies in the blood, may serve equally well as a marker of progression. Other related markers include HIV p24 antigen, serum neopterin, β_2-microglobulin, soluble interleukin 2 receptors and IgA. The conversion of a patient's viral phenotype from non-syncytia inducer (NSI) to syncytia inducer (SI) has been suggested as a viral indicator of more rapid disease progression, but this hypothesis remains controversial.

Antiretroviral therapy and widespread prophylaxis against PCP have substantially changed the natural history of HIV infection. Whereas the median survival from AIDS was 9 months in one study, the median survival of treated patients ranges from 2 to 3 years. Intervention has also delayed the onset of clinical AIDS and resulted in an increase in AIDS-indicator illnesses that are seen with more severe immuno-suppression, such as disseminated *Mycobacterium avium intracellulare* (MAI) infections. Various forms of tuberculosis, including those caused by drug-resistant mycobacterial strains, have emerged as important infections in AIDS patients in recent years.

Neurological disease HIV is a neurotropic virus, and HIV infection may lead to primary disease both within the CNS and of peripheral nerves and muscle. The most severe manifestation of CNS disease is the constellation of syndromes comprising the AIDS dementia complex (ADC), also known as HIV encephalopathy. This condition, which presents as a chronic progressive dementia (Price et al. 1988), is a late complication of HIV infection that develops in 15–20% of people with severe immunodeficiency (CD4 cell counts <200).

Early on, patients have some insight and complain of difficulties and slowness in thinking. Lack of concentration, poor memory and cognitive loss may be recognized by both patient and family. Rarely, CNS disease may present with an apparent agitated psychosis. Motor dysfunction may lead to poor balance, clumsiness and difficulty in walking. Finally, social withdrawal follows, culminating in a terminal apathetic vegetative state complicated by double incontinence.

It is necessary to exclude other secondary opportunistic CNS infections. Prominent among these are cryptococcal meningitis, cytomegalovirus (CMV) and herpes simplex virus (HSV) infection, toxoplasmosis and intracranial lymphoma. Spinal cord disease secondary to vacuolar myelopathy, peripheral neuropathy and myopathy may also be important manifestations of HIV disease. A clinical diagnosis of ADC in HIV-infected people is made by exclusion of other causes of encephalopathy.

IMMUNOPATHOLOGY OF HIV INFECTION

Immune system Early after HIV infection, enlargement of the lymph nodes frequently develops and may persist for a long time. Although usually symmetrical, generalized and stable, the lymphadenopathy may fluctuate; before the natural history of HIV infection was understood, the more florid cases of HIV-related lymphadenopathy posed a diagnostic need to exclude acute lymphoma. Many patients underwent biopsy with little diagnostic return. The most common finding in such biopsies was follicular hyperplasia, although in a few patients follicular involution and cellular depletion were also prominent. The 'latent' period of early infection, inferred from the apparent low viral activity and burden seen in the peripheral blood, seems to be a misnomer. A high viral activity and viral burden are paradoxically now recognized in the lymph nodes; numerous HIV-specific and non-specific immune responses are capable of controlling the virus to some degree. Progression to the more advanced stages of HIV infection reflects a loss of this ability to control the virus.

CNS disease Infection of the CNS with HIV occurs early after infection and may be the result of the initial viraemia or the traffic into the brain of infected monocytes and macrophages that behave as a 'Trojan horse'. The initial pathological abnormalities are found in the cerebral white matter and the deep subcortical structures and thalamus. Mild to moderate cortical atrophy with ventricular dilatation is visible on gross examination. Pallor of the myelin is prominent and most commonly seen in the periventricular and central white matter. In areas of pallor there is reactive astrocytosis and perivascular cuffing, surrounded by foci of demyelination and vacuolation. As the severity of disease increases, these foci become scattered more widely throughout the brain, together with glial nodules and multinucleated giant cells. HIV genome, antigens and virions can be shown in these cells by various techniques and seem to be a reliable histological indicator of CNS infection. There is some evidence that the number of multinucleated giant cells is related to the severity of the pathological changes, although not necessarily to the clinical severity.

5 EPIDEMIOLOGY

Both HTLV and HIV cause persistent infections, which result in a long period for opportunities of transmission to other hosts. HTLV and HIV are exogenous retroviruses and there is no evidence of integration into germ cell DNA. Successful infection depends on integration into host somatic cell DNA.

5.1 Prevalence of HTLV infections

HTLV-I infection is highly endemic in southern Japan and in many countries of the Caribbean basin. Reported seroprevalence in the general populations of these areas ranges from 5% to 20%. In both Japan and the Caribbean, HTLV-I seropositivity increases with age, and in older age groups rates are usually higher for women. In the Caribbean, HTLV-I seropositivity rates are significantly higher among black people than among other ethnic groups. HTLV-I infection is also endemic in parts of Melanesia, Africa, some Central and South American countries and in isolated areas of Asia (Kaplan and Khabbaz 1993). Molecular epidemiological studies have identified 5 types of HTLV-I strains circulating in different populations. In the USA and in Europe, HTLV-I infections are seen primarily in immigrants from areas where HTLV-I is endemic and in people who have had sexual contact with individuals from the Caribbean basin or Japan. HTLV-I accounts for a small proportion of HTLV seropositivity among injecting drug users.

HTLV-II infection is highly prevalent among

injecting drug users in the USA and Europe. Infection also seems to be endemic in several American Indian populations. HTLV-II infection has been reported among Pygmies in Central Africa and more recently among Mongolians in Asia. About two-thirds of US volunteer blood donors seropositive for HTLV-I/II are infected with HTLV-II. Molecular typing techniques have distinguished at least 2 types of HTLV-II strains, and it is likely that additional subtypes exist.

5.2 Risk factors and modes of transmission

HTLV-I and II infections are transmitted from mother to child, by sexual contact, by blood transfusion and by the sharing of contaminated needles. Mother-to-child transmission occurs primarily through breast-feeding. In areas where HTLV-I is endemic, 25% of breast-fed infants born to HTLV-I-seropositive mothers acquire infection. Intrauterine or perinatal transmission of HTLV-I occurs less frequently; 5% of children born to infected mothers, but not breast-fed, acquire infection. Sexual transmission of HTLV-I seems to be more efficient from males to females than from females to males. In the USA, 25–30% of sex partners of HTLV-I/II-seropositive blood donors are also seropositive. The most commonly reported risk factor among HTLV-II-infected female US blood donors is sexual contact with an injecting drug user. Transmission of HTLV-I and HTLV-II by blood transfusion occurs with transfusion of cellular blood products (whole blood, red blood cells and platelets) but not with the plasma fraction or plasma derivatives from HTLV-I-infected blood. Although seroconversion rates of 44–63% have been reported among recipients of HTLV-I-infected cellular components in areas where HTLV-I is endemic, lower rates (20%) have been reported in the USA. Differences in transmission rates may be partly due to differences in the preparation and duration of storage of various blood products.

5.3 Prevalence of HIV infections

In contrast with HTLV, HIV was introduced into the human population perhaps as recently as the mid-1960s. In the decade and a half since the initial recognition of the AIDS epidemic, the epidemiology of HIV infection has changed world-wide: HIV infection has become a widespread pandemic. Differences in access to healthcare and varying prevention and intervention strategies continue to affect the evolving epidemic, both in the developing and in the more developed world.

By December 1994, a cumulative total of 1 025 073 cases of AIDS had been reported to the World Health Organization (WHO 1995). This number is believed to be an underestimate of the total number of AIDS cases world-wide, due to under-reporting, especially in developing countries. The estimated number of HIV-infected people world-wide was 18 million through 1994. The WHO estimates that by the year 2000 there will be 10 million cases of AIDS and 20–40 million cases of HIV infection, 90% of which will probably have occurred in the developing world.

In the USA and in Europe the largest numbers of incident HIV infections and AIDS cases are currently seen among injecting drug users (IDUs), and increasing transmission is occurring via heterosexual contact. In the USA the largest number of AIDS cases reported to CDC continues to be among homosexual/bisexual men (52% of the total number of cases reported through June 1995: CDC unpublished data). Although this number largely reflects the high incidence of infection among homosexual/bisexual men a decade ago, incident HIV infections continue to occur in this risk group, especially among younger homosexual/-bisexual men. The proportion of AIDS cases reported among IDUs and among heterosexual contacts of cases is increasing. The incidence of AIDS among women has increased more rapidly than for men, from 8% in 1988 to 14% through June 1995. About half of all cases of AIDS among women in the USA have been attributed to IDUs and a third to heterosexual contact. In parallel with the increase in AIDS among women, an increasing number of children with AIDS, acquired mostly perinatally, are being reported. The rates of AIDS in the USA are also increasing disproportionately among blacks and Hispanics compared with whites. HIV seroprevalence surveys conducted by CDC in general have shown trends and patterns similar to those seen through AIDS surveillance: higher rates of HIV infection among men than women, among blacks and Hispanics than whites and among people 20–45 years of age.

In northern Europe, as in North America, the majority of AIDS cases have occurred in homosexual/bisexual men, whereas the predominant risk group in southern Europe has been IDUs. World-wide, sub-Saharan Africa has been the region most affected by AIDS, and prevalence rates there exceed 40% for adults in some areas. In Africa, AIDS is a heterosexual disease, and the overall ratio of males to females who are affected is equal. Associations with other sexually acquired infections, including genital ulcers, are prominent, and HIV prevalence rates of 75% have been reported among female prostitutes. Recently, a group 'O' subtype of HIV-1 has been identified in Africa that shows as much genomic diversity from HIV-1 as it does from HIV-2. HIV-2 in West Africa seems to have spread more slowly than HIV-1. It is interesting that co-infection with HIV-1 and 2 in some areas of West Africa seems to be less common than infection with HIV-1, suggesting the possibility of some cross-protection by HIV-2.

The past 5 years have witnessed considerable spread of HIV in southern and southeast Asia. Molecular epidemiological studies, which have identified at least 9 different subtypes of HIV-1 world-wide, suggest a separate introduction of HIV-1 in IDUs in Thailand and in female prostitutes in Thailand and India. HIV prevalence is increasing rapidly among female prostitutes in Asia.

The epidemiology of AIDS in Latin America and

the Caribbean basin is diverse and changing. Homosexual/bisexual men remain an important risk group, but increasing prevalence among IDUs has been observed since the late 1980s.

5.4 Modes of transmission/risk categories for HIV

Sexual transmission

World-wide, HIV infection is undoubtedly a sexually transmitted disease (STD). The exchange of body fluids during sexual intercourse is the apparent mode of transmission. Both the fluid and cellular components of semen contain HIV, as do endocervical secretions. Sexual behaviours are important determinants of HIV transmission. Sexual practices, including the practice of anal intercourse and vaginal intercourse during menses, sexual mixing patterns and level of condom use, have all been recognized as factors affecting spread. Biological factors also seem to affect the efficiency of transmission; these factors include the level of viraemia, infectivity and virulence of a particular HIV strain, and the presence of STDs such as genital ulcers (Plummer et al. 1991).

Transmission by blood

Recipients of unscreened blood and blood products from HIV-infected donors are at high risk of HIV infection. The likelihood of HIV infection occurring in a recipient of HIV-positive blood is close to 100%. The virus is present both in white cells and in the plasma. A single infected unit included in a plasma pool (often contributed by 20 000 or more donors) has the potential to infect all recipients of the pool, a situation similar to that seen with HBV. Consequently, the prevalence of HIV infection is high (60% or more in some clinics) among haemophiliac recipients of commercial clotting factor concentrates made before heat-inactivation was introduced. Plasma products, such as immunoglobulins prepared by using one of several fractionation processes, have not been associated with transmission of HIV. In countries where screening of blood for HIV has been instituted, the risk for HIV transmission through screened blood has been estimated to be 1/36 000 to 1/225 000 per unit transfused. This residual risk is due to antibody-negative infected donors in the 'window' period prior to seroconversion. Transmission of HIV by transplantation of vascular organs such as liver, heart, kidneys and bone marrow has occurred.

Transmission through injecting drug use

Among IDUs, HIV is transmitted by parenteral exposure to HIV-infected blood through the use of contaminated needles or other injection equipment. Factors associated with HIV infection in IDUs include duration (years) of injection, frequency of needle sharing, number of needle-sharing partners, number of injections and the use of 'shooting galleries'. In addition, unsafe sexual practices may contribute some infections among IDUs (Nelson et al. 1991).

Perinatal transmission

Mother-to-child transmission plays a major role in HIV infections in children. In prospective studies of infants born to HIV-infected women, transmission rates have ranged from 13% to 40%. Because maternal antibody crosses the placenta to the fetus and is present during the child's first few months of life, diagnosis of HIV infection is difficult in infants and must rely on the detection of viral antigen, viral genome by PCR or isolation of infectious virus. Perinatal infection can occur from transmission in one of the following ways:

1 **In utero**, implying transplacental passage of virus. Virus has been isolated and genome demonstrated in the products of conception from as early as 8 weeks' gestation and in placental tissue infected in vivo and in vitro.

2 **During birth**, implying infection during parturition as a result of transplacental bleeding or contact of abrasions with virus-containing fluids during passage along the birth canal. Transmission during birth seems to account for a large proportion of perinatal transmission, although it may be less frequent with caesarian than with vaginal delivery.

3 **Postnatally**, implying acquisition of infection from the mother. Instances of HIV transmission via breast milk from mothers who were infected by blood transfusion after delivery have been described and virus has been isolated from milk. Prospective cohort studies that compared breast-fed and bottle-fed infants estimated the attributable risk for transmission through breast milk to be 14–29%. Substitution of breast milk with formula or other appropriate food mixtures is recommended for the seropositive mother, but only if facilities are available for safe bottle-feeding.

(See section 5, p. 795, also Chapter 41.)

The risk of perinatal transmission varies with the disease state of the mother and is highest during acute primary infection and with advanced symptomatic disease (European Collaborative Study 1992). Markers of increased likelihood of perinatal transmission include high CD8+ lymphocytes and low CD4 T cell counts.

Transmission in health care settings

Skin, mucous membrane and needlestick exposures to blood and other body fluids are not infrequent in the healthcare setting. The average risk of seroconversion after a needlestick injury with HIV-positive blood is c. 0.3% (Tokars et al. 1993). Transmission of HIV after mucous membrane or cutaneous exposure seems to be much rarer. Transmission of HIV from a healthcare worker to patients has been described in a dental practice in Florida, USA. Transmission of HIV from patient to patient through the reuse of improperly decontaminated needles and syringes has been reported in Romania.

THE ORIGIN OF HIV

Besides HIV-1 and HIV-2, there is a related group of monkey lentiviruses, the simian immunodeficiency viruses (SIVs). Sequence analysis and comparisons of

HIV-1 and HIV-2 and representatives of the SIV group (defined in terms of the animals from which the viruses were isolated) do not give a precise indication of the evolutionary relationship between them. These analyses suggest that there may be 3 subgroups of related lentiviruses: HIV-1; HIV-2, SIVmn (isolate from sooty Mangabey monkey) and SIVagm (isolate from African green monkey); and SIVmand (isolate from mandrill monkey) (Gardner, Endres and Barry 1994).

One hypothesis about the origin of HIV is that HIV-2 arose through a zoonotic infection from monkeys and is of low pathogenicity in humans, whereas HIV-1 speciated recently from chimpanzees and is of high pathogenicity in humans. The contrary view is that HIV-2 infected humans as recently as HIV-1. Another hypothesis is that both HIV-1 and HIV-2 arose from an archetypal retrovirus carried in the common ancestor of Old World primates, which has endured independently in human and non-human species. According to this hypothesis the human virus has been maintained as an infection of low pathogenicity over a long period in different geographically isolated human populations, the developing pandemic representing the escape of both HIV-1 and HIV-2 from isolated populations through recent changes in social, sexual and migratory behaviour.

6 LABORATORY DIAGNOSIS

The diagnosis of HTLV and HIV infections relies primarily on serological testing for the detection of virus-specific antibody. Detection of circulating virus antigen or genome and, rarely, virus isolation may be used in conjunction with antibody detection.

6.1 HTLV infection

Detection of antibody

Several serological assays are available for screening for HTLV-I/II. These include enzyme-linked immunosorbent assays (ELISAs), particle agglutination assay and the immunofluorescent assay (IFA). All these assays have good sensitivity but are not specific and therefore result in a high frequency of false reactions, necessitating confirmation with additional, more specific, assays. In the USA, ELISAs that use HTLV-I whole-virus lysate as antigen have been licensed by the US Food and Drug Administration. These tests vary in their sensitivity to detect antibodies to HTLV-II. An additional ELISA that contains HTLV-I lysate and recombinant *env* p21e seems to have better sensitivity for the detection of HTLV-II. Particle agglutination is the standard screening assay used in Japan. IFA has had limited use as a research screening test. Specimens that are reactive by the screening assays are also tested by supplementary serological tests, such as the Western blot and the radioimmunoprecipitation assay (RIPA), which are capable of identifying antibodies to specific HTLV gene products. Both *gag* and *env* reactivity are sought. Western blots and ELISAs that use or incorporate recombinant env proteins or type-specific

synthetic peptides have recently simplified HTLV testing algorithms and also allowed serological differentiation between HTLV-I and HTLV-II infection (Fig. 38.8a) (Khabbaz, Heneine and Kaplan 1994).

DETECTION OF VIRUS

The isolation of HTLV from infected individuals depends on the activation of T lymphocytes and on cell culture conditions that allow long-term growth of lymphocytes. Co-cultivation with uninfected target cells (e.g. mitogen-stimulated peripheral blood mononuclear cells (PBMCs)) seems to improve the sensitivity for HTLV isolation. Detection of proviral DNA by PCR amplification is a highly sensitive molecular technique for detecting HTLV-I and HTLV-II provirus in infected cells, including PBMCs from asymptomatic HTLV-infected individuals and CSF from HAM/TSP patients (Fig. 38.8b). PCR is also useful for studying in vivo viral load and tissue distribution.

6.2 HIV infection

Detection of antibody

Infection after exposure to HIV is not inevitable. When it does follow, there is an initial period of viral replication during which antibody is undetectable. This period is termed a 'diagnostic window' and people at this early stage of infection may be difficult to identify. Once a patient has produced antibody, often within 1 month of infection and usually within 3 months, the diagnosis is easy and centres on the detection of anti-HIV. It is very rare for a person to seroconvert after 6 months of HIV infection, and only a few such instances have been documented.

Antibody to HIV can be detected by a number of methods, of which solid-phase ELISAs are by far the most widely used. Several formats are currently used. In early antiglobulin assays, use was made of whole-virus lysate antigens also containing antigens from cell cultures in which the viruses were grown. These tests were widely used and gave inaccurate estimates for the prevalence of HIV infection, particularly in African countries. More recently, the use of recombinant antigens and chemically synthesized peptides, usually gag and env, first of HIV-1 only and now of both HIV-1 and HIV-2, have produced assays that are highly sensitive and specific. Competitive assays, in which serum antibody and enzyme-labelled specific antibody compete for binding sites, at first used crude viral antigen captured onto a human antibody. Modifications, first using monoclonal anti-HIV for antigen capture and later using recombinant antigens or direct binding of viral antigens to the solid phase, have made competitive assays extremely sensitive as well as specific.

Agglutination assays, including particle and latex agglutination assays, antibody capture assays and solid-phase immunoassays, are also used to diagnose HIV infection. In the USA, a plasma or serum sample that is reactive by ELISA is usually retested in duplicate, and a repeat reactive sample is confirmed with a supplementary test (Western blot or IFA). The Western blot has the advantage of detecting antibodies to indi-

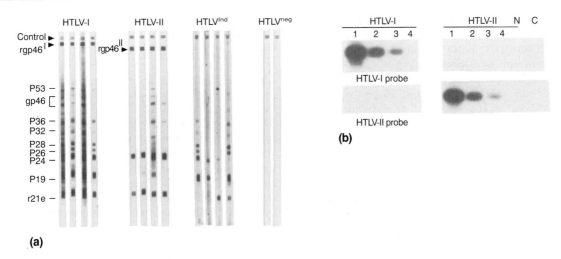

Fig. 38.8 (a) HTLV-I, HTLV-II, HTLV-indeterminate and HTLV-seronegative serum samples on Western blot spiked with recombinant proteins p21e, gp46I (HTLV-I-specific), and gp46II (HTLV-II-specific) (Genelabs Diagnostics). (b) Generic PCR amplification of HTLV-I and HTLV-II by SK110/SK111 and differentiation by type-specific probing. Numbers 1, 2, 3 and 4 refer to lysates of uninfected Hut-78 cells containing 1500, 150, 2 and 0 HTLV-I-infected (MT-2) or HTLV-II (MO-T) cells, respectively. C, reagent cocktail control; N, Hut-78. The HTLV-I-specific probe is SK112, and the HTLV-II probe is SK188.

vidual viral proteins. Antibodies to gag proteins appear first after seroconversion and may, in some individuals, become undetectable after symptoms begin. The criteria for the interpretation of Western blot results generally call for the presence of 2 or more antibody bands. Indeterminate Western blot results, containing one or more viral bands but insufficient to call positive, are usually followed up with repeat testing in 2–3 months. Stable indeterminate Western blot results are seen in 10–15% of people and do not represent infection. In addition to serum and plasma, antibodies to HIV have been sought in direct blood spots, saliva and urine (George and Schochetman 1994).

Sensitivity and specificity

Antibody tests can give false reactions, for a number of reasons. For example, false-positive reactions by ELISA have been caused by heat-inactivation of sera and by cross-reactive antibodies, including HLA class II antigens present on H9 cells. Some early assays for anti-HIV were of low sensitivity and gave negative results for sera from patients whose antibody levels had fallen in the late stages of severe disease. Current assays do not have this problem, and the failure to detect antibody now most probably indicates an absence of retrovirus infection. However, assays with narrow specificity may not detect antibody to a related virus; thus, tests for anti-HIV-1 alone may fail to identify all patients infected with HIV-2, and vice versa. Combined assays capable of detecting antibody to both viruses are now available.

Currently available screening assays are highly sensitive (>99.8%) and specific (>99.8%). However, the predictive value of a positive result is also affected by the overall seropositivity rate of the population tested, and in populations with low prevalence of HIV it is expected to be low.

Detection of virus

Virus isolation is not routinely used for diagnosis. Because virus can be cultured from only a small proportion of infected patients, failure to isolate an agent means little. However, collection of virus strains for certain characterization requires isolation. To support replication of HIV, peripheral blood leucocytes are stimulated in culture with phytohaemagglutinin (PHA) and IL-2, often in co-cultivation with human umbilical cord lymphocytes. The supernatant fluid of the cultures is tested regularly for as long as 28 days for evidence of RT activity and the expression of viral antigen. Typical syncytial cells may develop and virus can then sometimes, but by no means always, be passed into established cell lines, which are easier to maintain than umbilical cord cells. As shown by Ho and colleagues, under appropriate conditions it is possible to isolate virus from serum or plasma (Ho, Mougil and Alam 1989). Their method obviates the need for cryopreservation of leucocytes from infected patients and can be used routinely.

As an alternative to virus isolation, the detection of HIV genomic RNA has recently emerged as an important new tool to quantify circulating virus copies and also to predict clinical outcome. Several methods are available to quantify viral load directly from plasma, for example branched DNA (bDNA) or quantitative PCR (QC-PCR), all of which rely on the integrity of the genomic sequence. In addition to genome sequence-based identification, another method (amplified reverse transcriptase, AMP-RT), which directly measures RT activity of the virion, has received attention (Heneine et al. 1995). With this method the advantage is that the unique viral enzyme (RT) can be measured. RT activity generally reflects the infectious nature of the virus and can be used with genomic tests to differentiate between defective and infectious particles. The detection of circulating viral antigen may also be useful in diagnosis. People infected with HIV, particularly early in the course of infection, may have circulating p24 antigen, RT or virion RNA in their sera. The presence of p24 antigen may identify an infected person before the antibody response occurs. It is unlikely that assays for this antigen will ever replace those for antibody as a routine test. However, in the USA a decision has recently been made to add p24 antigen testing to the testing of volunteer blood donors in an attempt to reduce the diagnostic window period.

A situation in which virion detection may be of value is in monitoring the responses of HIV-infected patients to azidothymidine (AZT). In this circumstance, the quantitative measurement of virus levels may be useful in gauging the degree of virus suppression achieved.

As mentioned above, the detection of specific viral genes by probing and by amplification through PCR has been applied to the detection of HIV provirus. This technique has the theoretical advantage of being able to detect the virus before the onset of antibody production, either at the time of the early 'diagnostic window' or during extended periods of viral latency. PCR is an extremely powerful tool, and studies using this method contribute greatly to our understanding of viral variability and pathogenicity. However, routine diagnostic usefulness remains to be determined. As with other assays, a method of such extreme sensitivity is liable to give false-positive results and care is needed to prevent contamination of specimens while performing PCR. Despite this concern, PCR will probably have an important place in reference diagnostic testing, particularly in investigations of infants born to infected mothers and of patients who seem, on the basis of serology, to be doubly infected.

Testing and counselling

Testing for HIV infection should be voluntary, with informed consent obtained in accordance with local laws. Confidentiality and the prevention of discrimination toward people who test positive must be ensured. Mandatory testing is valuable in the context of tissue and organ donation. The confirmation of HIV infection can be devastating to the patient and must be explained with great care. It is necessary to discuss with the patient the implications of a positive finding before the test is done. The counselling for HIV-seropositive people should be tailored for each individual and should include interpretation of the test results and a discussion of the implications of the positive test result. The responsibility for handling this information lies ultimately with the clinician who is caring for the patient. Anyone who tests seropositive for HIV needs a medical evaluation, including immunological monitoring, and access to medical and therapeutic services, including antiretroviral therapy, prophylaxis against certain opportunistic infections, vaccinations and treatment of any other sexually transmitted diseases.

7 TREATMENT AND CONTROL

7.1 Antiretroviral therapy

A number of different antiretroviral agents have been developed and newer approaches are being evaluated for clinical use against HIV. Of these, the RT inhibitor AZT has been the most widely used. Major toxicities of AZT include neutropenia, anaemia and myopathy. Several other nucleotide analogues that act as chain terminators in the synthesis of the DNA provirus have also proved to be effective and selective inhibitors of reverse transcription and of HIV replication. These compounds, which include didanosine (DDI), zalcitabine (ddC) and stavudine (d4T), differ from each other and from AZT mainly by their major toxicities. Pancreatitis is the major toxicity associated with DDI, whereas peripheral neuropathy is most commonly seen with ddC and d4T. Non-competitive inhibitors of RT include nevirapine and delavirdine. These latter compounds seem to be specific for HIV-1 and do not inhibit HIV-2 or other lentiviruses. In general, all RT inhibitors are limited by their low potency, their side effects and the development of resistance. Protease inhibitors such as saquinavir have the advantage of being able to inhibit HIV replication in cells that are chronically infected. Gene therapy with compounds that inhibit the regulatory genes of HIV and the use of antisense oligonucleotides are under investigation. Approaches aimed at enhancing the host responses to HIV, such as replenishment of autologous CD8–cytotoxic/suppressor T lymphocytes or autologous CD4 cells are also being evaluated. Furthermore, therapies that target cellular structures or factors required to replicate HIV, such as anti-TNF-α, cyclosporin A and cellular transcriptional inhibitors, are being investigated (Butera and Folks 1992).

Studies of AIDS patients have demonstrated that AZT delays the development of opportunistic infections and prolongs survival. How early to start AZT remains controversial. Most clinical experts, however, agree on recommending AZT when the CD4 cell count drops below 500 (Sande et al. 1993). The development of clinically significant AZT resistance (heralded by a drop in CD4 counts), the development of opportunistic infections, and progressive weight loss and constitutional symptoms, seem to comprise a good indication for the need to change treatment. Various alternative treatment strategies have been recommended and it is widely believed that combination regimens may be superior to single antiretroviral agents. There are no clear guidelines for determining when to change treatment for patients who are clinically stable on AZT monotherapy. Viral markers, such as the level of HIV RNA, and drug resistance may eventually provide guidance for individualizing treatment for such patients.

Recently, AZT treatment started at 14–34 weeks' gestation reduced perinatal transmission of HIV by 60% among women who had received no antiretroviral therapy during the current pregnancy, who had no clinical indications for antenatal antiretroviral therapy, and who had CD4 counts above 200 at the time of entry into the study. In the USA, recommendations have been issued for the use of AZT in HIV-infected pregnant women to reduce perinatal transmission (CDC 1994b). (See also Chapter 46, section 3.2, p. 057.4.)

7.2 Prophylaxis against opportunistic infections

Since the start of the AIDS epidemic, important advances have been made in preventing or delaying many opportunistic infections. A decline in the percentage of AIDS patients who develop PCP and longer survival of patients with AIDS have resulted from the use of chemoprophylaxis against PCP. Agents exist that prevent *Mycobacterium avium* complex (MAC), toxoplasma, CMV and fungal infections. For the individual patient, the use of these agents must take into account the risk of developing a particular opportunistic infection, drug toxicities, drug interactions, potential for developing resistance and cost considerations. Comprehensive guidelines have been developed for the prevention of opportunistic infections in people infected with HIV (Kaplan 1995). These guidelines take into consideration the level of immunosuppression at which opportunistic disease is most likely to occur, the incidence and severity of the diseases, and the feasibility, efficacy and cost of the preventive measure. Recommended prevention strategies include vaccination against some agents, avoiding exposure to some and chemoprophylaxis.

In adults and adolescents, PCP prophylaxis is recommended for anyone with a history of PCP, with CD4 counts of <200, with unexplained fever lasting more than 2 weeks or with a history of oropharyngeal candidiasis. In neonates, PCP prophylaxis is recommended at 4–6 weeks of age for all infants who have been exposed perinatally to HIV. Decisions about continuing PCP prophylaxis after 12 months of age should take into account CD4 measurements and history of previous PCP infection (CDC 1995).

7.3 Prospects of vaccine development

T cells from peripheral blood and from the lungs (obtained by alveolar lavage) of HIV-infected patients express HLA class-restricted cytotoxicity for a number of HIV-related antigens in cell culture. The cytotoxicity mediated by CD8+, antigen-specific cells is directed predominantly against structural antigens but also against some regulatory proteins, such as nef. Specific receptor sites on these antigens for both helper and cytotoxic T cell functions have been suggested.

B cell epitopes have been mapped for HIV-1, initially using predictions from sequence analysis; the models suggest that as many as 11 sites in the env sequence may be recognized by B cells. In practice, smaller numbers of epitopes are recognized: 4 in gp120 and 5 in gp41. These sites are relatively well conserved in diverse isolates and can be shown regularly to bind antibody in the sera of HIV-infected patients, indicating their antigenicity in vivo. Antibodies raised against synthetic oligopeptides, containing the amino acid sequences defined by these sites, may be biologically active though their neutralization appears to be strain-specific. Studies of the binding natural antibodies and those raised against synthetic oligopeptides have localized a major strain-specific site to a loop structure, V3, in the variable region of env gp120. It is interesting that this site is identified with a T cell epitope and is a dominant site for neutralizing antibodies.

On the one hand, disease progresses and infection and infectivity persist in the face of brisk cellular and antibody immune responses to many HIV antigens. In addition, animals induced to produce antibody to synthetic and cell culture-derived antigens are not protected against live virus challenge (e.g. SIV) in spite of their antibody. On the other hand, an unprecedented knowledge of the lymphocyte target sites on HIV proteins means that it may be possible to tailor a vaccine, synthetic or recombinant, that could induce true immunity to infection. It is unlikely that such vaccines would affect the outcome in the individual already infected with HIV; however, reducing the initial viraemia due to a vaccine may be able to prolong disease progression. Field trials with humans have thus far been designed to examine the immune responses to antigens; trials to examine protective efficacy against infection are still quite some time away.

7.4 Safety precautions

IN LABORATORIES

Virus culture Both HIV and HTLV are considered to be biosafety level 3 pathogens and should be propagated only in laboratories appropriate for their containment (US Department of Health and Human Services 1993). The main hazards are inoculation or the contamination of mucous membranes or open cuts with virus-containing fluids. Avoidance of the use of sharp instruments and potentially breakable glassware, including glass Pasteur pipettes, is of major importance. For handling infected cultures, it is usual to have class I exhaust-protective flow cabinets or class II biosafety cabinets with a comparable protection factor. Disposable gowns and gloves should be worn at all times in the laboratory. The room should be secure, permitting minimal traffic, and, in the event of a spillage, disinfection with a 10–30% chlorine-based solution should be used.

Samples from patients Specimens from patients known or suspected to be infected with HIV should be handled with care to minimize the risk of accidental contamination or inoculation. There is no need to conduct their analysis in P3 level containment; a modified P2 environment (i.e. a P2 facility with P3 practice) is adequate. It is considered necessary at least to have designated areas within the laboratory and at best a designated room for handling such samples, and for staff to be suitably experienced in laboratory procedures. An exhaust-protective biosafety cabinet is not obligatory and does little to protect against accidental inoculation. Nevertheless, it does provide (simply but expensively) a designated work area for handling potentially infected specimens. In the long term it is better to bring all laboratory practices up to a standard at which such samples pose no additional risks.

IN WARDS

Clinical practices in the vicinity of HIV-infected patients must be designed to minimize the risk of exposure to blood and blood-containing fluids. It is prudent to consider all fluids shed by an HIV-infected patient as potential transmitters of virus and to avoid personal contamination. Such universal standards should be applied to the handling of all patients,

regardless of the perceived risk of infection. For surgeons, adherence to the principles of wearing gloves, avoidance of optional procedures known to favour accidents, and protection of the eyes and mouth are now all increasingly common features of everyday surgical and dental practice. All hospitals should have protocols for the sterilization of non-disposable equipment, particularly that used for HIV-infected patients. Fortunately, the infectivity of these enveloped viruses and of virus-infected cells is labile. Washing with hot water, detergents, chemical disinfectants (e.g. hypochlorite) or aqueous aldehyde solutions and disinfection with ethylene oxide are of known efficacy in inactivating HIV.

REFERENCES

Antoni BA, Stein SB et al., 1994, Regulation of human immunodeficiency virus infection: implications for pathogenesis, *Adv Virus Res*, **44**: 53–145.

Baltimore D, 1995, The enigma of HIV infection, *Cell*, **82**: 175–6.

Barré-Sinoussi F, Chermann JC et al., 1983, Isolation of a T-lymphotropic retrovirus from a patient at risk for acquired immune deficiency syndrome (AIDS), *Science*, **220**: 868–71.

Butera ST, Folks TM, 1992, Application of latent HIV-1 infected cellular models to therapeutic intervention, *AIDS Res Hum Retroviruses*, **8**: 991–5.

Centers for Disease Control and Prevention, 1992, 1993 revised classification system for HIV infection and expanded surveillance case definition for AIDS among adolescents and adults, *Morbid Mortal Weekly Rep*, **41**: 1–19.

CDC, 1994a, Revised classification system for HIV infection in children less than 13 years of age, *Morbid Mortal Weekly Rep*, **43**: 1–10.

CDC, 1994b, Recommendation of the US Public Health Service Task Force on the use of zidovudine to reduce perinatal transmission of HIV, *Morbid Mortal Weekly Rep*, **43**: 1–20.

CDC, 1995, Revised guidelines for prophylaxis against *Pneumocystis carinii* pneumonia for children infected with or perinatally exposed to HIV, *Morbid Mortal Weekly Rep*, **44**: 1–11.

Cease KB, Berzofsky JA, 1994, Towards a vaccine for AIDS: the emergence of immunobiology-based vaccine development, *Annu Rev Immunol*, **12**: 923–89.

Clavel F, Guetard D et al., 1986, Isolation of a new human retrovirus from West African patients with AIDS, *Science*, **233**: 343–6.

Coffin JM, 1995, HIV population dynamics in vivo: implications for genetic variation, pathogenesis, and therapy, *Science*, **267**: 483–9.

Dalgleish AG, Beverley PC et al., 1984, The CD4 (Tr) antigen is an essential component of the receptor for the AIDS retrovirus, *Nature (London)*, **312**: 776–7.

Embretson J, Zupancic M et al., 1993, Massive covert infection of helper T lymphocytes and macrophages by HIV during the incubation period of AIDS, *Nature (London)*, **362**: 359–62.

European Collaborative Study, 1992, Risk factors for mother-to-child transmission of HIV-1, *Lancet*, **339**: 1007–12.

Gardner MB, Endres M, Barry P, 1994, The simian retroviruses: SIV and SRV, *The* Retroviridae, vol 3, ed Levy JA, Plenum Press, New York, 133–276.

George JR, Schochetman G, 1994, Detection of HIV infection using serologic techniques, *AIDS Testing*, eds Schochetman G, George JR, Springer-Verlag, New York, 62–104.

Gitlin SD, Dittmer J et al., 1993, The molecular biology of human T-cell leukemia viruses, *Human Retroviruses*, ed Cullen BR, Oxford University Press, New York, 159–92.

Heneine W, Yamamoto S et al., 1995, Detection of reverse transcriptase by a highly sensitive assay in sera from persons infected with human immunodeficiency virus type 1, *J Infect Dis*, **171**: 1210–16.

Ho DD, Mougil T, Alam M, 1989, Quantitation of human immunodeficiency virus type 1 in the blood of infected persons, *N Engl J Med*, **321**: 1621–5.

Ho DD, Neumann AU et al., 1995, Rapid turnover of plasma virions and CD4 lymphocytes in HIV-1 infection, *Nature (London)*, **373**: 123–6.

Kaplan JE, Khabbaz RF, 1993, The epidemiology of human T-lymphotropic virus type I and II, *Rev Med Virol*, **3**: 137–48.

Kaplan JE, 1995, USPHS/IDSA guidelines for the prevention of opportunistic infections in person infected with HIV: an overview, *Clin Infect Dis*, **21, suppl 1**: S12–31.

Khabbaz RF, Heneine W, Kaplan JE, 1994, Testing for other human retroviruses: HTLV-I and HTLV-II, *AIDS Testing*, eds Schochetman G, George JR, Springer-Verlag, New York, 206–23.

Levy JA, 1993, Pathogenesis of human immunodeficiency virus infection, *Microbiol Rev*, **57**: 183–289.

Li CJ, Dezube BJ et al., 1994, Inhibitors of HIV-1 transcription, *Trends Microbiol*, **2**: 164–9.

Mahnke C, Kashaiya P et al., 1992, Human spumavirus antibodies in sera from African patients, *Arch Virol*, **123**: 243–53.

Martin MA, 1993, The molecular and biological properties of the human immunodeficiency virus, *The Molecular Basis of Blood Diseases*, eds Stamatoyannopoulos G, Nienhuis AW et al., WB Saunders, Philadelphia, 863–908.

Maurer B, Flugel RM, 1988, Genomic organization of the human spumaretrovirus and its relatedness to AIDS and other retroviruses, *AIDS Res Human Retroviruses*, **4**: 467–73.

Miyoshi I, Kubonishi I et al., 1981, Type C virus particles in a cord T-cell line derived by co-cultivating normal human cord leukocytes and human leukaemic T cells, *Nature (London)*, **294**: 770–1.

Nelson KE, Vlahov D et al., 1991, Sexually transmitted diseases in a population of intravenous drug users: association with seropositivity to HIV-1, *J Infect Dis*, **164**: 457–63.

Pantaleo G, Graziosi C et al., 1993, HIV infection is active and progressive in lymphoid tissue during the clinically latent stage of disease, *Nature (London)*, **362**: 355–8.

Plummer FA, Simonsen JN et al., 1991, Cofactors in male/female sexual transmission of HIV type 1, *J Infect Dis*, **163**: 233–9.

Poiesz BJ, Ruscetti FW et al., 1980, Detection and isolation of type C retrovirus particles from fresh and cultured lymphocytes of a patient with cutaneous T-cell lymphoma, *Proc Natl Acad Sci USA*, **77**: 7415–19.

Price RW, Sidkis JJ et al., 1988, The AIDS dementia complex, *AIDS and the Nervous System*, eds Rosenblum ML, Levy RM et al., Raven Press, New York, 203–19.

Redfield RR, Wright DC, Tramont EC, 1986, The Walter Reed staging classification for HTLV-III/LaV infection, *N Engl J Med*, **314**: 131–2.

Sande MA, Carpenter CJ et al., 1993, The National Institute of Allergy and Infectious Diseases State of the Art Panel on antiretroviral therapy for adult HIV-infected patients, *JAMA*, **270**: 2583–9.

Stein DS, Korvick JA, Vermund SH, 1992, CD4+ lymphocyte cell enumeration for prediction of clinical course of human immunodeficiency virus disease: a review, *J Infect Dis*, **165**: 352–63.

Subbramanian RA, Cohen EA, 1994, Molecular biology of the human immunodeficiency virus accessory proteins, *J Virol*, **68**: 6831–5.

Tokars JI, Marcus R et al., 1993, Surveillance of HIV infection and zidovudine use among health care workers after occu- pational exposure to HIV-infected blood, *Ann Intern Med*, **118**: 913–19.

US Department of Health and Human Services, 1993, Labora- tory biosafety criteria, *Biosafety in Microbiological and Biomedical Laboratories*, eds Richmond JY, McKinney RW, US Govern- ment Printing Office, Washington DC, 16–43.

Wei X, Ghosh SK et al., 1995, Viral dynamics in human immuno- deficiency virus type 1 infection, *Nature (London)*, **373**: 117– 22.

Weiss RA, Teich NM et al., 1985, *RNA Tumor Viruses*, Cold Spring Harbor Laboratory, Cold Spring Harbor NY.

World Health Organization, 1995, AIDS – global data, *Wkly Epide- miol Rec*, **70**: 5–7.

Yarchoan R, Venzon DJ et al., 1991, CD4 count and the risk for death in patients infected with HIV receiving antiretroviral therapy, *Ann Intern Med*, **115**: 184–9.

Chapter 39

PRIONS OF HUMANS AND ANIMALS

Stanley B Prusiner

1 PROPERTIES OF PRIONS

1.1 Introduction

Prions differ from all other known infectious pathogens in several respects. First, prions do not contain a nucleic acid genome that codes for their progeny. Viruses, viroids, bacteria, fungi and parasites all have nucleic acid genomes that code for their progeny. Secondly, the only known component of the prion is a modified protein that is encoded by a cellular gene. Thirdly, the major, and possibly only, component of the prion is the scrapie isoform of the prion protein (PrP^{Sc}) which is a pathogenic conformer of the cellular isoform PrP^C.

The fundamental event in prion diseases seems to be a conformational change which occurs during the conversion of PrP^C into PrP^{Sc}. PrP^C has been identified in all mammals and birds examined to date, and it is anchored to the external surface of cells by a glycolipid moiety. Its function is unknown (Stahl et al. 1987). All attempts to identify a post-translational chemical modification that distinguishes PrP^{Sc} from PrP^C have been unsuccessful to date (Stahl et al. 1993). PrP^C contains c. 45% α-helix and is virtually devoid of β-sheet (Pan et al. 1993). Conversion to PrP^{Sc} creates a protein that contains c. 30% α-helix and 45% β-sheet. The mechanism by which PrP^C is converted into PrP^{Sc} remains unknown but PrP^C seems to bind to PrP^{Sc} to form an intermediate complex during the formation of nascent PrP^{Sc}. Transgenic (Tg) mouse studies have demonstrated that PrP^{Sc} in the inoculum interacts preferentially with homotypic PrP^C during the propagation of prions (Prusiner et al. 1990, Scott et al. 1993).

The human prion diseases are frequently referred to as kuru, Creutzfeldt–Jakob disease (CJD), Gerstmann–Sträussler–Scheinker (GSS) disease and fatal familial insomnia (FFI) whilst the most common

prion diseases of animals are scrapie of sheep and goats, and bovine spongiform encephalopathy (BSE) or 'mad cow' disease (Table 39.1). Kuru was the first of the human prion diseases to be transmitted to experimental animals, and it has often been suggested that kuru spread among the Fore people of Papua New Guinea by ritualistic cannibalism (Gajdusek, Gibbs and Alpers 1966, Gajdusek 1977). The experimental and presumed human-to-human transmission of kuru led to the belief that prion diseases are infectious disorders caused by unusual viruses similar to those causing scrapie in sheep and goats. Yet a paradox was presented by the occurrence of CJD in families, first reported almost 70 years ago (Kirschbaum 1924, Meggendorfer 1930), which appeared to be a genetic disease. The significance of familial CJD remained unappreciated until mutations in the protein coding region of the PrP gene on the short arm of chromosome 20 were discovered (Sparkes et al. 1986, Hsiao et al. 1989, Prusiner 1994). The earlier finding that brain extracts from patients who had died of familial prion diseases inoculated into experimental animals often transmit disease posed a conundrum that was resolved with the genetic linkage of these diseases to mutations of the PrP gene (Masters, Gajdusek and Gibbs 1981a, Prusiner 1989, Tateishi et al. 1992). It seems likely that progressive subcortical gliosis will be found to be caused by prions (Neumann and Cohn 1967, Lanska et al. 1994). In families with this disease no PrP gene mutation has been found, raising the possibility that another gene product such as protein X, which is thought to mediate the conversion of PrP^C into PrP^{Sc}, can also feature in the pathogenesis of the inherited prion diseases.

The most common form of prion disease in humans is sporadic CJD. Many attempts to show that the sporadic prion diseases are caused by infection have been unsuccessful (Malmgren et al. 1979, Brown et al. 1987, Harries-Jones et al. 1988, Cousens et al. 1990). The

Table 39.1 Human prion diseases

Disease	Aetiology
Kuru	Infection
Creutzfeldt–Jakob disease:	
Iatrogenic	Infection
Sporadic	Unknown
Familial	PrP mutation
Gerstmann–Sträussler– Scheinker disease	PrP mutation
Fatal familial insomnia	PrP mutation

discovery that inherited prion diseases are caused by germ-line mutation of the PrP gene raised the possibility that sporadic forms of these diseases might result from a somatic mutation (Prusiner 1989). The discovery that PrP^{Sc} is formed from the cellular isoform of the prion protein, PrP^{C}, by a post-translational process (Borchelt et al. 1990) and that overexpression of wild type (wt) PrP transgenes produces spongiform degeneration and infectivity *de novo* (Westaway et al. 1994b) has raised the possibility that sporadic prion diseases result from the spontaneous conversion of PrP^{C} into PrP^{Sc}.

CJD has a world-wide incidence of c. 1 case per 10^6 population annually (Masters et al. 1978). Less than 1% of CJD cases are infectious and most of those seem to be iatrogenic. Between 10 and 15% cases of prion disease are inherited whilst the remaining cases are sporadic. Kuru was once the most common cause of death among New Guinea women in the Fore region of the Highlands (Gajdusek and Zigas 1957, Gajdusek and Zigas 1959, Gajdusek, Gibbs and Alpers 1966) but has virtually disappeared with the cessation of ritualistic cannibalism (Alpers 1987). Patients with CJD frequently present with dementia but c. 10% of patients exhibit cerebellar dysfunction initially. People with either kuru or GSS usually present with ataxia whereas those with FFI manifest insomnia and autonomic dysfunction (Hsiao and Prusiner 1990, Brown 1992, Medori et al. 1992b).

PrP^{CJD} has been found in the brains of most patients who died of prion disease. The term PrP^{CJD} is preferred by some investigators when referring to the abnormal isoform of HuPrP in human brain. In this chapter, PrP^{Sc} is used interchangeably with PrP^{CJD}. PrP^{Sc} is always used after human CJD prions have been passaged into an experimental animal, because the nascent PrP^{Sc} molecules are produced from host PrP^{C} and the PrP^{CJD} in the inoculum serves only to initiate the process. In the brains of some patients with inherited prion diseases as well as Tg mice expressing mouse (Mo) PrP with the human GSS point mutation (Pro→Leu), detection of PrP^{Sc} has been problematic despite clinical and neuropathological hallmarks of neurodegeneration (Hsiao et al. 1990, 1994). Horizontal transmission of neurodegeneration from the brains of patients with inherited prion diseases to inoculated rodents has been less frequent than with

sporadic cases (Tateishi et al. 1992). Whether this distinction between transmissible and non-transmissible inherited prion diseases will persist is unclear. Tg mice expressing a chimaeric Hu/Mo PrP gene are highly susceptible to Hu prions from sporadic and iatrogenic CJD cases (Telling et al. 1994). These Tg(MHu2M) mice should make the use of apes and monkeys for the study of human prion diseases unnecessary and allow for tailoring the PrP^{C} translated from the transgene to match the sequence of the PrP^{CJD} in the inoculum. The use of mice expressing MHu2MPrP transgenes with mutations may enhance the ability to transmit cases of the inherited human prion diseases.

Scrapie is the most common natural prion disease of animals. An investigation into the aetiology of scrapie followed the vaccination of sheep for louping-ill virus with formalin-treated extracts of ovine lymphoid tissue unknowingly contaminated with scrapie prions (Gordon 1946). Two years later, more than 1500 sheep developed scrapie from this vaccine. Although the transmissibility of experimental scrapie became well established, the spread of natural scrapie within and among flocks of sheep remained puzzling. Parry argued that host genes were responsible for the development of scrapie in sheep. He was convinced that natural scrapie is a genetic disease which could be eradicated by proper breeding protocols (Parry 1962, 1983). He considered its transmission by inoculation to be of importance primarily for laboratory studies and communicable infection of little consequence in nature. Other investigators viewed natural scrapie as an infectious disease and argued that host genetics only modulates susceptibility to an endemic infectious agent (Dickinson et al. 1965).

The offal of scrapie-infected sheep in Great Britain is thought to be responsible for the current epidemic of BSE (Wilesmith et al. 1992b). Prions in the offal from scrapie-infected sheep seem to have survived the rendering process that produced meat and bone meal (MBM). The MBM was fed to cattle as a nutritional supplement. After BSE was recognized, MBM produced from domestic animal offal was banned from further use. Since 1986, when BSE was first recognized, >160 000 cattle have died of BSE. Whether humans will develop CJD after consuming beef from cattle with BSE prions is of considerable concern (Chazot et al. 1996, Will et al. 1996).

As we learn about the molecular and genetic characteristics of prion proteins, our understanding of prions and their place in biology will undoubtedly undergo considerable change. Indeed, the discovery of the PrP, the identification of pathogenic PrP gene mutations, the profound differences in the structures of PrP^{C} and PrP^{Sc}, as well as studies of the process by which nascent PrP^{Sc} is formed, have already forced us to think about the modification of proteins from viewpoints not previously considered.

1.2 Development of the prion concept

HYPOTHESES ON THE NATURE OF THE SCRAPIE AGENT

The published literature contains a fascinating record of the structural hypotheses for the scrapie agent, proposed to explain the unusual features first of the disease and later those of the infectious agent. Among the earliest hypotheses was the notion that scrapie was a disease of muscle caused by the parasite *Sarcosporidia* (M'Gowan 1914, M'Fadyean 1918). With the successful transmission of scrapie to animals, the hypothesis that scrapie is caused by a 'filterable' virus became popular (Cuillé and Chelle 1939, Wilson, Anderson and Smith 1950). With the findings of Tikvah Alper and her colleagues that scrapie infectivity resists inactivation by UV and ionizing irradiation (Alper, Haig and Clarke 1966, Alper et al. 1967), a myriad hypotheses on the chemical nature of the scrapie agent emerged.

BIOASSAYS OF PRION INFECTIVITY

The experimental transmission of scrapie from sheep (Gordon 1946) to mice (Chandler 1961) gave investigators a more convenient laboratory model, which yielded considerable information on the nature of the unusual infectious pathogen that causes scrapie (Alper et al. 1966, 1967, Gibbons and Hunter 1967, Pattison and Jones 1967, Millson, Hunter and Kimberlin 1971, Alper, Haig and Clarke 1978). Yet progress was slow because quantification of infectivity in a single sample required holding 60 mice for one year before accurate scoring could be accomplished (Chandler 1961).

Attempts to develop a more economical bioassay by relating the titre to incubation times in mice were unsuccessful (Eklund, Hadlow and Kennedy 1963, Hunter and Millson 1964); however, some investigators used incubation times to characterize different 'strains' of scrapie agent whilst others determined the kinetics of prion replication in rodents (Dickinson and Meikle 1969, Dickinson, Meikle and Fraser 1969, Kimberlin and Walker 1978, 1979). Yet these investigators refrained from trying to establish quantitative bioassays for prions based on incubation times despite the successful application of such an approach for the measurement of picorna and other viruses 3 decades earlier (Gard 1940). After scrapie incubation times were reported to be c. 50% shorter in Syrian hamsters than in mice (Marsh and Kimberlin 1975), studies were undertaken to determine if the incubation times in hamsters could be related to the titre of the inoculated sample. Once it was found that there was an excellent correlation between the length of the incubation time and the dose of inoculated prions, a more rapid and economical bioassay was developed (Prusiner et al. 1980a, 1982b). This improved bioassay for the scrapie agent in Syrian golden hamsters accelerated purification of the infectious particles by a factor of nearly 100.

THE PRION CONCEPT

Once an effective protocol was developed for preparation of partially purified fractions of scrapie agent from hamster brain, it became possible to demonstrate that the procedures that modify or hydrolyse proteins produce a diminution in scrapie infectivity (Prusiner 1981, 1982). At the same time, tests done in search of a scrapie-specific nucleic acid were unable to demonstrate any dependence of infectivity on a polynucleotide (Prusiner 1982), in agreement with earlier studies reporting the extreme resistance of infectivity to UV irradiation at 254 nm (Alper et al. 1967).

On the basis of these findings, it seemed likely that the infectious pathogen capable of transmitting scrapie was neither a virus nor a viroid. For this reason the term 'prion' was introduced to distinguish the proteinaceous infectious particles that cause scrapie, CJD, GSS and kuru from both viroids and viruses (Prusiner 1982). Hypotheses for the structure of the infectious prion particle included (1) proteins surrounding a nucleic acid encoding them (a virus), (2) proteins associated with a small polynucleotide and (3) proteins devoid of nucleic acid (Prusiner 1982). Mechanisms postulated for the replication of infectious prion particles ranged from those used by viruses to the synthesis of polypeptides in the absence of nucleic acid template to post-translational modifications of cellular proteins. Subsequent discoveries have narrowed hypotheses for both prion structure and the mechanism of replication.

Considerable evidence has accumulated over the past decade supporting the prion hypothesis (Prusiner 1991). Furthermore, the replication of prions and their mode of pathogenesis also seem to be without precedent. After a decade of severe criticism and serious doubt, the prion concept is now enjoying considerable acceptance.

1.3 Discovery of the prion protein

Once the dependence of prion infectivity on protein was clear, the search for a scrapie-specific protein intensified. Although the insolubility of scrapie infectivity made purification problematic, we took advantage of this property along with its relative resistance to degradation by proteases to extend the degree of purification (Prusiner et al. 1980a, 1981). In subcellular fractions from hamster brain enriched for scrapie infectivity, a protease-resistant polypeptide of 27–30 kDa (later designated PrP 27–30) was identified; it was absent from controls (Bolton, McKinley and Prusiner 1982, Prusiner et al. 1982a, McKinley, Bolton, Prusiner 1983). Radioiodination of partially purified fractions revealed a protein unique to preparations from scrapie-infected brains (Bolton, McKinley and Prusiner 1982, Prusiner et al. 1982a).

Purification of PrP 27–30 to homogeneity allowed determination of its NH$_2$-terminal amino acid sequence (Prusiner et al. 1984). These studies were particularly difficult because multiple signals were found in each cycle of the Edman degradation. Whether multiple proteins were present in these 'purified fractions' or a single protein with a ragged NH$_2$ terminus was resolved only after data from 5 different preparations were compared. When the signals in each cycle were grouped according to their intensities of strong, intermediate and weak, it became clear that a single protein with a ragged NH$_2$ terminus was being sequenced. Determination of a single, unique sequence for the NH$_2$ terminus of PrP 27–30 permitted the synthesis of an isocoding mixture of oligonucleotides that was subsequently used to identify incomplete PrP cDNA clones from hamster (Oesch et al. 1985) and mouse (Chesebro et al. 1985). cDNA clones encoding the entire open reading frames (ORFs) of Syrian hamster (SHa) and MoPrP were subsequently recovered (Basler et al. 1986, Locht et al. 1986).

PrP is encoded by a chromosomal gene and not by a nucleic acid within the infectious scrapie prion particle (Oesch et al. 1985, Basler et al. 1986). Levels of PrP mRNA remain unchanged throughout the course of scrapie infection – an unexpected observation which led to the identification of the normal PrP gene product, a protein of 33–35 kDa, designated PrP^C (Oesch et al. 1985, Basler et al. 1986). PrP^C is protease-sensitive and soluble in non-denaturing detergents whereas PrP 27–30 is the protease-resistant core of a 33–35 kDa disease-specific protein, designated PrP^{Sc}, which is insoluble in detergents (Meyer et al. 1986). Progress in the study of prions was greatly accelerated by the discovery of PrP and determination of its N-terminal sequence (Bolton, McKinley and Prusiner 1982, Prusiner et al. 1982a, 1984). Indeed, all of the elegant molecular genetic studies in humans and animals as well as many highly informative transgenetic investigations have their origin in the purification of PrP 27–30 (Prusiner et al. 1983) and the determination of its N-terminal sequence (Prusiner et al. 1984).

PrP GENE STRUCTURE AND ORGANIZATION

The entire ORF of all known mammalian and avian PrP genes is contained within a single exon (Fig. 39.1) (Basler et al. 1986, Westaway et al. 1987, Hsiao et al. 1989, Gabriel et al. 1992). This feature of the PrP gene eliminates the possibility that PrP^{Sc} arises from alternative RNA splicing (Basler et al. 1986, Westaway et al. 1987, 1991); however, mechanisms such as RNA editing or protein splicing remain a possibility (Blum, Bakalara and Simpson 1990, Kane et al. 1990). The 2 exons of the SHaPrP gene are separated by a 10 kb intron: exon 1 encodes a portion of the 5′ untranslated leader sequence whilst exon 2 encodes the ORF and 3′ untranslated region (Basler et al. 1986). The Mo and sheep PrP genes are comprised of 3 exons with exon 3 analogous to exon 2 of the hamster (Westaway et al. 1991, 1994a). The promoters of both the SHa and Mo PrP genes contain multiple copies of G–C rich repeats and are devoid of TATA boxes. These G–C nonamers represent a motif that may function as a canonical binding site for the transcription factor Sp1.

Mapping PrP genes to the short arm of Hu chromosome 20 and the homologous region of Mo chromosome 2 argues for the existence of PrP genes prior to the speciation of mammals (Sparkes et al. 1986). Hybridization studies demonstrated <0.002 PrP gene sequences per ID50 unit in purified prion fractions, indicating that a nucleic acid encoding PrP^{Sc} is not a component of the infectious prion particle (Oesch et al. 1985). This is a major feature that distinguishes prions from viruses, including retroviruses that carry cellular oncogenes and from satellite viruses that derive their coat proteins from other viruses previously infecting plant cells.

Although PrP mRNA is constitutively expressed in the brains of adult animals (Chesebro et al. 1985, Oesch et al.

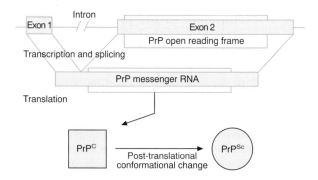

Fig. 39.1 Structure and organization of the chromosomal PrP gene. In all mammals examined the entire ORF is contained within a single exon. The 5′ untranslated region of the PrP mRNA is derived from either one or 2 additional exons (Basler et al. 1986, Puckett et al. 1991, Westaway et al. 1991, 1994a). Only one PrP mRNA has been detected. PrP^{Sc} is thought to be derived from PrP^C by a post-translational process (Basler et al. 1986, Borchelt et al. 1990, Caughey and Raymond 1991, Borchelt et al. 1992, Taraboulos et al. 1992b). The amino acid sequence of PrP^{Sc} is identical to that predicted from the translated sequence of the DNA encoding the PrP gene (Basler et al. 1986, Stahl et al. 1993), and no unique post-translational chemical modifications have been identified that might distinguish PrP^{Sc} from PrP^C. Thus, it seems likely that PrP^C undergoes a conformational change as it is converted to PrP^{Sc}.

1985), it is highly regulated during development. In the septum, levels of PrP mRNA and choline acetyltransferase increased in parallel during development (Mobley et al. 1988). In other brain regions, PrP gene expression occurred at an earlier age. In situ hybridization studies show that the highest levels of PrP mRNA are found in neurons (Kretzschmar et al. 1986a).

1.4 PrP amyloid

The discovery of PrP 27–30 in fractions enriched for scrapie infectivity was accompanied by the identification of rod-shaped particles in the same fractions (Prusiner et al. 1982a, 1983). Both by rotary shadowing and by negative staining, the fine structure of these rod-shaped particles failed to reveal any regular substructure. Indeed, it was the irregular ultrastructure of the prion rods that differentiated them from viruses, which have regular, distinct structures (Williams 1954), and made them indistinguishable ultrastructurally from many purified amyloids (Cohen, Shirahama and Skinner 1982). This analogy was extended when the prion rods were found to display the tinctorial properties of amyloids (Prusiner et al. 1983). These findings were followed by the demonstration that amyloid plaques in the brains of humans and other animals with prion diseases contain PrP, as determined by immunoreactivity and amino acid sequencing (Bendheim et al. 1984, DeArmond et al. 1985, Kitamoto et al. 1986, Roberts et al. 1988, Tagliavini et al. 1991).

The formation of prion rods requires limited proteolysis in the presence of detergent (McKinley et al. 1991a). Thus, the prion rods in fractions enriched for scrapie infectivity are largely, if not entirely, artefacts of the purification protocol. Solubilization of PrP 27–30 into liposomes with retention of infectivity (Gabizon, McKinley and Prusiner 1987) demonstrated that large PrP polymers are not required for infectivity, and permitted the immunoaffinity co-purification of PrP^{Sc} and infectivity (Gabizon et al. 1988, Gabizon and Prusiner 1990). In scrapie-infected mouse neuroblastoma cells, immunocytochemical studies demonstrated PrP^Sc confined largely to secondary lysosomes; there was no ultrastructural evidence for polymers of PrP (McKinley et al. 1991b). In Tg(SHaPrP) mice inoculated with SHa prions, numerous amyloid plaques were found but none was observed if these mice were inoculated with Mo prions, indicating that amyloid formation is not an obligatory feature of prion diseases (Prusiner et al. 1990, Prusiner and DeArmond 1994). In accord with these Tg(SHaPrP) mouse studies, PrP plaques are consistently found in some inherited prion diseases (Ghetti et al. 1989) but absent in others (Hsiao et al. 1991a).

1.5 Formation of PrP^Sc

Whether PrP^C is the substrate for PrP^Sc formation or a restricted subset of PrP molecules are precursors for PrP^Sc remains to be established. Several experimental results argue that PrP molecules destined to become PrP^Sc exit to the cell surface, as does PrP^C (Stahl et al. 1987) prior to its conversion into PrP^Sc (Caughey and Raymond 1991, Borchelt, Taraboulos and Prusiner 1992, Taraboulos et al. 1992b).

Like other glycophosphatidylinositol (GPI)-anchored proteins, PrP^C seems to re-enter the cell through a subcellular compartment bounded by cholesterol-rich, detergent-insoluble membranes which might be caveolae or early endosomes (Fig. 39.2) (Keller, Siegel and Caras 1992, Anderson 1993, Shyng, Heuser and Harris 1994, Gorodinsky and Harris 1995, Taraboulos et al. 1995). Within this cholesterol-rich, non-acidic compartment, GPI-anchored PrP^C seems to be either converted into PrP^Sc or partially degraded (Taraboulos et al. 1995). The partially degraded fragment of PrP^C seems to be the same as the protein previously designated PrP^C-II in partially purified fractions prepared from Syrian hamster brain (Haraguchi et al. 1989, Pan, Stahl and Prusiner 1992). After denaturation PrP^Sc, like PrP^C, can be released from the cell membranes by digestion with phosphatidylinositol-specific phospholipase C, suggesting that PrP^Sc is tethered only by the GPI anchor (Borchelt et al. 1993). In scrapie-infected cultured cells, PrP^Sc is trimmed at the N terminus to form PrP 27–30 in an acidic compartment (Caughey et al. 1991a, Taraboulos et al. 1992b). Whether this acidic compartment is endosomal or lysosomal where PrP 27–30 accumulates (McKinley et al. 1990) remains to be determined. In contrast to cultured cells, the N-terminal trimming of PrP^Sc is minimal in brain, where little PrP 27–30 is found (McKinley et al. 1991a). Deleting the GPI addition signal resulted in greatly diminished synthesis of PrP^Sc (Rogers et al. 1993). In contrast to PrP^C, PrP^Sc accumulates primarily within cells, where it is deposited in cytoplasmic vesicles, many of which seem to be secondary lysosomes (Taraboulos, Serban and Prusiner 1990, Caughey et al. 1991a, McKinley et al. 1991b, Borchelt et al. 1992, Taraboulos et al. 1992b). Studies of scrapie-infected brains suggest that PrP^Sc accumulates within either lysosomes or late endosomes (Laszlo et al. 1992, Arnold et al. 1995).

Although most of the difference in the mass of PrP 27–30 predicted from the amino acid sequence and observed after post-translational modification is due to complex-type oligosaccharides (Haraguchi et al. 1989), these sugar chains are not required for PrP^Sc synthesis in scrapie-infected cultured cells, based on experiments with the asparagine-linked glycosylation inhibitor tunicamycin and site-directed mutagenesis studies (Taraboulos et al. 1990).

SEARCH FOR A CHEMICAL MODIFICATION

The discovery that the entire ORF of the PrP gene is contained within a single exon, first in Syrian hamsters and later in humans and other animals, argued that PrP^Sc is not generated by alternative splicing (Basler et al. 1986, Goldmann et al. 1988, 1991b, Hsiao et al. 1989, Westaway et al. 1994a, 1994c). This prompted us to search for a post-translational chemical modification to explain the differences in the properties of these 2 PrP isoforms (Stahl et al. 1993). PrP^Sc was analysed by mass spectrometry and gas phase sequencing in order to identify any amino acid substitutions or post-translational chemical modifications. The amino acid sequence was the same as that deduced from the translated ORF of the PrP gene, and no candidates for post-translational chemical modifications that might differentiate PrP^C from PrP^Sc were found (Stahl et al. 1993). These findings forced consideration of the possibility that conformation distinguishes the 2 PrP isoforms.

STRUCTURES OF PURIFIED PrP^C AND PrP^Sc

To gather evidence for or against the hypothesis that a conformational change features in PrP^Sc synthesis, we purified both PrP^C and PrP^Sc using non-denaturing procedures and determined the secondary structure of each (Turk et al. 1988, Pan et al. 1993). Fourier transform infrared (FTIR) spectroscopy demonstrated that PrP^C has a high α-helix content (c. 40%) and no β-sheet (3%), findings that were confirmed by circular dichroism measurements (Fig. 39.3) (Pan et al. 1993). In contrast, the β-sheet content of PrP^Sc was c. 40% and the α-helix c. 30% as measured by FTIR (Pan et al. 1993) and CD spectroscopy (Safar et al. 1993a). That N-terminally truncated PrP^Sc derived by limited proteolysis and designated PrP 27–30 has a high β-sheet content was initially inferred from the green-gold birefringence of the prion rods after staining with Congo red (Prusiner et al. 1983). Subsequently, spectroscopy showed that PrP 27–30 when polymerized into rod-shaped particles with ultrastructural appearance of amyloid (Fig. 39.4) contains c. 50% β-sheet and c. 20% α-helix (Caughey et al. 1991b, Gasset et al. 1993, Safar et al. 1993b). Fibre diffraction studies have also demonstrated the high β-sheet content of PrP 27–30, and synthetic peptide studies suggest that the putative helical regions H1 and H2 are converted into β-sheets (Nguyen et al. 1995, Zhang et al. 1995). In contrast to PrP 27–30 which did polymerize into rod-shaped amyloids, neither purified PrP^C nor PrP^Sc formed aggregates detectable by electron microscopy (Fig. 39.4) (McKinley et al. 1991a, Pan et al. 1993).

Although the foregoing studies argue that the conversion of α-helices into β-sheets underlies the formation of PrP^Sc, we cannot eliminate the possibility that an undetected chemical modification of a small fraction of PrP^Sc initiates this process. Because PrP^Sc seems to be the only component of the 'infectious' prion particle, it is likely that this conformational transition is a fundamental event in the propagation of prions. In support of the above statement is the finding that denaturation of PrP 27–30 under conditions which reduced scrapie infectivity resulted in a concomitant diminution of β-sheet content (Gasset et al. 1993, Safar et al. 1993b).

CONVERSION OF PrP^C INTO PrP^Sc

Studies with Tg(SHaPrP) mice have provided some information about the process in which PrP^C is converted into PrP^Sc through the formation of a PrP^C/PrP^Sc complex (Prusiner et al. 1990). The level of PrP^C expression seems to be directly proportional to the rate of PrP^Sc formation and, thus, inversely related to the length of the incubation

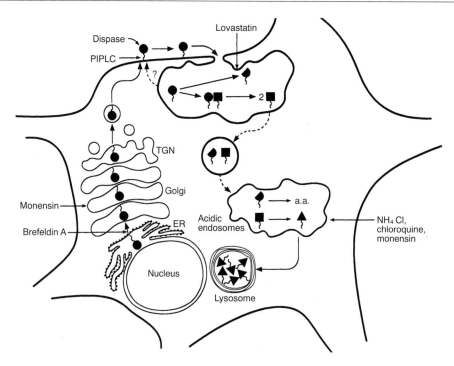

Fig. 39.2 Pathways of prion protein synthesis and degradation in cultured cells. PrP^{Sc} is denoted by squares; circles denote PrP^C. Before becoming protease-resistant, the PrP^{Sc} precursor transits through the plasma membrane and is sensitive to dispase or PIPLC added to the medium. PrP^{Sc} formation probably occurs in a compartment accessible from the plasma membrane, such as caveolae or early endosomes, both of which are non-acidic compartments. The synthesis of nascent PrP^{Sc} seems to require the interaction of PrP^C with existing PrP^{Sc}. In cultured cells, but not brain, the N terminus of PrP^{Sc} is trimmed to form PrP 27–30; PrP^{Sc} then accumulates primarily in secondary lysosomes. The inhibition of PrP^{Sc} synthesis by brefeldin A demonstrates that the endoplasmic reticulum (ER)–Golgi is not competent for its synthesis and that transport of PrP down the secretory pathway is required for the formation of PrP^{Sc}.

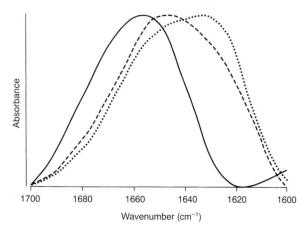

Fig. 39.3 Fourier transform infrared spectroscopy of prion proteins. The amide I′ band (1700–1600 cm^{-1}) of transmission FTIR spectra of PrP^C (solid line), PrP^{Sc} (dashed line) and PrP 27–30 (dotted line). These proteins were suspended in a buffer in D$_2$O containing 0.15 M sodium chloride/10 mM sodium phosphate, pD 7.5 (uncorrected)/0.12% ZW. The spectra are scaled independently to be full scale on the ordinate axis (absorbance). (Reproduced from Pan et al. 1993.)

time. Formation of the PrP^C/PrP^{Sc} complex was facilitated when the amino acid sequences of the 2 PrP isoforms were the same; SHaPrP differs from MoPrP at 16 positions out of 254. Differences in amino acid sequence delayed prion formation, resulting in a prolongation of the incubation time (Scott et al. 1989).

Although some investigators have reported the in vitro formation of PrP^{Sc} by mixing a 50-fold excess of PrP^{Sc} with [^{35}S-]PrP^C, their conclusions assume that protease-resistant PrP^C is equivalent to PrP^{Sc} (Kocisko et al. 1994). It is interesting that the binding of PrP^C to PrP^{Sc} depends on the same residues (Kocisko et al. 1995) that render Tg(MH2M) mice susceptible to SHa prions (Scott et al. 1993) and it seems to be strain-dependent (Bessen et al. 1995). Although we were able to confirm the binding of PrP^C to PrP^{Sc} in the presence of a large excess of PrP^{Sc} (see Figs 39.3a and 39.4b), we were unable to reproduce the renaturation of PrP^{Sc} from guanidium hydrochloride as judged by a restoration of protease resistance (Kaneko et al. 1995). Mixing equimolar amounts of PrP^C and PrP^{Sc} did not result in the conversion of PrP^C into PrP^{Sc} (Raeber et al. 1992).

1.6 Propagation of prions

Because our initial transgenetic studies had shown that the 'species barrier' between mice and SHa for the transmission of prions can be abolished by expression of a SHaPrP transgene in mice (Scott et al. 1989), Tg mice expressing HuPrP were constructed. These Tg(HuPrP) mice inoculated with Hu prions failed to develop CNS dysfunction more frequently than non-Tg controls (Telling et al. 1994). Faced with this apparent dichotomy, we constructed mice expressing a chimaeric Hu/mouse (Mo) PrP transgene designated MHu2M because earlier studies had shown that chimaeric SHa/Mo PrP transgenes supported transmission of either Mo or SHa prions (Scott et al. 1992, 1993). The Tg(MHu2M) mice expressing the chimaeric transgene were highly susceptible to Hu prions, suggesting that Tg(HuPrP) mice have considerable difficulty converting HuPrP^C into PrP^{Sc} (Telling

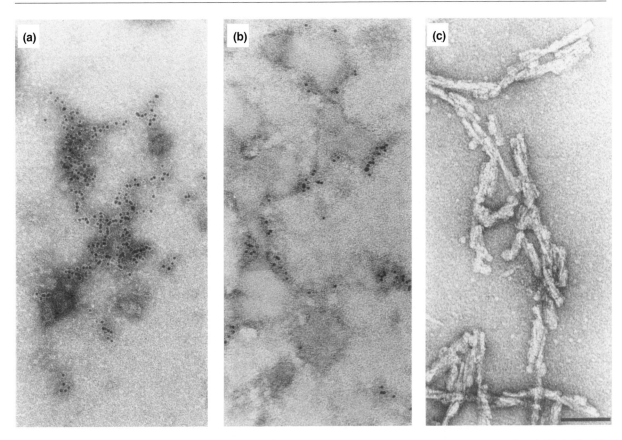

Fig. 39.4 Electron micrographs of negatively stained and immunogold-labelled prion proteins: (a) PrP^C and (b) PrP^{Sc}. (c) Prion rods composed of PrP 27–30 were negatively stained with uranyl acetate. Bar = 100 nm. (Reproduced from Pan et al. 1993.)

et al. 1994). Although MoPrP and HuPrP differ at 28 residues, only 9 or perhaps fewer amino acids in the region between codons 96 and 167 feature in the species barrier in the transmission of Hu prions into mice, as demonstrated by the susceptibility of Tg(MHu2M) mice to Hu prions.

When Tg(HuPrP) mice were crossed with gene targeted mice in which the MoPrP gene had been disrupted (Prnp$^{0/0}$) (Büeler et al. 1992), they were rendered susceptible to Hu prions. These findings suggested that Tg(HuPrP) mice were resistant to Hu prions because MoPrP^C inhibited the conversion of HuPrP^C into PrP^{Sc}; once MoPrP^C was removed by gene ablation, the inhibition was abolished (Telling et al. 1995). Whereas earlier studies argued that PrP^C forms a complex with PrP^{Sc} during the formation of nascent PrP^{Sc} (Prusiner et al. 1990), these findings suggested that PrP^C also binds to another macromolecule during the conversion process. We called this second macromolecule 'protein X' with the proviso that a second binding site on PrP^{Sc} might also function as protein X (Fig. 39.5). Like the binding of PrP^C to PrP^{Sc} which is most efficient when the 2 isoforms have the same sequence (Prusiner et al. 1990), the binding of PrP^C to protein X seems to exhibit the highest affinity when these 2 proteins are from the same species.

1.7   Transgenetics and gene targeting

Ablation of the PrP gene (Prnp$^{0/0}$) affected neither development nor behaviour of the mice (Büeler et al. 1992, Manson et al. 1994a). In fact, Prnp$^{0/0}$ mice have remained healthy for over 2 years. Prnp$^{0/0}$ mice are resistant to prions and do not propagate scrapie infectivity (Büeler et al. 1993, Prusiner

et al. 1993b, Sailer et al. 1994). Prnp$^{0/0}$ mice were sacrificed 5, 60, 120 and 315 days after inoculation with Rocky Mountain Laboratory prions passaged in CD-1 Swiss mice. Except for residual infectivity from the inoculum detected at 5 days after inoculation, no infectivity was detected in the brains of Prnp$^{0/0}$ mice (Table 39.2).

Prnp$^{0/0}$ mice crossed with Tg(SHaPrP) mice were rendered susceptible to SHa prions but remained resistant to Mo prions (Büeler et al. 1993, Prusiner et al. 1993b). Since the absence of PrP^C expression does not provoke disease, it is likely that scrapie and the other prion diseases result not from an inhibition of PrP^C function due to PrP^{Sc} but rather from the accumulation of PrP^{Sc} which interferes with some as yet undefined cellular process.

Mice heterozygous (Prnp$^{+/0}$) for ablation of the PrP gene had prolonged incubation times when inoculated with Mo prions (Fig. 39.6) (Prusiner et al. 1993b, Büeler et al. 1994, Manson et al. 1994b). The Prnp$^{+/0}$ mice developed signs of neurological dysfunction at 400–460 days after inoculation. These findings are in accord with studies on Tg(SHaPrP) mice in which increased SHaPrP expression was accompanied by diminished incubation times (Fig. 39.7b) (Prusiner et al. 1990).

Because Prnp$^{0/0}$ mice do not express PrP^C, we reasoned that they might more readily produce α-PrP antibodies. Prnp$^{0/0}$ mice immunized with Mo or SHa prion rods produced α-PrP antisera that bound Mo, SHa and Hu PrP (Prusiner et al. 1993b). These findings contrast with earlier studies in which α-MoPrP antibodies could not be produced in mice, presumably because the mice had been rendered tolerant by the presence of MoPrP^C (Barry and Prusiner

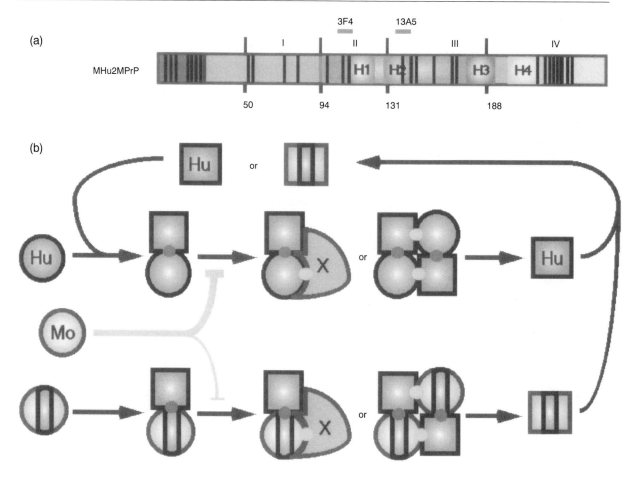

Fig. 39.5 The chimaeric Hu/Mo PrP transgene and a model for the formation of PrP^{Sc}. (a) Schematic representation of the open reading frame (ORF) of the PrP gene, showing the 28 differences between the Hu and Mo PrP (vertical blue lines). The ORF of HuPrP encoded a protein of 253 amino acids, and that of MoPrP 254 residues. The 4 putative α-helical regions of PrP^{C} are designated H1 (red), H2 (green), H3 (light blue) and H4 (yellow). In segments II and III, a DNA fragment from the HuPrP gene (cyan rectangle) was substituted for MoPrP (mauve rectangle). The signal peptide at the N terminus is denoted by the purple rectangle. The signalling sequence at the C terminus, which is removed on addition of the GPI anchor, is denoted by the yellow rectangle. (b) A possible model for the formation of PrP^{Sc}. PrP^{C} is represented by circles and PrP^{Sc} by squares. HuPrP is cyan and MoPrP is mauve. The site for binding of PrP^{Sc} to PrP^{C} is denoted by the orange disk and the site for binding of PrP^{C} to protein X by the yellow disk. When present, MoPrP^{C} inhibits the formation of HuPrP^{Sc} more than it inhibits the production of MHu2MPrP^{Sc} as denoted by the yellow effector lines. An alternative model for the formation of PrP^{Sc} is shown where protein X is PrP^{Sc}. If this is the case, the yellow disk designates the binding of the C terminal domain of PrP^{C} to PrP^{Sc}. Although a tetrameric intermediate is shown, a dimeric intermediate is also possible where the same molecule of PrP^{Sc} binds a molecule of PrP^{C} at 2 sites. See also Plate 39.5.

1986, Kascsak et al. 1987, Rogers et al. 1991). That Prnp$^{0/0}$ mice readily produce α-PrP antibodies is consistent with the hypothesis that the lack of an immune response in prion diseases is due to the fact that PrP^{C} and PrP^{Sc} share many epitopes. Whether Prnp$^{0/0}$ mice produce α-PrP antibodies that specifically recognize conformational dependent epitopes present on PrP^{Sc} but absent from PrP^{C} remains to be determined.

MODELLING OF GSS IN TRANSGENIC MICE

The codon 102 point mutation found in GSS patients was introduced into the MoPrP gene and Tg(MoPrP-P101L)H mice were created expressing high (H) levels of the mutant transgene product. The 2 lines of Tg(MoPrP-P101L)H mice designated 174 and 87 spontaneously developed CNS degeneration, characterized by clinical signs indistinguishable from experimental murine scrapie and neuropathology consisting of widespread spongiform morphology and astro-

cytic gliosis (Hsiao et al. 1990) and PrP amyloid plaques (Fig. 39.8) (Hsiao et al. 1994). By inference, these results indicate that PrP gene mutations cause GSS, familial CJD and FFI.

Brain extracts prepared from spontaneously ill Tg(MoPrP-P101L)H mice transmitted CNS degeneration to Tg196 mice and some Syrian hamsters (Hsiao et al. 1994). The Tg196 mice express low levels of the mutant transgene product and do not develop spontaneous disease. Many Tg196 mice and some Syrian hamsters developed CNS degeneration between 200 and 700 days after inoculation, whereas inoculated CD-1 Swiss mice remained well. Serial transmission of CNS degeneration in Tg196 mice required about one year whereas serial transmission in Syrian hamsters occurred after c. 75 days (Hsiao et al. 1994). Crossing the Tg196 mice with Prnp$^{0/0}$ mice produced recipient Tg196/Prnp$^{0/0}$ mice that developed CNS degeneration in >95% of the inoculated animals in c. 190 days. Serial transmission of CNS degeneration in Tg196/ Prnp$^{0/0}$ mice required c. 220 days whilst serial

Table 39.2   Prion titres in brains of Prnp[0/0] and Prnp[+/0] mice

Mouse	Log scrapie prion titres (ID50 units/ml ± SE)[a] at time of sacrifice after inoculation with RML scrapie prions				
	5 days	60 days	120 days	315 days	500 days
Prnp[+/+]	<1	3.9 ± 0.4	6.4 ± 0.3	...	...
	<1	4.8 ± 0.3	7.1 ± 0.1	...	...
	<1	4.6 ± 0.2	6.6 ± 0.2	...	...
Prnp[+/0]	<1	<1	5.1 ± 0.2	...	...
	0.6 ± 0.7	<1	5.2 ± 0.6	...	...
	1.2 ± 0.1[b]	3.4 ± 0.2	2.8 ± 0.1	...	...
Prnp[0/0]	<1[c]	<1	<1	<1	<1
	<1[d]	<1	<1	<1	<1
	...	<1	...	...	<1
	...	...	...	...	<1

[a]Titres are for 10% (w/v) brain homogenates. Log titres of <1 reflect no signs of CNS dysfunction in CD-1 mice for >250 days after inoculation except as noted.
[b]3 of 9 mice developed scrapie between 208 and 210 days after inoculation.
[c]2 of 9 mice developed scrapie between 208 and 225 days after inoculation.
[d]2 of 10 mice developed scrapie between 208 and 225 days after inoculation.

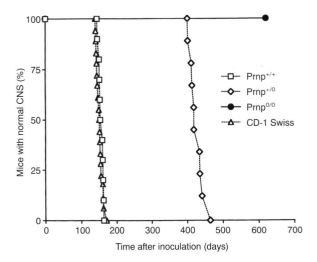

Fig. 39.6   Incubation times in PrP gene ablated Prnp[+/0] and Prnp[0/0] mice as well as wt Prnp[+/+] and CD-1 mice inoculated with RML mouse prions. The RML prions were heated and irradiated at 254 nm prior to intracerebral inoculation into CD-1 Swiss mice (open triangles), Prnp[+/+] mice (open squares), Prnp[+/0] mice (open diamonds) or Prnp[0/0] mice (solid circle).

transmission in Syrian hamsters occurred after c. 75 days (Telling et al. 1996).

Although brain extracts prepared from Tg(MoPrP-P101L)H mice transmitted CNS degeneration to inoculated recipients, little or no PrP[Sc] was detected by immunoassays after limited proteolysis. Undetectable or low levels of PrP[Sc] in the brains of these Tg(MoPrP-P101L)H mice may be due to low titres of infectious prions, the protease sensitivity of MoPrP[Sc] (P101L), or both. Although no PrP[Sc] was detected in the brains of inoculated Tg196 mice exhibiting neurological dysfunction by immunoassays after limited proteolysis, PrP amyloid plaques as well as spongiform degeneration were frequently found. The neurodegeneration in inoculated Tg196 mice seems likely to result from a modification of mutant PrP[C] that is initiated by mutant PrP[Sc] present in the brain extracts prepared from ill Tg(MoPrP-P101L)H mice. In support of this explanation are the findings in some of the inherited human prion diseases as described below (p. 821) where neither protease-resistant PrP (Brown et al. 1992a, Medori et al. 1992a) nor transmission to experimental rodents could be demonstrated (Tateishi et al. 1992). Furthermore, transmission of disease from Tg(MoPrP-P101L)H mice to Tg196 mice but not to Swiss mice is consistent with earlier findings which demonstrate that homotypic interactions between PrP[C] and PrP[Sc] markedly enhance the formation of PrP[Sc]. Why Syrian hamsters are more permissive than Swiss mice for prion transmission from Tg(MoPrP-P101L)H mice is unknown. Presumably, transmission to hamsters reflects the differences in tertiary structure between the 2 substrates SHaPrP[C] and MoPrP[C].

In other studies, modifying the expression of mutant and wtPrP genes in Tg mice permitted experimental manipulation of the pathogenesis of both inherited and infectious prion diseases. Although overexpression of the wtPrP-A transgene c. 8-fold was not deleterious to the mice, it did shorten scrapie incubation times from c. 145 to c. 45 days after inoculation with Mo scrapie prions (Telling et al. 1996). In contrast, overexpression at the same level of a PrP-A transgene mutated at codon 101 produced spontaneous, fatal neurodegeneration at between 150 and 300 days of age in 2 new lines of Tg(MoPrP-P101L) mice designated 2866 and 2247. Genetic crosses of Tg(MoPrP-P101L)2866 mice with gene targeted mice lacking both PrP alleles (Prnp[0/0]) produced animals with a highly synchronous onset of illness at 150–160 days of age. The Tg(MoPrP-P101L)2866/Prnp[0/0] mice had numerous PrP plaques and widespread spongiform degeneration, in contrast to the Tg2866 and 2247 mice that exhibited spongiform degeneration but only a few PrP amyloid plaques. Another line of mice, designated Tg2862, overexpress the mutant transgene c. 32-fold and develop fatal neurodegeneration at between 200 and 400 days of age. Tg2862 mice exhibited the most severe spongiform degeneration and had numerous, large PrP amyloid plaques. Whilst mutant PrP[C](P101L) clearly produces neurodegeneration, wtPrP[C] profoundly modifies both the age of onset of illness and the neuropathology for a given level of transgene

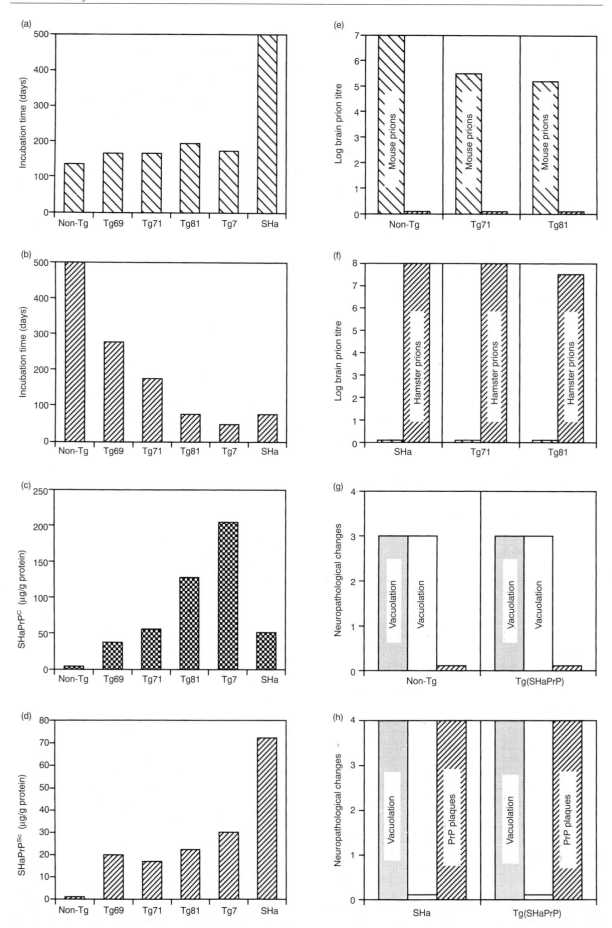

Fig. 39.7 Transgenic (Tg) mice expressing Syrian hamster (SHa) prion protein exhibit species-specific scrapie incubation times, infectious prion synthesis and neuropathology (Prusiner et al. 1990). (a) Scrapie incubation times in non-transgenic mice (Non-Tg) and 4 lines of Tg mice expressing SHaPrP and Syrian hamsters inoculated intracerebrally with c. 10^6 ID50 units of Chandler Mo prions serially passaged in Swiss mice. The 4 lines of Tg mice have different numbers of transgene copies: Tg69 and 71 mice have 2–4 copies of the SHaPrP transgene, whereas Tg81 have 30–50 and Tg7 mice have >60. Incubation times are the number of days from inoculation to onset of neurological dysfunction. (b) Scrapie incubation times in mice and hamsters inoculated with c. 10^7 ID50 units of Sc237 prions serially passaged in Syrian hamsters and as described in (a). (c) Brain SHaPrP^C levels in Tg mice and hamsters. SHaPrP^C levels were quantified by an enzyme-linked immunoassay. (d) Brain SHaPrP^{Sc} in Tg mice and hamsters. Animals were killed after exhibiting clinical signs of scrapie. SHaPrP^{Sc} levels were determined by immunoassay. (e) Prion titres in brains of clinically ill animals after inoculation with Mo prions. Brain extracts from non-Tg, Tg71 and Tg81 mice were bioassayed for prions in mice (left) and hamsters (right). (f) Prion titres in brains of clinically ill animals after inoculation with SHa prions. Brain extracts from Syrian hamsters as well as Tg71 and Tg81 mice were bioassayed for prions in mice (left) and hamsters (right). (g) Neuropathology in non-Tg mice and Tg(SHaPrP) mice with clinical signs of scrapie after inoculation with Mo prions. Vacuolation in grey (left) and white matter (centre); PrP amyloid plaques (right). Vacuolation score: 0 = none; 1 = rare; 2 = modest; 3 = moderate; 4 = intense. (h) Neuropathology in Syrian hamsters and transgenic mice inoculated with SHa prions. Degree of vacuolation and frequency of PrP amyloid plaques as described in (g). (Adapted from Prusiner 1991.)

expression. These findings and those from other studies (Telling et al. 1994) suggest that mutant and wtPrP interact, perhaps through a chaperone-like protein, to modify the pathogenesis of the dominantly inherited prion diseases.

1.8 Prion diversity

The diversity of scrapie prions was first appreciated in goats inoculated with 'hyper' and 'drowsy' isolates (Pattison and Millson 1961b). Scrapie isolates or 'strains' from goats with a drowsy syndrome transmitted a similar syndrome to inoculated recipients; whereas those from goats with a 'hyper' or ataxic syndrome transmitted an ataxic form of scrapie to recipient goats. Subsequently, studies in mice demonstrated the existence of many scrapie 'strains' in which extracts prepared from the brains of mice inoculated with a particular preparation of prions produced a similar disease in inoculated recipients (Dickinson and Fraser 1979, Bruce and Dickinson 1987, Kimberlin, Cole and Walker 1987, Dickinson and Outram 1988). Whilst the clinical signs of scrapie for different prion isolates in mice tended to be similar, the isolates could be distinguished by the incubation times, the distribution of CNS vacuolation that they produced and whether or not amyloid plaques formed.

That such isolates could be propagated through multiple passages in mice suggested that the scrapie pathogen has a nucleic acid genome that is copied and passed on to nascent prions (Dickinson, Meikle and Fraser 1968, Bruce and Dickinson 1987). But no evidence for scrapie-specific nucleic acid encoding information that specifies the incubation time and the distribution of neuropathological lesions has

emerged from considerable efforts using a variety of experimental approaches. In striking contrast, mice expressing PrP transgenes have demonstrated that the level of PrP expression is inversely related to the incubation time (Prusiner et al. 1990). Furthermore, the distribution of CNS vacuolation and attendant gliosis are a consequence of pattern of PrP^{Sc} deposition which can be altered by both PrP genes and non-PrP genes (Prusiner et al. 1990). These observations taken together begin to build an argument for PrP^{Sc} as the informational molecule in which prion 'strain'-specific information is encrypted. Deciphering the mechanism by which PrP^{Sc} carries information for prion diversity and passes it onto the nascent prions is a challenging goal. Whether PrP^{Sc} can adopt multiple conformations, each of which produces prions exhibiting distinct incubation times and patterns of PrP^{Sc} deposition remains to be determined (Cohen et al. 1994).

PRION STRAINS AND VARIATIONS IN PATTERNS OF DISEASE

Scrapie was first transmitted to sheep and goats by intraocular inoculation (Cuillé and Chelle 1939) and later by intracerebral, oral, subcutaneous, intramuscular and intravenous injections of brain extracts from sheep developing scrapie. Incubation periods of 1–3 years were common and often many of the inoculated animals failed to develop disease (Dickinson and Stamp 1969, Hadlow et al. 1980, Hadlow, Kennedy and Race 1982). Different breeds of sheep exhibited markedly different susceptibilities to scrapie prions inoculated subcutaneously, suggesting that the genetic background might influence host permissiveness (Gordon 1966).

The lengths of the incubation times have been used to distinguish prion strains inoculated into sheep, goats, mice and hamsters. Dickinson and his colleagues developed a system for 'strain typing' by which mice with genetically determined short and long incubation times were used in combination with the F1 cross (Dickinson, Meikle and Fraser 1968, Dickinson and Meikle 1971, Dickinson et al. 1984). For example, C57BL mice exhibited short incubation times of c. 150 days when inoculated with either the Me7 or the Chandler isolates; VM mice inoculated with these same isolates had prolonged incubation times of c. 300 days. The mouse gene controlling incubation times was labelled *Sinc* and long incubation times were said to be a dominant trait because of prolonged incubation times in F1 mice. Prion strains were categorized into 2 groups based on their incubation times: (1) those causing disease more rapidly in 'short' incubation time C57BL mice and (2) those causing disease more rapidly in 'long' incubation time VM mice. Noteworthy are the 22a and 87V prion strains that can be passaged in VM mice while maintaining their distinct characteristics.

MOLECULAR BASIS OF PRION STRAINS

The mechanism by which isolate-specific information is carried by prions remains enigmatic; indeed, explaining the molecular basis of prion diversity seems to be a formidable challenge. For many years some investigators argued that scrapie is caused by a virus-like particle containing a scrapie-specific nucleic acid that encodes the information expressed by each isolate (Bruce and Dickinson 1987). To date, no such polynucleotide has been identified, despite using a wide variety of techniques, including measurements of the nucleic acids in purified preparations. An alternative hypothesis has been suggested that PrP^{Sc} alone is capable of transmitting disease but the characteristics

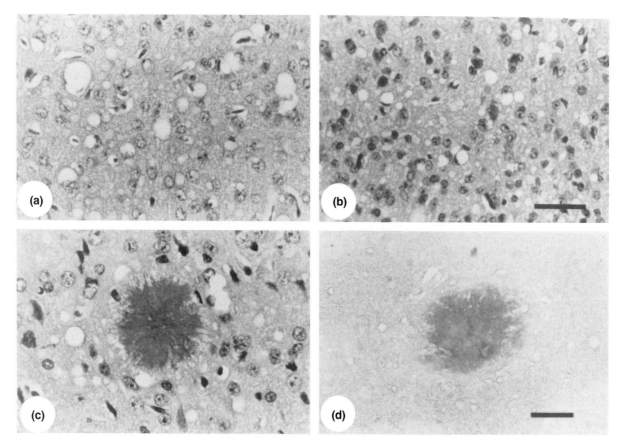

Fig. 39.8 Neuropathology of Tg(MoPrP-P101L) mice developing neurodegeneration spontaneously. The mice harbour transgenes carrying the PrP point mutation found in GSS(P102L) of humans. (a) Vacuolation in cerebral cortex of a Swiss CD-1 mouse that exhibited signs of neurological dysfunction at 138 days after intracerebral inoculation with c. 10^6 ID50 units of RML scrapie prions. (b) Vacuolation in cerebral cortex of a Tg(MoPrP-P101L) mouse that exhibited signs of neurological dysfunction at 252 days of age. (c) Kuru-type PrP amyloid plaque stained with periodic acid–Schiff in the caudate nucleus of a Tg(MoPrP-P101L) mouse that exhibited signs of neurological dysfunction. (d) PrP amyloid plaques stained with α-PrP antiserum (RO73) in the caudate nucleus of a Tg(MoPrP-P101L) mouse that exhibited signs of neurological dysfunction. Bar in B also applies to A = 50 μm. Bar in D also applies to C = 25 μm. (Reproduced from Prusiner 1993.)

of PrP^{Sc} might be modified by a cellular RNA (Weissmann 1991). This accessory cellular RNA is postulated to induce its own synthesis upon transmission from one host to another but there is no experimental evidence to support its existence. In fact, recent studies comparing the resistance of 2 prion strains show that each exhibits the same resistance to inactivation by irradiation at 254 nm (S Prusiner, H Serban and J Cleaver, unpublished data).

Two additional hypotheses not involving a nucleic acid have been offered to explain distinct prion isolates: a non-nucleic acid second component might create prion diversity, or post-translational modification of PrP^{Sc} might be responsible for the different properties of distinct prion isolates (Prusiner 1991). Whether the PrP^{Sc} modification is chemical or only conformational remains to be established, but no candidate chemical modifications have been identified (Stahl et al. 1993). Structural studies of GPI anchors of 2 SHa isolates have failed to reveal any differences; it is interesting that c. 40% of the anchor glycans have sialic acid residues (Stahl et al. 1992). A portion of the PrP^C GPI anchors also have sialic acid residues;

PrP is the first protein found to have sialic acid residues attached to GPI anchors.

Multiple prion isolates might be explained by distinct PrP^{Sc} conformers that act as templates for the folding of *de novo* synthesized PrP^{Sc} molecules during prion 'replication'. Although it is clear that passage history can be responsible for the prolongation of incubation time when prions are passed between mice expressing different PrP allotypes (Carlson et al. 1989) or between species (Prusiner et al. 1990), many scrapie strains show distinct incubation times in the same inbred host (Bruce et al. 1991).

2   CLINICAL AND PATHOLOGICAL ASPECTS OF PRION DISEASES

2.1   Scrapie

EXPERIMENTAL SCRAPIE

For many years, studies of experimental scrapie were performed exclusively with sheep and goats, which required incubation periods of 1–3 years. A crucial methodological advance in experimental studies of scrapie was created by the demonstration that scrapie could be transmitted to mice (Chandler 1961, 1963) which could be used for endpoint titrations of particular samples. In addition, pathogenesis experiments were performed directed at elucidating factors governing incubation times and neuropathological lesions (Eklund, Kennedy and Hadlow 1967, Dickinson, Meikle and Fraser 1968, Fraser and Dickinson 1968).

Natural scrapie in sheep and goats

Even though scrapie was recognized as a distinct disorder of sheep with respect to its clinical manifestations as early as 1738, the disease remained an enigma, even with respect to its pathology, for more than 2 centuries (Parry 1983). Some veterinarians thought that scrapie was a disease of muscle caused by parasites, whilst others thought that it was a dystrophic process (M'Gowan 1914). An investigation into the aetiology of scrapie followed the vaccination of sheep for louping-ill virus with formalin-treated extracts of ovine lymphoid tissue unknowingly contaminated with scrapie prions (Gordon 1946). Two years later, more than 1500 sheep developed scrapie from this vaccine.

Communicability

Scrapie of sheep and goats seems to be unique among the prion diseases in that it seems to be readily communicable within flocks. Although the transmissibility of scrapie seems to be well established, the mechanism of the natural spread of scrapie among sheep is so puzzling that it bears close scrutiny. The placenta has been implicated as one source of prions accounting for the horizontal spread of scrapie within flocks (Pattison and Millson 1961a, Pattison 1964, Pattison et al. 1972, Onodera et al. 1993). Whether this view is correct remains to be established. In Iceland, scrapie-infected flocks of sheep were destroyed and the pastures left vacant for several years; however, reintroduction of sheep from flocks known to be free of scrapie for many years eventually resulted in scrapie (Palsson 1979). The source of the scrapie prions that attacked the sheep from flocks without a history of scrapie is unknown.

Genetics of sheep

Parry argued that host genes were responsible for the development of scrapie in sheep. He was convinced that natural scrapie is a genetic disease which could be eradicated by proper breeding protocols (Parry 1962, 1983). He considered its transmission by inoculation to be of importance primarily for laboratory studies and communicable infection of little consequence in nature. Other investigators viewed natural scrapie as an infectious disease and argued that host genetics only modulates susceptibility to an endemic infectious agent (Dickinson et al. 1965). The incubation time gene for experimental scrapie in Cheviot sheep, called *Sip*, is said to be linked to a PrP gene (Hunter et al. 1989); however, the null hypothesis of non-linkage has yet to be tested and this is important, especially in view of earlier studies which argue that susceptibility of sheep to scrapie is governed by a recessive gene (Parry 1962, 1983).

Polymorphisms at codons 136 and 171 of the PrP gene in sheep that produce amino acid substitutions have been studied with respect to the occurrence of scrapie in sheep (Clousard et al. 1995). In Romanov and Ile-de-France breeds of sheep, a polymorphism in the PrP ORF was found at codon 136 (A→V) which seems to correlate with scrapie (Laplanche et al. 1993b). Sheep homozygous or heterozygous for Val at codon 136 were susceptible to scrapie whereas those that were homozygous for Ala were resistant. Unexpectedly, only one of 74 scrapied autochthonous sheep had a Val at codon 136; these sheep were from 3 breeds denoted Lacaune, Manech and Presalpes (Laplanche et al. 1993a).

In Suffolk sheep, a polymorphism in the PrP ORF was found at codon 171 (Q→R) (Goldmann et al. 1990a, 1990b). Studies of natural scrapie in the USA have shown that c. 85% of the afflicted sheep are of the Suffolk breed. Only those Suffolk sheep homozygous for Gln (Q) at codon 171 had scrapie although healthy controls with QQ, QR and RR genotypes were found (Westaway et al. 1994c). These results argue that susceptibility in Suffolk sheep is governed by the PrP codon 171 polymorphism. Whether the PrP codon 171 or 136 polymorphisms in Cheviot sheep have the same profound influence on susceptibility to scrapie as has been found for codon 171 in Suffolks is unknown (Goldmann et al. 1991a, Hunter et al. 1991).

2.2 Bovine spongiform encephalopathy

Epidemic of 'mad cow' disease

In 1986 an epidemic of a previously unknown disease appeared in cattle in Great Britain (Wells et al. 1987). This disease was initially named bovine spongiform encephalopathy (BSE) but is frequently called 'mad cow' disease. BSE was shown to be a prion disease by demonstrating protease-resistant PrP in brains of ill cattle (Hope et al. 1988, Prusiner et al. 1993a). Based mainly on epidemiological evidence, it has been proposed that BSE represents a massive common source epidemic which has caused more than 160 000 cases to date. In Britain, cattle, particularly dairy cows, were routinely fed meat and bone meal (MBM) as a nutritional supplement (Dealler and Lacey 1990, Wilesmith and Wells 1991, Wilesmith et al. 1988, 1992a, 1992b). The MBM was prepared by rendering the offal of sheep and cattle using a process that involved steam treatment and hydrocarbon solvent extraction. The extraction process produced a protein and fat rich fractions; the protein or greaves fraction contained about 1% fat from which the MBM was prepared. In the late 1970s, the price of tallow prepared from the fat fraction fell, making it no longer profitable to use hydrocarbons in the rendering process. The resulting MBM contained about 14% fat and it is postulated that the high lipid content protected scrapie prions in the sheep offal from being completely inactivated by steam.

Since 1988, the practice of using dietary protein supplements for domestic animals derived from rendered sheep or cattle offal has been forbidden in the UK. Curiously, almost half of the BSE cases have occurred in herds where only a single affected animal has been found; several cases of BSE in a single herd are infrequent (Wilesmith et al. 1988, Dealler and Lacey 1990, Wilesmith and Wells 1991). In 1992, the

BSE epidemic reached a peak, with over 35 000 cattle afflicted (Fig. 39.9). In 1993, fewer than 32 000 cattle were diagnosed with BSE and in 1994 the number was c. 22 000. The 1994 statistics argue that the epidemic is now under control as a result of the 1988 food ban.

Crossing a species barrier

Assuming the above postulate is correct, only sheep prions were present initially in the contaminated MBM. Because the species barrier depends, at least in part, on the amino acid sequences of PrP in the donor host and recipient, the similarity between bovine and sheep PrP was probably an important factor in initiating the BSE epidemic. Bovine PrP differs from sheep PrP at 7 or 8 residues, depending on the breed of sheep (Goldmann et al. 1991b, Prusiner et al. 1993a). As the BSE epidemic expanded, infected bovine offal began to be rendered into MBM that contained bovine prions.

Transmission of BSE to experimental animals

Brain extracts from BSE cattle have transmitted disease to mice, cattle, sheep and pigs after intracerebral inoculation (Fraser et al. 1988, Dawson, Wells and Parker 1990, Dawson et al. 1990, Bruce et al. 1993). Transmissions to mice and sheep suggest that cattle preferentially propagate a single 'strain' of prions. Seven BSE brains all produced similar incubation times as measured in each of 3 strains of inbred mice (Bruce et al. 1993).

Of particular importance to the BSE epidemic is the recent transmission of BSE to the non-human primate marmoset after intracerebral inoculation followed by a prolonged incubation period (Baker, Ridley and Wells 1993). The potential parallels with kuru of humans, confined to the Fore region of New Guinea (Gajdusek, Gibbs and Alpers 1966, Gajdusek 1977), are worthy of consideration. Once the most common cause of death among women and children in that region, kuru has almost disappeared with the cessation of ritualistic

cannibalism (Alpers 1987). Although it seems likely that kuru was transmitted orally, as proposed for BSE among cattle, some investigators argue that other routes of transmission were important because oral transmission of kuru prions to apes and monkeys has been difficult to demonstrate (Gajdusek 1977, Gibbs et al. 1980).

There is no example of zoonotic transmission of prions from animals to humans based on many epidemiological studies that have attempted to implicate scrapie prions from sheep as a cause of CJD (Malmgren et al. 1979, Harries-Jones et al. 1988, Cousens et al. 1990). Whether BSE poses any risk to humans is unknown, but 5 teenagers and 10 young adults in Britain and France have died of atypical CJD during 1995 and 1996 (Anonymous 1993a, 1993b, Sawcer et al. 1993, Chazot et al. 1996, Will et al. 1996).

Oral transmission of BSE prions

Besides BSE, 4 other animal diseases seem to have arisen from the oral consumption of prions. It has been suggested that an outbreak of transmissible mink encephalopathy in 1985 arose from the use for feed of a cow with a sporadic case of BSE (Marsh et al. 1991). The source of prions in chronic wasting disease of captive mule, deer and elk is unclear (Williams and Young 1980, 1982). The prion-contaminated MBM thought to be the cause of BSE is also hypothesized to be the cause of feline spongiform encephalopathy (FSE) and exotic ungulate encephalopathy. FSE has been found in almost 30 domestic cats in Great Britain as well as in a puma and a cheetah (Willoughby et al. 1992). Three cases of FSE in domestic cats have been transmitted to laboratory mice and PrP^{Sc} has been identified in their brains by immunoblotting (Pearson et al. 1992). Prion disease has been found in the brains of the nyala, greater kudu, eland, gembok and Arabian oryx in British zoos; all of these animals are exotic ungulates. Of 8 greater kudu born into a herd maintained in a London zoo since 1987, 5 have developed prion disease. Except for the first case, none of the other 4 kudu was exposed to feeds containing ruminant-derived MBM (Kirkwood et al. 1993). Brain extracts prepared from a nyala and a greater kudu have been transmitted to mice (Kirkwood et al. 1990, Cunningham et al. 1993). PrP of the greater kudu differs from the bovine protein at 4 residues; Arabian oryx PrP differs from the sheep PrP at only one residue (Poidinger, Kirkwood and Almond 1993).

2.3 Human prion diseases

The human prion diseases are manifest as infectious, inherited and sporadic disorders, and are often referred to as kuru, CJD, GSS and FFI, depending upon the clinical and neuropathological findings (see Table 39.1).

Diagnosis of human prion diseases

Human prion disease should be considered in any patient who develops a progressive subacute or

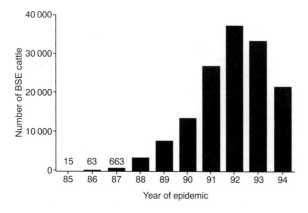

Fig. 39.9 Annual incidence of bovine spongiform encephalopathy in Great Britain. All cases were confirmed clinically and neuropathologically. (Statistics compiled by John Wilesmith of the Central Veterinary Laboratory at Weybridge, England.)

chronic decline in cognitive or motor function. Typically adults between 40 and 70 years of age, patients often exhibit clinical features helpful in providing a premorbid diagnosis of prion disease, particularly sporadic CJD (Roos, Gajdusek and Gibbs 1973, Brown et al. 1986a). There is as yet no specific diagnostic test for prion disease in the cerebrospinal fluid. A definitive diagnosis of human prion disease, which is invariably fatal, can often be made from the examination of brain tissue. Since 1992, knowledge of the molecular genetics of prion diseases has made it possible, using peripheral tissues, to diagnose inherited prion disease in living patients.

A broad spectrum of neuropathological features in human prion diseases precludes a precise neuropathological definition. The classic neuropathological features of human prion disease include spongiform degeneration, gliosis, and neuronal loss in the absence of an inflammatory reaction. When present, amyloid plaques that stain with α-PrP antibodies are diagnostic.

The presence of protease-resistant PrP (PrP^{Sc} or PrP^{CJD}) in the infectious and sporadic forms and most of the inherited forms of these diseases implicates prions in their pathogenesis. The absence of PrP^{CJD} in a biopsy specimen may simply reflect regional variations in the concentration of the protein (Serban et al. 1990). In some patients with inherited prion disease, PrP^{Sc} is barely detectable or undetectable (Little et al. 1986, Brown et al. 1992b, Manetto et al. 1992, Medori et al. 1992a); this situation seems to be mimicked in transgenic mice that express a mutant PrP gene and spontaneously develop neurological illness indistinguishable from experimental murine scrapie (Hsiao et al. 1990, 1994).

In humans and Tg mice that have no detectable protease-resistant PrP but express mutant PrP, neurodegeneration may, at least in part, be caused by abnormal metabolism of mutant PrP. Because molecular genetic analyses of PrP genes in patients with unusual dementing illnesses are readily performed, the diagnosis of inherited prion disease can often be established where there was little or no neuropathology (Collinge et al. 1990), atypical neurodegenerative disease (Medori et al. 1992a) or misdiagnosed neurodegenerative disease (Heston, Lowther and Leventhal 1966, Azzarelli et al. 1985), including Alzheimer's disease.

Although horizontal transmission of neurodegeneration to experimental hosts was for a time the 'gold standard' of prion disease, it can no longer be used as such. Some investigators have reported that transmission of the inherited prion diseases from humans to experimental animals is frequently negative when using rodents, despite the presence of a pathogenic mutation in the PrP gene (Tateishi et al. 1992), whilst others state that this is not the case with apes and monkeys as hosts (Brown et al. 1993). The discovery that Tg(MHu2M) mice are susceptible to Hu prions (Telling et al. 1994) promises to make feasible transmission studies that were not practical in apes and monkeys (Brown et al. 1994b).

The hallmark common to all of the prion diseases, whether sporadic, dominantly inherited or acquired by infection, is that they involve the aberrant metabolism of the prion protein (Prusiner 1991). Making a definitive diagnosis of human prion disease can be rapidly accomplished if PrP^{Sc} can be detected immunologically. PrP^{Sc} can often be detected by either dot-blot method or Western immunoblot analysis of brain homogenates in which samples are subjected to limited proteolysis to remove PrP^{C} before immunostaining (Bockman et al. 1985, 1987, Brown et al. 1986b, Serban et al. 1990). The dot-blot method exploits enhancement of PrP^{Sc} immunoreactivity following denaturation in the chaotropic salt, guanidinium chloride. Because of regional variations in PrP^{Sc} concentration, methods using homogenates prepared from small brain regions can give false negative results. Alternatively, PrP^{Sc} may be detected in situ in cryostat sections bound to nitrocellulose membranes followed by limited proteolysis to remove PrP^{C} and guanidinium treatment to denature PrP^{Sc}, and thus enhance its avidity for α-PrP antibodies (Taraboulos et al. 1992a). Denaturation of PrP^{Sc} in situ prior to immunostaining has also been accomplished by autoclaving fixed tissue sections (Kitamoto et al. 1992).

In the familial forms of the prion diseases, molecular genetic analyses of PrP can be diagnostic and can be performed on DNA extracted from blood leucocytes *ante mortem*. Unfortunately, such testing is of little value in the diagnosis of the sporadic or infectious forms of prion disease. Although the first missense PrP mutation was discovered when the 2 PrP alleles of a patient with GSS were cloned from a genomic library and sequenced (Hsiao et al. 1989), all subsequent novel missense and insertional mutations have been identified in PrP ORFs amplified by polymerase chain reaction (PCR) and sequenced. The 759 base pairs encoding the 253 amino acids of PrP reside in a single exon of the PrP gene, providing an ideal situation for the use of PCR. Amplified PrP ORFs can be screened for known mutations using one of several methods, the most reliable of which is allele-specific oligonucleotide hybridization. If known mutations are absent, novel mutations may be found when the PrP ORF is sequenced.

When PrP amyloid plaques in brain are present, they are diagnostic for prion disease as noted above (see p. 813). Unfortunately, they are thought to be present in only c. 10% of CJD cases but, by definition, in all cases of GSS. The amyloid plaques in CJD are compact (kuru plaques). Those in GSS are either multicentric (diffuse) or compact. The amyloid plaques in prion diseases contain PrP (Kitamoto et al. 1986, Roberts et al. 1986, 1988). The multicentric amyloid plaques that are pathognomonic for GSS may be difficult to distinguish from the neuritic plaques of Alzheimer's disease except by immunohistology (Ghetti et al. 1989, Nochlin et al. 1989, Ikeda et al. 1991). In the GSS kindreds the diagnosis of Alzheimer's disease was excluded because the amyloid plaques failed to stain with β-amyloid antiserum but stained with PrP antiserum. In subsequent studies, missense mutations were found in the PrP genes of these kindreds.

In summary, the diagnosis of prion or prion protein disease may be made in patients on the basis of (1) the presence of PrP^{Sc}, (2) mutant PrP genotype or (3) appropriate immunohistology, and should not be excluded in patients with atypical neurodegenerative diseases until one or preferably 2 of these examinations have been performed.

2.4 Infectious prion diseases

IATROGENIC CREUTZFELDT–JAKOB DISEASE

Accidental transmission of CJD to humans seems to have occurred by corneal transplantation (Duffy et al. 1974), contaminated EEG electrode implantation (Bernouilli et al. 1977) and surgical operations using contaminated instruments or apparatus (Table 39.3) (Masters and Richardson 1978, Kondo and Kuroina 1981, Will and Matthews 1982, Davanipour et al. 1984). A cornea unknowingly removed from a donor with CJD was transplanted to an apparently healthy recipient who developed CJD after a prolonged incubation period. Corneas of animals have significant levels of prions (Buyukmihci, Rorvik and Marsh 1980), making this situation seem quite probable. The same improperly decontaminated EEG electrodes that caused CJD in 2 young patients with intractable epilepsy caused CJD in a chimpanzee 18 months after their experimental implantation (Bernouilli et al. 1979, Gibbs et al. 1994).

Surgical procedures may have resulted in accidental inoculation of patients with prions during their operations (Gajdusek 1977, Will and Matthews 1982, Brown, Preece and Will 1992), presumably because some instrument or apparatus in the operating theatre became contaminated when a CJD patient underwent surgery. Although the epidemiology of these studies is highly suggestive, no proof for such episodes exists.

Since 1988, 11 cases have been recorded of CJD after implantation of dura mater grafts (Otto 1987, Thadani et al. 1988, Masullo et al. 1989, Nisbet, Mac-Donaldson and Bishara 1989, Miyashita et al. 1991, Willison, Gale and McLaughlin 1991, Brown, Preece and Will 1992, Martínez-Lage et al. 1993). All of the grafts were thought to have been acquired from a single manufacturer whose preparative procedures were inadequate to inactivate human prions (Brown, Preece and Will 1992). One case of CJD occurred after repair of an eardrum perforation with a pericardium graft (Tange, Troost and Limburg 1989).

Thirty cases of CJD in physicians and healthcare workers have been reported (Berger, David 1993); however, no occupational link has been established (Ridley and Baker 1993). Whether any of these cases represents infectious prion diseases contracted during care of patients with CJD or processing specimens from these patients remains uncertain.

HUMAN GROWTH HORMONE THERAPY

The possibility of transmission of CJD from contaminated human grown hormone (HGH) preparations

Table 39.3 Infectious prion diseases of humans

Diseases	No. of cases
Kuru (1957–1982)	
Adult females	1739
Adult males	248
Children and adolescents	597
Total	2584
Iatrogenic Creutzfeldt–Jakob disease	
Depth electrodes	2
Corneal transplants	1
Human pituitary growth hormone	55
Human pituitary gonadotropin	5
Dura mater grafts	11
Neurosurgical procedures	4
Total	78

References are cited in the text (p. 820).

derived from human pituitaries has been raised by the occurrence of fatal cerebellar disorders with dementia in >55 patients ranging in age from 10 to 41 years (see Table 39.3) (Brown 1985, Buchanan, Preece and Milner 1991, Fradkin et al. 1991, Brown et al. 1992). Although one case of spontaneous CJD in a 20 year old woman has been reported (Packer et al. 1980, Brown 1985, Gibbs et al. 1985), CJD in people under 40 years of age is very rare. These patients received injections of HGH every 2–4 days for 4–12 years (Gibbs et al. 1985, Koch et al. 1985, Powell-Jackson et al. 1985, Titner et al. 1986, Croxson et al. 1988, Marzewski et al. 1988, New et al. 1988, Anderson, Allen and Weller 1990, Billette de Villemeur et al. 1991, Macario et al. 1991, Ellis, Katifi and Weller 1992). It is interesting that most of the patients presented with cerebellar syndromes that progressed over periods varying from 6 to 18 months. Some patients became demented during the terminal phases of their illnesses. This clinical course resembles kuru more than ataxic CJD in some respects (Prusiner, Gajdusek and Alpers 1982). Assuming that these patients developed CJD from injections of prion-contaminated HGH preparations, the possible incubation periods range from 4 to 30 years (Brown, Preece and Will 1992). The longest incubation periods are similar to those (20–30 years) associated with recent cases of kuru (Gajdusek et al. 1977, Prusiner, Gajdusek and Alpers 1982, Klitzman, Alpers and Gajdusek 1984). Many patients received several common lots of HGH at various times during their prolonged therapies, but no single lot was administered to all the American patients. An aliquot of one lot of HGH has been reported to transmit CNS disease to a squirrel monkey after a prolonged incubation period (Gibbs et al. 1993). How many lots of the HGH might have been contaminated with prions is unknown.

Although CJD is a rare disease with an annual incidence of approximately one per million population (Masters and Richardson 1978), it is reasonable to assume that CJD is present with a proportional frequency among dead people. About 1% of the population dies each year and most CJD patients die within one year of developing symptoms. Thus, we estimate that one per 10^4 dead people have CJD. Since 10 000 human pituitaries were typically processed in a single HGH preparation, the possibility of hormone preparations contaminated with CJD prions is not remote (Brown et al. 1985, 1994a, Brown 1988).

The concentration of CJD prions within infected human pituitaries is unknown; it is interesting that widespread degenerative changes have been observed in both the hypothalamus and pituitary of sheep with scrapie (Beck, Daniel and Parry 1964). The forebrains from scrapie-infected mice have been added to human pituitary suspensions to determine if prions and HGH co-purify (Lumley Jones et al. 1979). Bioassays in mice suggest that prions and HGH do not co-purify with currently used protocols (Taylor et al. 1985). Although these results seem reassuring, the relatively low titre of the murine scrapie prions used in these studies may not have provided an adequate test

(Brown 1985). The extremely small size and charge heterogeneity exhibited by scrapie (Alper, Haig and Clarke 1966, Prusiner et al. 1978, 1980b, 1983, Bolton, Meyer and Prusiner 1985) and presumably CJD prions (Bendheim et al. 1985, Bockman et al. 1985) may complicate procedures designed to separate pituitary hormones from these slow infectious pathogens. Even though additional investigations argue for the efficacy of inactivating prions in HGH fractions prepared from human pituitaries using 6 M urea (Pocchiari et al. 1991), it seems doubtful that such protocols will be used for purifying HGH, because recombinant HGH is available.

Molecular genetic studies have revealed that most patients developing iatrogenic CJD after receiving pituitary-derived HGH are homozygous for either Met or Val at codon 129 of the PrP gene (Collinge, Palmer and Dryden 1991, Brown et al. 1994a, Deslys, Marcé and Dormont 1994). Homozygosity at the codon 129 polymorphism has also been shown to predispose individuals to sporadic CJD (Palmer et al. 1991). It is interesting that valine homozygosity seems to be over-represented in these HGH cases compared to the general population.

Five cases of CJD have occurred in women receiving human pituitary gonadotropin (Cochius et al. 1990, Cochius, Hyman and Esiri 1992, Healy and Evans 1993).

2.5 Inherited prion diseases

FAMILIAL PRION DISEASE

The recognition that c. 10% of CJD cases are familial (Kirschbaum 1924, Meggendorfer 1930, Stender 1930, Davison and Rabiner 1940, Jacob, Pyrkosch and Strube 1950, Friede and DeJong 1964, Rosenthal et al. 1976, Masters et al. 1979, 1981a, Masters, Gajdusek and Gibbs 1981b) posed a perplexing problem once it was established that CJD is transmissible (Gibbs et al. 1968, Gibbs and Gajdusek 1969). Equally puzzling was the transmission of GSS to non-human primates (Gibbs et al. 1968, Gibbs and Gajdusek 1969, Masters et al. 1981a) and mice (Tateishi et al. 1979), because most cases of GSS are familial (Gerstmann, Sträussler and Scheinker 1936). Like sheep scrapie, the relative contributions of genetic and infectious aetiologies in the human prion diseases remained a conundrum until molecular clones of the PrP gene became available to probe the inherited aspects of these disorders.

PrP MUTATIONS AND GENETIC LINKAGE

The discovery of the PrP gene and its linkage to scrapie incubation times in mice (Carlson et al. 1986) raised the possibility that mutation might feature in the hereditary human prion diseases. A proline (P)→leucine (L) mutation at codon 102 was shown to be linked genetically to development of GSS with a logarithm of odds (LOD) score exceeding 3 (Fig. 39.10) (Hsiao et al. 1989). This mutation may be due to the deamination of a methylated CpG in a germline PrP gene resulting in the substitution of a thymine (T) for cytosine (C). The P102L mutation has

been found in 10 different families in 9 different countries, including the original GSS family (Doh-ura et al. 1989, Goldgaber et al. 1989, Kretzschmar et al. 1991, Kretzschmar et al. 1992, Goldhammer et al. 1993). Amyloid plaques isolated from patients with GSS (P102L) were composed of PrP molecules with an L at residue 102 based on protein sequencing of purified peptides (Kitamoto et al. 1991). Patients with GSS who have a P→L substitution at PrP codon 105 have also been reported (Kitamoto et al. 1993).

Some patients with a mutation at codon 117 have a dementing or telencephalic form of GSS (Doh-ura et al. 1989, Hsiao et al. 1991b) whereas others have an ataxic form of the disease (Mastrianni et al. 1995). In both forms of GSS (A117V), PrP amyloid plaques were found as well as spongiform degeneration. The factor or factors that determine the different phenotypes of this disease are unknown.

Patients with PrP mutations at codons 198 and 217 (Hsiao et al. 1992) were once thought to have familial Alzheimer's disease, but are now known to have prion diseases on the basis of PrP immunostaining of amyloid plaques and PrP gene mutations (Farlow et al. 1989, Ghetti et al. 1989, Nochlin et al. 1989, Giaccone et al. 1990). A genetic linkage study of this family produced a LOD score exceeding 6 (Dlouhy et al. 1992). Patients with the codon 198 mutation resulting in a phenylalanine (F)→serine (S) substitution (Hsiao et al. 1992) have numerous neurofibrillary tangles (NFT) that stain with antibodies to tau (τ) protein and have amyloid plaques (Farlow et al. 1989, Ghetti et al. 1989, Nochlin et al. 1989, Giaccone et al. 1990) that are composed largely of a PrP fragment extending from residues 58 to 150 (Tagliavini et al. 1991). Because the F198S mutation is not contained within the major PrP peptide of the amyloid plaques, patients heterozygous at codon 129 were chosen to determine whether this peptide is derived from the mutant protein. Like the results of studies with GSS (P102L) (Kitamoto et al. 1991) and GSS (Y145Stop) (Kitamoto, Iizuka and Tateishi 1993), protein sequencing revealed that the PrP peptides are derived exclusively from the mutant protein (Tagliavini et al. 1994). Similar results were found with PrP peptides from a patient of Swedish ancestry with the codon 217 mutation resulting in a glutamine (Q)→arginine (R) substitution (Hsiao et al. 1992). The neuropathology of patients with the codon 217 mutation was similar to that of patients with the codon198 mutation (Ikeda et al. 1991).

One patient with a prolonged neurological illness spanning almost 2 decades who had PrP amyloid plaques and NFTs had an amber mutation of the PrP gene resulting in a stop codon at residue 145 (Kitamoto et al. 1993, Kitamoto and Tateishi 1994). Staining of the plaques with α-PrP peptide antisera suggested that they might be composed exclusively of the truncated PrP molecules. That a PrP peptide ending at residue 145 polymerizes into amyloid filaments is to be expected since an earlier study noted above showed that the major PrP peptide in plaques from patients with the F198S mutation was an 11 kDa PrP peptide beginning at codon 58 and ending at c. 150 (Tagliavini et al. 1991). A synthetic PrP peptide containing residues 90–145 was found to adopt an α-helical or β-sheet structure depending on the solvent as determined by 2-dimensional magnetic resonance imaging, FTIR spectroscopy and fibre diffraction (Nguyen et al. 1995, Zhang et al. 1995).

An insert of 144 bp at codon 53 containing 6 octarepeats has been described in patients with CJD from 4 families all

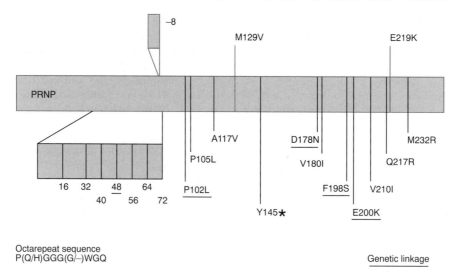

Fig. 39.10 Human prion protein gene (PRNP). The open reading frame (ORF) is denoted by the large grey rectangle. Human PRNP wild type coding polymorphisms are shown above the rectangle, and mutations that segregate with the inherited prion diseases are depicted below. The wild type human PrP gene contains 5 octarepeats [P(Q/H)GGG(G/–) WGQ] from codons 51–91 (Kretzschmar et al. 1986b). Deletion of a single octarepeat at codon 81 or 82 is not associated with prion disease (Laplanche et al. 1990, Puckett et al. 1991, Vnencak-Jones and Phillips 1992); whether this deletion alters the phenotypic characteristics of a prion disease is unknown. There are common polymorphisms at codons 117 (Ala→Ala) and 129 (Met→Val); homozygosity for Met or Val at codon 129 seems to increase susceptibility to sporadic CJD (Palmer et al. 1991). Octarepeat inserts of 16, 32, 40, 48, 56, 64 and 72 amino acids at codons 67, 75 or 83 are designated by the small rectangle below the ORF. Point mutations are designated by the wild type amino acid preceding the codon number and the mutant residue follows; e.g. P102L. These point mutations segregate with the inherited prion diseases and significant genetic linkage (underlined mutations) has been demonstrated where sufficient specimens from family members are available. The single letter code for amino acids is as follows: A, Ala; D, Asp; E, Glu; F, Phe; I, Ile; K, Lys; L, Leu; M, Met; N, Asn; P, Pro; Q, Gln; R, Arg; S, Ser; T, Thr; V, Val; and Y, Tyr.

residing in southern England (Fig. 39.10) (Crow et al. 1990, Owen et al. 1989, 1990b, 1991, Collinge et al. 1992, Poulter et al. 1992). This mutation must have arisen through a complex series of events, because the human PrP gene contains only 5 octarepeats, indicating that a single recombination event could not have created the insert. Genealogical investigations have revealed that all 4 families are related, arguing for a single founder born more than 2 centuries ago (Crow et al. 1990). The LOD score for this extended pedigree exceeds 11. Studies from several laboratories have demonstrated that 2, 4, 5, 6, 7, 8 or 9 octarepeats in addition to the normal 5 are present in individuals with inherited CJD (Owen et al. 1989, 1990b, 1992, Goldfarb et al. 1991a, Brown 1993), whereas deletion of one octarepeat has been identified without the neurological disease (Laplanche et al. 1990, Vnencak-Jones and Phillips 1992, Palmer et al. 1993).

For many years the unusually high incidence of CJD among Israeli Jews of Libyan origin was thought to be due to the consumption of lightly cooked sheep brain or eyeballs (Herzberg et al. 1974, Kahana et al. 1974, Kahana, Zilber and Abraham 1991). Recent studies have shown that some Libyan and Tunisian Jews in families with CJD have a PrP gene point mutation at codon 200 resulting in a glutamate (E)→lysine (K) substitution (Goldfarb et al. 1990c, Gabizon et al. 1991, Hsiao et al. 1991a). One patient was homozygous for the E200K mutation but her clinical presentation was similar to that of heterozygotes (Hsiao et al. 1991a), arguing that familial prion diseases are true autosomal dominant disorders. The E200K mutation has also been found in Slovaks originating from Orava in north central Czechoslovakia (Goldfarb et al. 1990c), in a cluster of familial cases in Chile (Goldfarb et al. 1991b) and in a large German family living in the USA (Bertoni et al. 1992). It is likely that the E200K

mutation has arisen independently multiple times by the deamidation of a methylated CpG as described above the codon 102 mutation (Hsiao et al. 1989, 1991a). In support of this hypothesis are records of Libyan and Tunisian Jews, indicating that they are descendants of Jews who settled on the island of Jerba off the southern coast of Tunisia around 500 BC and not from Sephardim (Udovitch and Valensi 1984). Although genetic linkage was established for the P102L mutation (Hsiao et al. 1989), some investigators continued to hold the view that an environmental co-factor was necessary and that mutant PrP genes render individuals susceptible to the ubiquitous 'scrapie virus' (Aiken and Marsh 1990, Kimberlin 1990, Chesebro 1992). This 'virus' also provided an explanation for what was mistakenly interpreted as incomplete penetrance of the codon 200 mutation in familial CJD (Goldfarb et al. 1990a, 1991b, Gajdusek 1992). From life-table analyses, we now recognize that, if carriers with the codon 200 mutation live long enough, they eventually develop prion disease (Fig. 39.11) (Chapman et al. 1994, Spudich et al. 1995).

Many families with CJD have been found to have a point mutation at codon 178, resulting in an aspartate (D)→asparagine (N) substitution (Fink et al. 1991, Goldfarb et al. 1991c, 1992a, Haltia et al. 1991, Brown et al. 1992a). In these patients as well as those with the E200K mutation, PrP amyloid plaques are rare; the neuropathological changes generally consist of widespread spongiform degeneration. Recently a new prion disease called fatal familial insomnia (FFI), which presents with insomnia, was described in 3 Italian families with the D178N mutation (Lugaresi et al. 1986, Medori et al. 1992a). The neuropathology in these patients with FFI is restricted to selected nuclei of the thalamus. It is unclear whether all patients with the D178N mutation or

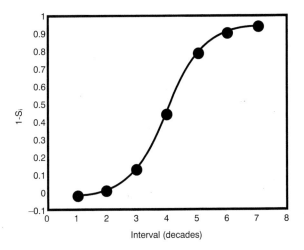

Fig. 39.11 Cumulative probability of developing CJD (1-S_i) as a function of age in the PrP-E200K carriers. Intervals are the ages of the carriers in decades.

only a subset present with sleep disturbances. It has been proposed that the allele with the D178N mutation encodes an M at position 129 in FFI whereas a V is encoded at position 129 in familial CJD (Goldfarb et al. 1992b). The discovery that FFI is an inherited prion disease clearly widens the clinical spectrum of these disorders and raises the possibility that many other degenerative diseases of unknown aetiology may be caused by prions (Johnson 1992, Medori et al. 1992a). The D178N mutation has been linked to the development of prion disease with a LOD score exceeding 5 (Petersen et al. 1992). Studies of PrPSc in FFI and familial CJD caused by the D178N mutation reveal that, after limited proteolysis, the molecular weight of the FFI PrPSc is c. 2 kDa smaller (Monari et al. 1994). Whether this difference in protease resistance reflects distinct conformations of PrPSc that give rise to the different clinical and neuropathological manifestations of these inherited prion diseases remains to be established.

A valine (V)→isoleucine (I) mutation at PrP codon 210 produces CJD with classic symptoms and signs (Pocchiari et al. 1993, Ripoll et al. 1993). The V210I mutation is thought to be incompletely penetrant, like the E200K mutation was previously thought to be (Chapman et al. 1994, Spudich et al. 1995). It seems likely that, if a sufficiently large number of people with the V210I mutation could be analysed, complete penetrance that is age-dependent would be found.

Other point mutations at codons 208 and, possibly, 232 also segregate with inherited prion diseases (Kitamoto et al. 1993, Kitamoto and Tateishi 1994, Mastrianni et al. 1995). The codon 208 mutation results in the substitution of arginine (R) for histidine (H). A patient with this mutation presented with a progressive dementia and widespread myoclonus was subsequently observed. The diagnosis of CJD was confirmed at autopsy. Patients with the codon 232 mutation present with dementia; this mutation is particularly notable, because it lies within the C-terminal signal sequence that is removed from PrP when the GPI anchor is attached (Stahl et al. 1992).

2.6 PrP gene polymorphisms

POLYMORPHISMS AT CODONS 129 AND 219

At PrP codon 129, an amino acid polymorphism for the M→V has been identified (see Fig. 39.10) (Owen

et al. 1990a). This polymorphism seems able to influence prion disease expression, not only in inherited forms but also in iatrogenic and sporadic forms of prion disease. A second polymorphism resulting in an amino acid substitution at codon 219 (E→K) has been reported in the Japanese population, in which the K allele occurs with a frequency of 6% (Kitamoto and Tateishi 1994).

DOES HOMOZYGOSITY AT CODON 129 PREDISPOSE TO CJD?

Studies of caucasian patients with sporadic CJD have shown that most are homozygous for M or V at codon 129 (Palmer et al. 1991). This contrasts with the general population, in which frequencies for the codon 129 polymorphism in caucasians are 12% V/V, 37% M/M and 51% M/V (Collinge et al. 1991). In contrast, the frequency of the V allele in the Japanese population is much lower (Doh-ura et al. 1991, Miyazono et al. 1992) and heterozygosity at codon 129 (M/V) is more frequent (18%) in CJD patients than the general population, in whom the polymorphism frequencies are 0% V/V, 92% M/M and 8% M/V (Tateishi and Kitamoto 1993).

Although no specific mutations have been identified in the PrP gene of patients with sporadic CJD (Goldfarb et al. 1990b), homozygosity at codon 129 in sporadic CJD (Hardy 1991, Palmer et al. 1991) is consistent with the results of Tg mouse studies. The finding that homozygosity at codon 129 predisposes to CJD supports a model of prion production that favours interactions between PrP molecules that are homologous in the H1 and H2 regions (Telling et al. 1995).

3 CONCLUDING REMARKS

3.1 Do prions exist in lower organisms?

In *Saccharomyces cerevisiae*, ure2 and [URE3] mutants were described that can grow on ureidosuccinate under conditions of nitrogen repression such as glutamic acid and ammonia (Lacroute 1971). Mutants of URE2 exhibit mendelian inheritance, whereas [URE3] is cytoplasmically inherited (Wickner 1994). The [URE3] phenotype can be induced by UV irradiation and by overexpression of ure2p, the gene product of ure2; deletion of ure2 abolishes [URE3]. The function of ure2p is unknown but it has substantial homology with glutathione-*S*-transferase; attempts to demonstrate this enzymic activity with purified ure2p have been unsuccessful (Coschigano and Magasanik 1991). Whether the [URE3] protein is a post-translationally modified form of ure2p which acts upon unmodified ure2p to produce more of itself remains to be established.

Another possible yeast prion is the [PSI] phenotype (Wickner 1994). [PSI] is a non-mendelian inherited trait that can be induced by overexpression of *Sup35* (Cox, Tuite and McLaughlin 1988, Chernoff, Derkach and Inge-Vechtomov 1993). The production of [PSI] has recently been shown to require the molecular chaperone HSP104, suggesting that this protein functions in producing an altered form of *Sup35* (Chernoff et al. 1995). Both [PSI] and [URE3] can be cured by exposure of the yeast to 3 mM GdnHCl. The mechanism responsible for abolishing [PSI] and [URE3] with a low concentration of GdnHCl is unknown. In the filamentous fungus *Podospora anserina*, the het-s locus controls the vegetative incompatibility; conversion from the S^s to the s state seems to be a post-translational, autocatalytic process (Deleu, Clavé and Bégueret 1993).

If any of the examples above cited can be shown to function in a manner similar to prions in animals, many new, more rapid and economical approaches to prion diseases should be forthcoming.

3.2   Prions are not viruses

The study of prions has taken several unexpected directions over the past few years. The discovery that prion diseases in humans are uniquely both genetic and infectious has greatly strengthened and extended the prion concept. To date, 19 different mutations in the human PrP gene, all resulting in non-conservative substitutions, have been found to either be linked genetically to or segregate with the inherited prion diseases (see Fig. 39.10). Yet the transmissible prion particle is composed largely, if not entirely, of an abnormal isoform of the prion protein designated PrP^{Sc} (Prusiner 1991). These findings argue that prion diseases should be considered pseudoinfections, since the particles transmitting disease seem to be devoid of a foreign nucleic acid and thus differ from all known micro-organisms as well as viruses and viroids. Because much information, especially about scrapie of rodents, has been derived using experimental protocols adapted from virology, we continue to use terms such as infection, incubation period, transmissibility and endpoint titration in studies of prion diseases.

ACKNOWLEDGEMENT

Supported by grants from the National Institutes of Health (NS14069, AG08967, AG02132, NS22786 and AG10770) and the American Health Assistance Foundation, as well as by gifts from the Sherman Fairchild Foundation and the Bernard Osher Foundation.

REFERENCES

Aiken JM, Marsh RF, 1990, The search for scrapie agent nucleic acid, *Microbiol Rev*, **54**: 242–6.

Alper T, Haig DA, Clarke MC, 1966, The exceptionally small size of the scrapie agent, *Biochem Biophys Res Commun*, **22**: 278–84.

Alper T, Haig DA, Clarke MC, 1978, The scrapie agent: evidence against its dependence for replication on intrinsic nucleic acid, *J Gen Virol*, **41**: 503–16.

Alper T, Cramp WA et al., 1967, Does the agent of scrapie replicate without nucleic acid?, *Nature (London)*, **214**: 764–6.

Alpers M, 1987, Epidemiology and clinical aspects of kuru, *Prions – Novel Infectious Pathogens Causing Scrapie and Creutzfeldt–Jakob Disease*, eds Prusiner SB, McKinley MP, Academic Press, Orlando FL, 451–65.

Anderson JR, Allen CMC, Weller RO, 1990, Creutzfeldt–Jakob disease following human pituitary-derived growth hormone administration, *Br Neuropatholog Soc Proc*, **16**: 543.

Anderson RGW, 1993, Caveolae: where incoming and outgoing messengers meet, *Proc Natl Acad Sci USA*, **90**: 10909–13.

Anonymous, 1993a, The first victim of mad cow disease?, *Daily Mail*, 13 Sep: 1.

Anonymous, 1993b, Second farmer's death raises fear of 'mad cow' cover-up, *The Times*, 13 Sep: 4.

Arnold JE, Tipler C et al., 1995, The abnormal isoform of the prion protein accumulates in late-endosome-like organelles in scrapie-infected mouse brain, *J Pathol*, **176**: 403–11.

Azzarelli B, Muller J et al., 1985, Cerebellar plaques in familial Alzheimer's disease (Gerstmann–Sträussler–Scheinker variant?), *Acta Neuropathol (Berl)*, **65**: 235–46.

Baker HF, Ridley RM, Wells GAH, 1993, Experimental transmission of BSE and scrapie to the common marmoset, *Vet Rec*, **132**: 403–6.

Barry RA, Prusiner SB, 1986, Monoclonal antibodies to the cellular and scrapie prion proteins, *J Infect Dis*, **154**: 518–21.

Basler K, Oesch B et al., 1986, Scrapie and cellular PrP isoforms are encoded by the same chromosomal gene, *Cell*, **46**: 417–28.

Beck E, Daniel PM, Parry HB, 1964, Degeneration of the cerebellar and hypothalamo-neurohypophysial systems in sheep with scrapie; and its relationship to human system degenerations, *Brain*, **87**: 153–76.

Bendheim PE, Barry RA et al., 1984, Antibodies to a scrapie prion protein, *Nature (London)*, **310**: 418–21.

Bendheim PE, Bockman JM et al., 1985, Scrapie and Creutzfeldt–Jakob disease prion proteins share physical properties and antigenic determinants, *Proc Natl Acad Sci USA*, **82**: 997–1001.

Berger JR, David NJ, 1993, Creutzfeldt–Jakob disease in a physician: a review of the disorder in health care workers, *Neurology*, **43**: 205–6.

Bernouilli C, Siegfried J et al., 1977, Danger of accidental person to person transmission of Creutzfeldt–Jakob disease by surgery, *Lancet*, **1**: 478–9.

Bernouilli CC, Masters CL et al., 1979, Early clinical features of Creutzfeldt–Jakob disease (subacute spongiform encephalopathy), *Slow Transmissible Diseases of the Nervous System*, vol 1, eds Prusiner SB, Hadlow WJ, Academic Press, New York, 229–51.

Bertoni JM, Brown P et al., 1992, Familial Creutzfeldt–Jakob disease with the PRNP codon 200^{lys} mutation and supranuclear palsy but without myoclonus or periodic EEG complexes, *Neurology*, **42, suppl 3**: 350 [Abstr].

Bessen RA, Kocisko DA et al., 1995, Non-genetic propagation of strain-specific properties of scrapie prion protein, *Nature (London)*, **375**: 698–700.

Billette de Villemeur T, Beauvais P et al., 1991, Creutzfeldt–Jakob disease in children treated with growth hormone, *Lancet*, **337**: 864–5.

Blum B, Bakalara N, Simpson L, 1990, A model for RNA editing in kinetoplastid mitochondria: 'guide' RNA molecules transcribed from maxicircle DNA provide edited information, *Cell*, **60**: 189–98.

Bockman JM, Kingsbury DT et al., 1985, Creutzfeldt–Jakob disease prion proteins in human brains, *N Engl J Med*, **312**: 73–8.

Bockman JM, Prusiner SB et al., 1987, Immunoblotting of Creutzfeldt–Jakob disease prion proteins: host species-specific epitopes, *Ann Neurol*, **21**: 589–95.

Bolton DC, McKinley MP, Prusiner SB, 1982, Identification of a protein that purifies with the scrapie prion, *Science*, **218**: 1309–11.

Bolton DC, Meyer RK, Prusiner SB, 1985, Scrapie PrP 27–30 is a sialoglycoprotein, *J Virol*, **53**: 596–606.

Borchelt DR, Taraboulos A, Prusiner SB, 1992, Evidence for synthesis of scrapie prion proteins in the endocytic pathway, *J Biol Chem*, **267**: 16188–99.

Borchelt DR, Scott M et al., 1990, Scrapie and cellular prion proteins differ in their kinetics of synthesis and topology in cultured cells, *J Cell Biol*, **110**: 743–52.

Borchelt DR, Rogers M et al., 1993, Release of the cellular prion protein from cultured cells after loss of its glycoinositol phospholipid anchor, *Glycobiology*, **3**: 319–29.

Brown P, 1985, Virus sterility for human growth hormone, *Lancet*, **2**: 729–30.

Brown P, 1988, The decline and fall of Creutzfeldt–Jakob disease associated with human growth hormone therapy, *Neurology*, **38**: 1135–7.

Brown P, 1992, The phenotypic expression of different mutations in transmissible human spongiform encephalopathy, *Rev Neurol*, **148**: 317–27.

Brown P, 1993, Infectious cerebral amyloidosis: clinical spectrum, risks and remedies, *Developments in Biological Standardization*, ed Brown F, Karger, Basel, 91–101.

Brown P, Preece MA, Will RG, 1992, 'Friendly fire' in medicine: hormones, homografts, and Creutzfeldt–Jakob disease, *Lancet*, **340**: 24–7.

Brown P, Gajdusek DC et al., 1985, Potential epidemic of Creutzfeldt–Jakob disease from human growth hormone therapy, *N Engl J Med*, **313**: 728–31.

Brown P, Cathala F et al., 1986a, Creutzfeldt–Jakob disease: clinical analysis of a consecutive series of 230 neuropathologically verified cases, *Ann Neurol*, **20**: 597–602.

Brown P, Coker-Vann M et al., 1986b, Diagnosis of Creutzfeldt–Jakob disease by Western blot identification of marker protein in human brain tissue, *N Engl J Med*, **314**: 547–51.

Brown P, Cathala F et al., 1987, The epidemiology of Creutzfeldt–Jakob disease: conclusion of 15-year investigation in France and review of the world literature, *Neurology*, **37**: 895–904.

Brown P, Goldfarb LG et al., 1992a, Phenotypic characteristics of familial Creutzfeldt–Jakob disease associated with the codon 178[Asn] PRNP mutation, *Ann Neurol*, **31**: 282–5.

Brown P, Goldfarb LG et al., 1992b, Atypical Creutzfeldt–Jakob disease in an American family with an insert mutation in the PRNP amyloid precursor gene, *Neurology*, **42**: 422–7.

Brown P, Kaur P et al., 1993, Real and imagined clinicopathological limits of 'prion dementia', *Lancet*, **341**: 127–9.

Brown P, Cervenáková L et al., 1994a, Iatrogenic Creutzfeldt–Jakob disease: an example of the interplay between ancient genes and modern medicine, *Neurology*, **44**: 291–3.

Brown P, Gibbs CJ Jr et al., 1994b, Human spongiform encephalopathy: the National Institutes of Health series of 300 cases of experimentally transmitted disease, *Ann Neurol*, **35**: 513–29.

Bruce ME, Dickinson AG, 1987, Biological evidence that the scrapie agent has an independent genome, *J Gen Virol*, **68**: 79–89.

Bruce ME, McConnell I et al., 1991, The disease characteristics of different strains of scrapie in *Sinc* congenic mouse lines: implications for the nature of the agent and host control of pathogenesis, *J Gen Virol*, **72**: 595–603.

Bruce M, Chree A et al., 1993, Transmissions of BSE, scrapie and related diseases to mice, *Proceedings of the IXth International Congress of Virology, Glasgow, Scotland*, p. 93.

Buchanan CR, Preece MA, Milner RDG, 1991, Mortality, neoplasia and Creutzfeldt–Jakob disease in patients treated with pituitary growth hormone in the United Kingdom, *Br Med J*, **302**: 824–8.

Büeler H, Fischer M et al., 1992, Normal development and behaviour of mice lacking the neuronal cell-surface PrP protein, *Nature (London)*, **356**: 577–82.

Büeler H, Aguzzi A et al., 1993, Mice devoid of PrP are resistant to scrapie, *Cell*, **73**: 1339–47.

Büeler H, Raeber A et al., 1994, High prion and PrP[Sc] levels but delayed onset of disease in scrapie-inoculated mice heterozygous for a disrupted PrP gene, *Mol Med*, **1**: 19–30.

Buyukmihci N, Rorvik M, Marsh RF, 1980, Replication of the scrapie agent in ocular neural tissues, *Proc Natl Acad Sci USA*, **77**: 1169–71.

Carlson GA, Kingsbury DT et al., 1986, Linkage of prion protein and scrapie incubation time genes, *Cell*, **46**: 503–11.

Carlson GA, Westaway D et al., 1989, Primary structure of prion protein may modify scrapie isolate properties, *Proc Natl Acad Sci USA*, **86**: 7475–9.

Caughey B, Raymond GJ, 1991, The scrapie-associated form of PrP is made from a cell surface precursor that is both protease- and phospholipase-sensitive, *J Biol Chem*, **266**: 18217–23.

Caughey B, Raymond GJ et al., 1991a, N-terminal truncation of the scrapie-associated form of PrP by lysosomal protease(s): implications regarding the site of conversion of PrP to the protease-resistant state, *J Virol*, **65**: 6597–603.

Caughey BW, Dong A et al., 1991b, Secondary structure analysis of the scrapie-associated protein PrP 27–30 in water by infrared spectroscopy, *Biochemistry*, **30**: 7672–80.

Chandler RL, 1961, Encephalopathy in mice produced by inoculation with scrapie brain material, *Lancet*, **1**: 1378–9.

Chandler RL, 1963, Experimental scrapie in the mouse, *Res Vet Sci*, **4**: 276–85.

Chapman J, Ben-Israel J et al., 1994, The risk of developing Creutzfeldt–Jakob disease in subjects with the *PRNP* gene codon 200 point mutation, *Neurology*, **44**: 1683–6.

Chazot G, Broussolle E et al., 1996, New variant of Creutzfeldt–Jakob disease in a 26-year-old French man, *Lancet*, **347**: 1181.

Chernoff YO, Derkach I, Inge-Vechtomov SG, 1993, Multicopy *SUP35* gene induces de-novo appearance of psi-like factors in the yeast *Saccharomyces cerevisiae*, *Curr Genet*, **24**: 268–70.

Chernoff YO, Lindquist SL et al., 1995, Role of the chaperone protein Hsp104 in propagation of the yeast prion-like factor [psi+], *Science*, **268**: 880–4.

Chesebro B, 1992, PrP and the scrapie agent, *Nature (London)*, **356**: 560.

Chesebro B, Race R et al., 1985, Identification of scrapie prion protein-specific mRNA in scrapie-infected and uninfected brain, *Nature (London)*, **315**: 331–3.

Clousard C, Beaudry P et al., 1995, Different allelic effects of the codons 136 and 171 of the prion protein gene in sheep with natural scrapie, *J Gen Virol*, **76**: 2079–101.

Cochius JI, Hyman N, Esiri MM, 1992, Creutzfeldt–Jakob disease in a recipient of human pituitary-derived gonadotrophin: a second case, *J Neurol Neurosurg Psychiatry*, **55**: 1094–5.

Cochius JI, Mack K et al., 1990, Creutzfeldt–Jakob disease in a recipient of human pituitary-derived gonadotrophin, *Aust N Z J Med*, **20**: 592–3.

Cohen AS, Shirahama T, Skinner M, 1982, Electron microscopy of amyloid, *Electron Microscopy of Proteins*, vol 3, ed Harris JR, Academic Press, New York, 165–206.

Cohen FE, Pan K-M et al., 1994, Structural clues to prion replication, *Science*, **264**: 530–1.

Collinge J, Palmer MS, Dryden AJ, 1991, Genetic predisposition to iatrogenic Creutzfeldt–Jakob disease, *Lancet*, **337**: 1441–2.

Collinge J, Owen F et al., 1990, Prion dementia without characteristic pathology, *Lancet*, **336**: 7–9.

Collinge J, Brown J et al., 1992, Inherited prion disease with 144 base pair gene insertion. 2. Clinical and pathological features, *Brain*, **115**: 687–710.

Coschigano PW, Magasanik B, 1991, The *URE2* gene product of *Saccharomyces cerevisiae* plays an important role in the cellular response to the nitrogen source and has homology to glutathione-S-transferases, *Mol Cell Biol*, **11**: 822–32.

Cousens SN, Harries-Jones R et al., 1990, Geographical distribution of cases of Creutzfeldt–Jakob disease in England and Wales 1970–84, *J Neurol Neurosurg Psychiatry*, **53**: 459–65.

Cox BS, Tuite MF, McLaughlin CS, 1988, The psi factor of yeast: a problem in inheritance, *Yeast*, **4**: 159–78.

Crow TJ, Collinge J et al., 1990, Mutations in the prion gene in human transmissible dementia, *Seminar on Molecular Approaches to Research in Spongiform Encephalopathies in Man*, Medical Research Council, London, 14 Dec 1990 [Abstr].

Croxson M, Brown P et al., 1988, A new case of Creutzfeldt–Jakob disease associated with human growth hormone therapy in New Zealand, *Neurology*, **38**: 1128–30.

Cuillé J, Chelle PL, 1939, Experimental transmission of trembling to the goat, *CR Seances Acad Sci*, **208**: 1058–60.

Cunningham AA, Wells GAH et al., 1993, Transmissible spongiform encephalopathy in greater kudu (*Tragelaphus strepsiceros*), *Vet Rec*, **132**: 68.

Davanipour Z, Goodman L et al., 1984, Possible modes of transmission of Creutzfeldt–Jakob disease, *N Engl J Med*, **311**: 1582–3.

Davison C, Rabiner AM, 1940, Spastic pseudosclerosis (disseminated encephalomyelopathy; corticopallidospinal degeneration). Familial and nonfamilial incidence (a clinicopathologic study), *Arch Neurol Psychiatry*, **44**: 578–98.

Dawson M, Wells GAH, Parker BNJ, 1990, Preliminary evidence of the experimental transmissibility of bovine spongiform encephalopathy to cattle, *Vet Rec*, **126**: 112–13.

Dawson M, Wells GAH et al., 1990, Primary parenteral transmission of bovine spongiform encephalopathy to the pig, *Vet Rec*, **127**: 338.

Dealler SF, Lacey RW, 1990, Transmissible spongiform encephalopathies: the threat of BSE to man, *Food Microbiol*, **7**: 253–79.

DeArmond SJ, McKinley MP et al., 1985, Identification of prion amyloid filaments in scrapie-infected brain, *Cell*, **41**: 221–35.

Deleu C, Clavé C, Bégueret J, 1993, A single amino acid difference is sufficient to elicit vegetative incompatibility in the fungus *Podospora anserina*, *Genetics*, **135**: 45–52.

Deslys J-P, Marcé D, Dormont D, 1994, Similar genetic susceptibility in iatrogenic and sporadic Creutzfeldt–Jakob disease, *J Gen Virol*, **75**: 23–7.

Dickinson AG, Fraser H, 1979, An assessment of the genetics of scrapie in sheep and mice, *Slow Transmissible Diseases of the Nervous System*, vol 1, eds Prusiner SB, Hadlow WJ, Academic Press, New York, 367–86.

Dickinson AG, Meikle VM, 1969, A comparison of some biological characteristics of the mouse-passaged scrapie agents, 22A and ME7, *Genet Res*, **13**: 213–25.

Dickinson AG, Meikle VMH, 1971, Host-genotype and agent effects in scrapie incubation: change in allelic interaction with different strains of agent, *Mol Gen Genet*, **112**: 73–9.

Dickinson AG, Meikle VMH, Fraser H, 1968, Identification of a gene which controls the incubation period of some strains of scrapie agent in mice, *J Comp Pathol*, **78**: 293–9.

Dickinson AG, Meikle VM, Fraser H, 1969, Genetical control of the concentration of ME7 scrapie agent in the brain of mice, *J Comp Pathol*, **79**: 15–22.

Dickinson AG, Outram GW, 1988, Genetic aspects of unconventional virus infections: the basis of the virino hypothesis, *Novel Infectious Agents and the Central Nervous System*, Ciba Foundation Symposium 135, eds Bock G, Marsh J, John Wiley, Chichester, 63–83.

Dickinson AG, Stamp JT, 1969, Experimental scrapie in Cheviot and Suffolk sheep, *J Comp Pathol*, **79**: 23–6.

Dickinson AG, Young GB et al., 1965, An analysis of natural scrapie in Suffolk sheep, *Heredity*, **20**: 485–503.

Dickinson AG, Bruce ME et al., 1984, Scrapie strain differences: the implications of stability and mutation, *Proceedings of Workshop on Slow Transmissible Diseases*, ed Tateishi J, Japanese Ministry of Health and Welfare, Tokyo, 105–18.

Dlouhy SR, Hsiao K et al., 1992, Linkage of the Indiana kindred of Gerstmann–Sträussler–Scheinker disease to the prion protein gene, *Nature Genet*, **1**: 64–7.

Doh-ura K, Tateishi J et al., 1989, Pro–Leu change at position 102 of prion protein is the most common but not the sole mutation related to Gerstmann–Sträussler syndrome, *Biochem Biophys Res Commun*, **163**: 974–9.

Doh-ura K, Kitamoto T et al., 1991, CJD discrepancy, *Nature (London)*, **353**: 801–2.

Duffy P, Wolf J et al., 1974, Possible person to person transmission of Creutzfeldt–Jakob disease, *N Engl J Med*, **290**: 692–3.

Eklund CM, Hadlow WJ, Kennedy RC, 1963, Some properties of the scrapie agent and its behavior in mice, *Proc Soc Exp Biol Med*, **112**: 974–9.

Eklund CM, Kennedy RC, Hadlow WJ, 1967, Pathogenesis of scrapie virus infection in the mouse, *J Infect Dis*, **117**: 15–22.

Ellis CJ, Katifi H, Weller RO, 1992, A further British case of growth hormone induced Creutzfeldt–Jakob disease, *J Neurol Neurosurg Psychiatry*, **55**: 1200–2.

Farlow MR, Yee RD et al., 1989, Gerstmann–Sträussler–Scheinker disease. I. Extending the clinical spectrum, *Neurology*, **39**: 1446–52.

Fink JK, Warren JT Jr et al., 1991, Allele-specific sequencing confirms novel prion gene polymorphism in Creutzfeldt–Jakob disease, *Neurology*, **41**: 1647–50.

Fradkin JE, Schonberger LB et al., 1991, Creutzfeldt–Jakob disease in pituitary growth hormone recipients in the United States, *JAMA*, **265**: 880–4.

Fraser H, Dickinson AG, 1968, The sequential development of the brain lesions of scrapie in three strains of mice, *J Comp Pathol*, **78**: 301–11.

Fraser H, McConnell I et al., 1988, Transmission of bovine spongiform encephalopathy to mice, *Vet Rec*, **123**: 472.

Friede RL, DeJong RN, 1964, Neuronal enzymatic failure in Creutzfeldt–Jakob disease. A familial study, *Arch Neurol*, **10**: 181–95.

Gabizon R, McKinley MP, Prusiner SB, 1987, Purified prion proteins and scrapie infectivity copartition into liposomes, *Proc Natl Acad Sci USA*, **84**: 4017–21.

Gabizon R, Prusiner SB, 1990, Prion liposomes, *Biochem J*, **266**: 1–14.

Gabizon R, McKinley MP et al., 1988, Immunoaffinity purification and neutralization of scrapie prion infectivity, *Proc Natl Acad Sci USA*, **85**: 6617–21.

Gabizon R, Meiner Z et al., 1991, Prion protein gene mutation in Libyan Jews with Creutzfeldt–Jakob disease, *Neurology*, **41**: 160.

Gabriel J-M, Oesch B et al., 1992, Molecular cloning of a candidate chicken prion protein, *Proc Natl Acad Sci USA*, **89**: 9097–101.

Gajdusek DC, 1977, Unconventional viruses and the origin and disappearance of kuru, *Science*, **197**: 943–60.

Gajdusek DC, 1992, Genetic control of de novo conversion to infectious amyloids of host precursor proteins: kuru–CJD–scrapie, *Current Topics in Biomedical Research*, eds Kurth R, Schwerdtfeger WK, Springer-Verlag, Berlin, 95–123.

Gajdusek DC, Gibbs CJ Jr, Alpers M, 1966, Experimental transmission of a kuru-like syndrome to chimpanzees, *Nature (London)*, **209**: 794–6.

Gajdusek DC, Zigas V, 1957, Degenerative disease of the central nervous system in New Guinea – the endemic occurrence of 'kuru' in the native population, *N Engl J Med*, **257**: 974–8.

Gajdusek DC, Zigas V, 1959, Clinical, pathological and epidemiological study of an acute progressive degenerative disease of the central nervous system among natives of the eastern highlands of New Guinea, *Am J Med*, **26**: 442–69.

Gajdusek DC, Gibbs CJ Jr et al., 1977, Precautions in medical care of and in handling materials from patients with transmissible virus dementia (CJD), *N Engl J Med*, **297**: 1253–8.

Gard S, 1940, Encephalomyelitis of mice. II. A method for the measurement of virus activity, *J Exp Med*, **72**: 69–77.

Gasset M, Baldwin MA et al., 1993, Perturbation of the secondary structure of the scrapie prion protein under conditions associated with changes in infectivity, *Proc Natl Acad Sci USA*, **90**: 1–5.

Gerstmann J, Sträussler E, Scheinker I, 1936, Über eine eigenartige hereditär-familiäre Erkrankung des Zentralnervensystems zugleich ein Beitrag zur frage des vorzeitigen lokalen Alterns, *Z Neurol*, **154**: 736–62.

Ghetti B, Tagliavini F et al., 1989, Gerstmann–Sträussler–Scheinker disease. II. Neurofibrillary tangles and plaques with PrP-amyloid coexist in an affected family, *Neurology*, **39**: 1453–61.

Giaccone G, Tagliavini F et al., 1990, Neurofibrillary tangles of the Indiana kindred of Gerstmann–Sträussler–Scheinker disease share antigenic determinants with those of Alzheimer disease, *Brain Res*, **530**: 325–9.

Gibbons RA, Hunter GD, 1967, Nature of the scrapie agent, *Nature (London)*, **215**: 1041–3.

Gibbs CJ Jr, Gajdusek DC, 1969, Infection as the etiology of spongiform encephalopathy, *Science*, **165**: 1023–5.

Gibbs CJ Jr, Gajdusek DC et al., 1968, Creutzfeldt–Jakob disease (spongiform encephalopathy): transmission to the chimpanzee, *Science*, **161**: 388–9.

Gibbs CJ Jr, Amyx HL et al., 1980, Oral transmission of kuru, Creutzfeldt–Jakob disease and scrapie to nonhuman primates, *J Infect Dis*, **142**: 205–8.

Gibbs CJ Jr, Joy A et al., 1985, Clinical and pathological features and laboratory confirmation of Creutzfeldt–Jakob disease in a recipient of pituitary-derived human growth hormone, *N Engl J Med*, **313**: 734–8.

Gibbs CJ Jr, Asher DM et al., 1993, Creutzfeldt–Jakob disease infectivity of growth hormone derived from human pituitary glands, *N Engl J Med*, **328**: 358–9.

Gibbs CJ Jr, Asher DM et al., 1994, Transmission of Creutzfeldt–Jakob disease to a chimpanzee by electrodes contaminated during neurosurgery, *J Neurol Neurosurg Psychiatry*, **57**: 757–8.

Goldfarb L, Korczyn A et al., 1990a, Mutation in codon 200 of scrapie amyloid precursor gene linked to Creutzfeldt–Jakob disease in Sephardic Jews of Libyan and non-Libyan origin, *Lancet*, **336**: 637–8.

Goldfarb LG, Brown P et al., 1990b, Creutzfeldt–Jakob disease and kuru patients lack a mutation consistently found in the Gerstmann–Sträussler–Scheinker syndrome, *Exp Neurol*, **108**: 247–50.

Goldfarb LG, Mitrova E et al., 1990c, Mutation in codon 200 of scrapie amyloid protein gene in two clusters of Creutzfeldt–Jakob disease in Slovakia, *Lancet*, **336**: 514–5.

Goldfarb LG, Brown P et al., 1991a, Transmissible familial Creutzfeldt–Jakob disease associated with five, seven, and eight extra octapeptide coding repeats in the *PRNP* gene, *Proc Natl Acad Sci USA*, **88**: 10926–30.

Goldfarb LG, Brown P et al., 1991b, Creutzfeldt–Jacob disease associated with the PRNP codon 200[Lys] mutation: an analysis of 45 families, *Eur J Epidemiol*, **7**: 477–86.

Goldfarb LG, Haltia M et al., 1991c, New mutation in scrapie amyloid precursor gene (at codon 178) in Finnish Creutzfeldt–Jakob kindred, *Lancet*, **337**: 425.

Goldfarb LG, Brown P et al., 1992a, Creutzfeldt–Jakob disease cosegregates with the codon 178[Asn] *PRNP* mutation in families of European origin, *Ann Neurol*, **31**: 274–81.

Goldfarb LG, Petersen RB et al., 1992b, Fatal familial insomnia and familial Creutzfeldt–Jakob disease: disease phenotype determined by a DNA polymorphism, *Science*, **258**: 806–8.

Goldgaber D, Goldfarb LG et al., 1989, Mutations in familial Creutzfeldt–Jakob disease and Gerstmann–Sträussler–Scheinker's syndrome, *Exp Neurol*, **106**: 204–6.

Goldhammer Y, Gabizon R et al., 1993, An Israeli family with Gerstmann–Sträussler–Scheinker disease manifesting the codon 102 mutation in the prion protein gene, *Neurology*, **43**: 2718–9.

Goldmann W, Hunter N et al., 1988, The PrP gene in natural scrapie, *Alzheimer Dis Assoc Disord* [Abstr suppl], **2**: 330.

Goldmann W, Hunter N et al., 1990a, Two alleles of a neural protein gene linked to scrapie in sheep, *Proc Natl Acad Sci USA*, **87**: 2476–80.

Goldmann W, Hunter N et al., 1990b, The PrP gene of the

sheep, a natural host of scrapie, *VIIIth International Congress of Virology*, Berlin, 26–31 Aug, 284 [Abstr].

Goldmann W, Hunter N et al., 1991a, Different scrapie-associated fibril proteins (PrP) are encoded by lines of sheep selected for different alleles of the *Sip* gene, *J Gen Virol*, **72**: 2411–7.

Goldmann W, Hunter N et al., 1991b, Different forms of the bovine PrP gene have five or six copies of a short, G–C-rich element within the protein-coding exon, *J Gen Virol*, **72**: 201–4.

Gordon WS, 1946, Advances in veterinary research, *Vet Res*, **58**: 516–20.

Gordon WS, 1966, Variation in susceptibility of sheep to scrapie and genetic implications, *Report of Scrapie Seminar*, ARS 91-53, US Department of Agriculture, Washington DC, 53–67.

Gorodinsky A, Harris DA, 1995, Glycolipid-anchored proteins in neuroblastoma cells form detergent-resistant complexes without caveolin, *J Cell Biol*, **129**: 619–27.

Hadlow WJ, Kennedy RC, Race RE, 1982, Natural infection of Suffolk sheep with scrapie virus, *J Infect Dis*, **146**: 657–64.

Hadlow WJ, Kennedy RC et al., 1980, Virologic and neurohistologic findings in dairy goats affected with natural scrapie, *Vet Pathol*, **17**: 187–99.

Haltia M, Kovanen J et al., 1991, Familial Creutzfeldt–Jakob disease in Finland: epidemiological, clinical, pathological and molecular genetic studies, *Eur J Epidemiol*, **7**: 494–500.

Haraguchi T, Fisher S et al., 1989, Asparagine-linked glycosylation of the scrapie and cellular prion proteins, *Arch Biochem Biophys*, **274**: 1–13.

Hardy J, 1991, Prion dimers – a deadly duo, *Trends Neurosci*, **14**: 423–4.

Harries-Jones R, Knight R et al., 1988, Creutzfeldt–Jakob disease in England and Wales 1980–1984: a case–control study of potential risk factors, *J Neurol Neurosurg Psychiatry*, **51**: 1113–9.

Healy DL, Evans J, 1993, Creutzfeldt–Jakob disease after pituitary gonadotrophins, *Br J Med*, **307**: 517–8.

Herzberg L, Herzberg BN et al., 1974, Creutzfeldt–Jakob disease: hypothesis for high incidence in Libyan Jews in Israel, *Science*, **186**: 848.

Heston LL, Lowther DLW, Leventhal CM, 1966, Alzheimer's disease: a family study, *Arch Neurol*, **15**: 225–33.

Hope J, Reekie LJD et al., 1988, Fibrils from brains of cows with new cattle disease contain scrapie-associated protein, *Nature (London)*, **336**: 390–2.

Hsiao K, Prusiner SB, 1990, Inherited human prion diseases, *Neurology*, **40**: 1820–7.

Hsiao K, Baker HF et al., 1989, Linkage of a prion protein missense variant to Gerstmann–Sträussler syndrome, *Nature (London)*, **338**: 342–5.

Hsiao KK, Scott M et al., 1990, Spontaneous neurodegeneration in transgenic mice with mutant prion protein, *Science*, **250**: 1587–90.

Hsiao K, Meiner Z et al., 1991a, Mutation of the prion protein in Libyan Jews with Creutzfeldt–Jakob disease, *N Engl J Med*, **324**: 1091–7.

Hsiao KK, Cass C et al., 1991b, A prion protein variant in a family with the telencephalic form of Gerstmann–Sträussler–Scheinker syndrome, *Neurology*, **41**: 681–4.

Hsiao K, Dlouhy S et al., 1992, Mutant prion proteins in Gerstmann–Sträussler–Scheinker disease with neurofibrillary tangles, *Nature Genet*, **1**: 68–71.

Hsiao KK, Groth D et al., 1994, Serial transmission in rodents of neurodegeneration from transgenic mice expressing mutant prion protein, *Proc Natl Acad Sci USA*, **91**: 9126–30.

Hunter GD, Millson GC, 1964, Studies on the heat stability and chromatographic behavior of the scrapie agent, *J Gen Microbiol*, **37**: 251–8.

Hunter N, Foster JD et al., 1989, Linkage of the gene for the scrapie-associated fibril protein (PrP) to the *Sip* gene in Cheviot sheep, *Vet Rec*, **124**: 364–6.

Hunter N, Foster JD et al., 1991, Restriction fragment length polymorphisms of the scrapie-associated fibril protein (PrP) gene and their association with susceptiblity to natural scrapie in British sheep, *J Gen Virol*, **72**: 1287–92.

Ikeda S, Yanagisawa N et al., 1991, A variant of Gerstmann–Sträussler–Scheinker disease with β-protein epitopes and dystrophic neurites in the peripheral regions of PrP-immunoreactive amyloid plaques, *Amyloid and Amyloidosis 1990*, eds Natvig JB, Forre O et al., Kluwer Academic, Dordrecht, 737–40.

Jacob H, Pyrkosch W, Strube H, 1950, Die erbliche Form der Creutzfeldt–Jakobschen Krankheit, *Arch Psychiatr Zeitschr Neurol*, **184**: 653–74.

Johnson RT, 1992, Prion disease, *N Engl J Med*, **326**: 486–7.

Kahana E, Zilber N, Abraham M, 1991, Do Creutzfeldt–Jakob disease patients of Jewish Libyan origin have unique clinical features?, *Neurology*, **41**: 1390–2.

Kahana E, Milton A et al., 1974, Creutzfeldt–Jakob disease: focus among Libyan Jews in Israel, *Science*, **183**: 90–1.

Kane PM, Yamashiro CT et al., 1990, Protein splicing converts the yeast TFP1 gene product to the 69-kD subunit of the vacuolar H⁺-adenosine triphosphatase, *Science*, **250**: 651–7.

Kaneko K, Peretz D et al., 1995, Prion protein (PrP) synthetic peptides induce cellular PrP to acquire properties of the scrapie isoform, *Proc Natl Acad Sci USA*, **32**: 11160–4.

Kascsak RJ, Rubenstein R et al., 1987, Mouse polyclonal and monoclonal antibody to scrapie-associated fibril proteins, *J Virol*, **61**: 3688–93.

Keller GA, Siegel MW, Caras IW, 1992, Endocytosis of glycophospholipid-anchored and transmembrane forms of CD4 by different endocytic pathways, *EMBO J*, **11**: 863–74.

Kimberlin RH, 1990, Scrapie and possible relationships with viroids, *Semin Virol*, **1**: 153–62.

Kimberlin RH, Cole S, Walker CA, 1987, Temporary and permanent modifications to a single strain of mouse scrapie on transmission to rats and hamsters, *J Gen Virol*, **68**: 1875–81.

Kimberlin RH, Walker CA, 1978, Pathogenesis of mouse scrapie: effect of route of inoculation on infectivity titres and dose–response curves, *J Comp Pathol*, **88**: 39–47.

Kimberlin RH, Walker CA, 1979, Pathogenesis of mouse scrapie: dynamics of agent replication in spleen, spinal cord and brain after infection by different routes, *J Comp Pathol*, **89**: 551–62.

Kirkwood JK, Wells GAH et al., 1990, Spongiform encephalopathy in an arabian oryx (*Oryx leucoryx*) and a greater kudu (*Tragelaphus strepsiceros*), *Vet Rec*, **127**: 418–20.

Kirkwood JK, Cunningham AA et al., 1993, Spongiform encephalopathy in a herd of greater kudu (*Tragelaphus strepsiceros*): epidemiological observations, *Vet Rec*, **133**: 360–4.

Kirschbaum WR, 1924, Zwei eigenartige Erkrankungen des Zentralnervensystems nach Art der spastischen Pseudosklerose (Jakob), *Z Ges Neurol Psychiatr*, **92**: 175–220.

Kitamoto T, Iizuka R, Tateishi J, 1993, An amber mutation of prion protein in Gerstmann–Sträussler syndrome with mutant PrP plaques, *Biochem Biophys Res Commun*, **192**: 525–31.

Kitamoto T, Tateishi J, 1994, Human prion diseases with variant prion protein, *Philos Trans R Soc Lond (Biol)*, **343**: 391–8.

Kitamoto T, Tateishi J et al., 1986, Amyloid plaques in Creutzfeldt–Jakob disease stain with prion protein antibodies, *Ann Neurol*, **20**: 204–8.

Kitamoto T, Yamaguchi K et al., 1991, A prion protein missense variant is integrated in kuru plaque cores in patients with Gerstmann–Sträussler syndrome, *Neurology*, **41**: 306–10.

Kitamoto T, Shin R-W et al., 1992, Abnormal isoform of prion proteins accumulates in the synaptic structures of the central nervous system in patients with Creutzfeldt–Jakob disease, *Am J Pathol*, **140**: 1285–94.

Kitamoto T, Ohta M et al., 1993, Novel missense variants of prion protein in Creutzfeldt–Jakob disease or Gerstmann–Sträussler syndrome, *Biochem Biophys Res Commun*, **191**: 709–14.

Klitzman RL, Alpers MP, Gajdusek DC, 1984, The natural incubation period of kuru and the episodes of transmission in three clusters of patients, *Neuroepidemiology*, **3**: 3–20.

Koch TK, Berg BO et al., 1985, Creutzfeldt–Jakob disease in a young adult with idiopathic hypopituitarism. Possible relation to the administration of cadaveric human growth hormone, *N Engl J Med*, **313**: 731–3.

Kocisko DA, Come JH et al., 1994, Cell-free formation of protease-resistant prion protein, *Nature (London)*, **370**: 471–4.

Kocisko DA, Priola SA et al., 1995, Species specificity in the cell-free conversion of prion protein to protease-resistant forms: a model for the scrapie species barrier, *Proc Natl Acad Sci USA*, **92**: 3923–7.

Kondo K, Kuroina Y, 1981, A case–control study of Creutzfeldt–Jakob disease: association with physical injuries, *Ann Neurol*, **11**: 377–81.

Kretzschmar HA, Prusiner SB et al., 1986a, Scrapie prion proteins are synthesized in neurons, *Am J Pathol*, **122**: 1–5.

Kretzschmar HA, Stowring LE et al., 1986b, Molecular cloning of a human prion protein cDNA, *DNA*, **5**: 315–24.

Kretzschmar HA, Honold G et al., 1991, Prion protein mutation in family first reported by Gerstmann, Sträussler, and Scheinker, *Lancet*, **337**: 1160.

Kretzschmar HA, Kufer P et al., 1992, Prion protein mutation at codon 102 in an Italian family with Gerstmann–Sträussler–Scheinker syndrome, *Neurology*, **42**: 809–10.

Lacroute F, 1971, Non-Mendelian mutation allowing ureidosuccinic acid uptake in yeast, *J Bacteriol*, **106**: 519–22.

Lanska DJ, Currier RD et al., 1994, Familial progressive subcortical gliosis, *Neurology*, **44**: 1633–43.

Laplanche J-L, Chatelain J et al., 1990, Deletion in prion protein gene in a Moroccan family, *Nucleic Acids Res*, **18**: 6745.

Laplanche J-L, Chatelain J et al., 1993a, French autochthonous scrapied sheep without the 136Val PrP polymorphism, *Mamm Genome*, **4**: 463–4.

Laplanche JL, Chatelain J et al., 1993b, PrP polymorphisms associated with natural scrapie discovered by denaturing gradient gel electrophoresis, *Genomics*, **15**: 30–7.

Laszlo L, Lowe J et al., 1992, Lysosomes as key organelles in the pathogenesis of prion encephalopathies, *J Pathol*, **166**: 333–41.

Little BW, Brown PW et al., 1986, Familial myoclonic dementia masquerading as Creutzfeldt–Jakob disease, *Ann Neurol*, **20**: 231–9.

Locht C, Chesebro B et al., 1986, Molecular cloning and complete sequence of prion protein cDNA from mouse brain infected with the scrapie agent, *Proc Natl Acad Sci USA*, **83**: 6372–6.

Lugaresi E, Medori R et al., 1986, Fatal familial insomnia and dysautonomia with selective degeneration of thalamic nuclei, *N Engl J Med*, **315**: 997–1003.

Lumley Jones R, Benker G et al., 1979, Large-scale preparation of highly purified pyrogen-free human growth hormone for clinical use, *Br J Endocrinol*, **82**: 77–86.

M'Fadyean J, 1918, Scrapie, *J Comp Pathol*, **31**: 102–31.

M'Gowan JP, 1914, *Investigation into the Disease of Sheep Called 'Scrapie'*, William Blackwood, Edinburgh.

McKinley MP, Bolton DC, Prusiner SB, 1983, A protease-resistant protein is a structural component of the scrapie prion, *Cell*, **35**: 57–62.

McKinley MP, Taraboulos A et al., 1990, Ultrastructural localization of scrapie prion proteins in secondary lysosomes of infected cultured cells, *J Cell Biol*, **111**: 316a.

McKinley MP, Meyer R et al., 1991a, Scrapie prion rod formation in vitro requires both detergent extraction and limited proteolysis, *J Virol*, **65**: 1440–9.

McKinley MP, Taraboulos A et al., 1991b, Ultrastructural localization of scrapie prion proteins in cytoplasmic vesicles of infected cultured cells, *Lab Invest*, **65**: 622–30.

Macario ME, Vaisman M et al., 1991, Pituitary growth hormone and Creutzfeldt–Jakob disease, *Br Med J*, **302**: 1149.

Malmgren R, Kurland L et al., 1979, The epidemiology of Creutzfeldt–Jakob disease, *Slow Transmissible Diseases of the Nervous System*, vol 1, eds Prusiner SB, Hadlow WJ, Academic Press, New York, 93–112.

Manetto V, Medori R et al., 1992, Fatal familial insomnia: clinical and pathological study of five new cases, *Neurology*, **42**: 312–9.

Manson JC, Clarke AR et al., 1994a, 129/Ola mice carrying a null mutation in PrP that abolishes mRNA production are developmentally normal, *Mol Neurobiol*, **8**: 121–7.

Manson JC, Clarke AR et al., 1994b, PrP gene dosage determines the timing but not the final intensity or distribution of lesions in scrapie pathology, *Neurodegeneration*, **3**: 331–40.

Marsh RF, Kimberlin RH, 1975, Comparison of scrapie and transmissible mink encephalopathy in hamsters. II. Clinical signs, pathology and pathogenesis, *J Infect Dis*, **131**: 104–10.

Marsh RF, Bessen RA et al., 1991, Epidemiological and experimental studies on a new incident of transmissible mink encephalopathy, *J Gen Virol*, **72**: 589–94.

Martínez-Lage JF, Sola J et al., 1993, Pediatric Creutzfeldt–Jakob disease: probable transmission by a dural graft, *Childs Nerv Syst*, **9**: 239–42.

Marzewski DJ, Towfighi J et al., 1988, Creutzfeldt–Jakob disease following pituitary-derived human growth hormone therapy: a new American case, *Neurology*, **38**: 1131–3.

Masters CL, Gajdusek DC, Gibbs CJ Jr, 1981a, Creutzfeldt–Jakob disease virus isolations from the Gerstmann–Sträussler syndrome, *Brain*, **104**: 559–88.

Masters CL, Gajdusek DC, Gibbs CJ Jr, 1981b, The familial occurrence of Creutzfeldt–Jakob disease and Alzheimer's disease, *Brain*, **104**: 535–58.

Masters CL, Richardson EP Jr, 1978, Subacute spongiform encephalopathy Creutzfeldt–Jakob disease – the nature and progression of spongiform change, *Brain*, **101**: 333–44.

Masters CL, Harris JO et al., 1978, Creutzfeldt–Jakob disease: patterns of worldwide occurrence and the significance of familial and sporadic clustering, *Ann Neurol*, **5**: 177–88.

Masters CL, Gajdusek DC et al., 1979, Familial Creutzfeldt–Jakob disease and other familial dementias: an inquiry into possible models of virus-induced familial diseases, *Slow Transmissible Diseases of the Nervous System*, vol 1, eds Prusiner SB, Hadlow WJ, Academic Press, New York, 143–94.

Mastrianni JA, Iannicola C et al., 1995, Identification of a new mutation of the prion protein gene at codon 208 in a patient with Creutzfeldt–Jakob disease [Abstr], *Neurology*, **45, suppl**: 201.

Masullo C, Pocchiari M et al., 1989, Transmission of Creutzfeldt–Jakob disease by dural cadaveric graft, *J Neurosurg*, **71**: 954.

Medori R, Montagna P et al., 1992a, Fatal familial insomnia: a second kindred with mutation of prion protein gene at codon 178, *Neurology*, **42**: 669–70.

Medori R, Tritschler H-J et al., 1992b, Fatal familial insomnia, a prion disease with a mutation at codon 178 of the prion protein gene, *N Engl J Med*, **326**: 444–9.

Meggendorfer F, 1930, Klinische und genealogische Beobachtungen bei einem Fall von spastischer Pseudosklerose Jakobs, *Z Ges Neurol Psychiatr*, **128**: 337–41.

Meyer RK, McKinley MP et al., 1986, Separation and properties of cellular and scrapie prion proteins, *Proc Natl Acad Sci USA*, **83**: 2310–4.

Millson G, Hunter GD, Kimberlin RH, 1971, An experimental examination of the scrapie agent in cell membrane mixtures. II. The association of scrapie infectivity with membrane fractions, *J Comp Pathol*, **81**: 255–65.

Miyashita K, Inuzuka T et al., 1991, Creutzfeldt–Jakob disease in a patient with a cadaveric dural graft, *Neurology*, **41**: 940–1.

Miyazono M, Kitamoto T et al., 1992, Creutzfeldt–Jakob disease with codon 129 polymorphism (Valine): a comparative study of patients with codon 102 point mutation or without mutations, *Acta Neuropathol*, **84**: 349–54.

Mobley WC, Neve RL et al., 1988, Nerve growth factor increases mRNA levels for the prion protein and the beta-amyloid protein precursor in developing hamster brain, *Proc Natl Acad Sci USA*, **85**: 9811–5.

Monari L, Chen SG et al., 1994, Fatal familial insomnia and familial Creutzfeldt–Jakob disease: different prion proteins

determined by a DNA polymorphism, *Proc Natl Acad Sci USA*, **91**: 2839–42.

Neumann MA, Cohn R, 1967, Progressive subcortical gliosis, a rare form of pre-senile dementia, *Brain*, **90**: 405–18.

New MI, Brown P et al., 1988, Preclinical Creutzfeldt–Jakob disease discovered at autopsy in a human growth hormone recipient, *Neurology*, **38**: 1133–4.

Nguyen JT, Inouye H et al., 1995, X-ray diffraction of scrapie prion rods and PrP peptides, *J Mol Biol*, **252**: 412–22.

Nisbet TJ, MacDonaldson I, Bishara SN, 1989, Creutzfeldt–Jakob disease in a second patient who received a cadaveric dura mater graft, *JAMA*, **261**: 1118.

Nochlin D, Sumi SM et al., 1989, Familial dementia with PrP-positive amyloid plaques: a variant of Gerstmann–Sträussler syndrome, *Neurology*, **39**: 910–8.

Oesch B, Westaway D et al., 1985, A cellular gene encodes scrapie PrP 27–30 protein, *Cell*, **40**: 735–46.

Onodera T, Ikeda T et al., 1993, Isolation of scrapie agent from the placenta of sheep with natural scrapie in Japan, *Microbiol Immunol*, **37**: 311–6.

Otto D, 1987, Jacob–Creutzfeldt disease associated with cadaveric dura, *J Neurosurg*, **67**: 149.

Owen F, Poulter M et al., 1989, Insertion in prion protein gene in familial Creutzfeldt–Jakob disease, *Lancet*, **1**: 51–2.

Owen F, Poulter M et al., 1990a, Codon 129 changes in the prion protein gene in Caucasians, *Am J Hum Genet*, **46**: 1215–6.

Owen F, Poulter M et al., 1990b, An in-frame insertion in the prion protein gene in familial Creutzfeldt–Jakob disease, *Mol Brain Res*, **7**: 273–6.

Owen F, Poulter M et al., 1991, Insertions in the prion protein gene in atypical dementias, *Exp Neurol*, **112**: 240–2.

Owen F, Poulter M et al., 1992, A dementing illness associated with a novel insertion in the prion protein gene, *Mol Brain Res*, **13**: 155–7.

Packer RJ, Cornblath DR et al., 1980, Creutzfeldt–Jakob disease in a 20-year-old woman, *Neurology*, **30**: 492–6.

Palmer MS, Dryden AJ et al., 1991, Homozygous prion protein genotype predisposes to sporadic Creutzfeldt–Jakob disease, *Nature (London)*, **352**: 340–2.

Palmer MS, Mahal SP et al., 1993, Deletions in the prion protein gene are not associated with CJD, *Hum Mol Genet*, **2**: 541–4.

Palsson PA, 1979, Rida (scrapie) in Iceland and its epidemiology, *Slow Transmissible Diseases of the Nervous System*, vol 1, eds Prusiner SB, Hadlow WJ, Academic Press, New York, 357–66.

Pan K-M, Stahl N, Prusiner SB, 1992, Purification and properties of the cellular prion protein from Syrian hamster brain, *Protein Sci*, **1**: 1343–52.

Pan K-M, Baldwin M et al., 1993, Conversion of α-helices into β-sheets features in the formation of the scrapie prion proteins, *Proc Natl Acad Sci USA*, **90**: 10962–6.

Parry HB, 1962, Scrapie: a transmissible and hereditary disease of sheep, *Heredity*, **17**: 75–105.

Parry HB, 1983, *Scrapie Disease in Sheep*, ed Oppenheimer DR, Academic Press, New York.

Pattison IH, 1964, The spread of scrapie by contact between affected and healthy sheep, goats or mice, *Vet Rec*, **76**: 333–6.

Pattison IH, Jones KM, 1967, The possible nature of the transmissible agent of scrapie, *Vet Rec*, **80**: 1–8.

Pattison IH, Millson GC, 1961a, Experimental transmission of scrapie to goats and sheep by the oral route, *J Comp Pathol*, **71**: 171–6.

Pattison IH, Millson GC, 1961b, Scrapie produced experimentally in goats with special reference to the clinical syndrome, *J Comp Pathol*, **71**: 101–8.

Pattison IH, Hoare MN et al., 1972, Spread of scrapie to sheep and goats by oral dosing with foetal membranes from scrapie-affected sheep, *Vet Rec*, **90**: 465–8.

Pearson GR, Wyatt JM et al., 1992, Feline spongiform encephalopathy: fibril and PrP studies, *Vet Rec*, **131**: 307–10.

Petersen RB, Tabaton M et al., 1992, Analysis of the prion protein gene in thalamic dementia, *Neurology*, **42**: 1859–63.

Pocchiari M, Peano S et al., 1991, Combination ultrafiltration and 6 M urea treatment of human growth hormone effectively minimizes risk from potential Creutzfeldt–Jakob disease virus contamination, *Horm Res*, **35**: 161–6.

Pocchiari M, Salvatore M et al., 1993, A new point mutation of the prion protein gene in familial and sporadic cases of Creutzfeldt–Jakob disease, *Ann Neurol*, **34**: 802–7.

Poidinger M, Kirkwood J, Almond W, 1993, Sequence analysis of the PrP protein from two species of antelope susceptible to transmissible spongiform encephalopathy, *Arch Virol*, **131**: 193–9.

Poulter M, Baker HF et al., 1992, Inherited prion disease with 144 base pair gene insertion. 1. Genealogical and molecular studies, *Brain*, **115**: 675–85.

Powell-Jackson J, Weller RO et al., 1985, Creutzfeldt–Jakob disease after administration of human growth hormone, *Lancet*, **2**: 244–6.

Prusiner SB, 1982, Novel proteinaceous infectious particles cause scrapie, *Science*, **216**: 136–44.

Prusiner SB, 1989, Scrapie prions, *Annu Rev Microbiol*, **43**: 345–74.

Prusiner SB, 1991, Molecular biology of prion diseases, *Science*, **252**: 1515–22.

Prusiner SB, 1993, Transgenetics and cell biology of prion diseases: investigations of PrP^{Sc} synthesis and diversity, *Br Med Bull*, **49**: 873–912.

Prusiner SB, 1994, Inherited prion diseases, *Proc Natl Acad Sci USA*, **91**: 4611–4.

Prusiner SB, DeArmond SJ, 1994, Prion diseases and neurodegeneration, *Annu Rev Neurosci*, **17**: 311–39.

Prusiner SB, Gajdusek DC, Alpers MP, 1982, Kuru with incubation periods exceeding two decades, *Ann Neurol*, **12**: 1–9.

Prusiner SB, Hadlow WJ et al., 1978, Partial purification and evidence for multiple molecular forms of the scrapie agent, *Biochemistry*, **17**: 4993–7.

Prusiner SB, Groth DF et al., 1980a, Molecular properties, partial purification, and assay by incubation period measurements of the hamster scrapie agent, *Biochemistry*, **19**: 4883–91.

Prusiner SB, Groth DF et al., 1980b, Gel electrophoresis and glass permeation chromatography of the hamster scrapie agent after enzymatic digestion and detergent extraction, *Biochemistry*, **19**: 4892–8.

Prusiner SB, McKinley MP et al., 1981, Scrapie agent contains a hydrophobic protein, *Proc Natl Acad Sci USA*, **78**: 6675–9.

Prusiner SB, Bolton DC et al., 1982a, Further purification and characterization of scrapie prions, *Biochemistry*, **21**: 6942–50.

Prusiner SB, Cochran SP et al., 1982b, Measurement of the scrapie agent using an incubation time interval assay, *Ann Neurol*, **11**: 353–8.

Prusiner SB, McKinley MP et al., 1983, Scrapie prions aggregate to form amyloid-like birefringent rods, *Cell*, **35**: 349–58.

Prusiner SB, Groth DF et al., 1984, Purification and structural studies of a major scrapie prion protein, *Cell*, **38**: 127–34.

Prusiner SB, Scott M et al., 1990, Transgenetic studies implicate interactions between homologous PrP isoforms in scrapie prion replication, *Cell*, **63**: 673–86.

Prusiner SB, Fuzi M et al., 1993a, Immunologic and molecular biological studies of prion proteins in bovine spongiform encephalopathy, *J Infect Dis*, **167**: 602–13.

Prusiner SB, Groth D et al., 1993b, Ablation of the prion protein (PrP) gene in mice prevents scrapie and facilitates production of anti-PrP antibodies, *Proc Natl Acad Sci USA*, **90**: 10608–12.

Puckett C, Concannon P et al., 1991, Genomic structure of the human prion protein gene, *Am J Hum Genet*, **49**: 320–9.

Raeber AJ, Borchelt DR et al., 1992, Attempts to convert the cellular prion protein into the scrapie isoform in cell-free systems, *J Virol*, **66**: 6155–63.

Ridley RM, Baker HF, 1993, Occupational risk of Creutzfeldt–Jakob disease, *Lancet*, **341**: 641–2.

Ripoll L, Laplanche J-L et al., 1993, A new point mutation in the prion protein gene at codon 210 in Creutzfeldt–Jakob disease, *Neurology*, **43**: 1934–8.

Roberts GW, Lofthouse R et al., 1986, Prion–protein immunoreactivity in human transmissible dementias, *N Engl J Med*, **315**: 1231–3.

Roberts GW, Lofthouse R et al., 1988, CNS amyloid proteins in neurodegenerative diseases, *Neurology*, **38**: 1534–40.

Rogers M, Serban D et al., 1991, Epitope mapping of the Syrian hamster prion protein utilizing chimeric and mutant genes in a vaccinia virus expression system, *J Immunol*, **147**: 3568–74.

Rogers M, Yehiely F et al., 1993, Conversion of truncated and elongated prion proteins into the scrapie isoform in cultured cells, *Proc Natl Acad Sci USA*, **90**: 3182–6.

Roos R, Gajdusek DC, Gibbs CJ Jr, 1973, The clinical characteristics of transmissible Creutzfeldt–Jakob disease, *Brain*, **96**: 1–20.

Rosenthal NP, Keesey J et al., 1976, Familial neurological disease associated with spongiform encephalopathy, *Arch Neurol*, **33**: 252–9.

Safar J, Roller PP et al., 1993a, Conformational transitions, dissociation, and unfolding of scrapie amyloid (prion) protein, *J Biol Chem*, **268**: 20276–84.

Safar J, Roller PP et al., 1993b, Thermal-stability and conformational transitions of scrapie amyloid (prion) protein correlate with infectivity, *Protein Sci*, **2**: 2206–16.

Sailer A, Büeler H et al., 1994, No propagation of prions in mice devoid of PrP, *Cell*, **77**: 967–8.

Sawcer SJ, Yuill GM et al., 1993, Creutzfeldt–Jakob disease in an individual occupationally exposed to BSE, *Lancet*, **341**: 642.

Scott M, Foster D et al., 1989, Transgenic mice expressing hamster prion protein produce species-specific scrapie infectivity and amyloid plaques, *Cell*, **59**: 847–57.

Scott MR, Köhler R et al., 1992, Chimeric prion protein expression in cultured cells and transgenic mice, *Protein Sci*, **1**: 986–97.

Scott M, Groth D et al., 1993, Propagation of prions with artificial properties in transgenic mice expressing chimeric PrP genes, *Cell*, **73**: 979–88.

Serban D, Taraboulos A et al., 1990, Rapid detection of Creutzfeldt–Jakob disease and scrapie prion proteins, *Neurology*, **40**: 110–7.

Shyng S-L, Heuser JE, Harris DA, 1994, A glycolipid-anchored prion protein is endocytosed via clathrin-coated pits, *J Cell Biol*, **125**: 1239–50.

Sparkes RS, Simon M et al., 1986, Assignment of the human and mouse prion protein genes to homologous chromosomes, *Proc Natl Acad Sci USA*, **83**: 7358–62.

Spudich S, Mastrianni JA et al., 1995, Complete penetrance of Creutzfeldt–Jakob disease in Libyan Jews carrying the E200K mutation in the prion protein gene, *Mol Med*, **1**: 607–13.

Stahl N, Borchelt DR et al., 1987, Scrapie prion protein contains a phosphatidylinositol glycolipid, *Cell*, **51**: 229–40.

Stahl N, Baldwin MA et al., 1992, Glycosylinositol phospholipid anchors of the scrapie and cellular prion proteins contain sialic acid, *Biochemistry*, **31**: 5043–53.

Stahl N, Baldwin MA et al., 1993, Structural analysis of the scrapie prion protein using mass spectrometry and amino acid sequencing, *Biochemistry*, **32**: 1991–2002.

Stender A, 1930, Weitere Beiträge zum Kapitel 'Spastische Pseudosklerose Jakobs', *Z Neurol Psychiat*, **128**: 528–43.

Tagliavini F, Prelli F et al., 1991, Amyloid protein of Gerstmann–Sträussler–Scheinker disease (Indiana kindred) is an 11-kD fragment of prion protein with an N-terminal glycine at codon 58, *EMBO J*, **10**: 513–9.

Tagliavini F, Prelli F et al., 1994, Amyloid fibrils in Gerstmann–Sträussler–Scheinker disease (Indiana and Swedish kindreds) express only PrP peptides encoded by the mutant allele, *Cell*, **79**: 695–703.

Tange RA, Troost D, Limburg M, 1989, Progressive fatal dementia (Creutzfeldt–Jakob disease) in a patient who received homograft tissue for tympanic membrane closure, *Eur Arch Otorhinolaryngol*, **247**: 199–201.

Taraboulos A, Serban D, Prusiner SB, 1990, Scrapie prion proteins accumulate in the cytoplasm of persistently infected cultured cells, *J Cell Biol*, **110**: 2117–32.

Taraboulos A, Rogers M et al., 1990, Acquisition of protease resistance by prion proteins in scrapie-infected cells does not require asparagine-linked glycosylation, *Proc Natl Acad Sci USA*, **87**: 8262–6.

Taraboulos A, Jendroska K et al., 1992a, Regional mapping of prion proteins in brains, *Proc Natl Acad Sci USA*, **89**: 7620–4.

Taraboulos A, Raeber AJ et al., 1992b, Synthesis and trafficking of prion proteins in cultured cells, *Mol Biol Cell*, **3**: 851–63.

Taraboulos A, Scott M et al., 1995, Cholesterol depletion and modification of COOH-terminal targeting sequence of the prion protein inhibit formation of the scrapie isoform, *J Cell Biol*, **129**: 121–32.

Tateishi J, Kitamoto T, 1993, Developments in diagnosis for prion diseases, *Br Med Bull*, **49**: 971–9.

Tateishi J, Ohta M et al., 1979, Transmission of chronic spongiform encephalopathy with kuru plaques from humans to small rodents, *Ann Neurol*, **5**: 581–4.

Tateishi J, Doh-ura K et al., 1992, Prion protein gene analysis and transmission studies of Creutzfeldt–Jakob disease, *Prion Diseases of Humans and Animals*, eds Prusiner SB, Collinge J et al., Ellis Horwood, London, 129–34.

Taylor DM, Dickinson AG et al., 1985, Preparation of growth hormone free from contamination with unconventional slow viruses, *Lancet*, **2**: 260–2.

Telling GC, Scott M et al., 1994, Transmission of Creutzfeldt–Jakob disease from humans to transgenic mice expressing chimeric human–mouse prion protein, *Proc Natl Acad Sci USA*, **91**: 9936–40.

Telling GC, Scott M et al., 1995, Prion propagation in mice expressing human and chimeric PrP transgenes implicates the interaction of cellular PrP with another protein, *Cell*, **83**: 79–90.

Telling GT, Haga T et al., 1996, Interactions between wild-type and mutant prion proteins modulate neurodegeneration in transgenic mice, *Genes Dev*, **10**: 1736–50.

Thadani V, Penar PL et al., 1988, Creutzfeldt–Jakob disease probably acquired from a cadaveric dura mater graft. Case report, *J Neurosurg*, **69**: 766–9.

Titner R, Brown P et al., 1986, Neuropathologic verification of Creutzfeldt–Jakob disease in the exhumed American recipient of human pituitary growth hormone: epidemiologic and pathogenetic implications, *Neurology*, **36**: 932–6.

Turk E, Teplow DB et al., 1988, Purification and properties of the cellular and scrapie hamster prion proteins, *Eur J Biochem*, **176**: 21–30.

Udovitch AL, Valensi L, 1984, *The Last Arab Jews: The Communities of Jerba, Tunisia*, Harwood Academic Publ, London.

Vnencak-Jones CL, Phillips JA, 1992, Identification of heterogeneous PrP gene deletions in controls by detection of allele-specific heteroduplexes (DASH), *Am J Hum Genet*, **50**: 871–2.

Weissmann C, 1991, A 'unified theory' of prion propagation, *Nature (London)*, **352**: 679–83.

Wells GAH, Scott AC et al., 1987, A novel progressive spongiform encephalopathy in cattle, *Vet Rec*, **121**: 419–20.

Westaway D, Goodman PA et al., 1987, Distinct prion proteins in short and long scrapie incubation period mice, *Cell*, **51**: 651–62.

Westaway D, Mirenda CA et al., 1991, Paradoxical shortening of scrapie incubation times by expression of prion protein transgenes derived from long incubation period mice, *Neuron*, **7**: 59–68.

Westaway D, Cooper C et al., 1994a, Structure and polymorphism of the mouse prion protein gene, *Proc Natl Acad Sci USA*, **91**: 6418–22.

Westaway D, DeArmond SJ et al., 1994b, Degeneration of skeletal muscle, peripheral nerves, and the central nervous system in transgenic mice overexpressing wild-type prion proteins, *Cell*, **76**: 117–29.

Westaway D, Zuliani V et al., 1994c, Homozygosity for prion protein alleles encoding glutamine-171 renders sheep susceptible to natural scrapie, *Genes Dev*, **8**: 959–69.

Wickner RB, 1994, [URE3] as an altered URE2 protein: evidence for a prion analog in *Saccharomyces cerevisiae*, *Science*, **264**: 566–9.

Wilesmith J, Wells GAH, 1991, Bovine spongiform encephalopathy, *Curr Top Microbiol Immunol*, **172**: 21–38.

Wilesmith JW, Wells GAH et al., 1988, Bovine spongiform encephalopathy: epidemiological studies, *Vet Rec*, **123**: 638–44.

Wilesmith JW, Hoinville LJ et al., 1992a, Bovine spongiform encephalopathy: aspects of the clinical picture and analyses of possible changes 1986–1990, *Vet Rec*, **130**: 197–201.

Wilesmith JW, Ryan JBM et al., 1992b, Bovine spongiform encephalopathy: epidemiological features 1985 to 1990, *Vet Rec*, **130**: 90–4.

Will RG, Matthews WB, 1982, Evidence for case-to-case transmission of Creutzfeldt–Jakob disease, *J Neurol Neurosurg Psychiatry*, **45**: 235–8.

Will RG, Ironside JW et al., 1996, A new variant of Creutzfeld–Jakob disease in the UK, *Lancet*, **347**: 921–5.

Williams ES, Young S, 1980, Chronic wasting disease of captive mule deer: a spongiform encephalopathy, *J Wildl Dis*, **16**: 89–98.

Williams ES, Young S, 1982, Spongiform encephalopathy of Rocky Mountain Elk, *J Wildl Dis*, **18**: 465–71.

Williams RC, 1954, Electron microscopy of viruses, *Adv Virus Res*, **2**: 183–239.

Willison HJ, Gale AN, McLaughlin JE, 1991, Creutzfeldt–Jakob disease following cadaveric dura mater graft, *J Neurol Neurosurg Psychiatry*, **54**: 940.

Willoughby K, Kelly DF et al., 1992, Spongiform encephalopathy in a captive puma (*Felis concolor*), *Vet Rec*, **131**: 431–4.

Wilson DR, Anderson RD, Smith W, 1950, Studies in scrapie, *J Comp Pathol*, **60**: 267–82.

Zhang H, Kaneko K et al., 1995, Conformational transitions in peptides containing two putative α-helices of the prion protein, *J Mol Biol*, **250**: 514–26.

Part IV

Syndromes caused by a range of viruses

Chapter 40

Infections of the central nervous

system

Sibylle Schneider-Schaulies, Lee M Dunster and V ter Meulen

1	Interaction of viruses with the human CNS	3 Conclusions and outlook
2	Viruses and associated CNS disorders in humans	

Viral infections of the central nervous system (CNS) represent clinically important, often life-threatening complications of systemic viral infections. Except for rabies, they do not result *per se* from a pathogen-specific tropism for neural tissue, as most viruses associated with CNS disorders frequently infect humans without involvement of this organ. Some of these viruses cause clinically significant diseases only when invasion of the CNS takes place, for example certain entero- or arthropod-borne viruses. Other agents such as herpes simplex or mumps viruses usually induce a mild illness, which may follow a more severe course when infecting the CNS. The establishment of a CNS viral infection depends not only on the biological properties of the invading agent but also on the breakdown of the host defence mechanisms that normally protect CNS cells from infection. Moreover, the degree of damage to CNS tissues is influenced by several special features that set the CNS apart from other tissues. Brain cells are not unusual in their fine structure, but they are unique in the high degree of cell differentiation and the interaction between cell types as revealed by the synapses between neurons and the relationship between myelin sheath and axons. These peculiarities, together with the existence of a blood–brain barrier in the absence of lymphatic tissue in the CNS, play a major role in the development of neurological disease.

Since the mid-1980s, virological, immunological and molecular biological studies have provided important information on the aetiology and pathogenesis of many acute and chronic disorders of the CNS associated with viral infections of animals and humans. In addition, information obtained from in vitro studies of persistently infected cells in culture has helped our understanding of the processes involved in a wide range of virus-induced neurological diseases. Although many unresolved problems still remain, great progress has been made in molecular virology and neuroimmunology. Many sensitive techniques have been developed that allow a better characterization of the virus–cell and virus–host interactions occurring in CNS infections. In particular, probes with high specific activity have emerged as essential tools in the search for aetiological agents and in the identification of infected cell populations in the CNS.

Rather than give a complete account of all virus infections of the CNS, this chapter concentrates on the virus infections that either have furthered our understanding of the aetiology and pathogenesis of the disease processes or have helped to unravel the nature of virus–host interactions. Rabies is dealt with separately in Chapter 33 and prion diseases in Chapter 39.

1   INTERACTIONS OF VIRUSES WITH THE HUMAN CNS

1.1   Pathways of virus spread to the nervous system

Successful infection of the CNS by virus depends on a number of factors, and it is the direct interplay between the host's immune system in controlling or attenuating infection on the one hand, and the neurotropism and neurovirulence of the infecting virus on the other, that has profound consequences for the host. Virus invasion of the CNS can be established via any of the commonly recognized routes for infection: vector-borne, faecal–oral, direct contact and aerosol.

Vector-borne

The most common route of infection associated with severe disorders of the CNS is via the bite of an infected arthropod vector which delivers virus inoculum through the dead keratinized layer of the skin into the dermis or blood stream. The human skin forms a formidable barrier to invading pathogens; the outer (dead) layer does not support virus replication and so must be breached for infection of living cells to occur. Viruses belonging to the families *Alphaviridae*, *Bunyaviridae* and *Flaviviridae* are usually transmitted to humans through the bite of an infected mosquito or tick, after the virus has replicated to high titres in the salivary glands of the insect. A number of the arthropod-borne viruses (arboviruses) are highly pathogenic and the CNS is often involved. Of the viruses commonly associated with CNS disease, Japanese encephalitis virus, a flavivirus, is the most important, with thousands of reported infections each year and an associated case fatality rate of c. 10% (see section 2.4, p. 855). Infection with arboviruses is limited geographically to areas supporting the virus vector, hence outbreaks of disease are often limited to particular regions; distinct seasonal patterns of disease are also encountered that relate to vector densities.

Faecal–oral

The faecal–oral route has long been established as an important mode of transmission of numerous enteroviruses and classically with epidemics of poliomyelitis. Enteric viruses, which replicate primarily in the alimentary tract, are shed in faecal matter which in turn may contaminate food and water supplies, particularly in areas of poor sanitation. These viruses are able to resist and survive gastric acidity. Enteric viruses are responsible for large epidemics of disease which, unlike the arboviruses mentioned above, are not restricted geographically. Within Europe enteroviruses are the leading cause of CNS disturbances although 90% of these infections are clinically inapparent. Of the remainder, symptoms may range from paralytic poliomyelitis to non-paralytic meningitis as well as the more rare encephalitides.

Direct contact

Direct contact (sexual, prenatal or by mechanical means, e.g. by needle, bite), as a mode of transmission for a number of viruses that cause CNS disease, is by nature a particularly emotive subject. Infection by direct contact involves the transfer of virus-infected cells or body fluids. These viruses include HIV-1 and 2, herpes simplex virus (HSV), rabies virus, and cytomegalovirus (CMV). More rarely, infection of the CNS with rabies virus or CMV has been reported following corneal tissue grafts. Vertical transfer of virus, commonly HSV, CMV, rubella, HTLV-I and HIV-1, from mother to fetus, may lead to severe CNS disease in newborns. In addition, breast-feeding by infected mothers is associated with HTLV-I, HIV and CMV infections in newborns.

Respiratory

Establishment of CNS infection via the respiratory tract is not widely recognized as a common event. The exception to this generalization is mumps virus when, during epidemics of parotitis, c. 0.1–10% of infected individuals develop quite severe meningitis. Infection of the CNS by rabies virus has been documented following the inhalation of virus-laden aerosols by visitors to bat caves, where the virus is mantained in the bat population, or in laboratory workers exposed to high concentrations of virus. Aerosols may also be associated with the transmission of other potentially neurotropic pathogens such as measles and varicella-zoster viruses.

Regardless of the site of entry, for successful infection of the host by a virus, a period of replication at this initial site is required and the virus must also evade local phagocytic cells that are an early form of host defence. The possible exception to the above concerns arthropod-borne viruses, which are often inoculated directly into the blood stream and initial replication is usually established in lymphatic tissue. Replication of virus at the site of entry or in lymphatic tissue increases the viral load and allows the establishment of viraemia. Once in the blood stream, virus is able to disseminate throughout the host and infection of susceptible secondary organs and tissues can take place. The ability of the immune system to terminate virus infection rapidly before significant viraemia levels are reached largely dictate the outcome of a number of potential viral diseases of the CNS. Two main routes for the invasion of the CNS by virus are recognized: the haematogenous route and the neural route.

ENTRY INTO THE CNS

The haematogenous route

The blood stream, with its extensive network of vessels serving every part of the body, forms the perfect dissemination vehicle for invading viruses. The extent to which tissues and organs become exposed to virus depends on the length of time that a high viral load is maintained in the blood stream and the efficiency with which the immune system can clear virus. Whether infection will be established by the virus depends on a number of factors, including the presence of specific cellular receptors for virus (see section 1.2, p. 837). Before virus can enter the CNS, the so-called blood–brain barrier (BBB) must be circumvented. The BBB comprises endothelial cells of the cerebral microvasculature, astrocyte foot processes and the basal lamina, which together are a formidable barrier. However, the CNS is accessible to activated lymphocytes and macrophages which, if infected with virus, afford access to this normally protected environment. Circumvention of the BBB by the transport of virus within infected cells is thought to be highly significant for CNS infection with mumps and measles viruses (Wolinsky, Klassen and Baringer 1976, Fournier et al. 1985) and HIV (Haase 1986). Direct infection of the endothelial cells of the BBB is the common method by which poliovirus traverses the

CNS, although direct infection of peripheral nerves by this virus in establishing CNS disease has not been definitively excluded. The choroid plexus is widely believed to be an important portal of entry for blood-borne virus to the CNS. This is based largely on the fine structure analysis of the choroid plexus itself, in which fenestrated endothelium and a sparse basement membrane combine to form a more permeable region. The choroid plexus is a major target of replication or tissue transport of mumps and arboviruses (or both) which subsequently infect ependymal cells lining the ventricles and finally the underlying brain tissue.

The neural route

A number of viruses establish CNS infection by directly infecting the nerves of the CNS. Viruses such as HSV, poliovirus and rabies (Sabin 1956, Martin and Dolvio 1983, Iwasaki et al. 1985) infect peripheral nerve endings and, by retrograde axonal transport, spread through the CNS. Entry into neurons is believed to occur via receptor-mediated endocytosis, after which virus is transported in vesicles. The exact mechanism of transport of virus within nerves remains to be established, although movement is known to occur via fast axonal transport (Kristensson 1982) which involves the passage of viral material in vesicles along microtubules. Viral replication occurs once virus particles reach the neuronal cell body and newly synthesized virion components accumulate at postsynaptic sites. It is interesting that high concentrations of receptors for certain viruses occur at synaptic terminals, which may in turn enhance virus spread. The site of inoculation can influence the ultimate distribution of lesions in the CNS, especially for viruses that spread along neural routes. For example, HSV infection of the genitourinary tract establishes latency of virus in the sacral ganglia, whereas infection with HSV orally establishes latency in the trigeminal ganglia. At the time of primary infection, HSV is transported from the mucous membrane by retrograde axonal transport, whereas during periods of reactivation virus is transported to the periphery by anterograde flow. Once the CNS has been invaded, advancement of infection by many neurotropic viruses occurs through cell-to-cell spread of virus although the more pathogenically important mode of spread is via the axoplasm of neurons. Viruses that are able to spread within neurons may also have the potential to spread from nerve cell to nerve cell (transneuronal transport). This seems to occur primarily at synapses (trans-synaptic transport).

The factors influencing the release of virus from presynaptic nerve terminals and the uptake of progeny at postsynaptic terminals are unknown. It is important to note that direct infection of peripheral nerve endings by virus may also take place during the viraemic phase of infection. For example, during the high titre viraemia found in clinically apparent infections of humans with the flavivirus Japanese encephalitis (JE) virus, the possibility that neurons of the olfactory bulb will be infected is enhanced. Retrograde transport of virus within specialized neurons is then possible. The olfactory mucosa itself offers a unique pathway for the spread of viruses into the CNS, where the apical processes of receptor cells penetrate beyond the surface of the epithelium as olfactory rods. However, olfactory uptake and spread is not a common route of virus infection of the CNS (Johnston 1994). Once in the CNS, the cellular tropism and neurovirulence of virus and its ability to avoid the immune response will largely determine the outcome of disease.

1.2   Tropism and neurovirulence

CELLULAR RECEPTORS AND HOST FACTORS

The ability of a virus to infect specific cell populations of the CNS defines its neurotropism, which is influenced either by host cell expression of receptors or by viral genes important for viral replication. In general, the distribution of specific virus cell receptors within a host governs the susceptibility of tissue(s) or organs, or both, to virus infection. The interaction of a specific receptor on a host cell with a viral cell attachment protein regulates viral entry and is a major determinant of viral tropism. In recent years, many cell surface proteins have been identified as viral receptors that normally serve various physiological functions. Some of these receptors have also been defined in the nervous system (a summary of the major receptors defined so far is given in Table 40.1).

Besides the viral receptor the virus attachment protein itself plays a central role in the initial interaction of the virus with its target cell. Numerous virus–cell attachment proteins have been identified by analysis of genetic recombinants, genetic reassortants and mutant viruses (Kennedy 1990). This approach has been used, for example, to define the neurotropism of serotype 3 reovirus, which has been mapped to the *S1* gene that encodes the σ1 protein (Tyler 1991). Similarly, neutralization escape mutants of rabies virus, with a single amino acid substitution in the envelope glycoprotein G that serves in viral cell attachment, revealed a lower virulence when compared to the parent virus (Tyler 1990). A more detailed molecular view of a ligand in virus receptor molecular interactions was obtained with the x-ray crystallographic analysis of the poliovirus virion. The analysis has shown that a series of peaks in the VP1 capsid proteins surrounded by a broad valley composed of VP1 and VP3 forms the receptor-binding pocket (Almond 1991). It is thought that other picornaviruses may have cell attachment proteins of similar topology. An exception to this is foot-and-mouth disease virus (FMDV), an aphthovirus, for which the virus attachment protein (VAP) is exposed on VP1 (Mason, Reider and Baxt 1994). Mutations occurring in the VAP may be responsible for altered tropism of virus or even defective virus that is no longer able to bind to its receptor. This may be manifested by attenuation of virus infectivity and is thought to be important in relation to the immunogenicity of vaccines.

In further attempts to unravel which factors govern neurovirulence of poliovirus, a combination of nucleotide sequencing and gene cloning identified the genetic differences between wild type and live attenuated vaccine strains of poliovirus (Almond 1991). Of the changes detected, the most significant were localized in the 5' non-translated

Table 40.1 List of viruses associated with CNS disease and their receptors

Virus (family)	Receptor	References
Picornaviridae		
Polioviruses	PVR (immunoglobulin-like)	Koike et al. 1990
		Mendelson, Wimmer and
		Racanielle 1989
Echovirus 1, 8	VLA-2 (α-chain)	Bergelson et al. 1992, 1993
Echovirus 22	$\alpha_v\beta_3$ (vibronectin)	Roivainan et al. 1991
Coxsackievirus 9		
Echovirus 7 (6, 11, 12, 20, 21?)	Decay-accelerating factor	Bergelson et al. 1994
	(CD55)	
Rhabdoviridae		
Rabies virus	Acetylcholine receptor (α-1)	Lentz 1990
Paramyxoviridae		
Measles virus	Membrane co-factor protein	Dörig et al. 1993
	(CD46)	Naniche et al. 1993
Lentiviridae		
HIV-1, 2	CD4	Dalgleish et al. 1984
		Klatzmann et al. 1984
HIV-1	Galactosylceramide	Harouse et al. 1991
Herpesviridae		
Human CMV	Heparan sulphate	Compton et al. 1993
HSV	Heparan sulphate	WuDunn and Spear 1989

region (NTR) at positions 480, 481 and 472 of poliovirus serotypes 1, 2 and 3, respectively. These mutations were associated with the ability of virus to replicate in the brains of mice or neuroblastoma cells in culture (La Monica, Almond and Racaniello 1987). A more detailed investigation of both the structure and the related function of mutated 5′ NTR regions of poliovirus revealed that attenuating mutations in vaccine strains act through the disruption of a stem–loop structure in the region of nucleotide positions 470–540. Computer-generated analysis has hinted that the greater the disruption of the system structure, the greater the temperature sensitivity and the degree of attenuation. Further analysis of the intracellular protein interactions associated with this poliovirus stem–loop structure may provide an explanation of why motor neurons are the specific targets of these viruses.

In addition to viral factors, host factors also influence viral tropism and virulence and modulate the viral pathogenesis of CNS infections. In this context, a lack of enzymatic activity required for maturational cleavage of viral proteins or completion of the virus replicating cycles will lead to incomplete infection of target cells, thereby limiting tropism and spread of virus. Moreover, it has been observed that many neurotropic viruses more readily invade the CNS of the young owing to an immature immune response, reduced capacity to produce interferon and dependence of susceptibility of viral infection on the stage of cell differentiation as well as the age-specific nature and distribution of receptor proteins (Coyle 1991). Bias of infection for a particular gender has also been noted. The CNS disorder tropical spastic paraparesis/HTLV-I associated myelopathy (TSP/HAM), for which HTLV-I is the proposed aetiological agent, has a prevalence in females with the female/male ratio of 1.6 : 1. Also of interest is the finding that polymorphous host genes can modulate the severity of most virus infections and that a particular locus seems to govern resistance to a specific pathogen. Human chromosome 21 is important in the susceptibility of individuals to influenza A and B infections

(Reeves et al. 1988). Genes controlling any of the numerous host-encoded post-translational modifying mechanisms may affect maturation of virus. Polymorphous resistant genes may act at different levels: at the target cell level where control of protein processing may be modulated, or at the whole organism level where antiviral effector mechanisms are regulated.

NEUROVIRULENCE AND VIRAL GENE EXPRESSION

Neurovirulence is the capacity of a virus to multiply and to extend infection after it has invaded the nervous system. This property together with the effectiveness of the host immune response determine the degree of tissue damage. Many viruses contain genetic elements, referred to as promoters or enhancers, that increase the transcription of specific genes. It is interesting that virus enhancers may exhibit cell or tissue specificity, and possibly species specificity, thus promoting or limiting virus infection. It has recently been proposed that HIV may contain cell type-specific enhancer regions within the long-terminal repeat (LTR) sequence and that differences within the LTR region could account for altered tropism of HIV in relation to macrophage or lymphocyte infection (Corboy et al. 1992). Important roles for viral enhancer elements in determining cell type-specific gene expression have also been described for papovaviruses. In the case of JC virus infection of the CNS in progressive multifocal leucoencephalopathy, an enhancer element confers tissue-specific expression in human oligodendrocytes (Feigenbaum et al. 1987).

The available data suggest that, in general, the outer capsid or envelope glycoproteins of neurotropic viruses are probably important determinants of virulence. This assumption is based, for instance, on the observation that amino acid sequence changes, of proteins or genetic reassortments between virulent and avirulent strains of a given neurotropic virus, can lead to an attenuated infection. On the other hand, not all changes in viral genes result in attenuation, as mutations causing reversions to neurovirulence have been seen in poliovirus isolates from vaccine recipients (Almond 1987). Moreover, when one region of a viral protein is linked to neurotropism and neurovirulence, changes in that protein could have dramatic effects on the resulting infections, as documented in studies of Theiler's murine encephalomyelitis virus infections (Nash 1991). Taken together, the interplay of host and viral factors determines tropism and virulence of viruses infecting the CNS.

1.3 Virus–cell interactions in the CNS

The interaction of infectious viruses with susceptible cells leads in general to cell destruction and is largely determined by the genetic constitution of the host cell and by the type of viral agent. This destruction can occur following cytolysis, persistent or even latent infection, cell transformation or be caused by infection-independent mechanisms. After infectious virus has reached the CNS, disease develops only if viral spread is accomplished and sufficient numbers of susceptible cells are infected resulting in brain dysfunction. In this respect, a number of unique features of the CNS are noteworthy. First, the CNS contains a highly differentiated cell population with complex functionally integrated cell-to-cell connections and highly specialized cytoplasmic membranes. This probably results in the great variability in virus receptor sites and their density on cells. Second, CNS tissue is unique in its high metabolic rate and a low regenerative capacity. Although persistent infection by a noncytopathogenic virus in cells of tissue with a low energy requirement and a high rate of regeneration may be tolerated, in CNS tissue such infections may interfere with normal cell functions, especially when neurons are affected. Third, the brain's relative isolation from the immune system is another feature that plays an important role in the establishment and pathogenesis of CNS infections.

ACUTE INFECTIONS

Acute infections lead to cell death and the release of progeny virus. Cell destruction is induced by the products of the viral genome or their effect on the regulatory mechanism of the cell. For some viruses, such as herpes and poliomyelitis virus, the molecular events during a lytic infection have been well described for tissue culture systems and it may be inferred that similar processes occur during CNS infections. One of the most severe acute viral infections of the CNS is caused by herpes simplex virus (HSV), which results mainly from the primary infection. Productive replication in brain tissue leads to cell destruction, which in its extent and pathology depends on the neuroinvasiveness and neurovirulence of the virus and on the effec-

tiveness of the host defence mechanisms. Extensive molecular biological studies have defined several regions on the viral genome as specific contributors to these processes (Stevens 1993). Among the HSV genes, 37 seem not to be necessary for HSV replication in tissue culture, and are referred to as 'supplemental essential genes'. They may be linked to the properties of neuroinvasiveness and neurovirulence by allowing the virus to invade the CNS, to replicate in a variety of different brain cells and to spread efficiently from cell to cell. Another destructive disease of nervous tissue occurs after poliovirus infection (Melnick 1990). Poliovirus, of which 3 serotypes exist, is a member of the *Enterovirus* genus, which contains an RNA genome of a single-stranded positive-sense molecule that closely resembles a cellular mRNA in structure and function (Kitamura et al. 1981). Following primary replication of poliovirus in the tonsils, the lymph nodes of the neck, Peyer's patches in the small intestine or its spread along the axons of peripheral nerves, poliovirus may enter the brain and the spinal cord. Here, neuronal tissue can be damaged or completely destroyed as a consequence of intracellular replication. The anterior and, in severe cases, the posterior horn cells of the spinal cord are most prominently involved, resulting in a flaccid paralysis.

PERSISTENT INFECTIONS

Within the group of viruses that can establish persistent infections, a variety of virus-cell and virus-host interactions exist that lead to a number of different disease processes.

1 Latent viral infections are characterized by intermittent episodes of viral replication and formation of infectious virus (recurrence). This may either remain clinically silent or result in clinical disease (recrudescence). In between these episodes, the virus remains within the host in a quiescent form.
2 In chronic viral infections, virus can be reproducibly and continuously recovered from the host, with or without development of clinical disease. Disease may be caused by the replication of virus or by immunopathological mechanisms.
3 In slow virus infections, a long incubation period of months to years is followed by a slow, progressive disease course that is usually fatal. The concentration of virus in the CNS increases until disease becomes clinically apparent.

The establishment and maintenance of persistent or latent infections in the CNS may be governed by viral factors or host cell factors, or both, depending on the individual virus–host cell relationships. As a general mechanism, virus-induced apoptosis may be an important pathogenic mechanism of CNS damage. In contrast, virus-mediated inhibition of the apoptotic pathway has been linked to the establishment of persistent infections in brain cells (Levine et al. 1991). In the human nervous system, only the latent and the slow virus type of infection are found. The classic latent infection is caused by HSV types 1 and 2. HSV is transmitted from human to human by skin or mucous membrane contact, and is able to remain latent in the nervous system for the lifetime of the host. Its occurrence is not restricted to sensory neurons and it has also been detected in neurons of peripheral nerve ganglia, the adrenal medulla, retina and the CNS (Stevens 1993). The establishment of the latent phase is controlled and executed by the neuron rather than by the virus itself, and HSV gene expression is almost completely abolished except for the expression of a set of so-called latency associated transcripts (LATs). No infectious virus can be isolated during latency. Although the underlying molecular events that trigger viral reactivation are still unknown, clinical observations indicate that recurrence is associated with physical or emotional stress, immune suppression, UV light or nerve damage. HSV in latently infected neurons is refractive to the immune system and cannot be cleared from those cells. The role of the immune system in controlling HSV infection is not entirely clear, because recurrences can be observed even in the presence of an apparently normal cell-mediated and humoral immune response. Although there seems to be no impact on nerve function during silent periods of latency, reactivation of HSV leads to the destruction of infected neurons.

The best studied slow virus disease of humans associated with a conventional virus is subacute sclerosing panencephalitis (SSPE) (ter Meulen, Stephenson and Kreth 1983). The disease develops after the establishment of a persistent measles virus (MV) infection in brain cells months to years after acute measles. How and when the virus reaches the CNS, and the mechanisms that trigger the disease, remain unknown. In brain material obtained *post mortem*, the accumulation of viral nucleocapsids in virtually any CNS cell population together with a general failure to reisolate infectious virus point to the presence of a defective viral replication cycle. This has been intensively investigated during the last decade. In general, gene functions required for intracellular amplification of the viral genome are functionally maintained whereas those associated with viral maturation and budding are highly restricted. This allows the virus to survive and replicate intracellularly while evading immune surveillance. In fact, an exceedingly high humoral immune response against MV proteins, except for the matrix (M) protein, in both serum and CSF of patients with SSPE is pathognomonic.

INFECTION-INDEPENDENT MECHANISMS

Viral invasion of the CNS may not always lead to infection of susceptible cells, but it may trigger pathological changes in the absence of viral spread. This is particularly important in parainfectious conditions, such as acute measles encephalitis in which the presence of the infectious agent cannot be unequivocally demonstrated or HIV in which the infected CNS cells can support only minimal viral replication. As detailed in section 2.5 (p. 857), the latter virus–host relationship has been studied intensively. As is apparent from tissue culture studies and animal experiments, HIV gene products such as gp120 and nef, as well as soluble factors and nitric oxide released from virus-infected microglial cells, may contribute to the pathogenesis of HIV brain infections. This occurs by the induction of neuronal damage and the functional impairment of both neuronal and macroglial cells that *per se* seem not to be susceptible to viral infection. Moreover, recent experimental evidence suggests that some viruses may trigger apoptosis in neural cells, thus leading to rapid destruction of the host cell before virus is efficiently replicated (Levine et al. 1991).

IMPACT ON SPECIFIC NEURAL CELL FUNCTIONS

The interaction of a virus with the CNS may cause severe dysfunction of the infected cell, even if only restricted areas of the CNS are involved. In rat astrocytoma cells persistently infected with MV, a strong reduction in the cAMP response to catecholamines was observed, the density of β-adrenergic receptors was decreased by 50% and their G protein coupling was affected (Halbach and Koschel 1979, Koschel and Münzel 1980). The endothelin-1-induced Ca^{2+} signal was absent in the same cells, 95% of the binding sites for endothelin-1 being lost (Tas and Koschel 1991).

A further example of the direct disturbance of brain cell functions is infection with rabies virus (RV). This virus causes a non-lytic infection of brain cells that rapidly leads to the death of the infected individual. In contrast to the limited cytopathology, death seems to result from interference of the virus with neuronal cell functions in vital centres of the brain that regulate sleep, body temperature and respiration (Tsiang 1993). The uptake and release of γ-aminobutyric acid (GABA) was reduced by 45% in the cortical neurons of rabies-infected embryonic rats (Ladogana et al. 1994) and binding of 5-hydroxytryptamine to serotonin receptor subtypes was reduced by 50% in infected rat brains (Ceccaldi et al. 1993). It is conceivable that disturbances of specialized receptor sytems for neurotransmitter and neurohormone turnover, as well as for the generation of chemical signals and electrical potentials, might be the main cause of death in this viral infection, rather than cytopathic effects or immunopathogenesis. (See also Chapter 33.)

INDUCTION OF CYTOKINE EXPRESSION IN THE BRAIN

Cytokines are produced in response to viral infection in the CNS and are secreted either from infected brain cells or from lymphomononuclear cell infiltrates. Virus-induced cytokine patterns in CSF and in brain tissue of both humans and experimentally infected animals have been intensively studied. Although individual variations may be observed between different virus infections, there seems to be a common set of cytokines present in the CNS, as in the periphery. These include type I (IFN-α/β) and type II (IFN-γ) interferons, the proinflammatory cytokines interleukin (IL)-1 and tumour necrosis factor (TNF)-α, IL-6 and, generally in lower amounts, IL-2 (Maudsley, Morris and Tomkins 1989, Plata-Salaman 1991). For example, in CSF of SSPE patients elevated levels of IFN-α/β are observed and brain cells staining for IFN-γ and TNF-α have been detected in autopsy material (Joncas et al. 1976, Cosby et al. 1989, Hofmann et al. 1991). In the brains of HIV-1 infected patients, where CD4+ microglial cells may constitute the only cell population supporting viral replication, these cells are the source of intrathecal synthesis of IL-1, IL-6, granulocyte macrophage colony stimulating factor (GM-CSF) and TNF-α (Merrill and Chen 1991). The multiple effects of cytokines in the CNS may be beneficial in stimulating immunological surveillance and intracellular viral resistance (mainly type I and II IFNs and TNF-α) (Schijns et al. 1991, Shankar et al. 1992). This occurs by recruiting and activating cells of the immune system as well as by inducing MHC molecules (Campbell 1991, Plata-Salaman 1991) or antiviral proteins such as MxA, P1 kinase (now referred to as PKR) or 2′,5′-A synthetase in brain cells that directly interfere with intracellular viral replication (Staeheli 1990). Triggering of immune responses and inflammatory reactions by proinflammatory cytokines such as IL-1 and TNF-α, together with the induction of neurotoxins (Giulian, Vaca and Noonan 1990) and reactive oxygen intermediates (Nathan 1992), may, however, also contribute directly to the immunopathology observed in most viral CNS conditions. Proinflammatory cytokines such as IL-1 or TNF-α produced by immune cells or by CNS cells in response to infection may be essential to the process of neuronal destruction (Quagliarello et al. 1991, Selmaj 1992), as indicated by the meningitis and BBB damage that followed injection of these cytokines into rat brains. Moreover, it has been shown for experimental allergic encephalitis that neurospecific T cells recruit activated inflammatory cells through the action of TNF-α and IFN-γ (Ruddle et al. 1990). In addition, these cytokines can prime macrophages for the production of inducible reactive oxygen and nitrogen intermediates (Ding, Nathan and Stuehr 1988), which are thought to play an important role in cytotoxicity (Nathan 1992).

Direct analysis of cytokine expression in human CNS diseases is often difficult to perform, because the production of cytokines may be localized, the levels may be very low and cytokines normally are rather unstable once secreted. Moreover, the role of cytokines in the development of viral CNS infection and in viral neuropathogenesis cannot be studied in humans for obvious reasons, so suitable animal models must be used. For example, experimentally induced CNS infections with Borna disease virus (BDV) in rats represent a recent example of an animal model to study the role of cytokines in neurological disorders (Stitz, Dietzschold and Carbone 1995). BDV is a negative-strand RNA virus that has been associated with CNS conditions in a variety of species, possibly including humans (Bode 1995). Induction of IL-1α, IL-2, IL-6, TNF-α and IFN-γ mRNA synthesis has been found in rat brains 2 weeks after intranasal infection, and IL-2 as well as IFN-γ mRNA expression correlated well with the appearance of CD4+ and CD8+ lymphocytes during the early stages of BDV infection (Shankar et al. 1992). Moreover, mRNA levels for inducible nitric oxide synthetase (iNOS) were up-regulated (Koprowski et al. 1993). It is interesting that the levels of iNOS mRNA correlated not only with the

degree of neurological involvement and CNS inflammation but also with the levels of TNF-α, IL-1 and IL-6 mRNA (Selmaj 1992), potential mediators of iNOS expression (Nathan 1992). In the chronic phase of the BDV infection of the CNS, levels of IL-1, IL-6 and TNF-α decreased dramatically, whereas mRNA levels for IFN-γ were greatly elevated, probably indicating that IFN-γ may act to reduce inflammation and to improve neurological signs during the transition phase from acute to chronic disease. In fact, IFN-γ has a pronounced synergistic effect in the TNF- and IL-1-mediated induction of manganese superoxide dismutase, which has been linked to protection of uninfected cells from reactive oxygen toxicity during immune responses (Harris et al. 1991). (See also Chapter 11, section 5.)

MHC EXPRESSION IN THE BRAIN AND ITS RELATION TO VIRAL INFECTION

An effective immunological response to viral infections of the CNS is undoubtedly hampered by the relative lack of MHC and adhesion molecule expression in this tissue (e.g. intercellular adhesion molecule 1, ICAM-1). MHC class I expression is believed to be virtually absent from the surface of neurons, whereas MHC class II expression is probably confined to microglia and to astrocytes after induction. These represent the most important antigen-presenting cells in the CNS. Much attention has been focused on the ability of certain cytokines such as IFN-γ and TNF-α to induce and up-regulate MHC and ICAM-1 expression on glial cells (Frohman et al. 1989). However, the presence of these factors in the CNS indicates that an inflammatory process had already been initiated, which is not likely to occur soon after the virus has entered the CNS. In support of this notion, IFN-γ and TNF-α independent up-regulation of MHC class I expression on a variety of cell types (reviewed in Maudsley, Morris and Tomkins 1989) and also MHC class II induction on otherwise negative cells (including astrocytes) have been described as more or less direct consequences of viral infection (Massa, Dörries and ter Meulen 1986, Massa et al. 1987). In addition, rapid augmentation of ICAM-1 expression has been found after MV infection of primary rat astroglial cells (Kraus et al. 1992). The mechanisms underlying virus-induced alterations of MHC expression on brain cells are not clear. As revealed by the latter study, MV infection alone was sufficient to increase astrocyte MHC class I and ICAM-1 expression, most probably mediated by MV-induced release of type I IFN.

Although it is certain that induction or augmentation (or both) of immunoregulatory surface molecules on the surface of brain cells is a prerequisite for an efficient immune response, their role in neuropathogenesis is unclear. For instance, MHC class II expression was readily inducible in the SJL and CBA mouse strains, which are susceptible to experimentally induced CNS infections with Theiler's virus, but not in the resistant Balb/c mice (Nash, Leyung and Wildy 1985). In contrast, BN rats, which live well with experimental coronavirus JHM or MV infections, showed a constitutive high MHC class II expression in the brain, whereas in Lewis rats, in which MHC class II expression occurs as a consequence of the viral infection, immunopathological (autoimmune) processes are observed in a significant proportion of animals. This illustrates that the early presence of immunoregulatory molecules in the brain may provide protection, whereas the same process could lead to pathology and disease when MHC molecules are expressed several days or weeks later (Sedgwick and Dörries 1991). Induction of MHC molecules on neural cells is, however, not sufficient to result in elimination of virus, as illustrated by observations in brain tissue from patients with progressive multifocal leucoencephalopathy (PML), a slow papovavirus infection predominantly involving oligodendrocytes. Here, both MHC class I and II are expressed in the lesions, yet viral clearance does not occur, probably because there are no reactive T cells generated by the immunosuppressed patients. This may allow the establishment of persistence and ultimately chronic viral infection with progressive disease (Achim and Wiley 1992).

1.4 The immune response to viral infections in the CNS

PASSAGE OF EFFECTOR LYMPHOCYTES INTO THE CNS

The blood–brain barrier (BBB) is the sentinel in the development of an inflammatory response in the CNS. Adhesion of lymphocytes and their subsequent migration through the capillary endothelium is essential for the development of an inflammatory reaction. Adhesion molecules expressed on the brain capillary endothelium act as important ligands to receptors on the surface of lymphocytes, and mediate both adhesion and subsequent migration (Cross 1992) (Fig. 40.1). Two families of molecules on the endothelium are well known in the initiation of adhesion. The inital binding seems to be mediated by those belonging to the selectin (CD62) family (E-selectin, L-selectin and P-selectin). The second family comprises the Ig superfamily of adhesion molecules such as ICAM-1 (CD54) and VCAM-1 (CD106) that bind to integrin molecules on lymphocytes (Springer 1994).

Migration is mediated by the secretion of chemoattractant molecules released by the endothelium as well as by astrocytes and microglial cells (Ransohoff et al. 1993). Because adhesion to the capillary endothelium is an important step before cell migration, it follows that factors influencing the expression of the receptor molecules on the capillary endothelium or on the lymphocyte surface are likely to influence the extent and severity of the inflammatory response. Proinflammatory cytokines such as IL-1, TNF-α and IFN-γ increase the expression of the Ig superfamily of adhesion receptors. In fact, ICAM-1 is expressed on CNS microvessels in experimental allergic encephalomyelitis (EAE) and its expression coincides with inflammatory cell infiltration (Canella, Cross and Raine 1991). Furthermore, in the human brain, ICAM-1 is expressed on vessels in viral encephalitic lesions (Sobel, Mitchell and Fondren 1990). Studies in vitro have shown that antibodies to proinflammatory cytokines, or cytokines that have an antagonistic affect such as transforming growth factor β2 (TGF-β2), alter the adhesion of lymphocytes to the capillary endothelium (Fabry et al. 1995). The anti-inflamma-

tory properties of TGF-β have been exploited in the amelioration of 2 distinct T cell-mediated EAEs (Racke et al. 1991, 1993), and it can interfere with the adhesion of lymphocytes to endothelial cells, possibly inhibiting the entry of effector cells into the CNS (Cai, Falanga and Chin 1991, Gamble and Vadas 1991). In support of this suggestion, TGF-β treatment in EAE does not influence the appearance of sensitized cells in peripheral blood and lymph nodes but does prevent accumulation of T cells in the brain and spinal cord. This suggests that the protective effect of TGF-β is exerted at the level of the target organ, the CNS, its vascular endothelium, or both (Santambrogio et al. 1993). The migration of T cells into the CNS has been widely accepted. It has been shown that T cells require prior activation to cross BBB (Hickey, Hsu and Kimura 1991). However, once the BBB was breached, no activation-dependent differences in the homing pattern of T lymphocytes were observed (Trotter and Steinman 1985). In EAE, the migration of a few specifically sensitized lymphocytes into the CNS can initiate autoimmune reactions (Werdelin and McCluskey 1971). After this step, lymphokines and chemokines are produced and released at the inflammatory site, leading to the influx of non-specific lymphocytes and monocytes.

THE HUMORAL IMMUNE RESPONSE IN THE CNS

The control of virus infection depends on efficient generation of both humoral and cell-mediated immune responses. Antibodies, which attack predominantly extracellular virus particles released from infected cells, are required to limit the spread of some viruses in the host. For example, it seems that the humoral immune reaction is essential in controlling poliovirus infections. For infections with other viruses such as varicella-zoster, cytomegalovirus or measles virus, T cell responses may be more important than antibody. In this context it is important to remember that the immune response to viral infections of the CNS is initiated in peripheral lymphoid tissue with subsequent entry of activated (end-differentiated) T cells into the meninges, brain parenchyma and cerebrospinal fluid (Sedgwick et al. 1991a, 1991b).

Inhibition of virus entry into the brain and blockade of intracerebral viral spread

Specific antibodies are the main tool of the infected host in preventing extracellular viral spread from primary sites of infection to other organs during viraemia (Sissons and Oldstone 1985). Virtually all viral CNS infections are preceded by primary peripheral infection, so it is obvious that virus neutralization and opsonization during viraemia comprise one of the most efficient defence reactions preventing viral entry into the CNS. Agammaglobulinaemic patients suffer more frequently from persistent CNS infections than do fully immunocompetent hosts (Smith, De Girolami and Hickey 1992), and peripheral virus-specific antibodies usually prevent neuroinvasion in perinatal viral hosts that do not display full immune competence.

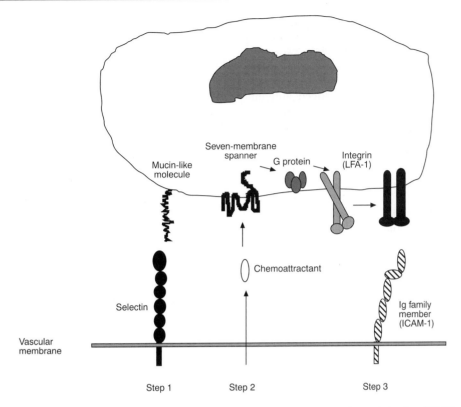

Fig. 40.1 Sequential steps in the traffic of leucocyte adhesion to the vascular endothelium. Selectins (CD62) on the surface of vascular endothelial cells initially interact with carbohydrate residues, often displayed on mucin-like molecules on flowing leucocytes to mediate a labile adhesion (step 1). This interaction brings leucocytes into close proximity with chemoattractants (released from the endothelial cells lining the vessel wall) which bind to receptors that span the membrane 7 times on the surface of leucocytes. Binding of chemoattractants to their receptors subsequently triggers activation of G proteins, which then transduce signals to activate integrin adhesiveness (e.g. by activating leucocyte function antigen 1, LFA-1) (step 2). The interaction of the latter with surface proteins of the Ig superfamily (expressed on the endothelial cells, such as intercellular adhesion molecule 1, ICAM-1) mediates strong adhesion, leading to an arrest of the rolling leucocyte (step 3). Following directional cues from chemoattractants and using integrins for traction, leucocytes then cross the endothelial lining of the blood–brain barrier and enter the CNS.

For example, lethal encephalomyelitis experimentally induced by the murine coronavirus JHM (JHMV) in newborn or suckling rats is prevented by nursing the babies from JHMV immunized mothers (Wege et al. 1983), and teratogenic effects induced by lymphocytic choriomeningitis virus (LCMV) in neonates are not observed when they are nursed by immunized mothers or injected with LCMV-specific neutralizing monoclonal antibodies (Baldrige and Buchmeier 1992, Baldrige et al. 1993). Moreover, experimental virus infections of the CNS in immunocompetent hosts usually remain subclinical, provided high titres of virus-neutralizing antibodies are mounted (Jubelt et al. 1991, Rima et al. 1991).

Nevertheless, in some instances, viruses escape extracerebral neutralization and invade the CNS. If retrograde transport occurs along the axons of peripheral nerves, the virus is inaccessible for an immune system. Neither virus-specific antibodies nor cytotoxic T lymphocytes (CTLs) can prevent the axonal transport of the virus to the CNS, particularly because nerve cells are thought to be unable to up-regulate MHC class I molecules (Momburg et al. 1986). Using leucocytes as 'Trojan horses' is another way to escape

neutralization by antibodies, although this hypothesis has so far not been supported by direct experimental evidence. Viral infection of peripheral recirculating monocytes may enhance invasion of the perivascular space in the CNS, because, in contrast to ramified microglia, the perivascular type of this cell is frequently exchanged by peripheral monocytes (Sedgwick et al. 1991a, 1991b, 1993).

Once in its target cell, the virus continues replicating and spreading in the CNS, until immune effector cells are recruited into the brain parenchyma. Plasma cells of the B lymphocyte lineage home to virus-infected sites in the tissue (Dörries et al. 1991), where they secrete virus-specific antibodies (Schwender, Imrich and Dörries 1991) and cytotoxic T lymphocytes provide an early virus-specific defence mechanism in the brain parenchyma. Although the latter may efficiently lyse virus-infected cells, formation of secondary virus-infected foci in the tissue by extracellular spread of the virus is prevented only when virus-specific antibodies are secreted intracerebrally in close proximity to infected sites. This has been confirmed in several animal models of virus-induced encephalitis. In addition to extracellular spread, virus-specific antibodies may inhibit dissemination from cell to cell, for example by interfering with cell fusion (Dietzschold et al. 1992). Moreover, antiviral antibodies may be directly involved in attenuating intracellular viral replication in vivo and in vitro. This concept, known as antibody-induced antigenic modulation (Fujinami and Oldstone 1980), has been established for MV infections in brain cells and mice with subacute combined immunodeficiency (SCID) infected with Sindbis virus (Levine et al. 1991).

Although it is generally assumed that the protective effect of a virus-neutralizing antibody in the CNS is mainly due to binding of its Fab part to viral epitopes necessary for infection of the target cell, the Fc part of the antibody molecule may also contribute. A monoclonal antibody specific for the yellow fever virus (YFV) non-structural protein NS1 protects mice from encephalitis only when given as an intact molecule, but not as an F(ab)2 fragment, which normally neutralizes YFV efficiently in vitro. Moreover, only monoclonal antibodies of the IgG2a subclass efficiently prevented acute encephalitis in this virus system, indicating that only binding of a distinct IgG subclass to NS1 allows recognition by FcR expressing cells. Similar observations have been made for Semliki Forest virus (SFV) infection of mice, in which IgG2a is the dominant subclass in the CSF, as well as for LCMV-induced encephalitis, which can be prevented with an IgG2a monoclonal antibody (Baldrige and Buchmeier 1992). In rabies virus-infected mice, however, protection from lethal disease is achieved by both IgG1 and IgG2a subclasses (Dietzschold et al. 1992).

Successful action of the humoral immune response requires very rapid migration of virus-specific plasma cells into the brain parenchyma. This is usually achieved if viral CNS infection occurs concomitantly with the acute peripheral infection and pre-existing plasma cells can immediately enter the brain tissue. When viral CNS infection occurs late after primary infection, the immune response has to be initiated in local secondary lymphatics such as the cervical lymph nodes. The period until humoral effector systems reach the brain parenchyma may be determined by the genetic background of the host, as documented for coronavirus JHM-induced encephalomyelitis in 2 genetically different rat strains (Schwender, Imrich and Dörries 1991).

Equally important for controlling virus-induced CNS infection are the specificity and effectiveness of the recruited humoral response. The effect of a late or a rather unspecific recruitment of humoral immunity to the CNS facilitates viral spread within the CNS. Consequently, large infected areas will result in a vigorous infiltration of virus-specific T cells, leading to enhancement of neurological disease. This intimate relation between virus-specific humoral response and T cell-mediated immunopathology was shown in acute LCMV-induced encephalitis of mice. In this model, mice injected with neutralizing antibodies before and shortly after viral infection were protected from lethal encephalitis and CTL responses were diminished as compared with unprotected mice (Wright and Buchmeier 1991).

Enhancement of viral pathogenesis by humoral effector systems

Humoral immunity is not generally thought to contribute to the pathology of viral CNS infection. Nevertheless, there are theoretical considerations and experimental data obtained in vitro that do not strictly rule out disease-enhancing properties of humoral immune responses. As in the periphery, intrathecal antibody synthesis could help to augment viral pathogenesis by antibody-dependent enhancement (ADE); i.e. antibody-complexed viral particles can be taken up by cells either by binding to Fc receptors (FcR) or, in the case of activation of the complement cascade, by attachment via the C3 receptor. In vitro, the latter seems to occur more readily than FcR binding. In both cases, cells of the monocyte/macrophage lineage are prime targets for ADE (Homsy et al. 1989), indicating that in the CNS ADE could occur with microglial cells. Furthermore, activation of macrophages or microglia may be triggered by engagement of the FcR, which is expressed to high densities on these cells, leading to indirect tissue destruction. Binding of immune complexes to the FcR can stimulate the release of toxic substances from macrophages, causing destruction of healthy cells surrounding the infected areas. This assumption is supported by the observation in vitro of macrophage-dependent oligodendroglia cell degeneration in mixed glial cell cultures when they are treated with immune complexes formed by canine distemper virus (CDV) and CDV-specific antibodies (Botteron et al. 1992).

Theoretically, the presence of virus-specific antibodies in the CNS may allow a complement-dependent immunological effector mechanism to operate: the antibody-activated cytolytic action of complement. So far, there are very few in vivo data supporting this hypothesis. Activation of the complement cascade in the CSF has been demonstrated in patients suffering from HIV-1 infection (Reboul et al. 1989). There is, however, no evidence for antibody-mediated tissue destruction in the CNS of AIDS patients (Lenhardt and Wiley 1989). Although not proven, there is some reason to suggest that complement-mediated lysis could contribute to the pathogenesis of SSPE, caused by a persistent MV infection of the human CNS. The major receptor for MV on most cell types (including brain cells) is CD46, a surface molecule whose normal function is to protect uninfected cells from non-specific lysis by activated complement (Liszweski, Post and Atkinson 1991). As with a variety of other virus–receptor interactions, including CD4-HIV, CD46 is down-regulated after MV infection or after surface contact with the MV haemagglutinin (Dörig et al. 1993, Naniche et al. 1993, Schneider-Schaulies et al. 1995). In both conditions, an enhanced sensitivity to complement-mediated lysis in CD46 modulated cells has been shown in vitro (Schnorr et al. 1995). Because extremely high titres of anti-MV-antibodies in the CSF are pathognomonic in SSPE, and both sera and CSF of SSPE patients reveal high complement activity (Oldstone et al. 1975), this mechanism may contribute to the pathology of SSPE. However, as haemagglutinin is expressed in very limited amounts in brain tissue in SSPE, it is unclear whether complement-mediated lysis really plays a role in vivo.

Viral persistence and virus-specific antibodies

Incomplete elimination of virus from the CNS may result in persistent infection that is usually accompanied by a long-lasting intrathecal antibody synthesis with specificity for viral proteins (Tyor et al. 1992). Over time there is selection of high avidity antiviral antibodies, and the respective clones are preferentially recruited to the CNS. In this case, isoelectric focusing of CSF specimens will show a restricted 'oligoclonal pattern' of antibody clones compared to the polyclonal distribution detectable in paired serum specimens. The presence of these oligoclonal bands can therefore be used as a diagnostic marker in viral infections of the CNS (Felgenhauer and Reiber 1992).

In addition to intrathecal virus-specific antibody synthesis being a reliable indicator of viral infection of the CNS, the long-lasting presence of antiviral antibodies at high titres may contribute to the selection of virus variants. In fact, changes in the neural cell tropism have been shown for the neurotropic JHMV grown in the presence of virus-neutralizing monoclonal antibodies (Buchmeier et al. 1984). This observation was extended by work in a rat model of MV-induced encephalitis (Liebert and ter Meulen 1987). Obviously, only rapid and effective elimination of virus-infected CNS cells will prevent the potentially dangerous development of viral variants with altered neurotropism.

THE CELL-MEDIATED IMMUNE RESPONSE

In vivo, antibody-mediated antiviral mechanisms either act predominantly on the virus itself or interact with cell surface molecules without damaging the cell's integrity. T cell-mediated immune protection is usually mediated by cell destruction. Because a timely T cell immune response encounters a small number of infected cells, the disease should be limited in most acute viral encephalitides, and the benefits will outweigh the harmful effects of the cell-mediated immune response. Paradoxically, the host's immune response to viral infection, which is usually protective outside the CNS, can be destructive when operating within this isolated compartment with such a low regenerative capacity. Cell lysis, complement activation and cytokines may themselves cause pathological changes while helping to clear virus, particularly during a persistent infection.

The role of CD4+ and CD8+ T cells

Although both CD4+ and CD8+ T cells can be relatively easily isolated and grown in culture from the CSF of patients with viral encephalitis and meningoencephalitis, their relative contributions to antiviral defence are uncertain. As is apparent in some animal models, the presence and function of CD4+ cells are more important than CD8+ T cells in viral CNS infections. This is in contrast to the situation in peripheral tissues in which, for example, during acute and chronic viral hepatitis cytotoxic MHC class I-restricted CD8+ T cells attack virus-infected hepatocytes and thus mediate protection as well as cell destruction (Almond et al. 1991).

Although there is still some controversy, results obtained in the Theiler's virus model in mice indicate that the ability to generate CD8+ T cells is not essential for viral clearance. In both C57BL/10 mice, which

develop an acute encephalitis followed by subsequent clearance of virus from the CNS, and SJL mice, which experience a persistent viral infection with demyelination lesions, there are CD8+ CTLs in the CNS (Lindsley, Thiemann and Rodriguez 1991). Furthermore, β2-microglobulin-deficient transgenic mice that lack MHC class I and, therefore, functional CD8+ cells, develop persistent encephalitis with extensive demyelination. However, neither antibody titres nor viral persistence was significantly affected (Pullen et al. 1993).

Consistent with these findings, CD4+ cells proved indispensable in achieving viral clearance from the CNS of rats after transfer into animals experimentally infected with MV, whereas CD8+ cells were not vital for recovery from the acute infection. It must be remembered, however, that in different species different virus-specific immune effector cells are generated in the control of viral infections in the periphery; even within a single species there is no unique T cell subset used for antiviral defence. In many murine virus infections, including HSV, influenza A virus, LCMV and mouse poxvirus, CD8+ CTLs are important in combating infection (Moskophidis et al. 1987, Nash et al. 1987, Ahmed, Butler and Bhatti 1988, Askonas, Taylor and Esquivel 1988). However, the clearance of murine hepatitis virus from the brain by CD8+ T cells depends on CD4+ help (Williamson and Stohlman 1990), and in the protective immunity to retroviruses both CD8+ and CD4+ T cells were only partially effective whereas the combination of both led to full protection (Hom et al. 1991). In contrast, recovery from acute murine CMV infection can proceed in the absence of the CD8+ subset and it is mediated by CD4+ T cells that develop a compensatory protective activity absent from normal mice (Jonjic et al. 1990). CD4+ T cells seem to be required for maintenance of the spontaneous recovery from Friend virus-induced leukaemia (Robertson et al. 1992). These examples illustrate that there is no general assignment of a determinative role in vivo to either T lymphocyte subset in the recovery from viral infections. It seems, however, that in the CNS antiviral cell-mediated activity is largely dependent on CD4+ T cells.

Mechanisms of T cell-mediated antiviral activity

The mechanism of the antiviral activity of CD4+ T cells in vivo has not been completely elucidated. A detailed characterization in vitro revealed that all protective T cell lines produce large amounts of IL-2, IFN-γ and TNF-α but not IL-4 or IL-6, defining them as Th1 cells (Liebert and Finke 1995). If cytokines secreted by Th1 cells were important, 2 requirements should be met: virus-primed T cells have to invade the CNS and home in on sites of infection; and blocking cytokine function should abolish protection. Adoptive transfer experiments in MV-infected rats as well as in mice, using a genetic marker, revealed that MV-specific CD4+ T cells from a donor animal enter the brain of the host. These cells accumulated in infected areas, where they represented ≤5% of all infiltrating T cells in immunocompetent animals. Furthermore, the neutralization of IFN-γ by administering antibodies rendered all mice susceptible to MV-induced acute encephalitis, suggesting that cytokines may indeed play an important role in the immune surveillance of the CNS. The mechanism of cytokine activity may be to assist in recruiting effector cells into the CNS (see also section 1.3, p. 839). The main source of IFN-γ and TNF-α in MV infection of the murine CNS seems to be CD4+ T cells.

In the Theiler's murine encephalomyelitis virus (TMEV) encephalitis model in mice, susceptibility to infection is associated with MHC, and maps to the class I locus H-2D that is highly up-regulated in the CNS, in contrast to the H-2K locus (Nash et al. 1987). In susceptible strains, CD8+ T cells apparently fail to recognize viral antigens in the context of MHC class I, so the virus persists and eventually causes disease. After depletion of CD8+ T cells in vivo, virus clearance is delayed and demyelinating disease develops, indicating that CD8+ T cells are not involved in demyelination and are not vital for recovery from acute infection. In contrast, depletion of CD8+ cells after the acute phase does reduce disease. Observations made in β2-microglobulin-deficient transgenic mice, however, suggest that CD8+ T cells may play a role in clearing viral persistence from glial cells (Pullen et al. 1993). Depletion studies of CD4+ cells in the TMEV model suggest that the major role of CD4+ T cells in picornavirus infections is probably controlling the early stages of infection by providing B cell help and thus enabling the production of neutralizing antibody (Virelizier 1989). TMEV-specific proliferation of CD4+ MHC class II restricted T cells was found in both resistant and susceptible strains (Clatch, Lipton and Miller 1987).

There is a strong correlation in a number of susceptible strains between demyelination and a CD4+ T cell-mediated DTH response, and one DTH T cell epitope in susceptible mice has been mapped to the VP2 protein (Geretry et al. 1994). The incidence of demyelinating disease was reduced following suppression of MHC II restricted CD4+ T cell function after viraemia. After TMEV infection and initial T cell infiltration into the CNS, MHC class II induction on astrocytes is a key step in allowing local antigen presentation and amplification of immunopathological responses within the CNS and, hence, the development of demyelinating disease (Borrow and Nash 1992). A bystander effect caused by the induction of mononuclear cell infiltration and activation of macrophages, which in turn can lead to damage on myelin sheaths, is probably responsible for the observed immunopathology.

For a full account of the immune response to viral infections, see Chapter 10.

Virus-induced cell-mediated autoimmune reactions against brain antigens

Another possibility involves T cells reactive against brain cell antigens, which could be induced during the course of infection and may exacerbate current pathology or initiate new lesions. The frequency of induction of T cells reactive against brain antigens and their role in the pathology of human viral CNS infections are unclear. One study suggests that a significant proliferative response of isolated peripheral lymphocytes occurs against myelin basic protein (MBP) in patients with acute measles encephalomyelitis (Johnston et al. 1984). Moreover, MBP was detected in CSF from such patients as a consequence of myelin breakdown. MBP-specific lymphoproliferative responses have also been seen after post-infectious encephalomyelitis following rubella, varicella and respiratory infection and in patients with post-exposure rabies immunization (Johnston and Griffin 1986). The latter disorder is probably the human equivalent of

EAE, because these patients received rabies vaccine prepared in brain tissue. Continuing the analogy to EAE, it is not surprising that an MBP-specific lymphoproliferative response in these virus infections is considered to be of pathogenic importance. In experimental CNS infections, autoimmune T cells do not seem to be involved in the induction of demyelination in Theiler's virus in mice, as tolerance induced to myelin antigens blocked the induction of EAE but did not affect the development of demyelinating disease (Kennedy et al. 1990). However, in rats infected with JHMV or MV, MBP-reactive CD4+ T cells were detected that could transfer EAE to naive uninfected animals (Watanabe, Wege and ter Meulen 1983, Liebert, Linington and ter Meulen 1988). There are several possibilities of how a virus could induce strong cell-mediated immunity (CMI) responses to brain antigen:

1 When enveloped viruses multiply in living cells, they may incorporate host antigens into their envelope. In this context these antigens might then be recognized by the host and thus elicit an immune reaction.

2 Viruses with a tropism for lymphocytes and macrophages might be involved in the destruction of lymphocyte subpopulations or the generation/expansion of autoreactive lymphocyte clones. The prime example is Epstein–Barr virus (EBV), which infects and transforms B lymphocytes that may secrete autoantibodies reacting with cellular constituents.

3 Immune responses raised against certain viral antigens may cross-react with normal host cell antigens and lead to autoimmunity by molecular mimicry (Oldstone 1989). In fact, computer analysis has revealed that several viruses contain part of the human MBP in their genome, and immunization of rabbits with a synthetic peptide from such a sequence from hepatitis B polymerase led to a CMI response to myelin and to the induction of EAE lesions in these animals (Fujinami and Oldstone 1985). Moreover, it was found that synthetic peptides derived from common viruses and are based on motifs required for MHC-II binding and T cell receptor recognition can activate human T cell lines specific for MBP (Wucherpfennig and Strominger 1995). These observations support the hypothesis that a range of viruses could be involved in the initiation of autoimmune processes.

1.5 Consequences of antiviral mechanisms in the CNS

In summary, immune responses generated in the periphery encounter great difficulties when combating CNS virus infections. If neurons are infected, direct interaction of T cells with the infected host cell is not possible, not least because of the lack of MHC expression. This would, in any case, not be desirable because any immune response, although beneficial in the periphery, would inflict enormous damage when attacking cells that lack the capacity to regenerate. Hence, rapid elimination of infected cells is necessary. In contrast, the development of a delayed immune response may allow the virus to spread in the CNS and, even if ultimately effective against the virus, may be destructive to the host. Thus, precautions are built into the system to prevent potentially damaging and disease-inducing immune responses during persistent infections in which the virus, at least temporarily, does not destroy its host cell.

The fine regulation of intracerebral immune surveillance has yet to be elucidated. However, it is clear that a delicate balance is normally maintained between the morphological and functional integrity of the CNS and the ability of the immune system to combat virus and eliminate infected cells. At present the evidence indicates that:

1 The immune response to viral infections of the CNS is initiated in peripheral lymphoid tissues, followed by entry of activated end-differentiated T and B cells into the CSF, meninges and brain parenchyma.

2 During viral infections, different sets of cytokines are induced.

3 Together with interferon-induced proteins, these factors contribute to the establishment of persistent infections, which may depend on downregulation of replication of certain viruses by lack of factors or the restriction of viral gene expression, or both.

4 During viral infections, MHC class I or II antigens are expressed on astrocytes and oligodendrocytes, and extensively on microglial cells which present viral antigen produced by infected cells.

5 Full development of the inflammatory response requires virus-specific T cells; natural killer (NK) cells, γ/δ T cells, mononuclear phagocytes, B cells and plasma cells participate in a bystander response.

6 In many viral systems, including the experimental coronavirus JHM and MV models, T cells are required for viral elimination, but clearance of virus may also depend on the timely presence of virus-specific antibodies.

7 When a virus infection encounters an unprimed immune system, a synergistic interaction of all major cell types of the immune system is required both for limiting virus spread within the CNS and, ultimately, for eliminating virus from brain cells.

8 However, immunopathology, autoimmunity or both may result from inopportune or inefficient T cell responses generated after the viral agent has succeeded in establishing a persistent infection in brain cells as a result of immune-mediated damage during attempted viral clearance.

2   VIRUSES AND ASSOCIATED CNS DISORDERS IN HUMANS

As mentioned on p. 835, except for rabies virus, human pathogenic viruses do not reveal *per se* a tro-

pism for the CNS but rather cause CNS diseases in the course of an infection in the periphery. A summary of the relative frequencies of the ability of human pathogenic viruses to cause CNS diseases is given in Table 40.2. For example, CNS involvement is quite frequent with mumps virus infections, whereas the proportion of patients with measles developing CNS complications is generally small. The same applies to EBV infections, which are ubiquitous and normally clinically inapparent, CNS complications being observed only rarely. The following sections thus focus on viral infections of the CNS that are of major clinical interest and have been investigated in more detail.

2.1   Papovaviruses

PROGRESSIVE MULTIFOCAL LEUCOENCEPHALOPATHY

Progressive multifocal leucoencephalopathy (PML) is a demyelinating disease of the CNS, resulting from infection of oligodendrocytes with JC virus, a papovavirus (Richards 1988) (see Chapter 16). Viral particles with typical papovavirus morphology were detected by electron microscopy in the brains of patients dying of PML (ZuRhein and Chou 1965). JCV (named after the initials of the patient from whom it was first isolated) was subsequently cultivated and identified in 1971 (Padgett et al. 1971). Until the AIDS epidemic, experience with this disease was limited. Once regarded by most neurologists as a clinical curiosity, PML has now been recognized as an AIDS-associated disorder. Current estimates suggest that c. 4–5% of all HIV-infected people will develop PML (Berger et al. 1987). In AIDS patients, as in those with other underlying diseases, PML usually progresses inexorably to death within a mean of 4 months. More than 80% succumb within 1 year of diagnosis. However, on rare occasions, individuals with PML experience both clinical and radiographic recovery, including full neurological recovery, in the absence of specific therapeutic intervention.

Pathogenesis

The spread of JCV is thought to occur via the respiratory route (Shah 1990). To date, no disease has been convincingly associated with the acute infection. Usually, asymptomatic persistent infections with JCV (and the closely related BK virus) are established; consequently, 80–90% of the healthy adult population have IgG antibodies against JCV (Padgett and Walker 1983). Kidney, CNS and, in some cases, peripheral blood mononuclear cells have been identified as sites of persistent infection (Houff et al. 1988, Arthur, Dagostin and Shah 1989, Elsner and Dörries 1992, Schneider and Dörries 1993, Dörries et al. 1994). It is not yet entirely clear how these persistent infections are established and maintained. Although heterogeneity within the JCV control regions in brain isolates could be defined, these changes could be linked neither to the persistent phenotype of the infection nor to the efficiency and frequency of reactivation (Elsner and Dörries 1992). On the other hand, it has

Table 40.2 Viruses causing acute meningoencephalitis and acute encephalitis in humans

Frequent	Infrequent	Rare
Herpes simplex types 1 and 2	Varicella-zoster	Adenovirus
Mumps	Measles	Epstein–Barr virus
Enteroviruses	Rubella	Reovirus
Arboviruses	Influenza A and B	Parainfluenza 1–3
Rabies	Cytomegalovirus	Respiratory syncytial virus
		Human parvovirus
		Lymphocytic choriomeningitis virus

been suggested that cell type specificity of JCV in vitro and in vivo are controlled by host and viral transcription factors that actively regulate JCV gene expression by interacting with the control region (Feigenbaum et al. 1987, Chowdhury et al. 1990, Lynch and Frisque 1991, Ranganathan and Khalili 1993). Reactivation of viral replication leading to PML is almost exclusively confined to immunosuppressed individuals (Walker and Frisque 1986), strongly suggesting that the host's immune system plays a major role in controlling viral replication in persistence. However, there is no evidence as to how the immune response controls virus persistence and prevents reactivation. Because only a minority of patients with underlying cellular immunodeficiency ultimately develop PML, it is possible that the presence of JCV and immunosuppression alone are not sufficient for its development.

The AIDS epidemic has dramatically altered the epidemiology of PML, transforming the male/female ratio of PML from 1 : 1 to 5 : 1 by 1987 (Holman et al. 1991). Instead of affecting chiefly elderly people, PML has become a disease of the young and middle-aged affected with AIDS. It is interesting that this disease rarely occurs in immunosuppressed children with HIV infection (Berger et al. 1992), perhaps as a result of the smaller percentage of children infected with JCV. The high prevalence of antibodies in the adult population and the rarity of PML in children supports the contention that PML results from reactivation of JCV in individuals who have become immunosuppressed. Until the early 1980s (before the AIDS epidemic), the vast majority of patients with PML had lymphoproliferative disorders leading to immunosuppression such as Hodgkin's disease, chronic lymphocytic leukaemia and lymphosarcoma, tuberculosis, lupus erythematosus or sarcoidosis (Brooks and Walker 1984). In contrast, AIDS has been estimated to be the underlying disease behind PML in 55–85% of all current cases in which PML was reported within 1 year after initial diagnosis of AIDS (Gullota et al. 1992, Kaye et al. 1992, Major et al. 1992).

Clinical disease and pathology

The clinical hallmark of PML is the presence of focal neurological changes associated with radiographic evidence of white matter lesions, depending on the location of the CNS infection. Cardinal features of PML, apparent on clinical examination, include an insidiously progressive psychomotor slowing, impaired

memory and apathy. The most common presentations include weakness, visual deficits and cognitive abnormalities, which occur in approximately one-third of patients (Brooks and Walker 1984). Weakness is typically a hemiparesis, but monoparesis, hemiplegia and quadriparesis may be observed as the disease progresses. Other motor disturbances include limb and trunk ataxia, resulting most often from cerebellar involvement. Nearly one-third of patients have cerebellar signs at the time of diagnosis (von Einsiedel et al. 1993). Extrapyramidal disease is rare at onset, but bradykinesia and rigidity may be detected in a substantial minority of patients with advanced disease. Dystonia and severe dysarthria have also been observed as a consequence of lesions in the basal ganglia. Neuro-ophthalmic symptoms occur in 50% of patients and are the presenting manifestation in 30–45%. The most common visual deficits are homonymous hemianopia or quadrantanopia due to lesions of the optic tracts. The spectrum of cognitive changes observed is quite broad. Unlike the slowly evolving global dementia of the HIV-associated dementia complex, the mental impairments of PML often advance more rapidly and typically occur in conjunction with focal neurological deficits. Cognitive abnormalities include personality and behavioural changes, poor attention, loss of motor persistence, memory impairment, dyslexia, dyscalculia, and the alien hand syndrome.

Neuropathologically, the cardinal feature of PML is demyelination, i.e. the loss of oligodendroglial cells and myelin sheaths (Fig. 40.2). Demyelination is typically multifocal, but may also be unifocal on rare occasions. Although these lesions may develop in any location in the white matter, they have a predilection for the parieto-occipital regions. Not infrequently, lesions involve a number of organs, including the cerebellum, brainstem and, less commonly, the spinal cord (Bauer, Chamberlin and Horenstein 1969, von Einsiedel et al. 1993, Kuchelmeister, Gullotta and Bergmann 1993). The lesions range in size from 1 mm to several centimetres, the larger lesions resulting from coalescence of many smaller ones.

Other histopathological hallmarks of PML include hyperchromatic, enlarged oligodendroglial nuclei and enlarged bizarre astrocytes with lobulated hyperchromatic nuclei (Fig. 40.2). The abnormal astrocytes may undergo mitosis and have quite a malignant appearance. Hybridization in situ for JCV DNA allows detec-

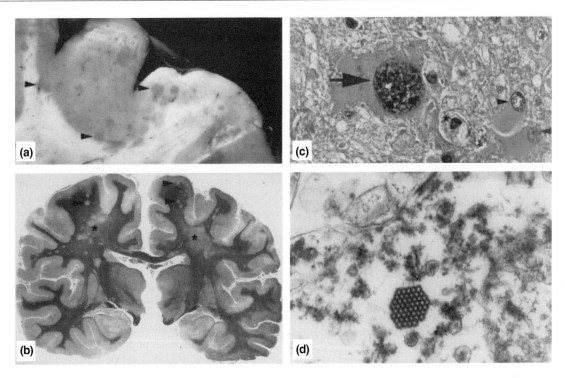

Fig. 40.2 (a) Close-up of the cortex of a patient who died from PML. Several small foci of demyelination are situated mainly at the border between the grey and the white matter. (b) Whole mount of the cerebrum of the same patient, stained with a myelinotropic dye. Again, there are several round areas of demyelination, as well as larger polycyclical (several circular confluent) regions of confluent foci in the central white matter. (c) Swollen, grotesquely deformed oligodendrocyte with a very large nucleus (×400). For comparison, see the 2 reactive astrocytes at the right of the picture (arrowed). (d) Electron micrograph showing papovaviruses within the affected oligodendrocytes. (Courtesy of Dr Adriano Aguzzi.)

tion of virions (c. 28–45 nm diam.) in the nuclei of infected oligodendroglial cells. Virions are detected less frequently in reactive astrocytes and only rarely in macrophages engaged in removing the affected oligodendrocytes (Mazlo and Tariska 1992). The subcellular distribution of virions, particularly in cells usually not involved in papovavirus infection (the nucleus and cytoplasm of neurons), has been reported in 2 cases (Boldorini et al. 1993). Although neuropathological findings do not reveal fundamental differences between cases of AIDS and non-AIDS PML, the former group more frequently presents with extensive lesions of a particularly destructive, necrotizing character.

PML in the absence of AIDS may be associated with a slight elevation in the CSF protein, a mild lymphocytic pleocytosis and the presence of MBP. In HIV-infected patients with PML, the CSF abnormalities typically reflect those observed as a consequence of the HIV infection, including mononuclear pleocytosis, elevated protein and borderline low glucose.

Until recently, confirmation of PML relied exclusively on demonstrating typical histopathological changes and detecting JCV in brain samples obtained from biopsies or at autopsy, using conventional techniques including electron microscopy, virus isolation, immunocytochemistry, and detection of viral DNA by in situ hybridization or PCR. The recent application of PCR to CSF samples is promising in enabling premortem diagnosis with less invasive procedures than brain biopsy (Orefice et al. 1993, Weber et al. 1994)

and is likely to prove a sensitive and highly specific diagnostic tool for PML.

2.2 Alphaherpesviruses

Of the numerous herpesviruses so far characterized, 8 have been isolated from humans. Among these, 3 members of the subfamily *Alphaherpesvirinae*, HSV-1, HSV-2 and varicella-zoster virus (VZV) (Chapter 18), have been identified as aetiological agents in the pathogenesis of human disease processes in both the peripheral and the CNS. HSV is responsible for the viral encephalitis with the highest fatality rate, and has also been implicated in the pathogenesis of other CNS disorders such as multiple sclerosis (Kastrukoff, Lau and Kim 1987) and Alzheimer's disease (Ball 1982). HHV-6, HHV-7 (Chapter 19) and HHV-8 have been isolated from human peripheral blood mononuclear cells (PBMCs) during recent years. Their association with human CNS diseases has not yet been fully defined, although a pathogenic role of HHV-6 has been suggested for multiple sclerosis (Challoner et al. 1995).

Alphaherpesviruses have a variable host range and short replication cycles, and spread rapidly in infected cell cultures, resulting in complete cell destruction. Paradoxically, they can establish latent, life-long infections in their natural hosts, including those with natural or vaccine-induced immunity. These latent infections occur primarily, but not exclusively, in neural tissue of sensory and autonomic nerve ganglia and the CNS.

HSV: VIRUS–HOST CELL AND HOST RELATIONSHIP

Following infection, HSV-1 and HSV-2 replicate at the mucocutaneous surface before entering nerve axons. Virus then moves centripetally via retrograde fast axonal transport to cell bodies of neurons in sensory and autonomic nerve ganglia and, in some cases, to the CNS (Fig. 40.3). Following retrograde transport, the virus replicates in the sensory ganglia, which innervate the site of infection. In experimental work in animals, there is evidence of lytic virus infection in neurons and accessory cells, and the virus can be recovered from ganglionic homogenates. Once replication in the sensory ganglia is complete, antiviral drugs cannot eliminate the virus if it enters its latent state. In acutely infected ganglia, 2 types of virus–neuron interaction can occur, resulting in either lytic or latent infection. Cellular factors involved in repressing immediate early gene expression may be paramount in this. After acute ganglionic infection subsides, virus persists in neurons, probably for the lifetime of the host. Infectious virus cannot be recovered from ganglionic homogenates during the latent phase of infection, but can be isolated from ganglionic explant cultures. Periodically, latent virus is reactivated either spontaneously or by a variety of stimuli. During this reactivation process, virus (or perhaps subviral particles) is transported centrifugally via the nerve cell axon to the original peripheral infection site, where virus replication can then recur.

The exact role of the cell in establishing latent HSV-1 infections is still unclear, because of the small number of latently infected cells present in vivo as well as the difficulty of establishing authentic in vitro latency systems. The dependence of latency on the presence of nerve growth factor (NGF) in primary cultures of sympathetic and sensory neurons has been described (Wilcox and Johnson 1988, Wilcox et al. 1990). Moreover, neurons in culture express factors that inhibit expression of HSV-1 immediate early genes (Ash 1986, Kemp, Dent and Latchman 1990, Wheatley et al. 1991, Lillycrop, Estridge and Latchman 1993) and therefore arrest HSV-1 replication at an early stage, before irreversible cell damage.

Some molecular aspects of HSV latency and reactivation have been described. The genome persists as a circularized or a linear concatenated structure that is not integrated into the cellular DNA in human and mouse tissue (Rock and Fraser 1983, 1985, Mellerick and Fraser 1987). The viral DNA is not extensively methylated, and estimates suggest that 20–30 copies of the viral genome may be present in individual cells (Stevens 1989). A set of RNAs is produced in latently infected neurons, where they are the only viral transcripts detectable (latency associated transcripts, LATs) (reviewed in McGeoch, Barnett and MacLean 1993, Rock 1993, Feldman 1994) (Fig. 40.4). They extend from a region in IR_L (large internal repeat region) without an assigned coding role into an oppositely orientated coding region. This region encodes at least one immediate early gene product. The larg-

est LAT species run into IR_S. Mutations in the region encoding LATs have been reported as affecting entry into or reactivation from the latent state. It seems that LAT elements have been conserved in evolution, thus strongly suggesting that there are important functions whose nature is unresolved. As there are no compelling signs of the presence of protein-encoding sequences within the LATs, they might act as antisense inhibitors of HSV-1 gene expression.

Primary CNS infection with HSV

Infection with HSV-1, generally limited to the oropharynx, can be transmitted by respiratory droplets or through direct contact of a susceptible individual with infected secretions. Thus, initial replication of virus occurs in the oropharyngeal mucosa. The trigeminal ganglia become colonized and harbor latent virus. HSV-2 infection is usually the consequence of transmission via a genital route. In these circumstances, virus replicates in the vaginal tract or on penile skin and eventually seeds the sacral ganglia. After recovery from primary infection, only a small percentage of individuals experience recurrent infections (Whitley 1985). HSV encephalitis is mainly associated with HSV-1 infection, whereas ascending myelitis or meningitis is linked mainly to HSV-2 (Shyu et al. 1993). Of these clinical entities, encephalitis is the most common and most severe HSV infection of the CNS. The clinical course is variable, depending on the location, as well as the acuteness of the infection.

HSV infections of the newborn can be aquired in utero, intrapartum (75–80% of all cases) or postnatally (see also Chapter 41). The clinical presentation of infection reflects the site and extent of viral replication. Neonatal HSV infection is almost invariably symptomatic and frequently lethal. Intrauterine infection is apparent at birth and is characterized by severe manifestations, such as microcephaly or hydrocephaly. Intrapartum or postnatally acquired HSV infections may lead to encephalitis or disseminated infection that involves multiple organs, including acute brain infections. In infants with disseminated infections, the virus probably seeds the brain by a blood-borne route, resulting in multiple areas of cortical haemorrhagic necrosis. In contrast, infants who present only with encephalitis probably develop brain disease as a consequence of retrograde axonal transmission of virus to the CNS. Clinical manifestations of encephalitis with or without associated disseminated disease include seizures (both focal and generalized), lethargy, irritability, tremors, poor feeding, temperature instability, a bulging fontanelle and pyramidal tract signs. Cultures of CSF yield virus in 25–40% of cases. Likely findings on CSF examination include pleocytosis and proteinosis, which increase with progressive disease. Death occurs in 50% of untreated infants with localized CNS disease and is usually related to brainstem involvement. With rare exceptions, survivors are left with neurological impairment.

Clinical manifestations of HSV encephalitis in older children and adults reflect the areas of pathology in the brain. These include primarily a focal encephalitis associated with fever, altered consciousness, bizarre behaviour, disordered mentation and localized neuro-

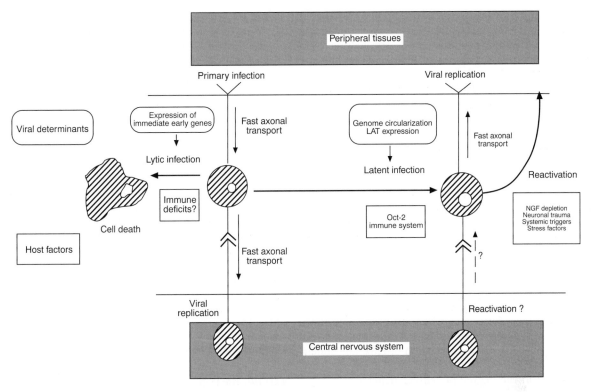

Fig. 40.3 Schematic representation of mechanisms of HSV-1 replication in the nervous system. After primary infection at peripheral tissues, the virion travels via fast axonal transport to peripheral sensory ganglia (PSG). Under conditions favouring viral replication (e.g. immune disruption), expression of HSV-1 immediate early genes followed by a complete viral replication cycle will ensue, leading to neuronal cell death. Again by fast axonal transport, the virus may seed the CNS, causing an acute, lytic infection (primary HSV-1 encephalitis). By contrast, in the presence of an effective immune system, viral replication will be prevented in PSG and probably CNS neurons (due at least in part to host cell factors such as neuronal-specific Oct-2 transcription factor). This may lead to either an abortive (not reactivatable) or a latent infection that is characterized by the circularization of the viral genomic DNA and a marked restriction of viral gene expression where no immediate early genes, but only latency-associated transcripts (LATs), are expressed. Under specific systemic (e.g. menstruation) and local triggering conditions, the latent genome can reactivate in PSG, travel to the periphery and replicate there. The ability of reactivated HSV-1 to invade the CNS is uncertain, as is reactivation from latent infections established in the CNS. NGF, neuronal growth factor.

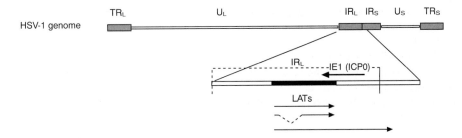

Fig. 40.4 The HSV-1 genome is a linear DNA molecule containing unique long (U_L) and short (U_S) regions bounded by the terminal and internal repeat regions (TR and IR, respectively). The region encoding the major species of latency-associated transcripts (LATs) that are expressed during viral latency is located within the IR_L region (as indicated by the black bar in the enlarged section). As also indicated, some LATs extend from the LAT locus into the IR_S region. The major LAT species expressed partly overlap with viral genes encoded in the opposite direction on the genome, as exemplified for the immediate early 1 gene (IE1 or ICP0). LATs may interfere with the expression of these genes because they are antisense to their mRNAs, leading to the formation of dsRNA molecules.

logical signs. These clinical findings are generally associated with neurodiagnostic evidence of localized temporal lobe disease. Histopathological findings include widespread areas of haemorrhagic necrosis, mirroring the area of infection, with oligodendrocytic involve-

ment, gliosis and, frequently, astrocytosis late in the disease course (Fig. 40.5). Primary HSV-2 infections can, independent of gender, be associated with fever, dysuria, localized inguinal adenopathy and malaise. The severity of primary infection and its association with complications are statistically higher in women than in men, for unknown reasons. Systemic complaints are common in both sexes, approaching 70% of all cases. The most common complications include aseptic meningitis (c. 20%). Following primary genital herpetic infection, sacral radiculomyelitis (which can lead to neuralgias) and meningoencephalitis can also occur. The relationship between HSV infections of the brain and chronic degenerative disease and psychiatric disorders requires further investigation.

Latent infection by HSV

Despite the wide range of anti-HSV immune responses to the initial infection, the non-replicating latent virus can persist in the ganglia for the lifetime of the patient. Whether latency *per se* causes any neurological injury is unknown, but it is well recognized that latent HSV is the source of virus responsible for recurrent infections in the peripheral nervous system. It is assumed that latent virus is reactivated to a replication-competent form and transported via sensory nerves to cutaneous or ocular sites where further replication results in recurrent HSV infections. The pathological changes induced by the replication of HSV are similar in both primary and recurrent infection, but vary according to the degree of cellular damage.

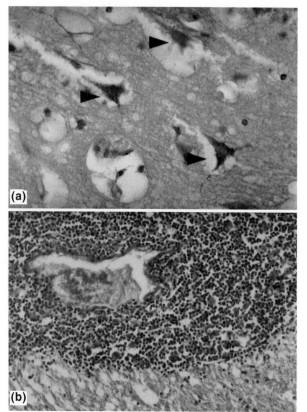

Fig. 40.5 Herpes simplex type 1 encephalitis. (**a**) Strongly positive intraneuronal staining with anti-HSV-1 immunostain (arrowed) (×400). (**b**) Massive accumulation of inflammatory cells (predominantly lymphocytes) in the neighbourhood of small vessels ('cuffing') (×50). (Courtesy of Dr Adriano Aguzzi.)

HSV encephalitis in immunocompetent individuals is about 1 million-fold less frequent than the peripheral disease (Whitley 1985). The source of virus behind HSV-1 encephalitis in immunocompetent individuals is unclear, as the ability of HSV-1 to reactivate in the CNS seems to be extremely limited. Despite the presence of HSV-1 nucleic acid in the human brain (Fraser et al. 1981, Steiner and Kennedy 1995), there is no convincing evidence of recurrent encephalitis induced by HSV-1, and attempts to reactivate it from explanted CNS tissue have generally failed. On rare occasions, reactivated virus may be transported from the trigeminal ganglia to the cerebral cortex, resulting in HSV encephalitis (Johnston 1982). However, not all cases of HSV encephalitis are caused by the strain responsible for cold sores in an individual (Whitley et al. 1982). Therefore, it is assumed that, in about half of the patients, HSV encephalitis occurs as a primary infection (Whitley 1990). Moreover, even with a history of a prior HSV-1 infection, a second primary infection with another HSV-1 strain may be responsible for the encephalitis.

Diagnosis and treatment of HSV encephalitis

The severity of HSV-associated CNS complications warrants the application of rapid and specific diagnostic approaches in order to achieve effective treatment. Seroconversion or an increase in serum antibody titre are not diagnostic of CNS infection. Serological diagnosis requires proof of intrathecal synthesis of virus-specific antibodies, which is evident only when the quantity of specific antibodies in the CNS cannot be explained by transport of antibodies from the periphery across the BBB into the CNS. Classically, CNS HSV IgG antibody is distinguished from peripheral blood-derived HSV antibody appearing in the CSF by calculation of an antibody index (CSF HSV IgG : serum HSV IgG/CSF albumin : serum albumin); HSV antibody index values >1.5 are considered indicative of intrathecal Ig synthesis. Several approaches are available to determine intrathecal antibody synthesis, including techniques such as ELISA, isoelectric focusing (IEF) or Western blotting using protein antigens (virus-purified or expressed as recombinant proteins) (Klapper and Cleator 1992). For the detection of viral antigens or nucleic acids, brain biopsies stained with virus-specific antibodies or hybridized with virus-specific probes have been used successfully (with a sensitivity of 80–85% and a specificity of 100%). More recently, PCR-based analysis of CSF samples has been widely used as a less invasive, highly sensitive method more appropriate for clinical application for the diagnosis of HSV encephalitis, particularly in the acute phase of disease in the absence of virus-specific antibodies and in suspicious relapses (Kühn et al. 1991, Pohl-Koppe et al. 1992).

Confirmed or even suspected diagnosis of HSV encephalitis requires the immediate administration of aciclovir, a potent therapeutic antiviral drug that specifically interferes with HSV polymerase function and is highly effective in reducing both mortality and morbidity. In fact, the early and systemic application of aciclovir has reduced the mortality of HSV encephalitis from 70% to 20% of the affected patients.

The currently accepted antiviral treatment is a 10 day intravenous course of aciclovir, which may, in the case of suspicious relapses, be extended to 21 days, although there is no evidence that under-treatment causes relapse. The use of steroid treatment in HSV encephalitis is a matter of controversy. As brain oedema is believed to represent the major cause of mortality associated with herpes encephalitis, reduction of intracranial pressure is another important consideration in the overall treatment.

VARICELLA-ZOSTER CNS COMPLICATIONS

As the name implies, varicella-zoster virus (VZV) causes 2 distinct clinical symptoms: chickenpox and shingles. Chickenpox (varicella) is a ubiquitous, highly contagious disease that spreads rapidly in a susceptible population and is seen predominantly in childhood as the manifestation of primary infection with this virus. In contrast, shingles (herpes zoster) is the manifestation of a recurrent VZV infection. It usually occurs in older or immunocompromised individuals and is characterized by a painful vesicular eruption, generally limited to a single dermatome.

VZV: virus–host relationship

As with HSV, a primary infection with VZV is thought to pass centripetally from skin and mucosal lesions to the corresponding sensory ganglia via contiguous sensory nerve endings and sensory nerve fibres. At the same time, some seeding of ganglia might also occur through direct spread of the virus owing to a varicella-associated viraemia. Once in the ganglion, the virus sets up a latent infection in the neuronal cells without replicating or damaging them.

Immune responses to VZV may play a role in maintaining the latent state and certainly seem to be responsible for preventing clinically apparent reactivation. Reactivation of VZV occurs only rarely, usually once in an individual's lifetime. The main factors that trigger reactivation include generalized immunosuppression such as HIV infection or certain cancers (e.g. Hodgkin's disease), suggesting that alteration in the host immunity to VZV may allow the development of zoster. Accumulating evidence points to CMI as the principal factor in the appearance of zoster. Zoster is seen most frequently in cases where CMI is lost (e.g. in bone marrow transplantation), and is accompanied by acute inflammation of the corresponding sensory nerve and ganglion. Acute lymphocytic inflammation, focal haemorrhage and neuronal destruction have also been described. In addition, the sensory nerve shows degeneration and demyelination both peripherally and centrally, and the presence of viral antigen in neuronal and satellite cells and within the corresponding sensory nerves has been described.

VZV latency and reactivation are quite different from HSV latency and reactivation (reviewed by Hay and Ruyechan 1994). In contrast to HSV, VZV seems able to establish ganglionic latency in non-neural cells (satellite cells that surround the neurons) and to express several lytic cycle viral genes while latent; these genes probably represent very early events in viral multiplication. LAT-like molecules have not been described in these infections, but VZV has no genomic region directly corresponding to LAT. The proposed block at the molecular level, however, may be quite weak, allowing small amounts of virus to be produced on a regular basis.

VZV: CNS involvement

CNS involvement in varicella is seen in about one case per 1000. It occurs most often in children aged 5–14 years. The pathogenesis of the neurological complications of varicella is not well understood. Direct invasion of the CNS is seen in some cases, particularly with disseminated visceral infection, whereas other CNS manifestations seem to be immunomediated in origin. Involvement of the ganglia and nerves precedes the development of cutaneous lesions. Similar changes are often observed in adjacent ganglia. The inflammatory and degenerative changes can be traced peripherally to the cutaneous lesions and centrally into the adjacent segments of the spinal cord or brainstem. The myelitis is generally unilateral and predominantly involves the posterior horns. Degeneration with neuronal necrosis and neuronophagia may also involve the posterior columns and the grey matter. A mild lymphocytic meningitis is frequently present and most intense in the involved area. Anterior nerve root degeneration can be associated with a motor neuron radiculitis. VZV can be isolated from CSF and nerve tissue, which suggests that these changes represent direct viral invasion. CNS involvement is responsible for 20% of the admissions to hospital. The most common presentation is acute cerebellitis, which appears towards the end of the first or the beginning of the second week after the onset of rash and is usually transient. A more serious form of encephalitis occurring earlier during the course of varicella is a progressive encephalopathy with loss of conciousness and convulsions. If brain swelling cannot be reduced the patient may assume a decorticate position. Less common neurological presentations seen in varicella include meningoencephalitis, transverse myelitis, peripheral neuritis and Reye's syndrome.

In contrast to neuralgia, the most common and important clinical manifestation of herpes zoster encephalitis is a rare complication. Typically, the rash involves cranial or upper cervical nerves, and little is known about its pathogenesis. Lesions of disseminated herpes zoster are identical to those of fatal varicella. In zoster meningoencephalitis there are lesions ranging from mononuclear infiltration of the meninges to necrotizing encephalitis with axonal degeneration, macrophage infiltration and characteristic intranuclear inclusions and viral particles in the glial cells

2.3 Enteroviruses

GENERAL CONSIDERATIONS

The genus *Enterovirus* belongs to the family *Picornaviridae* (Chapter 25). It contains a number of viruses that give rise to infections of the CNS, notably polioviruses, enteroviruses, Coxsackie and echoviruses. Epidemics of poliovirus, for instance, were once a worldwide scourge of the world, but with widespread vaccination, this disease has largely disappeared from developed countries. However, aseptic meningitis due to other enteroviruses is now the frequent neurological infection of viral origin. It may occur sporadically or in epidemic form with significant morbidity and, depending on specific host factors, mortality. Enteroviruses multiply in the lymphoid tissue of the alimentary tract and cause a wide range of syndromes. The extent to which enteroviruses are responsible for CNS disease is very difficult to gauge because of both under-reporting and the subclinical nature of infection in c. 90% of cases. Children are the main targets of enterovirus infection and also serve as a mode for virus dissemination. In general, gender does not seem to predispose to a certain type of disease, although cases of childhood paralytic poliomyelitis are twice as common in males as in females.

POLIOMYELITIS

General considerations

Natural infection with poliovirus occurs via the oral route whereupon virus replicates in the tonsils, the lymphatic tissue which drains the neck, Peyer's patches and the small intestine. Whether infection of lymphoid tissue such as the tonsils is achieved after initial replication of virus in the gut and subsequent viraemia or during the initial infection following ingestion is a topic of debate. It is generally held that, for successful invasion of the CNS by poliovirus, a viraemic phase is required, although some evidence suggests that direct infection of the CNS can take place via nerve endings in the gut.

Pathogenesis and pathology

Once poliovirus has gained access to the CNS, the outcome of disease can be devastating and is based largely on the highly cytopathic nature of poliovirus replication. The majority of infections (90–95%) are, however, silent, although virus may be recovered in the stools or throat swabs of infected persons. Abortive infections (4–8%) include self-limiting forms of poliovirus infection and may present as an upper respiratory tract infection, gastroenteritis or an influenza-like illness. Non-paralytic poliomyelitis (1–2%) presents initially as an abortive infection that is followed by invasion of the CNS by virus. Accompanying the assault on the CNS by virus are symptoms of aseptic meningitis with back pain and muscle spasms. Paralytic poliomyelitis/polio encephalitis (0.1–2%), like non-paralytic poliomyelitis, will generally present as an abortive infection during the prodromal stages of infection, although there is often no evidence of an early phase of infection. The illness may be biphasic (often seen in children) with meningeal irritation and, finally, onset of asymmetric flaccid paralysis (when whole muscle groups are involved) or paresis (when muscle group involvement is somewhat limited). Poliomyelitis can be divided into 3 basic

types (spinal, bulbar and bulbospinal) depending on the site of nerve cell involvement. Bulbar paralysis is more common in children and generally does not involve the limbs, whereas adults presenting with bulbar poliomyelitis typically have limb paralysis.

The gross pathology of poliovirus infection has been widely studied (Bodian and Horstmann 1965). Classically, there is extensive damage to the large anterior horn cells of the spinal cord. When paralysis is associated with poliomyelitis, cervical and lumbar areas (which serve limbs) are particularly affected. In fatal cases of poliomyelitis, there may also be involvement of the brainstem motor nuclei, as seen in bulbar poliomyelitis, or of nerve cells of the motor cortex or thalamus and hypothalamus. After infection of cells of the CNS by poliovirus, the earliest histological change is vascular engorgement, rapidly followed by perivascular infiltration. The infiltrate comprises mainly lymphocytes and, to some degree, polymorphonuclear neutrophils, plasma cells and microglia. Cell damage is largely due to cytolytic replication of poliovirus within cells. Infected nerves swell and undergo satellitosis before being phagocytosed by mononuclear cells. Viral destruction of cells results in degeneration of axons and axon sheaths, followed by atrophy of the affected area and astrocytic scarring. Flaccid paralysis accompanies these changes, followed by a widespread atrophy of muscle no longer innervated by affected nerves. Death is often due to respiratory failure as a result of respiratory paralysis or secondary complications (e.g. bacterial pneumonia). People affected by poliovirus may have additional muscle weakness later in life as part of the post-polio syndrome (Stone 1994). The basis for such a condition may be age-related or, as has been hypothesized following the discovery of intrathecal antibody to poliovirus, due to persistence of virus in neural cells, although this is still unproven (Munsat 1991).

ENTEROVIRUS

General considerations

Of the numerous serotypes of enteroviruses that are recognized, 2 deserve special recognition with respect to disease involvement of the CNS: enterovirus serotypes 70 and 71 (for review, see Yin-Murphy 1994). Both are transmitted by the faecal–oral route, although ocular infections with enterovirus 70 may be mediated by facecloths and bath towels, etc. Although enterovirus 70 has a marked predilection for epithelial cells of the conjunctiva, the fact that patients may exhibit signs of CNS involvement suggests neurotropism. However, enterovirus 70 has yet to be isolated from the CSF or CNS of infected patients.

Pathogenesis and pathology

The 3 forms of CNS disease caused by enterovirus 70 are (1) the spinal form, (2) the cranial form and (3) a combination of the spinal and cranial forms. The spinal form is by far the most commonly encountered and is characterized by an asymmetrical flaccid paralysis or paresis with one or more limbs involved. Paralysis is the manifestation of infection of the anterior horn cells of the spinal cord by enterovirus 70. Atrophy of affected muscle groups resembles poliomyelitis. In the cranial form, acute motor cranial nerve palsy is seen which may involve single nerves or groups of nerves. In the spinal cord there is marked degeneration of anterior horn cells and neuroglial cell proliferation. Immunofluorescence staining for enterovirus 70 antigen reveals the presence of virus in the microglial or neuronal cells, or both.

Although expression of clinical disease of the CNS by enterovirus 70 is somewhat rare, enterovirus 71 has caused epidemics of aseptic meningitis and encephalitis. Originally described in California, the virus has been associated with neurological disease on a worldwide scale. The major clinical manifestation is that of aseptic meningitis which may often be concomitant with encephalitis, bulbospinal disturbances and polyneuritis. Studies in primates with strains of virus isolated from patients with CNS disease show degeneration and necrosis of the neurons and neuronophagia by polymorphonuclear and mononuclear cells. Analysis of the CNS reveals predominantly perivascular cuffing in the lumbar and cervical cord, with minor involvement of specific areas of the brain (including the medulla oblongata and midbrain).

Coxsackie viruses

Coxsackie viruses also enter the host primarily via the oral route and follow essentially the same path as poliovirus, with replication in the Peyer's patches of the alimentary tract. Most infections are clinically silent, although some individuals exhibit greater susceptibility to infection with Coxsackie viruses than others (a male/female infection ratio of 1.5 : 2.0 is observed for clinical disease). The reasons for this discrepancy remain elusive. Nervous system involvement has been documented for coxsackieviruses A7 and A9, and for coxsackieviruses B1–6, which induce a poliovirus-like paralysis. Encephalitis, ataxia and paralysis of the cranial nerves are rare. Both coxsackieviruses A and B are responsible for aseptic meningitis, although echoviruses (see below) are more frequently involved. Pathological changes with encephalitic and poliomyelitis cases in laboratory animals include brown fat necrosis and myocarditis, which is widespread in animals infected with coxsackie B virus.

Echoviruses

Echoviruses have been associated with a number of syndromes, including aseptic meningitis, encephalitis, paralysis, ataxia and Guillain–Barré syndrome, to list those affecting the CNS. Humans are the only recognized host for echoviruses and several epidemics of disease have been attributed to them. Assigning a particular serotype to a specific syndrome has not been possible, although Guillain–Barré syndrome has been linked to infection with echovirus 9. In addition, echovirus 4 has been isolated from patients with bilateral limb paralysis. Similar syndromes have been noted for adults and children infected with echovirus serotypes 9, 14 and 30. Primary infection results in replication of virus in the alimentary tract, after which

other organs are seeded following an initial viraemia. The nature of the secondary target is largely random. Occasional peripheral neuropathies have been documented following expression of virus in the CNS. Initial clinical symptoms of CNS invasion by echoviruses can mimic bulbospinal poliomyelitis, although the major clinical manifestation is that of lymphocytic meningitis. Neonatal infection with echoviruses may lead to encephalitis with white matter sclerosis. In general, infection of newborns and younger children with echovirus is more severe than in older people.

2.4   Flaviviruses

General considerations

There currently exist c. 70 registered flaviviruses (Chapter 29), of which about 50% are associated with human disease (Karabatsos 1985). Of those that cause significant CNS disease, Japanese encephalitis virus, which causes epidemics over much of Asia, carries the highest mortality rate of any flavivirus. In epidemics, mortality rates range from 10–20% in most outbreaks to >30% (Umenai et al. 1985, Bu'Lock 1986). Mosquito-borne JE virus continues to threaten large populations, even though massive vaccination campaigns have been undertaken. Vaccination may, however, be undermined to a large degree by the high antigenic variation in different subtypes of JE virus (Susilowati et al. 1981). Other mosquito-borne flaviviruses that tend to involve the CNS include St Louis encephalitis (SLE) and Murray Valley encephalitis (MVE). SLE became a serious public health problem in the USA in the 1960s and continues to cause concern during sporadic outbreaks (Kokernot et al. 1969). MVE causes epidemics in Australia, disease occurring intermittently in areas that have experienced periods of high rainfall. Epidemics in the southern hemisphere are usually recorded from January to March and coincide with high population levels of the mosquito vector (Shope 1980).

Tick-borne encephalitis virus (TBE) has long been recognized as a public health problem of eastern Europe. In Russia, the virus caused high mortality in the 1930s, prompting a great effort to isolate the causative agent and to produce a vaccine (Silber and Soloviev 1946). A number of subtypes of TBE have been defined in different geographical locations, including eastern subtypes such as Sofyn, the agent of Russian spring–summer encephalitis (RSSE) (Silber and Soloviev 1946), and western subtypes, such as Hypr (Blaskovic, Pucekova and Kubinyi 1967) and Neudörfl (Ackerman et al. 1986).

Japanese encephalitis
General considerations

Japanese encephalitis (JE) occurs in epidemic form in temperate areas of Asia and the northern parts of tropical southeast Asia. With respect to number of cases and associated morbidity and mortality, JE is the most important of the arbovirus encephalitides.

JE is transmitted to humans via the bite of an

infected mosquito (*Culex* spp.). After an initial viraemic phase, the virus may enter the CNS. Highly variable neurovirulence is observed for JE isolates when inoculated into mice, but to what degree this is applicable to infections of humans is unknown. Amino acid substitutions in the envelope (E) protein have been shown to drastically alter the neuropathogenicity of JE for mice, indicating that the initial interaction of virus with its receptor is an important determinant of virulence.

Pathogenesis and pathology

How JE invades the CNS is unknown, but the major areas of the brain infected by virus include the cerebral cortex, cerebellum and spinal cord. Once in the CNS, JE virus replicates very efficiently in neurons and it is the destruction of these cells by virus that is directly related to the manifestation of encephalitis. After a variable incubation period of 6–16 days, the disease may be asymptomatic or fulminant in course. Death may be rapid, occurring 10 days after onset in some cases. The reason for such differences in disease outcome remains a mystery. For patients who develop encephalitis, the disease pattern begins with headache and gastroenteritis, proceeding to the onset of high fever and alterations in sensory perception (including confusion or delirium which may result in coma). Seizures are uncommon in adults but are often (20% or more) seen in children. Facial motor weakness is often observed and upper motor neuron paralysis and paresis are common.

The brain and meninges of JE patients show oedema, congestion and focal haemorrhages. Microscopically, there is degeneration and necrosis of neurons with accompanying neuronophagia in the cerebral cortex, cerebellum and spinal cord. There is marked destruction of Purkinje cells in the cerebellum, as well as perivascular cuffing and inflammatory infiltrates in surrounding neural tissue. JE antigen is usually not detected in glial cells. The highest concentration of infected neurons is in the thalamus and brainstem. Neurological sequelae are common (up to 70%) in survivors of symptomatic JE infection and are particularly severe in children. Such sequelae include convulsive disorders, motor abnormalities, impaired intellect and emotional disturbances.

St Louis encephalitis

General considerations

St Louis encephalitis (SLE) is a mosquito-borne flavivirus that occurs in both endemic and epidemic forms in the USA and represents the most important arbovirus disease of North America. The virus is transmitted by the *Culex* spp.

Pathogenesis and pathology

Clinically, infection with SLE can range from inapparent infections to fulminant encephalitis and death. Patients usually present with or progress rapidly to one of 3 established syndromes: febrile headache, aseptic meningitis or encephalitis. The febrile headache is often accompanied by vomiting and nausea. Analysis of the CSF may reveal pleocytosis. There are no apparent signs of meningeal involvement or neurological abnormalities. Aseptic meningitis presents as an acute febrile illness with signs of meningeal irritation and pleocytosis in the CSF. Encephalitis attributed to SLE infection also includes meningoencephalitis and encephalomyelitis. Alterations in the state of consciousness or localized neurological abnormalities, or both, may be seen. Brinker and co-workers (1979) analysed data from 18 reports of patients with SLE. It is estimated that 70–80% of patients suffer from headache, nuchal rigidity and an altered level of consciousness. Almost 50% display tremors, pathological reflexes and confusion. Some 20–30% of patients exhibit multiple cranial nerve abnormalities, hypoactive deep tendon reflexes, positive Babinski signs or myalgia. More significantly, 11–20% of those infected have VIIth cranial nerve lesions, lower motor neuron lesions, hyperactive deep tendon reflexes or myoclonus and progress to coma. Up to 10% exhibit convulsions, paresis, photophobia, nystagmus or ataxia. There is a striking increase in case fatality rates for SLE infection, depending on age. A fatality rate of c. 2% is observed for young adults, rising to 22% for the elderly. Of those infected with SLE, c. 50% with fatal disease die within one week after onset of symptoms.

Murray Valley encephalitis

General considerations

Antigenically, Murray Valley encephalitis (MVE) virus is closely related to both JE and SLE viruses. In a number of respects, the clinical presentation of patients suffering from MVE is similar to JE infection. Clinically, the disease begins with a prodrome of fever, headache, photophobia, myalgia, nausea and vomiting. There are often early signs of CNS involvement that include drowsiness, speech difficulties, disorientation and ataxia. Patients who do not progress to coma generally have a favourable prognosis, but may display sequelae including tremors, incontinence, stiffened limbs and neck, and speech impediments. Patients who enter coma often develop respiratory paralysis necessitating mechanical aid for breathing. Fatalities are usually the result of secondary infection or extensive brain destruction accompanied by decerebrate rigidity.

Tick-borne encephalitis

General considerations

The tick-borne encephalitis (TBE) complex of the family *Flaviviridae* comprises 14 antigenically related viruses, 8 of which are significant human pathogens. The 2 most important pathogens are Russian spring–summer encephalitis (RSSE) and Central European encephalitis (CEE). These differ in pathogenicity, the former being associated with much higher rates of morbidity and mortality.

Pathogenesis and pathology

RSSE is characterized by a gradual onset following 10–14 days' incubation after the transmission of virus from the bite of an infected tick. The patient suffers a prodromal phase of severe headache, nausea, photophobia, weakness, fever and chills. The body temperature may rise as high as 41°C and the fever lasts 5–7 days. These symptoms are followed by neck stiffness, sensory changes, visual disturbances and variable neurological dysfunction including paresis, paralysis, sensory loss and convulsions (Silber and Soloviev 1946). The more severe cases can develop central paralysis or involve the brainstem or spinal cord, which may lead to bulbospinal or spinal paralysis. In fatal cases, death occurs within the first week after onset with case fatality rates of c. 30% (Gresikova and Beran 1981). Disease is more severe in children than in adults. Recovery from infection is protracted with neurological sequelae in 30–69% of survivors, manifested by residual flaccid paralysis of the shoulders and arms. These sequelae probably reflect permanent damage to neurons.

In comparison to RSSE, infection with CEE subtypes of virus is much milder, with a number of abortive infections. Classically, CEE is a biphasic illness with a prodromal period resembling influenza that either resolves completely or is followed by sudden onset of encephalitis. Onset of illness is often rapid with fever, severe headache, photophobia, nuchal rigidity, nausea and vomiting. Patients who present with brainstem involvement or have ascending paralysis generally have a poor prognosis. Although case fatality rates range between 1% and 5%, 20% of survivors suffer minor neuropsychiatric sequelae (Radsel-Medvescek et al. 1980). It is interesting that a small percentage of patients who recover from CEE have a progressive chronic encephalitis with remissions and relapses (Silber and Soloviev 1946).

There are swelling, congestion and petechial haemorrhages in the brain, similar to other flavivirus encephalitides. There is also meningeal and perivascular inflammation with neuronal degeneration and necrosis, neuronophagia and glial nodule formation in the cerebellar cortex, brainstem, basal ganglia and spinal cord. Far Eastern subtypes have a tropism for neurons of the grey matter of the medulla oblongata and upper cervical cord. The predominance of lower motor neuron paralysis of the upper extremities, observed in many cases of encephalitis, may be explained by the vulnerability of the anterior horn cells of the cervical cord to virus infection.

2.5 Retroviruses

General considerations

In this section, 2 retroviruses (see also Chapter 38) that cause distinct syndromes affecting the CNS are considered. The first of these, human immunodeficiency virus (HIV), is the agent of the aquired immune deficiency syndrome (AIDS). The second, human T cell leukaemia virus I (HTLV-I), has been linked with a specific disease on the grounds of the distribution of infected individuals and clustering of infection. Both viruses have a prolonged incubation period (average of 8–10 years for HIV and up to 40

years for HTLV-I-associated myelopathy). Some similarities exist between modes of transmission via transfer of body fluids containing free virus or, more often, infected cells. HIV and HTLV-I both have a primary tropism for lymphocytes.

Neuro-AIDS

Over the past decade, HIV has provided the scientific community, both academic and clinical, with numerous challenges. A number of these challenges have been resolved to a large degree, but the control of HIV by vaccine remains the primary goal of scientists world-wide. Despite the enormous and somewhat staggering amount of data available on virtually every aspect of HIV infection, one particular area remains rather obscure: the neurological disturbances associated with HIV infection. Specifically, it is unclear whether HIV infection is directly responsible for the pathological changes observed (due to replication of the virus leading to cytopathic effects) or if it causes pathology indirectly (e.g. induction of cytokines). Lastly, neurological complications could also reflect a secondary infection with opportunistic pathogens secondary to immunodeficiency.

Exactly how HIV gains access to the CNS is unknown. In early acute infections, HIV can be detected as free virus in the CSF of patients without any apparent neurological disturbances. Crossing of the BBB is believed to occur through passage in infected peripheral blood macrophages, which then allows infection of brain macrophages. In addition, activated T cells have been documented in the CNS which have presumably entered the nervous system through endothelial cell spaces. Recent evidence points to infection of brain capillary endothelium as an initial point of infection. The mechanism by which HIV infects cells of the CNS is also speculative, because a number of cells of the CNS do not express CD4, the major receptor for HIV in peripheral infection. HIV can infect brain-derived glial cells, and brain capillary endothelial cells (CD4 negative). In the light of the extensive pathology associated with some HIV-related neurological conditions, the degree of replication of HIV in CD4– cell lines is, paradoxically, generally low. Although an alternative receptor for entry of HIV into CD4– cells has not been conclusively defined, galactosylceramide (GalC) has been proposed to fulfil such a function in brain-derived cells (Harouse et al. 1991). In contrast to HTLV-I (see 'HTLV-I and HTLV-I-associated myelopathy/tropical spastic paraparesis', p. 859), distinct differences in tropism between strains of HIV can be demonstrated. In general, macrophage-tropic strains of virus replicate more efficiently in cells of neural origin than strains of lymphotropic nature. Once an HIV strain has been transmitted to the CNS, adaptation of the virus may take place. This assumption is confirmed by PCR studies which showed that viruses isolated from the blood and brain of a single host behave differently.

Pathology of neuro-AIDS

AIDS itself is often characterized by a high prevalence of marked and extensive neurological disturbances. In numerical terms, it is suggested that as many as 80% of AIDS patients will have neuropathological abnormalities at postmortem and that as many as half of these patients will have suffered neurological disturbances prior to death. Transient neurological disturbances can also be detected at the time of seroconversion and may include aseptic meningitis (characterized by headache, fever and cellular pleocytosis of the CSF), acute encephalopathy and myelopathy. All these disturbances are usually self-limiting during early infection. As HIV infection progresses to AIDS, a new spectrum of neurological complications may emerge, which are globally described as the AIDS dementia complex (ADC) (Cortegis 1994). The primary stages of ADC show mild impairment of memory, as well as loss of concentration and ability to process information. Symptoms may then progress to severe cognitive dysfunction and possibly paralysis. Morphologically, features associated with ADC include either a diffuse leucoencephalopathy with severe reduction in myelin or areas of discrete demyelination and multinucleated giant cells (Fig. 40.6). Clinically, ADC is suspected in AIDS patients presenting with memory loss, disturbances in concentration, depression and motor complaints. Specific afflictions associated with ADC include peripheral neuropathy, cerebral tumours and vascular lesions. Peripheral neuropathies are often observed in severely immunosuppressed patients who present with painful paraesthesiae. These neuropathies are due to axonal degeneration of small myelinated and unmyelinated fibres as a result of exposure to toxic factors (see below). It is interesting to note that the inflammatory neuropathies, including demyelinating polyneuropathy are identical in clinical course to Guillain–Barré syndrome or chronic inflammatory demyelinating polyneuropathy (Cornblath et al. 1987, Tyor et al. 1995). In the latter condition, the nerves show perivascular lymphocytic and monocytic infiltrates, believed to be mediated by T cells and macrophages. Cerebrovascular complications such as vasculitis and haemorrhages are often found in areas of cerebral tumour or demyelination (Snider et al. 1983). Haemorrhages may occur due to alterations in coagulation (Snider et al. 1983).

Mechanism of CNS distubances in neuro-AIDS

The mechanism by which HIV infection causes the clinical disorder of ADC is still highly hypothetical. Direct viral infection of susceptible cells of the CNS may induce syncytia formation, producing multinucleated giant cells. Multinucleated giant cells are usually formed by macrophages or microglial cells and are considered a hallmark of subacute encephalitis in HIV-infected brains and spinal cord, but not in peripheral nerves (Cornblath et al. 1987) (Fig. 40.6). As only a restricted number of cells of the CNS are susceptible to infection by HIV, secondary mechanisms of cellular injury may be paramount in producing neurological disturbances in AIDS patients.

The release of soluble cellular factors by cells in response to viral assault or to binding of virus proteins may be an important facet of the disease process of HIV. The fact that brain atrophy in patients with AIDS is symmetrical supports the concept.

Infection of monocytes or macrophages by HIV is known to stimulate the synthesis and release of a number of cytokines, including interleukins (ILs), TNF-α and interferons. These are characteristically detected in high levels in the CSF of AIDS patients. Release of cytokines and lymphokines is not limited to cells of the macrophage/monocyte lineage. Astrocytes and microglial cells can also be induced to secrete IL-1, IL-6 and TNF-α. Altered concentrations of the above substances may be toxic to surrounding cells, particularly neurons, because they perturb normal cellular functions, such as metabolism and intercellular communication. During trauma or disease (e.g. bacterial infection), both IL-1 and TNF-α cause lesions in the white matter and astrogliosis, as well as vascular changes, including vascular permeability, neuroinvasion and necrosis of blood vessels. In one study, the most notable change associated with HIV dementia with AIDS was mRNA up-regulation for TNF-α. TNF-α levels were higher in patients with advanced dementia and those with multinucleated giant cells or diffuse myelin pallor (Wilt et al. 1995). The release of cytokines could also make the BBB more permeable to inflammatory cells which may then infiltrate the CNS to establish additional neurological sequelae. Although significant levels of quinolinic acid have been reported in the CNS of HIV-1 seropositive patients, whether there is a direct causal relationship to the observed neurological findings remains questionable. Induction of TGF-β by macrophages and astrocytes has also been linked to CNS disorders (Wahl et al. 1991). This connection was based on findings that TGF-β is expressed in the brains of HIV-infected patients and that purified human monocytes infected with HIV exhibited an increased propensity to secrete TGF-β. Supporting the role of secreted factors in the neuropathology of HIV infection is the observation that macrophages infected with HIV secrete soluble factors, in contrast to non-infected macrophages that are destructive to human brain cells in vitro (Pulliam et al. 1991). The principal question often raised when discussing the importance of secreted factors in neuro-AIDS, is whether the concentration of these various factors is sufficiently high to induce disease in vivo.

Autoimmunity is also thought to be important in the process of HIV-induced neurological disease and may be based on the partial identity between viral antigens and antigenic determinants on cells (i.e. molecular mimicry). An autoimmune process was proposed following the observation that small demyelinated regions of the brain seem similar to those in post-infectious encephalomyelitis or experimental allergic encephalitis (EAE) (Kumar et al. 1989). AIDS patients with peripheral neuropathy have autoantibodies to an unidentified protein on the surface of neurons. In addition, fluorescence studies have shown antibody attached to the perineurium in tissues from AIDS patients. AIDS patients suffering from peripheral neuropathy who undergo subsequent plasmaphaeresis obtain relief of symptoms similar to that observed in the autoimmune conditions of Guillain–Barré syndrome and thrombocytopenic purpura. Autoantibodies to peripheral nerves are associated with peripheral neuropathy. A likely target in the nervous system is the myelin sheath of nerves. Antibody levels to myelin basic protein have been described in CSF of AIDS patients that correlate directly with the severity of dementia (Liuzzi et al. 1994). Cross-reactivity of anti-gp41 antibodies with certain

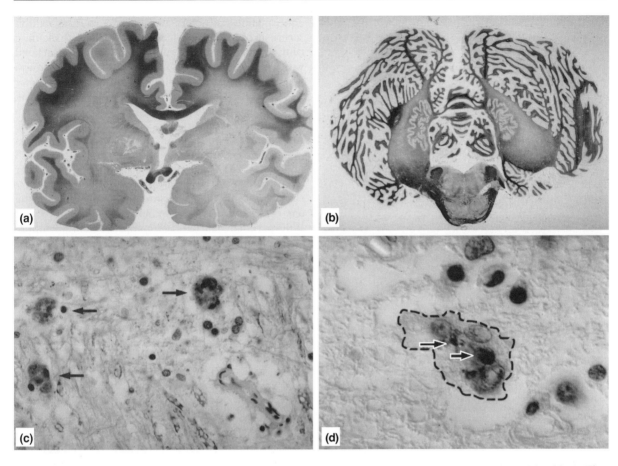

Fig. 40.6 HIV encephalopathy. (**a**) Whole mount of a brain slice, stained with a myelinotropic dye (Luxol-fast blue). The hallmark of HIV leucoencephalopathy is diffuse reduction of myelin stain in the central white matter. (**b**) Whole mount of the cerebellum of the same patient. Leucoencephalopathy is evident in the deep cerebellar white matter. (**c**) High power micrograph of HIV leucoencephalopathy, showing loss of myelin and typical multinucleated giant cells (arrows) (×200). (**d**) Immunostaining of a multinucleated giant cell for the HIV protein p24, showing granular immunoreactivity (arrows) (×400). (Courtesy of Dr Adriano Aguzzi.)

proteins of astrocytes could compromise the function of these cells. Moreover, cross-reaction of anti-V3 antibody with human brain proteins may also be an important part of the pathogenic process. Further brain-reactive proteins in the sera of infected patients may lead to immune complex disease.

A number of HIV products (e.g. gp120) are toxic to cultured human brain cells in vitro. The mechanism for these cellular disturbances is unknown, but may be due to the induction of IL-6 and TNF-α by gp120. It has been suggested that toxicity may occur via the NMDA receptor involving quinolinic acid. NMDA antagonists have been shown to reduce toxic effects attributed to gp120 interaction (Lipton et al. 1991). The same viral protein can also affect the permeability of the cell membrane, leading to ion influx/efflux and loss of electrical potential. In addition, HIV proteins gp41 and tat have been shown to be toxic for cultured cells; tat exhibits some homology with a neurotoxin and induces cellular aggregation and fascicle formation in primary rat cortical brain cells (Garry and Koch 1992). In addition, tat may induce differentiation of these cells (Kolson et al. 1993). The clinical relevance of these findings, however, remains unclear. When discussing HIV infection, it is also important to consider that neurotropic effects may reflect infection with an additional agent. A number of studies have shown the presence of viruses such as CMV (Fig. 40.7), herpes and

papovaviruses in the CNS of AIDS patients, and have led to the suggestion that secondary infections are the primary cause of neurological disturbances.

HTLV-I AND HTLV-I-ASSOCIATED MYELOPATHY/TROPICAL SPASTIC PARAPARESIS

General considerations

HTLV-I was established as the probable agent of acute T cell leukaemia (ATL) on the basis of epidemiological surveys linking virus prevalence to ATL cases. In addition, a correlation between tumour cells and a monoclonal or oligoclonal pattern of viral genome integration, infection of lymphocytes in vitro resulting in immortalized T cells, and the recent establishment of HTLV-I oncogenic animal model systems have been reported (Cann and Chen 1990). However, in 1985, it was discovered that a number of HTLV-I-seropositive patients in the Caribbean and Japan were suffering from a chronic myelopathy. Since then, increasing evidence has accumulated linking HTLV-I infection with what is now termed HTLV-I-associated myelopathy

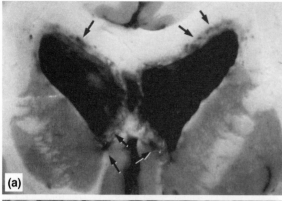

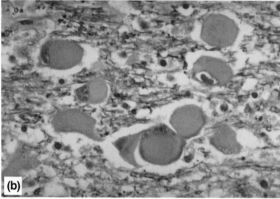

Fig. 40.7 Cytomegalovirus encephalitis in an AIDS patient. (a) Typical CMV-induced damage with areas of necrosis and microhaemorrhage located in subependymal positions (arrows). (b) Focus of CMV encephalitis within the corpus callosum (×400). Characteristic cytomegalic cells with large inclusion bodies representing viral products. (Courtesy of Dr Adriano Aguzzi.)

(HAM) or tropical spastic paraparesis (TSP), collectively known as HAM/TSP.

Pathogenesis and pathology

HAM/TSP presents as a clinical disease very distinct from ATL. The disorder is characterized by weakness and spasticity of the extremities, hyper-reflexia, peripheral sensory loss and chronic inflammation. Development of HAM/TSP correlates with the presence of lesions in the white matter of the spinal cord, including demyelination and axonal changes. In the subacute disease there is progressive paralysis of lower extremities and associated impotence, incontinence and sensory symptoms, paradoxically, often with minimal sensory findings on examination. Lesions are localized primarily in the thoracic spinal cord with little, if any, cerebral involvement. In cases of late disease, hyalinization of vessels with necrosis and demyelination of the spinal cord, particularly in the throracic region, is observed. Because many patients are infected through breast-feeding from infected mothers or via sexual transmission, the virus is thought to be transmitted by infected lymphocytes. The incubation period is particularly long, with onset often in the 4th or 5th decade of life.

Gross examination of the brain reveals no apparent

abnormalities, although the majority of cases exhibit severe atrophy of the spinal cord and some thickening of the meninges. These clinical findings are associated with HAM/TSP patients with a long history of illness, whereas in cases with a clinical history of one year or less the spinal cord often seems normal (Fukura et al. 1989). The overriding finding in HAM/TSP cases is a chronic inflammatory process involving grey and, more often, white matter of the spinal cord. This results in perivascular infiltrates throughout the CNS and in varying degrees of primarily white matter destruction (Wu et al. 1993). The inflammatory process varies in cellular constituents, depending on the age of the lesions in the spinal cord. New lesions with little parenchymal damage comprise mainly lymphocytes of the CD4+ lineage and monocytes, whereas older lesions with diffuse gliosis characteristically contain lipid-rich macrophages and CD8+ lymphocytes in the parenchyma or perivascular spaces with relatively sparse CD4+ lymphocytes and monocytes (Iwazaki 1990). As genetic analysis of virus isolated from ATL and HAM/TSP patients has not revealed the presence of determinants for neurotropism, the basis for such a major difference in disease pattern remains a mystery at present. HTLV-I sequence analysis of PBMCs of HAM/TSP patients demonstrates a pattern of polyclonal integration, in contrast to an oligoclonal or monoclonal pattern associated with ATL patients. Most HAM/TSP patients have higher titres of anti-HTLV-I antibody than asymptomatic HTLV-I patients. Nevertheless, despite a strong immunological response to HTLV-I, HAM/TSP patients have a much larger population of infected cells than HTLV-I carriers. Additional studies have shown a continuing state of lymphocyte activation in HAM/TSP patients, reflected by the large number of circulating mononuclear cells able to undergo spontaneous proliferation, or by an increase of anti-HTLV-I antibody in serum and CSF.

It has proved particularly difficult to isolate or convincingly demonstrate the presence of HTLV-I antigen or mRNA in the CNS of HAM/TSP patients. To date, the only evidence for the presence of virus has been through the detection of HTLV-I proviral DNA by PCR (Lehky and Jacobson 1995). An autoimmune basis for HAM/TSP has been proposed after isolation of circulating MHC class I restricted CTLs from HAM/TSP patients. The CTLs show specific activity against HTLV-I tax protein (Elovaara et al. 1993). In vitro, HTLV-I infects human glial cells with a resulting induction of MHC class II expression on these cells. This could result in functional disruption and development of lesions in the CNS. The occurrence of lesions outside the spinal cord is apparently rare, although perivascular mononuclear cell infiltration in the brain has been reported (Iwazaki 1990).

To help researchers and clinicians in understanding the disease process involved in HAM/TSP, a rat animal model has been developed in which the characteristics and distribution of lesions in the rat CNS are uncannily similar to those observed in human cases. The rat model of disease was produced after inoculation of MT-2 cells (human lymphoid cells that are persistently infected with HTLV-I) into neonatal Wistar–King–Aptekman (WKA) rats (Ishiguro et al. 1992). Sixteen months later the rats developed spastic paraparesis. Subsequent histological analysis revealed characteristic HAM/TSP-like lesions in the CNS in a distribution corresponding to human disease. Despite immunological and pathological observations in HAM/TSP, however, the role of HTLV-I in the pathogenesis of this disorder remains elusive.

2.6 Paramyxoviruses

The 2 paramyxoviruses liable to cause disease of the CNS are mumps and measles viruses, both members of the subfamily *Paramyxovirinae* (Chapter 23).

CNS MANIFESTATIONS OF MUMPS VIRUS INFECTION

Mumps is a highly communicable and generally self-limited infection caused by mumps virus (MuV). It occurs in epidemics among susceptible school-aged children and is clinically characterized by non-suppurative salivary gland enlargement. Although parotitis is the most obvious manifestation, mumps is clearly a systemic infection that can involve virtually all organs, including the CNS. Indeed, CNS involvement during acute mumps infection occurs with such high frequency that it should be considered a primary manifestation, rather than a complication. The spectrum of CNS infections caused by mumps virus ranges from aseptic meningitis, which is very common but usually mild, to fulminant encephalitis, which is very rare but potentially fatal. The term 'mumps meningoencephalitis' is often used to designate overlap syndromes that have features of both these typical forms.

Pathogenesis and pathology

Mumps is a highly contagious infection that is transmitted from human to human (the only known natural host) by droplets. Infected individuals may transmit the virus for about 10–16 days. During the incubation period (which averages 18 days), primary viral replication takes place in epithelial cells of the upper respiratory tract, followed by spread of the virus to regional lymph nodes and subsequent viraemia with systemic dissemination.

Symptomatic CNS involvement occurs in 10–20% of mumps cases (Russell and Donald 1958). The vast majority of cases of CNS MuV infections are uncomplicated aseptic meningitis, whereas symptomatic encephalitis occurs in <0.1% of cases (Klemola et al. 1965, Levitt et al. 1970). The incidence of CNS inflammation as evidenced by pleocytosis in the CSF (observed in only 60% of the cases) is actually much higher than the incidence of clinical meningoencephalitis (Bang and Bang 1943).

Although differences in neurotropism among MuV isolates have been demonstrated in animal models, there is no direct evidence that cases of human mumps encephalitis are caused by virus strains with enhanced neurotropism or virulence.

MuV spreads readily to the CNS either as free plasma virus or within infected mononuclear cells (Fleischer and Kreth 1982). Initially, viral replication occurs in choroidal epithelial cells with shedding of progeny virus into the CSF (Herndon et al. 1974). The development of mumps encephalitis probably results from a direct extension of virus from ependymal cells into neurons within the brain parenchyma, as has been demonstrated in experimentally induced mumps encephalitis in hamsters (Wolinsky et al. 1974). Because of the low case/fatality ratio, autopsy reports describing the pathological findings in mumps meningoencephalitis are rare and variable (reviewed in Gnann 1991). Histological changes are seen in the white matter of the cerebral hemispheres and cerebellum, and in the white and grey matter of the brainstem and the spinal cord. The most commonly recorded features are diffuse oedema of the brain, limited mononuclear cell infiltration of the meninges, perivascular infiltration with mononuclear cells, glial cell proliferation, focal areas of neuronal cell destruction, and localized demyelination. A few cases of purported chronic mumps encephalitis have been described, but available data are insufficient to support a role for mumps virus in chronic CNS infection (Ito et al. 1991).

Clinical findings

Patients with symptomatic mumps CNS infection most often present with fever, vomiting and headache. Other frequent findings include nuchal rigidity, lethargy and abdominal pain (possibly from pancreatitis). Defervescence is usually the first sign of clinical recovery, which is normally complete within 7–10 days. Patients with simple mumps aseptic meningitis have signs of meningeal irritation, however, with normal cortical functions. Cases of mumps encephalitis present with seizures, markedly depressed level of consciousness and focal neurological signs. Typical findings also include psychiatric disturbances, lethargy and stupor. CNS symptoms appear about 5 days after onset of parotitis, although CNS symptoms may accompany or even precede the development of salivary gland enlargement. No association between the parotitis and the frequency or severity of CNS manifestation has been established. Other neurological manifestations of mumps include cases of myelitis and polyneuropathy.

Confirmation of CNS involvement in patients with mumps is based on examination of the CSF. CSF findings do not differ significantly between mumps patients with meningitis and those with encephalitis. MuV can be isolated from CSF in 30–50% of patients with CSF pleocytosis (Björvatn and Wolontis 1971, Wolontis and Björvatn 1973). The spinal fluid opening pressure is normal. Infiltrating cells are predominantly lymphocytes, but significant amounts of polymorphonuclear leucocytes may be seen in the early stages of infection. CSF pleocytosis resolves slowly, and complete normalization of the spinal fluid may require several weeks (Azimi et al. 1975). No correlation has been established between the magnitude of the CSF pleocytosis and the severity of clinical illness.

MEASLES VIRUS INFECTIONS OF THE CNS

Measles virus (MV) is a highly contagious agent that leads to a well defined acute disease in unvaccinated individuals, followed by seroconversion and a lifelong immunity against reinfection. As hallmarks of acute measles, a transient, marked lymphopenia and immunosuppression are observed, which favour the establishment and fatal outcome of opportunistic infections, and are the main reasons for the annual death toll of more than 1.5 million children worldwide, particularly in third world countries (Clements and Cutts 1995). MV infections have also been linked aetiologically to the establishment of CNS disease processes that include an early acute measles encephalitis and 2 late complications: SSPE and measles inclusion body encephalitis (MIBE). Moreover, some studies have suggested a pathogenic role of MV for other disease processes, including multiple sclerosis (ter Meulen and Katz 1997), chronic liver disease (Robertson et al. 1987, Andjaparidzne et al. 1989), Paget's disease (Basle, Fournier and Rozenblatt 1986), otosclerosis (McKenna and Mills 1989) and, more recently, Crohn's disease (Wakefield et al. 1993). However, none of these diseases has been linked unequivocally to measles virus.

Virus–host interactions

Acute MV infections are characterized by the marked tropism of the virus for PBMCs, including both lymphocytic and monocytic cells (Borrow and Oldstone 1995). The virus is present in a highly cell-associated form and is efficiently spread via infected PBMCs, in which both viral nucleic acid and proteins can easily be detected and from which infectious virus can be recovered. Patients with a history of acute measles develop a lifelong immunity against reinfection. CNS involvement with acute measles is fairly common, as EEG and CSF changes are found in half of all patients with acute measles (Gibbs et al. 1959, Reinicke, Mordhorst and Ingerslev 1974). It is not entirely clear what pathogenic role MV plays in the development of acute measles encephalitis. MV has been occasionally recovered from CSF samples (McLean et al. 1966) and brain tissue of patients (ter Meulen et al. 1972), including the detection of MV-specific nucleic acids by PCR techniques (Nakayama et al. 1995). Because there is no evidence that MV is regularly present in the nervous system and because there is an aberrant immune reaction to brain antigens, acute measles encephalitis is considered an autoimmune disease (Griffin 1995).

In contrast, SSPE and MIBE develop months to years after acute measles on the basis of a persistent MV infection in neurons and glial cells (reviewed by Schneider-Schaulies and ter Meulen 1992). In contrast to MIBE in which a low or no antibody reaction to MV is detectable as a result of an underlying immunosuppression, in SSPE exceedingly high titres of anti-MV antibodies against the major structural proteins of MV (except for the M protein) are present both in serum and in CSF samples of the patients. No specific defects have been detected concerning cell-mediated immunity. Yet in both CNS diseases, MV nucleocapsid structures are present within infected cells, as confirmed by neuropathological studies (ter Meulen, Stephenson and Kreth 1983). However, rescue of infectious virus in tissue culture is rarely possible, indicating that the viral replication cycle is defective, rather than being capable of reactivation as seen with HSV. As with other persistent infections, MV gene expression is markedly restricted during persistence. Viral envelope proteins are generally expressed at extremely low levels, whereas internal proteins required for intracellular viral reproduction (N, P) can be detected easily. As characterized mainly in autopsy material, this is generally achieved by particular restrictions of the viral envelope-specific mRNAs (M, F and H) and by mutations within the envelope-specific genes that interfere with a functional expression of the corresponding proteins (reviewed in Billeter et al. 1994) (summarized in Fig. 40.8). It is significant for the pathogenesis that mutations introduced into the envelope gene reading frames are of 2 types: point mutations, caused by the naturally high infidelity of the viral polymerase during transcription/replication; and clustered hypermutations, ascribed to a cellular unwinding/modifying enzyme complex. Functional alterations or complete abolition of the MV envelope proteins seem to readily explain why the formation of infectious virus particles, viral budding and the formation of giant cells are not encountered in persistent MV CNS infections. Moreover, important antigenic structures are mainly lacking on the surface of infected cells, which thus escape detection by the MV-specific humoral immune response.

The pathogenesis of persistent MV CNS infection is not well understood. It is not clear how and how frequently MV is transported into the CNS during acute measles. Infected PBMCs have been proposed as potential carriers, but have not been positively identified. Moreover, a recent PCR study confirmed the presence of MV-specific nucleic acids in autopsy brain material obtained from patients with no history of measles-associated CNS illness (Katayama et al. 1995), suggesting that persistent MV infections of the brain may be more frequent than initially thought and may stay clinically inapparent throughout life.

Although it is not understood what triggers the development of a MV CNS disease, some progress has been made in understanding which factors lead to and maintain the establishment of a persistent MV infection in brain cells. Increasing evidence suggests that MV that infects brain cells is primarily non-defective and that host factors initially attenuate viral gene expression on both transcriptional and translational levels (reviewed by Schneider-Schaulies et al. 1994). In addition, MV-specific double-stranded RNA intermediates, as formed accidentally during viral transcription and replication, serve as targets for a cellular enzyme (dsRNA adenosine deaminase activity,

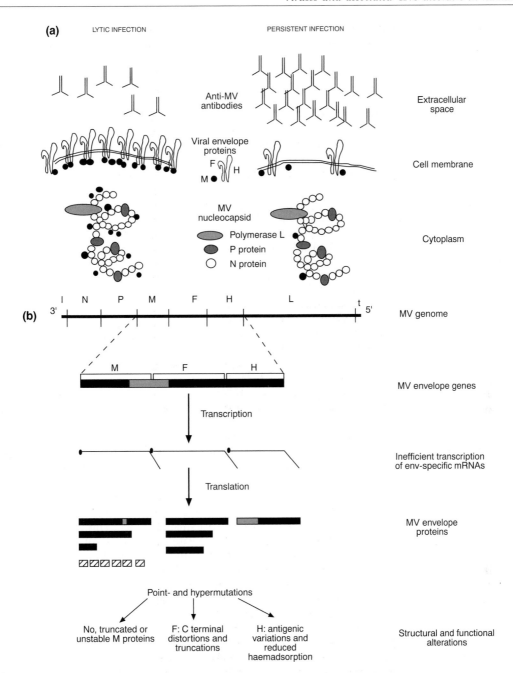

Fig. 40.8 Mechanisms of measles virus persistence in the human CNS. (**a**) During acute infection, the viral ribonucleocapsid particle (RNP) consisting of the genomic RNA encapsidated by the N protein and the transcriptase complex (L and P proteins) is amplified intracellularly. Concomitantly, the viral glycoproteins F and H (expressed as complexes) are expressed at the surface of the infected cell with the M protein underlying their integration sites. In persistent infections, the RNP structures are easily detected in large amounts in the cytoplasm (and the nucleus) of the infected brain cell. The expression of both the glycoproteins and the M protein is generally low or even absent. Pathognomonic for SSPE, a humoral hyperimmune reaction to viral antigens (mainly to N and H protein) is observed both in CSF and in serum. (**b**) The structural genes of MV are encoded in a linear arrangement along the MV genome: l represents the leader, t the trailer region that contains the viral promoter sequences and encapsidation sites. In persistent infections, the expression of the MV envelope genes *M*, *F* and *H* (shown enlarged, the grey region indicates a 1 kb non-coding region separating the *M* and *F* reading frames) is greatly reduced by different mechanisms: (1) the frequency of the corresponding mRNAs is very low, and (2) their reading frames are more or less affected by mutations that lead to complete abolition or truncated or distorted expression of the corresponding gene product. Most mutations have been encountered within the *M* genes, and all F proteins characterized so far have truncated C termini. Both point mutations (introduced by the viral polymerase) and hypermutations (clustered transitions most probably introduced by a cellular enzyme complex; see Fig. 40.9) have been described.

DRADA) present in large amounts in brain cells in vitro. This enzyme introduces up to 50% of nucleotide transitions within a given double-stranded target RNA, thus profoundly altering the coding sequences (Billeter et al. 1994) (Fig. 40.9). There is still, however, some controversy about whether mutations within the viral genome are a prerequisite for the establishment of persistent MV infection in brain cells, whether mutant viruses have a selective advantage in replication and spread in the brain, or if mutations are important for the long-term maintenance of MV persistence. The last possibility is weakened by the high variability of the mutations encountered in individual patients with SSPE and MIBE, and also by the finding that, at least in an animal model, persistent MV CNS infections have been established in the absence of detectable mutations.

Measles encephalitis

Acute encephalitis in the course of measles is observed in 0.5–1 per 1000 cases (Katz 1995). In general, about 15% of cases are fatal, and 20–40% of those who recover are left with lasting neurological sequelae. Encephalitis usually develops within about 8 days after the onset of measles. Occasionally, it may also occur during the prodromal stage. Measles encephalitis is characterized by resurgence of fever, headache, seizures, cerebellar ataxia and coma. As commonly seen in post-infectious encephalitis induced by other viruses, demyelination, perivascular cuffing, gliosis and the appearance of fat-laden macrophages near the blood vessel walls are detectable histopathologically. Petechial haemorrhages may be present and, in some cases, inclusion bodies have been observed in brain cells. CSF findings in measles encephalitis usually consist of mild pleocytosis and absence of MV-specific antibodies. Long-term sequelae include selective brain damage with retardation, recurrent convulsive seizures, hemiplegia and paraplegia.

Measles inclusion body encephalitis

MIBE has been recognized only recently and is confined to immunosuppressed children with, for example, leukaemia undergoing axial irradiation therapy. The incubation period ranges from weeks to several months. The condition commences with convulsions, myoclonic jerks as seen in SSPE. The seizures are often focal and localized to one site; other findings include hemiplegia, coma or stupor. However, the disease course is more rapid than SSPE and proceeds to death within weeks or a few months. Characteristically, no or only low titres of MV-specific antibodies are mounted in the serum and CSF of patients.

Subacute sclerosing panencephalitis

SSPE is a rare, fatal, slowly progressive degenerative disease of the CNS. It is generally seen in children and young adults aged 6–8 years after acute measles, with an overall incidence of 1 in 1 million cases. Boys are more likely than girls to develop SSPE, and half the patients have contracted measles before the age of 2 years. No unusual features of the acute measles have ever been demonstrated. The course of SSPE is variable and usually starts with a generalized intellectual deterioration, which may last for weeks or months, until definite neurological signs or motor dysfunctions such as dyspraxia, generalized convulsions, aphasia, visual disturbances and mild repetitive simultaneous myoclonic jerks appear. Viral invasion of the retina leads, in 75% of cases, to a chorioretinitis, often affecting the macular area, followed by blindness. Finally, the disease proceeds to progressive cerebral degeneration, leading to coma and inevitable death. The illness generally lasts for 1–3 years, but more rapid forms have been described. Neuropathological findings include a diffuse encephalitis affecting both the grey and white matter, characterized by perivascular cuffing and diffuse lymphocytic infiltrations. Gliosis is usually observed. Fibrous astrocytes, neurons and oligodendroglial cells contain large aggregates of intranuclear inclusion bodies that contain MV nucleocapsid structures visible on immunohistological examination. Giant cell formation or membrane changes consistent with virus maturation have not been detected.

Characteristic EEG changes are usually the first diagnostic hint and are regarded as characteristic and even pathognomonic for SSPE. They consist of periodic, high-amplitude slow wave complexes that are synchronous with myoclonic jerks recurring at 3.5–20 second intervals. These periodic complexes (Radermecker) are remarkably stereotypical in an individual patient, in that their form remains identical in any given lead. They are bilateral, usually synchronous and symmetrical. Moreover, they usually consist of 2 or more delta waves and are biphasic, triphasic or polyphasic in appearance. This EEG pattern, however, is variable within the course of the disease and from one patient to another, and may disappear as the disease progresses. Other important pathognomonic findings are the very high titres of measles antibodies in the blood – except those against the M protein – and a pronounced increase in the gammaglobulin in the CSF. In the CSF, the humoral immune response is oligoclonally restricted, as revealed by isoelectric focusing (Dörries and ter Meulen 1984). This indicates that antibodies are synthesized intrathecally by a restricted number of plasma cells that have invaded the CNS.

3 CONCLUSIONS AND OUTLOOK

The observation that viruses can induce slowly progressive neurological diseases with diverse pathology has led to speculations that many other neurological diseases of unknown cause may have a viral aetiology, the prime candidate being multiple sclerosis. This potential, together with epidemiological, neuropathological, immunological and clinical findings, has encouraged extensive virological studies in pursuit of relevant infectious agents. Although several claims have been made for viruses isolated from multiple sclerosis patients, no infectious agent has yet been

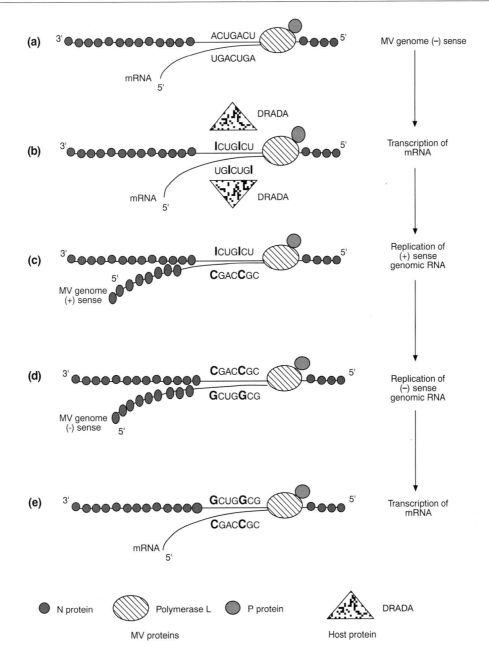

Fig. 40.9 DRADA (dsRNA adenosine deaminase activity): a cellular enzyme altering viral sequences. DRADA, initially detected and described in vitro in extracts of frog oocytes, is able to introduce clustered transitions into dsRNA structures both in vivo and in vitro. Increasing evidence suggests that unencapsidated viral dsRNAs (step **a**), accidentally formed during transcription/replication of negative-strand RNA viruses, may serve as targets for this cellular enzyme activity (step **b**) that deaminated adenosine (A) to inosine (I) residues. During replication of the positive-strand genome, a cytidine (C) residue will be introduced instead of the expected uridine (U) into the positive-strand intermediate (step **c**); upon replication of this altered (+) genome, G will be introduced into the (–) genomic RNA (step **d**) which will in turn lead to the introduction of C into the mRNA (step **e**), replacing the initial U (step **a**). Although DRADA is mainly found in the nucleus, some activity has been consistently detected in the cytoplasm, in particular of neural cells.

linked to the disease. Other diseases such as amyotrophic lateral sclerosis, continuous focal epilepsy or Alzheimer's disease also reveal certain features that would be compatible with a viral infection. Recently, Borna disease virus (BDV), which has been linked to a variety of neurological diseases in several animal hosts, has also been associated with certain psychiatric disorders in humans such as schizophrenia and manic-depression, because BDV-specific nuclei acids in

PBMCs of patients and BDV-specific antibodies have occasionally been detected (Bode 1995). No direct evidence is yet available to support the possibility that viruses cause these diseases, but their involvement cannot be ruled out

Better understanding of the pathogenesis of viral CNS infections is a prerequisite to obtaining new and more effective means to prevent disease (e.g. the development of potent vaccines that would prevent the virus from entering the nervous system). However, each virus has different protection requirements. On the other hand, neurotropic virus infections also offer interesting possibilities for studying the structure and function of the nervous system, as in studies using neurotropic rabies or HSV for tracing neural pathways (Kuypers and Ugolini 1990). Moreover, neurotropic viruses are also used as vehicles to bring foreign genes to the CNS. Gene therapy approaches have been used in animal experiments to reduce tumour growth in brain tissue (Tapscott et al. 1994). It is therefore conceivable that a controlled viral infection of the CNS might be used for the selective expression of, for example, pharmacological agents or neurotransmitters in order to influence functional aspects of the CNS. Thus, studies of viral infections of the CNS offer new perspectives, leading to a better understanding of the pathogenesis of disease.

ACKNOWLEDGEMENT

The work in the authors' laboratory was supported by the Deutsche Forschungsgemeinschaft and the Bundesministerium für Forschung und Technologie.

REFERENCES

Achim CL, Wiley CA, 1992, Expression of major histocompatibility complex antigens in the brains of patients with progressive multifocal leukoencephalopathy, *J Neuropathol Exp Neurol*, **51**: 257–63.

Ackerman R, Kruger K et al., 1986, Spread of early summer meningoencephalitis in the Federal Republic of Germany, *Dtsch Med Wochenschr*, **111**: 927–33.

Ahmed R, Butler LD, Bhatti L, 1988, T4⁺ T helper cell function in vivo: differential requirement for induction of antiviral cytotoxic T cell and antibody response, *J Virol*, **62**: 2102–6.

Almond JW, 1987, The attenuation of poliovirus neurovirulence, *Annu Rev Microbiol*, **41**: 153–80.

Almond JW, 1991, Poliovirus neurovirulence, *Semin Neurosci*, **3**: 101–8.

Almond PS, Bumgardner GL et al., 1991, Immunogenicity of class I⁺, class II⁻ hepatocytes, *Transplant Proc*, **23**: 108–9.

Andjaparidze OG, Chaplygina NM et al., 1989, Detection of measles virus genome in blood leucocytes of patients with certain autoimmune diseases, *Arch Virol*, **105**: 287–91.

Arthur RR, Dagostin S, Shah K, 1989, Detection of BK virus and JC virus in urine and brain tissue by the polymerase chain reaction, *J Clin Microbiol*, **27**: 1174–9.

Ash RJ, 1986, Butyrate-induced reversal of herpes simplex virus restriction in neuroblastoma cells, *Virology*, **155**: 584–92.

Askonas BA, Taylor PM, Esquivel F, 1988, Cytotoxic T cells in influenza infection, *Ann NY Acad Sci*, **532**: 230–44.

Azimi PH, Shaban S et al., 1975, Mumps meningoencephalitis: prolonged abnormality of cerebrospinal fluid, *JAMA*, **234**: 1161–2.

Baldridge JR, Buchmeier MJ, 1992, Mechanisms of antibody-mediated protection against lymphocytic choriomeningitis virus infection: mother-to-baby transfer of humoral protection, *J Virol*, **66**: 4252–7.

Baldridge JR, Pearce BD et al., 1993, Teratogenic effects of neonatal arenavirus infection on the developing rat cerebellum are abrogated by passive immunotherapy, *Virology*, **197**: 669–77.

Ball MJ, 1982, Limbic predilection in Alzheimer dementia: is reactivated herpesvirus involved?, *Can J Neurol Sci*, **9**: 303–6.

Bang HO, Bang J, 1943, Involvement of the central nervous system in mumps, *Acta Med Scand*, **113**: 487–505.

Basle MF, Fournier JG, Rozenblatt S, 1986, Measles virus RNA detected in Paget's disease bone tissue by in situ hybridisation, *J Gen Virol*, **67**: 907–13.

Bauer W, Chamberlin W, Horenstein S, 1969, Spinal demyelination in progressive multifocal leucoencephalopathy, *Neurology*, **19**: 287–94.

Bergelson JM, Finberg RW, 1993, Integrins as receptors for virus attachment and cell entry, *Trends Microbiol*, **1**: 287–9.

Bergelson JM, Shepley MP et al., 1992, Identification of the integrin VLA-2 as a receptor for echovirus 1, *Science*, **255**: 1718–20.

Bergelson JM, Chan M et al., 1994, Decay accelerating factor (CD55), a glycosylphosphatidyl-anchored comlement regulatory protein, is a receptor for several echoviruses, *Proc Natl Acad Sci USA*, **91**: 6245–50.

Berger JR, Kaszovitz B et al., 1987, Progressive multifocal leukoencephalopathy associated with human immunodeficiency virus infection. A review of the literature with a report of sixteen cases, *Ann Intern Med*, **107**: 78–87.

Berger JR, Scott S et al., 1992, Progressive multifocal leukoencephalopathy in HIV-infected children, *AIDS*, **2**: 837–41.

Billeter MA, Cattaneo R et al., 1994, Generation and properties of measles virus mutations typically associated with subacute sclerosing panencephalitis, *Ann NY Acad Sci*, **724**: 367–77.

Björvatn B, Wolontis S, 1971, Mumps meningoencephalitis in Stockholm November 1964–July 1971, *Scand J Infect Dis*, **5**: 253–60.

Blaskovic D, Pucekova G, Kubinyi L, 1967, An epidemiological study of tick-borne encephalitis in the Tribec region: 1956–63, *Bull W H O*, **36**: 89–94.

Bode L, 1995, Human infections with Borna disease virus and potential pathogenic implications, *Curr Top Microbiol Immunol*, **190**: 103–30.

Bodian D, Horstmann DM, 1965, Polioviruses, *Viral and Rickettsial Infections of Man*, 4th edn, eds Horsfall FL Jr, Tamm I, Lippincott, Philadelphia PA, 430–73.

Boldorini R, Cristina S et al., 1993, Ultrastructural studies in the lytic phase of progressive multifocal leukoencephalopathy in AIDS patients, *Ultrastruct Pathol*, **17**: 599–609.

Borrow P, Nash AA, 1992, Susceptibility to Theiler's virus-induced demyelinating disease correlates with astrocyte class II induction and antigen presentation, *Immunology*, **76**: 133–9.

Borrow P, Oldstone MBA, 1995, Measles virus–mononuclear cell interactions, *Current Top Microbiol Immunol*, **191**: 85–100.

Botteron C, Zurbriggen A et al., 1992, Canine distemper virus–immune complexes induce bystander degeneration of oligodendrocytes, *Acta Neuropathol (Berl)*, **83**: 402–7.

Brinker KR, Paulson G et al., 1979, St Louis encephalitis in Ohio, September 1975: clinical and EEG in 18 cases, *Arch Intern Med*, **139**: 561–6.

Brooks BR, Walker DL, 1984, Progressive multifocal leukoencephalopathy, *Neurol Clin*, **2**: 299–313.

Buchmeier M, Lewicki H et al., 1984, Murine hepatitis virus-4 (strain JHM) induced neurologic disease is modulated in vivo by monoclonal antibody, *Virology*, **132**: 261–70.

Bu'Lock FA, 1986, Japanese B encephalitis in India: a growing problem, *Q J Med*, **60**: 825–36.

Cai JP, Falanga V, Chin YH, 1991, TGF-β regulates the adhesive interactions between mononuclear cells and microvascular endothelium, *J Invest Dermatol*, **97**: 169–78.

Campbell IL, 1991, Cytokines in viral diseases, *Curr Opin Immunol*, **3**: 486–91.

Cann AJ, Chen ISY, 1990, Human T-cell leukemia virus types I and II, *Fields' Virology*, 2nd edn, eds Fields BN, Knipe DM et al., Raven Press, New York, 1501–28.

Cannella B, Cross AH, Raine CS, 1991, Adhesion-related molecules in the CNS: upregulation correlates with inflammatory cell influx during relapsing EAE, *Lab Invest*, **65**: 23–33.

Ceccaldi PE, Fillion MP et al., 1993, Rabies virus selectively alters 5-HT1 receptor subtypes in rat brain, *Eur J Pharmacol*, **245**: 129–38.

Challoner PB, Smith KT et al., 1995, Plaque-associated expression of human herpesvirus 6 in multiple sclerosis, *Proc Natl Acad Sci USA*, **92**: 7440–4.

Chowdhury M, Taylor JP et al., 1990, Regulation of the human neurotropic virus promoter by JCV-T antigen and HIV-1 tat protein, *Oncogene*, **5**: 1737–42.

Clatch RJ, Lipton HL, Miller SD, 1987, Class II restricted T cell responses in Theiler's murine encephalomyelitis virus (TMEV)-induced demyelinating disease. II. Survey of host immune responses and central nervous system virus titers in inbred mouse strains, *Microb Pathog*, **3**: 327–37.

Clements CJ, Cutts FT, 1995, The epidemiology of measles: thirty years of vaccination, *Curr Top Microbiol Immunol*, **191**: 13–33.

Compton T, Nowlin DM, Cooper NR, 1993, Initiation of human cytomegalovirus infection requires initial interaction with cell surface heparan sulphate, *Virology*, **193**: 834–42.

Corboy JR, Buzy JM et al., 1992, Expression directed from HIV long terminal repeats in the central nervous system of transgenic mice, *Science*, **258**: 1804–8.

Cornblath DR, McArthur JC et al., 1987, Inflammatory demyelinating peripheral neuropathies associated with human T-cell lymphotropic virus type III infection, *Ann Neurol*, **21**: 32–40.

Cortegis P, 1994, AIDS dementia complex: a review, *J Acquir Immune Defic Syndr*, **7**: 38–48.

Cosby SL, Macquaid S et al., 1989, Examination of eight cases of multiple sclerosis and 56 neurological and non-neurological controls for genomic sequences of measles virus, *J Gen Virol*, **70**: 2027–36.

Coyle P, 1991, Viral infections in the developing nervous system, *Semin Neurosci*, **3**: 157–63.

Cross AH, 1992, Immune cells traffic control and central nervous system, *Semin Neurosci*, **4**: 312–19.

Dalgleish AG, Beveriev PCL et al., 1984, The CD4 (T4) antigen is an essential component of the receptor for the AIDS retrovirus, *Nature (London)*, **312**: 763–7.

Dietzschold B, Kao M et al., 1992, Delineation of putative mechanisms involved in antibody-mediated clearance of rabies virus from the central nervous system, *Proc Natl Acad Sci USA*, **89**: 7252–6.

Ding AH, Nathan CF, Stuehr DJ, 1988, Release of reactive nitrogen and oxygen intermediates from mouse peritoneal macrophages: comparison of activating cytokines and evidence for independent production, *J Immunol*, **141**: 2407–12.

Dörig RE, Marcil A et al., 1993, The human CD46 molecule is a receptor for measles virus (Edmonston strain), *Cell*, **75**: 295–305.

Dörries R, ter Meulen V, 1984, Detection and identification of virus-specific oligoclonal IgG in unconcentrated cerebrospinal fluid by immunoblot technique, *J Neuroimmunol*, **7**: 77–89.

Dörries R, Schwender S et al., 1991, Population dynamics of lymphocyte subsets in the central nervous system of rats with different susceptibility to coronavirus-induced demyelinating encephalitis, *Immunology*, **74**: 539–45.

Dörries K, Vogel E et al., 1994, Infection of human polyomavirus JC and BK in peripheral blood leukocytes from immunocompetent individuals, *Virology*, **198**: 59–70.

von Einsiedel RW, Fife TD et al., 1993, Progressive multifocal leukoencephalopathy in AIDS: a clinicopathologic study and review of the literature, *J Neurol*, **240**: 391–406.

Elovaara I, Koenig S et al., 1993, High human T-cell lymphotropic virus type I (HTLV-I) specific precursor cytotoxic T-lymphocyte frequencies in patients with HTLV-I associated neurological disease, *J Exp Med*, **177**: 1567–73.

Elsner C, Dörries K, 1992, Evidence of human polyomavirus BK and JC infection in normal brain tissue, *Virology*, **191**: 72–80.

Fabry Z, Topham DJ et al., 1995, TGF-β2 decreases migration of lymphocytes in vitro and homing of cells into the CNS in vivo, *J Immunol*, **155**: 325–32.

Feigenbaum L, Khalili K et al., 1987, Regulation of the host range of human papovavirus JCV, *Proc Natl Acad Sci USA*, **84**: 3695–8.

Feldman LT, 1994, Transcription of the HSV-1 genome in neurons in vitro, *Semin Virol*, **5**: 207–12.

Felgenhauer K, Reiber H, 1992, The diagnostic significance of antibody specificity indices in multiple sclerosis and herpes virus induced diseases of the nervous system, *Clin Invest*, **70**: 28–37.

Fleischer B, Kreth HW, 1982, Mumps virus replication in human lymphoid cell lines and in peripheral blood lymphocytes: preference for T cells, *Infect Immun*, **35**: 25–31.

Fournier JG, Tardieu M et al., 1985, Detection of measles virus RNA in lymphocytes from peripheral blood and brain in perivascular infiltrates of patients with subacute sclerosing panencephalitis, *N Engl J Med*, **313**: 910–15.

Fraser NW, Lawrence NC et al., 1981, Herpes simplex virus type 1 DNA in human brain tissue, *Proc Natl Acad Sci USA*, **78**: 6461–5.

Frohman EM, Frohman TC et al., 1989, The induction of intercellular adhesion molecule 1 (ICAM-1) expression on human fetal astrocytes by interferon-gamma, tumor necrosis factor alpha, lymphotoxin and interleukin-1: relevance to intracerebral antigen presentation, *J Neuroimmunol*, **23**: 117–24.

Fujinami RS, Oldstone MBA, 1980, Alterations in expression of measles virus polypeptides by antibody: molecular events in antibody-induced antigenic modulation, *J Immunol*, **125**: 78–85.

Fujinami RS, Oldstone MBA, 1985, Amino acid homology and immune responses between the encephalitogenic site of myelin basic protein and virus: a mechanism for autoimmunity, *Science*, **230**: 1043–5.

Fukura H, Tashiro K et al., 1989, CT and MRI findings in HAM: a report on five cases, *Prog in CT*, **11**: 69–73.

Gamble JR, Vadas MA, 1991, Endothelial cell adhesiveness for human T lymphocytes is inhibited by TGF-β1, *J Immunol*, **146**: 1149–56.

Garry RF, Koch G, 1992, Tat contains a sequence related to snake neurotoxins, *AIDS*, **6**: 1541–2.

Geretry SJ, Karpus WJ et al., 1994, Class II-restricted T cell responses in Theiler's murine encephalomyelitis virus-induced demyelinating disease, *J Immunol*, **152**: 908–24.

Gibbs FA, Gibbs L et al., 1959, Electroencephalographic abnormality in 'uncomplicated' childhood diseases, *JAMA*, **171**: 1050–5.

Giulian D, Vaca K, Noonan CA, 1990, Secretion of neurotoxins by mononuclear phagocytes infected with HIV-1, *Science*, **250**: 1593–6.

Gnann JW, 1991, Meningitis and encephalitis caused by mumps virus, *Infections of the Central Nervous System*, eds Scheld WM, Whitley RJ, Durack DT, Raven Press, New York, 113–26.

Gresikova M, Beran GW, 1981, Tick-borne encephalitis., *CRC Handbook Series in Zoonoses*, section B: Viral Zoonoses vol I, ed Beran GW, CRC Press, Boca Raton FL, 201–8.

Griffin DE, 1995, Immune responses during measles virus infections, *Curr Top Microbiol Immunol*, **191**: 117–34.

Gullota F, Masini T et al., 1992, Progressive multifocal leukoencephalopathy in gliomas in an HIV-negative patient, *Path Res Pract*, **188**: 964–72.

Haase AT, 1986, Pathogenesis of lentivirus infections, *Nature (London)*, **332**: 130–6.

Halbach M, Koschel K, 1979, Impairment of hormone dependent signal transfer by chronic SSPE virus infection, *J Gen Virol*, **42**: 615–19.

Harouse JM, Bhat S et al., 1991, Inhibition of entry of HIV-1 in neural cell lines by antibodies against galactosyl ceramide, *Science*, **253**: 320–3.

Harris CA, Derbin KS et al., 1991, Manganese superoxide dismutase is induced by IFN-γ in multiple cell types: synergistic induction of IFN-γ and tumor necrosis factor of IL-1, *J Immunol*, **147**: 149–54.

Hay J, Ruyechan T, 1994, Varizella-zoster virus – a different kind of herpesvirus latency?, *Semin Virol*, **5**: 241–7.

Herndon RM, Johnston RT et al., 1974, Ependymitis in mumps virus meningitis, *Arch Neurol*, **30**: 475–9.

Hickey WF, Hsu BL, Kimura H, 1991, T-lymphocyte entry into the CNS, *J Neurosci Res*, **28**: 254–63.

Hofman FM, Hinton DR et al., 1991, Lymphokines and immunoregulatory molecules in subacute sclerosing panencephalitis, *Clin Immunol Immunopathol*, **58**: 331–42.

Holman RC, Janssen RS et al., 1991, Epidemiology of progressive multifocal leukoencephalopathy in the United States: analysis of national mortality and AIDS surveillance data, *Neurology*, **41**: 1733–6.

Hom RC, Finberg RW et al., 1991, Protective cellular retroviral immunity requires both CD4+ and CD8+ T cells, *J Virol*, **65**: 220–4.

Homsy J, Meyer M et al., 1989, The Fc and not CD4 receptor mediates antibody enhancement of HIV infection in human cells, *Science*, **244**: 1357–60.

Houff SA, Major EO et al., 1988, Involvement of JC virus-infected mononuclear cells from the bone marrow and spleen in the pathogenesis of progressive multifocal leukoencephalopathy, *N Engl J Med*, **318**: 301–5.

Ishiguro N, Abe M et al., 1992, A rat model of HTLV-I infection. Humoral antibody response, provirus integration and HAM/TSP-like myelopathy in seronegative HTLV-I carrier rats, *J Exp Med*, **176**: 981–9.

Ito M, Go T et al., 1991, Chronic mumps virus encephalitis, *Pediatr Neurol*, **7**: 467–70.

Iwasaki Y, 1990, Pathology of chronic myelopathy associated with HTLV-I infection (HAM/TSP), *J Neurol Sci*, **96**: 103–23.

Iwasaki Y, Liu D et al., 1985, On the replication and spread of rabies virus in the human central nervous system, *J Neuropathol Exp Neurol*, **44**: 185–95.

Johnston RT, 1994, Nervous system viruses, *Encyclopedia of Virology*, vol II, eds Webster RG, Granoff A, Academic Press, London, 907–14.

Johnston RT, Griffin DE, 1986, Virus-induced autoimmune demyelinating disease of the CNS, *Concepts in Viral Pathogenesis*, vol II, eds Notkins AL, Oldstone MBA, Springer Verlag, New York, 203–9.

Johnston RT, Griffin DE et al., 1984, Measles encephalomyelitis: clinical and immunological studies, *N Engl J Med*, **310**: 137–41.

Joncas JH, Robillard LR et al., 1976, Interferon in serum and cerebrospinal fluid in subacute sclerosing panencephalitis, *Can Med Assoc J*, **115**: 309–15.

Jonjic S, Pavic I et al., 1990, Efficacious control of cytomegalovirus infection after long-term depletion of CD8+ T lymphocytes, *J Virol*, **64**: 5457–64.

Jubelt B, Ropka SL et al., 1991, Susceptibility and resistance to poliovirus-induced paralysis of inbred mouse strains, *J Virol*, **65**: 1035–40.

Karabatsos N, 1985, Editorial, *International Catalogue of Arboviruses including other viruses of vertebrates*, The Subcommitte on Information Exchange of The American Society of Tropical Medicine and Hygiene, San Antonio TX, 3.

Kastrukoff LF, Lau AS, Kim SU, 1987, Multifocal CNS demyelination following peripheral inoculation with herpes simplex virus type 1, *Ann Neurol*, **22**: 52–9.

Katayama Y, Hotta H et al., 1995, Detection of measles virus nucleoprotein mRNA from autopsied brain tissues, *Arch Virol*, **76**: 3201–4.

Katz M, 1995, Clinical spectrum of measles, *Curr Top Microbiol Immunol*, **191**: 1–12.

Kaye BR, Neuwelt CM et al., 1992, Central nervous system systemic lupus erythematosus mimicking progressive multifocal leukoencephalopathy, *Ann Rheum Dis*, **51**: 1152–6.

Kemp LM, Dent CL, Latchman DS, 1990, Octamer motif mediates transcriptional repression of HSV immediate early genes and octamer-containing cellular promoters in neuronal cells, *Neuron*, **4**: 215–22.

Kennedy MK, Tan LJ et al., 1990, Inhibition of murine relapsing experimental autoimmune encephalomyelitis by immune tolerance to proteolipid protein and its encephalitogenic peptides, *J Immunol*, **144**: 909–15.

Kennedy PGE, 1990, The use of molecular techniques in studying viral pathogenesis in the nervous system, *Trends Neurosci*, **13**: 424–31.

Kitamura N, Semler BL et al., 1981, Primary structure, gene organization and polypeptide expression of poliovirus RNA, *Nature (London)*, **291**: 547–53.

Klapper PE, Cleator GM, 1992, The diagnosis of herpes encephalitis, *Rev Med Microbiol*, **3**: 151–8.

Klatzmann D, Champagne E et al., 1984, T lymphocyte T4 molecule behaves as the receptor for human retrovirus LAV, *Nature (London)*, **312**: 767–78.

Klemola E, Kaarinen L et al., 1965, Studies on viral encephalitis, *Acta Med Scand*, **177**: 707–16.

Koike S, Horie H et al., 1990, The poliovirus receptor protein is produced both as membrane bound and secreted forms, *EMBO J*, **9**: 3217–24.

Kokernot RH, Hayes J et al., 1969, St Louis encephalitis in the USA, *Am J Trop Med Hyg*, **18**: 750–71.

Kolson DL, Buchhalter J et al., 1993, HIV-1 Tat alters normal organization of neurons and astrocytes in primary rodent brain cell cultures, *AIDS Res Hum Retroviruses*, **9**: 677–85.

Koprowski H, Zeng YM et al., 1993, In vivo expression of inducible nitric oxid synthetase in experimentally induced neurological disease, *Proc Natl Acad Sci USA*, **90**: 3024–7.

Koschel K, Münzel P, 1980, Persistent paramyxovirus infections and behaviour of β-adrenergic receptors in C6 rat glioma cells, *J Gen Virol*, **47**: 513–17.

Kraus E, Schneider-Schaulies S et al., 1992, Augmentation of major histocompatibility complex class I and ICAM-1 expression on glial cells following measles virus infection: evidence for the role of type-1 interferon, *Eur J Immunol*, **22**: 175–82.

Kristensson K, 1982, Implications of axoplasmic transport for the spread of virus infections in the nervous system, *Axoplasmic Transport in Physiology and Pathology*, eds Weiss DG, Gorio A, Springer, New York, 153–8.

Kruypers HGJM, Ugolini G, 1990, Viruses as transneuronal tracers, *Trends Neurosci*, **13**: 71–5.

Kuchelmeister K, Gullotta F, Bergmann M, 1993, Progressive multifocal leukoencephalopathy (PML) in the acquired immune deficiency syndrome (AIDS). A neuropathological autopsy study of 21 cases, *Path Res Pract*, **189**: 163–73.

Kühn JE, Dahm C et al., 1991, Detection of herpes simplex virus (HSV) in clinical specimen by polymerase chain reaction (PCR), *Ärztl Laboratorium*, **37**: 69–73.

Kumar M, Resnick L et al., 1989, Brain reactive antibodies and the AIDS dementia complex, *J Acquir Immune Defic Syndr*, **2**: 469–71.

Ladogana A, Bouzamondo E et al., 1994, Modification of tritiated gamma-amino-*n*-butyric acid transport in rabies virus-infected primary cortical cultures, *J Gen Virol*, **75**: 623–7.

La Monica N, Almond JW, Racaniello VR, 1987, A mouse model for poliovirus neurovirulence identifies mutations that attenuate the virus for humans, *J Virol*, **61**: 2917–20.

Lehky TJ, Jacobson S, 1995, Induction of HLA class II in HTLV-I infected neuronal cell lines, *J Neurovirol*, **1**: 145–56.

Lenhardt TM, Wiley CA, 1989, Absence of humorally mediated damage within the central nervous system of AIDS patients, *Neurology*, **39**: 278–80.

Lentz TL, 1990, The recognition event between virus and host cell receptor: a target for antiviral agents, *J Gen Virol*, **71**: 751–66.

Levine B, Hardwick JM et al., 1991, Antibody-mediated clearance of alphavirus infection from neurons, *Science*, **254**: 856–60.

Levitt LP, Rich TA et al., 1970, Central nervous system mumps, *Neurology*, **20**: 829–34.

Liebert UG, Finke D, 1995, Measles virus infections in rodents, *Curr Top Microbiol Immunol*, **191**: 149–66.

Liebert UG, Linington C, ter Meulen V, 1988, Induction of auto-immune reactions to myelin basic protein in measles virus encephalitis in Lewis rats, *J Neuroimmunol*, **17**: 103–18.

Liebert UG, ter Meulen V, 1987, Virological aspects of measles virus induced encephalomyelitis in Lewis and BN rats, *J Gen Virol*, **68**: 1715–22.

Lillycrop KA, Estridge JK, Latchman DS, 1993, The octamer binding protein Oct-2 inhibits transactivation of the herpes simplex virus immediate-early genes by the virion protein Vmw65, *Virology*, **196**: 888–91.

Lindsley MD, Thiemann R, Rodriguez M, 1991, Cytotoxic T cells isolated from the central nervous systems of mice infected with Theiler's virus, *J Virol*, **65**: 6612–20.

Lipton SA, Sucher NJ et al., 1991, Synergistic effects of HIV coat protein and NMDA receptor-mediated neurotoxicity, *Neuron*, **7**: 111–18.

Liszewski MK, Post TW, Atkinson JP, 1991, Membrane cofactor protein (MCP or CD46): newest member of the regulators of complement activation gene cluster, *Annu Rev Immunol*, **9**: 431–55.

Liuzzi GM, Mastroianni CM et al., 1994, Myelin degrading activity in the CSF of HIV-1 infected patients with neurological diseases, *Neuroreport*, **6**: 157–60.

Lynch KJ, Frisque RJ, 1991, Factors contributing to the restricted DNA replicating activity of JC virus, *Virology*, **180**: 306–17.

McGeoch DJ, Barnett BC, MacLean CA, 1993, Emerging functions of alphavirus genes, *Semin Virol*, **4**: 125–34.

McKenna MJ, Mills BG, 1989, Immunohistochemical evidence of measles virus antigen in active otosclerosis, *Otolaryngol Head Neck Surg*, **101**: 415–18.

McLean DM, Best JM et al., 1966, Viral infection of Toronto children during 1965. II. Measles encephalitis and other complications, *Can Med Assoc J*, **94**: 905–10.

Major EO, Amemiya K et al., 1992, Pathogenesis and molecular biology of progressive multifocal leukoencephalopathy, the JC virus induced demyelinating disease of the human brain, *Clin Microbiol Rev*, **5**: 49–73.

Martin X, Dolvio M, 1983, Neuronal and transneuronal tracing in the trigeminal system of the rat using the herpes virus suis, *Brain Res*, **273**: 253–76.

Mason PW, Rieder E, Baxt B, 1994, RGD sequence of foot and mouth disease virus is essential for infecting cells via the natural receptor but can be by-passed by an antibody-dependent enhancement pathway, *Proc Natl Acad Sci USA*, **91**: 1932–6.

Massa PT, Dörries R, ter Meulen V, 1986, Viral antigens induce Ia antigen expression on astrocytes, *Nature (London)*, **320**: 543–6.

Massa PT, Schimpl A et al., 1987, Tumor necrosis factor amplifies measles virus-mediated Ia induction on astrocytes, *Proc Natl Acad Sci USA*, **84**: 7242–5.

Maudsley DJ, Morris AG, Tomkins PT, 1989, Regulation by interferon of the immune responses to viruses via the major histocompatibility complex antigens, *Immune Responses, Virus Infections and Disease*, eds Dimmock NJ, Minor PD, IRL Press, Oxford, 15–32.

Mazlo M, Tariska I, 1992, Progressive multifocal leukoencephalopathy: ultrastructural findings in two brain biopsies, *Acta Neuropathol (Berl)*, **56**: 323–39.

Mellerick DM, Fraser NW, 1987, Physical state of the latent herpes virus genome in a mouse model system: evidence suggesting an episomal state, *Virology*, **158**: 265–73.

Melnick JL, 1990, Enteroviruses: polioviruses, Coxsackieviruses, echoviruses and newer enteroviruses, *Fields' Virology*, 2nd edn, eds Fields BN, Knipe DM et al., Raven Press, New York, 549–604.

Mendelsohn CL, Wimmer E, Racaniello V, 1989, Cellular receptor for poliovirus: molecular cloning, nucleotide sequence, and expression of a new member of the immunoglobulin superfamily, *Cell*, **56**: 855–65.

Merrill JE, Chen ISY, 1991, HIV-1, macrophages, glial cells, and cytokines in AIDS nervous system disease, *FASEB J*, **5**: 2391–7.

ter Meulen V, Katz M, 1997, The proposed viral etiology of multiple sclerosis and related demyelinating diseases, *Multiple Sclerosis: clinical and pathogenetic basis*, eds Raine CS, McFarland H, Tourtellotte WW, Chapman & Hall, London, 287–305.

ter Meulen V, Stephenson JR, Kreth HW, 1983, Subacute sclerosing panencephalitis, *Comprehensive Virology*, eds Fraenkel-Conrat H, Wagner RR, Plenum Press, New York, London, 105–59.

ter Meulen V, Kackell Y et al., 1972, Isolation of infectious measles virus in measles encephalitis, *Lancet*, **2**: 1172–5.

Momburg F, Koch N et al., 1986, In vivo induction of H-2K/D antigens by recombinant interferon-γ, *Eur J Immunol*, **16**: 551–7.

Moskophidis D, Cobbold P et al., 1987, Mechanism of recovery from acute virus infection: treatment of lymphocytic choriomeningitis virus-infected mice with monoclonal antibodies reveals that Lyt-2⁺ T lymphocytes mediate clearance of virus and regulate the antiviral antibody response, *J Virol*, **61**: 1867–74.

Munsat TL, 1991, Poliomyelitis – new problems with an old disease, *N Engl J Med*, **324**: 1206–7.

Nakayama T, Mori T et al., 1995, Detection of measles virus genome directly from clinical samples by reverse transcriptase-polymerase chain reaction and genetic variability, *Virus Res*, **35**: 1–16.

Naniche D, Varior-Krishnan G et al., 1993, Human membrane cofactor protein (CD46) acts as a cellular receptor for measles virus, *J Virol*, **67**: 6025–32.

Nash AA, 1991, Virological and pathological processes involved in Theiler's virus infection of the central nervous system, *Sem Neurosci*, **3**: 109–16.

Nash AA, Leung KN, Wildy P, 1985, The T cell-mediated immune response of mice to herpes simplex virus, *The Herpesviruses*, 4th edn, eds Roizman B, Lopez C, Plenum Press, New York, 87–102.

Nash AA, Jayasuriya A et al., 1987, Different roles for L3T4⁺ and Lyt 2⁺ T cell subsets in the control of an acute herpes simplex virus infection of the skin and nervous system, *J Gen Virol*, **68**: 825–33.

Nathan C, 1992, Nitric oxide as a secretory product of mammalian cells, *FASEB J*, **6**: 3051–64.

Oldstone MBA, 1989, Molecular mimicry as a mechanism for the cause and a probe uncovering etiologic agent(s) of autoimmune disease, *Curr Top Microbiol Immunol*, **145**: 127–35.

Oldstone MBA, Bokisch VA et al., 1975, Subacute sclerosing panencephalitis: destruction of human brain cells by antibody and complement in an autologous system, *Clin Imm Immunopathol*, **4**: 52–8.

Orefice G, Campanella G et al., 1993, Presence of papovavirus-like particles in cerebrospinal fluid of AIDS patients with progressive multifocal leukoencephalopathy. An additional test for in vivo diagnosis, *Acta Neurol (Napoli)*, **15**: 328–32.

Padgett BL, Walker DL, 1983, Virologic and serologic studies of progressive multifocal leukoencephalopathy, *Prog Clin Biol Res*, **105**: 107–17.

Padgett BL, ZuRhein GM et al., 1971, Cultivation of papova-like virus from human brain with progressive multifocal leucoencephalopathy, *Lancet*, **1**: 1257–60.

Plata-Salaman CR, 1991, Imunoregulators in the central nervous system, *Neurosci Biobehav Rev*, **15**: 185–215.

Pohl-Koppe A, Dahm C et al., 1992, The diagnostic significance of the polymerase chain reaction and isoelectric focusing in herpes simplex virus encephalitis, *J Med Virol*, **36**: 147–54.

Pullen LC, Miller SD et al., 1993, Class I-deficient resistant mice intracerebrally inoculated with Theiler's virus show an increased T cell response to viral antigens and susceptibility to demyelination, *Eur J Immunol*, **23**: 2287–93.

Pullian L, Herndier BG et al., 1991, Human deficiency virus infected macrophages produce soluble factors that cause histological and neurochemical alterations in cultured human brains, *J Clin Invest*, **87**: 503–12.

Quagliarello VJ, Wispelwey B et al., 1991, Recombinant human IL-1 induced meningitis and blood–brain barrier injury in the rat, *J Clin Invest*, **87**: 1360–6.

Racke MK, Dhib-Jalbut S et al., 1991, Prevention and treatment of chronic relapsing EAE by transforming growth factor β1, *J Immunol*, **146**: 3012–19.

Racke MK, Sriram S et al., 1993, Long-term treatment of chronic relapsing EAE by transforming growth factor β2, *J Neuroimmunol*, **46**: 175–83.

Radsel-Medvescek A, Marolt-Gomiscek M et al., 1980, Late sequelae after tick-borne meningoencephalitis in patients treated at the Hospital for Infectious Diseases, University Medical Centre of Ljubljana, during the period 1974–1975, *Zentralbl Bakteriol*, **suppl 9**: 281–4.

Ranganathan PN, Khalili K, 1993, The transcriptional enhancer element, kappa B, regulates promoter activity of the human neurotropic virus JCV in cells derived from the CNS, *Nucleic Acids Res*, **21**: 1959–64.

Ransohoff RM, Hamilton TA et al., 1993, Astrocyte expression of MRNA encoding cytokines IP-10 and JE/MCP-1 in experimental autoimmune encephalomyelitis, *FASEB J*, **7**: 592–9.

Reboul J, Schuller E et al., 1989, Immunoglobulins and complement components in 37 patients infected by HIV-1 virus: comparison of general (systemic) and intrathecal immunity, *J Neurol Sci*, **89**: 243–52.

Reeves RH, O'Hara BF et al., 1988, Genetic mapping of the *Mx* influenza virus resistance gene within the region of mouse chromosome 16 that is homologous to human chromosome 21, *J Virol*, **62**: 4372–6.

Reinicke V, Mordhorst CA, Ingerslev N, 1974, Central nervous system affection in connection with ordinary measles, *Scand J Infect Dis*, **6**: 131.

Richards EP, 1988, Progressive multifocal leukoencephalopathy 30 years later, *N Engl J Med*, **318**: 315–16.

Rima BK, Duffy N et al., 1991, Correlation between humoral immune responses and presence of virus in the CNS in dogs experimentally infected with canine distemper virus, *Arch Virol*, **121**: 1–8.

Robertson DAF, Zhang SL et al., 1987, Persistent measles virus genome in autoimmune chronic active hepatitis, *Lancet*, **2**: 9–11.

Robertson MN, Spangrude GJ et al., 1992, Role and specificity of T-cell subsets in spontaneous recovery from Friend virus-induced leukemia in mice, *J Virol*, **66**: 3271–7.

Rock DL, 1993, The molecular basis of latent infections by alphaviruses, *Semin Virol*, **4**: 157–65.

Rock DL, Fraser NW, 1983, Detection of HSV-1 genome in central nervous system of latently infected mice, *Nature (London)*, **302**: 523–5.

Rock DL, Fraser NW, 1985, Latent herpes simplex virus type 1 DNA contains two copies of the virion DNA joint region, *J Virol*, **55**: 849–52.

Roivainen M, Hyypia T et al., 1991, RGD-dependent entry of coxsackievirus A9 into host cells and its bypass after cleavage of VP1 protein by intestinal proteases, *J Virol*, **65**: 4735–43.

Ruddle NH, Bergman CM et al., 1990, An antibody to lymphotoxin and tumor necrosis factor prevents transfer of experimental allergic encephalomyelitis, *J Exp Med*, **172**: 1193–200.

Russell RR, Donald JC, 1958, The neurological complications of mumps, *Br Med J*, **2**: 27–30.

Sabin AB, 1956, Pathogenesis of poliomyelitis. Reappraisal in the light of new data, *Science*, **123**: 1151–7.

Santambrogio L, Hochwald GM et al., 1993, Studies on the mechanism by which TGF-β protects against EAE, *J Immunol*, **151**: 1116–23.

Schijns VECJ, Van der Neut R et al., 1991, Tumour necrosis factor α, interferon-γ and interferon-β exert antiviral activity in nervous tissue cells, *J Gen Virol*, **72**: 809–15.

Schneider EM, Dörries K, 1993, High frequency of polyomavirus infection in lymphoid cell preparations after allogeneic bone marrow transplantation, *Transplant Proc*, **25**: 1271–3.

Schneider-Schaulies S, ter Meulen V, 1992, Molecular aspects of measles virus induced central nervous system diseases, *Molecular Neurovirology*, ed Roos RP, Humana, Clifton, 419–49.

Schneider-Schaulies S, Schnorr JJ et al., 1994, The role of host factors in measles virus persistence, *Semin Virol*, **5**: 273–80.

Schneider-Schaulies J, Schnorr JJ et al., 1995, Receptor usage and differential downregulation of CD46 by measles virus wild-type and vaccine strains, *Proc Natl Acad Sci USA*, **92**: 3943–7.

Schnorr JJ, Dunster LM et al., 1995, Measles virus-induced downregulation of CD46 is associated with enhanced sensitivity to complement-mediated lysis of infected cells, *Eur J Immunol*, **25**: 976–84.

Schwender S, Imrich H, Dörries R, 1991, The pathogenic role of virus-specific antibody-secreting cells in the central nervous system of rats with different susceptibility to coronavirus-induced demyelinating encephalitis, *Immunology*, **74**: 533–8.

Sedgwick JD, Dörries R, 1991, The immune system response to viral infection of the CNS, *Semin Neurosci*, **3**: 93–100.

Sedgwick J, Schwender S et al., 1991a, Isolation and direct characterization of resident microglia cells from the normal and inflamed central nervous system, *Proc Natl Acad Sci USA*, **88**: 7438–42.

Sedgwick JD, Mössner R et al., 1991b, MHC-expressing non-hematopoietic astroglial cells prime only CD8+ T lymphocytes: astroglial cells as perpetuators but not initiators of CD4+ T cell responses in the central nervous system, *J Exp Med*, **173**: 1235–46.

Sedgwick JD, Schwender S et al., 1993, Resident macrophages (ramified microglia) of the adult brown Norway rat central nervous system are constitutively major histocompatibility complex class II positive, *J Exp Med*, **177**: 1145–52.

Selmaj KW, 1992, The role of cytokines in inflammatory conditions of the central nervous system, *Semin Neurosci*, **4**: 221–9.

Shah KV, 1990, Polyomaviruses, *Fields' Virology*, 2nd edn, eds Fields BN, Knipe DM et al., Raven Press, New York, 1609–23.

Shankar V, Kao M et al., 1992, Kinetics of virus spread and changes in levels of several cytokine mRNAs in the brain after intranasal infection of rats with Borna disease virus, *J Virol*, **66**: 992–8.

Shope RE, 1980, Medical significance of togaviruses: an overview of disease in man and in domestic and wild animals, *The Togaviruses: Biology, Structure, Replication*, ed Schlesinger RW, Academic Press, New York, 47–77.

Shyu WC, Lin JC et al., 1993, Recurrent ascending myelitis: an unusual presentation of herpes simplex virus type 2 infection, *Ann Neurol*, **34**: 625–7.

Silber LA, Soloviev VD, 1946, *American Review of Soviet Medicine*, Special Supplement, American–Soviet Medical Society, New York, 1–50.

Sissons JGP, Oldstone MBA, 1985, Host response to viral infections, *Virology*, eds Fields BN, Knipe JM, Raven Press, New York, 265–79.

Smith TW, De Girolami U, Hickey WF, 1992, Neuropathology of immunosuppression, *Brain Pathol*, **2**: 183–94.

Snider WD, Simpson DM et al., 1983, Primary lymphoma of the nervous system associated with acquired immune-deficiency syndrome, *N Engl J Med*, **308**: 45.

Sobel RA, Mitchell ME, Fondren G, 1990, Intercellular adhesion molecule-1 (ICMA-1) in cellular immune reaction in the human CNS, *Am J Pathol*, **136**: 1309–16.

Springer TA, 1994, Traffic signals for lymphocyte recirculation and leukocyte emigration: the multistep paradigm, *Cell*, **76:** 301–3.

Staeheli P, 1990, Interferon-induced proteins and the antiviral state, *Adv Virus Res*, **38:** 147–200.

Steiner I, Kennedy PGE, 1995, Herpes simplex virus latent infection in the nervous system, *J Neurovirol*, **1:** 19–29.

Stevens JG, 1989, Human herpesviruses: a consideration of the latent state, *Microbiol Rev*, **53:** 318–32.

Stevens JG, 1993, HSV-1 neuroinvasiveness, *Intervirology*, **35:** 152–63.

Stitz L, Dietzschold B, Carbone KM, 1995, Immunopathogenesis of Borna disease, *Curr Top Microbiol Immunol*, **190:** 75–92.

Stone R, 1994, Post-polio syndrome: remembrance of viruses past, *Science*, **264:** 909.

Susilowati S, Okuno Y et al., 1981, Neutralisation antibody responses induced by Japanese encephalitis virus vaccine, *Biken J*, **24:** 137–43.

Tapscott SJ, Miller AD et al., 1994, Gene therapy of rat 9L gliosarcoma tumors by transduction with selectable genes does not require drug selection, *Proc Natl Acad Sci USA*, **91:** 8185–9.

Tas PW, Koschel K, 1991, Loss of the endothelin signal pathway in C6 rat glioma cells persistently infected with measles virus, *Proc Natl Acad Sci USA*, **88:** 6736–9.

Trotter J, Steinman L, 1985, Homing of Lyt-2$^+$ and Lyt-2$^-$ T cell subsets and B lymphocytes to the CNS of mice with EAE, *J Immunol*, **132:** 2919–25.

Tsiang H, 1993, Pathopysiology of rabies virus infection of the nervous system, *Adv Virus Res*, **42:** 375–411.

Tyler KL, 1990, Pathogenesis of viral infections, *Fields' Virology*, 2nd edn, eds Fields BN, Knipe DM et al., Raven Press, New York, 191–240.

Tyler KL, 1991, Pathogenesis of reovirus infections of the central nervous system, *Semin Neurosci*, **3:** 117–24.

Tyor WR, Wesselingh S et al., 1992, Long term intraparenchymal Ig secretion after acute viral encephalitis in mice, *J Immunol*, **149:** 4016–20.

Tyor WR, Wesselingh S et al., 1995, Unifying hypothesis for the pathogenesis of HIV-associated dementia complex, vacuolar myelopathy and sensory neuropathy, *J Acquir Immune Defic Syndr*, **9:** 379–88.

Umenai T, Krzyskov R et al., 1985, Japanese encephalitis: current worldwide status, *Bull W H O*, **63:** 625–31.

Virelizier JL, 1989, Cellular activation and human immunodeficiency virus infection, *Curr Opin Immunol*, **2:** 409–13.

Wahl SM, Allen JB et al., 1991, Macrophage and astrocyte-derived transforming growth factor β as a mediator of central nervous system dysfunction in acquired immune deficiency syndrome, *J Exp Med*, **173:** 981–91.

Wakefield AJ, Pittilo RM et al., 1993, Evidence of persistent measles virus infection in Crohn's disease, *J Med Virol*, **39:** 345–53.

Walker DL, Frisque RJ, 1986, The biology and molecular biology of JC virus, *The Papovaviridae*, ed Salzman NP, Plenum Press, London, New York, 327–77.

Watanabe R, Wege H, ter Meulen V, 1983, Adoptive transfer of EAE-like lesions from rats with coronavirus induced demyelinating encephalomyelitis, *Nature (London)*, **305:** 150–3.

Weber T, Turner RW et al., 1994, Specific diagnosis of progressive multifocal leukoencephalopathy by polymerase chain reaction, *J Infect Dis*, **169:** 1138–41.

Wege H, Watanabe R et al., 1983, Coronavirus JHM-induced demyelinating encephalomyelitis in rats: influence of immunity on the course of disease, *Prog Brain Res*, **59:** 221–31.

Werdelin I, McCluskey RT, 1971, The nature and the specificity of mononuclear cells experimental autoimmune inflammations and mechanisms leading to their accumulation, *J Exp Med*, **133:** 1242–9.

Wheatley SC, Dent CL et al., 1991, A cellular factor binding to the TAATGARAT DNA sequence prevents the expression of the HSV-1 immediate-early genes following infection of non-permissive cell lines derived from dorsal root ganglion neurons, *Exp Cell Res*, **194:** 78–82.

Whitley RJ, 1985, Epidemiology of herpes simplex viruses, *The Herpes Viruses*, 3rd edn, ed Roizman B, Plenum Press, New York, 1–44.

Whitley RJ, 1990, Herpes simplex viruses, *Fields' Virology*, 2nd edn, eds Fields BN Knipe, BM et al., Raven Press, New York, 1843–86.

Whitley RJ, Lakeman AD et al., 1982, DNA restriction-enzyme analysis of herpes simplex virus isolates from patients with encephalitis, *N Engl J Med*, **307:** 1060–2.

Wilcox CL, Johnson EM, 1988, Characterisation of nerve growth factor-dependent herpes simplex virus latency in neurons in vitro, *J Virol*, **62:** 393–9.

Wilcox CL, Smith RL et al., 1990, Nerve growth factor dependence of herpes simplex virus latency in peripheral sympathetic and sensory neurons, *J Neurosci*, **10:** 1268–75.

Williamson J, Stohlman S, 1990, Effective clearance of mouse hepatitis virus from the central nervous system both requires CD4$^+$ and CD8$^+$ T cells, *J Virol*, **64:** 4589–92.

Wilt SG, Milward E et al., 1995, In vitro evidence for a dual role of tumour necrosis factor-alpha in human immunodeficiency virus type 1 encephalopathy, *Ann Neurol*, **37:** 381–94.

Wolinsky JS, Klassen T, Baringer JR, 1976, Persistence of neuroadapted mumps virus in brains of newborn hamsters after intraperitoneal inoculation, *J Inf Dis*, **133:** 260–7.

Wolinsky JS, Baringer JR et al., 1974, Ultrastructure of mumps virus replication in newborn hamster central nervous system, *Lab Invest*, **31:** 402–12.

Wolontis S, Björvatn B, 1973, Mumps meningoencephalitis in Stockholm: November 1964–July 1971. II. Isolation attempts from the cerebrospinal fluid in a hospitalised group, *Scand J Infect Dis*, **2:** 261–71.

Wright KE, Buchmeier MJ, 1991, Antiviral antibodies attenuate T-cell-mediated immunopathology following acute lymphocytic choriomeningitis virus infection, *J Virol*, **65:** 3001–6.

Wu E, Dickson DW et al., 1993, Neuronoaxonal dystrophy in HTLV-I associated myelopathy/tropical spastic paraparesis: neuropathologic and neuroimmunologic correlations, *Acta Neuropath*, **86:** 224–35.

Wucherpfennig KW, Strominger JL, 1995, Molecular mimicry of T cell mediated autoimmunity: viral peptides activate human T cell lines specific for myelin basic protein, *Cell*, **80:** 695–705.

WuDunn D, Spear PG, 1989, Initial interaction of herpes simplex virus with cells is binding to heparansulfate, *J Virol*, **63:** 52–60.

Yin-Murphy M, 1994, Enteroviruses, *Encyclopedia of Virology*, eds Webster RG, Granoff A, Academic Press, London, 378–91.

ZuRhein GM, Chou SM, 1965, Particles resembling papovavirions in human cerebral demyelinating diease, *Science*, **148:** 1477–9.

VIRAL INFECTIONS OF THE FETUS AND NEONATE, OTHER THAN RUBELLA

G Enders

INTRODUCTION

1   GENERAL FACTORS IN TRANSMISSION OF INFECTION

The virus infections that may be transmitted from the mother during gestation or perinatally to the fetus or neonate are listed in Tables 41.1 and 41.2. The importance of the various infections depends both on the frequency of maternal infection in the epidemiological situations prevailing in different geographic areas and on the frequency and seriousness of the infections in the embryo, the fetus and the neonate. In this chapter, the various infections are discussed more in order of importance than on a taxonomic basis. Details of the viruses themselves are given in their respective chapters in this volume. A fuller description of infections in pregnancy is published elsewhere (Enders 1998).

Transmission of a virus to the products of conception may occur within the uterus, (**congenital** or **prenatal infection**), and during delivery or shortly thereafter (**perinatal infection**) (Table 41.3). Some viruses are transmitted only when the mother has an acute primary infection in pregnancy, others from chronically infected mothers. All such infections can be transmitted if maternal primary infection occurs shortly before delivery.

In certain viral infections the presence of antibodies in a woman before conception protects both her and the fetus against infection and disease. In the presence of certain vaccine-acquired antibodies (e.g. rubella, measles, mumps, varicella) silent reinfection of the mother may occur, but usually without causing infection or disease of the fetus. Antibodies to viruses that establish latent or chronic infection (e.g. herpesviruses, human immunodeficiency viruses) before conception cannot prevent reactivation or recurrence, with consequent risks of fetal or neonatal infection.

The consequences of maternal infection for the embryo, fetus or child are mainly determined by the gestational age and additional factors, such as the type of virus and its pathogenicity for the developing fetus. The effect of embryonic or fetal infection may be apparent as early as the 6th to 8th week of gestation (WG 6–8). The consequences of maternal infection may be: abortion (until WG 20); intrauterine death (after WG 21); stillbirth (after WG 37); prematurity; and the birth of infants with structural defects of various organs, growth deficits and other systemic abnormalities. Signs of disease may be absent at birth, but serious sequelae may become apparent months or years later. Structural defects may occur following early maternal infection at the time of organogenesis

Table 41.1 Virus infections in pregnancy with known consequences for the fetus and infant

Virus	Consequences for the fetus and infant	
	Congenital infection	Perinatal infection
Rubella	+	−
Cytomegalovirus	+	+
Varicella-zoster virus	+	+
Herpes simplex viruses 1, 2	+/−	+
Parvovirus B19	+	−
Human immunodeficiency viruses 1, 2	+/−	+
Hepatitis viruses B, C, D, G	+/−	+
Hepatitis virus E	+	+
Enteroviruses (excluding hepatitis A)	+/−	+
Lymphocytic choriomeningitis virus	+	−
Genital human papillomaviruses	+/−	+
Haemorrhagic fever viruses[a]	+	+

+, common; +/−, less common; −, none.
[a]Imported or in the respective geographic area.

(WG 3–8), for example in rubella. Maternal infection after WG 9 may lead to systemic abnormalities due to inhibition of organ development. Neonatal disease may also be caused by late intrauterine or perinatal infection.

The total rate of pregnancy loss after implantation due to all causes amounts to 31% (Wilcox et al. 1988). Among the factors – mostly of unknown nature – that can affect the outcome of pregnancy, only 5–10% are attributable to maternal microbial infections and, of these, c. 2% lead to congenital malformation or sys-

temic abnormalities. These low rates are due to the existence of complex mechanisms of protection. The placenta is a powerful barrier with a wide variety of macrophages and lymphocytes. It allows the transit of maternal IgG while preventing a large number of infective agents from reaching the embryo or the fetus. Furthermore, between the 3rd and 5th months of gestation the fetal immune systems, first humoral and then cellular, begin to develop (Lewis and Wilson 1995).

2 DIAGNOSTIC PROCEDURES

For the laboratory diagnosis of maternal, intrauterine and perinatally acquired infections, new techniques for detecting both viruses and their antibodies are becoming available (see Chapters 5 and 44). For detecting viruses and viral antigens, traditional methods have been replaced or supplemented by detection of specific nucleic acid by various molecular biological techniques such as the polymerase chain reaction (PCR). Whether the serological or virological route for diagnosis is pursued depends on the particular agent and on the availability of sensitive and specific assays for detecting it.

Unless stated otherwise, the techniques for diagnosing the various viral infections are the same as those used in non-pregnant people and are described in the relevant chapters in this volume.

Direct tests on the fetus commenced in 1983 (Daffos, Capella-Pavlovsky and Forestier 1983); the methods include ultrasound screening at low and high levels, detection of fetal infection by tests for specific IgM/IgA antibodies in the fetal blood, and detection of the agent in chorionic villi biopsies, amniotic fluid and fetal blood (Table 41.4). Tests for ensuring the purity of fetal blood samples are essential, and non-specific biological, biochemical and immunological factors reflecting fetal functions are also investigated (Forestier et al. 1988). The optimal time for chorionic villi sampling (CVS) is at about WG 11, when the risk of spontaneous abortion is lowest; CVS has, however, proved of lower efficacy than amniotic fluid or fetal blood sampling. The added risk of fetal complications

Table 41.2 Virus infections in pregnancy with possible/suspected consequences for the fetus and infant

Virus	Consequences for the fetus and infant		
	Congenital infection	Perinatal infection	Early postnatal infection
Measles virus	+/−	+/−	...
Mumps virus	−	+/−	...
Epstein–Barr virus	+/−	−	...
Influenza A virus	+/−	−	...
Human herpesvirus 6	+/−	−	...
Molluscum contagiosum virus	−	+/−	...
Hantavirus[a]	−	+/−	...
Dengue virus[a]	−	+/−	...
Respiratory syncytial virus	−	−	+

+, high risk; +/−, low risk; −, no risk.
[a]Imported or in the respective geographic area.

Table 41.3 Transmission of viral infections to embryo, fetus and neonate

Transmission	Mode	Time of gestation	Infections
Transovarian	Infected sperm	Early	Seldom: CMV, HIV-1
Intrauterine	Haematogenous transplacental	1st–39th week	Rubella, CMV, parvovirus B19, VZV, coxsackie and echoviruses, HIV-1,[a] HBV,[a] HCV[a]
	Local extension from foci of infection (e.g. ovaries)		
	Ascending from vaginal tract	Late, after rupture of membranes	CMV, HSV, HIV-1
Perinatal	Infected birth canal	Delivery	CMV, HSV, HIV-1, HBV, HCV, HPV
Early postnatal	Breast milk/environment	After birth	CMV, HSV, HBV, HIV-1, HCV?

[a]Possible, but rare.
CMV, cytomegalovirus; HBV, hepatitis B virus; HCV, hepatitis C virus; HIV, human immunodeficiency virus; HPV, human papillomaviruses; HSV, herpes simplex virus; VZV, varicella zoster virus.

after amniocentesis is 0.2–1% (Hanson et al. 1990) and the risk linked to fetal blood sampling by experienced teams is 0.5–1% (Maxwell et al. 1991).

Tests on the fetus have been applied to pregnancies complicated by infections with, for example, rubella, cytomegalovirus, parvovirus B19, varicella-zoster virus, *Toxoplasma gondii* and *Borrelia burgdorferi* infections (Enders and Jonatha 1987, Daffos et al. 1988, Enders 1994, Hohlfeld et al. 1994, Tercanli, Enders and Holzgreve 1996). They have proved helpful in rescuing many unaffected fetuses from being lost by termination of pregnancy.

To interpret the results obtained by tests on the fetus (Table 41.4) the pathogenicity of the agent for mother and fetus, the time of maternal infection during gestation and the specificity and sensitivity of the various methods must be considered. The ultrasound findings are of major importance when deciding to continue or terminate pregnancy. The predictive value of tests on the fetus can be fully estimated only by follow-up investigations: in cases of therapeutic abortion by detection of the virus or other agent in fetal tissue; or, if pregnancy continues, by tests for specific antibodies and agents in the infant.

In paediatric diagnosis, congenital infection can be assumed if either IgM antibodies or virus are detected in samples collected shortly after birth; perinatal infection is diagnosed if tests for IgM antibody and virus were negative soon after birth but positive in samples obtained 3–4 weeks later (Tables 41.5 and 41.6).

It should be remembered that, even though clinically apparent congenital virus infections are infrequent, there are some important ones whose risk can now be reduced by preventive measures (e.g. vaccination before pregnancy, safe sexual behaviour before and during pregnancy) and correct laboratory

Table 41.4 Prenatal diagnosis of fetal infection

Week of gestation	Investigation	Sample	Object of detection
≥11	Biopsy	Chorionic villi	Virus: by nucleic acid (PCR), antigen, culture
18–23	Amniocentesis	Amniotic fluid	
17–39	Ultrasonography of high level	...	Anatomical abnormalities
22–23	Cordocentesis and amniocentesis	Fetal blood (ensure purity of sample)	Specific IgM Total IgM mg/dl Other non-specific biological, biochemical markers
		Fetal blood Amniotic fluid	Virus: by nucleic acid (PCR), antigen, culture
≥24	If ultrasound is abnormal, investigation as for weeks 22–23		

PCR, polymerase chain reaction.

Table 41.5 Serological differentiation between congenital and perinatal infections

Type of infection	Transmission	Virus-specific antibodies		
		At birth	Neonate <4 weeks	Infant >4 weeks to 1 year
Congenital	Intrauterine	IgM +	IgM +	IgM +/−
		IgG +	IgG +	IgG +
Perinatal	Extrauterine	IgM −	IgM +/−	IgM +
		IgG +	IgG +	IgG +
None	None	IgM −	IgM −	IgM −
		IgG +	IgG +	IgG −

Adapted from Griffiths 1990.
+, positive; +/−, positive or negative; −, negative.

Table 41.6 Virological differentiation between congenital and perinatal infections

Type of infection	Transmission	Virus detection		
		At birth	Neonate	Infant
Congenital	Intrauterine	+	+	+/−
Perinatal	Extrauterine	−	+/−	+

Adapted from Griffiths (1990).
+, positive; +/−, positive or negative; −, negative.

diagnosis followed by intervention if appropriate. The value of TORCH screening (for **to**xoplasma, **r**ubella, **c**ytomegalovirus and **h**erpes) has been reassessed within the past few years (Editorial 1990, Sutherland 1993).

SPECIFIC INFECTIONS

3 CYTOMEGALOVIRUS

Cytomegalovirus (CMV), a gammaherpesvirus, is the most frequent cause of congenital infection in humans, with symptomatic disease at birth, and short- and long-term sequelae. Primary maternal CMV infection may cause congenital disease, whereas in recurrent infection, clinical manifestations are rare.

3.1 Effects on pregnancy, on the fetus and on the neonate

PROBABILITY OF CONTRACTING PRIMARY INFECTION IN PREGNANCY

Primary infections are defined by evidence of seroconversion, with detection of IgM antibody. The prevalence of antibody differs in various populations according to socioeconomic factors, race, geographic location and lifestyle (Istas et al. 1995); thus <40–60% (mean 45%) of pregnant and non-pregnant women aged 20–40 years from the middle- and upper socioeconomic groups have antibodies to CMV, compared with 85% of those from lower on the economic scale.

In developing countries more than 90% of young women are positive for CMV antibodies (Yow et al. 1988, Demmler 1991).

Primary CMV infections in adolescent women (aged 14–20) are acquired mainly by sexual/oral contact with saliva, genital secretions and semen (Shen et al. 1994), particularly in those of lower socioeconomic groups who change sex partners frequently (Istas et al. 1995). Women aged ≥25 years in the middle and upper socioeconomic classes, though not exempt from sexual promiscuity, may acquire infection predominantly by close contact with asymptomatic infants and toddlers excreting CMV in saliva and urine (Adler 1992, Stagno and Cloud 1994).

The annual rates of seroconversion in susceptible people range from 1% to 4% but are somewhat lower in women of higher income groups (2–3%) than in those of lower socioeconomic groups (c. 4%), including pregnant teenagers (Kumar et al. 1984). The rate of primary infection may increase, particularly in middle- and upper-class women, from 2.5% in the first pregnancy to c. 5% in the third to fourth pregnancy (Stagno et al. 1977). However, seronegative mothers whose children attend daycare centres have a 30% annual risk of acquiring a CMV infection (Adler 1992). This rate seems to be even higher if the CMV-infected infants are <20 months of age (see, e.g., Adler 1991, 1992, 1996). This underlines the increased risk for seronegative pregnant women, or for women planning pregnancy, of acquiring CMV infection when working in a child daycare setting. Adler (1992) found that the annual seroconversion rate in 202 seronegative carers was 11%, compared to

2.2% in an age-matched group of 219 seronegative women employed in a local hospital. Over all, c. 25% of serious congenital infections occurring each year in the USA can be attributed to exposure in daycare centres

RISK TO THE FETUS

The influence of primary CMV infection on fetal loss is not clear but in one study the numbers of spontaneous abortions in early gestation were higher (4/26; 15%) than in the control group (16/744; 2%) (Griffiths and Baboonian 1984). Primary infection in pregnancy, regardless of socioeconomic status, accounts for 30–35% of congenital infection; however, Stagno and colleagues (1986) found the congenital infection rate due to primary infection in low income groups to be less than that in high income groups (25% vs 65%).

Following primary infection in pregnancy the rate of transmission to the fetus is estimated as c. 40% (range 24–75%), compared to <2% in recurrent infection (Demmler 1991). In most studies, rates of viral transmission early or late in pregnancy are similar. However, some workers have reported a higher risk of congenital disease if primary infection occurs in the first or second trimester (Stagno, Pass and Cloud 1986).

3.2   Recurrent infection and reinfection

PREVALENCE

Recurrent infection as the cause of congenital CMV infection is generally recognized by the presence of specific IgG antibodies before conception and in some studies by the presence of IgG antibodies in the first 12 weeks of gestation without specific IgM antibodies and confirmation of infection in the offspring (Fowler et al. 1992). Recurrent infections are common, especially in highly immune populations as estimated by the rate of congenital infection. The risk of congenital infection after recurrent infection in pregnancy ranged from 1.5% in women of low socioeconomic background in the USA to c. 0.19% for women of middle to upper socioeconomic background in the USA (Stagno, Pass and Cloud 1986), Great Britain (Griffiths and Baboonian 1984) and Sweden (Ahlfors et al. 1984). In total, recurrent infection accounts for most subclinical congenital infection world-wide (Demmler 1994).

The most frequent mechanism for recurrent infection during pregnancy seems to be reactivation of latent virus. However, the possibility of reinfection by CMV strains other than the original infecting strain, particularly in women with multiple sexual partners, has been demonstrated by restriction enzyme analysis (Chou 1990).

Recurrent infection occurs most frequently in the late second and third trimester in seropositive women, when a marked transient depression of CMV-specific cellular immunity can be demonstrated (Gehrz et al. 1981). At the same time, the rate of viral shedding in cervicovaginal secretion and urine increases, rising from c. 2% in early pregnancy to c. 8% near term, which is comparable to the rate of genital excretion in the younger population in general. These findings suggest that productive CMV infection in seropositive women in early gestation is significantly suppressed by cellular immunity and hormonal changes. When these suppressing factors wane with advancing pregnancy, the rate of genital shedding steadily increases as a result of reactivation.

RISK TO THE FETUS

CMV-specific cellular immunity may also play a role in the risk of congenital infection. Women with recently acquired CMV infection in pregnancy who have a depressed lymphocyte transformation response seem to be at greater risk of delivering a congenitally infected child (Stern et al. 1986). Pre-existing IgG antibodies do not prevent congenital infection but may help to prevent serious disease.

In relation to CMV and pregnancy, it is interesting that the rates of viral shedding from female urinary and genital secretions, and in seminal fluid and semen of non-immunosuppressed men, is inversely related to age and ends at c. 35 years. It is plausible, therefore, that most congenital CMV infections without and with overt disease are in infants born to women aged <30 years (Fowler, Stagno and Pass 1993).

PATHOGENESIS OF FETAL INFECTION

It is assumed that, in primary maternal infection, transmission of virus to the fetus occurs most frequently during the viraemic phase by spread of infected leucocytes and macrophages across the placenta, followed by the events shown in Fig 41.1. Furthermore, placental and chorionic tissue may be directly infected, virus spreading to amniotic cells that are then ingested by the fetus. The virus replicates in the oropharynx and is then carried through the fetal blood circulation to target tissues such as the kidney. The renal tubular epithelium seems to be a major site of replication. Other modes of intrauterine transmission may include transovarian infection by infected semen (Shen et al. 1994); spread of virus from sites where it is replicating, for example the ovaries, endometrium and cervix (Mocarski et al. 1990, Reddehase et al. 1994); and in late pregnancy, by ascending infection from the vagina after premature rupture of the membranes.

In recurrent infection the mode of CMV transmission to the fetus is unknown. Because viraemia rarely occurs in seropositive immunocompetent women, the alternative modes of transmission described may be of significance for infection in utero. The hypothetical routes of intrauterine infections are shown in Figure 41.1.

The fetal cellular and humoral immune responses to intrauterine infection are limited (Lewis and Wilson 1995). Immune responses mediated by T cells (e.g. specific cytotoxic T lymphocytes) become detectable in fetal peripheral blood between WG 15 and 20. Fetal B cells synthesize IgM as early as WG 13, and IgG in WG 16 (Toivanen, Rossi and Hirvonen 1969).

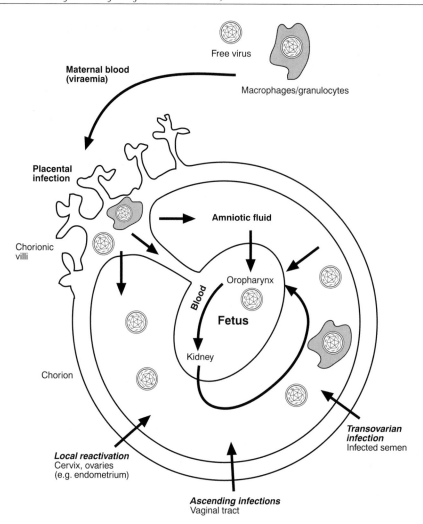

Fig. 41.1 The hypothetical routes of intrauterine cytomegalovirus infections.

In fetuses congenitally infected with CMV, specific IgM antibody in the blood is usually not detectable before WG 21, after which it appears in c. 50%, especially in fetuses with overt infection. After birth, 70% of symptomatic newborns are IgM antibody positive, compared with only 30% of asymptomatic infected neonates; IgM antibody may remain detectable for 3–4 weeks on average. IgG antibody measured in the cord blood or in the blood of the newborn is partly of maternal origin. An initial decrease of IgG antibody is followed by an increase and lifelong persistence at medium to low titres.

CONGENITAL DISEASE

Primary maternal infections are the main cause of overt congenital infection. In recurrent infections, however, congenitally infected newborns generally seem normal at birth, although there is a 5–8% risk of late sequelae, such as unilateral hearing loss (c. 5%) or microcephaly (2%) (Fowler et al. 1992).

Of the c. 1% of neonates congenitally infected with CMV (range in the USA 0.4–2.3%), up to 1 in 10 has signs at birth commonly associated with congenital CMV disease and about half of these have the classic stigmata of cytomegalic inclusion disease (CID). Another 5% present with milder or atypical involve-

ment and c. 90% are born with subclinical but chronic infection. Unusual manifestations such as hydrocephalus, haemolytic anaemia, pneumonitis and inguinal hernia (in males) have also been observed in congenitally infected neonates (Demmler 1994) (Table 41.7).

Sensorineural deafness, the most common handicap caused by congenital infection, usually passes unnoticed for the first 1–2 months of life, as does the less common chorioretinitis. Among the most severely affected infants mortality ranges between 12 and 30%. Most deaths occur in the neonatal period and are usually due to disseminated intravascular coagulation (DIC), hepatic dysfunction or bacterial superinfection. More than 90% of the survivors have major long-term sequelae. Those without physical signs at birth have a 10–17% risk of abnormal development, which usually presents during the first 2 years of life but may escape detection until school age (Table 41.8).

In 1970–1977 it became evident that women who were seropositive before they conceived might deliver consecutive infected babies (Stagno 1995). Rarely, congenital disease may also occur in infants of immunocompetent mothers (Rutter, Griffiths and Trompeter 1985, Nigro, Clerico and Mandaini 1993), but more such cases have been reported in immunosuppressed mothers with recurrent infection (Hayes,

Table 41.7 Clinical manifestations in newborns and infants with congenital CMV infection[a]

Clinical sign	Percentage (approx.)
Prematurity (<38 w)	34
Small for gestational age	40
Petechiae	51
Purpura	14
Jaundice	69
Hepatosplenomegaly	60
Neurological findings:	
One or more of the following	72
Microcephaly	50
Intracranial calcification	43
Lethargy/poor feeding	25
Convulsions	7
Elevated liver enzyme values	46
Thrombocytopenia	60
Death in the first 6 weeks	12

[a]According to/adapted from: Boppana et al. (1992), Ramsay, Miller and Peckham (1991), Dobbins, Stewart and Demmler (1991), Demmler (1994) and Stagno (1995).

Table 41.8 Long-term sequelae in infants with congenital cytomegalovirus infection

Sequelae	Signs of infection at birth (approx. percentage)	
	Present	Absent
Sensorineural hearing loss	58	7.4
Bilateral hearing loss	37	2.7
Speech difficulties	27	1.7
Chorioretinitis with/without optic drophy	20	2.5
Neurological findings:		
Microcephaly	37	1.8
Microcephaly with convulsions or paresis/paralysis	52	2.7
Convulsions	23	0.9
Paresis/paralysis	13	0
Death after the newborn period	6	0.3

According to/adapted from: Fowler et al. (1992), Istas et al. (1995), Pass, Fowler and Boppana (1991), Dobbins, Stewart and Demmler (1991), Demmler (1994) and Stagno (1995).

Symington and Mackay 1979, Laifer et al. 1995, Schwebke et al. 1995). Individual cases of congenital disease following maternal recurrent infection do occur, but seem to be exceptional when the mother is clinically normal.

PERINATAL AND EARLY POSTNATAL INFECTION

In perinatal and early postnatal infections mainly associated with recurrent maternal infection, virus is acquired by passage through the infected birth canal or from breast milk. There is a higher frequency of such infections in populations of low socioeconomic status, of high maternal seroprevalence and in which mothers usually breast-feed. Infection occurs in c. 60% of babies whose mothers shed CMV in their cervicovaginal secretions at the time of delivery. Transmission from the breast milk of seropositive mothers occurs in 30–70% of infants who have been breast-fed for more than one month (Stagno et al. 1980). In societies with higher socioeconomic status and lower seroprevalence (<40–60%) and a relatively low rate of breast-feeding as in, for example, western Europe and the USA, perinatal and early postnatal infections may be expected in c. 1–15% (Alford et al. 1990, Adler 1991).

In perinatally acquired infection, as in congenital infection, virus may be consistently excreted up to 6 years or longer in urine and into saliva for c. 2 years. The highest quantity is excreted during the first 6 months of life. Infants with perinatally acquired or inapparent congenital infection excrete significantly less virus than those with overt infection. The risks and benefits of horizontal CMV transmission in child daycare centres have been discussed in several reports (Dobbins et al. 1994, Stagno and Cloud 1994).

CLINICAL MANIFESTATIONS IN PERINATAL INFECTION

The incubation period for peri- and early postnatal infection is 4–12 weeks. There seem to be no short- or long-term clinical effects, apart from cases of CMV pneumonitis in early infancy. In term infants, disseminated disease may be prevented by the presence of maternal antibodies. In premature infants with low birth weight, perinatal infection (e.g. via breast milk) may cause disease characterized by hepatosplenomegaly, thrombocytopenia and neutropenia (Yeager et al. 1983) and an increased tendency to develop neuromuscular handicaps (Paryani et al. 1985). Shedding of virus from urine and saliva continues for years although in lower amounts than from infants with overt congenital infection.

Iatrogenic causes of early postnatal transfusion-associated CMV infection and disease, particularly in preterm seronegative infants, have been greatly reduced by the use of CMV antibody-negative blood or of de-glycerolized frozen red cells (Forbes 1989).

3.3 Diagnosis

DIAGNOSIS IN PREGNANCY

Primary or recurrent CMV infection in pregnancy is usually detected by chance, as the primary infection is generally asymptomatic or may cause non-specific symptoms. Fewer than 10% of adults present with a mononucleosis-like syndrome (Raynor 1993). Recurrent CMV infections are always asymptomatic if the pregnant woman is immunocompetent.

With the basic serological tests, primary infection can best be detected by seroconversion and rising IgG and IgM antibody titres within 2–4 weeks of onset. A less recent primary infection is indicated by a constant IgG titre and an elevated concentration of IgM antibodies, whereas normal or elevated IgG antibody values and medium to low concentrations of IgM antibody suggest a past primary or recurrent infection.

Serological tests that helped to distinguish primary from recurrent infections in pregnancy would be of major importance because of the greater risk to the fetus posed by maternal primary infection as opposed to recurrent infection (Boppana and Britt 1995). Such a test using recombinant β-gal fusion proteins (p52 and pp150) for quantitative detection of IgG antibody to either protein helped to support the diagnosis of primary infection (Enders and Daiminger 1996, personal observations). Assessment of the cellular immune response by CMV-specific lymphoproliferative assay in women with recent primary CMV infection is not used routinely to predict intrauterine transmission. The first study of this kind (Stern et al. 1986) revealed that newborns of women with a good lymphocyte response were not infected ($n = 8$), whereas mothers whose lymphocytes did not respond delivered infected babies (4/6). In a later study there was a fair, but not complete, correlation between a strong lymphocyte response and birth of non-infected infants (Fernando, Pearce and Booth 1993).

The detection of virus shedding in urine and cervical secretion in pregnant women is of little value for distinguishing primary from recurrent maternal infection or for predicting intrauterine infection (Raynor 1993).

DIAGNOSIS IN THE FETUS

Prenatal diagnosis of fetal CMV infection is increasingly used in asymptomatic and symptomatic pregnant women with seroconversion or suspicious serological markers for recent primary infection and in those with abnormal findings by ultrasound examination, whose immunological status is unknown. A variety of sonographic findings, generally beyond WG 22, have been reported, including: microcephaly, hydrocephalus, necrotic, cystic or calcified periventricular lesions in the brain, liver or placenta, oligohydramnios and intrauterine growth retardation (Lynch et al. 1991). Cases with isolated ascites and polyhydramnios, fetal meconium peritonitis, fetal abdominal echogenic mass and cerebral ventriculomegaly have also been reported.

Prenatal diagnosis relies on the detection of virus in amniotic fluid and fetal blood by the rapid shell vial technique and PCR (Revello et al. 1995). For detecting specific IgM antibodies, various commercial tests are used that differ in specificity and sensitivity (Landini 1993). In some studies, the detection of CMV was attempted only in amniotic fluid (Grose, Meehan and Weiner 1992), and rarely in chorionic villi (Dong et al. 1994). In several others, tests for virus were performed on amniotic fluid and fetal blood (Hogge, Buffone and Hogge 1993, Hagay et al. 1996), with or

without IgM antibody detection in the fetal blood and assessment of non-specific biological, biochemical and immunological markers for fetal function (Forestier et al. 1988).

The finding of virus in amniotic fluid obtained at WG 20 yielded the best results in detecting fetal infection (Donner et al. 1994, Hagay et al. 1996), but does not necessarily indicate congenital disease. Abnormal ultrasound findings beyond WG 21, combined with virus detection in fetal blood and amniotic fluid, are more significant for predicting congenital disease in the fetus. The finding of specific IgM antibody, elevated total IgM concentrations and abnormalities in non-specific markers provide additional evidence of congenital disease, but their absence does not preclude a decision to terminate pregnancy.

Most of the above-mentioned findings are supported by the author's own prospective series, including 173 pregnant women who underwent prenatal diagnosis with controlled outcome of pregnancy (Enders 1997, personal observations)

Hagay and colleagues (1996) concluded from the results of a meta-analysis that the accuracy of tests for diagnosing CMV infection in utero is as yet undetermined, and that the efficacy of routine antenatal screening for this purpose is limited. Nevertheless, our own experience suggests that prenatal diagnosis carried out with well controlled serological and virological techniques and with ultrasound screening has already saved a number of pregnancies with suspected primary infection that would otherwise have been terminated.

DIAGNOSIS IN INFANTS

A diagnosis of suspected congenital disease is confirmed by detection of virus in saliva, pharyngeal secretion, urine and, sometimes, in cerebrospinal fluid and by detection of IgM antibody in cord blood or blood of the newborn. Virological tests must be initiated within 2 weeks after birth to distinguish congenital from perinatally acquired infection. In asymptomatic infants of mothers with suspected primary or recurrent infection, urine and throat swab specimens at least should be tested to detect or exclude congenital infection. Antibody testing is less informative, because IgM antibody may be absent in >35%, particularly in asymptomatic infected infants or when maternal primary infection occurs very late in pregnancy. IgG antibodies may persist life-long. The presence of IgG antibody in asymptomatic infants ≥8 months of age may be due to congenital, perinatal or early postnatal infection (see also Table 41.4).

3.4 Management

MANAGEMENT IN PREGNANCY

Preventing primary CMV infection by taking hygienic precautions and altering their lifestyle is of interest only to women who want to become pregnant or are pregnant and known to be seronegative and at risk. For passive prophylaxis, several intravenous immunoglobulin preparations (IVIG) with known neutralizing antibody titres are available. They may be used in seronegative pregnant women with known contact with CMV, but their value in preventing primary infection is not established. The best approach for preventing disease due to CMV infection is vaccination before pregnancy. Clinical trials evaluating both Towne HCMV vaccine and the subunit glycoprotein B vaccine are in the early stages. To be effective, these vaccines should induce persisting titres of serum-neutralizing and mucosal antibodies comparable to those found after natural infection (Starr 1992, Adler et al. 1995, Wang et al. 1996). If safe and effective vaccines finally become available, they will have to be administered at a sufficiently young age to protect infants born to sexually active adolescents.

Treatment of pregnant women with suspected primary CMV infection with the antiviral drugs ganciclovir or foscarnet (both of which cross the placenta) is not recommended. Whether CMV-infected fetuses benefit from fetal intravascular administration of ganciclovir is uncertain (Revello et al. 1993).

MANAGEMENT OF THE NEONATE WITH CONGENITAL DISEASE

The effect of treatment with ganciclovir of infants with symptomatic congenital CMV and evidence of central nervous system involvement is under investigation in a controlled multicentre clinical trial in the USA (phase I data: Trang et al. 1993; phase II data: Whitley et al. 1997; phase III trial to determine clinical efficacy is ongoing: personal information by Demmler and Whitley). Both phases I and II data are favourable from the safety and antiviral standpoints.

Some reports treating selected infants with severe congenital CMV disease using different regimens of therapy suggest that acute symptoms (pneumonia, hepatitis) seem to resolve by early treatment (Hocker et al. 1990, Stronati et al. 1995, Nigro, Scholz and Bartmann, 1994). The availability of oral ganciclovir is a great advance in long-term treatment. Experience with foscarnet in the treatment of newborns is very limited.

The value of an anti-CMV monoclonal antibody preparation in infants with symptomatic congenital CMV infection without central nervous system involvement is under investigation.

SCREENING IN PREGNANCY AND PUBLIC HEALTH ASPECTS

Opinions vary on the value and cost-effectiveness of screening programmes for CMV. Recommendations for potentially child-bearing and pregnant women at occupational risk are also still under debate, but assessment of their immune response should be strongly encouraged. CMV antibody screening has not so far been introduced into prenatal programmes. Such programmes might, however, be helpful for the guidance of pregnant seronegative women in commonsense measures and for reassuring IgG positive/IgM negative women that there is little risk of the birth of a child with congenital disease. In cases of suspected primary infection, ultrasound screening

and prenatal diagnosis seem to be better options than immediate termination of pregnancy.

Caesarean section is not recommended because an infant possibly infected in utero does not profit by this mode of delivery; preventing perinatal infection at delivery is not an issue, as such infections usually carry no risk of disease, as does breast-feeding of term infants. In pre-term infants, especially those born to mothers who acquired CMV infection late in gestation, there may be a slight risk of overt disease. Breast-feeding should therefore be delayed until the milk has been tested for virus.

The public health impact of congenital CMV infection is enormous. As pointed out by Istas et al. (1995) much higher costs for affected infants must be expected when the late sequelae of congenital CMV infection (e.g. hearing defects and neurodevelopmental disorders) become more definitely associated with CMV congenital infection than they are at present (Table 41.9). In the USA the cost of congenital CMV disease was $315 000 per child in 1991 (Dobbins, Stewart and Demmler et al. 1991, Istas et al. 1995).

4 VARICELLA-ZOSTER VIRUS

Varicella-zoster virus (VZV) is an alphaherpesvirus that causes 2 main clinical syndromes: primary infection gives rise to varicella (chickenpox), and recurrent infection to herpes zoster (shingles). Varicella is highly contagious whereas herpes zoster is less so. Chickenpox in pregnancy may be associated with severe maternal disease, spontaneous abortion and, rarely, during the first 2 trimesters, with congenital varicella syndrome (CVS). Maternal varicella around term carries the risk of serious neonatal disease. Zoster at any time during pregnancy does not result in congenital anomalies or neonatal disease.

4.1 Infection in pregnancy

INCIDENCE

Varicella in pregnancy is relatively uncommon because in densely populated areas of the northern hemisphere c. 95% women of childbearing age are seropositive. However, this figure may be smaller in some populations (e.g. black women in the USA and in countries of the southern hemisphere) (Gray, Palinkas and Kelley 1990, Dworkin 1996). Asymptomatic reinfection is possible and second attacks of varicella have also been reported (Martin et al. 1994). Surveillance data in the UK suggest that the annual incidence of varicella in pregnancy is 3 per 1000. However, an upward shift of incidence to adults aged 15–44 years has been recognized in England (Miller, Vurdien and Farrington 1993) and in the USA (Gray, Palinkas and Kelley 1990, Choo et al. 1995). Zoster in pregnancy may have an annual incidence of 2 per 1000, similar to that in non-pregnant adults aged 15–40 years (Miller, Marshall and Vurdien 1993).

Table 41.9 Annual public health impact of congenital CMV infection and disease

	USA	UK	Germany
No. of live births/year	4 000 000	700 000	810 000
Rate of congenital infection (average)	c. 1%	c. 0.3%	c. 0.3%
No. of infected infants/year	40 000	2 100	2 430
No. of infants symptomatic at birth (c. 8%)	3 200	168	195
No. with sequelae (c. 90%)	2 880	152	175
No. with unusual signs at birth with unpredictable outcome (c. 5%)	2 000	105	122
No. of infants asymptomatic at birth (c. 87%)	34 800	1 827	2 115
No. with late sequelae (c. 15%)	5 220	275	318

Estimated figures for USA adapted from Demmler (1994), Stagno (1995), Istas et al. (1995); for UK adapted from Griffiths (1990); for Germany from Enders (unpublished).
CMV, cytomegalovirus.

ADVERSE EFFECTS IN PREGNANCY

VZV pneumonia seems to be the most common serious maternal complication in pregnancy (Haake et al. 1990, Katz et al. 1995). It usually develops within one week of the rash. The predominant signs and symptoms are fever, cough, dyspnoea and tachypnoea. The outcome is unpredictable and there may be rapid progress to hypoxia and respiratory failure. Pneumonia is regarded as a medical emergency requiring prompt diagnosis and treatment.

In pregnancies complicated by varicella, spontaneous abortion, stillbirth and prematurity do not seem to be significantly increased (Paryani and Arvin 1986, Balducci et al. 1992). In a prospective study of a total of 1373 VZV-complicated pregnancies, the incidence of fetal loss due to spontaneous abortion during the first 20 weeks and intrauterine death after the 20th week was 47 (3.6%) of 1291 live-born infants (Enders et al. 1994).

4.2 Effects on the fetus

CONGENITAL VARICELLA SYNDROME

The risk of CVS is an important concern. Since its first description by Laforet and Lynch (1947) more than 40 such cases have been reported. A causal association with maternal infection has been confirmed in only a few cases by isolation of VZV from skin lesions at birth (Da Silva, Hammerberg and Chance 1990), detection of genomic DNA in the fetal tissues of a live-born infant (Scharf et al. 1990) and in a fetus following intrauterine death during WG 23 (Puchhammer-Stöckl et al. 1994).

Clinical manifestations

The clinical manifestations of CVS range from severe multisystem involvement, resulting in death in the neonatal period, to dermatomal skin scarring, limb hypoplasia or both as the only defects. Table 41.10 shows the clinical features of CVS and their relative frequencies.

Pathogenesis of CVS

The precise mechanism of infection with VZV in utero is unknown. It is generally accepted that transplacental transmission of VZV may take place during the viraemic phase, resulting in congenital infection (Trlifojova, Brenda and Benes 1986). The pattern of defects in CVS, particularly the limb hypoplasia and scarring, suggests that they are due to intrauterine zoster. The extremely short period between reactivation and fetal infection may be the consequence of an inadequate cell-mediated immune response in early gestation (Higa, Dan and Manabe 1987).

The clinical consequences of congenital VZV infections depend on the stage of pregnancy at which maternal infection occurs (Table 41.11). Intrauterine varicella infection can, however, occur without clinical sequelae at any stage of pregnancy, the proportion rising from 5–10% in the first and second trimester to 25% towards WG 36 and reaching c. 50% when maternal varicella occurs 1–4 weeks before delivery (Miller, Cradock-Watson and Ridehalgh 1989). It seems possible that fetal infection early in pregnancy may result in clinical manifestations with healing of lesions before birth. Localized zoster in pregnancy could theoretically result in fetal infection, if the dermatomes involved were T10 to L1, as sensory nerves to the uterus originate from these segments; but no such cases have yet been documented (Miller, Marshall and Vurdien 1993).

The risk of zoster in infancy and childhood following maternal varicella in the second and third trimesters is estimated as c. 2–3% (Enders et al. 1994).

Risk of congenital varicella syndrome

Several workers undertook prospective studies to estimate the risk of CVS following maternal varicella infection at various stages of pregnancy (Enders 1984, Paryani and Arvin 1986, Balducci et al. 1992, Jones, Johnson and Chambers 1994, Pastuszak et al. 1994). One large survey included 1373 women who had varicella and 366 who had zoster (Enders et al. 1994). The overall risk during the first 20 weeks of gestation was c. 1%, the highest (2%) being observed between

Table 41.10 Congenital varicella syndrome

Main signs	Number of infants	
	$n = 37^a$	$n = 17^b$
Skin: dermatomal skin scarring, contractures	35 (95%)	13 (76%)
Limb hypoplasia	18 (49%)	9 (53%)
Eye: microphthalmia, chorioretinitis, cataract, Horner syndrome	24 (65%)	8 (47%)
Central nervous system: microcephaly, brain atrophy, paralysis, convulsions, encephalitis	18 (49%)	10 (59%)
Mental retardation	6 (16%)	5 (29%)
Other organ defects	5 (14%)	3 (18%)

[a]From world literature.
[b]Enders (personal observation): 9 from prospective study, 8 ascertained retrospectively.

Table 41.11 Clinical manifestations of congenital varicella infection following chickenpox in pregnancy

Stage of maternal infection	Sequelae
First and second trimester	Congenital varicella syndrome
Second and third trimester	Herpes zoster in infancy or childhood
Perinatal	Disseminated neonatal varicella

From Miller, Marshall and Vurdien (1993).

weeks 13 and 20. The latest gestational age at which CVS occurred was WG 19, which is consistent with the findings in one retrospective report (Alkalay, Pomerance and Rimoin 1987). Following localized zoster in pregnancy Enders et al. (1994) found no clinical or serological evidence of intrauterine infection in the infants. Only one infant with characteristic limb hypoplasia and skin scarring has been described following disseminated maternal zoster at WG 12 with presumed maternal viraemia (Higa, Dan and Manabe 1987).

4.3 Neonatal varicella

Severe neonatal disease is generally attributed to intrauterine infection and lack of maternal antibody. If the mother's rash appears more than 6 days before delivery, the infant invariably has maternal antibodies. When it is <6 days before delivery, only some infants have significant titres of antibody, whereas those born <3 days after onset of maternal rash, or infants whose mothers develop varicella after delivery are IgG negative. Infants at greatest risk of severe or fatal illness are those whose mother's rash appears 5 days before to 2 days after delivery (Gershon 1975, Miller, Cradock-Watson and Ridehalgh 1989). The interval between the onset of rash in the mother and infant is usually 12–13 days, but may be as brief as 2 days, suggesting transplacental infection. The clinical attack rate was estimated to be 17% (Meyers 1974) and the fatality rate 30% (Gershon 1975). According to a more recent prospective study the commonly cited fatality rate of 30% seems to be an overestimate due to selec-

tive reporting (Miller, Cradock-Watson and Ridehalgh 1989). Furthermore, a severe outcome of neonatal varicella is not limited to transplacentally acquired infection, but occasionally occurs in early postnatally acquired infection (minimum incubation period 8 days after birth) despite the use of varicella immunoglobulin (VZIG) even at high dosage. Early reactivation is not uncommon after neonatal varicella, giving rise to zoster within a few months or years of the primary infection. Further zoster episodes have not been reported in these children, suggesting that good cell-mediated immunity develops after reactivation.

Despite the potential for horizontal transmission of VZV from zoster cases, neonates do not seem to be at risk of infection if maternal zoster occurs around the time of delivery (Miller, Marshall and Vurdien 1993). The reason for this is the lower infectivity of zoster compared to chickenpox; furthermore, if the onset of maternal zoster is ≥4 days before delivery, the infant passively acquires antibody from the mother, whose own pre-existing immunity is reinforced as a result of her recent reactivation.

4.4 Diagnosis

DIAGNOSIS IN PREGNANCY

In typical cases of varicella and zoster a clinical diagnosis is usually sufficient. In pregnancy VZV infection should be verified serologically. To detect specific IgG and IgM antibodies the enzyme-linked immunosorbent assay (ELISA) is now the most widely used method, and for a very rapid determination of the immune status the latex agglutination test (LA) is also employed. Results with both tests correlate well with cell-mediated immunity as determined by lymphoproliferative assays (Weinberg et al. 1996). Virus detection is unnecessary in uncomplicated varicella, but is employed in cases of, for example, pneumonia and in prenatal diagnosis. VZV DNA has been detected in amniotic fluid and fetal blood by dot-blot hybridization (Gottard et al. 1991) but, at the time of writing, detection by nested PCR is the method of choice.

DIAGNOSIS IN THE FETUS

Prenatal diagnosis to exclude fetal infection with VZV is feasible but not generally recommended because of the low risk of CVS. Amniotic fluid taken at WG 18–20 and >4–6 weeks after the onset of maternal varicella is technically easy to obtain and yields the best results. Ultrasound screening is recommended between WG 19 and 23. If the findings are abnormal, fetal blood and amniotic fluid should be tested for VZV DNA; tests for fetal-specific IgM are not helpful. Major abnormalities such as limb hypoplasia or microcephaly can be recognized by ultrasound scan but seldom before WG 22–23; defects may not become evident until much later in pregnancy, when therapeutic abortion is not an option. These findings are substantiated by the author's own prospective series including thus far 115 women who underwent prenatal diagnosis with controlled outcome of pregnancy (Enders 1997, personal observations).

DIAGNOSIS IN INFANCY

Detection of virus in fetal or newborn tissues, blood and body fluid may now be achieved by finding VZV DNA with nested PCR (Mehraein et al. 1991, Puchhammer-Stöckl et al. 1994). The sensitivity of specific IgM as a marker of fetal infection is low, even in infants with CVS, and persisting IgG seems to be more indicative of congenital VZV, as shown in CVS cases assessed prospectively and retrospectively since 1980 (Enders et al. 1994). Only 14 of 31 cases (45.2%) had specific IgM antibodies at birth, whereas persistent IgG was found in 16 of 18 (88.9%) of the surviving infants tested. The specific IgM response in CVS differs therefore from that in congenital rubella syndrome with chronic multisystem infection, in which specific IgM is nearly always detectable at birth.

4.5 Management in pregnancy

PASSIVE PROPHYLAXIS WITH IMMUNOGLOBULIN

Protection from contact with infected individuals is of limited effect. For passive prophylaxis, 2 preparations of VZV immunoglobulins with defined antibody concentrations are available in Germany, one for intramuscular and the other for intravenous administration, with an IgG antibody concentration of c.2000 IU per adult dose. According to our experience in 196 pregnancies, even if VZIG is given in the recommended dosage and within 2–3 days of exposure, infection is prevented in only c. 45%. Of the remaining 55%, VZIG administration results in asymptomatic infection in c. 4% and in modified to normal disease in c. 50%. When VZIG is given 4–5 days after exposure, there is still a mitigating effect in 20% of patients. The only VZIG preparation available in the UK (distributed by the Public Health Laboratory Service for intramuscular administration) has a relatively low IgG antibody concentration (400–600 IU per adult dose). Its effect is to attenuate disease rather than to prevent infection (Miller, Marshall and Vurdien

1993). VZIG preparations for intramuscular application and recommendations for use are also available in the USA (CDC 1996a).

Passive immunization with VZIG should be recommended only for seronegative pregnant women directly exposed to an acute case of varicella. As a result of the findings in a prospective study that no case of CVS occurred in maternal varicella after WG 20 (Enders et al. 1994), VZIG is no longer recommended for exposed women after WG 22 (Table 41.12). VZIG is not normally used in seronegative pregnant women exposed to a case of zoster (Table 41.13).

ACTIVE PROPHYLAXIS WITH VACCINE

VZV live attenuated vaccine is now licensed for administration to anyone at risk. Pregnancy is mentioned among the contraindications. Because the virulence of the attenuated virus used in the vaccine is less than that of the wild type virus, the risk to the fetus, if any, should be even lower, and inadvertent administration is not a reason for termination of pregnancy. As a precaution, however, non-pregnant women who are vaccinated should avoid becoming pregnant for one month following each injection. In the USA, universal vaccination of children, adolescents and young adults with no history of varicella is now recommended (CDC 1996a), although such a programme remains controversial (Kennedy and McKendrick 1996). Recommendations for limiting nosocomial spread of varicella are given in Table 41.14.

ANTIVIRAL THERAPY

For antiviral chemotherapy of VZV infection, aciclovir (which has an excellent safety record), valaciclovir and famciclovir are available. The efficacy of intravenous aciclovir in the treatment of chickenpox in immunocompromised people is well established. Although it is not licensed for use in pregnancy, a follow-up of 460 women treated during the first trimester and 191 treated in the second or third trimester did not identify any association with fetal abnormalities (Kroon and Whitley 1995). In varicella complicated by, for example, pneumonia, early treatment with intravenous aciclovir at any stage of pregnancy is essential (Haake et al. 1990, Smego and Asperilla 1991).

4.6 Management of the neonate

For newborns of mothers who have varicella in the period from 4–5 days before to 2–7 days after delivery, treatment with VZIG is recommended to prevent neonatal infection or to modify the disease (see, e.g., Department of Health and Social Security, Joint Committee on Vaccination and Immunisation 1988). In addition, VZIG may also be recommended for premature infants with little or no IgG antibody who are exposed to acute cases of VZV at 1–4 weeks of age. If severe varicella develops despite treatment with VZIG, high-dose intravenous aciclovir is frequently given, but there are still very few data regarding its efficacy and safety. A fatal outcome despite prophylaxis with VZIG

Table 41.12   Management of varicella infection in pregnancy

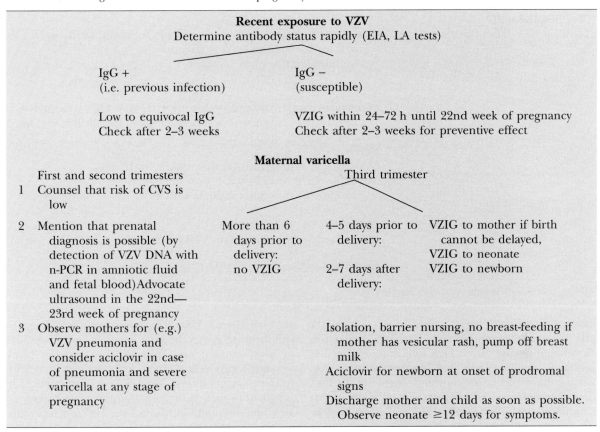

Modified from Riley (1994, table 6-2).
CVS, congenital varicella syndrome; EIA, enzyme-linked immunosorbent assay; LA, latex agglutination test; n-PCR, nested polymerase chain reaction; VZIG, varicella immunoglobulin.

Table 41.13   Management of zoster in pregnancy

Recent exposure to zoster lesion **Contagiousness is low** Determine VZV IgG antibody	
IgG +: No VZIG	IgG −: VZIG only if close contact until WG 22
Zoster in pregnancy	
1st–3rd trimester 1st,[a] 2nd, 3rd trimester	No VZIG Aciclovir if severe infection
4 days prior to delivery	No VZIG to newborn (even if maternal antibody is absent) Cover maternal zoster lesions Breast-feeding, if no vesicles in area of nipples; otherwise pump off breast milk

VZIG, varicella immunoglobulin; VZV, varicella-zoster virus; WG, week of gestation.
[a]Only in most severe cases.

and early treatment with aciclovir was reported by Holland, Isaacs and Moxon (1986). Its prophylactic use seems justified in high-risk cases in which maternal rash appears from 4 days before to 2 days after delivery (Sills et al. 1987).

5   HERPES SIMPLEX VIRUS TYPES 1 AND 2

Maternal herpes simplex virus (HSV) primary and recurrent genital infection, frequently asymptomatic,

Table 41.14 Limitation of nosocomial varicella transmission

For hospital staff	
Test for VZV IgG antibody	In personnel before working in maternity/newborn wards and wards for immunosuppressed patients
	Seropositive staff: remain on ward
In case of exposure, test for IgG antibody if immunity status is unknown	
	Seronegative staff: removal from work 8–21 days after exposure to a case of chickenpox **or** immediate vaccination with live vaccine ↓
	Vaccinees:
	Develop IgG antibody in low titre within 10–12 days
	Should avoid close association with susceptible high-risk individuals if they develop some vesicles
For pregnant women	
Shortly before and after delivery in contact with acute chickenpox	Determine IgG antibody titre
	Mother antibody-positive → no VZIG to neonate
	Mother antibody-negative → VZIG to neonate

VZIG, varicella immune globulin; VZV, varicella zoster virus.

may cause neonatal herpes, most often with type 2 (HSV-2). Although infrequent, neonatal herpes is a devastating disease with a high rate of morbidity and mortality despite early and appropriate therapy. Because its incidence is significantly higher in the USA than elsewhere, special efforts are being made in that country to establish a reliable and cost-effective strategy for prevention.

5.1 Infection in pregnancy

EPIDEMIOLOGY OF MATERNAL HSV INFECTION

In the past, c. 90% of herpetic genital infections were caused by HSV-2, but more recently HSV-1 has been implicated as the cause of up to 40% of cases of primary genital herpes in seronegative adults. However, the reactivation rate for genital HSV-2 is at least twice as high as for HSV-1, and so too are the risks of transmission by sexual intercourse and of neonatal herpes infection (Forsgren 1992, Koelle et al. 1992, Corey, Wald and Hobson 1996).

Seroprevalence studies with HSV type-specific antigens have demonstrated rates of HSV-1 infection of c. 30% in people aged 20–40 years in higher socioeconomic groups and c. 80% in those of lower socioeconomic groups (Corey and Spear 1986a, 1986b, Johnson et al. 1989). Thus people with higher living standards now acquire HSV-1 infection less frequently in childhood than they did in the past. The consequent lack of partial cross-protection may be one of the reasons for the higher frequency and severity of primary HSV-2 and HSV-1 genital infection (Koutsky et al. 1990, Bernstein 1991).

Most surveys of seroprevalence have shown a relatively low but increasing rate of HSV-2 infection during the last decade in the general adult population in the developed world; for example, in the USA from 16% in 1976–80 to c. 22% in 1989–91 (Johnson et al. 1989, 1994). HSV-2 seroprevalence in women of childbearing age in the USA varied from 10% to 35% in white women and from 35% to 60% in black women (Johnson et al. 1989, Arvin and Prober 1990). In more recent surveys, the HSV-2 seroprevalences in pregnant women in various countries ranged between 10% and 33%, and in most of the HSV-2 seropositive women, a large proportion (55–87%) had asymptomatic infections (Slomka 1996). This finding led to alterations to preventive strategies previously suggested (Prober et al. 1988, Randolph, Washington and Prober 1993).

CLASSIFICATION OF GENITAL HERPES INFECTION

Genital herpes infections are defined as primary, first episode non-primary or recurrent infections. **Primary** infections are those with seroconversion for either type 1 or type 2; in **first episode** infection, seroconversion occurs to one type in the presence of antibody to the other type; and in **recurrent** infection, homologous antibodies to the type in question are already present. The clinical signs of genital herpes are present in c. 25–30% of infected women (Table 41.15).

EFFECT ON PREGNANCY AND ITS OUTCOME

The form of genital infection at the time of delivery is of major importance, whereas primary or recurrent oropharyngeal type 1 infections are of little significance. Severe disease after primary oropharyngeal or genital infection in pregnancy is rare. Small numbers of cases of disseminated maternal infection have been reported by Wolf et al. (1992) and by Greenspoon et al. (1994). Before the availability of aciclovir therapy, the maternal mortality was >50%, and fetal death also occurred in >50% of cases but none of the surviving fetuses delivered by caesarean section had evidence of disease (Greenspoon et al. 1994).

Table 41.15 Clinical forms of genital herpes simplex infection and viral shedding

Primary infection: HSV-2, (HSV-1)	Seroconversion for either type 1 or 2
	Characteristic genital lesions, sometimes with systemic illness
	Low risk of disseminated severe disease
	Virus shedding in the cervix (c. 3 weeks) and in high concentration, often continuing after clinical healing
First episode non-primary infection: HSV-2, (HSV-1)	Seroconversion to one type in presence of antibody to the other type
	Significant to moderate local symptoms but little systemic illness
	Virus shedding often similar to that in primary infection
Recurrent infection: HSV-2, (HSV-1)	Homologous pre-existing antibody
	Usually minor or no local symptoms
	Viral shedding in low concentration during the very early phase for 2–5 days

(HSV-1) = less common.

Primary genital infections with HSV-2 up to mid-gestation have been associated with an increased rate of abortion (Nahmias et al. 1971), and in the second or third trimester with intrauterine growth retardation and prematurity (Brown et al. 1987). Furthermore, maternal primary, and less often first episode infection during the first or second trimester, may lead to congenital infection with severe disease evident at birth (Hutto et al. 1987).

RISK FACTORS IN MOTHER–INFANT TRANSMISSION

Most infants with neonatal herpes acquire infection by passage through an infected birth canal. Mothers with a known history of genital herpes and those with unrecognized genital herpes infection (c. 70%) are at risk of transmitting HSV to their infants. For the intrapartum route of transmission, the risk of neonatal infection depends on the form of maternal genital infection and is directly related to viral shedding into the cervicovaginal secretion at the onset of labour.

Brown and colleagues (1991) made a prospective study of the very important group of women who are asymptomatic at onset of labour. Viral shedding in the genital tract at the beginning of labour occurred in 56 of 15 923 women (0.35%). Of these, 51 shed HSV-2 and 5 HSV-1. Serological tests revealed that 35% of the women with HSV shedding at the onset of labour had recently acquired primary infection or first episode genital infection. Vertical transmission occurred in 12.5% in women with positive HSV cultures and in 0.02% of those with negative cultures, indicating that viral shedding is not always detectable. Neonatal herpes developed in 33% of the babies born to women with recent primary or first episode genital infections, but in only 3% of those born to mothers with recurrent asymptomatic infection. The incidence of neonatal herpes in this study population was 1 per 2000 live births.

Obviously, the risk of virus transmission to vaginally delivered infants is highest, being ≥30% in women with primary and first episode genital infection shortly (<2 weeks) before delivery, 3–5% in women with recurrent lesions and <3% in those with recurrent asymptomatic infection.

ADDITIONAL RISK FACTORS IN MOTHER–INFANT TRANSMISSION

Additional risk factors for virus transmission and neonatal disease are prolonged ruptured or leaky membranes (>6 h before delivery), increasing the risk of intrauterine infection by the ascending route. Fetal scalp electrode monitoring, forceps delivery or vacuum extraction may provide portals of virus entry in the newborn (Brown et al. 1991, Malm et al. 1991, Forsgren 1992).

5.2 Effects on the fetus and on the neonate

INCIDENCE OF NEONATAL DISEASE

Neonatal herpes in the USA occurs at an estimated annual rate of 1 per 3500–5000 deliveries, but may be as high as 1 per 2000 in certain population groups with high HSV-2 seroprevalence (e.g. Whitley 1994). For unknown reasons, the annual incidence is much lower in some other countries – e.g. the UK (1/40 000–60 000) and Sweden (1/15 000) – even though the seroprevalences of HSV-1 and HSV-2 in European countries are comparable with those in the USA. In general, a larger proportion of neonatal infections are caused by HSV-2 than HSV-1, but a nationwide survey indicated that in Japan twice as many infections are due to HSV-1 (Morishima et al. 1996).

PATHOGENESIS OF NEONATAL INFECTION

Of the reported neonatal herpes cases in the USA c. 4 % are acquired in utero, 86% intrapartum and 10% postnatally (Whitley 1993).

Transmission of infection in utero occurs transplacentally in <2% of cases, most probably in early to mid-gestation, because physical signs are present at birth and include some unusual stigmata (e.g. hydrocephalus, chorioretinitis); a further 2–3% arise late in gestation by the ascending route. In intrapartum transmission, the higher infection rate in infants born to mothers with primary or first episode genital herpes shortly before delivery, causing most cases of neonatal herpes, is related both to viral shedding in high concentration and to the absence of maternal neutralizing antibodies (see, e.g., Yeager et al. 1980, Brown et al. 1991, Whitley 1994). This is in contrast to recurrent infection, in which virus is shed for a shorter period in low amounts and maternal antibodies against the infecting type are passed to the newborn. Postnatal infections are acquired from maternal sources (oral, genital and breast lesions) or by close contact with people with herpetic lesions (e.g. of the mouth or fingers) or by nosocomial spread from other infected babies.

IMMUNE RESPONSE

In infected newborns the cellular immune response is suppressed and delayed as indicated by an absent or delayed T-lymphocyte proliferative response and decreased interferon-α and γ production in response to herpes simplex antigen (see, e.g., Kahlon and Whitley 1988, Cederblad, Riesenfeld and Alm 1989). The IgG antibody response is initially not recognizable because, in the first 6–8 weeks, it cannot be distinguished from maternal antibody. IgM antibodies develop within the first 2–3 weeks of illness and remain detectable for c. 6–8 weeks. IgG antibodies persist at medium to low titres for life. Transplacentally transferred neutralizing and antibody-dependent cell-mediated cytotoxic (ADCC) antibodies modify the severity of neonatal disease (Kohl et al. 1989).

CLINICAL MANIFESTATIONS

Neonatal herpes is almost invariably overt and frequently lethal. The most severely affected infants are those with infection acquired early in pregnancy (<2%) with physical signs apparent at birth. Lesions include skin vesicles or scarring, chorioretinitis, microcephaly and hydrocephaly (Hutto et al. 1987). So far, more than 30 such cases have been identified but the estimated incidence (1 per 200 000 live births) is low. Infants with intrauterine infections acquired late by the ascending route (2–3%) usually present only with skin or eye lesions at birth, without multi-organ involvement (Baldwin and Whitley 1989, Whitley 1993).

In a scheme based on large prospective studies, neonatal herpes cases are classified according to the 3 general patterns of infection, each occurring in about one third of cases (Forsgren 1992, Whitley 1994, Harrison 1995, Whitley and Arvin 1995) (Table 41.16).

In general, neonatal disease caused by HSV-1 has a better prognosis than that caused by HSV-2 (Forsgren 1992). However, in the national Japanese survey on neonatal herpes, although similar pattern of disease were evident, the type of virus had no significant effects on mortality, morbidity and response to treatment (Morishima et al. 1996).

5.3 Diagnosis in pregnancy and in the neonate

DIAGNOSIS IN PREGNANCY

Maternal infection with typical mucocutaneous lesions in the oropharynx and the genital tract is easily diagnosed but less typical, minor genital lesions need laboratory confirmation.

PCR is the most sensitive method for detecting both HSV-1 and HSV-2, and can be used at the onset of labour for a rapid decision on the mode of delivery, high levels of HSV DNA in the maternal secretion increasing the probability of transmission to the infant. Assessment of the type-specific antibodies to both HSV-1 and HSV-2 is essential for identifying mothers at risk of infecting their infants during delivery. The risk is highest in women with primary or first episode infection who seroconvert during pregnancy. ELISA and immunofluorescence tests with non-type-specific antigens detect seroconversion for IgG and IgM antibodies in primary oropharyngeal and genital infections and rises in specific IgG in genital first episodes; in recurrent infections (symptomatic or asymptomatic), there is no rise in specific IgG level and IgM is not detectable. The more cumbersome neutralization test, although not routinely used, is employed for determining the amount of protective antibodies in maternal and newborn blood.

None of the conventional tests, however, can accurately distinguish between type 1- and type 2-specific antibodies. This is possible only with assays (e.g. immunoblot, immunodot, gG2 indirect ELISA) employing native purified glycoprotein G antigen (gG-1 for HSV-1, gG-2 for HSV-2) (Svennerholm et al. 1984, Johnson et al. 1989, Eis-Hübinger et al. 1991, Forsgren 1992, Slomka 1996). HSV-2 type-specific IgM antibodies may also be detected more easily by such assays (Ho et al. 1993). It should be noted that the interval between onset of a primary or first episode genital infection to the detection of type-specific antibodies may range from 2 to 3 weeks for HSV-1 and from 2 to 4 weeks for HSV-2 (Ashley et al. 1988, Ho et al. 1993).

DIAGNOSIS IN INFANCY

Cases with skin vesicles are easily recognized; neonatal herpes should also be considered in the differential diagnosis of severe generalized disease or of encephalitis within the first month of life.

The most direct means of laboratory diagnosis is viral detection, especially by PCR, which is particularly useful for tests on CSF. Serology is of little help in the first weeks of life, for the reasons mentioned in 'Immune response' (p. 888). Testing the maternal serum together with acute phase and later sera of the infant is essential. A presumptive retrospective diagnosis of a child damaged by HSV-2 is obtained by demonstrating persistent IgG antibodies to HSV-2 or by isolating the virus from recurrent vesicles, because HSV-2 infections are rare before the onset of sexual activity (Malm et al. 1991).

Table 41.16 Classification, pattern and outcome of neonatal HSV disease

Disease	Onset of signs after birth	Mortality		Prognosis in survivors
		No therapy	**With therapy**	
Disseminated CNS, lung, liver, adrenals, SEM	6–12[a] days	>80%	>50%	40% develop normally
CNS Encephalitis/meningitis in 37–48% without SEM	16–18 days	>50%	15%	In c. 56% neurological and ophthalmological impairment and recurrent skin lesions
SEM	6–7 days	ND	0%	In ≥20% neurological impairment, recurrent skin lesions

ND, no data; SEM, skin/eye/mouth.
[a]Onset at 12 days is less frequent.

5.4 Management in pregnancy and of the neonate

At the first antenatal visit, a careful history should be taken of genital infections in the woman herself and her sexual partner, together with visual inspection of her genital tract both at this visit and at the onset of labour. If lesions are seen, swabs should be taken for virus detection, but a decision on caesarean section rests mainly on the presence of visible lesions. If serological tests are used, seroconversion to HSV-2 antibody-positive during pregnancy may be an indication for rapid virus detection by PCR and possible treatment; this approach might reduce the need for caesarean section.

Caesarean sections, considered at present as the only effective means of preventing neonatal herpes infection, are performed on up to 70% of women in the USA with a history of genital herpes, because of possible fetal infection and of medicolegal considerations. It is recommended generally for women with visible cervicovaginal lesions at onset of labour, irrespective of the antibody status or viral shedding, and is best performed before rupture of the membranes or <24 h thereafter. The procedure will, however, not always prevent neonatal herpes, even if performed before rupture of the membranes, and especially not after they have been ruptured for more than 4 h (Stone et al. 1989, Randolph, Washington and Prober 1993).

Prenatal diagnosis is not recommended because the fetus is rarely transplacentally infected until midgestation. Termination of pregnancy in women with disseminated disease is not an option.

For immunoprophylaxis, specific immunoglobulins, humanized murine and human monoclonal antibodies and hyperimmunoglobulin with high neutralizing activity (not yet commercially available) have been developed for administration to neonates lacking maternal antibodies. Vaccines for prevention and treatment, particularly of HSV-2 genital infections, have also been developed and a candidate subunit vaccine is on trial (Whitley and Arvin 1994).

Aciclovir or its derivatives are the mainstay of antiviral therapy for both topical and systemic application. Although this drug is not licensed for use in pregnancy, no association has so far been identified between its use in pregnancy and adverse effects in mother or child (Kroon and Whitley 1995).

In maternal primary disseminated infection, early intravenous treatment with aciclovir (5 or 10 mg/kg every 8 h) at any stage of pregnancy is recommended. Oral treatment with aciclovir (200 mg 5 times daily for 14 days) is considered beneficial for women with recognized primary or first episode genital infection in the later stages of pregnancy. This is also the case in maternal primary oral infection (e.g. gingivostomatitis) shortly before term, at delivery or in the neonatal period and in primary genital herpes in the neonatal period. To suppress viral shedding during labour in women with recurrent lesions in late pregnancy, prophylactic oral use (200 mg 4 times daily) c. 10 days before delivery is under trial (Stray-Pedersen 1990, Haddad et al. 1993) but is controversial for various reasons, such as potential renal toxicity for the fetus, occasional virus shedding despite suppressive treatment (Straus et al. 1989, Katz et al. 1995) and the question of its value. The need for suppressive therapy in the above-mentioned target group is limited, because there is only a low prospective risk to babies born to women with recurrent lesions, in contrast to those born to mothers with unrecognized primary and first episode genital infections (Whitley and Arvin 1994, Kroon and Whitley 1995).

The prophylactic administration of aciclovir to vaginally delivered asymptomatic newborns at risk of infection depends on the form of maternal infection and the infecting serotype. Follow-up for clinical and laboratory signs of infection is recommended up to 4 weeks after delivery (e.g. Forsgren 1992, Whitley 1994, Whitley and Arvin 1995).

6 PARVOVIRUS B19

Parvovirus B19 (B19), was discovered in the plasma of healthy blood donors in 1975, and recognized in 1983 as the cause of erythema infectiosum. Soon thereafter its causative role in hydrops fetalis and fetal death became evident. In addition, B19 is now associated with many haematological and non-haematological complications.

6.1 Postnatal infection

Postnatal infection is acquired through aerosol droplets by the respiratory route. The seroprevalence rate in childbearing age and in pregnancy ranges from <40% to 60% in individual countries and with regional differences. Transmission is greatest during viraemia and before clinical signs are apparent, complicating efforts to control transmission. During outbreaks the infection rate in susceptible adults is up to 50% within families and c. 20% for care workers and teachers, being highest for those in contact with younger and greater numbers of infected children (Gillespie et al. 1990).

6.2 Effects on the fetus

In pregnancy, c. 60% of infections are asymptomatic or overlooked (Enders and Biber 1990, Enders 1998). The first reports of fetal infection with B19 virus were published by Brown et al. in 1984. Schwarz and co-workers (1988) later demonstrated that maternal infection between WG 10 and 26 carries the main risk of fetal complications. The rates of transplacental transmission (derived from the persistence of IgG antibodies in children aged 1 year following maternal infection during pregnancy) have been estimated at c. 33% (Public Health Laboratory Service Working Party of Fifth Disease 1990) and c. 36% (Enders 1997, personal obsevations).

PATHOGENESIS OF FETAL INFECTION

The virus is transmitted to the fetus during the maternal viraemic phase, which starts c. 6 days after the infection is acquired and is highest, with 10^{11} DNA genome equivalents per millilitre of blood, shortly before the onset of symptoms and in asymptomatic people before detection of IgM antibodies.

The virus may cross the placenta at any time during pregnancy. B19 infects erythroid progenitor cells in which the virus replicates with lytic effects. Erythroblasts in the bone marrow and spleen as well as in the liver of the fetus are target cells. It is suggested that the fetus becomes susceptible to infection at 6 weeks of gestation, when the fetal liver contains erythroblasts. The pathogenesis of hydrops fetalis seems to be mainly due to inhibition of replication of erythroid progenitor cells, combined with a shortened fetal red cell life span of 45–70 days, leading to a deficiency of erythroblasts. Inhibition of fetal erythroid progenitor cells occurs mainly in the late pronormoblast stage in which intranuclear inclusions (Lantern cells) are com-

monly detected (Schwarz et al. 1991). There is considerable haemolysis in the B19-infected fetus with karyorrhexis of many infected cells and massive iron deposition in the liver and spleen. A drastic decline in reticulocytes precedes the decline of erythrocytes and haemoglobin concentration. Destruction of erythroid progenitor cells in addition to red cell aplasia produces a profound irreversible aplastic crisis in the fetus, with a resultant anaemia culminating in cardiovascular decompensation, hydrops, ascites and fetal death (CDC 1989).

FETAL COMPLICATIONS

Fetal complications, notably hydrops, occur most frequently 2–4 weeks (85%), 5–8 weeks (10%) after onset of maternal infection, less often between 9 and 12 weeks (4.3%) (Komischke, Searle and Enders 1997) and exceptionally as late as 18 weeks (Schwarz and Jäger 1995). Smoleniec and co-workers (1994) suggested that the risk of fetal complications might be higher in asymptomatic than in symptomatic maternal parvovirus infection, but this remains unconfirmed. It should be noted that hydrops sometimes resolves spontaneously without apparent ill-effects on the infant (Morey et al. 1991, Zerbini et al. 1993, Tercanli, Enders and Holzgreve 1996).

FETAL LOSS

The fetus seems to be at greatest risk of developing hydrops in the second trimester when the fetal red cell mass increases 3- to 4-fold, and at decreased risk in the third trimester when it is able to mount an immune response. The frequencies of fetal death reported in studies involving only small numbers of parvovirus-infected pregnant women were 1.66% (Gratacós et al. 1995), 2.5% (Rodis et al. 1990), 10% (CDC 1989) and 38% (Rodis et al. 1988). In 2 prospective multicentre studies (Public Health Laboratory Service Working Party on Fifth Disease 1990, Schwarz et al. 1990), including 184 and 120 pregnant women with clinically and serologically proven parvovirus infection, there were similar excess fetal losses of 11.8% and 11.7% in the second trimester. The risk of fetal death due to an infected pregnancy was estimated to be 9% (Public Health Laboratory Service Working Party on Fifth Disease 1990). In our large prospective study, the rate of hydrops fetalis and fetal loss is estimated as c. 17% and 12.3% (Enders 1997, personal observations).

DISEASE POSSIBLY DUE TO FETAL
PARVOVIRUS B19 INFECTION

In addition to the fetal complications described above, a few reports suggest that B19 virus may directly infect cells of mesoendodermal origin expressing the erythrocyte P antigen, the cellular receptor for B19 antigen (Brown, Anderson and Young 1993). Infection may lead, if the fetus survives, to specific and permanent organ defects. Most of those findings have been made in aborted fetuses with B19 infection and involvement of myocardial cells (Porter, Quantrill and Fleming 1988), eye anomalies and damage to other tissues (Weiland et al. 1987) or with bilateral cleft lip and palate, micrognathia and webbed joints (Tiessen et al. 1994).

Some abnormalities associated with prenatal infection in liveborn infants have also been reported. Brown and colleagues (1994) described 3 cases with chronic anaemia closely resembling congenital red cell aplasia or Diamond–Blackfan anaemia. In one instance hepatic disease was associated with intrauterine B19 infection in a premature newborn (Metzman et al. 1989). Furthermore, a case of 'prune belly' after maternal B19 infection and hydrops fetalis has been reported (Walther, Gloning and Schwarz 1994); and there is a more important preliminary report on 3 liveborn infants with severe nervous system anomalies following serologically confirmed maternal B19 infection (Conry, Török and Andrews 1993). Teratogenic effects and fetal damage caused by animal parvovirus in fetuses of different animal species are well known but have not so far been reported in humans.

6.3 Diagnosis

DIAGNOSIS IN PREGNANCY

B19 infection should be excluded in pregnant women who are contacts of patients with erythema infectiosum. In pregnant women with exanthems, lymphadenopathy or arthralgia, B19 infection as well as rubella must be considered. Anamnestic data about type and time of contact are helpful. In pregnant women with sonographic evidence of hydrops fetalis, B19 infection should be confirmed or excluded.

Detection of specific IgM with or without IgG antibody indicates acute B19 infection. In pregnancy this should be confirmed by testing a second serum. IgG antibodies (Ferguson, Walker and Cohen 1996) in the absence of IgM indicate previous infection (≥ 4 months) or protection (Searle, Guillard and Enders 1996).

Maternal B19 infection can be confirmed by PCR detection of B19 DNA when diagnostic interpretation of serological results is difficult. Large amounts of virus are still present in the blood shortly after onset of symptoms and can persist at low titres for 2–6 months (Musiani et al. 1995). When acute infection is diagnosed in pregnancy, weekly ultrasound monitoring up to 8–12 weeks after onset is recommended, to detect early signs of hydrops. If hydrops develops, the patient should be referred to a prenatal diagnostic centre for further tests and, if necessary, for intrauterine therapy.

DIAGNOSIS IN THE FETUS

Fetal infection is suspected most frequently when hydrops is diagnosed by ultrasound after a serologically confirmed recent parvovirus infection or at routine scan. Contrary to previous suggestions, the level of α-fetoprotein (AFP) in the maternal serum does not seem to be a reliable marker for early fetal involvement (Saller, Rogers and Canick 1993, Komischke, Searle and Enders 1997). Raised levels have, however, been observed shortly before intrauterine death. Hydrops fetalis is graded as mild, moderate or severe. Mild hydrops is not usually associated with significant anaemia (Hb 7.2–11.5 g/dl), and may resolve spontaneously over time (category I). Moderate hydrops fetalis is associated with Hb values of 5.7– 7.2 g/dl (category II). In cases with generalized hydrops, fetal Hb values range between 1.9 and 5.4 g/dl; without very early intervention, most cases end in intrauterine death (category III) (Tercanli, Enders and Holzgreve 1996).

Fetal blood sampling is performed in a prenatal diagnostic centre to determine reticulocyte and Hb values and to obtain amniotic fluid and fetal blood to confirm B19 infection by detecting viral DNA, IgM antibodies or both. To detect B19 DNA in fetal blood by PCR, it is important that heparin is not used for moistening the needle employed for cordocentesis, because this anticoagulant may inhibit Taq polymerase by binding to DNA (Beutler, Gelbart and Kuhl 1990, Schwarz et al. 1992) and can cause false negative results. The detection rate for B19 DNA by PCR in amniotic fluid, fetal blood and ascites in categories II and III is c. 70%. In most instances amniotic fluid and fetal blood of the same patients are both positive. In asymptomatic fetuses of mothers with serologically confirmed B19 infection, the detection rate for B19 DNA in amniotic fluid and fetal blood may still be as high as 20%. IgM antibody testing in fetal serum is of low diagnostic value, having a positivity rate of c. 15%.

6.4 Management

TREATMENT OF THE HYDROPIC FETUS

In B19 infection associated with fetal hydrops and moderate to severe anaemia, intrauterine transfusions with erythrocyte concentrates have been performed in various German prenatal diagnostic centres since 1986/7 and have seemed beneficial (Schwarz et al. 1988). In general, however, this treatment has been controversial. The findings in a recent study conducted in the UK during the epidemic year of 1993/4 indicate that intrauterine transfusion benefits some fetuses with hydrops arising from parvovirus infection. The surviving fetuses had no abnormalities related to B19 infection (Fairley et al. 1995).

MANAGEMENT IN PREGNANCY AND OF THE NEONATE

Efforts to prevent contact with infected individuals are of very limited effect. Prophylaxis with immunoglobulin may be effective, as it has been beneficial in patients with chronic parvovirus infection. A parvovirus vaccine is currently being developed and trials are underway (Bansal et al. 1993). Treatment, when needed, is symptomatic. Specific antiviral drugs are not available.

A pregnancy does not need to be terminated when B19 infection occurs, as there is little evidence of damage to fetuses that survive infection and are born alive. This is important for the justification of intrauterine treatment of infected fetuses. Infants of mothers with acute parvovirus B19 infection in pregnancy should be observed for abnormalities and for persistence of antibody at 10–12 months of age. Management following B19 exposure in pregnancy is described in Table 41.17.

Table 41.17 Management strategies for parvovirus B19 exposure in pregnancy

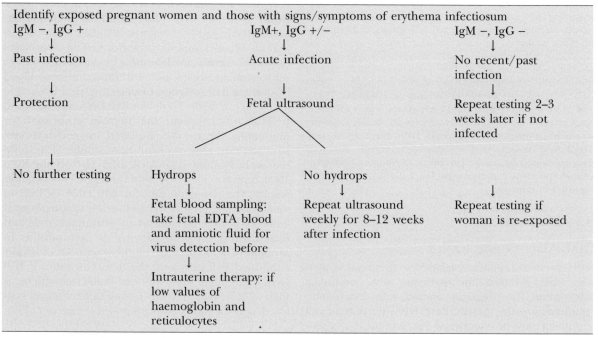

Identify exposed pregnant women and those with signs/symptoms of erythema infectiosum

IgM −, IgG +	IgM+, IgG +/−	IgM −, IgG −
↓	↓	↓
Past infection	Acute infection	No recent/past infection
↓	↓	↓
Protection	Fetal ultrasound	Repeat testing 2–3 weeks later if not infected

No further testing	Hydrops	No hydrops	Repeat testing if woman is re-exposed
	↓	↓	
	Fetal blood sampling: take fetal EDTA blood and amniotic fluid for virus detection before	Repeat ultrasound weekly for 8–12 weeks after infection	
	↓		
	Intrauterine therapy: if low values of haemoglobin and reticulocytes		

+, positive; +/−, borderline or negative; −, negative.

7 HUMAN IMMUNODEFICIENCY VIRUS

AIDS is caused by the lentiviruses, human immunodeficiency viruses 1 and 2 (HIV-1 and HIV-2); HIV-1 infection has become one of the leading causes of childhood mortality in some settings. Because females may be infected by heterosexual transmission, the number of HIV-1 positive pregnant women is increasing. Prenatal care is an important means of detecting HIV infection in pregnancy. Progress in diagnosis, therapy and interventional measures may perhaps further reduce the risk of vertical transmission.

7.1 Effects on pregnancy

Pregnancy does not seem to accelerate progression of HIV-1 disease (Berrebi et al. 1990). Fetal loss associated with early HIV transmission in utero may occur more often in pregnant women with AIDS than in HIV positive but asymptomatic women (Langston et al. 1995).

7.2 Maternal factors in mother–infant transmission

The main maternal factors associated with increased risk of vertical transmission are primary infection in pregnancy and advanced clinical disease, in which the virus load is usually high as measured by maternal plasma HIV-1 RNA levels. The critical threshold for transmission was estimated to be c.100000 RNA copies/ml of plasma (Fang et al. 1995). However, pregnant women with low copy numbers

(c.10000/ml) may also transmit HIV vertically although at lower frequency (Zöllner et al. 1996).

Other maternal factors that may increase the likelihood of transmission, either synergistically or independently, are low numbers of CD4+ lymphocytes, coexisting sexually acquired infection, drug abuse ('crack' cocaine), low vitamin A, chorioamnionitis, rupture of the membranes >4 hours before birth regardless of the mode of delivery, and premature delivery (e.g. Minkoff et al. 1995).

Rates of HIV transmission to the infant are decreased by zidovudine therapy of the mother and neonate (Connor et al. 1994); caesarean section before onset of labour or rupture of the membranes (e.g. Goedert et al. 1991, Schäfer and Friese 1996); the presence of maternal neutralizing antibodies (Scarlatti et al. 1993); delivery within 4 h after rupture of the membranes (Landesman et al. 1996); and, in African countries, by cleansing the birth canal in women delivering >4 h after rupture of the membranes, with transmission rates of 25% and 39% in the treated and control groups respectively (Biggar et al. 1996); and by not breast-feeding (CDC 1995b).

7.3 Routes of transmission

Transmission from the HIV-infected mother to the child may occur in utero or intrapartum or by breast-feeding.

Evidence of intrauterine infection by the transplacental route early in pregnancy has been provided by virus cultivation from the tissues of aborted first and second trimester fetuses (Lewis et al. 1990, Reynolds-Kohler et al. 1993, Langston et al. 1995). Intrauterine infection in early pregnancy is possible, but is more likely to occur shortly before delivery (Alimenti et al. 1991, Ehrnst et al. 1991, Douglas and King 1992). It is usually assumed to occur by haematogenous spread across the placenta. However, it may also spread from pelvic organs in which replication is occurring, and in late pregnancy by ascending infection from the vagina after rupture of the membranes.

The role of intrapartum transmission is supported by various observations. Comparison of 66 sets of twins, delivered either vaginally or by caesarean section, showed that 50% of first-born twins delivered vaginally were infected with HIV-1 compared with 38% of first-born twins delivered by caesarean section, and 19% of the second-born twins delivered by either route (Goedert et al. 1991). Two meta-analyses of prospective studies of perinatal HIV-1 transmission showed a lower rate of transmission to infants delivered by caesarean section than to those delivered vaginally (Villari et al. 1993, Dunn et al. 1994). This finding was confirmed by the European Collaborative Study (1994a) (caesarean section: 11.7% infected; vaginal delivery: 17.6% infected). Although the intrapartum route of HIV-1 transmission is recognized, the benefit of caesarean section in preventing transmission seems inconclusive without controls for key co-variates (CD4+ lymphocyte levels, viral load and time from rupture of membranes to delivery). This is supported by a study with control of the key co-variates (Landesman 1996), in which the benefit of caesarean section seemed to be small. A reduction of HIV-1 transmission from 18.7% to 13.9% among 487 women was observed when the membranes ruptured $\geq$4 h before delivery. The possibility of intrapartum transmission is further supported by studies in non-breast-fed infants with no virological HIV markers within the first 2 days after birth, but who were later shown to be infected (Dunn et al. 1994).

The early postnatal route of HIV-1 transmission is mainly by breast-feeding, and depends both on the HIV-1 virus load present in breast-milk and on the state of maternal immunosuppression and vitamin A deficiency (Nduati et al. 1995). Some milk factors protect against postnatal transmission, for example specific IgA and IgM and a molecule able to inhibit the binding of HIV to CD4+ lymphocytes. Breast-feeding may increase the rate of transmission by 10–20% (CDC 1995b). However, there are differences in the risk of mother-to-child transmission of HIV-1 by breast-feeding: in mothers infected before pregnancy the postnatal transmission rate was 8–18%, whereas in those infected while lactating it was 26% (Van de Perre 1995).

7.4 Rates of perinatal transmission

Transmission rates for HIV-1 range from 13% to 40% in studies in different geographic areas and socioeconomic conditions. In prospective studies, the perinatal transmission rate for 19 European countries was estimated to be 14% on average (European Collaborative Study 1992) and 25–35% in African countries (Peckham and Gibb 1995).

HIV-2 infections in pregnant women are rarely reported; limited data indicate very low transmission rates of nil to 1.2% (Adjorlolo-Johnson et al. 1994, De Cock et al. 1994).

7.5 HIV infection in infants

Two patterns of disease have been described for infants vertically infected with HIV-1. In one, infection progresses rapidly to AIDS within the first year of life in c. 25%. In the remainder it progresses more slowly and, of these, c. 25% remain asymptomatic until preadolescence (Blanche et al. 1990, Grubman et al. 1995). In the European Collaborative Study (1992) mortality in HIV-infected infants aged c. 1 year was 15%, and by the age of 5 years, 28%. The findings in Swiss and Italian studies were similar (Kind et al. 1992, Italian Register for HIV Infection in Children 1994). In Europe, the annual rate of progression to AIDS decreases after the first year of life to 6–8%, as does the mortality rate.

The more rapid progression of disease in vertically infected infants is explained by the relative immaturity of the immune system, the infectious dose, the route of infection (Wilfert et al. 1994) and infections with opportunistic organisms. In children infected with HIV-1 the wide range of clinical manifestations includes features of severe immunodeficiency, nonspecific symptoms and AIDS-related diseases. The prospects for survival of children with opportunistic infections, neurological disease and lymphoma are worse than for those with lymphocytic interstitial pneumonitis or bacterial infections (European Collaborative Study 1994b).

7.6 Diagnosis

Screening in pregnancy

Voluntary HIV screening in pregnancy has been implemented in the USA, Canada and western European countries in gynaecological, prenatal and other obstetric clinics, but for logistic, legal and cost-benefit reasons it is not sufficiently widespread (Evans et al. 1995, Ecker 1996, Landers and Sweet 1996). In Germany, HIV testing has, since 1987, been included in routine prenatal care if the pregnant woman gives her consent (Kassenärztliche Bundesvereinigung 1994). Although pregnant women remain at low risk of acquiring HIV-1 infection – 0.04% of 200 000 pregnancies from 1987 to 1997, including only 3 HIV-2 infections (Enders 1998) – prenatal screening is recommended. The prevalence may be higher in women who have not sought prenatal care, for example from some immigrant communities.

Antibody screening in pregnancy is performed with enzyme immunoassays (EIA), supplemented when appropriate by confirmatory tests, for example western blot, immunofluorescence, PCR and viral culture (CDC 1995b) (see also Chapter 38). In HIV-1-infected pregnant women the viral load in serum is determined by quantifying RNA and p24 antigen. The cellular immune status is determined by the CD4 T cell value and by the CD4/CD8 ratio.

TESTS ON THE FETUS

Tests on the fetus of an HIV-infected woman are not recommended, because most vertical HIV transmissions occur intrapartum, and only occasionally in early or late pregnancy. Furthermore, contamination with maternal blood during amnio- or cordocentesis may transmit the virus to the fetus, or may give false positive results.

NEONATAL AND PAEDIATRIC DIAGNOSIS

In HIV-1-infected newborns, congenital malformations or other signs of HIV infection are absent. However, significantly higher rates of prematurity, intra-uterine growth retardation and low birth weight have been found among them than among the uninfected HIV-1-exposed control group. Prematurity seems to be an important predictor of HIV-1 infection for seropositive infants (Abrams et al. 1995, Langston et al. 1995). According to the proposed definitions, intrauterine infection in live-born infants is confirmed by the detection of virus in peripheral blood mononuclear cells by culture or PCR within 48 h after birth. Intrapartum infection is presumed when test results are negative in the first week of life but become positive after 7–90 days in infants who are not breast-fed (Bryson et al. 1992, Report of a Consensus Workshop SI 1992). Early diagnosis of HIV infection in infants born to an HIV-seropositive mother cannot be made by the conventional serological tests because IgM or IgA antibodies are not detectable, but is confirmed by virus detection, by culture, PCR and p24 antigen assay (Burgard et al. 1992). The sensitivity of viral culture and PCR is about 40% at birth rising to 90% after 1–4 weeks (McIntosh et al. 1994). A positive p24 antigen test result at >1 month of age is strongly indicative of HIV infection, but a negative result within the first 4 weeks does not exclude it. IgA antibodies may be detectable at 3–6 months of age in about half of the infected infants. Emerging evidence suggests that recovery of a rapidly replicating syncytium-inducing virus from a neonate predicts fast progression of disease (De Rossi et al. 1993).

To confirm an early diagnosis, positive results on 2 consecutive blood specimens with one or more tests (e.g. PCR, viral culture or p24 antigen) are required. If 2 or 3 such tests are negative after 1–3 months of age and there are no other indicators of HIV disease, infection is unlikely in a non-breast-fed child despite the presence of IgG antibody. To confirm that a child is not infected with HIV, a final antibody test should be done at 15–18 months of age (Peckham and Gibb 1995).

A case of HIV clearance in a 3 month old infant was described by Bryson et al. (1995). Recently, additional cases of HIV clearance (i.e. transient HIV infections) were observed in infants born to HIV-infected mothers in 4 centres of the European Collaborative Study of children. Of 264 children, 9 who were initially positive

by virus culture or PCR subsequently seroreverted. Taking only those children who had 2 or more positive virus tests, 2.7% (6/219) cleared infection or tolerated the virus (Newell et al. 1996). These cases of infants with clearance of HIV infection are of significance and it is essential to exclude all possible diagnostic errors and to ensure that each reported case is adequately investigated and documented. In general, HIV clearance in individual cases is accepted but the reason has yet to be clarified (McMichael, Koup and Amman 1996). Current paediatric opinion is that children who serorevert are considered not to be infected with HIV-1.

7.7 Management of the mother

PREVENTION

The optimal preventive measure is the avoidance of unprotected sexual relations or sexual contact only with a partner known to be uninfected. Passive prophylaxis with immunoglobulin preparations is not effective, and vaccines for active prophylaxis are not yet available (Wood, Graham and Wright 1995).

CHEMOTHERAPY

Treatment of HIV-1-infected pregnant women is at present carried out with zidovudine (Connor et al. 1994, Matheson et al. 1995). Observation must be maintained for possible long-term adverse effects of the drug. Some of the promising newer therapeutic approaches with combinations of various nucleoside analogues (reverse transcriptase inhibitors), HIV-1 protease inhibitors (Perelson et al. 1996) and perhaps integrase inhibitors may also be candidates for use in pregnancy (Minkoff and Augenbraun 1997).

Appropriate counselling of the HIV-infected woman is a major task. This includes, for example, an explanation of the need for further testing, the possible benefit and side effects of zidovudine therapy, and the pros and cons of the mode of delivery. Termination of pregnancy is no longer suggested, as was done earlier when the risk of vertical transmission was estimated to be as high as 50% and when no antiviral drugs were available.

7.8 Management of the neonate

After delivery, isolation of mother and infant is recommended. Breast-feeding is contraindicated in countries where appropriate milk substitutes are available. In developing countries, however, breast-feeding is encouraged because artificial feeding in a poor hygienic environment greatly increases morbidity and mortality from diarrhoeal diseases and respiratory infections (Van de Perre 1995). Follow-up of infected or uninfected infants born to HIV-1-infected mothers is important, as outlined in the appropriate recommendations (e.g. CDC 1995b), including those for vaccination schedules (ACIP 1993).

8 HEPATITIS VIRUSES

The list of hepatitis viruses continues to expand. Of those so far identified, types B, C and E are of known significance in pregnancy and for the newborn (Table 41.18).

8.1 Hepatitis A virus

Hepatitis A (HAV) (enterovirus 72) is acquired by the faecal–oral route, and has an incubation period of c. 4 weeks.

INFECTION IN PREGNANCY AND IN NEONATES

Hepatitis A has no apparent adverse effect on the outcome of pregnancy. Transmission during birth (e.g. by exposure to maternal faeces or by breast-feeding) has not been identified in a number of studies (e.g. Zhuang 1989, CDC 1990, Ye 1990, Zhang, Zeng and Zhang 1990). In one investigation, neonatal infection was diagnosed in an infant born to a mother with hepatitis A 10 days after premature labour, the evidence indicating that he was infected by his mother before or during birth. HAV may spread within the neonatal intensive care unit, causing asymptomatic infection in neonates, and symptomatic or asymptomatic infection in staff members as a result of lapses in infection control precautions (Watson et al. 1993). Neonates, even when infected parenterally by transfusion with hepatitis A-contaminated blood (a rare event) rarely have biochemical evidence of hepatitis (Azimi et al. 1986). They are, however, a potential source of infection for non-immune staff members, as the virus is excreted in the stools of infected neonates and infants for up to 5 months (Rosenblum et al. 1991). This is much longer than in older children, except those in whom icteric hepatitis relapses, as has been reported in 3–20% of children (Sjogren et al. 1987).

CONTROL MEASURES

Infection can be controlled by adopting simple hygienic measures and by the sanitary disposal of excreta. Strict isolation of cases is not effective, as faecal shedding of the virus peaks during the prodromal phase. For pre- and postexposure prophylaxis, human normal immunglobulin preparations (HNIG) are in use and may be given to neonates born within 2 weeks of maternal illness; to neonates in an intensive care unit if a case occurs on the ward; and to non-immune staff members (Zhang, Zeng and Zhang 1990). Inactivated vaccines are effective, and will replace immunoglobulin for pre-exposure prophylaxis; they may also be useful for postexposure prophylaxis. Neither HNIG nor inactivated hepatitis A vaccines are contraindicated in pregnancy.

8.2 Hepatitis B virus

Hepatitis B virus (HBV), a hepadnavirus, is transmitted primarily by the parenteral route, by blood or by sexual contact through contaminated secretions from acutely infected patients or carriers, and by vertical transmission. Perinatal infection and infection during the first year of life have important consequences because 90% of these infants become chronic carriers, compared with only c. 10% of those infected after the age of 6 years. Such chronicity increases the risk of cirrhosis and hepatocellular carcinoma.

INFECTION IN PREGNANCY

Acute hepatitis B occurs in the USA in 1–2 per 1000 pregnancies, and chronic infection is present in 5–15 per 1000 pregnancies (Sweet 1990). Increases in fulminant cases and mortality rates due to acute HBV infection during pregnancy, as observed in some endemic areas, are probably due to poor health care and malnutrition (see, e.g., Christie et al. 1976). No such effects have been noted in countries with good living conditions (e.g. Shalev and Bassan 1982). No teratogenic effects have been associated with maternal HBV infection.

MOTHER–CHILD TRANSMISSION

Intrauterine infection by haematogenous transplacental transmission, possibly due to leakage of maternal blood to the fetus, has been suggested for some newborns of carrier mothers with evidence of HBV infection at birth (Lin et al. 1987, Ohto et al. 1987). In addition, 10% of neonates born to mothers with acute HBV infection in the first trimester have been found HBsAg positive at birth, suggesting intrauterine infection (CDC 1990, Sweet 1990). About 90% of vertical transmission, however, occurs as a consequence of intrapartum exposure to contaminated blood and genital secretions. The remaining cases result from the above-mentioned haematogenous transplacental transmission, breast-feeding and close postnatal contact between infant and the infected parent(s).

RATE OF TRANSMISSION

Of the offspring of women acutely infected in the third trimester, 80–90% are infected. The transmission rate from asymptomatic carrier mothers who are positive only for HBsAg is c. 10–20% in the absence of immune prophylaxis. Mothers positive for both HBsAg and HBeAg, and thus highly infectious, transmit the virus in 80–90% of cases (see, e.g., Stevens et al. 1979). For predicting persisting infection in infants and a possible failure of neonatal hepatitis B passive/active vaccination, the HBV DNA virus load in the maternal serum seems to be the most important factor (e.g. Burk et al. 1994, Del Canho et al. 1994).

OUTCOMES OF PERINATAL AND POSTNATAL INFECTION

Most infants born to carrier mothers are HBsAg negative at birth and, without immunoprophylaxis, seroconvert in the first 3 months after delivery. Perinatally and postnatally infected newborns and infants are asymptomatic. Fulminant hepatitis secondary to perinatal HBV infection has been reported in infants

Table 41.18 Effects of hepatitis A–G infection on pregnancy, on the fetus and the newborn

Hepatitis	Increased morbidity/mortality after acute infection	Increased incidence of abortion or IUD	Congenital defects	Vertical transmission			Postnatal disease	
				Intrauterine	Perinatal	Early postnatal infection	Early	Late
A (HAV)	No	Possible	No	Questionable[c]	No	Possible[b]	No	No
B (HBV)	No	No	No	Possible[b]	Yes	Yes	No	Yes
C (HCV)	No	No	No	Possible[b]	Yes	Possible	No	Yes
D (HDV) co-superinfection with HBV	No	No	No	Possible[b]	Yes only in HBsAg and HDV RNA positive mothers	N/A	No	N/A
E (HEV)	Yes mortality ±20% 3rd trimester	Yes 12%	No	Yes	Yes	N/A	Yes with increased mortality	N/A
G (HGV)	No[a]	No[a]	No[a]	N/A	Yes	N/A	No[a]	N/A

IUD, intrauterine death; N/A, data not yet available.
[a]Provisional.
[b]Possible but rare.
[c]1 case reported.

aged 2–6 months, particularly if the mother is anti-HBe positive and the infecting virus has undergone mutations in the pre-core region of its DNA (see, e.g., Carman et al. 1991, Omata et al. 1991, Terazawa et al. 1991, Schödel 1994, Weizsäcker et al. 1995). The risk of chronicity in perinatally and early postnatally infected infants and the rate of progression to liver disease or hepatocellular carcinoma are under observation. In studies of almost 350 Chinese and Italian children followed from one to 10 years, no progression of liver disease was noted although almost 50% had histological findings of chronic active hepatitis or cirrhosis at presentation (Bortolotti et al. 1986, Lok and Lai 1988); hepatocellular carcinoma may also follow perinatal or childhood HBV infection (Hsu et al. 1987).

DIAGNOSIS IN PREGNANCY

Screening in pregnancy for HBsAg detects both acutely infected and asymptomatic carrier women whose babies are at risk of perinatal infection. In most European countries universal antenatal screening is carried out and is also advocated in the USA and Canada (American College of Obstetricians and Gynecologists 1993) because selective screening has been of low efficiency (Boxall 1995). Antenatal screening is usually done early in pregnancy together with screening tests for blood group and syphilis (Grosheide et al. 1995). In Germany, selective HBsAg screening was introduced in 1987, but since 1994 has formed part of the obligatory prenatal care programme. Testing is performed in the third trimester with the same blood sample as provided for the second obligatory indirect Coombs' test (Kassenärztliche Bundesvereinigung 1994).

The screening procedures in pregnancy are as follows. If the test for HBsAg is negative, no further testing is done unless there is a clinical indication of hepatitis or suspicion of behavioural risk factors. If the result is positive, tests for HBeAg, anti-HBe, anti-HBc IgM and, less often, for quantifying HBV DNA are carried out. The HBsAg result is documented in the prenatal care notes and, if positive, the obstetrician is advised to administer active/passive hepatitis B immunization to the neonate within 12 hours after birth. If antenatal HBsAg screening is not documented, it will be done at delivery. In Germany, universal antenatal HBsAg screening was estimated to be cost-effective (Kassenärztliche Bundesvereinigung 1994).

MANAGEMENT IN PREGNANCY

Preventive measures are designed to prevent transmission by transfusion, transplantation, syringe-borne infection, frequent changes of sex partner and nosocomial infection between patients. Pregnant women in sexual or household contact with HBV-infected individuals should be offered active/passive immunisation after their HBsAg, anti-HBc and anti-HBs seronegativity is established. Specific antiviral drugs are not available. Treatment of chronic hepatitis B infection with interferon-α (IFN-α) and other recent

approaches to treatment (Ferrari et al. 1991, Pol et al. 1994) are not recommended for pregnant women. During pregnancy, acute HBV infection is treated by supportive measures as in non-pregnant patients. Caesarean section is not usually recommended, but may be performed in women with high serum levels of HBV DNA and HBeAg (Schalm and Pit-Grosheide 1989, Del Canho et al. 1994).

MANAGEMENT OF NEONATES

Until recently, active/passive hepatitis B immunization was carried out only in neonates born to HBsAg positive mothers identified during antenatal screening or at delivery. In most western countries those babies (term and preterm) are immunized within 12 h after birth with hepatitis B immunoglobulin (HBIG) and a low dose of hepatitis B vaccine, and again at 1 and 6 months of age; a test one month later for anti-HBs is recommended (e.g. American Academy of Pediatrics 1992, Robert Koch Institut 1995). Meanwhile, in the USA vaccination of all newborns is recommended regardless of the maternal HBsAg status, with anti-HBs testing of infants at age 7 months born to HBsAg positive mothers (Committee on Infectious Diseases 1994, Kim et al. 1995). Perinatal immune prophylaxis has been effective in Western populations, protecting 93–95% of infants one month after the third dose (antibody levels ≥10 mIU/ml). However, in areas with high HBV endemicity, use of the normal dose of vaccine instead of the low dose seems to be more effective in perinatal and infant vaccination (Lee 1995, Milne, Rodgers and Hopkirk 1995).

Lau and Wright (1994) found that c. 3% of babies become infected despite active/passive immunization at birth. These babies were born to chronic HBV-carrier mothers and the vaccine escape mutant was identified. If it could be verified that the inadequate immune response is due to an HBsAg escape mutant, the problem might be overcome by including the pre-S sequences in the vaccine (Schödel 1994).

To achieve a more rapid decline in the incidence of hepatitis B infection in Western countries, mainly in young adults, perinatal active/passive vaccination and vaccination of groups at risk because of their occupation, behaviour, contacts, travel etc. are not by themselves sufficiently effective. For this reason universal infant vaccination incorporated in the childhood immunization programme, booster vaccination at 13 years of age, and vaccination of previously unvaccinated adolescents have recently been introduced in various Western, Asian and African countries (CDC 1995a, Robert Koch Institut 1995, Ruff et al. 1995).

8.3 Hepatitis C virus

Hepatitis C virus (HCV), with >11 genotypes and >70 subtypes, is the aetiological agent of most non-A, non-B post-transfusion and sporadic hepatitis (Simmonds 1995, Maertens and Styver 1996). Acute HCV infections are asymptomatic in 75% of cases and in the remainder symptoms are mild, but >50% of infected adults develop chronic liver disease. Information on the perinatal implications of HCV is constantly expanding. Vertical transmission occurs generally at a low rate (<10%) and is favoured mainly by a high maternal virus load in the blood and such maternal risk factors as co-infection with HIV.

INFECTION IN PREGNANCY

The important risk factors for infection in pregnancy are intravenous drug abuse, sexual contact with intravenous drug users, high promiscuity and infection with other sexually transmitted diseases. Other risk factors are previous transfusions, transplantation and administration of blood products. In pregnant women at normal risk, antibody prevalence is 0.7–2.5%, being higher than in blood donors (c. 0.2–0.5%) in the same geographical area (Bohman et al. 1992, Marranconi et al. 1994, Pipan et al. 1996). In pregnant women from high-risk populations, antibody prevalence rates are >2.5%, irrespective of the geographic region.

At present, it is unknown whether pregnancy has an impact on the viral load and thus influences the clinical course of acute hepatitis C or the activity of chronic infection (Reth et al. 1995). Thus far, it seems that abortions or intrauterine deaths are not increased in acute or chronic HCV infection.

MOTHER–INFANT TRANSMISSION

Routes of transmission

Hepatitis C can be transmitted in utero, during parturition and by breast milk. Transmission by saliva and tears cannot be excluded. Intrauterine transmission is suggested in some reports because viral RNA was detected in cord or neonatal blood (e.g. Kurauchi et al. 1993, Kojima and Yamanaka 1994) but not always in follow-up sera of the infants. As in HBV infection, intrauterine transmission may occur late in pregnancy due to placental leakage in cases of threatened abortion and preterm labour (e.g. Lin et al. 1987). The major route, however, is intrapartum transmission, which probably occurs by contact with contaminated blood. This route is verified by detection of viral RNA in non-breast-fed infants >1 month old (e.g. Resti et al. 1995, Zanetti et al. 1995). Several studies of mother–infant pairs with follow-up of the infants show that the risk of vertical transmission is higher in mothers with acute infection in late pregnancy (Kuroki et al. 1991, Lynch-Salomon and Combs 1992) or chronic hepatitis (Degos et al. 1991); in high-risk mothers co-infected with HIV-1, HBV or both; and particularly if a high level of HCV RNA is present in maternal blood, with (Zanetti et al. 1995) or without (e.g. Ohto et al. 1994) behavioural risk cofactors.

Rates of vertical transmission and infection

Studies from 1990 to 1992 on vertical transmission in anti-HCV positive and HIV-1 negative mothers indicate that, on the basis of antibody persistence, the infection rate in infants followed up for 10–12 months was 4.5% (4/88) (Lynch and Ghidini 1993). In one of these studies, in which both HCV RNA detection and antibody persistence were used as markers of infection of infants, RNA was found not only in infants

who seroconverted or who had persisting antibody but also in those who became and remained antibody negative (Thaler et al. 1991). This puzzling observation was also made in later studies (e.g. Giacchino et al. 1995, Paccagnini et al. 1995) and may indicate false positive PCR results or seroreversion with clearance of infection, as has been found in a few infants born to HIV-1 positive mothers (Newell et al. 1996).

Table 41.19 summarizes the results of 4 prospective studies from 1994 to 1996 on vertical HCV transmission in low-risk HIV-negative mothers. All these studies indicate that infants are infected only by HCV RNA positive mothers, particularly those with a high virus load (Ohto et al 1994, Moriya et al. 1995). The investigation by Pipan et al. (1996) supports the efficiency of vertical transmission of HCV irrespective of the maternal viral load.

Table 41.20 summarizes the results of 4 prospective studies on the vertical transmission of HCV in mothers of high-risk groups with and without HIV-1 co-infection. Three of these studies show clearly a higher maternal HCV RNA positivity in HIV-1 co-infected mothers than in those with HCV RNA alone, and a higher rate of vertical transmission in the group positive for HIV-1 and HCV RNA. The study of Paccagnini et al. (1995) further indicates that HCV and HIV transmission, alone or in combination, can occur in infants born to co-infected mothers. In a smaller study in the UK no vertical transmission occurred in 12 HCV-infected high-risk pregnant women (Kudesia, Ball and Irving 1995), supporting observations (e.g. Zanetti et al. 1995, Zuccotti et al. 1995) that the risk of vertical transmission is low in mothers with behavioural risk factors but without HIV co-infection.

The outcomes of HCV-infected children in 4 of the above-mentioned studies are summarized in Table 41.21. Nearly all the infected infants showed signs of liver involvement during the follow-up period. Increased but fluctuating values of alanine aminotransferase (ALT) were usually detected, and histological evidence of liver disease. Tests for HCV RNA were repeatedly positive in all children aged ≥ 1 month; HCV antibodies persisted beyond 14 months of age in 12 infants; there was temporary seroreversion in 9 infants and loss of HCV antibodies in 6 infants aged 6–9 months despite persistence of HCV RNA.

Transmission via breast milk has been documented in some studies. Important factors seem to be the viral load and certain maternal factors (e.g. elevated liver enzymes, HIV co-infection, signs of active hepatitis). The virus load in breast milk is usually below the limit of detection by PCR, so it is presumed that breast-feeding carries a low risk of transmission (e.g. Gürakan, Oran and Yigit 1994, Lin et al. 1995, Zanetti et al. 1995, Zimmermann et al. 1995). A report of early postnatal transmission by saliva (Ogasawara et al. 1993) has not been substantiated.

In conclusion, mothers who are anti-HCV positive but HCV RNA negative and HIV-1 seronegative do not seem to infect their infants. The risk of vertical HCV transmission in HCV RNA positive mothers of low-risk groups is small: 0–10% compared to 25–44% in a high-

Table 41.19 Vertical transmission of hepatitis C from mothers of low-risk groups (HIV-1 negative)

Study	Year	Anti-HCV positivity in pregnancy	HCV RNA positivity at delivery	Rate of infected infants at follow-up born to mothers RNA positivity	RNA negativity
Ohto et al. (Japan)	1994	53/7698 (0.69%)	31/53 (58.5%)	3[a]/31 (9.7%)	0/22
Moriya et al. (Japan)	1995	163/16714 (0.98%)	87/163 (53%)	2/87 (2.3%)	...
Giacchio et al. (Italy)	1995	...	19/31 (61.3%)	2/19 (10.5%)	0/17
Pipan et al. (Italy)	1996	36/1388 (2.6%)	18/25 (72.0%)	0/18[b] (0%)	0/7

[a]Maternal high virus load.
[b]10/18 maternal high virus load.
HCV, hepatitis C; HIV, human immunodeficiency virus type 1.

risk group. Transmission occurs more frequently in HCV RNA positive mothers with a heavy virus load, with or without HIV-1 co-infection. In mothers with HIV-1 co-infection the HCV RNA virus load is usually higher than in those with HCV RNA positivity alone. The risk of transmission via breast milk is very low. The influence of HCV genotype on the risk of mother-to-infant transmission has been mentioned (e.g. Zuccotti et al. 1995), but needs further investigation. Infants with confirmed HCV infection are at risk of developing a chronic carrier state, with or without chronic liver disease.

The contribution of vertical transmission to community-acquired HCV infection in Western populations seems to be low (e.g. Alter et al. 1992, Goto et al. 1994) but may be important among children living in areas of high HCV prevalence (Chang et al. 1994).

DIAGNOSIS IN PREGNANCY

Laboratory tests for HCV infection in pregnancy are the same as for non-pregnant people. With regard to vertical transmission, a maternal viral load of more than 10^{6-7} genome equivalents/ml is considered high, 10^{4-6} as moderate and $<10^4$ as low or negative values. For quantitative and semi-quantitative HCV RNA assays, the detection limit varies considerably with the test kits now available.

DIAGNOSIS IN INFANCY

Infants born to anti-HCV positive and, particularly, to HCV RNA positive mothers should be tested at birth and every 3 months until the age of 15–20 months for anti-HCV and HCV RNA persistence. Liver function tests should be performed on HCV RNA positive infants at 2–3 monthly intervals and also on infants with antibodies persisting beyond 12 months of age.

MANAGEMENT

The possibility of sexual transmission exists, predominantly in cases of high promiscuity. Semen as a source of infection seems unlikely, and there is no need for concern about artificial insemination, because no or minimal quantities of HCV RNA have been detected in the semen or seminal fluid of HCV positive men (Hsu et al. 1991, Terada, Kawanishi and Katayama 1992). There is at present no contraindication to

pregnancy for HCV positive women or for anti-HCV negative women with an HCV positive partner.

The efficacy of passive prophylaxis for HCV by intravenous immunoglobulin seems limited (e.g. Krawczynski et al. 1996), and a vaccine is not yet available (Choo et al. 1994). Treatment with IFN-α alone or in combination with ribavirin (Di Bisceglie et al. 1995) is not indicated in pregnancy (McDonnell and Lucey 1995).

After delivery no special precautions (e.g. isolation) are needed. Breast-feeding by HCV positive mothers is not contraindicated, because of the generally low risk of early postnatal transmission, unless they have a high virus load in the serum. In them, breast milk may be quickly assessed for HCV RNA before routine breast-feeding is recommended (Pipan et al. 1996). Follow-up of infants born to anti-HCV and HCV RNA positive mothers is of great importance.

SCREENING TESTS

Universal screening of pregnant women with anti-HCV antibodies is not recommended (CDC 1991). Selective screening should be performed in women with behavioural risk factors, with known positive HIV or HBsAg status, in those with signs of hepatitis or with a history of transfusion or transplantation and in non-pregnant and pregnant women with an HCV positive partner. In cases of anti-HCV positivity, PCR for HCV RNA should be performed; if positive, the viral load should be estimated toward the end of pregnancy. If the virus load in the maternal serum is high, caesarean section has been suggested, to reduce the rate of vertical transmission (Paccagnini et al. 1995), but should rather be reserved for cases acquiring acute infection during the second and third trimester (Lin et al. 1996). There is no justification for therapeutic abortion because of maternal HCV infection.

8.4 Hepatitis D virus

Hepatitis D virus (HDV) is also known as delta agent. The RNA genome is enveloped by HBsAg, HBV acting as a helper virus for HDV. It is transmitted principally by blood and blood products, but also by sexual contact. There is considerable regional variation in its prevalence, HDV being more prevalent in areas with high endemicity of HBV. In areas with low HBV

Table 41.20 Vertical transmission of hepatitis C from mothers of high-risk groups

Study	Year	Anti-HCV pos. rate in pregnancy		HCV-RNA pos. rate at delivery		Rate of infected infants at follow-up born to mothers:				
						HIV pos.	HIV-neg.	HIV neg.	HCV-infected	
		HIV pos.	HIV neg.	HIV pos.	HIV neg.	RNA pos.	RNA pos.	RNA neg.	HIV pos.	HIV neg.
Zanetti et al. (Italy)	1995	22/116 (19%)	94/116 (81%)	18/22[a] (82%)	46/94 (49%)	8[b]/18 (44.4%)	0/46	0/52	...	...
Zuccotti et al. (Italy)	1995	20/37 (54%)	17/37 (46%)	13/20[c] (65%)	8/17 (47%)	4[d]/13 (31%)	2/8 (25%)	0/16	...	...
Paccagnini et al. (Italy)	1995	53/70[e] (76%)	17/70 (24%)	7/37[f] (19%)	2/37 (5.4%)	...	...	...	12/53 (23%)	2/17 (12%)
Kudesia et al. (UK)	1995	1/12[g] (8.3%)	11/12 (92%)	N/A	N/A	...	...	...	0[h]/1	0/8

[a]100% drug addicts.
[b]Maternal high viral load.
[c]80% drug addicts.
[d]2/4 simultaneously infected with HIV.
[e]93% drug addicts.
[f]Only 37 of 70 tested for HCV RNA.
[g]83% drug addicts.
[h]HIV but not HCV infected.
HCV, hepatitis C; HIV, human immunodeficiency virus type 1; N/A, not available.

Table 41.21 Outcome of hepatitis C infected infants born to mothers of low and high risk groups[a]

Study	Year	Infants age ≥8–>20 months at follow-up		
		HCV RNA pos.	Anti-HCV pos.	Abnormal ALT value
Ohto et al. (Japan)	1994	3	2/3	3/3
Giacchio et al. (Italy)	1995	2	2/2	2/2[d]
Zanetti et al. (Italy)	1995	8[b]	6/8	8/8
Paccagnini et al. (Italy)	1995	14[c]	11/14	10[e]/14

ALT, alanine aminotransferase; HCV, hepatitis C.
[a]See also Tables 41.19 and 41.20.
[b]3 HIV co-infected.
[c]4 HIV co-infected.
[d]Histological signs of liver disease: 2/2.
[e]Histological signs of liver disease: 4/10.

endemicity, HDV infections are generally limited to behavioural risk groups. Vertical transmission is possible.

INFECTION IN PREGNANCY AND IN THE NEONATE

A study in northern Italy demonstrated an incidence of anti-HDV antibody among HBsAg positive pregnant patients lower than that in a group of HBsAg positive patients with chronic liver disease (7% vs 20%) (Zanetti et al. 1982). Exacerbation of HDV infection during pregnancy has not been reported. Vertical transmission seems possible either during late pregnancy or intrapartum (Ramia and Bahakim 1988, Riongeard et al. 1992). Perinatal infection has been described in an infant born to a mother positive for both HBeAg and anti-HDV, but in none whose mothers were anti-HBe positive (Smedile et al. 1981). Prevalence rates of HDV as estimated by HDAg or anti-HDV antibody in hepatitis B-infected children range from 1.6% in Taiwan to 12.5% in parts of Italy, China and the Balkans, and up to 25% in the Amazon basin in Brazil (e.g. Chen, Zhang and Huang 1990, Torres and Mondolfi 1991).

PROPHYLAXIS

Measures to control the spread of HBV are also effective in preventing transmission of HDV infection to the infant. Administration of HBIG and HBV vaccine within 12–24 h after birth to newborns of HBsAg positive mothers seems to prevent both HBV and HDV infection (Silverman et al. 1991). Zanetti and colleagues (1982) reported serological evidence of HDV infection only in newborns who did not receive HBV immunoprophylaxis.

8.5 Hepatitis E virus

Hepatitis E virus (HEV) is transmitted enterically and is responsible for water-borne epidemics and sporadic outbreaks in developing countries. It is an important public health concern in Asia, Africa and Central America (Mast and Alter 1993). In contrast to hepatitis A, HEV affects mainly young adults and has considerable implications in pregnancy.

INFECTION IN PREGNANCY AND IN THE NEONATE

During epidemics the incidence of HEV infection in pregnant women is 9 times higher than in non-pregnant women or in men (Khuroo et al. 1981). Both in epidemics and in sporadic outbreaks, HEV causes fulminant hepatitis and maternal death, especially among women in the third trimester (Nanda et al. 1995). Mortality in pregnant women is as high as 20% compared to the overall mortality of 0.5–4% (Krawczynski 1993, Purdy and Krawczynski 1994). The reasons remain unknown, but it seems unlikely that HEV is the sole cause of liver failure in pregnant women (Fagan et al. 1994). Attempts to reproduce fulminant HEV hepatitis in pregnant rhesus monkeys were unsuccessful and there was no evidence of neonatal infection (Tsarev et al. 1995).

According to the early observations of Khuroo and co-workers (1981) even mild HEV infection during pregnancy seems to cause a high rate of abortion and intrauterine death and increased perinatal mortality in babies born to women with fulminant hepatitis. A more recent report suggests that, unlike other hepatitis viruses, HEV often causes intrauterine infection as well as substantial perinatal morbidity and mortality (Khuroo, Kamili and Jameel 1995). These observations require confirmation and further investigation of, for example, the pathogenesis of maternal and fetal infection (Scharschmidt 1995, Skidmore 1995).

PROPHYLAXIS

Faecally contaminated drinking water is the most common vehicle of transmission. Hygienic precautions (e.g. adequate heating of drinking water and food) are necessary in areas where HEV is endemic. Immunoglobulin prepared from plasma collected in industrialized countries is unlikely to contain sufficient specific antibody to prevent HEV infection (CDC 1993a). No vaccine or effective antiviral drugs exist.

8.6 Hepatitis G virus

An additional agent that may be responsible for as yet unexplained liver disease was discovered by molecular amplification and named hepatitis G virus (HGV) (Simons et al. 1995, Linnen et al. 1996). At present, HGV infection is mainly detected by reverse transcriptase polymerase chain reaction (RT-PCR) but serological assays are now also in use. The clinical importance of this agent is as yet unclear. No causal relationship between HGV and hepatitis has been established (Alter 1996, Alter et al. 1997). Mother-to-infant transmission has been demonstrated without evidence of disease manifestations.

INFECTION IN PREGNANCY AND IN THE NEONATE

Few data are yet available on vertical mother-to-child transmission and infection of the infant. Feucht and colleagues (1996) studied mothers belonging to a behavioural-risk group; 61 mother–infant pairs were investigated. In 6 of 30 mothers co-infected with HCV and 3 of 17 co-infected with HIV-1, HGV viraemia was detected by RT-PCR. Vertical transmission of HGV occurred in 3 of the 9 infants but co-transmission with HIV-1 or HCV could not be demonstrated. The rate of vertical transmission for HIV-1 was 11.8% (2/17) and for HCV 6.7% (2/30), corresponding with the reported vertical transmission rates of these viruses.

During follow-up of all 61 infants for vertical transmission of HGV, HCV and HIV-1 every 3 months for >1 year, none of the 3 HGV-infected infants or the 2 with HCV infection became icteric or showed other biochemical or clinical signs of hepatitis.

In another report on vertical transmission of HGV, 3 HGV positive pregnant women (1 co-infected with HCV, but all 3 negative for HIV-1) and their 3 infants were studied. All 3 women had elective caesarean delivery because of obstetric indications, and their infants were not infected with HGV or HCV during the 12 months of observation. These negative results may indicate that mother-to-infant transmission does not occur in women from low-risk populations or that caesarean delivery minimizes infection because there is less microtransfusion from mother to fetus compared with other modes of delivery (Lin et al. 1996).

9 ENTEROVIRUSES

There is no convincing evidence that maternal infection in early pregnancy with any of the picornaviruses is associated with teratogenic defects. Maternal poliomyelitis caused by wild type poliovirus is now largely of historical interest. In the pre-vaccination era, poliovirus infections in pregnancy could result in abortion, stillbirth and, rarely, in neonatal disease. Transplacental transmission of the virus to the fetus was demonstrated especially in maternal poliomyelitis in late pregnancy, but seldom in early pregnancy (Bates 1955, Carter 1956).

Maternal enterovirus infections with various Coxsackie and echoviruses may be followed by spontaneous abortion, intrauterine death, placentitis and multi-organ fetal infection, as demonstrated in various prospective studies (Basso et al. 1990, Garcia et al. 1991, Frisk and Diderholm 1992, Dommergues et al. 1994). Late intrauterine, intrapartum or early postnatally acquired infections are of particular importance (Enders 1998).

9.1 Coxsackie and echoviruses

CONGENITAL AND PERINATAL INFECTION

Clinical manifestations in the neonate or infant often include sepsis, meningoencephalitis, hepatitis, myocarditis and coagulation disorders (Kulhanjian 1992). Onset 1–2 days after birth suggests intrauterine or intrapartum transmission and disease is severe in c. 80% of cases. Onset 5–6 days after birth suggests that the infant has acquired infection by contact with infected mothers, siblings or an infected neonate in the maternity unit. The course of illness is less severe in such cases (Simoes and Abzug 1993).

Meningitis is a common manifestation of neonatal enterovirus infection: Shattuck and Chonmaitree (1992) found that enteroviruses were responsible as often as bacteria for meningitis in the first month of life. Data on the long-term prognosis of neonates with enteroviral meningitis are incomplete and contradictory. Children <2 years of age with enteroviral meningitis do not have long-term sequelae (Rorabough et al. 1992). Encephalitis occasionally occurs and in young infants may have neurological sequelae.

9.2 Management in pregnancy and of the neonate

Enterovirus infections in pregnancy occasionally cause abortion but are not teratogenic, and the mother should be reassured accordingly. Prenatal diagnosis seems not to be indicated (Enders 1998). Acute symptomatic infections toward the end of pregnancy, however, carry the risk of severe neonatal disease. The mother and child should be isolated at delivery; the baby can be breast-fed. The use of intravenous immunoglobulin up to the age of 14 days as a preventive measure for neonates exposed to infected infants did not confer significant benefit (Abzug et al. 1993). In hospitals, adequate hygienic measures must be observed because of the ready spread of these viruses in neonatal units.

10 POLIOVIRUS

Maternal, congenital and neonatal poliomyelitis caused by wild type poliovirus are largely of historical interest. Nevertheless, despite high vaccination coverage in both industrialized and developing countries, paralytic poliomyelitis continues to occur.

There is general agreement that vaccination with oral (OPV) or inactivated (IPV) poliovirus vaccines during pregnancy does not have any adverse effect on the fetus. In the recommendations of most European countries, revaccination with OPV in pregnancy is not contraindicated (with due regard to the specific contraindications for use of OPV). In contrast, the US Centers for Disease Control recommend that vaccination with OPV or IPV should be avoided in pregnant women, unless immediate protection against poliomyelitis is necessary (CDC 1996b).

11 LYMPHOCYTIC CHORIOMENINGITIS VIRUS

Lymphocytic choriomeningitis virus (LCMV) is an arenavirus, its reservoir being in animals, primarily rodents (mice and hamsters). The infected animals may be asymptomatic, but may excrete the virus for months. The illness in infected people is influenza-like and accompanied by fever, headache, nausea and myalgia lasting 5–10 days; a small proportion develop meningitis or choriomeningitis, which in adults usually resolves without sequelae.

11.1 Infection in pregnancy and of the fetus

Infection with LCMV in the first trimester of pregnancy may cause abortion (Ackermann, Stammler and Armbruster 1975, Biggar et al. 1975, Deibel et al. 1975), and infection of the fetus can result in congenital hydrocephalus, chorioretinitis, severe hyperbilirubinaemia and myopia (Sheinbergas 1975, Sheinbergas 1976). Although the number of published studies on intrauterine and perinatal infections is limited, the incidence of serious sequelae in infants seems to be high (Enders 1998).

Because healthy mice and hamsters shed LCMV chronically, pregnant women should avoid direct contact with these animals and their excreta.

12 HUMAN PAPILLOMAVIRUSES

Juvenile laryngeal papillomatosis (JLP) is associated most often with human papillomavirus (HPV) types 6 and 11; it is an uncommon but potentially serious problem, best treated by prevention if possible.

12.1 Infection in pregnancy

Growth of HPV warts is stimulated by several factors, including pregnancy. Some of the lesions may grow markedly during pregnancy, only to recede postpartum. This phenomenon is thought to be related to hormonal influences or to changes in local cellular immunity. Rarely, the lesions become so large as to obstruct the birth canal and extensive formation of HPV condylomata may lead to premature rupture of the membranes, chorioamnionitis and intrapartum infection of the fetus (Young, Acosta and Kaufman 1973).

12.2 Effects on the fetus and the neonate

Over all, the risk of perinatal transmission seems to be low, as indicated by a prospective cohort study (Watts et al. 1996). However, transmission from mother to fetus and to the newborn may occur both in clinically apparent and subclinical maternal infection, and may lead to intrauterine infections, perinatal infections or both. Approximately 50% of children with JLP are born to mothers with genital HPV (Quick et al. 1980, Nikolaidis et al. 1985), and HPV types 6 and 11, which are the most common in anogenital tract infections (Ferenczy 1989), are identified in >80% of JLP cases. Gastric and nasopharyngeal aspirates of babies born to mothers with genital tract HPV have been reported to contain HPV DNA (Ferenczy 1989, Sedlacek et al. 1989). The possibility of perinatal transmission is supported by the detection of DNA from HPV types 6, 11, 16 and 18 in foreskin specimens from neonates (Roman and Fife 1986).

12.3 Association with JLP

The long latent period from birth to development of JLP (>7 years) makes association with intrauterine or perinatal infection difficult because postnatally acquired infection cannot be excluded. For example, HPV may be transmitted on fomites after contact with individuals with warts (Patsner, Baker and Orr 1990) and sexual abuse may also result in postnatal infection (Fleming, Venning and Evans 1987). More recent data from Scandinavia indicate that, despite the increasing rate of genital HPV infections in pregnant women, the incidence of JLP remains very low (Lindbergh and Elbrond 1990).

12.4 Diagnosis

Clinical diagnosis can be made if the patient presents with warts, but many people with HPV infection have no evident warts. Women under treatment for cytologically and virologically proven HPV infection should be examined at intervals until lesions and HPV DNA are no longer detectable. Their partners should also be tested.

12.5 Management

The treatment of pregnant women with HPV lesions should be started as early as possible. and directed at elimination of the virus near term to diminish risk of the infant's acquiring HPV infection by passage through an infected birth canal. A new drug for reconstitutive immunotherapy (human leucocyte ultrafiltrate; LeukoNorm, CytoChemia) not contraindicated in pregnancy and applied for 10 weeks seems to be a promising tool for eliminating HPV 16 and 18 infection (Franke 1994, Spitzbart 1994). Prophylactic caesarean section in pregnant women with genital HPV infection is not advocated except in the rare event of large condylomata obstructing the birth canal.

Vaccines for prophylaxis and immunotherapy, employing, for example, recombinant self-assembling HPV major capsid proteins or E7 peptides, are under development (Hines et al. 1995, Borysiewicz et al. 1996).

13 MEASLES VIRUS

Infection in pregnancy with measles virus, a paramyxovirus, may be associated with increases in abortion, stillbirth and premature delivery, but not with congenital defects.

13.1 Infection in pregnancy

Measles in pregnancy has been uncommon in densely populated areas of the northern hemisphere owing to the high seroprevalence rate of ≥95% in adults with naturally acquired infection. Measles vaccination coverage of children is still incomplete in most countries, resulting in an increase in the incidence of measles in people aged ≥20 years and also in pregnancy. Early observations (e.g. Christensen et al. 1953) of a more severe course of measles in pregnant women, with higher incidences of complications and death than in non-pregnant women in the same age groups, are supported by recent studies in contemporary urban populations (Atmar, Englund and Hammill 1992, Eberhart-Phillips et al. 1993). The most common serious maternal complications are pneumonitis and hepatitis, which may be fatal in some cases. Following measles infections, particularly in the early third trimester, increased rates of spontaneous abortions or stillbirth within 14 days after onset of rash are probably secondary to placental injury from measles virus (Moroi et al. 1991), and increased rates of prematurity have been documented.

Since 1990, exposure to measles in utero as one of the risk factors for Crohn's disease has been suggested repeatedly (Ekbom et al. 1996). Large scale studies, however, are needed to prove this.

13.2 Infection of the neonate

In a prospective study, anatomical defects were not observed in infants of mothers who had measles in pregnancy (Eberhart-Phillips et al. 1993). Congenital measles is defined as disease developing in infants within the first 10–12 days of life. The rate of mortality, most commonly due to pneumonia, has been estimated to be as high as 30%. By contrast with observations in some very early reports, congenital measles was not noted within the first month of life in the above-mentioned study. One of the reasons may have been the administration of immunoglobulin to 72% of the 18 newborns whose mothers had active measles at the time of birth (Eberhart-Phillips et al. 1993). Measles developing >14 days after birth is considered to have been acquired postnatally; its course is usually mild.

13.3 Management in pregnancy and of the neonate

For confirming acute measles in pregnancy, tests (e.g. ELISA) for IgM and for rising IgG antibodies are indicated. Pregnant women infected with measles should be carefully observed for the development of either viral or secondary bacterial pneumonia. Such patients may require intensive care and should be hospitalized until the pneumonia has resolved. There is no indication for diagnostic tests on the fetus or for termination of pregnancy. There is no specific antiviral treatment.

PASSIVE IMMUNIZATION IN PREGNANCY

Following exposure to measles in pregnancy the immune status can be determined within 2 h by an ELISA test for IgG antibody. Even low titres of IgG antibodies protect against disease. Susceptible pregnant women should be given normal immunoglobulin 0.2 ml/kg body weight within 72 h of exposure. This may prevent measles or lessen its severity.

Vaccination with live monovalent measles or measles–mumps–rubella (MMR) vaccine is in principle contraindicated shortly before and during pregnancy. However, even if inadvertent vaccination has occurred, termination of pregnancy is not an option because no evidence has been obtained to substantiate the theoretical risk of fetal infection (CDC 1996c).

PASSIVE IMMUNIZATION OF THE NEONATE

Administration of 1–2 ml normal immunoglobulin (0.2 ml/kg body weight) prolongs the incubation time of onset of congenital or early postnatal measles. The neonate must be observed for congenital measles, which may be complicated by pneumonia, within the first 12 days of life.

14 MUMPS VIRUS

Primary infection with mumps virus, a paramyxovirus, in pregnancy does not seem to be associated with congenital anomalies although it was linked in some earlier studies to neonatal endocardial fibroelastosis and to hydrocephalus (St Geme, Noren and Adams 1966)

14.1 Infection in pregnancy

In densely populated areas of the northern hemisphere, >90% of adults ages 20 years or over possess mumps antibodies due to natural infection or vaccination. Primary symptomatic mumps virus infection occurs rarely in pregnancy and is no more severe than in non-pregnant women (Philip, Reinhard and Lachman 1959). An increased risk of spontaneous abortion in mumps-affected pregnancies compared with controls has been described, but effects on the incidence of stillbirth or prematurity have not (Siegel 1973).

14.2   Infection of the fetus and the neonate

Congenital mumps infections are uncommon (Rosen, Sternister and Klein 1989), but rare cases of perinatal mumps infections have been clearly documented. There are about 30 reports of symptomatic congenital mumps acquired from mothers who contracted the infection in the late third trimester or shortly before or after delivery. Only 3 of these infants developed typical, but uncomplicated, parotitis. However, congenital mumps infection may lead to, for example, transient splenomegaly and thrombocytopenia (Lacour et al. 1993) and to severe complications such as pneumonia and respiratory distress, even leading to death (Reman et al. 1986, Groenendaal et al. 1990).

14.3   Management in pregnancy and of the neonate

Diagnosis is usually made on a history of contact and the clinical findings; acute mumps may, however, be subclinical. Serological confirmation follows the lines described for measles (p. 904). Pregnant mumps-infected women need no medical intervention unless complications (e.g. meningitis) develop. Acute mumps in pregnancy is no indication for tests on the fetus or termination of pregnancy. There is no specific antiviral treatment.

If the onset of mumps occurs shortly before or after delivery, isolation of mother and baby is recommended, together with measures to prevent nosocomial spread (Sterner and Grandien 1990). Following exposure to mumps or inadvertent administration of mumps vaccine in pregnancy the mother should be reassured that no congenital defects are to be expected. By contrast with measles, the value of normal immunoglobulin in mumps prophylaxis is uncertain.

15   EPSTEIN–BARR VIRUS

There are very few reports of congenital anomalies caused by Epstein–Barr virus (EBV), a member of the *Gammaherpesvirinae.*

15.1   Infection in pregnancy

Few primary infections would be expected in pregnancy because of the high prevalence of antibodies ($\geq 90\%$) in the adult population. In several studies only 1–5% pregnant women were seronegative (e.g. Hunter et al. 1983, Le, Chang and Lipson 1983, Fleisher and Bolognese 1984). In acute maternal illness transplacental infection may be possible if infected B lymphocytes penetrate the placenta (Miller 1990), or by ascending infection from the cervix (Sixbey, Lemon and Pagano 1986). Reactivation of EBV infection in pregnancy is possible, but there seems to be no fetal risk.

15.2   Infection in the neonate

In 2 infants in whom serological evidence was suggestive of intrauterine EBV infection, CMV infection was also diagnosed. Many of the physical signs could be ascribed to CMV rather than to EBV infection (Joncas et al. 1981). In one other instance of multiple congenital defects, presumption of maternal EBV infection was based only on detection of EBV antigen in the lymphocytes of the neonate (Goldberg et al. 1981). Schuster et al. (1993) described a male infant with dystrophy, generalized hypotonia, hepatosplenomegaly, diffuse petechiae and haematomas, metaphysitis of the long bones, anaemia, hyperbilirubinaemia and elevated serum transaminases, lymphocytosis and thrombocytopenia. Serological studies suggested congenital EBV infection. Antibody evaluation in the maternal blood 3 weeks postpartum suggested acute EBV infection in late pregnancy. No mononucleosis-like symptoms were noted, but fetal retardation was observed by sonography 5 weeks before delivery.

The high excretion rate of EBV in the breast milk, which may be a source of early postnatal infection, has been noted (Junker et al. 1991).

15.3   Diagnosis in pregnancy and in the neonate

If acute mononucleosis occurs in pregnancy, serological tests should be carried out to verify EBV infection and to check for CMV infection. Tests on the fetus are not recommended. EBV infection in pregnancy is not an indication for termination. In the case of a symptomatic newborn of a mother with acute mononucleosis in pregnancy, laboratory tests for EBV should be carried out in addition to tests to exclude toxoplasmosis, rubella and CMV infection.

16   INFLUENZA A AND B

16.1   Infection in pregnancy

Influenza-associated excess mortality in pregnant women has not been reported except during the pandemic of 1918/19 and the epidemics of 1957/8 (ACIP 1997). Both events were also associated with increased risk of abortion, prematurity and stillbirth (Sterner, Grandien and Enocksson 1990). A significant increase in neonatal mortality was noted in 1970 after a major epidemic of influenza in the UK in 1969 (Wynne Griffith et al. 1972). In a series of 1350 cases of influenza in the USA the risk of abortion and prematurity was higher after infection in the first trimester (39%), but was also remarkably high for second and third trimester infections, 21% and 25% respectively. The risk was attributed to the high virulence of the circulating strain (Alberman and Peckham 1977).

Limited studies suggest that women in the third trimester of pregnancy and early puerperium, including those without underlying risk factors, might be at increased risk of serious complications, of which the most important is pneumonia (ACIP 1997).

In the UK, a cluster of spontaneous abortions and stillbirths was possibly associated with maternal influenza A infection. In women with influenza-like illness and positive serological findings, the rate of fetal loss was significantly higher than in women without influenza A infection (Stanwell-Smith et al. 1994).

EFFECTS ON THE FETUS

Early reports indicate that the influenza A virus can cross the placenta (McGregor et al. 1984), directing attention toward possible teratogenic effects (Coffey and Jessop 1963), but evidence for teratogenicity is inconclusive (Alberman and Peckham 1977, Fine et al. 1985).

16.2   Prophylaxis in pregnancy

Administration of influenza vaccine is considered safe at any stage of pregnancy. Pregnant women with conditions that increase their risk of complications from influenza should be vaccinated before the influenza season. In the USA, vaccination is recommended for women who would be in the third trimester of pregnancy or early puerperium during the influenza season.

Prophylaxis and treatment with the antiviral agents amantadine and rimantadine of high risk persons seem not to be contraindicated in pregnancy in the USA but are so far contraindicated in Europe (ACIP 1997).

17   HUMAN HERPESVIRUSES 6, 7 AND 8

For human herpesvirus (HHV) 6 the possibility of congenital infection by intrauterine transmission with infection of fetal organs and disease in the newborn has been reported. So far, there are no such reports for HHV-7 and 8.

17.1   Infection in pregnancy, of the fetus and of the neonate

Because of the high seroprevalence of HHV-6 IgG antibodies among adults, primary infection in pregnancy is rare, but there is uncertainty about the role of possible reactivation of the virus. Up to now only one case of exanthema subitum in a pregnant woman (Graham 1992) and one in a newborn have been described (Kawaguchi et al. 1992).

Congenital infection has been documented in 2 of 799 cord blood samples repeatedly positive for HHV-6 antibodies, but negative for HHV-6 genome and CMV IgM antibodies (Dunne and Demmler 1992); in 1 of 52 fetuses of mothers with HIV-1 infection who had decided to terminate their pregnancies, HHV-6-specific DNA was found in various fetal organs, in the peripheral blood mononuclear cells and in cerebrospinal fluid. In another report, HHV-6 IgM antibodies

were not detectable in the maternal or the fetal blood samples (Aubin et al. 1992). Further studies are needed to confirm possible congenital infection in primary, and perhaps reactivated, HHV-6 infection during pregnancy. The recent detection of HHV-6 DNA in acellular vaginal secretion suggests that HHV-6 virus is also transmissible by sexual contact and that newborns may be infected perinatally (Leach et al. 1994). HHV-6 transmission to the newborn via breast milk seems unlikely (Dunne and Jevon 1993).

17.2   Management

There are at present no indications for special measures, but the outcome of pregnancies affected by this virus should be monitored.

18   HANTAVIRUS

18.1   Infection in pregnancy and the effect on the fetus

The hantavirus enzootics and human disease have now been shown to have a worldwide distribution. The hantavirus pulmonary syndrome (HPS) may complicate pregnancy. The occurrence of rapidly progressing adult respiratory distress syndrome (ARDS) in the Four Corners area of southwestern USA was recognized before the identification of the predominant serogroup causing HPS, notably the Sin Nombre virus (SNV) (Khan, Ksiazek and Peters 1996). This severe infection has a case fatality rate of 50–75% (CDC 1993b).

HPS occurring during pregnancy may be life-threatening and may result in fetal hypoxaemic damage. Smith et al. (1990) reported on 14 obstetric patients, 6 (43%) of whom died as a result of ARDS. Mabie, Barton and Sibai (1992) reported a maternal mortality of 44% in 16 pregnant patients with ARDS and a perinatal mortality of 23%. Gilson et al. (1994) described 2 pregnant women with hantavirus pneumonitis, one complicated with ARDS. Her infant suffered from severe ARDS with long-term sequelae. As with the infants described in the other 2 reports, examination of the placenta and the infant's serum revealed no evidence of congenital or perinatal infection

Treatment of HPS is supportive; prompt delivery of mothers with hypoxia, lactacidaemia or both seems to be essential for maternal and fetal survival.

19   DENGUE VIRUS

There is only one report of vertical transmission of dengue in humans. A Thai woman with a febrile illness was delivered of a healthy infant by caesarean section. Although dengue virus was not isolated from the mother, the serological data are consistent with dengue as the cause of fever. The infant, who developed pyrexia on day 6 of life, presumably acquired his infection (due to dengue virus type 2) from his mother, although it cannot be excluded that he was infected by a mosquito on the first or second day of life (Thaithumyanon et al. 1994).

If travelling in areas where dengue virus is endemic, pregnant women should be warned of the possibility of an infection that may also affect the infant. If infection occurs, symptomatic treatment should be started immediately; careful monitoring of platelet counts and coagulative function is needed.

piratory tract diseases in infants and in young and school-aged children. Adenovirus DNA has been demonstrated by PCR in the amniotic fluid from some cases of hydrops (Tobiasch et al. 1994, Weiner, Towbin and Yankowitz 1995) but its significance is unknown. However, several cases of severe neonatal adenovirus disease, probably congenitally acquired, have been described (Montone et al. 1995).

20 ADENOVIRUS

Adenoviruses often cause acute upper and lower res-

REFERENCES

Abrams EJ, Matheson PB et al., 1995, Neonatal predictors of infection status and early death among 332 infants at risk of HIV-1 infection monitored prospectively from birth, *Pediatrics*, **96:** 451–8.

Abzug M, Keyserling H et al., 1993, Intravenous immune globulin treatment of neonatal enterovirus infection, *Pediatr Res*, **33:** 287A.

ACIP, 1993, Recommendations of the Advisory Committee on Immunization Practices (ACIP): use of vaccines and immune globulins in persons with altered immunocompetence, *Morbid Mortal Weekly Rep*, **42(RR-4):** 1–18.

ACIP, 1997, Prevention and control of influenza, *Morbid Mortal Weekly Rep*, **46:** 1–25.

Ackermann R, Stammler A, Armbruster B, 1975, Isolierung von Virus der Lymphozytären Choriomeningitis aus Abrasionsmaterial nach Kontakt der Schwangeren mit einem Syrischen Goldhamster (*Mesocricetus auratus*), *Infection*, 47–9.

Adjorlolo-Johnson G, De Cock KM et al., 1994, Prospective comparison of mother-to-child transmission of HIV-1 and HIV-2 in Abidjan, Ivory Cost, *JAMA*, **272:** 462–6.

Adler SP, 1991, Cytomegalovirus and child day care: risk factors for maternal infection, *Pediatr Infect Dis J*, **10:** 590–4.

Adler SP, 1992, Cytomegalovirus and pregnancy, *Curr Opin Obstet Gynecol*, **4:** 670–5.

Adler SP, 1996, Molecular epidemiology of cytomegalovirus: a study of factors affecting transmission among children at three day-care centers, *J Pediatr Infect Dis*, **10:** 584–90.

Adler SP, Starr SE et al., 1995, Immunity induced by primary human cytomegalovirus infection protects against secondary infection among women of childbearing age, *J Infect Dis*, **171:** 26–32.

Ahlfors K, Ivarsson S et al., 1984, Congenital cytomegalovirus infection and disease in Sweden and the relative importance of primary and secondary maternal infections. Preliminary findings from a prospective study, *Scand J Infect Dis*, **16:** 129–37.

Alberman E, Peckham CS, 1977, Long-term effects following infections in pregnancy, *Infections and Pregnancy*, ed Coid CR, Academic Press, London, 494–5.

Alford CA, Stagno S et al., 1990, Congenital and perinatal cytomegalovirus infections, *Rev Infect Dis*, **12:** 745–53.

Alimenti A, Luzuriaga K et al., 1991, Quantitation of human immunodeficiency virus in vertically infected infants and children, *J Pediatr*, **119:** 225–9.

Alkalay AL, Pomerance JJ, Rimoin DL, 1987, Fetal varicella syndrome, *J Pediatr*, **111:** 320–3.

Alter HJ, 1996, The cloning and clinical implications of HGV and HGBV-C, *N Engl J Med*, **334:** 1536–7.

Alter MJ, Margolis HS et al., 1992, The natural history of community acquired hepatitis C in the United States, *N Engl J Med*, **327:** 1899–905.

Alter HJ, Nakasuji Y et al., 1997, The incidence of transfusion-

associated hepatitis G virus infection and its relation to liver disease, *N Engl J Med*, **336:** 747–54.

American Academy of Pediatric ACOG, 1992, *Guidelines for Perinatal Care*, 3rd edn, AAP, ACOG, Elk Grove Village IL; Washington DC.

American College of Obstetricians and Gynecologists, 1993, Guidelines for hepatitis B virus screening and vaccination during pregnancy, *Int J Gynecol Obstet*, **40:** 172–4.

Arvin AM, Prober CG, 1990, Herpes simplex virus infections, *Pediatr Infect Dis J*, **9:** 764–7.

Ashley RL, Militoni J et al., 1988, Comparison of western blot (immunoblot) and glycoprotein G-specific immunodot enzyme assay for detecting antibodies to herpes simplex virus type 1 & 2 in human sera, *J Clin Microbiol*, **26:** 662–7.

Atmar RL, Englund JA, Hammill H, 1992, Complications of measles during pregnancy, *Clin Infect Dis*, **14:** 217–26.

Aubin J-T, Poirel L et al., 1992, Intrauterine transmission of human herpesvirus 6, *Lancet*, **340:** 482–3.

Azimi PH, Roberto RR et al., 1986, Transfusion-acquired hepatitis A in a premature infant with secondary spread in an intensive care nursery, *Am J Dis Child*, **140:** 23–7.

Balducci J, Rodis JF et al., 1992, Pregnancy outcome following first-trimester varicella infection, *Obstet Gynecol*, **79:** 5–6.

Baldwin S, Whitley RJ, 1989, Intrauterine herpes simples virus infection, *Teratology*, **39:** 1–10.

Bansal GP, Hatfield JA et al., 1993, Candidate recombinant vaccine for human B19 parvovirus, *J Infect Dis*, **167:** 1034–44.

Basso NG, Fonseca ME et al., 1990, Enterovirus isolation from foetal and placental tissues, *Acta Virol (Praha)*, **34:** 49–57.

Bates T, 1955, Poliomyelitis in pregnancy, fetus and newborn, *Am J Dis Child*, **90:** 189.

Bernstein DI, 1991, Effects of prior HSV-1 infection on genital HSV-2 infection, *Prog Med Virol*, **38:** 109–27.

Berrebi A, Kobuch WE et al., 1990, Influence of pregnancy on human immunodeficiency virus disease, *Eur J Obstet Gynecol Reprod Biol*, **37:** 211–17.

Beutler E, Gelbart T, Kuhl W, 1990, Interference of heparin with the polymerase chain reaction, *BioTechniques*, **9:** 166.

Biggar RJ, Woodall JP et al., 1975, Lymphocytic choriomeningitis virus outbreak associated with pet hamsters, *JAMA*, **232:** 494–500.

Biggar RJ, Miotti PG et al., 1996, Perinatal intervention trial in Africa: effect of a birth canal cleansing intervention to prevent HIV transmission, *Lancet*, **347:** 1647–50.

Blanche S, Tardieu M et al., 1990, Longitudinal study of 94 symptomatic infants with perinatal acquired human immunodeficiency virus infection: evidence for a bimodal expression of clinical and biological symptoms, *Am J Dis Child*, **144:** 1210–15.

Bohman VR, Stettler RW et al., 1992, Seroprevalence and risk factors for hepatitis C virus antibody in pregnant women, *Obstet Gynecol*, **80:** 609–13.

Boppana SB, Britt WJ, 1995, Antiviral antibody responses and intrauterine transmission after primary maternal cytomegalovirus infection, *J Infect Dis*, **171:** 1115–21.

Boppana SB, Pass RF et al., 1992, Symptomatic congenital cytomegalovirus infection: neonatal morbidity and mortality, *Pediatr Infect Dis J*, **11:** 93–9.

Bortolotti F, Calzia R et al., 1986, Liver cirrhosis associated with chronic hepatitis B virus infection in childhood, *J Pediatr*, **198:** 224–7.

Borysiewicz LK, Fiander A et al., 1996, A recombinant vaccinia virus encoding human papillomavirus types 16 and 18, E6 and E7 proteins as immunotherapy for cervical cancer, *Lancet*, **347:** 1523–7.

Boxall EH, 1995, Antenatal screening for carriers of hepatitis B virus, *Br Med J*, **311:** 1178–9.

Brown KE, Anderson SM, Young NS, 1993, Erythrocyte P antigen: cellular receptor for B19 parvovirus, *Science*, **262:** 114–17.

Brown KE, Green SW et al., 1994, Congenital anaemia after transplacental B19 parvovirus infection, *Lancet*, **343:** 895–6.

Brown T, Anand A et al., 1984, Intrauterine parvovirus infection associated with hydrops fetalis, *Lancet*, **2:** 1033–4.

Brown ZA, Vontver LA et al., 1987, Effects on infants of a first episode of genital herpes during pregnancy, *N Engl J Med*, **317:** 1246–51.

Brown ZA, Benedetti L et al., 1991, Neonatal herpes simplex virus infection in relation to asymptomatic maternal infection at the time of labor, *N Engl J Med*, **324:** 1247–52.

Bryson YJ, Luzuriaga K et al., 1992, Proposed definitions for in utero versus intrapartum transmission of HIV-1, *N Engl J Med*, **327:** 1236–7.

Bryson YJ, Pang S et al., 1995, Clearance of HIV infection in a perinatally infected infant, *N Engl J Med*, **332:** 833–8.

Burgard M, Mayaux M-J et al., 1992, The use of viral culture and p24 antigen testing to diagnose human immunodeficiency virus infection in neonates, *N Engl J Med*, **327:** 1192–7.

Burk RD, Hwang L et al., 1994, Outcome of perinatal hepatitis B virus exposure is dependent on maternal virus load, *J Infect Dis*, **170:** 1418–23.

Carman WF, Fagan EA et al., 1991, Association of a pre-core variant of HBV with fulminant hepatitis, *Hepatology*, **14:** 219–22.

Carter HM, 1956, Congenital poliomyelitis, *Obstet Gynecol*, **8:** 373.

CDC, 1989, Risks associated with human parvovirus B19 infection, *Morbid Mortal Weekly Rep*, **38:** 81–97.

CDC, 1990, Protection against viral hepatitis. Recommendations of the immunization practices advisory committee (ACIP), *Morbid Mortal Weekly Rep*, **39 (RR-2):** 1–26.

CDC, 1991, Public health service interagency guidelines for screening donors of blood, plasma, organs, tissues, and semen for evidence of hepatitis B and hepatitis C, *Morbid Mortal Weekly Rep*, **40:** 6–17.

CDC, 1993a, Hepatitis E among US travelers, 1989–1992, *Morbid Mortal Weekly Rep*, **42:** 1–4.

CDC, 1993b, Update: hantavirus pulmonary syndrome – United States, 1993, *Morbid Mortal Weekly Rep*, **42:** 816–20.

CDC, 1995a, Update. Recommendations to prevent hepatitis B virus transmission – United States, *Morbid Mortal Weekly Rep*, **44:** 574–5.

CDC, 1995b, US Public Health service recommendations for human immunodeficiency virus counseling and voluntary testing for pregnant women, *Morbid Mortal Weekly Rep*, **44:** 1–15.

CDC, 1996a, Prevention of varicella, *Morbid Mortal Weekly Rep*, **45:** 1–36.

CDC, 1996b, Poliomyelitis prevention, *Morbid Mortal Weekly Rep*, **45:** 8–10.

CDC, 1996c, Measles prevention: precautions and contraindications, *Morbid Mortal Weekly Rep*, **45:** 10–19.

Cederblad B, Riesenfeld T, Alm GA, 1989, Deficient herpes simplex virus-induced interferon alpha production by blood leukocytes of preterm and term newborn infants [published

erratum appears in *Pediatr Res* 1990: **27:** 507], *Pediatr Res*, **27:** 7–10.

Chang T-T, Liou T-C et al., 1994, Intrafamilial transmission of hepatitis C virus: the important role of inapparent transmission, *J Med Virol*, **42:** 91–6.

Chen GH, Zhang MD, Huang W, 1990, Hepatitis delta virus superinfection in Guangzhou area, *Chin Med J (Engl)*, **103:** 451–4.

Choo PW, Donahue JG et al., 1995, The epidemiology of varicella and its complications, *J Infect Dis*, **172:** 706–12.

Choo QL, Kuo G et al., 1994, Vaccination of chimpanzees against infection by the hepatitis C virus, *Proc Natl Acad Sci USA*, **91:** 1294–8.

Chou S, 1990, Differentiation of cytomegalovirus strains by restriction analysis of DNA sequences amplified from clinical specimens, *J Infect Dis*, **162:** 738–42.

Christensen PE, Schmidt H et al., 1953, An epidemic of measles in southern Greenland, 1951. Measles in virgin soil. II. The epidemic proper, *Acta Med Scand*, **144:** 430–49.

Christie AB, Allam AA et al., 1976, Pregnancy hepatitis in Libya, *Lancet*, **2:** 827–9.

Coffey VP, Jessop WJE, 1963, Maternal influenza and congenital deformities. A follow-up study, *Lancet*, **1:** 748–51.

Committee on Infectious Diseases, 1994, Update on timing of hepatitis B vaccination for premature infants and for children with lapsed immunization, *Pediatrics*, **94:** 403–4.

Connor EM, Sperling RS et al., 1994, Reduction of maternal–infant transmission of human immunodeficiency virus type 1 with zidovudine treatment, *N Engl J Med*, **331:** 1173–225.

Conry JA, Török T, Andrews PI, 1993, Perinatal encephalopathy secondary to in utero human parvovirus B19 (HPV) infection [abstract 736S], *Neurology*, **43:** A346.

Corey L, Spear PG, 1986a, Infections with herpes viruses II, *N Engl J Med*, **314:** 749–57.

Corey L, Spear PG, 1986b, Infections with herpes simplex viruses I, *N Engl J Med*, **314:** 686–91.

Corey L, Wald A, Hobson AC, 1996, Reactivation of herpes simplex virus type 2, *21st Herpesvirus Workshop, Chicago, July 27 – August 2 1996*, 263.

Da Silva O, Hammerberg O, Chance GW, 1990, Fetal varicella syndrome, *Pediatr Infect Dis J*, **9:** 854–5.

Daffos F, Capella-Pavlovsky M, Forestier F, 1983, Fetal blood sampling via the umbilical cord using a needle guided by ultrasound. Report of 66 cases, *Prenat Diagn*, **3:** 271–7.

Daffos F, Forestier F et al., 1984, Prenatal diagnosis of congenital rubella, *Lancet*, **2:** 1–3.

Daffos F, Forestier F et al., 1988, Prenatal management of 746 pregnancies at risk for congenital toxoplasmosis, *N Engl J Med*, **118:** 271–5.

De Cock KM, Zadi F et al., 1994, Retrospective study of maternal HIV-1 and HIV-2 infections and child survival in Abidjan, Cote d'Ivoire, *Br Med J*, **308:** 441–3.

De Rossi A, Giaquinto C et al., 1993, Replication and tropism of human immunodeficiency virus type 1 as predictors of disease outcome in infants with vertically acquired infection, *J Pediatr*, **123:** 929–36.

Degos F, Maisonneuve P et al., 1991, Neonatal transmission of HCV from mother with chronic hepatitis, *Lancet*, **338:** 758.

Deibel R, Woodall JP et al., 1975, Lymphocytic choriomeningitis virus in man. Serological evidence of association with pet hamsters, *JAMA*, **232:** 501–4.

Del Canho R et al., 1994, Failure of neonatal hepatitis B vaccination, the role of HBV-DNA levels in hepatitis B carrier mothers and HLA antigen, *J Hepatol*, **20:** 483–6.

Demmler GJ, 1991, Infectious Disease Society of America and Centers for Disease Control: summary of a workshop on surveillance for congenital cytomegalovirus disease, *Rev Infect Dis*, **13:** 315–29.

Demmler GJ, 1994, Cytomegalovirus, *Viral Diseases in Pregnancy*, ed Gonik B, Springer-Verlag, New York, Berlin, Heidelberg, 69–91.

Department of Health and Social Security, Joint Committee on Vaccination and Immunisation, 1988, *Immunisation against Infectious Disease*, HMSO, London, 115–17.

Di Bisceglie AM, Conjeevaram HS et al., 1995, Ribavirin as therapy for chronic hepatitis C, *Ann Intern Med*, **123**: 897–903.

Dobbins JG, Stewart JA, Demmler GJ, 1991, Surveillance of congenital cytomegalovirus disease, *Morbid Mortal Weekly Rep*, **41**: 35–44.

Dobbins JG, Adler SP et al., 1994, The risks and benefits of cytomegalovirus transmission in child day care, *Pediatrics*, **94**: 1016–18.

Dommergues M, Petitjean J et al., 1994, Fetal enteroviral infection with cerebral ventriculomegaly and cardiomyopathy, *Fetal Diagn Ther*, **9**: 77–8.

Dong ZW, Yan C et al., 1994, Detection of congenital cytomegalovirus infection by using chorionic villi of the early pregnancy and polymerase chain reaction, *Int J Gynaecol Obstet*, **44**: 229–31.

Donner C, Liesnard C et al., 1994, Accuracy of amniotic fluid testing before 21 weeks gestation in prenatal diagnosis of congenital cytomegalovirus infection, *Prenat Diagn*, **14**: 1055–9.

Douglas GC, King BF, 1992, Maternal–fetal transmission of human immunodeficiency virus: a review of possible routes and cellular mechanisms of infection, *Clin Infect Dis*, **15**: 678–91.

Dunn DT, Newell ML et al., 1994, Mode of delivery and vertical transmission of HIV-1: a review of prospective studies, *J Acquired Immune Defic Syndr*, **7**: 1064–6.

Dunne WM, Demmler GJ, 1992, Serological evidence for congenital transmission of human herpesvirus 6, *Lancet*, **340**: 121–2.

Dunne WM, Jevon M, 1993, Examination of human breast milk for evidence of human herpesvirus 6 by polymerase chain reaction, *J Infect Dis*, **168**: 250.

Dworkin RH, 1996, Racial differences in herpes zoster and age at onset of varicella, *J Infect Dis*, **174**: 239–40.

Eberhart-Phillips JE, Frederick PD et al., 1993, Measles in pregnancy: a descriptive study of 58 cases, *Obstet Gynecol*, **82**: 797–801.

Ecker JL, 1996, The cost-effectiveness of human immunodeficiency virus screening in pregnancy, *Am J Obstet Gynecol*, **174**: 716–21.

Editorial, 1990, TORCH syndrome and TORCH screening, *Lancet*, **335**: 1559–61.

Ehrnst A, Lindgren S et al., 1991, HIV in pregnant women and their offspring: evidence for late transmission, *Lancet*, **338**: 203–7.

Eis-Hübinger AM, Kleim JP et al., 1991, A related epitope is consistently present on glycoprotein C of herpes simplex virus type 1 and 2, *Acta Virol (Praha)*, **35**: 276–81.

Ekbom A, Daszak P et al., 1996, Crohn's disease after in-utero measles virus exposure, *Lancet*, **348**: 515–17.

Enders G, 1984, Varicella-zoster virus infection in pregnancy, *Progress in Medical Virology*, ed Melnick JL, Karger, Basel, 166–96.

Enders G, 1994, Pränatale Diagnostik: Meilensteine auf dem Gebiet der pränatalen Infektionsdiagnostik und der vorgeburtlichen Medizin, *Abbott Times*, **4 (1)**: 8–16.

Enders G, 1998, *Infektionen und Impfungen in der Schwangerschaft*, 3rd edn, Urban & Schwarzenberg, Munich, in press.

Enders G, Biber M, 1990, Parvovirus B19 infections in pregnancy, *Behring Inst Mitt*, **85**: 74–8.

Enders G, Jonatha W, 1987, Prenatal diagnosis of intrauterine rubella, *Infection*, **15**: 162–7.

Enders G, Miller E et al., 1994, Consequences of varicella and herpes zoster in pregnancy: a prospective study of 1739 cases, *Lancet*, **343**: 1547–50.

European Collaborative Study, 1992, Risk factors for mother-to-child transmission of HIV-1, *Lancet*, **339**: 1007–12.

European Collaborative Study, 1994a, Caesarean section and risk of vertical transmission of HIV-1 infection, *Lancet*, **343**: 1464–7.

European Collaborative Study, 1994b, Natural history of vertically acquired human immunodeficiency virus-1 infection, *Pediatrics*, **94**: 815–19.

Evans JA, Marriage SC et al., 1995, Unsuspected HIV infection presenting in first year of life, *Br Med J*, **310**: 1235–6.

Fagan EA, Menon T et al., 1994, Equivocal serological diagnosis of sporadic fulminant hepatitis E in pregnant Indians, *Lancet*, **344**: 342–3.

Fairley CK, Smoleniec JS et al., 1995, Observational study of effect of intrauterine transfusions on outcome of fetal hydrops after parvovirus B19 infection, *Lancet*, **346**: 1335–7.

Fang G, Burger H et al., 1995, Maternal plasma human immunodeficiency virus type 1 RNA level: a determinant and projected threshold for mother-to-child transmission, *Proc Natl Acad Sci USA*, **92**: 12100–4.

Ferenczy A, 1989, HPV-associated lesions in pregnancy and their clinical implications, *Clin Obstet Gynecol*, **32**: 191–9.

Ferguson M, Walker D, Cohen B, 1997, Report of a collaborative study to assess the suitability of the proposed International Standard for parvovirus B19 serum IgG, *Biologicals*, in press.

Fernando S, Pearce JM, Booth JC, 1993, Lymphocyte responses and virus excretion as risk factors for intrauterine infection with cytomegalovirus, *J Med Virol*, **41**: 108–13.

Ferrari C, Bertoletti A et al., 1991, Identification of immunodominant T cell epitopes of the hepatitis B virus nucleocapsid antigen, *J Clin Invest*, **88**: 214–22.

Feucht HH, Zöllner B et al., 1996, Vertical transmission of hepatitis G, *Lancet*, **347**: 615–16.

Fine PEM, Clarkson JA et al., 1985, *Infectious Disease during Pregnancy: a follow-up study of the long term effects of exposure to viral infections in utero*, Studies of medical and Population Subjects, 49, HMSO, London.

Fleisher G, Bolognese R, 1984, Epstein–Barr virus infections in pregnancy: a prospective study, *J Pediatr*, **104**: 374–9.

Fleming KA, Venning V, Evans M, 1987, DNA typing of genital warts and diagnosis of sexual abuse of children, *Lancet*, **2**: 454.

Forbes BA, 1989, Acquisition of cytomegalovirus infection: an update, *Clin Microbiol Rev*, **2**: 204–16.

Forestier F, Cox W et al., 1988, The assessment of fetal blood samples, *Am J Obstet Gynecol*, **158**: 1184–8.

Forsgren M, 1992, Herpes simplex virus infection in the perinatal period, *Rev Med Microbiol*, **3**: 129–36.

Fowler KB, Stagno S, Pass RF, 1993, Maternal age and congenital cytomegalovirus infection: screening of two diverse newborn populations, 1980–1990, *J Infect Dis*, **168**: 552–6.

Fowler KB, Stagno S et al., 1992, The outcome of congenital cytomegalovirus infection in relation to maternal antibody status, *N Engl J Med*, **326**: 663–7.

Franke W, 1994, Neue Ansätze bei der HPV-Therapie, *TW Gynäkologie*, **7**: 413–14.

Frisk G, Diderholm H, 1992, Increased frequency of coxsackie B virus IgM in women with spontaneous abortion, *J Infect*, **24**: 141–5.

Garcia AG, Basso NG et al., 1991, Enterovirus associated placental morphology: a light, virological, electron microscopic and immunohistologic study, *Placenta*, **12**: 533–47.

Gehrz RC, Christianson WR et al., 1981, Cytomegalovirus-specific humoral and cellular immune response in human pregnancy, *J Infect Dis*, **143**: 391–5.

Gershon AA, 1975, Varicella in mother and infant: problems old and new, *Infections in the Fetus and Newborn Infant*, eds Krugman S, Gershon AA, Alan R Liss, New York, 79–95.

Giacchino R, Picciotto A et al., 1995, Vertical transmission of hepatitis C, *Lancet*, **345**: 1122–3.

Gillespie SM, Carter ML et al., 1990, Occupational risk of human parvovirus B19 infection for school and day-care personnel during an outbreak of erythema infectiosum, *JAMA*, **263**: 2061–5.

Gilson GJ, Maciulla JA et al., 1994, Hantavirus pulmonary syndrome complicating pregnancy, *Am J Obstet Gynecol*, **171**: 550–4.

Goedert JJ, Duliège AM et al., 1991, High risk of HIV-1 infection for first-born twins. The international registry of HIV-exposed twins, *Lancet*, **338**: 1471–5.

Goldberg GN, Fulginiti VA et al., 1981, In utero Epstein–Barr virus (infectious mononucleosis) infection, *JAMA*, **246**: 1579–81.

Goto M, Fujiyama S et al., 1994, Intrafamilial transmission of hepatitis C virus, *J Gastroenterol Hepatol*, **9**: 13–18.

Gottard H, Rabensteiner A et al., 1991, Nachweis des Varizellen-virus mit der DNA-Sonde im fetalen Blut und im Frucht-wasser, *Geburtsh Frauenheilk*, **51**: 63–4.

Graham JM, 1992, Roseola infantum in pregnancy, *J Reprod Med*, **37**: 947–9.

Gratacós E, Torres P-J et al., 1995, The incidence of human par-vovirus B19 infection during pregnancy and its impact on perinatal outcome, *J Infect Dis*, **171**: 1360–3.

Gray GC, Palinkas LA, Kelley PW, 1990, Increasing incidence of varicella hospitalizations in the United States Army and Navy personnel: are today's teenagers more susceptible? Should recruits be vaccinated?, *Pediatrics*, **86**: 867–73.

Greenspoon JS, Wilcox JG et al., 1994, Acyclovir for disseminated herpes simplex virus in pregnancy – a case report, *J Reprod Med*, **39**: 311–7.

Griffiths PD, 1990, Virus infections of the fetus and neonate, other than rubella, *Topley & Wilson's Principles of Bacteriology, Virology and Immunity*, 8th edn, vol 4, *Virology*, eds Collier LH, Timbury MC, Edward Arnold, London, 533–45.

Griffiths PD, Baboonian C, 1984, A prospective study of primary cytomegalovirus infection during pregnancy: final report, *Br J Obstet Gynaecol*, **91**: 307–15.

Groenendaal F, Rothbarth PH et al., 1990, Congenital mumps pneumonia: a rare cause of neonatal respiratory distress, *Acta Pediatr Scand*, **79**: 1252–4.

Groothuis JR, Simoes EAF et al., 1995, Respiratory syncytial virus (RSV) infection in preterm infants and the protective effects of RSV immune globulin (RSVIG), *Pediatrics*, **95**: 463–7.

Grose C, Meehan T, Weiner C, 1992, Prenatal diagnosis of con-genital cytomegalovirus infection by virus isolation after amniocentesis, *Pediatr Infect Dis J*, **11**: 605–7.

Grosheide PM, Wladimiroff JW et al., 1995, Proposal for routine antenatal screening at 14 weeks for hepatitis B surface anti-gen, *Br Med J*, **311**: 1197–9.

Grubman S, Gross E et al., 1995, Older children and adolescents living with perinatally acquired human immunodeficiency virus infection, *Pediatrics*, **95**: 657–63.

Gürakan B, Oran O, Yigit S, 1994, Vertical transmission of hepa-titis C virus, *N Engl J Med*, **331**: 399.

Haake DA, Zakowski PC et al., 1990, Early treatment of acyclovir for varicella pneumonia in otherwise healthy adults: retro-spective controlled study and review, *Rev Infect Dis*, **112**: 788–98.

Haddad J, Langer B et al., 1993, Oral acyclovir and recurrent genital herpes during late pregnancy, *Obstet Gynecol*, **82**: 102–4.

Hagay ZJ, Biran G et al., 1996, Congenital cytomegalovirus infec-tion: a long-standing problem still seeking a solution, *Am J Obstet Gynecol*, **174**: 241–5.

Hanson FW, Happ RL et al., 1990, Ultrasonography guided early amniocentesis in singleton pregnancies, *Am J Obstet Gynecol*, **162**: 1376–81.

Harrison CJ, 1995, Neonatal herpes simplex virus (HSV) infec-tions, *Nebr Med J*, **10**: 311–15.

Hayes K, Symington G, Mackay IR, 1979, Maternal immuno-suppression and cytomegalovirus infection of the fetus, *Aust N Z J Med*, **9**: 430–3.

Higa K, Dan K, Manabe H, 1987, Varicella-zoster virus infections during pregnancy: hypothesis concerning the mechanisms of congenital malformations, *Obstet Gynecol*, **69**: 214–22.

Hines JF, Ghim S et al., 1995, Prospects for a vaccine against human papillomavirus, *Obstet Gynecol*, **86**: 860–6.

Ho DWT, Field PR et al., 1993, Detection of immunoglobulin

M antibodies to glycoprotein G-2 by western blot (immunoblot) for diagnosis of initial herpes simplex virus type 2 genital infections, *J Clin Microbiol*, **31**: 3157–64.

Hocker JR, Cook LN et al., 1990, Ganciclovir therapy of congeni-tal cytomegalovirus pneumonia, *Pediatr Infect Dis J*, **9**: 743–5.

Hogge WA, Buffone GJ, Hogge JS, 1993, Prenatal diagnosis of cytomegalovirus infection: a preliminary report, *Prenat Diagn*, **13**: 131–6.

Hohlfeld P, Daffos F et al., 1994, Prenatal diagnosis of congenital toxoplasmosis with a polymerase chain reaction test on amni-otic fluid, *N Engl J Med*, **331**: 695–9.

Holland P, Isaacs D, Moxon ER, 1986, Fatal neonatal varicella infection, *Lancet*, **2**: 1156.

Hsu HC, Wu MZ et al., 1987, Childhood hepatocellular carci-noma develops exclusively in hepatitis B surface antigen car-riers in three decades in Taiwan: a report of 51 cases strongly associated with rapid development of liver cirrhosis, *J Hepatol*, **5**: 260–7.

Hsu HH, Wright TL et al., 1991, Failure to detect hepatitis C virus genome in human secretions with polymerase chain reaction, *Hepatology*, **14**: 763–7.

Hunter K, Stagno S et al., 1983, Prenatal screening of pregnant women for infections caused by cytomegalovirus, Epstein–Barr virus, herpesvirus, rubella, and *Toxoplasma gondii*, *Am J Obstet Gynecol*, **145**: 269–73.

Hutto C, Arvin AM et al., 1987, Intrauterine herpes simplex virus infections, *J Pediatr*, **110**: 97–101.

Istas AS, Demmler GJ et al., 1995, Surveillance for congenital cytomegalovirus disease: a report from the National Congeni-tal Cytomegalovirus Disease Registry, *Clin Infect Dis*, **20**: 665–70.

Italian Register for HIV infection in children, 1994, Features of children perinatally infected with HIV-1 surviving longer than 5 years, *Lancet*, **343**: 191–5.

Johnson RE, Nahmias AJ et al., 1989, Seroepidemiologic survey of the prevalence of herpes simplex virus type 2 infection in the United States, *N Engl J Med*, **321**: 7–12.

Johnson RE, Lee F et al., 1994, US genital herpes trends during the first decade of AIDS: prevalences increased in young whites and elevated in blacks, *Sex Transm Dis*, **21**: 109.

Joncas JH, Alfieri A et al., 1981, Simultaneous congenital infec-tion with Epstein–Barr virus and cytomegalovirus, *N Engl J Med*, **304**: 1399–403.

Jones KL, Johnson KA, Chambers CD, 1994, Offspring of women infected with varicella during pregnancy: a prospective study, *Teratology*, **49**: 29–32.

Junker AK, Thomas EE et al., 1991, Epstein–Barr virus shedding in breast milk, *Am J Med Sci*, **302**: 220–3.

Kahlon J, Whitley RJ, 1988, Antibody response of the newborn after herpes simplex virus infection, *J Infect Dis*, **158**: 925.

Kassenärztliche Bundesvereinigung, 1994, Generelles Screening auf Hepatitis B in der Schwangerschaft, *Dtsch Ärztebl*, **91**: A-2778–9.

Katz VL, Kuller JA et al., 1995, Varicella during pregnancy. Maternal and fetal effects, *West J Med*, **163**: 446–50.

Kawaguchi S, Suga S et al., 1992, Primary human herpesvirus 6 infection (exanthem subitum) in the newborn, *Pediatrics*, **90**: 628–30.

Kennedy N, McKendrick MW, 1996, Controversies in varicella: vaccine and acyclovir, *Curr Opin Infect Dis*, **9**: 203–9.

Khan AS, Ksiazek TG, Peters CJ, 1996, Hantavirus pulmonary syndrome, *Lancet*, **347**: 739–41.

Khuroo MS, Kamili S, Jameel S, 1995, Vertical transmission of hepatitis E virus, *Lancet*, **345**: 1025–6.

Khuroo MS, Teli MR et al., 1981, Incidence and severity of viral hepatitis in pregnancy, *Am J Med*, **70**: 252–5.

Kim SC, Sinai LN et al., 1995, Universal hepatitis B immuni-zation (experience and reason – briefly recorded), *Pediatrics*, **95**: 764–5.

Kind C, Brandle B et al., 1992, Epidemiology of vertically transmitted HIV-1 infection in Switzerland: results of a nationwide prospective study, *Eur J Pediatr*, **151**: 442–8.

Koelle DM, Benedetti JK et al., 1992, Asymptomatic reactivation of herpes simplex virus in women after the first episode of genital herpes, *Ann Intern Med*, **116**: 433–7.

Kohl S, West MS et al., 1989, Neonatal antibody-dependent cellular cytotoxic antibody levels are associated with the clinical presentation of neonatal herpes simplex virus infection, *J Infect Dis*, **160**: 770.

Kojima T, Yamanaka T, 1994, Transmission routes of hepatitis C virus: analysis of anti-HCV-positive pregnant women and their family members, *Nippon Sanka Fujinka Gakkai Zasshi*, **46**: 573–80.

Komischke K, Searle K, Enders G, 1997, Maternal serum alpha-fetoprotein and human chorionic gonadotropin in pregnant women with acute parvovirus B19 infection with and without fetal complications, *Prenat Diagn*, in press.

Koutsky LA, Ashley RL et al., 1990, The frequency of unrecognised type 2 herpes simplex virus infection among women. Implications for the control of genital herpes, *Sex Transm Dis*, **17**: 90–4.

Krawczynski K, 1993, Hepatitis E, *Hepatology*, **17**: 932–41.

Krawczynski K, Alter MJ et al., 1996, Effect of immune globulin on the prevention of experimental hepatitis C virus infection, *J Infect Dis*, **173**: 822–8.

Kroon S, Whitley R, 1995, *Management Strategies in Herpes: can we improve management of perinatal HSV infections?*, PPS Europe, Worthing.

Kudesia G, Ball G, Irving W, 1995, Vertical transmission of hepatitis C, *Lancet*, **345**: 1122.

Kulhanjian J, 1992, Fever, hepatitis and coagulopathy in a newborn infant, *Pediatr Infect Dis J*, **11**: 1069–72.

Kumar ML, Gold E et al., 1984, Primary cytomegalovirus infection in adolescent pregnancy, *Pediatrics*, **74**: 493–500.

Kurauchi O, Furui T et al., 1993, Studies on transmission of hepatitis C virus from mother to child in the perinatal period, *Arch Obstet Gynecol*, **253**: 121–6.

Kuroki T, Nishiguchi S et al., 1991, Mother-to-child transmission of hepatitis C virus, *J Infect Dis*, **164**: 427–8.

Lacour M, Maherzi M et al., 1993, Thrombocytopenia in a case of neonatal mumps infection: evidence for further clinical presentations, *Eur J Pediatr*, **152**: 739–41.

Laforet EG, Lynch CL, 1947, Multiple congenital defects following maternal varicella: report of a case, *N Engl J Med*, **236**: 534–7.

Laifer SA, Ehrlich GD et al., 1995, Congenital cytomegalovirus infection in offspring of liver transplant recipients, *Clin Infect Dis*, **20**: 52–5.

Landers DV, Sweet RL, 1996, Reducing mother-to-infant transmission of HIV – the door remains open, *N Engl J Med*, **334**: 1664–5.

Landesman SH, Kalish LA et al., 1996, Obstetrical factors and the transmission of human immunodeficiency virus type 1 from mother to child, *N Engl J Med*, **334**: 1617–23.

Landini MP, 1993, New approaches and perspectives in cytomegalovirus diagnosis, *Progress in Medical Virology*, ed Melnick JL, Karger, Basel, 157–77.

Langston C, Lewis DE et al., 1995, Excess intrauterine fetal demise associated with maternal human immunodeficiency virus infection, *J Infect Dis*, **172**: 1451–60.

Lau JYN, Wright TL, 1994, Reply to Schödel F: emerging viral mutants in hepatitis B, *Lancet*, **343**: 355–6.

Le CT, Chang RS, Lipson MH, 1983, Epstein–Barr virus infections during pregnancy: a prospective study and review of the literature, *Am J Dis Child*, **137**: 466–8.

Leach CT, Newton ER et al., 1994, Human herpesvirus 6 infection of the female genital tract, *J Infect Dis*, **169**: 1281–3.

Lee SS, 1995, Hepatitis B vaccination strategy for newborn babies, *Lancet*, **346**: 900–1.

Lewis DB, Wilson CB, 1995, Developmental immunology and role of host defences in neonatal susceptibility to infection,

Infectious Diseases of the Fetus and the Newborn Infant, 4th edn, eds Remington JS, Klein JO, WB Saunders, Philadelphia, 20–98.

Lewis SH, Reynolds-Kohler C et al., 1990, HIV-1 in trophoblastic and villous Hofbauer cells, and haematologic precursors in eight-week fetuses, *Lancet*, **335**: 565–8.

Lin HH, Lee TY et al., 1987, Transplacental leakage of HBeAg-positive maternal blood as the most likely route in causing intrauterine infection with hepatitis B virus, *J Pediatr*, **111**: 877–81.

Lin HH, Kao JH et al., 1995, Absence of infection in breast-fed infants born to hepatitis C virus-infected mothers, *J Pediatr*, **126**: 589–91.

Lin HH, Kao JH et al., 1996, Least microtransfusion from mother to fetus in elective cesarean delivery, *Obstet Gynecol*, **87**: 244–8.

Lindbergh H, Elbrond O, 1990, Laryngeal papillomas: the epidemiology in a Danish subpopulation 1965–84, *Clin Otolaryngol*, **15**: 125–31.

Linnen J, Wages J et al., 1996, Molecular cloning and disease association of hepatitis G virus: a transfusion-transmissible agent, *Science*, **271**: 505–8.

Lok ASF, Lai CL, 1988, A longitudinal follow-up of asymptomatic hepatitis B surface antigen positive Chinese children, *Hepatology*, **8**: 1130–3.

Lynch L, Ghidini A, 1993, Perinatal infections, *Curr Opin Obstet Gynecol*, **5**: 24–32.

Lynch L, Daffos F et al., 1991, Prenatal diagnosis of fetal cytomegalovirus infection, *Am J Obstet Gynecol*, **165**: 714–18.

Lynch-Salamon DI, Combs CA, 1992, Hepatitis C in obstetrics and gynecology, *Obstet Gynecol*, **79**: 621–9.

McDonnell M, Lucey MR, 1995, Hepatitis C infection, *Curr Opin Infect Dis*, **8**: 384–90.

McGregor JA, Burns JC et al., 1984, Transplacental passage of influenza A/Bangkok (H_3N_2) mimicking amniotic fluid infections syndrome, *Am J Obstet Gynecol*, **149**: 856–9.

McIntosh K, Pitt J et al., 1994, Blood culture in the first 6 months of life for the diagnosis of vertically transmitted human immunodeficiency virus infection, *J Infect Dis*, **170**: 996–1000.

McMichael A, Koup R, Amman AJ, 1996, Transient HIV infection in infants, *N Engl J Med*, **334**: 801–2.

Mabie WC, Barton JR, Sibai BM, 1992, Adult respiratory distress syndrome in pregnancy, *Am J Obstet Gynecol*, **167**: 950–7.

Maertens G, Stuyver L, 1997, Genotypes and genetic variation of hepatitis C virus, *Molecular Medicine of Viral Hepatitis*, eds Zuckerman AJ, Harrison TJ, John Wiley, Chichester, 183–233.

Malm G, Forsgren M et al., 1991, A follow-up study of children with neonatal herpes simplex virus infections with particular regard to nervous disturbances, *Acta Pediatr Scand*, **80**: 226–34.

Marranconi F, Fabris P et al., 1994, Prevalence of anti-HCV and risk factors for hepatitis C virus infection in healthy pregnant women, *Infection*, **22**: 333–7.

Martin KA, Junker AK et al., 1994, Occurrence of chickenpox during pregnancy in women seropositive for varicella-zoster virus, *J Infect Dis*, **170**: 991–5.

Mast EE, Alter MJ, 1993, Epidemiology of viral hepatitis: an overview, *Semin Virol*, **4**: 274–83.

Matheson PB, Abrams EJ et al., 1995, Efficacy of antenatal zidovudine in reducing perinatal transmission of human immunodeficiency virus type 1, *J Infect Dis*, **172**: 353–8.

Maxwell DJ, Johnson P et al., 1991, Fetal blood sampling and pregnancy loss in relation to indication, *Br J Obstet Gynaecol*, **98**: 892–7.

Mehraein Y, Rehder H et al., 1991, Die Diagnostik fetaler Virusinfektionen durch In-situ-Hybridisierung, *Geburtsh Frauenheilk*, **51**: 984–9.

Metzman R, Anand A et al., 1989, Hepatic disease associated with intrauterine parvovirus B19 infection in a newborn premature infant, *J Pediatr Gastroenter Nutr*, **9**: 112–14.

Meyers JD, 1974, Congenital varicella in term infants: risk reconsidered, *J Infect Dis*, **129**: 215–17.

Miller E, Cradock-Watson J, Ridehalgh M, 1989, Outcome in newborn babies given anti-varicella-zoster immunoglobulin after perinatal maternal infection with varicella-zoster virus, *Lancet*, **2**: 371–3.

Miller E, Marshall R, Vurdien JE, 1993, Epidemiology, outcome and control of varicella-zoster virus infection, *Rev Med Microbiol*, **4**: 222–30.

Miller E, Vurdien JE, Farrington P, 1993, Shift in age in chickenpox, *Lancet*, **341**: 308–9.

Miller G, 1990, The switch between latency and replication of Epstein–Barr virus, *J Infect Dis*, **161**: 833–44.

Milne A, Rodgers E, Hopkirk N, 1995, Hepatitis B vaccination of babies in Melanesia, *Lancet*, **346**: 318.

Minkoff H, Augenbraun M, 1997, Antiretroviral therapy for pregnant women, *Am J Obstet Gynecol*, **176**: 478–89.

Minkoff H, Burns DN et al., 1995, The relationship of the duration of ruptured membranes to vertical transmission of human immunodeficiency virus, *Am J Obstet Gynecol*, **173**: 585–9.

Mocarski ES, Abenes GB et al., 1990, Molecular genetic analysis of cytomegalovirus gene regulation in growth, persistence and latency, *Curr Top Microbiol Immunol*, **154**: 46–74.

Montone KT, Furth EE et al., 1995, Neonatal adenovirus infection: a case report with in situ hybridization confirmation of ascending intrauterine infection, *Diagn Cytopathol*, **12**: 341–4.

Morey AL, Nicolini U et al., 1991, Parvovirus B19 infection and transient fetal hydrops, *Lancet*, **337**: 496.

Morishima T, Morita M et al., 1996, Clinical survey on neonatal herpes simplex virus (HSV) infection in Japan, *21st Herpesvirus Workshop, July 27–August 2*, 401.

Moriya T, Sasaki F et al., 1995, Transmission of hepatitis C virus from mothers to infants: its frequency and risk factors revisited, *Biomed Pharmacother*, **49**: 59–64.

Moroi K, Saito S et al., 1991, Fetal death associated with measles virus infection of the placenta, *Am J Obstet Gynecol*, **164**: 1107–8.

Musiani M, Zerbini M et al., 1995, Parvovirus B19 clearance from peripheral blood after acute infection, *J Infect Dis*, **172**: 1360–3.

Nahmias AJ, Josey WE et al., 1971, Perinatal risk associated with maternal genital herpes simplex virus infection, *Am J Obstet Gynecol*, **110**: 825.

Nanda SK, Ansari IH et al., 1995, Protracted viremia during acute sporadic hepatitis E virus infection, *Gastroenterology*, **108**: 225–30.

Nduati RW, John GC et al., 1995, Human immunodeficiency virus type 1-infected cells in breast milk: assocation with immunosuppression and vitamin A deficiency, *J Infect Dis*, **172**: 1461–8.

Newell ML, Dunn D et al., 1996, Detection of virus in vertically exposed HIV-antibody negative children, *Lancet*, **347**: 213–15.

Nigro G, Clerico A, Mandaini C, 1993, Symptomatic congenital cytomegalovirus infection in two consecutive sisters, *Arch Dis Child*, **69**: 527–8.

Nigro G, Scholz H, Bartmann U, 1994, Ganciclovir therapy for symptomatic congenital cytomegalovirus infection: a two-regimen experience, *J Pediatr* 124: 318–22.

Nikolaidis ET, Trost DC et al., 1985, The relationship of histologic and clinical factors in laryngeal papillomatosis, *Arch Pathol Lab Med*, **109**: 24–9.

Ogasawara S, Kage M et al., 1993, Hepatitis C virus RNA in saliva and breastmilk of hepatitis C carrier mothers, *Lancet*, **341**: 561.

Ohto H, Lin HH et al., 1987, Intrauterine transmission of hepatitis B virus is closely related to placental leakage, *J Med Virol*, **21**: 1–6.

Ohto H, Terazawa S et al., 1994, Transmission of hepatitis C virus from mothers to infants, *N Engl J Med*, **330**: 744–50.

Omata M, Ehata T et al., 1991, Mutations in the precore region of hepatitis B virus DNA in patients with fulminant and severe hepatitis, *N Engl J Med*, 1699–704.

Paccagnini S, Principi N et al., 1995, Perinatal transmission and manifestation of hepatitis C virus infection in a high risk population, *Pediatr Infect Dis J*, **14**: 195–9.

Paryani SG, Arvin AM, 1986, Intrauterine infection with varicella-zoster virus after maternal varicella, *N Engl J Med*, **314**: 1542–6.

Paryani SG, Yeager AS et al., 1985, Sequelae of acquired cytomegalovirus infection in premature and sick term infants, *J Pediatr*, **107**: 451–6.

Pass RF, Fowler KB, Boppana SB, 1991, Progress in cytomegalovirus research, *Proceedings of the Third International Cytomegalovirus Workshop*, Bologna, Italy, June 1991, ed Landini MP, Excerpta Medica, London, 3–10.

Pastuszak AL, Levy M et al., 1994, Outcome after maternal varicella infection in the first 20 weeks of pregnancy, *N Engl J Med*, **330**: 901–5.

Patsner B, Baker DA, Orr JWJ, 1990, Human papillomavirus genital tract infections during pregnancy, *Clin Obstet Gynecol*, **33**: 258–67.

Peckham CS, Gibb D, 1995, Mother-to-child transmission of the human immunodeficiency virus, *N Engl J Med*, **333**: 298–302.

Perelson AS, Neumann AU et al., 1996, HIV-1 dynamics in vivo: virion clearance rate, infected cell life-span, and viral generation time, *Science*, **271**: 1582–6.

Philip RN, Reinhard KR, Lachman DB, 1959, Observations on a mumps epidemic in a virgin population, *Am J Epidemiol*, **69**: 91–100.

Pipan C, Amici S et al., 1996, Vertical transmission of hepatitis C virus in low-risk pregnant women, *Eur J Clin Microbiol Infect Dis*, **15**: 116–20.

Pol S, Driss F et al., 1994, Specific vaccine therapy in chronic hepatitis B infection, *Lancet*, **344**: 342.

Porter HJ, Quantrill AM, Fleming KA, 1988, B19 parvovirus infection in myocardial cells, *Lancet*, **1**: 535–6.

Prober CG, Hensleigh PA et al., 1988, Use of routine viral cultures at delivery to identify neonates exposed to herpes simplex virus, *N Engl J Med*, **318**: 887–91.

Public Health Laboratory Service Working Party of Fifth Disease, 1990, Prospective study of human parvovirus (B19) infection in pregnancy, *Br Med J*, **300**: 1166–70.

Puchhammer-Stöckl E, Kunz C et al., 1994, Detection of varicella-zoster virus (VZV) DNA in fetal tissue by polymerase chain reaction, *J Perinat Med*, **22**: 65–9.

Purdy MA, Krawczynski K, 1994, Hepatitis E, *Gastroenterol Clin North Am*, **23**: 537–46.

Quick CA, Watts SL et al., 1980, Relationship between condylomata and laryngeal papillomata: clinical and molecular virological evidence, *Ann Otol Rhinol Laryngol*, **89**: 467–71.

Ramia S, Bahakim H, 1988, Perinatal transmission of hepatitis B virus-associated hepatitis D virus, *Ann Inst Pasteur Virol*, **139**: 285–90.

Ramsay MEB, Miller E, Peckham CS, 1991, Outcome of confirmed symptomatic congenital cytomegalovirus infection, *Arch Dis Child*, **66**: 1068–9.

Randolph AG, Washington AE, Prober CG, 1993, Caesarean delivery for women presenting with genital herpes lesions, *JAMA*, **270**: 77–82.

Raynor BD, 1993, Cytomegalovirus infection in pregnancy, *Semin Perinatol*, **17**: 394–402.

Reddehase MJ, Balthesen M et al., 1994, The conditions of primary infection define the load of latent viral genome in organs and the risk of recurrent cytomegalovirus disease, *J Exp Med*, **179**: 185–93.

Reman O, Freymuth F et al., 1986, Neonatal distress due to mumps, *Arch Dis Child*, **61**: 80–1.

Report of a Consensus Workshop SI, 1992, Early diagnosis of HIV infection in infants, *J Acquir Immune Defic Syndr*, **5**: 1169–78.

Resti M, Azzari C et al., 1995, Mother-to-infant transmission of hepatitis C virus, *Acta Paediatr*, **84**: 251–5.

Reth P, Sola R et al., 1995, The effect of pregnancy on the course of chronic hepatitis C [letter, in Spanish], *Gastroenterol Hepatol*, **18**: 162.

Revello MG, Percivalle E et al., 1993, Prenatal treatment of congenital human cytomegalovirus infection by fetal intravascular administration of ganciclovir, *Clin Diagn Virol*, **1**: 61–7.

Revello MG, Baldanti F et al., 1995, Polymerase chain reaction for prenatal diagnosis of congenital human cytomegalovirus infection, *J Med Virol*, **47**: 462–6.

Reynolds-Kohler C, Jahn G et al., 1993, Human immunodeficiency virus infection of foetal tissue, *Local Immunity in Reproduction Tract Tissues*, eds Griffin PD, Johnson PM, Oxford University Press, Oxford, 377–90.

Riley LE, 1994, Varicella-zoster virus, *Viral Diseases in Pregnancy*, ed Gonik B, Springer-Verlag, New York, Berlin, Heidelberg, 92–105.

Riongeard P, Sankale JL et al., 1992, Infection due to hepatitis delta virus in Africa: report from Senegal and review, *Clin Infect Dis*, **14**: 510–14.

Robert Koch Institut, 1995, Impfempfehlungen der Ständigen Impfkommission am Robert-Koch-Institut (STIKO), *InfFo*, **4**: i–xii.

Rodis JF, Hovick TJ et al., 1988, Human parvovirus infection in pregnancy, *Obstet Gynecol*, **72**: 733–8.

Rodis JF, Quinn DL et al., 1990, Management and outcomes of pregnancies complicated by human B19 parvovirus infection: a prospective study, *Am J Obstet Gynecol*, **163**: 1168–71.

Roman A, Fife K, 1986, Human papillomavirus DNA associated foreskins of normal newborns, *J Infect Dis*, **153**: 855–61.

Rorabough M, Berlin L et al., 1992, Absence of neurodevelopmental sequelae from aseptic meningitis, *Pediatr Res*, **31**: 177A.

Rosen A, Sternister W, Klein M, 1989, Präpartale Mumpsinfektion, ein Risiko für das Neugeborene?, *Z Geburtshilfe Perinatol*, **193**: 100–1.

Rosenblum LS, Villarino ME et al., 1991, An outbreak in a neonatal intensive care unit: risk factors for transmission and evidence of prolonged viral excretion among preterm infants, *J Infect Dis*, **164**: 476–82.

Ruff TA, Gertig DM et al., 1995, Lombok hepatitis B model immunization project: toward universal infant hepatitis B immunization in Indonesia, *J Infect Dis*, **171**: 290–6.

Rutter D, Griffiths P, Trompeter RS, 1985, Cytomegalic inclusion disease after recurrent maternal infection, *Lancet*, **2**: 1182.

Saller DN, Rogers BB, Canick JA, 1993, Maternal serum biochemical markers in pregnancies with fetal parvovirus B19 infection, *Prenat Diagn*, **13**: 467–71.

Scarlatti G, Albert J et al., 1993, Mother-to-child transmission of human immunodeficiency virus type 1: correlation with neutralizing antibodies against primary isolates, *J Infect Dis*, **168**: 207–10.

Schäfer APA, Friese K, 1996, Massnahmen zur Senkung des maternofetalen HIV-Transmissionsrisikos, *Deutsch Ärztebl*, **93**: 2234–6.

Schalm SW, Pit-Grosheide P, 1989, Prevention of hepatitis B transmission at birth, *Lancet*, **1**: 44.

Scharf A, Scherr O et al., 1990, Virus detection in the fetal tissue of a premature delivery with congenital varicella syndrome. A case report, *J Perinat Med*, **18**: 317–22.

Scharschmidt BF, 1995, Hepatitis E: a virus in waiting, *Lancet*, **346**: 519–20.

Schödel F, 1994, Emerging viral mutants in hepatitis B, *Lancet*, **343**: 355.

Schuster V, Janssen W et al., 1993, Konnatale Epstein–Barr-Virus-Infektion, *Monatsschr Kinderheilkd*, **141**: 401–4.

Schwarz TF, Jäger G, 1995, Das humane Parvovirus B19 und seine klinische Bedeutung, *Hautarzt*, **46**: 831–5.

Schwarz TF, Roggendorf M et al., 1988, Human parvovirus B19 infection in pregnancy, *Lancet*, **2**: 566–7.

Schwarz TF, Nerlich A et al., 1990, Parvovirus B19 infection in pregnancy, *Int J Exp Clin Chemother*, **3**: 219–23.

Schwarz TF, Nerlich A et al., 1991, Parvovirus B19 infection of the fetus: histology and in situ hybridization, *Am J Clin Pathol*, **96**: 121–6.

Schwarz TF, Jäger G et al., 1992, Diagnosis of human parvovirus B19 infections by polymerase chain reaction, *Scand J Infect Dis*, **24**: 691–6.

Schwebke K, Henry K et al., 1995, Congenital cytomegalovirus infection as a result of nonprimary cytomegalovirus disease in a mother with acquired immunodeficiency syndrome, *J Pediatr*, **126**: 293–5.

Searle K, Guilliard C, Enders G, 1996, Parvovirus B19 diagnosis in pregnant women – quantification of IgG antibody levels (IU/ml) with reference to the international parvovirus B19 standard serum, *Infection*, **25**: 32–4.

Sedlacek TV, Lindheim S et al., 1989, Mechanism for human papillomavirus transmission at birth, *Am J Obstet Gynecol*, **161**: 55–9.

Shalev E, Bassan HM, 1982, Viral hepatitis during pregnancy in Israel, *Int J Gynaecol Obstet*, **20**: 73–8.

Shattuck K, Chonmaitree T, 1992, The changing spectrum of neonatal meningitis over a fifteen-year period, *Clin Pediatr (Phila)*, **31**: 130–6.

Sheinbergas MM, 1975, Antibody to lymphocytic choriomeningitis virus in children with congenital hydrocephalus, *Acta Virol (Praha)*, **19**: 165–6.

Sheinbergas MM, 1976, Hydrocephalus due to prenatal infection with the lymphocytic choriomeningitis virus, *Infection*, **4**: 185–91.

Shen CY, Chang SF et al., 1994, Cytomegalovirus is present in semen from a population of men seeking fertility evaluation, *J Infect Dis*, **169**: 222–3.

Siegel M, 1973, Congenital malformations following chickenpox, measles, mumps, and hepatitis: results of a cohort study, *JAMA*, **226**: 1521–4.

Sills JA, Galloway A et al., 1987, Acyclovir in prophylaxis and perinatal varicella, *Lancet*, **1**: 161.

Silverman NS, Darby MJ et al., 1991, Hepatitis B prevalence in an unregistered prenatal population, *JAMA*, **266**: 282–5.

Simmonds P, 1995, Variability of hepatitis C virus, *Hepatology*, **21**: 570–83.

Simoes EAF, Abzug MJ, 1993, Enteroviruses: issues in poliomyelitis immunization and perinatal enterovirus infections, *Curr Opin Infect Dis*, **6**: 547–52.

Simons JN, Leary TP et al., 1995, Isolation of novel virus-like sequences associated with human hepatitis, *Nature Med*, **1**: 564–9.

Sixbey JW, Lemon SM, Pagano JS, 1986, A second site for Epstein–Barr virus shedding: the uterine cervix, *Lancet*, **2**: 1122–4.

Sjogren MH, Tanno H et al., 1987, Hepatitis A virus in stool during clinical relapse, *Ann Intern Med*, **106**: 221–6.

Skidmore S, 1995, Hepatitis E, *Br Med J*, **310**: 414–15.

Slomka MJ, 1996, Seroepidemiology and control of genital herpes: the value of type specific antibodies to herpes simplex virus, *CDR Rev*, **6**: R41–5.

Smedile A, Dentico P et al., 1981, Infection with HBV associated delta agent in HBsAg carriers, *Gastroenterology*, **81**: 992–7.

Smego RA, Asperilla MO, 1991, Use of acyclovir for varicella pneumonia during pregnancy, *Obstet Gynecol*, **78**: 1112–16.

Smith JL, Thomas F et al., 1990, Adult respiratory distress syndrome during pregnancy and immediately postpartum, *West J Med*, **153**: 508–10.

Smoleniec JS, Pillai M et al., 1994, Subclinical transplacental parvovirus B19 infection: an increased fetal risk?, *Lancet*, **343**: 1100–1.

Spitzbart H, 1994, Immunotherapy of gynaecological high risk human papilloma virus infections with a human leucocyte ultrafiltrate, *13th International Papillomavirus Congress*, Amsterdam, 8–12 October 1994.

St Geme JW J, Noren GR, Adams PJ, 1966, Proposed embryopathic relation between mumps virus and primary endocardial fibroelastosis, *N Engl J Med*, **275**: 339–47.

Stagno S, 1995, Cytomegalovirus, *Infectious Diseases of the Fetus and Newborn Infants*, 4th edn, eds Remington JS, Klein JO, WB Saunders, Philadelphia, 312–53.

Stagno S, Cloud GA, 1994, Working parents: the impact of day care and breast-feeding on cytomegalovirus infections in offspring, *Proc Natl Acad Sci USA*, **91:** 2384–9.

Stagno S, Reynolds SW et al., 1977, Congenital cytomegalovirus infection. Occurrence in an immune population, *N Engl J Med*, **296:** 1254–8.

Stagno S, Reynolds DW et al., 1980, Breast milk and the risk of cytomegalovirus infection, *N Engl J Med*, **302:** 1073–6.

Stagno S, Pass RF et al., 1986, Primary cytomegalovirus infection in pregnancy: incidence, transmission to fetus and clinical outcome, *JAMA*, **256:** 1904–8.

Stanwell-Smith R, Parker AM et al., 1994, Possible association of influenza A with fetal loss: investigation of a cluster of spontaneous abortions and stillbirths, *CDR Rev*, **4:** R28–32.

Starr SE, 1992, Cytomegalovirus vaccines: current status, *Infect Agents Dis*, **1:** 146–8.

Stern H, Hannington G et al., 1986, An early marker of fetal infection after primary cytomegalovirus infection in pregnancy, *Br Med J*, **292:** 718–20.

Sterner G, Grandien M, 1990, Mumps in pregnancy at term, *Scand J Infect Dis*, **71:** 36–8.

Sterner G, Grandien M, Enocksson E, 1990, Pregnant women with acute respiratory disease at term, *Scand J Infect Dis*, **71:** 19–26.

Stevens CE, Neurath RA et al., 1979, HBeAg and anti-HBe detection by radioimmunoassay: correlation with vertical transmission of hepatitis B virus in Taiwan, *J Med Virol*, **3:** 237–41.

Stone KM, Brooks CA et al., 1989, National surveillance for neonatal herpes simplex virus infections, *Sex Transm Dis*, **16:** 152–6.

Straus SE, Seidlin M et al., 1989, Effect of oral acyclovir on symptomatic and asymptomatic virus shedding in recurrent genital herpes, *Sex Transm Dis*, **16:** 107–13.

Stray-Pedersen B, 1990, Acyclovir in late pregnancy, *Lancet*, **2:** 756.

Stronati M, Revello MG et al., 1995, Ganciclovir therapy of congenital human cytomegalovirus hepatitis, *Acta Pediatr*, **84:** 340–1.

Sutherland S, 1993, *Torch Screening Reassessed*, 2nd edn, Public Health Laboratory Service, London.

Svennerholm B, Olofsson S et al., 1984, Herpes simplex virus type-selective enzyme linked immunosorbent assay with helix pomatia lectin-purified antigens, *J Clin Microbiol*, **19:** 235–9.

Sweet RL, 1990, Hepatitis B infection in pregnancy, *Obstet Gynecol Rep*, **2:** 128–39.

Terada S, Kawanishi K, Katayama K, 1992, Minimal hepatitis C infectivity in semen, *Ann Intern Med*, **117:** 171–2.

Terazawa S, Kojima M et al., 1991, Hepatitis B virus mutants with precore-region defects in two babies with fulminant hepatitis and mothers positive for antibody to hepatitis B antigen, *Pediatr Res*, **29:** 5–9.

Tercanli S, Enders G, Holzgreve W, 1996, Aktuelles Management bei mütterlichen Infektionen mit Röteln, Toxoplasmose, Zytomegalie, Varizellen und Parvovirus B19 in der Schwangerschaft, *Gynäkologe*, **29:** 144–63.

Thaithumyanon P, Thisyakorn U et al., 1994, Dengue infection complicated by severe hemorrhage and vertical transmission in a parturient woman, *Clin Infect Dis*, **18:** 248–9.

Thaler MM, Park CK et al., 1991, Vertical transmission of hepatitis C virus, *Lancet*, **338:** 17–18.

Tiessen RG, van Elsacker-Niele AM et al., 1994, A fetus with a parvovirus B19 infection and congenital anomalies, *Prenat Diagn*, **14:** 173–6.

Tobiasch E, Rabreau M et al., 1994, Detection of adeno-associated virus DNA in human genital tissue and in material from spontaneous abortion, *J Med Virol*, **44:** 215–22.

Toivanen P, Rossi T, Hirvonen T, 1969, Immunoglobulins in human fetal sera at different stages of gestation, *Experientia*, **25:** 527–8.

Torres JR, Mondolfi A, 1991, Protracted outbreak of severe delta hepatitis: experience in an isolated Amerindian population of the Upper Orinoco basin, *Rev Infect Dis*, **13:** 52–5.

Trang JM, Kidd L et al., 1993, Linear single-dose pharmacokinetics of ganciclovir in newborns with congenital cytomegalovirus infections, *Clin Pharmacol Ther*, **53:** 15–21.

Trlifojova J, Brenda R, Benes C, 1986, Effect of maternal varicella-zoster virus infection on the outcome of pregnancy and the analysis of transplacental virus transmission, *Acta Virol (Praha)*, **30:** 249–55.

Tsarev SA, Tsareva TS et al., 1995, Experimental hepatitis E in pregnant rhesus monkeys: failure to transmit hepatitis E virus (HEV) to offspring and evidence of naturally acquired antibodies to HEV, *J Infect Dis*, **172:** 31–7.

Van de Perre P, 1995, Postnatal transmission of human immunodeficiency virus type 1: the breast-feeding dilemma, *Am J Obstet Gynecol*, **173:** 483–7.

Villari P, Spino C et al., 1993, Cesarean section to reduce perinatal transmission of human immunodeficiency virus, *Online J Curr Clin Trials*, **2:** doc 74.

Wald A, Zeh J et al., 1995, Virologic characteristics of subclinical and symptomatic genital herpes infections, *N Engl J Med*, **333:** 770–5.

Walther J-U, Gloning KP, Schwarz TF, 1994, Prune belly nach Hydrops fetalis bei mütterlicher Parvovirus-B19-Infektion, *Monatsschr Kinderheilkd*, **142:** 592–5.

Wang JB, Adler SP et al., 1996, Mucosal antibodies to human cytomegalovirus glycoprotein B occur following both natural infection and immunization with human cytomegalovirus vaccines, *J Infect Dis*, **174:** 387–92.

Watson JC, Fleming DW et al., 1993, Vertical transmission of hepatitis A resulting in an outbreak in a neonatal intensive care unit, *J Infect Dis*, **167:** 567–71.

Watts DH, Koutsky LA et al., 1996, Risk of perinatal transmission of human papillomavirus (HPV) is low: results from a prospective cohort study, *Am J Obstet Gynecol*, **174:** 319.

Weiland HT, Vermey-Keers C et al., 1987, Parvovirus B19 associated with fetal abnormality [letter], *Lancet*, **1:** 682–3.

Weinberg A, Hayward AR et al., 1996, Comparison of two methods for detecting varicella-zoster virus antibody with varicella-zoster virus cell-mediated immunity, *J Clin Microbiol*, **34:** 445–6.

Weiner CP, Towbin JA, Yankowitz J, 1995, Detection of viral infection by polymerase chain reaction in pregnancies complicated by either nonimmune hydrops or hydramnios, *Ultrasound Obstet Gynecol*, **6:** 42.

von Weizsäcker F, Pult I et al., 1995, Selective transmission of variant genomes from mother to infant in neonatal fulminant hepatitis B, *Hepatology*, **21:** 8–13.

Whitley RJ, 1993, Neonatal herpes simplex virus infections, *J Med Virol*, **1:** 13–21.

Whitley RJ, 1994, Herpes simplex virus infections of women and their offspring: implications for a developed society, *Proc Natl Acad Sci USA*, **91:** 2441–7.

Whitley RJ, Arvin A, 1994, *Seminars in Pediatric Infectious Diseases*, ed Baker CJ, WB Saunders, Philadelphia, vol 5, 56–64.

Whitley RJ, Arvin AM, 1995, Herpes simplex virus infections, *Infectious Diseases of the Fetus and Newborn Infant*, 4th edn, eds Remington JS, Klein JO, WB Saunders, Philadelphia, 354–76.

Whitley RJ, Cloud G et al., 1997, Ganciclovir treatment of symptomatic congenital cytomegalovirus infection: results of a phase II study, *J Infect Dis*, in press.

Wilcox AJ, Weinberg CR et al., 1988, Incidence of early loss of pregnancy, *N Engl J Med*, **319:** 189–94.

Wilfert CM, Wilson C et al., 1994, Pathogenesis of pediatric human immunodeficiency virus type 1 infection, *J Infect Dis*, **170:** 286–92.

Wolf H, Kuehler O et al., 1992, Leberdystrophie bei disseminierter Herpes-simplex-Infektion in der Schwangerschaft, *Geburtsh Frauenheilk*, **52:** 123–5.

Wood AJJ, Graham BS, Wright PF, 1995, Drug therapy: candidate AIDS vaccines, *N Engl J Med*, **333:** 1331–9.

Wynne Griffith G, Adelstein AM et al., 1972, Influenza and infant mortality, *Br Med J*, **2:** 553–6.

Ye JY, 1990, Outcome of pregnancy complicated by hepatitis A in the urban districts of Shanghai, *Chung-Hua Fu Chan Ko Tsa Chih*, **25:** 219–21.

Yeager AS, Arvin AM et al., 1980, Relationship of antibody to outcome in neonatal herpes simplex virus infections, *Infect Immun*, **29:** 532–8.

Yeager AS, Palumbo PE et al., 1983, Sequelae of maternally derived cytomegalovirus infections in premature infants, *Pediatrics*, **102:** 451–6.

Young RL, Acosta A, Kaufman RH, 1973, The treatment of large condylomata acuminata complicating pregnancy, *Obstet Gynecol*, **41:** 65–73.

Yow MD, Williamson DW et al., 1988, Epidemiologic characteristics of cytomegalovirus infection in mothers and their infants, *Am J Obstet Gynecol*, **158:** 1189–95.

Zanetti AR, Tanzi E et al., 1995, Mother-to-infant transmission of hepatitis C virus, *Lancet*, **345:** 289–91.

Zanetti RA, Gerroni P et al., 1982, Perinatal transmission of the hepatitis B virus and of the HBV-associated delta agent from mothers to offspring in northern Italy, *J Med Virol*, **9:** 139–48.

Zerbini M, Musiani M et al., 1993, Symptomatic parvovirus B19 infection of one fetus in a twin pregnancy, *J Clin Infect Dis*, **17:** 262–3.

Zhang RL, Zeng JS, Zhang HZ, 1990, Survey of 34 pregnant women with hepatitis A and their neonates, *Chin Med J (Engl)*, **103:** 552–5.

Zhuang YL, 1989, Acute hepatitis A in pregnancy: a report of 43 cases, *Chung-Hua Fu Chan Ko Tsa Chih*, **24:** 136–8.

Zimmermann R, Perucchini D et al., 1995, Hepatitis C virus in breast milk [letter], *Lancet*, **345:** 928.

Zöllner B, Feucht HH et al., 1996, HIV quantification: useful for prediction of vertical transmission?, *Lancet*, **347:** 899.

Zuccotti GV, Ribero ML et al., 1995, Effect of hepatitis C genotype on mother-to-infant transmission of virus, *J Pediatr*, **127:** 278–80.

VIRUS INFECTIONS IN IMMUNOCOMPROMISED PATIENTS

A Simmons

1 **Introduction**	3 **HIV-infected children**
2 **HIV-infected adults**	4 **Immune deficiencies not caused by HIV**

1 INTRODUCTION

Perturbations of immunity can influence the pathogenesis of viral infections in several ways. Prominent among these is increased frequency or severity of disease, exemplified *par excellence* by the debilitating manifestations of many herpesvirus infections in immunocompromised hosts. However, not all viral infections are exacerbated by immunosuppression and the acute stages of some diseases, such as hepatitis B, may be unusually mild. This is presumably because immunologically mediated lysis of infected cells contributes more than virally induced cell damage to the pathogenesis of some diseases in normal hosts.

Diagnosis of viral infections in immunocompromised patients can be difficult. Total and differential leucocyte counts tend to be unhelpful, clinical signs and symptoms of infection are often atypical, and symptoms produced by the host's immune response (e.g. the rash of measles) may be absent. Serology has little role in diagnosis because patients with dysfunctional immunity do not usually mount appropriate immune responses rapidly enough to influence decisions about management. The mainstay of diagnosis is detection of virus in appropriate clinical specimens: rapid procedures, such as direct antigen detection, nucleic acid detection and culture amplified enzyme immunoassays, have increased the usefulness of laboratory diagnosis enormously (Simmons 1996). In some situations (e.g. post-transplantation) regular surveillance cultures may be helpful: virus shedding may precede the onset of symptoms, and initiation of therapy as soon as virus is detected may prevent extensive tissue damage.

The AIDS pandemic has created an explosive increase in the number of profoundly immunocompromised people world-wide. The clinical manifestations of viral infections in HIV-infected individuals often differ significantly from the signs and symptoms caused by the same viruses in patients with other types of immune deficiency. Accordingly, a significant part of this chapter is devoted specifically to patients infected with HIV.

2 HIV-INFECTED ADULTS

The progressive decline in immunological function associated with HIV infection is usually monitored by measuring the absolute CD4+ T cell count. In general, significant opportunistic viral infections (Table 42.1) are not seen until CD4+ T cells fall below $200/mm^3$ and the most severe problems are associated with CD4 cell counts of $<100/mm^3$. Herpesviruses, particularly cytomegalovirus and herpes simplex viruses types 1 and 2, are common causes of serious disease in profoundly immunosuppressed HIV-infected individuals and therefore herpesviruses receive particular attention here. Infections caused by papillomaviruses and enteric viruses are also given special consideration. Where appropriate, the discussion includes diagnosis and treatment of first episode disease, prophylaxis against recurrence and, finally, measures to prevent acquisition of infection in previously unexposed individuals.

2.1 Herpesvirus infections

Several genetically distinct herpesviruses have been isolated from humans. Some, namely herpes simplex viruses types 1 and 2 (HSV-1 and HSV-2), varicella-zoster virus (VZV), Epstein–Barr virus (EBV) and cytomegalovirus (CMV) have been recognized for decades. In contrast, human herpesviruses types 6 and 7

Table 42.1 Opportunistic viral infections in HIV-infected patients

Virus	Prominent clinical manifestations	References
Adenovirus	Gastroenteritis	Khoo and Bailey 1995
Retrovirus	Gastroenteritis	Grohmann et al. 1993
BK virus	Nephropathy, encephalitis	Vallbracht et al. 1993
Herpesviruses:		
Cytomegalovirus	Retinitis, gastrointestinal disease, encephalitis, adrenalitis	Peters et al. 1991; Drew 1988
Epstein–Barr virus	Oral hairy leucoplakia, lymphoma	Andersson 1991
Herpes simplex virus type 1	Mucocutaneous lesions, keratoconjunctivitis	Stewart et al. 1995
Herpes simplex virus type 2	Genital and perianal ulceration	Stewart et al. 1995
Human herpesvirus type 6	Pneumonitis, disseminated infection	Knox and Carrigan 1994
Human herpesvirus type 8	Kaposi's sarcoma?	Chang et al. 1994
Varicella-zoster virus	Retinitis, recurrent dermatomal zoster, disseminated zoster, pneumonia, prolonged varicella	Buchbinder et al. 1992; Kelly et al. 1994
Hepatitis B virus	Increased rate of chronic infection	Hadler et al. 1991
Human papillomavirus	Recurrent and persistent anogenital warts, premalignant and malignant tumours, oral lesions	Palefsky 1991
Human parvovirus B19	Persistent anaemia, red cell aplasia	Frickhofen et al. 1990
Influenza virus	Increased severity of illness	Safrin, Rush and Mills 1990
JC virus	Progressive multifocal leucoencephalopathy	Berger et al. 1987
Measles virus	Encephalitis, pneumonia	Mustafa et al. 1993
Molluscum contagiosum virus	Disseminated cutaneous lesions	Epstein 1992
Parainfluenza virus	Exacerbation of respiratory symptoms	Hague et al. 1992
Picobirnavirus	Gastroenteritis	Grohmann et al. 1993
Respiratory syncytial virus	Increased mortality, prolonged viral shedding	Chandwani et al. 1990

(HHV-6 and HHV-7) are relatively recent discoveries and the latest addition to the list, referred to here as human herpesvirus type 8 (HHV-8), is of particular interest in the present context because it is found in Kaposi's sarcoma cells (Chang et al. 1994).

Most well characterized herpesviruses establish latent infections from which disease can periodically reactivate. In some cases, there are prolonged periods of asymptomatic virus shedding. Human herpesvirus infections are generally acquired in early childhood and therefore most of the clinical problems associated with herpesviruses in adults are the result of reactivations. With the exception of varicella and herpes zoster, primary and recurrent human herpesvirus infections are often clinically inapparent and transmission of infection commonly occurs during periods of asymptomatic virus shedding.

The herpesviruses that cause greatest morbidity among HIV-infected people are HSV, CMV, VZV and EBV. Significant morbidity has not been attributed to HHV-6 or HHV-7, and it remains to be shown whether HHV-8 has a causal relationship with Kaposi's sarcoma.

HERPESVIRUSES AS CO-FACTORS IN PROGRESSION OF HIV-RELATED DISEASE

Aside from their direct clinical impact, it has been suggested that herpesviruses could be co-factors in the development of AIDS, i.e. herpesviruses might accelerate progression toward immunodeficiency and death by influencing the pathogenesis of HIV infection at the molecular or cellular level. Epidemiological data supporting this hypothesis are limited. A study of HIV-infected haemophiliacs suggested more rapid progression to AIDS in CMV-seropositive compared with CMV-seronegative patients (Webster et al. 1989) but this result could not be confirmed in a similar study elsewhere (Rabkin et al. 1993). Probably the best way to address the hypothesis is to study the effect of herpesvirus-specific antiviral drugs on HIV progression. There have been several clinical trials in which patients have been treated prophylactically with the anti-herpes compound aciclovir (acyclovir), in addition to zidovudine. Cooper et al. (1993) and Youle et al. (1994) showed, independently, that combination therapy increased survival time compared with zidovudine alone. However, neither study showed a decrease in deaths related to any of the known human herpesviruses and the explanation for the apparent benefit of combination therapy remains obscure.

Although the proposal that herpesviruses promote the development of AIDS is in the realms of speculation, several molecular mechanisms can be envisaged by which HIV replication, or reactivation of latent provirus, could be enhanced. For instance, all human herpesviruses encode proteins called transactivators, which up-regulate viral gene expression during replication. Some herpesvirus transactivators are 'promiscuous', i.e. they can up-regulate expression not only of herpesvirus genes but also of genes belonging to other viruses or host cells. In vitro, several herpesvirus transactivators have been shown to interact with the HIV long terminal repeat, which is the main region of the HIV genome responsible for controlling gene expression. Thus, co-infection of a cell with a herpesvirus and HIV could, in principle, result in enhanced HIV replication. Alternatively, reactivation of latent HIV might be stimulated by superinfection with a herpesvirus. The best candidates for herpesviruses that might enhance HIV replication are CMV and HHV-6, because these viruses are commonly found in the same tissues as HIV in autopsy specimens. Therefore, co-infection of, for example, lymphocytes with HIV and either CMV or HHV-6 is a theoretical possibility. Furthermore, HHV-6 infection has been shown to transactivate the HIV *tat* gene in vitro.

Promiscuous transactivation of various cellular genes could also, in principle, promote the spread of HIV. For example, up-regulation of CD4, the cell surface receptor for HIV, might facilitate the spread of HIV from cell to cell. Similarly, up-regulation of cell surface Fc receptors, a property of most herpesviruses, could enable antibody-coated HIV particles to enter CD4– cell types, thereby expanding the pool of HIV-infected cells.

Co-infection of a cell with more than one type of virus raises the possibility of phenotypic mixing and the formation of virus pseudotypes. This phenomenon is well established in vitro and can be manipulated to the extent that HIV genomes can be packaged into the capsids of vesicular stomatitis virus. Formation of pseudotypes comprising HIV genomes packaged into particles containing herpesvirus glycoproteins has not been documented in vivo, but, nevertheless, pseudotype formation remains a theoretical way in which HIV genomes could gain entry into a wide variety of otherwise resistant cell types.

HERPES SIMPLEX VIRUSES TYPES 1 AND 2

Herpes simplex is one of the commonest infections of humans. HSV-2 is transmitted almost exclusively by sexual contact; consequently, HSV-2 seropositivity is rare before the onset of sexual activity. The epidemiology of HSV-1 is more diverse; infection is commonly acquired during infancy or childhood from infected oral secretions, but sexual transmission of HSV-1 is becoming increasingly common. HSV patently infects primary sensory neurons innervating the portal of entry, creating a reservoir of infection that can periodically give rise to recrudescent disease. The generally early acquisition of HSV means that most episodes of herpes simplex seen in the clinic are recrudescences.

In the context of HIV infection, HSV causes a wide spectrum of disease, including genital herpes, perioral and facial herpes, perianal lesions, proctitis, conjunctivitis and keratitis, aseptic meningoencephalitis, herpetic whitlow, autonomic nervous system dysfunction and acute necrotizing retinitis. In profoundly immunocompromised patients, with CD4 cell counts of $<100/\text{mm}^3$, extensive and chronic mucocutaneous ulceration is a frequently encountered and troublesome clinical problem, particularly in the genital and perianal regions (Safrin et al. 1991). In the absence of a normal inflammatory response, the lesions tend to respond slowly or poorly to antiviral therapy and they are often indolent or atypical in appearance.

In addition to prolonged mucocutaneous ulceration, there are several other severe manifestations of HSV infections in AIDS patients that merit further consideration. HSV may invade the oesophagus or other parts of the gastrointestinal tract, giving rise to symptoms that reflect the region of the gut that is infected. Disseminated infection is rare but life-threatening. Many organs may be involved, including the lungs, liver and adrenals. Prolonged ulcerative lesions and visceral disease are AIDS-defining illnesses.

There is evidence to suggest that genital ulceration facilitates sexual transmission of HIV and, in industrialized nations, the commonest cause of genital ulceration is HSV. By extrapolation, it has been proposed that genital herpes promotes the spread of HIV, but direct evidence in support of this hypothesis is lacking.

Prevention of exposure

Strictly speaking, strategies designed to prevent exposure to HSV apply only to those rare individuals who are HSV-seronegative. However, first episode genital infections caused by HSV-2 in people previously exposed only orally to HSV-1 may be symptomatic; i.e. prior HSV-1 infection is only partially cross-protective against HSV-2. Furthermore, in HIV-infected people, exogenous reinfection of the genital tract with different strains of HSV-2 is a possibility. With these considerations in mind, it is recommended that all HIV-infected people use latex condoms during sexual contact. Condom usage is essential irrespective of whether the sexual partner has noticeable herpetic lesions, because HSV is frequently shed from the genital tract asymptomatically.

Treatment and suppression of symptoms

Herpes simplex virus replication is inhibited by aciclovir and its pro-drug, valaciclovir. Aciclovir is available in oral and intravenous formulations; the appropriate route of administration and dose depend on the severity of lesions and the degree of immunological impairment. Primary genital herpes can be managed with oral aciclovir unless immune function is profoundly impaired or lesions are unusually severe, in which case intravenous aciclovir is required. Recurrent genital herpes in patients with early HIV infection generally resolves spontaneously. In this group of patients, the approach to management is the same as for immunocompetent people: symptomatic relief of mild, infrequent outbreaks or, in selected patients who experience clear prodromal symptoms, episodic aciclovir. Continuous administration of aciclovir should be considered for patients with frequent episodes or when lesions tend to heal slowly (Safrin et al. 1991). In advanced HIV infection, when immune suppression is profound, herpetic lesions often require prolonged therapy with high doses of aciclovir; treatment failure is not uncommon, even when the drug is administered intravenously (Whitley and Gnann 1992). In this patient population, emergence of aciclovir-resistant viral strains, which are also resistant to the related nucleoside analogue, ganciclovir, is an increasingly recognized problem (Chatis and Crumpacker 1992). There are few avenues available for the treatment of recalcitrant lesions caused by aciclovir-resistant virus, the main option being intravenous foscarnet.

Aciclovir resistance

Aciclovir is a nucleoside analogue which, when phosphorylated, inhibits DNA replication. The drug is phosphorylated by an HSV-encoded enzyme, thymidine kinase (TK), hence it is active only in HSV-infected cells. Emergence of HSV strains resistant to aciclovir is rare in immunocompetent hosts, even after long-term suppressive therapy. The situation is different in immunocompromised hosts, particularly patients with advanced HIV infection, in whom aciclovir resistance is a significant clinical problem.

HSV becomes resistant to aciclovir by way of viral TK mutations that decrease the ability of the virus to phosphorylate the drug. Such mutations can also affect the ability of TK to phosphorylate nucleosides required for virus replication. However, TK-altered HSV strains are able to grow in most cell types, because cellular kinases substitute for viral TK. Consequently, aciclovir-resistant viruses may cause aggressive mucocutaneous lesions. However, non-dividing cells, notably neurons, express unusually low amounts of endogenous kinases and, in these cells, replication of aciclovir-resistant HSV strains is, fortuitously, inhibited. This has important practical consequences: HSV must replicate in neurons in order to reactivate from latency and, therefore, the latency/reactivation cycle is broken for aciclovir-resistant viruses. The subtle influence of viral TK on the pathogenesis of herpes simplex may explain, in part, why aciclovir resistance is largely confined to patients treated over long periods for recalcitrant cutaneous lesions.

VARICELLA-ZOSTER VIRUS

Varicella is a common disease of childhood that is generally benign in immunocompetent hosts. In industrialized nations, seropositivity to VZV is >90% by the age of 15 years and therefore varicella is uncommon in adults. This is fortunate, because the clinical impact of varicella in adults with impaired cellular immunity is high. Clinical manifestations include extensive, often haemorrhagic, cutaneous lesions and pneumonitis.

VZV establishes latency in sensory ganglia in much the same way as herpes simplex, although it has been suggested that the virus may be dormant in satellite glia rather than in neurons (Croen et al. 1988). Recurrent VZV infection (herpes zoster, or shingles) is characterized by a blistering dermatomal rash and pain. HIV infection has a substantial impact on the incidence of VZV recurrence. HIV-infected adults are 9 times more likely than the general population to develop herpes zoster (Holmberg et al. 1995) and the annual incidence of the disease is 7 times higher in HIV-infected adults than in the general population. HIV-positive homosexual men are 17 times more likely to develop zoster than demographically matched HIV-negative subjects (Buchbinder et al. 1992).

The clinical manifestations of recurrent VZV infections in HIV-infected patients depend on the degree of immunological impairment. In the early stages of HIV infection, the signs and symptoms resemble herpes zoster in immunologically normal hosts. In contrast, repeated episodes of severe, prolonged and sometimes atypical disease are characteristic of advanced HIV infection. A few patients develop VZV retinitis, which has a particularly poor prognosis if the CD4 cell count is $<50/\text{mm}^3$. In some cases, atypical herpes zoster may require laboratory tests for confirmation of the diagnosis, in which case material from a recently erupted lesion should be sent for virus culture, rapid antigen detection or, if available, culture amplified enzyme immunoassay. *Ante mortem* diagnosis of herpes zoster is particularly difficult when atypical manifestations of the disease, such as retinitis, meningoencephalitis, optic neuritis and visceral involvement, occur in the absence of cutaneous lesions.

Prophylaxis and treatment

Most adults with no history of chickenpox have antibodies to VZV, and serological tests are useful for determining whether an HIV-infected patient is truly at risk of acquiring primary VZV infection. Seronegative patients should avoid contact with varicella- and herpes zoster; if contact is documented, they should receive varicella-zoster immunoglobulin (VZIG) within 96 hours of exposure. The prophylactic effect of varicella vaccine, administered to susceptible HIV-infected people before CD4+ cells become depleted, has yet to be fully evaluated.

Most cases of herpes zoster respond well to high dose oral aciclovir. Disseminated, recurrent or unusually severe cases should be treated intravenously. Aciclovir-resistant VZV strains have been isolated from severely immunocompromised people on long-term suppressive therapy (Lyall et al. 1994). The usual cause of resistance is mutation of the viral TK gene; aciclovir-resistant VZV remains sensitive to intravenous foscarnet (Balfour and Benson 1994).

CYTOMEGALOVIRUS

CMV infection is extremely common and is generally acquired before HIV. Therefore primary CMV infections are rare among HIV-infected adults. Reactivation of CMV does not cause illness in immunocompetent adults. In contrast, when cellular immunity is impaired, reactivation has many potential clinical manifestations, including retinitis, oesophagitis, colitis, pneumonitis and CNS disease. The spectrum of disease caused by recurrent CMV infection is significantly different in HIV-infected people compared with transplant recipients. For instance, necrotizing retinitis and CNS disease, common complications of CMV infection in advanced AIDS (Drew 1988, Jacobson and Mills 1988), are very unusual in the transplant setting. Conversely, CMV pneumonitis is unusual in HIV-infected adults but is not uncommon in transplant recipients.

CMV is frequently present in body fluids of AIDS patients and it is often difficult to establish a causal relationship between CMV and disease. Detection of CMV in affected organs provides circumstantial evidence that disease is CMV-related, but this approach frequently fails. CMV is often detected in bronchoalveolar lavage specimens from AIDS patients but this alone is not predictive of CMV pneumonitis; histological examination of cells or tissue for characteristic cytomegaly is required to establish the diagnosis.

Prevention, pre-emptive therapy and treatment

Immunization is not an option currently available for protection against primary CMV infection in immunocompromised people. Measures to prevent exposure apply to only a small proportion of HIV-infected adults and include counselling that CMV is present in genital secretions. Blood products should be obtained from CMV-seronegative donors.

Most adults are already infected with CMV when HIV infection is diagnosed, and ways to prevent subsequent development of CMV disease are being explored. Anti-CMV drugs are too toxic for continuous administration and therefore true prophylaxis awaits the development of safer, orally active compounds. In the meantime, ways of predicting the onset of CMV disease are being sought in order to allow pre-emptive therapy to be commenced before irreversible damage has been done. Unfortunately, CMV viraemia is no more predictive of CMV disease than CD4 T cell counts; most patients who develop CMV disease have <200 CD4 cells/mm^3, and the risk increases as the CD4 count falls. The greatest risk is in patients with <50 CD4 cells/mm^3, in whom the median time to development of retinitis is 6 months. Oral administration of ganciclovir to patients with <100 CD4 cells/mm^3 delays the onset of CMV disease and increases survival.

Intravenous ganciclovir and foscarnet are the mainstays of treatment for established disease, especially retinitis. Both drugs are toxic, so it is usual to reduce the dosage to maintenance levels after an initial period of induction. Without maintenance, relapse is inevitable; even on maintenance, relapse is common, necessitating periods of reinduction.

Epstein–Barr virus

HIV infection promotes the development of a variety of EBV-related diseases. Oral hairy leucoplakia is an EBV-associated hyperkeratotic disease of the tongue that is very common in HIV-infected patients but very rare otherwise. It responds to aciclovir but relapses if therapy is stopped. Lymphomas occur with greatly increased frequency in HIV-positive individuals, and a high proportion of the tumours, which tend to be monoclonal, contain cells expressing EBV antigens. Despite intensive chemotherapy, the prognosis is poor, especially in patients with low CD4 cell counts.

Herpesviruses 6, 7 and 8

HHV-6 and HHV-7 are ubiquitous, closely related betaherpesviruses, and most humans are infected with these agents in early childhood. Primary infection may be asymptomatic or cause roseola infantum. It is probable that both viruses establish latent infections in lymphoid tissues; in immunocompromised people, latent infection may reactivate and disseminate. HHV-6 is also known to be resident in the brain. In AIDS patients, HHV-6 has been detected in a wide variety of tissues *post mortem* and may cause fatal pneumonitis (Knox and Carrigan 1994). Further work is required to clarify its clinical impact.

HHV-8 is found in Kaposi's sarcoma but not in normal skin. On the basis of nucleotide sequence analysis, this newly discovered agent is a gammaherpesvirus. Establishing whether HHV-8 plays an aetiological role in Kaposi's sarcoma is a research priority because antiviral therapy may be possible.

2.2 Human papillomavirus infections

Of the 70 or so known human papillomaviruses (HPVs), more than 25 have been detected in the genital region. Some HPVs, notably types 16 and 18, are associated with precancerous intraepithelial neoplasias of the cervix, vagina, vulva, penis and anus. HIV-induced immune dysfunction increases the prevalence of detectable genital HPV infection and HPV-associated intraepithelial neoplasia (Northfelt and Palefsky 1992), as does iatrogenic immunosuppression (Penn 1986). However, the association between HIV and HPV is not explicable solely on the basis of immunosuppression, because HPV DNA is detectable with increased frequency in the genital tracts of women with early HIV infection, before there is a measurable decline in the CD4 cell count. Both direct interaction between HIV and HPV and the common risk factors for their acquisition may contribute to the association between HIV infection and HPV-related disease.

In HIV-infected women, cervical intraepithelial neoplasia (CIN) recurs more frequently than expected after treatment (Maiman et al. 1990), and recurrence is related to severity of immunosuppression. Although CIN does not seem to progress unusually rapidly to invasive cancer, the latter is an AIDS-defining condition according to the Centers for Disease Control and Prevention guidelines.

2.3 Enteric infections

Diarrhoea is very common among HIV-infected patients. Potential viral causes include astroviruses, adenoviruses, picobirnavirus and caliciviruses (Grohmann et al. 1993), on the basis that they are detected more frequently in patients with diarrhoea than in patients without diarrhoea. CMV is also associated with gastrointestinal disease in HIV-infected adults (Laughon and Druckman 1988).

Picobirnaviruses

Picobirnaviruses are small, bisegmented, double-stranded RNA viruses that have been detected in a wide variety of vertebrates, including pigs, in which they are associated with diarrhoea (Gatti and de Castro 1989). They can be grown in mammalian cell cultures, suggesting that they are vertebrate viruses rather than viruses of other intestinal organisms such as protozoa. It is not known with certainty whether picobirnaviruses cause diarrhoea in humans but their detection in a significant proportion of faecal specimens from HIV-infected patients with diarrhoea raises this possibility. Development of serological tests might help to determine the prevalence of picobirnavirus infections in the human population.

Enteric adenoviruses

Reported rates of faecal carriage of adenoviruses among patients with advanced HIV infection are very high (Cunningham et al. 1988). Adenovirus infections of the gastrointestinal tract are frequently asymptomatic, and when symptoms are noted they are often mild. In immunocompetent people, adenoviruses associated with diarrhoea usually belong to subgenera A, C or F, but in HIV antibody-positive patients at least one report suggests that the most predominant faecal isolates belong to subgenus D (Khoo and Bailey 1995). There is some suggestion that prolonged infections in patients with CD4 cell counts <200/mm³ may allow antigenic drift and genetic recombination between different serotypes (Hierholzer and Adrian 1988).

3 HIV-INFECTED CHILDREN

The impact of opportunistic viral infections on HIV-infected children has yet to be fully determined. However, as in adults, herpesviruses are a major problem.

3.1 Herpesvirus infections

There are marked differences in the clinical manifestations of herpesvirus infections in HIV-infected children compared with adults. In part, the differences depend on whether HIV infection precedes primary infections with herpesviruses.

Herpes simplex viruses

In children, herpes simplex is almost always limited to the oropharynx. Oesophagitis is rare, as is dissemination or invasion of the CNS. Furthermore, there is no evidence suggesting that neonatal herpes is more common among the offspring of HIV-infected mothers. The diagnostic method of choice is detection of virus or viral antigens in material collected from newly erupted lesions. Treatment follows guidelines similar to those applied to herpes simplex in adults: oral or intravenous aciclovir according to the severity of disease and suppressive therapy with oral aciclovir for frequently recurrent episodes.

Varicella-zoster virus

Only a small number of cases of varicella in HIV-infected children have been reported in the literature. Some cases run an uneventful course whereas others may be prolonged or complicated by sepsis, pneumonia or cerebral vasculitis. Recurrent varicella- and herpes zoster have been documented. The severity of complications seems to be inversely related to the CD4 cell count (Jura et al. 1989). Diagnosis is usually possible on clinical grounds. Atypical disease may require laboratory confirmation by detection of VZV in material collected from a freshly erupted vesicle.

Prophylaxis and treatment

Serological tests may be required to identify children who are susceptible to primary infection with VZV. Seronegative children should avoid contact with chickenpox and herpes zoster; when exposure is documented, VZIG may be useful. However, even when VZIG is given within 96 hours of exposure, protection is not guaranteed (Srugo et al. 1993). It has yet to be determined whether it is safe to give varicella vaccine to HIV-infected children.

Aciclovir is effective in the treatment of varicella in HIV-infected children (Jura et al. 1989). Intravenous therapy is recommended, particularly for children with poor immune function.

Cytomegalovirus

CMV infection is very common among infants whose mothers are HIV antibody-positive. Furthermore, maternal HIV infection seems to increase the prevalence of congenital CMV. CMV-related disease is an important AIDS indicator event in HIV-infected children, and dissemination of CMV in children with advanced HIV infection carries a high mortality. There is evidence to suggest that HIV-related disease develops up to 3 times more rapidly in CMV-infected infants compared with uninfected infants. Therefore prophylaxis is a desirable but currently unattainable goal.

There are differences in the clinical manifestations of CMV infection in HIV-infected children and adults that most probably represent the different outcomes of primary and recurrent infections, respectively. Pneumonitis and hepatitis, the commonest diseases caused by CMV in HIV-infected children, are probably the result of primary infection. In contrast, CMV retinitis, which is common in adults and rare in children, is thought to follow reactivation of latent virus in the immune host.

Diagnosis of CMV disease is notoriously difficult,

owing to the high prevalence of asymptomatic infection by the age of 2 years. Detection of CMV in urine is common and not indicative of CMV disease. Detection of CMV in the diseased organ (by culture, viral antigen detection, culture amplified antigen detection or polymerase chain reaction) is currently the best diagnostic approach but the predictive value of a positive result is not absolute.

Prophylaxis and treatment

Ganciclovir and foscarnet have both been used to treat CMV disease in children. Toxicity is less of a problem in children compared with adults but both drugs must be given intravenously, creating problems with compliance. Realistically, neither drug is suitable for prophylactic use.

Epstein–Barr virus

EBV DNA has been detected in the lungs of HIV-infected patients with lymphoid interstitial pneumonitis (LIP). LIP is rare in HIV-infected adults but is one of the commonest complications of HIV infection in infants under the age of 2 years. Clinical manifestations of LIP include lymphadenopathy, parotitis, bronchospasm, tachypnoea and sleep apnoea. Serum immunoglobulin levels may be unusually high, with an associated hyperviscosity syndrome. Chest infections may complicate the disease and therefore immunization against bacterial pathogens is recommended. Diagnosis rests on sequential clinical assessments and chest x-ray changes over a period of 2 months, together with lung biopsy if necessary. Further work is merited to determine whether EBV, the host response to it, or other viruses, play an aetiological role in LIP because, if this is the case, specific therapy may be possible. Corticosteroids and zidovudine have been reported to be useful in the management of the disease.

3.2 Respiratory syncytial virus infections

Pneumonitis, rather than bronchiolitis or wheezing, seems to be a prominent clinical manifestation of RSV in HIV-infected children (Chandwani et al. 1990). Bronchiolitis is thought to be the result of immune-mediated damage to the lung, which might explain its rarity in immunocompromised hosts. In infants with low CD4 cell counts, RSV pneumonia may be life-threatening as a result of secondary bacterial infection (Chandwani et al. 1990). Pre-emptive antibacterial therapy may therefore be worthwhile in severely immunocompromised children who fail to respond promptly to ribavirin.

4 Immune deficiencies not caused by HIV

Malignant tumours, cytotoxic chemotherapy or radiotherapy, and congenital disorders may all profoundly compromise the immune system, predisposing patients to unusually severe or prolonged infections with a wide range of viruses.

4.1 Herpesvirus infections

It has been known for a long time that herpesviruses are important opportunistic pathogens in patients with disorders of cellular immunity. The potential manifestations of infection are diverse and sometimes life-threatening.

Herpes simplex

The frequency and severity of recurrent episodes of herpes simplex are increased in patients with dysfunctional immunity, particularly allograft recipients (Naraqi et al. 1977, Rand et al. 1977, Meyers, Flournoy and Thomas 1980), those with malignancy or those receiving anti-tumour chemotherapy (Muller, Herrmann and Winkelmann 1972) and patients with Wiskott–Aldrich syndrome (St Geme et al. 1965). In allograft recipients, herpes simplex most commonly presents in the second week after transplantation.

Shedding of HSV may be asymptomatic or may present as vesicles or ulcers. Lesions may be widespread and persistent, and may involve the oesophagus or rectum, causing pain and gastrointestinal disturbances. Ulcers may become indolent and, in immobile patients, perianal ulcers may be confused with pressure sores. Major manifestations of visceral infection are pneumonia and hepatitis.

Virus detection is the mainstay of laboratory diagnosis. In the case of a superficial infection, the specimen required is material collected from the base of the lesion. To diagnose HSV pneumonia, broncho-alveolar lavage fluid or, preferably, a lung biopsy specimen is necessary. Virus culture is probably the most sensitive diagnostic procedure in routine use but it can take up to 7 days before a characteristic cytopathic effect (CPE) develops. More rapid procedures include direct detection of viral antigens and culture-amplified enzyme immunoassays, in which inoculated cell cultures are tested for the presence of viral antigens after 24–48 hours, in order to prevent the development of cytopathology.

Prophylaxis and treatment

To prevent reactivation of HSV caused by iatrogenic immunosuppression, bone marrow recipients are often given aciclovir prophylactically, commencing at the start of induction chemotherapy. However, some transplant units believe it is more cost effective to treat episodes as they arise.

Intravenous aciclovir is recommended for the treatment of all HSV disease in profoundly immunocompromised patients, irrespective of whether the infection is localized or disseminated at the time of diagnosis. Oral aciclovir may be appropriate for localized herpes simplex in patients who are not severely immunocompromised, with the caveat that intestinal absorption of the drug may be reduced by irradiation of the gut or systemic chemotherapy.

Varicella

Varicella is an aggressive and potentially fatal disease in people with severe cellular immune defects. The rash may be florid or haemorrhagic, and visceral manifestations include hepatitis, pneumonitis and encephalitis. Most cases of varicella can be diagnosed on clinical grounds but, occasionally, virus culture or antigen detection tests are required, particularly to distinguish the disease from disseminated herpes simplex.

Treatment and prophylaxis

Intravenous aciclovir is of proven efficacy for the treatment of visceral disease caused by VZV in children with malignant disease (Schulman 1985). The drug is beneficial in immunocompromised children presenting at the time of emergence of rash (Nyerges et al. 1988) and treatment should begin as soon as possible after rash eruption to be effective in reducing the incidence of visceral complications.

For prevention of varicella, live attenuated varicella vaccine (Oka strain) is safe and effective when given to children with leukaemia (in remission) or other malignancies, provided that anti-cancer chemotherapy is suspended from 1 week before to 1 week after vaccination. Passive immunization with VZIG is useful for seronegative people known to have been exposed to varicella. VZIG is potentially beneficial when given within 96 hours of exposure but protection is not a certainty.

Herpes zoster

Herpes zoster (recrudescent VZV infection) is common in immunocompromised children and adults and, unlike zoster in immunocompetent people, episodes may be recurrent. After bone marrow transplantation, 30% of patients develop herpes zoster within a year, with a peak incidence in the fourth month (Locksley et al. 1985). The disease is also common in renal transplant recipients (Naraqi et al. 1977) and in patients with Hodgkin's disease (Schulman 1985).

Infection may be confined to a single dermatome or may involve overlapping or non-contiguous dermatomes. Cutaneous dissemination of infection is not uncommon and, in severely immunocompromised patients, life-threatening visceral dissemination may occur.

Treatment and prophylaxis

Oral aciclovir, valaciclovir or famciclovir may be used to treat localized herpes zoster in patients who are not severely immunocompromised (e.g. those on maintenance chemotherapy). Treatment should be commenced as soon as possible after eruption of the rash. In profoundly immunocompromised patients and in patients with signs of disseminated disease, intravenous aciclovir is currently the treatment of choice.

At the present time it is not feasible or cost effective to prevent herpes zoster in immunocompromised patients by continuous administration of antiviral compounds. This situation might change in the future if safe and inexpensive oral compounds with high activity against VZV become available. There is interest in determining whether herpes zoster can be prevented in immunocompetent adults by vaccination with the Oka strain of VZV. If this approach proves to be effective, it may be applicable to some immunocompromised patients, given that vaccination of leukaemic children during periods of remission safely protects them against varicella.

Cytomegalovirus infections

Cytomegalovirus infection is usually asymptomatic in the immunocompetent host. Primary infection is acquired at any time throughout life; by 40 years of age, c. 70% of the general population are infected. Primary infection or reinfection of an immune host may be acquired as a result of transfusion of CMV-seropositive blood or blood products, or receipt of a kidney from a seropositive donor. However, reactivation of latent virus is the cause of most CMV infections in immunocompromised hosts. CMV is a major cause of morbidity and mortality in allograft recipients (Peterson et al. 1980, Meyers, Flournoy and Thomas 1982). Characteristically, reactivation is detected in the second and third months after bone marrow transplantation.

CMV causes a wide range of clinical syndromes in people with dysfunctional immunity, prominent among which are hepatitis, gastrointestinal disease and pneumonitis. The last is thought to be immunologically mediated (Grundy, Shanley and Griffiths 1987) and responds poorly to specific antiviral therapy. In bone marrow recipients, graft-versus-host disease is a risk factor for development of CMV pneumonitis. Reactivation of CMV may be manifest as fever without localizing signs of infection, creating considerable difficulty in diagnosis. Surveillance cultures of urine, saliva and blood, taken twice weekly, are useful in this respect, because virological evidence of active infection precedes disease.

Diagnosis of CMV disease requires detection of virus in material from the affected organ. For diagnosis of CMV pneumonitis, a transbronchial biopsy is a suitable specimen. Detection of virus in buffy coat cells may be a useful adjunct to diagnosis when material cannot be obtained from the affected organ. In order to be useful in patient management, virus detection must be rapid. On average, 16 days are required to identify CMV in conventional cell cultures, making virus culture impractical when decisions have to be made about therapy. Rapid diagnosis depends on direct immunohistochemical detection of viral antigen in biopsy material (Volpi et al. 1983) or culture amplified antigen detection methods. The latter approach is both rapid and sensitive and is based on the principle that a few cells in an inoculated monolayer express immediate early CMV antigens, which can be detected, for instance, by enzyme immunoassay, within 24–48 hours of infection.

Epstein–Barr virus infections

Primary EBV infection is very common in early childhood and adolescence, and more than 90% of the adult population are EBV-seropositive. EBV replicates in B lymphocytes and pharyngeal epithelial cells and the virus is transmitted in saliva. In the normal host, lytic infection is kept under control by cytotoxic T lymphocytes (CTLs) with specificity for virally encoded antigens. After recovery from primary infection, EBV persists in a latent form in B lymphocytes. In renal allograft recipients and other profoundly immunosuppressed patients, lytic infection is not adequately controlled, leading to frequently recurrent or persistent virus shedding and an unusually high virus load in the blood. In one report, EBV was detected in throat washings from more than 80% of seropositive renal transplant patients (Chang et al. 1978).

There has been considerable debate as to whether EBV can persist in epithelial cells in addition to lymphoid tissue. Current evidence suggests that lymphocytes are the only true reservoir of EBV. Carriage of EBV is lost following ablation of lymphoid tissue in EBV-seropositive patients undergoing bone marrow transplantation (Gratama et al. 1990). Furthermore, the characteristic pattern of viral gene expression associated with latency is not evident in epithelial cells at sites of oral hairy leucoplakia (Sandvej et al. 1992).

Primary EBV infections may be asymptomatic or cause infectious mononucleosis (IM). The clinical features of reactivated infection are poorly characterized: fever and hepatitis have been implicated as potential manifestations of recrudescent disease but undoubtedly most reactivations must be asymptomatic. Primary and recurrent infections are associated with B cell lymphomas in transplant recipients (Hanto et al. 1982, Ho et al. 1985), and EBV nuclear antigen and EBV DNA can be detected in the tumour cells. The incidence of lymphomas in transplant patients has increased substantially with the use of more aggressive immunosuppressive regimens, and recipients of bone marrow, heart and liver grafts are most at risk. Rapidly progressive lymphomas that develop early after transplantation are most commonly the result of primary rather than recurrent EBV infections, acquired either from the graft or from transfused blood. Lymphoma tends to be a late complication of recurrent EBV infection. Post-transplant lymphomas are resistant to standard anti-tumour chemotherapies, and aciclovir is not beneficial.

All post-transplantation lymphomas contain EBV DNA. The higher the virus load in the blood, the greater is the risk of developing lymphoma (Riddler, Breinig and McKnight 1994, Savoie et al. 1994), consistent with the hypothesis that failure to control lytic infection predisposes to the outgrowth of malignant cells. Tumours are often multifocal and particularly affect the gastrointestinal tract, liver and CNS. They may progress from a polyclonal to a monoclonal phenotype, presumably representing dominance by the most rapidly growing cell in the original tumour. Different tumours in the same patient commonly have different clonal origins.

The lymphoma cells have several properties in common with EBV-transformed lymphoblastoid cell lines, suggesting that EBV may be the only factor underlying tumour development in vivo. Chromosomal translocations of the Burkitt's lymphoma type and *c-myc* rearrangements have been reported but are rare. Tumours may regress with improved

immune function (Starzl et al. 1984), suggesting that they remain sensitive to attack by EBV-specific CTLs. The possibility of treating post-transplant lymphomas by adoptive transfer of CTLs is being explored.

X-linked lymphoproliferative syndrome

X-linked lymphoproliferative syndrome (XLPS) is a rare form of immunodeficiency that selectively predisposes affected males to life-threatening EBV-related disease (Purtilo et al. 1975). About 75% of those affected die within a few weeks of primary EBV infection. The remainder have a greatly increased risk of developing lymphomas or hypogammaglobulinaemia.

Many patients with XLPS fail to control the initial proliferation of EBV-transformed B cells associated with acute IM, despite the presence of reactive T cells. This may result in a disease resembling immunoblastic lymphoma in transplant patients. Infiltration of organs by lymphocytes is a common cause of death in these individuals. Alternatively, the initial proliferation of B cells and reactive T cells may abate, to be followed by widespread infiltration and destruction of lymphoid tissues and bone marrow by phagocytic cells (Sullivan and Woda 1989). This type of pathology is indistinguishable from the virus-associated haemophagocytic syndrome.

The genetic defect responsible for XLPS is closely linked to 2 X chromosome markers, DXS42 and 37. Several phenotypic defects have been identified in XLPS patients and carriers, including failure to develop antibodies to EBV nuclear antigens. IgM to IgG switching is defective and the ability of T cells to produce interferon-γ is reduced. It has been postulated that patients with XLPS have a critical defect in their ability to support the activity of EBV-specific cytotoxic T lymphocytes.

4.2   Papillomavirus infections

Warts are common in patients with dysfunctional cellular immunity, including those with leukaemia or lymphoma and renal transplant recipients (Koranda et al. 1974). Most infections probably represent reactivations of latent virus.

EPIDERMODYSPLASIA VERRUCIFORMIS

Epidermodysplasia verruciformis (EV) is a rare disease that is first manifest in infancy or childhood by the development of multiple warts that do not regress spontaneously. Patients with EV have a poorly understood immunological defect that predisposes them, apparently quite specifically, to papillomavirus disease. There is often a family history of the disease but its pattern of inheritance is not clear. Parental consanguinity is common, suggesting that the trait is recessive.

A mixture of typical flat warts and reddish-brown plaques is characteristic. The lesions are caused by a wide variety of papillomavirus types, most of which rarely cause warts in the general population. Some of the warts, particularly those in areas of the body exposed to the sun, progress to intraepithelial or invasive squamous carcinomas (Jablonska and Majewski 1994).

4.3 Enteric viruses

Many viruses have been associated with gastroenteritis. In immunocompetent hosts, illness is usually mild and shedding of virus in the faeces is transient. In contrast, enteric viruses cause significant morbidity in immunocompromised patients. Rotaviruses, adenoviruses, astroviruses, caliciviruses and small round viruses have all been associated with severe or persistent diarrhoea in patients with perturbed immune function (Chrystie et al. 1982, Pedley et al. 1984, Oishi et al. 1991, Cox et al. 1994, Flomberg et al. 1994), bone marrow recipients being particularly at risk. A nosocomial outbreak of rotavirus infection, with severe diarrhoea, has been documented in renal transplant recipients (Peigue-Lafauille et al. 1991). Although enteroviruses are not usually associated with gastrointestinal disease, coxsackie A viruses have been implicated as causes of diarrhoea in the contexts of hypogammaglobulinaemia (Johnson et al. 1982) and bone marrow transplantation (Townsend et al. 1982).

Enteroviral meningoencephalitis

Severe and persistent enterovirus infections are seen in patients with congenital hypogammaglobulinaemia, despite regular immunoglobulin replacement therapy. This finding is unusual in that hypogammaglobulinaemic patients respond normally to other viral infections. The most frequent complication is chronic, often fatal, meningoencephalitis. Patients may present with neck stiffness, headache, lethargy, weakness or seizures, with or without fever. These features are often associated with a dermatomyositis-like syndrome, characterized by oedema of the extremities, sometimes with an erythematous or violaceous rash overlying groups of muscles. Echovirus types 2, 3, 5, 9, 11, 17, 19, 24, 25, 30 and 33, and coxsackie B3 have been isolated from the cerebrospinal fluid or brain tissue, and occasionally from muscle, in these patients (Mease, Ochs and Wedgwood 1981, Cooper et al. 1983). Respiratory illness caused by enteroviruses has also been described, and evidence of disseminated infection has been found in fatal cases.

4.4 Measles

Dysfunctional cellular immunity predisposes to persistence of measles virus with potentially lethal consequences. Two complications, namely giant cell pneumonia and measles inclusion body encephalitis (MIBE), are recognized, neither of which is seen in immunocompetent hosts. Giant cell pneumonia usually presents 2–3 weeks after exposure to measles. The characteristic measles rash may be absent, in which case the diagnosis may remain obscure until postmortem. Laboratory approaches to diagnosis include detection of virus or viral antigens in nasopharyngeal fluid, bronchoalveolar lavage fluid or lung tissue and demonstration of multinucleated giant cells with characteristic inclusion bodies in histological sections of lung.

MIBE usually arises within 6 months of exposure to measles virus and is occasionally accompanied by giant cell pneumonia or retinopathy. The disease may be rapidly progressive and has a poor prognosis; rapid deterioration leads to death within a few weeks of onset. The underlying pathology is one of gliosis. Intracytoplasmic and intranuclear inclusion bodies are present in glial cells and neurons, and inflammatory cell infiltration of the brain is minimal. Defective measles virus has been detected in the brains of MIBE patients and it is possible that the disease is an accelerated version of subacute sclerosing panencephalitis (Ohuchi et al. 1987).

Measles vaccine contains live attenuated virus and is not generally recommended for administration to immunocompromised patients. The current vaccination programme for normal children reduces the number of susceptible patients among those who subsequently develop dysfunctional immunity, and may reduce the chance of exposure in non-immune individuals. Measles in previously vaccinated hosts has, however, been reported. Administration of normal human immunoglobulin after exposure to measles virus has some beneficial effect, but may not prevent complications, particularly MIBE (Kay and Rankin 1984). There is as yet no specific antiviral therapy with proven efficacy for the treatment of measles or its complications in immunocompromised hosts, but sporadic case reports suggest that aerosolized ribavirin might be of some benefit to patients with pneumonitis.

4.5 Polyomavirus infections

BK virus (BKV) and JC virus (JCV) are human polyomaviruses which, according to serological studies, are ubiquitous. It was thought that active, persistent infections were rare in immunocompetent hosts, but recent data suggest that urinary excretion of JCV is common in older people and pregnant women.

About half of renal transplant recipients have serological or other evidence of prior exposure to polyomavirus (Hogan et al. 1980, Gardner et al. 1984), in keeping with the high seropositivity rate in the general population. BKV and JCV are commonly detected in the urine of transplant patients, suggesting that immunosuppression allows latent infections to reactivate. Primary and reactivated infections are usually asymptomatic, although ureteric stenosis has been reported and there may be an association with impaired graft function. Infections are frequent in the second month after renal transplantation, but late infections, occurring several months or even years later, are not unusual.

Urinary excretion of BKV and JCV is also common after bone marrow transplantation (O'Reilly et al. 1981) and has been reported in association with leukaemia, lymphoma, solid tumours and Wiskott–Aldrich syndrome. Infection is generally asymptomatic, although deterioration in renal and hepatic function has been observed; BK viruria following bone marrow transplantation may be associated with haemorrhagic cystitis (Rice et al. 1985).

Polyomavirus infections of the urinary tract may be diagnosed by electron microscopy or by demonstrating characteristic intranuclear inclusions in exfoliated urinary epithelial cells. The presence of polyomavirus antigens within these cells can be confirmed by immunofluorescence. BK virus can be isolated in cell cultures, such as human embryo lung fibroblasts.

PROGRESSIVE MULTIFOCAL LEUCOENCEPHALOPATHY

JCV is the cause of progressive multifocal leucoencephalopathy (PML), a rare neurological disease characterized by multiple foci of demyelination throughout the CNS. PML has a global distribution and, in patients who do not have AIDS, it is most common in people over the age of 50. The disease is seen in patients with a wide variety of disorders associated with impaired immune function but very rarely in immunocompetent hosts. JCV is found in the nuclei of oligodendrocytes in affected areas of the brain, and viral DNA is present in the cerebrospinal fluid (Gibson et al. 1993). The clinical features of PML are gradual deterioration of cerebral function, progressing to dementia, blindness, paralysis and eventual coma and death, usually within 6 months of onset.

PML affects only a minority of immunocompromised patients infected with JCV, and virus has been detected in the brains of normal individuals. The factors predisposing to PML are unclear. It has been suggested that JCV may adapt itself for growth in the nervous system during the course of infection. In support of this hypothesis, structural alterations in the archetypal regulatory region of the JCV genome have been found in JCV DNA from PML brains. Structural variations in the regulatory region have also been reported among viral DNAs from different organs in the same infected patient (Loeber and Dorries 1988). However, the issue of virus adaptation to different tissues is controversial because different organs have been shown to be infected with the same JCV subtype and PML isolates can be the same subtype as urinary isolates (Myers, Frisque and Arthur 1989).

Diagnosis of PML is based on the characteristic clinical picture, and should be confirmed by brain biopsy. The histological appearances are typical and polyomavirus particles can be demonstrated by electron microscopy. Immunofluorescence microscopy of acetone-fixed brain tissue may reveal the presence of polyomavirus antigens. Virus may also be isolated in primary cultures of human fetal glial cells.

No agent has proven efficacy for the treatment of polyomavirus infections; reduction of immunosuppressive therapy, when practicable, may be beneficial.

REFERENCES

Andersson JP, 1991, Clinical aspects of Epstein–Barr virus infection, *Scand J Infect Dis*, **80 (suppl)**: 94–104.

Balfour HH, Benson C, 1994, Management of acyclovir resistant herpes simplex and varicella-zoster virus infections, *J Acquired Immune Defic Syndr*, **7**: 254–60.

Berger JR, Kaszovita B et al., 1987, Progressive multifocal leukoencephalopathy associated with human immunodeficiency virus infection, *Ann Intern Med*, **107**: 78–87.

Buchbinder SP, Katz MH et al., 1992, Herpes zoster and human immunodeficiency virus infection, *J Infect Dis*, **166**: 1153–6.

Chandwani S, Borkowsky W et al., 1990, Respiratory syncytial virus infection in human immunodeficiency virus-infected children, *J Pediatr*, **117**: 251–4.

Chang RS, Lewis JP et al., 1978, Oropharyngeal excretion of Epstein–Barr virus by patients with lymphoproliferative disorders and by recipients of renal homografts, *Ann Intern Med*, **88**: 34–40.

Chang Y, Cesarman E et al., 1994, Identification of herpesvirus-like DNA sequences in AIDS-associated Kaposi's sarcoma, *Science*, **266**: 1865–9.

Chatis PA, Crumpacker CS, 1992, Resistance of herpesviruses to antiviral drugs, *Antimicrob Agents Chemother*, **36**: 1589–95.

Chrystie K, Booth IW et al., 1982, Multiple faecal virus excretion in immunodeficiency, *Lancet*, **1**: 282.

Cooper JB, Pratt WR et al., 1983, Coxsackie B3 producing fetal meningoencephalitis in a patient with X-linked agammaglobulinaemia, *Am J Dis Child*, **137**: 82–3.

Cooper DA, Pehrson O et al., 1993, The efficacy and safety of zidovudine alone or as cotherapy with acyclovir in the treatment of patients with AIDS and AIDS related complex: a double blind randomised trial, *AIDS*, **7**: 197–207.

Cox GJ, Matsui SM et al., 1994, Etiology and outcome of diarrhoea after bone marrow transplantation: a prospective study, *Gastroenterology*, **107**: 1398–407.

Croen KD, Ostrove JM et al., 1988, Patterns of gene expression and sites of latency in human nerve ganglia are different for varicella-zoster and herpes simplex viruses, *Proc Natl Acad Sci USA*, **85**: 9773–7.

Cunningham AL, Grohmann GS et al., 1988, Gastrointestinal viral infections in homosexual men who were symptomatic and seropositive for human immunodeficiency virus, *J Infect Dis*, **158**: 386–91.

Drew WL, 1988, Cytomegalovirus infection in patients with AIDS, *J Infect Dis*, **158**: 449–56.

Epstein WL, 1992, Molluscum contagiosum, *Semin Dermatol*, **11**: 184–9.

Flomberg B, Babbitt J et al., 1994, Increasing incidence of adenovirus disease in bone marrow transplant recipients, *J Infect Dis*, **169**: 775–81.

Frickhofen N, Abkowitz JL et al., 1990, Persistent B19 parvovirus infection in a patient infected with human immunodeficiency virus infection type 1 (HIV-1): a treatable cause of anaemia in AIDS, *Ann Intern Med*, **113**: 926–33.

Gardner SD, Mackenzie EFC et al., 1984, Prospective study of the human polyomaviruses BK and JC and cytomegalovirus in renal transplant recipients, *J Clin Pathol*, **37**: 578–86.

Gatti MSV, de Castro AFP, 1989, Viruses with bisegmented double-stranded RNA in pig faeces, *Res Vet Sci*, **47**: 397–8.

Gibson PI, Knowles WA et al., 1993, Detection of JC virus DNA in the cerebrospinal fluid of patients with progressive multifocal leukoencephalopathy, *J Med Virol*, **39**: 278–81.

Gratama JW, Oosterveer MAP et al., 1990, Eradication of Epstein–Barr virus by allogeneic bone marrow transplantation: implications for site of viral latency, *Proc Natl Acad Sci USA*, **85**: 8693–9.

Grohmann GS, Glass RI et al., 1993, Enteric viruses and diarrhea in HIV-infected patients, *N Engl J Med*, **329**: 14–20.

Grundy JE, Shanley JD, Griffiths PD, 1987, Is cytomegalovirus interstitial pneumonitis in transplant recipients an immunopathological condition? *Lancet*, **2**: 996–8.

Hadler SC, Judson FN et al., 1991, Outcome of hepatitis B virus infection in homosexual men and its relation to prior human immunodeficiency virus infection, *J Infect Dis*, **163**: 454–9.

Hague RA, Burns SE et al., 1992, Virus infections of the respiratory tract in HIV-infected children, *J Infect*, **24**: 31–6.

Hanto DW, Frizzera G et al., 1982, Epstein–Barr virus-induced

B-cell lymphoma after renal transplantation, *N Engl J Med*, **306:** 913–18.

Hierholzer JC, Adrian T, 1988, Analysis of antigenically intermediate strains of subgenus B and D adenovirus isolates from AIDS patients, *Arch Virol*, **103:** 99–115.

Ho M, Miller G et al., 1985, Epstein–Barr virus infections and DNA hybridization studies in post-transplantation lymphoma and lymphoproliferative lesions: the role of primary infection, *J Infect Dis*, **152:** 876–86.

Hogan TF, Borden EC et al., 1980, Human polyomavirus infections with JC virus and BK virus in renal transplant patients, *Ann Intern Med*, **92:** 373–8.

Holmberg SD, Buchbinder SP et al., 1995, The spectrum of medical conditions and symptoms before AIDS in HIV-infected homosexual and bisexual men, *Am J Epidemiol*, **141:** 395–404.

Jablonska S, Majewski S, 1994, Epidermodysplasia verruciformis, *Human Pathogenic Papillomaviruses*, ed zur Hausen H, Springer-Verlag, Heidelberg, 157–75.

Jacobson MA, Mills J, 1988, Serious cytomegalovirus disease in the acquired immune deficiency syndrome (AIDS). Clinical findings, diagnosis, and treatment, *Ann Intern Med*, **108:** 585–94.

Johnson JP, Yolken RH et al., 1982, Prolonged excretion of group A coxsackievirus in an infant with agammaglobulinaemia, *J Infect Dis*, **146:** 712.

Jura E, Chadwick EG et al., 1989, Varicella-zoster virus infections in children infected with human immunodeficiency virus, *Pediatr Infect Dis J*, **8:** 586–90.

Kay HEM, Rankin A, 1984, Immunoglobulin prophylaxis of measles in acute lymphoblastic leukaemia, *Lancet*, **1:** 901–2.

Kelly R, Mancao M et al., 1994, Varicella in children with perinatally acquired human immunodeficiency virus infection, *J Pediatr*, **124:** 271–3.

Khoo SH, Bailey AS, 1995, Adenovirus infections in human immunodeficiency virus-positive patients: clinical features and molecular epidemiology, *J Infect Dis*, **172:** 629–37.

Knox KK, Carrigan DR, 1994, Disseminated active HHV-6 infections in patients with AIDS, *Lancet*, **343:** 577–8.

Koranda FC, Dehmel EM et al., 1974, Cutaneous complications in immunosuppressed renal homograft recipients, *JAMA*, **229:** 419–24.

Laughon BE, Druckman DA, 1988, Prevalence of enteric pathogens in homosexual men with and without AIDS, *Gastroenterology*, **94:** 984–93.

Locksley RM, Flournoy N et al., 1985, Infection with varicella-zoster virus after marrow transplantation, *J Infect Dis*, **152:** 1172–81.

Loeber G, Dorries K, 1988, DNA rearrangement in organ-specific variants of polyomavirus JC strain, *J Virol*, **62:** 1730–5.

Lyall EGH, Ogilvie MM et al., 1994, Acyclovir resistant varicella-zoster and HIV infection, *Arch Dis Child*, **70:** 133–5.

Maiman M, Fruchter RG et al., 1990, Human immunodeficiency virus and cervical neoplasia, *Gynec Oncol*, **38:** 377–82.

Mease PJ, Ochs HD, Wedgwood RJ, 1981, Successful treatment of echovirus meningoencephalitis and myositis-fasciitis with intravenous immune globulin therapy in a patient with X-linked agammaglobulinemia, *N Engl J Med*, **304:** 1278–80.

Meyers JD, Flournoy N, Thomas ED, 1980, Infection with herpes simplex virus and cell mediated immunity after marrow transplant, *J Infect Dis*, **142:** 338–46.

Meyers JD, Flournoy N, Thomas ED, 1982, Non-bacterial pneumonia after allogeneic marrow transplantation: a review of ten years experience, *Rev Infect Dis*, **4:** 1119–32.

Muller SA, Herrmann EC, Winkelmann RK, 1972, Herpes simplex infections in hematologic malignancies, *Am J Med*, **52:** 102–14.

Mustafa MM, Weitman SD et al., 1993, Subacute measles encephalitis in the young immunocompromised host: report of two cases diagnosed by polymerase chain reaction and

treated with ribavirin, and review of the literature, *Clin Infect Dis*, **16:** 654–60.

Myers C, Frisque RJ, Arthur RR, 1989, Direct isolation and characterization of JC virus from urine samples of renal and bone marrow transplant patients, *J Virol*, **63:** 4445–9.

Naraqi S, Jackson GG et al., 1977, Prospective study of prevalence, incidence and source of herpesvirus infections in patients with renal allografts, *J Infect Dis*, **136:** 531–40.

Northfelt DW, Palefsky JM, 1992, Human papillomavirus-associated anogenital neoplasia in persons with HIV infection, *AIDS Clinical Review*, eds Velberding P, Jacobson MA, Marcel Dekker, New York, 241–59.

Nyerges G, Meszner Z et al., 1988, Acyclovir prevents dissemination of varicella in immunocompromised children, *J Infect Dis*, **157:** 309–13.

Ohuchi M, Ohuchi R et al., 1987, Characterisation of measles virus isolated from the brain of a patient with immunosuppressive measles encephalitis, *J Infect Dis*, **156:** 436–41.

Oishi I, Kimura T et al., 1991, Serial observation of chronic rotavirus infection in an immunodeficient child, *Microbiol Immunol*, **35:** 953–61.

O'Reilly RJ, Lee FK et al., 1981, Papovavirus excretion following marrow transplantation: incidence and association with hepatic dysfunction, *Transplant Proc*, **13:** 262–6.

Palefsky J, 1991, Human papillomavirus infection among HIV-infected individuals: implications for development of malignant tumors, *Hematol Oncol Clin N Am*, **5:** 357–70.

Pedley S, Hundley F et al., 1984, The genomes of rotaviruses isolated from chronically infected immunodeficient children, *J Gen Virol*, **65:** 1141–50.

Peigue-Lafeuille H, Henquell C et al., 1991, Nosocomial rotavirus infections in adult renal transplant recipients, *J Hosp Infect*, **18:** 67–70.

Penn I, 1986, Cancers of the anogenital region in renal transplant recipients. Analysis of 65 cases, *Cancer*, **58:** 611–16.

Peters BS, Beck EJ et al., 1991, Cytomegalovirus infection in AIDS. Patterns of disease, response to therapy and trends in survival, *J Infect*, **23:** 129–37.

Peterson PK, Balfour HH et al., 1980, Cytomegalovirus disease in renal allograft recipients: a prospective study of the clinical features, risk factors and impact on renal transplantation, *Medicine (Baltimore)*, **59:** 283–300.

Purtilo DT, Cassel C et al., 1975, X-linked recessive progressive combined variable immunodeficiency (Dunan's disease), *Lancet*, **1:** 935–41.

Rabkin CS, Hatzakis A et al., 1993, Cytomegalovirus infection and risk of AIDS in human immunodeficiency virus-infected haemophilia patients, *J Infect Dis*, **168:** 1260–3.

Rand KH, Rasmussen LE et al., 1972, Cellular immunity and herpesvirus infections in cardiac-transplant patients, *N Engl J Med*, **296:** 1372–7.

Rice SJ, Bishop JA et al., 1985, BK virus as a cause of haemorrhagic cystitis after bone marrow transplantation, *Lancet*, **2:** 844–5.

Riddler SA, Breinig MC, McKnight JLC, 1994, Increased levels of circulating Epstein–Barr virus (EBV)-infected lymphocytes and decreased EBV nuclear antigen antibody responses are associated with the development of post-transplant lymphoproliferative disease in solid organ transplant recipients, *Blood*, **84:** 972–84.

Safrin S, Rush JD, Mills J, 1990, Influenza in patients with human immunodeficiency virus infection, *Chest*, **98:** 33–7.

Safrin S, Ashley R et al., 1991, Clinical and serologic features of herpes simplex virus infection in patients with AIDS, *AIDS*, **5:** 1107–10.

Sandvej K, Krenacs L et al., 1992, Epstein–Barr virus latent and replicative gene expression in oral hairy leukoplakia, *Histopathology*, **20:** 387–95.

Savoie A, Perpete C et al., 1994, Direct correlation between the load of Epstein–Barr virus infected lymphocytes in the peripheral blood of paediatric transplant patients and risk of lymphoproliferative disease, *Blood*, **83:** 2715–22.

Schulmann ST, 1985, Acyclovir treatment of disseminated varicella in childhood malignant neoplasms, *Am J Dis Child*, **139:** 137–40.

Simmons A, 1996, Rapid diagnosis of viral infections, *Practical Medical Microbiology*, 14th edn, eds Collee JG, Fraser AG et al., Churchill Livingstone, London, 655–73.

Srugo J, Israele V et al., 1993, Clinical manifestations of varicella-zoster virus infections in human immunodeficiency virus-infected children, *Am J Dis Child*, **147:** 742–5.

St Geme JW, Prince JT et al., 1965, Impaired cellular resistance to herpes simplex virus in Wiskott–Aldrich syndrome, *N Engl J Med*, **273:** 229–34.

Starzl TE, Nalesnik MA et al., 1984, Reversibility of lymphomas and lymphoproliferative lesions developing under cyclosporin A-steroid therapy, *Lancet*, **1:** 583–7.

Stewart JA, Reef SE et al., 1995, Herpesvirus infections in persons infected with human immunodeficiency virus, *Clin Infect Dis*, **21, suppl 1:** 114–20.

Sullivan JL, Woda BA, 1989, X-linked lymphoproliferative syndrome, *Immunodefic Rev*, **1:** 325–47.

Townsend TR, Yolken RA et al., 1982, Outbreak of coxsackie A1 gastroenteritis: a complication of bone-marrow transplantation, *Lancet*, **1:** 820–3.

Vallbracht A, Löhler J et al., 1993, Disseminated BK type polyomavirus infection in an AIDS patient with central nervous system disease, *Am J Pathol*, **143:** 29–39.

Volpi A, Whitley RJ et al., 1983, Rapid diagnosis of pneumonia due to cytomegalovirus with specific monoclonal antibodies, *J Infect Dis*, **147:** 1119–20.

Webster A, Lee CA et al., 1989, Cytomegalovirus infection and progression towards AIDS in haemophiliacs with human immunodeficiency virus infection, *Lancet*, **2:** 63–6.

Whitley RJ, Gnann JW Jr, 1992, Acyclovir: a decade later, *N Engl J Med*, **327:** 782–9.

Youle MS, Gazzard BG et al., 1994, Effects of high dose oral acyclovir on herpesvirus disease and survival in patients with advanced HIV disease: a double-blind placebo-controlled study, *AIDS*, **8:** 641–9.

Part V

Principles of diagnosis and control

Chapter 43

Safety in the Virology Laboratory

Michael P Kiley and Graham Lloyd

1   INTRODUCTION

Most current safety legislation is based on the principles laid down in a variety of government regulations, which may differ slightly from country to country. Examples of such regulations include the Health and Safety at Work Act 1974 in the UK, the Occupational Safety and Health laws in the USA and Labour Canada regulations, all of which place a duty of care on employers in relation to the safety of their employees and others. The laws also require employees to co-operate with employers and place a duty on them to avoid putting themselves, colleagues or others at potential risk. Therefore, overall safety in the virology, or any other, laboratory is the responsibility of all laboratory workers. People in a supervisory or managerial position are responsible for the health, safety and welfare of all staff and visitors in laboratories under their jurisdiction. The emphasis in this chapter, though, is the unique subset of safety issues resulting from the operation of a microbiology laboratory using pathogenic or potentially pathogenic agents. The ability to perform accurate risk assessments (job hazard analysis), based on factual information, is of key importance.

In his review of laboratory-acquired infections, Pike (1979) concluded 'the knowledge, the techniques and the equipment to prevent most laboratory infections are available'. Over the last decade safety-related technology has advanced significantly, developing biosafety systems that provide a safer working environment. Despite these advances, laboratory accidents still occur at a disturbing rate; unfortunately, as in the past, the most common cause of such accidents is human error. New, sophisticated biosafety systems and improved training methods are necessary to cope with the increased challenges raised by the emergence and re-emergence of significant pathogenic viruses such as arenaviruses, dengue viruses, Ebola, hantavirus, the new hepatitis viruses and HIV. The fundamental concepts on which to construct a laboratory safety programme must therefore ensure minimal risk to both laboratory workers and the community. These concepts include both the proper use and maintenance of new safety equipment and, especially, a greater appreciation of good laboratory practice and proper risk assessment.

A safety programme must be based on: a sound understanding of the microbiological properties of the agent to be manipulated; a microbiological risk assessment programme (Advisory Committee on Dangerous Pathogens 1996 [UK]); an understanding of the protective potential of scientific equipment and facilities; comprehensive personnel training and development appropriate to the studies to be undertaken; and use of guidelines and protocols, with the understanding that both must be flexible and dynamic. Any understanding of the properties of a micro-organism must include its virulence, means of spread, tropism, infectious dose and environmental stability. For a safety programme to be effective, it must have the support of laboratory workers and managers. Laboratory management have the ultimate responsibility of providing a safe working environment as described above.

This chapter discusses the typical components of a prudent virology laboratory safety programme. Topics include facilities, containment criteria, work practices, biohazard surveillance, waste management and training. It must be repeated, though, that the cornerstone of any worthwhile safety programme is accurate risk assessment and management that is based on full understanding of the infectious and pathogenic potential of the agents under investigation.

Information on laboratory safety and biosafety may be found in a variety of national and international guidelines or codes of practice (National Institute of Health 1987 [Japan], Ministry of Health 1988 [Sweden], Association Française de Normalisation 1990, Standards Association of Australia 1991, US Department of Health and Human Services 1993, World Health Organization 1993, Advisory Committee on Dangerous Pathogens 1995a, 1995b [UK], Health and Welfare Canada 1996).

2 HISTORICAL PERSPECTIVE

The risk of infection is higher in virology laboratories than in the general population, although the risk of exposure to infectious agents is somewhat less than among other groups of healthcare workers.

To determine the essential components of a laboratory safety programme it is first necessary to assess the 'risk' of infection associated with working in a virus laboratory. Pike (1979) compiled the best collection of data to date dealing with accidental infections of laboratory workers with pathogenic micro-organisms. The analysis was based on global data relating to laboratory-acquired infections recorded from the beginning of the century. Although much of the data covers the period before the age of chemotherapy and biosafety cabinets, it still gives some idea of the potential risk to people working in laboratories. The study concluded that most of the reported infections occurred mainly in research rather than clinical laboratories. However, the data did not provide any information about the changing pattern of laboratory techniques or the relative importance of different groups of infectious agents responsible for the infections.

Examination of these data, as well as analysing more recent anecdotal and unpublished information, has demonstrated a major shift away from bacteria and rickettsiae as the chief causes of laboratory-acquired infections. Most such infections reported in the recent past have been of viral origin (see Table 43.1). The trend is generally a decrease in aerosol infections and an increase in blood-borne diseases.

The overall decrease in aerosol infections in the laboratory is probably due to the development of biosafety cabinets and an increased awareness of the routes of infection and of the need for safe practices in the laboratory. The discovery of antiviral drugs, as well as the increase in the number of vaccines available, has also played a role in the decrease in illness due to laboratory infections. Despite these general trends, though, laboratory-acquired infections still occur regularly; however, because of the lack of a worldwide reporting system and the absence of adequate medical surveillance, their true extent may never be known. In some countries, for example the UK (Health and Safety Executive 1986), microbiological accidents must be reported.

Table 43.1 lists some of the laboratory-acquired infections in virology laboratories reported since 1970. These are merely examples that emphasize the need for a strong and continuing biosafety programme in all virus laboratories. The Subcommittee of Arbovirus Laboratory Safety (1980) collated a number of reports relating to arbovirus incidents involving laboratory workers: Crimean–Congo haemorrhagic fever (8 cases, 1 death); Chikungunya fever (39 cases); Japanese encephalitis (22 cases); Argentinian haemorrhagic fever (21 cases); Kyasanur Forest disease (133 cases); Marburg fever (31 cases, 5 deaths); Rift Valley fever (47 cases); West Nile fever (18 cases); western equine encephalitis (7 cases, 2 deaths); yellow fever (38 cases, 8 deaths); and numerous others.

It should be noted that most of the incidents could have been prevented by the use of common, readily available, biosafety practices. An example of this was seen during the investigation into the cause of several laboratory-acquired dengue virus infections which occurred over a brief period in the late 1980s. It was determined that each infection was due to entry of the virus through a skin abrasion or wound and that these infections could have been prevented by the use of common safety practices such as covering exposed skin or by wearing gloves.

3 COMPONENTS OF A BIOSAFETY PROGRAMME

Rules and regulations about the use, management and disposal of hazardous and carcinogenic chemicals in the laboratory have been in place for some time. The US Fire Protection Agency, US Occupational Safety and Health Administration (OSHA) regulations, UK Health and Safety Executive and Labor Canada are agencies that enforce the regulations which are backed by law. Before 1989, the criteria for working safely with biological materials consisted of a series of guidelines and recommendations issued by such organisations as the US Centers for Disease Control (CDC) and the National Institutes of Health (NIH), the UK Public Health Laboratory Service (PHLS) or professional groups. The Canadian MRC/HWC guidelines were published in 1990.

The concern for laboratory safety generated by the appearance of the human immunodeficiency virus (HIV) as well as the continuing problem of hepatitis B infections among healthcare workers and potential infections from emergent and re-emergent pathogens have led to the adoption of regulations to reduce occupational exposure to blood-borne pathogens. These regulations have taken various forms, such as the UK Management of Health and Safety at Work Regulations 1992, Control of Substances Hazardous to Health Regulations (COSHH) 1994, Categorisation of Biological Agents According to Hazard and Categories of Containment 1995, Workplace (Health, Safety and Welfare) Regulations 1992, Safe Working and the Prevention of Infection in Clinical Laboratories 1991; the European Directives to Member States, relating to the protection and exposure of workers to biological

Table 43.1 Examples of recent laboratory-acquired viral infections

Agent	Country/Date	Laboratory type	Infection route
Dengue (Kiley, unpublished)	USA 1988	Research	Direct
Ebola (Emond et al., 1977)	UK 1976	Research	Needle-stick
Hantaan (Desmyter et al. 1983)	Belgium 1983	Animal house	Aerosol
Hantaan (Lloyd and Jones 1986)	UK 1976	Research	Aerosol
Junin (Weissenbacher et al. 1978)	Argentina 1978	Research	Aerosol (?)
Lassa (Leifer, Gocke and Bourne 1970)	USA 1969	Research	Direct
Marburg (Martini et al. 1969)	Germany 1968	Tissue culture	Direct
	Yugoslavia 1968		
Sabià (Ryder and Gordsman 1995)	USA 1994	Research	Aerosol

agents 1990; the US OSHA Bloodborne Pathogens Standard (29 CFR part 1910.1030); and the Canadian WHIMIS Biosafety Guidelines. They include most of the information in earlier guidelines with recommendations that stress the importance of employee training and education, the use of safety equipment and the duty of an employer to provide a safe working environment. Although the new regulations cover many areas relating to laboratory safety, they should viewed only as a starting point. A comprehensive laboratory safety programme relating to work with biological agents should ensure that:

1 Senior management support it.
2 Full and proper risk policies and procedures are in place, and take into account the agent (virulence, transmissibility, routes of infection); the work being considered; and the codes of practice needed to prevent exposure.
3 Laboratories, their equipment and other facilities are properly maintained for the safe conduct of the work.
4 Laboratories undergo regular safety audits to ensure compliance with agreed protocols and the identification of new problems.
5 Laboratory workers are provided with suitable safety information, safety instruction and training as part of their continuing professional development.
6 An effective infection control programme, including monitoring of exposure, health surveillance and listing of employees working with class 3 and 4 organisms, is developed and implemented.

All staff, regardless of their position, have a duty to protect themselves, their colleagues and the community from any hazard arising from their work.

3.1 Developing a laboratory safety programme

Each safety programme, while having similar objectives, will vary according to the type of institution involved and any unique features present in the local regulations. Factors to be considered include the scope of the work done, the level of technical expertise of laboratory staff, the availability of personal protective equipment (laboratory coats and gowns, gloves,

eye protection, respiratory protective equipment, ear defenders) and laboratory hardware designed to ensure a safe work environment. Of equal importance is engineering support to ensure the proper installation and maintenance of biosafety cabinets and fume hoods, eye washes, and the proper air balance. It is also crucial that staff understand, and use, the correct procedures for operating laboratory equipment.

4 MICROBIOLOGICAL RISK ASSESSMENT AND INFECTION CONTROL

The exact incidence of occupational infection among laboratory workers is unknown. A number of published reports detail individual or small group outbreaks of laboratory-acquired infections, retrospective studies and anecdotal information but there has been no report that has succeeded in determining the population at risk for any of these incidents. The overall mortality of reported cases is c. 4% but this number is probably very high considering the unknown denominator and the great number of unreported illnesses.

All virology laboratories should provide safe working conditions for all staff. In order to accomplish this goal it is essential to understand and determine the possible risks involved in the manipulation and propagation of viruses (including genetically manipulated viruses), the propagation of viruses in cell cultures and undertaking viral immunoassays. In addition, the potential hazards of chemicals and radiological products used must be taken into account during the risk assessment to reduce exposure to non-microbiological hazards.

It is increasingly recognized that a structured microbiological risk assessment (MRA) is necessary to identify and characterize microbiological hazards associated with laboratory working practices. Such formal risk assessments underpin current legislation in the UK (Health and Safety Executive 1994); Europe (EC Directive 90/679); Canada (Workplace Hazardous Materials Information System (WHIMIS), 1987) and the USA (OSHA). Although such legislation requires employees to make suitable assessments of risk, they do not offer any formal guidelines on conducting risk analysis. Several agencies have begun to produce risk assessment guidelines on specific viruses: for example, HIV ([UK] Departments of Health 1990); hepatitis ([UK] Public Health Service 1992); and bovine spongiform encephalitis ([UK] Health and Safety Executive 1996). For the process to be meaningful, it is important that formal risk analysis be undertaken on laboratory work practices, including the following:

1 Risk assessment that identifies the source(s) of the hazard(s) and quantifies the risk of each hazard within the conditions examined.
2 Identification of the gravity of the risk, to guide the management of that risk.
3 A formal record of the assessment and recommendation of working practice that is communicated to all staff.
4 A regular review process.

For any risk assessment to be acceptable, some attempt at measurement or quantification of the risk(s) must be made. This relies on available experimental data, case and epidemiological information and population studies including mathematical modelling, all of which relate to different aspects of risk.

It is important when establishing an infection control/medical surveillance programme that the institution's authorities understand the relative risks that their employees face. This requires information about infectious agents and other potential sources of risk that are likely to be found at their institution. Laboratories should be especially alert if dealing with large numbers and wide varieties of clinical or veterinary materials received for laboratory diagnosis or research.

Knowledge of infectious disease processes is the cornerstone of an infection control programme. People must be identified whose duties include routine and anticipated tasks involving or potentially involving exposure to infectious material. Particular duties must be evaluated for their 'infectious potential'. It is the job that is rated and not the individual, although anyone who is highly susceptible to infection should be excluded from duties that are not a risk to the normal population. Especially vulnerable are people whose immune system has been compromised, for whatever reason. The infectious potential of any job is usually determined by asking a series of questions about the work involved. For example, does the individual routinely come in contact with virus-containing blood or blood products? Does the individual routinely handle incoming shipments of potentially infectious material? Other information required may include the type of laboratory equipment that is used, the nature of the materials used and whether test samples are inactivated.

Once it has been determined that a worker is at risk, a written infection control plan for that position must be considered. This plan should contain an exposure determination (the criteria used to evaluate the position), a schedule and method for meeting any relevant safety standards and the content of any training to be undertaken. A well structured and recorded training programme is vitally important to overall laboratory safety. Training should include familiarization with the nature of laboratory pathogens, and proper and safe use of laboratory equipment. A laboratory safety manual (or code of laboratory practice) must be developed and available to all employees and should include all approved laboratory protocols as well as a list of duties and

responsibilities. One of the responsibilities of any laboratory worker should be to report any incident that might have the potential for an occupational exposure, according to a defined incidence policy.

Any infection control policy should include medical surveillance. This should incorporate a medical evaluation including an occupational/medical history and a physical examination covering conditions that a physician feels might interfere with a worker's ability to use personal protective equipment. It is also essential to ensure that all workers are adequately immunized.

A major goal of an effective medical surveillance policy is to educate workers of the need, and indeed the requirement, to report an occupational exposure. Employees should also have the right to a confidential medical evaluation and follow-up after reporting such an incident. Elements of such a follow-up include documentation of the events surrounding the exposure, the source (if known) and the route of exposure. For incidents involving possible exposure to HIV or Lassa virus, a quick decision may be necessary as to whether to begin AZT or other treatment regimen, or ribavirin treatment. It is therefore prudent to have an established policy covering the various possibilities within any establishment handling viruses. Continuing follow-up, including counselling and illness reporting, should also be part of the programme.

A surveillance policy designed for reporting illnesses away from the work-site should also be developed. A typical plan should include employees carrying an information card that will notify treating physicians that the patient may be at risk of certain diseases because of his or her occupation. The card would also contain a means for contacting the employee's institution if it is deemed necessary, such as a physician noting symptoms compatible with a disease related to that person's work. The system is important for two reasons:

1 It is essential for an employer to know if more than one employee has contracted a similar disease, because this may be an indication of a common occupational source.
2 Maintenance of a good reporting system helps to determine any source of infection. Experience has taught us that examination of most laboratory accident reports seldom pinpoints the source of occupationally acquired illnesses.

It is evident that a good infection control/medical surveillance programme requires well designed and clearly written procedures and policies. It is also essential that the policy be made known to all employees at their induction and any modifications circulated as part of a continuing process of awareness. Results of investigations of laboratory incidents, with a guarantee of anonymity, should be widely published for educational purposes. Laboratory workers should be made to appreciate the ultimate goal and benefit of policy and not be made to fear it.

All workers in microbiology laboratories should provide a baseline serum sample; consideration should be given to establishing a system whereby employees are tested at quarterly intervals for evidence of infection by any agents used in the laboratory, the purpose being to detect silent infections. Although this policy has not been adopted in all parts of the world, knowledge of such subclinical infections can lead to examination of safety procedures, which may result in changes that will eliminate the potential for infections with clinical, and therefore possibly political, consequences. A major laboratory has recently been able to detect silent infections with a virus with known pathogenic relatives that were being studied there. Procedural and protocol changes have eliminated the potential for what could have been a very serious incident.

4.1 Definition of hazard groups

The classification of microbial pathogens is based on the inherent hazard of the organism. The corresponding levels of containment set out in Table 43.2 are intended to compensate for microbial risks encountered when working with pathogens as defined in the various hazard groups. 'Hazard' is taken as expressing the level of danger associated with the nature of the organism and 'risk' as the probability that in some circumstances the dangers will be manifested as an infection. The more inherently infectious the microbe, the higher the risk. In reality there are different levels of risk arising from work with viruses, depending on such factors as the immune status of the individual, the dose, the route and the site of infection.

Categorizing any virus into the currently recognized 4 hazard groups depends on whether the organism is: (1) infectious for people; (2) hazardous to laboratory workers; (3) transmissible to the community; and (4) susceptible to effective prophylaxis or treatment.

All pathogenic viruses (and other micro-organisms) are assigned to one of the higher hazard groups according to the infective hazard they pose for healthy workers. The categorization does not allow for any additional risks that an organism can present to people who may be more severely affected for other reasons, such as pre-existing disease, compromised immunity, pregnancy or the effects of medication.

The hazard group assigned to a particular organism indicates the minimum level of containment under which it must be handled. It should be noted that viruses listed under one category may require a containment level different from that normally assigned. The decision may be influenced by the techniques used (animal infection, virus concentration procedures or production of an aerosol). It should also be noted that some organisms are subject to monitoring by national departments of agriculture and fisheries.

5 STANDARD MICROBIOLOGICAL CODE OF SAFETY PRACTICES

The importance of establishing good laboratory practices cannot be overstated. Previous investigations of laboratory accidents indicate that failures in good laboratory practice are frequently the direct cause of accidents. Information derived from the investigation of laboratory accidents, practical experience obtained from working in microbiological laboratories and the application of informed risk assessment have contributed to the development of a list of good working practices.

1 Management practice should ensure that all laboratory personnel are competent and understand the biological and other hazards found in a laboratory, and are fully trained to the biohazard level required before undertaking any work.

2 The laboratory director should be the individual responsible for granting or limiting access to the laboratory. In general, people who are at increased risk of infection or for whom infection may be particularly dangerous should not be allowed in the laboratory. Some other situations, such as a pregnancy, will have to be considered on an individual basis. Children under the age of 16 should not be allowed in the laboratory. Animals not involved in laboratory procedures should never be allowed in the laboratory.

3 A laboratory code of practice should be available, read and signed before a new member of staff commences work.

4 Laboratories should have a designated biological safety officer and/or a safety committee whose responsibilities include ensuring that all work is carried out in accordance with established safety practices.

5 Laboratories must be kept clean, neat and orderly, and all materials or equipment not pertinent to the work should be kept to the minimum.

6 Access to the laboratory must be strictly limited to authorised personnel (especially biosafety level 3 and 4 (BL3 and 4) laboratories). The laboratory door should remain closed and an international biohazard sign should be prominently displayed on the door, indicating that the room contains potentially infectious material. When an infectious agent (or agents) used in the laboratory requires special provisions for entry (e.g. vaccination), the relevant information must be included in the sign, together with the name of the individual responsible for the laboratory.

7 Work surfaces should be decontaminated daily, and immediately following any spill involving potentially infectious material.

8 All procedures should minimize the production of aerosols. This usually requires the development of standard operating practice and risk assessments for all laboratory procedures, and the timely review of these procedures to ensure that they are abreast of current technology and take advantage of the latest innovations in safety.

9 Procedures that have the potential for producing an infectious aerosol should be undertaken within a biosafety cabinet. **It is essential that all people who use such cabinets understand the principles of their operation.**

10 Laboratory coats, gowns, smocks or uniforms should be worn in the laboratory, and removed before leaving the laboratory for other areas. Although a regular laboratory coat is sufficient for most clinical/diagnostic laboratory situations, a rear-closing, solid-front gown is required when practising BL3 procedures.

11 Face and eye protection or other such devices

Table 43.2 Comparative categorization of biological agents and categories of containment

Country/Organization	Disease	Facility
Australia	Biosecurity level 1	Biosecurity level 1
	Biosecurity level 2	Biosecurity level 2
	Biosecurity level 2(E)	Biosecurity level 2(E)
	Biosecurity level 3	Biosecurity level 3
	Biosecurity level 3(E)	Biosecurity level 3(E)
	Biosecurity level 3(Z)	Biosecurity level 3(Z)
	Biosecurity level 4	Biosecurity level 4
Canada	Risk group 1	Containment level 1
	Risk group 2	Containment level 2
	Risk group 3	Containment level 3
	Risk group 4	Containment level 4
European Directive	Group 1	Containment level 1
	Group 2	Containment level 2
	Group 3	Containment level 3
	Group 4	Containment level 4
UK	Hazard group 1	Laboratory containment 1
	Hazard group 2	Laboratory containment 2
	Hazard group 3	Laboratory containment 3
	Hazard group 4	Laboratory containment 4
USA	Class 1	Biosafety 1
	Class 2	Biosafety 2
	Class 3	Biosafety 3
	Class 4	Biosafety 4
	Class 5[a]	Biosafety 3 or 4[b]
WHO	Risk group 1	Basic biosafety level 1
	Risk group 2	Basic biosafety level 2
	Risk group 3	Containment biosafety level 3
	Risk group 4	Maximum containment 4

E, exotic; Z, zoonotic
[a]Non-indigenous pathogens
[b]Facility use dependent upon virus and work involved.

must be worn when it is necessary to protect from splashes, impacting objects, harmful substances and UV light, especially if the work is carried out on the open bench.

12 Gloves must be worn for all procedures that might involve contact between broken skin or mucous membranes and potentially infectious material, toxins or infected animals. This usually means wearing gloves for most laboratory work, including drawing blood. Gloves used in the laboratory are generally made of latex or a vinyl compound (usually polvinylchloride, PVC), and there seems to be no difference in barrier effectiveness between gloves made of either material. When choosing gloves, consideration should be given to the toxic products (e.g. vinyl chloride and hydrochloric acid) produced when PVC gloves are incinerated.

13 Mechanical pipetting devices should be used; mouth pipetting should never be permitted. Modern mechanical pipetting devices are available for almost any laboratory situation.

14 Eating, drinking, smoking, application of cosmetics or storage of food should be strictly prohibited in laboratory work areas.

15 Staff must wash their hands immediately after handling any infectious materials or animals and when leaving the laboratory. For this purpose sinks, preferably with foot or elbow controls and located near the exit door, should be provided in each laboratory. Because of the number of times hands are washed it is probably best to use a mild soap with a lanolin base; although these soaps are not disinfectants, their use should remove most surface microbes from the skin.

16 All contaminated or infectious liquid or solid materials must be decontaminated before disposal or cleaning for reuse. Contaminated materials that are autoclaved or incinerated at a site away from the laboratory must be packaged and labelled properly for transport and have the outside of the container disinfected chemically.

17 Accidents and incidents should be immediately reported to and recorded by the person responsible for the work and to the proper safety and occupational health authorities.

18 Appropriate medical surveillance and treatment should be provided.

19 Hypodermic needles, syringes and needles, and scalpels, collectively referred as 'sharps', are the

main source of accidents. It is therefore especially important that laboratory workers, as well as others, use and dispose of these items with extreme caution. Needles and syringes should be restricted to parenteral injection and aspiration of fluids from laboratory animals. Only needle-locking syringes or disposable syringe–needle units should be used. Needles should not be recapped or removed by hand; attempts to perform these procedures are a major cause of needle-stick injuries. Whenever a person's free hand is near a syringe and needle in the other hand, the potential for an accident is very high. Several recent needle-stick injuries have occurred when used syringes, capped or uncapped, were placed in the pocket of a laboratory coat and either the individual wearing the coat or a colleague was subsequently stuck. Hypodermic needles and syringes should not be used as substitutes for pipetting devices in the manipulation of infectious fluids. Once used, needles should be promptly placed in a puncture-proof container and decontaminated, preferably by incineration or autoclaving, before disposal.

20 Any soiled 'sharp', except non-disposable items, should be placed in a sharps disposal container. Needles should be placed in such a container uncapped along with used scalpels and other sharps. The sharps container itself must be of rigid construction and leak-proof. The top opening should be large enough so that the used sharps can be dropped into the container without the need to overfill it. These containers should have a top that closes easily and tightly when it is full, and they should be placed at convenient locations throughout the laboratory. When full, a container should be decontaminated by autoclaving and then it and its contents should be incinerated.

21 In modern laboratories instrumentation is a potential source of laboratory accidents. These accidents may involve chemical or electrical hazards or the possibility of infection with a biological agent. Centrifuges – ultra, high speed or clinical – are always a potential source of aerosols. Care should be taken to load and unload centrifuge tubes containing infectious or harmful material in a biosafety cabinet. It is also prudent to use sealed tubes or safety heads while centrifuging such dangerous material. Automated analysers are another potential source of danger in the laboratory. Blood or serum samples are often introduced into the instrument under pressure, which can increase the potential for aerosolization. The level of containment of such equipment will depend on the risk assessment and the infectious nature of the material.

22 A programme for insect and rodent control should be in place.

23 If an autoclave is not present in the laboratory, all potentially infectious material for decontamination must be taken out of the laboratory in containers that preclude both aerosolization and leakage of the contents.

6 BIOSAFETY LABORATORIES

Working with potentially infectious viruses in the microbiological laboratory requires an appreciation both of work practices and of the facilities needed to make such laboratories a safe environment. Guidelines on the safe handling of pathogens have evolved over the last decade and have reached the point where there is general agreement on the basic principles of biosafety in the laboratory (Table 43.3). Four biosafety levels have been described (BL1 through BL4), which comprise combinations of laboratory practices and procedures, safety equipment and laboratory facilities appropriate for the operations performed and the hazard posed by the infectious agent. Essentially, the numerical designation of a safety level increases with an increase in the risks involved in working with an agent.

The levels of containment are intended to reflect the risks encountered when working with biological agents as categorized in the various hazard groups. All laboratories in which there is likely to be exposure to human pathogens (whether or not they are to be propagated or concentrated) require a minimum of BL2 containment. When there is a likelihood or strong indication that material (specimens or samples) contains BL3 or BL4 agents, additional controls are necessary.

Many national guidelines list the essential laboratory procedures that are basic to good laboratory practice (Table 43.4). It must be emphasized that good microbiological practice is fundamental to laboratory safety and cannot be replaced by specialised equipment or safety barriers, which can only supplement it.

6.1 Biosafety level 1

BL1 practices, safety equipment and laboratory facilities require no special engineering features for work with organisms that present no danger to humans. Examples of laboratories that may be operated at this level include undergraduate training and teaching laboratories. In these laboratories work is undertaken with well characterized agents that are most unlikely to cause disease in normal healthy adult humans. Many agents not normally able to produce disease in healthy individuals may produce severe illness in elderly people, the immunodeficient or the immunosuppressed, and can cause allergic or toxogenic responses, so appropriate precautions must be taken. Also, vaccine strains that, because they are attenuated in virulence, do not usually produce disease in healthy individuals may produce severe disease in some individuals. The latter two categories of organisms should be manipulated under BL2 conditions.

Work is generally conducted on the bench, and specialized containment equipment is not normally required. Laboratory personnel should have specific

Table 43.3 General summary of relation between hazard groups and biosafety level, work practices and containment level

Hazard group	Biosafety level (BL)	Working practices and procedures (use)	Engineering considerations
1	BL1	Standard microbiological practices (SMP)	No special engineering requirements; containment achieved by adherence to standard laboratory practice
2	BL2	BL1 work practice, *plus*: Limit access Limit aerosols Biohazard signs Laboratory code of practice Protective personal equipment (PPE): gloves, laboratory coats, face protection as needed Infectious waste decontaminated	Procedures that produce potentially infectious aerosols performed in a biological safety cabinet (BSC) On-site autoclave required
3	BL3	BL2 work practice, *plus*: All virus material contained Restricted access PPE: gloves, protective laboratory clothing, respiratory protection as needed	Inward airflow Air-lock facility Exhaust air discharged from laboratory via HEPA filtration (optional)
4	BL4 (maximum containment)	BL3 work practice, *plus* Change of clothing before entry Shower on exit All waste autoclaved before leaving facility Regular engineering and biosafety maintenance	HEPA-filtered supply and exhaust air Work undertaken in BSC class III cabinets or BSC II using an air-supplied positive full-body pressure suit in an airtight laboratory All waste decontaminated

Table 43.4 Summary of basic laboratory containment requirements at different containment levels

Containment requirements	Containment levels			
	1	2	3	4
Laboratory site: isolation	No	No	Partial	Yes
Laboratory: sealable	No	No	Yes	Yes
Ventilation:				
Inward airflow/negative pressure	Opt	Opt	Yes	Yes
Through safety cabinet	No	Opt	Opt	No
Mechanical: direct	No	Opt	Opt	No
Mechanical: independent	No	No	Opt	Yes
Airlock	No	No	Yes	Yes
Airlock: with shower	No	No	No/Opt	Yes
Effluent treatment	No	No	Yes	Yes
Autoclave site:				
On site	No	No	No	No
En suite	No	Yes	Yes	No
In laboratory: free-standing	No	No	Opt	No
In laboratory: double-ended	No	No	Rec	Yes
Microbiological safety cabinet/enclosure	No	Opt	Yes	Yes
Biosafety cabinet	NR	I	I/III	III I/II[a]

[a]Class I and II biological safety cabinets permitted with use of positive-pressure suits
NR, not required; Opt, optional; Rec, recommended.

training in the procedures undertaken within the laboratory and be supervised by experienced senior staff. The following laboratory facilities and basic work practices apply to viruses assigned to BL1.

LABORATORY FACILITIES

Laboratories should be designed so that the floors, walls and ceilings are easy to clean. Bench tops should be impervious to water and resistant to acids, alkalis, organic solvents and moderate heat. Laboratory furniture should be of similar resistant materials and be arranged so as not to obstruct workers while performing their duties. Equipment should be placed where it is easily accessible for cleaning and, if it is likely to produce an aerosol, in the safest possible location. Attention should be paid to door swings because a door opening in the wrong direction has the potential to knock items from someone's hands. Equipment must not be placed near thermostats, because it may interfere with temperature control. Floors should be non-skid, to reduce the likelihood of slipping. Handwashing facilities must be provided, preferably near the point of exit.

6.2 Biosafety level 2

Conditions described for BL2 are usually applicable to clinical, diagnostic, research and teaching facilities in which work is done with a wide variety of microorganisms that cause human disease and may be a hazard to laboratory workers but unlikely to spread to the community. Laboratory exposure rarely produces infection, and effective prophylaxis or treatment is usually available. Many of the agents that require BL2 containment are already present in the community, and community vaccination programmes for them are routine.

Hepatitis A virus, herpes simplex types 1 and 2, measles, Epstein–Barr virus and certain viral vaccines are among those that can be manipulated at the BL2 level. Generally the agents that are assigned to this level cause blood-borne diseases and do not have a history of infection via the respiratory route. It is not surprising, then, that the usual routes of laboratory-acquired infections with agents in this group are auto-inoculation, ingestion and mucous membrane exposure to the infectious agent. Procedures with agents assigned to this level that have a high probability of aerosol production should be conducted in primary containment equipment (e.g. Class 2 biosafety cabinet) or similar devices.

The competence expected of laboratory workers is greater than that of a newly qualified graduate. Personnel at this level need to be familiar with the institution's safety policy, to have received training in the handling of the viruses and be supervised by a competent senior member of staff.

LABORATORY DESIGN

The laboratory requiring BL2 containment is generally similar in construction and design to a BL1 facility. It also incorporates criteria for microbiological practices in association with additional primary and secondary containment facilities (Fig. 43.1).

The equipment is selected according to the following principles:

1 Designed to prevent or limit exposure of the operator to infectious material.
2 Constructed of materials that are resistant to corrosion and meet structural requirements.
3 Installed to aid operation, maintenance, cleaning, decontamination and safety testing
4 Complies with safety specifications.

Laboratories that anticipate working with potentially infectious material should use a biosafety cabinet, isolator or other suitable containment. Standard laboratory working practice is undertaken at this level, with additional features that reflect the higher containment level (see Tables 43.3 and 43.4). Procedures with the potential for creating infectious aerosols should be conducted within a biosafety containment cabinet. These include grinding, blending, vigorous shaking or mixing, sonic disruption and opening containers of infectious materials. Intranasal inoculation of animals and harvesting infectious tissues from animals or eggs should also be done in a biosafety cabinet or equivalent. Any work with high concentrations of infectious agents should be carried out in a containment cabinet. The reduction of aerosols is also a consideration when working with many of the analytical machines found in any virology laboratory. Special precautions should be taken with machines such as cell sorters and when loading analytical machines where the sample may be under pressure and more likely to produce an aerosol. In many cases a splash-guard may suffice.

There may be occasions when agents routinely manipulated at BL2 may require BL3 containment, or at least BL3 practices. This usually occurs when the procedures produce concentrations significantly exceeding the physiological concentration of the agent in nature. A higher biosafety level should also be considered for studies involving animals.

6.3 Biosafety level 3

All the laboratory design features and working practices required for BL2 are applicable to BL3, with special emphasis on some of them. The work practices, safety equipment and facilities for BL3 apply when working with indigenous or exotic agents and when aerosol infection is a significant possibility resulting in disease that may have serious, or even lethal, consequences. Agents for which BL3 safeguards are routinely recommended include *Hantavirus* (Hantaan, Seoul, Sin Nombre) and St Louis encephalitis virus. Two of the more exotic agents that require BL3 containment are Rift Valley fever virus and yellow fever virus, haemorrhagic fever viruses from Africa that can be worked with at this level provided workers are immunized.

Although autoinoculation, ingestion and mucous membrane contamination are hazards with these agents the major concern is aerosol infection. The

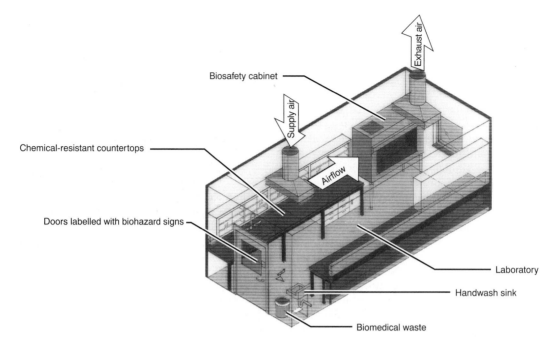

Fig. 43.1 A schematic of a generic BL2 laboratory design. (Courtesy of Smith Carter, architects, engineers, planners, interior designers.)

requirements for BL3 are more stringent than those for BL2 and are aimed at controlling aerosol production and possible spread into the community.

The laboratory staff must understand the safety procedures as well as the risks involved in working with the agents used in their laboratory. Training, including the use of specialized equipment, should be done by competent scientists who have experience of working with the viruses contained at this level.

LABORATORY DESIGN

The laboratory has engineering and design features and physical containment equipment additional to those found at BL2 (see Tables 43.3 and 43.4). Principal differences from BL2 requirements are that the laboratory must be separated from other laboratory space by an anteroom and that personnel access is strictly controlled. The laboratory must be maintained at an air pressure negative to the atmosphere (maintain a verifiable inward directional air flow) and extracted air must be HEPA filtered (in some countries) and discharged to the outside so that it is dispersed clear of adjacent buildings or air intakes (Fig. 43.2).

Laboratory practices

All work involving infectious material is undertaken within biosafety cabinets by staff wearing full frontal gowns, gloves and eye protection. Alternatively, some laboratories prefer to use class III cabinets. Contaminated solid materials that are to be decontaminated at a site away from the laboratory are sealed in a leak-proof container before being removed to an autoclave and then incineration. Contaminated liquids are autoclaved or disinfected in the laboratory area. An auto-

clave should be available in the laboratory or laboratory suite.

6.4 Biosafety level 4

This containment level is to be used when working with viruses that cause severe human disease (some with a high mortality rate), and present a serious hazard to laboratory workers for which there is no vaccine or generally no reliable treatment. A variety of agents causing haemorrhagic fevers, including Lassa, Marburg, Ebola, Congo–Crimean haemorrhagic fever and related viruses, are those most commonly studied at BL4.

LABORATORY DESIGN

The laboratory is either a separate building or an isolated zone equivalent to a separate building within a building. Mainly because of their high construction and operational costs, there are fewer than 10 BL4 laboratories in the world.

There are 2 operational designs that provide efficient primary containment. The first and oldest system is based on protecting the worker from exposure by containing the agent within a series of interconnecting air-tight class III biosafety cabinets (Fig. 43.3).

Each cabinet is equipped with its own HEPA filtered air supply and extracts exhaust air via HEPA filters in series, and can be independently sealed and fumigated without interference with the rest of the system. All equipment (refrigerators, freezers, microscopes, centrifuges and incubators) is built as an integral part of the system. All staff have a complete change of clothing and shower after each day's work. All work is conducted through glove ports. The cabinet system is

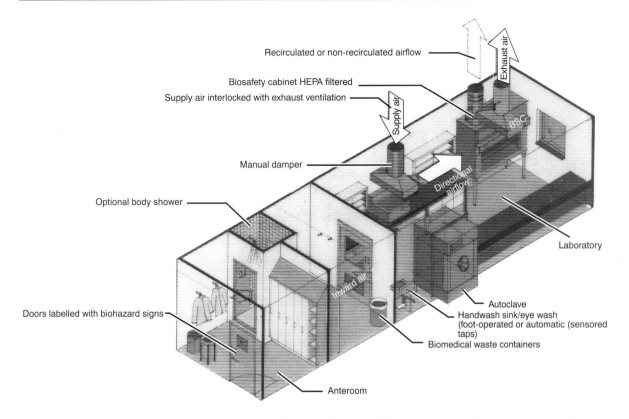

Fig. 43.2 A schematic of a generic BL3 laboratory design. (Courtesy of Smith Carter, architects, engineers, planners, interior designers.)

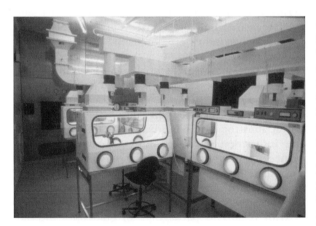

Fig. 43.3 Cabinet-line BL4 laboratory.

connected to a double-ended high-containment auto-clave, through which all liquid and solid waste is decontaminated before being removed for inciner-ation. A chemical 'dunk tank' or formaldeclave is located at the other end of the system, through which suitably packaged material can be taken in or out of the system. The whole system is incorporated within a laboratory providing environmental protection and operating an interlocking HEPA filtered supply and exhaust air system.

The alternative system, 'the suit laboratory' isolates the workers from the laboratory environment by means of fully encapsulating suits supplied with air from outside the laboratory (Fig. 43.4). By the use of

special construction techniques (impermeable sur-faces and welded ductwork) the laboratory facility pro-vides the biosafety barrier that ensures the protection of the exterior environment. Work with infectious material is carried out within class II biosafety cabi-nets. Air from the room and biosafety cabinets is removed via HEPA filtration, the HEPA filters are also an integral component of the supply air ductwork. A special chemical shower must be provided to decon-taminate the surface of the suit before the worker leaves the area. A double-doored autoclave is provided for decontaminating waste materials to be removed from the suit area. When necessary, appropriate material may be removed from the laboratory, without heat treatment, by proper packaging and removal through the chemical shower or a dunk tank.

Laboratory practices

Basic work practices are undertaken in the same man-ner in both systems. Because of the complexity of the work, a detailed code of practice should be developed and form part of an individualized training pro-gramme. On entering, staff should put on a complete change of clothing; before leaving, they must shower before putting on their own clothing. Entry and exit of personnel and supplies must only be through an air-lock or pass-through system. All fluid effluents from the facility, including shower water, must be rendered safe before final release.

A regular, rigorous, preventative maintenance pro-gramme for the engineering controls, air flow, auto-

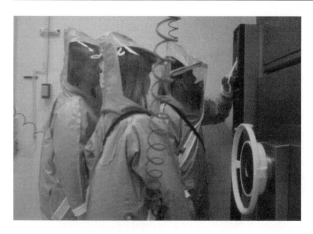

Fig. 43.4 BL4 suit laboratory.

clave, safety cabinets etc. should be developed to ensure continued integration of the facilities and suitability of the safety procedures. Within the UK the Health and Safety Commission institute regular safety inspections of the facilities, safety management and procedures.

7 LABORATORY WASTE

The general principle involved in the treatment of laboratory waste is that all infectious or potentially infectious laboratory waste must be rendered non-infectious before leaving the laboratory. An alternative is to develop a system whereby infectious material can be safely delivered to an off-site disposal facility.

In general, local regulations cover the disposal of infectious waste. There are different interpretations of what constitutes 'infectious waste', so this must be considered when developing a waste management programme. A programme designed to minimize the production of regulated waste will reap cost savings because regulated waste is far more costly to dispose of.

8 PACKING AND SHIPPING OF INFECTIOUS MATERIALS

The safe shipment of infectious substances or diagnostic specimens within or between countries is important for everyone involved with the process. Although no reports of illness have been attributed to the transportation of such materials, there are numerous areas of conflicting guidelines throughout the world. Because these packages have the potential for harbouring infectious agents and move in public places during their journey, their transportation is strictly regulated. Postal and transport authorities have always been aware of the potential hazards to their employees of infectious material transported and handled by them.

In many countries such material is sent through the mail, and local regulations apply; guidelines are often issued (e.g. the *Post Office Guide* in the UK and the *Postal Service Manual* in the USA). The USPS require-

ments for the mailing of 'diseased tissue, blood, serum, and cultures of pathogenic micro-organisms' are listed in their Postal Service Manuals.

The US Department of Transportation, the UK's Health and Safety Executive and Canada's Transport Canada have a major responsibility for safe transportation and provide the authorisation for the movement of hazardous materials within their respective countries and to foreign countries. The importation of infectious agents that are predominately pathogenic to animals also needs to take into account various national regulations and permit requirements. (UK: Importation of Animal Pathogens Order 1980; Canada: Animal Disease Protection Act; USA: USDA, APHIS 9 CFR Parts 94 and 95). Workers sending infectious material to other laboratories should ensure that those laboratories have the facilities to work with the agent. This applies particularly to the transfer of viruses in hazard groups 3 and 4. In the USA new regulations have just been enacted on this aspect (42 CFR Part 72, sections 6 and 7).

An agreement between the Universal Postal Union (UPU), the International Air Transport Association (IATA) and the International Civil Aviation Organization (ICAO) led to new regulations for overseas mail. The IATA/ICAO guidelines and procedures also should be considered because they were designed to facilitate the safe shipment of infectious substances while ensuring the safety of the transport personnel and the general public. The regulations define the terms 'diagnostic specimen', 'biological product' and 'aetiological agent', and give minimum packaging requirements and volume limits for each.

The regulations define a diagnostic specimen as 'any human or animal material including, but not limited to, excreta, secretions, blood and its components, tissue, and tissue fluids, being shipped for the purposes of diagnosis (excluding live infected animals)'. These must be transported under ICAO/IATA packing instruction 602. Infectious substances are 'substances containing viable micro-organisms or toxins known or suspected to cause diseases in animals or humans (including HIV)' and are transported according to ICAO/IATA packing instruction 650.

With regard to packaging, all guidelines indicate that no one may knowingly transport or cause to be transported, directly or indirectly, any diagnostic specimens or biological product which they reasonably believe may contain an aetiological agent unless such material is packaged to withstand leakage of contents, shocks, pressure changes and other conditions incident to ordinary handling in transportation. The major decision to be made, then, when determining the transport requirements for any sample is whether it contains an aetiological agent. It is prudent to be conservative in this matter and assume that each specimen may contain an agent unless you are certain that it does not.

The current packaging requirement is for triple packaging. A securely closed, water-tight primary container is enclosed in a second, durable water-tight container, with enough material in the space between them to absorb all of the contents of the primary container in the event of leakage. Each set of primary and secondary containers is then enclosed in an outer shipping container constructed of fibreboard, cardboard, wood or other material of equivalent strength. An aetiological agent/biomedical material sticker is required for the outer mailing package. Any packaging requiring solid carbon dioxide (dry ice) should ensure that it permits the release of carbon dioxide gas to prevent the build-up of pressure.

On 1 January 1995, IATA (a voluntary organization of air carriers) issued requirements for packaging, and has established a certification procedure for packaging companies who wish to provide packages to ship 'infectious material' on aircraft. Certification of packaging is now a requirement.

9 SUMMARY

A variety of publications already cover the many topics involved in general safety, laboratory safety and biosafety. In this chapter we have tried to make virologists aware of the range of guidelines and regulations that affect work in a virology laboratory. But we have also attempted to present the issue of biosafety from the view of the scientist. Virological scientific programmes need to be conducted in an efficient and safe manner. Because it is the scientists who should have the best knowledge of the nature of the agents under investigation, including factors such as pathogenic potential, they should play a pivotal role in the development of continuing biosafety policy.

The biosafety professionals have knowledge of the guidelines and regulations that apply to the operation of a virology laboratory. They also have knowledge of the latest in biosafety technology and practices that have been developed around the world. In addition, occupational safety and health professionals generally have information in such areas as transportation of specimens and requirements for importation of agents, which can help the laboratory function more efficiently.

A good working relationship between scientists and biosafety professionals can go a long way to ensure that the primary mission of the laboratory, the programme, can be conducted efficiently and safely.

REFERENCES

Advisory Committee on Dangerous Pathogens [UK], 1995a, *Categorisation of Biological Agents according to Hazard and Categories of Containment*, 4th edn, HMSO, London.

Advisory Committee on Dangerous Pathogens [UK], 1995b, *Protection against Blood-borne Infections at Work – HIV and hepatitis*, HMSO, London.

Advisory Committee on Dangerous Pathogens [UK], 1996, *Microbiological Risk Assessment. An interim report*, HMSO, London.

Association Française de Normalisation, 1990, *Liste des espèces microbiennes communement reconnues comme pathogènes pour l'homme [List of microbial species known to be pathogenic for man]*, AFNOR, Paris.

Departments of Health [UK], 1990, *Guidance for Clinical Health Care Workers: protection against infection with HIV and hepatitis viruses*, HMSO, London.

Desmyter J, LeDuc JW et al., 1983, Laboratory rat associated outbreak of haemorrhagic fever with renal syndrome due to hantaan-like virus, *Lancet*, **2**: 1445–8.

EC Directive, 1990, *Protection of Workers from Risks related to Exposure to Biological Agents at Work*, 90/679/EEC.

EC Directive, 1993, *Biological Agents Directive*, 93/88/EEC.

Emond RTD, Evans B et al., 1977, A case of Ebola virus infection, *Br Med J*, **2**: 541–4.

Health and Safety Executive [UK], 1986, *A Guide to the Reporting of Injuries, Diseases and Dangerous Occurrences Regulations (RIDDOR)*, HMSO, London.

Health and Safety Executive [UK], 1994, *Control of Substances Hazardous to Health Regulations (COSHH)*, HMSO, London.

Health and Safety Executive [UK], 1996, *BSE (Bovine Spongiform Encephalopathy): background and general occupational guidance*, HMSO, London.

Health and Welfare Canada, 1996, *Laboratory Biosafety Guidelines*, 2nd edn, Laboratory Centre for Disease Control, Health Protection Branch, Ottawa.

Labour Canada, 1987, *Workplace Hazardous Materials Information System (WHIMIS)*, Canada Labour Code, Bill C-70, Ottawa.

Leifer E, Gocke DJ, Bourne H, 1970, Lassa fever. A new virus disease of man from West Africa. II. Report of a laboratory acquired infection, *Am J Trop Med Hyg*, **19**: 677–9.

Lloyd G, Jones N, 1986, Infections of laboratory workers with Hantaan virus acquired from immunocytomas propagated in laboratory rats, *J Infect*, **12**: 117–25.

Martini GA, Knauff HG et al., 1969, A hitherto unknown infectious disease contracted from monkeys, *German Med Mth*, **8**: 457–69.

Ministry of Health [Sweden], 1988, *Arbetarskyddsstyrelsens kungörelse med foreskrifter om mikroorganismer samt allmana rad om tillämpningen av foreskrifterna. [Statement of the Workers' Protection Board containing regulations on micro-organisms, with general advice on their application]*, Ministry of Health, Stockholm.

National Institutes of Health, 1987, *Regulations on the Safety Control of Laboratories Handling Pathogenic Agents*, National Institute of Health, Tokyo.

Pike RM, 1979, Laboratory-associated infections: incidence, fatalities, causes and prevention, *Annu Rev Microbiol*, **33**: 41–66.

Public Health Laboratory Service, 1992, Exposure to hepatitis B virus: guidance on post-exposure prophylaxis, *Commun Dis Rep*, **2**: 9.

Ryder RW, Gordsman EJ, 1995, Laboratory acquired Sabià virus infection [letter], *N Engl J Med*, **333**: 1716.

Standards Association of Australia, 1991, *Australian Standard AS 2243*, Part 3: Microbiology, SAA, Sydney NSW.

Subcommittee Arbovirus Laboratory Safety, 1980, Laboratory safety for arboviruses and certain other viruses of vertebrates, *Am J Trop Med Hyg*, **29**: 1359–81.

US Department of Health and Human Services, 1993, *Biosafety in Microbiological and Biomedical Laboratories*, HHS Publication No (CDC) 93-8395, 3rd edn, Centers for Disease Control and National Institutes of Health, Washington DC.

Weissenbacher MC, Grela ME et al., 1978, Inapparent infections with Junin virus among laboratory workers, *J Infect Dis*, **137**: 309–13.

World Health Organization, 1993, *Laboratory Biosafety Manual*, 2nd edn, WHO, Geneva.

FURTHER READING

Health and Safety Commission, 1994, *Control of Substances Hazardous to Health Regulations. Approved Code of Practice*, HMSO, London.

Health and Safety Executive, 1992, *Workplace (Health, Safety and Welfare) Regulations 1992. Approved Code of Practice*, HMSO, London.

Health Services Advisory Committee, 1991, *Safe Working and the Prevention of Infection in Clinical Laboratories*, HMSO, London.

Health and Safety Commission, 1992, *Management of Health and Safety at Work Regulations 1992. Approved Code of Practice*, HMSO, London.

Lee HV, Johnson KM, 1982, Laboratory acquired infections with Hantaan virus the etiologic agent of Korean haemorrhagic fever, *J Infect Dis*, **146:** 645–51.

National Research Council USA, 1989, *Biosafety in the Laboratory. Prudent practices for the handling and disposal of infectious materials*, National Academy Press, Washington DC.

THE LABORATORY DIAGNOSIS OF VIRAL INFECTIONS

Pekka E Halonen and C R Madeley

1	Introduction	4	Detection of antibody responses
2	Principles of diagnosis	5	Specimen collection and transport
3	Detection of virus	6	Selection of diagnostic methods

1 INTRODUCTION

There are 4 main reasons for diagnosing viral infections: to decide on specific treatment; as a basis for management such as termination of pregnancy; to provide epidemiological information; or to provide a definite diagnosis and prognosis. Of these the first, second and fourth require a quick answer within the working day. For the third a more complete identification is needed, usually at serotype level, but speed is less important except for 'new' strains of influenza.

The true value of a definite diagnosis is to allow savings on antibiotics not used, investigations not needed and hospital-days saved through earlier discharge. These apply particularly to respiratory infections but, in addition, inappropriate use of antibiotics in gut infections can do serious damage.

With the increasing availability of kits, some basic diagnostic virology is being done in microbiology laboratories and specialist virology laboratories are needed to evaluate these. To do this requires experienced staff using validated techniques regularly. This chapter outlines those techniques in current use but touches little on commercial kits, because it would not be possible to cover the alternatives comprehensively.

2 PRINCIPLES OF DIAGNOSIS

Figure 44.1 illustrates a typical virus infection. Not all will be as straightforward as this but the diagram illustrates some of the important principles of diagnosis. It is a graph of quantity (y axis) against time (x axis) but the figures mark events not a time-scale.

At point 1, the patient becomes infected by the virus. This is followed by a very variable incubation

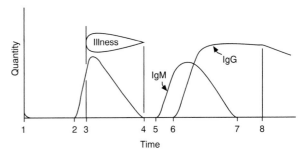

Fig. 44.1 Outline of a typical acute uncomplicated virus infection (not to scale). See text for details.

period (measured in days to years) at the end of which symptoms and signs appear (point 3). Shortly before this (point 2) the virus will become detectable as a result of multiplication. After point 3 the patient will become ill as virus multiplication reaches a peak, followed in most cases by recovery as the virus declines and the body's defence mechanisms overcome the invader. By point 4 recovery is well advanced and the virus is no longer detectable. The appearance of specific antibody follows about a week to 10 days later, initially short-term of the IgM class (point 5) and then long(er) term of the IgG class (point 6) which will, in most cases, indicate development of immunity and resistance to reinfection. Other antibodies, such as locally secreted IgA mucosal antibody, play a part in inhibiting virus but are not used routinely at present for diagnosis. Similarly, cell-mediated immunity (CMI) is important in recovery from virus infections but assays to measure it are not yet routinely available.

Experience of diagnosis, especially when the patient is immunocompromised, will show the sequence outlined in Fig. 44.1 to be a gross oversimplification.

Nevertheless this concept indicates an **early phase** (up to point 4) and a **later phase** (from point 5 onwards). It is appropriate to look during the early phase for virus or viral components, and during the later phase for an immune response, if any, to such components. Thereafter the presence of specific IgG class antibody confirms past experience of the virus (generally equated with immunity) and forms the basis of screening tests. Prolonged or recurrent virus replication will blur this simple concept but it indicates that waiting for an immune response will be of little value in deciding whether to treat most acute infections. It will be too late and the response may not occur at all in immunocompromised patients.

The main exception in which antibody detection is of practical value in management is when virus replication is continuing and so the detection of IgM class antibody may be helpful. Some respiratory infections caused by non-viral agents (Q fever, chlamydiae and mycoplasmas) are traditionally diagnosed in virology laboratories. Because they have a more insidious onset, respond to antibiotics and are difficult to isolate, antibody tests provide the only practical route to diagnosis.

In this chapter we concentrate on newer and widely used diagnostic techniques. Less space has been given to some of the well established techniques that either are being superseded (e.g. animal and egg inoculation) or are well covered by existing standard textbooks (neutralization, haemagglutination inhibition, complement fixation). These tests are mentioned only briefly although complement-fixation tests (CFTs) are still widely used in the absence so far of an equally useful alternative. For more details of these aspects the reader is referred to Lennette and Lennette (1995).

As indicated in section 6 (see p. 960), the choice of test depends on local needs and the breadth of experience of the laboratory staff. Nevertheless, the increasing availability of system-based commercial assays heralds new approaches that will have to be evaluated. Diagnostic virology does not stand still; new and better techniques should find their place in the laboratory.

3 DETECTION OF VIRUS

3.1 Electron microscopy

The electron microscope is the only instrument with which we can see virus particles directly. One typical particle makes the diagnosis but not all viruses are instantly recognizable and it is the number of particles with consistent identifying features that is finally convincing. Nevertheless, electron microscopy (EM) is the only currently available catch-all technique: there is no need for a decision on which virus to seek. This is particularly valuable in viral diarrhoeas, the context in which the EM is most frequently used. Table 44.1 lists the viruses, the diseases and the specimens in which viruses may be detected by EM, and shows that virus may be present in EM-detectable concentrations in

specimens other than faeces though the latter will provide >80% of the workload.

The limitations of EM are, first, the cost of providing the instrument, maintaining it and the labour of a trained operator and, secondly, its apparent insensitivity. Diagnostic EM requires a stable instrument that is easy to use and capable of straightforward transmission EM at about 50 000 × magnification. This can be provided by a relatively cheap good-quality second-hand microscope and does not require the latest state-of-the-art machine. Good immediate maintenance is essential, as is a good operator. However, even more than other tests in diagnostic virology, EM should be used as much as possible. If it is, a workload of about 3000 specimens a year will make the cost of EM competitive with other tests, especially in that it may be able to detect up to 9 different viruses in one examination.

In many virus infections, particularly those of the skin or gut, vast numbers of virus particles are present in the available specimens. Hence a good specimen taken early in the infection will allow the diagnosis to be made easily. Later in the disease, and in specimens from some outbreaks of diarrhoea and vomiting, the levels are lower and the diagnosis is more difficult to make. In these cases, enhancement (by antibody, if available) or other techniques may be necessary (Doane and Anderson 1987).

The negative contrast ('negative staining') method is the fastest way, other than latex agglutination, to make a virus diagnosis. Thin section and scanning EM techniques are of very limited value in routine diagnosis (Oshiro and Miller 1992).

The essence of negative contrast preparation is to obtain a concentrated aqueous suspension of virus from the specimen, free of as much salt and protein as possible. This is mixed with an equal volume of a solution of a heavy metal salt (usually 2–3% phosphotungstic acid, PTA, adjusted to a pH of 7.0 with 1N KOH). One drop of the mixture is placed on a carbon–Formvar-coated 400 mesh copper grid and the surplus drawn off with the torn edge of a piece of filter paper. The preparation is allowed to dry briefly and is then examined, first at low magnification to confirm a reasonable density of material on the grid and then at about 50 000 × to look for virus. Representative examples of any virus found should be photographed for future reference. An atlas of virus micrographs is helpful in recognizing individual viruses (Doane and Anderson 1987, Madeley and Field 1988, Palmer and Martin 1988).

Different laboratories have evolved their own detailed methods of preparing specimens; there is no best one. Some useful principles are:

1 Preparation: remove salt and soluble protein by differential (low speed and high speed) centrifugation (Madeley and Field 1988) or precipitation with ammonium sulphate (Caul, Ashley and Egglestone 1978) or hydroxyapatite (Codd and Narang 1986). This is more important than just concentrating the virus.

2 Include a wetting agent (e.g. 0.1% bacitracin) in the diluent used to make the suspension to be mixed with the stain.

3 Potassium phosphotungstate will disrupt membranes. This is important in diagnosing herpes infections, in which only the internal icosahedral capsid can be ident-

Table 44.1 Detection of viruses in diagnostic electron microscopy

Body system/Disease	Specimen	Viruses detectable
Gut Diarrhoea and vomiting	Faeces	Rotavirus Adenovirus Astrovirus Calicivirus Norwalk/SRSV SRV Coronavirus (faecal) Torovirus Picobirnavirus
Skin Vesicular rashes	VF	Herpes simplex Varicella-zoster
Vesicular lesion Warty lesions	VF/crust/scraping Molluscum body[a] Biopsy	Orf, pseudocowpox Molluscum contagiosum Papilloma
Urine Congenital CMV	Urine	Cytomegalovirus
CNS Meningitis	CSF	Enterovirus Mumps Varicella-zoster

CSF, cerebrospinal fluid; SRSV, small round structured virus; SRV, small round virus; VF, vesicular fluid.
[a]Squeezed out of molluscum lesions.

ified with certainty. Leaving the stain in contact with the specimen for about 20 min before putting the mixture onto the grid may convert an apparent negative to a positive.

4 Always use separate forceps for each grid and disinfect them by boiling after use. Cross-contamination can occur very easily.

5 Drift (movement of the specimen), uncorrected astigmatism and poor focusing will ruin photographs taken. Wait for any movement to cease before taking the micrograph. Learn to correct astigmatism and to focus correctly.

6 Calibrate the microscope's magnification using fixed beef liver catalase crystals (Wrigley 1968). The manufacturer's figures may be wrong by as much as 10%, although most modern microscopes are very stable and the true figure, once established, varies little.

Good micrographs provide teaching material and illustrations for chapters and papers.

ENHANCEMENT

Enhancement, broadly, is the use of antibody either to improve the sensitivity of the test or to help identify the virus or serotype (or both) involved. EM is labour-intensive; using antibody, provided the appropriate one is available, adds to the labour-intensiveness but may be essential in some cases. Antibody can be used to clump the virus (this can be difficult to control) or to coat the grid (solid phase immune electron microscopy, SPIEM) to make it 'sticky' for the virus concerned. This may increase the number of visible virus particles 10- to 100-fold, but introduces bias toward that one virus. SPIEM may be used to type

some viruses if this cannot be done otherwise but it is too time consuming for routine use.

An experienced operator should be encouraged to keep in practice with a good workload. Any temptation to screen out common faecal viruses such as rotaviruses and adenoviruses, for which other tests are available, should be resisted. Regular positives of any kind maintain the confidence and morale of the microscopist.

3.2 Antigen detection

IMMUNOFLUORESCENCE

The use of antibodies labelled with a fluorescent dye to identify viral antigens directly in specimens is over 40 years old. However, practical problems in obtaining antisera of adequate titre and specificity to make the technique work satisfactorily has limited the number of laboratories using immunofluorescence (IF) to a few whose staff had the resources and determination to make the necessary high-quality polyclonal sera (usually in rabbits). Most preferred the indirect sandwich method with the binding of rabbit antibodies to viral antigens revealed by a conjugated anti-rabbit globulin. Such conjugates were often made commercially but there were very few antiviral sera of high enough titre to be acceptable because the cost was prohibitive.

Where the reagents were carefully prepared and assessed, the results were reliable and could be obtained within the working day, making them available in time to influence decisions on treatment. The data on this approach to IF were collected by Gardner and McQuillin (1980). Their methods were copied in some other laboratories but directly conjugated monoclonal antibodies have recently made available satisfactory reagents that can be used directly off the shelf. These are commercially produced and most are of high quality although, even with an enhancing mountant (see p. 951), they are slightly (c. 5%) less sensitive than good polyclonal sera. In 1996 they are not available for all viruses that may be detected directly by IF (Table 44.2).

There are two components to successful IF: (1) an appropriate and adequate specimen that is prepared suitably; and (2) the staining and microscopy system.

Specimens

Because particulate fluorescence outside cells is difficult to interpret, a satisfactory specimen must contain a good number of virally infected cells, which will require some skill and persistence to obtain, particularly from the upper respiratory tract. From elsewhere (e.g. in biopsies) cells must be collected only from an infected part of the tissue.

Aspirated nasopharyngeal secretions (NPSs) will contain sufficient infected cells (if collected thoroughly from the posterior nasopharynx) but will also contain mucus, which autofluoresces and can obscure the infected cells. It must be removed by diluting the secretions in phosphate-buffered saline, pipetting them briskly to break up the mucus and then sedimenting the cells in a bench centrifuge. The resuspended cells are then put on 'wells' in Teflon-coated slides, air-dried and fixed in cold (4°C) acetone. Fixation both attaches the cells to the slide and opens them to penetration by antibodies by lysing the cell membrane. As many wells as possible are prepared in

this way to allow each to be 'stained' with a different antibody and to provide spares for reagent evaluation (see below).

Cells from skin scrapings, biopsies or postmortem tissues are similarly spread on wells to leave individual cells separate when seen under the microscope. It is impossible to interpret the results on clumps of cells.

The collection and preparation of specimens for IF is discussed in greater detail by Gardner and McQuillin (1980), Foot and Madeley (1992) and Madeley (1992).

Staining and microscopy

Antisera, whether polyclonal or monoclonal, are not necessarily suitable for IF even if they have high titres of antibody in other assays. They must be shown to be suitable on known positive clinical **specimens**. (Fixed spare slides of positive specimens may be stored at −40°C). Infected cell cultures may be useful for initial screening but the final assessment must be made on validated positive specimens. This also applies to commercial monoclonal sera, and intending purchasers should satisfy themselves that this validation has been done.

The serum at optimal working dilution is layered onto the appropriate cell spread, allowed time (usually 30 min at 37°C) to react and thoroughly washed before a labelled conjugated antiglobulin is added, reacted and washed as before. If conjugated antiviral serum (as are most commercial monoclonal preparations) is used this second layer is not necessary.

After a final rinse in distilled water to prevent salt crystallizing on the slide, it is air-dried and is ready for examination. With good quality polyclonal antisera a coverslip is not necessary but the lower sensitivity of monoclonal sera can be partly compensated by using

Table 44.2 Viruses detectable by immunofluorescence

Viruses	Specimens	Commercial monoclonal conjugates available
Respiratory viruses		
Respiratory syncytial virus		Yes
Influenza A	Nasopharyngeal secretions (NPS,NPA)[a]	Yes
Influenza B		Yes
Parainfluenza viruses types 1–4		Yes (as group antiserum)
Adenovirus	Bronchoalveolar lavage (BAL)	No[b] (as group antiserum)
Varicella-zoster		No
Herpes simplex	Lung biopsy	No[b]
Cytomegalovirus		No[c]
Measles		No
Skin infections		
Varicella-zoster	Lesion scrapings	No
Herpes simplex		No[b]
Cell cultures		As above, plus adenovirus
All the above		and herpes simplex

[a]Endotracheal secretions from intubated patients may also be used. Sputum contains other debris and may be less suitable though obtained more easily from adults.
[b]Available but not yet licensed for direct use.
[c]Not yet available commercially.

a fluorescence-enhancing mountant, such as Imagen® Mounting Medium (Dako). Evans blue, as a counterstain, helps to highlight infected cells in the preparation.

A suitable microscope is one fitted with epifluorescence and interference filters, a ×50 oil immersion objective and a ×10 eyepiece. Each preparation should be examined thoroughly and individually, and experience from looking at known positives provides good preparation for looking at unknowns.

The advantages of the technique are its speed and certainty, while at the same time providing feedback to the viewer on the quality of the original specimen. It is easy to collect poor quality specimens, which will, of course, often give false negative results. The disadvantages are that IF is labour-intensive, depends on properly evaluated antisera (as do other similar immunoassays) and provides traps for the overenthusiastic and inexperienced operator. However, the last problem can be overcome by thorough training of new staff.

We have used IF routinely since 1968, using polyclonal rabbit antisera prepared in-house. Latterly, commercially produced monoclonal conjugates have been used to provide quicker answers although negatives have been re-tested with the polyclonal reagents. More elaborate (and potentially more sensitive) variants such as anti-complement ones (Leland 1992) have not been used because they are too elaborate and not robust enough for large volume day-to-day work in a busy laboratory.

A variety of viruses cause respiratory infections. They cannot be distinguished clinically and there is a need to identify the culprit viruses in all such illnesses, even when one is particularly in season, if the full epidemiological picture is to be visible. However, not all viruses are present at the same time and to be economic the antisera to be used should be tailored to their prevalence. This requires a close watch on published epidemiological data, allied to experience.

SOLID-PHASE IMMUNOASSAYS

Radioimmunoassays (RIAs) and enzyme immunoassays (EIAs) have been used successfully for the detection of viral antigens for over 20 years. Applications in diagnostic virology have included detecting HBsAg in serum, gastroenteritis viruses in stool specimens, herpes simplex virus and varicella-zoster virus in vesicle fluid, and HIV in blood (Arstila and Halonen 1988).

The basic principle of EIAs is to bind antigen to a solid phase (polystyrene plate or bead) and detect its presence with a detector antiviral antibody and an antiglobulin antibody to which an enzyme (usually horseradish peroxidase or alkaline phosphatase) has been conjugated. Successive bonds mean that the enzyme is tethered to the solid phase only if the virus antigen is present (Fig. 44.2). After thorough washing, a colourless substrate is added and the enzyme acts on it to produce a clearly visible coloured product whose presence (indicating a positive result) can be read by eye or a spectrophotometer. Difficulties in binding

antigen direct from the specimen have prompted variations such as using a capture antibody (Fig. 44.2) to pull it onto the plate or bead.

The route to success with such assays is attention to detail. The constituents and their concentration in diluents and wash buffers used to rinse the solid phase, and the surface properties of the latter, are critical and must be carefully evaluated. The more complex (i.e. the more components) the assay, the more likely are non-specific results, particularly with polyclonal antibodies.

The scope of these assays has been extended with the development of monoclonal antibodies. Every combination of capture, detection and indicator (antiglobulin) antibodies has been used with a variety of labels, simple and complex. The procedures have been simplified to reduce the number of steps in the assay and to improve its sensitivity, particularly in commercially produced systems. The concept lends itself well to automation, and the alternatives available to detect different viruses increase daily.

Candidate monoclonal antibodies for use in these tests must be put through the same rigorous evaluation on genuine specimens as applied to IF (see p. 950) (Arstila and Halonen 1988). Only a proportion will be found suitable.

Further modifications of solid-phase antigen detections are time-resolved fluoroimmunoassay (TR-FIA) and biotin EIA. Combined with the one-incubation

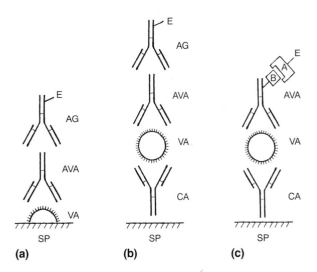

Fig. 44.2 Enzyme immunoassay formats used to detect viral antigen in specimens taken from the patient. (a) Specimen of viral antigen (VA) is bound to the solid phase (SP) nonspecifically and detected by a polyclonal antiviral antibody (AVA). The subsequent binding of an enzyme (E)-labelled antiglobulin (AG) is revealed by adding a colourless substrate which the enzyme converts to a coloured product to give a positive signal readable on an automatic spectrophotometer. (b) Very similar to (a) except that a capture antiviral antibody (CA) is used to make the solid phase 'sticky' to the viral antigen and this antibody must be made in a species different from that of the AVA. (c) Another way to improve performance by using a CA and an AVA linked to the enzyme by biotin–avidin (B, A) 'bridges', thereby binding more enzyme to small amounts of antigen.

principle the sensitivity of these tests is improved; the tests are also more practical, with fewer incubation and washing steps (Halonen, Obert and Hierholzer 1985, Walls et al. 1986, Hierholzer, Anderson and Halonen 1990, Scalia et al. 1995). In the test format specimens are added simultaneously with the labelled Europeum (Eu)-chelate or biotin detector antibody to the wells of polystyrene strips already coated with capture antibody. After a short incubation, the wells are washed and the enhancement solution (TR-FIA) or peroxidase-labelled avidin (biotin-EIA) is added. The test format allows the antigen in the specimen and the detector antibody to react quickly and efficiently in liquid phase, and later the formed antigen–antibody complex binds to capture antibody on solid phase.

The advantages of EIAs and related techniques are: (1) specimen transportation is not critical because intact cells are not required; (2) treatment of the specimen is not elaborate; (3) automation allows the test to handle larger numbers; and (4) the cut-off level can be set in advance and the results assessed by computer. The disadvantages of EIAs in antigen detection are the absence of quality control on the specimens and the lack of commercial monoclonal antibodies that have been evaluated for this particular use.

Commercial kits and systems

These are now becoming available in a variety of formats. It is beyond the scope of this chapter to review all the kits and machine systems on which to run them. They will not be equally good, neither will they give equal value for money. Purchasers should satisfy themselves that such kits work by comparing them with other existing established methods, although this will be difficult for smaller laboratories lacking, for example, cell culture facilities. More formal validation arrangements will probably become necessary.

Latex agglutination and immunochromatography

Small latex spheres coated with antibody can be agglutinated with the viral antigen present in stool extracts, for example (Hughes et al. 1984). The level of rotavirus or adenovirus antigen present in many stools is high enough to give adequate sensitivity although some stools will also cause the control spheres (coated with pre-immune serum) to agglutinate non-specifically.

These simple commercially produced assays, intended for use at the bedside or in the doctor's office, still require an extract of the stool to be made and are relatively expensive if used on small numbers. Early versions required experience to read them reliably but this aspect has improved. Their place in routine diagnosis is unclear at present although their speed (about 5 min) makes them useful for specimens received at the end of the working day. Currently they are available only for rotavirus and adenovirus, so they are unsuitable for investigating all but a small handful of outbreaks of diarrhoea and vomiting.

Under development are extensions of this principle in which the reagents are placed on a test card. An extract of the specimen is placed on an indicated spot or in a well and the antigens migrate with the aid of a solvent, towards an antibody elsewhere on the card where combination produces a colour change (enzymatically mediated) with the addition of the necessary substrate. Alternatively, this may be mediated by antibody-coated coloured beads that capture the antigen as it rehydrates them. They then migrate toward a second tethered antibody that will anchor the colour in a reading window to give a positive result (Bunce, Thorpe and Keen 1991).

These ingenious developments have been used so far on classic antigen–antibody reactions and depend on labelled antibody to provide the positive signal. They do not use any new principles, although the old ones are applied in novel ways to provide easy-to-use assays requiring no elaborate equipment. In contrast, nucleic acid detection systems approach virus, diagnosis differently.

3.3 Nucleic acid detection

Detection of viral genomic DNA/RNA directly in clinical specimens is a new, sensitive diagnostic technique that has great potential in certain virus infections, and particularly when diagnosis is possible neither by culture nor by antigen detection or is impractical. In some virus infections viral DNA can be detected directly by hybridization but usually the polymerase chain reaction (PCR) (Saiki et al. 1988) or another form of amplification reaction is required.

Hybridization

Blot and in situ hybridizations are standard diagnostic methods for the detection of papilloma viruses in genital and other specimens (Wagner et al. 1984). The presence of viral DNA is usually confirmed with radioactive-labelled probes but enzyme-labelled probes may also be used. For blot hybridization, total DNA is extracted from the specimen and, after boiling to separate the strands and cooling, they are immobilized on a filter and detected with the probe, usually made from a selected region of the DNA. The sensitivity of adenovirus detection in stool specimens by blot hybridization using a full length radioactive probe (Hyypia et al. 1984) or astrovirus detection by a subgenomic probe (Willcocks et al. 1991) is comparable with a highly sensitive EIA but antigen detection offers a more practical approach. For in situ hybridization the intracellular target DNA is fixed to a microscope slide as a thin section of tissue, but this is too cumbersome for daily use except in a histopathology laboratory.

Nucleic acid amplification techniques

The place of PCR and similar techniques, such as the ligase chain reaction (LCR) (Birkenmeyer and Mushahwar 1991) or nucleic acid sequence based amplification (NASBA) (Compton 1991), is still being assessed but commercial kits are already available. New developments both in preparation of the specimen and in details of the techniques are frequent, and this is in a state of flux in 1996. These techniques are sensitive but expensive; they are very liable to cross-contamination because they can amplify very small amounts of nucleic acid. However, PCR is valuable in pinpointing herpes simplex or varicella-zoster virus DNA in the CSF from patients with encephalitis due to either virus (Aurelius et al. 1991, Puchhammer-Stöckl et al. 1991). This approach is very helpful in diagnosing infections that are otherwise very difficult to confirm. PCR is also finding a place in the diagnosis, or confirmation of the presence, of cytomegalovirus, enteroviruses, hepatitis B and C, human immunodeficiency virus, papovaviruses and rhinoviruses. Some helpful guidance on technique is given, for example, by Becker and Darai (1995).

The extreme sensitivity of PCR brings both technical and interpretation problems. Extraction of the viral DNA or RNA from the specimen must be reliable and must remove inhibitors of the enzyme used in amplification. It may be necessary to add primers for another marker DNA (such as for β-globin) to confirm that no inhibitors are present (Saiki et al. 1988). RNA cannot be amplified directly by PCR (though it can by NASBA) and has to be reverse-transcribed into DNA first, adding to the complexity of the system.

After 30–40 cycles of annealing, extension and denaturing to give, typically, an amplification of more than 10^6-fold, the product is identified by its size after electrophoresis on an agarose gel or by liquid phase hybridization in microtitre plates (Fig. 44.3). The probe used may be labelled radioactively or, more probably, with an enzyme joined by a biotin/streptavidin link (Jansen and Ledley 1989).

The significance of detecting small copy numbers of a viral genome will vary with the virus and the circumstances. In some, such as papilloma virus DNA in cervical biopsies, it will depend on the genotype, whereas absence of cytomegalovirus DNA in buffy coat white cells post-transplant will rule out virus activity at that time. The presence of hepatitis C genomic RNA in serum will help to resolve ambiguous serological results. Other examples will emerge with time. The significance of a positive result must be carefully assessed and hasty conclusions avoided.

An alternative approach to nucleic acid detection is to use a short probe similar to that used in hybridization to bind to the target and then to amplify a marker instead. This is the basis for the branched chain DNA assay. The original viral genome segment of DNA or RNA is denatured to a single strand but is not then itself amplified, thus avoiding the dangers of cross-contaminating other specimens with newly produced amplicons. Branched chains of non-specific DNA are tethered to the target sequence which is itself anchored to a polystyrene solid phase by short sequences of complementary (probe) DNA. The branched chains are then labelled with a chemiluminescent marker which can be assayed in an automated reader. The branched chain assay shows promise but its role is still being evaluated, particularly in estimates of viral load in patients with HIV and hepatitis C infections.

3.4 Culture

Fertile hens' eggs

These are used much less than they were, although they remain important for work with influenza viruses. There are several reasons for this: expense, tighter regulations over the use of embryo tissues, the eradi-

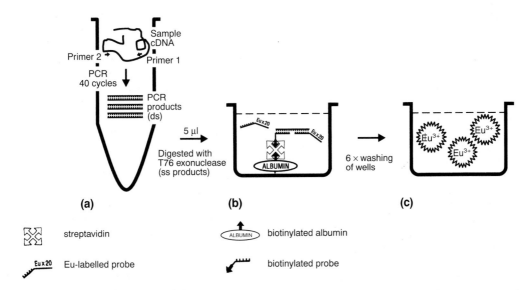

Fig. 44.3 Principle of liquid phase hybridization by time-resolved fluorometry in detection of PCR products: (a) PCR; (b) liquid phase hybridization and collection of hybrids on solid phase; (c) development of fluorescence by enhancement solution. After 40 cycles the double-stranded (ds) PCR products are digested into single strands (ss) and the final detection is done by TR-FIA in microtitre wells coated first with biotinylated albumin, followed by streptavidin and biotinylated probe. The single-stranded PCR product and the Eu-labelled probe are added simultaneously into the microtitre wells with these 3 layers of reagents, incubated for 1 h, washed carefully and, after the enhancement solution is added, fluorescence is measured with a single-photon-counting fluorometer.

cation of smallpox, the development of simpler and more reliable methods for typing herpes simplex and the development of molecular techniques. Where egg inoculation is retained, it is to prepare influenza virus for strain characterization or vaccine production, for making teaching material and as an extra method for isolating 'difficult' wild strains of influenza A or B.

For details of work with fertile hens' eggs, see Chapter 5 and Lennette and Lennette (1995).

CELL CULTURES

The propagation and identification of viruses is described in detail in Chapter 5. The availability of cell cultures in which to grow virus has been the main way to distinguish between laboratories capable of providing a widely based diagnostic service and those offering just a testing service. Cell culture allows the diagnostic net to be cast more widely; it will provide more virus to examine in greater depth and to develop new tests. It opens many new possibilities, but at a price. Cell culture is neither easy nor cheap and needs constant attention to prevent contamination and to remain adequately sensitive.

No single cell type will support the growth of all viruses. The secret of growing those such as hepatitis B and C viruses has yet to be found and some laboratories are better than others at growing some fastidious viruses such as rhinoviruses.

Three kinds of cells are used in diagnosis: primary cells, semi-continuous and continuous. Primary cells are from disaggregated adult tissues, often from the kidneys of various species of monkey. They are very limited in their ability to divide before they deteriorate, and may already contain passenger viruses such as simian virus (SV) 5, SV40 or mycoplasmas. These contaminants interfere very little with their ability to grow wild viruses but will contaminate any isolates made. The short lifespan of these cells means that continuing supplies of the original tissue will have to be available, now usually provided by a central institute or a commercial company. This makes primary cells expensive but they are the most sensitive for several common viruses such as influenza virus and parainfluenza viruses.

Semi-continuous cells are fetal in origin, may divide up to about 70 times and are generally free of passenger viruses. Fetal diploid cells or cord blood cells of human origin are essential to grow cytomegalovirus, herpesviruses 6 and 7 and varicella-zoster virus, which will not replicate in any other cells. A source of fresh fetal tissues will be needed occasionally.

Continuous cells are usually derived from malignant tissue but can be maintained in culture indefinitely provided they remain uncontaminated. They may be human (HeLa, HEp-2, G293, etc.), mouse (L), monkey (Vero, LLC-MK2, etc.), hamster (BHK-21 clone 13) or rabbit (RK13) in origin.

It is usual to keep one or 2 continuous cell lines (usually HeLa, HEp-2, G293 or Vero) available in the laboratory as well as semi-continuous diploid cells (MRC-5, WI-38 or equivalent) and primary (usually monkey: rhesus or baboon), to isolate the variety of

viruses likely to be circulating at any one time. The detailed choice of which cells to keep will therefore vary between the tropics and temperate climes. Respiratory specimens are usually incubated both in stationary cultures at 37°C and in roller drums at 33°C (Hamparian 1979). The lower temperature and the constant rolling of the inoculum over the cells increases the number of positives.

The duration of incubation and the number of times the material is passaged or the medium is changed varies from laboratory to laboratory. Any manipulation (passage or changing the medium) increases the cost of the test, and opening the culture (usually in 4×0.5 in. (10×1.25 cm) silicone rubber-stoppered test tubes) risks (cross-)contamination.

Cells are usually grown to near-confluence in medium containing 10% calf serum but this is changed to serum-free (and therefore antibody-free) maintenance medium before the specimen is added. The cultures are examined microscopically and unstained either daily or on alternate days for evidence of cytopathic effect. Toxic effects and bacterial/fungal contamination from the specimen may make passage or re-inoculation from the original specimen necessary.

The slow growth of, particularly, cytomegalovirus (CMV) has prompted an alternative approach. Normal culture may not be positive for up to 4 weeks but some viral antigens (immediate early) will be expressed intracellularly before this. Coverslip (shell-vial) cultures can be fixed after 1, 2 or 7 days and stained with a suitable mouse monoclonal antibody and a conjugated anti-mouse globulin (Stirk and Griffiths 1987). We have found a peroxidase label to be more sensitive than a fluorescent one. This has the additional advantage of providing a permanent preparation that can be read on an ordinary light microscope.

Although some workers claim that they can read and identify cytopathic effects (CPEs) due to a variety of viruses directly in cell cultures, it is prudent to confirm and identify the isolates. This will allow the isolate to be typed, which is discussed further in the next section.

RAPID IDENTIFICATION OF ISOLATES

Immunoperoxidase (IP) or immunofluorescence (IF) staining with monoclonal antibodies of cell cultures inoculated with respiratory specimens increases the sensitivity of culture. The results, including the serotypic identification of the isolate, may be available in 48 hours, and are read more easily and quickly than by looking for CPE by microscopy (Ziegler et al. 1988, Waris et al. 1990). The virus is grown in Costar 24-well polystyrene plates which allow a large number of specimens to be processed easily, increased sensitivity being provided by centrifuging the specimens onto the cell cultures. The method is used in Turku, Finland, for CMV, herpes simplex, respiratory syncytial virus (RSV), parainfluenzas, influenza A and B and adenoviruses. Rapid identification of isolates can be used for type- and subtype-specific identification of influenza viruses directly from clinical specimens after overnight incubation in MCDK cultures (Ziegler et al. 1995).

3.5 Enzyme detection

Virus replication involves a variety of enzymes, some of which may be unique to the virus concerned. However, it is only with viruses that are too difficult to grow, such as hepatitis B and human immunodeficiency virus (HIV), that diagnostic tests have been based on virus-coded enzymes. Detection of the DNA polymerase of hepatitis B in serum is an indication of continuing virus replication (Hollinger and Dienstag 1985) as is the detection of HIV reverse transcriptase (RT) (Gupta et al. 1987). The latter assay is now being used to assess HIV load (Pyra, Boni and Schubach 1994, Heneine et al. 1995).

4 DETECTION OF ANTIBODY RESPONSES

Detection of antibody response to a virus is the second approach to virus diagnosis (see Fig. 44.1) but the inevitable delay until (usually) serum antibody appears limits its value to a few respiratory infections by treatable non-viral organisms. Nevertheless, demonstrating seroconversion, a rise in antibody titre or the presence of IgM class antibody is widely used in diagnostic laboratories. Such tests are usually cheap and can be performed on readily available specimens. Serological tests to detect virus-specific IgG (long-term antibody) are currently the only practical way to gauge immune status, to indicate the prevalence of infection in the community and to estimate the success rate of vaccines. With the need to assess antibodies in intravenous drug users and children, from neither of whom is it easy to obtain blood, the use of saliva is increasing (Parry, Perry and Mortimer 1987). Made up from crevicular fluid (a serum transudate) as well as salivary gland secretions, its composition is closer to serum than to mucosal fluid which contains local secretory antibody (IgA).

EIAs are slowly replacing older methods for antibody detection such as complement fixation, haemagglutination inhibition, immunofluorescence and neutralization assays. Because it is possible to automate EIAs and there has been an increase in the availability of commercial versions, interest in them has grown. The results of EIAs can often be read by an automatic spectrophotometer and appear as a list of absorption values that may be transformed mathematically. Evaluating the significance of these results requires expertise. Understanding possible problems, the limitations of the tests and the reasons for non-specific results requires detailed knowledge of the immunological principles used, whether they are prepared in-house or bought commercially.

Individual laboratories have been experimenting with EIAs but a full range of suitably evaluated antigens has yet to appear commercially. Where they have

been explored more fully, IgG EIAs have seemed to be satisfactory and on paired serum specimens have been more sensitive than single IgM assays in the diagnosis of acute respiratory infections (Koskinen, Vuorinen and Meurman 1987, Vuorinen and Meruman 1989, Nohynek et al. 1991). Nevertheless, IgM assays have been useful in showing recent or continuing virus activity.

4.1 Solid-phase immunoassays

The sensitivity and specificity of EIAs is influenced strongly by the conditions and reagents used. The quality and purity of the antigens, assay buffers, washes and the enzyme-labelled anti-human immunoglobulins, variations in the materials and equipment (including microtitre strips or plates, automatic pipettors, washers and spectrophotometers) will affect the quality of the test profoundly and may cause daily fluctuations in the results. Indirect assays used for IgG or total Ig detection are particularly sensitive to the quality of the antigens used to coat the solid phase. With more highly purified antigens, fewer non-specific reactions occur but it becomes more difficult to identify the rare specimens that still react non-specifically. For most routine purposes, antigens from infected cell lysates provide satisfactory results in tests prepared in the laboratory whereas non-specifically reacting specimens can be identified by using mock-infected lysate antigens as negative controls (Forghani and Schmidt 1979). Genetically engineered antigens are used increasingly in commercial kits, but they may be difficult to purify adequately for assays prepared in-house (Harmon et al. 1989). The concentrations of detergent and protein in assay buffers are directly related; if higher concentrations of protein are used, more detergent is required.

Many EIA formats have been developed but usually work best if kept simple. However, three basic ones have been more widely used: indirect, capture and competition (Fig. 44.4). They have been developed to use either microtitre plates or, more economically, strips that fit into a template to form part of a whole plate.

INDIRECT EIA

An optimal concentration of antigen is coated onto the solid phase, washed thoroughly, sealed and stored at 4°C for weeks or months until required. The optimal concentration of antigen is determined by a chessboard titration against dilutions of control positive and negative sera.

Antibody may be estimated by testing a dilution series (which is cumbersome) or by the colour density at one dilution compared to a standard curve (Fig. 44.5), though with some viruses, such as RSV, 2 dilutions may have to be tested to give a clear result. Note that results in the 'grey zone' will be ambiguous, being neither clearly positive nor negative.

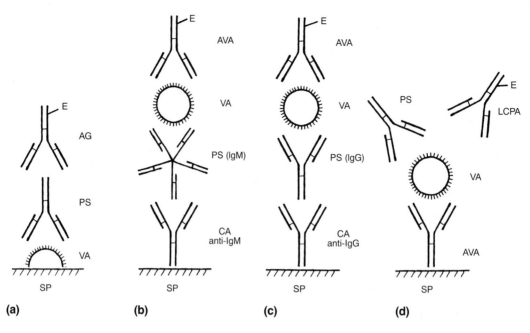

(a)   (b)   (c)   (d)

Fig. 44.4   Common enzyme immunoassay formats used to detect antiviral antibody. (a) Indirect technique in which viral antigen (VA) is bound to the solid phase (SP). Antibody in the patient's serum (PS) binds to it and is revealed by an enzyme (E) label attached to an anti-human globulin antibody (AG). (b) IgM-capture assay: an anti-IgM-capture antibody (CA) is attached to the solid phase (SP) and captures the IgM fraction of the antibody in the patient's serum (PS). Viral antigen (VA) binds only to specific IgM and is revealed by an antiviral antibody (AVA) labelled with an enzyme (E). This label may be replaced by a radioisotope to make a IgM-antibody capture radioimmune assay (MACRIA). (c) Similar format for a IgG-capture assay, except that the capture antibody (CA) is anti-IgG and the fraction captured from the serum is IgG. Because the proportion of specific IgG will be small these tests lack sensitivity but use, again, of a radioisotope label improves sensitivity in a IgG-capture antibody RIA (GACRIA). (d) Competitive or blocking test in which antibody in the patient's serum (PS) binds to viral antigen (VA) captured onto the solid phase (SP) by a bound antiviral antibody (AVA). The patient's antibody then blocks the binding of a labelled competing positive antibody (LCPA). Failure to convert the substrate to a coloured product indicates a positive (blocking) activity by the patient's antibody.

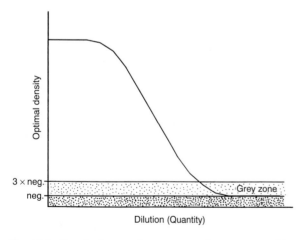

Fig. 44.5   Standard curve for an enzyme immunoassay. The colour developed by the tethered enzyme depends on how much of the latter is bound. As the antibody becomes more dilute there is no longer enough enzyme to give a colour deeper than the negative (neg.) background but a 'grey' zone of ambiguity will 'blur' a sharp endpoint.

COMPETITIVE EIA

In competitive (or blocking, or inhibition) EIAs the antibody in the patient's serum competes with labelled antibody. In this test format the results are highly specific but some practical problems, such as the production of a suitable labelled antibody, has limited its use in tests developed in-house. In these assays, a positive is an absence of a signal, a result also achieved if one component is omitted in error.

CAPTURE EIA

The solid phase is coated with an anti-human antibody specific for one class of antibody, usually IgM. It adsorbs the appropriate immunoglobulins from the patient's serum and any specific viral antibodies are then detected by adding first antigen and then a labelled antibody to the virus. Preformed antigen–labelled antibody complexes cannot be used because rheumatoid factor then causes non-specific reactions. As long as the antigen and labelled antiviral antibody are added separately, and the wells washed thoroughly between each addition, the test does not pick up rheumatoid factor, and this format is now used widely for IgM assays. However, other rare serum factors may also cause non-specific reactions. Capture EIAs are insensitive for IgG because the proportion of specific viral antibody relative to the total IgG adsorbed is small (Erdman et al. 1991).

IgG ANTIBODY AVIDITY TEST

The avidity (strength of binding) of the antibody present in a patient's serum increases with time, and low avidity indicates that recent infection after IgM is no longer detectable. Such low avidity antibody can be dissociated/denatured by 8M urea washes during assay. This property has been used to solve problems with rubella (Thomas and Morgan-Capner 1988), varicella-zoster (Kangro, Manzoor and Harper 1991) and RSV (Meurman, Waris and Hedman 1992).

4.2 Conventional techniques

These include such widely used assays as complement fixation (CFT), neutralization and haemagglutination inhibition (HI). All have drawbacks and are slowly being superseded. They have been described in detail by Lennette and Lennette (1995), but their strengths and weaknesses are discussed below.

COMPLEMENT FIXATION TEST

This is a complex system whose components must be carefully balanced. This has made the test fragile but its continued use suggests it has some virtues; 2 in particular have kept it in regular use.

1 Because it can be partly automated and validated and antigens are widely available, it can be used to screen sera against several viruses when there is more than one possible aetiology.
2 The CFT detects short-term antibody present for up to a year after the original stimulus. Consequently, a considerable number of convalescent phase antisera can be screened simultaneously against a battery of antigens; only a small proportion will be positive and require further testing. However, detection of only short-term antibody makes CF almost useless for immunity screening and some sera also give false positive results because they can fix complement in the absence of antigen (anticomplementary sera).

More precise possibilities, such as antibody-class specific EIAs outlined above (p. 956) cannot offer the screening advantage of CFTs. Machine-based EIAs will be able to offer more consistent and generally reliable results against, at first, a narrower spectrum of viral antigens. Because they detect longer-term antibody they will present more problems of interpretation.

NEUTRALIZATION

This requires both a titrated stock of virus and an assay system (usually cell culture) that estimates residual infectivity. It has the advantage of directly measuring the amount of antibody in serum that neutralizes infectivity but at the price of maintaining a supply of infectious virus and of a test that takes several days to complete.

A standard amount of virus is mixed with increasing dilutions of the patient's serum, allowed time to react and the mixtures added to susceptible cell cultures. Cytopathic effects or other indicators of virus growth are recorded and the highest dilution of serum inhibiting all or most of the virus is taken as the titre.

Neutralization has been used routinely to assess antibody to polioviruses and Coxsackie B viruses but is now being replaced by EIAs, reflecting the practical problems of using it routinely. Few virologists use neutralization if there is a satisfactory alternative.

HAEMAGGLUTINATION INHIBITION

This assay, which can be used only with viruses that have a haemagglutinin (many, but not all), has 3 important characteristics. First, it detects long-term antibody, making it suitable for immunity screening. Secondly, it is type specific, which limits its use largely to viruses (such as rubella) with only one serotype. Thirdly, it is sensitive to non-specific inhibitors in serum that will give false positive results if not removed.

Single radial haemolysis (SRH) is a development of HI, in which the virus–red cell combination is immobilized in an agarose gel. The test sera are added to wells cut in the gel and antibody diffuses radially. With the addition of complement to the system the antibodies lyse the red cells around the well, producing a circular zone of haemolysis whose area is proportional to the amount of antibody (Kurtz et al. 1980). SRH detects long-term antibody and has been widely used in screening the sera of pregnant women for evidence of rubella immunity. A large number of sera can be screened simply, reliably, cheaply and quickly (overnight), although skill in filling the wells accurately is required. The results are to an extent quantitative (though usually reported only as 'immune', 'susceptible' or 'borderline') when compared to a standard serum. For this purpose it is satisfactorily sensitive, though repeat or other tests will be necessary on some borderline sera.

The main drawback to SRH is that the test plates have to be prepared by the laboratory staff and have not been available commercially because of storage problems.

IMMUNOFLUORESCENCE

By using prepared slides on which infected cell cultures have been fixed, antibody in patients' sera can be detected by its binding to viral antigens and demonstrated by a conjugated antiserum to human serum antibody. The test can be made specific for IgG or IgM class antibody by the conjugate used, and this system has been employed widely to detect antibody to Epstein–Barr (EB) virus (Hotchin and Crawford 1991). Monospot or Paul–Bunnell tests are non-specific, and it has proved difficult to develop a reliable EIA for EB virus. IF is labour-intensive and very sensitive to rheumatoid factor in IgM tests. Nevertheless, it has been useful in laboratories that are already heavily committed to IF for viral antigen detection, to whom IF gives fewer problems. Commercially produced slides are now available and IF is currently the best approach to detecting antibody to the more recently recognized herpesviruses, HHV-6 and HHV-7 (Okuno et al. 1989).

LATEX AGGLUTINATION

Virus antigen is coated onto latex particles, and antibodies in the serum specimens form bridges between the particles to agglutinate them. Positive reactions can be seen by naked eye or hand lens. The antigen–antibody combination takes place quickly and can be read in a few minutes. Commercially produced versions commonly use slides marked with test circles into which the serum specimens, followed by the latex reagent, are placed and mixed. After tilting and rotating the test slides for 5 min they can be read and compared with control latex coated with normal cell extracts. A recent modification provides dried latex reagent on the test circle and only the specimen has to be added to it.

Commercial latex agglutination tests are available for a number of viral antibody assays, including rubella in which the cut-off has been adjusted to the internationally agreed level of immunity. The sensitivity of latex agglutination is not a limiting factor in antibody tests, as it may be in antigen tests, because there will be a high enough concentration of specific viral antibodies in most positive-test serum specimens.

4.3 IgM assays

IgM assays have the theoretical advantage of requiring only one serum specimen to show recent infection, but this should be taken just after the acute stage of the disease (when the clinicians may not remember to take it). Tests for IgM antibody are usually confined to the occasions when detecting IgM antibody will resolve uncertainties. Examples include high HI/SRH titre against rubella which could be due to recent infection, uncertainties over glandular fever, congenital CMV infection, etc.

Both indirect and captive EIAs have been used for IgM as outlined above. Although they have more steps, capture assays are preferable because they have fewer problems with rheumatoid factor (Meurman 1983). When extra sensitivity is required, a radio-label has been preferred (M-antibody capture radioimmunoassay, MACRIA) (Mortimer et al. 1981). Antinuclear antibodies may also cause problems but, fortunately, these non-specific reactions are very rare. An experienced virologist can interpret the results correctly by testing paired serum specimens in multiple dilutions.

4.4 Interpretation of antibody assays

Viruses infect individuals but do not always make them ill and, if they do, not always in a typical way. Hence virus diagnosis has some similarities to detective work: the clues have to be recognized and all the information synthesized into as logical and as complete an interpretation as possible; virologists rarely have the complete picture before them. Most of what they know about the patient will come from the request form, which is often both incomplete and inaccurate. Virologists should therefore make regular contact with their clinical colleagues to discuss the results of testing. This is particularly important with serology. All that can be said with certainty about the presence of antibody is that it is produced in response to an antigenic stimulus. It does not indicate where in the body this stimulus occurred nor how major it was. Antibody induced to an enterovirus may indicate a silent infection in the gut, meningitis, myocarditis, intercostal

myalgia or a skin rash. Distinguishing them requires an alert and sceptical mind.

Only the clinician in charge of the patient has the most complete set of information about the illness, including bacteriological results, clinical chemistry data, x-ray appearances etc., as well as the virological results. The virologist has a duty to put the latter in as complete a context as possible. This will mean discussing preliminary positive results with the clinician, especially if they are unexpected.

Virologists who report all apparently positive results as significant will be embarrassed sooner or later. For example, it is not uncommon for the sera of middle-aged or elderly patients to have a moderate titre of measles antibody by CF; this may be genuine but the patients are not febrile nor do they have a rash and there is no apparent cause. Virologists must try to marry their results to the clinical picture in the individual patient but this will not always be complete or even possible. The reasons for this are several: (1) the timing of the specimens; (2) non-specific stimuli; (3) cross-reactions; and (4) anamnestic responses.

The timing of the specimens

For a clear serological result, 2 specimens of serum are needed: one (acute) taken at acute onset of the illness and another (convalescent) taken 10–14 days later. Seroconversion or a rise in titre, accompanied by the appearance of specific IgM antibody, confirms that an appropriate stimulus coincided with the disease. Frequently, neither acute nor convalescent sera are taken at the optimum times, the clear response pattern being blurred as a result.

Non-specific stimuli

There may be a polyclonal stimulus in glandular fever giving several apparently positive results (Linde et al. 1990).

Cross-reactions

These are common between mumps and para-influenzas, among enteroviruses and between HHV-6 and CMV (Linde et al. 1990, Sutherland et al. 1991). They are generally low-titred but underline the need to carry out a screen of tests against several antigens to establish the reaction pattern of single sera.

Anamnestic responses

With both influenza and enteroviruses, infection may provoke a reactivation of antibody production to previously experienced strains of that virus ('original antigenic sin') (Ginsberg 1988). This applies mainly to strain-specific tests, but may occur even with group-specific tests such as complement fixation.

In any serological test, the level of antibody found has to be viewed in the context of the patient's illness together with isolation/identification and other serological results. Isolates are not always confirmed by a rise in antibody level, nor vice versa. Low, slow and sluggish rises in antibody (e.g. 1/10 rising to 1/40 over one month) should be regarded critically, although the old and the immunocompromised (for whatever reason) will react less well or not at all.

EIAs have a 'grey zone' close to the cut-off level (see Fig. 44.5). This will remain no matter how carefully it is defined, and repeat testing may only make the uncertainty greater; all other tests will have similar zones of ambiguity at low titre. There are 2 ways to resolve this: use another test on the first specimen, either in the laboratory or by using a reference laboratory, or ask for another specimen, in the reasonable hope that the titre will have altered enough to give a definite result. Earlier textbooks gave roughly the same weight to a falling titre as a rising one. We are not convinced by falling titres except over a period of several months.

Viruses are usually good antigens inducing a brisk antibody response. The main exceptions are hepatitis B and C, neither of which induces early brisk and reliable responses (except to the core antigen of hepatitis B).

The clinician may be the person best placed to assess the significance of serological results but it is very much the responsibility of the virologist to point out any that are questionable.

5 SPECIMEN COLLECTION AND TRANSPORT

Good specimens are the basis of good virus diagnosis.

Table 44.3 Recommended diagnostic specimens and tests by presenting symptoms

Symptoms/Disease	Specimens[a]	Tests[b]	Alternatives	Sera[c]
URTI[d]	NPA N/S, T/S	EIA IF Culture	System EIAs[e]	P
LRTI[f]	NPA N/S, T/S (Sputum) BAL Lung biopsy	EIA IF Culture	EIAs	P, S
Diarrhoea and vomiting	Faeces (Vomitus)	EM EIA Latex agglutination (Culture)	Latex agglutination PAGE[g]	
Encephalitis, meningitis, paralysis (flaccid)	CSF Stool	PCR Culture	...[k]	P, CSF
PUO[h]	NPA N/S, T/S Faeces	IF EIA EM Culture	Paul–Bunnell	S, P
Vesicular rash/lesion	VF Scraping (NPA)	EM IF EIA	...	P
Maculo-papular rash	NPA Faeces	IF Culture Hybridization	...	P
Hepatitis	...	...	PCR (hepatitis C)	S
Mumps	T/S	Culture	...	P
Mononucleosis	...	...	Paul–Bunnell	S, P
HFRS[i]	...	...	...	S, P
Haemorrhagic fever	T/S	Culture	...	S, P
Skin 'tumours'[j]	Biopsy	EM Hybridization PCR	...	

Entries in parentheses in columns 2 and 3 are less suitable.
[a] For virus isolation or identification: BAL, bronchoalveolar lavage; CSF, cerebrospinal fluid; NPA, nasopharyngeal aspirate (secretions); N/S, nose swab; T/S, throat swab; VF, vesicular fluid.
[b] EIA, enzyme immunoassay; EM, electron microscopy; IF, immunofluorescence.
[c] CSF, tested for antibody – no tests available routinely; P, paired sera, 10–14 days apart; S, single serum, taken as early as possible.
[d] URTI, upper respiratory tract infection, including laryngitis and croup.
[e] Commercially produced machine-based assays and devices.
[f] LRTI, lower respiratory tract infection, including bronchiolitis and pneumonia.
[g] PAGE, polyacrylamide gel electrophoresis with silver staining.
[h] PUO, pyrexia of unknown origin, and feverish illnesses in pregnancy.
[i] HFRS, haemorrhagic fever with renal syndrome, nephropathia epidemica.
[j] For example, molluscum contagiosum, warts; will include some lesions on mucosal surfaces.
[k] Not suitable.

People taking specimens should collect as much as possible, preferably from the site where disease is present, and get them to the laboratory as quickly as possible. This topic has been discussed in detail in a previous publication (Madeley 1992) but some general comments can be made here.

5.1 The specimen

The bigger the quantity obtained the better, particularly if the specimen may have to be tested for several viruses by EM, IF or EIA. Few laboratories find themselves with too much, but many receive poor specimens, either taken from the wrong site or of too small a quantity.

Wherever possible the specimen should be taken from the lesion but this is not always feasible (e.g. from peripheral lung, heart or brain). In these cases, bronchoalveolar lavage, faecal or CSF specimens will be helpful but the results will require interpretation. For IF the specimen must contain infected cells. This means that nasopharyngeal secretions (NPSs), for example, must be collected thoroughly and from the posterior nasal cavity (lined with ciliated columnar 'respiratory' cells) and not from the anterior nares (lined with squamous epithelium). Similarly, skin scrapings should be taken from the active edge of the lesion. Taking NPSs and scrapings may be uncomfortable for the patient but confirming the diagnosis can justify the discomfort.

Swabs should be taken firmly and thoroughly, and adequate quantities of urine, faeces and, as far as possible, CSF should be sent. It is impossible to send too much.

The supporting information should be equally complete. Clinical details should be accurate and relevant. The duration of the illness is an important factor in interpreting the results, especially in serology.

5.2 Transport to the laboratory

Once outside the body, viruses will decay with time. Hence the sooner the specimen reaches the laboratory the better. The rate of decay can be reduced by (1) lowering the temperature and (2) adding virus transport medium (VTM).

LOWERING THE TEMPERATURE

Transport on wet (not dry) ice prolongs survival and can be achieved by the use of wide-mouthed vacuum flasks which, though expensive to buy, can be cycled very successfully between wards and laboratory (in the same or different hospitals). Freezing the specimen should be avoided as this readily inactivates respiratory viruses in particular. Specimens waiting for transport should be kept at 4°C in the ward refrigerator.

ADDING VTM

This contains a sterile buffered salt solution, protein (usually as bovine serum albumin), antibiotics and an indicator. It does not need to be added to NPS, faeces, urine or CSF but swabs should be broken off into a vial of VTM.

Skin scrapings can be spread in a drop of saline on a marked area on a microscope slide (or in a 'well' on a Teflon-coated one) and air-dried before transport by courier or by post. Alternatively, the scrapings may be put in VTM but as large a number of cells as practicable should be collected.

6 SELECTION OF DIAGNOSTIC METHODS

The selection of diagnostic methods for each virus infection often depends on the type, the location and previous experience of the laboratory, the expertise available, the number of specimens tested daily, etc. Cost considerations have become important with regard to the purchase of commercial kits. Major regional virus laboratories will be more interested in epidemiological aspects than individual hospital-based ones, although there is, and should be, considerable overlap between them. These factors make it difficult to give any definitive guidance on which methods to select. Table 44.3 provides some general suggestions but it should be read in the context of local needs.

REFERENCES

Arstila P, Halonen P, 1988, Direct antigen detection, *Diagnosis of Infectious Diseases: Principles and Practices*, vol 2, *Viral, Rickettsial and Chlamydial Diseases*, eds Lennette EH, Halonen P, Murphy FA, Springer-Verlag, New York, 60–75.

Aurelius E, Johansson B et al., 1991, Rapid diagnosis of herpes simplex encephalitis by nested polymerase chain reaction assay of cerebrospinal fluid, *Lancet*, **337:** 189–92.

Becker Y, Darai E, eds, 1995, *PCR: Protocols for Diagnosis of Human and Animal Virus Diseases*, Springer-Verlag, New York.

Birkenmeyer LG, Mushahwar IK, 1991, DNA probe amplification methods, *J Virol Methods*, **35:** 117–26.

Bunce R, Thorpe G, Keen L, 1991, Disposable analytical devices permitting automatic, timed, sequential delivery of multiple reagents, *Anal Chim Acta*, **249:** 263–9.

Caul EO, Ashley CR, Egglestone SI, 1978, An improved method for the routine identification of faecal viruses using ammonium sulphate precipitation, *FEMS Microbiol Lett*, **4:** 1–4.

Codd A, Narang HK, 1986, An ion-exchange capture technique for routine identification of faecal viruses by electron microscopy, *J Virol Methods*, **14:** 229–35.

Compton J, 1991, Nucleic acid sequence-based amplification, *Nature (London)*, **350:** 91–2.

Doane F, Anderson N, 1987, *Electron Microscopy in Diagnostic Virology: a practical guide and atlas*, Cambridge University Press, Cambridge.

Erdman D, Anderson D et al., 1991, Evaluation of monoclonal antibody-based capture enzyme immunoassay for detection of specific antibodies to measles virus, *J Clin Microbiol*, **29:** 1466–71.

Foot AMB, Madeley CR, 1992, Collection of respiratory specimens for immunofluorescence, *Immunofluorescence Techniques in Diagnostic Microbiology*, ed Caul EO, Public Health Laboratory Service, London, 21–32.

Forghani B, Schmidt NJ, 1979, Antigen requirements, sensitivity and specificity of enzyme immunoassays for measles and rubella viral antibodies, *J Clin Microbiol*, **9:** 657–64.

Gardner PS, McQuillin J, 1980, Rapid virus diagnosis, *Application of Immunofluorescence*, 2nd edn, Butterworths, London, 317.

Ginsberg HS, 1988, Orthomyxovirus, *Virology*, 2nd edn, ed Dulbecco R, Ginsberg HS, JB Lippincott, Philadelphia PA, 217–37.

Gupta P, Balachandran R et al., 1987, Detection of human immunodeficiency virus by reverse transcriptase assay, antigen capture assay and radioimmunoassay, *J Clin Microbiol*, **25:** 1122–5.

Halonen P, Obert G, Hierholzer J, 1985, Direct detection of viral antigens in respiratory infections by immunoassays: a four year experience and new developments, *J Med Virol*, **4:** 65–83.

Hamparian VV, 1979, Rhinoviruses, *Diagnostic Procedures for Viral, Rickettsial and Chlamydial Infections*, 5th edn, eds Lennette EH, Schmidt NJ, American Public Health Association, Washington DC, 535–75.

Harmon MW, Jones I et al., 1989, Immunoassays for serological diagnosis of influenza type A using recombinant DNA produced nucleoprotein antigen and monoclonal antibody to human IgG, *J Med Virol*, **27:** 25–30.

Heneine W, Yamamoto S et al., 1995, Detection of reverse transcriptase by a highly sensitive assay in sera from persons infected with human immunodeficiency virus type 1, *J Infect Dis*, **171:** 1210–16.

Herrmann K, Erdman D, 1992, IgM determinations, *Clinical Virology Manual*, 2nd edn, eds Spector S, Lanez GJ, Elsevier Science, New York, 263–76.

Hierholzer JC, Anderson LJ, Halonen PE, 1990, Monoclonal time-resolved fluoroimmunoassay: sensitive systems for the rapid diagnosis for respiratory virus infections, *Medical Virology IV*, eds de la Maza M, Peterson EM, Plenum Press, New York, 17–45.

Hierholzer JC, Bingham PG et al., 1993, Time-resolved fluoroimmunoassay with monoclonal antibodies for rapid identification of parainfluenza type 4 and mumps viruses, *Arch Virol*, **130:** 335–52.

Hollinger FB, Dienstag JL., 1985, Hepatitis virus, *Manual of Clinical Microbiology*, 4th edn, eds Lennette EH, Balows A et al., American Society for Microbiology, Washington DC, 813–35.

Hotchin NA, Crawford DH, 1991, The diagnosis of Epstein–Barr virus-associated disease, *Current Topics in Clinical Virology*, ed Morgan-Capner P, Public Health Laboratory Service, London, 115–40.

Hughes JH, Tuomari AL et al., 1984, Latex immunoassay for rapid detection of rotavirus, *J Clin Microbiol*, **20:** 441–7.

Hyypia T, Stalåndske P et al., 1984, Detection of viral nucleic acids in cell cultures and in clinical specimens by spot hybridization, *Recent Advances in Virus Diagnosis*, Martinus Nijhoff, The Hague, 95–100.

Jansen R, Ledley F, 1989, Production of discrete high specific activity DNA probes using the polymerase chain reaction, *Gene Anal Tech*, **6:** 79–83.

Kangro H, Manzoor S, Harper D, 1991, Antibody avidity following varicella-zoster virus infection, *J Med Virol*, **33:** 100–5.

Koskinen P, Vuorinen T, Meurman O, 1987, Influenza A and B virus IgG and IgM serology by enzyme immunoassays, *Epidemiol Infect*, **99:** 55–64.

Kurstak E, Tijessen P et al., 1986, Enzyme immunoassays and related procedures in diagnostic medical virology, *Bull WHO*, **63:** 793–811.

Kurtz JB, Mortimer PP et al., 1980, Rubella antibody measured by radial haemolysis: characteristics and performance of a simple screening method for use in diagnostic laboratories, *J Hyg (Camb)*, **84:** 213–22.

Leland DS, 1992, Concepts of clinical virology, *Laboratory Diagnosis of Viral Infections*, 2nd edn, ed Lennette EH, Marcel Dekker, New York, 3–43.

Lennette EH, Lennette ET, eds, 1995, *Diagnostic Procedures for Viral, Rickettsial and Chlamydial Infections*, 7th edn, American Public Health Association, Washington DC.

Linde G, Fridell E et al., 1990, Effect of primary Epstein–Barr virus infections on human herpesvirus 6, cytomegalovirus, and measles virus immunoglobulin G titers, *J Clin Microbiol*, **28:** 211–15.

Madeley CR, 1992, Respiratory viruses, *Immunofluorescence Techniques in Diagnostic Microbiology*, ed Caul EO, Public Health Laboratory Service, London, 33–48.

Madeley CR, Field AM, 1988, *Virus Morphology*, 2nd edn, Churchill Livingstone, Edinburgh.

Meurman OH, 1983, Detection of antiviral IgM antibodies and its problems – a review, *Curr Top Microbiol Immunol*, **104:** 101–31.

Meurman O, Waris M, Hedman K, 1992, Immunoglobulin G antibody avidity in patients with respiratory syncytial virus infection, *J Clin Microbiol*, **30:** 1479–84.

Mortimer PP, Tedder RS et al., 1981, Antibody capture radioimmunoassay for anti-rubella IgM, *J Hyg (Camb)*, **86:** 139–53.

Nohynek H, Eskola J et al., 1991, The causes of hospital-treated lower respiratory tract infection in children, *Am J Dis Child*, **145:** 618–22.

Okuno T, Takahashi K et al., 1989, Seroepidemiology of human herpesvirus 6 infection in normal children and adults, *J Clin Microbiol*, **27:** 651–3.

Oshiro LS, Miller SE, 1992, Application of electron microscopy to the diagnosis of viral infections, *Laboratory Diagnosis of Viral Infections*, 2nd edn, Marcel Dekker, New York, 45–68.

Palmer E, Martin M, 1988, *Electron Microscopy in Viral Diagnosis*, CRC Press, Boca Raton FL.

Parry J, Perry KV, Mortimer PP, 1987, Scientific assays for viral antibodies in saliva: an alternative to tests on serum, *Lancet*, **330:** 72–95.

Puchhammer-Stöckl E, Popow-Kraupp T et al., 1991, Detection of varicella-zoster virus DNA by polymerase chain reaction in the cerebrospinal fluid of patients suffering from neurological complications associated with chickenpox or herpes zoster, *J Clin Microbiol*, **29:** 1513–16.

Pyra H, Boni J, Schubach J, 1994, Ultrasensitive retrovirus detection by a reverse transcription assay based on product enhancement, *Proc Natl Acad Sci USA*, **91:** 1544–8.

Saiki RK, Gelfano DH et al., 1988, Primer-directed enzymatic amplification of DNA with a thermostable DNA polymerase, *Science*, **239:** 487–91.

Scalia G, Halonen P et al., 1995, Comparison of monoclonal biotin–avidin enzyme immunoassay and monoclonal time-resolved fluoroimmunoassay in detection of respiratory virus antigens, *Clin Diagn Virol*, **3:** 351–9.

Stirk P, Griffiths P, 1987, Use of monoclonal antibodies for the diagnosis of cytomegalovirus infection by the detection of early antigen fluorescent foci (DEAFF) in cell culture, *J Med Virol*, **21:** 329–37.

Sutherland S, Christofinis G et al., 1991, A serological investigation of human herpesvirus 6 infections in liver transplant recipients and the detection of cross-reacting antibodies to cytomegalovirus, *J Med Virol*, **33:** 172–6.

Thomas HIJ, Morgan-Capner P, 1988, Rubella-specific IgG subclass avidity ELISA and its role in the differentiation between primary rubella and rubella reinfection, *Epidemiol Infect*, **101:** 591–8.

Vuorinen T, Meurman O, 1989, Enzyme immunoassays for detection of IgG and IgM antibodies to parainfluenza types 1, 2 and 3, *J Virol Methods*, **23:** 63–70.

Wagner D, Ikenberg H et al., 1984, Identification of human papillomavirus in cervical swabs by deoxyribonucleic acid in situ hybridization, *Obstet Gynecol*, **64:** 767–72.

Walls H, Johansson K et al., 1986, Time-resolved fluoroimmunoassay with monoclonal antibodies for rapid diagnosis of influenza infections, *J Clin Microbiol*, **24:** 907–12.

Waris M, Ziegler T et al., 1990, Rapid detection of respiratory syncytial virus and influenza A virus in cell cultures by immunoperoxidase staining with monoclonal antibodies, *J Clin Microbiol*, **28:** 1159–62.

Willcocks MM, Carter MJ et al., 1991, A dot-blot hybridization procedure for the detection of astrovirus in stool samples, *Epidemiol Infect*, **107**: 405–10.

Wrigley NG, 1968, The lattice spacing of crystalline catalase as an internal standard of length in electron microscopy, *J Ultrastruct Res*, **24**: 454–64.

Ziegler T, Waris M et al., 1988, Herpes simplex virus detection by microscopic reading after overnight incubation and immunoperoxidase staining, *J Clin Microbiol*, **26**: 2013–17.

Ziegler T, Hall H et al., 1995, Type- and subtype-specific detection of influenza viruses in clinical specimens by rapid culture assay, *J Clin Microbiol*, **33**: 318–21.

Chapter 45

IMMUNOPROPHYLAXIS OF VIRAL DISEASES

S C Hadler, S C Redd and R W Sutter

1 INTRODUCTION

Vaccines are among the most effective and cost-effective means for the prevention of disease. The development of viral vaccines predates the recognition of viral agents as causes of disease by over a century; their use has resulted in marked decreases in the incidence of or eradication of diseases that were important causes of human mortality. Vaccines are now available to prevent 14 viral diseases, and new generations of vaccines being developed through molecular techniques hold the promise of providing protection against others.

The modern era of vaccine development began with the demonstration by Jenner that inoculation with cowpox virus provided protection against smallpox and the subsequent recommendation for wide use of variolation to protect against this disease. The effective use of variola vaccine world-wide culminated, in 1977, in the certification of eradication of smallpox after a decade-long campaign co-ordinated by the World Health Organization (Fenner et al. 1988). By 1977, viral vaccines to prevent rabies, influenza, yellow fever, poliomyelitis, measles, rubella and mumps had also been developed and used with striking success to reduce the disease burden due to these viruses. Following the eradication of smallpox, global immunization programmes to prevent 6 childhood diseases, including poliomyelitis and measles, were implemented (Galazka 1994). A goal for global eradication of poliomyelitis by the year 2000 has been established, and implementation is now well underway, with eradication already certified in the Americas. A global strategy, which includes mass vaccination campaigns and intensive surveillance for acute flaccid paralysis in children, is being implemented in regions where polio is endemic (Hull et al. 1994). A regional campaign to eliminate measles is also underway in the Americas, and shows promise as a guide for future global efforts against this disease (de Quadros et al. 1996).

2 IMMUNOPROPHYLAXIS OF VIRAL INFECTIONS

The primary objectives of viral immunoprophylaxis are to prevent viral infection or to modify viral disease. Active immunoprophylaxis with viral vaccines stimulates the immune system to develop antibodies, cell-mediated immunity, or both, to prevent infection (e.g. measles, polio), and is usually given before exposure to disease. Vaccines (e.g. rabies, hepatitis B) may be effective in preventing disease after exposure, because the immune system is stimulated during the long incubation periods of these infections. Vaccines intended to modify the course of previously established infection (e.g. HIV infection, varicella vaccine to prevent herpes zoster recurrences) are currently undergoing clinical trials.

Passive immunoprophylaxis, using pooled immuno-globulins prepared from human or animal serum, provides temporary protection either against infection (pre-exposure prophylaxis for hepatitis A) or to prevent or modify infection after exposure (disease-specific immunoglobulins to prevent rabies, hepatitis B, varicella).

3 TYPES OF VIRAL VACCINES

The two classic approaches to active viral immunization include inactivated viruses or their purified components, and live attenuated vaccines. For some viral diseases, both approaches have been used (poliomyelitis, measles, influenza).

3.1 Inactivated viral vaccines

Inactivated vaccines may consist of whole virus particles, purified antigenic surface proteins or smaller peptide epitopes (Table 45.1). Inactivated whole virus vaccines are produced by the multiplication of virus in other animal species (e.g. rabies in mouse brain); in eggs, chick embryos or allantoic fluid (influenza, measles, mumps); or in cell culture (rabies in human diploid cells, polio), followed by purification and inactivation. Whole virus vaccines have the advantage of producing immune responses not only to surface proteins but also internal components, which may help eliminate viral infection. In the past, purified antigenic protein vaccines have been produced either by disruption of whole virus and purification of component proteins (split virus influenza) or by purification from the blood of virus carriers (plasma-derived hepatitis B vaccine). Newer generations of inactivated vaccines have been developed by inserting DNA that encodes antigenic viral proteins into other microorganisms (*Escherichia coli*, yeast, CHO cells, other viruses) and by producing recombinant proteins, which are subsequently purified (hepatitis B surface antigen and herpes simplex virus glycoprotein in yeast).

New approaches to development

Other methods for producing inactivated vaccines include the use of synthetic peptides and idiotypic antibodies. Synthetic peptides, initially produced in 1963, were thought to have great promise as vaccines, especially as DNA sequencing technologies permitted identification of the precise sequences of antigenic

sites of viral proteins (Brown 1988). The antigenic sites of viruses may be identified by determining the 3-dimensional structure of the virus, comparing sequences of mutant and wild type viruses or identifying hydrophilic regions of surface proteins and constructing peptides duplicating these sequences. Production of highly purified peptides is feasible, potentially inexpensive and results in a well defined product without risk of containing adventitious agents. The feasibility of inducing protection in an immunized animal model has been demonstrated by use of an icosapeptide of the surface protein of the foot-and-mouth disease virus (Murphy and Channock 1990). However, other efforts with human disease viruses have met with less success. Peptides are often poorly immunogenic, may stimulate development of binding but not neutralizing antibodies, do not generally induce T cell responses unless coupled to larger proteins, and cannot mimic conformational epitopes. Efforts to overcome these limitations include coupling to peptide carriers containing T cell epitopes to enhance immunogenicity and incorporating antigens into self-assembling particles. Although experimental vaccines have been produced (influenza, foot-and-mouth disease) and found to be protective in animals (canine parvovirus and mink enteritis virus), it is uncertain whether vaccines for use in humans will follow (Meloen et al. 1995).

Anti-idiotype vaccines are based on the principle that neutralizing antibodies to viral antigens contain the mirror image of these epitopes, known as idiotypes. Anti-idiotype antibodies can be generated that mimic the conformation of the original viral epitope, and can then be used to induce neutralizing antibodies in the host. Immunization with anti-idiotype antibody results in the development of neutralizing antibodies to several viruses (poliovirus, hepa-

Table 45.1 Currently available inactivated viral vaccines

Vaccine	Vaccine type	Uses
Inactivated polio	Killed whole virus	Immunization of immunocompromised people; universal childhood immunization (some developed countries)
Hepatitis B	Purified HBsAg produced by recombinant yeast, mammalian cells or from plasma	Routine childhood or adolescent immunization; immunization of high risk adults; postexposure immunization with HBIG
Influenza	Killed whole or split virus	Vaccination of high risk individuals or the elderly
Rabies	Killed whole virus	Postexposure vaccination of individuals, with HRIG; pre-exposure: veterinarians/travellers
Hepatitis A	Killed whole virus	Pre-exposure vaccination: high risk people and travellers
Japanese B encephalitis	Killed whole virus	Pre-exposure vaccination of travellers to endemic areas; routine or mass vaccination in endemic areas
Tick-borne encephalitis	Killed whole virus	Pre-exposure vaccination of travellers to endemic areas; (?)routine or mass vaccination in endemic areas

titis B surface antigen (HBsAg), rabies) and protection against disease in animal models (Dalgliesh and Kennedy 1988). However, the levels of antibodies induced have been less than those induced by the original antigen, and the practicality of this approach remains to be demonstrated.

INACTIVATION OF VIRAL VACCINES

Inactivated whole virus vaccines produced in culture, animal tissues or human serum must be subjected to steps that can inactivate the original virus as well as any adventitious agents that may be present in the initial substrate. Formalin has been most commonly used to ensure inactivation of residual viral activity in such vaccines. A balance between the concentration of formalin and the duration of treatment is needed to eliminate residual infectivity of the virus without destroying immunogenicity. Inadequate inactivation of poliovirus by formalin resulted in an outbreak of paralytic poliomyelitis due to inactivated polio vaccine soon after its introduction in the USA (Nathanson and Langmuir 1963). Review of this incident subsequently led to improvement in methods of viral purification and of formalin inactivation procedures. Other inactivating agents that may be used include heat, acetylethyleneimine and β-propiolactone. These inactivating agents may also provide protection against adventitious agents which can replicate in the cell or animal substrates used to produce vaccines. However, this protection depends on the sensitivity of the agent to the inactivation process. The failure of formalin to inactivate SV40 virus contamination in inactivated polio vaccine originating from monkey kidney cell substrate raised concern about the safety of this vaccine (Melnick and Stinebaugh 1962), although subsequent epidemiological studies failed to show adverse effects in recipients (Mortimer et al. 1982).

DNA VACCINES

DNA vaccines represent a new and highly promising strategy for vaccine development. DNA-encoding antigenic portions of viruses – envelope, core or nucleoprotein – are inserted into a plasmid, which can be injected directly into the host as 'naked' DNA free of protein or nucleoprotein complexes. Host cells take up the DNA and may express the encoded proteins. Because the proteins are produced intracellularly, they enter the major histocompatibility complex (MHC) class I pathway and stimulate a strong cell-mediated immune response (CMI), in contrast to inactivated vaccines, which enter the MHC class II pathway and produce primarily an antibody response (Fynan et al. 1995, McDonnell and Askari 1996). This predominantly cell-mediated immune response may assist in immune control of both acute and chronic viral infections. Multivalent vaccines could be constructed that provide protection against several diseases simultaneously.

A prototype naked DNA vaccine using the core nucleoprotein of influenza virus has been developed that protects mice from lethal doses of both homologous and heterologous strains of influenza virus. This vaccine induces both humoral antibody and CMI. Although antibodies to surface glycoproteins protect against infection from the homologous strain, it is likely that CMI provides protection against heterologous strains. Development of DNA vaccines that stimulate CMI to conserved internal proteins is a promising approach to the prevention or treatment of infections with viruses that rapidly mutate their surface antigens, such as hepatitis C and human immunodeficiency virus (HIV). Candidate vaccines to prevent hepatitis B, HIV and other viruses are under development.

Key concerns about these vaccines include possible mutagenesis if the DNA plasmid is inserted into the host genome; the potential for developing tolerance to the antigen because of ongoing production in host cells; and the potential for immune attack on the cells producing the encoded antigen.

3.2 Live attenuated viral vaccines

Currently available live attenuated virus vaccines have been prepared by 2 approaches: (1) from related species of virus (jennerian approach: vaccinia to prevent smallpox; rhesus rotavirus), and (2) by serial passage of virus through live organisms or through one or more cell culture lines (Table 45.2). Examples of the latter include yellow fever vaccine, developed via passage of wild virus in mice and subsequently in chick embryos; and polio (types 1 and 3) and measles vaccines, initially passaged in monkey kidney cells and chick embryo fibroblasts respectively. Concern about the presence of adventitious viruses in animal derived cell lines (SV40 virus in monkey kidney cell lines) has led to increased use of human diploid cell lines for producing live virus vaccines (rubella, varicella, polio). Several cell lines (WI-38 and MRC-5) are now commonly used. The World Health Organization has established guidelines for assessing the safety of vaccines produced in human cell lines (World Health Organization 1987).

Live attenuated vaccines may also be produced via genetic reassortment. Among viruses with multiple-strand genomes, reassortants that combine the genomes encoding antigenic surface proteins from wild virus strains with genomes from attenuated or related strains of virus (cold-adapted influenza; rhesus- or bovine-based rotavirus vaccines) have been developed and shown to be effective (Murphy 1993, Kapikian 1994).

NEW APPROACHES TO DEVELOPMENT

Other approaches to the development of live virus vaccines include directed mutagenesis, use of strains of viruses from related species, and use of viral vectors such as vaccinia and canarypox. Methods for direct mutagenesis include growth in low temperatures (25 or 32–34°C) to select temperature-sensitive or cold-adapted strains that do not grow well at human body temperature (Murphy and Channock 1990). Molecular biological techniques, combined with better understanding of molecular aspects of viral replication, can be used to develop specific mutations, such as deletion

Table 45.2 Currently available live attenuated viral vaccines

Vaccine	Vaccine type	Uses
Oral polio	Attenuated trivalent	Routine childhood immunization; mass campaigns
Measles	Attenuated (Schwarz, Moraten, others)	Routine childhood immunization; mass campaigns
Rubella	Attenuated (RA 27/3)	Routine childhood immunization; adolescent girls; susceptible women of childbearing age
Mumps	Attenuated (Urabe or Jeryl Lynn)	Routine childhood immunization
Measles, mumps, rubella (MMR)	Attenuated	Routine childhood immunization (1 or 2 doses)
Varicella	Attenuated (Oka)	Routine childhood immunization (USA); vaccination of susceptible people
Yellow fever	Attenuated (17D)	Routine immunization or mass vaccination in endemic areas; vaccination of travellers to endemic areas
Smallpox (limited availability)	Vaccinia virus	Vaccination of research workers
Under development		
Rotavirus	Rhesus or bovine reassortants (4 serotypes)	(?)Routine childhood immunization
Influenza	Cold adapted/reassortants	(?)Immunization of high risk children/adolescents

mutants, which are unlikely to revert to wild strains. Vaccines that are being developed from related animal viruses include rhesus rotavirus as a candidate strain to prevent human rotavirus type 3, combined with reassortants that incorporate the surface protein genes for human rotavirus types 1, 2 and 4 (Kapikian 1994). Bovine parainfluenza virus type 3 induces neutralizing antibodies to human parainfluenza virus type 3, and is a candidate vaccine to prevent this disease. Large viruses such as vaccinia and other orthopoxviruses can incorporate DNA that encodes essential proteins from other viruses (e.g. hepatitis B, rabies, measles haemagglutinin or fusion proteins), attached to viral promoters that ensure adequate production of these antigens (Perkus 1985, Moss et al. 1988). Vaccination results in replication of the parent virus, production of the encoded viral proteins and stimulation of both humoral and cell-mediated immunity. Although there has been some success in inducing immune response to the encoded proteins (HBsAg, influenza A, herpes simplex glycoprotein, rabies) and protection has been induced in experimental animals, concern about the potential for serious adverse events following vaccinia vaccination and limited success in inducing a strong antibody response have slowed development of vaccinia-recombinants for humans. The use of canarypox virus, which undergoes only abortive infection in humans, may overcome concerns about the safety of such vaccines, and candidate vaccines have induced high levels of antibody against rab-

ies glycoprotein and the measles haemagglutinin gene in humans.

RISK OF ADVENTITIOUS AGENTS

Possible contamination with adventitious agents is also a concern with live virus vaccines (Waters et al. 1972). A series of tests for potential contaminating agents is undertaken during vaccine development, safety testing and postlicensing monitoring of vaccines (World Health Organization 1987). However, concerns regarding agents not detectable by current methods continue to arise despite the apparent safety of these vaccines.

3.3 Immunological basis of response to active immunization

Development of an immune response generally requires the interaction of T lymphocytes with antigen processing and presenting cells (dendritic or macrophages) (McDevitt 1980, Lanzavecchia 1985, Claman 1992). T cell response is induced following the uptake of antigen by mononuclear phagocytes or dendritic cells, and can be enhanced by use of an adjuvant; the antigen is processed and presented, in association with MHC antigens, to T-helper cells. T cells recognize polypeptide antigens of 8–20 amino acids in size, presented in association with specific MHC molecules; the type of MHC molecule with which the antigen is presented by antigen-processing cells depends on the source and processing of the polypeptide. These in turn determine the primary type of T cell response, either cytotoxic or helper. Presentation to T-helper cells results in secretion of immune mediators (cytokines) that can stimulate the maturation of naive T cells and communicate between leucocytes (via interleukins) to regulate the immune response (Baker 1975, Reinherz and Schlossman 1980, Arai et al. 1990). (See also Chapter 11.)

Antigens from inactivated vaccines are absorbed into vacuoles, and processed and presented with MHC class II antigens; antigens from live attenuated vaccines or vectored vaccines, produced within the cell, are processed in microtubules and presented with MHC class I antigens. Depending on the antigen and its MHC presentation, T lymphocytes differentiate into either T-helper type 1 cells (Th1, stimulated by MHC I associated antigen), which mediate CMI, or T-helper 2 (Th2, with MHC II), which assist B cells in developing antibody production. Each of these subsets produces different interleukins and other immune mediators responsible for modulating the immune response.

An antibody response to an initial dose develops 2–6 weeks after immunization with inactivated antigens but may be incomplete even after 2 doses; after effective priming, booster responses occur within 4–14 days. The initial response is usually IgM antibodies, followed within weeks by IgG antibodies. Response to live vaccines requires a cycle of replication of the vaccine virus, and a period of several weeks or months for full development of the immune response. Response to measles vaccination is usually maximal by 6 weeks, but in younger children antibody titres may continue to rise for several months after vaccination.

3.4 Immune response to inactivated and live attenuated vaccines

INACTIVATED VACCINES

Inactivated or purified viral vaccines induce responses only to the components present in the vaccine. Multiple doses, usually 3 or more, are necessary to induce a satisfactory response that will persist for long periods; booster doses may be necessary to ensure lasting protection. Most inactivated vaccines are given parenterally, and induce either no mucosal antibody or lower levels than live attenuated vaccines administered by the oral or nasal routes. Inactivated vaccines may have limited ability to induce T cell-mediated immunity, which is induced more strongly by antigens produced intracellularly as occurs with replication of live viral vaccines.

The advantages of inactivated vaccines are the absence of risk of disease due to the vaccine virus, given adequate inactivation; greater thermal stability and ease of handling in routine vaccination programmes; and a lower risk of contamination with active adventitious agents than in live attenuated vaccines. Nevertheless, examples of both inadequate inactivation and presence of active adventitious agents

were documented in the past in inactivated polio vaccine (IPV) (Nathanson and Langmuir 1963, Mortimer et al. 1982), although these problems have not been observed with hepatitis B, hepatitis A, or any other recently developed inactivated vaccines. Inactivated vaccines can be given safely to people with immunosuppressive conditions.

A disadvantage of inactivated vaccines is the possible potentiation of the disease that the vaccine is intended to prevent. The original killed measles vaccines induced a detectable immune response, but recipients exposed to wild measles virus developed atypical measles with systemic symptoms and giant cell pneumonia (Annunziato et al. 1982). Subsequent analyses indicated that the formalin treatment destroyed the antigenicity of the measles fusion protein, resulting in an unbalanced response (to haemagglutinin only). Similar accentuation of respiratory syncytial virus disease in recipients of a formalin-inactivated vaccine was observed in early trials, and later shown in experimental animals to result from stimulation of formation of binding but not neutralizing antibodies to the surface F and G glycoproteins (Murphy and Channock 1990).

LIVE ATTENUATED VACCINES

Live attenuated vaccines have the advantage of inducing a complex immunological response simulating natural infection. Replication of the vaccine organism and processing of antigens mimic those of the natural organism, and both humoral and cell-mediated responses are generated to a variety of antigens. Because these antigens are similar or identical to those of the wild organism, responses are usually more effective and cross-reactive than those induced by inactivated vaccines. In addition, mucosal antibody may be stimulated directly by such vaccines when administered through oral or nasal routes (McGhee et al. 1992). Administration of oral or nasal live vaccines is more convenient than injection of inactivated vaccines. Immunity induced by one dose of a live attenuated vaccine is long lasting, possibly life-long. However, the strength of humoral response is usually less than that of natural infection, and detectable antibodies may wane with time and result in some loss of protection. Induction of immunity by live vaccines can be inhibited by passively acquired antibody, whether from transplacental acquisition from the mother or from receipt of immunoglobulin-containing blood products; thus, achieving optimal response relies on ensuring that passive antibody (e.g. of maternal origin or acquired through administration of blood products) has declined to an adequate degree. In addition, because the response may be incomplete (90–95%) after a single dose, 2 or more doses may be necessary to induce sufficient immunity to protect both the individual and the community.

The potential disadvantages of live vaccines include residual virulence of the vaccine in both healthy and immunocompromised hosts; possible contamination with adventitious agents; possible interference of response by other viral infections; and greater lability of the vaccine. Potential reversion to virulence has been well demonstrated with oral polio vaccine, paralytic poliomyelitis occurring in either vaccinees or their contacts at a rate of c. 1 per 2.5 million vaccine doses distributed, with greatest risk after the first vaccine dose (Strebel et al. 1992). Persistent viral infection may occur in immunocompromised people after inadvertent use of measles and oral polio vaccines, and may rarely occur in healthy adults given rubella vaccine (Institute of Medicine 1991, 1993). However, measles vaccine has not been linked to the development of subacute sclerosing panencephalitis. Early lots of oral polio vaccine and yellow fever vaccine were contaminated with SV40 and avian leucosis viruses, respectively. Although these were not linked with any long-term consequences (Waters et al. 1972), cell substrates used for vaccine production are now tested to ensure that these and other known pathogenic viruses are not present. Nevertheless, it may not be possible to ensure the absence of any adventitious agents in live virus vaccines. The stability of live virus vaccines depends on appropriate handling. Such vaccines require a sound cold chain, with storage at either 0–4°C (measles; measles, mumps, rubella (MMR)) or –15°C (polio, varicella), which can increase the cost of vaccination and impede their use in developing countries.

3.5 Determinants of response to viral vaccines

Vaccine and host characteristics are the primary determinants of vaccine response. Response may be affected by vaccine dosage, adjuvant, route and site of administration, number and timing of doses, and vaccine handling. Vaccine doses are determined before licensing to ensure a high level of response; adjuvants such as aluminium hydroxide, used only with inactivated antigens, stimulate a better response with a lower dose of antigen. The route of administration – intradermal, subcutaneous, intramuscular or mucosal – can determine both the strength and the nature of the immune response. Mucosal administration (intranasal or oral) stimulates higher levels of mucosal immunity (IgA antibodies), which may inhibit disease transmission with greater effectiveness than parenteral administration, which induces limited or no mucosal response (McGhee et al. 1992). Intradermal vaccination with low doses may induce antibody responses similar to those induced by intramuscular or subcutaneous administration of recommended doses, but is more difficult to deliver precisely and achieves less predictable responses. Intramuscular injections should be given in the anterior thigh (infants) or deltoid (older children and adults); injection into the buttocks produces a lower response (well documented in adults), probably owing to delivery of the vaccine into adipose tissue (Centers for Disease Control and Prevention 1994b). The timing of vaccine doses is important: a minimum interval of 1 month between primary doses is usual for inactivated vaccines; delay of a third or reinforcing dose for

6 or more months after the first enhances the response and duration of antibody persistence, and is preferred unless high risk of disease necessitates shorter intervals. Intervals of 4–6 weeks are considered necessary to ensure optimal response to successive doses of live virus vaccines. The recommended routes and sites of administration and the timing of doses are devised to ensure optimal effectiveness in disease prevention and should therefore be used.

HOST FACTORS

Host factors that affect immune response include genetic factors (MHC polymorphism), age, nutritional and immune status, gender, pregnancy and smoking. Although genetic factors such as MHC polymorphism are known to affect response at a molecular level, they have a limited effect on population response to available vaccines. Age is an important factor in response to immunization. Newborn infants generally do not develop as strong a response to inactivated vaccines as older infants or children (hepatitis B), and with certain vaccines maternal antibody may inhibit it (IPV, hepatitis A). For live vaccines such as measles, inhibition of the response by maternal antibodies determines the optimal timing for vaccination in early childhood. The response to vaccines is excellent in young and adolescent children and in young adults, but decreases with increasing age. Male gender in adults and pregnancy have minor negative effects on antibody response of limited clinical significance; smoking decreases response to many antigens, and may increase the risk of non-response when other negative factors are present (Hadler and Margolis 1992). Extreme debilitation, acquired or congenital immunodeficiency disorders, diseases or treatments that cause immunosuppression, and some chronic diseases (renal disease, diabetes) can decrease immune response. For people with such conditions, inactivated vaccines are recommended despite lower effectiveness but may require higher or more frequent doses to achieve optimal response; live vaccines are often contraindicated owing to the risk of disseminated disease and possible death due to the vaccine organism (Centers for Disease Control and Prevention 1993b).

3.6 Measurement of response

Ideally, reliable laboratory tests should be available to measure the presence and strength of each of the major effectors of protection against the disease. In practice, tests for the presence of antibody are usually available (e.g. radioimmunoassay (RIA), enzyme immunoassay (EIA), complement fixation, immunofluorescent techniques) but these often do not measure the presence of functional (neutralizing or opsonizing) antibody. Tests for CMI are generally available only in research facilities. For some diseases, such as hepatitis B, polio and measles there are reliable tests for neutralizing antibodies and the levels needed to confer protection are known; however, only for hepatitis B are inexpensive tests available widely. For other diseases such as rubella, commercial tests are available, often using EIA methods, but specificity is often less well defined, and sensitivity is lower than that of neutralization assays. Development of better laboratory methods to measure protection and to permit rapid diagnosis of acute disease will remain a priority of disease control programmes.

4 PRELICENSING VACCINE EVALUATION

Licences are granted only after extensive review of safety and efficacy data. Before licensing, vaccines are studied first in animals and then in small numbers of humans to determine safety, immunogenicity and optimal dosages and schedules (phase I and II trials). Phase III trials examine safety and efficacy in larger numbers (1000–10 000) of subjects. Nevertheless, prelicensing trials are limited in their ability to detect rare adverse reactions (frequency less than 1 per 1000–10 000 doses) to vaccination, or adverse events in specific risk groups. Phase IV trials postlicensing may include larger numbers of vaccinees and can better define the frequency of uncommon adverse events. Linking the records of vaccination and of medical outcome in large numbers of children in health maintenance organizations (HMOs) or other providers of comprehensive medical care can provide a way to assess causality of temporally related adverse events. In addition, postmarketing surveillance permits detection of new or unanticipated adverse events; reporting of such events observed after vaccination is required in many countries.

5 PRINCIPLES OF IMMUNIZATION PROGRAMMES

The development of successful disease control programmes requires safe and effective vaccines and effective public health strategies to prevent disease. Strategies for vaccine use are based on knowledge of epidemiology, consideration of whether eradication or reduction of disease is the primary goal, and the potential for implementing effective programmes to deliver vaccines either to the entire population or to target groups (Table 45.3). Among the critical aspects of disease epidemiology are: (1) whether the disease causes infection universally in humans (e.g. poliomyelitis, measles, rubella, varicella, hepatitis B in some populations) or only in specific groups (hepatitis B in developed countries; rabies; yellow fever); (2) the primary age groups affected; (3) the primary reservoir for infection, including whether an animal reservoir exists (rabies, yellow fever) or infection occurs naturally only in humans (hepatitis B, hepatitis A, measles, mumps, rubella, poliomyelitis); and (4) whether the virus causes only acute infection or results in chronic or latent infection. Strategies targeted at eradication may be considered for diseases without substantial animal reservoirs or chronic or latent infection in humans, whereas reduction must be the initial

goal when animal (rabies) or human reservoirs (hepatitis B, varicella) exist (Centers for Disease Control and Prevention 1993c). Mathematical modelling of the possible impact of vaccines on disease incidence may be helpful for selecting immunization strategies (Fox et al. 1972, Anderson and May 1990, Halloran et al. 1994).

Considerations of cost-effectiveness of vaccination programmes also have become increasingly important when developing vaccination strategies. Universal use of vaccines to prevent polio, measles, mumps and rubella saves money when direct costs of health care are considered (Hatziandreu et al. 1994). Studies showing that universal use of varicella and hepatitis B vaccines resulted in savings in combined direct (health care) and indirect costs influenced the development of policy for the use of these vaccines throughout the USA (Lieu et al. 1994, Margolis et al. 1995).

Programmes based on universal vaccination of infants or young children have been implemented successfully (poliomyelitis, measles) in both developed and developing countries (Hinman and Orenstein 1994). Alternative approaches include universal vaccination of adolescents (rubella, hepatitis B), universal vaccination of all or some adults (influenza) and vaccination only of certain target groups or exposed people (rabies, hepatitis B, influenza). Mass immunization campaigns targeted at specific age groups are important in efforts to reduce the incidence of disease rapidly and in elimination programmes for poliomyelitis and measles (Hull et al. 1994, de Quadros et al. 1996).

5.1 Vaccine schedules

Childhood immunization programmes are now recommended in all countries and have resulted in substantial declines in the occurrence of vaccine-preventable diseases in both developed and developing countries (Galazka 1994, Centers for Disease Control and Prevention 1994a). Childhood immunization schedules are usually established by national governments or advisory bodies. In the USA, policy is established by the Advisory Committee on Immunization Practices (ACIP) of the US Public Health Service and the Committee on Infectious Diseases of the American Academy of Pediatrics (AAP), in consultation with the American Academy of Family Physicians (Centers for Disease Control and Prevention 1994b, Committee on Infectious Diseases 1994, Gindler et al. 1995). Effective January 1997, the unified childhood immunization schedule recommends use of vaccines to prevent 6 viral diseases: measles, mumps, rubella, polio, hepatitis B and varicella (Fig. 45.1). With recommended universal hepatitis B vaccination of children, immunization can start at birth or any time up to 2 months of age. Routine doses are scheduled at 2, 4 and 6 months of age (diphtheria and tetanus toxoids and pertussis vaccine, DTP; *Haemophilus influenzae* type b, Hib; polio vaccine (either oral polio vaccine (OPV) or inactivated polio vaccine (IPV)

Table 45.3 Approaches to control of viral diseases with vaccines

Disease	Proportion of population infected	Primary age of infection[a]	Chronic carrier	Animal reservoir	Eradicable with vaccine	Type of vaccination programme
Polio	High	Child	No	No	Yes	Child; mass campaigns
Smallpox[b]	High	Child	No	No	Yes	Child; containment
Measles	Universal	Child	No	No	Yes	Child
Rubella	Universal	Child/adult	No	No	Yes	Child; adolescent girls/women
Varicella	Universal	Child/adult	Yes[d]	No	Possible[c]	Child; adult (susceptible)
Hepatitis B	Variable	Child/adult	Yes	No	Possible[c]	Infant; adolescent; high risk adult
Influenza	High	All	No	H + A[e]	No	High risk persons (e.g. elderly)
Yellow fever	None to high	All	No	Yes	No	High risk; universal
Rabies	Very low	All	No	Yes	No	High risk; postexposure

[a]Prior to wide use of vaccine.
[b]Smallpox was certified as eradicated in 1977.
[c]Potentially eradicable after several generations of vaccination or if human carriage of virus can be eliminated.
[d]Latent infection.
[e]Human + animal.

or sequential IPV–OPV); and hepatitis B). MMR is recommended at 12–15 months of age. Booster doses of DTP and polio vaccine are recommended at school entry, with the second MMR dose given at either primary or secondary school entry.

During the early adolescent years (age 11–16), immunization status should be assessed to ensure that the second dose of MMR has been given, to provide the primary series of hepatitis B vaccine to children who have not already received it and to ensure immunity to varicella.

In the UK, recommendations for immunization are issued and periodically updated by the Departments of Health (Department of Health et al. 1996).

Routine childhood vaccinations and schedules vary in other countries (Hinman and Orenstein 1994). Polio and measles vaccination are almost universal, and rubella, mumps and hepatitis B vaccination are offered by many developed and some developing countries. The World Health Organization recommends that all countries provide immunization to prevent 6 diseases, including polio and measles, vaccinations being given at birth, at 6, 10 and 14 weeks of age, and at 9 months of age (Table 45.4). Hepatitis B vaccination, beginning at birth or 6 weeks of age, is recommended in all areas where hepatitis B virus (HBV) infection is endemic (>2% HBV carriers) (Kane 1993), and yellow fever vaccination is recommended at 9 months of age in areas where this disease occurs.

Vaccination of adults is also recommended in many countries. Influenza vaccination is recommended for high-risk groups and in some countries for all elderly people (>64 years in the USA) (Table 45.5) (Centers for Disease Control and Prevention 1991c, Hinman and Orenstein 1994). In addition, vaccination of adults at risk for hepatitis B, hepatitis A, measles, mumps, rubella and varicella may be recommended on the basis of licensing of vaccines and the burden of disease in a risk group as well as a lack of history of previous disease or immunization.

SIMULTANEOUS ADMINISTRATION OF VACCINES

All childhood vaccines may be given simultaneously if necessary, on the basis of data from many studies showing that most vaccines can be given at the same time without compromising safety or immunogenicity. Thus, DTP, Hib, OPV, hepatitis B, MMR and varicella vaccines may be given simultaneously or within any interval of each other (King and Hadler 1994). Interference between live virus vaccines other than OPV (e.g. MMR) can, theoretically, occur if they are given not simultaneously but within close intervals; live virus vaccines should either be given simultaneously or at least 1 month apart. Interference has been found between certain vaccines for travellers (cholera and yellow fever) (Centers for Disease Control and Prevention 1994b). Immunoglobulins or blood products containing immunoglobulins inhibit the response to cer-

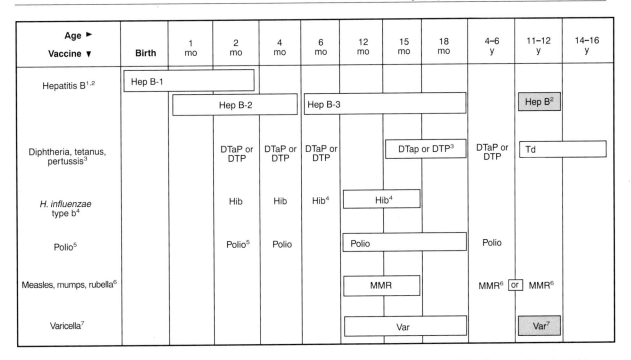

Fig. 45.1 Recommended childhood immunization schedule, USA, January to December 1997. (Approved by the Advisory Committee on Immunization Practices, the American Academy of Pediatrics and the American Academy of Family Physicians.) This schedule indicates the recommended age for routine administration of currently licensed childhood vaccines. Some combination vaccines are available and may be used whenever administration of all components of the vaccine is indicated. Providers should consult the manufacturers' package inserts for detailed recommendations. Vaccines are listed under the routinely recommended ages. Open bars indicate the range of acceptable ages for vaccination. Shaded bars indicate 'catch-up' vaccination: at 11–12 years of age, hepatitis B (Hep B) vaccine should be administered to children not previously vaccinated, and varicella virus vaccine should be administered to unvaccinated children who lack a reliable history of chickenpox.

1 Infants born to HBsAg-negative mothers should receive the first dose of vaccine at birth or by 2 months of age, and a second dose ≥1 month later. Infants born to HBsAg-positive mothers should receive 0.5 ml hepatitis B immunoglobulin (HBIG) within 12 h of birth, and a dose of vaccine at a separate site. The second dose is recommended at 1–2 months of age and the third at 6 months of age. For infants born to mothers whose HBsAg status is unknown at time of delivery, blood should be drawn at the time of delivery to determine the mother's HBsAg status; if it is positive, the infant should receive HBIG as soon as possible (no later than 1 wk of age). The dosage and timing of subsequent vaccine doses should be based upon the mother's HBsAg status.

2 Children and adolescents who have not been vaccinated against heptitis B in infancy may begin the series during any childhood visit. Those who have not previously received 3 doses of hepatitis B vaccine should initiate or complete the series at the age of 11–12 years. The second dose should be administered at least 1 month after the first dose, and the third dose at least 4 months after the first dose and at least 2 months after the second dose.

3 DTaP (diphtheria and tetanus toxoids and acellular pertussis vaccine) is the preferred vaccine for all doses in the vaccination series, including completion of the series in children who have received ≥1 dose of whole-cell DTP vaccine. Whole-cell DTP is an acceptable alternative to DTaP. The fourth dose of DTaP may be administered as early as the age of 12 months, provided 6 months have elapsed since the third dose, and if the child is considered unlikely to return at the age of 15–18 months Td (tetanus and diphtheria toxoids, adsorbed, for adult use) is recommended at the age of 11–12 years if at least 5 years have elapsed since the last dose of DTP, DTaP or DT. Subsequent routine Td boosters are recommended every 10 years.

4 Three *Haemophilus influenzae* type b (Hib) conjugate vaccines are licensed for infant use. If PRP-OMP is administered at 2 and 4 months of age, a dose at 6 months is not required. After completing the primary series, any Hib conjugate vaccine may be used as a booster.

5 Two poliovirus vaccines are currently licensed in the USA; inactivated poliovirus vaccine (IPV) and oral poliovirus vaccine (OPV). The following schedules are all acceptable by the Advisory Committee on Immunization Practices, the American Academy of Pediatrics and the American Academy of Family Physicians, and parents and providers may choose among them: (1) IPV at the ages 2 and 4 months, OPV at the ages 12–18 months and 4–6 years; (2) IPV at the ages 2, 4, 12–18 months and 4–6 years; (3) OPV at the ages 2, 4, 6–18 months and 4–6 years. The Advisory Committee on Immunization Practices routinely recommends schedule 1. IPV is the only poliovirus vaccine recommended for immunocompromised persons and their household contacts.

6 The second dose of MMR is routinely recommended at 4–6 or 11–12 years of age, but may be administered at any time provided at least 1 month has elapsed since the first dose, and that both doses are administered at or after 12 months of age.

7 Susceptible children may receive Varicella vaccine (Var) during any visit after the first birthday, and unvaccinated persons who lack a reliable history of chickenpox should be vaccinated at 11–12 years of age. Susceptible persons older than 13 years should receive 2 doses, at least 1 month apart

Table 45.4 Vaccine schedule for expanded programme on immunization

Age	Vaccine(s)
Birth	TOPV, BCG, Hep B
6 weeks	TOPV, DTP, Hep B
10 weeks	TOPV, DTP, Hep B
14 weeks	TOPV, DTP, Hep B
9 months	Measles

BCG, bacillus Calmette–Guérin; DTP, diphtheria and tetanus toxoids and pertussis vaccine; Hep B, hepatitis B; recommended in HBV-endemic areas, 3 dose series beginning at birth; TOPV, trivalent oral polio vaccine dose at birth (optional).

tain live virus vaccines (MMR, varicella). The duration of inhibition of response is related to the dose of immunoglobulins, and algorithms have been devised for calculating appropriate delays of MMR or measles vaccination after administration of such products (Siber, Werner and Halsey 1993). In general, MMR vaccines should be delayed at least 3 months after giving the usual doses of immunoglobulin (to prevent hepatitis A) or blood products, and for longer after higher doses (e.g. ⩾10 months after 2 g/kg IVIG for treatment of Kawasaki disease).

5.2 Vaccination in special situations

VACCINATION OF PREMATURE INFANTS

Infants born prematurely, regardless of birth weight, should be vaccinated at the same chronological age and with the same schedule as full-term infants. Some studies suggest that response to hepatitis B vaccine may be diminished in infants with birth weights below 2000 g; in an infant born to an HBsAg-negative mother, vaccination can be initiated either when the infant reaches 2000 g or at 2 months of age with administration of other childhood vaccines (Centers for Disease Control and Prevention 1994b, Committee on Infectious Diseases 1994).

VACCINATION OF PREGNANT WOMEN

The risk from vaccination during pregnancy is largely theoretical. The benefit of vaccinating a pregnant woman may outweigh the risk when the probability of exposure is high and when infection might cause harm to the mother or the infant, but the vaccine is unlikely to do so (Centers for Disease Control and Prevention 1994b). Hepatitis B and influenza vaccines may be given to those at high risk of these diseases. Live virus vaccines such as MMR and varicella are contraindicated in pregnant women on theoretical grounds; however, as no case of congenital rubella syndrome has been reported after MMR vaccination among over 200 susceptible women exposed during the first trimester of pregnancy, inadvertent vaccination is not a reason to interrupt pregnancy (Centers for Disease Control and Prevention 1989b). Pregnant women may receive OPV and yellow fever vaccines if there is a risk of exposure. Vaccination of family members with live virus vaccines does not pose a risk to pregnant women. Breast-feeding does not affect adversely the responses to live or killed vaccines.

VACCINATION OF PEOPLE WITH ALTERED IMMUNOCOMPETENCE

People with altered immunocompetence require special consideration for vaccination (Centers for Disease Control and Prevention 1993b). Such individuals are often at increased risk of serious adverse consequences of disease; they may also be at increased risk of serious consequences of vaccination or of a poor response. Important groups of immunocompromised people include those with congenital immunodeficiency diseases; acquired immunodeficiency due to infection (AIDS); haematopoietic or disseminated malignancy; immunosuppression because of administration of chemotherapy, systemic corticosteroids, radiation or other toxic drugs; and other chronic conditions, including splenectomy and diabetes. All such people can be vaccinated safely with killed vaccines, which are usually recommended in the same doses and schedules as for immunocompetent individuals. Certain vaccines (e.g. influenza) may be specifically indicated for such people. The response to both killed and live vaccines, however, may be suboptimal, and

Table 45.5 Vaccines recommended for adults in the USA

Age group	Vaccine/Toxoid							Pneumococcal polysaccharide
	Td	Measles	Mumps	Rubella	Varicella	Hepatitis B	Influenza	
18–40 y	All	High risk	High risk	High risk	Susceptible	High risk	High risk	High risk
41–64 y	All	...	...	...	Susceptible	High risk	High risk	High risk
65+ y	All	...	...	...	...	...	All	All

Td: Tetanus and diphtheria toxoids; booster doses recommended every 10 years.
Measles and mumps: indicated for unvaccinated or susceptible people born after 1956, particularly college students and healthcare workers.
Rubella: indicated for susceptible college students, healthcare workers and women of childbearing age.
Varicella: indicated for susceptible adults, particularly healthcare workers and close contacts of immunocompromised people.
Hepatitis B: indicated for people in high risk groups (e.g. healthcare workers, sexually active people with multiple partners, injecting drug abusers; see p. 980).
Influenza and pneumococcal polysaccharide vaccines: indicated for people under age 65 with high risk conditions (cardiac, pulmonary, metabolic, renal disease, etc.).

higher doses or an increased number of doses may be needed to ensure protection. Live viral vaccines are generally not recommended for any of these groups, except for people with chronic medical conditions (e.g. diabetes), because of a known or theoretical risk of disseminated infection due to the vaccine. An exception is the recommendation of MMR vaccine for persons with HIV infection without severe immunocompromise, because of the high risk of serious consequences of wild measles infection (Onorato, Markowitz and Oxtoby 1988, Centers for Disease Control and Prevention 1996d).

INTERNATIONAL TRAVELLERS

International travellers may be at increased risk of exposure to vaccine-preventable diseases, even in developed countries. All children, adolescents and adults planning international travel should be up to date for all routine childhood immunizations. Other viral vaccines that should be considered before travel include hepatitis A and B vaccines, yellow fever, Japanese encephalitis and rabies (if exposure to rabid animals is anticipated). The need for these vaccines should be determined by consulting specific guidelines for travellers (Centers for Disease Control and Prevention 1994c).

5.3 Vaccine safety and vaccine injury compensation

Viral vaccines, like other vaccines, usually cause only minor local and systemic adverse reactions, such as induration and pain at the injection site, fever and malaise. Serious or life-threatening reactions can occur after some viral vaccines, such as paralytic poliomyelitis following oral polio vaccine, disseminated measles vaccine virus infection in immunocompromised children, or encephalitis following yellow fever vaccine in young children. The Institute of Medicine (IOM) in the USA has reviewed available information regarding the possible causality of serious adverse events following each of the licensed childhood vaccines (Institute of Medicine 1991, 1993). For many events, information was considered insufficient to determine causality. However, the panels were able to classify some events definitively, as summarized in Table 45.6. These comprise the most comprehensive compilation of data on vaccine safety, although controversy still persists about some events. Re-analysis of additional data suggests that the available evidence does not support causation by oral polio vaccine of Guillain–Barré syndrome (Rantala, Cherry and Shields 1994).

Contraindications and precautions for each viral vaccine are usually described in the recommendations for use and in vaccine package inserts. For inactivated vaccines, anaphylactic reaction to a constituent or to a previous dose is usually the only contraindication, whereas, for live virus vaccines, any condition that results in immunocompromise (blood dyscrasias, HIV infection, steroid or chemotherapy, etc.) contraindicates use of the vaccine. Pregnancy is usually a contraindication for live vaccines that might be teratogenic (rubella, varicella), but not for inactivated vaccines. Potential recipients should be questioned regarding the presence of such conditions before any vaccine is administered.

Because viral vaccines may, rarely, cause serious adverse events, some countries have established programmes to compensate people who develop permanent injury following vaccination (Centers for Disease Control and Prevention 1988). A specific table of injuries may describe conditions for which compensation is routinely provided; in addition, anyone who can provide medical evidence of causality may be compensated. In the USA, this programme is funded by a special excise tax on each dose of vaccine to which the programme applies (DTP, OPV, MMR at present; Hib, hepatitis B, and varicella vaccines to be added).

5.4 Surveillance for vaccine-preventable diseases and adverse events

Monitoring the impact of vaccination programmes and of the safety of vaccines is critical for refining immunization strategies and for assuring the public and medical community that vaccines are safe. Surveillance has shown the high effectiveness of universal childhood vaccines; reductions of over 95% in the incidence of disease have been observed in the USA for polio, measles, mumps and rubella compared to the prevaccine era (Centers for Disease Control and Prevention 1995).

Surveillance for communicable diseases is maintained in each country, and may include any or all vaccine-preventable diseases (Wharton and Strebel 1995). These data should be monitored to assess the effectiveness of the vaccines and of the vaccination programme. For each reported case of disease, confirmation by laboratory testing and determination of vaccination status are essential to monitor whether continuing infections are due to failure to deliver vaccine or to lack of vaccine efficacy. As the elimination of particular indigenous diseases approaches (targeted for 1996 for measles in the USA), determination of chains of transmission, whether the case is indigenous or imported, and rapid implementation of control measures also become crucial. All healthcare providers are urged to report every suspected case of vaccine-preventable disease promptly to the local or national authorities. Monitoring the efficacy of vaccines after licensing is essential, particularly during outbreaks in highly vaccinated populations, to reassess effectiveness in wide use and to maintain public confidence in vaccination (Orenstein, Bernier and Hinman 1988).

Monitoring of adverse events after vaccination is also usually required in each country; in the USA it is the joint responsibility of the Food and Drug Administration (FDA) and the Centers for Disease Control (CDC). Physicians are required by law to report certain events that occur after vaccination, and should report all suspected adverse reactions after vaccination to the Vaccine Adverse Events Reporting System

Table 45.6 Summary of Institute of Medicine findings on the relationship of adverse events to individual vaccines

Vaccine	Establishes causation	Favouring causation	Favouring rejection of causation
Measles (see also MMR)	Death from measles vaccine strain in immunocompromised people	Anaphylaxis	None
MMR (see also measles, mumps and rubella)	Anaphylaxis Thrombocytopenia	None	None
Mumps (see MMR)	None	None	None
OPV	Poliomyelitis in recipient or contact Death from polio vaccine strain in immunocompromised people	Guillain–Barré syndrome	None
IPV	None	None	None
Hepatitis B	Anaphylaxis	None	None
Rubella[a] (see also MMR)	Acute arthritis	Chronic arthritis	None

[a]Reviewed by an earlier committee. Initial report categories corresponding to those table headings were 'Evidence indicates a causal relationship', 'Evidence is consistent with a causal relationship', and 'Evidence does not indicate a causal relationship'.

(VAERS) (Centers for Disease Control and Prevention 1988, Chen et al. 1994).

5.5 Vaccine handling and storage

Vaccines are perishable products that require specific care in handling and storage; ensuring that a vaccine maintains potency and safety is a responsibility shared by the manufacturer and everyone handling the vaccine. Live attenuated vaccines are more susceptible to rises in temperature than are inactivated vaccines or toxoids. Adjuvanted inactivated vaccines must be protected from freezing to ensure potency. Vaccines that are exposed to damaging environmental conditions may suffer loss of potency without a change in appearance. A vaccine quality control programme should be established in each clinical practice, focusing on education of personnel, maintenance of equipment and adherence to routine daily monitoring of vaccines (Committee on Infectious Diseases 1994).

6 PASSIVE IMMUNOPROPHYLAXIS

Passive immunoprophylaxis consists of the use of purified antibodies prepared from animal or human serum to prevent infection or to modify the course of infection, when given either before or after exposure. The use of such antibodies was developed in the late nineteenth century, when sera from hyperimmunized horses and rabbits were used to treat diphtheria and tetanus. Although the use of antibiotics has largely reduced the use of passive immunoprophylaxis for bacterial infections (except tetanus, diphtheria and replacement prophylaxis for those who are a- or hypo-

gammaglobulinaemic or immunocompromised), passive prophylaxis has maintained a role in preventing the serious consequences of a number of viral infections.

Immunoglobulin preparations currently used for viral immunoprophylaxis or treatment are prepared from human serum by the modified Cohn fractionation technique, using cold ethanol precipitation (Cohn et al. 1946, Oncley et al. 1949). This yields 3 fractions, enriched in cryoprecipitates, globulins and albumin, respectively, determined by the specific ethanol concentration, temperature, pH and ion and protein concentrations. Immunoglobulin prepared by Cohn fractionation consists of mainly IgG types 1, 2 and 3, but is relatively depleted in IgG4. Immunoglobulin preparations maintain the properties of complement activation and opsonization associated with Fc receptors, and may also have immunomodulatory functions, which appear to play only a minor role in viral infections.

6.1 Types of immunoglobulin

Three types of immunoglobulin products are used for viral immunoprophylaxis: pooled human immunoglobulin (prophylaxis for hepatitis A, measles) for intramuscular use; specific immunoglobulins (hepatitis B immunoglobulin (HBIG), rabies immunoglobulin (HRIG), varicella-zoster immunoglobulin (VZIG), etc. used to prevent the respective diseases); and intravenous immunoglobulin, used for immunoprophylaxis of immunodeficient people (Table 45.7) (Siber and Snydman 1989). Pooled human immunoglobulin is generally prepared from large pools of donors (>1000) who are not screened for specific antibodies; however, the final immunoglobulin preparation is required to have minimal levels of antibodies to measles and polio (neutralizing), diphtheria (antitoxin) and to hepatitis B surface antigen (anti-HBs). Antibodies to other viral pathogens, including enteroviruses, hepatitis A (HAV) and respiratory syncytial virus (RSV), are also present, although titres may vary widely in different lots. Owing to the relatively high frequency of hepatitis A infection in the general population, anti-HAV titres in immunoglobulin lots produced in the USA have remained relatively constant, although they have decreased in recent years in Great Britain.

Specific immunoglobulins are produced from a smaller donor pool that has either been screened for high titres of the specific antibody (varicella-zoster, RSV, cytomegalovirus (CMV) or been boosted by vaccination of donors (hepatitis B, rabies) to ensure high levels of antibody.

Intravenous immunoglobulin preparations are suitable for administering the larger doses needed by certain groups of immunodeficient patients. To prevent the occurrence of immunoglobulin aggregates, which could activate complement and cause serious reactions if given intravenously, techniques to break them down have been developed, including pepsin or plasmin digestion, reduction and alkylation, β-propiolactone treatment, or ultrafiltration and diafiltration (Waldvogel 1981). These are intended to ensure that >80% of IgG is present in monomeric form and that minimal aggregates of dimeric or larger forms exist. These treatments are designed to limit cleavage of the Fc fragment and reduction in the physiological effects that depend on Fc binding.

6.2 Uses of passive immunoprophylaxis

Immunoglobulin preparations may be used as pre-exposure prophylaxis, given before anticipated exposure to a specific viral agent or as postexposure prophylaxis, either to prevent clinical disease (measles, hepatitis B, rabies) or to modify the course of infection (varicella) (Table 45.7).

PRE-EXPOSURE PROPHYLAXIS

Pre-exposure prophylaxis with immunoglobulin is now limited to hepatitis A prevention. Immunoglobulin is about 80% effective when given in a dose of 0.02 ml/kg for short-term protection to travellers to countries where HAV is endemic, or 0.06 ml/kg for protection for up to 6 months. In developed countries, hepatitis A vaccine will probably greatly reduce the need for passive prophylaxis.

IVIG is the treatment of choice for preventing bacterial and viral infections in people with primary immunodeficiency disorders associated with low serum IgG levels (Committee on Infectious Diseases 1994). The frequency of treatment is tailored to the severity of each patient's symptoms. Although this procedure may be most valuable in preventing bacterial infections, IVIG also reduces the risk of viral infections, including measles, enteroviruses and RSV IVIG is recommended to prevent infection in children with paediatric acquired immunodeficiency syndrome (AIDS) and people with chronic lymphocytic leukaemia, and is being studied for use in premature babies (<1500 g), multiple myeloma and bone marrow transplantation (Siber and Snydman 1989). Specific CMV IVIG is partially effective in preventing seri-

Table 45.7 Immunoglobulins currently available for use in viral diseases

Preparation	Route of injection	Uses
Human immunoglobulin (NHIG)	Intramuscular	Pre- and postexposure prophylaxis for hepatitis A; postexposure prophylaxis for measles; treatment of hypogammaglobulinaemia
Hepatitis B immunoglobulin (HBIG)	Intramuscular	Postexposure prophylaxis for hepatitis B (with hepatitis B vaccine): perinatal, sexual, blood/body fluid exposure
Human rabies immunoglobulin (HRIG)	Intramuscular + intralesion	Postexposure prophylaxis for rabies (with rabies vaccine)
Varicella-zoster immunoglobulin (VZIG)	Intramuscular	Postexposure prophylaxis for susceptible infants, immunocompromised people, adults
Vaccinia immunoglobulin	Intramuscular	Treatment of complications of vaccinia (disseminated vaccinia)
Immunoglobulin (IVIG)	Intravenous	Treatment of a- and hypogammaglobulinaemia; treatment of viral infections in immunocompromised
Respiratory syncytial immunoglobulin (RSV IVIG)	Intravenous	Prevention of respiratory syncytial virus infection in premature infants and children with pulmonary dysplasia
Cytomegalovirus immunoglobulin (CMV IVIG)	Intravenous	Prevention of serious CMV infection in transplant patients (experimental)

ous outcomes of CMV infection in recipients of solid organ or bone marrow transplants.

A high titre RSV IVIG has recently been licensed in the USA to prevent RSV infection in children with bronchopulmonary dysplasia and in premature babies (<35 weeks' gestation). It is 40–53% effective in preventing the most serious complications of RSV disease in these children, and is given in monthly doses of 750 mg/kg to those <24 months of age at high risk during the RSV season (November through April in the USA) (Siber et al. 1992).

POSTEXPOSURE PROPHYLAXIS

Immunoglobulin (0.02 ml/kg) is recommended for postexposure prophylaxis to prevent hepatitis A in susceptible people with household or other close exposure if it can be given within 2 weeks of exposure. Immunoglobulin prophylaxis may modify hepatitis A disease without preventing virus excretion, and therefore should only be given to food handlers with the caution that strict hygieneic precautions should be followed for 6 weeks. Some experts prefer not to give immunoglobulin to food handlers. Immunoglobulin may also be given to prevent measles (0.5 ml/kg) in susceptible people at high risk of severe measles (<12 months of age, immunocompromised) if it is given within one week of exposure. Postexposure prophylaxis with specific immunoglobulins is recommended to prevent hepatitis B, rabies and varicella infection. Hepatitis B immunoglobulin (HBIG) is generally given with hepatitis B vaccine to provide passive–active prophylaxis, which may enhance short-term protection and ensure long-lasting immunity: indications for HBIG include perinatal exposure to an HBsAg positive mother (given as soon as possible after birth); sexual exposure to an HBsAg positive person; and needlestick, blood or other percutaneous exposure to HBsAg positive blood or body secretions (Centers for Disease Control and Prevention 1991b). Rabies immunoglobulin is also given as passive–active immunization with rabies vaccine after exposure to a rabies-infected animal. VZIG is indicated for susceptible people at high risk of severe varicella who have household or other sustained contact (at least 1 h direct contact) with an infected individual. Those with highest priority include neonates exposed to maternal varicella (manifest between 2 days before and 5 days after birth), susceptible immunocompromised people and premature infants born to varicella-susceptible mothers (Centers for Disease Control and Prevention 1996a). It may also be used for exposed adults, although pre-exposure use of varicella vaccine should greatly reduce the use of VZIG over all and particularly in this population.

THERAPEUTIC USES

Immunoglobulin products may, rarely, be used to treat diseases. Vaccinia immunoglobulin (VIG) is a well established treatment for people with serious complications of vaccinia immunization (disseminated disease, vaccinia necrosum). IVIG has also been used experimentally with apparent success to treat parvo-

virus B19 aplastic crises and RSV infection (Siber and Snydman 1989).

Immune plasma is still used very occasionally to treat established infections with rare infections such as those due to haemorrhagic fever viruses (Maiztegui, Fernandez and DeDamilano 1979, Peters, Johnson and McKee 1991). Such experimental treatment employs convalescent serum from a previously infected patient but poses the risk of serious adverse events, including immune complex deposition and serum sickness.

6.3 Adverse reactions

Immunoglobulin products for intramuscular use prepared by Cohn fractionation are very safe, with few adverse events and no apparent risk of transmission of blood-borne diseases. Adverse reactions to intramuscular immunoglobulin are uncommon and usually mild, consisting of local pain or low grade fever (Barundun and Morell 1981, Siber and Snydman 1989). Allergic reactions may, rarely, occur; the risk is greater in people with isolated IgA deficiency. The risk of systemic reactions is greater with IVIG, primarily in people with a- or hypogammaglobulinaemia who are beginning therapy. The reaction may be reduced by decreasing the rate of administration or by premedication with antihistamines, analgesics (aspirin or paracetamol/acetaminophen) or steroids.

Intramuscular IgG produced in developed countries has never been implicated in the transmission of blood-borne diseases such as hepatitis B, HIV infection or hepatitis C, even before the screening of donor blood for these agents. This elimination of infectious agents is probably due to a combination of exposure to high concentrations of ethanol (20–25%) and the presence of antiviral antibodies that neutralize activity or enhance the removal of virus during precipitation and centrifugation (Wells et al. 1986, Cuthbertson et al. 1987). All plasma donors in developed countries are now screened for these agents. Several incidents of transmission of HCV infection by intravenous immunoglobulin preparations have been reported, the most recent in the USA after screening of plasma donors for HCV antibodies was initiated (Rousell 1988, Williams et al. 1988b, Centers for Disease Control and Prevention 1994d). Although this step was intended to eliminate most HCV-positive plasma donors, the removal of HCV antibodies may have permitted HCV not complexed with antibodies to remain in the final product. This potential hazard has been recognized and methods of manufacture modified to eliminate the risk by heat or chemical inactivation. Rarely, immunoglobulin produced in less developed countries has transmitted blood-borne disease, possibly owing to inadequate quality control (Siber and Snydman 1989).

7 VACCINES RECOMMENDED FOR ROUTINE USE IN CHILDREN

7.1 Measles, mumps and rubella

The live attenuated vaccines for measles, mumps and rubella are frequently, though not universally, administered as a single combined product. The administration of a combined product is more common in developed countries. The immune response to each component vaccine is similar whether a combined or single product vaccine is administered. Simultaneous administration of measles, mumps, rubella (MMR) vaccine (or individual component vaccines) and other childhood vaccines does not alter the immune responses to any of them. Vaccination with MMR and its component vaccines is contraindicated for pregnant women and for people with moderate or severe febrile illnesses, with a previous anaphylactic reaction to any of the components of the vaccine, or with immunocompromising conditions (Centers for Disease Control [and Prevention], 1989a, 1989c, 1990b). Recent studies suggest that anaphylactic reactions to eggs are not contraindications to vaccination with measles, mumps or MMR vaccines (James et al. 1995).

As well as providing universal immunization of children with a first dose, many developed countries have also implemented a schedule calling for a second dose of MMR vaccine. This may be administered at times ranging from 18 months to 11–12 years of age (Hinman and Orenstein 1994). The aim is to induce protective immunity in children who have not responded to the first dose of the measles component, but there is the added benefit of increasing the proportion of people immune to mumps and rubella (Centers for Disease Control 1989a). Among people who develop antibodies following vaccination, protection from all 3 vaccines is assumed to be life-long, although disease has been observed among people responding to measles vaccine (Mathias et al. 1989).

MEASLES

Within a few years of the initial isolation of the measles virus by Enders and Peebles (1954), an attenuated vaccine was developed by serial passage of the virus in chick embryo fibroblasts. The first measles vaccine was approved for use in 1963. The most common strains of measles vaccine in current use include the Moraten and Schwarz strains (Markowitz and Katz 1994). An inactivated measles vaccine was withdrawn from production following reports of an atypical measles syndrome characterized by high fever, pneumonia and an unusual rash that occurred after exposure to wild type measles virus (Annunziato et al. 1982).

In different countries, measles vaccine may be routinely administered at 9 months, 12 months (Hinman and Orenstein 1994) or 12–15 months of age (Centers for Disease Control and Prevention 1994b). The maternal antibodies to measles transferred to the fetus across the placenta are sufficient to prevent or reduce the immune response to vaccination in young children (Albrecht et al. 1977). Selecting the most appropriate age for vaccination against measles requires balancing the likelihood of a child retaining maternal antibodies against the possibility of being without antibody protection and being exposed to measles. The rates of seroconversion range from c. 80–85% in 9 month old children to 95% and higher in 15 month old children (Halsey 1983).

Measles vaccine is extremely safe, although 5–15% of children who receive it have a raised temperature 7–12 days after immunization (Centers for Disease Control 1989a). A smaller proportion develop a rash, usually c. 10 days after immunization. Rarely, the raised temperature provokes a febrile convulsion. Serious adverse events that are even less common include thrombocytopenia (1 per 25 000–40 000 doses) and anaphylaxis (Institute of Medicine 1993).

The worldwide administration of measles vaccine has sharply reduced both the number of cases and the number of deaths attributed to measles; in 1990 the use of measles vaccine among children aged 12–23 months was 80%. It is estimated that, in 1993, there were 44.5 million cases of measles and 1.19 million deaths throughout the world; in the pre-vaccine era as many as 125 million cases and 7 million deaths may have occurred globally (World Health Organization 1995).

Because measles infection results in lifelong protective immunity, there is no carrier state and humans are the only host, measles is theoretically eradicable (Centers for Disease Control and Prevention 1993c). In 1967, elimination of measles was achieved in The Gambia, and sustained for a 4-year period (Foege 1971). Since that time, 2 strategies for its elimination have evolved: one based on routine 2 dose vaccination and another on routine vaccination with supplemental mass vaccination campaigns. Finland and the USA have implemented elimination programmes based on a routine 2 dose programme. In Finland, the programme achieved elimination (Peltola et al. 1994), and in the USA, indigenous transmission was interrupted in 1993 (Rota et al. 1996). The UK and most countries in the Americas have used supplemental mass vaccination against measles (de Quadros et al. 1996, Anonymous 1994), the incidence of which has generally decreased by >90% following these campaigns.

Further progress in the control of measles depends on other countries implementing accelerated activities to achieve its elimination. Molecular epidemiological techniques will take on increasing importance in tracking the transmission of the measles virus and identifying importations (Rota et al. 1996). Whether mass vaccination using currently available vaccines as implemented in the western hemisphere would interrupt transmission in urban centres of Africa and Asia, where substantial measles transmission occurs among children under 9 months of age, is a very important unresolved issue.

MUMPS

The mumps virus was first cultured in 1945 in chick embryos, leading to the development of vaccines that were first licensed in the Soviet Union and the USA in the 1960s (Cochi, Wharton and Plotkin 1994). Several strains of mumps virus have been used to produce vaccine; until recently, the most widely used have been the Jeryl Lynn, Urabe and Hoshino. All produce seroconversion rates of 90–95%, although recent outbreaks among immunized school-age children in the USA have produced estimates of vaccine efficacy of c. 85% (Cheek et al. 1995).

Mumps vaccine is well tolerated and, except for aseptic meningitis, few adverse events have been directly associated with vaccination. Aseptic meningitis has been associated with vaccination with the Urabe strain of mumps vaccine (Miller et al. 1993). Many developed countries, including Japan, the UK and other European countries, have removed the Urabe mumps vaccine from the market. These adverse events have had a detrimental effect on vaccination programmes, in particular reducing acceptance of the combined MMR vaccine. The Jeryl Lynn strain has not been associated with aseptic meningitis and remains the mumps vaccine of choice throughout the world.

Widespread vaccination has greatly reduced the reported incidence of mumps in every country that has introduced it. As a disease without a carrier state and without a non-human host, the highly efficacious vaccine makes mumps, like measles, potentially eradicable (Centers for Disease Control and Prevention 1993c). It is not yet known whether a single dose can provide adequate population immunity to eradicate mumps.

Rubella

The mild febrile rash illness due to rubella is important because of the congenital rubella syndrome (CRS). Women infected with rubella during the first trimester of pregnancy frequently give birth to babies with characteristic birth defects. The association between rubella and this congenital syndrome was first recognized as a triad of ocular abnormalities, cardiac defects and deafness in newborns in Australia in 1941 (Gregg 1941). Subsequent studies have expanded the list of abnormalities in the CRS to include mental retardation, hepato- and splenomegaly, as well as thrombocytopenia, hypothyroidism and diabetes mellitus. Infection in the first trimester of pregnancy results in the highest frequency of, and most devastating, abnormalities, although infection in the third trimester may cause cataracts (Centers for Disease Control and Prevention 1990b). (See also Chapter 41.)

In the years following the isolation of the virus in 1962, several vaccines were developed. The RA27/3 vaccine strain is now the most commonly used throughout the world (replacing the Cendehill and HPV 77 vaccines in the USA), although the T0-336 and BRD-2 strains are used in Asia and have potency similar to the RA27/3 strain (Plotkin 1994). Rubella vaccine induces an effective immune response in >95% of recipients, which seems to be less affected by maternal antibody than is the response to measles vaccine.

Rubella vaccination is usually well tolerated

although arthritis or arthropathy may occur. This side effect is more common in susceptible adult women than in children or adult men (Centers for Disease Control and Prevention 1990b, Institute of Medicine 1991). Joint symptoms are usually self-limited, although chronic arthritis associated with rubella vaccine has been reported (Tingle, Allen and Petty 1986). Symptoms may be less common following vaccination with RA27/3 than after vaccination with other strains. Some workers have found no association with rubella vaccination and the subsequent development of persistent joint symptoms. Inadvertent rubella vaccination during pregnancy has not been associated with congenital defects, but vaccination is contraindicated in pregnancy (Centers for Disease Control 1989b).

Two distinct but not exclusive strategies have been implemented to control rubella and CRS. Some countries have opted to immunize only women of childbearing age, in practice girls 12–13 years of age, just before their reproductive years. With complete implementation of the programme, virus continues to circulate among unvaccinated children and men, providing periodic boosting of immunity in vaccinated women. In theory, the control of CRS is achieved by protecting all women who might become pregnant. In the UK, an immunity level of 97% was found to be inadequate to prevent all cases of CRS (Miller 1991). The second strategy is universal vaccination of children. The ultimate aim here is the elimination of rubella transmission and the reduction of CRS by vaccination-induced immunity and herd immunity (Centers for Disease Control and Prevention 1990b). Currently, most developed countries combine the 2 strategies, through universal immunization of children at 12–15 months of age with MMR vaccine or measles, rubella vaccine and immunization of susceptible women with rubella vaccine (Hinman and Orenstein 1994).

Rubella, like measles, has only a human host and no chronic carrier state, so can theoretically be eradicated. Mathematical modelling suggests that a single dose of vaccine, given universally, should be sufficient to eliminate rubella. To date, only Finland has declared success in this effort (Peltola et al. 1994). The major constraints to eradication are a perceived lack of importance because of the mild clinical syndrome and the difficulty in maintaining surveillance for a disease in which half the cases may lack any clinical symptoms. In developing countries, inadequate surveillance for CRS has meant that its importance is not known. Consequently, few medium or low income countries currently vaccinate against rubella, and rubella is not included in the World Health Organization's Expanded Programme on Immunization.

7.2 Poliomyelitis

Poliomyelitis was a widespread cause of childhood morbidity and mortality in the pre-vaccine era (Strebel et al. 1992). In 1949, the discovery that poliovirus could be propagated in non-nervous human tissue permitted the large-scale production necessary for vaccine manufacture (Enders, Weller and Robbins 1949). Two standard approaches were pursued: inactivation and attenuation of poliovirus.

Following large-scale field trials of inactivated poliovirus vaccine (IPV) developed by Jonas Salk, IPV became, in 1955, the first poliovirus vaccine to be licensed in the USA (Francis et al. 1957, Salk, Drucker and Malvin 1994). IPV contains formalin-inactivated poliovirus types 1, 2 and 3. In 1961, monovalent oral poliovirus vaccines (OPV) developed by Albert Sabin were licensed. Two years later, a balanced formulation of the 3 monovalent vaccines (trivalent OPV) became available and rapidly replaced IPV as the vaccine of choice for preventing poliomyelitis in the USA and in most other countries. OPV contains live attenuated polioviruses of the 3 poliovirus serotypes formulated ratio 10 : 1 : 6, with 10^6 median tissue culture infective dose (TCID50) of poliovirus type 1, 10^5 TCID50 of poliovirus type 2 and $10^{5.8}$ TCID50 of poliovirus type 3 (Centers for Disease Control 1982). In the 1980s, enhanced-potency IPVs (eIPV) were developed; eIPV containing 40 : 8 : 32 D-antigen units of poliovirus types 1, 2 and 3, respectively, was licensed in the USA in 1987 (Centers for Disease Control 1987).

In most industrialized countries, including the USA before 1997, and virtually all developed countries, the vaccine of choice for the prevention of poliomyelitis is OPV (Centers for Disease Control 1982, Hinman and Orenstein 1994). The primary series in the USA consists of 3 doses of OPV given at 2, 4 and 6–18 months of age, followed by a supplemental dose at school entry (i.e. 4–6 years). The primary series of IPV consists of 3 doses given at 2, 4 and 12–18 months, followed by a fourth, supplementary, dose of IPV at school entry. Until 1997, IPV in the USA was indicated primarily for immunologically abnormal infants and their family contacts, and for unvaccinated adults (Centers for Disease Control 1987). Following primary reliance on OPV between 1961 and 1996, the USA revised its poliomyelitis prevention policy effective early 1997. Recognizing the absence of indigenous wild poliovirus circulation since 1979, the occurrence of 8–9 cases of VAPP annually in the USA and the rapid progress in global polio eradication, a policy to increase the use of IPV was adopted. Three options for polio vaccination are now considered acceptable: OPV alone, IPV alone and sequential IPV (doses at 2 and 4 months old) followed by OPV (doses at 12–18 months and 4–6 years). The sequential schedule ensures development of both humoral and mucosal immunity while reducing the risk of VAPP, and is recommended by the ACIP (McBean and Modlin 1987; Centers for Disease Control and Prevention 1997). IPV has been used exclusively in many northern European countries, including Finland, Sweden and the Netherlands, and has led to eradication in these countries. More recently, Canada, France and Norway recommended an all-IPV schedule to reduce the risk of vaccine-associated paralytic poliomyelitis (Hinman and Orenstein 1994). In addition, Denmark, Estonia, Hungary and Israel use sequential schedules of IPV and OPV.

The Expanded Programme on Immunization of the World Health Organization recommends a schedule of 4 OPV doses administered at birth (zero week), 6, 10 and 14 weeks to ensure earlier protection against poliomyelitis in infants residing in the developing world; polio continues to be endemic in many of these countries. Many developing countries also recommend a dose of OPV in the second year of life.

The objective of the routine series of poliovirus vaccine is to induce humoral immunity for individual protection against poliomyelitis and mucosal immunity for community protection against its circulation. In industrialized countries, 3 doses of OPV or IPV result in seroconversion or seroprevalence levels of >90% to all 3 poliovirus serotypes. In developing countries, the immunogenicity of OPV is substantially lower, with median seroconversion levels of 72%, 95% and 65% (Patriarca, Wright and John 1991) to poliovirus types 1, 2 and 3, respectively, following the administration of 3 doses of OPV. The lower immunogenicity of OPV in developing countries may be due to interference by concurrent enterovirus infection, diarrhoea, nonspecific inhibition or other factors. In addition, the immunogenicity of OPV may be lower under programme conditions because of suboptimal storage, handling and administration. The immunogenicity of IPV does not seem to differ in industrialized and developing countries. Whereas OPV and IPV induce a similarly high level, the humoral immune response in infants residing in industrialized countries, the intestinal mucosal immunity induced by OPV is clearly superior to that induced by IPV in limiting the replication and excretion of circulating poliovirus (Sutter and Patriarca 1993).

The widespread use of IPV, starting in 1955, led to a major reduction in the incidence of poliomyelitis in the USA: from 57 879 cases in 1952 to 5485 cases by 1957. The widespread use of OPV led to the elimination of indigenous circulation of wild poliovirus in the 1960s. The last endemic and epidemic cases of poliomyelitis were reported in 1979. Since 1980, aside from a few imported cases of poliomyelitis, only c. 8 cases of vaccine-associated paralytic poliomyelitis (VAPP) are reported each year in the USA (Strebel et al. 1992). Of these 8 VAPP cases, c. 3 cases each occur in OPV recipients and in people in contact with OPV recipients and 2 cases in immunologically abnormal people.

The occurrence of VAPP is the most serious adverse event following use of OPV and has been reported from most industrialized countries (Esteves 1988, Joce et al. 1992, Strebel et al. 1992). The risk of VAPP in the USA has been relatively stable for the last 30 years. Among immunocompetent people, the highest risk of VAPP is in recipients of the first dose of OPV (one VAPP case per 1.5 million infants) and in unvaccinated contacts (one VAPP case per 2.2 million contacts) of recently vaccinated infants. However, the risk of VAPP is highest in the presence of immunological abnormality (either congenital or acquired), particularly people with B cell deficiencies. In Romania, a country that had reported very high rates of VAPP for many years, a case–control study suggested that the apparently increased incidence was primarily due to multiple intramuscular injections of antibiotics following administration of OPV (Strebel et al. 1995). IPV is not known to cause serious adverse reactions.

Progress toward poliomyelitis control in industrialized and developing countries prompted the member countries of the World Health Organization (WHO) Region of the Americas to adopt the goal, in 1985, of regional elimination of poliomyelitis from the western hemisphere by the year 1990. Following the implementation of key strategies (see p. 980), the last case of poliomyelitis associated with wild poliovirus isolation was reported from Peru in September 1991, and the region was certified free of indigenous wild poliovirus by an International Certification Commission in September 1994 (Pan American Health Organization 1994). In 1988, the World Health Assembly, the governing body of WHO, adopted the goal of global eradication of poliomyelitis by the year 2000 (Expanded Programme on Immunization 1995). A unique partnership of governmental and private organizations is supporting this initiative; Rotary International, a private organization, is providing close to $400 million and immeasurable volunteer time to achieve the goal of eradication.

The poliomyelitis eradication initiative relies on 3 strategies: (1) high routine coverage with OPV; (2) supplemental immunization, including national immunization days (NIDs) twice a year to vaccinate all children in order to eliminate the remaining poliovirus reservoirs; and (3) enhanced epidemiological and virological surveillance to detect cases immediately, institute control measures and eventually assist in eliminating wild poliovirus circulation (Hull et al. 1994).

Progress toward eradication can be measured both by outcome evaluation (e.g. the incidence of poliomyelitis) and by process evaluation (e.g. the number of countries conducting NIDs). World-wide, the reported number of poliomyelitis cases has decreased by 76%, from 35 251 cases in 1988 to 8549 cases in 1994. Substantial decreases in the incidence of poliomyelitis have been reported from the Western Pacific region of WHO, including China, the Philippines, Vietnam, Cambodia and Laos, and from the European and eastern Mediterranean regions of WHO; polio-free zones have begun to emerge in southern and northern Africa, Europe and east Asia. During the same period, the number of countries conducting NIDs has increased from 15 to 63. In 1995, about half of the world's children <5 years of age received supplemental OPV doses administered during NIDs.

The progress so far toward global eradication of poliomyelitis suggests that this objective may be within reach by the year 2000. However, increased efforts are necessary to ensure that adequate resources are made available to eliminate the remaining poliovirus reservoirs, particularly those in southern Asia and Africa.

7.3   Hepatitis B vaccine

Hepatitis B vaccines initially consisted of HBsAg particles purified from the plasma of HBV carriers. Plasma-derived vaccines produced in several countries were highly effective in preventing hepatitis B, were used in developed countries throughout the early 1980s and continue to be used in some developing countries (Szmuness et al. 1981, Kane 1993). In 1985, the first recombinant HB vaccines became available. These consist of purified HBsAg produced by recombinant DNA technology in yeast or in mammalian cells. Newer generation vaccines, which include the pre-S1 or pre-S2 antigens, or both, in addition to HBsAg have also been developed but have not replaced the vaccines based solely on HBsAg (Hadler and Margolis 1992).

Hepatitis B vaccine is usually given as a 3 dose series. The licensed schedule includes doses at 0, 1 and 6 months, with an alternative schedule of 4 doses given at 0, 1, 2 and 12 months. However, schedules that vary the timing of the second and third doses to permit integration into the routine childhood immunization schedule have been highly immunogenic (Centers for Disease Control and Prevention 1991b). Dosages vary by age, vaccine and whether the child is born to an HBsAg-positive mother; in the USA, dosages for infants and children are one-quarter to one-half those required for adults.

The response to a 3 dose series is excellent in all age groups, with anti-HBs produced in 85–99% of vaccinees; response is highest in children aged 2–19 years, and decreases with increasing age (Hadler and Margolis 1992). People with immunocompromising conditions such as renal failure have poorer responses, and higher dosages are recommended. Placebo-controlled trials both in high risk children in HBV-endemic countries and in high risk adults in the USA and elsewhere have shown short-term efficacy of 80–95% (Szmuness et al. 1981, Stevens et al. 1992). Long-term follow-up of both children and adults for up to 11 years has demonstrated protection against serious consequences of infection (chronic carriage and chronic liver disease) in virtually all people who respond to the initial series (anti-HBs $\geqslant$10 miu/ml) (Hadler and Margolis 1992, West and Calendra 1996). Although booster doses are not recommended for any age group, the need for them continues to be evaluated.

Hepatitis B vaccine causes few adverse reactions, mainly fever and soreness at the injection site. Rarely, anaphylaxis can occur, and contraindicates additional doses of vaccine. Serious neurological injuries such as Guillain–Barré syndrome have been reported following vaccination (primarily after plasma-derived vaccine, no longer used in the USA), but there is insufficient evidence to link it with the vaccine (Centers for Disease Control and Prevention 1991b).

In developed countries, including the USA and Europe, hepatitis B vaccine was initially recommended only for infants of HBV-carrier mothers and high risk adults; however, in the USA, the lack of impact on its incidence led to the development of a comprehensive strategy for eliminating hepatitis B (Centers for Disease Control and Prevention 1991b). The components of this strategy now being implemented include: (1) universal screening of pregnant women for HBsAg, and providing hepatitis B immunoglobulin and initiating hepatitis B vaccination within 12 hours of birth for infants born to hepatitis B-carrier mothers; (2) universal vaccination of all infants, beginning either at birth or by 2 months of age when other routine childhood vaccines are initiated; (3) vaccination of all previously unvaccinated children at 11–12 years of age; and (4) vaccination of children, adolescents and adults in high risk groups, including people who live in households with HBsAg carriers; children ≤11 years old of immigrants from areas of high HBV endemicity; people who abuse drugs parenterally; the sexually active, whether homosexual or heterosexual; and those at occupational risk. The recommendation for universal vaccination of infants (initiated in 1991) was based on several considerations: the low dose of vaccine required for this age group; the feasibility of integration into the routine childhood immunization schedule; the need to prevent chronic infection in high risk children; and data suggesting that protection against disease persists to the age when high risk behaviours begin.

Vaccination of all previously unvaccinated adolescents at 11–12 years of age is now recommended in the USA, and is the primary strategy for hepatitis B control in Canada and some countries in Europe (Committee on Infectious Diseases 1994, Hinman and Orenstein 1994). This approach has the advantage of ensuring that adolescents will be protected before beginning high risk behaviours, that immunity will be high and that a booster dose of vaccine will not be needed. A key challenge is providing the 3 dose vaccine series to this age group in the absence of regular preventive healthcare visits. The vaccination of adolescents has been implemented successfully in British Columbia via school-based programmes (Dobson, Schiefle and Bell 1995).

In developing countries with high HBV endemicity, including eastern and southern Asia and Africa, universal vaccination of infants is the primary strategy for disease control (Kane 1993). In countries in which >2% of the population are HBV carriers, hepatitis B vaccine is recommended to be integrated into the schedule of the Expanded Programme on Immunization, the initial dose being given as soon after birth as possible. By 1995, 80 countries had routine immunization programmes, based mainly on universal vaccination of infants (Global Programme for Vaccines and Immunization 1995). In countries with extremely low HBV endemicity (Scandinavia, Great Britain), strategies continue to rely on vaccination of high risk adults.

7.4 Varicella vaccine

Live attenuated varicella-zoster vaccine was developed in the late 1970s, has been available in Japan and

Korea and some European countries for many years, and was licensed for primary prevention of varicella in American children and adults in March 1995. This vaccine, developed from the Oka strain of varicella virus, is over 95% effective in providing protection for 1–2 years (Kuter et al. 1991, Bernstein et al. 1993). Protection against infection appears to wane over time, with long-term efficacy against infection estimated to be 70–90% for 7–9 years after vaccination (Centers for Disease Control and Prevention 1996a). However, the 1–4% of children and adults who experience breakthrough infection annually develop mild disease with an average of ≤50 lesions (compared to 300 lesions in typical varicella). Trials of this vaccine for protection against the development of varicella-zoster disease are currently being planned.

For primary prevention, varicella vaccine is given as a single dose for children age 12 months to 12 years, and 2 doses separated by at least 1 month for older children and adults (Centers for Disease Control and Prevention 1996a). Varicella vaccine may be given simultaneously with all other childhood vaccines. For adolescents and adults, serological screening of people without a history of varicella is likely to be cost-effective, because 70–91% of them will be immune to varicella.

Varicella vaccine induces a mild varicelliform rash and fever in 5–10% of vaccinees. It is contraindicated in people who are immunocompromised, except for children with acute lymphocytic leukaemia, for whom the vaccine is available in the USA through an Investigational Drug Protocol, in pregnant women and in anyone who has an anaphylactic reaction to varicella vaccine or any component, including gelatin. Vaccination should be delayed for 5 months after the administration of immunoglobulin or blood products, because the response to vaccine administered within this interval is unknown. The risk of herpes zoster after varicella vaccination appears to be lower than after natural varicella infection.

Strategies for the use of varicella vaccine include voluntary vaccination of susceptible people, particularly adults at high risk of serious disease, and universal vaccination. The former has been used in Japan and Korea for many years without known adverse consequences, but provides protection only to those who are vaccinated.

Universal vaccination is intended to reduce disease transmission greatly and provide herd immunity to those who remain unvaccinated, and is the strategy recently adopted by the USA (Centers for Disease Control and Prevention 1996a). Varicella vaccine is recommended for all children at 12–18 months of age and for all susceptible older children (with no prior history of varicella). All children who have not had natural varicella infection should be vaccinated at 11–12 years of age. Varicella vaccine is also recommended for susceptible healthcare workers and others in close contact with immunocompromised people who might experience severe varicella if infected; it should be considered for susceptible adults who may have contact with infected children and any adults with no prior history of varicella. The hazards of this strategy are that only a fraction of the population will be vaccinated, reducing but not eliminating disease transmission and resulting in delayed exposure and development of more serious disease in adulthood (Halloran et al. 1994). Uncertainty about the quality of long-term protection by vaccine, of the importance of exposure to natural disease in maintaining vaccine-induced protection and of the risk of varicella-zoster in vaccinees have generated controversy about this policy.

8　OTHER VIRAL VACCINES

8.1　Hepatitis A vaccine

Both killed and live attenuated hepatitis A vaccines have been under development since the 1980s (D'Hondt 1992). Killed vaccines produced in tissue culture, purified and inactivated with formalin became available in the early 1990s, but live attenuated vaccines have not yet achieved an appropriate balance of attenuation and protection necessary for licensing. Inactivated hepatitis A vaccines are highly immunogenic and over 95% effective in preventing hepatitis A infection when given as a 2–3 dose series to children or a 2 dose series to adults (Werzberger et al. 1992, Innis et al. 1994). The duration of protection is not known but, on the basis of high antibody levels induced by the vaccine, is expected to exceed 5 years (Van Damme et al. 1994). This vaccine may also provide protection postexposure, and be useful in controlling hepatitis A outbreaks in well defined populations.

Licensed hepatitis A vaccine is given as a 2 or 3 dose series, with doses at 0 and 6–12 months (or 0, 1 and 6–12 months) to children ≥2 years of age, and as a 2 dose series given 6–12 months apart to adults (Centers for Disease Control and Prevention 1996b). The known adverse reactions are limited to pain at the injection site. Hepatitis A vaccine may be given simultaneously with other childhood vaccines or vaccines for international travellers. The administration of passive immunoglobulin or maternal antibody interferes with response to the first dose of vaccine, but differences in final antibody response after the multidose series seem unlikely to be of clinical importance.

Hepatitis A vaccine is recommended for people at high risk of infection, particularly those travelling to or working in countries where hepatitis A is highly endemic. Primary groups recommended to receive hepatitis A vaccine in the USA include native Americans and other groups that experience cyclic hepatitis A epidemics, haemophiliacs, homosexual men and users of illicit drugs and people with cirrhosis (Centers for Disease Control and Prevention 1996b). Vaccination also may be considered for the prevention or control of community-wide outbreaks, although the data on effectiveness in this situation are limited. Ultimately, universal vaccination may be necessary to reduce the burden of disease in some developed coun-

tries such as the USA; however, this will probably require a less costly preparation and its incorporation into combination childhood vaccines.

8.2　Influenza virus vaccines

The influenza vaccines now available are prepared from inactivated whole or disrupted (split) influenza viruses (Centers for Disease Control and Prevention 1996c). Because of the frequent antigenic changes in influenza viruses, the antigenic content of both types of vaccine is changed annually to optimize protection against the influenza type A and B strains expected to circulate during the following winter and spring. Influenza viruses of type A (N1H1 and H3N2) and B are selected according to their immunological match with circulating strains, grown in chicken embryos, inactivated with formalin and combined into vaccine.

The efficacy of vaccine is related to the degree of match between the vaccine and the circulating influenza viruses. In recent years, efficacy has been estimated to be 60–80% in younger adults, but lower in older adults. Protection against serious complications, including hospitalization and death, is higher than against uncomplicated influenza (Nichol et al. 1994, Gross et al. 1995). When major antigenic shifts occur, vaccine effectiveness may be substantially less. Annual vaccination is necessary to ensure protection against the current strains.

For previously unvaccinated children 6 months to 8 years of age, 2 doses of vaccine, given at 4 week intervals, are recommended (Centers for Disease Control and Prevention 1996c). For other groups, only a single dose is necessary. Children <13 years of age should be given only split virus vaccine because of its lower reactogenicity, whilst others may be given either vaccine. About 3–5% of vaccinees experience local tenderness or fever after vaccination. The occurrence of Guillain–Barré syndrome within 6 weeks of influenza vaccination was observed in adults after the swine influenza vaccine campaign in 1976, but was not observed subsequently until 1990, when a case–control study suggested a slightly elevated risk in 18–64 year olds but not in those over 65 years of age (Schonberger et al. 1979, Chen et al. 1992). Given the substantial benefits of influenza vaccination among the target populations, the risk, if any, of Guillain–Barré syndrome is exceeded by the benefits. A previous anaphylactic reaction to egg protein is the only contraindication to influenza vaccination.

Vaccination is intended to reduce the complications and mortality due to influenza infection. Annual immunization is recommended for those at highest risk of these complications (Centers for Disease Control and Prevention 1996c). In most developed countries, vaccination is recommended for people with certain chronic medical conditions, including cardiovascular and pulmonary disorders, asthma, other medical disorders such as metabolic disease (including diabetes mellitus), renal disease, haemoglobinopathies (including sickle cell disease), and for people with immunosuppressive disorders or treatments and children on long-term aspirin therapy. In many countries, annual vaccination is recommended for all adults aged ≥65. Although immunogenicity and efficacy have not been established in all these groups, the risk from vaccine virus is non-existent because vaccine is inactivated. Healthcare workers and people caring for those at high risk should also be vaccinated. Many countries have developed plans to prepare for pandemic influenza, which occurs every 10–40 years and can have devastating mortality. Such plans include the rapid production and availability of vaccine to ensure the vaccination either of people at highest risk or of the entire population.

Cold-adapted live attenuated influenza vaccines have been under development for many years, and have been used in Russia since 1977 (Murphy 1993, Maassab, Shaw and Heilman 1994). These incorporate influenza virus strains attenuated through growth at 25°C, but with reduced growth at 37°C. The genes for relevant circulating influenza strains can be incorporated into these vaccines by reassortment, and the vaccine is administered intranasally. In controlled trials, these vaccines have been as or slightly less effective than inactivated influenza vaccines. However, they have not yet been licensed for wide use in the USA and Europe.

8.3 Japanese encephalitis vaccine

Japanese encephalitis (JE) vaccine is a purified preparation of whole virus grown in mouse brain and inactivated with formalin. When given as a 3 dose series, the vaccine has 91% efficacy in adults (Hoke et al. 1988). Antibody persists for at least 2 years; the need for booster doses is uncertain. Primary immunization consists of 3 doses given at 0, 7 and 30 days; the third dose may be given at 14 days if the schedule does not permit the longer interval (Centers for Disease Control and Prevention 1993a). The dose for young children (1–3 years) is 0.5 ml, and that for older children and adults is 1.0 ml. No data are available on safety and immunogenicity in children <1 year of age. Adverse events include local reactions (20%) and minor systemic symptoms (10%). Generalized allergic reactions (angioedema, urticaria) may occur in 1–6 per 1000 vaccinees; more rarely, respiratory distress and hypotension have been reported. Rare neurological events have been reported but causation by vaccine has not yet been established.

JE vaccine is recommended for travellers or residents in areas where the disease is endemic (south and east Asia), who potentially will be exposed during the transmission season particularly in rural areas when travelling for 30 or more days (Centers for Disease Control and Prevention 1993a). JE vaccine is used routinely in many of these countries.

8.4 Rabies vaccine

The first attenuated and inactivated rabies vaccines were developed by Pasteur from desiccated infected rabbit brains. Subsequent vaccines were developed from virus harvested from the brains of rabbits, sheep or goats, but caused neuroparalytic disease due to residual myelin derivatives in about 1 per 2000 recipients. Vaccines developed from duck embryos reduced the risk of serious adverse events about 10-fold (Hattwick 1974). However, these vaccines have now been replaced by those grown in diploid human cell lines (World Health Organization 1984). Rabies virus is harvested from cell culture and inactivated with β-propiolactone. This vaccine (human diploid cell strain: HDCS) is highly immunogenic when given as a multidose series, either alone (pre-exposure) or with human rabies immunoglobulin (HRIG) (post-exposure). The vaccine schedules for pre-exposure prophylaxis is a 3 dose series at weekly intervals. For people at high continuing risk of infection (e.g. veterinarians, travellers to endemic areas), testing for the presence of neutralizing antibody should be done at 2 year intervals and booster doses given if inadequate antibody is present; alternatively, booster doses may be given at 2 year intervals without testing. Postexposure prophylaxis includes a 5 dose series: the first dose with HRIG, half infiltrated at the site of the bite and half given intramuscularly elsewhere, followed by additional vaccine doses 3, 7, 14 and 28 days later (Centers for Disease Control and Prevention 1991a). Although episodes of rabies have rarely followed the use of HDCS alone, there have been no reports of vaccine failure with HDCS given with HRIG (Devriendt et al. 1982, Centers for Disease Control and Prevention 1991a).

HDCS causes few adverse events. Type III hypersensitivity similar to serum sickness can occur with repeated doses. Although cases of neurological disease such as Guillain–Barré syndrome have been reported following HDCS, these are not conclusively linked to the vaccine. New vaccines under investigation include recombinant vaccines containing the surface glycoprotein produced in *E. coli*, mammalian or yeast cells, or vectored into vaccinia and canarypox viruses.

8.5 Yellow fever vaccine

Yellow fever (YF) vaccine, available since the 1930s, is the live attenuated 17D strain of YF virus. A single dose, given subcutaneously, is highly effective in inducing protection that may last for 10 or more years; booster doses are recommended only at 10 year intervals (Centers for Disease Control and Prevention 1990a). YF vaccine causes local and limited systemic symptoms in 2–5% of recipients 5–10 days after vaccination. Serious reactions including encephalitis are rare; the risk is highest in children 4–9 months of age, and the vaccine is contraindicated in those younger than 10 months. YF vaccine should not be administered to pregnant women; however, if a pregnant woman is travelling to an endemic area and cannot avoid potential exposure, YF vaccine may be given. YF vaccine is contraindicated in people with anaphylactic allergy to egg or who are immunocompromised. The response to YF vaccine can be inhibited by cholera vaccine; these vaccines should be given at least 3 weeks apart. Because cholera vaccine is rarely indicated, YF should be given first.

Vaccine is recommended for travellers 9 months of age and older going to areas where YF is endemic, and may be required for entry into such countries. YF vaccine is used in endemic areas, and may be given in mass campaigns, which are often stimulated by the occurrence of outbreaks. The incorporation of YF vaccine into the routine childhood immunization schedule at 9 months of age is recommended by the Expanded Programme on Immunization, but requires wider availability of affordable vaccine in many developing countries.

9 NEW VIRUS VACCINES

9.1 Rotavirus vaccines

Live attenuated rotavirus vaccines have been developed from rotaviruses of other species, using a jennerian approach enhanced with modern virological techniques. Current vaccines now in phase III efficacy trials are derived from rhesus and bovine rotaviruses, which have minimal pathogenicity for humans (Kapikian 1994, Clark et al. 1996). Taking advantage of the segmented genome of rotavirus, reassortants have been developed that retain most of the genome of the parent virus, but include one or both of 2 key surface glycoproteins – VP7 and VP4 – of the human viruses. Multivalent vaccines were developed following the recognition that rotavirus disease is caused by 4 major serotypes, and that monovalent vaccines, although effective against the same serotype, had little or no effect against the others (Glass, Gentsch and Smith 1994).

The rhesus rotavirus based vaccine (RRV-TV) currently in trials is tetravalent, and includes the parent virus, which provides protection against rotavirus type 3, and reassortants that include the VP7 surface protein from human rotavirus types 1, 2 and 4, respectively. The bovine rotavirus based vaccine (WC-3) also is tetravalent, and includes 3 reassortants containing VP7 from human rotaviruses types 1, 2 and 3, and a fourth containing VP4 common to human rotaviruses type 1, 2 and 3 (G6); this vaccine provides protection only against human rotavirus types 1, 2 and 3. The vaccines are grown in diploid fetal rhesus lung or rhesus kidney cells.

The use of multivalent rotavirus vaccines given as a multidose series is being studied. Two or 3 doses of 10^5 (RRV-TV) or 10^7 (WC179-9) pfu are given during infancy with other childhood vaccines (at 2, 4 and 6 months of age in the USA). Clinical trials of the tetravalent vaccines in developed countries have indicated 49–67% efficacy in preventing rotavirus diarrhoea, and 75–87% efficacy in preventing severe diarrhoea causing dehydration or requiring hospitalization (Bernstein et al. 1995, Rennels et al. 1996). Adverse events observed in clinical trials have included fever >38°C (15% vs 7% in placebo recipients); fewer than 20% of vaccinees excreted rotavirus after vaccination.

Efficacy trials with these vaccines in less developed countries are underway.

On the basis of observed efficacy and the substantial burden of disease in infants, it is anticipated that rotavirus vaccines will be cost-effective when used in infants in developed countries such as the USA, and will probably be incorporated into the routine childhood immunization schedule (Glass, Gentsch and Smith 1994). Low cost vaccines will be necessary to ensure that such vaccines can be used in developing countries, where the burden of rotavirus disease is largest. Additional approaches to the development of rotavirus vaccines include the use of human strains isolated from infants without diarrhoea, viruses attenuated by cold adaptation and self-assembling particles produced in baculovirus into which rotavirus VP7 genes have been cloned.

9.2 Human immunodeficiency virus vaccines

Intensive efforts are underway to develop vaccines to prevent or modify the course of human immunodeficiency virus (HIV) infection (Hoth et al. 1994, Dolin 1995, Graham and Wright 1995). The development and testing of vaccines have been hampered by a lack of complete understanding of the correlates of immunity to HIV infection and the lack of animal models that mimic both infection and disease. Nevertheless, studies of HIV vaccines in primates (chimpanzees) and human volunteers and of vaccines to prevent simian immunodeficiency virus (SIV) infection, as a possible model for HIV vaccines, have progressed to phase II trials.

The main approaches to the development of HIV vaccine include: the use of inactivated whole HIV (pursued less actively because of concerns of possible residual infectivity); vaccines in which the surface glycoproteins gp120 or gp160 are produced in recombinant systems such as mammalian cells, yeast or insect cells; vectored recombinant constructs in which genes encoding gp120 or gp160 are inserted into vaccinia or canarypox virus; use of subunit peptides, either alone or boosted using a vectored virus; and core protein/peptide vaccines. Various recombinant vaccines have been tested in over 1500 human volunteers in the USA and elsewhere.

Recombinant gp120 vaccines have progressed to phase II trials. These vaccines are given at 0, 1, 6 and 12+ months. These schedules produce antibody detectable by Western blot or ELISA in virtually all recipients after 3 doses. However, functional antibody responses are less complete; neutralizing antibodies to homologous strains can be detected in virtually all recipients, but less frequently and of lower titre to other laboratory HIV strains, and to wild HIV isolates. Cell-mediated responses include lymphoproliferative responses and CD4 cytotoxic lymphocytes (CTLs) detectable in some vaccine recipients. The vaccines have been well tolerated, with minor local reactions and no evidence of systemic reactions.

Live vectored vaccines produced in vaccinia have also been tested widely, but have had disappointing immunogenicity even in vaccinia-naive subjects. Current approaches are to provide an initial dose of the live vector vaccine followed by a dose of the recombinant protein itself, and this has induced neutralizing antibodies and MHC class I restricted CTL activity in some subjects.

In phase II clinical trials, some vaccinated subjects have subsequently developed HIV infection, suggesting that the vaccines are not fully protective, but these studies were not designed to provide estimates of vaccine efficacy. The study of people who develop infection despite vaccination may provide information on the nature of the protective immune response.

REFERENCES

Albrecht P, Ennis FA et al., 1977, Persistence of maternal antibody in infants beyond 12 months: mechanism of measles vaccine failure, *J Pediatr*, **91:** 715–18.

Anderson RM, May RM, 1990, Immunization and herd immunity, *Lancet*, **335:** 641–5.

Annunziato D, Kaplan MH et al., 1982, Atypical measles syndrome: pathologic and serologic findings, *Pediatrics*, **70:** 203–9.

Anonymous, 1994, National measles and rubella immunization campaign, *Communicable Dis Rep Weekly*, **4 (31):** 149–50.

Arai K, Lee F et al., 1990, Cytokines: coordinators of immune and inflammatory responses, *Annu Rev Biochem*, **59:** 783–836.

Baker PJ, 1975, Homeostatic control of antibody responses. A model based on the recognition of cell-associated antibody by regulatory T-cells, *Transplant Rev*, **26:** 3–20.

Barundun S, Morell A, 1981, Adverse reactions to immunoglobulin preparations, *Immunotherapy. A Guide to Immunoglobulin Prophylaxis and Therapy*, ed Nydegger UE, Academic Press, New York, 223–7.

Bernstein HH, Rothstein EP et al., 1993, Clinical survey of natural varicella compared with breakthrough varicella after immunization with live attenuated Oka/Merck varicella vaccine, *Pediatrics*, **92:** 833–7.

Bernstein DI, Glass RI et al., 1995, Evaluation of rhesus rotavirus monovalent and tetravalent reassortant vaccines in US children, *JAMA*, **273:** 1191–6.

Brown F, 1988, Use of peptide vaccines for immunization against foot and mouth disease, *Vaccine*, **6:** 180–2.

Centers for Disease Control, 1982, Recommendation of the Immunization Practices Advisory Committee (ACIP). Poliomyelitis prevention, *Morbid Mortal Weekly Rep*, **31:** 22–31.

Centers for Disease Control, 1987, Recommendation of the Immunization Practices Advisory Committee (ACIP). Poliomyelitis prevention: enhanced potency inactivated poliomyelitis vaccine – supplementary statement, *Morbid Mortal Weekly Rep*, **36:** 795–8.

Centers for Disease Control, 1988, National Childhood Vaccine Injury Act: requirements for permanent vaccination records and for reporting of selected events after vaccination, *Morbid Mortal Weekly Rep*, **37:** 197–200.

Centers for Disease Control, 1989a, Recommendation of the Immunization Practices Advisory Committee (ACIP). Measles prevention, *Morbid Mortal Weekly Rep*, **38 (S-9):** 1–18.

Centers for Disease Control, 1989b, Rubella vaccination during pregnancy: United States, 1971–88, *Morbid Mortal Weekly Rep*, **38:** 289–93.

Centers for Disease Control, 1989c, Recommendation of the Immunization Practices Advisory Committee (ACIP). Mumps vaccine, *Morbid Mortal Weekly Rep*, **38:** 388–92, 397–400.

Centers for Disease Control and Prevention, 1990a, Recommendation of the Immunization Practices Advisory Committee (ACIP). Yellow fever vaccine, *Morbid Mortal Weekly Rep*, **39 (RR-6):** 1–6.

Centers for Disease Control and Prevention, 1990b, Recommendation of the Immunization Practices Advisory Committee (ACIP). Rubella prevention, *Morbid Mortal Weekly Rep*, **39 (RR-15):** 1–18.

Centers for Disease Control and Prevention, 1991a, Rabies prevention: United States, 1991. Recommendations of the Immunization Practices Advisory Committee, *Morbid Mortal Weekly Rep*, **40 (RR-3):** 1–19.

Centers for Disease Control and Prevention, 1991b, Recommendations of the Immunization Practices Advisory Committee. Hepatitis B virus: a comprehensive strategy for eliminating transmission in the United States through universal childhood vaccination, *Morbid Mortal Weekly Rep*, **40 (RR-13):** 1–25.

Centers for Disease Control and Prevention, 1991c, Recommendations of the Advisory Committee on Immunization Practices. Update on adult immunization, *Morbid Mortal Weekly Rep*, **40 (RR-12):** 1–94.

Centers for Disease Control and Prevention, 1993a, Recommendations of the Immunization Practices Advisory Committee (ACIP). Inactivated Japanese encephalitis virus vaccine, *Morbid Mortal Weekly Rep*, **42 (RR-1):** 1–15.

Centers for Disease Control and Prevention, 1993b, Recommendations of the Advisory Committee on Immunization Practices (ACIP). Use of vaccines and immune globulins in persons with altered immunocompetence, *Morbid Mortal Weekly Rep*, **42 (RR-4):** 1–18.

Centers for Disease Control and Prevention, 1993c, Recommendations of the International Task Force for Disease Eradication, *Morbid Mortal Weekly Rep*, **42 (RR-16):** 1–38.

Centers for Disease Control and Prevention, 1994a, Reported vaccine preventable diseases, United States 1993, and the Childhood Immunization Initiative, *Morbid Mortal Weekly Rep*, **43:** 57–61.

Centers for Disease Control and Prevention, 1994b, Recommendation of the Immunization Practices Advisory Committee (ACIP). General recommendations on immunization, *Morbid Mortal Weekly Rep*, **43 (RR-1):** 1–38.

Centers for Disease Control and Prevention, 1994c, *Health Information for International Travel, 1994*, US Government Printing Office, Washington DC.

Centers for Disease Control and Prevention, 1994d, Outbreak of hepatitis C associated with intravenous immunoglobulin administration: United States, October 1993–June 1994, *Morbid Mortal Weekly Rep*, **43:** 505–9.

Centers for Disease Control and Prevention, 1995, Summary of notifiable diseases, United States, 1994, *Morbid Mortal Weekly Rep*, **44 (53):** 3.

Centers for Disease Control and Prevention, 1996a, Varicella prevention. Recommendations of the Advisory Committee on Immunization Practices, *Morbid Mortal Weekly Rep*, **45 (RR-11):** 1–36.

Centers for Disease Control and Prevention, 1996b, Prevention of Hepatitis A through active or passive immunization. Recommendations of the Advisory Committee on Immunization Practices, *Morbid Mortal Weekly Rep*, **45 (RR-15):** 1–30.

Centers for Disease Control and Prevention, 1996c, Recommendations of the Immunization Practices Advisory Committee (ACIP). Prevention and control of influenza, *Morbid Mortal Weekly Rep*, **45 (RR-5):** 1–24.

Centers for Disease Control and Prevention, 1996d, Measles pneumonitis following measles-mumps-rubella vaccination of a patient with HIV infection, 1993, *Morbid Morality Weekly Rep*, **45:** 603–6.

Centers for Disease Control and Prevention, 1997, Poliomyelitis prevention in the United States: introduction of a sequential schedule of inactivated poliovirus vaccine (IPV) followed by oral poliovirus vaccine (OPV), *Morbid Mortality Weekly Rep*, **46 (RR-2)**: 1–26.

Cheek JE, Baron R et al., 1995, Mumps outbreak in a highly vaccinated school population, *Arch Pediatr Adolesc Med*, **149**: 774–8.

Chen R, Kent J et al., 1992, Investigation of a possible association between influenza vaccination and Guillain–Barré syndrome in the United States, 1990–1991 [abstract], *Post Marketing Surveillance*, **6**: 5–6.

Chen RT, Rastogi SC et al., 1994, The vaccine adverse events reporting system (VAERS), *Vaccine*, **12**: 542–50.

Claman HN, 1992, The biology of the immune response, *JAMA*, **268**: 2790–6.

Clark HF, Offit PA et al., 1996, The development of multivalent bovine rotavirus (strain WC3) reassortant vaccine for infants, *J Infect Dis*, **174, suppl 1**: S73–80.

Cochi SL, Wharton M, Plotkin SA, 1994, Mumps vaccine, *Vaccines*, 2nd edn, eds Plotkin SA, Mortimer EA Jr, WB Saunders, Philadelphia, 277–301.

Cohn EJ, Strong LE et al., 1946, Preparation and properties of serum and plasma proteins. IV. A system for the separation into fractions of protein and lipoprotein components of the biological tissues and fluids, *J Am Chem Soc*, **68**: 459–75.

Committee on Infectious Diseases, American Academy of Pediatrics, 1994, *Report of the Committee on Infectious Diseases*, 23rd edn, American Academy of Pediatrics, Elk Grove Village IL.

Cuthbertson B, Perry RJ et al., 1987, The viral safety of intravenous immunoglobulin, *J Infect*, **15**: 125–33.

Dalgleish AC, Kennedy RC, 1988, Anti-idiotype antibodies as immunogens: idiotype-based vaccines, *Vaccine*, **6**: 215–20.

Devriendt J, Staroukine M et al., 1982, Fatal encephalitis apparently due to rabies occurrence after treatment with human diploid cell vaccine but not rabies immune globulin, *JAMA*, **248**: 2304–6.

D'Hondt E, 1992, Possible approaches to develop vaccines against hepatitis A, *Vaccine*, **10, suppl 1**: S48–52.

Dobson S, Schiefle D, Bell A, 1995, Assessment of a universal, school based hepatitis B vaccination program, *JAMA*, **274**: 1209–13.

Dolin R, 1995, Human studies in the development of human immunodeficiency virus vaccines, *J Infect Dis*, **172**: 1175–83.

Enders JF, Peebles TC, 1954, Propagation in tissue cultures of cytopathogenic agents from patients with measles, *Proc Soc Exp Biol Med*, **86**: 277–86.

Enders JF, Weller TH, Robbins FC, 1949, Cultivation of the Lansing strain of poliomyelitis virus in cultures of various human embryonic tissues, *Science*, **109**: 85–7.

Esteves K, 1988, Safety of oral poliomyelitis vaccine: results of a WHO enquiry, *Bull W H O*, **66**: 739–46.

Expanded Programme on Immunization, Global Programme for Vaccines and Immunization, World Health Organization, and Centers for Disease Control, 1995, Progress toward global poliomyelitis eradication, 1985–1994, *Morbid Mortal Weekly Rep*, **44**: 273–5, 281.

Fenner F, Henderson DA et al., 1988, *Smallpox and Its Eradication*, World Health Organization, Geneva.

Foege WH, 1971, Measles vaccination in Africa, *Proceedings of the International Conference on the Application of Vaccines Against Viral, Rickettsial and Bacterial Diseases in Man*, PAHO scientific publication 226, Pan American Health Organization, Washington DC, 207–12.

Fox JP, Elveback L et al., 1972, Herd immunity: basic concept and relevance to public health immunization practices, *Am J Epidemiol*, **94**: 179–89.

Francis T, Napier JA et al., 1957, *Evaluation of the 1954 Field Trial of Poliomyelitis Vaccine. Final Report*, Poliomyelitis Vaccine Evaluation Center, Department of Epidemiology, School of Public Health, University of Michigan, Ann Arbor.

Fynan EF, Webster RG et al., 1995, DNA vaccines: a novel approach to immunization, *Int J Immunopharmacol*, **17**: 79–83.

Galazka AM, 1994, Achievements, problems and perspectives of the expanded program on immunization, *Int J Med Microbiol*, **281**: 353–64.

Gindler J, Hadler SC et al., 1995, Recommended childhood immunization schedule, United States, 1995, *Clin Pediatr*, **34**: 66–72.

Glass RI, Gentsch J, Smith JC, 1994, Rotavirus vaccines: success by reassortment?, *Science*, **265**: 1389–91.

Global Programme on Vaccines and Immunization, 1995, *Programme Report, 1994*, 95.1, World Health Organization, Geneva.

Graham BS, Wright PF, 1995, Candidate AIDS vaccines, *N Engl J Med*, **333**: 1331–8.

Gregg NA, 1941, Congenital cataract following german measles in the mother, *Trans Ophthalmol Soc Aust*, **3**: 35–46.

Gross PA, Hermogenes AW et al., 1995, The efficacy of influenza vaccine in elderly persons. A meta-analysis and review of the literature, *Ann Intern Med*, **123**: 518–27.

Hadler SC, Margolis HS, 1992, Hepatitis B immunization: vaccine types, efficacy, and indications for immunization, *Current Topics in Clinical Infectious Diseases*, eds Remington JS, Swartz MN, Blackwell Scientific, Boston MA, 283–308.

Halloran ME, Cochi SL et al., 1994, Epidemiologic effects of routine immunization with varicella vaccine in the United States, *Am J Epidemiol*, **140**: 81–104.

Halsey NA, 1983, The optimal age for administering measles vaccine in developing countries, *Recent Advances in Immunization. A bibliographic review*, PAHO publication 451, eds Halsey NA, de Quadros CA, Pan American Health Organization, Washington DC, 4–17.

Hattwick MAW, 1974, Human rabies, *Public Health Rev*, **3**: 229–74.

Hatziandreu EJ, Palmer CS et al., 1994, *A Cost Benefit Analysis of the Diphtheria–Tetanus–Pertussis Vaccine*, Battelle, Arlington VA.

Hinman AR, Orenstein WA, 1994, Public health considerations, *Vaccines*, 2nd edn, eds Plotkin SA, Mortimer EA Jr, WB Saunders, Philadelphia, 903–32.

Hoke CH, Nisalak A et al., 1988, Protection against Japanese encephalitis by inactivated vaccines, *N Engl J Med*, **319**: 609–14.

Hoth DF, Bolognesi DP et al., 1994, HIV vaccine development: a progress report, *Ann Intern Med*, **8**: 603–11.

Hull HF, Ward NA et al., 1994, Paralytic poliomyelitis: seasoned strategies, disappearing disease, *Lancet*, **343**: 1331–7.

Innis BL, Snitbhan R et al., 1994, Protection against hepatitis A by an inactivated vaccine, *JAMA*, **271**: 1363–4.

Institute of Medicine, 1991, *Adverse Effects of Pertussis and Rubella Vaccines*, eds Howson CP, Howe CJ, Fineberg HV, National Academy Press, Washington DC.

Institute of Medicine, 1993, *Adverse Events Associated with Childhood Vaccines. Evidence bearing on causation*, eds Stratton KR, Howe CJ, Johnston RB, National Academy Press, Washington DC.

James JM, Burks W et al., 1995, Safe administration of the measles vaccine to children allergic to eggs, *N Engl J Med*, **332**: 1262–6.

Joce R, Wood D et al., 1992, Paralytic poliomyelitis in England and Wales, 1985–1991, *Br Med J*, **305**: 79–82.

Kane MA, 1993, Progress in control of hepatitis B infection through immunization, *Gut*, **34, suppl 2**: S10–12.

Kapikian AZ, 1994, Rhesus rotavirus-based human vaccines and observations on selected non-Jennerian approaches to rotavirus vaccination, *Viral Infections of the Gastrointestinal Tract*, 2nd edn, ed Kapikian AZ, Marcel Dekker, New York, 443–69.

King GE, Hadler SC, 1994, Simultaneous administration of childhood vaccines: an important public health policy that is safe and efficacious, *Pediatr Infect Dis J*, **13**: 394–407.

Kuter BJ, Weibel RE et al., 1991, Oka/Merck varicella vaccine in healthy children: final report of a 2 year efficacy study and 7 year follow-up studies, *Vaccine*, **9**: 643–7.

Lanzavecchia A, 1985, Antigen-specific interaction between T and B cells, *Nature (London)*, **314:** 537–9.

Lieu TA, Cochi SL et al., 1994, Cost-effectiveness of a routine varicella vaccination program for US children, *JAMA*, **271:** 375–81.

McBean AM, Modlin JF, 1987, Rationale for the sequential use of inactivated poliovirus vaccine and live attenuated poliovirus vaccine for routine poliomyelitis immunization in the United States, *Pediatr Infect Dis J,* **6:** 881–7.

McDevitt HO, 1980, Regulation of the immune response by the major histocompatibility complex system, *N Engl J Med,* **303:** 1514–17.

McDonnell WM, Askari FK, 1996, DNA vaccines, *N Engl J Med,* **334:** 42–5.

McGhee JR, Mestecky J et al., 1992, The mucosal immune system: from fundamental concepts to vaccine development, *Vaccine,* **10:** 75–88.

Maassab HF, Shaw MW, Heilman CA, 1994, Live influenza virus vaccine, *Vaccines,* 2nd edn, eds Plotkin S, Mortimer EA Jr, WB Saunders, Philadelphia, 781–801.

Maiztegui JI, Fernandez NJ, DeDamilano AJ, 1979, Efficacy of immune plasma in treatment of Argentinian heamorrhagic fever and association between treatment and a late neurological syndrome, *Lancet,* **2:** 1216–17.

Margolis HS, Coleman PJ et al., 1995, Prevention of hepatitis B virus transmission by immunization. An economic analysis of current recommendations, *JAMA,* **274:** 1201–8.

Markowitz LE, Katz SL, 1994, Measles vaccine, *Vaccines,* 2nd edn, eds Plotkin S, Mortimer EA Jr, WB Saunders, Philadelphia, 229–76.

Mathias RG, Meekison WG et al., 1989, The role of secondary vaccine failures in measles outbreaks, *Am J Public Health,* **79:** 475–8.

Melnick JL, Stinebaugh S, 1962, Excretion of vacuolating SV40 virus (papovavirus group) after ingestion as contaminant of oral polio vaccine, *Proc Soc Exp Biol Med,* **109:** 965–8.

Meloen RH, Casal JI et al., 1995, Synthetic peptides vaccines: success at last, *Vaccine,* **13:** 885–6.

Miller E, 1991, Rubella in the United Kingdom, *Epidemiol Infect,* **107:** 31–42.

Miller E, Goldacre M et al., 1993, Risk of aseptic meningitis after measles, mumps, and rubella vaccine in UK children, *Lancet,* **341:** 979–82.

Mortimer EA, Lepow ML et al., 1982, Long-term follow-up of persons inadvertently inoculated with SV40 as neonates, *N Engl J Med,* **305:** 1517–18.

Moss B, Fuerst TR et al., 1988, Roles of vaccina virus in the development of new vaccines, *Vaccine,* **6:** 161–3.

Murphy BR, 1993, Use of live attenuated cold-adapted influenza A reassortant virus vaccines in infants, children, young adults, and elderly adults, *Infect Dis Clin Pract,* **2:** 174–81.

Murphy BR, Chanock RM, 1990, Immunization against viruses, *Fields' Virology,* 2nd edn, eds Fields BN, Knipe DM et al., Raven Press, New York, 469–502.

Nathanson N, Langmuir AD, 1963, The Cutter incident. Poliomyelitis following formaldehyde-inactivated poliovirus vaccination in the United States during the spring of 1955, *Am J Hygiene,* **78:** 16–28, 29–60.

Nichol KL, Margolis KL et al., 1994, The efficacy and cost effectiveness of vaccination against influenza among elderly persons living in the community, *N Engl J Med,* **331:** 778–84.

Oncley JL, Melin M et al., 1949, The separation of antibodies, isoagglutinins, prothrombin, plasminogen and β-lipoproteins into sub-fractions of human plasma, *J Am Chem Soc,* **71:** 541–50.

Onorato IM, Markowitz LE, Oxtoby MJ, 1988, Childhood immunization, vaccine-preventable diseases and HIV infection, *Pediatr Infect Dis J,* **7:** 588–95.

Orenstein WA, Bernier RH, Hinman AR, 1988, Assessing vaccine efficacy in the field, *Epidemiol Rev,* **10:** 212–41.

Pan American Health Organization, 1994, Certification of polio-myelitis eradication – the Americas, 1994, *Morbid Mortal Weekly Rep,* **43:** 720–2.

Patriarca PA, Wright PF, John TJ, 1991, Factors affecting the immunogenicity of oral poliovirus vaccine in developing countries: a review, *Rev Infect Dis,* **13:** 926–39.

Peltola H, Heinonen OP et al., 1994, The elimination of indigenous measles, mumps, and rubella from Finland by a 12-year, two-dose vaccination program, *N Engl J Med,* **331:** 1397–402.

Perkus ME, Piccini A et al., 1985, Recombinant vaccinia virus: immunization against multiple pathogens, *Science,* **229:** 981–4.

Peters CJ, Johnson ED, McKee KT Jr, 1991, Filoviruses and management of viral hemorrhagic fevers, *Textbook of Human Virology,* 2nd edn, ed Belshe RB, Mosby Yearbook, St Louis MO, 699–712.

Plotkin SA, 1994, Rubella vaccine, *Vaccines,* 2nd edn, eds Plotkin SA, Mortimer EA Jr, WB Saunders, Philadelphia, 303–6.

de Quadros C, Olive JM et al., 1996, Measles elimination in the Americas. Evolving strategies, *JAMA,* **275:** 224–9.

Rantala H, Cherry JD, Shields WD, 1994, Epidemiology of Guillain–Barré syndrome in children: relationship of oral polio vaccine administration to occurrence, *J Pediatr,* **124:** 220–3.

Reinherz EL, Schlossman SF, 1980, Regulation of the immune response – inducer and suppressor T lymphocyte subsets in human beings, *N Engl J Med,* **303:** 370–3.

Rennels MB, Glass RI et al., 1996, Safety and efficacy of high-dose rhesus–human rotavirus vaccines – report of the national multicenter trial, *Pediatrics,* **97:** 7–13.

Rota JS, Heath JL et al., 1996, Molecular epidemiology of measles virus: identification of pathways of transmission and implications for measles elimination, *J Infect Dis,* **173:** 32–7.

Rousell RH, 1988, Clinical safety of intravenous immune globulin and freedom from transmission of viral disease, *J Hosp Infect,* **12, suppl D:** 17–27.

Salk J, Drucker JA, Malvin D, 1994, Noninfectious poliovirus vaccine, *Vaccines,* 2nd edn, eds Plotkin SA, Mortimer EA Jr, WB Saunders, Philadelphia, 205–27.

Schonberger LB, Bregman DJ et al., 1979, Guillain–Barré syndrome following vaccination in the National Influenza Immunization program, United States, 1976–1977, *Am J Epidemiology,* **110:** 105–23.

Siber GR, Snydman DR, 1989, Use of immunoglobulin in the prevention and treatment of infections, *Current Topics in Clinical Infectious Diseases,* eds Remington JS, Swartz MN, Blackwell Scientific, Boston MA, 208–56.

Siber GR, Werner BC, Halsey NA, 1993, Interference of immune globulins with measles and rubella immunization, *J Pediatr,* **122:** 204–11.

Siber GR, Lesczynski J, Pena-Cruz et al., 1992, Protective activity of a human respiratory syncytial virus immmune globulin prepared from donors screened by a microneutralization assay, *J Infect Dis,* **165:** 456–63.

Stevens CE, Toy PT et al., 1992, Prospects for control of hepatitis B virus infection: implications of childhood vaccination and long term protection, *Pediatrics,* **90:** 170–3.

Strebel PM, Sutter RW et al., 1992, Epidemiology of poliomyelitis in the United States one decade after the last reported case of indigenous wild virus-associated disease, *Clin Infect Dis,* **14:** 568–79.

Strebel PM, Ion-Nedelcu I et al., 1995, Intramuscular injections within 30 days of immunization with oral poliovirus vaccine – a risk factor for vaccine-associated paralytic poliomyelitis, *N Engl J Med,* **332:** 500–6.

Sutter RW, Patriarca PA, 1993, Inactivated and live, attenuated poliovirus vaccines: mucosal immunity, *Measles and Poliomyelitis. Vaccines, Immunization, and Control,* ed Kurstak E, Springer-Verlag, Vienna, 279–94.

Szmuness W, Stevens CE et al., 1981, A controlled clinical trial of the efficacy of hepatitis B vaccine (Heptavax B): a final report, *Hepatology,* **1:** 377–85.

Tingle AJ, Allen M, Petty RE, 1986, Rubella associated arthritis.

I. Comparative study of joint manifestations associated with natural rubella infection and RA 27/3 rubella immunization, *Ann Rheum Dis*, **45:** 110–14.

Van Damme P, Thoelen S et al., 1994, Inactivated hepatitis A vaccine: reactogenicity, immunogenicity, and long-term antibody persistence, *J Med Virol*, **44:** 446–51.

Waldvogel FA, 1981, *Immunotherapy: a Guide to Immunoglobulin Prophylaxis and Therapy*, ed Nyedegger UE, Academic Press, London, 357.

Waters TD, Anderson PS Jr et al., 1972, Yellow fever vaccination, avian leukosis virus and cancer risk in man, *Science*, **177:** 76–7.

Wells MA, Wittek AE et al., 1986, Inactivation and partition of human T-cell lymphotropic virus type III during ethanol fractionation of plasma, *Transfusion*, **26:** 210–13.

Werzberger A, Mensch B et al., 1992, A controlled trial of a formalin inactivated hepatitis A vaccine in healthy children, *N Engl J Med*, **327:** 453–7.

West DJ, Calendra GB, 1996, Vaccine induced immunologic memory for hepatitis B surface antigen: implications for policy on booster vaccination, *Vaccine*, **12:** 1019–27.

Wharton M, Strebel PM, 1995, Vaccine preventable diseases, *From Data to Action. CDC's Public Health Surveillance for Women, Infants and Children*, eds Wilcox LS, Marks JS, US Department of Health and Human Services, Atlanta GA, 281–90.

Williams PE, Hague RA et al., 1988a, Treatment of human immunodeficiency virus antibody positive children with intravenous immunoglobulin, *J Hosp Infect*, **12, suppl D:** 67–73.

Williams PE, Yap PL et al., 1988b, Non-A non-B hepatitis transmission by intravenous immunoglobulin, *Lancet*, **2:** 501.

World Health Organization, 1984, WHO Expert Committee on Rabies. Seventh Report, *Technical Report Series*, **709:** 1–104.

World Health Organization, 1987, Acceptability of cell substrates for production of biologicals, *Technical Report Series*, **747:** 1.

World Health Organization, 1988, *Report of the Forty-first World Health Assembly*, WHO, Geneva.

World Health Organization, 1995, *Expanded Programme on Immunization Information System*, WHO, Geneva, 95.2.

Chapter 46

ANTIVIRAL CHEMOTHERAPY

H J Field and R J Whitley

1 Introduction	4 Problems in antiviral chemotherapy
2 Discovery and assessment of new antiviral compounds	5 Combination chemotherapy for viral infections
3 Mechanism of action of important antiviral compounds	6 Conclusions and future prospects

1 INTRODUCTION

Over the last 2 decades there has been a revolution in antiviral chemotherapy. Viruses are obligate intra-cellular parasites that are completely dependent on an intact host cell to provide the ribosomal machinery for protein synthesis. As such, it was considered by many that 'selective toxicity' towards viruses was unattainable and that the cost of interfering with virus replication would necessarily be unacceptable damage to the host. Indeed, lack of susceptibility to antibiotics was considered to be one of the hallmarks of a virus. This gloomy prospect has been transformed by a series of discoveries that led to effective and safe systemic chemotherapy for several virus infections. The mechanisms of action and mode of application of some of the best known are covered in this chapter.

1.1 Achieving selective toxicity against human viruses

Although the potential toxicity of antiviral compounds remains important, over the last 2 decades the pre-scription of safe systemic antiviral chemotherapy has gradually come to be taken for granted. This revolution was largely brought about by the development of the nucleoside analogue, acyclovir (now to be known as aciclovir), which has become one of the world's best known medicines with more than 33 million patients treated (Darby 1995). Such is the confidence in its safety that it has been administered prophylactically for over 10 years to individuals, apparently without ill-effects, to suppress recurrences of genital herpes (Whitley and Gnann 1992, Tilson, Engle and Andrews 1993). The confidence generated by this one compound provides a completely new background to our current thinking about the devel-

opment of antiviral chemotherapy and the scope for future therapeutic strategies.

1.2 The importance of specific diagnosis and early therapy

Useful inhibitors are generally specific for one family of virus and, in some cases, to individual members of that family (e.g. particular members of the *Herpesviridae*). Initiating the appropriate therapy therefore depends on rapid and accurate diagnosis, and much tissue damage will sometimes be done before this has been achieved. For many acute respiratory infections with short incubation periods (e.g. those due to rhinoviruses) the small window of opportunity for intervention by chemotherapy following diagnosis is an important barrier to the development of new compounds. However, experience with aciclovir has demonstrated that therapy can be beneficial, even when the infection has progressed for several days, although, as we shall see, early therapy is of paramount importance in determining the outcome when treating herpes zoster, herpes simplex encephalitis and the complications of cytomegalovirus infection. In several virus infections, however, the slow development of clinical signs allows ample opportunity, following diagnosis, to benefit the patients including those with human immunodeficiency virus (HIV) causing AIDS, the hepatitis viruses and papilloma-virus infections

1.3 The importance of an intact immune system

Another widely held view at the outset of antiviral chemotherapy was that an intact immune system would be a prerequisite for clearing infection. Experience with several good virus inhibitors has shown that this is not necessarily true. Indeed, some of the most spectacular successes with antiviral chemotherapy or prophylaxis have been obtained using aciclovir in severely immunosuppressed patients suffering from herpesvirus infections (Meyers et al. 1982). A particular problem in such patients, however, is their tendency to develop infections resistant to antiviral therapy.

2 DISCOVERY AND ASSESSMENT OF NEW ANTIVIRAL COMPOUNDS

2.1 Molecular targets for inhibition

The obligate parasitic mode of viral replication determines that it shall pass through a series of stages common to all viruses: adsorption; entry; uncoating of the nucleic acid; expression of the genome; transcription and translation of proteins; replication of nucleic acids; assembly and release of mature progeny (Fig. 46.1).

So far, most, if not all, the useful inhibitors of viruses are targeted to one or another of these steps. The mechanism of action of many compounds in current use involves interference with nucleic acid metabolism; they include the many nucleoside analogues that inhibit herpesviruses and nucleoside and non-nucleoside analogues that interact with HIV reverse

transcriptase (reviewed by De Clercq 1992). Several compounds that inhibit influenza effect the disassembly of particles by blocking a virus protein complex that acts as an ion channel (Wang et al. 1993). Most viruses induce one or more proteases involved in processing virus polypeptides into functional components. The HIV protease was the first such enzyme to be targeted, and novel inhibitors of the proteases of many other viruses are now being developed (Mills 1993). Finally, a series of inhibitors of picornaviruses act by binding directly to the virion capsid, thus blocking the interaction between the virion and the receptor on the cell surface that facilitates its entry and disassembly (Rossmann 1990).

2.2 Drug discovery

SERENDIPITOUS DISCOVERY

In the early days, most new antiviral compounds were discovered by chance (often referred to as serendipity); indeed, several of the earliest antiviral compounds (e.g. idoxuridine) originated from cancer research where there was an interest in using nucleoside analogues to interfere with DNA synthesis and hence to inhibit the rapid division of tumour cells (Darby 1994).

RATIONAL DRUG DESIGN

With thorough understanding of the molecular basis of the replication of many important viruses, the avail-

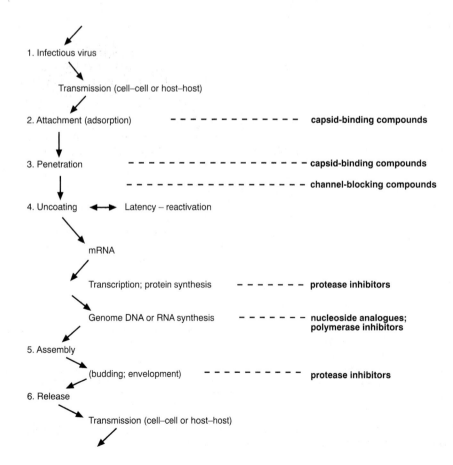

Fig. 46.1 Sites of action for several important classes of virus inhibitors. The sites at which the current successful antiviral compounds act are shown in the right hand column.

ability of the entire nucleotide sequences of their genomes and, in some cases, the 3-dimensional protein structure derived from x-ray diffraction analysis, compounds can be designed to interact with specific targets involved in the virus replication cycle. In practice, the most useful molecular targets are virus-induced enzymes which often have properties differing from those of counterpart enzymes induced by the host cell. The best known examples are thymidine kinase (TK) and DNA polymerase (DNApol) induced by some herpesviruses and reverse transcriptase and protease induced by retroviruses. Knowledge of such enzymes enables the establishment of biochemical screens to test many thousands of potential inhibitors and to develop structure–activity relationships. When the enzyme concerned can be crystallized and its 3-dimensional structure solved, the synthesis of appropriate molecules to interact with particular sites on that enzyme can be attempted. This approach is being pursued in relation to the picornavirus capsid-binding molecules, HIV reverse transcriptase, protease, and many other potential virus targets (Laver and Air 1990). Although the discovery of future antiviral compounds will rely heavily on these methods, the development of successful drugs still depends on finding molecules with the appropriate pharmacokinetic properties and lack of toxicity, and which can be synthesized cheaply in large quantities from available precursors; thus few new successful antiviral agents are likely to be developed.

2.3 Methods for detecting the inhibition of molecular targets directly

Virus enzyme screens

Viruses induce enzyme activities in the infected cells and there are now many examples of the assay of such enzymes in vitro and the screening of potential inhibitors for activity (Öberg 1983b). DNA and RNA polymerases have been the best-studied systems, particularly in herpes and retroviruses respectively. The herpesvirus TK was one of the earliest viral enzymes to be studied, because, as well as being a target for inhibition itself (Wright 1994), it is responsible for the phosphorylation of many nucleoside analogues that then become DNA polymerase inhibitors. In recent years the availability of the complete nucleotide sequences of a growing list of viruses has enabled identification of further enzymes and other proteins as specific targets for screening novel compounds.

Effective concentration (EC50) and toxic concentration

Antiviral compounds are usually assessed at an early stage for their ability to inhibit viral growth in tissue culture. The virus is generally titrated by means of cytopathic effect, plaque production or some other measure. The percentage reduction is usually plotted against the $\log_{10}$ of the drug concentration. The concentration of compound that reduces the titre of virus by 50% is measured and is usually expressed as the

effective dose 50 concentration (ED50), inhibitory concentration (IC50) or something similar (Fig. 46.2) (Newton and Field 1988).

Although the ED50 provides the most reproducible value, in some cases the ability to reduce virus yield by 90% (ED90) is regarded as a more realistic measurement and is sometimes quoted. When expressing results it is important to state the type of cell culture used for the test and the multiplicity of infection, because the species of origin, the tissue from which the cells are derived and whether the cells are resting or dividing can all influence the result. The multiplicity of infection may also be important: plaque reduction tests are necessarily conducted at low multiplicity but those based on reduction of cytopathic effect or virus yield may be carried out at different multiplicities and this can profoundly affect the result (Harmenberg, Wahren and Öberg 1980, Harmenberg et al. 1985).

A number of important human viruses that are targets for chemotherapy have yet to be grown in convenient tissue culture systems, which presents a major difficulty in the identification and early development of inhibitors. Examples are human papillomaviruses (Stanley 1993) and hepatitis C (Murphy 1993).

The quantification of viral toxicity is very much more difficult to assess in tissue culture and many methods have been employed (Dayan and Anderson 1988, Newton and Field 1988). They include effects on cell division; cell generation time over several rounds of replication (Field and Reading 1987); cell replication measured by thymidine uptake; cell volume; and various other more subjective measurements of cytopathic effect. Several assays employ vital dyes to assess cell viability and in these cases colorimetric apparatus can be used to automate the readings (McLaren, Ellis and Hunter 1983). Further tests have been devised to assess genetic damage (Evans 1983) and effects on DNA repair systems (Collins, Downes and Johnson 1984).

An important consideration for both toxicity and antiviral activity in cell culture is that cells from species

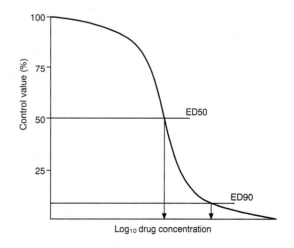

Fig. 46.2 Determination in cell culture of effective dose (ED50, ED90) for an inhibitor.

other than humans are often employed and may give different results (Harmenberg, Abele and Malm 1985). Furthermore, cells adapted for tissue culture may provide misleading data in comparison with those actually involved in the natural pathogenesis (Perno and Calio 1994). Experimental work with differentiated cells (e.g. human macrophages or neuroblastomas) or organ fragments (e.g. tracheal rings or ganglion explants) have been used in attempts to circumvent these difficulties. Although these methods can provide additional information the results may be difficult to interpret (reviewed by Field 1983).

Structure–activity relationships

Having established that a particular chemical inhibitor has a useful selective index against a particular virus or family of viruses, many closely related chemical analogues are synthesized, if possible. These are then screened for antiviral and toxic activity. It often emerges that particular features of the molecule are important and further modifications may be attempted in order to improve or refine the properties of the leading drug for further development. The analysis of such series led to the concept of structure–activity relationship (SAR) and this has been most important in the development of many new drugs. Examples of such series are the 5-substituted 2′-deoxyuridine inhibitors of herpesviruses (De Clercq et al. 1982) and the non-nucleoside reverse transcriptase inhibitors and peptidomimetic protease inhibitors of HIV (Roberts et al. 1990).

ANIMAL MODELS

Animal infection models were essential to the programme of development of all the major compounds in clinical use. This is less true of compounds active against HIV because there is a paucity of suitable models (Koch and Ruprecht 1992).

Infection models for herpes simplex dating back to the 1920s (Goodpasture and Teague 1923) have been developed in mice, rabbits and guinea-pigs. There is thus a very large amount of published information on the pathogenesis of experimental infections, which aids the interpretation of the different models and the extent to which the results can be extrapolated to humans (reviewed by Field and Brown 1989). Table 46.1 indicates some of the most important models for studying herpes simplex as a cause of labial, genital and ocular lesions, and of encephalitis and disease in the immunocompromised host. Such models have been used to provide further evidence of efficacy, to compare different compounds and to study therapeutic regimens. However, their particular strength is the ability to investigate complex features of pathogenesis and their interaction with potential inhibitors. For example, the effects of antiviral compounds on the establishment, maintenance and reactivation of latency are extremely difficult to study in humans (reviewed by Darby and Field 1984).

Many viruses, including other herpesviruses (e.g. human cytomegalovirus and varicella-zoster), have a restricted host range and cannot establish infections in laboratory animals comparable with those in humans. It is, however, sometimes possible to do so using a different member of the same family of viruses, for example murine cytomegalovirus (Sandford et al. 1985) and feline immunodeficiency virus (North et al. 1993). Clearly, the range of questions that may be asked of such models may be limited, but they can provide powerful systems for studying both the dynamics of drug resistance developing during therapy and countermeasures (e.g. the use of combinations or alternations of drugs).

Animals also play a vital role in the study of toxicity, and a number of statutory tests, both short- and long-term, are carried out in several species in attempts to evaluate the risks of side effects before new compounds enter clinical trials.

Selective index and therapeutic index

The ratio of the 50% toxic concentration to the 50% virus inhibitory concentration for the compound is often termed the **selective index**. When this is close to unity, the compound is generally taken to be toxic and is very unlikely to become useful. Conversely, a high selective toxicity index suggests a potentially useful compound. It should be stressed, however, that this ratio can be extremely misleading. For example, trifluorothymidine (Kaufman and Heidelberger 1964) has a selective index close to unity yet has been licensed as a topical agent against ocular herpes simplex, for which it has enjoyed some success (Kaufman 1979). There are, of course, many compounds with high selective indices in vitro that demonstrate toxicity only when tested in vivo. Thus, when possible, compounds are tested in animals infected with the target virus itself or a suitable relative for comparison. If inhibition of virus growth and of clinical signs are observed with doses that are tolerated by the host, an estimate of **therapeutic index** (the ratio of the toxic dose to the therapeutic dose) can be made (Field 1988a). This value is generally obtained in suitable animal models; it may remain theoretical for humans.

CLINICAL TRIALS

The evaluation of a potential antiviral drug in humans generally proceeds through several phases, numbered I to IV (Rees and Brigden 1988). Although the boundaries are not always exact, this terminology is widely employed.

Phase I studies

The evaluation begins with the administration of the drug to a limited number of healthy volunteers. It is normally given in small single doses at first, increasing by stages to multiple doses in an attempt to mimic the probable clinical use of the compound. During these studies the pharmacokinetics, pharmacology and metabolism of the compound are closely monitored. If these results are favourable the investigation may proceed to studies on virus-infected patients.

Table 46.1   Examples of the many animal models used to study and evaluate inhibitors of herpes simplex virus

Type of disease	Animal species	Route of inoculation
Orofacial herpes	Guinea-pig	Flank
	Mouse	Ear pinna
		Flank
		Lip
		Foot pad
	Hairless mouse	Flank
	Nude mouse/human skin	
Genital herpes	Guinea-pig (female)	Vagina
Ocular herpes	Rabbit	Cornea
	Mouse	Cornea
Herpes encephalitis	Mouse	Nares
		Vagina
		Cerebrum
		Tail vein
		Peripheral nerve (sciatic)
		Peritoneal cavity
	Rabbit	Olfactory bulb
Disease in immunocompromised host	Mouse (x-irradiated, cyclosporin-treated; nude etc.)	Various routes

Phase II studies

The compound is administered to diseased patients, and data similar to those in phase I are obtained. This is important because the metabolism of the drug in disease may differ from that in healthy subjects. Phase II studies are often open, uncontrolled investigations in limited numbers of patients (<100) and offer little opportunity for estimation of clinical efficacy. One should be wary of claims of therapeutic benefit derived from such studies.

Phase III studies

In this type of study the drug is usually compared against placebo or existing therapies. The main aim is to establish the therapeutic spectrum of the drug and the benefits to be gained from therapy compared with the risks associated with its use (the risk/benefit ratio). These studies require 100–1000 patients.

Phase IV studies

These are generally defined as investigations conducted after obtaining marketing approval. Phase IV studies increase experience of treating patients and provide more information about safety and efficacy. Different formulations, dosages, durations of therapy, drug interactions and comparisons or combinations with other drugs may be evaluated and special problems such as the selection of drug-resistant mutants detected.

There are many reports of antiviral compounds that demonstrate good selective indices against particular viruses in cell culture and, in some cases, high therapeutic indices in animal models. Most of these compounds, however, lack the pharmacokinetic properties appropriate for use in humans and only a minority have proved clinically useful.

In practice, most compounds described during the preclinical investigation as active in enzyme screens, cell culture and animal models fail to pass through all the phases of clinical studies and many are withdrawn during these evaluations. Nevertheless, for severe and life-threatening diseases, the degree of toxicity allowed to certain compounds may be quite high. They include zidovudine for treating HIV infections and ganciclovir for treating cytomegalovirus in immuno-suppressed patients.

The remainder of this chapter is confined to the relatively small group of compounds that are currently used for chemotherapy of virus infections or are likely to become clinically useful in the near future.

3   MECHANISM OF ACTION OF IMPORTANT ANTIVIRAL COMPOUNDS

Of the innumerable compounds known to inhibit one or other of the viruses, only very few have proved useful for treating human infections. The compounds that have been licensed for use in one or more indications were dominated by those for use against herpesviruses, especially herpes simplex, although recently this emphasis has given way to the many new therapies for patients infected with HIV and suffering from AIDS.

3.1   Inhibitors of herpesviruses

Herpes simplex virus offered one of the most attractive targets for chemotherapy, and thousands of compounds have been discovered that inhibit it selectively. The infections are extremely common and lesions are prone to recur. The clinical signs are very characteristic, and specific diagnosis (including self-diagnosis) is possible and can often be made when prodromal symptoms appear (Griffiths 1995). Mucocutaneous and ocular lesions offer the possibility of topical application. Finally, the lesions are almost always self-limiting; in some cases this makes it difficult to prove a clinical benefit or, indeed, a lack of benefit.

ACYCLOVIR; ACICLOVIR; A PARADIGM FOR SELECTIVE TOXICITY

Acyclovir (first published under the name acycloguanosine and now as aciclovir, ACV) is a nucleoside analogue structurally related to the natural nucleoside guanosine (Fig. 46.3) (Elion et al. 1977, Schaeffer et al. 1978, reviewed by Elion 1993). To become active, the nucleoside must be converted by 3 phosphorylation steps to ACV mono-, di- and then triphosphate (Fig. 46.4) (Fyfe et al. 1978).

ACV is a poor substrate for cellular enzymes, and uninfected human cells convert very little ACV to its triphosphate (ACV-TP). In contrast, the herpes simplex virus-induced enzyme thymidine kinase (TK) can, albeit with relatively low efficiency, convert ACV to ACV monophosphate (ACV-MP). Thus the herpes simplex virus TK recognizes ACV as thymidine but the fact that cellular enzymes convert ACV monophosphate (ACV-MP) successively to the di- and triphosphate only within virus-infected cells accounts for the

extremely high selective index of the compound (Darby 1995). ACV-TP enters the cellular nucleotide pool where it competes with guanosine triphosphate as a substrate for herpes simplex DNA polymerase. It is a particularly potent inhibitor of herpes simplex virus DNA polymerase (the inhibition constant, K_i, versus the natural substrate, deoxyguanosine, is c. 0.01 μM) and this appears to provide further selectivity, because cellular DNA polymerases are much less sensitive to inhibition. As the ACV residue is linked to the growing chain of virus DNA, it forms a chain terminator since there is no 3′-OH group on the ACV sugar moiety to link to the next residue in the growing chain of virus DNA (Fig. 46.5) (Furman et al. 1979). ACV may thus be described as an obligate chain terminator.

In summary, ACV is taken up only by herpes simplex virus-infected cells and strongly inhibits virus DNA synthesis, thus preventing the production and release of infectious virus progeny.

Clinically, ACV is licensed world-wide in topical, oral and intravenous formulations. Generally, the drug is effective when given systemically for primary and recurrent genital herpes simplex virus infections (Bryson et al. 1983, Mertz et al. 1984, Goldberg et al. 1993), mucocutaneous herpes simplex in immunocompromised hosts and life-threatening infections, e.g. encephalitis and neonatal disease (Whitley et al. 1986, 1991). It is also an effective therapy for chickenpox (Balfour et al. 1990, Dunkle et al. 1991, Wallace

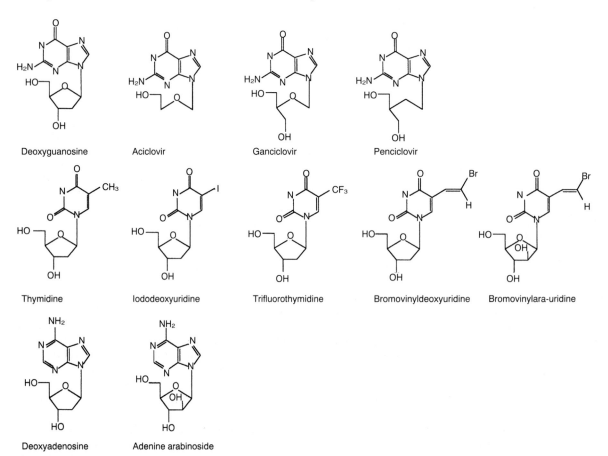

Deoxyguanosine   Aciclovir   Ganciclovir   Penciclovir

Thymidine   Iododeoxyuridine   Trifluorothymidine   Bromovinyldeoxyuridine   Bromovinylara-uridine

Deoxyadenosine   Adenine arabinoside

Fig. 46.3 Nucleoside analogues related to the natural nucleosides: deoxyguanosine, thymidine and deoxyadenosine.

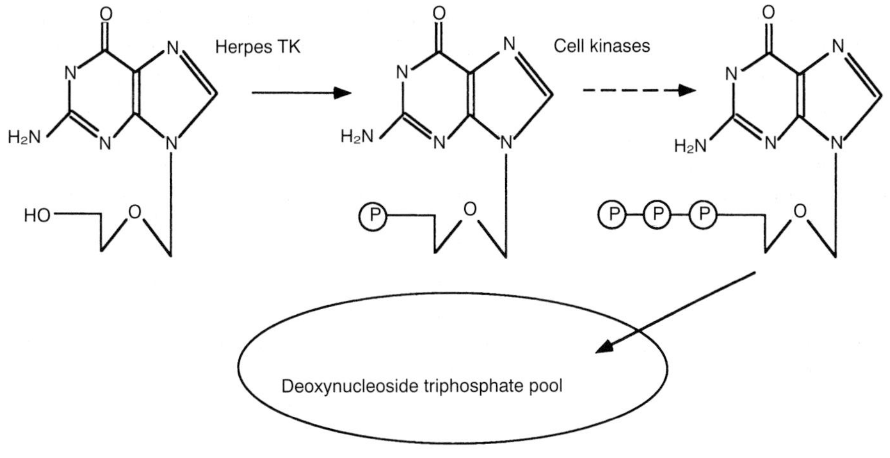

Fig. 46.4 The mechanism of action of aciclovir: activation.

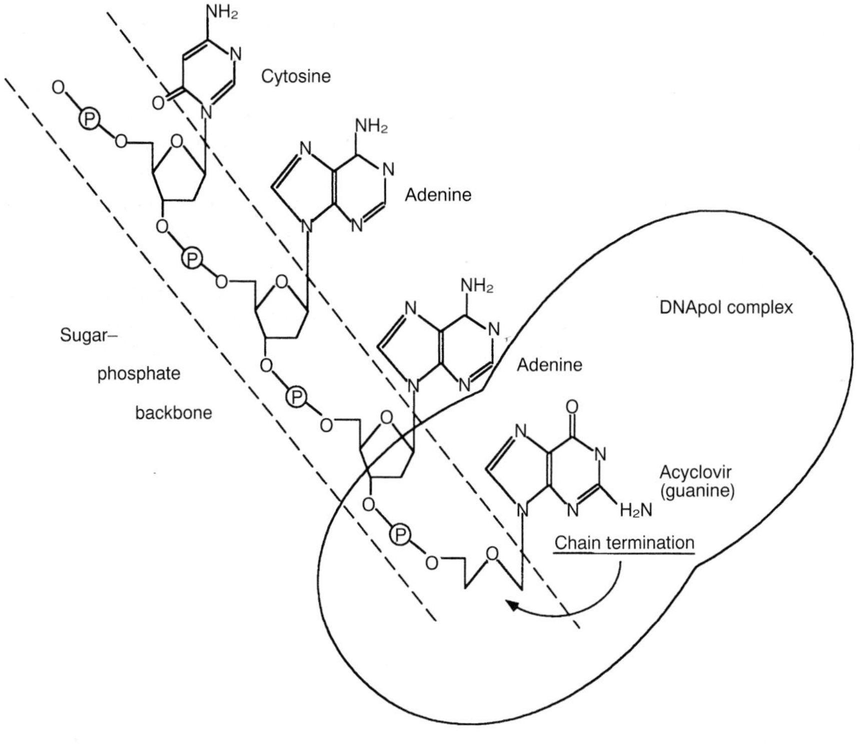

Fig. 46.5 The mechanism of action of aciclovir: inhibition of DNA synthesis and chain termination.

et al. 1992) and herpes zoster in normal (Crooks, Jones and Fiddian 1991) and immunocompromised hosts (Griffiths 1995).

NUCLEOSIDE ANALOGUES RELATED TO ACICLOVIR

Following the discovery and development of ACV, many other nucleoside analogues with similar modes of action were described. Some have high selective indices similar to or higher than that of ACV and several have been developed for clinical use. Each new compound, even those with close structural similarities with ACV (e.g. ganciclovir and penciclovir), has individual properties that differ from those of ACV, although the differences may be very subtle (Darby 1995). It is most important that this is kept in mind when comparing the antiviral efficacy and potential toxicity of such compounds with those of ACV.

Ganciclovir

Figure 46.3 shows that ganciclovir (GCV) is closely similar to ACV, with an additional carbon atom in the sugar moiety and the presence of a 3′-OH group (Smee et al. 1983). The compound therefore differs from ACV in that further extension of the DNA chain is possible after incorporation of GCV-TP. Although the compound shows significant toxicity in humans, its spectrum of action is wider than that of ACV and includes human cytomegalovirus (Freitas et al. 1985, Matthews and Boehme 1988). Unlike herpes simplex virus, human cytomegalovirus does not encode a TK. Studies of viruses with acquired resistance to GCV have, however, revealed that a previously unsuspected virus enzyme is responsible for the metabolic conversion from GCV to GCV-MP (Litter, Stuart and Chee 1992, Sullivan et al. 1992). The enzyme is a product of cytomegalovirus gene *UL97*, a discovery that focused attention on this gene which codes for a protein with close homology to several eukaryotic protein kinases. Once formed in the cytomegalovirus-infected cells, GCV-TP inhibits cytomegalovirus DNA polymerase and virus replication is prevented.

Clinical use of GCV has focused on patients at high risk for cytomegalovirus disease (Fan-Harvard, Nahata and Brady 1989, Levinson and Jacobson 1992). Thus, individuals with AIDS benefit from GCV therapy of retinitis and gastrointestinal disease. Oral administration of GCV delays onset of end-organ disease in patients with AIDS who have CD4 counts $<200/\mu l$. Similarly, GCV delays the onset of cytomegalovirus disease in organ transplant recipients. Poor bioavailability and the problem of toxicity limit the value of the compound.

Penciclovir

Penciclovir (PCV) is another nucleoside analogue in which the base, guanine, is normal but the sugar moiety has a structural modification (Boyd et al. 1987). The structural similarity to ACV is apparent (see Fig. 46.3); there is, however, no oxygen atom in the acyclic 'sugar' moiety although an OH group exists in the position equivalent to that of the $3'$-OH group in the normal nucleoside, guanosine. Like ACV, PCV is converted to its monophosphate by the herpes simplex virus or varicella-zoster virus TK (Vere Hodge and Cheng 1993), and PCV-TP inhibits the viral DNA polymerase but with the possibility of internal incorporation of PVC residues into viral DNA and further chain extension (Vere Hodge and Perkins 1989). The initial conversion of PVC to its monophosphate is more efficient than the phosphorylation of ACV, but the PCV-TP formed in infected cells is less active than ACV-TP as an inhibitor of herpes simplex virus DNA polymerase (Table 46.2) (Earnshaw, Bacon and Darlison 1992).

The triphosphate of PCV has a significantly longer intracellular half-life than ACV-TP (Vere Hodge and Perkins 1989). Although the full implications of this observation have yet to be elucidated, it does seem that the compound may have more long-lasting inhibitory effects in infected tissues; this supposition is supported by tests in animals that compared FCV and VACV (Sutton and Kern 1993, Field et al. 1995). It remains to be seen whether this biochemical feature will translate into clinical benefit in humans. Although the compound seems to have a very high selective index, the bioavailability is poor and the drug chosen initially for clinical development is a prodrug of PCV termed famciclovir.

It has become clear that, as well as good activity against members of the *Herpesviridae*, PCV is also highly active against hepatitis virus B (Boker et al. 1994, Locarnini et al. 1994). Thus far, no mechanism of action for this unexpected activity has been reported; it is, however, likely to involve specific inhibition of the hepatitis B virus-induced DNA polymerase although there is no explanation as yet for the phosphorylation of PCV in the infected hepatocytes.

Brivudin; bromovinyl deoxyuridine

Historically, brivudin, or bromovinyl deoxyuridine (BVDU), was discovered at about the same time as ACV (De Clercq et al. 1979) and, in vitro, appeared to be even more active than ACV against herpes simplex type 1 (De Clercq et al. 1980). In the event the drug proved less useful than was hoped. It is much more closely related to the natural substrate for TK (i.e. thymidine) and the modification is the bromovinyl group in the 5 position of the pyrimidine ring (see Fig. 46.3). The mechanism of action resembles that of ACV except that the conversion of BVDU-MP to BVDU-DP seems also to be achieved by the herpes simplex virus TK (Descamps et al. 1982). The virus (but not cellular) TK thus possesses a thymidylate kinase activity. BVDU is significantly less active against herpes simplex type 2, probably because of the lack of conversion of the monophosphate to the diphosphate by the herpes simplex virus type 2 TK (De Clercq et al. 1981). A limitation of the compound in vivo is attack by phosphorylases that convert BVDU to bromovinyl ara-uracil, which is inactive. This, and concern about toxicity, has limited the development of the compound for clinical use; even so, the principles discovered during the development of this drug and SAR studies have led to several compounds (e.g. bromovinyl ara-uridine) that seem more promising.

Sorivudine; bromovinylarabinosyl-uracil; brovavir

The mechanism of action of sorivudine, or bromovinylarabinosyl-uracil (BVaraU) (see Fig. 46.3), seems similar to that of BVDU (Yokota et al. 1989, Machida 1990); its spectrum of action is, however, different and it seems to be some 2000-fold more active than ACV or BVDU against varicella-zoster virus repli-

Table 46.2 Comparison of key biochemical properties of the guanosine analogues aciclovir and penciclovir which are produced in vivo by their respective prodrugs, valaciclovir and famciclovir

	Famciclovir	**Valaciclovir**
	Oral absorption and blood pharmacokinetics of **PCV** and **ACV** are similar	
	Penciclovir	Aciclovir
HSV1 thymidine kinase	High affinity (K_i = **1.5** μM)	Low affinity (K_i = 173 μM)
HSV1 DNA polymerase	Low affinity (K_i = 8.5 μM)	High affinity (K_i = **0.07** μM)
Stability of triphosphate	Long ($t_{1/2}$ = **10** h)	Short ($t_{1/2}$ = 0.7 h)
DNA chain terminating	Rapid	Obligate

cation in cell culture (ED50 = 0.001 μM, compared with 14 μM for ACV) (Machida and Nishitani 1990). Like BVDU, however, the compound is poorly active against herpes simplex type 2. It is an extremely good substrate for varicella-zoster TK and its antiviral activity is attributed to the inhibition by BVaraU-TP of varicella-zoster DNA polymerase; the compound is thought not to be incorporated into virus DNA. Unfortunately, one of the metabolites is bromovinylarabinosyl-uracil (BVU), a potent inhibitor of dihydrothymine dehydrogenase which is responsible for degrading drugs such as 5-fluorouracil that are used in cancer chemotherapy. Although this interaction was predicted, a number of deaths have occurred as a result of co-administration of the 2 drugs (Meeting Report 1995) (see section 4.2, p. 1005). As a consequence, the compound will not be licensed in the USA.

VIDARABINE; ADENINE ARABINOSIDE

Vidarabine, or adenine arabinoside (AraA), was an important landmark in the development of antiviral chemotherapy (Schabel 1968), being among the early compounds that achieved proven clinical benefit with relatively little acute toxicity, particularly in the systemic treatment of severe herpes simplex infections (Whitley et al. 1977). The compound is a close analogue of adenine except that the OH group in the 2′ position on the 'sugar' moiety is in the unnatural 'arabinosyl' configuration (see Fig. 46.3). The nucleotides formed from the phosphorylation of AraA have the potential to interfere with many different steps in the metabolism of DNA and its precursors, for example blocking of S-adenosyl homocysteine hydrolase (Hersfield 1979). The relative importance of these effects is unknown but, as with the other nucleoside analogues, the primary target for AraA-TP seems to be the herpes simplex virus-induced DNA polymerase. The compound has low toxicity and may be used systemically, but its poor solubility necessitates the intravenous administration of large quantities of fluids. Secondly, its activity in vivo is limited by rapid deamination of AraA by adenosine deaminase, yielding arabinosyl-hypoxanthine which has no antiviral activity (Whitley et al. 1980a). Attempts to circumvent this problem by the administration of AraA-MP have enjoyed little success (Whitley et al. 1980b). Today, vidarabine has largely been replaced in the physician's armoury for systemic therapy by more active and less toxic medication.

IDOXURIDINE

The pyrimidine analogue, idoxuridine (IDU), was one of the first specific antiviral compounds to be discovered (Prusoff 1959) and is the best known example of the 5-substituted 2′-deoxyuridine analogue series (see Fig. 46.3); it is thus similar to BVDU. However, IDU does not possess the high selectivity associated with the more modern drugs. This 'first generation' nucleoside analogue is readily phosphorylated by cellular enzymes and thus can be converted to the active nucleotide in normal, as well as in virus-

infected, cells although the conversion is much more efficient in the latter. The IDU-TP inhibits viral (and cellular) DNA synthesis, but a major part of the antiviral action may be due to incorporation of the analogue into viral nucleic acids and subsequent perturbation of virus gene expression (De Clercq 1982). The exact mechanism of action is unknown but some selectivity is assumed to result from the comparatively greater accumulation of IDU-TP in infected cells. IDU is, however, severely toxic upon systemic administration and is useful only as a topical agent, for which it continues to be useful both for herpes zoster and herpes simplex virus keratitis. Skin penetration is a problem for topical administration and, in an attempt to overcome this obstacle, formulations have been prepared in dimethyl sulphoxide (DMSO) for treating zoster (Dawber 1974; reviewed by Spruance 1994). Notwithstanding its traditional use for treating herpes simplex virus in humans, the potential long-term genetic toxicity of this compound remains a major concern.

TRIFLURIDINE; TRIFLUOROTHYMIDINE

Like IDU, trifluridine, or trifluorothymidine (TFT) (see Fig. 46.3), synthesized in 1964 (Heidelberger, Parsons and Remy 1964), is also highly toxic and is unsuitable for systemic use. Even to demonstrate its selective antiviral effect in cell culture requires the use of cells lacking TK that are resistant to its toxic effects (Field, McMillan and Darby 1981). However, the compound is very soluble and has found a particular use in the topical treatment of ocular infections (Wellings et al. 1972). The very rapid hydrolysis of TFT to harmless metabolites probably accounts for the lack of toxicity in this application (Dexter et al. 1972). It is the treatment of choice for herpes simplex keratoconjunctivitis (reviewed by Bigar 1979). The compound is reported to be effective against drug-resistant strains and remains in the armoury of antiherpes drugs despite its toxicity in vitro.

NUCLEOSIDE ANALOGUE PRODRUGS

An important limitation of many nucleoside analogues is their poor bioavailability following oral administration. The development of orally bioavailable compounds that are converted in vivo to yield the relevant nucleoside analogues thus represents a major advance. A similar strategy is being explored for many compounds, but the first 2 drugs of this type to be licensed for use in humans are derived from ACV and PCV.

Valaciclovir

Valaciclovir (VACV) is the L-valyl ester of aciclovir (Fig. 46.6) which, following oral administration, is cleaved in the gut and liver by an enzyme referred to as valaciclovir hydrolase to yield ACV and the natural amino acid L-valine, little VACV being detected in plasma (Beauchamp et al. 1992). Multiple oral doses of VACV (>1 g 4 times daily) result in plasma ACV concentrations similar to those achieved with intravenous ACV (5 or 10 mg/kg 3 times daily) but without the sharp peak concentrations (Carrington 1994, Crooks 1995). Once formed and distributed to the infected tissues, the mode of action is, of course, identical to that of simple ACV. This compound offers a formulation that is more convenient to administer for the treatment of herpes zoster than ACV (Murray 1995).

Famciclovir

The concept that led to VACV also resulted in famciclovir (FCV) (Vere Hodge et al. 1989), the diacetyl ester of 6-deoxy-penciclovir (Fig. 46.6). In this case 2 enzymes are involved, first in removing one ester preferentially, then the second, followed by oxidation by aldehyde oxidase to yield PCV (Vere Hodge 1993). The only degradation products from this reaction are harmless carboxylic acid and PCV and, as with VACV, little FCV is detected in plasma. Ease of administration provides a distinct advantage over ACV in the treatment of herpes zoster (Carrington 1994).

NUCLEOTIDE ANALOGUES

A series of acyclic purine nucleoside phosphonates was first described in 1986 (De Clercq et al. 1986). Several of the compounds showed a wide spectrum of activity against viruses, including both DNA and RNA viruses. Unlike the natural nucleotides, the acyclic nucleotide phosphonates resist phosphorolytic cleavage by cellular esterases and are, as such, taken up by the cells intact. Several compounds in this series seem to have potential as future antiviral drugs; one of the most promising examples is the next to be described.

Cidofir; hydroxyphosphonylmethoxycytosine

Unlike the nucleoside analogues described above, cidofovir, or hydroxyphosphonylmethoxycytosine (HPMPC) (Fig. 46.7), does not require specific conversion to the monophosphate to initiate its inhibitory effects. Although the mechanism of action has not been completely elucidated, it seems that the crucial target is again the virus-specific DNA polymerase (Votruba et al. 1987). HPMPC has another particularly important feature, viz. a very long tissue half-life; it has been shown in many animal models that long intervals between doses can be allowed without loss of antiviral effect. Thus, as little as one dose per week has been employed in humans with apparent success (Snoeck et al. 1993). The compound suffers from toxic side effects, particularly a nephrotoxicity, although this can be minimized by co-administration of the drug probenecid (which competitively inhibits the transport of drugs through the glomeruli) and intravenous hydration. HPMPC has been used to combat sight-threatening cytomegalovirus retinitis in AIDS patients.

PYROPHOSPHATE ANALOGUES

A series of compounds has been known for many years whose members interact directly with herpesvirus DNA polymerase at the pyrophosphate binding site. This was first shown with phosphonacetic acid (Purifoy, Lewis and Powell 1977). In the event this was not a useful drug, but the closely related compound phosphonoformate (Fig. 46.7) has been developed for use in humans (reviewed by Öberg 1983a).

Foscarnet; phosphonoformic acid

Forscarnet, or phosphonoformate (PFA), seems to have a relatively simple mode of action, being a direct inhibitor of herpes simplex DNA polymerase (Leinback et al. 1976). The compound suffers from some toxic features, and its tendency to accumulate in bone (Crisp and Clissold 1991) is of particular concern. It does, however, offer an alternative strategy for treating both infections with ACV-resistant strains of herpes simplex and cytomegalovirus retinitis in AIDS patients (Fanning et al. 1990).

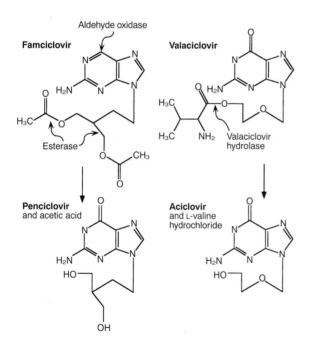

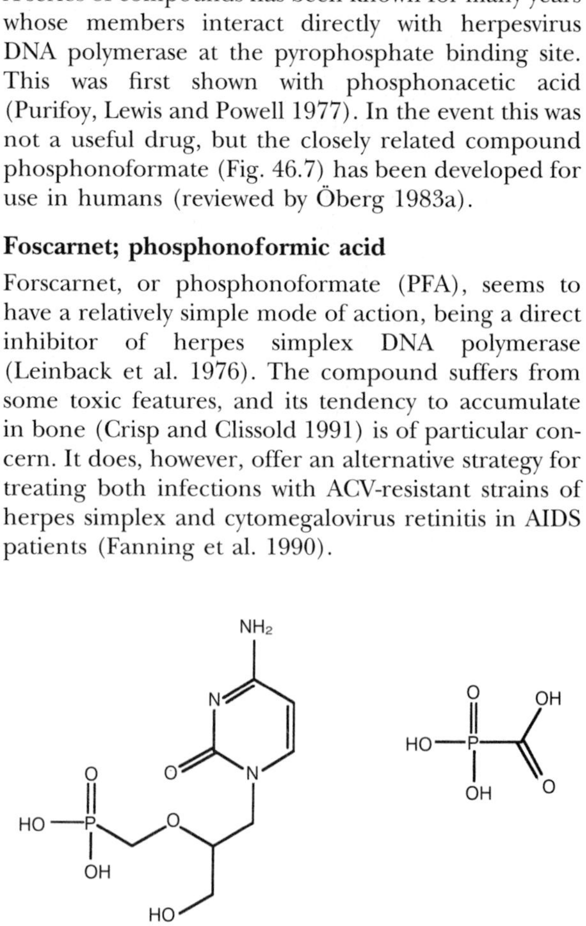

Fig. 46.6 The nucleoside analogue prodrugs famciclovir and valaciclovir showing their conversion to the active metabolites, penciclovir and aciclovir respectively.

Fig. 46.7 Two effective inhibitors of herpesvirus DNA polymerase: a member of the phosphonyl group, HPMPA, and a pyrophosphate analogue, foscarnet.

3.2 Inhibitors of human immunodeficiency virus

REVERSE TRANSCRIPTASE INHIBITORS

The emergence of HIV as a major pathogen resulted in an unprecedented effort to develop new antiviral agents. The earliest compounds to enjoy limited therapeutic success were all nucleoside analogues; the first to be widely prescribed was 3'-azido-3'-deoxythymidine (azidothymidine).

Zidovudine; azidothymidine

Zidovudine, or azidothymidine (AZT), is a close analogue of thymidine (Fig. 46.8) (Mitsuya et al. 1985) and is readily phosphorylated in actively dividing cells. The drug is initially phosphorylated by cellular TK, the rate-limiting step being its conversion to the diphosphate by cellular thymidylate kinase. AZT-TP competitively inhibits HIV reverse transcriptase with respect to thymidine triphosphate (TTP) and, because the 3'-azido group prevents the formation of 5',3'-phosphodiester linkages, AZT-TP acts as a chain terminator of DNA synthesis (Darby 1995). The compound, via its metabolites, also inhibits a variety of cellular enzymes, including DNA-polymerase-γ, which undoubtedly contributes to the range of toxic effects associated with prolonged clinical use of the drug (Fischl et al. 1987). It was the first drug to be used against HIV, and is still accepted as conferring at least transient benefit.

Stavudine; didehydrodideoxyuridine

Stavudine, or 2',3'-didehydro-2'-deoxythymidine (D4T), is similar to AZT in that it is a thymidine nucleoside analogue (Fig. 46.8) (Baba et al. 1987). It readily enters cells but, in contrast to AZT, the rate-limiting step is the initial phosphorylation by cellular TK. Once formed, D4T-TP is rapidly converted to the di- and triphosphate derivatives. The mechanism of action at the level of reverse transcriptase seems to be similar to that of AZT (reviewed by Hitchcock 1991); toxicity in the form of peripheral neuropathy is, however, more common. The clinical use of D4T is increasing world-wide.

Didanosine; dideoxyinosine

Didanosine, or 2',3'-dideoxyinosine (DDI), is a purine nucleoside analogue (Fig. 46.8) (Mitsuya and Broder 1986) which is taken up intracellularly and converted by 5' nucleotidase to DDI-MP and further metabolized by cellular enzymes to DDA-TP, which has a prolonged intracellular half-life (8–24 h). Again, the molecular target for the drug action is the HIV reverse transcriptase (reviewed by McClaren et al. 1991). Clinical trials have been conducted in AIDS patients (Darbyshire and Aboulker 1992, Kahn et al. 1992) but the clinical use of DDI has been limited by its oral formulation which may cause gastrointestinal discomfort.

Zalcitabine; dideoxycytidine

Zalcitabine, or 2',3'-dideoxycytidine (DDC) (Fig. 46.8), is active against HIV-1 and 2 and against some strains that are resistant to AZT (Mitsuya and Broder 1986). The drug seems to be similar in potency to AZT (Bozzette et al. 1995).

Lamivudine; thiacytidine

Finally, in this series of nucleoside analogue inhibitors of reverse transcriptase, lamivudine, or 2'-deoxy-3'-thiacytidine (3TC) (Fig. 46.8), is synergistic with AZT in vitro and is active against HIV-resistant strains (Soudeyns et al. 1991). It seems to be relatively non-toxic but is less active than AZT in monotherapy. This drug is of particular interest for combination studies with AZT and a protease inhibitor. It should be noted that 3TC is also an active inhibitor of hepatitis B DNA polymerase in vitro (Doong et al. 1991) and against hepatitis B infection in vivo (Honkoop and de Man 1995).

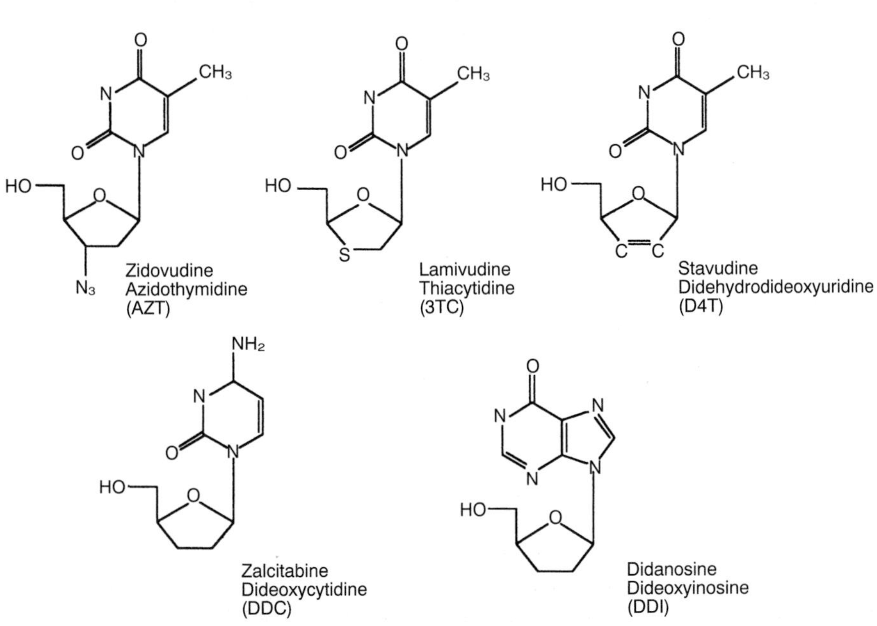

Fig. 46.8 Five nucleoside analogue inhibitors of HIV reverse transcriptase that are currently in use in humans, alone and in combination.

NON-NUCLEOSIDE REVERSE TRANSCRIPTASE INHIBITORS

The intensive screening of compounds for anti-HIV activity led to the discovery of several families of inhibitors that, although they differ from one another in structure, share the property of inhibiting reverse transcriptase by binding to sites other than that which normally interacts with the nucleosides. Some act at concentrations in the nanomolar range and are cytotoxic only at 10 000- to 100 000-fold higher concentrations. HIV-1 (but, notably, not HIV-2) reverse transcriptase is the target sensitive to inhibition. Enzyme studies, however, indicated that such compounds inhibit reverse transcriptase in a non-competitive fashion (De Clercq 1992). The site on the enzyme at which these compounds bind has been termed the TIBO site (Pauwels et al. 1990) and certain other compounds (e.g. HEPT, an acyclic uridine derivative) seem to interact with the same site (Baba et al. 1989) (TIBO and HEPT are discussed below). These compounds have been collectively described as allosteric inhibitors. The rapid selection of drug resistance seems to be a major limitation of the success of these compounds, which, however, are likely to have an important role when used in combination both with other non-reverse transcriptase inhibitors and with other classes of inhibitor.

TIBO, nevirapine and HEPT

A series of nucleoside inhibitors have been discovered that are tetrahydro-imidazo[4,5,1-jk][1,4]-benzodiazepin-2H(1H)-thione derivatives (Fig. 46.9) (Debyser et al. 1991). This almost unpronounceable name is usually shortened to TIBO. This benzodiazepine-like drug was the first of the non-nucleoside reverse transcriptase inhibitors to be identified (De Clercq 1992). Early trials showed a large but transient reduction in viral load. The drug is of relatively low toxicity but oral bioavailability is poor. Nevirapine is another non-competitive inhibitor of reverse transcriptase that interacts with tyrosine residues on the enzyme (Merluzzi et al. 1990) and yet another series of compounds of this general type, hydroxyethoxymethylphenylthiothymine derivatives, has been given the acronym HEPT (Miyasaka et al. 1989).

PROTEASE INHIBITORS

HIV encodes an enzyme that specifically cleaves protein precursors in the maturation of gag and pol polyproteins (Pearly and Taylor 1987). Inhibition of this enzyme results in the production of non-infectious virus (Kohl et al. 1988). This virus-induced enzyme has no known cellular function, but a number of highly specific inhibitors of HIV whose action is based on inhibition of the HIV protease have been reported (De Clercq 1995).

Saquinavir

This was the first active virus protease inhibitor to be described (Fig. 46.10). It is a peptide-based transition-state mimetic of an Asn.Phe.( )Pro. substrate sequence, in which ( ) indicates the cleavage site (Fig. 46.10) (Roberts et al. 1990).

Saquinavir is an extremely active inhibitor of HIV replication in cell culture, with a very high selective index. The drug has already advanced to phase III clinical studies and experience shows it to be well tolerated, although, as with other anti-HIV compounds, drug resistance does occur. Its pharmacokinetic properties are, however, not ideal for use in vivo and many alternative HIV protease inhibitors are currently under development (Roberts 1995). Furthermore, viruses of many other families encode proteases, including pathogens as diverse as polio, hepatitis C, influenza and herpes simplex viruses, against which a similar approach is being directed. The potential for these compounds to be valuable inhibitors seems to be great but their ultimate success in clinical use cannot yet be predicted.

3.3 Inhibitors of orthomyxo- and paramyxoviruses

AMANTADINE AND RIMANTADINE

The compound amantadine (Fig. 46.11) has long been known as a specific inhibitor of influenza virus A although influenza B and C are not affected. The mechanisms of action of amantadine, and subsequently of rimantadine which is very similar but with superior pharmacological properties (Hayden et al. 1981, 1985), have only been elucidated within the past few years (Hay 1992).

Following attachment to host cell plasma membrane receptors by means of the envelope glycoprotein spikes, or haemagglutinin (HA), influenza virus is taken up by cells into clathrin-coated pits. The virus, at this early stage of its replication cycle, is contained within lysosomes. Low pH within the lysosome results in conformational changes in the HA which exposes the amino-terminus region of the HA2; this region is hydrophobic and triggers a fusion between the endosomal membrane and the virus envelope, releasing the nucleocapsid into the cytoplasm of the

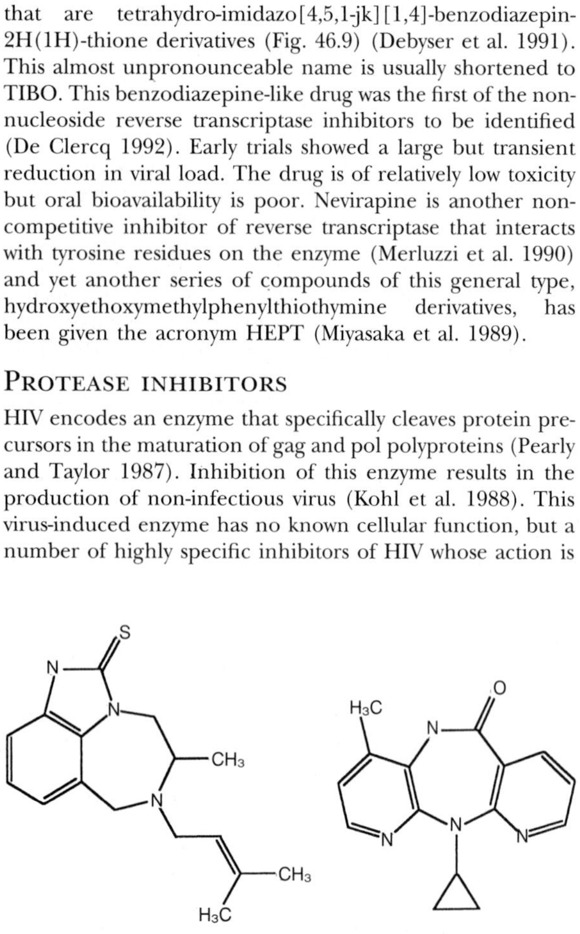

Fig. 46.9 Two non-nucleoside inhibitors of HIV reverse transcriptase that are in use in humans, alone or in combination.

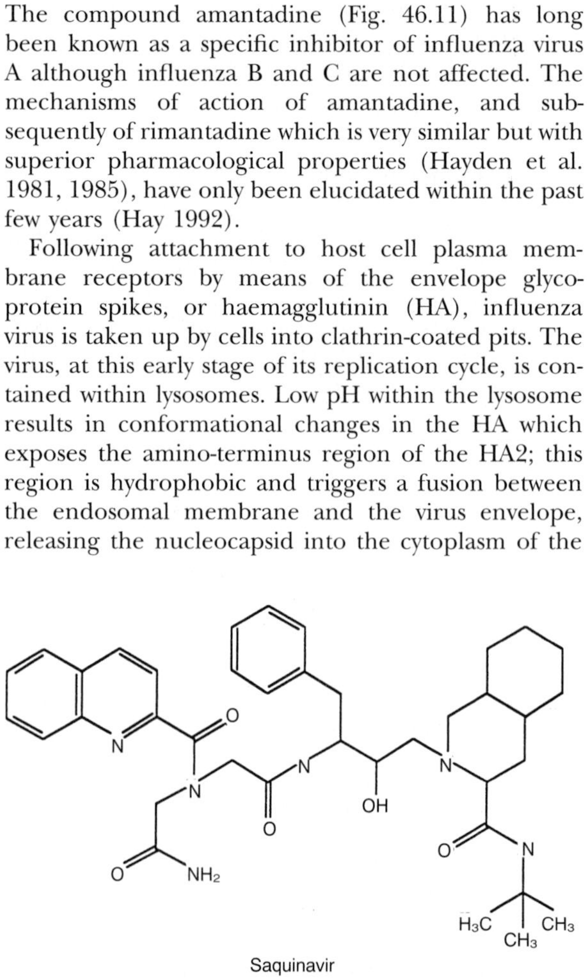

Fig. 46.10 The first peptide-mimetic HIV protease inhibitor to be tested in human trials.

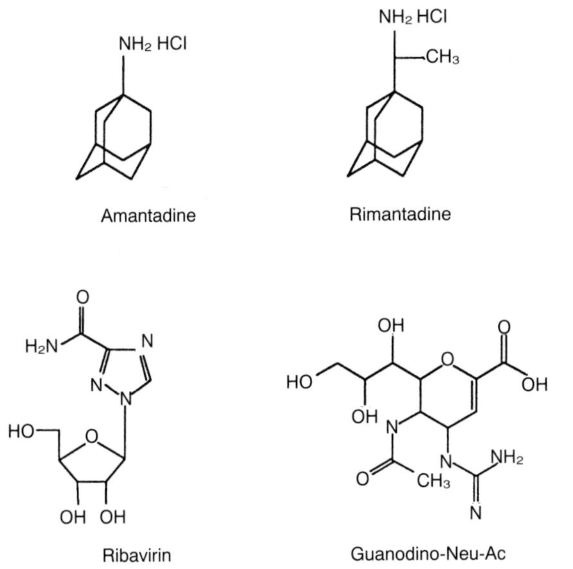

Fig. 46.11 Four compounds used for chemotherapy of influenza virus and (for ribavirin) of respiratory syncytial virus.

host cell. Originally, amantadine was thought to work simply by raising lysosomal pH, thereby interfering with the conformational change leading to virus fusion with membrane. It now appears that the process of inhibition is more subtle. The M2 protein in the nucleocapsid seems to form a polymeric tube-like structure which behaves as an ion channel through which protons pass. Amantadine and rimantadine seem to act by binding to M2, possibly being inserted into the channel itself, and thus interfering with the penetration of hydrogen ions into the virion; a process essential for uncoating the single-strand RNA genome (Wang et al. 1993). Resistant mutations map to the *M2* gene and such variants may ultimately limit the success of chemotherapy (Hayden 1994). Both amantadine and rimantadine have a basket-like hydrocarbon structure and further active compounds of this type are under study. The knowledge of how these compounds interact with the M2 proton channel should enable the rational design of further influenza inhibitors of this type.

4-Guanidino-Neu5Ac2en

The neuraminidase component of the of influenza virion functions by removing sialic (neuraminic) acid residues from virus glycoproteins and cell receptors – a process that seems to facilitate release and spread of virus budding from infected cells. Working from the crystallographic structure of the enzyme, inhibitors have been designed, and one of these, 4-guanodino-Neu5Ac2en (Fig. 46.11), has high binding affinity and specificity for the virus enzyme (von Itzstein et al. 1993). The compound is undergoing clinical trials, suggesting that it has promise for use against human influenza. Resistant variants (some of which contain mutations that map to HA) have been detected; their clinical significance is unknown.

Ribavirin

Ribavirin is an inhibitor of paramyxoviruses, particularly respiratory syncytial virus; its history has been controversial since its discovery was reported in 1972 (Sidwell et al. 1972). The compound is a guanosine analogue (Fig. 46.11); evidence has been obtained for at least 3 distinct modes of action and the important molecular targets have yet to be confirmed (reviewed by Sidwell et al. 1985). It is a structural analogue of guanosine and is converted successively to the mono-, di- and triphosphate derivatives by cellular enzymes. The inhibition of virus is not, however, reversed by adding guanosine, suggesting a more complicated mode of action (Gilbert and Knight 1986). The enzyme inosine monophosphate dehydrogenase is effectively inhibited in vitro by ribavirin monophosphate, with a resulting decrease in pool size of GTP. However, this is not thought to be the single inhibitory factor. It is of interest that ribavirin-resistant mutants have been very difficult, if not impossible, to isolate in the laboratory. This may be because the compound interferes with multiple virus targets; alternatively, there may be one or more important cellular effects that are not virus-specific. Clinically, aerosolized ribavirin has been reported to be efficacious for treating respiratory syncytial virus infection of infants (Sidwell et al. 1985); however, the results of more recent clinical trials cast doubt on the value of this agent (Wald, Dashefsky and Green 1988).

3.4 Inhibitors of picornaviruses

Pirodavir and WIN-54954

The *Picornaviridae* are among the smallest of the RNA viruses and cause a wide range of human and animal diseases. Among the *Picornaviridae* are the rhinoviruses, and those seeking to develop antiviral chemotherapy are often reproached with failure to 'cure the common cold'. A steadily increasing number of compounds have been reported as potent inhibitors of rhinoviruses; they comprise an assorted collection that fall into one of 2 classes, with different antiviral targets. The first class (non-capsid binding) includes compounds such as enviroxime (Fig. 46.12) (De Long 1984). Compounds of this type seem to act shortly after uncoating, inhibiting the formation of the virus RNA-dependent RNA polymerase complex.

The second class of compounds (capsid binding) has a quite different target of inhibition. Picornaviruses possess a capsid comprising 3 types of protein subunit (VP1, VP2 and VP3) assembled into an icosahedral shell. The virions are not enveloped and therefore rely on receptor sites on their protein shell to engage and dock on to protein receptor molecules in the plasma membrane of the host cell. X-ray crystallographic studies revealed that attachment of the virus is mediated by a canyon-shaped receptor site which encircles each of the 12 pentameric vertices of the icosahedral capsid. It has also been shown that certain inhibitory compounds, e.g. pirodavir and WIN-54954, work by binding into a hydrophobic pocket (the 'win pocket') situated in VP1 beneath the canyon floor (Fig. 46.13) (Rossmann 1990). It is suggested that this pocket forms a natural molecular hinge in the protein which may give flexibility to the molecule during disassembly and assembly of the icosahedral structure required when uncoating, and again during production of

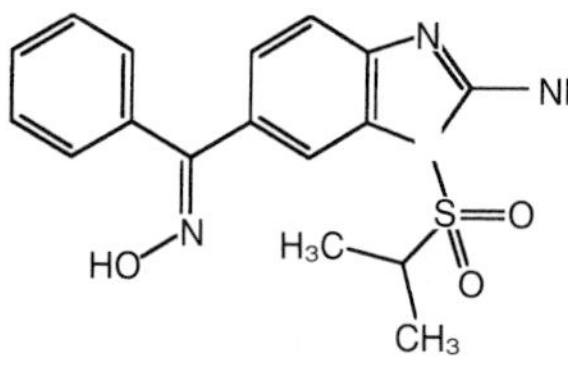

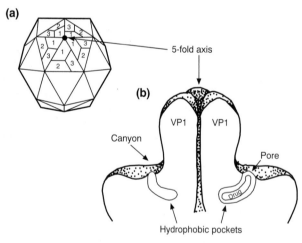

Enviroxime

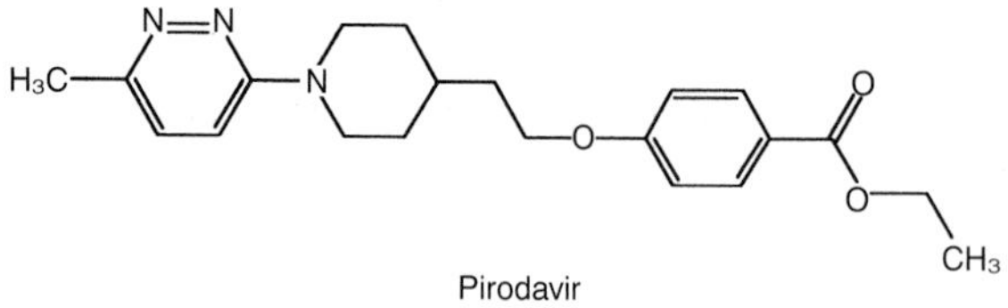

Pirodavir

Fig. 46.12 Two examples of compounds that have been tested against rhinovirus infection in humans.

new virus particles. When the inhibitor is bound into the pocket it may have 2 effects. First it can interfere with virus attachment to the cell receptor. Secondly, and more important, it may interfere with uncoating (Woods et al. 1989, Andries et al. 1992).

3.5 Other virus targets and future prospects

HEPATITIS VIRUSES

Among the hepatitis viruses, hepatitis B and C have

attracted particular attention as targets of antiviral therapy. These viruses establish chronic infections and are associated with both cirrhosis and hepatic carcinoma. Leucocyte and lymphoblastoid interferons, of both human and recombinant origin, have been reported as effective in decreasing viral replication in patients (Hoofnagle 1994). The best clinical results have been obtained with α interferons, but relapse often occurs when medication is discontinued. However, interferon is not effective for treating perinatally acquired hepatitis B infections. Treatment with nucleoside analogues (e.g. fialuridine, ribavirin, lamivudine and famiciclovir) has also been investigated (Honkoop and de Man 1995). Because of the worldwide burden of disease, these viruses are ideal candidates for new therapies.

PAPILLOMAVIRUSES

Human papillomavirus infections most often cause genital warts or juvenile laryngeal papillomatosis, and interferons have been extensively evaluated for treating such infections (see Chapter 16) The local (intralesional) therapy of genital warts refractory to cytodestructive therapy is effective. The association between genital warts and cervical carcinomas provides further impetus for the development of antiviral agents to treat diseases associated with these viruses. Recently there has been much interest in a new compound, 1-(2-methylpropyl)-1H-imidazo[4,5-C]quinolin-4-amine), given the generic name imiquimod (Fig. 46.14) (Miller et al. 1995). The activity seems to result from interferon-α induction and, if so, would place this compound among the immunomodulators, which are in general beyond the scope of this chapter.

4 PROBLEMS IN ANTIVIRAL CHEMOTHERAPY

4.1 Viral evolution and resistance

Drug resistance in viruses generally implies the emergence of strains for which the ED50 significantly

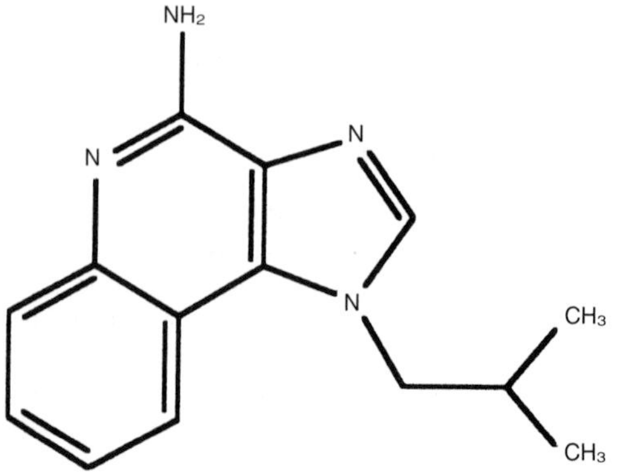

(a)

5-fold axis

(b)

VP1   VP1

Canyon

Pore

Drug

Hydrophobic pockets

Fig. 46.13 The proposed mechanism of action for capsid-binding inhibitors of picornaviruses, including rhinoviruses. (a) Icosahedral capsid of a rhinovirus, depicting the arrangement of the 3 capsid proteins about a 5-fold axis. (b) Three of the 5 VP1 proteins at the 5-fold axis. A typical rhinovirus inhibitor is binding to the hydrophobic pocket at the base of the canyon, probably reducing the flexibility of the VP1 protein and affecting receptor binding and uncoating. An amino acid substitution in the region forming the pocket may lead to resistance because of the lost ability to bind drug. (Field and Goldthorpe (1985), with permission).

NH₂

Imiquimod

Fig. 46.14 Structure of imiquimod, a cytokine inducer active against papillomavirus infection.

exceeds the inhibitory concentration normally achieved in vivo with a therapeutic dose (Field 1988b). When possible, a drug-resistant variant is compared directly with its drug-sensitive parent, but in clinical practice the latter may not be available.

It has been shown repeatedly that point mutations, or small groups of mutations, can readily lead to substantial increases in resistance to various specific antiviral drugs (Coen 1986, Field and Owen 1988, Mellors, Larder and Schinazi 1995). Given the relatively large replication potential of viruses coupled with mutation rates that may exceed $1/10^4$ bases per replication cycle (Coen 1991), it was predicted that drug resistance might render all specific antiviral drugs useless. In the event, resistance has not been an overwhelming problem, at least among the herpesviruses. It seems that drug-resistance mutations are typically associated with attenuation of the virus (Field, Darby and Wildy 1980). For herpes simplex virus such strains have usually become a problem only in immunocompromised patients (Field and Goldthorpe 1989, Darby 1995). Resistance does, however, seem to be a major problem in HIV infections, although, in this case, immunosuppression is a central part of the pathogenesis. Nevertheless, in these circumstances resistance has an important role in limiting the continued effectiveness of the inhibitor (Bean et al. 1987, Ljungman et al. 1990, Safrin et al. 1994). There is currently much interest in the use of drug combinations or alternations as an approach to this problem in the treatment of AIDS.

Although drug resistance may be seen as a depressing setback after many years of otherwise successful development of a new drug, it does have useful aspects: the isolation of resistant variants defines the compound as having a virus-specific mode of action; it enables the molecular targets for drug action to be identified with certainty; and, particularly when such targets are unsuspected, it may reveal hitherto unknown targets for the design of further inhibitors. Finally, when the precise mechanisms of drug resistance are elucidated, this information may provide a rationale for alternative therapeutic strategies to minimize or circumvent the impact of drug resistance in the patient.

HERPES SIMPLEX VIRUS AND VARICELLA-ZOSTER VIRUS

Selection for resistance in the laboratory

Much early work on drug resistance in viruses employed herpes simplex virus as a model in which drug-resistant variants could be selected with extreme ease in the laboratory. A single passage of virus in the presence of a subinhibitory concentration of the compound (e.g. aciclovir, penciclovir or brivudin) results in significant decrease in sensitivity to the respective compound (Larder and Darby 1984). Clinical isolates, including those obtained from normal patients who have never received chemotherapy, seem to contain a small proportion (perhaps 0.1%) of pre-existing drug-resistant mutants (Paris and Harrington 1982) that

can continue to multiply when selective pressure is applied.

In cell cultures, the kinetics and yields of such mutants are similar to those of their parental strains, but they are usually more or less attenuated when tested in animal models (Field, Darby and Wildy 1980, reviewed by Field 1989). Similar results have been obtained with varicella-zoster virus although the virus is more difficult to culture in vitro and there are no convenient models to test drug-resistant strains for virulence (Kimberlin et al. 1995).

Biochemical characterization of drug-resistant strains

Analysis of mutants selected for resistance to any of the common nucleoside analogues or to phosphonacetic acid shows them all to have changes in one of 2 sites: either the TK or DNA polymerase genes (Collins and Darby 1991). In some cases, both sites contain a mutation. The possibilities are summarized in Table 46.3.

It is important to stress that herpesvirus TK is not essential for growth of virus in cell culture, at least in actively dividing cells; therefore, many different mutations, including base substitutions, insertions or deletions, may give rise to lack of functional enzyme and hence to drug resistance. In contrast, DNA polymerase is always essential for virus replication and only particular base substitutions leading to subtle changes in the protein are possible without compromising the normal function of the enzyme.

Several laboratory mutants of each type shown in Table 46.3 have been fully characterized (Larder and Darby 1984, Coen 1986). The mutant proteins (TK or DNA polymerase) undergo changes in their enzymatic properties and DNA sequencing has identified the specific base substitutions of other changes that give rise to the drug-resistant phenotype; thus, the origin of resistance is fully explained (Collins and Darby 1991). Furthermore, several drug-resistant strains obtained from clinical isolates, almost all from immunocompromised patients following drug failure, proved to have genotypes identical to the previously characterized laboratory-selected strains (Larder and Darby 1984).

Although the biochemical picture appears to be complete, it is not yet clear exactly why drug-resistant strains seem to be so very rare among clinical isolates. After more than 10 years of widespread use of ACV there is still no evidence of a reduction of sensitivity among clinical isolates (Darby 1995). The proportion of drug-resistant strains has remained constant at <3%. These results are confirmed by several very large surveys of clinical isolates; such surveillance is continuing but, so far, there is fortunately no evidence of the emergence of drug resistance to ACV (Collins and Ellis 1993). It is likely, however, that rare viruses will emerge in which the drug-resistance mutations occur among a constellation of other changes that result in a highly pathogenic and transmissible virus. We must therefore remain vigilant for such events.

Table 46.3 Nature of herpes virus drug-resistant mutants so far isolated

Genetic locus	Genetic change	Resistance	Frequency in clinical isolates
TK (TK⁻)	Base: substitution insertion deletion Mutations in promoter site	Little or no TK enzyme to phosphorylate thymidine or thymidine analogue	Relatively common (in mixtures) but usually attenuated
TK (Tkʳ)	Base substitution	Altered TK substrate specificity; reduced phosphorylation of inhibitor but whole or partial phosphorylation of thymidine analogue	Quite rare
DNApolʳ (DNApolʳ)	Base substitution	Low affinity for nucleoside analogue triphosphate	Very rare

Resistance to herpes simplex in the immunocompromised patient

Drug resistance to ACV has been encountered among immunocompromised patients, of whom several large surveys suggest that c. 5% shed resistant virus (Wade et al. 1982, Englund et al. 1990). All 3 mechanisms of drug resistance have been observed (Table 46.3) and, in some cases, clinical isolates comprise mixtures of sensitive and resistant viruses, perhaps with more than one type of resistant virus present (Martin et al. 1985, Christophers and Sutton 1987, Sacks et al. 1989). Viruses that are resistant through lack of TK are, naturally, cross-resistant to other drugs that depend on virus TK for activation, whereas viruses of the TKʳ phenotype show varying patterns of cross-resistance. Foscarnet selects for resistance only at the DNA polymerase locus and is a possible alternative for therapeutic use when resistance develops to the nucleoside analogues. However, multiple drug resistance has occurred in some patients (Crumpacker et al. 1982). In summary, although drug resistance in the immunocompetent patient does not seem to be a problem at present, it may be prove a very serious matter in the individual patient with defective immunity.

DRUG RESISTANCE IN HUMAN CYTOMEGALOVIRUS

Human cytomegalovirus infection is one of the major virological problems in the immunocompromised patient and, unfortunately, drug resistance has emerged as a significant additional problem in these cases (Drew et al. 1991). Viruses that have acquired resistance to GCV have been encountered, and analysis of these strains led to the discovery of a hitherto unsuspected site of action of the drug (Drew et al. 1991, Drew, Miner and Saleh 1993). The drug-resistance mutations were traced to gene *UL97*, which, as mentioned under 'Ganciclovir' (p. 995), encodes a protein kinase function (Littler, Stuart and Chee 1992, Sullivan et al. 1992). Although this finding confirms a serious problem in these patients that renders

the therapy ineffective, at a biochemical level it is an exciting discovery because it has revealed a new potential molecular target for the design of new inhibitors against this and other viruses (Birch and Mills 1994, Biron 1994). The hope is that, from this early setback with GCV, new and more effective inhibitors will be born.

DRUG RESISTANCE IN HIV

At first it was difficult to show the development of resistance to the early drugs directed against HIV. Unfortunately, this turned out to be due to a technical problem and, once the methods for detection were improved, drug resistance was revealed as a universal feature of all chemotherapeutic strategies so far employed against this infection.

Drug resistance in HIV results from point mutations leading to alterations in the affinity of reverse transcriptase for the inhibitor, although this has, in many cases, been very difficult to prove by testing the enzyme functions for reduced sensitivity to inhibition in vitro. Development of resistance was first shown for zidovudine (Larder, Darby and Richman 1989, Larder and Kemp 1989), and subsequently for all other nucleoside inhibitors. Resistance to the non-nucleoside reverse transcriptase inhibitors apparently occurs even more readily and the resistant strains are cross-resistant (Richman et al. 1991, Condra et al. 1992). Resistance to the various proteinase inhibitors has also been clearly demonstrated (Otto et al. 1993, Kaplan et al. 1994, Mellors, Larder and Schinazi 1995).

Particular mutations (and in some cases sequences of mutations) lead to progressively more resistant virus populations in the patient. Knowledge of resistance patterns to individual drugs enables rational strategies for combinations of drugs or for the sequential use of different compounds. This approach offers perhaps the most optimistic outlook for HIV chemotherapy but, given the ability for genetic variation and the fact that many drug-resistant mutations do not apparently reduce the pathogenicity of the virus, it is not exactly clear why drug resistance in HIV has quickly emerged as being much more serious than that of herpes simplex virus in immunocompetent individuals.

RESISTANCE IN ORTHOMYXOVIRUSES

Influenza A virus has long been known to develop resistance to amantadine (Cochran et al. 1965, Oxford, Logan and Potter 1970). Resistance was mapped first to the haemagglutinin and subsequently to the *M2* gene (Lamb, Zebedee and Richardson 1985, Hay et al. 1986) which codes for a component of the nucleocapsid. Of the 2 sites, changes in the M2 protein are the more important (Hay et al. 1985). Analyses of such drug-resistant mutants were of paramount importance in defining the mechanism of action of amantadine and similar compounds (Field and Owen 1988) (see section 3.3, p. 1000).

Although drug resistance is readily selected for in cell culture, there are too few surveys available to assess the impact of resistance in humans to amantadine. The rapid development of resistance following transmission to susceptible birds was, however, reported following the experimental infection and therapy of chickens with fowl plague (Webster, Kawaoka and Bean 1986), and more recently a similar rapid development of drug resistance has been observed in humans infected with influenza A (Belshe et al 1989, Hayden et al 1989, 1991, Hayden 1994).

RESISTANCE IN PICORNAVIRUSES

The action of capsid-binding molecules that interact with rhinoviruses is readily reversed by the growth of mutants with point mutations in the genes coding for the capsid proteins concerned (Ninomiya et al. 1985). The patterns of cross-resistance have been widely studied (Yasin et al. 1990a) and in some cases cross-resistance to the effects of neutralizing antibodies occurs (Dutko et al. 1990, Rossmann 1990). Such antibodies also depend on capsid-binding at a nearby site in order to achieve neutralization. Although the study of such resistance is very useful in elucidating precise virus-inhibitor mechanisms, its implication for the future use of anti-picornavirus compounds of this type is far from clear. Resistance has the potential to arise very rapidly in vitro, and the unresolved question is whether such resistant variants will have impaired pathogenicity or reduced ability to spread. One trial suggested that this may indeed be the case (Dearden et al. 1989, Yasin et al. 1990b); however, there is as yet far too little information to predict the possible impact of drug resistance in the clinic were such compounds to become widely used (Al-Nakib 1993).

4.2 The problem of toxicity of antiviral compounds

As stated at the outset of this chapter, the principal obstacle to the development of antiviral compounds has been to obtain selective toxicity. Having established by tests in vitro and toxicity tests in a variety of animal species that a compound has a high selective index, there may still remain problems that are encountered only when the compounds are administered to humans. In some cases the toxic effects may, of course, be caused by minor metabolites of the original compound.

Nucleoside analogues often cause a variety of acute effects, including malaise, weight loss, tremors, mutism, peripheral neuropathy, acute liver and kidney damage as well as the more common complaints of nausea and vomiting. In some cases these effects have been related to the inhibition of cellular enzymes, particularly mitochondrial enzymes, by the antiviral compounds. Amantadine administration is associated with reversible neurological change (rimantadine is used successfully in the control of Parkinson's disease) and these effects are thought to relate to the release and uptake of dopamine in the central nervous system (Mizoguchi et al. 1994). To these problems must be added the long-term concern regarding possible teratogenicity and genetic damage caused by agents that interact with DNA (Griffiths 1995). The latter can theoretically occur when nucleoside analogues are incorporated into host cell DNA or, indirectly, as a result of inhibition of DNA repair systems (Darby 1995).

'Familiarity breeds contempt' and there have been 2 incidences of toxicity in patients that resulted in deaths, reminding us of the need for constant attention to the potential that antiviral agents have for producing serious side effects.

TWO EXAMPLES OF SEVERE TOXICITY PROBLEMS IN HUMANS

Fialuridine toxicity

Fialuridine (1-2′-deoxy-2′-fluoro-1-β-D-arabinofuranosyl-5-iodouracil; FIAU) is an orally bioavailable compound active against hepatitis B (Fried et al. 1992). Pilot studies with a 4-week course were encouraging and showed that significant reduction in virus replication could be achieved. However, further trials with a longer treatment period were stopped after 12 weeks when patients developed myopathy, lactic acidosis, peripheral neuropathy, pancreatitis and liver failure; there were several deaths (Meeting Report 1995). The mechanism for this unexpected delayed toxicity seems to be a consequence of FIAU incorporation into mitochondrial DNA.

Sorivudine, BVaraU: toxic interactions with 5-fluoruracil

Sorivudine, or BVaraU, is a potent inhibitor of varicella-zoster (see section 3.1, p. 993) and the drug is currently undergoing clinical trials. It was licensed in Japan in 1993 but the licence was withdrawn when several deaths occurred in patients also receiving 5-fluorouracil. The toxicity resulted from the formation of the metabolite bromovinyluracil (Ashida et al. 1993) which inhibits dihydrothymine dehydrogenase, normally responsible for degrading 5-fluorouracil. This drug interaction led to the accumulation of 5-uracil in cancer patients receiving both drugs, and thus to fatal bone marrow suppression.

4.3 The problem of virus latency

Herpesvirus latency

Several viruses are capable of establishing latency in infected cells. This is a particular feature of all the herpesviruses, and both herpes simplex and varicella-zoster can remain latent in neurons for the lifetime of the infected individual (Wildy et al. 1982). Periodic reactivations may cause clinical recurrences. In some cases they are subclinical but, whether or not disease is apparent, the infection may be transmitted during the episode to a susceptible contact. Because, during the latent phase, the virus does not seem to express the genes coding for virus proteins, including TK and DNA polymerase, it is unaffected by any of the conventional nucleoside analogues or drugs that rely on viral protein targets. Latency is generally held to be established within a few days of the start of the primary infection and, in some cases, the foci of latent infection are thought to be present a few hours after the first round of virus replication at the mucosal site. The implication is that chemotherapy cannot be started early enough to prevent the establishment of latency; even if it is successful in limiting the clinical signs of disease during the primary infection, the virus will persist, to reactivate later (Darby and Field 1984). However, ACV does suppress recurrent infections and patients have taken suppressive therapy for this purpose over periods up to 10 years (Douglas et al. 1984, Straus et al. 1984, Goldberg et al. 1993). Furthermore, prophylaxis can prevent episodes of herpes resulting from reactivation in immunosuppressed patients. The problem of eradicating herpesvirus DNA harboured in latently infected cells is one for which there is no obvious solution.

Retrovirus latency

HIV can establish a different kind of latency in which the viral DNA, always formed as an intermediate during replication, may become stably integrated into the chromosome of the host cell. In some cases the cells survive infection and continue to harbour the viral genes, which are not expressed or are expressed at a very low level with the potential to become active later. The drugs so far used to treat HIV infections have not been successful in producing a prolonged inhibition of virus replication. The existence of latently infected cells is not thought to be important in limiting the success of available drugs and it remains to be seen whether such cells will present an additional problem when, using more effective compounds, the virus has been eradicated from cells actively involved in viral replication. Clearly, both latency and drug resistance represent major obstacles to the long-term success of antiviral chemotherapy that only became apparent as the original problems of toxic side effects were so successfully overcome.

5 COMBINATION CHEMOTHERAPY FOR VIRAL INFECTIONS

As with the treatment of some bacterial diseases, especially mycobacterial infections, combinations of drugs have proven exceedingly valuable. The recognition that monotherapy of HIV infections has not resulted in a cure has led to numerous clinical trials evaluating various combinations of antiretroviral therapy (e.g. zidovudine plus didanosine; zidovudine plus lamivudine) (Schinazi 1991, 1995). Similarly, for life-threatening herpesvirus infections (e.g. encephalitis or neonatal herpes), combination therapies will be tested, including the combined use of drugs and immunoglobulins or cytokines, including interferons.

6 CONCLUSIONS AND FUTURE PROSPECTS

The rapid application of molecular biology to the study of viruses most assuredly will lead to the development of novel antiviral drugs. Already, the identification of protease in a variety of viruses other than HIV has led to a great increase in research directed toward the synthesis of peptidomimetics that inhibit these enzymes. Hepatitis C, HSV, cytomegalovirus etc. are prime targets. In HSV alone, many genes provide targets for debilitation of viral replication; they include both those essential for viral replication and others that are not. The application of antisense RNA, triplex-forming oligonucleotides, ribozymes and direct DNA targeting, although intellectually appealing, poses drug delivery problems that have yet to be overcome in clinical practice.

REFERENCES

Al-Nakib W, 1993, Drug resistance in rhinoviruses, *Int Antiviral News*, **1**: 100.

Andries K, Dewindt B et al., 1992, In vitro activity of pirodavir (R 77975), a substituted phenoxy-pyridazinamine with broad-spectrum antipicornaviral activity, *Antimicrob Agents Chemother*, **36**: 100–7.

Ashida N, Ljichi K et al., 1993, Metabolism of 5′-ether prodrugs of 1-beta-D-arabinofuranosyl-E-5-(2-bromovinyl)uracil in rats, *Biochem Pharmacol*, **46**: 2201–7.

Baba M, Pauwels R et al., 1987, Both 2′,3′-dideoxythymidine and its 2′,3′-unsaturated derivative (2′,3′-dideoxythymidinene) are potent and selective inhibitors of human immunodeficiency virus replication in vitro, *Biochem Biophys Res Commun*, **142**: 128–34.

Baba M, Tanaka H et al., 1989, Highly specific inhibition of human immunodefiency virus type 1 by a novel 6-substituted acyclouridine derivative, *Biochem Biophys Res Commun*, **165**: 1375–81.

Balfour HH Jr, Kelly JM et al., 1990, Acyclovir treatment of varicella in otherwise healthy children, *J Pediatr*, **116**: 633–9.

Bean B, Fletcher C et al., 1987, Progressive mucocutaneous herpes simplex infection due to acyclovir-resistant virus in an immunocompromised patient: correlation of viral susceptibilities and plasma levels with response to therapy, *Diagn Microbiol Infect Dis*, **7**: 199–204.

Beauchamp LM, Orr GF et al., 1992, Amino acid ester prodrugs of acyclovir, *Antiviral Chem Chemother*, **3**: 157–64.

Belshe RB, Burk B et al., 1989, Resistance of influenza A virus to amantadine and rimantadine: results of one decade of surveillance, *J Infect Dis*, **159**: 430–5.

Bigar F, 1979, Clinical experiences with trifluorothymidine in herpes simplex keratitis, *Adv Ophthalmol*, **38**: 110–15.

Birch C, Mills J, 1994, Cytomegalovirus and drug resistance, *Int Antiviral News*, **2**: 119–20.

Biron K, 1994, Ganciclovir resistance of cytomegalovirus: mechanisms and prospects for rapid detection, *Int Antiviral News*, **2**: 117–18.

Boker KHW, Ringe B et al., 1994, Prostaglandin E plus famciclovir – a new concept for the treatment of severe hepatitis B after liver transplantation, *Transplantation*, **57**: 1706–8.

Boyd MR, Bacon TH et al., 1987, Antiherpesvirus activity of 9-(4-hydroxy-3-hydroxymethylbut-1-yl)guanine (BRL39123) in cell culture, *Antimicrob Agents Chemother*, **31**: 1238–42.

Bozzette SA, Kanouse DE et al., 1995, Health status and function with zidovudine or zalcitabine as initial therapy for AIDS: a randomized controlled trial. Roche 3300/ACTG Study Group, *JAMA*, **273**: 295–301.

Bryson YJ, Dillon M et al., 1983, Treatment of first episodes of genital herpes simplex virus infection with oral acyclovir. A randomized double-blind controlled trial in normal subjects, *N Engl J Med*, **308**: 916–21.

Carrington D, 1994, Prospects for improved efficacy with antiviral prodrugs: will valaciclovir and famciclovir meet the clinical challenge?, *Int Antiviral News*, **2**: 50–3.

Christophers J, Sutton RNP, 1987, Characterization of acyclovir-resistant and sensitive clinical isolates of herpes simplex virus from an immunocompromised patient, *J Antimicrob Chemother*, **20**: 389–98.

Cochran KW, Massab HR et al., 1965, Studies on the antiviral activity of amantadine hydrochloride, *Ann N Y Acad Sci*, **130**: 432–9.

Coen DM, 1986, General aspects of virus drug resistance with special reference to herpes simplex virus, *J Antimicrob Chemother*, **18, suppl B**: 1–10.

Coen DM, 1991, Antiviral drug resistance, *Ann N Y Acad Sci*, **616**: 224–37.

Collins A, Downes CS, Johnson RT, eds, 1984, *DNA Repair and its Inhibition*, IRL Press, Oxford.

Collins P, Darby G, 1991, Laboratory studies of herpes simplex virus strains resistant to acyclovir, *Rev Med Virol*, **1**: 19–28.

Collins P, Ellis MN, 1993, Sensitivity monitoring of clinical isolates of herpes simplex virus to acyclovir, *J Med Virol*, **41, suppl 1**: 58–66.

Condra JH, Emini EA, 1992, Identification of the human immunodeficiency virus reverse transcriptase residues that contribute to the activity of diverse nonnucleoside inhibitors, *Antimicrob Agents Chemother*, **36**: 1441–6.

Crisp PL, Clissold SP, 1991, Foscarnet, *Drugs*, **41**: 104–29.

Crooks RJ, 1995, Valaciclovir – a review of its potential in the management of genital herpes, *Antiviral Chem Chemother*, **6, suppl 1**: 39–44.

Crooks RJ, Jones DA, Fiddian AP, 1991, Zoster-associated chronic pain: an overview of clinical trials with acyclovir, *Scand J Infect Dis*, **suppl 80**: 62–8.

Crumpacker CS, Schnipper LE et al., 1982, Resistance to antiviral drugs of herpes simplex virus isolated from a patient treated with acyclovir, *N Engl J Med*, **306**: 343–6.

Darby G, 1994, A history of antiherpes research, *Antivir Chem Chemother*, **5, suppl 1**: 3–9.

Darby G, 1995, In search of the perfect antiviral, *Antiviral Chem Chemother*, **6, suppl 1**: 54–63.

Darby G, Field HJ, 1984, Latency and acquired resistance – problems in chemotherapy of herpes infections, *Pharmacol Ther*, **23**: 217–51.

Darbyshire JH, Aboulker J-P, 1992, Didanosine for zidovudine-intolerant patients with HIV disease, *Lancet*, **340**: 1346–7.

Dawber R, 1974, Idoxuridine in herpes zoster: further evaluation of intermittent topical therapy, *Br Med J*, **2**: 526–7.

Dayan AD, Anderson D, 1988, Toxicity of antiviral compounds, *Antiviral Agents: the development and assessment of antiviral chemotherapy*, vol I, ed Field HJ, CRC Press, Boca Raton FL, 111–25.

De Clercq E, 1982, Specific targets for antiviral drugs, *Biochem J*, **205**: 1–13.

De Clercq E, 1995, Antiviral chemotherapy: where do we stand and what can we expect?, *Int Antiviral News*, **3**: 52–4.

De Clercq E, Descamps J et al., 1979, (E)-5-(2-bromovinyl)-2′-deoxyuridine: a potent and selective antiherpes agent, *Proc Natl Acad Sci USA*, **76**: 2947–51.

De Clercq E, Descamps J et al., 1980, Comparative efficacy of antiherpes drugs against different strains of herpes simplex virus, *J Infect Dis*, **141**: 563–74.

De Clercq E, Verhelst G et al., 1981, Differential inhibition of herpes simplex viruses type 1 (HSV-1) and type 2 (HSV-2), by (E)-5-(2-X-vinyl)-2′-deoxyuridines, *Acta Microbiol Acad Sci Hung*, **28**: 307–12.

De Clercq E, Balzarini J et al., 1982, Antiviral, antimetabolic, and cytotoxic activities of 5-substituted 2′-deoxycytidines, *Mol Pharmacol*, **21**: 217–23.

De Clercq E, Holy A et al., 1986, A novel selective broad-spectrum anti-DNA virus agent, *Nature (London)*, **323**: 464–7.

De Long DC, 1984, Effect of enviroxime on rhinovirus infections in humans, *Microbiology*, eds Leive L, Schlessinger D, American Society of Microbiology, Washington DC, 431–4.

Dearden C, Al-Nakib W et al., 1989, Drug-resistant rhinoviruses from the nose of experimentally treated volunteers, *Arch Virol*, **109**: 71–81.

Debyser Z, Pauwels R et al., 1991, An antiviral target on reverse transcriptase of human immmunodeficiency virus type 1 revealed by tetrahydroimidazo-[4,5,1-jk][1,4]benzodiazepin-2(1H)-one and thione derivatives, *Proc Natl Acad Sci USA*, **88**: 1451–5.

Descamps J, Sehgal RK et al., 1982, Inhibitory effect of E-5-(2-bromovinyl)-1-beta-D-arabinofuranosyluracil on herpes simplex virus replication and DNA synthesis, *J Virol*, **43**: 332–6.

Dexter DL, Wolberg WH et al., 1972, The clinical pharmacology of 5-trifluoromethyl-2′-deoxyuridine, *Cancer Res*, **32**: 247.

Doong SL, Tsai CH et al., 1991, Inhibition of the replication of hepatitis B virus in vitro by 2′,3′-dideoxy-3′-thiacytidine and related analogues, *Proc Natl Acad Sci USA*, **88**: 8495–9.

Douglas JM, Critchlow C et al., 1984, A double-blind study of oral acyclovir for suppression of recurrences of genital herpes simplex virus infection, *N Engl J Med*, **310**: 1551–6.

Drew WL, Miner RC, Saleh E, 1993, Antiviral susceptibility testing of cytomegalovirus: criteria for detecting resistance to antivirals, *Clin Diagn Virol*, **1**: 179–85.

Drew WL, Miner RC et al., 1991, Prevalence of resistance in patients receiving ganciclovir for serious cytomegalovirus infection, *J Infect Dis*, **163**: 716–19.

Dunkle LM, Arvin AM et al., 1991, A controlled trial of acyclovir for chickenpox in normal children, *N Engl J Med*, **325**: 1539–44.

Dutko FJ, Diana GD, 1990, Quantitative structure–activity relationships and biological consequence of picornavirus capsid-binding compounds, *Use of X-ray Crystallography in the Design of Antiviral Agents*, eds Laver WG, Air GM, Academic Press, San Diego CA, 187–98.

Earnshaw DL, Bacon TH, Darlison SJ, 1992, Penciclovir: mode of action of penciclovir in MRC-5 cells infected with herpes simplex virus (HSV-1), HSV-2 and varicella-zoster virus, *Antimicrob Agents Chemother*, **36**: 2747–57.

Elion GB, 1993, Acyclovir: discovery, mechanism of action and selectivity, *J Med Virol*, **suppl 1**: S2–6.

Elion GB, Furman PA et al., 1977, Selectivity of action of an antiherpetic agent 9-(2-hydroxyethoxymethyl)guanine, *Proc Natl Acad Sci USA*, **74**: 5716–20.

Englund JA, Zimmerman ME et al., 1990, Herpes simplex virus resistant to acyclovir: a study in a tertiary care center, *Ann Intern Med*, **112**: 416–22.

Evans HJ, 1983, Cytogenetic methods for detecting effects of chemical mutagens, *Ann N Y Acad Sci*, **407**: 131.

Fan-Havard P, Nahata MC, Brady MT, 1989, Ganciclovir: a review of pharmacology, therapeutic efficacy and potential use for treatment of congenital cytomegalovirus infections, *J Clin Pharm Ther*, **14:** 329–40.

Fanning MM, Read SE et al., 1990, Foscarnet therapy of cytomegalovirus retinitis in AIDS, *J Acquired Immune Defic Syndr*, **3:** 472–9.

Field HJ, ed, 1983, *Antiviral Agents: the development and assessment of antiviral chemotherapy*, vols I, II, CRC Press, Boca Raton FL.

Field HJ, ed, 1988a, Animal models in the evaluation of antiviral chemotherapy, *Antiviral Agents: the development and assessment of antiviral chemotherapy*, vol I, CRC Press, Boca Raton FL, 67–84.

Field HJ, ed, 1988b, The development of antiviral drug resistance, *Antiviral Agents: the development and assessment of antiviral chemotherapy*, vol I, CRC Press, Boca Raton FL, 127–49.

Field HJ, 1989, Persistent herpes simplex virus infection and mechanisms of virus drug resistance, *Eur J Clin Microbiol Infect Dis*, **8:** 671–80.

Field HJ, Brown GA, 1989, Animal models for antiviral chemotherapy, *Antiviral Res*, **12:** 165–80.

Field HJ, Darby G, Wildy P, 1980, Isolation and characterization of acyclovir-resistant mutants of herpes simplex virus, *J Gen Virol*, **49:** 115–24.

Field HJ, Goldthorpe SE, 1989, Antiviral drug resistance, *Trends Pharm Sci*, **10:** 333–7.

Field H, McMillan A, Darby G, 1981, The sensitivity of acyclovir-resistant mutants of herpes simplex virus to other antiviral drugs, *J Infect Dis*, **143:** 281–5.

Field HJ, Owen LJ, 1988, Virus drug resistance, *Antiviral Drug Development*, eds De Clercq E, Walker RT, Life Sciences Series A 143, Plenum Press, New York, 203–36.

Field HJ, Reading MJ, 1987, The inhibition of bovine herpesvirus-1 by methyl 2-pyridyl ketone thiosemicarbazone and its effects on bovine cells, *Antiviral Res*, **7:** 245–56.

Field HJ, Tewari D et al., 1995, Comparison of efficacies of famciclovir and valaciclovir against herpes simplex virus type 1 in a murine immunosuppression model, *Antimicrob Agents Chemother*, **39:** 1114–19.

Fischl MA, Richman DD et al. and AZT Collaborative Working Group, 1987, The efficacy of azidothymidine (AZT) in the treatment of patients with AIDS and AIDS-related complex: a double blind, placebo-controlled trial, *N Engl J Med*, **317:** 185–91.

Freitas VR, Smee DF et al., 1985, Activity of 9-(1,3-dihydroxy-2-propoxymethyl)guanine compared with that of acyclovir against human, monkey and rodent cytomegaloviruses, *Antimicrob Agents Chemother*, **28:** 240–5.

Fried MW, Dibisceglie AM et al., 1992, FIAU, a new oral antiviral agent, profoundly inhibits HBV DNA in patients with chronic hepatitis B, *Hepatology*, **16:** 127A.

Furman PA, St Clair MH et al., 1979, Inhibition of herpes simplex virus induced DNA polymerase activity and viral DNA replication by 9-(2-hydroxyethoxymethyl)guanine, *J Virol*, **32:** 72–7.

Fyfe JA, Keller PM et al., 1978, Thymidine kinase from herpes simplex virus phosphorylates the new antival compound 9-(2-hydroxyethoxymethyl)guanine, *J Biol Chem*, **253:** 8721–7.

Gilbert BE, Knight V, 1986, Biochemistry and clinical applications of ribavirin, *Antimicrob Agents Chemother*, **30:** 201–5.

Goldberg LH, Kaufman R et al., 1993, Long-term suppression of recurrent genital herpes with acyclovir: a 5-year bench mark. Acyclovir study group, *Arch Dermatol*, **129:** 582–7.

Goodpasture EW, Teague O, 1923, Transmission of the virus herpes febrilis along nerves in experimentally infected rabbits, *J Med Res*, **44:** 139–84.

Griffiths PD, 1995, Progress in the clinical management of herpesvirus infections, *Antiviral Chem Chemother*, **6:** 191–209.

Harmenberg J, Abele G, Malm M, 1985, Deoxythymidine pools in animal and human skin with reference to antiviral drugs, *Arch Dermatol Res*, **277:** 402–3.

Harmenberg J, Wahren B, Öberg B, 1980, Influence of cells and virus multiplicity on the inhibition of herpesvirus with acycloguanosine, *Intervirology*, **14:** 239–44.

Harmenberg J, Wahren B et al., 1985, Multiplicity dependence and sensitivity of herpes simplex virus isolates to antiviral compounds, *J Antimicrob Chemother*, **15:** 567–73.

Hay AJ, 1992, The action of adamantanamines against influenza A viruses: inhibition of the M2 ion channel protein, *Semin Virol*, **3:** 21–30.

Hay AJ, Wolstenholme AJ et al., 1985, The molecular basis of the specific anti-influenza action of amantadine, *EMBO J*, **4:** 3621–4.

Hay AJ, Zambon MC et al., 1986, Molecular basis of resistance of influenza A viruses to amantadine, *J Antimicrob Chemother*, **18, suppl B:** 19–29.

Hayden FG, 1994, Amantadine and rimantadine resistance in influenza A viruses, *Curr Opinion Infect Dis*, **7:** 674–7.

Hayden FG, Gwaltney JM et al., 1981, Comparative toxicity of amantadine hydrochloride and rimantadine hydrochloride in healthy adults, *Antimicrob Agents Chemother*, **19:** 226–33.

Hayden FG, Minocha A et al., 1985, Comparative single dose pharmacokinetics of amantadine hydrochloride and rimantadine hydrochloride in young and elderly adults, *Antimicrob Agents Chemother*, **28:** 216–21.

Hayden FG, Belshe RB et al., 1989, Emergence and apparent transmission of rimantadine-resistant influenza A virus in families, *N Engl J Med*, **321:** 1696–702.

Hadyen FG, Sperber SJ et al., 1991, Recovery of drug-resistant influenza A virus during therapeutic use of rimantadine, *Antimicrob Agents Chemother*, **35:** 1741–7.

Heidelberger C, Parsons DG, Remy D, 1964, Synthesis of 5-trifluoromethyluracil and 5-trifluoromethyl-2′-deoxyuridine, *J Med Chem*, **7:** 1.

Hersfield MS, 1979, Apparent suicide inactivation of human lymphoblast S-adenosyl homocysteine hydrolase by 2′-deoxyadenosine and adenine arabinoside, *J Biol Chem*, **254:** 223.

Hitchcock MJM, 1991, 2′,3′-Didehydro-2′,3′-dideoxythymidine (D4T), an anti-HIV agent, *Antivir Chem Chemother*, **2:** 125–32.

Honkoop P, de Man RA, 1995, Clinical aspects of nucleoside analogues for chronic hepatitis B, *Int Antiviral News*, **3:** 78–80.

Hoofnagle JH, 1994, Therapy of acute and chronic viral-hepatitis, *Adv Intern Med*, **39:** 241–75.

von Itzstein M, Wu W-Y et al., 1993, Rational design of potent sialidase-based inhibitors of influenza virus replication, *Nature (London)*, **363:** 418–23.

Kahn JO, Lagakos SW et al., 1992, A controlled trial comparing continued zidovudine with didanosine in human immunodeficiency virus infection, *N Engl J Med*, **327:** 581–7.

Kaplan AH, Michael SF et al., 1994, Selection of multiple human immunodeficiency virus type 1 variants that encode viral proteases with decreased sensitivity to an inhibitor of the viral protease, *Proc Natl Acad Sci USA*, **91:** 5597–601.

Kaufman HE, 1979, Antiviral update, *Ophthalmology*, **86:** 131–6.

Kaufman HE, Heidelberger C, 1964, Therapeutic antiviral action of 5-trifluormethyl-2′-deoxyuridine in herpes simplex keratitis, *Science*, **145:** 585–6.

Kimberlin DW, Kern ER et al., 1995, Models of antiviral resistance, *Antiviral Res*, **26:** 415–22.

Koch JA, Ruprecht RM, 1992, Animal models for anti-AIDS therapy, *Antiviral Res*, **19:** 81–109.

Kohl NE, Emini EA et al., 1988, Active human immunodeficiency virus protease is required for viral infectivity, *Proc Natl Acad Sci USA*, **85:** 4686–90.

Lamb RA, Zebedee SL, Richardson CD, 1985, Influenza virus M2 protein is an integral membrane protein expressed on the infected cell surface, *Cell*, **40:** 627–33.

Larder BA, Darby G, 1984, Virus drug-resistance: mechanisms and consequences, *Antiviral Res*, **4:** 1–42.

Larder BA, Darby G, Richman DD, 1989, HIV with reduced sensitivity to zidovudine (AZT) isolated during prolonged therapy, *Science*, **243:** 1731–4.

Larder BA, Kemp SD, 1989, Multiple mutations in HIV-1 reverse transcriptase confer high-level resistance to zidovudine (AZT), *Science*, **246:** 1155–8.

Laver GW, Air GM, eds, 1990, *Use of X-ray Crystallography in the Design of Antiviral Agents*, Academic Press, London.

Leinback SS, Reno GM et al., 1976, Mechanisms of phosphonoacetate inhibitions on herpes virus-induced DNA polymerase, *Biochemistry*, **15:** 426–30.

Levinson ML, Jacobson PA, 1992, Treatment and prophylaxis of cytomegalovirus disease, *Pharmacotherapy*, **12:** 300–18.

Littler E, Stuart AD, Chee MS, 1992, Human cytomegalovirus open reading frame encodes a protein that phosphorylates the antiviral nucleoside analogue ganciclovir, *Nature (London)*, **358:** 160–2.

Ljungman P, Ellis MN et al., 1990, Acyclovir-resistant herpes simplex virus causing pneumonia after marrow transplantation, *J Infect Dis*, **162:** 711–15.

Locarnini SA, Shaw T et al., 1994, Antiviral activity of penciclovir, a novel antiherpesvirus compound, against duck hepatitis B in vitro, *Antiviral Res*, **23, suppl 1:** S79.

McLaren C, Ellis MN, Hunter GA, 1983, A colorimetric assay for the measurement of the sensitivity of herpes simplex virus to antiviral agents, *Antiviral Res*, **3:** 223–34.

McLaren C, Datema R et al., 1991, Didanosine, *Antivir Chem Chemother*, **2:** 321–8.

Machida H, 1990, In vitro anti-herpes virus action of a novel antiviral agent, brovavir (BV-araU), *Chemotherapy (Tokyo)*, **38:** 256–61.

Machida H, Nishitani M, 1990, Drug susceptibilities of isolates of varicella-zoster virus in a clinical study of oral brovavir, *Microbiol Immunol*, **34:** 407–11.

Martin JL, Ellis MN et al., 1985, Plaque autoradiographic assay for the detection and quantitation of thymidine kinase-deficient and thymidine kinase-altered mutants of herpes simplex in clincial isolates, *Antimicrob Agents Chemother*, **28:** 181–7.

Matthews T, Boehme R, 1988, Antiviral activity and mechanism of action of ganciclovir, *Rev Infect Dis*, **10, suppl 3:** S490–4.

Meeting Report, 1995, 8th International Conference on Antiviral Research, *Int Antiviral News*, **3:** 101.

Mellors JW, Larder BA, Schinazi RF, 1995, Mutations in HIV-reverse transcriptase and protease associated with drug resistance, *Int Antiviral News*, **3:** 8–13.

Merluzzi VJ, Hargrave KD et al., 1990, Inhibition of HIV-1 replication by a non-nucleoside reverse transcriptase inhibitor, *Science*, **250:** 1411–33.

Mertz GJ, Critchlow CW et al., 1984, Double-blind placebo-controlled trial of oral acyclovir in first-episode genital herpes simplex virus infection, *JAMA*, **252:** 1147–51.

Meyers JD, Wade JC et al., 1982, Multicenter collaborative trial of intravenous acyclovir for treatment of herpes simplex virus infection in the immunocompromised host, *Am J Med*, **73:** 229–35.

Miller R, Birmachu W et al., 1995, Imiquimod: cytokine induction and antiviral activity, *Int Antiviral News*, **3:** 111–13.

Mills JS, 1993, Discovery of the HIV proteinase inhibitor Ro 31-8959: a paradigm for drug discovery, *Int Antiviral News*, **1:** 18–19.

Mitsuya H, Broder S, 1986, Inhibition of the in vitro infectivity and cytopathic effect of human T-lymphotrophic virus type III/lymphadenopathy-associated virus (HTLV-III/LAV) by 2′,3′-dideoxynucleosides, *Proc Natl Acad Sci USA*, **83:** 1911–15.

Mitsuya H, Weinhold KJ et al., 1985, 3′-Azido-3′-deoxythymidine (BWA 509U): an antiviral agent that inhibits infectivity and cytopathic effects of human T-lymphotropic virus type III lymphadenopathy associated virus in vitro, *Proc Natl Acad Sci USA*, **82:** 7096–100.

Miyasaka T, Tanaka H et al., 1989, A novel lead for specific anti-HIV-1 agents: 1-[(2-hydroxyethoxy)methyl]-6-(phenylthio)-thymine, *J Med Chem*, **32:** 2507–9.

Mizoguchi K, Yokoo H et al., 1994, Amantadine increases the extracellular dopamine levels in the striatum by re-uptake

inhibition and by *N*-methyl-D-aspartate antagonism, *Brain Res*, **662:** 255–8.

Murphy VF, 1993, Molecular targets for novel antiviral agents in the treatment of hepatitis C virus infection, *Int Antiviral News*, **1:** 115–17.

Murray AB, 1995, Valaciclovir – an improvement over aciclovir for the treatment of zoster, *Antiviral Chem Chemother*, **6, suppl 1:** 34–8.

Newton AA, 1988, Tissue culture methods for assessing antivirals and their harmful effects, *Antiviral Agents: the development and assessment of antiviral chemotherapy*, vol I, ed Field H, CRC Press, Boca Raton FL, 2–66.

Ninomiya Y, Aoyama M et al., 1985, Comparative studies on the modes of action of the antirhinovirus agents Ro 09-0410, Ro 09-0179, RMI-15,731, 6-dichloroflavan, and enviroxime, *Antimicrob Agents Chemother*, **27:** 595–9.

North TW, Remington KM et al., 1993, Feline immunodeficiency virus: a unique model for studies of viral resistance to AIDS chemotherapy, *Int Antiviral News*, **1:** 71–2.

Öberg B, 1983a, Antiviral effects of phosphonoformate (PFA, foscarnet sodium), *Pharmacol Ther*, **19:** 387–415.

Öberg B, 1983b, Inhibitors of virus-specific enzymes, *Problems of Antiviral Therapy*, eds Stuart-Harris CH, Oxford J, Academic Press, London, 35–69.

Otto MJ, Garber S et al., 1993, In vitro isolation and identification of human immunodeficiency virus (HIV) variants with reduced sensivity to C-2 symmetrical inhibitors of HIV type 1 protease, *Proc Natl Acad Sci USA*, **90:** 7543–7.

Oxford JS, Logan IS, Potter CW, 1970, The in vivo selection of an influenza A2 strain resistant to amantadine, *Nature (London)*, **226:** 82–3.

Paris DS, Harrington JE, 1982, Herpes simplex virus variants resistant to high concentrations of acyclovir exist in clinical isolates, *Antimicrob Agents Chemother*, **22:** 71–7.

Pauwels R, Andries K et al., 1990, Potent and selective inhibition of HIV-1 replication in vitro by a novel series of tetrahydro-imidazo[4,5,1-jk][1,4]-benzodiazepin-2(1H)-one and -thione (TIBO) derivatives, *Design of Anti-AIDS Drugs*, ed De Clercq E , Pharmacochemistry Library, 14, Elsevier, Amsterdam, 103–22.

Pearly LH, Taylor WR, 1987, A structural model for the retroviral protease, *Nature (London)*, **329:** 351–4.

Perno C-F, Calio R, 1994, Evaluation of anti-HIV compounds in monoctye/macrophages: importance and clinical implications, *Int Antiviral News*, **2:** 88–9.

Prusoff WH, 1959, Synthesis and biological actiivities of iododeoxyuridine, an analogue of thymidine, *Biochim Biophys Acta*, **39:** 295–6.

Purifoy DJM, Lewis RB, Powell KL, 1977, Identification of the herpes simplex virus DNA polymerase gene, *Nature (London)*, **269:** 621–3.

Rees PJ, Brigden WD, 1988, Problems of assessing antiviral agents in man, *Antiviral Agents: the development and assessment of antiviral chemotherapy*, vol I, ed Field HJ, CRC Press, Boca Raton FL, 85–109.

Richman D, Shih CK et al., 1991, Human immunodeficiency virus type 1 mutants resistant to nonnucleoside inhibitors of reverse transcriptase arise in tissue culture, *Proc Natl Acad Sci USA*, **88:** 11241–5.

Roberts NA, 1995, Progress of saquinavir (Ro 31-8959) in clinical trials, *Int Antiviral News*, **3:** 2–3.

Roberts NA, Martin JA et al., 1990, Rational design of peptide-based HIV proteinase inhibitors, *Science*, **248:** 358–61.

Rossmann MG, 1990, Neutralizing rhinoviruses with antiviral agents that inhibit attachment and uncoating, *Use of X-ray Crystallography in the Design of Antiviral Agents*, eds Laver WG, Air GM, Academic Press, San Diego CA, 115–37.

Sacks SL, Wanklin RJ et al., 1989, Progressive esophagitis from acyclovir-resistant herpes simplex. Clinical roles for DNA polymerase mutants and viral heterogeneity, *Ann Intern Med*, **111:** 893–9.

Safrin S, Elbeik T et al., 1994, Correlation between response to acyclovir and foscarnet therapy and in vitro susceptibility result for isolates of herpes simplex virus from human immunodeficiency virus-infected patients, *Antimicrob Agents Chemother*, **38**: 1246–50.

Sandford GP, Wingard JR et al., 1985, Genetic analysis of the susceptibility of mouse cytomegalovirus to acyclovir, *J Virol*, **53**: 104–13.

Schabel GM Jr, 1968, The antiviral activity of 9-beta-D-arabinofuranosyladenine (araA), *Chemotherapy (Basel)*, **13**: 321–38.

Schaeffer HJ, Beauchamp L et al., 1978, 9-(2-hydroxyethoxymethyl)guanine activity against viruses of the herpes group, *Nature (London)*, **272**: 583–5.

Schinazi RF, 1991, Combined chemotherapeutic modalities for viral infections: rationale and clinical potential, *Synergism and Antagonism in Chemotherapy*, eds Chou T-C, Rideout DC, Academic Press, Orlando FL, 109–82.

Schinazi RF, 1995, A brighter future for nucleoside antiviral agents, *Int Antiviral News*, **3**: 45–6.

Sidwell R, Revankar G, Robins R, 1985, Ribavirin: review of a broad-spectrum antiviral agent, *International Encyclopedia of Pharmacology and Therapeutics*, vol 2, section 116; viral chemotherapy, ed Shugar D, Pergamon Press, Oxford, 49–108.

Sidwell RW, Huffman JH et al., 1972, Broad-spectrum antiviral activity of virazole: 1-beta-D-ribofuranosyl-1,2,4-triazole-3-carboxamide, *Science*, **177**: 705.

Smee DF, Martin JC et al., 1983, Antiherpes activity of the acyclic nucleoside 9-(1,3-dihydroxy-2-propoxymethyl)guanine, *Antimicrob Agents Chemother*, **23**: 676–82.

Snoeck R, Neyts J, De Clercq E, 1993, Strategies for the treatment of cytomegalovirus infections, *Multidisciplinary Approach to Understanding Cytomegalovirus Disease*, eds Michelson S, Plotkin SA, Elsevier, Amsterdam, 269–78.

Soudeyns H, Yao X-J et al., 1991, Anti-human immunodeficiency virus type 1 activity and in vitro toxicity of 2′,3′-dideoxy-3′-thiacytidine (BCH-189) a novel heterocyclic nucleoside analog, *Antimicrob Agents Chemother*, **35**: 1386–90.

Spruance SL, 1994, Topical therapy of mucocutaneous herpesvirus infections, *Int Antiviral News*, **2**: 86–7.

Stanley M, 1993, In vitro culture systems for papillomaviruses, *Int Antiviral News*, **1**: 85–6.

Straus SE, Takiff HE et al., 1984, Suppression of frequently recurring genital herpes. A placebo-controlled double-blind trial of oral acyclovir, *N Engl J Med*, **310**: 1545–50.

Sullivan V, Talarico CL et al., 1992, A protein kinase homologue controls phosphorylation of ganciclovir in human cytomegalovirus-infected cells, *Nature (London)*, **358**: 162–4.

Sutton D, Kern ER, 1993, Activity of famciclovir and penciclovir in HSV-infected animals: a review, *Antiviral Chem Chemother*, **4, suppl 1**: 37–46.

Tilson HH, Engle CR, Andrews EB, 1993, Safety of acyclovir: a summary of the first 10 years' experience, *J Med Virol*, **suppl 1**: S67–3.

Vere Hodge RA, 1993, Famciclovir and penciclovir. The mode of action of famciclovir including its conversion to penciclovir, *Antiviral Chem Chemother*, **4**: 67–84.

Vere Hodge RA, Cheng YC, 1993, The mode of action of penciclovir, *Antiviral Chem Chemother*, **4**: 13–24.

Vere Hodge RA, Perkins RM, 1989, Mode of action of 9-(4-hydroxy-3-hydroxymethylbut-1-yl)guanine (BRL 39123) against herpes simplex virus in MRC-5 cells, *Antimicrob Agents Chemother*, **33**: 223–9.

Vere Hodge RA, Sutton D et al., 1989, Selection of an oral prodrug (BRL 42810; famciclovir) for the antiherpesvirus agent BRL 39123 [9-(4-hydroxy-3-hydroxymethylbut-1-yl)guanine; penciclovir], *Antimicrob Agents Chemother*, **33**: 1765–73.

Votruba I, Bernaerts R et al., 1987, Intracellular phosphorylation of broad-spectrum anti-DNA virus agent (S)-9-(3-hydroxy-2-phosphonylmethoxypropyl)adenine and inhibition of viral DNA synthesis, *Mol Pharmacol*, **32**: 524–9.

Wade JC, Newton B et al., 1982, Intravenous acyclovir to treat mucocutaneous herpes simplex virus infection after marrow transplantation: a double blind trial, *N Engl J Med*, **96**: 265–9.

Wald ER, Dashefsky B, Green M, 1988, Ribavirin: case of premature adjudication, *J Pediatr*, **112**: 154–8.

Wallace MR, Bowler WA et al., 1992, Treatment of adult varicella with oral acyclovir. A randomized placebo-controlled trial, *Ann Intern Med*, **117**: 358–63.

Wang C, Takeuchi K et al., 1993, Ion channel activity of influenza A virus M2 protein: characterization of the amantadine block, *J Virol*, **67**: 5585–94.

Webster RG, Kawoaka Y, Bean WJ, 1986, Vaccination as a strategy to reduce the emergence of amantadine and rimantadine resistant strains of A/chick/Pennsylvania/83 (H5N2) influenza virus, *J Antimicrob Chemother*, **18, suppl B**: 157–64.

Wellings PC, Awdry PN et al., 1972, Clinical evaluation of trifluorothymidine in the treatment of herpes simplex corneal ulcers, *Am J Ophthalmol*, **73**: 932.

Whitley R, Gnann JW, 1992, Acyclovir: a decade later, *N Engl J Med*, **327**: 782–9.

Whitley RJ, Soong S-J et al. and Collaborative Study Group, 1977, Adenine arabinoside therapy of biopsy-proved herpes simplex encephalitis, *N Engl J Med*, **297**: 289–94.

Whitley R, Alford C et al., 1980a, Vidarabine: a preliminary review of its pharmacological properties and therapeutic use, *Drugs*, **20**: 267–82.

Whitley RJ, Tucker BC et al., 1980b, Pharmacology, tolerance, and antiviral activity of vidarabine monophosphate in humans, *Antimicrob Agents Chemother*, **18**: 709–15.

Whitley RJ, Alford CA et al., 1986, Vidarabin vs acyclovir therapy in herpes simplex encephalitis, *N Engl J Med*, **314**: 144–9.

Whitley R, Arvin A et al., 1991, A controlled trial comparing vidarabine with acyclovir in neonatal herpes simplex virus infection. Infectious Diseases Antiviral Collaborative Study Group, *N Engl J Med*, **324**: 444–9.

Wildy P, Field HJ, Nash AA, 1982, Classical herpes latency revisited, *Virus Persistence*, SGM Symposium 33, eds Mahy BWJ, Minson AC, Darby GK, Cambridge University Press, Cambridge, 133–67.

Woods MG, Diana GD et al., 1989, In vitro and in vivo activities of WIN 54954, a new broad-spectrum antipicornavirus drug, *Antimicrob Agents Chemother*, **33**: 2069–74.

Wright GE, 1994, Herpesvirus thymidine kinase inhibitors, *Int Antiviral News*, **2**: 84–6.

Yasin SR, Al-Nakib W, Tyrrell DA, 1990a, Pathogenicity for humans of human rhinovirus type 2 mutants resistant to or dependent on chalcone Ro 09-0410, *Antimicrob Agents Chemother*, **34**: 936–66.

Yasin SR, Al-Nakib W, Tyrrell DAJ, 1990b, Isolation and preliminary characterization of chalcone Ro 09-0410-resistant human rhinovirus type 2, *Antiviral Chem Chemother*, **1**: 149–54.

Yokota T, Konno K et al., 1989, Mechanism of selective inhibition of varicella-zoster virus replication by 1-beta-D-arabinofuranosyl-E-5-(2-bromovinyl)uracil, *Mol Pharmacol*, **36**: 312–16.

Chapter 47

EMERGENCE AND RE-EMERGENCE OF VIRAL INFECTIONS

Brian W J Mahy and Frederick A Murphy

1 Introduction
2 The virus: variation and the emergence of new viral phenotypes
3 The individual host: susceptibility/resistance factors favouring the emergence of viral diseases
4 The host population: individual and societal behavioural factors favouring the emergence of viral diseases

5 The environment: ecological and zoonotic factors favouring the emergence of viral diseases
6 The prevention and control of new, emerging and re-emerging viral diseases

1 INTRODUCTION

1.1 The emergence of new diseases

New or previously unrecognized viral diseases are constantly being identified. In most cases, there is no way to predict when or where the next important new viral pathogen will emerge. Neither is there any way to predict the ultimate importance of a virus as it first emerges: it may be the cause of a geographically limited curiosity, of intermittent outbreaks of disease or of a new epidemic. New viral diseases seem to be emerging with increasing frequency, as suggested by published reports of cases, outbreaks and epidemics and by the rate of identification of new pathogenic viruses. The list of newly emergent viruses of humans and animals is impressive (Tables 47.1 and 47.2).

1.2 Determinants contributing to the emergence of new diseases

Many different elements can contribute to the emergence of a new viral disease. These include: (1) virological determinants such as mutation, recombination, reassortment, natural selection, fitness adaptation and evolutionary progression; (2) individual host determinants such as specific risk behaviours, innate resistance and acquired immunity, physiological factors such as age, nutritional status and pregnancy; (3) host population determinants such as behavioural, societal,

transport, commercial and iatrogenic factors; and (4) environmental determinants such as ecological and zoonotic influences. These determinants need to be understood if we are to develop control measures to prevent occurrence and spread of disease within human or animal populations. In this chapter we consider the underlying causes for emergence and re-emergence and illustrate them with selected examples.

1.3 Initial recognition of new, emerging diseases

Since 1986, following upon the development of the polymerase chain reaction and other biotechnological methods, we have seen a dramatic increase in the direct detection of viruses in diseased tissues and tissue culture cells. As a consequence, several new viruses have been recognized (Table 47.3). In fact, viruses have been described and named solely on the basis of genomic sequences amplified by reverse transcription and polymerase chain reaction from diseased postmortem tissue. Bayou virus is a case in point (Khan et al. 1995). The diversity of human papillomaviruses has been recognized, even though culture of these viruses has not been accomplished and serotyping is not possible; individual papillomaviruses that are associated with specific diseases or syndromes can be distinguished on the basis of their genome nucleotide sequence.

Table 47.1   Some of the most important new, emerging and re-emerging human virus pathogens

Crimean–Congo haemorrhagic fever virus[a]	Tick-borne; severe human disease with 10% mortality; widespread across Africa, the Middle East and Asia
Dengue viruses[a]	Mosquito-borne; the cause of millions of cases of febrile disease in the tropics, and of dengue haemorrhagic fever, a life-threatening disease, especially in children
Ebola[a] and Marburg[a] viruses	Natural reservoirs unknown; Ebola and Marburg viruses are the causes of the most lethal haemorrhagic fevers known
Group A, B and C rotaviruses	Rotavirus enteric disease is the second leading cause of death among infants in the world
Guanarito virus[a]	Rodent-borne; the newly discovered cause of Venezuelan haemorrhagic fever
Hantavirus[a]	Rodent-borne; the cause of important rodent-borne haemorrhagic fever in Asia and Europe
Hepatitis C virus	Newly identified; the cause of much severe, chronic liver disease in the USA
Hepatitis delta virus	An unusual 'helper' virus that makes hepatitis B more lethal
Hepatitis E virus	Newly identified; the cause of epidemic hepatitis, especially in Asia; recently recognized as widespread along the US–Mexico border; the infection has a high mortality rate in pregnant women
Hepatitis G virus	Newly identified; a possible cause of a small proportion of transfusion-related hepatitis world-wide
Human herpesviruses 6 and 7	Newly identified; the cause of a substantial proportion of febrile disease in children
Human herpesviruses 8	Newly identified; associated, possibly causally, with Kaposi's sarcoma
Human immunodeficiency viruses (HIV-1 and HIV-2)	The causes of AIDS, still emerging in many parts of the world
Human papillomaviruses	Over 70 viruses; some associated with cervical, oesophageal and rectal cancers
Human parvovirus B19	The cause of roseola in children; a possible cause of fetal damage when pregnant women become infected
Human T-lymphotropic viruses (HTLV-I and HTLV-II)	The cause of an adult leukaemia and neurological disease, especially in the tropics
Influenza viruses	The cause of thousands of deaths every winter in the elderly; the cause of the single most deadly epidemic ever recorded – the worldwide epidemic of 1918, in which over 20 million people died
Japanese encephalitis virus	Mosquito-borne; very severe, lethal encephalitis; now spreading across southeast Asia; great epidemic potential
Junin virus[a]	Rodent-borne; the cause of Argentine haemorrhagic fever
Lassa virus[a]	Rodent-borne; a very important, severe disease in West Africa; imported into a Chicago hospital in 1990
Machupo virus[a]	Rodent-borne; the cause of Bolivian haemorrhagic fever
Measles virus	Re-emerging in several countries with poor vaccine coverage
Norwalk and related viruses	Major causes of outbreaks of severe diarrhoea
Polioviruses	The cause of poliomyelitis; still an important problem in developing countries of Africa and Asia; targeted by WHO for worldwide eradication by the year 2000
Rabies virus	Transmitted by the bite of rabid animals; raccoon epidemic spreading across northeastern USA
Rift Valley fever virus[a]	Mosquito-borne; the cause of one of the most explosive epidemics ever seen in Africa
Ross River virus	Mosquito-borne; the cause of epidemic arthritis; has moved across the Pacific region several times
Sabía virus	Rodent-borne; virus from Brazil; newly discovered cause of haemorrhagic fever, including 2 laboratory-acquired cases
Sin Nombre virus	Emerging as the major cause of severe, often fatal, acute respiratory distress syndrome in the the USA
Venezuelan encephalitis virus	Mosquito-borne; the cause of recent major epidemics in Central and South America
Yellow fever virus[a]	Mosquito-borne; one of the most deadly diseases in history

[a]The viruses that cause haemorrhagic fevers in humans.

Table 47.2 Some of the most important new, emerging and re-emerging virus pathogens of animals

African horse sickness viruses	Mosquito-borne; a historic problem in southern Africa; now becoming entrenched in the Iberian peninsula; a major threat to horses world-wide
African swine fever virus	Tick-borne and also spread by contact; an extremely pathogenic virus; recently present in Europe and South America; a major threat to swine in North America
Avian influenza viruses	Spread by wild birds; a major threat to the poultry industry of the USA
Bluetongue viruses	*Culicoides*-borne; the isolation of several strains in Australia has become an important non-tariff trade barrier issue
Bovine spongiform encephalopathy agent	Recognized in 1986; the cause of a major epidemic in cattle in the UK, resulting in major economic loss and trade embargo
Canine parvovirus	A new virus, having mutated from feline panleucopenia virus; the virus has rapidly swept round the world, causing a pandemic of severe disease in dogs
Chronic wasting disease of deer and elk	A spongiform encephalopathy agent of unknown source, discovered in captive breeding herds in the USA
Dolphin, porpoise and phocine (seal) morbilliviruses	Epidemic disease first identified in 1988 in European seals; was first thought to be derived from a land animal morbillivirus, such as canine distemper or rinderpest, but now it is realized that there are several important, emerging pathogens endangering these species
Equine morbillivirus	A new virus; the cause of fatal acute respiratory distress syndrome in horses (and humans), in Queensland, Australia, in 1994
Feline immunodeficiency virus and simian immunodeficiency viruses	Important new viruses, the one affecting cats in nature and the other serving as an important model in AIDS research
Foot-and-mouth disease viruses	Still considered the most dangerous exotic viruses of animals in the world because of their capacity for rapid transmission and great economic loss; still entrenched in Africa, the Middle East and Asia
Lelystad virus (mystery swine disease)	A new virus, causing an important disease, porcine reproductive and respiratory syndrome (PRRS) in swine in Europe and the USA
Malignant catarrhal fever virus	An exotic, lethal herpesvirus of cattle; an important non-tariff trade barrier issue throughout the world
Myxoma virus	Used to control rabbits in Australia, but with diminishing success; a proposal has been advanced that genetically engineered myxoma virus carrying a gene for a sperm antigen be distributed to sterilize infected surviving rabbits
Rabbit haemorrhagic disease virus	Being investigated as new way to control rabbits in Australia
Rinderpest virus	Still considered very dangerous, with potential for causing great economic loss; still entrenched in Africa and Asia

Papillomavirus genome DNA is a small circular molecule that is easily cloned from biopsy specimens of infected tissues. Originally these viruses were classified by DNA hybridization, and considered to be different types if they shared less than 50% homology. With the advent of simpler methods for DNA sequencing, this proved to be inconsistent, and a papillomavirus type is now defined as new when the genome DNA is more than 10% dissimilar in the combined nucleotide sequences of 3 genes, *E6*, *E7* and *L1*. This requires determination of 2.4 kbp of sequence (one-third of the genome) for each new isolate. More than 70 human papillomaviruses have now been recognized as types by this method, and divided into supergroups. For example, 54 papillomavirus types of genital origin form one supergroup by sequence analysis, and another includes 24 types associated with epidermodysplasia verruciformis and other cutaneous

lesions (Chan et al. 1995). Molecular techniques have also been important in the recognition of so-called non-A non-B hepatitis viruses.

In 1989 Bradley and co-workers (Choo et al. 1989) cloned a new hepatitis virus, now known as hepatitis C virus, from the blood of a chimpanzee that had been experimentally infected with factor VIII that was known to transmit non-A non-B hepatitis (Matsuura and Miyamura 1993). RNA extracted from the chimpanzee blood was reverse-transcribed to make cDNAs using random primers. The DNA was cloned in the bacteriophage λgt 11 expression vector, and the resultant bacterial colonies were screened using sera from patients with non-A non-B hepatitis. After screening thousands of clones in this way, one was found that reacted with antibodies in the sera of infected patients. DNA from the positive clone was then used to screen other clones by

Table 47.3   Emerging human viral disease: recognition by molecular techniques

Virus	Disease	Method
Human papillomaviruses (more than 70 types)	Warts, anogenital cancer Laryngeal papillomatosis	Cloning and restriction analysis or sequencing of viral DNA from infected tissues
Hepatitis C virus	PT-hepatitis, often chronic, leading to carcinoma	Cloning, sequencing, expression and immunoselection with specific sera
Hepatitis E virus	Acute epidemic hepatitis, usually water-borne	Cloning, sequencing, expression and immunoselection with specific sera
Hepatitis G virus	?PT-hepatitis	Cloning, sequencing, expression and immunoselection with specific sera
Hepatitis viruses GBV-A, GBV-B and GBV-C	?PT-hepatitis	Cloning, sequencing, expression and immunoselection with specific sera
Sin Nombre virus	Hantavirus pulmonary syndrome	Reverse transcription and polymerase chain reaction amplification from infected human and rodent tissues and sequence analysis
Bayou virus	Hantavirus pulmonary syndrome	Reverse transcription and polymerase chain reaction amplification from infected human tissues and sequence analysis

PT, parenterally transmitted.

DNA hybridization, and eventually the full length sequence of hepatitis C virus was determined. We now recognize multiple genomic variants of the original virus (see Chapter 35). Hepatitis E virus was isolated in a similar manner, and is now recognized as the most important agent of explosive epidemics of hepatitis in Asia and South America (see Chapter 34). Since the discovery of hepatitis C, additional viruses with similar characteristics (member viruses of the family *Flaviviridae*), also associated with human hepatitis, have been found using molecular techniques (Muerhoff et al. 1995, Linnen et al. 1996).

Recognition may be triggered by a variety of circumstances, such as the occurrence of a specific outbreak which leads to intensive investigation, or isolation of the agent and subsequent development of laboratory methods permitting specific diagnosis. New diseases that are clinically unique, such as acquired immunodeficiency syndrome (AIDS), are more likely to be recognized earlier than diseases that closely resemble well established clinical entities, such as hepatitis, diarrhoea or encephalitis. One example of 'delayed emergence' owing to late recognition is California encephalitis, caused by La Crosse virus. This virus was first isolated in 1964 from a fatal case of encephalitis in a child who had been hospitalized and died in 1960 in La Crosse, Wisconsin, USA. Using this isolate as a source of antigen, retrospective serological surveys showed that the virus was an important cause of disease previously listed under the heading 'viral meningitis of undetermined aetiology'. Since that time, La Crosse encephalitis has been reported each year from the midwestern region of the USA, at an average annual incidence of c. 75 cases, with no evidence of increasing or decreasing occurrence over the last 25 years. This is consistent with an endemic infection that had been occurring regularly for many decades, i.e. long before the mid-1960s when the virus came to light.

2   THE VIRUS: VARIATION AND THE EMERGENCE OF NEW VIRAL PHENOTYPES

2.1   The variety and diversity of viruses

As knowledge of the molecular structure and replication of viruses has increased, we have learned that the viruses that we know to be responsible for human and animal diseases represent only a small fraction of a large, diverse global virus population. Currently, some 3600 virus species are recognized taxonomically, but international reference centres and culture collections keep track of more than 30 000 viral strains (Murphy et al. 1995). This number continues to increase because, each time a potential host species or a new disease is studied in detail, new viruses are found. In addition, the evolution of viruses during replication generates many genetic variants.

2.2 Polygenic basis for viral variation

There are several genetic mechanisms that drive virus evolution: discussed below are mutation (section 2.3), recombination (section 2.5) and reassortment of genes (section 2.6, p. 1016). However, many of the most important variances among viruses are polygenic, and of ancient derivation, the result of natural selection. Classic examples of such variation were the definition many years ago of smallpox virus variants, variola major (Indian subcontinent and Europe, mortality up to 30%) and variola minor (South America, mortality c. 1%) (Fenner et al. 1988) and naturally occurring attenuated poliovirus variants, some of which inspired the development of Sabin live-attenuated polio vaccines (Sabin 1981). Only recently has it been possible to begin to explain such phenotypic differences from a molecular genetic perspective.

2.3 Mutation

The replication of viruses involves copying the genome nucleic acid millions of times; mistakes in the copying process introduce mutations (see Chapter 2). When such mutations lead to new phenotypic characters that enable the virus to replicate in a new host or cell type, to replicate to a higher titre or at a faster rate, or to better escape host defences, the potential exists for emergence of a new viral disease. Genetically, mutational changes affecting phenotype may be minimal, involving one or a few nucleotides, or they may be large and complex, involving the addition of new genes into viral genomes. In any case, it is the expression of genotypic change as a new phenotype that is important in nature, and usually it is phenotypic change affecting transmission that is at the heart of the emergence of a new disease. Mutations that affect antigenic determinants on the viral surface proteins may be selected for, especially when viruses replicate in the presence of antibody. This has been clearly documented in the case of influenza. New antigenic variants of influenza virus occur so pervasively that they require reformulation of vaccine on an annual basis.

The emergence of variants by the accumulation of point mutations is termed antigenic drift (see Chapter 22). Such mutations may dramatically alter viral pathogenicity, but more importantly they result in new viral surface epitopes that the population does not recognize. In 1983, an outbreak of avian influenza A virus (H5N3) in Pennsylvania spread through the poultry industry of the region, leading to the destruction of 17 million fowl and a loss of about US$60 million. When the virus was sequenced, it was found to have acquired a single point mutation that altered the cleavability of its haemagglutinin, thereby greatly increasing its pathogenicity. A dramatic example of the emergence of a new virus by mutation is afforded by canine parvovirus (Parrish 1990, 1994). Serological evidence suggests that this virus made its first appearance as a new pathogen of dogs in 1976. The virus was isolated in 1978 as the cause of severe enteritis,

sometimes fatal, that occurred in dogs in North America, Europe and Australia. Outbreaks of sudden death in puppies due to myocarditis were also linked to the new virus. Soon after its isolation, it became clear from antigenic analysis and restriction endonuclease mapping that the canine virus was closely related to feline panleucopenia virus, a pathogen that had been recognized since the 1920s. Sequence analysis of isolates of the canine virus revealed that it differed from feline panleucopenia virus in only 6 nucleotides, and probably originated as a result of 2 amino-acid changes in the viral capsid, which for the first time allowed the feline virus to replicate in dog cells. The rapidity with which canine parvovirus disease spread round the world has not been explained, but the extreme physical stability of the virus probably made fomite carriage by humans very efficient.

2.4 The special case of high frequency mutation and quasispecies formation in RNA viruses

Given their great potential for generating new genotypes, the RNA viruses seem to represent an enormous and continuous risk with regard to the emergence of new epidemic diseases, but in fact the frequency of emergence of such new diseases is lower than might be expected (see Chapter 2). New genotypes are tested severely by natural selection and few represent a better fit than current wild types. Better fit and better adaptation to an econiche require that a new genotype or a new virus has certain improved traits, such as improved transmissibility, improved capacity to move through the host population, and perhaps even improved capacity for surviving 'lean times' such as those presented by a highly immune population. There is no doubt that the mode of transmission is the critically important element in this regard; viruses transmitted by the respiratory route fit their econiches very well indeed, and represent the threats to our civilization of major epidemic or pandemic disease (Mims 1991). However, as we are learning from the insidious spread of human immunodeficiency virus (HIV) in Africa and Asia, other transmission patterns can be equally deadly.

2.5 Recombination

Genetic recombination involves an interaction between viral genomes during mixed infection of a cell, giving rise to progeny having a genome with characteristics derived from both parental genotypes. Recombination is observed with both DNA and RNA viruses, but surprisingly few examples have been documented of emergence of new viruses through this mechanism. For example, although experimental evidence exists for recombination in vivo among herpesviruses, and many individuals are dually infected by more than one herpesvirus, no herpesvirus disease manifestation in humans has ever been attributed to recombinational events (Javier, Sedarati and Stevens

1986). Western equine encephalitis (WEE) virus is a recombinant, its 2 glycoprotein genes being derived from a Sindbis-like virus progenitor and the remainder of its genome derived from Eastern equine encephalitis virus (Hahn et al. 1988). It is estimated that 2 cross-over events were required to produce WEE from its progenitors, and that this probably occurred during persistent infection in a mosquito host more than 1000 years ago (Strauss and Strauss 1994). Recombination is also well documented between serotypes of polioviruses, for example after administration of trivalent Sabin vaccine to infants. This confirms the potential for generation of recombinant viruses with altered pathogenicity or altered host range, yet it is surprising that so few examples have been found.

2.6 Reassortment

Closely related viruses that have segmented genomes often undergo genetic recombination during dual infections. This special case of recombination in which whole genome segments are recombined is termed reassortment. Different influenza A viruses can reassort their genome segments, forming viable progeny; when this results in replacement of the haemagglutinin or neuraminidase genes it is termed 'antigenic shift'. No reassortment occurs between influenza A and influenza B viruses; the basis for this restriction is not known. Each of the major human influenza pandemics of this century (1918, 1957 and 1968) was caused by reassortment of genome segments between an existing human virus and an avian virus (Webster and Kawaoka 1994). Swine probably provide an important intermediate host in the stabilization of reassortants between avian and human influenza viruses. Reassortment between animal and human viruses also seems to be important in generating new pathogenic strains of rotaviruses (Gentsch et al. 1993).

2.7 Epidemic potential of newly evolved viruses

The epidemic potential of newly emergent viruses varies, depending upon the mode of transmission, the immunological and genetic susceptibility of the host population, the size of the population at risk, and other epidemiological and pathogenetic factors. Epidemic potential is greatest for an agent that is readily transmitted from host to host, particularly via the respiratory route. Conversely, zoonotic agents and arthropod-borne agents are usually limited in their geographic range, although the latter are certainly not limited in their capacity for causing very large epidemics.

Certain kinds of phenotypic change are most notable in the epidemic potential of particular viral diseases. A change in host range can permit a virus to spread into a new species with devastating consequences. An increase in virulence (based on any of several mechanisms) can convert a non-pathogenic or trivially pathogenic virus into one with devastating pathogenic qualities. A change in antigenic signature can permit a virus to infect a population already immune to parental strains of the same virus.

3 THE INDIVIDUAL HOST: SUSCEPTIBILITY/RESISTANCE FACTORS FAVOURING THE EMERGENCE OF VIRAL DISEASES

In many ways, the influence of the host on the emergence of viral diseases is more pervasive than that of the virus. The host brings a much more complex genome to the battle between virus and host that involves the qualities of the virus that are crucial for its transmission and survival, as described in section 2.4 (p. 1015), and the resistance of the host. These host factors are usually categorized under (1) innate resistance, mostly dependent on poorly understood non-specific resistance factors, (2) acquired resistance (e.g. macrophages and the cellular and humoral immune responses), and (3) physiological factors affecting resistance (e.g. age, nutritional status, hormonal effects especially in pregnancy, fever). When host resistance is optimal, infection may be subclinical or abortive, but when host response is inadequate qualitatively or quantitatively, disease is the usual outcome. Furthermore, when an overly exuberant immune response occurs there can be immunopathological disease.

3.1 The host immune response

Studies with inbred mice have identified a large repertoire of genes that confer survival potential on the host. Most of these genes are specific for a single family of viruses, although a few map to the major histocompatibility locus and encode proteins that influence host immune responses to multiple agents. Polygenic resistance characteristics are less well understood, but seemingly even more important. For example, line-breeding and inbreeding experiments led to the development of the classic strains of mice that are exquisitely sensitive to certain viruses: these mice have been used for many years to isolate arboviruses, rabies virus and picornaviruses. The genes selected for in these mice may be unknown, but the implication is that many genes may affect host resistance to viral infections.

POLIOVIRUSES

It is likely that poliomyelitis has occurred as a sporadic disease since ancient times. During the eighteenth and first half of the nineteenth centuries a few clusters of cases were reported, but from about 1905 onwards epidemics were reported annually in the USA. The same pattern of emergence of poliomyelitis as an epidemic disease has been repeated many times since, first in developed and then in developing countries. What accounts for this emergence of epidemic poliomyelitis? There is no evidence that it was due to the appearance of virus strains of increased virulence. Epidemiological data suggest that there is a correlation between age at the time of infection and risk of paralytic disease. It was proposed by Nathanson and Martin (1979) that the appearance of epidemic poliomyelitis was due, paradoxically, to improvements in public sanitation and personal hygiene, which led to a reduction in virus transmission. A delay in the age of initial infection, beyond the age when infants are protected by passively acquired maternal antibody, is postulated to have increased the risk of clinical disease. An intrinsically lower case : infection ratio in infancy compared to early childhood may represent a secondary contributing factor.

3.2 Persistent infection and chronic shedding

The dynamics of emergence of a new viral disease can vary greatly, depending on the incubation period, whether the infection is rapidly self-limiting or persistent and whether the resulting disease (and shedding pattern) is acute or chronic. When associated with a short incubation period and acute disease, emergence can be a dramatic event. However, when the emerging agent is associated with a long incubation period, the resulting epidemic may rise over a period of years before it reaches a peak. Furthermore, a long interval between infection and disease occurrence may obscure the identification of the causal agent and its mode of transmission. Finally, if the disease is chronic, the impact on the healthcare system may spread over decades rather than weeks, with major economic consequences beyond those ordinarily associated with an acute epidemic.

HIV AND AIDS

The premier example of an emergent long incubation period disease is AIDS. In fact, the length of the incubation period, which averages 8–10 years, repeatedly led to underestimates of the true spread and penetration of the epidemic (Fig. 47.1). Associated with this was uncertainty regarding the proportion of infections that would lead to death. The long incubation period led to the initial assumption that only a small proportion of infections, perhaps no more than 10%, would be fatal; projections of total AIDS incidence were correspondingly low. Also important was a failure to appreciate the impact of lifelong persistence of infection and virus shedding. It proved difficult to devise a model of the number of potentially infectious individuals in the population at any given time, and their impact on transmission dynamics. Finally, it was not appreciated that the chronic nature of AIDS would produce a vast new burden upon the healthcare system.

3.3 Altered host resistance and coincident change in viral virulence

The best documented example of coincident change in host and virus leading to the emergence of a variant disease involves the rabbit and myxoma virus. The disease, myxomatosis of rabbits, is caused by the poxvirus, myxoma virus; it occurs naturally as a mild infection of rabbits in South America and California (*Sylvilagus* spp.) where it produces a skin tumour from which virus is transmitted mechanically by biting insects. However, in the European rabbit (*Oryctolagus cuniculus*), myxoma virus causes a lethal infection, a finding that led to its use for biological control of wild rabbits in Australia. The European rabbit was introduced into Australia in 1859 for sporting purposes and rapidly spread to become the major animal pest of agricultural and pastoral industries. Myxoma virus was successfully introduced into this rabbit population in 1950; when originally introduced the virus produced case-fatality rates of over 99%. This highly virulent virus was readily transmitted by mosquitoes. Farmers operated 'inoculation campaigns' to introduce the virus into wild rabbit populations.

It might have been predicted that the disease, and with it the virus, would disappear at the end of each summer, owing to the greatly diminished numbers of susceptible rabbits and mosquitoes during the winter. This must have occurred often in localized areas, but it did not happen over the continent as a whole. The capacity of virus to survive the winter conferred a great selective advantage on viral mutants of reduced lethality: during this period, when mosquito numbers were low, rabbits infected by such mutants survived in an infectious condition for weeks instead of a few days and thereby contributed disproportionately to the progeny pool. Within 3 years such 'attenuated' mutants became the dominant strains throughout Australia. Thus the original highly lethal virus was progressively replaced by a heterogeneous collection of strains of lower virulence, but most of them were still virulent enough to kill 70–90% of genetically unselected rabbits.

Rabbits that recover from myxomatosis are immune to reinfection. However, because most wild rabbits have a life-span of less than a year, herd immunity is not an important factor in the epidemiology of myxomatosis. Selection for more genetically resistant animals operated from the outset. In areas where repeated outbreaks occurred, the genetic resistance of surviving rabbits increased progressively. The early appearance of the viral strains of lower virulence, which allowed 10% of genetically unselected rabbits to recover, was an important factor in allowing the number of genetically resistant rabbits to increase. In areas where annual outbreaks occurred, the case-fatality rate fell from 90% to 25% within 7 years. Subsequently, in areas where there were frequent outbreaks, somewhat more virulent strains of virus became dominant, because they produced the kind of disease that was best transmitted in populations of genetically resistant rabbits. Thus, the ultimate balance struck between myxoma virus and Australian rabbits involved adaptations of virus and host populations, reaching a dynamic equilibrium that finds rabbits still greatly reduced compared with their pre-myxomatosis numbers, but too numerous for the wishes of farmers and conservationists.

3.4 Crossing the species barrier

The ability of animal viruses to cross the species barrier as a result of mutations has been documented in several cases (Table 47.4) but there are no clear examples among important human viral pathogens.

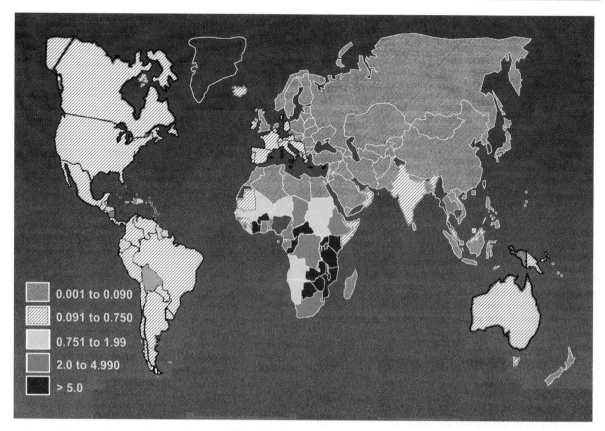

Fig. 47.1 Global prevalence of HIV infection in adults, by country. The different shades indicate the percentage HIV prevalence rate in sexually active adults as at the end of 1994. Fifteen countries, all in sub-Saharan Africa, had more than 5 infections per 100 people. (Data from WHO Global Programme on AIDS.)

Legend:
- 0.001 to 0.090
- 0.091 to 0.750
- 0.751 to 1.99
- 2.0 to 4.990
- > 5.0

Table 47.4 Emerging viral diseases: examples of probable interspecies transfer

Year	Virus	Disease	Species transfer	Cause
1978	Canine parvovirus	Pandemic enteritis, myocarditis	Cat to dog	Mutation of feline panleucopenia virus
1986	BSE agent	Bovine spongiform encephalopathy	Sheep to cattle	Changes in cattle food rendering process
1988	Phocid distemper virus 1	Fatal respiratory disease (distemper)	Harp seals to harbour seals	Migration of harp seals due to climatic conditions
	Phocid distemper virus 2	Fatal respiratory disease (distemper)	Dogs to Siberian seals	Contact between different marine species or contact with terrestial animals (dogs)
1990	Lelystad virus	Porcine reproductive/respiratory syndrome (PRRS)	Rodent to pig	?Mutation of rodent virus
1994	Equine morbillivirus	Acute respiratory distress syndrome (ARDS)	Unknown native mammal to horses	?Mutation of unknown virus

The human immunodeficiency viruses (HIV-1 and HIV-2) may be examples of species cross-over, however.

HIV-1 AND HIV-2

Both HIV-1 and HIV-2 viruses have a narrow host range, seemingly limited to humans. The viruses can experimentally infect certain non-human primates, in which replication usually occurs without apparent disease. However, simian lentiviruses (simian immunodeficiency viruses, SIVs) can be recovered from a range of African monkey species. Phylogenetic analysis points strongly to a simian origin of HIV-1 and HIV-2 (Doolittle 1989, Myers, MacInnes and Korber 1992). The viruses seem to have arisen as causes of immunodeficiency in humans and primates at about the same time, and there is evidence that SIVs can infect humans (Gao et al. 1992, Khabbaz et al. 1994). There is also clear overlap between the areas in Africa where HIV-2 was first detected and the range of known SIV-infected monkey species (Smallman-Raynor and Cliff 1991). However, it is impossible with existing data to pinpoint the location, the time or the putative mutational changes that led to the emergence of HIV as an epidemic disease in humans (Nathanson et al. 1993).

EQUINE MORBILLIVIRUS

In 1994 a horse trainer and a stablehand in Queensland, Australia, became ill while nursing a sick horse that had recently been brought onto the property. The disease spread to other horses in the stables, and 14 of 21 infected horses died from a pulmonary disease with haemorrhagic manifestations that was caused by a previously unknown morbillivirus. Although the stablehand survived the infection, the trainer died. One year later another horse farmer died of encephalitis caused by the same virus acquired from another sick horse that died in 1994. The 3 human infections were isolated cases, and no disease or antibody seroconversion was detected in the surrounding populations of humans or horses. The reservoir of the infection, which may have been an animal or arthropod vector species, has not been determined. However, whatever the source of the virus, its transmission to humans did not result in a spreading infection as occurred among the horses in the stable.

Many zoonotic viruses can cross the species barrier and infect humans, but transmission to humans represents a 'dead end' for the virus because no further transmission occurs. Many of these viruses are arthropod-borne, including alphaviruses such as Eastern and Western equine encephalitis viruses, flaviviruses such as Murray Valley, Japanese and St Louis encephalitis viruses, and bunyaviruses such as La Crosse virus and Rift Valley fever virus. Other viruses are transmitted directly to humans from zoonotic animal reservoirs, most commonly from rodent reservoirs. Examples include bunyaviruses such as Hantaan (agent of haemorrhagic fever with renal syndrome), Seoul, Puumala (agent of nephropathia epidemica) and Sin Nombre (agent of hantavirus pulmonary syndrome) viruses, and arenaviruses such as Machupo (agent of Bolivian haemorrhagic fever) and Junin (agent of Argentine haemorrhagic fever) viruses. Historically, each of these viruses has been responsible for the emergence of a 'new' human disease.

4 THE HOST POPULATION: INDIVIDUAL AND SOCIETAL BEHAVIOURAL FACTORS FAVOURING THE EMERGENCE OF VIRAL DISEASES

Several influences pertaining to human behaviour (individual and societal behaviour) have favoured the emergence of new virus diseases; all of these influences seem to have accelerated over the last century. The global human population has continued to grow inexorably, bringing increasingly larger numbers of people into close contact. There have been successive revolutions in the speed of transportation, making it possible to circumnavigate the globe in less than the incubation period of most viral infections (Murphy and Nathanson 1994). For this reason, viral diseases occurring anywhere in the world can no longer be presumed to stay confined to their country or continent of origin. The death of a patient from Lassa fever in a hospital in Chicago in 1989 provided sobering testimony to the distance and speed that exotic viruses can move around the world (Holmes et al. 1990). The patient, an American citizen who had visited Nigeria to attend his mother's funeral, became ill 2 days after his return to Chicago. A total of 102 people had contact with him in the hospital. Fortunately, none of these contacts became infected. However, the incident illustrates the potential vulnerability of populations remote from the normal locale of geographically limited diseases.

4.1 The influence of individual behavioural factors

There are diverse influences pertaining to the behaviour of individuals that can lead to the emergence of new diseases or new patterns of disease transmission. Many diseases that depend upon such factors are emergent or re-emergent. Behavioural influences include: (1) risk factors leading to sexually transmitted diseases (e.g. multiple sex partners, homosexual risk behaviours); (2) risk factors associated with day care; (3) behavioural risk factors favouring the transmission of childhood diseases in the community; and (4) risk factors pertaining to food preparation and storage in the home.

SEXUALLY TRANSMITTED DISEASES

After declining over many years in developed countries, sexually transmitted diseases are now increasing at epidemic rates in urban populations in Europe, the USA and many developing countries. Changes in sexual attitudes and behaviour in such populations, combined with injectable drug use, have led to rapid amplification of certain viral diseases that are spread sexually or by blood contact. This is especially disturbing because many of the sexually transmitted diseases enhance the risk of transmission of each other (via new bacteria and viruses entering through established lesions). Thus, the risk of transmission is increased beyond expected rates and 'curable' diseases, such as gonorrhoea and syphilis, support the spread of 'incurable' diseases, such as genital herpes and HIV infection/AIDS. The major societal failing in this regard stems from declining support for public health programmes, but in some instances emergence reflects advances in our ability to detect new viruses. One example is the emergence through recognition of human papillomavirus infection, genital papillomatosis and cervical cancer. Multiple risk factors contribute to cervical cancer; these include behavioural (sexual behaviour), dietary, hormonal and viral risk factors (Reeves et al. 1994). There are several theories but no real proof as to how these risk factors, in concert, lead to cervical neoplasia. Now that one risk factor for cervical cancer is known to be infection with certain types of human papillomaviruses, DNA probes for these viruses are being added to cytological screening programmes.

DAY CARE AND VIRAL INFECTIONS

Shifts in the structure of the family in all developed countries have resulted in a dramatic increase in the proportion of children in day care; currently, 11 million children in the USA spend a large part of their time in day care. This trend is likely to continue in the USA; by the year 2000 it is estimated that more than 75% of mothers with children under 6 years of age will be working outside the home. Viral diseases represent the most important problems in day care, respiratory and diarrhoeal illnesses being most common. Children attending day care facilities may also become silent reservoir hosts for some agents of disease, such as hepatitis A virus and several enteroviruses. Depending on the disease, children attending day care have a 2- to 18-fold increased risk of becoming ill compared with children at home. The most common viral diarrhoeal pathogens acquired in day-care centres are rotaviruses. Rotaviruses infect every child in its first 3–4 years of life; this leads, in the USA, to an estimated 3 million cases of diarrhoea, 500 000 doctor visits, 70 000 hospitalizations for 300 000 inpatient days and 75–125 deaths, and the costs for hospital care total US$200–400 million per year. World-wide, nearly one million children die each year of rotavirus diarrhoea. Yet as late as 1973 the human rotaviruses were unknown, even though they are now relatively easy to detect. There are probably several more viruses causing diarrhoea that have yet to be discovered.

4.2 The influence of societal, commercial and iatrogenic factors

There are diverse societal, commercial and medical care factors that lead to the emergence of new diseases or new disease patterns. Again, many diseases that depend on such factors are emergent or re-emergent. Such risk factors include: (1) those associated with the commercial food industries, from sources on the farm to processing, transportation, wholesaling and retailing; (2) those associated with water supply, (3) those associated with pharmaceuticals and biologicals; (4) those causing iatrogenic diseases.

DISEASES ASSOCIATED WITH ADVANCED MEDICAL CARE

Diseases such as those associated with immunosuppressive therapy, organ transplantation (including xenotransplantation), blood banking and kidney dialysis are all increasing substantially in all developed countries. Since the early 1980s there has been an unprecedented rise in opportunistic infections associated with immunosuppression. A rapid increase in organ transplantation practices with associated immunosuppressive drug treatment has combined with the emerging

AIDS epidemic to create a large, highly susceptible population at risk for a variety of viral diseases (see Chapter 42). In many cases viruses cause diseases of greatly increased severity in such individuals. These include diseases caused by DNA viruses, such as cytomegalovirus, Epstein–Barr virus, varicella-zoster virus, human herpesvirus type 6, human papillomaviruses, human parvovirus B19, human polyomaviruses JC and BK, adenoviruses, hepatitis B virus and molluscum contagiosum virus, and RNA viruses such as measles, hepatitis C, influenza, respiratory syncytial and parainfluenza viruses. Human herpesvirus 8, which is strongly associated with and may be the cause of Kaposi's sarcoma, is an example of an emerging virus that might not have been recognized except for its association with HIV and its immunosuppressive effects (Chang et al. 1994). As the number of HIV-infected people throughout the world continues to expand, it is likely that new viral diseases, or new manifestations of old viral diseases, will continue to emerge as a consequence of immunosuppression.

MODERN AGRICULTURAL AND FOOD INDUSTRY PRACTICES AND VIRAL INFECTIONS

Changes in every aspect of the food industry, from on-the-farm technologies to processing technologies, favour the emergence of new viral disease problems. Animal husbandry has changed in ways that increase stress and promote viral transmission and endemic infection cycles. Large numbers of animals are being confined in limited space and at very high density, cared for by a few, inadequately trained workers. Elaborate housing systems are used, but with inadequate evaluation of systems for ventilation, feeding, waste disposal and cleaning. In addition, some diseases are favoured by the global expansion of agricultural markets, involving the global transport of animals, animal products, and animal semen and embryos. Yet other diseases can emerge as a consequence of changes in processing and distribution systems.

LIVESTOCK DISEASES

We usually think of the importance of livestock diseases in terms of financial losses, because the capacity of the commercial livestock food and fibre industries of developed countries are such that surpluses are a greater problem than are shortages. However, in developing countries this is not the case: livestock diseases, especially new, emerging or re-emerging diseases, cause immediate human suffering by substantially compromising scarce human food resources, especially the supply of high-quality protein.

4.3 Epidemiological considerations

Perpetuation of a virus in nature depends on the maintenance of serial infections, i.e. a chain of transmission; the occurrence of disease is neither required nor necessarily advantageous. Although clinical cases may be somewhat more productive sources of virus than inapparent or mild infections, the latter are generally more numerous and do not restrict the movement of infectious individuals, and thus provide a major mechanism of viral dissemination and emergence.

Epidemics are classically divided according to their means of spread into 2 major categories, propagated and common source (Nathanson 1996).

PROPAGATED EPIDEMICS AND CRITICAL COMMUNITY SIZE

In propagated epidemics, spread from host to host continues to expand as long as each infection gives rise to more than one new infection. The rate of transmission depends on a number of variables, such as the density of the population, the proportion of the population that is susceptible, the degree and duration of contagiousness, and the frequency of contacts leading to transmission. The classic large epidemics of viral diseases have all been propagated epidemics.

For viruses that produce acute self-limiting infections to survive, the susceptible host population must be both large and relatively dense. Such viruses may disappear from a population because they exhaust the supply of susceptible hosts as they acquire immunity to reinfection. Persistent viruses, on the other hand, may survive in very small populations, sometimes by spanning generations. Depending on the duration of immunity and the pattern of virus shedding, the critical community size varies considerably with different viruses.

MEASLES

Much was learned about the dynamics of the viral transmission chain by Panum, who studied the devastating measles epidemic of 1846 in the Faroe Islands; this was at a time when even the concept of a virus was unknown (Panum 1939). With an incubation period of about 12 days, maximum viral excretion for the next 6 days and solid immunity to reinfection, between 20 and 30 susceptibles would need to be infected in series to maintain measles transmission for a year. Since nothing like such precise one-to-one transmission occurs, many more than 30 susceptibles are needed to maintain endemicity. Analyses of the incidence of measles in different size communities have shown that a population of about half a million people is needed to ensure a large enough annual input of new susceptibles, provided by the annual birth cohort, to maintain measles indefinitely as an endemic disease. Because infection depends on close contact, the duration of epidemics of measles is correlated inversely with population density. If a population is dispersed over a large area, the rate of spread is reduced and the epidemic will last longer, so the number of susceptible persons needed to maintain endemicity is reduced. On the other hand, in such a situation a break in the transmission cycle is much more likely. If a large proportion of the population is initially susceptible, the intensity of the epidemic builds up very quickly, often reaching almost 100%. Virgin-soil epidemics in isolated communities have had devastating consequences owing to lack of medical care and the disruption of work capacity. In large urban communities, before the era of vaccination, measles epidemics occurred every 2–3 years, each time exhausting available susceptibles; this epidemic cycle occurred on a continental scale. Before the introduction of vaccine, the cyclic occurrence of measles epidemics was influenced by several variables besides the build-up of susceptibles; these included the dynamics of re-introduction of the virus and seasonal influences.

COMMON SOURCE EPIDEMICS

Common source epidemics occur when a virus is disseminated from a single focus; they usually result from contamination of air, food, water, drugs, biomedical devices or the like. If a virus is introduced from a common source into a large population, disease can emerge on an epidemic scale. A recent example is the epidemic of bovine spongiform encephalopathy now underway in the UK (see Chapter 39).

HEPATITIS B

In the early stages of World War II, it was decided to immunize large numbers of American troops with 17D yellow fever vaccine. In order to stabilize the infectivity of the live attenuated 17D virus, protein was added to the final vaccine formulation. To prevent serum sickness, human serum was selected as the protein source. Almost 1000 donors were used; unfortunately, at least one donor was a carrier of hepatitis B virus. Consequently, in the spring of 1942 over 400 000 troops received contaminated vaccine, causing about 20 000 cases of hepatitis (Sawyer et al. 1944). Although the onset of disease was spread over a considerable time, when plotted according to the interval from administration of the vaccine the timeline formed a classic log-normal curve, thereby providing statistical proof of the association of the epidemic with the administration of the vaccine. This epidemic clearly established hepatitis B as a distinct entity, separable from hepatitis A (e.g. different mean incubation periods: 3 months for hepatitis B, one month for hepatitis A).

5 THE ENVIRONMENT: ECOLOGICAL AND ZOONOTIC FACTORS FAVOURING THE EMERGENCE OF VIRAL DISEASES

Ecological factors pertaining to unique environments and geographic isolation often underpin the emergence of new viruses and thereby new viral diseases. Such factors favour the adaptation of viruses to new econiches. When ecosystems are altered, viral infections of humans and animals follow. Population movements and the intrusion of humans and domestic animals into new arthropod habitats have resulted in many new emergent disease episodes. The classic example of this was the emergence of yellow fever when susceptible humans entered the Central American jungle to build the Panama Canal; there are many contemporary examples suggesting that similar events will continue to happen, in most cases in unanticipated circumstances. Deforestation has been the key to the exposure of farmers and domestic animals to new arthropods and the viruses they carry. The occurrence of Mayaro virus disease in Brazilian wood-cutters as they cleared the Amazonian forest in recent years is a case in point. Increased long-distance transportation facilitates the carriage of exotic arthropod vectors around the world. The carriage of the Asian mosquito, *Aedes albopictus*, a vector for dengue and California encephalitis viruses, into the USA in the water contained in imported used tyres represents an unsolved problem of this kind. Increased long-distance transportation of livestock facilitates the carriage of viral agents and arthropods (especially ticks) around the world. The introduction of the tick-borne agent, African swine fever virus, from Africa into Portugal

(1957), Spain (1960) and South America (1960s and 1970s) is thought to have occurred in this way; it is just a matter of time until this virus makes further international forays.

Changed routes of long-distance bird migrations, brought about by new water impoundments, represent an important yet still untested additional risk of introduction of arboviruses into new areas. This may be a key to the movement of Japanese encephalitis virus into new areas of Asia. Ecological factors pertaining to environmental pollution and uncontrolled urbanization are contributing to many new, emergent disease episodes. Arthropod vectors breeding in accumulations of water (tin cans, old tyres, etc.) and sewage-laden water are a problem world-wide. Environmental chemical toxicants (herbicides, pesticides, residues) can also affect vector–virus relationships directly or indirectly. For example, mosquito resistance to' all licensed insecticides in parts of California is a known direct effect of unsound mosquito abatement programmes, augmented indirectly by uncontrolled pesticide usage against crop pests. Ecological factors relating to water use (i.e. increasing irrigation and the expanding re-use of water) are becoming important aspects in the emergence of viral disease. The problem with primitive water and irrigation systems that are developed without attention to arthropod control is exemplified in the emergence of Japanese encephalitis in new areas of southeast Asia and the Indian subcontinent. Global warming, affecting sea level, estuarine wet-lands, swamps and human habitation patterns, may be affecting arthropod vector relationships throughout the tropics; however, data are scarce and many programmes to study the effect of global warming have not included the participation of viral disease experts.

DENGUE

Dengue is one of the most rapidly emerging diseases in the tropical parts of the world, millions of cases occurring each year. For example, Puerto Rico had 5 dengue epidemics in the first 75 years of this century, but has had 6 epidemics since 1986, at an estimated cost of over US$150 million. At the same time, a record number of cases have occurred elsewhere in the Americas; Brazil, Bolivia, Colombia, Paraguay, Ecuador, Venezuela, Nicaragua and Cuba have experienced major dengue epidemics. These epidemics have involved multiple virus types; of the 4 dengue virus types, 3 are now circulating in the Caribbean region. These are the circumstances that lead to dengue haemorrhagic fever: the lethal end of the dengue disease spectrum. Dengue haemorrhagic fever first occurred in the Americas in 1981; since then, most countries have reported cases, and since 1990 over 3000 cases have been reported each year.

Why is dengue emerging, especially in the Americas? The answer is simple: urban mosquito habitats are expanding (the vector mosquito, *Aedes aegypti*, is extremely well adapted to human proximity), mosquito density is increasing and mosquito control is failing. This is occurring not just in the least developed countries but also in many developed countries. Financial resources for public health are severely limited and, too often, mosquito control, which is very expensive, falls off the bottom of the priority list. Meanwhile, mosquito control is becoming more expensive as older,

cheaper chemicals lose effectiveness or are banned as damaging to the environment. As mosquito control fails, dengue follows quickly.

YELLOW FEVER

An even more frightening situation associated with failing mosquito control is that yellow fever virus, which is transmitted by the same mosquito vector as dengue, *Ae. aegypti*, might also re-emerge. Where dengue occurs, the conditions are also appropriate for yellow fever (initiated by importation via an infected person or an infected mosquito). It is one of the mysteries of tropical medicine that yellow fever does not occur more often where vector density and a susceptible human population coexist. In fact, no one knows where, when or even if yellow fever virus will re-emerge in the kinds of epidemics that were the scourge of tropical and subtropical cities of the western hemisphere and Africa throughout the seventeenth, eighteenth and nineteenth centuries; however, because this virus is so dangerous, the possibility is constantly on the mind of national and international health officials.

HANTAVIRUSES AND HAEMORRHAGIC FEVER WITH RENAL SYNDROME

The first well characterized hantavirus disease was Korean haemorrhagic fever, which emerged during the Korean war of 1950–52. Thousands of United Nations troops developed a mysterious disease marked by fever, headache, haemorrhage and acute renal failure; the mortality rate was 5–10%. Despite much research, the agent of this disease remained unknown for 26 years; then, in 1976, a new virus, named Hantaan virus, was isolated in Korea from fieldmice. The discovery of this virus was, however, just 'the tip of an iceberg.' In subsequent years, related viruses have been found in many parts of the world in association with different rodents and as the cause of human diseases with more than 150 different local names. It has been found in recent years that, from an ecological perspective, there are 7 or 8 different subgroups of viruses and 3 different transmission patterns: rural, urban and laboratory acquired. From a clinical perspective, 2 disease patterns are described, one marked by severe disease (haemorrhagic fever with renal syndrome, with significant mortality) and the other by mild disease (febrile disease, without mortality). The rural, severe disease is widespread in the Far East (e.g. Korean haemorrhagic fever in Korea; 'epidemic haemorrhagic fever' in China, causing more than 100 000 cases per year). A similar rural, severe disease is emerging in the Balkans (mortality rate c. 20%).

HANTAVIRUSES AND ACUTE RESPIRATORY DISTRESS SYNDROME

In May 1993, a new hantavirus disease was recognized in the southwestern region of the USA. The disease appeared as an acute respiratory distress syndrome. Clinical signs include fever, headache and cough, followed by acute pulmonary congestion and oedema leading to hypoxia, shock and, in many cases, death. Within a short time, cases were found in 23 States. By October 1996, more than 160 cases had been confirmed, with 75 deaths. At the beginning of the investigation in 1993, even though the causative virus had not been isolated, serological tests (using surrogate antigens from related hantaviruses) and molecular biological tests were developed and used to prove that the aetiological agent was a previously unknown Hantavirus, now named Sin Nombre virus. Viral RNA was amplified from patients' specimens by the polymerase chain reaction (PCR), followed by sequencing. Comparing sequences obtained from specimens from different areas indicated that several different variant viruses (seemingly at least 5 variants), all new and previously unknown, were active in the USA. PCR sequences were extended until much of the genome of the new viruses had been sequenced; these sequences were then used in expression systems to produce homologous antigens for further studies and diagnostic services. The same serological and molecular biological methods were applied to large numbers of rodents collected in the areas where patients lived; this proved that at least 8 species of rodents were involved, the primary reservoir host in the southwest being *Peromyscus maniculatus*, the deer mouse (c. 30% of this species were found to harbour the viruses in several areas of southwestern USA). These viruses, like other hantaviruses, do not cause disease in their reservoir rodent hosts, but virus is shed in the saliva, urine and faeces of these animals, probably for their entire lives. Human infection occurs by inhalation of aerosols or dust containing infected dried rodent saliva or excreta. These viruses have probably always been present in the large area of the western region of the USA inhabited by *Peromyscus* species; they were recognized in 1993 only because of the number and clustering of human cases, which in turn were probably caused by a great increase in rodent numbers consequent on an increase in piñon seeds and other rodent food. As a result of this kind of rapid field and laboratory investigation, the public is being advised about reducing the risk of infection, mostly by reducing rodent habitats and food supplies in and near homes and taking precautions when cleaning rodent-contaminated areas.

RABIES

Rabies can serve as an example of ecological factors relating to the adaptation and emergence of viruses in new econiches. The most dramatic illustration of this in recent years has been the appearance of epidemic raccoon rabies in northeastern USA. The epizootic has been traced to the importation of raccoons from Florida to West Virginia in 1977. This epidemic demonstrates dramatically how human disturbance of the environment, in this instance involving the transportation of wild animals, can lead to emergence of a disease in a previously unaffected area. A key to our understanding of this episode was the discovery that rabies virus is not one virus; rather, it is a set of different genotypes, each transmitted within a separate reservoir host niche. In North America, there are about 6 terrestrial animal genotypes, one involving the skunk in the north-central states, one the skunk in the south-central states, one the Arctic fox and red fox in Alaska and Canada, one the grey fox in Arizona, one the coyote and feral dog in southern Texas and northern Mexico, and one the raccoon in southeastern, mid-Atlantic and now northeastern states. 'Raccoons-bite-raccoons-bite-raccoons' and after some time their virus becomes a distinct genotype, highly adapted to the host cycle and inefficient if introduced into another host cycle. When this discovery was made (using monoclonal antibody and molecular biological methods), many mysteries of rabies ecology were clarified.

6 THE PREVENTION AND CONTROL OF NEW, EMERGING AND RE-EMERGING VIRAL DISEASES

Since 1991 we have witnessed the emergence or re-emergence of a surprisingly large number of human viral diseases (Fig. 47.2). When a new virus disease is suspected, a complex continuum of prevention and control activities may be called into action, but, given financial and resource constraints, decisions must be made and priorities must be set. The full continuum comprises the following activities and resources, which may be divided into investigative and interventional phases.

THE INVESTIGATIVE PHASE

1 The disease must be characterized (usually the work of clinicians and pathologists).
2 There is nearly always need for epidemiological field investigation to assess the risk to the population (usually the work of medical epidemiologists).
3 The agent must always be sought. When a new virus is suspected, it must be isolated, identified, characterized.
4 There is usually need for diagnostics development, to provide and authenticate primary, reference and confirmatory tests.
5 An integrated research programme is usually needed (but not always implemented), covering sciences as diverse as molecular virology, pathogenesis, pathophysiology, immunology, ecology, epidemiology, sociology and behaviour, vector biology, etc.

THE INTERVENTIONAL PHASE

1 There is always a need for comprehensive communications systems.
2 There is often need for technology transfer (transfer of diagnostics technology to local agencies and transfer of information pertinent to vaccine and drug development to the commercial sector).
3 There is usually need for training and clinical continuing education.
4 Comprehensive public health systems may need to be adapted to the disease at hand. This may involve new public education programmes, new vital record and disease register systems, rapid case reporting, new surveillance systems, expanded laboratory diagnostics services, new staffing and staff support, new logistical systems (facilities, equipment, supplies, transport), and the like.
5 There may be a need for new policy decisions, new risk management decisions. These may involve new legislation and regulations, new law enforcement action, and even new administrative and management systems.
6 There may be need for new clinical medical systems (isolation of cases by quarantine, barrier nursing, physical biocontainment, and extra disinfection and sterilization). There may be need for new patient management systems and even need for improving the general health of the population at risk (better nutrition, housing, primary medical care).
7 There may be need for specialist systems, such as vector control, reservoir host control, environmen-

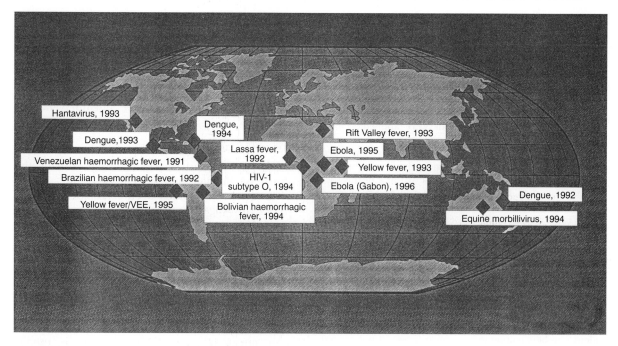

Fig. 47.2 Recent emergence and re-emergence of human viral diseases. VEE, Venezuelan equine encephalitis.

tal control (water, animal and arthropod habitats, etc.) and sanitary engineering (to provide safe food and water, sewage treatment, etc.).

8 In the largest epidemics there are also global issues to be dealt with, such as control of international movement of people and animals, establishment of international disease control task forces, and the like. Finally, there is the global issue of adequate funding for such programmes.

All these activities must be integrated to construct a comprehensive view of the immediate problem at hand and a strategy and programmes for its control. Today, this kind of integrated investigative, problem-solving activity is usually thought to be the sole responsibility of government agencies, but, in fact, many professionals from throughout the health sector have played central roles in recent episodes. As it turns out, assessing risk and guiding intervention involve quite diverse activities; for example, in some cases complex field studies of the incidence of infection in the general population or in a selected subpopulation are necessary to determine risk factors for infection, mode of transmission, targets for intervention, etc., whereas in other cases, studies of the pathogenetic mechanisms underpinning the clinical presentation in the individual patient might hold the key. Today, in nearly every instance, important clues lie in characterizing the molecular structure and replication strategy of the virus and the cellular pathobiology of the infection.

REFERENCES

Chang Y, Cesarman E et al., 1994, Identification of herpes-like DNA sequences in AIDS-associated Kaposi's sarcoma, *Science*, **266:** 1865–9.

Chan S-Y, Delius H et al., 1995, Analysis of genomic sequences of 95 papillomavirus types: uniting typing, phylogeny and taxonomy, *J Virol*, **69:** 3074–83.

Choo QL, Kuo G et al., 1989, Isolation of a cDNA clone derived from a blood-borne non-A, non-B viral hepatitis genome, *Science*, **244:** 359–62.

Doolittle RF, 1989, Immunodeficiency viruses: the simian–human connection, *Nature (London)*, **339:** 338–9.

Fenner F, Henderson DA et al., 1988, *Smallpox and its Eradication*, World Health Organization, Geneva.

Gao F, Yue L et al., 1992, Human infection by genetically diverse SIVsm-related HIV-2 in West Africa, *Nature (London)*, **358:** 495–9.

Gentsch JR, Das BK et al., 1993, Similarity of the VP4 protein of human rotavirus strain 116E to that of the bovine B223 strain, *Virology*, **194:** 424–30.

Hahn CS, Lustig S et al., 1988, Western equine encephalitis virus is a recombinant virus, *Proc Natl Acad Sci USA*, **85:** 5997–6001.

Holmes GP, McCormick JB et al., 1990, Lassa fever in the United States. Investigation of a case and new guidelines for management, *N Engl J Med*, **323:** 1120–3.

Javier RT, Sedarati F, Stevens J, 1986, Two avirulent herpes simplex viruses generate lethal recombinants in vivo, *Science*, **234:** 746–8.

Khabbaz RF, Heneine W et al., 1994, Brief report: infection of a laboratory worker with simian immunodeficiency virus, *N Engl J Med*, **330:** 172–7.

Khan AS, Spiropoulou CF et al., 1995, Fatal illness associated with a new hantavirus in Louisiana, *J Med Virol*, **46:** 281–6.

Linnen J, Wages J et al., 1996, Molecular cloning and disease association of hepatitis G virus: a transfusion transmissible agent, *Science*, **271:** 505–8.

Matsuura Y, Miyamura T, 1993, The molecular biology of hepatitis C virus, *Semin Virol*, **4:** 297–304.

Mims CA, 1991, The origin of major human infections and the crucial role of person-to-person spread, *Epidemiol Infect*, **106:** 423–33.

Muerhoff AS, Leary TP et al., 1995, Genomic organization of GB viruses A and B: two new members of the flaviviruses associated with GB agent hepatitis, *J Virol*, **69:** 5621–30.

Murphy FA, Nathanson N, 1994, The emergence of new viral diseases: an overview, *Semin Virol*, **5:** 87–102.

Murphy FA, Fauquet CM et al., 1995, *Virus Taxonomy*, Sixth Report of the International Committee on Taxonomy of Viruses, Springer-Verlag, New York.

Myers G, MacInnes K, Korber B, 1992, The emergence of simian/human immunodeficiency viruses, *AIDS Res Hum Retroviruses*, **8:** 373–86.

Nathanson N, 1996, Epidemiology, *Fields' Virology*, 3rd edn, eds Fields BN, Knipe D, Raven Press, New York, 251–71.

Nathanson N, Martin JR, 1979, The epidemiology of poliomyelitis: enigmas surrounding its appearance, epidemicity, and disappearance, *Am J Epidemiol*, **110:** 672–92.

Nathanson N, McGann KA et al., 1993, The evolution of viral diseases: their emergence, epidemicity, and control, *Virus Res*, **29:** 3–20.

Panum PL, 1939, Observations made during the epidemic of measles in the Faroe Islands in the year 1846, *Med Classics*, **3:** 839–86.

Parrish CR, 1990, Emergence, natural history and variation of canine, mink and feline parvoviruses, *Adv Virus Res*, **38:** 403–50.

Parrish CR, 1994, The emergence and evolution of canine parvovirus – an example of recent host range mutation, *Semin Virol*, **5:** 121–32.

Reeves WC, Gary HE Jr et al., 1994, Risk factors for genital papillomavirus infection in populations at high and low risk for cervical cancer, *J Infect Dis*, **170:** 753–8.

Sabin AB, 1981, Paralytic poliomyelitis: old dogma and new perspectives, *Rev Infect Dis*, **3:** 543–64.

Sawyer WA, Meyer KF et al., 1944, Jaundice in army personnel in the western region of the United States and its relation to vaccination against yellow fever, *Am J Hyg*, **39:** 337–87.

Smallman-Raynor M, Cliff A, 1991, The spread of human immunodeficiency virus type 2 into Europe: a geographic analysis, *Int J Epidemiol*, **20:** 480–9.

Strauss JH, Strauss EG, 1994, The alphaviruses: gene expression, replication and evolution, *Microbiol Rev*, **58:** 491–562.

Webster RG, Kawaoka Y, 1994, Influenza – an emerging and re-emerging disease, *Semin Virol*, **5:** 103–11.

INDEX

Note: Page numbers in *italics* refer to major discussions. *vs* denotes differential diagnosis or comparisons.

Since the main subjects of this volume are viruses and viral infections, entries have been kept to a minimum under these terms and readers are advised to seek more specific entries.

Entries referring to the properties and characteristics of viruses are listed separately from those referring to the infections, e.g. Hepatitis A is separated from Hepatitis A virus (HAV); Enteroviruses is separated from Enterovirus infections. Cross-references are not always inserted and are assumed. Transmission of a virus/virus infection is included in the entry for the virus, whilst references to specific vaccines are included under the entries for the specific infection.

Phages are listed under Bacteriophage.